PRIMARY
CARE

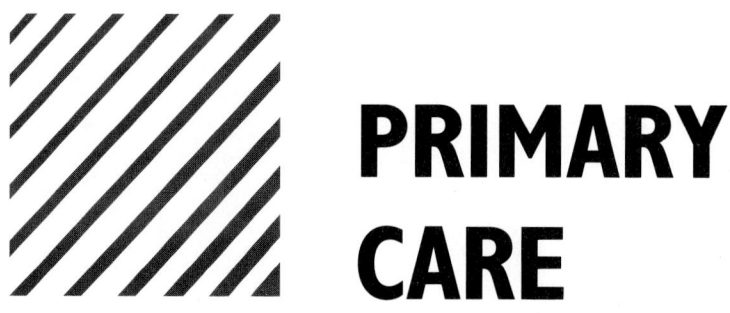

PRIMARY CARE

JOANNE K. SINGLETON, PhD, RN, CS, FNP

Assistant Professor
Pace University
Lienhard School of Nursing
Department of Graduate Studies
Pleasantville, NY
and
Clinical Instructor (Voluntary)
Department of Family Practice
SUNY–Health Science Center at Brooklyn
Brooklyn, NY

SAMUEL A. SANDOWSKI, MD

Assistant Professor
Department of Family Practice
Medical Director
Family Practice Center
State University of New York
Health Science Center at Brooklyn
Brooklyn, NY

CAROL GREEN-HERNANDEZ, PhD, RN, CS, ANP/FNP

Associate Professor and Director of Primary Care
Nurse Practitioner Program
Department of Nursing
University of Vermont
Burlington, VT
and
Family Nurse Practitioner in Private Practice
Burlington, VT

THERESA V. HORVATH, PA-C, MPH

Assistant Professor and Director
Physician Assistant Program
Mercy College
Dobbs Ferry, NY

ROBERT V. DiGREGORIO, PharmD

Associate Professor of Pharmacy Practice
Arnold and Marie Schwartz College of Pharmacy and
Health Sciences
Long Island University
Brooklyn, NY
and
Clinical Coordinator for Pharmacy and Emergency Services
The Brookdale University Hospital and Medical Center
Brooklyn, NY

STEPHEN PAUL HOLZEMER, PhD, RN

Dean
School of Nursing
Long Island College Hospital
Brooklyn, NY
Curriculum Consultant
Baccalaureate Nursing Education
St. Francis College
Brooklyn, NY

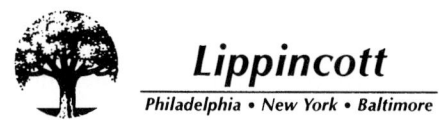

Lippincott

Philadelphia • New York • Baltimore

Acquisitions Editor: Lisa Stead
Editorial Assistant: Claudia Vaughn
Associate Managing Editor: Barbara Ryalls
Senior Production Manager: Helen Ewan
Senior Production Coordinator: Nannette Winski
Design Coordinator: Nicholas Rook/Brett Mac Naughton
Indexer: Ann Cassar
Compositor: Maryland Composition Co.
Printer: Courier Westford

9 8 7 6 5 4 3 2 1

Library of Congress Cataloging-in-Publication Data

Primary care / [edited by] Joanne K. Singleton . . . [et al.].
    p.   cm.
    Includes bibliographical references and index.
    ISBN 0-7817-1041-3 (alk. paper)
    1. Primary care (Medicine)   I. Singleton, Joanne K.
    [DNLM: 1. Primary Health Care.   WB 110P9523 1999]
RA427.9.P74   1999
616—dc21
DNLM/DLC
for Library of Congress   98-42214
                                   CIP

We dedicate this book to students' and providers' spirit of inquiry in the challenge of participating with patients, their families, and communities in interdisciplinary relationship-centered care.

JKS, SAS, CG-H, TVH, RDG, SPH

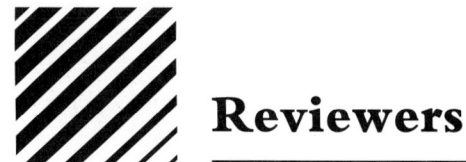

Reviewers

Lisa Andrist, PhD, RNC, WHNP
Assistant Professor, Graduate Program In Nursing
Coordinator, Adult/Womens' Health Nurse Practitioner
  Track
Massachusetts General Hospital Institute of Health
  Professions
Boston, MA

Susan Appling, RN, MS, CRNP
Assistant Professor, School of Nursing
Nurse Practitioner, Breast Center
Johns Hopkins University
Baltimore, MD

Kathleen Lent Becker, MS, CRNP
Assistant Professor
Johns Hopkins University
School of Nursing
Baltimore, MD

Clarice Begemann, MSN, MPPM, FNP, RN, CS
Family Nurse Practitioner, Fair Haven Community Health
  Center
Program Instructor, School of Nursing
Yale University
New Haven, CT

Pamela Betta, PhD, RN, CS
Tallahassee, FL

Susan Buchholtz, EdD, RN, ANP
Department of Pre-surgical Testing
Northshore University Medical Center at Forrest Hills
Forrest Hills, NY

Leann Busby, MSN, RNC, FNP
Assistant Professor
Vanderbilt University School of Nursing
Nashville, TN

Ruth Cox, PhD, LMP, ARNP, CFNP
Family Nurse Practitioner Specialty Director
Assistant Professor
University of Alabama, Birmingham
Birmingham, AL

Margaret Clayton, MS, RN, CS, FNP
Raleigh, NC

Eileen Crutchlow, EdD, FNP, APRN
Associate Professor
Department of Nursing
Southern Connecticut State University
New Haven, CT

Debbie Daly-Gawanda, MS, RN
Assistant Professor of Community Health Nursing
College of Nursing
Rush University
Director, Employee Health Services
Rush-Presbyterian-St. Luke's Medical Center
Chicago, IL

William E. Dudley, II, MD
Dover, NH

Thomas Egan, PharmD, BCPS, FASCP
President
Clinical Pharmacotherapeutics, Inc.
Gibbsboro, NJ

Linda Fahey, MN, ANP-C
Professor, Nursing Department
California State University, Los Angeles
Los Angeles, CA

Kathryn Fiandt, ARNP, DNS
Assistant Professor, College of Nursing
Coordinator, Family Nurse Practitioner Program
University of Nebraska Medical Center
Omaha, NE

Catherine Foster, BSN, MSN, CNP
Graduate Faculty, Nurse Practitioner Programs
Nurse Practitioner
College of Nursing and Health
University of Texas, El Paso
El Paso, TX

Diana French, PhD, MSN, FNP-C, GNP-C
Associate Professor
School of Nursing
Medical College of Ohio
Toledo, OH

Nancy Giordano, EdD, RN, NP
Coordinator of the Nurse Practitioner Program
College of New Rochelle
New Rochelle, NY

Joanne Haeffele, MS, RN, CS, FNP
Family Nurse Practitioner, Adjunct Faculty
Westminster College
Brigham Young University
Salt Lake City, UT

Mary Jane Hanson, PhD, RN, CRNP, CS
Assistant Professor, Department of Nursing
Director of Graduate Nursing Program
University of Scranton
Scranton, PA

Judy Herrmann, MSN, RN, CS
Education Specialist
Education Service
Cincinnati VA Medical Center
Cincinnati, OH

Joan King, PhD, RN, ANP, ACNP
Faculty, School of Nursing
Specialty Director for ANCP
Vanderbilt University
Nashville, TN

Mary Neiheisel, BSN, MSN, EdD, CSN, FNP-C
Professor of Graduate Nursing
College of Nursing
University of Southwestern Louisiana
Lafayette, LA

Carol Patten, PhD, CCRN, CRNP
CRNP at Family Nurse Practice Clinic
Associate Professor, Nursing
Carlow College
Pittsburgh, PA

Betty Porter, EdD, ARNP, FNP-C
Chair, Department of Nursing and Allied Health Sciences
Family Nurse Practitioner
Morehead State University
Morehead, KY

James Ressler, PA-C
Associate Faculty
Senior Physician Assistant
Department of Orthopaedic Surgery
University of California, San Francisco
San Francisco, CA

Jessica Shank Coviello, RN, MSN, CS
Lecturer, Yale University School of Nursing
ANP-Connecticut Heart Group
New Haven, CT

Benita Walton-Moss, DNS, RNCS, FNP
Assistant Professor, School of Nursing
Coordinator, Family Nurse Practitioner Program
The Catholic University of America
Washington, DC

Dale Welch, RN, CS, ANP, MSN
Nurse Practitioner, Internal Medicine, Kaiser Permanente
Clinical Instructor, George Washington University
Affiliate Faculty, George Mason University
Fairfax, VA

Altan Yenicay, MD
New York, NY

Jeffery Yeres, DDS
New York, NY

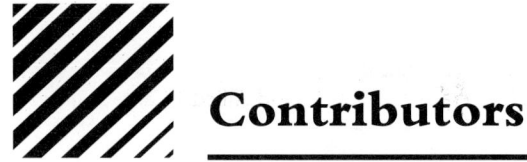

Contributors

Dalia Abdelmacksoud, PharmD
Graduate Assistant
Arnold & Marie Schwartz College of Pharmacy and Health Sciences
Long Island University
Brooklyn, NY

Cathy S. Alexander, MD
Director of Clinical Affairs
Chase-Brexton Health Services, Inc.
Baltimore, MD

Matthew R. Anderson, MD
Assistant Professor, Department of Family Medicine
Albert Einstein College of Medicine
Bronx, NY

Daisy A. Arce, MD
Clinical Assistant Instructor
Department of Family Practice
State University of New York
Health Science Center at Brooklyn
Brooklyn, NY

Alice M. Arden, RN, MA, ANP, CS
Adult Nurse Practioner
Cardiac Catheterization Lab
Department of Cardiology
The New York Hospital
Cornell Medical Center
New York, NY

Sanjiv Bansal, MD
Chief Resident
Department of Orthopaedics
State University of New York
Health Science Center at Brooklyn
Brooklyn, NY

Karen Benker, MPH, MD
Teaching Fellow
Department of Family Practice
Assistant Clinical Professor
Department of Preventive Medicine and Community Health
State University of New York
Health Science Center at Brooklyn
Brooklyn, NY

Charles Berk, MD
Faculty
Department of Family Medicine
State University of New York, Downstate
Brooklyn, NY

John Bisson, MD
Clinical Assistant Professor of Urology
Department of Surgery
College of Medicine
University of Vermont
Burlington, VT

Gail Breen, PharmD, BCPS
Assistant Professor of Clinical Pharmacy
Philadelphia College of Pharmacy and Science
Philadelphia, PA

Carol Buck-Rolland, RN, MS, PNP, OGNP
Faculty Nurse-Practitioner
Primary Care Program
University of Vermont
Burlington, VT
Clinical Site and Child Development
Planned Parenthood
Burlington, VT

Harry L. Bush, Jr., MD
Associate Professor of Surgery
Department of Surgery
Cornell University Medical College
New York, NY

Charlotte C. Cabello, MSN, RN
Clinical Nurse Manager
GI Care Center
Department of Nursing
Mount Sinai Medical Center
New York, NY

Raffi Calikyan, MD
Fellow
Department of Pulmonary and Critical Care
State University of New York
Health Science Center at Brooklyn
Brooklyn, NY

Francis Cannizzo, Jr., MD, PhD
Resident
Department of Surgery
State University of New York
Health Science Center at Brooklyn
Brooklyn, NY

Dennis A. Cardone, DO, CAQSM
Assistant Professor
Department of Family Medicine
Director
Sports Medicine Center
University of Medicine and Dentistry of New Jersey
New Brunswick, NJ

Wanda J. Cennerazzo, MA, C-ANP
Certified Adult Nurse Practioner, Outreach Coordinator
Department of Surgery
The New York Presbyterian Hospital, Cornell Campus
New York, NY

Judy Cheng, PharmD
Assistant Professor of Pharmacy Practice
Division of Pharmacy Practice
Arnold and Marie Schwartz College of Pharmacy and Allied Health Sciences
Brooklyn, NY

Alfonso Ciervo, MD
Chief Resident in Surgery
Department of Surgery
State University of New York
Health Science Center at Brooklyn
Brooklyn, NY

Henry Cohen, MS, PharmD
Associate Professor of Pharmacy Practice
Arnold and Marie Schwartz College of Pharmacy and Allied
    Health Sciences
Long Island University
Coordinator of Clinical Pharmacy Services
Departments of Pharmacy and Medicine
Kingsbrook Jewish Medical Center
Clinical Associate Professor of Pharmacology and Medicine
State University of New York
Health Science Center at Brooklyn
Brooklyn, NY

Paul H. Cohen, MD
Assistant Professor of Medicine
Division of Digestive Diseases
Department of Medicine
State University of New York
Health Science Center at Brooklyn
Brooklyn, NY

Catherine M. Concert, MS, RN, CS, FNP
Administrative Supervisor
Wyckoff Heights Medical Center
Brooklyn, NY

Carmel Dato, RN, MS, CS
Instructor
School of Nursing
Long Island University
Brooklyn, NY

Gwyneth Davis, MD
Residency Director and Assistant Professor
Department of Family Practice
State University of New York
Health Science Center at Brooklyn
Brooklyn, NY

Spiro Demetis, MD, FCCP
Assistant Professor of Medicine
Division of Pulmonary and Critical Care Medicine
Director of Medical Firm B
State University of New York
Health Science Center at Brooklyn
Brooklyn, NY

Joseph DeRose, Sr., MD
Associate Professor of Medicine and Family Practice
State University of New York
Health Science Center at Brooklyn
Brooklyn, NY

Joseph DeRose, Jr., MD
Cardiovascular Research Fellow
Columbia University College of Physicians and Surgeons
New York, NY

Marielaina S. DeRose, MD
Senior Resident
Columbia Presbyterian Medical Center
Department of Medicine
Columbia University College of Physicians and Surgeons
New York, NY

Maria Procopio Dugan, DO
Assistant Professor
Department of Family Practice
State University of New York
Health Science Center at Brooklyn
Brooklyn, NY

Linda Efferen, MD, FACP, FCCP
Assistant Professor of Medicine
Acting Chief
Division of Pulmonary and Critical Care Medicine
State University of New York
Health Science Center at Brooklyn
Brooklyn, NY

Felix Enabosi, OT, PhD
Director of Rehabilitation Services
Dr. Susan Smith McKinney Nursing and Rehabilitation Center
Brooklyn, NY

Edgar Fayans, DDS, FADSA
Associate Chairman, Dental & Oral Surgery
The Dr. Samuel Cranin Dental Center
The Brookdale University Hospital and Medical Center
Brooklyn, NY
and
Assistant Professor
New York University College of Dentistry
New York, NY
Assistant Professor
University of Pennsylvania School of Dental Medicine
Philadelphia, PA

Dennis E. Feierman, MD, PhD
Assistant Professor of Anesthesiology
Department of Anesthesiology
The Mt. Sinai Medical Center
New York, NY

Eva Fischer, MD
Assistant Professor of Surgery
Director, Physician Assistant Program
The New York Hospital
Cornell Medical Center
New York, NY

Jane Gannon, CNM, MSN
Staff Nurse-Midwife, Clinical Assistant Professor
Fletcher Allen Health Care/Women's Health Care Service
Claire M. Lintilhac Nurse-Midwifery Service
University of Vermont
Burlington, VT

Goldie Gianoulis-Alossandratos, RN, MS, FNP
Dermatology Nurse Practitioner and Nurse Manager
Department of Dermatology at Beth Israel Medical Center
New York, NY

Lawrence Glaubiger, MD, FACP
Assistant Professor of Medicine
Pulmonary and Critical Care
Brooklyn Veterans' Administration Hospital
State University of New York
Health Science Center at Brooklyn
Brooklyn, NY

Richard W. Golub, MD, FACS
Assistant Professor of Surgery
Department of Surgery
State University of New York
Health Science Center at Brooklyn
Brooklyn, NY

Joseph A. Grillo, PharmD
Assistant Professor
Shenandoah University
School of Pharmacy
Winchester, VA

B. Mayer Grob
Assistant Professor
Department of Urology
State University of New York
Health Science Center at Brooklyn
Brooklyn, NY

Seth P. Harlow, MD
Assistant Professor of Surgery
College of Medicine
University of Vermont
Burlington, VT

Michael T. Harris, MD
Assistant Clinical Professor of Surgery
Mount Sinai School of Medicine
New York, NY

Albert E. Heurich, MD
Associate Professor of Clinical Medicine
Department of Medicine
State University of New York
Health Science Center at Brooklyn
Brooklyn, NY

Joanne Hickey, PhD, RN, CS, ACNP, CNRN, FAAN
Professor of Clinical Nursing
Acute and Continuing Care
The University of Texas, Houston
School of Nursing
Houston, TX

Ann Higgins, MS, RN, ANP
Adult Nurse Practioner
Family Care Center
Long Island College Hospital
Brooklyn, NY

Valerey Hughes, RN, BSN
HIV Clinician
AIDS Center Program
Lenox Hill Hospital
New York, NY

Steven Kaner, MD
Assistant Professor of Clinical Medicine
Department of Internal Medicine
State University of New York
Health Science Center at Brooklyn
Medical Director
Dr. Susan Smith McKinney Nursing and Rehabilitation Center
Brooklyn, NY

Duke Kasprisin, MD
National Medical Officer
American Red Cross—Tissue Services
Washington DC

Karen Anderson Keith, PhD, RN, CS
Associate Professor
Family Nurse Practitioner Program
Department of Graduate Studies
Lienhard School of Nursing
Pace University
Pleasantville, NY

Robert Keith, PA-C
Assistant Director of HIV Services
Daniel C. Lecht Assessment Clinic
Gouverneur Hospital
New York, NY

Debbie Kosko, MN, FNP-C
Instructor
School of Nursing
Johns Hopkins University
Baltimore, MD

Timothy F. Landers, RN, CS, CRNP, MA, MS
Nurse Practitioner
Caroline Health Services
Denton, MD

Nuria Lawson, MD
Chief Resident
State University of New York
Health Science Center at Brooklyn
Brooklyn, NY

Steven Lowy, MD
Larchmont, NY

Richard MacDougall, RPA-C
Physician Assistant
Diabetes and Endocrinology
St. Francis College
Loretto, PA

RosaLinda Marguiles, BSN, MPH, RNC
Education Specialist
GI Care Center
The Department of Nursing Education
Mt. Sinai Medical Center
Brooklyn, NY

James F. Marion, MD
Clinical Instructor of Medicine
Division of Gastroenterology
Mount Sinai School of Medicine
New York, NY

Edwin J. Masters, MD
Chairman, Department of Family Practice
Southeast Missouri Hospital
Cape Giradeau, MO

Jay Mazel, MD
Fellow, Arrhythmia Services
Department of Cardiovascular Medicine
Yale University—New Haven Hospital
New Haven, CT

Mary McCormack, RN-C, FNP-C, MSN, MPH
Family Nurse Practitioner
Family Care Center
Long Island College Hospital
Brooklyn, NY

Salah Mesad, MD
Senior Epilepsy and Neurophysiology Fellow
Department of Neurology
New York University Medical Center
New York, NY

Nancy Schlapper Morris, PhD, RNCS, ONC, ANP
Assistant Professor
School of Nursing
University of Vermont
Burlington, VT

Candis Morrison, PhD, RN
Assistant Professor
Johns Hopkins University School of Nursing
Nurse Practitioner
Johns Hopkins Oncology Center
Baltimore, MD

Hyman B. Muss, MD
Director, Hematology/Oncology
Department of Medicine
University of Vermont
Fletcher Allen Health Care
Burlington, VT

Muriel Helene Nathan, MD, PhD
Assistant Professor, Endocrinology
Department of Medicine
University of Vermont
Fletcher Allen Health Care
Burlington, VT

Tracey Offerdahl, PharmD
Assistant Professor of Clinical Pharmacy
Philadelphia College of Pharmacy
University of the Sciences in Philadelphia
Philadelphia, PA

Elaine B. Owen, RNCS, MSN, AOCN
Advanced Practice Nurse Practitioner
Mountainview Medical
Montpelier, VT

Thomas F. Panetta, MD
Professor of Surgery and Radiology
Chief, Division of Vascular Surgery
State University of New York
Health Science Center at Brooklyn
Brooklyn, NY

Harry Pomeranz, PA-C, MPH
Faculty
Department of Physician Assistant Education
State University of New York at Brooklyn
Health Science Center at Brooklyn
Brooklyn, NY

Ian Rabinowitz, MD
Assistant Professor
Hematology/Oncology Division
Department of Medicine
University of New Mexico
Albuquerque, NM

Eileen M. Reilly, RN, MS, FNP, CS
Coordinator for Vascular Surgery
Department of Surgery
The New York Hospital
Cornell University Medical College
New York, NY

Joseph Reilly, PharmD
Assistant Professor of Pharmacy Practice
Arnold & Marie Schwartz College of Pharmacy & Health
   Sciences
Long Island University
Brooklyn, NY

David Resch, MD
Assistant Professor
Departments of Internal Medicine and Psychiatry
Chief
Division of Internal Medicine and Psychiatry
Southern Illinois University School of Medicine
Springfield, IL

Ellen R. Rich, PhD, RN, CS, FNP
Assistant Professor and Chairperson
Family Nurse Practitioner Program
Lienhard School of Nursing
Pace University
Pleasantville, NY

Stephen Richardson, MD, FACP
Associate Professor of Medicine
New York University School of Medicine
New York, NY

Virginia E. Robertson, MD
Assistant Attending Physician
Department of Family Practice
Long Island College Hospital
Brooklyn, NY
and
Clinical Assistant Professor
State University of New York
Health Science Center at Brooklyn
Brooklyn, NY

Aymarah M. Robles, MD, FACP
Assistant Professor of Medicine
State University of New York
Health Science Center at Brooklyn
Brooklyn, NY

Peter Sanna, RPA, C, MPH
Administrator
Department of Medicine
Beth Abraham Health Services
Bronx, NY

Pamela Sass, MD
Assistant Professor
State University of New York
Health Science Center at Brooklyn
Brooklyn, NY

Joseph Scarpa, MD, CMD
Director of Medical Services
Department of Medicine
Beth Abraham Health Services
Bronx, NY

Naomi Schlesinger, MD
Assistant Professor of Clinical Medicine
Division of Allergy, Immunology and Rheumatology
University of Medicine and Dentistry
Newark, NJ

Bayo Sedenu, PT, PhD
Director of Physical Therapy
Dr. Susan Smith McKinney Nursing and Rehabilitation Center
Brooklyn, NY

Miriam Shustik, MD, ABFP
Clinical Instructor
Department of Family Medicine
Warren Hospital
Robert Wood Johnson Medical School
University of Medicine and Dentistry of New Jersey
New Brunswick, NJ
and
Clinical Instructor
Department of Family Medicine
St Luke's Hospital
University of Pennsylvania
Philadelphia, PA

Ofer Shustik, MD, ABFP
Palmer Family Practice
Easton, PA

Diane M. Snow, RN, PhD, CARN, PMHNP
Specialist and Acting Director
Psychiatric-Mental Health Nurse Practitioner Program
School of Nursing
University of Texas at Arlington
Arlington, TX

Alfred F. Tallia, MD, MPH
Associate Professor and Vice Chairman of Family Medicine
Robert Wood Johnson Medical School
University of Medicine and Dentistry of New Jersey
New Brunswick, NJ

James Tazelaar, MS, FNP-C
Orthopaedic Nurse Practitioner
Orthopaedic Service
Veterans' Administration Hospital
White River Junction, VT

Elena M. Umland, PharmD
Assistant Professor of Clinical Pharmacy
Department of Pharmacy Practice and Pharmacy
  Administration
Philadelphia College of Pharmacy and Science
Philadelphia, PA

William Urban, MD
Assistant Professor of Orthopaedic Surgery and Rehabilitative
  Medicine
Director of Sports Medicine
State University of New York Health Science Center at
  Brooklyn
Brooklyn, NY

Sanjeev Vaderah, MD
Clinical Instructor
Division of Cardiovascular Medicine
Department of Medicine
State University of New York
Health Science Center at Brooklyn
Brooklyn, NY

Deborah Wachtel, RNP, MPH, OGNP
Clinical Research Nurse Practitioner
General Clinical Research Center
Burlington, VT
Women's Health Nurse Practitioner
Fletcher Allen Health Care
Burlington, VT

Hillary Wall-Grillo, PharmD
Assistant Clinical Professor of Pharmacy Practice
Clinical Coordinator for Adult Internal Medicine
Department of Clinical Pharmacy Practice
St. John's University
Jamaica, NY

Steve Weintraub, BS, DO
Attending Physician
Department of Family Medicine
Helene Fuld Medical Center
Orthopaedic Consultant
Medical Center of Ocean County
Clinical Assistant Professor & Sports Medicine Fellowship
  Faculty
Department of Sports Medicine
Robert Wood Johnson University Hospital
New Brunswick, NJ

Willem Wisselink, MD
Assistant Professor of Surgery
State University of New York
Health Science Center at Brooklyn
Brooklyn, NY
Chief
Section of Endovascular Surgery
Veterans Administration Medical Center
Brooklyn, NY

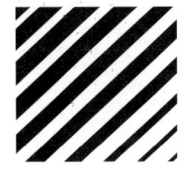

Clinical Consultants

Christine Alicea, BS, RN
Pleasantville, NY

Kathleen Lent Becker, MS, CRNP
Assistant Professor
Adult Nurse Practitioner
Johns Hopkins University School of Nursing
Baltimore, MD

Theresa M. Bertozzi, MS, RN, CS, FNP
IV Specialist, Home Care
Valhalla, NY

Susan Buchholtz, EdD, RN, CS, ANP
Department of Pre-Surgical Testing
Northshore University Medical Center at Forrest Hills
Forrest Hills, NY

Nancy Giordano, EdD, RN, CS, WNP
Coordinator, Nurse Practitioner Program
College of New Rochelle
New Rochelle, NY

Philip Grover, DC
Doctor of Chiropractic Medicine
Pittsfield, MA

Aliza Holtz, PhD
Research Consultant
New York, NY

Susan L. W. Krupnick, MSN, RN, CARN, CS
Psychiatric Liaison, Clinical Nurse Specialist
Baystate Medical Center
Springfield, MA

Lynda Mackin, RN, C, MS, ANP
Assistant Clinical Professor
Department of Physiological Nursing
University of California, San Francisco
San Francisco, CA

Marilyn Morley, BS, RN, CARN
Psychiatric Nurse Consultant
Brightwaters, NY

Nancy Murphy, BS, RN
New York, NY

Holly Nadal, LMT
Licensed Massage Therapist
New York, NY

Sandra M. Nettina, RN, C, MSN, ANP
Adjunct Faculty
George Washington University, Washington, DC
and George Mason University, Fairfax, VA
Adult Nurse Practitioner
Laurel, MD

Yoshiaki Omura, MD, ScD, FACA, FICAE
Director of Medical Research, Heart Disease Research
Foundation, NY
President, International College of Acupuncture and Electro-
Therapeutics, NY
Visiting Research Professor, Dept. of Electrical Engineering,
Manhattan College, NY
Professor, Dept. of Non-Orthodox Medicine, Ukrainian
National Medical University, Kiev, Ukraine
Adjunct Professor, Dept. of Physiology, Showa University
School of Medicine, Tokyo, Japan

Ellen Rich, PhD, RN, CS, FNP
Family Nurse Practitioner & Certified Biofeedback Therapist
Pace University, Health Care Unit
Pleasantville, NY

Margaret Rowlett, ARNP, BS
Women's Health Nurse Practitioner
Certified Clinical Aromatherapist, Instructor Status
St. Johnsbury, VT

Daniel B. Rukstalis, MD
Chief of Urology
Department of Surgery
Allegheny University of the Health Sciences
Philadelphia, PA

Joan Wanveer
Brooklyn, NY

Tad Wanveer, LMT
Licensed Massage Therapist
Craniosacral Therapist
New York, NY

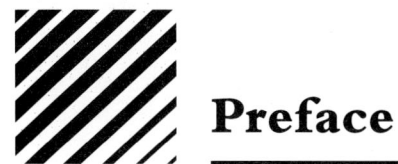

Preface

All books begin with an idea; this one is no different. Its development began with the recognized need for a book that would offer comprehensive, integrated information on the care of patients with prevalent diagnoses, primarily of a chronic nature, seen in primary care. Primary care is complex and encompassing, and care is given by many different types of providers—nurse practitioners, physicians, physician assistants, nurse midwives, and clinical PharmDs, who work together in both formal and informal interdisciplinary groups. All primary care providers are not the same. We come from different disciplines, and no one owns all this knowledge. While the disciplines have shared knowledge, each brings their own ways of applying that knowledge to practice.

Health care is experiencing a shift from a reactive disease orientation to one of proactive primary health care. Patient participation, to the best extent possible, is critical to this changing health paradigm. Interdisciplinary practice enriches not only the experience of delivering primary care, but broadens our knowledge base and supports relationship-centered care.

In Section 1 the framework for primary care is presented. Chapter 1 elucidates our philosophy and identifies concepts essential for achieving interdisciplinary relationship-centered primary care. Building upon this, the remaining chapters in Section 1 describe a framework for providers to facilitate com-

prehensive assessment and management that includes family and cultural assessment; health promotion and disease prevention, including information on complementary approaches to care; nutritional assessment; violence exposure and vulnerability assessment; and community assessment. Section 2 presents comprehensive, integrated information on prevalent primary care diagnoses of adult primary care patients. As appropriate for each condition, the following are included: Anatomy, Physiology, and Pathology; Epidemiology; Diagnostic Criteria; History and Physical Exam; Diagnostic Studies; Treatment Options, Expected Outcomes, and Comprehensive Management; Teaching and Self-Care; Community Resources; Referral Points and Clinical Warnings; and an Editor's Note on Selected Complementary Approaches. At the end of the book are three appendices. Appendices A and B offer additional information on specific vitamins, minerals, herbs and supplements, and the selected complementary modalities. Appendix C discusses preoperative evaluation.

This book is intended to assist faculty and students in the primary care disciplines in teaching and learning, support experienced practitioners, and facilitate specialized health care providers as they make the transition to providing primary care.

JKS and the Editorial Group

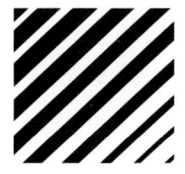

Personal Thank-You's

❧❧❧❧❧❧❧❧❧

Behind a successful woman is often a supportive man. I am fortunate to be such a woman, and thank Rolf. His untiring love and counsel encouraged me to stay focused on the work at hand.
My son Andrew, thanks for always helping out, and,
Lily, always a pleasant distraction and calming influence.

JKS

❧❧❧❧❧❧❧❧❧

My wife Ofra for all of her support, encouragement, love and devotion
My daughters, Sarit, Yaara, and Sapir for their inspiration
and patience through all the endless nights and missed weekends
My father, sister, and grandmother, for helping me to get to where I am

SAS

❧❧❧❧❧❧❧❧❧

To Ed, Ian, and Gillian, as always and in always. . .

CG-H

❧❧❧❧❧❧❧❧❧

I wish to thank
Linda Efferen, whose work on this project always surpassed expectation
Joanne Singleton, who was a constant buoy in rough currents, and
Mark Gombiner, who is the best writer I know.

THV

❧❧❧❧❧❧❧❧❧

To my son Adam who taught me that blankies are more effective than analgesics,
and to the rest of my family for their faith in my abilities.

RDG

❧❧❧❧❧❧❧❧❧

John Shannon Keogh
Carolyn A. Fish (in memory)
Barbara McCampbell Holzemer

SPH

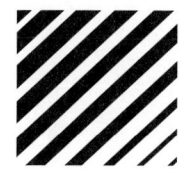

The Editors wish to say "Thank You"

ঌঌঌঌঌঌঌঌ

Lisa Stead, our Editor who really walked the walk with us on this journey. . . Lisa, you're an amazing person and editor, it's been real. . . !

ঌঌঌঌঌঌঌঌ

Claudia Vaughn, our Editorial Assistant, whose cheery voice and enduring optimism that "everything is okay" helped carry us through this project

ঌঌঌঌঌঌঌঌ

RK, for his negotiating savvy, administrative assistance, and constant unwavering support

ঌঌঌঌঌঌঌঌ

Our contributors, for sharing their knowledge, experience, and insights

ঌঌঌঌঌঌঌঌ

Harriet Feldman, PhD, RN, FAAN, Dean, Pace University, Lienhard School of Nursing—thanks for your encouragement and support

ঌঌঌঌঌঌঌঌ

Maureen Anello, Pace University, Lienhard School of Nursing, NYC Campus—thanks for helping to move things along

ঌঌঌঌঌঌঌঌ

Pace University's Security Guards, NYC Campus, 41 Park Row—thanks for watching over us those late nights

ঌঌঌঌঌঌঌঌ

Miriam T. Vincent, MD, Associate Professor and Interim Chairperson, SUNY–Health Science Center Brooklyn, Department of Family Practice—thanks for your support and encouragement

ঌঌঌঌঌঌঌঌ

Patricia Winstead-Fry, RN, PhD, Interim Dean, University of Vermont, School of Nursing—thanks for your support and encouragement

ঌঌঌঌঌঌঌঌ

Linda Rubino—thanks for helping to keep things on the straight and narrow

❧❧❧❧❧❧❧❧

Patricia Blagman, EdD, RN—thanks for sharing your knowledge of therapeutic touch

❧❧❧❧❧❧❧❧

Cathleen Besch, MS, RN, CS, FNP

Madelyn Goldthwaite, RN, OGNP
thanks for your assistance

❧❧❧❧❧❧❧❧

Christina Whited, for her insight

❧❧❧❧❧❧❧❧

To all our families, friends, colleagues, students, and patients, who in so many different
ways offered kind words and gestures of support to us throughout this project,
thank you.

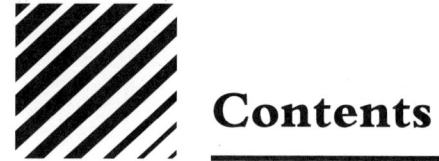

Contents

PART

One

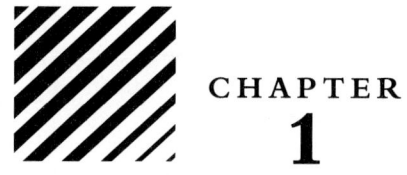

CHAPTER

1

The Structure of Primary Care

Joanne K. Singleton, PhD, RN, CS, FNP, Carol Green-Hernandez, PhD, RN, CS, FNP/ANP, and Stephen Paul Holzemer, PhD, RN

Health care delivery in the United States reflects a history of change in response to science, technology, and the cost of health care. Helping people meet their health needs is the central mission of all health disciplines. How this is accomplished, however, continues to change with the times. Lacking a scientific basis, health care before the 20th century was able to offer little more than caring and attention to personal health in the home setting.

The scientific basis for health care became more formalized after 1900 with the inclusion of sciences in the medical and nursing curricula. Health was defined as the presence or absence of disease, and the development of technology was directed at treating and curing diseases. This necessitated the movement of the delivery of care into the hospital setting, where patients were seen as passive recipients of specialized, technologic care that focused on their physical and biologic needs.

In the early years of the 20th century, great advances were made in the control of infectious diseases. As a result, specialization and technology became more highly regarded than caring and personal care. Although it was recognized that with these changes something had been lost (Flexner, 1930), health care continued to proceed in that direction. Highly specialized care dominated, yet it lacked oversight of the appropriate use of services, the need for services, or the cost of those services.

This view persisted until it was acknowledged in the past decade that the health care needs of the United States, access to services, and the ability to pay for them in the current fee-for-service system of reimbursement had changed. Health care needs of Americans were changed by the profound advances made in the control of infectious diseases and the use of technology. This resulted in people living longer, and with this came the advent of chronic diseases.

In the fee-for-service system, economic incentive was based on the use of services. Ultimately, this led to inappropriate use and over-use of services, resulting in health care costs that are approaching one trillion dollars each year in the United States. Despite this enormous expenditure, almost 40 million Americans are without health insurance. Access to health care, in the absence of universal health care coverage, remains an issue of national concern. The cost of health care, access to health care, types of services, and delivery of those services have become common topics of conversation both inside and outside the health care arena. Each proposed solution poses different challenges.

Today's view of health must acknowledge the juxtaposition of multiple factors that may influence and predispose a person to illness(es). These factors include the complex interdependent biologic, psychological, social, and spiritual needs of the person. The integrated needs of the individual places the person within the context of their family and community. It also recognizes that health is not simply the presence or absence of disease, it is an ongoing process that can be fostered through activities directed at health promotion and disease prevention. Health as a dynamic state of being is active, and as such, for individuals to actualize their health potential, they must engage in the process of health. This necessitates a change in perspective from the individual as a passive recipient of care to the individual as an active participant in their own health.

To meet these needs, health care delivery in the United States is shifting to primary care, in which providers address a wide range of health care needs and facilitate health care delivery.

Primary care in this book is recognized as the provision of integrated, accessible health care services by providers who are accountable for addressing a large majority of personal health care needs. These providers develop sustained partnerships with patients and practice within the context of family and community (Donaldson et al, 1996). This concept of primary care allows patients and providers to enter relationships where patients, families, and communities have the opportunity to become full participants in health care decision making.

In today's health care environment, economic considerations loom. Capitation of services through managed care is one current response to cost containment. Capitated reimbursement means that there are fixed prepaid fees for each enrollee. That fee must cover the entire range of services the enrollee is entitled to through the plan. If enrollees use more services than covered by the plan, providers are at risk for absorbing those costs. The objective is for providers to have the incentive to keep their enrollees healthy. More than 50 million Americans are insured through managed care plans, and this number is expected to increase to 100 million by the year 2000 (Bodenheimer, 1996).

It is unclear how systems of care will adapt, and how providers will be able to deliver effective, comprehensive care in capitated managed care or other fiscally restructured environments. One key issue is whether financial incentives can safely guide clinical decision making.

Professional standards may be challenged through the managed care approach. Despite these changes, providers must rigorously adhere to practice standards and maintain the integrity of their clinical relationships. The patient must remain the focus of care, regardless of whatever changes are occurring in health care. Providers need to work together to develop creative strategies to sustain and nurture relationship-centered care.

Foundational to the therapeutic nature of patient–provider interactions is the relationship that develops between patient and provider. This relationship is believed to be central to improved patient outcomes and patient–provider satisfaction (Tresolini, 1994). Relationship-centered care redefines the therapeutic value of patient–provider interactions, recognizing the importance of the health care relationships formed by providers with families and communities. Primary care providers can use this time of change in the delivery of health care as an opportunity to work with each other and their patients to create comprehensive, interdisciplinary, relationship-centered primary care networks that improve outcomes and satisfaction for both patients and providers.

This chapter identifies concepts essential for achieving relationship-centered primary care. The idea of caring and trust as the foundation of primary care is explored. Building upon this, a framework for providers to facilitate comprehensive assessment and management is presented. This foundation and framework creates a structure for providers and patients to work together as architects in the redesign of health care.

THE FOUNDATION OF PRIMARY CARE: CARING AND TRUST

Effective relationship-centered primary care demands increased attention to the interpersonal aspects of health care relationships. Valuing professional caring is central to this kind of relationship. Professional caring is comprised of feelings and behaviors within the relationship. It requires the provider to enter and sustain relationships with their patients, as well as with colleagues, as opposed to simply performing tasks or techniques. A caring relationship creates the climate for trust to develop, and for the patient and provider to use their personal resources most effectively toward positive patient outcomes (Green-Hernandez, 1997).

Both patients and providers bring expertise to the care planning. Ideally, they meet and work together to create acceptable plans of primary care. Providers bring expertise in their discipline of study. Patients bring knowledge of their subjective experience of illness, or their health care needs that reflect aspects such as family history, culture, values, and beliefs as they relate to health care.

In situations where the patient is unwilling or unable to enter into a relationship with the provider, various standards of assessment are used to provide safe and prudent primary care. When patients refuse care or do not follow jointly agreed-upon plans of care, the primary care relationship must be reevaluated. In relationship-centered care, providers recognize that a patient may need to work with a different provider, and so must strive to actively refer the patient to someone with whom the patient can work with effectively. While the patient is waiting for the referral appointment, the referring provider is responsible for constructing a "safety net" to ensure that the patient has services available during this time.

Learning How to Give Caring

Fundamental to providers learning how to give caring is their ability to challenge traditional stereotyping or labeling of the patient as a chief complaint, a diagnosis, a disease, or a passive recipient of care. For a partnership to be formed, the provider must see the patient first as a person. In so doing, the provider appreciates and respects the patient's individuality and subjective response to the presenting health care need(s). It must also

be recognized that the patient's subjective response to illness or a health care problem will be influenced by values and beliefs, which may differ from those of the provider.

Seeing the patient as a person requires communication, which is essential to learning how to give caring (Green-Hernandez, 1997). Communication goes beyond the spoken word. It involves one person sending a message and another receiving that message. Through communication both providers and patients let each other know that they are willing and available to enter into a caring partnership. Providers must be open to receiving a response from patients about their willingness and level of ability to participate in their own care. With this understanding, the provider and the patient will be able to define what the patient's health care needs are, and how they will be met. This partnership will be defined and redefined over time.

An ongoing concern of providers is the brevity of health care encounters. How realistic is it in a 10- to 15-minute visit to communicate to a patient one's willingness and availability to enter into a caring partnership? Regardless of the length of visit, providers still retain control over how they interact with patients. Simple approaches to interactions with patients, such as those in Table 1-1, communicate caring and therapeutic intent. These are some of the many approaches that will communicate to the patient that they are the focus of the encounter. This caring process is a reflection of using the time the provider has with the patient for the patient (Green-Hernandez, 1997; Singleton, 1993).

Re-Visioning Compliance

From the previous discussion, it follows that providers who learn how to give caring have effectively learned how to use themselves therapeutically. To do this, providers must recognize the importance of what they bring to relationship-centered care. This requires both introspection and learning how to use

---

TABLE 1-1

Initiating the Encounter
Greet the patient by name.
Offer a handshake or a touch on the arm.
Establish eye contact, if culturally appropriate.

During the Encounter
Sit nearby without invading the patient's personal space.
Have only the patient's chart on your desk.
Take only urgent or emergency phone calls.
Have all the supplies and equipment in the room needed for the visit to avoid leaving the room once you've begun the encounter.
Review with the patient the last visit and what has transpired in the interim.
Do not do things to patients without explaining what you are doing.
When discussing the patient's care with others, such as the patient's family or a health care colleague, in the presence of the patient, do not exclude the patient from the conversation.
Your tone of voice, volume and speed of verbal communication, and nonverbal behaviors, such as eye contact, nervousness, or hyperactive behaviors, can influence communication.
Ask questions that allow the patients to explain their experiences.
Do not put words in the patient's mouth.
Remember to address the patient's reason for the visit and concerns.

Ending the Encounter
Ask the patient if there is anything else they would like to discuss.
Discuss treatment and management, including options.
Once a plan is agreed upon, discuss and identify how it will be carried out.

the different strategies discussed to be reflective practitioners. These practitioners reflect on their practice, using patient encounters to critique themselves in order to be more effective in their use of self. Reflective practice is a skill that requires conscious self-study and development over time.

Learning how to care necessitates changing preexisting perspectives that may be detrimental to the patient–provider relationship. One such critical perspective that must be revisited is that of paternalistic relationships, in which the provider uses power and authority to prescribe care, seeking compliance from the patient. In these scenarios, true communication does not take place. These patients are at risk for being labeled "noncompliant" if they do not carry out the provider's orders. Because of the lack of communication, it is unlikely that any understanding will be gained of why the patient did not follow through with the plan of care. With the exception of situations that involve the immediate safety or protection of the patient, provider, family or community, the word "noncompliant" expresses an attitude inconsistent with relationship-centered care. Providers who value relationship-centered care continue to work toward replacing this word with the word and perspective of participation, reflecting a changing paradigm from paternalism to caring. Thus trusting partnerships are developed.

TRUST

Trust is an attitude that one has in regard to another. Attributes of trust include reliability, confidence, vulnerability, and fragility (Johns, 1996). Trust must be reciprocal and reflexive. Patients should have trust in providers and in themselves to participate in meeting their own health care needs. Patients will trust providers who are reliable and in whom they have confidence. Providers need to trust that patients will participate in decision making related to health care. Providers must also trust in their own technical and professional ability to provide and coordinate the care of patients.

Trust is essential in the patient–provider relationship and may be instrumental in influencing patient outcomes. Elements that may facilitate patients in developing trust in their providers include technical proficiency and professional competence.

Technical Proficiency

Technical proficiency results from developing the psychomotor skill repertoire required for practice. There are skills that will be common to all primary care providers and others that may be specific to providers working with different patient populations, or to the focus and scope of services in their primary care practice group. Providers need to identify the skills necessary to their practice. Learning and performing skills helps providers to gain a feeling of technical competence (Green-Hernandez, 1997). Necessary skills will change over time, both in how they are performed and in the skills required. Providers must keep abreast of these changes to maintain technical proficiency.

Professional Competence

Professional competence is predicated on developing essential skills, including learning how to give caring, technical proficiency, and effectiveness in coordinating care. Coordinating care of patients may include interdisciplinary consultation, referral, or comanagement with the interdisciplinary team. Professional competence is the culmination of achieving and balancing these skills (Green-Hernandez, 1997).

Interdisciplinary Practice

The relationships among provider and colleagues, although different from provider–patient relationships, are central to providing primary care. Relationships among interdisciplinary colleagues can offer valuable perspectives on assisting patients in meeting their health care needs. Providers must trust the contributions that can be made through consultation with or referral to their interdisciplinary colleagues. For this trust to develop, providers have to believe that interdisciplinary practice will improve patient outcomes. They also need to be willing to gain greater understanding of, insight into, and respect for other disciplines, and the contribution they can make to patient outcomes (Singleton & Green-Hernandez, 1998).

Barriers to interdisciplinary education and practice are identified as negative attitudes and inaccurate perceptions of faculty and providers toward the benefits of interdisciplinary education and practice (Baldwin, 1994; Grant, Finocchio, and the California Primary Care Consortium Committee on Interdisciplinary Collaboration, 1995). It is interesting to note, and certainly holds hope, that students of the health care disciplines view interdisciplinary education and clinical practice experiences positively and actively seek to participate in them. Several benefits of interdisciplinary practice have been identified. These include greater patient satisfaction, better outcomes, and cost efficiency (Baldwin, 1994). Without confronting these barriers, the benefits of interdisciplinary primary care will not be realized.

A caring, trusting patient–provider relationship is the foundation for a relationship-centered approach to proactive primary care. Through this approach, providers come to truly know their patients. This facilitates accurate and comprehensive assessment of the patient. Relationship-centered care incorporates more than traditional, formalized assessment. From its initiation, the patient is recognized as having expert knowledge of their health care need(s). Through empowering the patient in a health care system that traditionally disempowers, negotiation of care occurs through active participation with the patient.

THE FRAMEWORK FOR PRIMARY CARE

The framework for primary care presented in this book offers a comprehensive view of assessing and working with patients, with the goal of developing over time an inclusive management plan. Through this framework, proactive primary care is achieved by assessing such factors as family, culture, nutrition, and community, health promotion and disease prevention, and violence exposure and vulnerability, while being knowledgeable about the common conditions, primarily of a chronic nature, seen in primary care. As appropriate for each condition, this book discusses:

- Anatomy, physiology, and pathology
- Epidemiology
- Diagnostic criteria
- History and physical exam
- Diagnostic studies
- Treatment options, expected outcomes, comprehensive management, including: teaching and self-care community resources health promotion and disease prevention
- Referral points and clinical warnings
- Selected complementary health care approaches related to the condition. While there are self-care recommendations

specific for each condition, an important consideration for providers is how, at a time when a typical patient visit is 10 to 15 minutes, can the provider maximize patient education to encourage self-care?

Maximizing Self-Care

In its most simplistic sense, self-care means taking care of one-self. The processes involved, commitment and motivation of individuals in taking care of themselves, are not yet well understood. Motivation, however, is recognized as a complex phenomenon which is internally driven. While providers may not be able to directly motivate their patients to care for themselves, they can create a climate to encourage motivation. Educating patients is an important strategy providers can use to encourage patients in self-care and to achieve positive health outcomes. To effectively use health education as a strategy, patients should be approached based on their learning styles.

Assessing Learning Style for Health Education

Much is written concerning how best the primary care provider can offer health education in a busy office or clinic setting. The realities of managing this process can be especially challenging when there is little time for teaching during the visit, let alone time for assessing learning needs regarding growth and development, health promotion, disease prevention, and illness/disease management. The following section provides a guide for assessing a patient's learning style, while also providing several suggested teaching intervention techniques.

Basic Necessities for Health Education

The patient and family's understanding is critical to their success in participating in developing and carrying out a plan. The evaluation component of the plan's outcome is tied to this comprehension. Key areas of knowledge to be evaluated include:

- The disease process and course
- Symptoms and symptom management
- Self-care strategies for symptom control
- Whom to call if a problem arises
- Medication administration
- Use of medical equipment
- Possible food–drug interactions
- When and how to seek further care
- Prior experience with the health care team

Learning style is not a one-dimensional concept. It is made up of many elements, including the learner's reading comprehension and verbal understanding levels, developmental level, learning style, and emotional status. Basic personality and learning style also influence the learner's ability to take in and use new information. A further complication to learning ability may be the fact that, when uninvited information is given (information the patient may not wish to hear or is unwilling to hear), its acceptance and integration may not take place.

Reading Levels and Content Understanding

Twenty percent of the U.S. population is functionally illiterate. They are unable to read most magazines and newspapers, which are written at the 9th- to 12th-grade level, let alone read or interpret basic written instructions. Another 30% have marginal reading skills and may be able to follow very basic written directions, if clearly and simply worded. This is problematic for providers, as most written health care literature available to patients is generally written at least at the 6th-grade level. Literacy poses serious implications for health care delivery, as poor understanding of health and illness results in poor patient participation in health care regimens.

Reading competency is categorized based on ascending complexity from level one through five. Approximately 20% of adults read at the lowest literacy level, which corresponds to below the 5th-grade level. Levels two to three in reading function approximates 8th- to 9th-grade reading competency and is the average level for most North Americans. Exceptions to this include nearly 40% of individuals who are over age 65, as well as minority populations living in inner cities, who read below level one (Doak, Doak & Root, 1996).

Understanding health and the role of personal choice in its management is further influenced by patients' health values. Individuals of low literacy exhibit more risk-taking behavior and experience increased health care costs over their lifetimes (Doak, Doak & Root, 1996). Table 1-2 presents some of the basic differences between poor and skilled readers, with suggestions on how a primary care provider can help the former to take in and understand the context for those written health teaching materials one provides.

While primary care providers acknowledge the importance of the patient's level of understanding, testing reading skills and comprehension levels in patients is beyond the resources of providers. A logical strategy is for the provider to present written material to the patient. Until one is sure that the patient is capable of reading and understanding the material, the wise practitioner works with the patient in reading some of the materials together, using the above directives provided in Table

TABLE 1-2	Differences Between Good and Poor Readers—and How You Can Manage the Problems	
Skilled Readers	**Poor Readers**	**Managing the Problems**
Interpret meaning	Take words literally	Explain the meaning
Read with fluency	Read slowly, miss meaning	Use common words, examples
Get help for uncommon word	Skip over the word	Use examples, review
Grasp the context	Miss the context	Tell context first, use visuals
Persistent reader	Tire quickly	Short segments, easy layout

Doak et al, (1996).

1-2 to ensure that the content is usable for the patient. For patients who are not able to read and comprehend the health materials, a capable and responsible family member may assist in the patient's participation. Providers may wish to supplement commercially available written literature with their own written materials. Table 1-3 provides a clear framework for creating these kinds of materials for patients with low literacy skills.

Meeting Learning Needs

"The teachable moment" means that the provider uses every possible opportunity to convey the message. In primary care, this message focuses on all aspects of health promotion and disease prevention. Teaching–learning can be contagious. A health message may reach a patient because of its relevance to the patient or to the patient's family and friends. Having a selection of pamphlets available to patients in the waiting room helps to ensure that they pass on the "correct" version of this message. Teaching messages can be reinforced in the waiting room through use of colorful health posters and a variety of pamphlets. Non-English versions should be displayed if appropriate to the patient population.

Consider assigning different clinic staff with the responsibility of periodically changing posters as well as replenishing and updating health teaching literature, so that frequent clinic users will be exposed to more than one or two ongoing messages. Ongoing messages may include, for example, posters and literature related to smoking and alcohol use, safer sex, healthy babies, diabetes, cholesterol, and heart disease. Ideally, posters should be changed every few months. These simple acts can add interest to the patient's wait, while reinforcing the messages providers wish to convey. People will peruse material new to them the first time. After that initial exposure, their interest must continue to be piqued if health messages are to be reinforced.

These strategies can also find their way into examining rooms or cubicles. Consider posting materials on wall space and ceilings. A cheerful poster displayed in an unexpected spot can be an especially powerful teaching strategy.

"The teachable moment" presents itself in many ways. For primary care providers, learning to make the most of a teachable moment may be the critical element in creating a climate to encourage patients in health promotion and disease prevention self-care.

SUMMARY

Current changes in health care needs, how health is viewed, and the delivery of services all point to the importance of patients being actively involved in meeting their health care needs. This calls for challenging traditional ways of thinking, changing views, shedding preassigned roles, and rethinking patient–provider roles and relationships. There is a moral imperative for primary care providers to work as partners with patients, helping them meet their health care needs through developing and maintaining relationship-centered, proactive primary care.

References

Baldwin, D. (1994). The role of interdisciplinary education and teamwork in primary care and health care reform. Dept. of Human Services. Bureau of Health Professions, HRSA March 1994; Order No. 92-1009 (P).

Bodenheimer, T. (1996). The HMO backlash: Righteous or reactionary. *N Engl J Med, 355,* 1601–1604.

Doak, C.C., Doak, L.G., & Root, J.H. (1996). *Teaching patients with low literacy skills.* Philadelphia: Lippincott-Raven.

Donaldson, M.S., Yordy, K.D., Lohr, K.N., & Vanselor, N.A. (Eds). (1996). *Primary care: America's health in a new era.* Washington DC: Nation Academy Press.

Grant, R., Finocchio, L, and the California Primary Care Consortium Committee on Interdisciplinary Collaboration (1995). *Interdisciplinary collaborative teams in primary care; A model curriculum and resource guide.* San Francisco: Pew Health Professions Commission.

Green-Hernandez, C. (1997). Application of caring theory in primary care: A challenge for advanced practice. *Nursing Science Quarterly, 21*(4), 77–82.

Johns, J. (1996). A concept analysis of trust. *J Advanced Nursing, 24,* 76–83.

Singleton, J.K., Green-Hernandez. (1998). Interdisciplinary education and practice: Has its time come? *Journal of Nurse Midwifery, 43*(1).

Singleton, J.K. (1993). *Nursing Interventions to Encourage Residents' Self Care in Long Term Care: An Ethnography,* University Microfilm International.

Tresolini, C.P., & the Pew-Fetzer Task Force. (1994). *Health professions education and relationship-centered care.* San Francisco: Pew Health Professionals Commission.

Bibliography

American Medical Association, Center for Health Policy Research (1992). *Socioeconomic characteristics of medical practice.* Chicago: American Medical Association.

Doak, L.G., & Doak, C.C. (1980). Patient comprehension profiles: Recent findings and strategies. *Patient Counseling and Health Education, 2*(3), 101–106.

Lawrence, D. (1993) Physician assistants and nurse practitioners: Their impact on health care access, costs, and quality. *Health Medical Care Service Review, 1*(2), 1–12.

Lipson, J., Dibble, S., & Minarik, P. (1996). *Culture & nursing care: A pocket guide.* San Francisco: UCSF Press.

National Association of County Health Officials. (1994) *Providing culturally appropriate services.* Washington DC: Author.

Pullen, C., & Edwards, J. (1994). A comprehensive primary care delivery model. *J Professional Nursing, 10*(4), 201–208.

US Congress, Office of Technology Assessment (1990). *Health care in rural America,* OTA-H-434. Washington DC: US Government Printing Office.

TABLE 1-3	Guidelines for Health Education Methods and Materials

- Set Realistic objective(s)
  Limit the objective to what the majority of the target population needs now. Use a planning sheet to write down the objective and key points.

- To change health behaviors, focus on behaviors and skills
  Emphasize behaviors and skills rather than facts. Consider the sequence for the topics shown in Box 2-1. Otherwise, consider placing the key points first and last.

- Present context first (before giving new information)
  State the purpose or use for new content information before presenting it. Relate new information to the context of patients' lives.

- Partition complex instructions
  Break instruction into easy-to-understand parts. Provide opportunities for small successes.

- Make it interactive
  Consider including an interaction after each key topic. The patient must: write, tell, show, demonstrate, select, or solve a problem.

Doak et al, (1996).

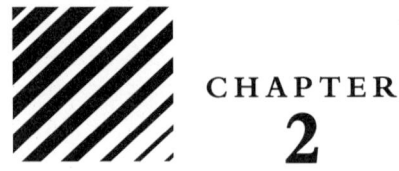

CHAPTER
2

Family and Cultural Assessment Measures in Primary Care

Carol Green-Hernandez, PhD, FNS, ANP/FNP-C

Primary care that is truly family-focused uses the family unit as a basis for data gathering in assessing and meeting patient needs. Successful implementation and evaluation of management interventions can occur when the patient is a partner in the entire primary care process. This chapter will illuminate the challenge to primary care of placing family and culture in context with demographics, geography, and economic influences. Models for family assessment, and for family-focused cultural assessment, will be presented as tools for data collection in primary care. This assessment data is foundational to the patient's health history. As an antecedent to this content, values clarification will be discussed as a strategy that can help the provider in giving patient-centered care that is salient for both provider and patient.

VALUES CLARIFICATION IN PRIMARY CARE

The primary care provider may find that clarifying their own values and beliefs can assist in discerning possible sources for prejudicial assessment of patients. Values clarification may prove especially helpful when caring for patients whose values, beliefs, and health behaviors differ from those of the provider. After clarifying what is important for oneself, the provider can sift out values and beliefs that are congruent with those of their patient. Areas of value digression might be found between the patient and the provider. But the process of self-reflection in values clarification can help the provider to avoid out-and-out conflict with the patient when strong differences in beliefs emerge. Clearly, such conflict can jeopardize a therapeutic relationship, the purpose of which is to facilitate patient health rather than serving as a foundation for a "bully pulpit." Values clarification can help the provider to deliver primary care unburdened by anger or betrayal if a patient chooses to ignore the health plan. A sample values clarification tool and directions for its use are found in Appendix 2-1.

Values clarification can empower provider and patient alike. The goal, of course, is to create and maintain primary care that is relationship-centered for provider and patient. Such care must be both legal and ethical, while promoting self-actualization of the patient and family (Green-Hernandez, 1997). This means that the provider is sensitive to both verbal and nonverbal cues and behaviors, including body stance, positioning, and use of eye contact. Similarly, maintenance of body space and use of touch can signal respect or its lack. Patients are not passive recipients of primary care—they are in fact active partners in that care. By using relationship-centered care as a basis for communicating and working with patients, the provider can

avoid some of the value-laden problems that often emerge in the course of primary care that is provider-controlled. The patients' feelings, values, and beliefs, including those pertaining to health, are integral to all care management strategies in primary care.

When values conflict between provider and patient and/ or the family, referral to a different provider may need to be considered if consensus on treatment options cannot be reached. This is exemplified by a case where a provider advises adoption to a young unmarried woman who is unexpectedly pregnant, and who asks for abortion services. If the provider does not subscribe to reproductive choice, this value can impact a patient's decision-making capability to the extent that she follows through on a pregnancy against her will. This scenario's implications may not end there. Her family may pressure her to keep the baby, leading her to abandon plans to complete her education. Conversely, she may follow-through on adoption, but may later regret this decision. This scenario is one that is very real. Because there are no easy answers to many of the dilemmas faced in primary care, it is incumbent on the provider to examine personal values and beliefs before addressing patient care.

TAKING VALUES CLARIFICATION TO THE FAMILY

Like all open living systems, the family is an evolving entity. Today a family may be headed by an emancipated minor, a single parent, two or more unrelated individuals, same-sex heads-of-household, as well as the so-called "traditional," nuclear family. The concept of a "typical" family eludes characterization. The family is what its members envision it to be, with the group defining membership as the key to family composition. This vision for family demography impacts family functioning. It is this impact, and the implications it holds for health promotion and illness management, that presents an important challenge to primary care providers.

FAMILY-CENTERED PRACTICE

Traditionally, the practice of primary care treated the patient as an individual who required treatment. The family was treated as an extension of the patient insofar as the individual's illness might be communicated to other members. Some enlightened providers were also concerned about the impact of illness or treatment requirements on family members but, by and large, care delivery was individual- rather than family-focused. In Western medicine, this tradition was further underscored by society's cultural belief in the primacy of individual rights and freedoms.

Today the practice of primary care is experiencing a realignment toward family-centered health care. This is a clear and important difference from specialty practice, whose emphasis is the individual. There are two paths toward family-centered practice, each with its own distinct, theoretical underpinnings. The first is a traditional path, which centers on individual-focused care. The second path uses a family systems framework. This path is seen as the most inclusive of individual and family members. It is based on respect for the primacy of the individual. The family systems path is seminal to primary care practice that is relationship-centered. The provider must keep in mind that confidentiality in dealing with an individual family member must be at the forefront of relationship-centered care. Family-centered practice does not imply abandoning the legal and ethical responsibilities the provider owes to the patient.

The Traditional Path in Primary Care

This first and earliest practice model sees the family as comprised of individuals. The outcome of care delivered within an individual-focused model uses family studies as well as developmental and social learning theory in organizing, explaining, and predicting care needs for that individual (Wright & Leahey, 1993). This model is exemplified by the anticipatory guidance given to the caretaking adult of the patient with dementia, or to the parent of a teenager at the time of her pre-college physical. The focus of concern is the patient or the family, rather than an integration of the patient and the family. The traditional path approaches patient management from the perspective of either the patient or the family, rather than focusing on the family as a whole.

The Family Systems Path in Primary Care

The second path for primary care is delivered within a family systems framework. The family systems path targets each individual family member as well as the family as a whole, at one and the same time (Wright & Leahey, 1993). The family systems path is optimum in a practice that is relationship-centered. What happens to the patient is seen as happening to the family as a unit. Primary care delivered to the individual impacts the family as well. Whether integrating health promotion or confronting illness management, family members experience together the provider's professional caring for, communication with, and treatment of one of its members. This is the optimal model for the practice of relationship-centered primary care. This model is not seen as an evolutionary product of the first, individual-focused path but, rather, as an alternate route that can form a strong basis for humanistic primary care. The Family Systems framework guides how this care impacts family functioning from the perspective of each family member as an individual and as a member of a unique group. Family members' feelings and responses to the patient's health status and care management are recognized as important to the family's interactional function. Care given to one member is evaluated within the context of other family members' responses to and connectedness with the patient, while keeping in mind that the community is part of that connectedness. This kind of care delivery model is inherently more holistic than the traditional family

practice model, in which care is individual-focused. Conversely, a Family Systems framework guides the provider in treating the patient as a being who is interconnected with others in the family and, in a broader way, with the community.

■ ■ ■ **CLINICAL PEARLS**

Care that is family-focused does not imply that all members are always entitled to know every aspect of each other's primary care issues. The primary care provider must sometimes walk a fine line, balancing family support with individual privacy needs.

FAMILY SYSTEMS IN PRACTICE

The following three examples will introduce the idea of a Family Systems perspective for practicing primary care. Their presentation exemplifies the interconnectedness that emerges from giving primary care that uses Family Systems as a practice foundation. These three case presentations then will be placed within the context of family assessment.

Case # 1

A young woman is diagnosed with breast cancer. The provider works with her and her husband in deciding upon referral options for cancer treatment and community resources. This management of her primary care needs does not occur in isolation. The young woman's church, neighbors, co-workers, and parents of her children's friends all share in her family's fear and anxiety. Many people come forward to volunteer their help in her and her family's care. Many others in the community may forge new bonds in helping the family meet financial and family-management challenges associated with her cancer treatment.

Case # 2

A respected elderly man in the community is diagnosed with dementia of the Alzheimer's type. The primary care provider is concerned with how this diagnosis impacts both the patient and the family's functioning. The provider works with the wife and an adult son in developing a management plan. Because of the provider's referral to the local home care or community-based organization, a plan of care is set up to develop and implement a respite network. Friends and neighbors have expressed an interest in helping the family with respite activities. Their contributions are included in the management plan. The outcome of this management plan is a coordination of efforts that support the patient's primary care needs, while assisting his family in providing for round-the-clock care.

Case # 3

A recent flu epidemic ultimately takes the life of an 18-year-old patient with asthma. The provider practices primary care within a Family Systems perspective. This means that the provider's work does not end with the teen's death. In practicing relationship-centered primary care that is family-focused, the provider collaborates with other providers in assessing intervention needs of the victim's family and close friends. This assessment can serve as a springboard for community involvement. In this instance, the following autumn the local high school's PTA coordinates with local health authorities to set up a free influenza immunization clinic for the entire community. All of this is done in the teen's memory.

THE FAMILY ASSESSMENT

Family assessment data can help the provider deliver individualized primary care. Such data can enhance the provider's understanding of the family and its needs from individual as well as interpersonal perspectives. Data collected within this context frames a Family Assessment. This data adds a critical dimension to one's interactions with the patient and their family. The Family Assessment is a tool that provides contextual details about the objective information obtained in the genogram, which was collected during the patient's history. Family Assessment also can clarify immediate and extended familial relationships as well as social and community networks that might impact family-focused care. These assessment data help the provider work as a partner with the family in meeting their primary care needs (Artinian, 1994).

There are several published family assessment tools. Appendix 2-2 presents a sample Family Assessment tool designed and used by the author. This instrument can be used as is, or modified to fit practice needs. Regardless of which tool one ultimately uses, several areas are key to collecting data that is complete. It is important to note the role played by culture and ethnic traditions in family functioning. Important areas for collecting data in family assessment are summarized in Table 2-1.

TABLE 2-1	Areas for Family Assessment

- Information about the family, including immediate as well as extended members. It is important to include persons who, although perhaps not legally related, may still be considered by the patient as part of the family matrix. Include valued pets.

- Affectional and social networks of informal significance to the patient should be identified. Constructing a matrix delineating the patient's sources for immediate social support can be valuable in times of crisis. Its ready availability can enhance care delivery. Distant or extended sources for social support should also be identified because, in time of crisis, the more sources of assistance known, the better the provider will be able to facilitate their implementation.

- Clarification of life events of significance to the patient and family should also be attempted, including births, deaths, marriages, remarriages, and informal domestic arrangements of past and present.

- Delineation of neighborhood factors of importance to the patient and family, including safety, stability, and social as well as economic variables that may affect the patient's and the family's health and well-being.

- How do family members make decisions affecting the group? Does each member have input? What resources (financial, emotional, spiritual, professional, etc.) do they believe are available to them?

- What satisfaction do they derive from family life? What stresses?

- What does each member feel he or she contributes to the family?

- What is of importance to the family? Do they feel supported or guided by a higher power? What beliefs and value structure guides them?

- What roles do gender and birth order play in family functioning, including member status? Are these variables sources for conflict? (The provider must be clear about personal beliefs and values when collecting and analyzing these data. Differences—and even obvious conflicts—between personal and professional beliefs and values must be clarified to maximize the provider's capability to analyze and use these data in a nonjudgmental, effective way.)

- What (if any) change in cultural or ethnic identity has been lost to or assimilated by a country's larger context for cultural expression? If loss has occurred, does this affect individual and family function and, in the wider arena, community identity? How are health beliefs, health values, and, in turn, health function affected?

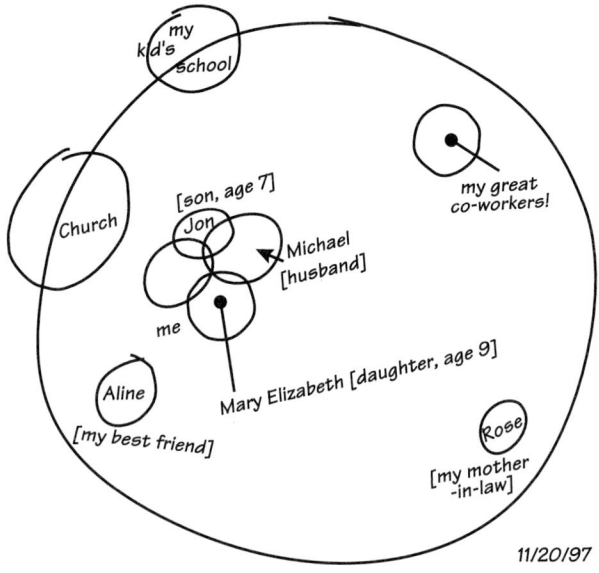

I have great people I work with. I have a very close family. I'm blessed that way. My best friend is just down the road — we'd do anything for each other. We're active in the church and our kid's school.

FIGURE 2-1 Family Circle diagram for a young woman with breast cancer.

A Family Circle is the first step in Family Assessment. As such, this data should be appended to the family assessment. The process for gathering a Family Circle diagram is quick and straightforward (Thrower et al, 1982). The provider gives the patient a pen and paper, prompting them to date it and then draw a circle which represents the family. The patient draws smaller circles inside and/or outside this larger circle, representing the patient, individual family members, and, if desired, any significant relationships including pets. As it is constructed by the patient, the circle illustrates the emotional relationships inherent in their family matrix. A Family Circle diagram serves as a visual aid for a patient's perception of the direction and importance of relationships at the point in time in which it

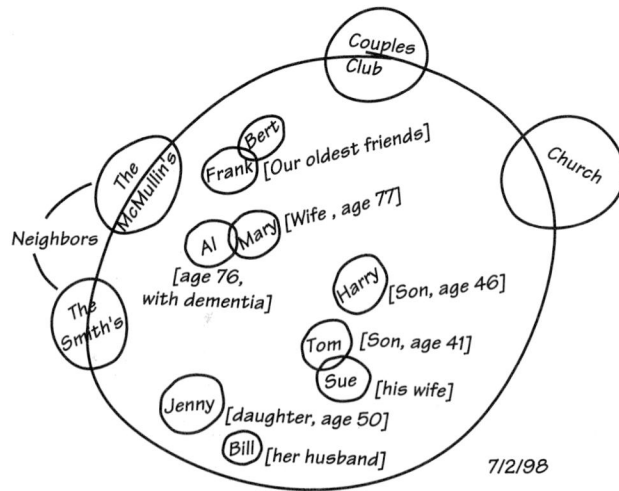

FIGURE 2-2 Family Circle diagram for the family of an elderly person with dementia.

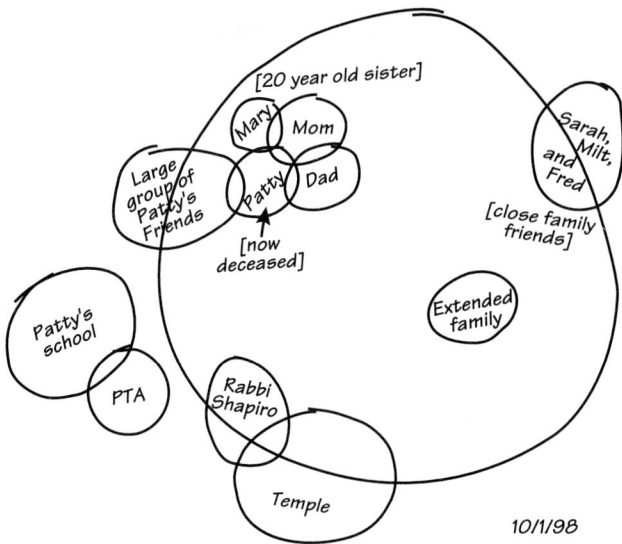

FIGURE 2-3 Family Circle diagram for an adolescent with asthma.

was drawn. Each circle's size can be interpreted to mean an individual's significance, while distance between circles may indicate the extent of affection felt for or closeness to that family member. The patient may want to write a brief statement which describes their feelings about the circles and their meaning. The provider and patient then discuss the Family Circle diagram together, with the patient confirming and/or explaining the Circle's interpretation. This subjective data can be extremely valuable to the provider's overall Family Assessment. Figure 2-1 illustrates a Family Circle for Case # 1, that of the family of the young woman diagnosed with breast cancer. Figure 2-2 presents the family in Case # 2, with the elderly man with dementia. Figure 2-3 represents the family of the young patient with asthma presented in Case # 3. The role of community resources is demonstrated in each Family Circle diagram.

Commonalities exist among these circles in their depiction of the family and its relationship to the wider community. Differences in the community's influence on family functioning also are evident. In Figure 2-1, the family's reliance on community resources is not as great as in Figures 2-2 and 2-3. The volunteer community's response to the family with elder-support needs (see Fig. 2-2) is more directly focused toward helping the family cope with its respite needs. The response of the last scenario demonstrates efforts in meeting both family needs and those of the wider community (see Fig. 2-3).

CULTURAL ASSESSMENT

At its most basic, cultural assessment is a clinical method for collecting and using data that support the provider's understanding of the historical perspective and world view of the patient and family. Familial patterns of expression are a part of a person's culture and ethnic identity. These patterns can be placed within the context of the community at large. Cultural assessment is a logical outgrowth of family assessment. In all but homogeneous groups, both family and cultural assessments are logical precursors to a community appraisal. Family and cultural evaluations are a logical base for community assessment, as in a locale peopled by those sharing the same ethnic

and cultural heritage. This is exemplified by a rural community of people sharing a similar birthplace, ethnic heritage, and means of livelihood. The assessment for this community would differ from that done on an urban area whose residents come from a variety of ethnic traditions and are of varying socioeconomic levels.

Just as identifying the importance of ethnic heritage is important in cultural assessment, so too is recognizing the role played by geographic place, whether urban, suburban, or rural. For example, rural dwellers share a rural cultural base that differs from that of urban or suburban areas. Non-native residents of each of these regions may appreciate and even try to assimilate into its culture, but cannot fully leave behind their geographic culture of origin. This last factor will be discussed later in this chapter.

The Meaning of Culture

The first step in undertaking a cultural assessment is clarifying the notion of culture and its meaning. Culture embodies the beliefs, values, attitudes, customs, and ethnicity of a group. Although perhaps similar in outlook to those of other people, cultural practices may be unique because they derive from a group's particular world view. Cultural practices and beliefs continue to evolve over time. Were they to remain completely static, their relevance would lessen, for people naturally grow and change with life experiences and outside influences.

Culture informs beliefs, attitudes, and values. Culture can exert a powerful influence on family functioning. Gender roles and the relevance of birth order can impact an individual's health behavior as well as response to life cycle events, including childbirth, aging, and illness. Life cycle events influence the individual's as well as the family's evolvement. For example, the "sandwich generation" describes adult children who must balance caring for ailing parents against nurturing their own young children, often while working full-time outside the home.

The notion of what is family varies from one culture to another, even when taken within the context of the so-called dominant culture of a country. For example, cultural themes that were perpetuated by the television media of the 1950s and 1960s supported the view that family structure was nuclear and parented by a heterosexual, legally-married couple. Extended family and friends' roles frequently were enacted indirectly rather than directly. Of course the reality is more complex than this view. Multiculturalism is just that—many-cultured.

The so-called dominant culture of many Western countries is actually a montage of different cultures, each having different beliefs and values about family functioning. For example, families of African heritage often delineate family from a framework of both related and unrelated individuals, in a kin and community structure. Church or mosque may also serve as a central anchoring point for this family. The family of English heritage may indeed most value the traditional nuclear structure. Families of Native North American, Hispanic, Mediterranean, and Semitic backgrounds may function from a span of three or even four generations, and can include very close friends. Church, temple, or mosque may be at the core for families of these backgrounds, and as such actually may serve the broader role of community (Szapocznik & Kurtines, 1993; Markowitz, 1994). In addition to the kin/close friend networks of the preceding examples, many families of Asian ancestry include forebears as well as descendants in their vision of a kinship network (Berg & Jaya, 1993). Further enriching this picture of ethnic diversity in modern life is the realization that some cultures assign decision-making to authority figures such as a family or clan elder.

In the larger context of a nation's culture, individual rights and privileges of a particular culture or ethnic group may sometimes be superseded by those of the dominant culture. This broader cultural view may conflict with an ethnic group's traditional view.

Culture and Family: Clarifying the Influence of One's Origins

Geographic and regional differences can influence both the provider's and the patient's values and beliefs about health, wellness, and personal responsibility in health management. But in addition, the provider's own cultural beliefs and practices—not to mention family structure—may agree, disagree, or even strongly conflict with those of the patient and their family. Sometimes the provider's ethnic and cultural values may so conflict with those of the patient that care delivery is perceived to be compromised. For example, a clinical plan for hypertension management may be doomed to failure if not prescribed within a cultural context that recognizes and values a patient's dietary heritage. In relationship-centered primary care, the provider might better ensure success by working with the patient to develop a management plan that reflects their dietary customs. Asking why this patient does not just accept the standard hypertension management prescription and follow it, when, in fact, that plan may be culturally incongruent can mean the difference between working with rather than against the patient. In respecting rather than rejecting cultural differences, the provider can work with the patient to integrate cultural and ethnic traditions into a management plan that works. The successful provider aims to deliver primary care that is relationship-centered, and inclusive of patient and family cultural values. Primary care that is culturally sensitive can better ensure positive health outcomes, while affording the opportunity to deliver care that is patient-specific and, hence, more salient for the provider, patient, and family.

Value Orientations in Family Life

Despite differences in the expression of family life in different cultures and/or in different geographic regions of a country, five value orientations have been identified that are shared universally by human families (Table 2-2). An awareness of these

TABLE 2-2	The Five Universal Value Orientations of Human Families

- A temporal focus for life, at least in relation to important milestones. For some ethnic or cultural groups, this focus may be seasons of the year; the progression of the calendar may be important to others.
- Preferred or habitual blueprints for action in relationships
- Standards for behavior in relation to others
- Connections to the world around us, within us, and beyond us
- Beliefs about the innate nature of human beings

(Adapted from Ho, M.K. (1987). *Family therapy with ethnic minorities*. Rockville, MD: Aspen)

TABLE 2-3	Topics to Explore in Cultural Assessments

- Country of origin (or, if native-born, region). How long has the patient lived in this country/region?
- Ethnic group and strength of ethnic feelings
- Sources of social support, including family and friends (if applicable, ethnic community ties)
- Verbal and reading capability, and in what language
- Method for nonverbal communication
- Religion—its relevance and practice demands
- Food choices—any taboos?
- Personal economics—sufficient to meet the patient's needs?
- Health and illness notions and customs
- Beliefs, values, and customs surrounding birth, death, and sickness

(Adapted from Lipson, J.G., & Meleis, A.I. (1985), in Lipson, J.G., Dibble, S.L., & Minarik, P.A. (1996). *Culture and nursing care: A pocket guide*. San Francisco: UCSF Nursing Press)

value orientations can help the provider to deliver primary care that is sensitive to the patient's core beliefs and values.

Using Value Orientation Data in the Cultural Assessment

Acknowledgment of the five value orientations can enhance the practice of primary care in today's complex, multicultural and multiethnic society. Value orientations underscore the cultural assessment. A cultural assessment can clarify the provider's picture of the patient's values and beliefs. Lipson et al (1996) cite 10 topical areas that should underscore the cultural assessment (Table 2-3).

Verbal and Nonverbal Communication in Cultural Assessment

When faced with a patient whose language skills and abilities differ from those of the provider, it may be necessary to use nonverbal communication, including pantomime, to communicate information. If nonverbal means prove inadequate, it may be necessary to use a language interpreter. Ideally, this role is served by a non-family member whose language skill can interface effectively with that of the provider, and whose language skill will be acceptable to both provider and patient. A non-family member may be better able to communicate information in a non-judgmental manner. Information that is perceived as embarrassing or private is less likely to be deleted from such a transmission.

When a family member or close friend provides the interpretation, be aware that the communication may have been "edited" by either the translator or the patient. Family translation also lends itself to possible violations of patient confidentiality. If family or close friends must be used for translation, guard against possible "editing" by closely observing both patient and translator, in turn, as they speak. Avoid using staff members who have expertise in translation unless such service is a part of their work assignment. Translating takes time and as such might place an employee under an undue burden, relative to the employer's work expectations. In the case of the patient who is hearing-challenged, endeavor to obtain the services of a credentialed sign language interpreter.

Communication is clearly improved when the provider approaches every interaction with an awareness of the patient's cultural and ethnic beliefs and values. Clinical practice can be enhanced when the provider knows cultural expectations about the use of touch or eye contact, personal space, and conversational pacing. It is also helpful to understand the patient's awareness of time and whether or not family members expect to be included in any examination or health teaching activities.

Culture, Geography, Education, and Economic Class

Besides culturally-ascribed beliefs and values, adult expectations are directly influenced by childhood experiences. Where one grew up, and at what educational or socioeconomic level, can have a powerful influence on expectations one has for the community and its goods and services. The act of growing up and moving to a different geographic locale may not change the powerful influence of childhood experiences.

Clearly, cultural incongruence can emerge when the provider's geographic, social, educational, and economic background differ from that of the community where he or she practices. This incongruence is also possible when a patient lives in a community that does not share their world view of the types and kinds of services needed and how they should be delivered. Does the patient expect services that include house calls? Should care delivery be contractual, where both provider and patient agree on points of management? Or does the patient expect that the provider will direct needs assessment and care delivery? How these questions are answered depends upon a variety of factors, including cultural and ethnic heritage, past and current socioeconomic background, geographic origin, and educational level of both provider and patient. Health beliefs and values are shaped by the foregoing and, further, are influenced by past and present experiences of both traditional and complementary health care and its delivery.

The Demographics of Geography: Rural Versus Urban and Suburban

Traditionally, a dearth of services in rural, agrarian areas (few people, fewer services) meant that rural dwellers needed to develop skills in self-reliance, as much out of necessity as out of any sense of stubborn independence. A person's measure might derive more from physical endurance and native intuition than from social, educational, or economic advantages. Because cultural outcomes are at least in part a product of a lived world view, rural culture can be seen to reflect the traits of uncomplaining acceptance of that which one cannot change for oneself. Energy and purpose may emanate as much from the individual as from the wider community.

Urban life brings with it a cultural context that is distinctly different from that of its rural counterpart. A wide array of services of all sorts emerges in a nonagrarian society. Competition for services may be replaced by their oversupply, necessitating further service differentiation. The result is increased demand for services and, hence, other-reliance rather than self-reliance, as in the traditional rural model (Kaslow et al, 1995). Similar to urban life, modern suburban culture is fast-paced and replete with ready availability of goods and services.

Residents of both urban and suburban areas generally expect ready availability of and variety in goods and services. This expectation extends to health care delivery, and crosses socioeconomic lines. Creative yet cost effective models for urban/suburban primary care acknowledge this consumer expectation. In contrast, this expectation is typically missing among native residents of rural areas, where people are less accustomed to their providers making frequent specialty referrals or prescribing nonroutine, diagnostic testing. This, of course, is in part because of the lesser availability of referral services, including more of the so-called state-of-the-art diagnostics (Vermont AHEC Proposal, 1996; American Medical Association, 1992).

The Demographics of Education and Economic Class: The Potential for Cultural Conflict

The geographic locale of where one grew up can exert a powerful influence on one's world view. If a provider "moves away" from this place, one may find that local customs and values are different from those of the childhood region. In such a case, rather than ignore that differences exist, the provider may find it helpful to examine values and beliefs that emanate from where one grew up. Even before one becomes enmeshed in the community, identify for example how holidays are celebrated. Is the community ethnically homogeneous, or is it diverse? How does the community celebrate religious, patriotic, and other events? Do people reside nearby who share the provider's ethnic or religious background? How are local schools and services similar to or different from those available to the provider while growing up? For example, an urban or suburban youngster might spend leisure time in adult-supervised activities, including shopping or museum exploration. A rural child might spend long hours alone, exploring woods and fields. Urban residents do not typically hunt wild game for leisure, let alone winter food. Native-born rural youngsters typically learn to hunt or have family members who do so. These childhood experiences have a direct bearing on adult patterns of behavior.

Of course providers can successfully practice in an area where they are not native. They may want to begin their practice career by reviewing their total life experiences, educational and economic heritage, and family customs. This process may assist the provider in discerning similarities and differences that exist in values and traditions where they now practice. Such examination can assist the provider in clarifying personal expectations, as well as helping to shed light on those of colleagues and patients.

Demographics, including perceptions of socioeconomic status and class as well as educational levels, impact health care and health promotion delivery. Table 2-4 illustrates how some

TABLE 2-4	Differences Between Rural and Urban/Suburban Practice

- Rural providers tend to have less access to office support services.
- Rural providers see more patients per week than their urban/suburban colleagues (126.1 rural visits/week versus 111.8 visits/week in urban/suburban areas of less than 1,000,000, and 100.6/week in areas over 1,000,000).

(Source: American Medical Association, Center for Health Policy. (1992). *Socioeconomic characteristics of medical practice.* Chicago: American Medical Association)

TABLE 2-5	**Key Demographic Differences Between Rural and Urban/Suburban Residents**

- Rural dwellers have lower income levels ($24,000) than urban/suburban families ($33,000) (US Congress, Office of Technology Report, 1990). These figures factor in the much lower incomes of the urban poor but do not clearly demarcate them.

- 13% of rural people are over age 65, compared to 10.7% of their urban/suburban peers.

- 9% of rural dwellers are college graduates, compared to nearly 13% of urban/suburbanites.

- 14.5% of rural dwellers lack health insurance, compared to 12% in urban/suburban areas.

(Source: American Medical Association, Center for Health Policy. (1992). *Socioeconomic characteristics of medical practice*. Chicago: American Medical Association)

of these differences impact the practice of primary care in rural versus urban/suburban areas. This table demonstrates that less time and resources are available for health promotion in rural office practice. Compounding these problems is the fact that rural dwellers tend to delay provider visits for many reasons. Table 2-5 summarizes key demographic differences between rural and urban/suburban residents.

■ ■ ■   CLINICAL PEARLS

The provider's application of primary care that is relationship-centered will be more successful and more salient if they enter into practice in a community with respect and honor. These attributes flow from the provider's efforts to learn about that community's values. Astute providers inform themselves about local ethnic groups, values and beliefs, festivals, and ethnic or religious traditions.

SUMMARY

Ideally, the practice of primary care that is relationship-centered is underscored by family and cultural assessments. This process begins with the provider's acknowledgment of one's own cultural heritage and the influence of geography, education, and socioeconomic factors on personal development. This process can support the provider's creation of therapeutic relationships with patients and their families, helping one to give care that is not value-laden. Patient and family needs can be better met when addressed from their own unique life perspectives, supported by understanding family, cultural, and ethnic influences on health beliefs, values, and behaviors.

References

American Medical Association, Center for Health Policy Research. (1992). *Socioeconomic characteristics of medical practice*. Chicago: American Medical Association.

Artinian, N.T. (1994). Selecting a model to guide family assessment. *Dimensions of Critical Care Nursing, 14*(1), 4–13.

Berg, I.K., & Jaya, A. (1993). Different and the same: Family therapy with Asian-American families. *Journal of Marital and Family Therapy, 19*, 31–38.

Green-Hernandez, C. (1997). Application of caring theory in primary care: A challenge for advanced practice. *Nursing Administration Quarterly, 21*(4), 77–82.

Kaslow, N.J., Celano, M., & Dreelin, E.D. (1995). A cultural perspective on family theory and therapy. *Psychiatric Clinics of North America, 18*(3), 621–633.

Lipson, J.G., Dibble, S.L., & Minarik, P.A. (eds). (1996). *Culture and nursing care: A pocket guide*. San Francisco: UCSF Nursing Press.

Markowitz, L. (1994). The cross-currents of multiculturalism. *Family Therapy Networker, 4*, 18–27.

Szapocznik, J., & Kurtines, W.M. (1993). Family psychology and cultural diversity. *American Psychologist, 48*, 400–407.

Thrower, S.M., Bruce, W.E., & Walton, R.F. (1982). The family circle method for integrating family systems concepts in family medicine. *Journal of Family Practice, 15*, 451.

University of Vermont College of Medicine. (1996). *Vermont AHEC proposal* (unpublished proposal). Burlington, VT: The University of Vermont.

Wright, L.M., & Leahey, M. (1993). Trends in nursing of families. In Wegner, G.D., & Alexander, R.J. (eds). *Readings in family nursing*. Philadelphia: JB Lippincott.

APPENDIX 2-1

Values Clarification Tool

The individual is asked to respond in writing to each question in turn:

1. Write down three things you enjoy doing.
2. Record a place—either real or imaginary—that you go to when you're feeling sad.
3. What is your most important *personal* achievement?
4. Record the three most pressing problems you face now, ordering them from worst to least.
5. Now, assume that you have only 1 year to live. You won't be handicapped or in pain because of your terminal status, however. What will you do this last year? How will you use your time and abilities?
6. Now, assume that your last year is at an end. Write down three words you'd like others to remember you by. Write down one word you do not want used to describe you after your death.

Interpretation of this tool:

- When you're having a hard time of it, plan to do some of the activities you enjoy, or go (either physically or mentally) to your "get-away" place.

- For item 4: You may not be able to solve your most difficult problem, but it's possible that you will be able to solve the second one in a reasonable time frame, such as 3 to 6 months. You may be able to resolve your least difficult issue now. Keep in mind that these are guidelines rather than an exact timetable for problem resolution.

- For item 6: Seek out friends and family who personify these attributes. Steer clear of anyone whose temperament puts you in mind of the characteristic you identified as unacceptable to you.

(Adapted from *Personal Coat of Arms*, in King, E.C. (1984). *Affective Education in Nursing*, p. 31. Rockville, MD: Aspen)

FAMILY ASSESSMENT TOOL

Cultural heritage

For each family member:

Age
Relationship
Degree of contact

Religion (if applicable)

Religious practices (if applicable)

Values

What's important to each member?
Any conflict in values, as between role in home, among family, compared to workplace?
If yes, has this conflict been resolved?
If not, how is the family member managing?

Ethnic/cultural traditions (if applicable)

Coping patterns

- day-to-day

Stress management

- day-to-day
- in times of increased stress

Caring for self

- How does each family member feel about himself or herself?
- What does each member do to take care of himself or herself?
- Does everyone do self-caring activities (eg, setting aside some time for self each day)?
  > if yes, kinds of activities and their frequency
  > if not, why not

Caring for others of importance to the family's members

- How does the family feel about them?
- Do family members help with any of their care?
  > if yes, how do they feel about this?
  > How are they managing?
- Does the family want to continue in these activities?
  > if yes, does anyone need any help?
- Is the family aware of resources and support services if needed or desired?

Family management

- Who is responsible for
  > housework
  > house maintenance (inside and out)
  > yard work
  > finances
  > pets (if applicable)
  > children (if applicable)
  > parent care (if applicable)

Family communication

- How does everyone communicate with each other?
- How do members feel about family communication?

Family support

- How do members feel about each other?
- Is there a particular member they turn to in times of need?
  > if yes, who?
- Does the family perceive that there are other resources available to them if needed?
  > if yes, who or what?

Income needs

- Which family member's income provides financial support?
- Are there gaps between family members' income needs and income available?
  > if yes, explain
- What are the usual work schedules for employed members?
- Is there any flexibility in these schedules?

School supports

- Which (if any) members attend school?
  > if any, full-time or part-time?
  > what are their schedules?
  > any flexibility in these schedules?
- Any problems associated with schooling?
- What school supports are available if needed?

Social and community supports

- What social activities do members engage in?
- Any problems or stressors associated with these activities?
- What social and community resources are available if needed?

Logistical needs

- Does the family have reliable transportation available to them?
  > if yes, and if not private transport, what is the schedule?
  > is there off-hour (ie, nights, weekends, holidays) availability?
- What is the average distance the family travels for health care, including the primary care office? Medical emergency services?

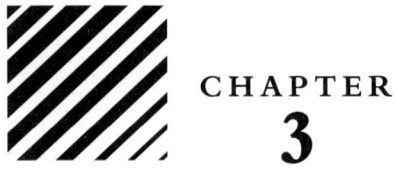

CHAPTER

3

Health Promotion and Disease Prevention

Robert V. DiGregorio, Pharm D, RPh and Joanne K. Singleton PhD, RN, CS, FNP

Health promotion and disease prevention have often been over-shadowed by the efforts of the practitioner to restore health and manage disease states. Primary care providers recognize that the old adage "an ounce of prevention is worth a pound of cure" is not only a truism, but imparts significant health, as well as, financial benefits. For example, smoking cessation programs, which may prevent a variety of diseases, could eliminate many of the more than 400,000 deaths and reduce the associated health care costs of more than $65 billion per year in the U.S. Health promotion, however, is often confused with traditional preventive medicine which has focused on disease prevention and has not fully integrated the concept of overall wellness. While health promotion is about disease prevention, it goes much further. This chapter will discuss health promotion from the perspective of relationship-centered care, including screening for early indicators of disease and advocating for overall wellness.

HEALTH PROMOTION IN RELATIONSHIP-CENTERED CARE

The expanded definition of health promotion includes areas of wellness such as injury prevention, healthy eating and reducing stress, to name a few. The concept of overall wellness and health promotion can be easily coupled to the concept of relationship-centered care when viewed as a process of empowerment. Health promotion is a process that enables individuals to improve their quality of life through a partnership with their families and health care providers who assist the individual in making informed decisions about their health. Once the decisions are made by the individual patient and their family, the health care provider moves into a position that provides support for and encourages participation in the individual's plan for healthy living. Described in this chapter are various aspects of health promotion that could be considered in health-promotion or wellness plans that providers develop with their patients.

The concept of relationship-centered health promotion is echoed in the current national health and wellness initiative, *Healthy People 2000* (U.S. Department of Health and Human Services [DHHS], 1992) and the *Guide to Clinical Preventive Services* (U.S. Preventive Services Task Force [USPSTF], 1996). The central purpose of *Healthy People 2000* was to increase the proportion of Americans who live long and healthy lives by maintaining a full range of functional capacity throughout their life. The lifestyle promoted in this initiative enables an individual to enter into satisfying relationships with others, pursue career goals, and enjoy recreational activities. The impetus to accomplish these goals and modify behaviors comes from the increasingly health-conscious, responsible public in partner-

ship with their health-care providers. Other goals of *Healthy People 2000* included reducing health disparities among Americans and achieving access to preventive services for all Americans. It is interesting, and disappointing, to note that as the year 2000 approaches, the three primary goals of *Healthy People 2000* have not been fully met. These ambitions must therefore continue into the 21st century.

The *Guide to Clinical Preventive Services* reflects relationship centered care. It provides through detailed guidelines for health care providers in their role as counselors, health facilitators, and patient educators. Many patients read magazines and pamphlets pertaining to their health and are aware of the risks involved with certain behaviors. Despite their knowledge, they continue to partake in a variety of risky behaviors. Information and knowledge are important for promoting a healthy lifestyle: patients need to motivate themselves and rely more on an overall strategy for changing less-than-optimal health behaviors. Strategies for changing health behaviors can be incorporated into routine health visits, and are outlined in Table 3-1.

Implementing patient counseling in the practice setting raises important issues for providers. Issues regarding the value of screening and the appropriate time to screen patients are discussed below and in the individual chapters in Part 2 . Other issues may arise as barriers to implementing counseling interventions, such as insufficient reimbursement, patient volume requirements, provider uncertainty about how to counsel effectively, varying interest on the part of patient or staff, and lack of an organizational system of support to facilitate the delivery of patient education (USPSTF, 1996; MacLean, 1996). Many of these issues are addressed by the government publication "Put Prevention into Practice" (PPIP), the U.S. Public Health Service's prevention implementation program (DHHS, 1994). PPIP and the strategies provided in this chapter can serve as tools to assist the provider in developing an ongoing dialogue to encourage patients at every visit to change their personal health practices.

EVIDENCE-BASED HEALTH SCREENING

Effectiveness should be the most basic requirement for providing any health care service. This includes health-promotion activities, where the health care provider has the ethical responsibility to "do no harm" to patients. Effectiveness is usually determined from compilations of data or evidence from large randomized clinical trials. The ability to track down, critically appraise and incorporate this evidence into clinical practice has been referred to as "evidence-based medicine." Evidence of effectiveness alone, however, is not a sufficient reason to perform a particular screening. Factors other than effectiveness,

TABLE 3-1	Strategies Useful in Changing Health Behaviors
Strategy	**Method**
1. Listen	The provider should elicit the patient's health care beliefs and concerns and incorporate them into the wellness plan. Cultural sensitivity is also extremely important.
2. Explain	Fully inform patients of the purposes, benefits, and time frame to reach the goals of the particular intervention.
3. Set reasonable goals	Start slow; small changes are easier to accomplish than large ones.
4. Be thorough	Be specific and thorough when instructing patients on how to carry out their agreed-on regimen. Patients are less likely to participate in their regimen if they are uncertain of what to do once they leave the provider's office or clinic.
5. Establish new behaviors	It is easier to add new positive behaviors than to eliminate established behaviors.
6. Link behaviors	Combine old and new behaviors so that the patient simply adds another step into an already established practice or routine rather than creating a whole new practice.
7. Be definitive	Be sympathetic and supportive while conveying firm, definitive messages to the patient.
8. Use an open-ended approach	Patients should be encouraged to describe how they will incorporate their behavior modification into their daily routine. Meanwhile, the provider should be on the lookout for barriers to success for the patient.
9. Mix resources	In addition to verbal communication, use written materials and integrate support groups, counseling, audiovisual aids, etc.
10. Involve office staff	Staff members and the overall office environment should communicate consistent positive health care messages.
11. Refer	If a provider is too busy to work with the patient, the patient should be referred. Patient education and counseling can be provided by many different health care providers, as well as community agencies, voluntary health organizations, instructional materials, and other patients.
12. Follow up	Provider-initiated contact is more effective than patient-initiated contact.

reflecting the trade-offs and broad implications of screening, are relevant to the goals of health promotion.

When deciding on a particular screening instrument, providers must decide to what degree the information from the screening procedure is accurate and reliable. The provider and patient must also determine how the data gained from the screening process will ultimately be applied to patient care. For example, obtaining mammographies in younger women is the subject of great controversy (Schmidt, 1995; Leitch, 1995). Mammographic screening, yielding false-positive findings, has caused many women to undergo breast biopsies that uncovered normal tissue. In retrospect, these biopsies were not only unnecessary, but also subjected the women to a painful, invasive procedure and the accompanying anxiety of a possible breast cancer diagnosis. If a younger woman understood this possibility prior to requesting or submitting to a mammogram, she might opt to wait and simply continue to conduct monthly breast self exams with annual clinical breast examinations. Considerable controversy also exists with regard to screening asymptomatic patients for colorectal cancer (Hart et al, 1995) and prostate cancer (Mandelson et al, 1995).

Misinterpretation of screening tests, based on false-positive and false-negative findings, may lead to over- or undertreating patients. While false-positive results may cause undue anxiety and diagnostic work-up for a patient, a false-negative finding can give a patient a false sense of security as well as delay treatment. Providers must understand the sensitivity, specificity, and reliability, underlying disease prevalence and relative cost of screening before incorporating a screening process into a patient's wellness plan.

Sensitivity

The ability of a particular test to detect an abnormal condition is referred to as the sensitivity of the test. A test that detects minute variations from the normal condition would be described as a highly sensitive test. Even highly sensitive tests, however, do not always confirm specific disease states. For example, current technology allows for the measurement of gamma glutamyl transferase (GGT) levels within 1 unit/L; thus, a GGT level of 1 unit above normal could be detected. However, this elevated level does not differentiate between alcoholism, hepatitis, smoking, lupus, or a biliary obstruction. In fact, it may not indicate any abnormal condition. The smell of a patient's clothing may, on the other hand, reveal the unmistakable odor of cigarette smoke. Of course, this rudimentary test would not reveal how much the person smokes or even if the smell was from the individual or second hand.

Specificity

Specificity refers to the ability of a test or screening procedure to identify the exact problem or condition. In the above example, GGT was a highly sensitive but nonspecific screening test. Examples of highly specific screening tests include: blood pressure measurement for hypertension, ejection fraction for cardiac function, prostate-specific antigen for prostate cancer, and blood cultures for infectious pathogens. It is important to consider that a positive finding in a highly specific test does not necessarily confer a disease. The possibility of second-hand smoke in the above example illustrates this scenario. Another example of specificity without diagnostic merit would be the use of a blood level to determine drug toxicity. While an elevated level may certainly be specific to the drug product in question, not every patient with an elevated level will exhibit toxic effects. A summary of specificity and sensitivity measures is shown in Table 3-2.

Reliability

Tests used in screening procedures may be highly sensitive and specific, yet remain unreliable. Reliability takes into account the accuracy and precision of the test. Test results may indicate a specific finding marginally above the norm, but because of technical error, expired reagents, or faulty test techniques, it may be inaccurate. Variability in the performance of the test procedure or examination can lead to unreliable results by compromising precision or reproducibility. Blood pressure readings taken incorrectly (eg, the arm is not at heart level), by inexperienced individuals, or the use of electronic blood pressure measuring devices may increase the amount of blood pressure screening and monitoring data available to providers; however, this data may be imprecise, inaccurate and therefore unsuitable for making health care decisions.

Cost Factors

In an ideal world of unlimited resources, patients would have infinite access to their health care providers, health technology, and health care products. However, resources are increasingly limited, and the utility of screening for conditions, simply because the technology exists, is not appropriate. Even screening that is relatively free may lengthen a health care visit and prevent another patient from obtaining care that day. Extremely specific, sensitive and reliable testing may be available but not utilized due to disproportionally high costs as compared to an older, less expensive test. Screening for cervical cancer with newer test methods rather than Pap smears is a good example of this phenomenon. For each screening test, the cost of evaluating all susceptible individuals must be weighed against the prevalence of the condition and the cost of treating the condition. In some cases, the relatively low prevalence and low cost

of treating a disease may make implementing such a screening program unrealistic. Likewise, therapy leading to an individual's complete cure of a disease may cost less than screening or immunizing an entire population.

SCREENING

As a form of health promotion and disease prevention, screening can be as simple as questioning a patient about the common warning signs or symptoms of a disease state, or as complex as subjecting the patient to invasive examinations or testing procedures. The most common areas of health screening include the prevention and early identification of coronary artery disease and a variety of cancers. The warning signs and symptoms and current approaches to this type of screening are covered in detail in the individual chapters of Part 2. Screening for high-risk behaviors, injury prevention, and complementary approaches to wellness are discussed in this chapter.

GROWTH AND AGING IN HEALTH PROMOTION

Primary care providers must use their time wisely to provide counseling on high-risk behaviors. It may be inappropriate to counsel certain age groups on certain behaviors. If morbidity and mortality data are considered, a provider might decide that counseling a 70-year-old female of a 45-year marriage on birth control and sexually transmitted diseases might not be prudent. Likewise, counseling the 20-year-old college student of the dangers of falls and this year's influenza vaccine may be equally pointless. Realistic expectations for health promotion during routine health examinations are outlined by specific age groups in Tables 3-3 and 3-4.

Developing health-promotion and disease-prevention plans with patients requires consideration of growth, development, and maturation across the adult lifespan. Milestones of the young adult, middle adult, and older adult stages help to provide a framework for health-promotion and disease-prevention activities.

Young Adult

The young adult stage spans the ages of 18 to 35 years. The physical and emotional changes that occur during this time, and the style of learning, through experimentation and experience, focus health-promotion and disease-prevention activities. Generally, by the age of 20, physical growth is complete. This pe-

TABLE 3-2	Decision Theory Based on Sensitivity, Specificity, and Reliability of Screening Procedures	
	No Disease	**Disease**
Negative test	Accurate screening	False negative (test inaccurate or hyposensitive)
Positive test	False positive (hypersensitive or nonspecific test used)	Accurate screening

$$\text{Sensitivity} = \frac{\text{true positives}}{\text{true positives} + \text{false negatives}}$$

$$\text{Specificity} = \frac{\text{true negatives}}{\text{true negatives} + \text{false positives}}$$

riod is often described as the healthiest time of life. Maintaining proper functioning is a goal for this period of time that will impact the person not only as a young adult, but throughout adult life. Toward this end, health-promotion and disease-prevention activities should be focused on developing healthy lifestyle behaviors, early detection of health problems, prevention of accidents, injuries, and, the morbidity and mortality associated with violence.

Middle Adult

Middle adulthood spans the ages of 35 to 65. This period of time is marked by biologic changes. It may also be a time of turmoil, reassessment, and change. Leading causes of death during this time are heart disease, lung cancer, cerebrovascular disease, breast cancer, colorectal cancer, and, obstructive lung disease. Genetics, as well as other factors that health promotion and disease prevention activities can be directed toward, such as nutrition and exercise, contribute to these conditions.

Older Adult

By the year 2030, it is projected that 18% of the population will be over age 65. Within the older adult age group is the fastest growing segment of the population, those over the age of 85. It is expected that by the year 2000 this group will have increased by 70% (U.S. Senate Special Committee on Aging, 1991). Physiologic aging is universal, progressive, decremental,

TABLE 3-3	Health-Promotion Activities by Age Group: 11–24 Years
Awareness of leading causes of death	Unintentional injuries/motor vehicle accidents Homicide Suicide Malignant neoplasms Heart disease
Screening	Height & weight Blood pressure Pap test (women) Chlamydia screen (women <20 years) Rubella serology or vaccination history (women >12 years) Assess for problem drinking
Counseling	Injury prevention (helmet use, seat belt use, smoke detectors) Safe storage of firearms Avoid tobacco use Avoid underage drinking & illicit drug use Avoid alcohol or drug use while driving, swimming, boating, etc. Sexually transmitted infection prevention Diet & exercise Dental health
Immunizations	Tetanus–diphtheria Hepatitis MMR Varicella Rubella
Chemoprophylaxis	Multivitamin with folate (for women planning pregnancy)

(Adapted from USPSTF, 1996)

TABLE 3-4	Health-Promotion Activities by Age Group: 25–64 years
Awareness of leading causes of death	■ Malignant neoplasms ■ Heart disease ■ Unintentional injuries/motor vehicle accidents ■ HIV infection ■ Suicide & homicide
Screening	■ Blood pressure ■ Height & weight ■ Total blood cholesterol (men 35–65, women 45–65) ■ Pap test (women) ■ Fecal occult blood test and/or sigmoidoscopy (>50 years) ■ Mammogram and clinical breast exam (women 50–69 years) ■ Assess for problem drinking ■ Rubella serology or vaccination history (women of childbearing age)
Counseling	■ Substance abuse ■ Tobacco cessation ■ Avoid alcohol or drug use while driving, swimming, boating, etc. ■ Diet & exercise ■ Adequate calcium intake (women) ■ Regular physical activity ■ Injury prevention (helmet use, seat belt use, smoke detectors) ■ Safe storage of firearms ■ Sexually transmitted infection prevention ■ Dental health
Immunizations	■ Tetanus-diphtheria boosters ■ Rubella (women of childbearing age)
Chemoprophylaxis	■ Multivitamin with folate (for women planning pregnancy) ■ Discuss hormone prophylaxis (perimenopausal women)

(Adapted from USPSTF, 1996)

and intrinsic (Goldman, 1986). Age-related changes are inevitable but occur with variability. Chronic illness and functional disabilities are interrelated and increase with age. Thirty-three percent of those over 65 years have some type of functional limitation related to a chronic condition (US Public Health Service, 1991).

Accidents are a common problem of the elderly. With physiologic aging come decreased sensory acuity, reaction time, muscle strength, and impaired balance. As a result, in those over 70 years of age, falls are the greatest cause of accidents, with 50% of the falls caused by environmental factors (U.S. Public Health Service, 1991). Risk factors for falls include: functional status and use of assistive devices, polypharmacy, and medical history. Providers should evaluate the fall potential of patients and develop strategies for fall prevention which may include minimizing environmental risks, teaching or reteaching adaptive behavior, and reducing accompanying risk factors such as changes in visual acuity.

The leading causes of death is this age group are heart disease, cancer, cerebrovascular accident, chronic obstructive pulmonary disease, pneumonia, influenza, and injury. Alcohol and drug abuse, homelessness, and physical abuse are also concerns

TABLE 3-5	Adult Immunization Guidelines			
Vaccine	**Schedule**	**Booster**	**Indications**	**Precautions**
Rabies	Three doses at 0, 7, 21–28 d (1 mL IM deltoid)	3 y if antibodies decline	>30-day stay in SE Asia	(HCDV) Start chloroquine >3 wk after series complete
Tetanus-diphtheria	Three doses at 0, 1, and 6–12 mo (0.5 mL SQ or IM)	5 y	Nonimmune	
Varicella	Two doses at 0, 1–2 mo (0.5 mL SQ)	10 y	13 y old; likely exposure in nonimmune adult	Concurrent aspirin use; neomycin allergy; immunocompromise; planning pregnancy
Yellow fever	One dose (0.5 mL SQ)	10 y	Travel to equatorial Africa and S. America. Required by some countries.	Egg allergy; immunocompromise; pregnancy; age < 1 y
Cholera	Two doses >1 week apart (0.5 mL SQ or IM)	6 mo	Decreased gastric acidity, hx of gastric resection, achloryhydria	Pregnancy; age <6 mo
Hepatitis A	Two doses at 0 and 6–12 mo (1 mL IM)	6–12 mo	Travel >3 times/5 y or for >30 days to endemic area	Age <2 y
Hepatitis B	Three doses at 0, 1, 6 mo (1 mL IM)	Unknown	Child, adolescent, sexually active, or travel >6 mo to endemic area	N/A
Immunoglobulin	One dose 0.02 mL/kg IM/3 mo protection; 0.06 mL/kg IM divided/5 mo protection	3–5-mo intervals, as per initial dose	Single visit <3 mo to endemic area	Give measles >2 wk before or >3 mo after immunoglobulin.
Influenza	One dose (0.5 mL IM or SQ)	Annual	>64 y, travel to tropics or to Southern Hemisphere April–September; immunocompromise	Egg allergy (anaphylaxis)
Japanese B encephalitis	Three doses at 0, 7, and 30 days (1 mL SQ)	3 y	>30 days to SE Asia, especially rice paddies and pig farms	Pregnancy; age <1 y
Measles	One dose, assuming childhood immunizations (0.5 mL SQ)	None	One dose needed at 12 y old, one dose as adult if born between 1957 and 1980	Immunocompromise; pregnancy; immunoglobulin; egg allergy (if measles/mumps/rubella)
Meningococcus (*Neisseria meningitidis*)	One dose (0.5 mL SQ)	None	Travel to sub-Saharan Africa December–June	
Plaque	Three doses. 1st dose 1 mL IM. 2d dose 0.2 mL IM. 3d dose 0.2 mL IM 3–6 mo after 2d dose.	2 y	Field researchers with high exposure to rodents in Africa, Asia, S. America	Pregnancy
Pneumococcus	One dose	6 y for high-risk persons	>64 y or <65 with heart disease, lung disease, diabetes, kidney disease, or other chronic conditions	

These guidelines are routinely updated; please refer to the National Immunization Program Internet site (http://www.cdc.gov/nip) for the most current immunization guidelines.

(Adapted from *MMWR*, 44:942–943, 1996)

in the older adult population that must be considered in health-promotion and disease-prevention activities.

Health Care Decisions

When patients are in good health, matters related to their ability to make health care decisions are generally not of concern. It is, however, important for primary care providers to discuss with patients their right to direct the kind of health care they would or would not want, in the event that they are unable to do so.

Advance directives are broadly defined to include living wills and appointment of a health care agent. A living will is a document created by an individual to authorize in advance withholding or withdrawing artificial life-support measures in the case of terminal or debilitating illness, injury, or irreversible coma, it is signed, dated and witnessed. All but three states, Massachusetts, Michigan, and New York, have living will statutes.

Appointing a health care agent differs from state to state and may be referred to as: Durable Power of Attorney for Health Care; Health Care Power of Attorney; Appointment of a Health Care Agent; or, health care proxy. Regardless of state mandates, the objective of appointing a health care agent is the same: allowing an individual to appoint someone they trust to control their health care through the individual's written instructions.

Competent adults have the right to create an advance directive regarding treatment decisions, including life-sustaining measures. There are state-mandated forms for advance directives that the patient completes. Patients have the right to change their health care agent, and/or change their written instructions, or cancel their advance directive, at will. If the patient has both a living will, and an appointed health care agent, usually the appointment of the health care agent takes precedence.

Discussing advance directives with patients is an important part of proactive primary care. Encouraging patients to appoint a health care proxy and knowing whom the patient has appointed are essential to respecting a patient's wishes should they be unable to make their own health care decisions.

Adult Immunizations

Most immunizations are completed during a person's childhood health visits. For many individuals, the need for adult immunizations is limited to booster injections of tetanus (usually combined with diphtheria as Td) and measles vaccine (for adults born after 1956 without evidence of immunity or who attend high school or college). After age 65, influenza and pneumococcal inoculations are indicated as discussed in the following sections. Other conditions exist where adults may need to receive immunizations, including foreign travel or immigration to a foreign country, working in high-risk areas (including health-care workers), during periods of immunosuppression, and for missed childhood immunizations. A summary of the adult immunization guidelines can be found in Table 3-5. Travel guidelines are updated routinely. Before foreign travel, travelers should consult their primary care provider for the latest guidelines. Patients may also contact the Centers for Disease Control and Prevention directly or through the Internet to access these guidelines.

INFLUENZA

Each year in the United States, approximately 20,000 individuals die from influenza; 80% to 90% of these deaths are in persons aged 65 or older (Plichta, 1996). Influenza vaccines vary from year to year, therefore, immunization against influenza should be administered annually. Patients should receive the influenza vaccine beginning in September. Patients who receive their vaccination as late as December or January may still be protected. Patients who receive their vaccination during a flu outbreak should also receive antiviral prophylaxis with amantadine or rimantidine for 2 weeks.

PNEUMOCOCCAL DISEASE

Pneumococcal disease is the most common cause of hospitalization and death in persons age 65 years or older (Plichta, 1996). Pneumococcal vaccine has a varied effectiveness depending on the age and immunologic status of the patient, with patients under 55 years old deriving the most benefit (Plewa, 1990). Pneumococcal vaccine is given only once, but may be repeated for high-risk patients every 5 to 6 years.

TETANUS

Tetanus guidelines were established in the 1950s for childhood immunization. This decreased the incidence of tetanus among children and young adults. Older adults, however, have been shown to have nonprotective tetanus antibody titers in many cases (Alagappan et al, 1997). It is believed that this lack of protective titer may be caused by the failure to receive the initial tetanus vaccination or booster immunizations every 5 to 10 years. A cost-effective approach to tetanus vaccination in this population includes combining tetanus with diphtheria (Td)at least every 10 years for adult patients.

IDENTIFYING AND MODIFYING HIGH-RISK BEHAVIORS

High-risk behavior has been associated with a multitude of disease states and injuries. In many cases individuals are involved with multiple high-risk behaviors, such as smoking and drinking, driving while intoxicated (often without the protection of a seat belt). The possible combinations and permutations of high-risk behaviors is almost endless. In addition to the possibility of contracting disease or incurring injury, the injuries sustained while engaging in high-risk behaviors may be more severe, lead to longer hospitalizations and subsequently higher health care costs. In one study, total hospital costs were 7% higher for motorists not wearing seat belts and motorcyclists not wearing helmets than for their matched counterparts who used protective equipment (Mackersie et al, 1995).

High-risk sexual behavior, the use of alcohol, drugs and tobacco, and other injury-prone behavior was addressed in the national health promotion initiative, *Healthy People 2000.* Whether or not the public has significantly modified these behaviors and reduced morbidity and mortality has not yet been determined; however, at least one study of New Jersey college students determined that the national objectives for tobacco and cocaine use will be met. Unfortunately, the same study determined that the national targets set for condom and birth control use, alcohol and marijuana use, and seat belt and helmet use are not likely to be met (Lewis, 1996).

Smoking

Cigarette smoking has been linked to serious pulmonary, cardiovascular, and oncologic problems and remains the most important modifiable cause of premature mortality in the United States (MMWR, 1994; DHHS, 1996). It has been estimated that more than 420,000 Americans die each year (20% of all deaths) as a result of smoking (DHHS, 1996). In 1997, after cigarette manufacturers faced the public in a series of legal actions, major regulatory concessions were made and the tobacco industry agreed to spend $368 billion dollars, over the next 25 years to foster health promotion. While both the public and the tobacco industry have taken more responsibility for their actions and the associated health problems, approximately 25% of Americans, or 46 million, still smoke. While the percentage of Americans who smoke continues to decline, the nation's goal of reducing smoking prevalence to no more than 15% of adults, and decreasing the number of new smokers, by the year 2000 will not be reached (USDHHS, 1992). Substantial efforts to help smokers quit must continue well into the new millennium.

As a smoker quits, the health care risks associated with smoking decline drastically. The risk of lung cancer drops by 50% after 10 years of abstinence, the risk of mouth and throat cancers drops by 50% in 5 years, the risk of a myocardial infarction is reduced by 50% in 1 year. After 10 to 15 years, many of the risks associated with smoking are reduced to the same frequency as nonsmokers. Effective counseling and therapy for the cessation of smoking may be the single most important health-promoting activity that health care providers undertake.

Guidelines for primary care providers on smoking cessation have been published (USDHHS, 1996). Counseling, support systems and pharmacotherapy are described in these guidelines. Keys to successful smoking cessation programs and newer pharmacotherapy, introduced after the guidelines were originally published, are summarized in Tables 3-6 and 3-7.

Problem Drinking

Alcohol is virtually a ubiquitous substance. A variety of alcohol-containing products are used in religious and cultural ceremonies. Drunkenness is often the subject of comedians, movies, songs, and other versions of pop culture. Drinking alcohol is so prevalent in our society that it is practically considered a rite of passage into adulthood. Research has even shown that one to three glasses of red wine per day may prevent coronary artery disease (Gaziano et al, 1993). But there is also a negative side to alcohol. More than 100,000 deaths are attributed to alcohol

TABLE 3-6	Compelling Reasons to Quit Smoking

1. Tobacco is one of the most potent human carcinogens.
2. Smoking promotes atherosclerosis.
3. Smoking is a risk factor for pulmonary disease.
4. Nicotine is addictive.
5. Tobacco use may increase the risk of osteoporosis.
6. Smoking affects the health of nonsmokers.
7. Cigarettes are the cause of more than 25% of the deaths from house fires.

(Adapted from USPTF, 1996)

each year; almost half of which are related to injuries, motor vehicle accidents, drownings, murders, suicides and deaths from fires. (CGPHS). The remaining deaths are related to the pathophysiologic changes induced by chronic alcohol exposure, including: hypertension, cirrhosis, stroke, hepatic cancer, esophageal cancer and bleeding, chronic malnourishment, vitamin deficiencies, pancreatitis and cardiomyopathy.

Identifying alcohol dependence can be a difficult task in primary care. Physical examination may reveal signs of alcoholism (eg, enlarged liver, ascites, spider angiomas) that warrant immediate intervention. Identification of asymptomatic individuals, however, is of equal importance. Despite the need for providers to inquire about alcohol consumption, patients are often reluctant to discuss problem drinking openly with their providers. Other screening methods, such as the use of questionnaires may be useful for this purpose. Controversy exists over which questionnaire is the most sensitive and specific. Providers should consider using a short screening questionnaire such as the Alcohol Use Disorders Identification Test (AUDIT), or others, to uncover information related to the drinking quantity, frequency and impact of drinking on the individual patient. Alcohol usage leading to significant hazards has been defined as five drinks (12 ounces of beer/5 ounces of wine/1.5 ounces of spirits) per day in men or two drinks per day in women. (USPSTF, 1996). The use of serum markers to identify alcohol dependence is not routinely used. Serum GGT levels rise with alcohol use, but an elevated level is not specific for alcoholism. Serum carbohydrate-deficient transferrin (CDT) may have greater potential as a alcohol marker but has not been universally accepted. (Sillanaukee, 1996)

If problem drinking is identified, several approaches to care may be considered. The first step should include counseling by the primary care provider regarding the health risks of problem drinking. If it is acceptable to the patient, family support should be incorporated into the treatment plan. Additionally, outside support groups such as Alcoholics Anonymous (AA), Al-Anon, and AlaTeen can be used. Pharmacotherapy, including benzodiazepines and naltrexone, may be utilized to decrease intake by limiting the symptoms of alcohol withdrawal. Disulfiram has traditionally been used to discourage alcohol ingestion by making the patient experience unpleasant gastrointestinal and cutaneous effects when alcohol is taken concurrently with the medication. Success with disulfiram has been extremely limited and is not currently recommended.

Illicit or Recreational Drugs and Abuse of Legalized Medications

The use of illicit or recreational drugs and abuse of legalized medications represents a serious concern for society. Illicit drug use is a problem centered around 18- to 25-year-olds, with 14% of individuals in this age group, and only 3% of the population over 35 years of age, reporting recent drug use. (DHHS, 1993) Marijuana remains the primary drug of use, with more than 5 million regular users, but cocaine, heroin, amphetamines, benzodiazepines, steroids, and "designer drugs" are also frequently used. While the occasional use of marijuana has not yet been definitively linked to serious health risks, users of cocaine and other drugs are not as safe. Even occasional use of cocaine may provoke ischemia, myocardial infarction, arrhythmias, seizures, and death. Illicit drugs are often mixed or

TABLE 3-7	Guidelines for Successful Smoking Cessation Programs
Principles of smoking cessation in primary care	1. Every smoker should be offered cessation therapy at each visit. 2. The tobacco use status of each patient should be recorded in the patient's medical record. 3. As little as 3 minutes of counseling can be effective as cessation therapy. 4. Better results are obtained with more intensive therapy. 5. Nicotine replacement therapy, social support, and skills training should be incorporated into cessation therapy. 6. Health care systems should allow for follow-up at each visit.
The three-step plan	1. Establish an office-wide mechanism to determine tobacco use status and record findings. 2. Advise tobacco users to abstain. 3. Assist the patient in accomplishing this goal.
Intensive cessation programs	1. Intensive programs, run by specialists, are highly effective. 2. Programs generally run four to seven sessions over 2 weeks. 3. Every smoker should be offered nicotine replacement therapy (unless contraindicated). 4. Individual or group counseling should accompany the program. 5. Counseling should offer problem-solving skills, social support, and positive reinforcement.

Treatment strategies	Pharmacotherapies can be used alone or in combination.
	Pharmacotherapy should be combined with counseling.
	Nicotine replacement therapy:
	  1. The transdermal system, or patch, requires daily application to a hairless area of the torso for 8 weeks. Sites should be rotated, reusing sites once per week.
	  2. Gum therapy involves chewing and "parking" the gum between the cheek and gum every 30 minutes, with a new piece of gum every 1–2 hours. Therapy is less effective than the patch and may take up to 3 months with the 4-mg dose.
	  3. Use of the nasal spray
	
	Buproprion therapy:
	(contraindicated with seizure disorders, anorexia nervosa, bulimia, or concurrent buproprion or MAOI therapy)
	  1. Begin therapy with 150 mg/day for 3 days while patient is still smoking.
	  2. Increase to 150 mg BID (maximum 300 mg/day).
	  3. Set a target date for cessation approximately 10 days after initiating therapy.
	  4. Continue therapy for 7–12 weeks.
	  5. If cessation is not accomplished in 7 weeks, therapy is not likely to be successful.
	  6. Tapering off therapy is not necessary.

Follow-up	1. First follow-up within 1–2 weeks 2. Second follow-up in a month 3. Congratulate success or solicit a new commitment if patient lapsed.
Relapse prevention	1. Congratulate and stress the importance of remaining abstinent. 2. Review positive health benefits available after cessation. 3. Review the patient's success in quitting. 4. Ascertain difficulties patient may be having maintaining abstinence. 5. Anticipate problems that may lead to relapse, such as weight gain, depression, nicotine withdrawal, and lack of support.

(Adapted from USDHHS. [1996])

"cut" with toxic agents including pesticides, quinine, and other drugs. The effects of the adulterants may be just as dangerous as the "marketed agent." Designer drugs come with endless possibilities of untoward effects. Coupled with the inherent dangers of the drugs themselves, the associated motor vehicle injuries, homicides, suicides and other criminal activity associated with illicit drug use cannot be underestimated.

The American Medical Association (1988) and the American Academy of Family Physicians (1994) agree that screening for drug abuse should be incorporated into each patient's primary care visit. This screening should identify the quantity and frequency of drug use as well as any effects of drug use on the patient's life and relationships. Success with this type of screening is limited and health care providers should also consider physical signs of drug abuse. Such physical signs may include weight loss, malnutrition, "track" marks, nasal and sinus problems, respiratory problems, and tachycardia.

There is always a temptation to use laboratory testing to confirm suspicion of drug abuse. Such testing is readily available and reliable. False-positive and false-negative test results are rare but possible, and usually are related to the use of other medications, food interactions, or deliberate tampering with the specimen. Despite the availability of such testing and the widespread use of this testing by employers, primary care providers should not employ such testing unless the patient consents to the evaluation. Failure to respect a patient's right to autonomy and confidentiality may lead to severe repercussions in their job, loss of credibility in the community, damage in their personal relationships, and may threaten the patient–provider relationship.

For those patients who are identified and are willing to listen, providers should encourage limiting or stopping drug use. Patients may be referred to support groups, as well as inpatient and outpatient drug treatment programs. Patients should be counseled about the risk of other disease states, such as HIV infection and hepatitis with intravenous drug use, cardiovascular disease with cocaine and stimulant use, and glomerular disease with anabolic steroid use. If the patient agrees, family and friends may be asked to intervene and participate in the process of becoming drug-free.

Misuse and Abuse of Medications

Inappropriate usage of medications can be described as the nation's "other drug problem." The misuse of prescription and over-the-counter medications contributes to an increase in morbidity, mortality, and health-care costs (Johnson & Bootman, 1995). Variations of the term "compliance" have often been used to describe the appropriate use of a medication by a patient. Patients are often labeled as noncompliant or overcompliant for choosing to use medications in a manner other than that recommended by their health care providers or product labeling. While this concept is one of tremendous importance, the term "compliance" does not foster a patient-centered approach to health care. Since the use of the term compliance imparts a message of paternalistic health care, use of the term has been avoided in this text; instead the authors and contributors have opted to describe how a patient may optimally *participate* in their health care by using medications rationally.

The assumption in patient-centered care is that patients are involved in making the choices for their therapy and are involved in a partnership with their provider for successful therapy. Providers must acknowledge and accept that patients are affected by the act of prescribing in a variety of ways. Often overlooked are the reasons for misuse of medications, including adverse effects of a selected regimen, cost of the regimen, inconvenience of multiple daily dosing, a lack of well-defined symptoms, and the psychological components of taking medications and being "sick." Patients may be reluctant to discuss their choice to underuse or discontinue their medications because of the possible embarrassment of revealing side effects (eg, impotence with antihypertensives), unwillingness to disclose financial problems, or for fear of disappointing their provider. Overuse of medications may be related to less-than-expected efficacy or refractory disease (eg., overuse of ergotamine or sumatriptan for migraine headaches). Rather than discussing these issues with their health-care providers, many patients have resorted to alternative therapies or discontinued therapy altogether. To encourage rationale and appropriate medication use and participation in therapeutic care plans, providers should provide patients with information regarding the available treatment options (pharmacotherapeutic, surgical, and complementary) for their condition, as well as specific information on the therapy chosen. Counseling and follow-up are appropriate for all members of the health-care team; however, if a patient has concerns that cannot be addressed in the time frame of an office visit, or if the quest for information is beyond the scope of the provider's expertise, the patient should be referred to additional resources for the information.

Sexually Transmitted Infections

A discussion of health promotion and disease prevention as related to the spread of sexually transmitted infections (STIs) may be found in Chapter 69.

INJURY PREVENTION

Unintentional injuries are the fifth leading cause of death in the United States (USPSTF, 1996). Motor vehicle accidents, falls, and poisonings are the three leading causes of death in this category. Other fatal and nonfatal household injuries include firearm injuries, bicycle injuries, drownings, burns and other fire related injuries. General guidelines for household safety are listed in Table 3-8. Specific recommendations for preventing motor vehicle, bicycle, and in-line skating injuries are described below.

Motor Vehicle Accidents

Motor vehicle accidents were the eighth leading cause of death in 1993. (USPSTF, 1996) While many of these deaths may have been attributed to alcohol or drug use, more than half of these deaths could have been prevented with the proper use of automotive restraints. (USPSTF, 1996) Current restraint systems include shoulder/lap belts and supplemental restraint systems (SSRs; airbags).

New York was the first state to enact mandatory safety belt legislation in late 1984 (States et al, 1990). Since 1984, 43 states enacted similar legislation. Until 1997, SRS were not mandatory in U.S. automobiles. Beginning in 1997, coincident with mandatory inclusion of SRS in new automobiles, injuries related to SRS were reported. These SRS related injuries included 80 deaths, mostly involving children and low weight adults. (MMWR, 1996) SRS-related deaths have caused debate over the relative benefits of SRSs and may lead to switching to systems that will enable drivers to prevent activation of the SRS. Despite this controversy, the use of automotive safety devices has reduced the likelihood of hospital admission, surgery, severe injuries, and death in several studies. (Henry, 1996; Lund,

TABLE 3-8	Checklist for Household Safety

☐ Install & test smoke detectors (combination of photoelectric and ionization models preferred).

☐ Review fire escape plans and meeting point.

☐ Cease or decrease cigarette smoking to decrease incidence of fires.

☐ Set hot-water thermostats to 120°F or less to prevent scalding.

☐ Install & test carbon monoxide detectors.

☐ Place all medications, poisons, chemicals, and matches in childproof containers and out of reach.

☐ Post the phone number for the nearest Poison Control Center.

☐ Keep a 30-mL bottle of syrup of ipecac on hand in case of poisoning (contact Poison Control Center before use).

☐ Learn cardiopulmonary resuscitation skills.

☐ Install fences with self-locking gates around swimming pools.

☐ Learn to use automated external defibrillators.

☐ Install window guards for young children.

☐ Use protective equipment when doing household repairs.

☐ Remove, or unload and lock all firearms.

☐ Learn to swim.

☐ Wear personal flotation devices when boating.

☐ Wear protective sporting equipment, including helmets.

☐ Wear fluorescent orange clothing when hunting.

1995; Loo, 1996) Thus, patients should be encouraged and reminded to use these devices. An appropriate time to include this information in the visit may be when alcohol use is discussed, so that driving under the influence of alcohol may also be addressed.

Bicycle Injuries

Bicycles are owned by approximately 30% of Americans, with approximately 1000 annual deaths related to cycling injuries (MMWR, 1995). Almost two thirds of these deaths are attributed to head injuries in unprotected cyclists. (JAMA, 1996; Frank et al, 1995; Thompson et al, 1996). Bicycle helmets, regardless of design (as long as they are approved by either ANSI, the Snell Memorial Foundation or the American Society for Testing and Materials) provide significant protection against these fatal head injuries. (Thompson, 1996) However, despite widespread availability of inexpensive bicycle helmets, many cyclists choose to ride without a helmet. Interestingly, most of these high-risk cyclists are not children, but adults in their 20s. Counseling adults who ride bicycles on the routine use of bicycle helmets may be an important part of a routine health visit. Additional efforts should be made by health providers to promote community and statewide educational efforts to promote helmet use. These efforts may be in the form of community lectures on injury prevention, providing educational materials in the office waiting area and supporting local and state legislation for the mandated use of helmets.

In-Line Skating Injuries

In-line skating, also known as roller-blading, has become an extremely popular recreational activity. The popularity of this activity nearly doubled from an estimated 12.6 million skaters in 1993 to an estimated 22.5 million skaters in 1995 (Schieber, 1995; Schieber, 1996). As might be expected, along with this increase in participation came an increase in related injuries, as demonstrated by an increase from 31,000 to approximately 100,000 injuries in respective years (Schieber, 1995). Most skaters have had no formal training in the sport (Adams, 1996) and several studies have shown that 30% to 75% of skaters did not wear any form of protective gear (Adams, 1996; Schieber, 1996; Young, 1995; Orenstein, 1996). Most accidents and injuries have been associated with loss of balance, excessive speed, and collisions. The majority of injuries were fractures and dislocations of the wrist and distal arm. Throughout the studies, those who wore protective gear had fewer injuries and required less hospitalization than those that wore no protective gear. Based on these data, it would be prudent to advise such protective equipment, encouraging the use of wrist and elbow guards at a minimum, to patients when discussing their physical activity.

COMPLEMENTARY HEALTH CARE APPROACHES

The traditional Western, or allopathic approach to health care is increasingly becoming integrated with other healing traditions. These other healing traditions, often categorized as alternative, complementary, or unconventional therapies, are based on whole systems, and the belief that human beings are more than the sum of their parts. In this paradigm the body, mind, and spirit are united.

The integration of these approaches comes from both patients' and providers' beliefs in and knowledge of these complementary healing traditions. Patients may choose to incorporate other approaches for health promotion or disease prevention, and to treat complex conditions that require multifaced approaches. Providers may offer or recommend other approaches that can complement Western or conventional health care and benefit their patients.

One third of adult Americans regularly use what have been referred to as unconventional therapies for health problems, generally in addition to conventional therapies, and often without informing their providers (Eisenberg et al, 1993). Many of these so-called unconventional therapies, however, may be a longstanding part of health care treatment in other cultures. In 1992, the Office of Alternative Medicine (OAM) was established within the National Institutes of Health to identify and evaluate these practices by supporting and conducting research and disseminating information about these therapies. Through this effort, scientific information will develop providing evidence for the efficacy of various unconventional therapies.

In supporting patients within the context of family and community, providers work with patients to develop the most appropriate and cost-effective care, which may include complementary health care approaches. Providers are challenged to work with patients to develop a plan that is responsive to the patient's multiple needs, while at the same time is not harmful to the patient. Initiating a nonjudgmental discussion with patients is the best place to begin this conversation, as it is recognized that although a significant number of patients use complementary approaches, the majority of patients do not discuss this with their provider. This should become a routine part of history taking, and ongoing conversations with patients in order to remain informed about their use of these therapies. One reason why providers may not ask patients about their use of complementary approaches is their own lack of knowledge of these approaches. The following section will help to familiarize the reader with selected complementary approaches. In evaluating alternative/complementary therapies, providers can contact, The National Institutes of Health's Office of Alternative Medicine for reliable information, as well as searching the National Library of Medicine's MEDLINE database for specific types of alternative/complementary therapies.

Overview of Complementary Health Care Approaches

Complementary approaches that are based on the interrelatedness of the mind's ability to affect body functions include meditation, biofeedback, and imagery.

While there are many forms of meditation they result in similar physical and psychological changes. Through focused effort on one thought, or sound, or one's own breathing, the mediator can quiet the mind, and with regular practice can produce positive effects. The benefits of meditation, have been shown over time in a number of well-designed clinical trials. Through meditation, stress of both body and mind can be reduced. Meditation has been shown to help lower blood pressure in hypertensive patients (Alexander et al, 1996); reduce health care use, and chronic pain, and increase longevity and quality of life (Kabat-Zinn et al, 1985, 1986); reduce serum cholesterol levels (Cooper & Aygen, 1978); and reduce substance abuse (Sharma et al, 1991).

Biofeedback uses monitoring devices to feed back physiologic information to patients that they might otherwise be unaware of. Biofeedback instruments mirror physiologic events such as muscle contraction and relaxation, skin temperature, brain waves, and galvanic skin response. Through repetitive training patients can learn to modulate bodily processes previously thought to be involuntary. Developed in the 1960s, the effectiveness of biofeedback training has been demonstrated in a wide range of conditions, including Raynaud's syndrome/disease and some types of urinary and fecal incontinence (for which it is the preferred treatment), bronchial asthma, drug and alcohol abuse, tension and migraine headaches, cardiac arrhythmias, essential hypertension, irritable bowel, muscle strengthening and rehabilitation, epilepsy, hot flashes associated with menopause, chronic pain syndromes, and anticipatory nausea and vomiting related to chemotherapy, and for general stress management (Basmajian, 1989).

Imagery requires the individual's attention and concentration on imagining through multiple senses. It is used to facilitate changes in behavior, attitude or physiologic reactions. The use of this approach is based on the belief that images have an effect on health, either direct or indirect. Imagery has been found to be effective in immunology, alleviating nausea and vomiting in patients receiving chemotherapy, to relieve stress, and to control pain (Achterberg & Ryder, 1989).

Commonly known nonallopathic systems of healing include: traditional Chinese medicine; Ayurvedic medicine, homeopathic medicine, and naturopathic medicine. These systems of practice may improve U.S. health care by the identification of their outcomes through research. Each of these systems is based on standards of practice that are grounded in different traditions.

Traditional Chinese medicine is an ancient tradition of the Chinese culture and the philosophies of Taoism, Confucianism, and Buddhism. This system is applied to health promotion, as well as treatment of illness, respecting the interrelatedness of the person and nature. It is characterized by the diagnosis of disturbances in the flow of energy, or *chi*. Diagnosis requires observation, questioning and listening, and palpation of pulses. Acupuncture and acupressure are two well known treatments used by Asian medicine practitioners.

Acupuncture is based on ancient Chinese philosophy and healing practices in which health is believed to be affected by internal energy forces, chi, and external forces, such as nutrition, environment, weather, and exercise. These factors are balanced by acupuncture. Chi flows through energy pathways or meridians. An imbalance is caused by blockage or stagnation of a meridian. Energy is stimulated by the insertion of needles into specific meridians which disperses or activates chi which helps to restore health. Adjunct therapies such as diet, herbs, acupressure, massage, and moxibustion (application of heat to acupuncture points) may also be used. Treatment is based on history and physical exam using one of the models within traditional Chinese medicine. The approach may vary based on the background of the practitioner, and the patient's diagnosis. For chronic conditions, a series of 10 treatments is usually prescribed, whereas minor injuries may be as few as one to four treatments (Reed, 1994). Scientific evaluation of acupuncture while not statistically conclusive does show that it is the most researched of the alternative therapies, and suggests indications in which it may be beneficial. Its use in chronic pain management and drug addiction has shown positive results. Acupressure, another intervention used in this tradition, is the direct application of pressure by the therapist's fingers or hands to energy points. It may be used for overall health, or for first-aid or symptomatic relief (Reed, 1994). Acupuncturists have educational and certification requirements, and in most states a license to practice is required.

Life-knowledge, or Ayurvedic medicine, is the ancient medicine of India. Its approach to treatment is through lifestyle changes and natural therapies. Diagnosis is made thought the evaluation of the three doshas, which is accomplished by pulse palpation of the radial artery. Treatment includes the use of herbs and other therapies, such as yoga, breathing practices, diet and meditation. Ayurvedic practitioners in India receive training recognized by the state alongside of those training in conventional Western and homeopathic medicine. Studies of the physiologic effects of yoga and meditation have shown improvements in patients with chronic conditions such as rheumatoid arthritis, asthma, chronic bronchitis, eczema, psoriasis, hypertension, constipation, headaches, chronic sinusitis, and non-insulin-dependent diabetes mellitus (Janssen, 1989). Additionally, studies of Ayurvedic herbal preparations and therapies have shown potential benefits in the prevention and treatment of breast, lung and colon cancers (Sharma et al, 1990). The National Cancer Institute has included two Ayurvedic herbal compounds on its list of potential chemoprotective agents and has funded studies on them (Reed, 1994).

Homeopathic medicine developed from the work of Samuel Hahnemann in the late 1700s. It is based on his personal experience of taking quinine bark, which was used for the treatment of malaria. After taking it, he suffered from classic malarial symptoms. From this he developed the principle of similars, "like cures like." In other words, if a substance is given to someone without the disease, it can cause its symptoms, whereas if the person has the disease it can cure it. Furthermore, Hahnemann found that by significantly diluting the substance in a water–alcohol solution and vigorously shaking the solution, the substance could be "potentialized," still having an effect while decreasing side effects. Homeopathic remedies are often diluted to a concentration that may exclude any actual molecules of the original compound, while still retaining properties of that compound. It is currently used for health promotion, disease prevention, and acute and chronic conditions. Homeopathy was widely practiced in the United States until the early 1900s, when guidelines for funding medical schools approved by the AMA were put forward. It remained widely practiced in other countries, and has over the past 15 years become popular again in the U.S. Clinical trials have shown a positive effect from the use of homeopathic medicines on allergic rhinitis (Reilly et al, 1994), fibrositis (Fisher et al, 1989), influenza (Ferely et al, 1989), and osteoarthritis (Kleijnen et al, 1991).

Herbal products have also experienced a resurgence in use in the past several years, with more than 16% of Americans currently using these products. Herbal remedies are natural pharmaceutical products, from plant or animal origin, studied by pharmacognosists. Documented use of herbal remedies dates back to the year 78 AD and perhaps even earlier to the Babylonians. Herbal products have been used successfully for the treatment of many disease states and were the primary source of pharmaceuticals until only a few decades ago. Several antibiotics, digoxin, quinine, insulin, and many other pharmaceuticals still are derived from natural sources.

However, the market for herbal remedies is not for those products made available through FDA approved sources. Rather, most herbal products are marketed as food supplements and sold through health food stores, mail order advertisements, and infomercials. While many of these products may have a therapeutic benefit, several also have the potential for severe, if not life-threatening, toxicity. Additionally, herbal products are not required to have childproof packaging and do not undergo purity testing. Many products are imported from the Far East and have been known to be contaminated, mislabeled, and adulterated with other products. In some cases, herbal products have been adulterated with synthetic pharmaceuticals to increase their yield on the market, obliterating the whole concept of natural products. More data are becoming available on the safety and toxicity of these products and primary care providers should stay abreast of new developments in this area. Patients must also be cautioned regarding the potential toxicity of some of these agents.

Naturopathic medicine was developed in the early 1900s, but declined shortly thereafter because of the belief that disease could be eradicated through the use of pharmaceutical drugs rather than natural therapies. It has also seen a resurgence in the past 2 decades, and today reflects an integration of natural therapies that may include, botanicals, nutrition, homeopathy, acupuncture, traditional Oriental medicine, hydrotherapy, and naturopathic manipulative therapy with conventional medical science and standards of care. Research in this area has focused on natural treatments for women's health problems. Positive effects have been found in the use of a botanical formula for the reduction of menopausal symptoms (Hudson & Standish, 1993).

The use of a practitioner's hands for either touch or manipulation can be traced back to the earliest days of health care. Manual healing methods include approaches such as chiropractic manipulation, massage therapy, pressure point therapy, and craniosacral therapy.

Chiropractic medicine is grounded in the principles of natural healing. It is based on the relationship between structure, primarily that of the spine, and function. This basis is used to diagnose and treat structural problems. Chiropractic physicians use manual procedures and interventions rather than surgery or pharmaceuticals. Manipulation has been found to be effective in back pain (Handelman, et al, 1992). Chiropractic services are covered by most third-party payers.

Massage therapy dates back to Hippocrates. Through scientific manipulation of soft tissue, the soft tissue is neutralized through a variety of manual techniques. Massage affects the circulatory, lymphatic, musculoskeletal, and nervous systems. Its aim is to aid the body in healing itself and improving health and well-being. There are more than 80 different types of massage therapy, divided into two different groupings–traditional European and contemporary Western massage. Swedish massage is the main example of traditional European massage in which five soft tissue manipulation approaches are used. They include gliding strokes or effleurage, kneeing or petrissage, friction or rubbing, percussion or tapotement, and vibration. In contemporary Western massage, a wide range of approaches are used including deep-tissue massage, sports massage, neuro-

muscular massage, and manual lymph drainage. Massage has been found to be effective in the treatment of acute and chronic pain, inflammation, anxiety, depression, insomnia, grand mal seizures, muscle spasm, chronic lymph edema, soft-tissue dysfunctions, and psychoemotional states (Rubik et al, 1994). Licensure for massage therapists is currently required in 19 states and some localities, with more expected to require licensure. A national certification exam was put in place in 1992, and has been adopted by some states as their licensing exam.

Pressure point therapies are used to reduce pain and to treat other diseases. Release points, which include oriental meridians, and neurologic release points have pressure applied to them by the therapists fingers. Pressure point therapies include: reflexology, both hand and foot; traditional Chinese massage, of the hand, palm and fingers and acupressure, shiatsu being the most widely know.

Craniosacral therapy is a gentle, light touch (pressure usually does not exceed 5 g of force), noninvasive manipulative technique that was developed from the work of William Sutherland, D.O. Sutherland based his "cranial osteopathy" on the essential feature of the constant rhythmic motion associated between the central nervous system and associated structures (the cranial structure, internal cranial membranes, dural tube, spinal column to the sacrum), and his belief in the importance of this motion to life and health. Gentle manipulation of the skull eases pressure and increases the mobility of the cranial bones, which allows for remodeling and enhanced adaptation and functioning. John Upledger, D.O., in the late 1970s, investigated the scientific basis of the craniosacral system, and from this research developed CranioSacral Therapy™, which goes beyond the work of Sutherland and focuses on manipulating the underlying membranes. CranioSacral Therapy™ is used to evaluate and treat problems involving the brain and spinal cord, such as chronic pain, headache, temporomandibular joint syndrome, mood disorders, dyslexia, autism, stroke, epilepsy, cerebral palsy, dizziness, tinnitus, edema, hypertension, hypotension, and some muscular conditions (Burton Goldberg Group, 1994). Contraindications to craniosacral therapy include acute intracranial hemorrhage, intracranial aneurysm, recent skull fracture, and herniation of the medulla oblongata (Upledger & Vredevoogd, 1997).

Therapeutic touch (TT) is a biofield therapy. It is a form of energy healing through which the vibrational component to the patient's universal energy field is corrected. Although called therapeutic "touch," actually touching the patient is not necessary for this type of energy healing. TT was developed by Dolores Kreiger, Ph.D., R.N., a nurse educator and researcher, and Dora Kuntz, a healer, in 1972. It is a contemporary interpretation of ancient healing traditions of laying on of the hands and has been practiced for the past 25 years by nurses, as well as other health professionals and caregivers. Treatment begins with the practitioner centering oneself. Once centered the practitioner assesses the energy field by moving their hands gently down the front of the patient's body and then down the back. This is done in one of the patient's energy fields which is 2″ to 4″ away from the body. Slowly and smoothly, as if smoothing out a cloth, the practitioner moves their hands over the patient's body. Through this assessment, the practitioner and patient sense each others' energy fields. Vibrational alterations are assessed, and the practitioner then concentrates on directing energy to those specific locations. TT is holistic and its out-

TABLE 3-9	Selected Resources for the Promotion of Health Activities
U.S. Public Health Service	(202) 690-6867
Agency for Health Care Policy and Research	(301) 594-1364 or http://www.ahcpr.gov/
Centers for Disease Control and Prevention	(404) 639-3286 or http://www.cdc.gov/
Food and Drug Administration	(301) 443-1130 or http://www.fda.gov/
Health Resources and Services Administration	(301) 443-3376
National Institutes of Health	(310) 496-5787
Office of Disease Prevention and Health Promotion	(202) 205-5968
Travel Gopher	gopher://gopher.moon.com:7000/11h/travel.health
Tulane Tropical Medicine Web Page	http://www.tropmed.tulane.edu
Preventive Medicine Web Page (with links)	http://www.monash.edu.au/health/links.htm

comes encompass multiple aspects of the patient's health. Specific therapeutic intentions of TT include promotion of relaxation (Kreiger, 1993), pain relief (Hinze, 1988; Keller & Bzdek, 1986), reducing anxiety (Kramer, 1990), and general well-being (Quinn, 1992).

Another ancient approach used to complement, support, and enhance allopathic treatments is aromatherapy. Its origins can be traced back 18,000 years and its use spans every continent and many civilizations. During the 1920s, a French chemist, Rene Gottefose, coined the term "aromatherapie" and revived interest in the use of essential oils. Since that time, there has been continued research into the healing properties of essential oils. Essential oils are volatile, aromatic substances extracted by various methods from natural botanicals. They contain a mixture of complex chemicals, and it is from these chemicals that an essential oil gives its therapeutic properties. Essential oils enter the body through the olfactory and integumentary systems by inhalation, massage, compresses, and baths. A clinical aromatherapist, trained in the safe and controlled use of essential oils can play a vital complementary role in health and well-being.

CONCLUSION

Health promotion, disease prevention, and overall wellness strategies are of paramount importance in the practice of primary care. While the activities described in this chapter have been extensive, providers are encouraged to undertake as many of these activities as time permits in a routine health visit. In many cases, the choice of topics can be limited by age group or special population. In cases where many important areas need to be discussed but time is limited, the provider is encouraged to enlist other providers, provide written information, and use office staff to disseminate the promotional activities. Resouces for obtaining information on health promotion are listed in Table 3-9.

References

Achterberg, J., & Ryder, M.S. (1989). The effect of music-mediated imagery on neutrophils and lymphocytes. *Biofeedback Self Regul 14*, 247–257.

Adams, S.L., Wyte, C.D., Paradise, M.S., & del Castillo, J. (1996). A prospective study of inline skating. *Acad Emerg Med.*

Alagappan, K., Rennie, W., Narang, V., & Auerbach, C. (1997). Immunologic response to tetanus toxoid in geriatric patients. *Ann Emerg Med, 30*, 459–462.

Alexander, C.N., Schneider, R.H. (1996). Trial of stress reduction for hypertension in older African Americans. *Hypertension, 28*(2), 228.

American Academy of Family Physicians. (1994). Age charts for periodic health examination. Kansas City, MO: American Academy of Family Physicians.

American Medical Association. (1988). Drug abuse in the United States: A policy report. Report of the board of trustees. Chicago: American Medical Association.

Anonymous. (1996). Update: Fatal air bag-related injuries to children—United States, 1993–1996. *MMWR, 45*(49), 1073–1076.

Anonymous. (1995). Injury-control recommendations: Bicycle helmets. National Center for Injury Prevention and Control, Centers for Disease Control and Prevention. *MMWR, 44*(RR-1), 1–17.

Basmajian, J.V. (1989). *Biofeedback: Principles and practice for clinicians.* Baltimore: Williams & Wilkins.

Burton Goldberg Group. (1994). *Alternative medicine: The definitive guide.* Tiburon, CA: Future Medicine Publishing.

Cooper, M., & Aygen, M. (1978). Effect of meditation on blood cholesterol and blood pressure. *Journal of the Israel Medical Association, 95*, 1–2.

Eisenberg, D., Kessler, R., Foster, C., Norlock, F., Culkins, D., & Delbanco, R. (1993). Unconventional medicine in the United States. *N Engl J Med, 328*, 246–252.

Ferely, J.P., Smirou, D., D'Adhemar, R.R., & Balducci, F. (1989). A controlled evaluation of a homeopathic preparation in the treatment of influenza-like syndromes. *Br J Clin Pharmacol, 27*, 329–335.

Fisher, P., Greenwood, A., & Huskisson, E.C. (1989). Effect of homeopathic treatment on fibrositis (primary fibromyalgia). *Br Med J, 299*, 365–366.

Frank, E., Frankel, P., Mullins, R.J., & Taylor, N. (1995). Injuries resulting from bicycle collisions. *Academic Emergency Medicine, 2*(3), 200–203.

Gaziano, J.M., Buring, J.E., Breslow, J.L., et al. (1993). Moderate alcohol intake, increased levels of high-density lipoprotein and its subfractions, and decreased risk of myocardial infarction. *N Engl J Med, 329*(25), 1829–1834.

Goldman, J. (1986). Decline in organic function with age. In Rossman, I. (ed.) *Clinical Geriatrics*, 3d ed. Philadelphia: JB Lippincott.

Hart, A.R., Wicks, A.C.B., & Mayberry, J.F. (1995). Colorectal cancer screening in asymptomatic populations. *Gut, 36*, 590–597.

Henry, M.C., Hollander, J.E., Alicandro, J.M., Cassara, G., O'Malley, S., & Thode, H.C. Jr. (1996). Prospective countywide evaluation of the effects of motor vehicle safety device use on hospital resource use and injury severity. *Annals of Emergency Medicine, 28*(6), 627–634.

Hinze, M. (1988). *The effects of therapeutic touch and acupressure on experimentally-induced pain.* Doctoral dissertation, University of Texas, Austin.

Hudson, T., & Standish, L. (1993). Clinical and endocrinologic effects of a menopausal formula. Presented at American Association of Naturopathic convention, Portland, OR.Janssen, G.W. (1989). The application of Maharisihi Ayur-Veda in the treatment of ten chronic diseases: A pilot study. *Nederlands Tijdschrift Voor Intergrale Geneeskunde, 5,* 586–594.

Johnson, J.A., & Bootman, J.L. (1995). Drug-related morbidity and mortality: A cost-of-illness model. *Arch Intern Med, 155*(18), 1949–1956.

Kabat-Zinn, J., Lipworth, L., Burney, R., et al. (1985). The clinical use of mindfulness meditation for the self-regulation of chronic pain. *J Behav Med, 8,* 163–190.

Kabat-Zinn, J., Lipworth, L., et al. (1986). Four-year follow-up of a meditation-based program for the self-regulation of chronic pain. *Clin J Pain, 2,* 150–173.

Keller, E., & Bzdek, V. (1986). Effects of therapeutic touch on tension headache pain. *Nursing Research, 35,* 101–110.

Kleijnen, J., Knipschild, P., & Riet, G. (1991). Clinical trials of homeopathy. *Br Med J, 302,* 316–323.

Kramer, N. (1990). Comparison of therapeutic touch and casual touch in stress reduction of hospitalized children. *Pediatric Nursing, 15,* 483–485.

Kreiger, D. (1993). *Therapeutic touch: How to use your hands to help or heal.* Englewood Cliffs, NJ: Prentice Hall.

Leitch, M.A. (1995). Controversies in breast cancer screening. *Cancer, 76*(10), 2064–2069.

Lewis, D.F., Goodhart, F., & Burns, W.D. (1996). New Jersey college students' high-risk behavior: Will we meet the health objectives for the year 2000? *Journal of Americam College Health, 45*(3), 119–126.

Loo, G.T., Siegel, J.H., Dischinger, P.C., Rixen, D., Burgess, A.R., Addis, M.D., O'Quinn, T., McCammon, L., Schmidhauser, C.B., Marsh, P., Hodge, P.A., & Bents, F. (1996). Airbag protection versus compartment intrusion effect determines the pattern of injuries in multiple trauma motor vehicle crashes. *Journal of Trauma, 41*(6), 935–951.

Mackersie, R.C., Davis, J.W., Hoyt, D.B., Holbrook, T., & Shackford, S.R. (1995). High-risk behavior and the public burden for funding the costs of acute injury. *Arch Surg, 130*(8), 844–849.

MacLean, C.D. (1996). Principles of cancer screening. *Med Clin North Am, 80*(1), 1–13.

Mandelson, M.T., Wagner, E.H., & Thomson, R.S. (1995). PSA screening: A public health dilemma. *Ann Rev Public Health, 16,* 283–306.

MMWR. (1994). Medical care expenditures attributable to cigarette smoking–US, 1993. *MMWR, 43*(26), 469–472.

MMWR. (1996). Immunization guidelines from the Centers for Disease Control. *MMWR, 44,* 942–943.

Orenstein, J.B. (1996). Injuries and small-wheel skates. *Ann Emerg Med, 27*(2), 204–209.

Plewa, M.C. (1990) Altered host response and special infections in the elderly. *Emerg Med Clin North Am, 8*(2), 193–205.

Plichta, A.M. (1996). Immunization: Protecting older patients from infectious disease. *Geriatrics, 51,* 47–52.

Quinn, J. (1992). The senior's therapeutic touch program. *Holistic Nursing Practice, 7,* 32–37.

Reed, J.C. (1994). Alternative systems of medical practice. In *Alternative medicine: Expanding medical horizons.* Washington DC: U.S. Government Printing Office.

Reilly, D.T., Taylor, M.A., & Beattie, N.G. (1994). Is evidence of homeopathy reproducible? *Lancet, 344,* 1601–1606.

Rubik, B., Pavek, R., & Greene, E. (1994). Alternative systems of medical practice. In *Alternative medicine: Expanding medical horizons.* Washington DC: U.S. Government Printing Office.

Schieber, R.A., Branche-Dorsey, C.M., Ryan, G.W., Rutherford, G.W. Jr., Stevens, J.A., & O'Neil, J. (1996). Risk factors for injuries from in-line skating and the effectiveness of safety gear. *N Eng J Med, 335*(22), 1630–1635.

Schieber, R.A., & Branche-Dorsey, C.M. (1995). In-line skating injuries. Epidemiology and recommendations for prevention. *Sports Medicine, 19*(6), 427–432.

Schmidt, R.A. (1995). Screening mammography below age 50: is it worth it? Meeting abstract: 12th Annual International Breast Cancer Conference, Miami, FL.

Sharma, H.M., Triguna, B.D., & Chopra, D. (1991). Marharishi Ayur-Veda: Modern insights into ancient medicine. *JAMA, 265,* 2633–2637.

Sharma, H.M., Dwivedi, C., Satter, B.C., Gudehihihlu, H.A.., Malarkey, W., & Tejwani, G.A. (1990). Antineoplastic properties of Maharishi 4 against DMBA-induced mammary tumors in rats. *J Pharmacology Biochemistry Behavior, 35,* 767–773.

Sillanaukee, P. (1996). Laboratory markers of alcohol abuse. *Alcohol Alcoholism, 31*(6), 613–616.

States, J.D., Annechiarico, R.P., Good, R.G., et al. (1990). A time comparison study of the New York State safety belt use law, utilizing hospital admission and police accident report information. *Accident Analysis & Prevention, 22*(6), 509–521.

Thompson, D.C., Rivara, F.P., & Thompson, R.S. (1996). Effectiveness of bicycle safety helmets in preventing head injuries. A case-control study. *JAMA, 276*(24), 1968–1973.

Upledger, J.E., & Vredevoogd, M.F. (1997). *Your Inner Physician and You: Craniosacral Therapy,* Berkley, CA: North Atlantic.

U.S. Department of Health and Human Services. (1992). *Healthy People 2000: National health promotion and disease prevention objectives.* Washington DC: DHHS.

U.S. Department of Health and Human Services, Substance Abuse and Mental Health Services Administration. (1993). *National household survey on drug abuse: Population estimates.* Washington DC: DHHS.

U.S. Department of Health and Human Services. (1994). *Put prevention into practice.* Washington DC: DHHS.

U.S. Department of Health and Human Services. (1996). *Smoking cessation: A guide for primary care providers.* Washington DC: DHHS.

U.S. Preventive Services Task Force. (1996). *Guide to clinical preventive services,* 2d ed. Washington DC: DHHS.

U.S. Public Health Service. (1991). *Chronic and other disabling conditions impair the quality of life of many Americans.* Washington D.C.: U.S. Public Health Service, Office of Disease Prevention and Health Promotion.

U.S. Senate Special Committee on Aging. (1991). *Aging America: Trends and projections.* Washington DC: U.S. Government Printing Office.

Young, C.C., & Mark, D.H. (1995). In-line skating. An observational study of protective equipment used by skaters. *Archives of Family Medicine, 4*(1), 19–23.

Bibliography

Buckle, J. (1997). *Aromatherapy in nursing.* San Diego: Singular Publishing.

Handelman, S., Chipman-Smith, D., & Peterson, D.M. (1992). *Guidelines for chiropractic quality assurance and practice parameters.* Gaithersburg, MD: Aspen.

Mojay, G. (1996). *Aromatherapy for health.* New York: Holt.

Price, S. (1994). *Practical aromatherapy.* London: Harper Colliers.

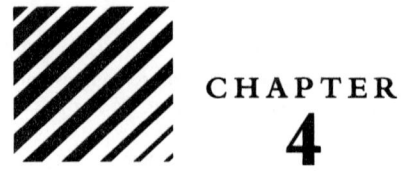

Violence Screening and Primary Care

Theresa Horvath, PA-C, MPH

Screening and appropriate intervention by primary health care providers can play an important role in reducing the widespread problem of physical violence. Screening may be especially beneficial in combating domestic violence, which is more difficult to detect and more likely to be repeated than random acts of violence perpetrated by strangers. There is an acute need for the identification and treatment of domestic violence situations because of the far-reaching and often catastrophic effects they may have on the entire family structure.

Firearm ownership compounds the problems of violence both within the family and among strangers. Guns greatly increase the risk that serious injury will result from physical conflict. Further, firearms are associated with greater rates of successful suicide and accidental injury for both their owners and other family members, particularly children.

Screening for violent behavior is an especially demanding task. Unlike screening for purely medical conditions, violence screening is often more time-consuming and may uncover other complex, underlying problems requiring timely intervention. Nevertheless, the potential impact of screening and subsequent intervention for reducing morbidity and death from trauma for the entire family justifies the difficulty of this task.

PROBLEMS OF HISTORY-TAKING IN VIOLENCE SCREENING

Opportunities for preventive violence counseling and crisis intervention in the primary care setting are often missed. Providers may lack sufficient knowledge or may have values, biases, or experiences that leave them lacking in the confidence to explore violence-related issues with their patients. Moreover, some providers have experienced violence themselves, provoking feelings of guilt or inadequacy about handling these issues and rendering them unable to aid their patients.

By the same token, patients who are either targets or perpetrators of violent behavior are often ashamed and hide their histories from health care providers. A person abused by violence may present with focal, unrelated symptoms, such as gastrointestinal distress, pelvic pain, or diffuse, chronic symptoms that defy a clear diagnosis. Perpetrators, on the other hand, may exhibit uncontrolled anger or threatening behavior or may appear inappropriately solicitous toward the provider.

Anticipation of the relationship between these presentations and violence may lead a provider to explore nonverbal clues, despite the seemingly unrelated symptoms bringing a patient for care. Eliciting a history of violence may reveal other related illnesses, such as underlying depression or substance abuse.

Besides patients' reticence to disclose their history, the sensitivity of issues related to violence may impede successful intervention. Although primary care providers have grown accustomed to addressing other confidential behaviors such as sexual practices, eating disorders, or drug use, patients may still feel threatened, frightened, or intruded on by frank, pointed questions. This is one reason why suggestions for behavior modification are often met with little enthusiasm.

For some patients, the wish to engage in a romantic relationship, parent a child, or own a gun without interference is akin to the democratic notion of a right. Strong feelings concerning the intrusion of government or cultural mores may impede a working relationship between the patient and the provider. This dilemma is compounded by legal requirements that, in cases such as suspected child abuse, compel the provider to set aside the wishes of the patient and comply with legislative mandates.

Balancing the needs of the patient and legislative mandates presents a challenge for practitioners of relationship-centered care. At times, a provider will learn information that will lead to removal of children from a patient's home or will provoke the break-up of a romantic relationship. A provider may be conflicted as to what constitutes an appropriate response to information elicited, especially within a relationship ostensibly inspired by trust.

There are two factors to consider in this unique dilemma. First, adult patients who are not yet ready to confront the impact of their violent behavior will not respond honestly to pointed questions, no matter how skillful the interviewer. Those who are willing to change violent behavior patterns often have anticipated the personal risks involved. Second, the patient may experience a sense of relief after making the decision to seek help, allowing the provider to be a source of continued support and guidance.

In cases of child abuse, the role of the provider is more complicated and may create a dilemma, especially if a situation arises where the needs of a child and an adult conflict—for instance, if both are patients of the same provider. But because children are physically and emotionally vulnerable to adults and cannot protect or advocate for themselves within the social service agencies or medical or school arenas where the violence is likely to be discovered, a child's needs must prevail. An important exception is suspected abuse between adult children and elderly parents, in which case the elder is the more vulnerable and most often the victim.

Regardless of initial impediments, violence screening becomes more effective after acquiring four skills:

- Adopting an interview style that imparts an air of seriousness and acceptance without being dismissive or confrontational
- Ascertaining which information is helpful to elicit

- Learning effective ways to intervene once a history of violence is elicited
- Developing adequate follow-up mechanisms.

DOMESTIC VIOLENCE

Domestic violence has been defined as a pattern of assault or coercion used by an adult or adolescent to force a partner to comply with the other partner's wishes (Neufeld, 1996). Although abuse of men by women is known, women are overwhelmingly the targets of violence by men. Reports estimate between 2 and 4 million women are beaten by a male intimate every year, accounting for 85% to 90% of all cases of partner abuse.

Homicide is the greatest danger in battering relationships. Among all women homicide victims, Bailey et al (1997) reported that 82% were slain by someone they knew, most often by firearms. The mere presence of a gun in the home is strongly associated with domestic violence and is a predictor that violence will result in the homicide of a woman. A woman's chances of becoming a homicide victim in a domestic dispute are also increased if she lives alone, abuses illicit drugs or alcohol (although violence is most strongly associated with alcohol abuse by the batterer), has a history of prior domestic violence, or lives with someone with a record of arrest.

Pregnant woman are at special risk for violence. An unplanned or unwanted pregnancy can renew or escalate an existing battering relationship (Gazmararian et al, 1995). Furthermore, women assaulted during pregnancy are twice as likely to have preterm labor and are at increased risk for chorioamnionitis as well (Berenson et al, 1995).

Violence within lesbian and gay relationships is compounded by a number of factors. Many gay men and lesbians forego police intervention for fear of harassment or ridicule from insensitive law enforcers. Even when police have been called, gay and lesbian partnerships have not been seen as families by many official agencies and therefore have been omitted from reporting mechanisms documenting heterosexual abuse. The extent of underreporting of gay and lesbian domestic violence is not known. The inability to define the extent of the problem has left a void in the identification of the particular risk factors and interventions within these communities. This problem is compounded by a reluctance among some health care workers to address the problem honestly, excluding gay and lesbian patients from the majority of health education efforts.

Role of the Primary Health Care Provider

A primary care provider may be the first "official" who identifies a patient in a violent relationship. A careful history and a physical examination offer the opportunity to identify or validate physical abuse. Careful and precise documentation of physical injuries, including measurement of lacerations, abrasions, and ecchymoses, may be needed in legal actions. Equally important is the support patients receive when their concern is echoed by a provider. On the other hand, failure to diagnose abuse, especially when injuries are present, may further isolate and dishearten a patient seeking help. The risk associated with misdiagnosis is considerable, similar to many purely medical conditions.

Once providers begin to look for family violence among their patients, they are often amazed how prevalent the problem is. Diffuse symptoms such as chronic persistent pelvic pain, headache, backache, or abdominal pain may indicate hidden physical or sexual abuse. The presence of a sexually transmitted disease or HIV infection, especially in a woman engaged in a steady, long-term romantic relationship, raises the possibility that she is physically or sexually abused.

Another factor that can lead to untimely diagnosis of and intervention for domestic violence is provider bias. Unlike screening for child abuse, which relies heavily on physical findings and is widely practiced in all sectors of health care, domestic violence does not have many of the "hard" signs that providers rely on. Further, particular features of domestic violence screening may result in a delay in or omission of initiating this discussion:

- Underestimation of a patient's risk
- Fear of offending or harming a relationship with a patient
- Lack of proof that a violent relationship exists, fostering disinclination to delve into sensitive areas
- Reluctance to commit to a time-consuming and difficult visit
- Fear that a provider is wasting time if suggestions are not taken by the patient (Neufeld, 1996).

There are also more personal reasons why a provider may avoid a frank discussion about abuse. Women providers especially may have had personal experiences with domestic violence themselves. Among medical students and faculty members, 17% of women and 3% of men in one report experienced physical or sexual abuse by a partner as adults (deLahunta & Tulsky, 1996). Rates of partner abuse among providers are comparable to those in the general population. Self-care measures, including the recognition of personal issues when counseling patients and therapeutic counseling or other support for the provider, may be needed in these cases.

Biases against screening for domestic violence can be overcome by incorporating a screening mechanism into every examination. Using a regular set of questions will ensure that all patients are asked the same questions, regardless of the impression they have made on the provider.

CHILD ABUSE

Screening for child abuse is infrequently performed by providers caring for adults. However, primary care providers may have reason for concern about the battering potential of adult patients toward their children. Intervention may be sought as a result of either an observed interaction between a patient and child, or historical factors elicited in an examination.

A history of violence in the home of origin is closely tied with adult battering behavior. Women who experienced violence as children or witnessed domestic abuse between their parents are more likely to become subject to violence in their adult lives. Further, they are at greater risk for physically abusing their children, especially if they were abused as children themselves. Asking patients if they are concerned about the way they discipline their children, or if they feel they use undue force, may be a way to begin a dialogue on this sensitive subject.

Violence between parents is a strong predictor of child abuse by the abusive parent. There is a direct relation between the severity of spousal violence and the likelihood of child abuse. If only one act of spousal abuse occurs, there is a 5% chance that a child will be battered. If more than 50 incidences between adults occur, there is a 30% likelihood of child abuse when a woman is abusive, and abuse is nearly certain if the batterer is a man (Ross, 1996). Identification of domestic violence within a household necessitates careful screening of all children who live there.

A more difficult problem exists when an adult physically or emotionally abuses a child in the midst of an examination. Responding to the act without losing the trust of the patient can take great skill. Reprimanding, counseling, or advising in these situations is likely to be fruitless, especially if there is a cultural difference between the provider and the patient. Cultures vary widely on what constitutes sufficient discipline. Providers, however, are bound to a standard of acceptable behavior set forth by regulatory agencies. Mandated courses on child abuse, as well as special offices established in many hospitals, should provide the boundaries needed for emergency intervention.

If a witnessed incident does not meet the criteria for emergency intervention, a team response may be most helpful. If social work services are available, they can determine what type of intervention would be most appropriate. Community-based family therapy or family-based behavioral science may also be of use.

Responding to child abuse may take a commitment of time and energy. The development of parent education classes or continued support groups for young or first-time mothers and fathers may address some of the issues on a wider scale. The initiation of a community dialogue involving parents, community leaders, and primary care providers may establish an arena to air differences and plan successful interventions jointly.

ELDER ABUSE

Those who are infirm or disabled may suffer abuse from those who care for them. Many members of this population are 65 years and older, and their children often care for them. As with all other types of family abuse, elder abuse is underreported, but it is estimated that 10% of all adults age 65 or older are abused every year. Men appear to be abused more frequently than women, although abuse is reported in women more frequently. This is caused partly by some men's reluctance to admit weakness or vulnerability. Those who need a great deal of physical care, or care in excess of what the family can provide, are especially at risk. Abuse is more likely if the caregiver comes from a violent family or has mental illness or severely impaired coping mechanisms resulting from drug or alcohol abuse. Further, caregivers are more likely to be abusive if they are coping with other emotional stresses such as loss of a job, chronic illness, or a poor preillness relationship with the elder, or if they themselves fear aging. Abusive adults can be spouses or adult children as well as strangers. An abusive caregiver is likely to be dependent on the elder for money or housing (Greenberg, 1996).

Elder abuse is classified into six categories. It may take such severe forms as physical or sexual abuse or may manifest in other harmful ways, such as neglect, psychological abuse, financial exploitation, or a violation of civil rights. Elder neglect is the deliberate or unintentional loss of maintenance care. The caregiver may not provide basic needs such as food preparation,

housekeeping, or adequate care for bedridden adults. Neglect is sometimes intentional, especially when the adult child feels this is an appropriate outlet for unresolved conflicts with the elder. It may be insidious, as when foods are prepared that the elder cannot eat or does not like. Further psychological abuse may involve withholding family social activities from elders, calling them names, or otherwise demeaning them.

Screening for elder abuse is similar to screening for other types of domestic violence. A simple history is taken, eliciting information about past harm caused by another person, especially someone living with the patient, or fear that harm might be done if the caregiver's wishes were not met. As in spousal abuse, it may be difficult to remove the caregiver from the examination, in which case nonverbal cues must be monitored.

A thorough examination is performed, with special attention paid to signs of trauma and the patient's cognitive functioning and mental status. As in spouse abuse, all irregularities are described, documented, measured, and if possible photographed. Physical signs of abuse may necessitate hospitalization. These signs may not be obvious in cases of neglect, and metabolic problems such as dehydration should be investigated. Admitting an elder to the hospital under a medical diagnosis should be considered if the patient's safety is a concern. Finally, the abuse must be reported to the state adult protective service agency. Further help can be found from national organizations for the elderly, listed at the end of this chapter.

RISKS OF WEAPON OWNERSHIP

Gun ownership is widely associated with high rates of homicide, suicide, and accidental death. Although there is an increased risk for adults who are severely depressed or demented, or veterans suffering from posttraumatic stress syndrome, those overwhelmingly vulnerable to firearm-induced death are children and young men, aged 15 to 24.

Adolescents and young adults use guns for power and prestige and usually obtain their own weapons without adult guidance or permission. However, children are in danger of injury by guns owned by adults, often their parents. Screening for weapon ownership of adults, therefore, may prevent injury for the whole family.

Accidental Gun Injury

Forty percent of families in the United States own a gun. Some use guns for hunting or collect them, but most gun owners keep a gun in the home for protection. Ironically, owning a gun in and of itself can place family members at risk for injury and death. Firearms are second only to motor vehicle accidents as the leading cause of fatal injury nationwide. Accidents involving improper cleaning, storage, or handling of guns can harm adults, but improper storage can especially harm children. Even some adults may not be aware that a gun kept in their home may be loaded, and children often cannot consider the lethal potential of a gun when found in the confines of their normally safe home.

Young children enjoy exploring the environment around them, raising the specter of potential harm in the home. Campaigns within pediatrics and family practice have heightened parents' awareness of safety measures such as using electrical outlet covers and safety latches on cabinets to protect toddlers and preschoolers. However, safe storage of guns has not gained the popularity in patient education that other home safety measures have, despite the fact that a child younger than 10 years old is 2.5 times more likely to be killed by a gun than by swallowing poison (Webster, 1992).

Finding a gun may be a risk even for older children who are aware of the potential harm of firearms. Popular movies and television shows have contributed to a fascination with guns in this country and contribute to the excitement generated by the destruction wrought and power gained by guns, especially for boys. Many are curious and eager to explore a gun and will do so when given access to one.

There are misconceptions regarding what constitutes safe storage. Keeping guns out of reach of children has some of the same pitfalls as storing poisons on a top shelf. If children know a gun is there, they may be tempted to find a way to get it. Therefore, recommended ways to store guns safely include trigger locks, portable lockboxes, and most importantly separation of guns from ammunition (Denno et al, 1996). Guns kept loaded are a severe risk for injury should they be accidentally discovered. Studies have shown that loaded guns are more likely to be kept in the homes of nonwhite families living without children in the southern United States. Owning a handgun (as opposed to a rifle) for protection, instead of for sport, increases the likelihood that it is stored loaded. Also, guns that are not kept in a locked place are more likely to be loaded (Weil & Hemenway, 1992).

Few providers discuss with their patients the need to keep firearms unloaded and locked away. However, many patients report that they would be receptive to provider advice about firearm safety. Several obstacles have been reported by providers that impede screening for guns:

- Inadequate time during a primary care visit for counseling
- Insufficient awareness of the relative risk of firearm injury and death
- Lack of knowledge about proper firearm counseling
- Not wanting to be seen as an antigun zealot.

Firearm screening may be accomplished by adding just one question: "Is there a gun in your home?" If the answer is yes, discussing safe, locked storage and keeping bullets away from guns may take only a few minutes. In many ways, this is the most efficacious violence screening in primary care.

Suicide and Gun Use

Depressed persons who have access to firearms are more likely to succeed if they attempt to kill themselves. Suicide is the eighth leading cause of death in the United States, and 60% of suicides are caused by firearms (Price et al, 1997). Within subgroups, this percentage is higher. Among the elderly, for instance, white men have higher suicide rates than women, younger men, or other racial and ethnic subgroups, and firearms account for 80% of the deaths. These men tend to be age 65 to 84, live in nonurban areas, and have less than a high-school education. Marital status did not play a role (Kaplan et al, 1996). Among women, successful suicide in the home was influenced by living alone, having a history of mental illness, and having a gun in the home (Bailey et al, 1997).

Among adolescents, the mere presence of a firearm in the home makes it twice as likely that a teenager will commit suicide, although those who suffer from depression or alcohol or drug use or have other emotional problems are at increased

risk (Camosy, 1966). For adolescents, the type of weapon, separation of the weapon from ammunition, or locking weapons did not play a role in the rates of successful suicide. One reason for this difference is that young adults are more likely than others to follow their impulses. Having the means to carry out suicidal ideation, if only fleeting, makes a gun in the home of an adolescent a great risk, regardless of how it is stored.

Gun legislation and limiting access to handguns have been suggested as ways to combat high rates of gun-inflicted suicide. Although these ideas have been proposed around the world, they have met with the most resistance in the United States, even though most agree that the presence of a gun in the home of a depressed person presents a danger. Counseling depressed patients and their family members about gun removal from the home should be considered.

Adolescent and Young Adult Gun Use

Young people aged 15 to 24 are at an especially high risk for morbidity and death from violence: homicide is the second leading cause of death for them. For men in this age group, the homicide rate is 20 times higher in the United States than in most other industrialized nations. Eighty-five percent of adolescent homicides occur with guns (Federal Bureau of Investigation, 1993). Also, 60% of all those aged 15 to 19 years old who commit suicide use a gun (Rosenberg et al, 1997). Young men die from gunshot wounds six times as often as young women. White males are four times as likely to commit suicide with guns as African American men are, whereas African American men are nine times as likely to die in a gun-related homicide as white males (MMWR, 1992; Fingerhut, 1993).

Besides being male and African American, there are other predictors for risk of gun-induced homicide:

- **Location.** Within the United States, homicides of young African American men are concentrated in New York, Florida, Michigan, Missouri, California, and the District of Columbia. The homicide rate in these areas for African American men age 15 to 24 exceeds 100 per 100,000 population (Public Health Reports, 1991).
- **History of fighting.** Injuries sustained in non-gun-related interpersonal violence predispose a young man to carry a gun. Twenty-five percent of young men and 5% of young women reported having carried a gun in one Washington D.C. survey.
- **History of arrest.** This is the single best predictor for gun carrying among men. Further, 100% of those with a drug-related arrest record have been found to carry guns subsequently.

Guns are not the only potentially fatal weapons used by young people. A survey of 295 seventh- and eighth-grade students in Washington D.C. reported that 47% of young men and 37% of young women had carried a knife for protection at some time; 20% of both groups regularly armed themselves with knives (Webster, 1993; Webster et al, 1993).

VIOLENCE INTERVENTION

Concrete measures can be used to aid in violence screening and intervention. For domestic violence, the widely used SAFE questionnaire may be used to screen patients for the presence

TABLE 4-1	SAFE Questions

STRESS/SAFETY

What stress do you experience in your relationships?

Do you feel safe in your relationships (marriage)?

Should I be concerned for your safety?

AFRAID/ABUSED

Are there situations in your relationships where you have felt afraid?

Has your partner ever threatened or abused you or your children?

Have you been physically hurt or threatened by your partner?

Has your partner forced you to have sexual intercourse that you did not want?

FRIENDS/FAMILY

If you have been hurt, are your friends or family aware of it?

Do you think you could tell them if it did happen?

Would they be able to give you support?

EMERGENCY PLAN

Do you have a safe place to go and the resources you (and your children) need in an emergency situation?

If you are in danger now, would you like help in locating a shelter?

Would you like to talk with a social worker, a counselor, or me to develop an emergency plan?

or degree of abuse (Table 4-1). If, as the result of screening, further intervention is needed, Table 4-2 lists some national organizations that can advise a patient or provider should emergency intervention be needed. Familiarity with local organizations and support groups can further aid in intervention.

Reporting agencies for child and elder abuse should be known to all members of a medical staff. Hospital-sponsored courses on child abuse detection and reporting may provide helpful information, and instructors may be a continuing resource for advice in difficult or unclear situations.

Public health measures such as population surveillance, identification of personal risk factors, early detection, and effective intervention can greatly affect the course of violence intervention. Trends will emerge that reflect impediments to successful intervention. These might include the culture of a community, such as local customs, geographic barriers, or the prevalence of drug use. Once these factors are identified and accounted for, it is then possible to intervene on a wider scale, using broad-based education for the entire population, not only those at risk.

Although intervention for many types of violence is best served by broad-based educational campaigns, such as for safe gun storage, most primary care providers concentrate on surveillance, detection, and intervention during individual provider–patient encounters. When screening identifies large numbers of people at risk for violence, providers can look for and join or initiate community efforts to curtail violence.

Intervention for Young Adult Gun Use

Young men age 15 to 24 are an extremely challenging patient population with which to work, mostly because these adolescents and young adults feel invulnerable to injury or harm. This feeling is common to some extent in all young people, but some subgroups, such as those who are poor or members of racial or ethnic minorities, may feel especially fearless and therefore are at greater risk. There are three reasons for this:

- Poorer neighborhoods lack opportunities taken for granted in more prosperous communities. Substandard schools impede a successful academic career, and withdrawal of commerce from poorer neighborhoods leads to low rates of employment. Dangerous risk-taking is attractive if young adults feel they have few options, or that their lives cannot be influenced by their own choice.

- Drug use, accompanied by the violence inherent in users and especially sellers of drugs, is pervasive in some communities. Ample opportunity exists to become a member of a violent drug community or to fall victim to it simply by living in close proximity to it.

- Suitable role models and mentors are scarcer in these neighborhoods. Some older adults also have long histories of risk-taking and violent behavior. These community members are seen by some as successful and powerful,

TABLE 4-2	Resources for Violence Prevention

RESOURCES FOR VICTIMS OF DOMESTIC VIOLENCE

PHYSICAL AND SEXUAL ABUSE IN CHILDREN

C. Henry Kemp National Center for the Prevention and Treatment of Child Abuse & Neglect: 303-321-3963

National Committee to Prevent Child Abuse: 312-663-3520

National Clearinghouse on Child Abuse and Neglect Information: 703-385-7565

PARTNER ABUSE

National Domestic Violence Hotline: 800-799-SAFE

GROUPS THAT OFFER MORE INFORMATION ON VIOLENCE PREVENTION

Adolescent Violence Prevention Resource Center: 1-800-225-4276

National Child Safety Council: 1-800-327-5107

National Citizens' Crime Prevention Campaign: 1-800-937-7383

National Mental Health Association: 1-800-969-6642

National Resource Center on Domestic Violence: 1-800-537-2238

Toughlove International (for parents of troubled children): 1-800-333-1069

RESOURCES FOR GUN SAFETY INFORMATION

Organization/Program	Telephone Number
Adolescent Violence Prevention Resource Center:	617-969-7100
American Academy of Family Physicians and U.S. Preventive Services Task Force: Clinician's Handbook of Preventive Services:	800-274-2237
American Academy of Pediatrics:	800-433-9016
Center to Prevent Handgun Violence:	202-289-7319
Handgun Epidemic Lowering Plan (HELP Network) of Concerned Professionals:	312-880-3826
Johns Hopkins University Center for Gun Policy and Research:	410-955-7625
National Crime Prevention Council:	202-466-6272
National Rifle Association: Eddie the Eagle Gun Safety Program:	800-231-0752
Physicians for a Violence-Free Society:	214-590-8807

and the desire to emulate them may push a young man to take risks beyond what he normally would.

Conflict resolution programs and violence prevention curricula have been used in many school and community settings, but the effectiveness of these measures has been unconvincing (Webster, 1993). The focus of these programs has been on the individual, particularly on anger control and negotiation skills. Studies have shown that violent conflicts among young adults begin over issues of respect, status, and dominance, gang issues, and lovers. The social and community aspects of violent conflict have been ignored.

Young men under age 24 are among the least likely to present for primary health care. Should health care be sought, counseling efforts to cease violent activity may not compete with the pervasive social, economic, and cultural factors reinforcing gun use as a status symbol.

Community organizing may have a greater impact than individual counseling or screening for this problem. Civic groups have been formed in urban areas to combat a variety of social ills; one focus is on reducing gun use in their neighborhoods. Health care workers have also developed organizations that provide health education to young adults about the effects of firearm injury. Working with community organizations, or iniwtiating one if none exists, may have the best effect in communities where gun-related morbidity and death are prevalent.

COMMUNITY RESOURCES

- National 24-Hour Domestic Violence Hotline: 1-800-799-SAFE; TDD: 1-800-787-3224; http://www.inetport.com/ndvh/
- Safety Net: http://www.cybergirl.com/planet/dv/nyc.html: Offers a domestic violence handbook, domestic violence projects and organizations, New York City shelter number, state coalitions, and links to additional Internet resources
- Center for Children in Crisis, 2112 S. Congress Ave., West Palm Beach, FL 33406; 561-641-1500; http://www.shadow.net/cpt/
- Center for Prevention of Sexual and Domestic Violence, 936 N. 34th St., #200, Seattle, WA 98103; 206-634-1903; http://www.cpsdv.org
- Violence Prevention Special Interest Group/National Network for Family Resilience, University of Wyoming, P.O. Box 3354, Laramie, WY 82071; 307-766-5689
- Victim Services Domestic Violence Shelter Tour: http://www.dvsheltertour.org: Provides essential information for battered women; offers a tour of a domestic violence shelter; offers help in local areas and links to additional Internet resources
- National Coalition Against Domestic Violence, P.O. Box 18749, Denver, CO 80218; 303-839-1852 or 1-800-333-7233

CONCLUSION

Domestic violence produces significant injury and death, although all types are underreported because of the complicated emotional relationships inherent in families. Provider reluc-tance to screen for family violence further endangers persons at risk. The use of screening tools and participation in community organizations can identify those in need of aid. Familiarity with national and local crisis intervention agencies can be used to provide help when needed. All types of abuse must be reported to state protective services. The risk of death is compounded by gun ownership. Safe storage and patient education may reduce accidents. The presence of a gun in the home compounds existing problems of domestic violence, depression, dementia, or mental illness.

References

Bailey, J.E., Kellermann, A.L., Somes, G.W., Banton, J.G., Rivara, F.P., & Rushforth, N.P. (1997). Risk factors for violent death of women in the home. *Archives of Internal Medicine, 157*(7), 777–782.

Berenson, A.B., Wiemann, C., Wilkinson, G.S., Jones, W.A., & Anderson, G.D. (1995). Perinatal morbidity associated with violence experienced by pregnant women. *American Journal of Obstetrics and Gynecology, 172*(5), 1644–1645.

Camosy, P.A. (1996). Incorporating gun safety into clinical practice. *American Family Physician, 54*(3), 971–975.

deLahunta, E.A., & Tulsky, A.A. (1996). Personal exposure of faculty and medical students to family violence. *JAMA, 275*(24), 1903–1906.

Denno, D.M., Grossman, D.C., Britt, J., & Bergman, A.B. (1996). Safe storage of handguns: What do the police recommend? *Archives of Pediatric and Adolescent Medicine, 150*(9), 927–931.

Fingerhut, L.A. (1993). Firearm mortality among children, youth and young adults 1–34 years of age: Trends and current status, United States 1985–1990. *Advance data, 231*(1), 1–20.

Gazmararian, J.A., Adams, M.M., Saltzman, L.E., et al. (1995). The relationship between pregnancy intendedness and physical violence in mothers of newborns. The PRAMS Working Group. *Obstetrics & Gynecology, 85*(6), 1031–1038.

Greenberg, E.M. (1996). Violence and the older adult: The role of the acute care nurse practitioner. *Critical Care Nursing Quarterly, 19*(2), 76–84.

Kaplan, M.S., Adamek, M.E., & Geling, O. (1996). Sociodemographic predictors of firearm suicide among older white males. *Gerontologist, 36*(4), 530–533.

Neufeld, B. (1996). SAFE questions: Overcoming barriers to the detection of domestic violence. *American Family Physician, 53*(8), 2575–2580.

Price, J.H., Everett, S.A., Bedell, A.W., & Telljohann, S.K. (1997). Reduction of firearm-related violence through firearm safety counseling. The role of family physicians. *Archives of Family Medicine, 6*(1), 79–83.

Rosenberg, M.L., Fenley, M.A., Johnson, D., & Short, L. (1997). Bridging prevention and practice: Public health and family violence. *Academic Medicine, 72*(1 Suppl), S13–18.

Ross, S.M. (1996). Risk of physical abuse to children of spouse abusing parents. *Child Abuse & Neglect, 20*(7), 589–598.

Webster, D.W. (1993) The unconvincing case for school-based conflict resolution programs for adolescents. *Health Affairs,* 126–141.

Webster, D.W., Gainer, P.S., & Champion, H.R. (1993). Weapon carrying among inner-city junior high school Students: Defensive behavior vs. aggressive delinquency. *American Journal of Public Health, 83*, 1604–1608.

Weil, D.S., & Hemenway, D. (1992). Loaded guns in the home. Analysis of a national random survey of gun owners. *JAMA, 267*, 3033–3037.

Bibliography

Dubowitz, H., King, H. (1995). Family Violence. A child-centered, family focused aprroach. *Pediatric Clinics of North America*, *42*(1)(, 153–163.

Kellermann, A.L., Rivara, F.P., Somes, G., et al. (1992). Suicide in the home in relation to gun ownership. *N Engl J Med, 327*(2), 467–472.

O'Donnell, C.L. (1995). Firearm Deaths Among Children and Youth. *American Psychologist, 50*(9), 771–776.

Rosenblatt, D.E. (1997). Elder mistreatment. *Critical Care Nursing Clinics of North America, 9*(2), 183–192.

Steiner, R.P., Vansickle, K., Lippmann, S.B. (1996). Domestic Violence. Do you know when and how to intervene? *Postgraduate Medicine, 100*(1), 103–116.

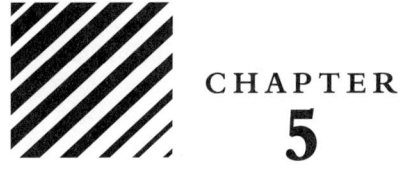

CHAPTER
5

Nutritional Assessment

Samuel Sandowski, MD

The old adage "you are what you eat" is a mainstay of nutritional education. This chapter will elaborate on the importance of nutrition in primary care as well as explain the methodology and techniques used in assessing nutritional status and prescribing diets. As with all aspects of primary care, nutrition must be individualized. Cultural, religious, economic, and social values must be accounted for in nutrition evaluations.

IMPORTANCE OF NUTRITION IN PRIMARY CARE

Nutritional assessment is an integral part of the primary care provider's role. In addition to assessing the patient's overall nutritional status, the provider must also identify any existing or potential deficiency states. Total calorie malnutrition (marasmus) or protein calorie deficiency alone (kwashiorkor) may be seen. Patients may be deficient in only one nutrient, vitamin, mineral, or essential element. These deficiencies are often first noted and addressed by the primary care provider.

Patients' concerns must also be addressed. A patient with a desire to lose weight and start an exercise program is a common scenario in "health-conscious America." The patient who asks the provider if it is "okay" to have his or her family on a vegetarian diet is quite common too.

Food faddisms are constantly changing. Patients often approach their providers with questions such as "Is garlic really healthy?" or "Will vitamin E prevent aging and cancer?" Providers must also be familiar with the latest antiobesity and anorectic medications, especially if the media informs the public before the medications are FDA-approved.

Providers must counsel patients about specific illnesses. Diabetes mellitus, hypertension, coronary artery disease, renal disease, liver disease, obesity, anemia, gastrointestinal disturbances, and hypercholesterolemia are but a few disease states in which nutrition is intimately related to both the disease process and the treatment. Nutritional factors are the second leading cause of preventable deaths in the United States (cigarette smoking is the first) (McGinnis & Foese, 1993).

Patients often take supplements without the provider's knowledge. Supplementation refers to extra sources (ie, outside standard diet) for nutrition, whether it be vitamins and minerals, high-calorie shakes, or even parenteral nutrition. Many vitamins in excess are excreted in the urine, but overdoses and megadoses of the fat-soluble vitamins (A, D, E, K) are potentially toxic. Excess of minerals may be toxic as well.

NUTRITIONAL ASSESSMENT

The basic parts of the nutritional assessment include the history, the physical exam, laboratory studies, and calculation of the patient's needs. The difficult part is finding an appropriate prescription, one that reflects the patient's physical needs as well as their willingness and ability to participate.

The Dietary History

The dietary history is part of a comprehensive history. It includes several aspects of the patient's life, reflecting the biopsychosocial model of health care in addition to the actual food intake.

BIOLOGIC

This part of the history should include hard-core medical data including age, gender, allergies, medical illnesses, and past surgeries. In addition, usual weight and recent weight changes should be included, as should recent changes in appetite, as well as past patterns of dieting. Bowel patterns, dentition, dysphagia, and current medications should be inquired about as well. Use of supplements, vitamins, and herbs must also be explored.

PSYCHOSOCIAL

Psychosocial factors are critical to assessing both nutritional status and the patient's ability to make changes in their diet. These include questions such as where and with whom does the patient eat? Who does the shopping and who prepares the food? Can the patient afford to buy foods different than those he or she currently purchases? What religious dietary restrictions and cultural preferences apply?

Food Intake Records

There are several methods to evaluate a patient's food intake. Three common ways are 24-hour food recall, food diaries, and food frequency questionnaires. Each method can be useful, but because each has flaws, a combination of these three methods may be recommended.

The 24-hour food recall requires the patient to remember, or recall what has been eaten over the past 24 hours. This is often done by the patient describing the last things eaten first and working backwards. Foods and beverages, methods of preparation, and portion sizes must be noted. Though this is a quick and easy method, a one-day history may not be representative of the patient's usual diet. Multiple 24-hour food recalls, however, may be more accurate than a food diary (Buzzard et al, 1996).

The food diary, an accurate method of evaluating a patient's intake, may be rather cumbersome and time-consuming. The patient writes down all that he or she eats and drinks over a given number of days. Again, portion sizes and methods of preparation must be noted. It is true that the patient may change eating patterns while maintaining a food record, but then again, does this mean we have succeeded in having our patients educated and change their eating behaviors?

Food frequency questionnaires will question the patient about how often they eat certain foods. This may identify potential deficiencies in a particular food group. However, portion sizes (described below) are often not accounted for or understood by the person completing the questionnaire. Also, if a food that a patient usually eats is not listed, this will skew the results. For example, when trying to assess fat consumption, asking the patient how often they eat cakes and ice cream, but not asking about chocolates, will not accurately reflect fat intake. An example of a food frequency questionnaire is shown in Figure 5-1.

Exchange Lists and Portion Sizes

The American Dietetic Association has a list of food exchanges. The list includes foods grouped into the following food groups:

Think about your eating habits over the past year or so. Indicate how often you usually eat the foods listed within the 15 groups of foods described in the FOODS column by putting an "x" in the appropriate column under the heading "FREQUENCY OF CONSUMPTION."

Once you have completed this, please turn the page over for further instructions.

Frequency of Consumption

FOODS	Never, or less than once per MONTH (0)	2–3 times per MONTH (1)	1–2 times per WEEK (2)	3–4 times per WEEK (3)	5 times per WEEK (4)	FOOD SCORE
Hamburgers or cheeseburgers						
Beef, such as steak, roasts						
Fried chicken						
Hot dogs, franks						
Cold cuts, luncheon meats						
Salad dressings, mayonnaise (not diet)						
Margarine or butter						
Eggs						
Bacon or sausage						
Cheese or cheese spread						
Whole milk						
French fries						
Potato or corn chips, popcorn						
Ice cream						
Doughnuts, pastries, cake, cookies						

Total Score _____

FIGURE 5-1 Dietary Fat Intake Self-Assessment Form.*

* This form was developed and tested by the National Cancer Institute.

TABLE 5-1	Food Exchanges and their Nutritional Values

STARCHES/BREADS

One exchange contains 15 g carbohydrate, 3 g protein, a trace of fat, and 80 calories.

One starch exchange often equals one slice of bread or one third to one half a cup of a starchy vegetable.

MEAT

Lean: One exchange contains 7 g protein, 3 g fat, and 55 calories.

Medium-fat: One exchange contains 7 g protein, 5 g fat, and 75 calories.

High-fat: One exchange contains 7 g protein, 8 g fat, and 100 calories.

One meat exchange often equals 1 ounce of cooked meat.

VEGETABLES

One exchange contains 5 g carbohydrate, 2 g protein, and 25 calories.

One vegetable exchange often equals 1/2 cup cooked vegetables or 1 cup raw vegetables.

FRUIT

One exchange contains 15 g carbohydrate and 60 calories. Sizes of fruit exchanges vary depending on the type of fruit, but 1/2 cup of fruit juices often equals one fruit exchange.

MILK

Skim: one exchange contains 12 g carbohydrate, 8 g protein, and 90 calories.

Low-fat: One exchange contains 12 g carbohydrates, 8 g protein, 5 g fat, and 120 calories.

Whole: One exchange contains 12 g carbohydrate, 8 g protein, 8 g fat, and 150 calories.

One exchange of milk equals 1 cup.

FAT

One exchange contains 5 g fat and 45 calories. One fat exchange varies (eg, 1 teaspoon of butter or 2 tablespoons of gravy).

starches/breads, meats, vegetables, fruits, milk/dairy and fats (Table 5-1). An exchange is a measured amount of food that would be of equal caloric value as another food in that same group. For example, one exchange from the starch/breads group is equal to 80 kcal. Therefore, one slice of bread or half a cup of cooked pasta are each one exchange, or 80 kcal. Based on the number and type of exchanges one eats, the total calories as well as the amount of carbohydrate, protein, and fat consumed can be calculated.

Portion sizes refer to the amount a patient eats of a particular food. A portion size in many diet plans does not necessarily mean one food exchange; often a portion of meat is equal to about 3 meat exchanges. A quick and easy way to estimate appropriate portion sizes is using a fistful (about half a cup) and palm size (about 3 meat exchanges).

Physical Examination

The physical examination is as important as a good history. Height and weight must be recorded. Weight alone is an incomplete assessment. A 5′ tall woman weighing 100 pounds may be appropriate. However, a 6′ tall male at this weight would be grossly malnourished. For a complete nutritional assessment, a complete physical must be done. The provider must note the hair, skin, eyes, mouth, tongue, teeth, glands, nails, heart, abdomen, bones and joints, and muscles of the extremi-

ties and must perform a complete neurologic exam (Table 5-2).

Laboratory Studies

Many different laboratory values are used as potential nutritional assessors. Often looked at are albumin and cholesterol. Both of these tend to fall when patients become malnourished. However, these are not pathognomonic for nutritional deficiencies. Some people tend to have low total cholesterol levels without any deficiencies. In addition, total cholesterol levels may fall with disease states regardless of nutritional status. Albumin too tends to fall with acute stress and trauma, as well as with certain diseases, such as protein-losing enteropathies and nephropathies. Prealbumin, which has a shorter half-life than albumin, may be a better tool to assess the patient's prognosis and nutritional state (Bernstein & Pleban, 1996; Mears, 1996). Transferrin, another acute-phase reactant also may be useful in assessing nutritional status and is one of the factors in calculating the prognostic nutritional index (PNI), an assessment tool used in helping predict prognosis, morbidity, and mortality of preoperative patients.

Another laboratory value often considered is the complete blood count (CBC). Anemia may reflect an iron-deficient state if the mean corpuscular volume (MCV) is low. If the MCV is elevated, this may represent deficiency in vitamin B_{12} or folate, or it may suggest alcoholism. A low lymphocyte count may reflect malnutrition. Deficiency in vitamin K prolongs the prothrombin time (PT) (ie, increase the INR), and bleeding time is prolonged with vitamin C deficiency. Direct screening for specific vitamin deficiencies are not done routinely and should be obtained only if there is a high index of suspicion.

Calculations

IDEAL BODY WEIGHT

Once patients have been assessed, their nutritional needs must be calculated. An ideal body weight (IBW) is calculated based on a person's gender, height and body frame. These IBWs were set by Metropolitan Life Insurance Company (Table 5-3) using a select cohort, and this should noted when addressing patients. A simple bedside calculation for IBW for men can be calculated as follows: Ideal body weight = 106 lbs for the first 5′ and 6 lbs for each additional inch. For women, the formula is: ideal body weight = 100 lbs for the first 5′ and 5 lbs for each additional inch. These are for medium frame adults and should be adjusted plus or minus 10% for larger or smaller body frames.

In bed-ridden, elderly, or kyphotic patients who have difficulty standing erect, the patient's height can be calculated measuring the knee height. The knee height is the distance, in centimeters, from the bottom of the foot to the top of the knee (ie, distal femur) when the knee is flexed at 90 degrees. The formula for knee height is:

Men:

$$Ht\ (cm) = 64.19 - (0.04 \times age) + (2.02 \times knee\ height)$$

Women:

$$Ht\ (cm) = 84.88 - (0.24 \times age) + (1.83 \times knee\ height)$$

BODY FRAME

Body frame is measured by bone width. Using calipers, the widest point between the medial and lateral condyles of the elbow is measured. Others use wrist circumference to assess

TABLE 5-2	Physical Examination Findings with Nutritional Deficiencies	
Organ	**Finding**	**Deficiency State**
Skin	Sebhorreic dermatitis	Essential fatty acids, vitamin B_6, zinc, biotin, niacin
	Hyperpigmentation	Niacin, vitamin B_{12}
	Follicular keratosis	Essential fatty acids
	Petechia	Vitamin C, vitamin K
	Xerosis	Essential fatty acids, vitamin A
	Pallor	Vitamin B_{12}, iron, folate
	Poor wound healing	Protein, zinc, vitamin C
Nails	Koilonychia (spoon nails)	Iron
Hair	Dull, brittle, easily pluckable	Protein
Mouth	Cheilosis, angular stomatitis	Protein, niacin, riboflavin
Tongue	Glossitis	Niacin, riboflavin (magenta-colored tongue), vitamin B_{12} (beefy-red, fissured tongue), vitamin B_6, folate, zinc, iron (atrophic papillae)
	Bleeding gums	Vitamin C
Eyes	Photophobia	Riboflavin
	Bitot's spots	Vitamin A
	Poor night vision	Vitamin A
Heart	Arrhythmia	Iron, vitamin B_{12}, folate (secondary to anemia), hypokalemia, hyperkalemia, hypocalcemia, hypercalcemia, hypomagnesemia
	Cardiomyopathy	Selenium, protein, thiamine, excessive alcohol
	Congestive heart failure	Thiamine
Musculoskeletal	Rickets (beading on ribs, frontal bossing, bowing of legs)	Vitamin D
	Osteomalacia	Vitamin D
	Osteoporosis	Vitamin D, calcium
	Muscle atrophy	Protein
	Muscle cramps	Hypokalemia, hyponatremia, hypophosphatemia
Abdomen	Hepatomegaly	Protein deficiency
Thyroid	Goiter	Iodine
Nervous system	Lethargy	Protein, calories, hyponatremia
	Confusion/dementia	Thiamine, niacin, folate, vitamin B_{12}, magnesium
	Neuropathy	Niacin, folate, vitamin B_{12}

body frame. Tables for elbow breadth and wrist circumference have been established, taking into account height (Fig. 5-2).

ADJUSTED BODY WEIGHT

Adjusted body weight (ABW) is a technique used to personalize IBW. Goals of weight change become more realistic, taking into account the patient's present weight. The formula for adjusted body weight is: ABW = ([present body weight − ideal body weight] / 4) + ideal body weight.

BODY MASS INDEX

Body mass index (BMI) is a value based on both weight and height. It is equal to weight/height^2 in kg/m^2. Often considered "ideal" is a BMI of 19–25 (National Center for Health Statistics, 1995). A BMI of more than 27.8 for men and 27.3 for women may increase the risk of morbidity and mortality.

BODY FAT ESTIMATES

It is worthwhile to note that a person's height and weight alone may still not be enough for assessment. With recent fads in body building and steroid abuse, certain patients may be "overweight" based on ideal body weight, but they may have a low percentage of total body fat. Body composition can be measured by many sophisticated techniques, but simple bedside calculations can be measured by midarm circumference and triceps and subscapular skin folds. The midarm circumference is the circumference, in centimeters, of the left arm, halfway between the elbow and shoulder, with the arm fully extended. The triceps skin fold is measured by separating the skin and the subcutaneous fat away from the triceps muscle on the left arm and measuring the thickness (Fig. 5-3). Skinfold measurements can be located on the graph in Figure 5-4 and a patient's percentile for body fat can be estimated. Other methods for determining body fat include underwater weighing (in submersion tanks), bioelectrical impedance, potassium-40 counting, and dual photon absorptiometry.

CALORIC EXPENDITURE ESTIMATES

Accurate calculations in determining caloric requirements involve determining the basal metabolic rate (BMR), the thermogenic effect of food (TEF), and the activity factor.

Calories consumed = BMR + TEF + activity

The basal metabolic rate is the amount of calories required to

TABLE 5-3	Height and Weight for Men and Women		
Height Feet Inches	Small Frame	Medium Frame	Large Frame
WOMEN			
4'10"	102–111	109–121	118–131
4'11"	103–113	111–123	120–134
5'0"	104–115	113–126	122–137
5'1"	106–118	115–129	125–140
5'2"	108–121	118–132	128–143
5'3"	111–124	121–135	131–147
5'4"	114–127	124–138	134–151
5'5"	117–130	127–141	137–155
5'6"	120–133	130–144	140–159
5'7"	123–136	133–147	143–163
5'8"	126–139	136–150	146–167
5'9"	129–142	139–153	149–170
5'10"	132–145	142–156	152–173
5'11"	135–148	145–159	155–176
6'0"	138–151	148–162	158–179
MEN			
5'2"	128–134	131–141	138–150
5'3"	130–136	133–143	140–153
5'4"	132–138	135–145	142–156
5'5"	134–140	137–148	144–160
5'6"	136–142	139–151	146–164
5'7"	138–145	142–154	149–168
5'8"	140–148	145–157	152–172
5'9"	142–151	148–160	155–176
5'10"	144–154	151–163	158–180
5'11"	146–157	154–166	161–184
6'0"	149–160	157–170	164–188
6'1"	152–164	160–174	168–192
6'2"	155–168	164–178	172–197
6'3"	158–172	167–182	176–202
6'4"	162–176	171–187	181–207

Weights at ages 25-59 based on lowest mortality. Weight in pounds according to frame (in indoor clothing weighing 5 lbs. for men and 3 lbs. for women; shoes with 1" heels). Table supplied by MetLife: www.metlife.com ©1996–1997 Metropolitan Life Insurance Company

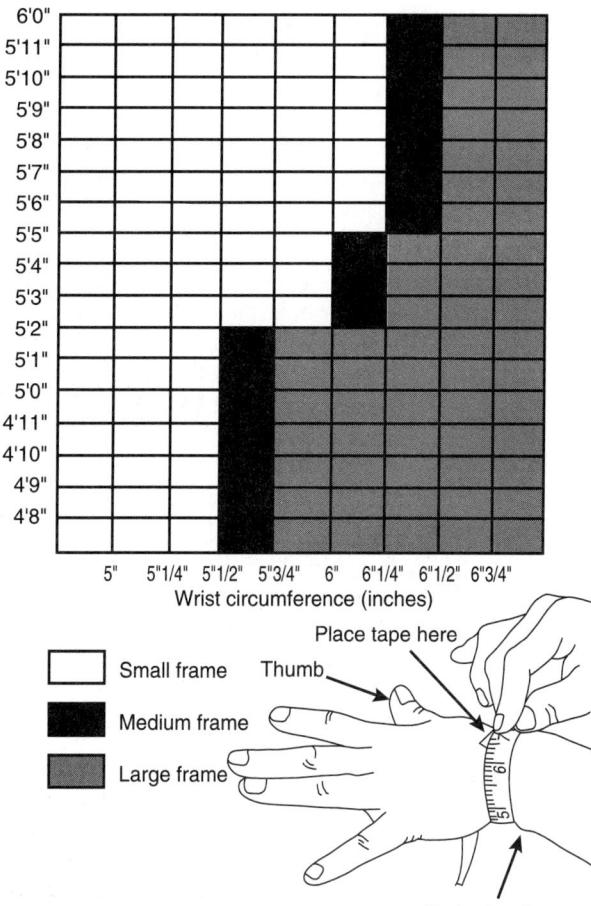

FIGURE 5-2 Finding body frame by wrist circumference.

RECOMMENDED DAILY ALLOWANCES

The recommended daily allowance (RDA) is a recommended amount of daily intake of a particular nutrient. These amounts do not reflect minimal amounts necessary, nor do they suggest ideal amounts to be consumed. The RDA represents a safe intake amount that will not cause deficiencies nor excesses. The RDAs vary based on age, gender, and particular states (eg, pregnancy).

sustain the body at a particular weight without any activity. It is based on age, height, gender, and current weight. One such formula is the Harris Benedict equation (Table 5-4). The digestion of food expends energy, and there is an increase in the metabolic rate after a meal. This is the thermogenic effect of food. Depending on the level of activity, an individual may require several thousand calories more than the BMR to sustain current body weight. Activity includes both voluntary activity, such as exercising, and involuntary activity. Stresses, such as burns and surgery, as well as illnesses are involuntary activities that may significantly increase the BMR and therefore increase calorie expenditure. Fever too may increase the BMR significantly. Table 5-5 lists different activities and their influence on the BMR.

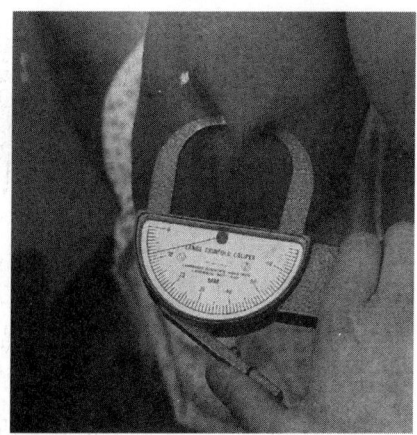

FIGURE 5-3 Measuring the triceps skinfold.

PUTTING IT INTO PRACTICE

Prescribing the diet is perhaps the most difficult part of nutritional assessment. In addition to identifying the patient's requirements, the patient's willingness to participate is essential. Usually the whole family is affected by one person's diet, whether the patient cooks for the family, or another family member cooks for the patient.

Steps in calculating a diet plan include:

1. What are the patient's calorie requirements?
2. From what sources should the patient receive calories (ie, carbohydrate, protein, fat)?

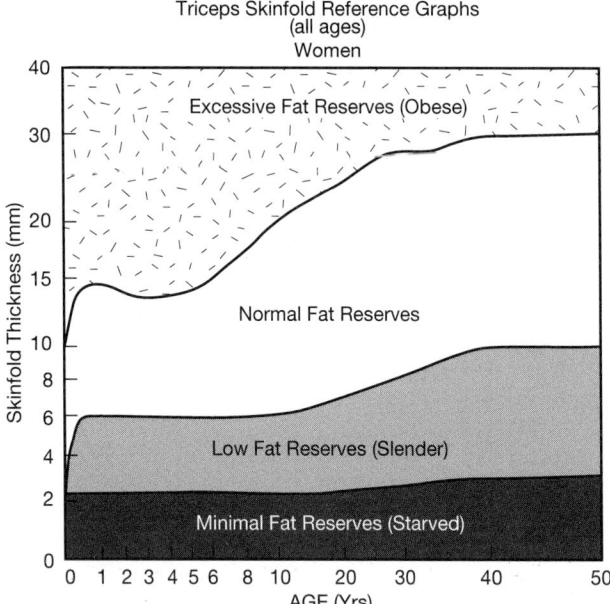

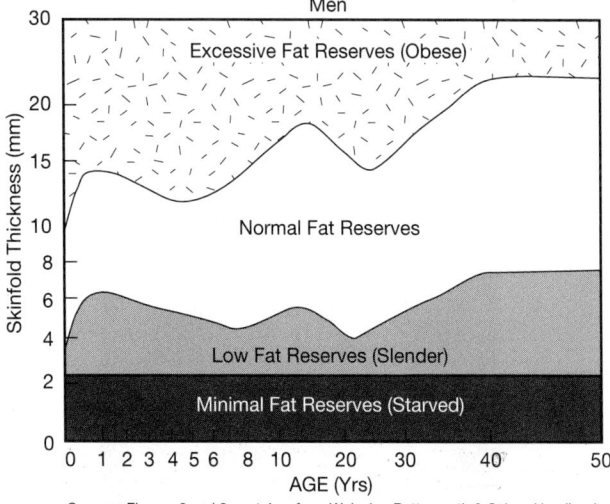

Source: Figures 2 and 3 are taken from Weinsier, Butterworth & Sahm: Handbook of Clinical Nutrition Birmingham, University of Alabama Dept. of Nutrition Sciences 1977

FIGURE 5-4 Triceps skinfold thickness and body fat composition. Figures from Weinsier and Butterworth. *Handbook of Clinical Nutrition.* The University of Alabama Department of Nutrition Sciences. (1981) Table from West, C., and Crowley, M. (1984) *Nutrition Priciples and Application in Health Promotion.* Philadelphia: J.B. Lippincott Company. *(continued)*

Triceps Skinfold

Percentiles for White Persons of the U.S. Hanes I (1971–1974)

Age In Years	Percentiles				
	10	25	50	75	90
Males					
1-1.9	7	8	10	12	14
5-5.9	6	8	9	11	14
10.10.9	6	8	10	14	18
15-15.9	5	6	8	11	18
25-34.9	6	8	12	16	20
45-54.9	6	8	12	15	20
Females					
1-1.9	7	8	10	12	14
5-5.9	7	8	10	12	15
10.10.9	8	10	12	17	23
15-15.9	10	12	17	21	25
25-34.9	12	16	21	27	34
45-54.9	16	20	25	30	36

Source: Nutrition Principles and Application in Health Promotion 2nd Edition. Carol West Suitor, Merrily Forbes Crowley, JB LIppincott Co. – 1984

FIGURE 5-4 *(Continued)*

TABLE 5-5	Activities Influencing the BMR
Activity	**Influence on BMR**
Burns	Increases BMR in direct proportion to the level of the burn
Surgery	Increases BMR in direct proportion to the level of the stress of surgery
Trauma	Increases BMR in direct proportion to the level of trauma
Exercise	Increases BMR from 400 to 4000 calories, depending on level of exercise
Fever	Increases BMR by 7% for each degree (Celsius) of fever
Surface area	Increases BMR
Lean body mass	Increases BMR
Thyrotoxicosis	Increases BMR
Age	Decreases BMR (because lean muscle mass decreases with age)
Starvation	Decreases BMR (to 25% by day 20 of fasting)

TABLE 5-4	The Harris Benedict Equation: Calculating the Basal Metabolic Rate (BMR)
Men: BMR =	$66.473 + (13.751 \times$ wt [kg]$) + (5.0033 \times$ ht [cm]$) - (6.755 \times$ age$)$
Women BMR =	$655.0955 + (9.563 \times$ wt [kg]$) + (1.8 \times$ ht [cm]$) - (4.675 \times$ age$)$

3. What other considerations and adjustments need to be made to the diet (eg, certain medical conditions, desire to gain/lose weight)?

The following example will show how to calculate a person's needs and formulate an appropriate diet:

Mr. Jones is a 50-year-old male who has a history of hypertension and a family history of coronary artery disease. He expresses a desire to lose weight. He is able and willing to exercise. Mr. Jones currently weighs 220 lbs (100 kg) and is 5'10" (180 cm) tall.

Calculating calories needed:

Based on the Harris Benedict equation, Mr. Jones' daily requirements (BMR) to maintain his current weight is: $66 + (13.7 \times 100 \, [kg]) + (5 \times 180 \, [cm]) - (6.8 \times 50 \, [yrs]) = 1996$ calories/day.

Considering stresses, exercise, and daily activities, assume Mr. Jones has a 25% increase in requirements above the BMR (or $1996 \times 1.25 = 2495$ calories/day).

Using bedside calculations, the requirement for a slightly active person is 25 cal/kg. Therefore Mr. Jones, who weighs 100 kg, would require about 2500 calories/day.

For Mr. Jones to lose 1 pound, he must expend 3500 calories. Assuming a weight loss of 1 pound/week, Mr. Jones needs to expend 3500 calories/week (or 500 calories/day) more than he takes in. Therefore, Mr. Jones should consume about 2000 calories/day (2500—500).

From where should the calories come?

Using the Dietary Guidelines for Americans (U.S. Department of Agriculture & U.S. Department of Health & Human Services, 1995), the American Heart Association Diet (Krauss & Deckelbaum, 1996), and the National Cholesterol Education Program Diet (NCEP) (the step I diet) (National Cholesterol Education Program, 1988), the following may be recommended for Mr. Jones:

- 60% (55%–60%) of the calories should come from complex carbohydrates (60% of 2000 calories = 1200 calories of complex carbohydrates/day. Since each gram of carbohydrates is about 4 calories, Mr. Jones needs: (1200 divided by 4) 300 grams of carbohydrates per day.
- 15% (10%–20%) of the calories come from protein (15% of 2000 calories = 300 calories of proteins/day. Since each gram of protein is about 4 calories, Mr. Jones needs: (300 divided by 4) 75 grams of protein per day. (Others use 0.8 g/kg/day, which would equal 80 grams of protein per day.)
- 9% (up to 15%) of the calories come from monosaturated fats (180 cal/day or 20 g/day).
- 8% (up to 10%) of the calories come from polyunsaturated fats (160 cal/day or about 18 g/day)
- 8% (up to 10%) of the calories come from saturated fats (160 cal/day or about 18 g/day)
- * The calculation of fat requirements was based on each gram of fat containing 9 calories.

Further recommendations include:

- Limiting daily cholesterol intake to less than 300 g/day
- Restricting sodium intake to less than 2.4 g/day (and ideally to less than 2.0 g/day)
- Limiting alcohol use (if Mr. Jones already drinks and has no contraindications) to 1 to 2 ounces of alcohol per day
- Consume 25–30 g of dietary fiber per day

With this information, the provider and Mr. Jones may build a menu. The menu designed will require much time and effort. It will require Mr. Jones to read labels and calculate how much of each nutrient he is consuming. However, Mr. Jones' diet can evolve in accordance with his taste, availability of food, religious, cultural, and family influences.

This type of participation requires much education and often requires dietitians to assist in the planning and preparation of the diet. However, it is the provider's responsibility to write the dietary prescription for the dietitian, just as would be done with a medication prescription for the pharmacist or a consultation request for a specialist. In a dietary prescription, caloric requirements, desired dietary goals for the patient, and a medical and surgical history must be included, as should current medications and other pertinent information.

Special Disease States and Nutritional Considerations

There are many different diets prescribed, including the American Heart Association (AHA) diet, the NCEP step I diets, the low-sodium diet, and the "renal diet." Any diet is reasonable to promote health, as long as it is well balanced, prescribes the appropriate amount of calories, allows for a variety of foods, and addresses any specific disease states as well as patient concerns.

Certain disease states may require specific dietary modifications.

CARDIOVASCULAR DISEASE

The example of Mr. Jones' diet above is a prudent diet for all people. It is also useful for patients with hypertension, coronary artery disease, and hyperlipidemia. Though some may argue that salt restriction to 2.0 to 2.4 grams per day is only warranted in salt-sensitive hypertensive patients, it is currently difficult to identify which patient is salt sensitive, and therefore a worthwhile generalized recommendation. Salt restriction is also warranted in patients with congestive heart failure.

For hypercholesterolemia, the NCEP recommends a step II diet if the step I diet (similar to the diet above) fails in reducing the cholesterol to acceptable levels. The step II diet is similar to the step I diet, except saturated fats are restricted to no more than 7% of the total daily caloric intake and cholesterol is restricted to no more than 200 g/day. Though some have advocated a very-low-fat diet, the AHA does not recommend that the daily fat intake fall below 15% of the daily caloric intake (Krauss & Deckelbaum, 1996).

The AHA further states that the use of supplements such as antioxidant vitamins A, C, and E for cancer prevention, vitamin B_6 and B_{12} to reduce homocysteine (associated with coronary artery disease, congestive heart failure, and peripheral vascular disease), omega-3 fatty acids for reducing thrombogenesis, and soy have not yet been proven in clinical studies and therefore can not yet be recommended.

The American Dietetic Association (ADA) parallels the recommendations of the AHA. They note the importance of a variety of foods, following the food pyramid (Fig. 5-5). They also recognize the need for patients to participate in the dietary planning, stating that there is not a single "diabetic diet," but rather goals and a prescription plan (Position Statement, 1994).

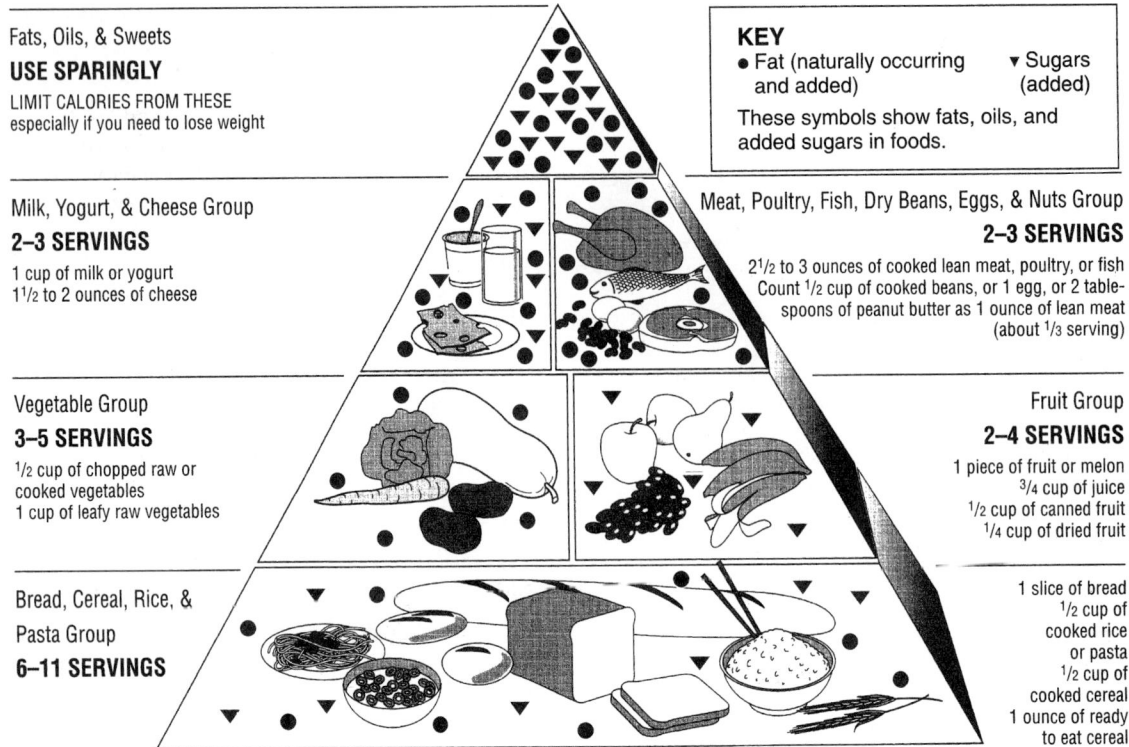

FIGURE 5-5 Food Guide Pyramid.

A recent study has shown that patients with diabetes mellitus and elevated triglycerides and VLDL may benefit from diets that have less complex carbohydrates and up to 20% of the total calories from monosaturated fats (Shad & Garg, 1996).

RENAL DIET

The "renal diet" is one that stresses low protein, low phosphorus, and low potassium. Protein restriction has often been shown to reduce the rate of decline of renal function (based on the glomerular filtration rate), although this has been disputed. However, even when disputed, protein restriction is recommended at 0.6 g/kg/day (Levey et al, 1996). Because of the risk of hyperkalemia, foods rich in potassium, such as avocados, dried apricots and peaches, tomatoes, potatoes, and bananas, may need to be avoided. Potassium should be restricted to 2 g/day. Phosphorus should also be restricted in the predialysis patient to 10 to 12 mg for each gram of protein per day. Calcium is often supplemented at 1000 to 1500 mg/day and the patient may also opt to take a multivitamin daily. Predialysis patients may require fluid and sodium restriction.

HEPATIC DIET

Patients with liver disease should be recommended a well-balanced diet with a variety of foods. A diet, such as Mr Jones' (above) may be suggested. However, when the patient develops hepatic encephalopathy, protein restriction to 0.6 g/kg is prudent. When ascites is present, fluid and sodium restriction is suggested.

VEGETARIAN DIET

The vegetarian diet implies that there are no animal ingredients in the foods consumed. Interpretation of this varies, and different definitions of vegetarian diets have evolved. The lactoveget

arians use milk, but not eggs, while the lacto-ovovegetarians use milk and eggs. Vegans do not use meat or any animal-derived products, including milk and eggs. A semivegetarian may omit just red meats or meats and poultry and still eat fish and seafood. Therefore, when learning that a patient is a "vegetarian," this must be further explored, so that an appropriate diet plan can be created.

TABLE 5-6	Sources for Potentially Deficient Nutrients in a Vegan Diet
Nutrient	**Source**
Vitamin D	Supplement
	Fortified soy milk
	Fortified rice milk
	Sunlight
Vitamin B$_{12}$	Supplement
	Fortified cereals
Calcium	Fortified soy milk
	Fortified rice milk
	Fortified orange juice
	Broccoli
	Cooked amaranth leaves
Iron	Leafy green vegetables
	Fortified cereals, breads, and grains
	Potato skins
	Soybeans (tofu)
	Spinach
Zinc	Leafy green vegetables
	Fortified cereals, breads, and grains
	Nuts
	Soybeans (miso)
	Palm hearts

Reasons for choosing a vegetarian diet vary. Some do it for spiritual reasons, while others feel this is a "healthier" diet. Regardless of the reason, the vegetarian diet can provide for a healthy diet. As with any other diet, there must be a balance and variety of foods, providing all essential vitamins and elements with the appropriate amounts of carbohydrates, fats, and proteins. Of particular concern is the intake of calcium, iron, zinc, vitamin B_{12} and vitamin D in the vegan's diet. Though vitamins D and B_{12} are often obtained through supplements, certain foods (Table 5-6) are good sources for calcium, iron, and zinc. Vegans are not more iron or zinc deficient than meat-eaters (Sizer & Whitney, 1997).

OBESITY

Obesity, a disease state, is included in the first part, and not in the second part of the book, where the other disease states are, because obesity has become extremely prevalent. It has been estimated that approximately one third of the U.S. population is obese (Kiczmarsk et al, 1994). It is even more prevalent among non-Hispanic Blacks and Mexican Americans (Update, 1997). With obesity being so common, it is becoming a norm.

Though exact cutoff points defining obesity have not been clearly established, obesity has been described as a BMI above 27 and/or weighing more than 20% over the IBW. Morbid obesity is when patient are more than 100% over their ideal body, more than 45.4 kg. above their IBW, or have a BMI greater than 35 (Sizer & Whitney, 1997). In addition to the psychologic and social stresses obesity may cause, morbid obesity is associated with, and may directly cause, many illnesses, including degenerative joint disease, hypertension, hypercholesterolemia, coronary artery disease, diabetes mellitus, sleep apnea and pulmonary hypertension. Nutritional disorders are second only to cigarette smoking as preventable causes of death. Although smoking cessation may cause a small increase in the prevalence of obesity, smoking cessation must be encouraged (Califano, 1995).

Pathophysiology

Obesity may be primary or secondary. However, the secondary disorders are rare and do not contribute significantly to the incidence of total obesity (West, 1996). Many theories have been developed as to the etiology of primary obesity.

POOR EATING HABITS

People with a caloric intake greater than their expenditure will gain weight. For every extra 3500 calories, a person will gain 1 pound. It is often difficult to calculate exact energy expenditures because individuals of the same height have different basal metabolic rates, different thermogenic effects of food, and different activity levels. Moreover, when estimating caloric intake, patients often underestimate. In addition, Americans are not eating prudent diets—they consume an excess of fats as a source for calories. Cultural and environmental influences greatly affect eating habits and patterns.

GENETICS

It is believed that people are genetically predisposed to be thin, average, or obese. The risk of being obese is 60% if one parent is obese and 90% if both parents are obese (Sizer & Whitney,

1997). Studies have shown a positive correlation of BMI between adopted children and their biologic parents. In addition, monozygous twins are twice as likely as dizygotic twins to have similar BMIs (Sorenson, 1995). The reason for this is unclear, but recently as many as six genes have been associated with obesity (Robert & Greenberg, 1996). Apolipoproteins, uncoupling protein, Na-K-ATPase, (beta) B3-adrenergic receptors, tumor necrosis factor (TNF), and lipoprotein lipase have all been associated with obesity (Robert & Greenberg, 1996).

One of the proteins recently associated with obesity is leptin. Leptin is a hormone secreted by adipose tissue, coded for on the obesity (ob) gene. It is believed that leptin affects the satiety center in the hypothalamus, making the individual feel full, and therefore decreases food intake. Initially it was believed that a lack of leptin was the reason for obesity. However, when obese humans were studied, increased leptin levels were found. This led to the belief that though leptin levels were adequate, receptors to leptin were deficient and/or ineffective in obese patients (Kricuciunas et al, 1996). It is postulated that the (db) gene codes for these leptin receptors.

Hypothalamic neuropeptide Y is another protein associated with obesity. It stimulates food intake and decreases thermogenesis, thereby promoting weight gain. Any trigger to enhance this neuropeptide may cause obesity. Decreasing neuropeptide Y levels, or blocking their effects, may be a mechanism to induce weight loss.

Physical Examination

Weight and height tables and BMI calculations are the criteria often used when studying obesity. However, these may be misleading. Certain patients, such as athletes and sports enthusiasts, may have a large amount of lean body mass (muscle) and therefore weigh more than the average for a given height. However, they are not obese. Body fat analysis (discussed above in nutritional assessment—body fat estimates) may be a better indication of obesity.

Two types of fat distribution patterns have been described: visceral fat and subcutaneous fat. Subcutaneous fat is stored diffusely under the skin, whereas visceral fat is stored in the abdomen. An excess in visceral fat causes central obesity. Central obesity may be noted by the waist-to-hip ratio. If the ratio of the waist measurement (in inches) to hip measurement (in inches) is greater than 0.8 (for women) and greater than 0.95 (for men) this suggests central obesity. The presence of central obesity poses a higher risk of morbidity and mortality than peripheral obesity or no obesity at all.

Treatment

The mainstays of treatment for obesity are diet and exercise. These modalities are essential regardless of any other adjunctive therapies, such as medications, surgery or complementary treatments. To lose weight, caloric expenditure must be greater than caloric intake. To lose 1 pound, 3,500 more calories must be expended than consumed. However, with all the different diet plans available, results of dieting and exercising have been disappointing (NIH, 1992).

"Dieting" has become a task and even a punishment for many patients. This makes long-term participation in any diet and exercise program difficult. Instead, the diet and exercise program must become part of the patient's lifestyle. A strong commitment must be made by the patient and the patient's family to incorporate such a change. The provider's role is to help direct the patient to an appropriate plan (for both exercise and diet) and to be supportive.

Over the years, many medications have been used to assist patients with weight loss. Amphetamines, dextroamphetamine, ephedrine, methamphetamine, fenfluramine, dexfenfluramine, fluoxetine, phentermine, sibutramine, and phenylpropanolamine are just a few of the agents tried. (Not all of these agents are FDA-approved and indicated for weight loss.) In general, the medications work by either increasing thermogenesis (metabolism), causing an increase in calorie expenditure, or affecting the satiety center, making the patient feel full and causing a decrease in calorie consumption. Some agents work by stimulating noradrenergic receptors and activity and increasing thermogenesis. Others work by increasing the release of serotonin and decreasing its reuptake (and probably enhancing satiety). Sibutramine's activity is caused by its ability to block the reuptake of both, serotonin and norepinephrine.

Dexfenfluramine has been shown to cause a statistically significant reduction in weight (Ryan, 1996). However, fenfluramine and dexfenfluramine pose serious side effects, including primary pulmonary hypertension, cardiac valve abnormalities, and possibly damage to serotonin neurons (Abenhain et al, 1996; McCann et al, 1997). These medications have been removed from the market by the FDA.

In general, medications have been approved for weight reduction only if the BMI is greater than 30, or the BMI is greater than 27 and there are comorbid conditions such as diabetes mellitus, hypertension, or hypercholesterolemia. The use of these drugs is short term; long-term trials (and effects) have not been studied.

For morbidly obese patients, a weight reduction of 5%, 10%, or even 15% may still not be enough. Several surgical procedures have been developed to cause weight loss. Four basic surgical approaches have been used: 1) induction of global malabsorption (no longer used); 2) limit oral intake per meal; 3) limit oral per meal and induce dumping; and 4) induce selective maldigestion and malabsorption (Balsinger et al, 1997). Global malabsorption caused many life-threatening complications and is no longer recommended. Oral intake is limited by gastroplasty (gastric stapling). This reduces one's intake of solid food, but high-fat liquid foods are easily ingested, and less than 40% of patients maintained a weight loss of at least 50% of their excess weight at the end of 3 years after surgery (Balsiger et al, 1997). Limiting oral intake and dumping is done by separating most of the stomach from the cardia, causing a functionally small stomach. The cardia is then attached to the jejunum. This causes earlier satiety and rapid transit of food. Complications may include malabsorption and diarrhea. Prolonged weight loss (>3 years) is usually achieved (Balsiger et al, 1997). Induced selective maldigestion and malabsorption is caused by a subtotal (80%) gastrectomy with a partial biliopancreatic bypass. In addition to early satiety (caused by the gastroplexy), bile and pancreatic enzymes are secreted into the terminal ilium, and their efficacy in digestion is significantly reduced. Combinations of these techniques are being tested, including laparoscopic approaches (Ryan, 1996).

References

Abenhain, L., Moride, Y., Brenot, F., et al. (1996). Appetite suppressant drugs and the risk of pulmonary hypertension. *N Engl J Med, 335*, 609–616.

Balsiger, B.M., Leon, E.L., & Sarr, M.G. (1997). Concise review for primary-care physicians. Surgical treatment of obesity: Who is an appropriate candidate? *Mayo Clin Proc, 72*, 551–558.

Bernstein, L., & Pleban, W. (1996). Prealbumin in nutritional evaluation. *Nutrition, 12*(4), 255–259.

Buzzard, I.M., Faucett, C.L., Jeffery, R.W., et al. (1996). Monitoring dietary change in a low-fat diet intervention study: Advantages of using 24-hour dietary recalls vs. food records. *J Am Dietetic Assoc, 96*(6), 574–579.

Califano, J.A. Jr. (1995). The wrong way to stay slim. *N Engl J Med, 333*(18), 1214–1216.

Kiczmarsk, R.J., Flegal, K.M., Campbell, S.M., & Johnson C.L. (1994). Increasing prevalence of overweight among US adults 1960–1991. NHANES III. *JAMA, 272*, 205–211.

Krauss, R.M., & Deckelbaum, R.J. (1996). Dietary guidelines for healthy American adults: A statement for health professionals from the Nutrition Committee, American Heart Association. *Circulation, 94*, 1795–1800.

Kricuciunas, A., Stephens, T.W., Nyce, M.R., et al. (1996). Serum immunoreactive leptin concentrations in normal-weight and obese humans. *N Engl J Med, 334*, 292–295.

Levey, A.S., Adler, S., Caggiula, A.S., et al. (1996). Effects of dietary protein restriction in the modification of diet in renal disease study. *Am J Kidney Dis, 27*(5), 652–663.

McCann, U.D., Lewis, S.S., Lewis, J.R., & Ricaurte, G.A. (1997). Brain serotonin neurotoxicity and primary pulmonary hypertension from fenfluramine and dexfenfluramine. *JAMA, 278*(8), 666–672.

McGinnis, J.M., & Foese, W.H. (1993). Actual causes of death in the United States. *JAMA, 270*, 2207–2212.

Mears, E. (1996). Outcomes of continuous process improvement of a nutritional care program incorporating serum prealbumin measurements. *Nutrition, 12*(7–8), 479–484.

National Center for Health Statistics. (1995). *Health, United States.* Hyattsville, MD: U.S. Public Health Service. DHHS Pub. No. (PHS) 95-1232.

National Cholesterol Education Program. (1988). Report of the NCEP Expert Panel on detection, evaluation and treatment of high blood cholesterol in adults. *Arch Intern Med, 148*, 39–69.

NIH Technology Assessment Conference Panel. (1992). Methods for voluntary weight loss and control. *Ann Intern Med, 116*, 942–949.

Position Statement. (1994). Nutritional recommendations and principles for people with diabetes mellitus. *Diabetes Care, 17*, 519–522.

Robert, S.B., & Greenberg A.S. (1996). The new obesity gene. *Nutrition Reviews, 54*(2), 41–49.

Ryan, D.H. (1996). Medicating the obese patient. *Endocrinol Metabol Clin North Am, 25*(4), 989–1004.

Shah, M., & Garg, A. (1996). High-fat and high-carbohydrate diets and energy balance. *Diabetes Care, 19*(10), 1142–1152.

Sizer, F., & Whitney, E. (1997). *Nutrition concepts and controversies,* 7th ed. Minneapolis/St. Paul: West/Wadsworth, pp. 335–370.

Sorenson, T.I.A. (1995). The genetics of obesity. *Metabolism: Clinical and Experimental, 44*(suppl 9), 4–6.

Update. (1997). Prevalence of overweight among children, adolescents and adults—United States 1988–1994. *JAMA, 277*(14), 1111.

U.S. Department of Agriculture and U.S. Department of Health and Human Services. (1995). *Nutrition and your health: Dietary guidelines for Americans.* Washington DC: U.S. Government Printing Office.

West, D.B. (1996). Genetics of obesity in humans and animal models. *Endocrinol Metabol Clin North Am, 25*(4), 801–813.

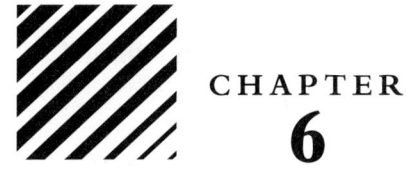

CHAPTER
6

Primary Care in the Community: Assessment and Use of Resources

Stephen Paul Holzemer, PhD, RN, Joanne K. Singleton, PhD, RN, FNP-C, and Carol Green-Hernandez, PhD, RN, FNP/ANP-C

One key aspect of integrated systems in primary care is the use of community assessment to guide the strategic use of resources. Participation in proactive primary care requires that providers know the actual and potential health-related problems in the community and know how to secure the resources to ameliorate them. Chapter 1 provided a context for examining the uncertainty of how systems of care will adapt to changes in the contemporary health care marketplace. This chapter promotes the importance of studying the community and its resources to meet the needs of people in changing care delivery systems.

Primary care providers from all disciplines are challenged to work together with their patients to create comprehensive primary care networks. Accurate and complete community assessment ensures that the picture of available health care resources is clear to both patients and providers. Evidence of a caring relationship between providers and patients can promote the public's confidence that resource allocation decisions have the potential to promote the primary care needs of patients, families, and communities (Donaldson et al, 1996).

The meaning of relationship-centered care for the community as a whole will be reviewed, and examples of aggregate-level interventions will be identified and discussed. The Alliance for Health model (Holzemer & Arnold, 1997) will be introduced as one model that could be helpful for providers to use when participating in community assessment, a critical process in obtaining appropriate resources for relationship-centered primary care delivery.

RELATIONSHIP-CENTERED CARE IN THE COMMUNITY

Primary care providers and patients are responsible for creating acceptable plans of primary care. These plans are a reflection of professional caring, which frames relationship-centered care. Relationship-centered care respects and promotes the work of both the patient and the provider to improve health (Green-Hernandez, 1997). These relationships are displayed at the community level in the form of aggregate data, or health indicators on a population level.

Aggregate health indicators include variables such as morbidity, mortality, clean air standards, statistics on civil disobedience and unrest, family and community violence rates, and patterns of providing primary care to groups of people who cannot pay for care. Each community will have similar and different health indicators that reflect an aggregate level of wellness.

Healthy communities are those where people, families, groups, and larger aggregates can work in harmony to create the primary care systems (with providers) that meet the needs of the public (Krout, 1994; National Association of County Health Officials, 1994; Pender, 1996; Tresolini & the Pew-Fetzer Task Force, 1994).

Primary care occurs within the relationship that develops between a health care provider or health care team and a patient, family, group, or community (the care recipient). The outcomes of these relationships are intended to heal or move the patient (and the community as a whole) toward improved health. The definition of healing or health differs according to patients' cultural or ethnic and spiritual beliefs as well as their experience in getting their health care needs met. The overall success that people, families, and groups have in meeting their health needs as a whole provides a picture of the health of a community.

Relationship-centered care respects the needs of patients and is within the legal and ethical mores of society. Providers use standards of care if the patient cannot make his or her ethical and legal wishes for care known. The following two situations examine the relationships between patients and providers. The relationships are examples of interaction on a one-to-one level. To reiterate, the overall sum of relationships between providers and patients is one way to illustrate a community's health. Community assessment, discussed later in this chapter, is a strategy to monitor the health of the relationships between the aggregate of patients and care providers.

In situation 1, the primary care provider is working with a patient who does not want to continue conventional treatment for her illness. The interaction between this provider and the patient can have an impact on the community. Allowing patients as a group to control decision making about care could be the first step in, for instance, negotiating hospice services for a growing elderly population, creating legislation to expand home care benefits for patients at the end of life, and changing the curricula in primary care programs to emphasize patient self-determination.

In situation 2, the patient continues to inject drugs and does not follow the health care goals set by him and the provider. The patient participates only sporadically in health care services, failing to establish a sound relationship with the provider because of his addictive behavior. Primary care providers are responsible for maintaining some level of a relationship even when the patient is not participating in his or her care. A population-focused intervention that could develop from a situation

---

SITUATION 1: MRS. DAREN IS READY TO DIE

Mae Daren is a 65-year-old widow who is ready to die. Her primary care provider is optimistic that Mrs. Daren will want to enjoy life more once her chronic obstructive pulmonary disease is better controlled by medication. Mrs. Daren refuses to enter the hospital and wishes to be maintained at home on low-dose oxygen therapy alone. Mrs. Daren has a living will that reflects her wishes.

Evidence of Relationship-Centered Care

The primary care provider in this situation has a challenge to make sure that Mrs. Daren is competent to make decisions about her care. The primary care provider should assess Mrs. Daren for confusion, depression, or a neurologic deficit that could impair judgment, review medication combinations that could affect pain relief or ease of respirations, and verify Mrs. Daren's decision with family members to elicit their support. The primary care provider then sets up home care services that will support the decision of Mrs. Daren to stay at home and makes a referral for hospice services as needed.

---

where provider–patient relationships are not working could include implementing a street-based mobile health care service, increasing the cadre of drug addiction counselors to provide more support to the drug-addicted population, and developing a system of recreation activities to discourage drug use in neighborhoods where prevalence is high.

These situations reflect the dynamic relationships between patients and their care providers. Patient–provider relationships extend to the community as a whole as primary care providers implement population-focused activities to improve the health of the public. Primary care providers should participate in creating a plan, in partnership with the public, that outlines how to allocate resources that will maintain the health of the community (Centers for Disease Control and Prevention & National Association of County Health Officials, 1994; Committee for the Study of the Future of Public Health, Institute of Medicine, 1988). A community may need more health-related teaching about issues important to the community. Resources might be needed to screen for or treat an emerging communicable disease.

SITUATION 2: MR. WHITE CHOOSES TO KEEP INJECTING DRUGS

Mark White is under the care of a primary care provider to monitor his diabetes and methadone maintenance. He is thought to be an active injection-drug user and is not following diabetic dietary guidelines even though he has access to government food coupons.

Evidence of Relationship-Centered Care

The provider facilitates getting Mr. White placed in drug rehabilitation. After many meetings with the interdisciplinary team, the primary care provider is unsuccessful in helping him participate more fully in his health care. The primary care provider makes every effort to invite Mr. White back into a therapeutic relationship when he comes to the primary care clinic for episodic, sporadic care.

ROLE OF COMMUNITY ASSESSMENT IN PRIMARY CARE

The relationships of primary care providers and patients on the whole can be examined through community assessment. The results of the community assessment, a picture of the community's health, can be used to allocate resources to improve the health of the community. The Alliance for Health model provides one blueprint to help students and primary care providers understand components of community health assessment and care delivery. This model offers a view of health and illness that incorporates the health care needs of the community as well as the process of obtaining sufficient resources to support systems of care delivery. The model identifies the relationship between the provider and the care recipient as critical to successful care delivery. Over time, providers and patients develop relationships that allow for sound, cost-effective decision making when these relationships foster cooperation.

Components of the Alliance for Health Model

The five components of the model represent core areas for assessment:

- Community-based needs
- Care management techniques
- Influences on resource allocation decisions
- Expertise of the interdisciplinary team
- Validation of services by the patient.

The model, shown in Figure 6-1, helps providers to view health concerns beyond a narrow, one-discipline perspective. Each of the five components of the model is considered essential to working in the community and making proper clinical judgments about the care that patients need. Primary care pro-

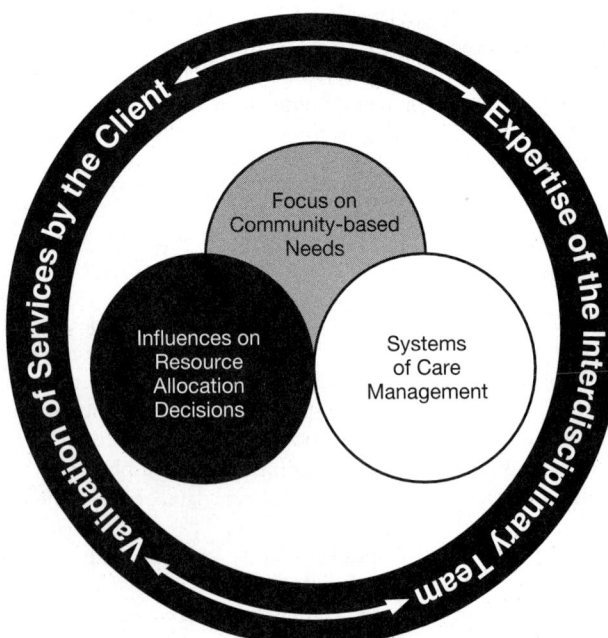

FIGURE 6-1 The Alliance for Health Model for Community Health Assessment and Care Delivery.

viders have a role in assessing each of the five essential components, although different providers will have special skills in one or more areas.

COMMUNITY-BASED NEEDS

Community-based needs include but are not restricted to the assessment and analysis of the sources of information found in Figure 6-2. Needs are identified by formal study of the community in a community assessment, as well as through the long-term relationship developed between professionals and the public.

The way community-based needs are met or not met is a reflection of how professionals and the public manage care and allocate resources. Because each community has unique health care needs, primary care providers must re-evaluate their assessment of community needs frequently.

CARE-MANAGEMENT TECHNIQUES

The management of health care is a complex phenomenon and includes the variables listed in Figure 6-2. Care management techniques develop and change according to the evolution of health care problems (community-based needs) and decisions about how populations allocate resources. Various communities may manage care differently; primary care providers need to be flexible about how they approach care-management issues.

INFLUENCES ON RESOURCE ALLOCATION DECISIONS

A number of variables influence resource allocation decision making; some of these variables are listed in Figure 6-2. In any community, one or more of these variables may influence resource allocation decisions at the same time. The major influences on how health care resources are allocated are associated

with care-management techniques and the volume and complexity of community-based needs.

When the resources to provide care are limited, rationing of high-technology care is required to provide a more comprehensive level of care. Care providers and recipients need to discuss how limited resources should be allocated in an ethical way. Without a guarantee of services (ie, national health plan) and with the free market, a two- or multiple-tiered system of health care will exist: people with financial means will have one level of care, and the poor will have another.

Primary care providers are partly responsible for the resources they allocate to provide care. Variables such as budget restrictions, the mission of organizations, and the preferences of more traditional gatekeepers (ie, administrators, physicians) affect the resource allocation decisions of primary care providers. However, the influences on resource allocation do not absolve primary care providers from providing resources to their patients appropriately. When systems allocate resources unfairly, providers have the responsibility to work to correct these systems.

The way patients are referred in the use of community resources is critical. Providers need to make sure that referring the patient to community resources is not a negative experience that could adversely affect primary care. Providers should not refer patients to resources that have not been validated as appropriate from financial, cultural, and functional perspectives. It is the responsibility of providers to evaluate the community resources being used by their patients.

EXPERTISE OF THE INTERDISCIPLINARY TEAM

The expertise of the interdisciplinary team depends on the involvement of all disciplines giving care. Although each team member will be somewhere on the continuum between expert and novice, the team as a whole needs to be competent to care for the public's health. With varied expertise, the team will have the resources to make referrals within and outside the group. Team members need to work together successfully to make a positive difference in the care people receive.

VALIDATION OF SERVICES BY THE PATIENT

Health care services need to be available, accessible, affordable, appropriate, adequate, and acceptable (Krout, 1994). Only patients can validate health-related services as being those that they want or need. Certain vulnerable populations such as prisoners, children, and people with severe disabilities need to have others act for them to validate services. If it is impossible to validate services with the patient or his or her health care proxy, the provider should offer services that reflect a general standard of care. Standards are generated by professionals who are charged with defining safe and prudent care.

COMPARISON OF TWO COMMUNITIES

Table 6-1 uses the components of the alliance model for community assessment to compare a fictitious inner-city community and a fictitious rural community. In this example, the inner-city community is made up of many city blocks; the rural community has borders that contain miles of land. Each of the components of the assessment reflects aspects of health or ill-

Community–Based Needs

Patterns of morbidity and mortality
Demographics (age, gender, education level, income, housing)
Environmental concerns
Public services (fire, police, sanitation, education, recreation, and sports)
Aesthetics (art, music, culture, religion)
Health–related facilities (hospitals, community–based organizations, subacute and custodial–care facilities, public health facilities, home care organizations)

Care Management Techniques

Mix of patient problems
Expectations of the public for care
Competence of professionals
Accepted standards of care
Use of interdisciplinary care plans or action plans

Influences on Resources Allocation Decisions

Patterns of resource allocation
Values and beliefs of the population
Reliance on local, regional, and federal government funding
Influence of special interest groups on resource
Patterns of insurance coverage

FIGURE 6-2 Community-based Needs, Care Management Techniques, and Influences on Resource Allocation Decisions..

TABLE 6-1	An Inner-City Community and a Rural Community	
Variable	**Community A**	**Community B**
COMMUNITY-BASED NEEDS	INNER-CITY COMMUNITY	RURAL COMMUNITY
Patterns of morbidity and mortality	In the inner-city community, the major causes of death and illness are HIV disease, violence, injection-drug use, and heart disease. Poor eating and exercise patterns are related to a sense of apathy and hopelessness in the community. Incidence of hypertension and high cholesterol levels are above state and national levels.	Major causes of illness and disability are cerebrovascular accident, cardiovascular problems, diabetes mellitus, and trauma from farm equipment and motor vehicle accidents.
Demographics (age, gender, education level, income, housing)	One fifth of residents do not live to the age of 25 years. One third are high-school dropouts and 45% live in subsidized housing. The unemployment rate is 60%.	The majority of residents over 70 years are women on fixed incomes. Residents under 65 years engage in farming and service-related occupations. Eight percent are college graduates; 67% completed high school.
Environmental concerns	Twenty percent of the public housing does not meet inspection codes. The general community spaces are not considered safe after sunset. The last major business in the area was closed for improper waste disposal.	Farmhouses and in-town homes are clean but sparsely decorated. Fresh-water wells provide the majority of drinking water. Most residents plant gardens for food. Regulation of pesticides is limited.
Public services (fire, police, sanitation, education, recreation, sports)	EMS response time is twice that of the city as a whole. Government services are lacking in many areas and satisfaction with services is poor. An evening sports program for children under 16 years is very popular and includes door-to-door transportation.	Health-related services (ie, ambulance, first aid) are provided by trained volunteers. Recreation and sports activities are primarily related to what is available on radio and television. The centralized school district covers a 30-mile area.
Aesthetics (art, music, culture, religion)	The neighborhood houses of worship provide the primary aesthetic support and socialization of new residents into the community.	The city large enough to support a museum and music hall is 250 miles away. A movie theater provides some entertainment for the community.
Health-related facilities (hospitals, community-based organizations, etc)	The geographic area has one 450-bed city-run acute care facility and two public health clinics (sexually transmitted disease and maternal-child care). There are no elder-care or psychiatric facilities in the community.	A skilled nursing facility and an emergency center are located in the community. Acute/intensive hospital care is located 75 miles away. Limited home care is provided by the public health department.
SYSTEMS OF CARE MANAGEMENT		
Mix of client problems	HIV and injection-drug use problems are twice the regional average. The community is considered the most dangerous in the category of violence to others.	Health problems are compounded among the under- or uninsured. Spouse abuse is thought to be 15% lower and depression 25% higher than in larger communities.
Expectations of the public for care	The community has a general feeling of apathy and hopelessness related to getting the care they need. Lay caregivers using herbal therapies provide some care in makeshift clinics.	Care expectations are restricted to the services that are available. Some people use fewer services because of long travel and the related loss of income.
Competence of professionals	The majority of primary care providers have extensive experience. The acute care providers have a 33% turnover rate. Lay community workers have an extensive orientation and evaluation program.	Twenty percent of the providers in the skilled nursing facility have formal geriatric certification. Primary care providers are difficult to attract and retain because of geographic isolation.

(continued)

TABLE 6-1	An Inner-City Community and a Rural Community *(Continued)*	
Variable	Community A	Community B
SYSTEMS OF CARE MANAGEMENT	**INNER-CITY COMMUNITY**	**RURAL COMMUNITY**
Accepted standards of care	The Joint Commission for the Accreditation of Health Care Organizations has placed the hospital on warning to lose accreditation because of unmet standards in obstetric care. The public health department has full accreditation from the Community Health Accreditation Program (CHAP) of the National League for Nursing.	The retirement facility is licensed by the state to operate. Complex care is usually not managed in the community; some members of the community are hesitant to report symptoms for this reason.
Use of interdisciplinary care (or action) plans	The quality care management team of the municipal hospital system is implementing interdisciplinary care plans in all areas except HIV care and psychiatric care. Some providers feel that the care requirements in these areas are changing so rapidly that care guidelines are not useful for these patients.	The geographic space between providers limits the use of interdisciplinary plans of care. Referral from provider to provider is the standard of practice.
INFLUENCES ON RESOURCE ALLOCATION		
Patterns of resource allocation	The inner-city community relies on services that require city budget approval yearly.	The area's residents are very conservative with resources. Residents have little influence on obtaining resources at the state level because of budgetary problems.
Values and beliefs of the population	The community relies on the leaders of their houses of worship for direction.	People in the rural area are politically conservative. Traditional family structures are valued by the residents.
Reliance on government funding	Funding for inner-city activities will soon be incorporated into block grants. Residents are suspicious about who will act as their advocates.	The community has basic needs covered by Medicare and Medicaid.
Influence of special-interest groups on resource allocation	The inner city provides little special-interest concerns except for developers who want to displace residents for more business development.	Conservative religious groups live in the rural area. Many attempts have been made to influence the primary and secondary school curricula with religious beliefs.
Patterns of insurance coverage	Sixty-six percent of residents are not insured.	The residents rely on Medicare and Medicaid to support their health-related needs.
EXPERTISE OF THE INTERDISCIPLINARY TEAM	Primary care providers in this community are expert providers, but the high turnover rate makes team cohesiveness problematic.	The community cannot support many specialists. The few primary care providers are well credentialed.
VALIDATION OF SERVICES BY THE PATIENT	As previously noted, the community (as patient) has little sustained interaction with primary care providers.	Town meetings to give health updates are well attended. Changes in service delivery are advertised in many local newspapers.

ness of the two communities. The communities have very different problems that require different solutions.

The comparison of the inner-city community with the rural community reveals few similarities. The states of health, support networks, and use of resources are very different. The successful primary care provider approaches each community as a unique set of problems and potentials. Strategies of intervention may vary, but the focus on improving health by strengthening the relationships between providers and patients is central to working with both communities.

Population-focused interventions for the inner-city community could include:

- Holding community discussion groups led by leaders of the houses of worship and lay caregivers
- Funding an antiviolence project (sponsored by local businesses) that is developed by members of the community to foster cooperation between segments of the community
- Developing a citizen patrol in high-crime areas

- Implementing a multineighborhood immunization project to improve immunization rates before children reach school age
- Organizing a summer camp program for preadolescents to foster reproductive responsibility.

Population-focused interventions for the rural community lacking access to primary care services could include:

- Inviting representatives from other rural areas to discuss issues such as providing support services for the community's elderly
- Establishing an agreement with health-related schools (ie, nursing, medicine) to set up a local primary care services network for people in underserved geographic areas
- Implementing a first-aid training workshop for each segment of the community
- Promoting the development of a plan for water storage in the event of well contamination
- Creating a network of friendly lay visitors to provide unskilled respite care for families with elderly members at home.

USING COMMUNITY RESOURCES TO IMPROVE THE HEALTH OF THE PUBLIC

Each community has resources to assist in providing primary care to patients. Finding the resources can be a challenge because sources of material and information change rapidly. The most important goal for the provider is to give the patient accurate and useful information. Although this sounds basic, many patients complain about the difficulty in obtaining resources that are useful. Table 6-2 provides guidelines for using community-based resources.

Lists of resources should be kept for patient use. Table 6-3 provides some examples of resources that providers or patients may use, including caregiver resources, audiovisual community resources, and publications and newsletters. Providers should keep in mind that after the patient reviews the material, he or she may need time to ask questions about the film, booklet, or handout used for teaching purposes. A list of frequently asked questions gives the provider suggestions for discussions with patients who deny having questions.

The key to efficient resource use is to have an idea about what resources are available well before they are needed. Because government entitlements and insurance benefits vary widely, it is important to seek information on how to secure community-based resources in advance. Files should be set up on local and state sources of assistance.

Because of the aging of the population, the fact that people are living longer with disabilities, and the increasing poverty in some parts of the country, most providers will care for patients receiving Medicare and Medicaid benefits. Medicare (Title XVIII of the Social Security Act) is a federal program designed to pay part of the health-related expenses for people who are 65 years of age or older or are disabled. Medicaid (Title XIX of the Social Security Act) is a federally aided, state-operated and state-administered program to provide health services for low-income persons. States determine patient eligibility, payment rates for providers, and administrative policies and procedures. Table 6-4 explains more about the services that are available through Medicare and Medicaid.

TABLE 6-2	Guidelines for Using Community-Based Resources

1. Make sure that the community-based agency/organization provides the services as described in any advertising material. The agency should be able to describe clearly the services it provides, including duration and cost.

2. Create a list of patients who are using or have used the services. Contact them periodically to evaluate services. Get permission for new users to call patients for their recommendation.

3. Investigate local consumer-based information services and organizations that provide support to patients. An example of a free medical library is:

Center for Medical Consumers
237 Thompson Street
New York, NY 10012
212-674-7105

4. Inquire about accreditation/quality assurance status for direct care providers:

Community Health Accreditation Program
61 Broadway
New York, NY 10006
phone 800-669-1656
    212-363-5555
fax 212-989-2272

(Accredits home care and community health agencies; the Benchmarks for Excellence program identifies services that are rated against other providers in the industry)

Joint Commission for the Accreditation of Health Care Organizations
1 Renaissance Boulevard
Oak Brook Terrace, IL 60181
phone 630-916-5600
fax 630-792-5005

(Accredits hospital-based home care departments, ambulatory care, behavioral health care, health care networks, and pathology and clinical laboratory services)

National Committee for Quality Assurance
2000 L. Street, NW
Suite 500
Washington, DC 20036
e-mail/web site http://www.ncqa.org
phone 800-839-6487
    202-955-3500
fax 202-955-3599

(Accredits health plans, health maintenance organizations, and managed care organizations)

5. Examine written material for accuracy of information, literacy concerns, and appropriateness from a cultural perspective. Local schools of nursing, social work, and patient education programs may be willing to work on such projects as part of a clinical experience. The following resource, or another like it, is one the provider may want to review:

Doak, C. C., Doak, L. G., & Root, J. H. (1996). *Teaching patients with low literacy skills* (2nd ed.). Philadelphia: J.B. Lippincott.

6. Order minimal amounts of printed material to decrease waste if the material becomes dated. This is especially true of material related to drug dosages and experimental treatment regimens. One resource for materials developed specifically for consumers is:

Consumer Information Center-7D-8
P.O. Box 100
Pueblo, CO 81002
phone 719-948-4000
fax 719-948-9724
e-mail/web site cic.info@pueblo.gsa.gov www.pueblo.gsa.gov

(This center of the U.S. General Services Administration provides a consumer information catalog of free and low-cost publications of consumer interest. Topics are health-related, of general interest, and very consumer-friendly.)

TABLE 6-3	Caregiver Resources, Audiovisual Resources, and Publications and Newsletters

CAREGIVER RESOURCES

National Association of Hospital Hospitality Houses
4013 W. Jackson Street
Muncie, IN 47304
phone 800-542-9730
      317-288-3226
e-mail/web site http://visit-usa.com/hhh

AUDIO AND VISUAL COMMUNITY RESOURCES

Descriptions of sample products and resources are included.

Academy for Educational Development
1255 23rd Street, NW
Suite 400
Washington, DC 20037
phone 202-884-8862
e-mail/web site http://www.aed.org

The Academy for Educational Development contracts with the Centers for Disease Control and Prevention to develop community-based health information materials, primarily for community planners and program managers. The Center for Community-Based Health Strategy can be accessed through their web site.

Alexander Graham Bell Association for the Deaf
3417 Volta Place, NW
Washington, DC 20007-2778
voice/TTY 202-337-5220
fax 202-337-8270
e-mail/web site agbell2@aol.com

This membership organization provides written and video materials addressing language development, parenting issues, medical interventions, and rehabilitation as these subjects relate to deafness.

Aquarius Productions, Inc.
5 Powderhouse Lane
P.O. Box 1159
Sherborn, MA 01770
phone 508-651-2963
fax 508-650-4216
e-mail/web site aqvideos@ix.netcom.com

Health and healing videos under the topics of mental health, learning and developmental disabilities, relaxation, and stress reduction. The following videos were reviewed: *Grown-Up Tears* provides very individualized stories about adults experiencing the death of their parents. How people and families cope with death is discussed. *Attention Deficit Disorder (Children)* reviews the therapeutic approaches to this problem. Showing how to work with people and families to improve attention and coping with problems is reviewed.

Fanlight Productions
47 Halifax Street
Boston, MA 02130
phone 800-937-4113
fax 617-524-8838
e-mail/web site fanlight@tiac.net
http://www.fanlight.com

The videotape *Hello In There: Understanding the Success of Person-Centered Care* is a short film about the need to truly get to know the patients cared for by providers. *Handbook for Viewers and Facilitators* offers suggestions for educating providers in creating relationships that respect the patient's special needs. Educating providers about the lives of patients improves the relationships that result between provider and patient.

Films for the Humanities & Sciences
P.O. Box 2053
Princeton, NJ 08543-2053
phone 609-275-1400
      800-257-5126
fax 609-275-3767

Basic and advanced educational material for professionals and lay people are available. Scientific and ethical problems are explored in video and CD-ROM format. The video *Alzheimer's disease: How families cope,* was an indepth examination into the physical and emotional impact of this disease on three families. The stresses on the lay caregiver in Alzheimer's disease are addressed with sensitivity and empathy.

(continued)

TABLE 6-3	Caregiver Resources, Audiovisual Resources, and Publications and Newsletters *(Continued)*

Health EDCO
P.O. Box 21207
Waco, TX 76702
phone 800-299-3366
fax 888-977-7653
e-mail/web site sales@wrsgroup.com
http://www.wrsgroup.com

Films, booklets, and anatomic models are available for patient teaching for a variety of ages. areas of concentration are women's health, lifestyle health, elementary health, and patient education. The videotape *Breast Health: Every Woman's Responsibility* is a short and comprehensive review of breast self-examination and diagnostic tests used to diagnose breast abnormalities. The dialogue is provided, for the most part, by breast cancer survivors in an open, nonthreatening way.

Krames Communications
1100 Grundy Lane
San Bruno, CA 94066-3030
phone 800-333-3032
fax 415-244-4512
e-mail/web site www.krames.com

A comprehensive listing of health education pamphlets on many diseases as well as health promotion topics are available. Booklets reviewed were on nasal allergies and migraine and tension headaches. The color drawings and graphics were clear and culturally sensitive. A number of the pamphlets are written in Spanish as well.

The National Center for Health Care Advances
A Division of NIMCO, Inc.
P.O. Box 9
102 Hwy 81 North
Calhoun, KY 42327-0009
phone 800-962-6662
        502-273-5050
fax 502-273-5844
e-mail/web site www.nimcoinc.com

A wide variety of video, CD-ROM, and anatomic models are available to provide education to beginning and more advanced practitioners. *Transplanting Miracles: Donor Crisis* discusses the need for more education in the area of transplantation and dispels myths. *Avoiding Medical Malpractice* examines the outcomes of real and perceived injury to patients and the legal outcomes.

Parlay International
5835 Doyle Street
Box 1817
Emeryville, CA 94662-0817
phone 510-601-1000
        800-457-2752
fax 510-601-1008

Health education resources come in the form of reproducible pages for teaching. *Children's Health* has 48 pages including topics such as lactose intolerance, lead poisoning, and safety. *Senior Health* has 55 pages including topics such as depression, elder abuse, becoming a grandparent, and dental care. Slides and color brochures can be used for more formal teaching. Educators who use the material are encouraged to make copies and alter information as needed.

Venture Publishing, Inc.
1999 Cato Avenue
State College, PA 16801
phone 814-234-4561
fax 814-234-1651
e-mail/web site VPUBLISH@VENTUREPUBLISH.COM

Publications in the area of recreation and leisure, long-term care, therapeutic recreation, activity programming, and private, public, and commercial recreation give providers guidance in program planning. *The ABC's of Behavior Change: Skills for Working With Behavior Problems in Nursing Homes* is a comprehensive training manual to guide classroom and on-the-job training for staff in long-term care facilities. The units focus on communication skills, observational skills, and interventions to decrease confused, depressed, agitated patient behaviors, and changing staff behaviors relating to these situations.

(continued)

TABLE 6-3	Caregiver Resources, Audiovisual Resources, and Publications and Newsletters *(Continued)*

Wisconsin Clearinghouse for Prevention Resources
University of Wisconsin-Madison
P.O. Box 1468
Madison, WI 53701-1468
phone 800-322-1468
fax 608-262-6346

Very specific, age-related material for ages 5 years to adult are available, examining individual, family, and community-wide health problems. Health promotion resources are well developed, with similar messages provided in different media. Poster, pamphlet, video, book, and CD-ROM materials provide flexible approaches to educating for one problem or developing a health-related curriculum. *The Mentor's Guide* and *The Mentor Program Handbook* are excellent resources for creating mentor programs for school-aged children and young adults. *How to Get Unstressed: The Bare Facts* is a comprehensive pamphlet on the causes of stress and how to avoid it or remove it from one's life. *Young Children & Drugs: What Parents Can Do* is a resource for parents to encourage discussion about avoiding drug use. Many materials are available in both Spanish and English.

PUBLICATIONS/NEWSLETTERS

HIV Frontline
World Health CME
41 Madison Avenue, 29th Floor
New York, NY 10010-2202
phone 212-679-6700

This newsletter is for professionals who counsel people living with HIV. The editorial board is interdisciplinary and the focus includes concerns of both patients and providers in HIV care.

Perspective on Aging
The National Council on the Aging, Inc.
409 Third Street SW
Washington, DC 20024
phone 202-479-6982

Published quarterly, this publication reflects the National Council on Aging (NCOA) philosophy of promoting the dignity, self-determination, well being, and contributions of older persons.

Consumer Choice News
The National Council on the Aging, Inc.
409 Third Street SW
Washington, DC 20024
phone 202-479-6982

This journal is a product of the National Institute on Consumer-Directed Long-term Services, a partnership between the NCOA and the World Institute on Disability.

Rural Health News
Maine Rural Health Research Center
Edmund S. Muskie School of Public Service
University of Southern Maine
P.O. Box 9300
Portland, ME 04104-9300
e-mail/web site www.muskie.usm.maine.edu/research

National rural health concerns are discussed from financial, policy, and current event perspectives. The focus is on tracking changes in rural health care across the country.

Prevention Report
Office of Disease Prevention and Health Promotion
U.S. Department of Health and Human Services
Humphrey Building, Room 738G
200 Independence Avenue SW
Washington, DC 20201
phone 202-205-8611
e-mail/web site http://odphp.osophs.dhhs.gov

Progress reports and programs of interest on national health issues are reported as they relate to *Healthy People 2000*. The goals for *Healthy People 2010* are reviewed and discussed.

(continued)

TABLE 6-3	**Caregiver Resources, Audiovisual Resources, and Publications and Newsletters** *(Continued)*

Issue Brief
Center for Studying Health System Change
600 Maryland Avenue SW
Suite 550
Washington, DC 20024-2512
phone 202-554-7549
fax 202-484-9258

This center is affiliated with Mathematical Policy Research, Inc. Current health care issues are discussed with the input of panels made up of experts across the country.

TABLE 6-4	**Medicare Part A and Part B Insurance**

Services	Benefit	Medicare Pays	You Pay
MEDICARE PART A			
Hospitalization	First 60 days	All but $736	$736
Semiprivate room and board,	61st–90th day	All but $184/day	$184/day
general nursing, and other	91st-150th day	All but $368/day	$368/day
hospital services and supplies	Beyond 100 days	Nothing	All costs
Skilled nursing facility care	First 20 days	100% approved amount	Nothing
Semiprivate room and board,	Additional 80 days	All but $92/day	Up to $92/day
skilled nursing and rehabilitation	Beyond 100 days	Nothing	All costs
services, and other services			
and supplies*			
Home health care	Unlimited as long as you	100% of approved amount:	Nothing for
Part-time or intermittent skilled	meet Medicare	80% of approved amount	services; 20%
care, home health aide	requirements for home	for DME	of approved
services, durable medical	health care benefits		amount for
equipment (DME) and supplies,			DME
and other services			
Hospice care	For as long as the MD	All but limited costs for	Limited cost
Pain relief, symptom	certifies need	outpatient drugs and	sharing for
management, and support		inpatient respite care	outpatient
services for terminally ill			drugs and
			respite care
Blood	Unlimited during a	All but first 3 pints/calendar	For first 3 pints†
When furnished by a hospital or	benefit period if	year	
skilled nursing facility during a	medically necessary		
covered stay			
MEDICARE PART B			
Medical expenses	Unlimited if medically	80% of approved amount	$100 deductible‡
MD's services, inpatient and	necessary	(after $100 deductible),	plus 20% of
outpatient medical and surgical		50% of approved amount	approved
services and supplies, physical		for most outpatient mental	amount and
and speech therapy, diagnostic		health services	limited charges
tests, DME, and other services			above federal
			cost limit, 50%
			for most mental
			health services
Clinical laboratory services	Unlimited if medically	Generally 100% of approved	Nothing for
Blood tests, urinalysis, and more	necessary	amount	services
Home health care	Unlimited as long as you	100% of approved amount:	Nothing for
Part-time or intermittent skilled	meet Medicare	80% of approved amount	services; 20%
care, home health aide	requirements for home	for DME	of approved
services, DME, supplies, and	health care benefits		amount for
other services			DME
Outpatient hospital treatment	Unlimited if medically	Medicare payment to hospital	20% of billed
Services for the diagnosis or	necessary	based on hospital costs	after the $100
treatment of an illness or injury			deductible

(continued)

TABLE 6-4	Medicare Part A and Part B Insurance *(Continued)*		
Services	Benefit	Medicare Pays	You Pay
MEDICARE PART B			
Blood	Unlimited if medically necessary	80% of approved amount (after $100 deductible) and starting with the 4th pint	First 3 pints plus 20% of approved amount for additional pints (after $100 deductible)

* Neither Medicare nor Medigap insurance will pay for most nursing home care.

† To the extent the three pints of blood are paid for or replaced under one part of Medicare during the calendar year, they do not have to be paid for or replaced under the other part.

‡ $100 deductible is paid once a year.

(Adapted from the 1996 Guide to Health Insurance for People with Medicare, Health Care Financing Administration, www.pueblo.gsa.gov)

TABLE 6-5	State Medicaid Contact Numbers

Alabama: phone 334-242-5600
fax 334-242-5097

Alaska: phone 907-465-3355
fax 907-465-2204

American Samoa:
phone 011-684-633-4590
fax 011-684-633-1869

Arizona:
phone 602-417-4000 ×4680
fax 602-252-6536

Arkansas: phone 501-682-8292
fax 501-682-1197

California: phone 916-654-0391
fax 916-657-1156

Colorado: phone 303-866-2859
fax 303-866-2993

Connecticut: phone 860-424-5053
fax 860-424-4958

Delaware: phone 302-577-4901
fax 302-577-4405

Washington, DC:
phone 202-727-0735
fax 202-610-3209

Florida: phone 904-488-3560
fax 904-488-2520

Georgia: phone 404-656-4479
fax 404-657-5238

Guam: phone 011-671-734-7269
fax 011-671-734-5901

Hawaii: phone 808-586-5391
fax 808-586-5389

Idaho: phone 208-334-5747
fax 208-334-0657

Illinois: phone 217-782-2570
fax 217-782-5672

Indiana: phone 317-233-4455
fax 317-232-7382

Iowa: phone 515-281-8794
fax 515-281-7791

Kansas: phone 913-296-5217
fax 913-296-4813

Kentucky: phone 502-564-4321
fax 502-564-3232

Louisiana: phone 504-342-3891
fax 504-342-3893

Maine: phone 207-287-2093
fax 207-287-2675

Maryland: phone 410-225-6505
fax 410-225-6489

Massachusetts: phone 617-348-5690
fax 617-348-5535

Michigan: phone 517-335-5001
fax 517-335-5007

Minnesota: phone 612-297-4113
fax 612-297-3230

Mississippi: phone 601-359-6059
fax 601-359-6048

Missouri: phone 573-751-6922
fax 573-751-6564

Montana: phone 406-444-4141
fax 406-444-1861

Nebraska: phone 402-471-9718
fax 402-471-9092

Nevada: phone 702-687-4176
fax 702-687-4733

New Hampshire:
phone 603-271-4353
fax 603-271-4376

New Jersey: phone 609-588-2600
fax 609-588-3583

New Mexico: phone 505-827-3106
fax 505-827-3185

New York: phone 518-486-4803
fax 518-486-6852

North Carolina: phone 919-733-2060
fax 919-733-6608

North Dakota: phone 701-328-2321
fax 701-328-1544

Northern Mariana Islands:
phone 011-670-234-8950 ext. 2905
fax 011-670-234-8931

Ohio: phone 614-644-0140
fax 614-752-3986

Oklahoma: phone 405-530-3439
fax 405-530-3470

Oregon: phone 503-945-5881
fax 503-373-7823

Pennsylvania: phone 717-787-1870
fax 717-787-4639

Puerto Rico: phone 809-765-1230
fax 809-250-0990

Rhode Island: phone 401-464-5274
fax 401-464-3350

South Carolina: phone 803-253-6100
fax 803-253-4137

South Dakota: phone 605-773-3495
fax 605-773-4855

Tennessee: phone 615-741-0213
fax 615-741-0882

Texas: phone 512-424-6517
fax 512-424-6585

Utah: phone 801-538-6406
fax 801-538-6099

Vermont: phone 802-241-2880
fax 802-241-2974

Virginia: phone 804-786-7933
fax 804-371-4981

Virgin Islands: phone 809-774-4624
fax 809-774-4918

Washington: phone 360-902-7855
fax 360-664-0788

West Virginia: phone 304-926-1700
fax 304-926-1776

Wisconsin: phone 608-266-2522
fax 608-266-1096

Wyoming: phone 307-777-7531
fax 307-777-6964

An example of resources that vary from state to state is found in the Medicaid program. Primary care providers need to be aware of what services are available for people who are disabled or financially disadvantaged. Table 6-5 provides the contact numbers for Medicaid state offices, which can provide information on service delivery.

SUMMARY

Primary care in the community is a reflection of the relationships between patients and their care providers. The relative health of that relationship affects the quality of the health care that is provided. Concerns about resource allocation suggest that a close professional relationship would be one where resource allocation decisions could be made as soundly as possible for the health of the community as a whole.

Community assessment is necessary in providing primary care so that resource allocation decisions can be made fairly and ethically. When used for community assessment, the Alliance for Health model provides a framework for examining community-based needs, care-management techniques, influences on resource allocation decisions, and the expertise of the interdisciplinary team. The model supports the validation of services by the patient as critical to the delivery of primary care.

Increased skill in community assessment can assist primary care providers in ensuring that the affordable, accessible care that people need will be available when they need it. Tapping community resources is part of community assessment. Making sure that providers know which services are appropriate for patients will strengthen the provider–patient relationship. Evaluation of community-based resources is an ongoing responsibility of providers. Involving patients in the evaluation process should give providers a clear picture of patients' satisfaction with the services provided (Adams & Anthony, 1997).

References

Adams, C.E., & Anthony, A.L. (Eds.). (1997). *Home health outcomes and resource utilization: Integrating today's critical priorities.* New York: National League for Nursing Press.

Centers for Disease Control and Prevention & National Association of County Health Officials. (1994). *Blueprint for a healthy community: A guide for local health departments.* Washington DC: National Association of County Health Officials.

Committee for the Study of the Future of Public Health, Institute of Medicine. (1988). *The future of public health.* Washington DC: National Academy Press.

Donaldson, M.S., Yordy, K.D., Lohr, K.N., & Vanselow, N.A. (Eds.). (1996). *Primary care: America's health in a new era.* Washington DC: National Academy Press.

Green-Hernandez, C. (1997). Application of caring theory in primary care: A challenge for advanced practice. *Nursing Administration Quarterly, 21*(4), 77–82.

Holzemer, S.P., & Arnold, J. (1997). Alliance for health: A model for community health assessment. In Klainberg, M., Holzemer, S.P., Leonard, M., & Arnold, J. (Eds.). *Community health nursing.* New York: McGraw-Hill.

Krout, J.A. (ed.). (1994). *Providing community-based services to the rural elderly.* Thousand Oaks, CA: Sage.

National Association of County Health Officials. (1994). *Providing culturally appropriate services.* Washington DC: Author.

Pender, N.J. (1996). *Health promotion in nursing practice,* 3d ed.). Stamford, CT: Appleton & Lange.

Tresolini, C.P., & the Pew-Fetzer Task Force. (1994). *Health professions education and relationship-centered care.* San Francisco: Pew Health Professions Commission.

PART

Two

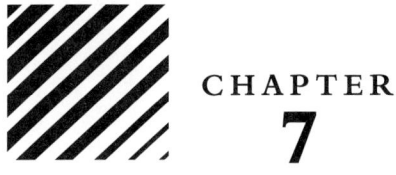

CHAPTER
7

Arrhythmia

Judy Cheng, PharmD, BCPS

An arrhythmia is defined as a disturbance of cardiac electrical conduction. The synchronous interaction between the electrical and the mechanical properties of the heart is important for the heart to function properly and to maintain adequate blood supply and perfusion to other vital body organs. The management of arrhythmias continues to evolve as results of many landmark studies are published.

With the original discovery of surface electrocardiogram (ECG) and the more recent availability of intracardiac recordings and programmed cardiac stimulation, there is considerable insight into cardiac electrophysiology. This technology has allowed for sophisticated classification of many arrhythmias.

Cardiac arrhythmias can be broadly classified into two groups: supraventricular (originate above the ventricle) and ventricular (originate from the ventricle) arrhythmias. Common supraventricular arrhythmias include atrial fibrillation, atrial flutter (Aflutter), paroxysmal supraventricular tachycardia (PSVT), sinus tachycardia, and bradycardia. Atrial fibrillation is probably the most common sustained cardiac arrhythmia encountered in primary care practice. The prevalence of atrial fibrillation increases with increasing age and the presence of structural heart disease. Atrial fibrillation is the major cause of stroke, especially in the elderly. Ventricular arrhythmias include ventricular premature beats (VPBs or PVC), monomorphic and polymorphic (such as torsades de pointes) ventricular tachycardia (VT), and ventricular fibrillation (VF).

Multiple antiarrhythmic agents are available for management of these disorders. Unfortunately, many problems are associated with these agents, proarrhythmia being the most significant since it has a potential effect on patient mortality. Fortunately, technical advances have been made in the development of nondrug therapies. Some examples include radiofrequency ablation, the internal cardioverter/defibrillator, and pacemakers.

This chapter will discuss the pathophysiology, management and social impact of arrhythmias in a primary care setting, with an emphasis on long-term management to prevent complications such as life-threatening ventricular arrhythmias, heart failure, or thromboembolic events.

ANATOMY, PHYSIOLOGY, AND PATHOLOGY

Anatomy and Physiology

CARDIAC ELECTRICAL CONDUCTION PATHWAY

The heart is an organ that is capable of producing an intrinsic electrical rhythm and has automaticity. This rhythm may be modified by the autonomic nervous system (sympathetic and parasympathetic nervous systems). In normal cardiac conduction, the electrical activity begins in the sinoatrial (SA) node, or the pacemaker of the heart. The SA node is located in the upper portion of the right atrium (Fig. 7-1).

In adults, the SA node fires at a regular rate of 60 to 100 beats per minute (bpm), which is defined as the normal sinus rhythm (NSR). Following discharge of the SA node, the electrical impulse is conducted through the right atrium, to the left atrium, then to the atrioventricular (AV) node. The impulse continues to conduct through the AV node, with a momentary delay, then to the bundle branches. From the bundle branches, the electrical activity is carried to the ventricular muscle by networks of Purkinje fibers. In abnormal cardiac conduction, enhanced automaticity and formation of re-entry circuits at certain foci of the heart (either SA node or other latent pacemakers) may lead to tachycardia.

Electrical impulses are capable of conduction through ion channels. The major ion channels include sodium and potassium channels (fast conduction channels), as well as calcium channels (slow conduction channels). They are labeled as fast and slow conduction channels based on the speed of ion influx and efflux. These conduction channels are distributed throughout the myocardium. However, most sodium and potassium channels are located in the atria and ventricular muscle, and most calcium channels are located at the SA and AV nodes respectively. The activity of antiarrhythmic agents is based on these sites of action. For instance, calcium channel blockers such as verapamil will exert their main action at the SA and the AV nodes. Class I antiarrhythmic agents, such as procainamide are sodium channel blockers, exert their action mainly on the atrial and the ventricular tissue.

ELECTROCARDIOGRAM

The electrocardiogram (ECG) complexes reflect the cardiac electrical activity. Electrical conduction of the heart is represented by waveforms on the ECG. The P wave represents atrial depolarization, the QRS complex represents ventricular depolarization and the T wave represents ventricular repolarization (Fig. 7-2). The atrial contraction follows the P wave and the ventricular contraction follows the QRS complex. There are three key intervals that play an important part in ECG interpretation. The PR interval, normally 0.12 to 0.20 seconds in duration, represents the travel of electrical impulse from the SA node through the AV node. A prolongation of the PR interval indicates a delay in AV nodal conduction, known as first-degree

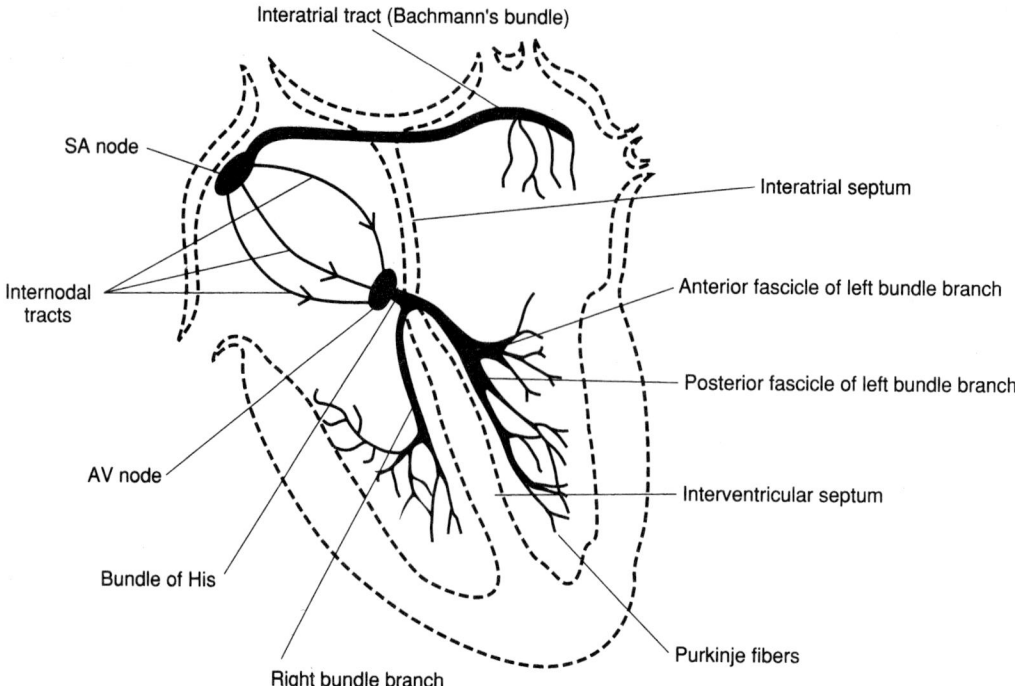

FIGURE 7-1 The electrical conduction pathway of the heart. (Huff, J. [1997]. ECG Workout: Exercises in Arrhythmia Interpretation, 3/e. Philadelphia: Lippincott-Raven Publishers.)

heart block. The QRS interval, normally less than 0.12 seconds in duration, represents the time required for the ventricle to depolarize. Prolongation of the QRS interval may indicate ventricular hypertrophy (it takes longer for a thicker piece of muscle to depolarize) or a defect in the conduction of the Purkinje fibers. The QT interval, normally 0.4 seconds or less, represents the time necessary for ventricular depolarization and repolarization. Prolongation of the QT interval (> 0.5 seconds) indicates prolongation of the relative refractory period. During this phenomenon the ventricles are especially vulnerable to extra stimuli. This increases the risk of developing life-threatening arrhythmias such as torsades de pointes.

Pathophysiology

The mechanisms of tachyarrhythmias (both supraventricular and ventricular) have been classified into two general categories; those resulting from an abnormal impulse generation and

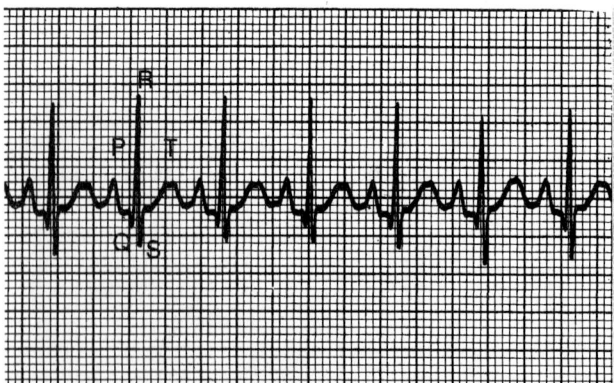

FIGURE 7-2 ECG waveforms and intervals of the cardiac cycle. (Huff, J. [1997]. ECG Workout: Exercises in Arrhythmia Interpretation, 3/e. Philadelphia: Lippincott-Raven Publishers.)

those resulting from an abnormal impulse conduction or reentrant tachycardia.

Automatic tachycardias depend on spontaneous impulse generation in latent pacemakers, which compete with the SA node for dominance of cardiac rhythm. If the rate of spontaneous impulse generation of the abnormally automatic tissue exceeds that of the SA node, then an automatic tachycardia may result. Trigger automaticity is also a possible mechanism for abnormal impulse generation. Trigger automaticity is the transient membrane depolarization that occurs during repolarization (early after-depolarization) or after depolarization (delayed after-depolarization) but before repolarization.

Reentry tachycardia involves indefinite propagation of the impulse and continued activation of previously refractory tissue. Three conduction requirements must be fulfilled for the formation of a viable reentrant focus. There must exist two pathways for impulse conduction with an area of unidirectional block (prolonged refractoriness) and slow conductions in the other pathway (Fig. 7-3).

A critically timed premature beat initiates reentry. The premature impulse enters both conduction pathways but encounters refractory tissue in one of the pathways at the area of the unidirectional block. The impulse subsides because it is still refractory from the sinus impulse. Although it fails to propagate in one pathway, the impulse will still proceed in a forward (antegrade) direction through the other pathway because of this pathway's relatively shorter refractory period. The impulse may then proceed through the loop of tissue and reenter the area of the unidirectional block in a backward (retrograde) direction. Because the antegrade pathway has slow conduction properties, the area of unidirectional block has time to recover its excitability. The impulse can proceed retrogradely through this (previously refractory) tissue and continue around the loop of tissue. The reentrant focus may excite surrounding tissue at a rate

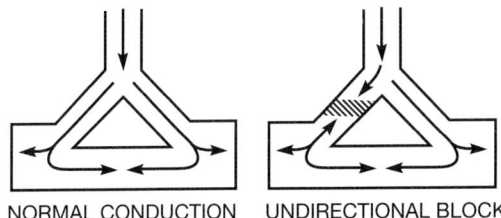

NORMAL CONDUCTION   UNDIRECTIONAL BLOCK

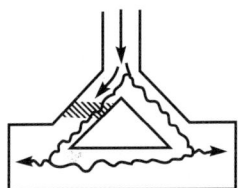

UNDIRECTIONAL BLOCK WITH SLOWED CONDUCTION

FIGURE 7-3 Mechanism of re-entry. (Bauman, J. (1983). Understanding and treating supraventricular arrhythmias. Clinical Pharmacology Therapeutics. 2:312–320.)

greater than that of the SA node, and a clinical tachycardia results. Bradycardia is usually due to sick sinus or AV nodal conduction delay or blockade.

Different precipitating factors of automaticity and reentry may lead to different types of bradyarrhythmias or tachyarrhythmias. Classifications of cardiac arrhythmias are summarized in Table 7-1. Pathophysiology of some of the more clinically significant arrhythmias are discussed in greater detail below.

SUPRAVENTRICULAR ARRHYTHMIA
Atrial Fibrillation and Atrial Flutter
In atrial fibrillation, reentry circuits are formed when the atrium is being stretched or disturbed. They take over the SA node and become multiple independent pacemakers of the heart. All of these pacemakers beating independently results in an overall atrial rate of 400 to 600 bpm. In atrial flutter, the mechanism is similar except that there is one instead of multiple reentry circuits.

Paroxysmal Supraventricular Tachycardia
Paroxysmal supraventricular tachycardias (PSVTs) include those arrhythmias caused by AV nodal reentry, SA nodal reentry, and intra-atrial reentry. AV nodal reentry is by far the most

TABLE 7-1	Classification of Cardiac Arrhythmias

SUPRAVENTRICULAR

Premature atrial contraction

Atrial fibrillation

Atrial flutter

Paroxysmal supraventricular tachycardia (Wolff-Parkinson-White syndrome, Lown-Ganong-Levine syndrome)

Sinus bradycardia

VENTRICULAR

Ventricular premature beats or premature ventricular contractions

Ventricular tachycardia

Ventricular fibrillation

Torsades de pointes

common form of PSVT. Lown-Ganong-Levine (LGL) syndrome is an example of AV nodal reentry PSVT. Wolff-Parkinson-White (WPW) syndrome is another type of PSVT that involves both the AV node (slow conduction pathway) and an extranodal AV connection (accessory fast conduction pathway). PSVT that involve accessory pathway may be the more common orthodromic (down AV node, up accessory pathway) or the less common antidromic (down accessory pathway, up AV node) type.

VENTRICULAR ARRHYTHMIAS
Ventricular Tachycardia
Ventricular tachycardia is defined as three or more repetitive VPBs, occurring at a rate greater than 100 bpm. VT can be subdivided into two major types, monomorphic VT which has a consistent QRS morphology, and polymorphic VT, which has varying QRS morphology. VT may occur acutely as a result of metabolic abnormalities, electrolyte abnormalities such as hypokalemia, ischemia, organic heart disease such as congestive heart failure (CHF), left ventricular aneurysm, or drug toxicities such as digoxin overdose. Ventricular tachycardia, if sustained for a prolonged period of time, can lead to hemodynamic collapse. Immediate treatment is required.

Ventricular Fibrillation
Ventricular fibrillation is an electrical anarchy of the ventricle, resulting in no blood pressure or cardiac output. VF is a medical emergency that requires advanced cardiac life support measures. VF is often preceded by VT. Ventricular fibrillation occurs most commonly in patients with ischemic heart disease, WPW, and less commonly, mitral valve prolapse.

Torsades de Pointes
Torsades de pointes is a rapid form of polymorphic VT associated with delayed ventricular repolarization (prolonged QT intervals). Table 7-2 lists the common causes of Torsades.

EPIDEMIOLOGY

The most common type of arrhythmia, other then atrial and ventricular premature contraction (which most people will experience during their lifetime), is atrial fibrillation. The best source of epidemiology data on atrial fibrillation is the Framingham study (Kannel et al, 1982; Wolf et al, 1987). It is important to realize that the Framingham population may not represent the ethnic and racial diversity in other parts of the country.

Among patients in the Framingham Heart Study, the cumulative 22-year incidence of new atrial fibrillation was 21.5 per 1000 men and 17.1 per 1000 women respectively. However, this incidence rose sharply with increases in age, from 0.5% for age 50 to 59 years to 8.8% for age 80 to 89 years. Excluding people with rheumatic heart disease, the 2-year incidence of developing atrial fibrillation in the Framingham study was 0.04% for men and 0% for women age 30 to 39 years but rose to 4.6% for men and 3.6% for women age 80 to 89 years. Heart failure and rheumatic heart disease were the most powerful predictive precursors for atrial fibrillation, with relative risk in excess of sixfold. Hypertension, a history of cerebrovascular disease, diabetes, and left ventricular hypertrophy were also found to be significantly associated with atrial fibrillation.

The clinical importance of atrial fibrillation, other than its difficult-to-tolerate signs and symptoms, such as palpitation,

TABLE 7-2	Causes of Torsades de Pointes

PHYSICAL CONDITIONS

Congenital long Q–T syndrome

Myocarditis

Ischemia

Severe bradycardia due to AV block, heart rate <50 bpm

Hypokalemia

Hypomagnesemia

Hypothyroidism

Cardiomyopathy

Subarachnoid hemorrhage

DRUGS

Antiarrhythmic agents
    Class IA (procainamide, quinidine)
    Class IC (flecainide, propafenone)
    Class III (amiodarone, sotalol, ibutilide)

Psychotropic agents
    Phenothiazines
    Tricyclic antidepressants
    Haloperidol

Toxins
    Organophosphate insecticides
    Arsenic

Antihistamines
    Terfenadine
    Astemizole

Antibiotics
    Pentamidine
    Erythromycin

dizziness, and fatigue, is its relation to a mortality rate doubled that of control subjects. Much of its morbidity and mortality related to atrial fibrillation is caused by stroke (Wolf et al, 1987). This is because atrial fibrillation creates turbulent flow in the cardiac chambers, promoting the formation of thrombi. Such thrombi, when dislodged from the cardiac chambers, may eventually lodge in another organ and lead to a thromboembolic event. Other morbidity and mortality related to atrial fibrillation include heart failure. The risk of stroke from atrial fibrillation is estimated to be 1.5% for those age 50 to 59 years and approaches 30% for those age 80 to 89.

The phase "lone atrial fibrillation" refers to atrial fibrillation in the subgroup of patients who do not have other underlying cardiac diseases. This type of atrial fibrillation accounts for 11.4 percent of all cases of atrial fibrillation. Studies have indicated that prognosis in this group of patients is good (Kopecky, 1987).

For ventricular arrhythmias, the incidence of VT is not as well defined. Drug-induced torsades occurs in approximately 5% to 20% of patients (McCollam & Parker, 1991). Approximately 2% to 11% of patients will experience VF within 24 hours after myocardial infarction (MI) (Bauman & Dekker Schoen, 1997).

DIAGNOSTIC CRITERIA

Supraventricular Arrhythmias

PREMATURE ATRIAL COMPLEXES

A premature atrial complex (PAC) is an electrical impulse originating in the atria other than the sinus node. Premature atrial complexes often occur without apparent cause and symptoms.

Commonly recognized clinical causes include the use of stimulants such as caffeine, tobacco, or alcohol.

The ECG criteria are:

- Rhythm: Irregular
- P waves: Different in morphology from those of sinus mode origin.

PAROXYSMAL SUPRAVENTRICULAR TACHYCARDIA

Paroxysmal supraventricular tachycardia is a clinical syndrome characterized by repeated episodes of atrial tachycardia with an abrupt onset (preceded frequently by a premature atrial contraction), lasting from a few seconds to many hours. They usually end abruptly and often can be terminated by vagal maneuvers. Possible causes of PSVT include physical and psychological stress, hypoxia, hypokalemia, and excessive use of caffeine or other stimulants. Primary cardiac causes include MI, congenital heart disease, and cardiomyopathy. Other causes include digitalis toxicity and chronic pulmonary disease. Patients may feel a sudden rapid palpitation and severe anxiety. Congestive heart failure, angina, and shock may occur as a result of a decreased cardiac output and an increased need for myocardial oxygen, if the tachyarrhythmia is persistent.

The ECG criteria are:

- *Rate*: The atrial rate is usually 160–240 beats/minute.
- *Rhythm*: Regular. The ventricular rate is most often regular with 1:1 AV conduction when the atrial rate is less than 200. When atrial rates above 200, 2:1 AV block is common. Higher-grade block may also occur.
- *P wave*: P waves may be difficult to identify because they can be buried in the preceding T wave. However, when visualized, their morphology is different from the sinus P waves.

Lown-Ganong-Levine (LGL) Syndrome

Lown-Ganong-Levine, one type of PSVT, is usually benign unless debilitating tachyarrhythmias occur. ECG criteria are normal except PR intervals are abnormally short but constant.

Wolff-Parkinson-White (WPW) Syndrome

WPW occurs mostly in younger patients (20–35 years old). It usually requires no intervention unless debilitating tachyarrhythmias occur.

ECG criteria are:

- Rate and rhythm: Within normal limits, however, WPW can predispose abrupt episodes of PSVT, atrial fibrillation and atrial flutter with rates up to 300 bpm.
- PR interval: Short
- QRS interval: Duration is prolonged. Beginning of the waveform is slurry (delta wave).

ATRIAL FIBRILLATION/ATRIAL FLUTTER

Atrial fibrillation is a type of supraventricular arrhythmia defined as an extremely rapid and disorganized atrial activation (400–600 atrial bpm). This occurs when other ectopic foci in the atrium take over the role of the sinus node as the pacemaker. Such disorganized atrial contractions lead to a supraventricular impulse penetrating the AV conduction system in variable degrees, resulting in a totally irregular, often rapid ventricular rate. Because the AV node is composed of mostly slow conduction channels compared to the atrial tissue, which is composed of mostly fast conduction channels, most of the supraventricular impulses are not conducted through the AV node. Therefore, although the atrial rates usually vary between 400 to 600 bpm, the ventricle responds at a considerably slower rate (120–180 bpm).

Atrial fibrillation is now believed to occur under certain distinct clinical circumstances:

- As a secondary arrhythmia in the absence of structural heart disease but in the presence of systemic abnormalities that predispose the patient to atrial fibrillation
- As a secondary arrhythmia associated with cardiac diseases that affects the atria
- As an idiopathic primary arrhythmia (lone atrial fibrillation)

The etiology of atrial fibrillation is categorized in Table 7-3 (Geraets & Kienzle, 1993).

Any situation that leads to an increase in atrial mass, atrial dilatation (in fluid overload states), myocardial injury (in coronary artery disease), increased vagal tone, or any other disturbance to the atria (open heart surgery) increases the risk of developing atrial fibrillation.

Atrial flutter is another form of supraventricular arrhythmia. Atrial flutter occurs less frequently than atrial fibrillation but has similar precipitating factors, consequences, and approach to treatment. This arrhythmia is characterized by rapid but regular atrial activation (250–350 bpm). This slower and regular atrial activity leads to a regular ventricular response and a pulse rate in dividends of 300 bpm (100 bpm for a 3:1 AV conduction, 150 bpm for a 2:1 AV conduction, and 300 bpm for a 1:1 conduction). Atrial flutter usually occurs in conjunction with atrial fibrillation; in this situation, the ventricular rate will be irregular.

TABLE 7-3	Etiologies of Atrial Fibrillation

SYSTEMIC ABNORMALITY

Hyperthyroidism

Pulmonary disease (asthma, chronic obstructive pulmonary disease, pneumonia, pulmonary emboli)

Cerebrovascular disease

Fluid overload state

Electrolyte abnormality

Febrile illness

Trauma and stress

Alcohol

Drugs: theophylline, caffeine

CARDIAC DISEASES

Cardiomyopathy

Rheumatic or nonrheumatic valvular disease

Tumor, lipomatous hypertrophy

Atrial septal defect

Coronary artery disease

Pericarditis

Cardiothoracic surgery

OTHER CAUSES

Hypertension

Increased vagal tone

Symptoms of atrial fibrillation and atrial flutter are similar. Patients often present complaining of palpitation, dizziness, fatigue, and dyspnea, especially if they have a rapid ventricular rate. Patients with a relatively slower ventricular rate may be asymptomatic. A prolonged uncontrolled ventricular rate may lead to cardiac decompensation or CHF. Atrial fibrillation is usually categorized as paroxysmal or chronic and the management approaches are different. Atrial flutter, on the other hand, is an unstable rhythm and rarely remains chronic.

ECG criteria for atrial fibrillation are:

- Rate: Atrial rate usually greater then 400 bpm. Ventricular rates usually range from 100 to 150 bpm but can be less than 100 bpm.
- Rhythm: Irregularly irregular
- P wave: No P wave

ECG criteria for atrial flutter are:

- Rate: Atrial rate is rapid and around 250 to 350 bpm. Ventricular rate depends on degree of AV block (usually between half to one quarter of the atrial rate).
- Rhythm: Regular
- P wave: Saw-toothed, referred to as "flutter wave"

BRADYARRHYTHMIAS

Bradyarrhythmia usually refers to sinus bradycardia. Sinus bradycardia is an arrhythmia where the sinus rate is below 60 bpm and all impulses come from the SA node. Sinus bradycardia is usually observed in athletes, most likely due to there increase in vagal tone. It is also noted during sleep, elevation of intracranial pressure, and situations with increased vagal tone such as straining of stool, vomiting, intubation, sick sinus syndrome, and hypothyroidism. Certain medications such as beta-blockers, calcium channel blockers and adenosine may also induce sinus bradycardia.

Ventricular Arrhythmias

VENTRICULAR PREMATURE BEATS (VPBs)

Ventricular premature beats are ectopic ventricular beats that occur earlier than the normally expected beat and is often followed by a compensatory pause. VPBs may be uniform, arising from the same ectopic focus (unifocal), or multiform (multifocal), arising from two or more different ventricular sites. Patients experiencing VPBs may be asymptomatic or may complain of "skipping beats." Depending on a patient's ventricular function and the duration and frequency of the VPBs, a decrease in cardiac output may result. VPBs are more dangerous if they occur in the presence of heart disease. Possible cause of VPBs include digitalis toxicity, hypokalemia, hypocalcemia, and the use of caffeine and other stimulants.

The ECG criterion is a QRS interval that is wide and bizarre in morphology. While most VPBs are benign, certain forms of VPBs may be predictive of potentially serious arrhythmic events (eg, sustained VT). Potentially dangerous VPBs include:

- Couplets, triplets, or more VPBs in a row
- Bigeminy (every other beat is a VPB) and trigeminy (every third beat is a VPB)
- Multifocal VPBs (VPBs with different morphology)
- More than six VPBs in a minute

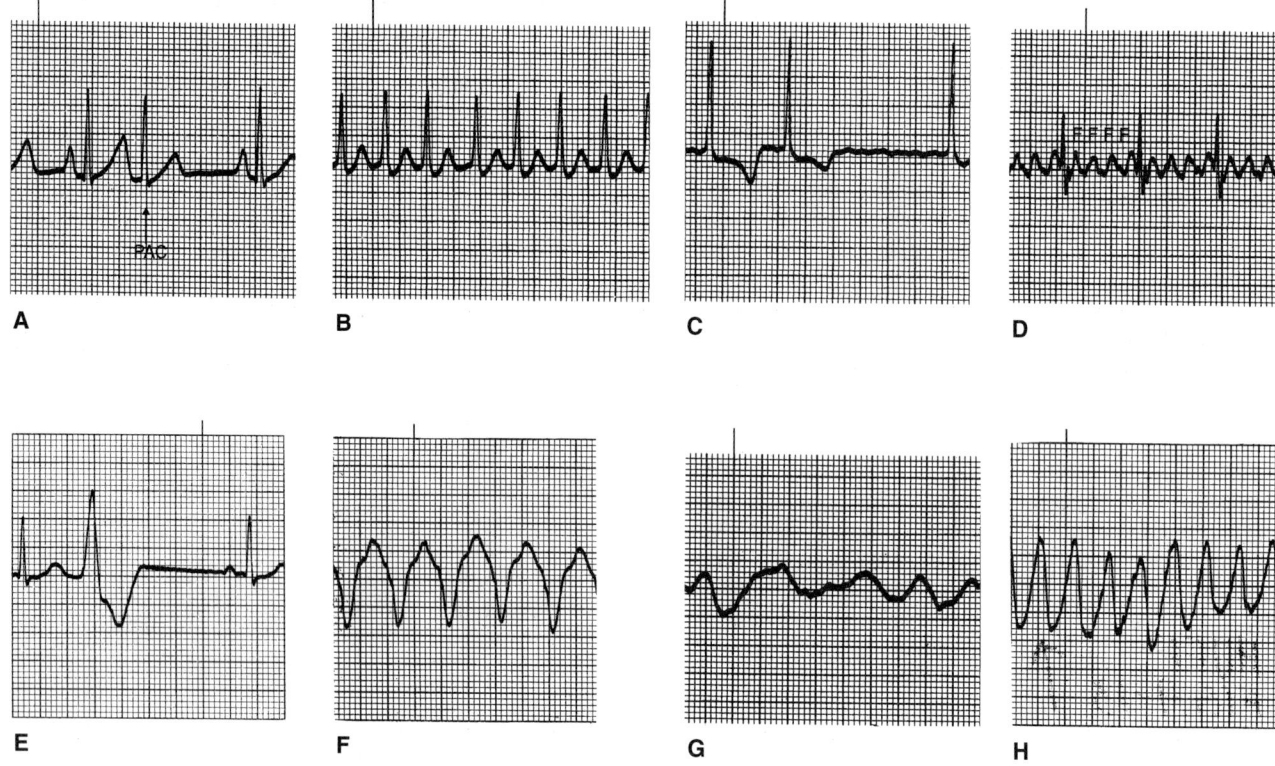

FIGURE 7-4 (**A**) Premature atrial complexes. (**B**) Supraventricular tachycardia. (**C**) Atrial fibrillation. (**D**) Atrial flutter. (**E**) Ventricular premature beats. (**F**) Ventricular tachycardia. (**G**) Ventricular fibrillation. (**H**) Torsades de pointes.

- R-on-T phenomenon: The VPB falls on the preceding beat's T wave. This type of VPB can lead to VT and VF.

VENTRICULAR TACHYCARDIA

Ventricular tachycardia is defined as premature ventricular complexes occurring in succession at a rate of more than 100 bpm. If sustained, cardiac output may drop drastically and the rhythm may deteriorate to VF. Common cardiac causes of VT include acute MI, coronary artery disease, rheumatic heart disease, and cardiomyopathy or heart failure. Other noncardiac causes include pulmonary embolism, electrolyte imbalance (eg, hypokalemia) and drug toxicity (eg, digitalis, procainamide, quinidine, and vasopressors such as epinephrine). If conscious, the patient may complain of palpitations, dizziness, and shortness of breath. Patients usually lose consciousness quickly if VT is rapid and sustained.

ECG criteria are:

- Rate: Atrial rate cannot be determined. Ventricular rate usually betwen 100 to 250 bpm.
- Rhythm: Usually regular; slight irregularity may occur.
- QRS complex: wide and bizarre.

VENTRICULAR FIBRILLATION

Ventricular fibrillation is an arrhythmia marked by rapid, disorganized depolarizations of the ventricles and characterized by a lack of organized electrical impulse, conduction, and ventricular contractions. Patients at risk of developing VF include those with acute MI, untreated VT, electrolyte imbalance (hypokalemia and alkalosis, hyperkalemia and hypercalcemia), electric

shock, and hypothermia. Patients are usually unconscious in this situation and there is an absence of pulse, heart sounds and blood pressure. ECG criteria are an indeterminate rate and a rapid and chaotic rhythm, with no pattern or regularity.

TORSADES DE POINTES

Torsades de pointes is a syndrome characterized by atypical polymorphic VT (the QRS polarity spiral around the isoelectric line) and a prolonged QT interval. Any condition that lead to prolonged QT intervals can precipitate torsades (see Table 7-2). Similar to VT, patients with torsades usually lose consciousness rapidly. If conscious, the patient may complain of palpitations, dizziness, chest pain, or shortness of breath.

ECG criteria are:

- Rate: Atrial rate cannot be determined, ventricular rate varies between 150 to 250 bpm.
- QRS interval: Usually wide with a phasic variation in its electrical polarity, shown by complexes that point downward for several beats, then upward and so on.
- QT intervals of the sinus beat preceding torsades are usually prolonged.

Figure 7-4 illustrates the appearance of the different arrhythmias on the surface ECG.

HISTORY AND PHYSICAL EXAMINATION

A complete medical history and physical examination are extremely important, once patients are stabilized hemodynamically, to rule out underlying causes of any arrhythmia. Elimination of the underlying causes (if possible) is the best management strategy for arrhythmia. The following is information that should be obtained from patients for arrhythmia evaluation:

- Past medical history
- Medication history
- Time of onset of arrhythmia and duration of symptoms
- Symptoms
- Complete physical examination
- Laboratory tests including electrolytes, complete blood count, blood urea nitrogen, serum creatinine, thyroid function test (especially for diagnosing supraventricular arrhythmia).

DIAGNOSTIC STUDIES

The following are diagnostic tests recommended to confirm the diagnosis and differentiate various forms of arrhythmias.

ECG and rhythm strips provide a significant amount of information for the diagnosis of different arrhythmias. They can also be used to confirm or rule out the diagnosis of ischemia/MI, which may induce arrhythmias.

A signal-averaged ECG amplifies the recording of a repetitive waveform from the regular surface ECG, usually the QRS complex, while simultaneously decreasing the random noise (such as skeletal muscle activity) recorded from the body surface. After amplification of the QRS complex, low-amplitude late potentials that occur in the terminal portion of the QRS complex can be detected. These late potentials are thought to be caused by areas of slow and fragmented conduction through damaged ventricular tissue (McCollam & Parker, 1991). The presence of late potentials indicates a high risk of developing VT.

Echocardiography (Echo) is useful to confirm the presence or absence of structural heart diseases, pericardial effusion, ventricular hypertrophy, or wall motion abnormalities. In addition, echo is useful to confirm or rule out intracardiac thrombi. Transesophageal echo, which gives a better view of the atrium, may be more useful if there is concern about a major atrial thrombus. Ruling out intracardiac thrombi is important, especially in the management of atrial fibrillation, when a therapeutic decision has to be made regarding restoration of NSR either electrically or pharmacologically (discussed below).

Holter monitoring or transtelephonic recordings are methods of continuous ECG monitoring used to capture nonsustained symptomatic or asymptomatic runs of arrhythmias.

Electrophysiologic testing (EP) is performed for the management of ventricular arrhythmias. EP is performed in a specialized cardiac catheterization laboratory by venous insertion of electrode catheters into the right side of the heart. Using these catheters, the electrical activity of the heart can be recorded and programmed stimulation can be performed in an attempt to induce the patient's problematic tachycardia (McCollam & Parker, 1991). EP testing can help to identify the site of origin of the arrhythmia, which is essential when surgical, electrical, or chemical ablative therapy is considered. EP also allows the evaluation of the effect of pharmacologic or nonpharmacologic therapy (such as an implantable cardioverter/defibrillator [AICD]).

Other diagnostic tests used to rule out possible etiologies of arrhythmias, such as thyroid function tests (for supraventricular tachycardia [SVT]), electrolytes, and complete blood count, should also be performed.

Special Diagnostic and Treatment Considerations

SUPRAVENTRICULAR ARRHYTHMIAS

To understand the different therapeutic options and specific treatment considerations for the management of supraventricular arrhythmias, one has to first define the goals of treatment.

Goals of Management of Supraventricular Arrhythmias

- *Rapid control of ventricular rate* to eliminate symptoms (such as palpitation [in tachycardia], fatigue, presyncope) and to prevent hemodynamic decompensation and complications.
- *Restoration of NSR*
- *Anticoagulation* (for atrial fibrillation) to prevent thromboembolic event

All three goals may not be achieved or need to be achieved in all patients. Patient cases need to be considered individually based on the underlying cause of the arrhythmia, the duration of arrhythmia, and age.

All patients who experience symptoms of palpitation, fatigue, dizziness and have ECG evidence of a rapid heart rate require some kind of ventricular rate control. Different pharmacologic agents are available to achieve this endpoint. However, based on the age of the patient, the underlying causes of supraventricular arrhythmias, and the presence of other coexisting cardiac conditions, the treatment of choice may be different. For instance, patients with a history of heart failure should use digoxin for rate control while younger patients, who usually have high sympathetic nervous activity, or patients with supraventricular tachyarrhythmias induced by hyperthyroidism, may respond best to beta-blocker therapy. Patients with antidromic WPW should avoid rate control agents that block or slow down AV node conduction. By decreasing AV node conduction, more impulses will be conducted through the fast bypass tract, worsening the tachyarrhythmia.

CLINICAL WARNING: Do not use beta-blockers or calcium channel blockers in antidromic WPW patients.

In the situation of atrial fibrillation, conversion of the irregular rhythm to NSR is important to prevent complications such as heart failure and thromboembolic events (eg, stroke). In terms of conversion of atrial fibrillation to NSR, different factors such as the duration of atrial fibrillation, the size of the atrium, other coexisting cardiac conditions, and the side effect profile of individual antiarrhythmic agents needs to be considered. For instance, in patients with chronic atrial fibrillation (duration >48 hours) and an atrial size of >0.5 cm by echocardiogram, the likelihood of conversion to NSR is slim (Van Gelder et al, 1991). The risk of using antiarrhythmic agents in an attempt to convert atrial fibrillation to NSR therefore outweighs the benefit. For patients with heart failure, amiodarone, which has relatively few negative inotropic effects compared to other alternative agents, should be used.

For adequately anticoagulating patients with atrial fibrillation to prevent thromboembolic events, the duration of atrial fibrillation and the age of the patient again play an important role in the decision. For patients with chronic atrial fibrillation, the likelihood that there is a thrombus in the ventricle is high. Therefore, if it is decided to attempt cardioversion, anticoagulation therapy needs to be administered for 3 weeks before conversion and continued for 4 weeks after restoration of NSR to prevent the precipitation of thromboembolic events during the cardioversion process, when the atrium regains its atrial "kick" (Laupacis et al, 1995). In terms of age, patients older than 75 years are generally more sensitive to the effect of anticoagulation therapy with warfarin. Therefore, a more conservative approach needs to be used when dosing older patients on warfarin. The next section will discuss these issues in greater detail.

VENTRICULAR ARRHYTHMIAS

Patients experiencing VT are generally more hemodynamically unstable than those with SVT. Treatments that lead to fast restoration of NSR are essential. Electrical cardioversion plays a major role in treating patients who are hemodynamically unstable. Because VT originates from the ventricle, agents that primarily target the AV node (eg, digoxin, calcium channel blockers, and beta-blockers) will not be effective in controlling the heart rate. Class I and III antiarrhythmic agents may be effective in restoring NSR.

Choice of agents depends on factors such as onset of action and route of administration of the antiarrhythmic agents, as well as the underlying cause and other concurrent diseases of the patient. For instance, lidocaine is usually used in patients for acute management of VT due to ischemic events such as acute MI. This is because lidocaine is one of the few antiarrhythmic agents that is available in intravenous (IV) form and has a rapid onset of action. Lidocaine is also particularly effective in treating arrhythmias that originate from ischemic tissue. For long-term control of recurrent VT in post MI patients, amiodarone, however, is the drug of choice. This is because amiodarone is the only antiarrhythmic agent that has been proven, not to increase mortality when used in post MI patients (Cairns et al, 1997; Julian et ala, 1997). Class IC agents, such as flecainide and morizicine, and pure class III agents, such as d-sotalol, have been proven to increase mortality when used in patients after MI (Echt et al, 1991; Cardiac Arrhythmia Suppression Trial, 1992; Waldo et al, 1996). For patients who have CHF and VT, amiodarone is the drug of choice because of its relative lack of negative inotropic effects compared to other antiarrhythmic agents.

TREATMENT OPTIONS, EXPECTED OUTCOMES, AND COMPREHENSIVE MANAGEMENT RECOMMENDATIONS

Prevention

PRIMARY PREVENTION

As previously mentioned, most arrhythmias usually occur as a secondary phenomenon associated with other cardiac diseases or systemic abnormalities. Therefore, primary prevention should focus on the prevention and proper management of these underlying abnormalities. Patients should be counseled on consuming a low-fat, low-cholesterol diet to prevent coronary artery disease and to reduce salt consumption to prevent hypertension. Because caffeine and alcohol consumption is also a major systemic cause of arrhythmias, decreased consumption of these agents should also be advocated. In the situation of postcardiac surgery atrial fibrillation, the use of beta-blockers perioperatively has been demonstrated to be beneficial in preventing this arrhythmia (Bauman & Dekker Schoen, 1997; Lauer et al, 1989). Correction of underlying structural abnormalities, such as heart valve replacement, if possible, may also prevent the onset of certain arrhythmias such as atrial fibrillation. In patients with heart failure, proper management to maintain normal fluid and electrolyte status will also prevent both SVT and VT. As previously mentioned, numerous medications and electrolyte abnormalities may induce arrhythmias. Therefore, maintaining normal electrolyte concentrations and avoiding arrhythmogenic agents, especially in patients with other underlying cardiac disorders, will help to prevent arrhythmias.

Secondary Prevention

EARLY DIAGNOSIS, PROMPT TREATMENT, AND DISABILITY LIMITATION

Supraventricular Arrhythmia

Patients who present with supraventricular arrhythmias may be asymptomatic or may complain of classic symptoms such as palpitations (in the case of tachyarrhythmias), shortness of breath, or dizziness. In patients with atrial fibrillation, it is common that the initial or presenting event in an asymptomatic patient is a cerebral or peripheral embolism. If suspected, an evaluation should be performed immediately to confirm the diagnosis to prevent disabling complications. Prolonged untreated SVT can lead to syncope, hypotension, and in the case of tachyarrhythmias heart failure as well. Prolonged continuous atrial fibrillation for more then 48 hours is considered chronic (Takahashi et al, 1981). Chronic atrial fibrillation creates turbulence in the cardiac chambers, which promotes thrombi formation and eventually leads to thromboembolic events. Prompt ventricular rate control and anticoagulation therapy when necessary in atrial fibrillation are essential for preventing devastating consequences.

Ventricular Arrhythmias

Patients with ventricular arrhythmias need to be treated promptly to reverse or prevent hemodynamic instability. However, once the patient is stabilized, it is crucial that further measures be instituted to prevent future similar events. Because most ventricular arrhythmias occur due to underlying causes such as ischemic heart disease, heart failure, or electrolyte or acid–base imbalance, trying to manage these conditions properly will help in preventing future events. For ventricular arrhythmias where underlying causes cannot be easily identified, or in situations where the recurrence rate is deemed to be significant, patients should be referred for EP testing to evaluate the inducibility of the arrhythmia. Secondary prevention management with either pharmacotherapy or devices such as defibrillators should be used in arrhythmias that are easily induced during EP testing.

Tertiary Prevention

Because most arrhythmias have different underlying causes, rehabilitation involves the proper management and recovery from the underlying diseases. Once triggering factors are eliminated or controlled, arrhythmias are usually controlled as well. However, patients who require long-term antiarrhythmic therapy will need to be monitored closely. Patients who have devices placed, such as a pacemaker or defibrillator, will need to be followed-up to ensure that the devices are functioning properly. Patients should also be warned about possible interference between pacemakers, defibrillators, and a strong magnetic field (Moser et al).

MEDICATION REGIMEN

Supraventricular Arrhythmias

Among the different types of supraventricular arrhythmias, PAC is a benign and self-limiting arrhythmia that does not require medical attention in most circumstances. Primary treatment of sinus bradycardia includes removal of the underlying cause (if identified) and placement of a pacemaker. Management of atrial fibrillation, flutter, and PSVT (the most common arrhythmias seen in the primary care setting), however, will be discussed in greater detail in the following sections.

ATRIAL FIBRILLATION/ATRIAL FLUTTER

The three main goals of atrial fibrillation management are control of ventricular rate, restoration of NSR and prevention of thromboembolic events. Patients' symptoms very often direct the therapeutic decision. For instance, in the setting of bothersome palpitations, rapid control of ventricular rate by applying treatment to block the AV node pharmacologically or nonpharmacologically is required. Restoration of NSR may be considered. In contrast, for patients with atrial fibrillation and a controlled ventricular rate, who experience other symptoms such as fatigue or shortness of breath, restoration and maintenance

of NSR should be the primary goal. Patients should always be evaluated for the necessity for anticoagulation based on the duration of atrial fibrillation.

Control of Ventricular Rate

Pharmacotherapeutic agents that slow down conduction and prolong refractoriness in the AV node are frequently used to control symptoms and improve hemodynamics in the setting of atrial fibrillation with rapid ventricular rate (heart rate >120 bpm or if patients are experiencing bothersome symptoms). Commonly used drugs include digoxin, beta-blockers, and calcium channel blockers. Table 7-4 compares and contrasts the advantages and disadvantages and side effects of these agents. Table 7-5 lists the initiating and maximum dosages of these agents. In the presence of severe symptoms, an IV formulation should be administered because of its fast onset of action for rapid control of a ventricular rate. Once patients are stabilized, oral agents can be used for chronic rate control if necessary. In the absence of significant symptoms related to a rapid response of atrial fibrillation, IV medications are not indicated because of the potential of side effects such as hypotension or precipitation of CHF. The choice of agent for each individual patient will be based upon their age and concurrent diseases. For most patients, calcium channel blockers (verapamil and diltiazem only; no dihydropyridines such as nifedipine) should be used as the drug of choice due to their excellent efficacy and relatively rapid onset of action (median time 4 minutes) (Prystowsky et al, 1996). If there is no response when the maximum dose is given, substitute with beta-blockers. In younger patients, who usually have higher sympathetic nervous activity, and patients who develop atrial fibrillation after cardiothoracic surgery, beta-blockers should be used as the drug of first choice. If patients also have heart failure, calcium channel blockers and

TABLE 7-4	Pharmacologic Agents Used for Ventricular Rate Control		
Pharmacologic Agent	Side Effects	Advantages	Disadvantages
Digoxin	Nausea, vomiting, yellow-green halo, cardiac arrhythmia	Use in patients with heart failure; no negative inotropic effects	Slow onset of action, ineffective in patients with increased sympathetic nervous activity
Calcium Channel Blockers			
Verapamil	Constipation, heart block, hypotension	Fast onset, effective	Cause hypotension, may induce or worsen heart failure
Diltiazem	Heart block, hypotension		
Beta-Blockers			
Propranolol Metoprolol Atenolol Esmolol	Hypotension, heart block, fatigue, masking hypoglycemic symptoms in diabetic patients, trigger bronchospasm in patients with asthma/COPD	Fast onset, effective in preventing postoperative atrial fibrillation, effective in patients with high sympathetic nervous activity	Contraindicated in patients with asthma/COPD, cause hypotension, may induce or worsen heart failure
Adenosine	Bronchospasm, heart block	Extremely fast onset of action	Short-acting (half-life: 10 seconds); not for long-term administration

TABLE 7-5	Dosages of Rate-Controlling Agents

DIGOXIN

Loading dose: Total of 1 mg IV, given as 0.5 mg IV × 1, then 0.25 mg IV in 4–6 hrs and another 0.25 mg IV in another 4–6 hrs
Maintenance dose: 0.125–0.5 mg daily IV or PO, adjusted according to serum concentration and patient response

CALCIUM CHANNEL BLOCKERS

Verapamil

Loading dose: 2.5 mg IV bolus over 2 min; may repeat in 5-min intervals until adequate heart rate has been achieved, a total of 15 mg has been administered, or hypotension or signs of CHF develop
Maintenance dose: 2.5–10 mg/hr IV infusion
Change to oral once patient can tolerate PO.

Diltiazem

Loading dose: 0.25 mg/kg IV over 2 min; if response is still inadequate after 15 min, give 0.35 mg/kg over 2 min.
Maintenance dose: 5–15 mg/hr continuous IV infusion
Change to oral when patient can tolerate PO. 5 mg/hr IV = 180 mg/d PO; mg/hr IV = 240 mg/d PO; 11 mg/hr IV = 360 mg/d PO.

BETA-BLOCKERS

Esmolol

Loading dose: 0.5 mg/kg IV over 1 min; may repeat (see titrating scheme below)
Maintenance dose: 50–300 μg/kg/min IV infusion
Dose initiation and titration: Bolus with 0.5 mg/kg over 1 min, then start infusion of 50 μg/kg/min. If response is inadequate after 5 min, rebolus with 0.5 mg/kg over 1 min, then titrate infusion to 100 μg/kg/min. Continue to rebolus with 0.5 mg/kg and increase maintenance infusion by increments of 50 μg/kg/min up to a maximum of 300 μg/kg/min.
Change to an oral beta-blocker once patient can tolerate PO (e.g., metoprolol PO 25–100 mg bid).

beta-blockers have negative inotropic effects and may decrease myocardial contraction; thus, digoxin should be the drug of choice. Digoxin usually has a slower onset of action compared to the other two classes of agents (up to 6 hours) (Prystowsky et al, 1996). Adenosine is another agent that has AV nodal blocking effects. It has extremely fast onset of action (in seconds). Adenosine is available only in an IV formulation. Due to its extremely short half-life (10 seconds), it is considered a very safe agent to use in emergency situations. It has no long-term role in rate control.

In regard to the duration of therapy, if the underlying cause is reversible, therapy should be continued until the underlying cause is treated (eg, rate control for atrial fibrillation induced by excessive alcohol consumption). If the underlying cause is also a long-term irreversible disease such as heart failure, then therapy for rate control may also be required chronically.

Restoration of Normal Sinus Rhythm

Restoration of NSR may improve symptoms and hemodynamics. This is particularly important in certain patient populations, such as those with heart failure, who do not tolerate symptoms associated with atrial fibrillation well. However, not every patient with atrial fibrillation can be successfully converted back to NSR. Factors that determine whether NSR can be restored include the duration of atrial fibrillation, the size of the atrium, and the underlying etiologies of atrial fibrillation. The longer the duration of atrial fibrillation, the less likely it is to be successfully restored to NSR. In new-onset atrial fibrillation, approximately 50% of patients will convert spontaneously

to NSR within 24 to 48 hours of presentation (Falk et al, 1987). The size of the atrium also determines the ease of restoration. Atrial size of more than 4.5 cm measured by echocardiography has a smaller chance of conversion to NSR. Underlying etiologies of atrial fibrillation will determine the duration of antiarrhythmic therapy that the patients may need. Atrial fibrillation from reversible causes usually requires short-term treatment only. In contrast, atrial fibrillation from chronic diseases such as coronary artery disease or CHF usually requires chronic maintenance therapy.

Antiarrhythmic agents that affect atrial electrophysiology can terminate or prevent atrial fibrillation. These include class I antiarrhythmics (sodium channel blockers) such as quinidine, procainamide, propafenone, and flecainide and class III antiarrhythmics (potassium channel blockers) such as amiodarone and sotalol. Table 7-6 summarizes some important properties of different antiarrhythmic agents.

Despite the numerous choices available, the efficacy of these agents is generally still poor. Only 30% of patients receiving procainamide will continue to remain in NSR in 1 year. Approximately 50% of patients will be maintained in NSR with the use of quinidine, propafenone, flecainide, and sotatol (Reimold et al, 1993; Juul-Moller et al, 1990). Amiodarone is considered the most effective agent for refractory, symptomatic recurrent atrial fibrillation; almost 70% of patients will remain in NSR after 1 year (Horowitz et al, 1985). Amiodarone has the most extensive side effect profile among all the antiarrhythmic agents. Some of the important side effects include corneal microdeposits, hypo- or hyperthyroidism, pulmonary fibrosis, hepatitis, nausea and vomiting, and photosensitivity. It is believed that with the dose commonly used to treat atrial fibrillation (200 mg/day), the incidence of these side effects may be lower than anticipated.

The choice of a specific agent depends on the individual patient's underlying disease and the anticipated duration of therapy required. If the patient has never received antiarrhythmic agents before and may only receive antiarrhythmic agents for a short period of time for atrial fibrillation, agents such as procainamide and quinidine can be used. Examples include postoperative atrial fibrillation or atrial fibrillation induced by pneumonia. If long-term maintenance therapy is required, or in the case of refractory atrial fibrillation, class III agents such as sotalol or amiodarone should be used.

Cardiac function is also a factor for consideration when choosing antiarrhythmic agents. Amiodarone is the agent of choice for patients with heart failure or post-MI. The reason for the former is due to its relative lack of negative inotropic effects compared to other antiarrhythmic agents (Singh et al, 1995; Hernan et al, 1994). Amiodarone is the only antiarrhythmic agent that has been proven not to increase mortality in post-MI patients (Pfisterer et al, 1993; Cairn et al, 1991).

Proarrhythmia is a side effect common to all antiarrhythmic agents, often making providers reluctant to use antiarrhythmics. The most common proarrhythmic event reported is torsades de pointes. Patients most at risk are those with ventricular dysfunction, hypokalemia, hypomagnesemia, or baseline prolongation of the QT interval on ECG. It is recommended that patients initially receive antiarrhythmic therapy in a hospital to prevent unexpected proarrhythmic effects. After therapy is stabilized, frequent monitoring of serum potassium concentration and ECG tracings are necessary to ensure safety. Although the mechanism is unclear, amiodarone has been reported as

TABLE 7-6	Classifications of Antiarrhythmic Agents Used for Atrial Fibrillation Management		
Drug	Usual Dosage	Advantages	Disadvantages
Sodium Channel Blockers			Poor effectiveness; most patients eventually return to atrial fibrillation.
Class IA			
Procainamide	PO: 50–100 mg/kg/d every 3–4 hrs (immediate-release form) or every 6–8 hrs (sustained-release form)	Available IV, fast onset	Nausea/vomiting, hypotension, lupus
Quinidine	PO: 19 mg/kg/d (immediate-release form every 6 hrs, extended-release form every 8–12 hrs)		Diarrhea; ↑ mortality
Disopyramide	PO: 5.6 mg/kg/d every 6 hrs (immediate-release form) or every 12 hrs (extended-release form)		Anticholinergic effect
Class IC			
Propafenone	150–300 mg every 8 hrs	More effective than class Ia agents	Exacerbates CHF
Flecainide	100–200 mg every 12 hrs		Exacerbates CHF; ↑ mortality post-MI
Potassium Channel Blockers		Very effective for refractory atrial fibrillation	
Class III			
Amiodarone	Loading dose: approximately 1 g total given as 200 mg PO t.i.d. for 1–3 weeks, then 200 mg/day		Extensive side effect profile
Sotalol	80–160 mg PO every 12 hrs		Proarrhythmia, exacerbates CHF, contraindicated in asthma and COPD
Ibutilide	0.01 mg/kg (up to 1 mg); repeat in 10 min if necessary		For acute conversion to NSR only. No PO form available. Not for long-term use.

the least proarrhythmic agent among all the antiarrhythmics (Lazzara, 1989).

Prevention of Thromboembolic Events
Stroke is the most devastating complication in atrial fibrillation. To prevent such an event, anticoagulation should be considered for any patient without contraindications, who has continuous atrial fibrillation for more than 48 hours and is 65 years or older, and younger patients with the following risk factors: previous thromboembolic events including transient ischemic attack, hypertension, or heart failure. Patients younger than 65 years old with paroxysmal atrial fibrillation (intermittent) should receive aspirin 325 mg/day if there are no concurrent risk factors. Otherwise, warfarin therapy should be considered. Anticoagulation with warfarin has been shown to significantly reduce the incidence of ischemic stroke (Laupacis, 1995). When warfarin therapy is used, doses should be titrated to achieve an International Normalized Ratio (INR) of 2 to 3 to achieve maximum efficacy and minimal risk of bleeding. If faster anticoagulation is necessary, or if the patient is admitted to the hospital, IV heparin therapy can be used first to achieve therapeutic anticoagulation within a short period of time while waiting for warfarin to exert its therapeutic effect (which may take 3–4 days).

Anticoagulation therapy needs to be continued for as long as the patient remains in atrial fibrillation (chronic atrial fibrillation). If cardioversion is attempted, either pharmacologically or electrically, anticoagulation therapy needs to be initiated and continued for 3 weeks before cardioversion (unless atrial fibrillation episodes are less than 48 hours) and continue for 4 weeks after NSR has been restored (Laupacis, 1995). This is to prevent the precipitation of thromboembolic events during cardioversion, when the atrium suddenly regains its atrial "kick" and dislodges any thrombi that may be present at the time of cardioversion. Figure 7-5 presents an algorithm for the management of atrial fibrillation and atrial flutter.

PAROXYSMAL SUPRAVENTRICULAR TACHYCARDIA
Similar to atrial fibrillation and atrial flutter, both pharmacologic and nonpharmacologic methods have been used to treat patients with PSVT. Because PSVT is usually a regular rhythm (unlike atrial fibrillation which is irregular), the main goal of PSVT management is simply to control ventricular heart rate. Depending on where the reentrant circuit and accessory pathways are located, medications used in the treatment of PSVT can be divided into three broad categories: those that directly or indirectly increase vagal tone to the AV node (such as digoxin);

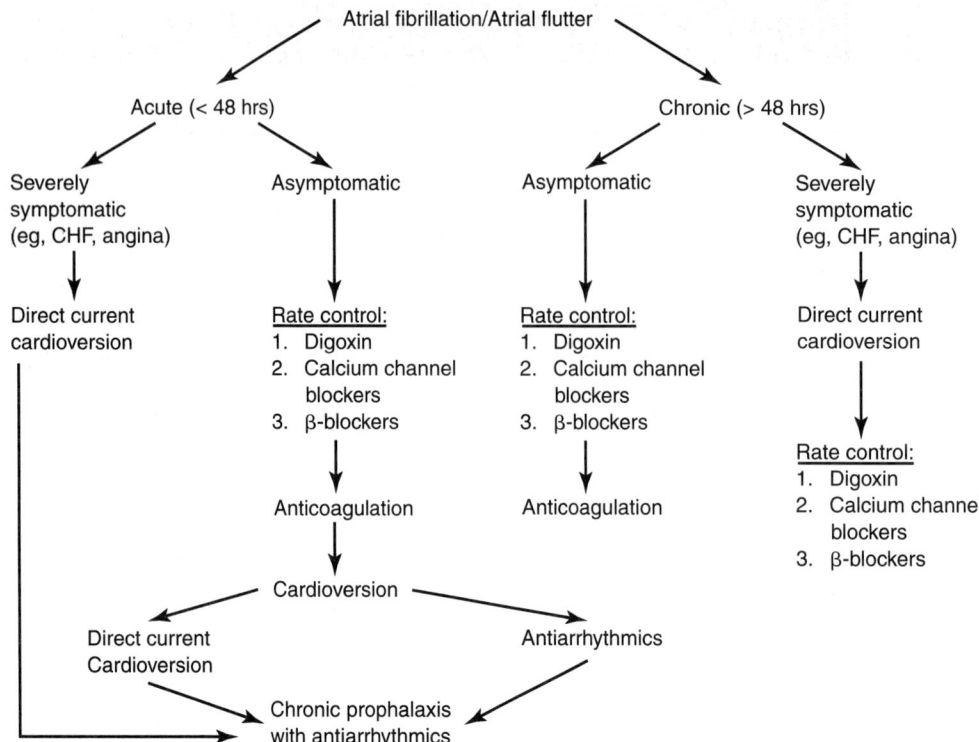

FIGURE 7-5 Algorithm of management of atrial fibrillation and atrial flutter.

those that depress conduction through slow, calcium-dependent tissue (such adenosine, beta-blockers, and calcium channel blockers); and those that depress conduction through fast, sodium-dependent tissue (such as class IA, IC, and III antiarrhythmic agents). In PSVT due to AV re-entry, type IA (eg, procainamide), IC (eg, flecainide), and III (eg, amiodarone) antiarrhythmic agents act primarily on the retrograde fast pathway. Digoxin and beta-blockers may work on either the retrograde fast or the antegrade slow limb. Verapamil, diltiazem and adenosine prolong conduction time and increase refractoriness primarily in the slow antegrade pathway of the reentrant loop.

As in any rapid reentrant tachycardia resulting in hemodynamic instability, synchronized direct cardioversion (DCC) is the treatment of choice. Patients with only mild to moderate symptoms usually do not require DCC; nondrug measures that increase vagal tone to the AV node can be used first. Carotid sinus massage, Valsalva maneuver or ice-water facial immersion are often successful in terminating PSVT (Fig. 7-6).

If vagal maneuvers fail, pharmacotherapy is indicated. Figure 7-6 presents an algorithm for the treatment of acute and chronic PSVT. In patients with narrow QRS intervals, IV verapamil, diltiazem, and adenosine are equally efficacious. Verapamil has an advantage in terms of cost, whereas adenosine may be safer because of its ultrashort duration of action (10 seconds). The most recent American Heart Association emergency care guidelines promote adenosine as the drug of first choice in patients with PSVT (Emergency Cardiac Care Committee, 1992). These recommendations are important especially when treating patients who present with wide QRS intervals, which can represent VT or PSVT due to antidromic AV reentry. In these situations, prolonged blockade of the AV node can lead to severe hemodynamic compromise. The short duration of action of adenosine will minimize this problem. An

alternative treatment for these types of patients would be type IA, IC, or III antiarrhythmic agents, which work on the fast, sodium- or potassium dependent extranodal pathway. Procainamide, amiodarone, and ibutilide are options in this case because of their availability in IV formulation, which allows for a faster onset of action.

Once the acute episode of PSVT is terminated, a decision for long-term preventive therapy must follow. Some patients do not require long-term therapy. Preventive treatment is indicated if frequent episodes occur that necessitate therapeutic intervention, or if infrequent but severely symptomatic symptoms occur. If preventive treatment is necessary, the actual mechanism of the PSVT needs to be defined to determine the most appropriate treatment. EP testing may help in defining the mechanism and distinguishing VT from PSVT. If PSVT is due to AV nodal reentry, digoxin, calcium channel blockers, and beta-blockers are agents of choice. Similar to atrial fibrillation and atrial flutter management, the choice of agent for individual patients will be based upon age and concurrent diseases. For most patients, calcium channel blockers (verapamil and diltiazem only, not dihydropyridines such as nifedipine) should be used as the drug of choice. If the PSVT is caused by AV re-entry, class IA, IC, and III agents should be used.

Ventricular Arrhythmias

VENTRICULAR PREMATURE CONTRACTIONS (VPBs) AND NON-SUSTAINED VENTRICULAR TACHYCARDIA

The occurrence of VPBs and nonsustained VT carries little or no risk to well-being. Treatment is unnecessary as long as the patient is asymptomatic. If the patient becomes symptomatic, beta-blockers can be used. Antiarrhythmic agents should be avoided for VPBs and nonsustained VT management due to

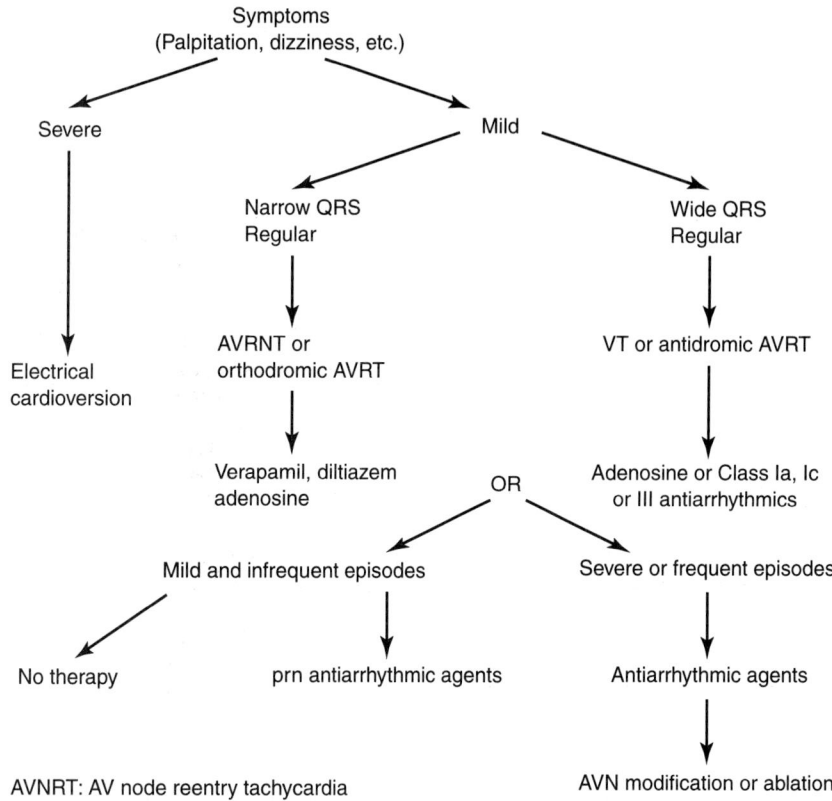

Symptoms
(Palpitation, dizziness, etc.)

Severe — Mild

Narrow QRS
Regular

Wide QRS
Regular

Electrical
cardioversion

AVRNT or
orthodromic AVRT

VT or antidromic AVRT

Verapamil, diltiazem
adenosine

OR

Adenosine or Class Ia, Ic
or III antiarrhythmics

Mild and infrequent episodes

Severe or frequent episodes

No therapy

prn antiarrhythmic agents

Antiarrhythmic agents

AVN modification or ablation

FIGURE 7-6 Algorithm of management of acute and chronic paroxysmal supraventricular tachycardia.

AVNRT: AV node reentry tachycardia
AVRT: AV reentry tachycardia
prn: as necessary

their association with an increased mortality rate (Echt et al, 1991; Cardiac Arrhythmia Suppression Trial, 1992).

VENTRICULAR TACHYCARDIA

Like other rapid tachycardias, the initial management of acute VT requires a quick assessment of the patient's hemodynamic status and symptoms. If the patient is hemodynamically compromised, DCC should be instituted to restore NSR immediately. The diagnosis of acute MI should be considered, since ischemia is the most common cause of VT. If VT is thought to be an isolated electrical event associated with a transient factor, lidocaine can be administered and continued for 24 to 48 hours until the patient is stable. No long-term therapy is needed in this case. Patients should be monitored for side effects of lidocaine, such as tinnitus, central nervous system stimulation (agitation, confusion), and seizures in severe cases.

For patients who have mild or no symptoms during an acute episode, antiarrhythmic agents can be used. Lidocaine is usually considered the drug of choice because of its high degree of effectiveness, quick onset, and ease of administration. If lidocaine fails to terminate the tachycardia, IV procainamide can be used. If patients have heart failure, IV amiodarone should be used after lidocaine, because of its relative lack of negative inotropic effects compared with other antiarrhythmic agents. DCC should be instituted if the patient's status deteriorates, VT degenerates to VF, or drug therapy has failed.

Once an acute episode of VT has been terminated, prevention of recurrence needs to be considered. The possibility of recurrence can often be confirmed by the use of EP testing. Patients with chronic recurrent sustained VT need to be treated

properly to prevent sudden cardiac death. Selection of appropriate therapy depends on specific patient factors and EP testing guidance results. Inability to induce sustained VT with EP testing indicates efficacy of pharmacotherapy. In rare circumstances, patients may require combination antiarrhythmic therapy with resistant VT. Figure 7-7 is an algorithm for VT management.

VENTRICULAR FIBRILLATION

Patients with VF should be managed according to the American Heart Association's recommendations for advanced cardiac life support (Emergency Cardiac Care Committee, 1992). DCC should be immediately instituted and repeated twice (if unsuccessful) before drug therapy. If DCC does not restore a stable rhythm, epinephrine (IV or endotracheally, if an IV line is not available) should be administered before the next DCC. If epinephrine (coupled with DCC) is unsuccessful, lidocaine and then bretylium should be given with DCC repeated as necessary. Figure 7-8 summarizes the advanced cardiac life support algorithm for VF.

Once a patient is resuscitated, antiarrhythmics should be continued until the patient's status is stable. If VF is due to acute MI, long-term antiarrhythmic agents are probably unnecessary. Otherwise, patients should undergo EP testing to determine the most appropriate long-term treatment. Selection for long-term preventive therapy is similar to VT.

TORSADES DE POINTES

Most patients with torsades require DCC for acute stabilization. After that, therapy is necessary to prevent recurrence. Elimination of the underlying cause, such as discontinuing all

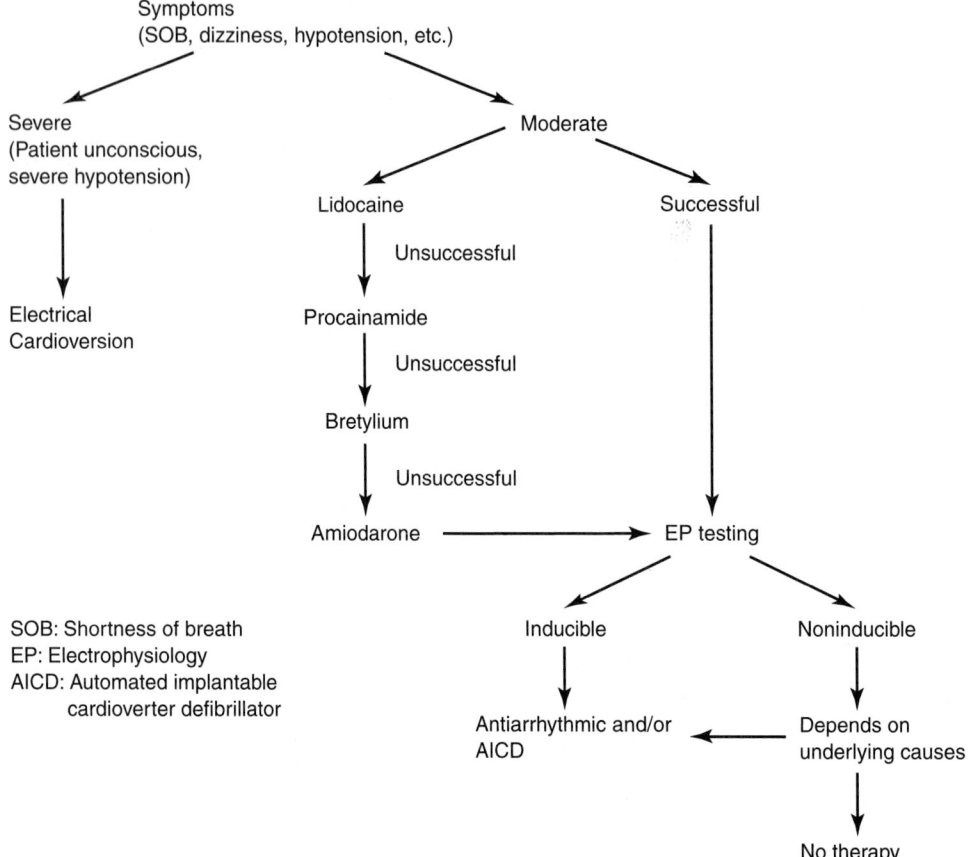

FIGURE 7-7 Algorithm of management of sustained VT.

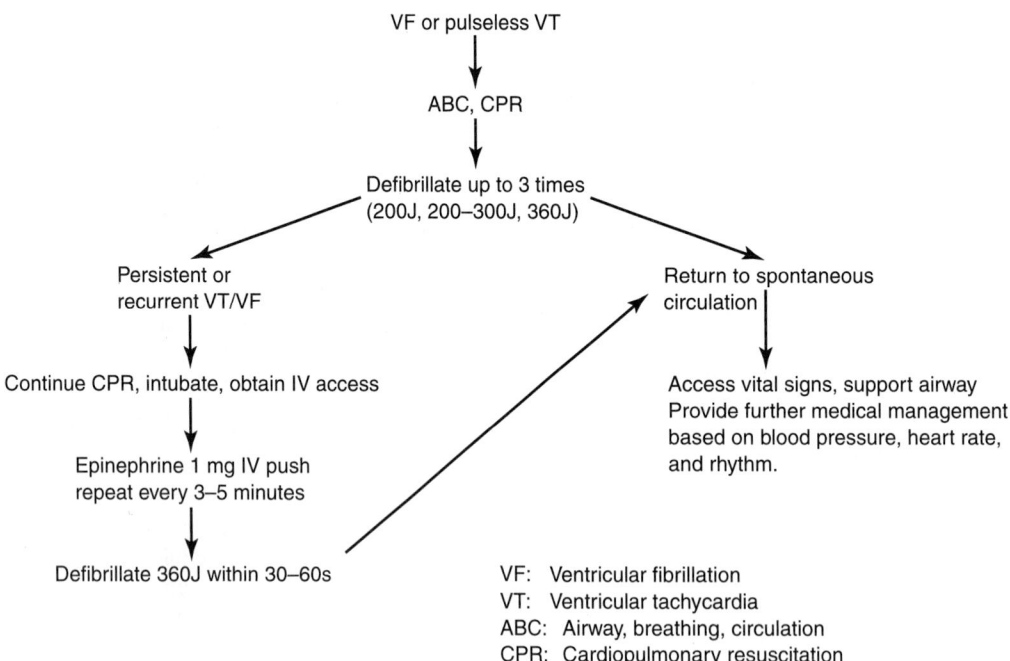

FIGURE 7-8 Algorithm of management of VF.

agents that can lead to prolongation of QT intervals, is the first essential step to prevention. Increasing baseline heart rate and shortening ventricular repolarization is considered preventive therapy. Initial treatments (other then DCC) include temporary transvenous pacing to 100 to 120 bpm. Intravenous magnesium therapy, independent to serum magnesium concentrations, also provides valuable adjunctive therapy.

NONPHARMACOLOGIC INTERVENTION

Supraventricular Tachycardia

Nonpharmacologic methods for management of SVT to control ventricular rate include vagal maneuvers (carotid massage), endocardial catheter ablation or modification of the AV junction and surgically induced AV block (Cardiac Arrhythmia Suppression Trial, 1992). Catheter ablation is recommended in patients who have not responded to or are intolerant of pharmacologic rate control. Nonpharmacologic therapy can also be used to restore NSR. Electrical cardioversion can be used in place of pharmacologic agents for conversion of atrial fibrillation to NSR. This is especially applicable to patients who are hemodynamically unstable and require immediate restoration of NSR. The problem of electrical cardioversion is the short duration of effects: patients often return to atrial fibrillation. Maintenance therapy with antiarrhythmic agents therefore is necessary for patients to remain in NSR. Atrial pacing and endocardial catheter ablation can also be used to prevent atrial fibrillation.

Ventricular Arrhythmia

The development of the automated implantable cardiovertor/defibrillator (AICD) has revolutionized the therapy of VT. An AICD is a device that is placed in the patient's thoracic cavity using transvenous insertion techniques. Newer AICDs provide, in a sequential fashion, programmed stimulation, overdrive pacing, and low-energy cardioversion before internal defibrillation is used. In addition, backup bradycardia pacing and an extended battery life have made these devices much more desirable for VT management. AICDs are recommended for patients with VT resistant to drug therapy or as a backup to drug therapy in the case of breakthrough arrhythmias. As AICD therapy continues to evolve, the exact role of AICD and pharmacotherapies may change.

Intracardial ablation of reentrant circuit in the ventricle has also been used for VT resistant to both pharmacologic and AICD therapy. Its effect on morbidity and mortality, however, still needs to be determined.

TEACHING AND SELF-CARE

After the diagnosis of arrhythmia is made, patients and their families or caregivers need to be counseled regarding:

- Nature of disease: Explanation of arrhythmia, etiology of disease, and expected symptoms
- Vagal maneuvers for patients with SVT: Patients should be taught to do unilateral carotid massage. This may help patients to control and relieve the bothersome symptoms they may experience as an outpatient during future SVT episodes.

- Medications: Effects of medications, dosing and side effects, and the importance of participating in the therapeutic plan should be stressed. Since there are numerous drug interactions for antiarrhythmic agents and warfarin, patients should be advised not to self-medicate before checking with their cardiologist, primary care provider, or community pharmacist.
- Dietary recommendations: Patients receiving antiarrhythmic agents should be advised to maintain a good level of potassium intake to prevent hypokalemia which may put them at risk for developing torsades. As well, patients should be advised not to consume alcohol because alcohol is a triggering factor for atrial fibrillation and will interact with warfarin. Patients who are receiving warfarin also need to be advised to maintain a constant consumption of foods rich in vitamin K such as dark green vegetables. Warfarin exerts its therapeutic effect by inhibiting the production of vitamin K-dependent clotting factors (factors II, VII, IX, and X). Therefore, varying the consumption of vitamin K drastically may produce fluctuation in the effect of warfarin.
- The overall care plan should include input from the patient to enhance the patient's participation in the plan.
- Basic cardiac life support/cardiopulmonary resuscitation: It is advisable that all patients and their family members learn basic cardiac life support to reduce the risk of sudden cardiac death.

COMMUNITY RESOURCES

No support groups are currently available for patients with arrhythmias. However, patients should be encouraged, if interested, to join support groups for their corresponding underlying diseases (eg, heart failure, stroke, or MI). More information regarding individual support groups or other general patient educational materials for heart disease can be obtained from The American Heart Association, 7272 Greenville Ave., Dallas TX 75231-4596 (1-800-AHA-4596; www.amhrt.org). The American Heart Association also sponsors numerous local basic cardiac life support (cardiopulmonary resuscitation) training programs for patients and their family members.

REFERRAL POINTS AND CLINICAL WARNINGS

The hemodynamic status of a patient is the major determinant of whether the patients should be referred to emergency care or a specialist. If the patient is hemodynamically unstable, indicated by one or more of the following clinical signs, immediate referral to emergency care or cardiac specialist is necessary:

- Profound hypotension (systolic blood pressure <90 mmHg)
- Development of signs and symptoms of progressive heart failure
- In the case of SVT, development of VT or VF, and in the case of VT, deterioration to VF
- Changes on ECG signifying myocardial ischemia
- Signs and symptoms of cerebrovascular accident (change in mental status, loss of sensation in extremities, sudden onset of blindness, slurred speech)
- Syncope
- Refractory to pharmacotherapy.

Otherwise, proper control of ventricular rate, anticoagulation to prevent thromboembolic events (in the case of atrial fibrillation) and an attempt at conversion of atrial fibrillation to NSR can be performed while investigating and eliminating the underlying cause of the different arrhythmias.

■ ■ ■   **CLINICAL PEARLS**

■ While the best source of epidemiology data on atrial fibrillation is the Framingham study, the study population may not represent the ethnic and racial diversity in other parts of the country.

■ A situation that will lead to an increase in atrial mass, atrial dilation (in fluid overload states), myocardial injury (in coronary artery disease), increased vagal tone or any other disturbance to the atria (open heart surgery) will increase the risk of developing atrial fibrillation.

■ Transesophageal echo, which gives a better view of the atrium, may be more useful if there is a concern for a major atrial thrombus.

■ Patients who have devices such as a pacemaker or defibrillator should be warned of possible interference between the device and a strong magnetic field.

■ It is recommended that patients initially receive antiarrhythmic therapy in the hospital to prevent expected proarrhythmic effects.

■ The occurrence of ventricular premature contractions and nonsustained ventricular tachycardia conveys little or no risk to the patient's well-being. Treatment is unnecessary as long as the patient is asymptomatic.

EDITOR'S NOTE:

COMPLEMENTARY APPROACHES

A general discussion of complementary approaches can be found in Chapter 3. The following, while not an exhaustive list, are some complementary approaches being used for this condition. Additional information on these approaches, including precautions, can be found in Appendices A and B. Providers need to assess for the use of complementary approaches as part of the patient's history, as they may impact conventional therapies, and patients may not volunteer this information unless specifically asked. Efficacy of many complementary approaches is not as well documented as that of conventional therapies. Providers need to read the literature before suggesting these complementary approaches.

■ Complementary Modalities
  Aromatherapy

References

Bauman, J.L., & Dekker Schoen, M. (1997). The arrhythmias. In: Dipiro, J.T., & Talbert, R.L. (Eds.). *Pharmacotherapy: A pathophysiologic approach*, 3d ed. Stamford: Appleton & Lange; 323–360.

Cairns, J., Connolly, S., Gent, M., & Roberts R. (1991). Post-myocardial infarction mortality in patients with ventricular premature depolarizations. *Circulation, 84*, 550–557.

Cairns, J., Connolly, S., Robin, R., et al. (1997). Randomized trial of outcome after myocardial infarction in patients with frequent or repetitive ventricular premature depolarizations: CAMIAC. *Lancet, 349*, 675–682.

Cardiac Arrhythmia Suppression Trial II Investigators. (1992). Effect of the antiarrhythmic agent moricizine on survival after myocardial infarction. *N Engl J Med, 327*, 227–233.

Echt, D., Philip, L., Mitchell, B., et al. (1991). Mortality and morbidity in patients receiving encainide, flecainide, or placebo. *N Engl J Med, 324*, 781–788.

Emergency Cardiac Care Committee and Subcommittee, American Heart Association. (1992). Guidelines for cardiopulmonary resuscitation and emergency care. *JAMA, 268*, 2219–2241.

Falk, R., Knowlton, A., Bernard, S., Gotlied, N., & Battinelli, N. (1987). Digoxin for converting recent-onset atrial fibrillation to sinus rhythm: A randomized, double-blinded trial. *Annals of Internal Medicine, 106*, 504–506.

Geraets, D., & Kienzle, M. (1993). Atrial fibrillation and atrial flutter. *Clinical Pharmacy, 12*, 721–735.

Hernan, D., Nul, D., Grancelli, H., et al. (1994). Randomized trial of low-dose amiodarone in severe congestive heart failure. *Lancet, 344*, 493–498.

Horowitz, L., Spielman, S., Greenspan, A., et al. (1985). Use of amiodarone in the treatment of persistent and paroxysmal atrial fibrillation resistant to quinidine therapy. *Journal of the American College of Cardiology, 57*, 124–127.

Julian, D., Camm, A., Janse, M., et al. (1997). Randomized trial of effect of amiodarone on mortality in patients with left-ventricular dysfunction after recent myocardial infarction: EMIAC. *Lancet, 349*, 667–674.

Juul-Moller, S., Edvardsson, N., & Rehnqvist-Anlberg, N. (1990). Sotalol versus quinidine for the maintenance of sinus rhythm after direct current conversion of atrial fibrillation. *Circulation, 82*, 1932–1939.

Kannel, W., Abbott, R., Savage, D., & McNamara, P. (1982). Epidemiologic features of chronic atrial fibrillation. *N Engl J Med, 306*, 1018–1022.

Kopecky, S.L., Gersh, B.J., McGoon, M.D., et al. (1987). The natural history of lone atrial fibrillation: A population-based study over three decades. *N Engl J Med, 317*, 669–674.

Lauer, M., Eagle, K., Buckley, M., & DeSanctis, R. (1989). Atrial fibrillation following coronary artery bypass surgery. *Progress in Cardiovascular Diseases, 31*(5), 367–378.

Laupacis, A., Albers, G., Dalen, J., Dunn, M., Feinberg, W., & Jacobson, A. (1995) Antithrombotic therapy in atrial fibrillation. *Chest, 108*(4), 352S–359S.

Lazzara R. (1989). Amiodarone and torsades de pointes. *Annals of Internal Medicine, 111*, 549–551.

McCollam, P.L., & Parker, R.B. (1991). Evaluation and treatment of ventricular arrhythmias. *Clinical Pharmacy, 10*, 195–205.

Moser, S., Crawford, D., & Thomas, A. (1989). Caring for patients with implantable cardioverter defibrillators. *Critical Care Nurse, 8*, 52–64.

Pfisterer, M., Kiowski, W., Brunner, H., Burckhardt, D., & Burkart, F. (1993). Long-term benefit of 1-year amiodarone treatment for persistent complex ventricular arrhythmias after myocardial infarction. *Circulation, 87*, 309–311.

Prystowsky, E., Benson, W., Fuster, V., et al. (1996). Management of patients with atrial fibrillation. *Circulation, 93*, 1262–1277.

Reimold, S., Cantillon, C., Friedman, P., & Antman, E. (1993). Propafenone versus sotalol for suppression of recurrent symptomatic atrial fibrillation. *American Journal of Cardiology, 71*, 558–563.

Singh, S., Fletcher, R., Fisher, S., et al. (1995). Amiodarone in patients with congestive heart failure and asymptomatic ventricular arrhythmia. *N Engl J Med, 333*, 77–82.

Takahashi, N., Seki, A., Imataka, K., & Fujii, J. (1981). Clinical features of paroxysmal atrial fibrillation. *Japan Heart Journal, 22*(2), 143–149.

Van Gelder, I., Crijns, H., Van Gilst, W., et al. (1991). Prediction of uneventful cardioversion and maintenance of sinus rhythm from direct-current electrical cardioversion of chronic atrial fibrillation and flutter. *American Journal of Cardiology, 68*, 41–46.

Waldo, A., Camm, A., deRuyter, H., et al. (1996). Effect of d-sotalol on mortality in patients with left ventricular dysfunction after recent and remote myocardial infarction. *Lancet, 348*, 7–12.

Wolf, P., Abbott, R., & Kannel, W. (1987). Atrial fibrillation: A major contributor to stroke in the elderly: The Framingham study. *Archives of Internal Medicine, 147*, 1561–1564.

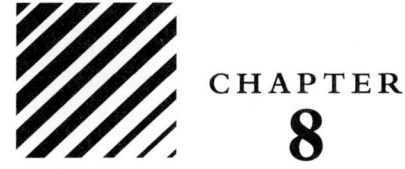

CHAPTER
8
Cardiomyopathies

Sanjeev Vaderah, MD

Cardiomyopathies are a heterogeneous group of disorders that directly affect the heart muscle and cause abnormal myocardial performance. Cardiomyopathies do not include myocardial disease from secondary causes such as valvular heart disease, hypertension, or coronary artery disease. Although some cases of cardiomyopathy have a specific cause such as sarcoid or viral myocarditis, most cases are idiopathic.

Cardiomyopathies may be grouped by etiology, as listed in Table 8-1, or classified by functional class. The functional classification places nearly all cardiomyopathies into one of three groups: dilated (or congestive), hypertrophic, or restrictive. This chapter will review cardiomyopathies using these three major functional classifications because diagnosis, therapy, and management are guided primarily by functional class regardless of etiology.

DILATED CARDIOMYOPATHY

Dilated cardiomyopathy is characterized by left or biventricular dilatation and systolic dysfunction. Idiopathic dilated cardiomyopathy refers to dilated cardiomyopathy in the absence of hypertension or coronary, valvular, or pericardial disease.

Anatomy, Physiology, and Pathology

Abnormalities of both cellular and humoral elements have been implicated in the pathogenesis of dilated cardiomyopathy. Cardioselective M7 antimitochondrial antibodies have been identified in cases of both dilated and hypertrophic cardiomyopathy. A genetic basis has been suggested based on the increased prevalence of HLA B27, HLA A2, HLA DQ4, and HLA DR4 antigens in cases of dilated cardiomyopathy (Anderson, 1984). Dilated cardiomyopathy can occur in healthy patients after a viral myocarditis, and enteroviral RNA sequences have been isolated from pathology specimens.

Ventricular dilatation is the chief morphologic feature. Cardiac mass is increased without ventricular wall thickening. Mural thrombi are often seen in both atria and ventricles. On histology, marked myocyte hypertrophy with large bizarre nuclei, myofilament loss, and varying degrees of replacement fibrosis are seen. These changes do not correlate with disease severity. Coronary arteries are normal (Fuster, 1994).

Epidemiology

The incidence varies from 3 to 10 per 100,000 population depending on the diagnostic criteria used (McKee et al, 1971; Torp, 1978). Dilated cardiomyopathy accounts for almost 20,000 deaths per annum. It can occur at any age, but the peak incidence is in the fourth and fifth decades. African American men have a 2.5 times higher risk than whites and women; this is unexplained by socioeconomic factors (Fuster, 1994).

Diagnostic Criteria

The echocardiogram is the best diagnostic tool. It typically shows dilated ventricles with global hypokinesis. Abnormal ventricular contractility is the *sine qua non* of idiopathic dilated cardiomyopathy and an ejection fraction less than 45% is generally required for diagnosis (Fuster, 1994).

History and Physical Examination

Dilated cardiomyopathy presents with symptoms of congestive heart failure (eg, exertional dyspnea, paroxysmal nocturnal dyspnea, orthopnea, peripheral edema). Abdominal pain from hepatic congestion may be present. Exertional chest pain indistinguishable from angina is present in almost a third of patients and may represent a reduced coronary reserve. Systemic and pulmonary emboli may also occur.

On the physical examination, resting tachycardia is commonly seen. Hemodynamics may be normal initially, but with the onset of heart failure, a narrow pulse pressure, pulsus alternans, and hypotension may be present. An S_4 and murmurs of mitral or tricuspid regurgitation (because of the effect of chamber dilatation on valvular annulus) are common, and with advanced disease an S_3 is heard. Cool, pale extremities are a subtle sign of systemic hypoperfusion.

Diagnostic Studies

The chest x-ray may show cardiomegaly, pulmonary vascular congestion, and pleural effusions. No characteristic abnormalities are present on the electrocardiogram; however, nonspecific ST–T changes and conduction abnormalities are commonly seen.

Echocardiography is an excellent tool for diagnosis. Ventricular mass, chamber dimensions, and cardiac function can all be accurately assessed noninvasively. Cardiac catheterization should be considered in most patients with risk factors for coronary artery disease or regional wall motion abnormalities on echocardiogram to exclude coronary artery disease, which may be reversible.

The main purpose of RV biopsy is to distinguish idiopathic dilated cardiomyopathy from myocarditis. However, given its low diagnostic yield and lack of effective therapy for myocarditis, its role in clinical management is being re-evaluated.

TABLE 8-1	Etiologic Classification of Cardiomyopathy

INFLAMMATORY
Viral
Postpartum
Bacterial
Lyme
Fungal
Giant cell

METABOLIC
Hypothyroid/hyperthyroid
Carcinoid
Uremia
Storage diseases
Hurler's, Hunter's, Gaucher's, Pompe's diseases
Deficiency states
Beriberi, selenium, hypophosphatemia

COLLAGEN VASCULAR DISEASES
Systemic lupus erythematosus
Rheumatoid arthritis
Kawasaki disease
Polyarteritis nodosa

TOXINS
Alcohol
Doxorubicin
Heavy metals

MISCELLANEOUS
Amyloid
Muscular dystrophy

Treatment Options and Expected Outcomes

A few causes of dilated cardiomyopathy (eg, endocrine and nutritional disorders) are reversible, and there are specific therapies for these. However, most cases are irreversible and therapy is supportive, identical to that for congestive heart failure.

Vasodilators, diuretics, and salt and fluid restriction are the mainstay of therapy. Angiotensin-converting enzyme (ACE) inhibitors have been shown to reduce the mortality rate. A combination of isosorbide and hydralazine has similar benefits in patients who cannot tolerate ACE inhibitors.

Digoxin is the drug of choice to control the heart rate in atrial fibrillation. There is controversy about the role of digoxin in patients in sinus rhythm. Digoxin reduces symptoms and may reduce hospitalizations for congestive heart failure exacerbation (Digitalis Investigators Group, 1997).

Data have suggested that beta-blockers may improve hemodynamics and reduce the mortality rate. Potential mechanisms for benefit are protection from catecholamine toxicity, upregulation of myocardial beta-receptors, reduction in heart rate, and reduction in afterload (Schalant,). Care must be taken to avoid precipitation of heart failure with beta-blockers. Carvedilol, an agent with both alpha- and beta-blocking properties, has demonstrated a significant reduction in the mortality rate from heart failure in clinical trials. Gradual increases in dosage and careful monitoring are mandatory whenever a beta-blocker is started in a patient with a dilated cardiomyopathy to avoid exacerbation of congestive hearth failure (Packer, 1996).

Although nonsustained ventricular tachycardia is commonly seen on Holter monitoring, routine antiarrhythmic therapy is not recommended. Patients with sustained ventricular tachycardia or syncope should undergo electrophysiologic stress testing and be considered for an automatic implantable cardioverter/defibrillator.

Chronic oral anticoagulation should be considered because of the high incidence of mural thrombi (*Circulation*, 1988), and the International Normalized Ratio (INR) should be maintained between 2 and 3.

Dilated cardiomyopathy is the most common indication for cardiac transplantation. This should be considered in younger patients with refractory heart failure and minimal comorbid conditions.

The prognosis of cardiomyopathy is variable and may depend on the underlying etiology. Stabilization or even improvement is seen in 20% to 50% of cases. With the onset of heart failure, the prognosis is similar to that of heart failure from other causes. The annual mortality rate is 25%, and the 5-year mortality rate is 40% to 80%. Specific indicators of a poor prognosis include persistent S_3 gallop, New York Heart Association class IV, low ejection fraction, severe ventricular dilatation, hyponatremia, and elevated ANF levels (Fuster, 1994; Braunwald,).

Teaching and Self-Care

Effective management of heart failure requires patient motivation and education. Patient participation in medication and diet regimens is important. Patients should be encouraged to stop smoking, drinking, and using illicit drugs. Patients with compensated heart failure can enroll in an exercise program. Increasing exertional dyspnea, progressive orthopnea, nocturnal frequency of urination, paroxysmal nocturnal dyspnea, and swelling of the legs are all signs of worsening heart failure, and patients should be advised to seek medical attention if they notice these signs.

HYPERTROPHIC CARDIOMYOPATHY

Hypertrophic cardiomyopathy is characterized by an abnormally hypertrophied, nondilated ventricle in the absence of any secondary precipitating factors, such as hypertension. Hypertrophy may be symmetrical, involving the entire ventricle proportionately, or may involve only the septum or the apex.

Anatomy, Physiology, and Pathology

The increased ventricular mass leads to impairment of cardiac function. The left ventricular (LV) outflow can become obstructed because the hypertrophied septum and the mitral valve obstruct the ventricular outflow tract during systole. The thickened myocardium also impairs ventricular relaxation and causes diastolic dysfunction. Increased metabolic demands and abnormal intramural arteries may result in myocardial ischemia. The hypertrophied and disorganized myocardium can also provide a substrate for initiation of a potentially lethal arrhythmia.

In about 55% of cases, the hypertrophy is diffuse and involves the septum and the free posterior and anterolateral walls. In other cases it is localized to the septum; an apical form has been described in Japanese patients. Chief histologic features include cardiac muscle cell disorganization, replacement fibrosis, and abnormal intramural coronary arteries.

Epidemiology

The exact incidence of hypertrophic cardiomyopathy is unknown, but it is estimated to be present in 0.1% to 0.2% of the general population (Spirito, 1989, 1997). Most cases go unrecognized. Hypertrophic cardiomyopathy can manifest at any age, including infancy. More than 50 mutations have been described in one of the four genes that encode for the cardiac sarcomeres. The precise molecular defect in hypertrophic cardiomyopathy can vary markedly among patients.

History and Physical Examination

Most patients are asymptomatic or mildly symptomatic and are often identified incidentally (eg, during screening of relatives of a known case). Patients present with dyspnea, chest pain, or postexertional syncope when the diastolic filling is reduced and outflow obstruction is increased. Arrhythmias such as atrial fibrillation are very common and result from chronically elevated left atrial pressures. Ventricular arrhythmias are less common but can result in sudden cardiac death.

On physical examination, a sustained apical impulse, a loud S_4, and a systolic ejection murmur may be present. The murmur increases in intensity with maneuvers that increase the gradient across the aortic valve, such as Valsalva, upright posture, sympathetic stimulation, and amyl nitrate administration, and decreases with squatting.

Diagnostic Studies

As in dilated cardiomyopathy, the echocardiogram is invaluable. It reveals a small, hypercontractile chamber and increased chamber thickness, in a symmetrical or asymmetrical distribution. The LV outflow tract becomes obstructed by the hypertrophied septum and systolic anterior motion of the mitral valve into the LV outflow tract during systole. Doppler studies across the aortic valve reveal a dynamic gradient that increases markedly with amyl nitrate administration. Left ventricular hypertrophy is invariably present on the electrocardiogram. Prominent septal Q waves may suggest myocardial infarction.

Treatment Options and Expected Outcomes

Beta-blockers and calcium channel blockers are the mainstay of therapy. They improve ventricular filling and decrease the gradient across the aortic valve. Neither one of these agents causes a reversal of hypertrophy. Prophylactic therapy with these agents in high-risk patients has not been studied (Spirito, 1989).

Prevention of sudden cardiac death is an important concern in the management of these patients. Because syncope may be caused by mechanisms other than arrhythmia in these patients, a single episode of syncope should be evaluated conservatively with Holter monitoring or a tilt-table test. Patients with repeated episodes of syncope without an identifiable etiology should be considered for invasive electrophysiologic testing. Electrophysiologic studies have not convincingly been shown to identify patients at risk for sudden cardiac death; however, patients at high risk for arrhythmias should receive antiarrhythmic therapy or have a cardioverter/defibrillator implanted.

Patients with a significant (>50 mmHg) gradient across the aortic valve and symptoms refractory to medical therapy are candidates for a myotomy or myomectomy. These procedures can result in complete resolution of the gradient.

Certain nonsurgical procedures have been tried with varying degrees of success. Dual chamber pacing may reduce the gradient and improve hemodynamics by altering contraction sequence patterns within the ventricle (Fananpazir, 1994). Embolization of the first major septal branch of the LAD with alcohol can also be performed to reduce septal contractility and minimize the outflow tract gradient. Patients with end-stage disease, as evidenced by LV thinning and chamber dilatation with systolic dysfunction, are treated with vasodilators and diuretics, as described above for dilated cardiomyopathies.

The 3% to 6% annual mortality rate is probably an overestimate. In unselected cases, the annual mortality rate is closer to 1%. Some patients remain asymptomatic throughout life, whereas others develop progressive symptoms.

Prevention

Although the disease cannot be prevented, symptoms may be reduced or prevented. The presence of certain features may portend a less benign course and can identify patients who require earlier intervention. These features include a family history of premature cardiac death from hypertrophic cardiomyopathy, nonsustained ventricular tachycardia, a significant gradient across the aortic valve (>50 mmHg), left atrial enlargement, and an abnormal blood-pressure response on exercise. These patients should avoid competitive sports and vigorous training but can participate in recreational sports. Asymptomatic patients, in the absence of these features, can be followed and need no restrictions on recreational sports and employment. They should, however, avoid intensive training and competitive sports (Spirito, 1989).

Genetic diagnosis in the future may be used to identify and possibly to alter the clinical course in patients with a more severe form of mutation (eg, Arg 403 Glu, which appears to be associated with reduced survival).

RESTRICTIVE CARDIOMYOPATHY

Restrictive cardiomyopathy is a disorder of cardiac muscle that results in increased stiffness, leading to impaired diastolic filling of the ventricles with normal or reduced ventricular volume and preserved ventricular function. It is the least common form of cardiomyopathy (Ableman, 1984). Its principal importance lies in properly distinguishing it from constrictive pericarditis.

Anatomy, Physiology, and Pathology

Restrictive cardiomyopathy may be idiopathic or secondary to infiltrative diseases, radiation, or drugs. The idiopathic form is characterized by a mild to moderate increase in the cardiac mass and biatrial enlargement. Thrombi may be present in the appendage. Patchy endomyocardial fibrosis is seen (Fuster, 1997).

Of the infiltrative disorders, amyloid is the most common—specifically primary amyloidosis. The abnormal increase in circulating amyloid IgG light chains leads to replacement of normal contractile elements in the myocardium by infiltrative

TABLE 8-2	Causes of Restrictive Cardiomyopathy

Idiopathic

Familial

Amyloidosis

Sarcoidosis

Gaucher's disease

Hemochromatosis

Glycogen storage disorders

Endomyocardial fibrosis

Radiation carcinoid

Posttransplant

Drugs (ergot, busulfan)

interstitial deposits. Amyloid deposition leaves the myocardium rubbery and noncompliant, with an increased wall thickness. The many causes of restrictive cardiomyopathy are listed in Table 8-2 and should be considered in the differential diagnosis.

History and Physical Examination

The primary diagnostic challenge is in distinguishing restrictive cardiomyopathy from constrictive pericarditis. In the history, tuberculosis, collagen vascular disorders, prior surgery, or pericarditis all favor constrictive pericarditis. On the physical examination, an S_3 is present in restrictive cardiomyopathy, a pericardial knock in constrictive pericarditis. Kussmaul's sign is seen more commonly in constrictive pericarditis.

On the electrocardiogram, low-voltage complexes, left axis deviation, and atrial fibrillation are commonly seen in restrictive cardiomyopathy. The presence of a bundle branch block favors the diagnosis of restrictive cardiomyopathy over constrictive pericarditis. On the chest x-ray, a normal-size cardiac silhouette with evidence of pulmonary vascular congestion is typical. The presence of pericardial calcification favors constrictive pericarditis. Occasionally a cardiac biopsy is used to distinguish restrictive cardiomyopathy from constrictive pericarditis.

Diagnostic Studies

Restrictive cardiomyopathy should be considered in patients with features of congestive hearth failure with normal systolic function and without evidence of cardiomegaly or hypertrophy. Jugular venous distention is common with a prominent x and y descents. Echocardiography shows a normal-size heart with no valvular lesions. Doppler echocardiography shows an increased E:A ratio on mitral inflow velocities. During cardiac catheterization, the classic feature is the "dip and plateau" pattern or the "square root sign" on the ventricular pressure tracing.

Treatment Options and Expected Outcomes

Preload reduction with diuretics and nitrates is used to relieve symptoms of pulmonary congestion. Excessive diuresis, however, can lead to reduced cardiac output. Digoxin is used with caution because it is potentially arrhythmogenic. Steroids may be used for patients with sarcoidosis and Löffler's syndrome. Cardiac transplantation may be considered in patients with the idiopathic form of the disease.

COMMUNITY RESOURCES

Resources include the following:

- The American Heart Association, 7272 Greenville Ave., Dallas, TX 75231; www.amhrt.org
- Heart Home Page: www.hearthome.com
- Community Outreach Health Information System: www.bu.edu/COHIS/cardvasc/cvd.htm
- Hypertrophic Cardiomyopathy Association: www.kanter.com/

CLINICAL WARNINGS AND REFERRAL POINTS

In several circumstances, patients with cardiomyopathies should be referred to other providers. If sustained ventricular tachycardia or syncope occurs, the patient should be referred to a cardiologist. Patients with refractory heart failure and minimum comorbid conditions should be referred to a cardiac surgeon for transplantation consideration.

■ ■ ■ CLINICAL PEARLS

- In patients with dilated cardiomyopathy, although non-sustained ventricular tachycardia is commonly seen on holter monitoring, routine antiarrhythmic therapy is not recommended.
- Patients with hypertrophic cardiomyopathy may be asymptomatic or mildly symptomatic and are often identified incidentally (i.e., during screening of relatives of a known case).
- Restrictive cardiomyopathy must be distinguished from constrictive pericarditis. On physical exam a S3 is present in restrictive cardiomyopathy while a pericardial knock is present in constrictive pericarditis.

EDITOR'S NOTE:
COMPLEMENTARY APPROACHES

A general discussion of complementary approaches can be found in Chapter 3. The following, while not an exhaustive list, are some complementary approaches being used for this condition. Additional information on these approaches, including precautions, can be found in Appendices A and B. Providers need to assess for the use of complementary approaches as part of the patient's history, as they may impact conventional therapies, and patients may not volunteer this information unless specifically asked. Efficacy of many complementary approaches is not as well documented as that of conventional therapies. Providers need to read the literature before suggesting these complementary approaches.

- Vitamins, minerals, herbs, supplements
  Carnitine
  Coenzyme Q10

References

Ableman, W.H. (1984). *Progress in Cardiovascular Diseases, 27,* 73–94.

Anderson, J.L. (1984). *American Journal of Cardiology, 33;* 1326–1330.

Braunwald, E. In *Heart Disease*, 4th ed, pp. 1398–1420

Digitalis Investigators Group. (1997). *N Engl J Med, 336,* 525–532.

Fananpazir, L. (1994). *Circulation, 90,* 2731.

Fuster, V. (1994). *N Engl J Med, 331,* 1564–1574.

Fuster, V. (1997). *N Engl J Med, 336,* 267–275.

McKee, P.A., et al. (1971). *N Engl J Med, 285,* 141–146.

Packer, M. (1996). *N Engl J Med, 334,* 1349–1355.

Schalant, R.L. In Hurst's *The Heart*, 8th ed, p. 1616.

Spirito, P, (1989). *N Engl J Med, 320,* 747–755.

Spirito, P. (1997). *N Engl J Med, 336,* 775–783.

Torp, A. (1978). *Postgraduate Medical Journal, 54,* 435–437.

(1988). *Circulation,* 1388.

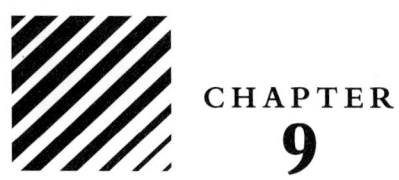

CHAPTER
9

Coronary Artery Disease in Primary Care

Joseph J. DeRose, Sr., MD, Joseph J. DeRose, Jr., MD, and Marielaina S. DeRose, MD

Mortality from cardiovascular disease has declined significantly from the early 1970s until today (National Institute of Health, 1994). In the period from 1980 to 1988 the age-adjusted ischemic heart disease death rate for patients older than 35 years of age fell 24%, from 588.3 to 448.8 per 100,000 (American Heart Association, 1991). Despite these marked reductions, coronary artery disease (CAD) remains the number-one cause of death in the United States for both men and women. Approximately 900,000 cases of acute myocardial infarction (MI) occur annually, resulting in nearly 250,000 deaths (Farmer & Gotto, 1997). The costs of traditional present care are estimated at $8 to $10 billion annually, and 50% of patients admitted to the hospital for possible acute ischemic CAD are found to have noncardiac causes. As such, CAD remains an enormous public health problem, and its evaluation and management remain a major clinical challenge.

Knowledge of the etiology, pathogenesis, clinical manifestations, diagnosis, and treatment of CAD has grown considerably. It remains the responsibility of the primary care provider not only to recognize patients with cardiac chest pain but also to identify and treat risk factors associated with CAD in asymptomatic patients. It is hoped that preventive guidelines will reduce both the morbidity and mortality rates of this disease.

ANATOMY, PHYSIOLOGY, AND PATHOLOGY

Coronary Anatomy

The right coronary artery and left coronary artery are the two major arterial trunks that originate from the aortic root to supply the myocardium. Functionally, the coronary circulation is divided into the right coronary artery, which perfuses the right ventricle; the left anterior descending branch of the left coronary artery, which supplies the anterior wall of the left ventricle and the anterior septum; and the circumflex branch of the left coronary artery, which perfuses the lateral wall of the left ventricle (Fig. 9-1). These are the three territories that clinicians frequently refer to as "triple-vessel disease" when describing coronary artery pathology.

The coronary circulation is referred to as "right dominant" when the major vessel supplying the posterior aspect of the left ventricle, the posterior descending artery, originates from the right coronary artery. In contrast, a "left dominant" coronary circulation is one in which the circumflex artery gives rise to the posterior descending artery. Seventy-five percent of patients have a right dominant circulation, 15% of patients are left dominant, and 10% of patients have a balanced coronary circulation (Kirklin & Barratt-Boyes, 1993).

The arteriosclerotic process usually affects multiple coronary arteries. Among all patients undergoing coronary angiography,

40% have all three vessels affected; approximately 30% have disease in two vessels. The main trunk of the left coronary artery has a significant stenosis in 10% to 20% of patients undergoing angiography (Gensini, 1975). The disease process usually affects the proximal portions of larger coronary arteries at or just beyond the sites of branching. When the disease is more extensive, the secondary distal branches of the larger coronary arteries may be affected, rendering them unsuitable for interventional or surgical revascularization procedures (Kirklin & Barratt-Boyes, 1993; Gensini, 1975).

Arterial Physiology

The arterial tree is more than just a series of conduits through which blood travels to the various organs. Rather, both normal and diseased arteries are capable of complex biologic processes involved in hemostasis, cytokine and growth factor secretion, permeability, metabolism of vasoactive substances, connective tissue formation, lipid metabolism, and cellular proliferation.

The normal artery is composed of three layers: intima, media, and adventitia. A single cell layer of endothelial cells lines the luminal aspect of the blood vessel and makes up the intima. Endothelial cell integrity is critical for maintaining a permeability barrier between the blood and the extracellular tissues. Endothelial cells are also responsible for providing an intraluminal nonthrombogenic surface. They secrete a wide range of vasoactive substances, including endothelial-derived relaxing factor, prostacyclin, endothelin, angiotensin-converting enzyme, and platelet-derived growth factor. A special capacity of endothelium particularly important in atherogenesis is its ability to modify lipoproteins. Low-density lipoproteins (LDLs) can be bound by LDL receptors on endothelial cells, internalized, and modified. Modified LDLs can then bind to scavenger receptors on the surface of macrophages to form foam cells, an important contributor to the atherosclerotic plaque (Krieger, 1995).

The muscular layer of the artery is termed the media and is composed of smooth muscle cells. These smooth muscle cells normally exist in a quiescent state and exhibit a contractile phenotype that is capable of altering blood vessel tone. Like endothelial cells, these smooth muscle cells exhibit LDL receptors and are capable of lipoprotein modification and presentation to macrophages. With overlying endothelial denudation or injury, medial smooth muscle cells are capable of responding to a variety of mitogens and chemoattractants. The quiescent contractile smooth muscle cell can then be stimulated to differentiate into a proliferative phenotype that can migrate into the intima, divide, and secrete extracellular matrix (Krieger, 1995; Ross, 1993).

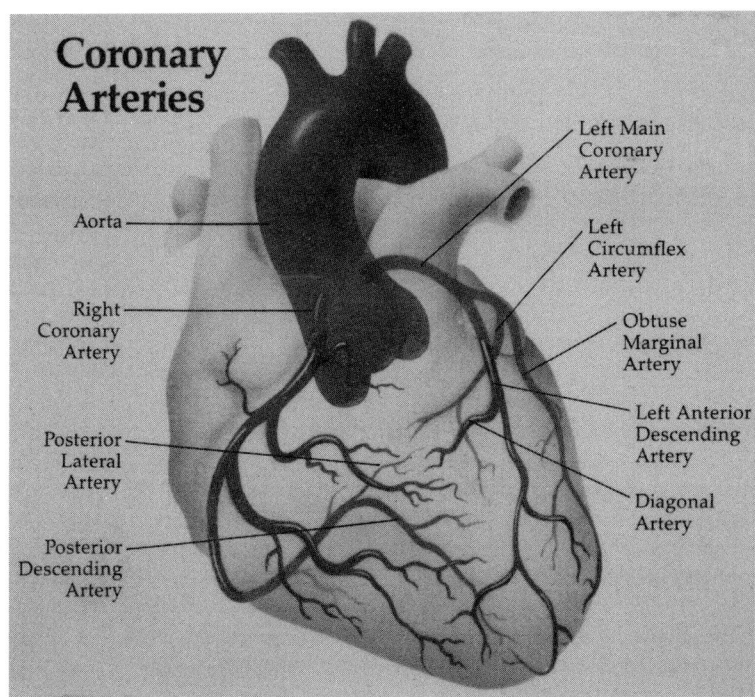

FIGURE 9-1 Coronary arterial anatomy. The three major arterial distributions include the right coronary artery, the left anterior descending artery, and the circumflex artery.

The outermost layer of the vessel wall, the adventitia, is composed of a thin layer of collagen and fibroblasts. Although once thought to be a biologically inactive layer, it is now being recognized that adventitial fibroblasts participate in the processes of atherogenesis and arterial restenosis. Differentiation of adventitial fibroblasts into myofibroblasts can result in remodeling of the vessel wall. Adventitial myofibroblasts may serve to decrease vessel size in the process of atherogenesis and arterial restenosis, not unlike their role in wound contraction during wound healing (Gibbons & Dzau, 1994).

Process of Atherogenesis

Endothelial injury is the inciting event in the generation of luminal stenosis. Disruption of the endothelial lining exposes the circulating blood elements to the underlying thrombogenic surface of the media. Platelets readily adhere to this surface and release mitogens and growth factors. Medial smooth muscle cells are stimulated to migrate into the intima, proliferate, and secrete extracellular matrix, resulting in intraluminal stenosis. Lymphocytes are also attracted to the site of injury, resulting in continued cytokine release and antigen presentation. This response to the injury process is responsible for restenosis after angioplasty and coronary artery bypass grafting (CABG), as well as the transplant atherosclerosis seen in immunologically injured endothelium of heart transplants (Ross, 1993; Gibbons & Dzau, 1994; Badimon et al, 1993).

The cause of endothelial injury in primary atherosclerosis is most commonly secondary to hyperlipidemia (Ross, 1993; Gibbons & Dzau, 1994). Circulating lipoproteins, especially LDLs, can be taken up by endothelial cells and medial smooth muscle cells. After modification and presentation, resident macrophages scavenge the modified LDLs and oxidize them. Lipid-laden macrophages in the subendothelium are responsible for the earliest lesion of arteriosclerosis, termed the fatty streak. Grossly, this appears as an area of yellow discoloration

on the luminal aspect of the artery. The fatty streak is seen as early as late childhood and young adulthood and is anatomically distributed in areas ultimately affected with progressive atherosclerosis.

Oxidation of LDLs by macrophages leads to toxic injury to the endothelium through generation of superoxide radicals. This endothelial injury, together with secretion of numerous growth factors by these activated macrophages, sets into motion the cascade of smooth muscle cell activation. The resulting lesion is a fibrous plaque composed of large numbers of intimal smooth muscle cells, collagen fibers, macrophages, and lymphocytes. Continued lipid uptake results in intracellular and extracellular accumulations of cholesterol esters. Progressive growth of the fibrous plaque results in slow stenosis of the arterial lumen and eventual occlusion.

Endothelial injury in atherogenesis may also occur in response to flow dynamics associated with hypertension, glycosylation associated with diabetes, superoxide production involved in cigarette smoking, and primary viral injury from cytomegalovirus infection (Badimon et al, 1993). Although the mechanisms of endothelial injury operating in these coronary risk factors are not clearly elucidated, the cascade of proliferation and the final pathologic pathway all remain the same.

Thrombosis and Plaque Stability

Continued injury to the endothelium results in worsening endothelial dysfunction. The permeability barrier created by the endothelium is lost, and the balance between intraluminal anticoagulant and procoagulant properties is disrupted (Loscalzo, 1992). Rupture of the endothelial lining of an atherosclerotic plaque can result in intramural hemorrhage, exposure of subintimal collagen, and intraluminal thrombosis. In contrast to the slow luminal reduction caused by the progressing atherosclerotic plaque, plaque rupture and thrombosis results in acute vessel closure. Without the time necessary for compensatory collateral formation and angiogenesis, plaque rupture results in acute myocardial ischemia and potential myocardial cell death.

Coronary Blood Flow and Myocardial Ischemia

Ischemia refers to the inadequate delivery of oxygen to the myocardium, accompanied by an inadequate removal of metabolites consequent to reduced perfusion. Myocardial ischemia is the result of an imbalance between myocardial oxygen demand and myocardial oxygen supply. The therapies for CAD are aimed at re-establishing this balance by decreasing myocardial oxygen consumption, increasing coronary blood flow, or both.

DETERMINANTS OF MYOCARDIAL OXYGEN CONSUMPTION

Cardiac energy generation is primarily aerobic, and therefore myocardial oxygen consumption is an accurate measure of total cardiac metabolism. Increases in cardiac oxygen consumption are primarily affected by changes in systolic wall tension, contractility, and heart rate (Ardehali & Ports, 1990; Rooke & Fiegel, 1984; Graham et al, 1968).

Systolic wall tension is determined by both stroke volume and systolic pressure generation. These determinants of wall tension have their clinical correlates in preload and afterload. Increases in either parameter result in a greater overall external workload and an increase in myocardial wall tension (Rooke & Fiegel, 1984). By the Laplace relation, myocardial wall tension is decreased by decreasing ventricular size and increased with ventricular dilatation.

Changes in contractility increase both systolic pressure generation and time to peak pressure generation; without significant changes in ventricular volume, these translate into increased myocardial wall tension and increased myocardial oxygen consumption (Ardehali & Ports, 1990; Rooke & Fiegel, 1984; Graham et al, 1968). Positive inotropic agents also enhance excitation–contraction coupling. Increased oxygen requirements then result from greater and more rapid calcium uptake by the sarcoplasmic reticulum. Finally, acceleration of the heart rate increases myocardial oxygen demand by increasing the frequency of tension development per unit of time and simultaneously by increasing contractility (Ardehali & Ports, 1990; Rooke & Fiegel, 1984). Myocardial ischemia is the result when any of these determinants cause increased myocardial metabolic demands without concomitant regulation of oxygen delivery.

DETERMINANTS OF MYOCARDIAL OXYGEN DELIVERY

Coronary blood flow is the major determinant of myocardial oxygen delivery. Perfusion of the coronary arteries occurs primarily during diastole because of myocardial compression of the intramyocardial and subendocardial arterioles during systole. Approximately 80% of coronary flow to the left ventricle and 50% of flow to the right ventricle occur during diastole. Coronary perfusion pressure, therefore, is determined by both mean aortic pressure and left ventricular end-diastolic pressure.

Autoregulation of the coronary circulation via neurohumoral mechanisms serves to maintain coronary flow fairly constant over a wide range of perfusion pressures. In the presence of fixed coronary stenoses, however, autoregulation cannot further increase regional blood flow to accommodate increases in myocardial oxygen demand. Coronary vessels with fixed atherosclerotic lesions are maximally dilated to maximize distal flow in the setting of luminal obstruction. With further metabolic demands, autoregulation is not possible and regional myocardial ischemia with resultant myocardial dysfunction occurs. Furthermore, in the setting of atherosclerosis, endothelial dysfunction results in impaired ability to generate vasoactive substances such as endothelial-derived relaxing factor and prostacyclin. This results in further impairment of smooth muscle relaxation as well as a loss of platelet aggregation inhibition.

EPIDEMIOLOGY AND RISK FACTORS

Risk factor assessment and modification are an integral part of the evaluation and treatment of patients with both known and suspected CAD. Unfortunately, risk factors are often misinterpreted as either necessary or sufficient causes of disease. The primary care provider must be mindful of the fact that risk factors represent associations that may or may not be causal. Risk factors can be divided into modifiable and nonmodifiable categories (Table 9-1). This characterization has clinical implications: only the former can be targeted for preventive measures. However, patients with strong nonmodifiable risk factors may warrant greater intensity of risk factor management because of an increased risk of CAD.

Nonmodifiable Risk Factors

AGE, GENDER, AND FAMILY HISTORY

CAD increases linearly with age. The prevalence of CAD is greater in men than women until age 75, at which point it equalizes. The incidence of CAD in persons younger than 55 years of age is three to four times greater in men than women.

The National Cholesterol Education Program defines family history of premature CAD as MI or sudden death in a father or first-degree male relative less than 55 years of age or in a mother or first-degree female relative less than 65 years of age (Summary of the Second Report of NCEP, 1993). Family history is one of the most powerful determinants of CAD independent of other risk factors (Rissanen, 1979; Friedlander, 1994;

TABLE 9-1	Risk Factors Associated With the Epidemiology of CAD

NONMODIFIABLE RISK FACTORS FOR CAD

Male sex

Age >45

Family history

Socioeconomic factors

MODIFIABLE RISK FACTORS FOR CAD

Serum lipid levels

Diabetes

Hypertension

Postmenopausal status

Physical activity

Obesity

Alcohol intake

Type A personality

Serum homocysteine levels

Hamstn & De Faire, 1987). Siblings of patients with CAD have an increased risk of dying (5.2 times higher) compared to a control population (Rissanen, 1979). The presence of this very strong nonmodifiable risk factor should prompt the physician to treat aggressively any concomitant risk factors in such a patient.

SOCIOECONOMIC FACTORS

A variety of psychosocial factors are associated with the development of CAD in the Western world. Social factors such as lower educational level and economic insecurity are associated with increased cardiac risk (Berkman et al, 1992; Kaplan & Keil, 1993). There is an inverse correlation between educational level and the age-adjusted mortality rate from CAD. Neither risk factor modification nor decreased MI rates have been uniform across all socioeconomic groups. The mechanism of increased risk among certain socioeconomic groups may be indirectly related to poor participation in a strict risk factor modification program. Some authors believe that the higher the level of education and socioeconomic status, the greater potential for lifestyle modification.

TEACHING AND SELF-CARE

Modifiable Risk Factors

LIPIDS

There is a well-established relation between total blood cholesterol and CAD, with a graded risk down to a cholesterol level of 180 mg/dL (Stamler et al, 1993a; Neaton & Wentworth, 1992). LDLs appear to be most strongly associated with the development of CAD. It has been estimated that with every 1% difference in LDL cholesterol, there is a 2% to 3% difference in the risk for CAD (Summary of the Second Report of NCEP, 1993). The National Cholesterol Education Program has stratified CAD risk according to LDL cholesterol level (Table 9-2) (Summary of the Second Report of NCEP, 1993).

The LDL cholesterol level increases with age and weight. Diets high in saturated fats and cholesterol similarly cause progressive increases in serum LDL concentrations. Conditions such as hypothyroidism, nephrotic syndrome, liver disease, and estrogen deficiency can also be accompanied by increases in serum LDLs. As referred to earlier, oxidative modification of LDLs plays an important role in the accelerated atherogenic process (Berliner et al, 1995; Morris et al, 1994).

There is a strong inverse epidemiologic association between high-density lipoprotein (HDL) cholesterol, and CAD. The Adult Treatment Panel II classified an HDL cholesterol level of less than 35 mg/dL as low and considered the presence of a high HDL cholesterol level to be a negative risk factor for

CAD (Summary of the Second Report of NCEP, 1993). For every 1 mg/dL decrease in HDL cholesterol, the relative risk for CAD increases by 2% to 3% (Gordon et al, 1989). HDL cholesterol levels are affected by genetics, tobacco use, obesity, and physical activity. There are no clinical trials that indicate a decreased risk of coronary disease secondary only to an increase in HDL cholesterol. This is most likely because lifestyle and dietary modifications affect multiple lipids simultaneously.

The relation between triglycerides and CAD remains controversial. A 1992 Consensus Development Conference defined a triglyceride level of 200 to 400 mg/dL as borderline high, 400 to 1000 mg/dL as high, and more than 1000 mg/dL as very high (NIH Consensus Development Panel, 1993). In univariate analysis, triglycerides predict coronary disease but lose their power when other lipids (especially HDL cholesterol) are factored into a multivariate analysis. It has been suggested that HDL and triglycerides should not be considered separately when evaluating cardiac risk. Low HDL levels are usually associated with high triglycerides because of the transfer of a cholesterol ester between HDL particles and triglyceride-rich lipoproteins. Lifestyle modifications including weight loss, dietary restriction, decrease in alcohol consumption, smoking cessation, and increased physical activity all decrease triglyceride levels. The reduction in triglyceride levels is associated with the greatest risk reduction in patients with the highest risk—those with low HDL or elevated LDL cholesterol levels.

Although LDL levels are directly associated with CAD, the combination of elevated LDL cholesterol, elevated triglycerides, and low levels of HDL cholesterol places the patient in the highest lipid risk stratification category (Manninen et al, 1992; Assman & Schulte, 1992).

DIABETES

Both insulin-dependent diabetes mellitus and non-insulin-dependent diabetes mellitus are major risk factors for the development of CAD. The National Diabetes Data Group defined diabetes as a fasting blood glucose level of more than 127 mg/dL (American Diabetes Association, 1997). Atherosclerosis accounts for 80% of all deaths related to diabetes, and 25% of all heart attacks in the United States occur in persons with diabetes (Diabetes Control & Complications Trial, 1993; Getz, 1993; Schwartz et al, 1992; Stamler, 1987; Butler et al, 1985). The First National Health and Nutrition Examination Survey (NAHANES I) revealed that age-adjusted death rates for men and women with diabetes were twice those seen in persons without diabetes, with 75% of the excess mortality attributed to CAD (Kleinman et al, 1988). The pathogenesis of atherosclerosis in persons with diabetes is multifactorial because there are multiple metabolic derangements in persons with diabetes, including hyperglycemia, insulin resistance, dyslipidemia, and increased platelet aggregation.

The pathogenic role of hyperglycemia is well supported. Observational studies have shown that better metabolic control lowers vascular risk in patients with insulin-dependent diabetes mellitus, but this has not been clearly shown in non-insulin-dependent diabetes mellitus (Diabetes Control & Complications Trial, 1993; Reichard et al, 1993). The secondary complications of diabetes are additive in the risk of atherosclerosis. The development of nephropathy leads to elevated blood pressure and dyslipidemia, which together compound the patient's cardiac risk.

TABLE 9-2	CAD Risk Stratification Based on Serum LDL Level as Designated by the National Cholesterol Education Program

Serum LDL Level	Risk Stratification
<130 mg/dL	Desirable
130–159 mg/dL	Borderline high risk
>160 mg/dL	High risk

HYPERTENSION

Hypertension is a major modifiable risk factor. Elevated shear stress and increased myocardial oxygen demand caused by hypertension have been implicated in atherogenesis and arterial injury. Nearly 50 million adult Americans suffer from hypertension, and the level of risk associated with elevated blood pressure varies substantially with gender, race, and age. Elderly people have a greater risk of cardiovascular events at every level of hypertension.

There is a continuous relation between both systolic and diastolic pressures and cardiovascular disease (Joint National Committee, 1993; Stamler et al, 1993b; MacMahon et al, 1990). A meta-analysis of several large prospective studies demonstrated a linear relation between hypertension and CAD, with a relative risk approaching three times the risk at the highest levels of blood pressure (MacMahon et al, 1990).

The risk of hypertension cannot be taken in isolation. It frequently coexists with other risk factors, including physical inactivity, obesity, alcohol use, hyperlipidemia, diabetes, and smoking. The presence of these CAD risk factors appears to be both causal and additive for hypertension.

TOBACCO

Cigarette smoking is an independent risk factor for cardiovascular disease. Several independent studies have demonstrated that smoking increases the cardiovascular mortality rate by 40% to 60% (*Reducing the health consequences of smoking*, 1989; Rigotti & Pasternak, 1996). Nicotine accelerates the process of atherosclerosis by a variety of mechanisms. Inhalation of cigarette smoke produces a transient and reversible prothrombotic increase in fibrinogen levels, increases platelet aggregation, and decreases the ability of endothelial cells to produce or release prostacyclin. Nicotine is also a potent agonist for the adrenergic nervous system, resulting in increased coronary tone and vasoconstriction. The enhanced vasoconstriction results in an imbalance between oxygen supply and demand and has been associated with silent myocardial ischemia (Deanfiels et al, 1986).

Tobacco smoke may augment cardiovascular death from other risk factors. Cigarette smoking adversely affects lipid profiles. Heavy smokers have lower levels of HDL cholesterol and higher levels of LDL cholesterol and triglycerides (Migas, 1988). Smoking has a variable effect on blood pressure. The acute inhalation results in a rise in blood pressure. Epidemiologic studies have shown that chronic smokers tend to have lower blood pressures than nonsmokers, possibly secondary to lower body weight (Green et al, 1986). The Hypertension Detection and Follow-up Program demonstrated that smokers had twice the mortality rate of nonsmokers (Langford et al, 1986). The incidence of MI is definitely diminished after smoking cessation. The risk reduction occurs early and may be demonstrated 12 months after cessation.

POSTMENOPAUSAL STATUS

CAD presents later in women than in men. Endogenous estrogen protects premenopausal women from coronary disease. Estrogen replacement therapy (ERT) confers a 50% reduction in the risk of developing CAD (Barrett-Conner & Bush, 1991). Estrogen favorably affects both HDL and LDL cholesterol. However, the beneficial effects of estrogen appear to be the result of more than just its improvement in the overall lipid profile. The nonlipid cardioprotective mechanisms of estrogen include direct actions on vessel walls, estrogen-associated calcium antagonist effects, estrogen-associated antioxidant effects, and estrogen-induced genetic changes. The initial clinical presentation of CAD is reduced by 30% to 70% in users of ERT (Barrett-Conner & Bush, 1994; Bush & Korenman, 1990). The Lipids Research Clinic Follow-Up Study demonstrated that after 9 years, estrogen users had a 64% lower risk of coronary death than nonusers (Bush et al, 1987). This was still significant after adjustments for known CAD risk factors, and 50% of the protection was afforded by estrogen-induced increases in HDL levels.

All studies on ERT have been observational in design, raising many questions regarding unrecognized biases that can account for the observed protective effect of estrogen. Some such biases include whether healthier women may be more likely to be prescribed estrogen or whether estrogen users may be more likely to participate in all prevention therapies. Proof of the protective benefit of estrogen awaits the results of prospective randomized clinical trials to answer these questions. One such study is the Women's Health Initiative, which is a long-range study enrolling more than 165,000 women. Preliminary results from this study are expected over the next several years.

PHYSICAL ACTIVITY

The role of physical activity in the prevention of CAD remains controversial. The exact mechanism of protection is multifactorial. Exercise is important in maintaining ideal body weight, muscle mass, and normal blood pressure as well as optimizing lipid levels. Regular aerobic exercise decreases both systolic and diastolic pressures, improves the myocardial oxygen supply/demand ratio, lowers triglycerides, raises HDL levels, and decreases platelet aggregation.

The greatest risk reduction is achieved in nonactive and moderately active persons. Intense exercise is associated with decreases in total and LDL cholesterol and increases in HDL cholesterol (Seiler et al, 1988). Patients who exercise regularly have a decreased incidence of sudden death, although sedentary patients who begin an exercise regimen may be at increased risk for acute MI or malignant ventricular arrhythmia. Therefore, a thorough physical examination is recommended for people older than 40 years before initiating a vigorous exercise program. Likewise, younger patients with hypertension, diabetes, and other associated CAD risk factors should undergo a thorough assessment before undertaking an aggressive exercise regimen, including a baseline electrocardiogram (ECG). A history of angina or an abnormal ECG result should prompt further diagnostic testing before initiating an intensive exercise program.

OBESITY

The definition of obesity is arbitrary, but it may be defined as an increase of 120% above ideal body weight for height. There is a linear relation between body mass and cardiovascular mortality (Manson et al, 1995). The precise role of obesity as an independent risk factor remains unclear. The increased risk of obesity with CAD is chiefly related to its close association with other risk factors. Obesity has a direct relation with all CAD risk factors except smoking. Obesity is positively correlated with hypertension, hypertriglyceridemia, and hyperinsulinemia and negatively correlated with HDL.

Central obesity is quantified as the waist/hip ratio and has been shown to increase CAD risk. An elevated waist/hip ratio has been associated with hypertension, hypercholesterolemia, elevated levels of fibrinogen, and hypertriglyceridemia. In men, the development of CAD is correlated with the abdominal distribution of fat independent of obesity. In women, abdominal fat deposition constitutes a greater risk than obesity. The waist/hip ratio appears to be a more significant predictor than the total degree of obesity. A waist/hip ratio of less than 0.9 for men and less than 0.8 for women is desirable (Freedman et al, 1990).

ALCOHOL

The effect of alcohol on coronary disease is dichotomous. Moderate consumption (one to three drinks per day) results in a 40% to 50% reduction of CAD compared to abstinence (Gaziano et al, 1993; Yano et al, 1977). However, excessive consumption results in an overall increased risk (Shaper et al, 1988). Alcohol increases the HDL cholesterol level, which accounts for half of the reduction in MI. However, no beneficial effect of alcohol has been demonstrated in angina pectoris (Yano et al, 1977). Its adverse effects include the development of alcoholic cardiomyopathy, hypertension, and cardiac arrhythmias.

TYPE A PERSONALITY

The most notorious psychosocial factor associated with CAD is the "Type A personality." Type A people are characterized as highly competitive, ambitious, and in constant struggle with their environment. There is an increased incidence in the development of angina pectoris but no subsequent increase in fatal cardiac events (Eaker et al, 1989; O'Connor et al, 1995). The increased rate of stable angina could not be explained by the presence of other cardiac risk factors. However, there are no data available that have clearly proven that this behavior itself, nor any modifications, changes the overall cardiac risk.

SERUM HOMOCYSTEINE

A newer, independent risk factor for atherosclerosis is an elevated plasma level of the amino acid homocysteine. A plasma homocysteine concentration of more than 15 μmol/L is referred to as hyperhomocysteinemia. Such elevated homocysteine levels can induce pathologic changes in the arterial wall, with a subsequent increased risk for CAD, peripheral vascular disease, cerebrovascular disease, and venous thrombosis. There is increasing evidence that homocysteine may affect the coagulation cascade and the resistance of the endothelium to thrombosis (Nygard et al, 1997). It may also interfere with the vasodilator and antithrombotic effects of nitric oxide. Although several epidemiologic studies have established the relation between total homocysteine level and CAD, studies are still ongoing to determine whether lowering homocysteine levels can prevent vascular occlusive events.

DIAGNOSTIC CRITERIA

The diagnosis of CAD is based on a history of chest pain or anginal equivalent pain together with diagnostic studies that demonstrate either functional or anatomic coronary obstruction. The diagnosis of MI is based on history, ECG changes, and myocardial fraction of creatine kinase. If two of these three criteria are positive, then the diagnosis of evolving MI is made.

New wall motion abnormalities on echocardiography may also be used as soft criteria for recent myocardial injury.

HISTORY AND PHYSICAL EXAMINATION

History

The diagnosis of CAD is based on a careful, skillful clinical history. Within the current atmosphere of health care cost containment, a concisely focused outlined history will obviate the need for more costly testing.

Typical stable angina pectoris is described as a viselike, constrictive, crushing, or squeezing type of retrosternal chest pain induced by exertion. In some patients the quality of discomfort is described as mild pressure or substernal burning. In each instance the symptoms reach their maximal intensity in a few minutes and then dissipate with the cessation of exercise. Typical angina pectoris is relieved within minutes of rest or by using nitroglycerin. The response to nitroglycerin usually occurs within 3 to 5 minutes and can be a very useful diagnostic test. Nonetheless, it has been clearly established that esophageal pain and other syndromes may also respond to nitroglycerin.

Typical angina may be induced by exertional activities such as walking against the wind, climbing stairs or hills, vigorous arm work, and sexual intercourse. The discomfort can likewise be incited by emotional stress (panic, fear, anger, or anxiety), or it may follow a heavy meal. Anginal pain may even occur nocturnally after lying down (angina decubitus) secondary to increased ventricular filling pressure. The duration of discomfort and its cessation are reproducible for each typical anginal syndrome.

Although the area of discomfort is classically retrosternal, radiation is very common. The regions of discomfort may manifest themselves anywhere between the mandible and the epigastrium. Discomfort can radiate to the shoulders, the jaw, the ulnar surface of the left arm, the right arm, and the outer surface of both arms.

Symptoms of myocardial ischemia other than typical anginal discomfort, such as dyspnea with minimal exertion, fatigue, and faintness, are referred to as anginal equivalents. These symptoms are common in the elderly and in patients at high risk for coronary heart disease. The symptoms may be caused by elevation of the left ventricular filling pressure and despite a normal ECG should alert the provider to probable severe ischemic heart disease.

Stable angina is a predictable pattern of chest discomfort with a similar degree of severity and classic precipitating factors occurring either recently or over several months. It maintains a constant threshold in severity and relief over time. The corresponding lesion is usually a stable, fixed atherosclerotic lesion that is flow-limiting only when myocardial metabolic demands reach a threshold.

Unstable angina refers to angina of recent onset, intensifying in nature with a lower level of exertion or occurring nocturnally without immediate relief by rest or with nitroglycerin. The underlying coronary lesion in this emergent situation is usually a critical stenosis with either acute coronary vasospasm or thrombus formation, resulting in intermittent or permanent vessel occlusion. This unstable pattern requires more aggressive attention and evaluation because 20% will progress to MI within a 3-month period.

Variant angina, originally described by Prinzmetal, refers to chest pain occurring almost exclusively at rest, not precipitated by physical exertion or emotional stress. It is associated with electrocardiographic ST-segment elevation. It has been demonstrated that variant angina is related to coronary artery spasm with subsequent myocardial ischemia. In addition, it may be associated with MI, ventricular tachycardia, and ventricular fibrillation as well as sudden death (Mark et al, 1984).

Finally, silent myocardial ischemia can occur in patients with angina at rest, unstable angina, and chronic stable angina. It has been clearly established that patients who are at high risk for CAD can be evaluated by 24-hour double-channel Holter monitoring or stress testing for silent but significant electrocardiographic ST-segment changes (Cohn, 1996). Prognostically, this may be the only way to limit sudden death from MI as well as to identify and avoid an initial or subsequent MI.

Other conditions that should be included in the differential diagnosis of angina include common painful esophageal reflux, achalasia, esophageal spasm, peptic ulcer, and biliary colic (Table 9-3). Chest wall discomfort with localized pain, tenderness, and swelling of the costal cartilages, described in 1931 as Tietze's syndrome, is a common additional differential diagnosis. Cervical radiculitis, chest wall spasm, and severe pulmonary hypertension associated with chest pain on exertion may all simulate anginal pain. Pulmonary embolism, acute pericarditis, mitral valve prolapse, and herpes zoster can all be included in the differential diagnosis. Although all of these can in most cases be readily distinguished from angina by a detailed history and a comprehensive physical examination, the physician must ensure that chronic coronary heart disease does not simultaneously exist with noncardiac disease.

Physical Examination

Although patients with chronic CAD and stable angina are often found to have an entirely normal physical examination, it is the responsibility of the primary care provider to perform a diligent and complete physical examination in all patients. The primary care provider can often identify useful clues to the

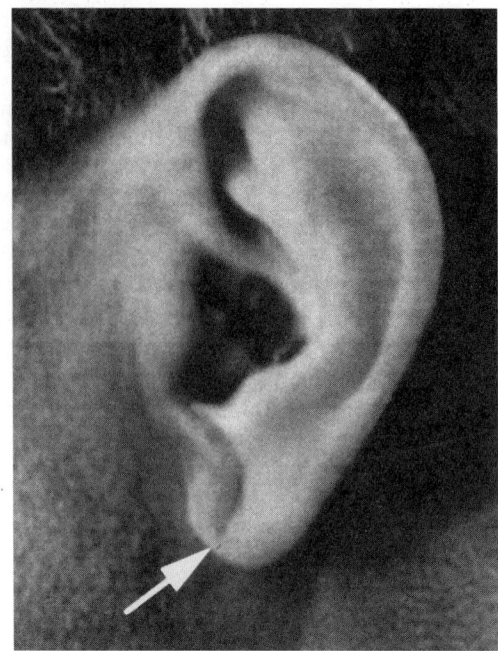

FIGURE 9-2 Photograph of diagonal earlobe crease, which may have a correlation with coronary artery disease.

diagnosis of CAD and identify patients who are at the highest risk for this disease.

The blood pressure may be chronically elevated. A diagonal earlobe crease may be identified that has had some correlation with CAD (except in Native American Indians and Asians) (Fig. 9-2). In the young, the diagonal earlobe crease is unilateral and becomes bilateral with advancing age (Tranchesi et al, 1992). Ophthalmologic examination may reveal a corneal arcus (Fig. 9-3). The size of the corneal arcus positively correlates with

TABLE 9-3	Differential Diagnosis of Chest Pain
CARDIAC	**GASTROINTESTINAL**
Coronary artery disease	Esophageal spasm
Aortic stenosis	Esophageal perforation
Pericarditis	Esophageal reflux
PULMONARY	Biliary colic
Pleuritis	Peptic ulcer disease
Pneumonia	Pancreatitis
Tracheobronchitis	**MUSCULOSKELETAL**
Pneumothorax	Costochondritis
Tumor	Cervical radiculopathy
VASCULAR	Subacromial bursitis
Aortic dissection	**OTHER**
Pulmonary embolism	Herpes zoster
Abdominal aortic aneurysm	Fibrocystic breast disease

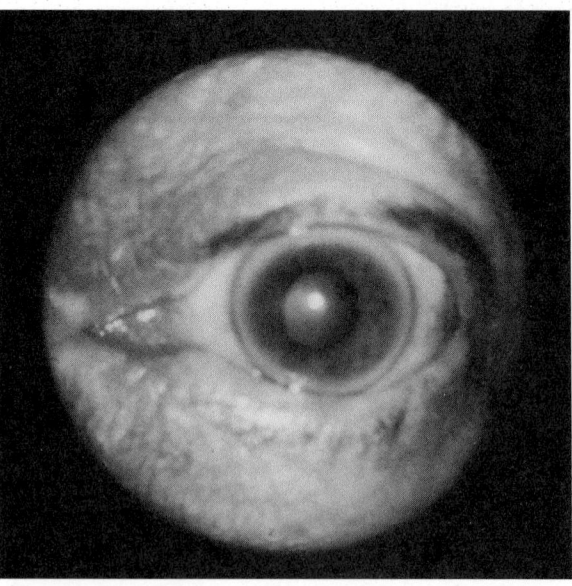

FIGURE 9-3 Photograph of corneal arcus. The size of the corneal arcus positively correlates with age, levels of total cholesterol, and low-density lipoproteins. (This photograph can also be found in color insert 23.)

age, levels of total cholesterol, and levels of LDL (Winder, 1983). The retina may reveal arteriolar atherosclerotic hypertensive or diabetic changes. The skin may demonstrate xanthelasma, which may be promoted by increased levels of triglycerides and a relative deficiency of HDLs (Winder, 1983).

Of utmost importance in the general physical examination is to check all arterial pulses and search for abnormalities in the venous system. The association between peripheral vascular disease and coronary heart disease is well documented. This is not confined only to patients with symptomatic disease, clinically overt peripheral vascular disease, or carotid artery disease, but is also seen in asymptomatic, ultrasonically proven, hemodynamically significant obstructive arterial disease. Examination of the patient's venous system can reveal previous venous CABG.

The cardiac examination may be most helpful during an episode of symptomatic angina because ischemia may produce transient left ventricular dysfunction with a third heart sound and bibasilar pulmonary rales. A softened mitral component of the first heart sound and paradoxical splitting of the second heart sound may occur during an anginal attack. A mid systolic click followed by a late systolic murmur may occur in patients with CAD related to transient papillary muscle dysfunction, with alteration in the alignment of the papillary muscles.

DIAGNOSTIC STUDIES

Noninvasive Testing

ELECTROCARDIOGRAPHY

Fifty percent of patients with chronic stable angina have normal ECG tracings at rest, but they may have severe CAD. However, the 12-lead ECG during a provoked episode of substernal chest pain or during an attack of angina may reveal downward or horizontal sloping depression of the ST segment, T-wave peak-ing, or inversion. These ECG changes accompanied by chest discomfort may signal the possibility of coronary stenosis.

EXERCISE ELECTROCARDIOGRAPHY

Exercise treadmill ECG has been the most studied noninvasive test for the evaluation of CAD in both men and women. Stress testing increases overall cardiac work and heart rate. This increased work results in an increase in myocardial oxygen demand and a subsequent requirement for increased oxygen delivery via an increase in coronary flow. If narrowed or obstructed lesions prevent the required increase in coronary blood flow, chest pain or ECG changes may arise. In both sexes the exercise ECG is most accurate in patients who are able to exercise to 85% of their maximal predicted heart rates (Severi & Michelassi, 1991). However, this goal can be modified based on the characteristics of the patient being evaluated. A young patient with a low risk for CAD will have a much more sensitive result should he or she reach the maximal heart rate target or exercise to exhaustion. An older, high-risk patient, on the other hand, may reveal clinically meaningful information at lower cardiac workloads.

Criteria for determining a positive ECG stress test vary among different institutions. Depression or downsloping of the ST segment 0.08 seconds after the J point of the ECG is the typical ischemic change sought as a positive result (Fig. 9-4). However, the degree of ST-segment depression defined as positive can range anywhere from 0.5 mV to 2 mV. Using the lower end of this range will produce a test that is more sensitive but less specific, whereas the higher end produces a result that is less sensitive but more specific. Most centers use a 1-mm ST depression as a criterion for positivity. If typical chest discomfort occurs during the test associated with an ST depression of more than 1 mm, the predictive value for the detection of CAD is 90% (Wilson et al, 1991). ST depressions of more than 2

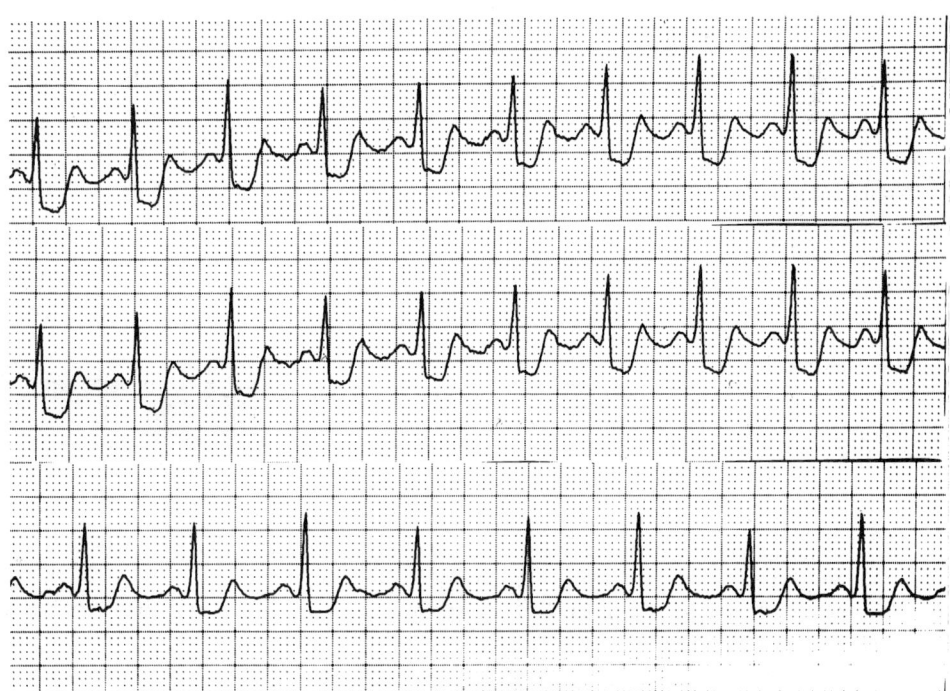

FIGURE 9-4 Downsloping of the ST segment 0.08 seconds after the J point of the ECG is the typical ischemic change sought as a "positive" result during exercise stress testing.

TABLE 9-4	Indications and Contraindications to Exercise Stress Testing	
Indications	**Contraindications**	
Diagnose the etiology of chest pain	Recent onset of unstable angina	
Assess prognosis	Uncontrolled hypertension	
Assess the need for angiography	Severe decompensated CHF	
Evaluate functional capacity	Significant ventricular arrhythmias	
Assess degree of ischemia after MI	Severe obstructive valvular disease	
Assess adequacy of revascularization after CABG	Associated cardiopulmonary conditions, including severe pulmonary hypertension, myocarditis, pericarditis, recent pulmonary embolism, rapid atrial fibrillation	
Ascertain the effects of medical, interventional, or surgical management of CAD		

mm in the setting of typical chest discomfort are virtually diagnostic of CAD.

The referring provider must be mindful of the fact that the results of exercise stress testing are likewise affected by the patient's pretest probability of having disease. In men with classic angina pectoris or a previous MI, a positive test result will accurately predict CAD about 85% of the time (Wilson et al, 1991; Weiner et al, 1979). Similarly, the results of exercise stress testing in women may be less sensitive than those obtained in men, given the lower prevalence of CAD in women younger than age 70. In the Coronary Artery Surgery Study, which included a large number of women, the sensitivity and specificity of the exercise ECG was 76% and 64%, respectively, for women, compared with 80% and 74% for men (Weiner et al, 1979). Asymptomatic, low-risk patients also have a significant false-positive rate that may range as high as 60% (Wilson et al, 1991; Weiner et al, 1979).

In general, exercise stress testing is used for prognosis, diagnosis, and assessment of the effectiveness of therapy (Table 9-4). Diagnostic interpretations must be performed with pretest probabilities of disease for each patient kept in mind. As a prognostic test, a submaximal ECG stress test can identify patients at high risk after MI. Likewise, a positive result after minimal exertion is frequently indicative of three-vessel disease and should prompt angiography if appropriate. Finally, documentation of improved exercise capacity and ischemic ECG changes after medical, interventional, or surgical therapy can guide future treatment plans.

Contraindications to exercise stress testing are listed in Table 9-4 and include any underlying condition that might preclude an appropriate increase in cardiac output after exercise. Recent onset of unstable angina or MI is an absolute contraindication to the maximal stress test, but submaximal exercise testing can be performed as early as 10 days after MI with relative safety (Gibbons et al, 1997).

RADIONUCLIDE STUDIES

Radionuclide imaging during stress and at rest has been the gold standard for assessing myocardial viability and can improve the accuracy of the diagnosis of CAD over the exercise test alone. Thallium-201 is rapidly extracted by viable myocardium and is one of the most commonly used radioisotopes. During exercise, thallium is preferentially distributed to coronary artery territories that are maximally dilated. Stenotic coronary arteries are not capable of dilating in response to exercise, and blood flow is therefore stolen from these areas. This appears as a perfu-

sion defect on a nuclear scan. At rest, the maximally dilated coronary arteries resume normal flow patterns and blood again flows through the stenotic lesions. In follow-up scans, the area of thallium defect will now appear perfused, and this reversible perfusion defect signifies an area of viable myocardium with disadvantaged flow. An irreversible perfusion defect is suggestive of a fixed obstructive lesion with no underlying viable myocardium (ie, myocardial scar). Several clinical studies have now shown that 35% to 60% of apparently fixed defects on repeat delayed (3 to 6 hours) thallium imaging involve substantial viable myocardium, and function can be restored by revascularization (Pohost & Johnson, 1992).

The addition of radionuclide imaging to ECG stress testing is expensive. It should be used only when the results are likely to add diagnostic information. Conditions such as mitral valve prolapse, left ventricular hypertrophy, and left bundle branch block, as well as digitalis use, may cause repolarization abnormalities that obscure stress-induced ECG changes. In such situations, radionuclide imaging can significantly increase the detection of inducible ischemia over stress testing alone. Other indications for thallium scanning include assessment of myocardial viability in patients undergoing revascularization risk stratification, as well as in patients before major noncoronary surgery and in patients after MI (Table 9-5) (Pohost & Johnson, 1992; Koss et al, 1987; Gould, 1989).

PHARMACOLOGIC STRESS TESTS

Dipyridamole and dobutamine tests are inexpensive and safe diagnostic tools with excellent specificity and good sensitivity. They are primarily used in patients who cannot exercise for ECG or radionuclide stress tests.

Dipyridamole works by increasing intracellular cyclic adenosine monophosphate levels and inhibiting the formation of

TABLE 9-5	Indications to Add Radionuclide Imaging to Standard ECG Stress Testing
■ Left ventricular hypertrophy	
■ Left bundle branch block	
■ Bifascicular block	
■ Baseline ECG repolarization abnormality	
■ Assess myocardial viability before revascularization	
■ Assess myocardial viability after MI	
■ Myocardial risk stratification before noncoronary surgery	

thromboxane A_2, a patent vasoconstrictor. When injected it acts as a coronary vasodilator. Stenotic coronary lesions are already maximally dilated and cannot respond to dipyridamole. Nonstenotic coronary arteries maintain their ability to vasodilate, and preferential flow down these newly dilated vessels results in coronary steal from the stenotic arteries. Dipyridamole infusion is contraindicated in patients with bronchospastic pulmonary disease as well as in patients who take xanthine derivatives or have recently ingested coffee.

Dobutamine is a synthetic beta-1 and beta-2 agonist. Dobutamine causes myocardial ischemia primarily through a marked increase in myocardial oxygen demand resulting from increased heart rate, blood pressure, and myocardial contractility. The increase in coronary blood flow achieved is comparable to that during physical exercise but slightly less than with dipyridamole. Dobutamine stress testing is an appropriate alternative in patients who cannot exercise and who have contraindications to dipyridamole. Dobutamine stress testing causes ventricular ectopy in 40% to 50% of patients; a recent history of tachyarrhythmias is a relative contraindication.

Either dobutamine or dipyridamole may be used in stress testing in lieu of treadmill exercise with an equal sensitivity. When coupled with thallium radionuclide imaging, CAD detection is similar to that of exercise thallium testing and is a powerful tool in patients who cannot exercise. Dobutamine and dipyridamole stress echocardiography has also been used in the diagnosis and management of CAD with similar sensitivities to stress thallium testing (Cates et al, 1989).

AMBULATORY 24-HOUR HOLTER MONITORING
Asymptomatic or silent ischemia in the high-risk patient can be detected during everyday activities by Holter monitoring. ST-segment depression at a low level of exercise (<120 beats per minute) of more than 2 mm in magnitude and lasting 6 minutes or more implies a high risk for MI (Cohn, 1996; Pepine et al, 1994a; Pepine et al, 1994b). The greatest likelihood of modifying an adverse outcome is to submit these patients to cardiac catheterization and often revascularization.

The ambulatory 24-hour ECG monitor has the ability to identify persons with and without typical anginal warning signs. These ischemic events are often silent and can go unnoticed until a fatal event occurs (Pepine et al, 1994b). Three groups of patients have been studied since 1981 to the present. The first group consists of patients who never had symptoms (type I), the second group consists of patients who are asymptomatic after MI but still manifest ischemia (type 2), and the third group includes patients who are symptomatic with only some of their ischemic episodes and who may or may not have had a prior MI (type 3).

In type I persons who are asymptomatic or mildly symptomatic, risk factor modification and aspirin should be considered. In this group, anti-ischemic medical therapy with atenolol (Atenolol Silent Ischemic Study) demonstrated event-free survival at 1 year, reduced daily like ischemia, and was associated with reduced risk for adverse outcome (Pepine et al, 1994a). In patients with type 2 silent ischemia, the post-MI mortality rate appears markedly higher than in patients without silent ischemia. In type 3 patients, 75% to 80% can be found to have silent ischemic episodes in addition to anginal attacks. Prognosis in these patients is extremely poor when episodes of silent ischemia fail to respond to high doses of anti-ischemic agents,

when triple-vessel coronary disease exists, and when left ventricular function is decreased.

Detection of asymptomatic silent ischemia in all three types can be effectively documented by Holter monitoring. Ischemic events have important prognostic significance and are often incidentally observed. High-risk patients should be vigorously pursued with this accurate, noninvasive test.

Coronary Arteriography

Cardiac catheterization and selective coronary arteriography is still the gold standard for visualization of the *in vivo* morphologic details of the coronary arteries. Access to the coronary circulation is usually achieved through the femoral artery. In patients with severe peripheral vascular disease, an alternative arterial entry using the radial or brachial artery can be used. Each coronary ostia is then selectively cannulated and an angiogram of each vessel is taken in several standard views.

Coronary angiography can detect as little as 20% narrowing of the main coronary arteries, as well as a critical stenosis of 70% or greater (de Bono, 1993). The cardiac catheterization assesses hemodynamic measurements, including left ventricular function, valve surface area, as well as valvular gradients. Indications for coronary angiography are continually changing. A broad list of indications for cardiac catheterization and coronary angiography is shown in Table 9-6. Relative contraindications include uncontrolled ventricular arrhythmias, uncorrected metabolic disturbances, decompensated heart failure, uncontrolled hypertension, elevated prothrombin time, severe allergy to contrast agents, and severe renal insufficiency.

The incidence of complications of coronary arteriography is low but is directly related to the skill and experience of the interventional cardiologist as well as to the severity of the cardiac condition. The incidence of death is 0.55% in patients with left main coronary artery disease, 0.33% in patients with an ejection fraction of less than 30%, and 0.29% in patients with

TABLE 9-6	Broad-Based Indications for Coronary Arteriography

PATIENTS WITH CHEST PAIN
1. Chronic chest pain
   Severe anginal pain unresponsive to medical therapy
   Atypical chest pain with uncertain diagnosis by noninvasive studies
2. Unstable angina
3. Prinzmetal's angina
4. Preoperative evaluation of valvular heart disease
5. Evaluation of recurrent angina after bypass surgery
6. Suspected anomalies of the coronary circulation

PATIENTS WITHOUT CHEST PAIN
1. Asymptomatic patients with abnormal ECGs
2. Persistent heart failure after MI
3. Unexplained ventricular failure as the main symptom
4. Preoperative evaluation of valvular disease
5. Intractable ventricular arrhythmias or history of cardiac arrest not associated with a recent MI
6. Suspected congenital anomalies of the coronary circulation
7. Evaluation of coronary circulation after bypass surgery

New York Heart Association functional class IV heart failure (de Bono, 1993).

Finally, it should be appreciated by the primary care provider who assesses the angiographic findings that the presence of CAD provides more clinical information than the severity of the obstruction itself. This lack of correlation with the angiographic findings of mild plaque disease and severe obstructive disease may be related to the inability of the arteriogram to identify unstable plaques that may be at high risk of rupture and to distinguish them from critically obstructive stenoses that are stabilized.

TREATMENT OPTIONS, EXPECTED OUTCOMES, COMPREHENSIVE MANAGEMENT

Medical

NITRATES

Numerous studies have documented the clinical effectiveness of nitrates in the management of chronic stable angina pectoris (Garlin & Sadock, 1994; Cohn et al, 1997; Bassan, 1990; Parker et al, 1995). Nitrates act as vasodilators by contributing nitric oxide, which allows for vascular smooth muscle relaxation. Nitrates have different effects on different smooth muscle beds. The vasodilator effects of nitrates can be demonstrated in coronary arteries and veins in both normal persons and in patients with ischemic heart disease. Veins are the most sensitive, and the consequences of venodilation are reduced workload and heart size with a reduction in ventricular preload. Arterial dilatation from nitrates occurs in normal and stenotic areas as well as in a previously constricted coronary artery, thereby leading to increased tissue perfusion. There is some evidence that collateral blood flow is increased through a variety of actions, including enlargement of the contributing artery and possible dilatation of the thin-walled collaterals themselves (Garlin & Sadock, 1994; Cohn et al, 1997). In chronic stable angina pectoris, nitrates reduce attacks and improve exercise tolerance.

There are many nitrate preparations as well as a variety of routes of administration. Sublingual nitroglycerin tablets, buccal, oral, and lingual sprays, and ointment forms are the drugs of choice for acute anginal episodes and can also be used prophylactically for known stable angina-provoking attacks. Adverse reactions include headache, flushing, and rarely hypotension. Methemoglobinemia is a rare complication of high doses of nitrates.

Isosorbide dinitrate is a longer-acting effective antianginal drug that can be administered orally, sublingually, in chewable form, or as a sustained-release tablet or capsule. Because partial or complete tolerance develops at a dose of 30 mg four times daily, a 10- to 12-hour nitrate-free interval should be followed (Bassan, 1990). Isosorbide-5-mononitrate is an active metabolite of isosorbide dinitrate that is also effective in the treatment of chronic stable angina. Single dosing has not demonstrated tolerance, but double dosing at 12-hour intervals does result in tachyphylaxis. There are several available mononitrates that provide a long period of improvement in ischemic attacks.

Topical nitroglycerin ointment (15 mg/inch) spread over a wide area of skin and covered with plastic is absorbed in 30 minutes and is effective for 4 to 6 hours. It is highly useful in patients with severe acute angina, as well as for prophylactic use in patients with nocturnal angina. Transdermal nitroglycerin therapy is more likely to retain effectiveness than oral or sustained-release tablets, provided that the patch is not applied for more than 12 out of 24 hours. In addition, the transdermal patch has been shown to increase exercise duration and maintains anti-ischemic effects for 12 hours (Parker et al, 1995).

Although nitrates have a proven symptomatic effect on both unstable and chronic stable angina, it is less clear whether nitrates have an effect on the mortality rate. Some investigators have shown that nitrates may decrease morbidity and even mortality rates after MI (Jugdutt & Warnica, 1988).

BETA-ADRENORECEPTOR BLOCKING AGENTS

Beta-adrenoreceptor blocking agents have anti-ischemic properties, are effective antihypertensives, and are antiarrhythmic. Beta-blockers reduce myocardial oxygen consumption by slowing the heart rate and thereby increasing diastolic coronary perfusion. They reduce myocardial oxygen demands during activity. The major factors influencing myocardial oxygen use include heart rate, blood pressure, and myocardial contractility. In the face of coronary artery insufficiency, beta-blockers positively alter the imbalance between supply and demand, leading to improvement in myocardial ischemia.

Of the many beta-blockers available in the United States, there are two major subtypes. Beta-1 receptors predominate in the heart and allow selective blockade of the cardiac beta-1 receptor. Cardioselective beta-blockers (acebutolol, atenolol, bisoprolol, betaxolol, esmolol, and metoprolol) reduce myocardial oxygen demand and may be advantageous in patients with sensitive airway disease, dyslipidemia, or diabetes mellitus. Nonselective beta-blocking drugs (propranolol, nadolol, penbutolol, pindolol, carvedilol, timolol, and carteolol) block beta-1 and beta-2 receptors. They are effective as anti-ischemic agents and may also reduce the risk of sudden cardiac death. However, the use of beta-2-blockers should be avoided in true asthmatics and diabetics. It should also be understood that even cardioselective beta-1-blockers in high doses lose their selectivity and therefore are contraindicated in the aforementioned disease states.

Some beta-blockers also cause vasodilatation. These include labetalol, carvedilol, and bucindolol. Agents with intrinsic sympathomimetic activity (acebutolol, carteolol, celiprolol, penbutolol, and pindolol) are partial beta agonists. They provide low-grade beta stimulation when sympathetic tone is low but behave more like conventional beta-blockers when adrenergic tone is high (eg, physical exercise or emotional stress). Compared to other beta-blockers, beta blockers with intrinsic sympathomimetic activity have not uniformly been shown to improve survival after MI.

Beta-blockers have demonstrated a primary preventive role in men with hypertension. In the Metoprolol Atherosclerosis Prevention in Hypertensives study, a 5-year follow-up of patients treated with metoprolol confirmed that the total mortality rate was significantly lowered in the patients treated with metoprolol. The reduction was primarily revealed by a 30% reduction in sudden cardiac deaths (Olsson et al, 1991). Data from other studies have also shown trends favoring the use of beta-blockers in primary prevention (Green, 1991; Wikstrand et al, 1992).

Randomized trials in acute MI, recent MI, stable angina, and silent ischemia have all consistently shown benefit from beta-blockers (Goldstein, 1996; Viscoli et al, 1993; Viskin et al, 1995). Therefore, beta-blockers should be given to all patients with unstable angina unless heart block, severe bradycardia, severe bronchospastic lung disease, or severe left ventricular dysfunction exists. Patients with a history of depression, Raynaud's phenomenon, or peripheral vascular disease are poor candidates for beta-blocker therapy.

CALCIUM CHANNEL BLOCKERS

There are three major classes of calcium antagonists: the dihydropyridines (eg, nifedipine), the phenylalkylamines (eg, verapamil), and the modified benzothiazepines (eg, diltiazem) (Weiner, 1988; Franz & Messerli, 1995).

Nifedipine is a potent systemic and coronary vasodilator of the calcium channel antagonists but has few negative inotropic characteristics. It works primarily by increasing myocardial oxygen delivery without much effect on myocardial oxygen consumption. Common side effects with this class of calcium channel antagonists include flushing, dizziness, headache, nausea, and diarrhea. Immediate-release products may cause a reflex tachycardia from excessive systemic vasodilatation. This may lead to an increase in myocardial oxygen demand, thus limiting use of the medication.

Verapamil has fewer peripheral vasodilatory properties than nifedipine but more negative inotropic properties. It also produces significant retardation of atrioventricular nodal conduction. Its antianginal efficacy stems not only from coronary vasodilatation but also from a reduction in myocardial contractility and subsequent myocardial oxygen demand.

Diltiazem produces retardation of atrioventricular nodal conduction, like verapamil, but has fewer negative inotropic effects. Its vasodilatory properties are in between those of nifedipine and verapamil.

Calcium channel blockers are selected and tailored based on individual patient characteristics. However, calcium channel blockers of all categories have demonstrated efficacy in most stable anginal syndromes (Mehta et al, 1981). Reductions in symptomatic and asymptomatic ischemia have been demonstrated, as well as a reduction in objective chest pain, reduced use of nitroglycerin, and improved exercise tolerance. Because of their potent coronary vasodilatory properties, calcium channel antagonists are the drugs of choice in the treatment of variant angina and vasospastic syndromes.

Calcium channel antagonists may also have an effect on the progression of atherosclerosis. The mechanism of action is not entirely understood but may involve inhibition of smooth muscle cell migration and proliferation (Lichtlen et al, 1990).

Caution needs to be taken in the use of calcium channel antagonists, with specific attention to concomitant cardiac actions of each agent. In patients with exertional angina pectoris, diltiazem and verapamil reduce sinus node activity, decrease atrioventricular conduction, and reduce heart rate and blood pressure, causing a limitation in exercise. In patients with left ventricular dysfunction, sinus bradycardia, sick sinus syndrome, atrioventricular block, and severe vasodilatation, the phenylalkylamines and the modified benzothiazepines should not be used. In patients who are hypotensive or who have severe aortic valve stenosis or unstable angina and are not simultaneously receiving a beta-blocker because of reflex-mediated increases in heart rate, calcium channel blockers can be harmful. Orthostatic hypotension and bradyarrhythmias may be seen with the use of the phenylalkylamines (verapamil) in patients older than age 70. Finally, calcium channel antagonists should be used cautiously in patients with an ejection fraction of less than 30%.

ASPIRIN

Aspirin has become a mainstay of treatment in unstable angina and in the prevention of progressive coronary disease in patients with chronic stable angina. Low-dose aspirin therapy selectively inhibits platelet cyclo-oxygenase, the enzyme that converts arachidonic acid into thromboxane A_2. Thromboxane A_2 causes platelet aggregation and degranulation and promotes thrombus formation. In unstable angina, aspirin therapy has been shown to reduce the mortality rate significantly (Lewis et al, 1983; RISC Group, 1990). Small amounts (81 mg/daily) have also been shown to be beneficial in reducing rates of MI and death in patients with stable, documented CAD.

CHOICE OF THERAPY

Many patients with myocardial ischemia are maintained on combination therapy. Antianginal drugs should be tailored to the type of anginal presentation. Acute anginal attacks should be initially treated with sublingual nitroglycerin, and patients should be maintained on sustained-release nitrate preparations. If exertional angina persists, beta-blockers can be added for a synergistic anti-ischemic effect. For patients with vasospastic or mixed angina, a calcium channel blocker and a nitrate are most effective. If double therapy fails to improve anginal pain, a third drug can be added for stabilization. These patients should be closely monitored, and revascularization may need to be considered.

Coronary Revascularization

Although decisions regarding percutaneous or surgical interventions are usually made in consultation with a cardiologist, the primary care provider must have an understanding of the potential benefits and limitations of the various coronary revascularization strategies to participate in the process of informing and directing his or her patient. A knowledge of individual patient concerns and expectations is also critical when both patient and physician are engaged in making these sometimes very difficult decisions.

PERCUTANEOUS TRANSLUMINAL CORONARY ANGIOPLASTY

Percutaneous transluminal coronary angioplasty (PTCA) refers to the technique of mechanical dilatation of stenotic coronary lesions by percutaneous guide-wire techniques. Access to the arterial tree is most commonly gained through the femoral artery, although severe iliofemoral or aortic atherosclerotic disease may at times necessitate arterial access through the brachial artery. After full heparinization, a flexible guide-wire is passed into one of the coronary ostia and directed across the appropriate target lesion. A balloon catheter can then be exchanged over this wire and positioned across the lesion. Inflation of the balloon results in "cracking" of the atherosclerotic plaque, with subsequent medial and adventitial stretching and luminal dilatation. Vascular sheaths are removed after the effect of heparin has worn off, and the patient is discharged on aspirin to protect against early thrombosis.

Indications and Results

In general, PTCA may be indicated when evidence of ongoing myocardial ischemia exists in the setting of epicardial coronary stenoses. This can be manifested as recurrent stable angina or persistent evidence of silent ischemia in patients who are on a maximal medical regimen. Likewise, patients manifesting recurrent chest pain or ventricular arrhythmias after MI may be candidates for PTCA. Finally, PTCA may be necessary when coronary stenoses and myocardial ischemia increase the risk of major noncardiac surgery (Bittl, 1997).

The acute success rate of PTCA is dependent on lesion anatomy. Discrete, short, concentric, smooth lesions can be dilated with a success rate of more than 85% and a low complication rate. In contrast, long, diffuse, eccentric, irregular, ostial lesions pose a more difficult technical challenge, with a concomitantly lower success rate and higher complication rate.

Decisions regarding the use of PTCA versus CABG are usually made based on the anatomic distribution of the coronary lesions. Typically, PTCA has been quite successful in the treatment of proximal single- and double-vessel disease. When high-risk anatomy exists in which acute vessel closure would be likely to result in hemodynamic collapse (ie, significant left main coronary artery disease), surgery is a more prudent option. Similarly, multivessel disease in the setting of poor ventricular function is usually more effectively approached with CABG, although cases should be assessed on an individual basis.

In patients with preserved ventricular function, diffuse multivessel disease can be treated with new and innovative PTCA techniques. The Bypass Angioplasty Revascularization Investigation (BARI) trial (1996) sought to identify whether an initial strategy of PTCA or CABG was more appropriate in this cohort of patients. In a prospective randomized study, these investigators reported an equal rate of MI, stroke, and 5-year survival among patients initially treated with PTCA or CABG. However, only 8% of patients initially treated with CABG required additional revascularization procedures, compared to 54% of patients initially treated with PTCA. Thirty-one percent of patients initially treated with PTCA eventually required CABG.

In the setting of multivessel disease and normal ventricular function, the primary care provider must take an active role in decision making regarding revascularization. The initial approach to revascularization must be based on the patient's current and projected future medical status as well as the patient's wishes and desires regarding surgery or repeat procedures.

Complications

Complications of PTCA can be separated into two categories: cardiac and extracardiac. Cardiac complications include arrhythmia, acute vessel occlusion, and vessel dissection. Vessel closure during angioplasty is unpredictable and still occurs at a rate of 2% to 8% (Ellis et al, 1997). The need for emergency CABG after PTCA occurs with an incidence of 2% to 3%. Extracardiac complications include dye-related reactions, arterial embolism, and local groin complications. Groin-related vascular complications range from groin hematoma to arteriovenous fistula and pseudoaneurysm formation. Approximately 3% of all percutaneous coronary interventions result in a vascular complication requiring surgical repair (Muller et al, 1992).

The primary chronic or late complication that continues to limit the effectiveness of PTCA remains arterial restenosis. Arterial injury sets into motion the complex cascade of medial smooth muscle cell proliferation and neointimal formation. The incidence of restenosis after PTCA is approximately 25% to 40% (Bittl, 1997; Serruys et al, 1994). No currently available therapy reduces the incidence of clinical restenosis, although intracoronary radiation and numerous pharmacologic therapies are the subjects of intense ongoing research.

INTRACORONARY STENTS

The widespread application of intracoronary stenting represents the most recent significant development in interventional cardiology. More than 12 different coronary stent designs are in clinical use and several more are under clinical investigation. Stents are distinguished by their type of delivery system (self-expanding versus balloon-expanding), their composition (stainless steel, titanium, biodegradable, polymeric), and their configuration (mesh structure, slotted, tube, coil). Intracoronary stenting is technically more challenging than standard PTCA, and the local introducer systems are larger and more complex (Cohn & Schwartz, 1996).

The indications for stenting are evolving, and randomized studies to assess its efficacy in different clinical situations are underway. Coronary stenting has been used most commonly in the treatment for restenosis after PTCA, as a "bail-out" procedure in the setting of acute vessel closure after unsuccessful PTCA, and in the treatment of difficult lesions associated with a low PTCA success rate (Cohn & Schwartz, 1996).

To date there have been two large, prospective, randomized trials comparing stents with PTCA for the treatment of *de novo* native vessel lesions, with specific attention to rates of restenosis: the Belgium Netherlands Stent Study (Benestent) and the Stent Restenosis Study (STRESS) (Serruys et al, 1994; Fischman et al, 1994). In both studies there were no differences in the rates of mortality, MI, or coronary bypass surgery over a 6-month follow-up period. However, both studies demonstrated an increased frequency of angina and need for target vessel revascularization in patients treated with PTCA. This was manifested as a significant reduction in the restenosis rate for stenting versus PTCA (27% versus 39%). In the most recent, ongoing randomized trial of stents and PTCA, a heparin-coated stent has demonstrated a 1-year restenosis rate as low as 18% (Macaya et al, 1996; Serruys et al, 1996). Although cardiac complications of PTCA and stenting were equal in both Benestent and STRESS, local vascular complications appear to be more common because of the larger introducer systems.

CORONARY ARTERY BYPASS GRAFTING

CABG refers to the surgical creation of a vascular anastomosis distal to the site of a coronary blockage to restore blood flow to the target area of perfused myocardium. Classically, CABG is performed by placing the patient on a heart-lung machine, arresting and preserving the heart with cardioplegia solution, and performing the coronary anastomosis on the still, nonbeating heart. The two primary conduits used are the saphenous vein, which is harvested from the leg, and the left internal mammary artery, which lies underneath the sternum. Proximal flow through a saphenous vein graft is created through a separate aortocoronary anastomosis, whereas the left internal mammary artery derives proximal flow via its native takeoff from the left subclavian artery.

In 10 years of follow-up, saphenous vein graft conduits have been found to be prone to intimal hyperplasia and atherosclerotic progression and have a patency rate of only 50% to 60%. Internal mammary artery grafts, on the other hand, appear to be fairly resistant to progression of atherosclerosis and intimal hyperplasia, with a 10- to 12-year patency rate of 90%. Alternative arterial conduits include the right internal mammary artery, the radial artery, and the right gastroepiploic artery. Although promising early results have been obtained with some of these alternative conduits, long-term follow-up has yet to be obtained.

Results and Indications

From historical studies, it has been accepted that CABG offers a survival advantage compared to medical therapy in patients with either left main disease or triple-vessel disease with depressed left ventricular function (Table 9-7) (Kirklin et al, 1991). In a comparison between CABG and PTCA, the BARI study (1996) also identified diabetic patients with triple-vessel disease and normal ventricular function to be a subgroup who achieved a survival advantage with an initial therapeutic intervention of surgery versus PTCA.

Patients with angina unresponsive to medical therapy also achieve a significant quality-of-life benefit from CABG. Percutaneous coronary interventions are likewise quite successful in achieving symptomatic relief in a number of different situations. The major area of controversy between these two approaches lies in the revascularization of patients with triple-vessel disease and preserved ventricular function. Although PTCA can suffice in 69% of these patients, 50% of patients or more will need multiple percutaneous procedures and 31% will eventually require CABG. Although repeat procedures are necessary only 8% of the time in this cohort after CABG, the increased morbidity of a surgical procedure can impair early quality of life. As such, intervention in these patients requires a dialogue among patient, cardiologist, and primary care provider.

Complications

The mortality rate for elective CABG ranges from 1% to 4%, with the risk of death increasing in the setting of multiple medical comorbidities, reoperation, congestive heart failure (CHF), and increasing age. Cardiac complications include arrhythmia, postoperative MI, conduction abnormalities, and pericarditis (Hammermeister et al, 1990).

Atrial fibrillation is the most common arrhythmia encountered after CABG and may occur in up to 30% of patients (Leitch et al, 1990). Prophylactic postoperative beta blockade can reduce the incidence of atrial fibrillation and is routinely used in patients without direct contraindications (Silverman et al, 1982). Perioperative MI is the result of inadequate intraoperative cardioprotection and occurs in up to 25% of patients,

TABLE 9-7	Indications for Coronary Artery Bypass Grafting

IMPROVED MORTALITY

- Left main coronary artery disease
- Triple-vessel disease with depressed left ventricular function
- Diabetes with triple-vessel disease and normal left ventricular function

IMPROVED QUALITY OF LIFE

- Triple-vessel disease and angina unresponsive to medical therapy
- ? Multivessel disease and normal left ventricular function

depending on the criteria used. Although such events are usually not accompanied by significant echocardiographic abnormalities, an increased incidence of ventricular arrhythmias can occur in such patients (Chaitman et al, 1983). Postpericardiotomy syndrome occurs in approximately 30% of patients after CABG and is manifested by fever, lethargy, and dull chest pain in the setting of a pericardial rub and pericardial effusion. Concomitant pleural effusions and pleuritic pain may also exist. The usual presentation is at 4 to 6 weeks after surgery, but patients can manifest symptoms as early as 1 week after surgery and as late as 6 months after CABG. Most patients are adequately treated with nonsteroidal anti-inflammatory agents, although severe cases require steroids and pericardial or pleural drainage.

Noncardiac complications after CABG are related to heart-lung bypass and aortic manipulation. The foreign surfaces of the bypass machine and the oxygenator cause a well-described systemic inflammatory response that can manifest as postoperative abnormalities in coagulation, renal function, and pulmonary function. Subtle changes in mood and psychological well-being are also an increasingly described phenomenon after cardiopulmonary bypass. These complications are usually treated supportively and may decrease in incidence with the use of new oxygenators and heparin-coated circuits.

Cerebral embolic events after CABG are most commonly the result of aortic cross-clamping and cannulation of the atherosclerotic aorta. Patients with extensive peripheral vascular disease are at highest risk for such intraoperative events. The use of intraoperative echocardiography to guide aortic manipulation may decrease the incidence of cerebral embolic events.

MINIMALLY INVASIVE CORONARY ARTERY BYPASS GRAFTING

New surgical approaches to coronary revascularization are under clinical investigation and have come under the title of "minimally invasive" approaches to CABG. One such approach aims at eliminating the systemic inflammatory response of cardiopulmonary bypass by performing CABG on the beating heart. The operation can be performed through a sternotomy or a small anterior thoracotomy, and various stabilization devices allow the anastomosis to be created. The aorta is not clamped and the left internal mammary artery is the primary conduit used (Subramanian, 1997).

A second approach involves placing the patient on cardiopulmonary bypass, arresting the heart, and clamping the aorta, all through percutaneous endoluminal techniques. The anastomoses are then performed through thoracoscopic ports in exactly the same manner as in conventional CABG. Although the patient is exposed to cardiopulmonary bypass, small incisions may allow for quicker recovery (Schwartz et al, 1997).

Both of these minimally invasive approaches use promising techniques that will add to the surgeon's armamentarium of surgical revascularization strategies. However, prospective, randomized studies and long-term follow-up are necessary to establish the efficacy of these approaches as standard therapies for CAD.

ACUTE MYOCARDIAL INFARCTION

Each year 900,000 people in the United States experience acute MI. Of these, roughly 225,000 die, including 125,000 who die "in the field" before obtaining medical care (Ryan et al, 1996). Because early reperfusion improves myocardial salvage as well as patient survival, patients with symptoms of acute MI should be quickly and aggressively evaluated. Treatments such as thrombolysis and angioplasty have become the cornerstone of acute therapy and the most important modalities of emergent management.

HISTORY AND PHYSICAL

Presentation

Because acute MI has a circadian pattern, most acute MIs occur between 6 AM and noon or within a few hours of arising from sleep. Other precipitating factors may be exertion, surgical procedures, pulmonary embolus, hypoglycemia, and emotional stress. Retrosternal chest pain described as viselike, constrictive, squeezing, or crushing with radiation to the left shoulder, arm, jaw, neck, right arm, epigastrium, and upper back are the most common symptoms. Other commonly associated symptoms include diaphoresis, lightheadedness, nausea, vomiting, and overwhelming weakness or fainting.

If there is no chest pain, a history of dyspnea and abdominal pain must be carefully evaluated. Clinical signs of CHF, pulmonary edema, changes in mental status, arrhythmias, syncope, or stroke may also be the presenting manifestations of acute MI. Because 25% of cases of acute MI occur silently, the careful evaluation of coronary risk factors and genetic history is extremely valuable.

Diagnostic Studies

Clinical presentation, ECG, and serum enzymes are the three most important clues to diagnosis. The physical examination may be normal, it may reveal only an S_4 gallop, or the patient may be in pulmonary edema or overt shock.

Elevations in creatine kinase and its isoenzyme (CPK-MB) 4 to 6 hours after the onset of pain remain the gold standard for the diagnosis of acute MI. Troponin T is an earlier and more specific marker for myocardial injury and is now also being used to diagnose acute MI (Adams et al, 1993).

The ECG can reveal several different patterns. The classical pattern of transmural infarction is ST-segment elevation, T-wave changes, and subsequent development of Q waves (Fig. 9-5). Nontransmural infarction reveals ST-segment depression with symmetrical T-wave inversion. New-onset bundle branch block, as well as nonspecific ST–T wave changes, can be the ECG presenting pattern. The localization of injury is based on the location of the ST-segment elevation and the Q waves. When acute MI is highly suspected but not seen on the ECG, the following diagnostic tests can be used: echocardiography, pyrophosphate infarct scintigraphy, radionuclide ventriculography, and thallium myocardial perfusion scanning.

Treatment Options, Expected Outcomes, Comprehensive Management

The management of evolving MI must be initiated rapidly to decrease the time to reperfusion. Guidelines for the management of acute MI have been outlined by the American Heart Association and the American College of Cardiology (Fig. 9-6) (Ryan et al, 1996).

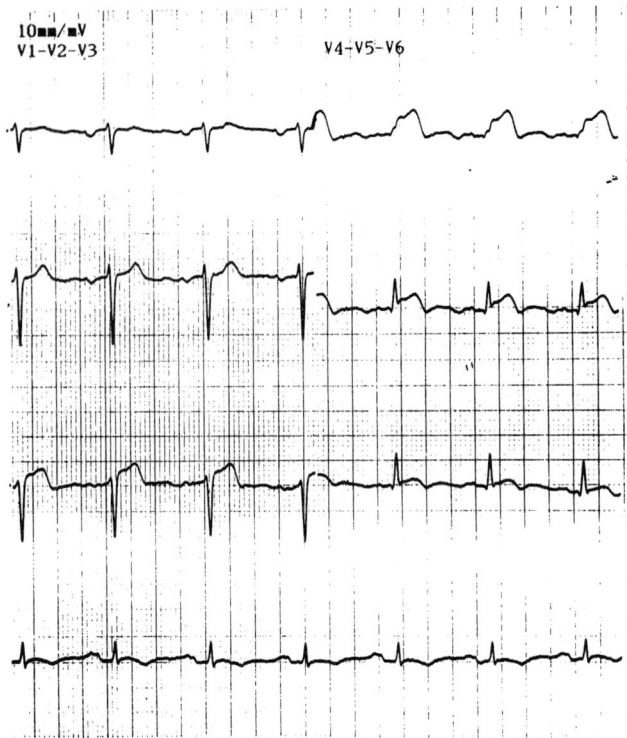

FIGURE 9-5 ECG of evolving acute transmural anterior wall myocardial infarction. Notice the elevated ST-T segments across the precordial leads.

MEDICAL

Initial treatment with a clearly defined evolving acute MI should be started without delay. Therapy should be aimed at controlling cardiac pain and reducing myocardial oxygen demand. Interventions to stabilize coronary plaque or to reduce thrombus formation may also be effective in limiting the progression of infarction.

Analgesics

For pain relief, intravenous (IV) morphine sulfate (2 to 5 mg initially) is the usual drug of choice. Meperedine (oral, subcutaneous, or IV; 50 to 100 mg) is an alternative drug for pain relief, especially in patients with bradycardia in the setting of an acute inferior wall MI. Diazepam (2 to 5 mg IV) is an excellent drug for relief of anxiety.

Nitrates

Nitrates have been reported to reduce infarct size and improve postinfarction ventricular remodeling in patients with acute MI (Derrida et al, 1978; Jugdutt & Warnica, 1988). Nitrates work primarily as venodilators and cause significant reductions in preload. Such reductions result in a decrease in left ventricular end-diastolic pressure and subsequent reductions in left ventricular wall tension and myocardial oxygen demand. Although nitrates also possess significant coronary vasodilatory properties, they rarely are capable of opening occluded arteries, and their primary anti-ischemic effects in acute MI are through reductions in preload. Because of their marked effects on venous return, nitrates should be used only with extreme caution in the setting of right ventricular infarction.

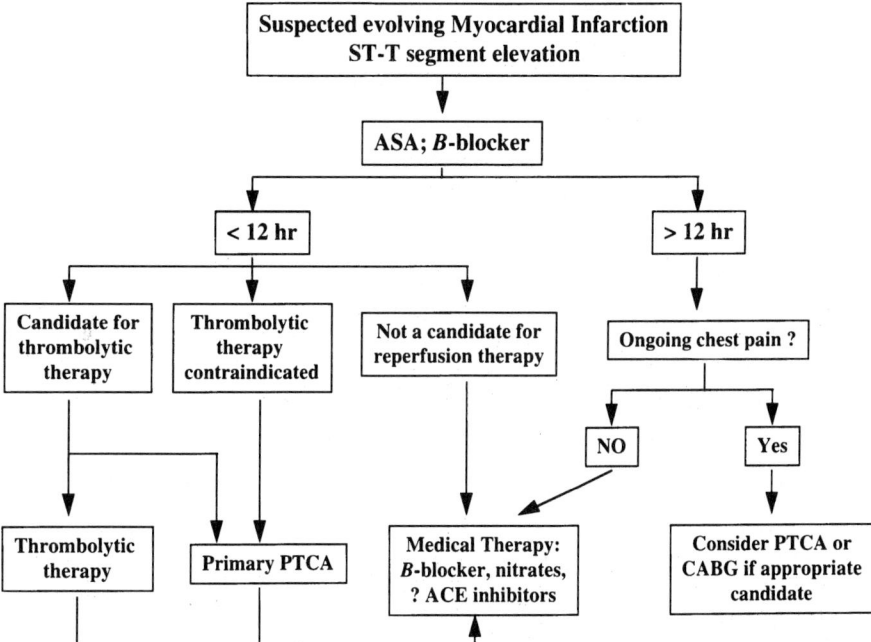

FIGURE 9-6 ACC/AHA algorithm for the management of patients with ST-segment elevation. (ACE = angiotensin-converting enzyme, ASA = acetylsalicylic acid, CABG = coronary artery bypass grafting, PTCA = percutaneous transluminal coronary angioplasty.)

IV nitroglycerin can be administered safely at an initial infusion rate of 5 μg/min with stepwise increments of 5 μg/min until the mean arterial blood pressure is reduced by 10%. Sublingual nitroglycerin can also be used in the setting of acute MI. However, the rate of absorption is difficult to predict with sublingual administration, and hypotension can develop rapidly. Tolerance to nitroglycerin can develop as early as 12 hours after the initial infusion and is manifested by increasing nitrate requirements.

Beta-Adrenoreceptor Blockade

Beta blockade causes a reduction in myocardial oxygen demand by reducing cardiac index, heart rate, blood pressure, and tension-time index levels. Beta-blockers have beneficial effects in both the acute and chronic treatment (secondary prevention) of acute MI. Four large randomized trials have been completed to date designed to test the effect of early beta blockade in MI (Roberts et al, 1984; International Collaborative Study Group, 1984; MIAMI Trial, 1985; ISIS-1, 1986). All four have shown a reduction in infarct size among beta-blocked patients compared to those receiving placebo. Furthermore, in a multicenter trial of more than 16,000 patients, early use of IV atenolol resulted in a significant reduction in the mortality rate when compared to placebo-treated patients (ISIS-1, 1986).

Beta-blockers have also demonstrated significant benefits in the months after MI. In this setting, beta-blockers have been shown to reduce the mortality rate by 15% to 25%, with benefits demonstrated for up to 2 years (Viscoli et al, 1993; Viskin et al, 1995). The greatest reduction in mortality is enjoyed by patients at highest risk after MI, including those with: an ejection fraction of less than 40% with compensated CHF; ventricular tachycardia or fibrillation; ongoing ischemia; frequent premature ventricular contractions; and recurrent MI.

Beta-blockers are recommended for all patients after Q-wave MI if no contraindications exist. Beta-blockers should not be administered in patients with bronchial asthma, second- or third-degree heart block, significant CHF, heart rate less than 50 beats per minute, or systolic blood pressure less than 90 mmHg.

Aspirin

Coronary thrombi frequently occur at sites of rupture or fissure of atherosclerotic plaques to produce the syndrome of acute MI. Such arterial thrombi are primarily composed of aggregated platelets. Knowledge of these pathologic mechanisms has led to a number of clinical trials evaluating the use of antiplatelet agents in lysing or preventing coronary thrombi. Landmark studies have shown that aspirin therapy reduces the incidence of both first-time and subsequent MI by as much as 20% (Lewis et al, 1983; Antiplatelet Trialists, 1994; ISIS-2, 1988). The Second International Study of Infarct Survival (ISIS-2) demonstrated a 44% reduction in the incidence of nonfatal MI and a 21% reduction in the incidence of fatal MI among 17,187 patients receiving either immediate aspirin therapy or placebo for acute cardiac chest pain. Aspirin alone was similar in efficacy to thrombolysis alone, and the administration of both was additive.

Based on this study, the American College of Chest Physicians has recommended that nonenteric-coated aspirin (160 to 325 mg) be chewed and swallowed immediately in patients experiencing acute MI (Dalen & Hirsch, 1995). Aspirin should also be continued indefinitely in patients after acute MI. A prior allergic response to aspirin, an ongoing history of ulcer disease, and a history of recent or ongoing systemic anticoagulation with warfarin therapy are contraindications to initiation of aspirin therapy in acute MI.

Angiotensin-Converting Enzyme Inhibitors

Several recent trials have demonstrated significant beneficial effects of therapy with angiotensin-converting enzyme (ACE) inhibitors after MI. The incidence of CHF appears to be reduced by 11% to 46%, and reductions in overall mortality as high as 29% have been demonstrated with ACE inhibitor therapy when compared to placebo (Ambrosioni et al, 1994; Pfeffer et al, 1992; Acute Infarction Ramipril Efficacy Study, 1993; Kober et al, 1995; Swedberg et al, 1992).

Based on this current evidence, ACE inhibitors are recommended in patients after MI who demonstrate ST-segment elevation in two or more anterior leads, have clinical symptoms of CHF, or have an ejection fraction of less than 40%. Early administration appears to be most beneficial, but treatment within the first hours of MI should be avoided because of the possibility of inducing hypotension (Swedberg et al, 1992).

Thrombolysis

The primary therapeutic objective in patients with evolving MI is restoration of normal antegrade flow in the occluded artery. Salvaging myocardium and limiting the extent of injury in patients with evolving MI can be accomplished with prompt initiation of thrombolytic therapy. The efficacy of thrombolysis in dissolving clot, however, is dependent on the time to initiation of treatment, with rates of normal flow restoration decreasing significantly if treatment is initiated more than 3 to 6 hours after the onset of pain (Muller & Topol, 1990).

The two most widely studied thrombolytic agents to date have been streptokinase and recombinant tissue-type plasminogen activator (t-PA). Streptokinase is a thrombolytic enzyme derived from the streptococcus bacteria that can be given as a one-time IV dose. It is the most inexpensive of clinically used thrombolytics, but repeat dosing is not possible secondary to antibody formation. t-PA is an endogenously produced enzyme that is released from the vascular endothelium. It is produced by recombinant techniques and costs approximately 20 times more than streptokinase. Nonetheless, the success rate of establishing normal flow appears to be slightly better than with streptokinase, and repeat dosing is possible.

The major side effect of thrombolytic therapy is intracranial bleeding, which occurs in 1% to 2% of patients. Approximately 10 to 15 additional new thrombolytic agents are currently under investigation, and these may have fewer bleeding complications. Nonetheless, thrombolytics should not be used in patients with known intracranial pathology or gastrointestinal bleeding or after head trauma.

In placebo-controlled, randomized trials, prompt thrombolysis has been shown to significantly reduce infarct size, improve left ventricular function, and reduce mortality (Fibrinolytic Therapy Trialists, 1994; GUSTO, 1993). Thrombolytic therapy is widely available and is easily and quickly administered. Such therapy can be given immediately on presentation and may be administered by a physician, nurse, or technician in the field before arriving at the hospital. However, many patients are ineligible for treatment because of bleeding risk, late presentation, or nondiagnostic ECG findings.

PERCUTANEOUS TRANSLUMINAL CORONARY ANGIOPLASTY

Whereas the mainstays of medical treatment for acute MI remain aspirin, heparin, and beta blockade, the role of interventional approaches remains unclear. Thrombolysis therapy has been successfully used now for more than 10 years in patients without contraindications to dissolve clot and re-establish flow in a recently occluded vessel. However, limitations to this therapy include the risk of cerebral bleeding and the need to administer therapy within 6 to 12 hours of the onset of pain. A vessel patency rate of only 50% has led to the introduction of early interventional techniques in the setting of acute MI.

In several prospective, randomized studies, PTCA has demonstrated a 90% success rate in achieving target vessel patency for acute MI. Although the mortality rate remains statistically unchanged in most studies with follow-up to 6 months, early PTCA appears to result in fewer future cardiac events and a lower need for repeat revascularization of the target vessel. The incidence of early reocclusion also appears to be significantly less in patients undergoing primary PTCA as compared to patients initially undergoing treatment with thrombolysis (Grines et al, 1993).

THROMBOLYSIS VERSUS PERCUTANEOUS TRANSLUMINAL CORONARY ANGIOPLASTY

The optimal strategy for establishing vessel patency in acute MI remains controversial. Thrombolysis can be initiated early, is inexpensive, and can be performed in any health care setting. PTCA has the advantage of re-establishing normal flow in more than 90% of occluded arteries and has a better long-term patency rate than thrombolysis. However, the need for access to a catheterization laboratory still limits its universal use.

The primary care provider is frequently the first to evaluate and diagnose acute MI. It is therefore incumbent on him or her to make rapid decisions, in consultation with a cardiologist, regarding the most appropriate initial therapeutic interventions for acute MI. Knowledge of ongoing trials is imperative for the primary care provider to participate in complex management decisions with patients.

CORONARY ARTERY BYPASS GRAFTING

Historically, CABG in the setting of acute MI has been associated with an increased mortality rate, and surgery is reserved for situations in which cardiogenic shock ensues despite maximal support. Surgical revascularization may safely take place 7 to 10 days after adequate medical treatment and diagnostic anatomic studies when indicated.

TEACHING AND SELF-CARE

Primary Prevention

The term "primary prevention" refers to risk factor screening and modification in patients with neither a history of CAD nor an unusually high risk for having CAD. Primary prevention emphasizes lifestyle modifications, including smoking cessation, maintenance of normal blood pressure, healthy diet (<10% of the total calories from saturated fats), exercise, and behavior modification. All modifications are designed to promote a healthy style of living with the hope of avoiding, or at least delaying, the development of atherosclerosis.

A clinical approach to prevention, either primary or secondary, includes accurate risk factor assessment, a specific treatment plan, long-term assessment, and an effective follow-up plan. The initial evaluation should include a careful medical history with emphasis on CAD risk factors, including age, gender, family history of CAD, socioeconomic status, tobacco use, and exercise history. In addition, a thorough physical examination should be performed with accurate measurement of height, weight, and blood pressure. Specific risk factor modifications are mentioned herein with attention to CAD prevention. More detailed descriptions of each condition can be found elsewhere in this text.

Randomized trials including both genders, all races, and a wide spectrum of pressures have demonstrated that small decreases in both systolic and diastolic blood pressure can reduce the incidence of CAD by up to 6% (Collins et al, 1990). A subset analysis of younger versus older patients revealed a similar percentage reduction in events but a greater absolute reduction in events in the elderly (Cutler et al, 1995). Most of the published trials have used beta-blockers, diuretics, or both as initial drug therapy. Before the initiation of drug therapy, lifestyle modifications should be instituted, including weight control, physical activity, and moderate intake of alcohol and sodium. Age, left ventricular hypertrophy, proteinuria, and the presence of vascular disease identify patients at higher risk. The modest efficacy demonstrated by blood-pressure reduction may underestimate the actual benefit that higher-risk populations might enjoy.

The actual blood-pressure measurement is usually chosen as the goal of therapeutic intervention. However, it may be necessary to pay attention to other physiologic endpoints. Optimal treatment may entail therapy that inhibits vascular wall thickening, normalizes arterial compliance, prevents or reverses left ventricular hypertrophy, corrects proteinuria, normalizes endothelial dysfunction, and reverses insulin resistance. Therefore, blood pressure alone may not be an adequate surrogate. The efficacy of various therapeutic regimens on these other endpoints, however, still needs to be established.

A nonfasting total cholesterol and HDL cholesterol should be obtained in all patients more than 20 years of age at least once every 5 years. The intensity of treatment of the individual patient depends on his or her risk status. Patients can be divided into three general risk categories: those with a high blood cholesterol level but low risk otherwise (fewer than two CAD risk factors), those with a high blood cholesterol level without a history of CAD but with more than two other CAD risk factors, and those with evidence of CAD and a high cholesterol level (Table 9-8). Primary prevention aimed at lowering the serum cholesterol level reduces both the incidence of CAD and the overall mortality rate (Shepherd et al, 1995; Shepherd, 1995). The West of Scotland Study, a large randomized trial comparing placebo versus pravastatin for elevated total cholesterol levels, demonstrated a 31% reduction in the relative risk of a definite coronary event (Shepherd, 1995). This reduction was apparent in the first 6 months and continued to increase throughout the 5 years of follow-up. There were no excess deaths from non-CAD causes. The treatment of hyperlipidemia is discussed in detail in Chapter 10.

Homocysteine levels should be modified in patients at high risk for CAD. Interventions aimed at reduction of homocysteine levels are straightforward and nontoxic. Hyperhomocysteinemia is corrected with a daily multivitamin plus an additional 800 μg of folate daily for 8 weeks. A persistently elevated homocysteine level after 8 weeks of therapy may be treated with 2 mg of folate daily. Eating fruits and green leafy vegetables can likewise help to lower homocysteine levels. Other dietary sources of folate include breakfast cereals, lentils, chickpeas, asparagus, spinach, and most beans.

Secondary Prevention

Conclusive evidence from population-based studies of reduction of all-cause mortality by modification of CAD risk factors has been lacking. However, significant reduction in CAD mortality and morbidity rates has been demonstrated. The benefit is greatest in patients with evidence of CAD or those who are at a mortality risk of 4% or greater per year. Secondary prevention refers to risk factor modification in patients who have had a prior clinical coronary event (ie, angina pectoris or acute MI). The objectives of risk reduction are to reduce mortality, ischemic symptoms, recurrent MI, and other manifestations of atherosclerosis and to improve overall general health. A thorough clinical approach should be the standard of care for all patients, as outlined for primary prevention. A guide to comprehensive risk reduction for patients with cardiovascular disease by the American Heart Association and endorsed by the American College of Cardiology is provided in Table 9-9.

Cigarette smoking is the single most obvious and important risk factor for coronary and vascular disease (Jonas et al, 1992). It must be eliminated in the management of all patients at high risk for, or with evidence of, CAD. Patients who continue to smoke after MI are at increased risk of death and reinfarction (English et al, 1940). Smoking has been clearly implicated in bypass graft atherosclerosis and thrombosis, with a twofold increase in the relative risk of death and an increase in the incidence of nonfatal MI and angina.

Hypertension should be rigorously controlled in patients with prior coronary events. Recommendations for treatment are similar to those outlined for primary prevention. Therapy should be aimed at lowering the systolic blood pressure to less than 140 mmHg and the diastolic blood pressure to less than 90 mmHg. Blood-pressure medication should be added to lifestyle modifications and diet if hypertension persists after 3 months or if the initial blood pressure exceeds 160 mmHg systolic or 100 mmHg diastolic.

TABLE 9-8	Treatment Decisions Regarding Lipid Management Based on Presenting CAD Risk and LDL Level		
Category	Starting LDL Level (mg/dL)	Initial Treatment	LDL Goal (mg/dL)
Without CAD and <2 risk factors	160–189	Dietary therapy	<160
	≥190	Drug therapy	<160
Without CAD and with ≥2 risk factors	130–159	Dietary therapy	<130
	≥160	Drug therapy	<130
With CAD	100–129	Dietary therapy	<100
	≥130	Drug therapy	<100

As recommended by the Second Report of the National Cholesterol Education Program.

TABLE 9-9	Guide to Comprehensive Risk Reduction for Patients With CAD as Outlined by the American Heart Association
Risk Intervention	**AHA Recommendations**
Smoking	Goal: Complete cessation Encourage patient and family to stop smoking. Provide counseling, nicotine replacement, and formal cessation programs as appropriate.
Lipid Management	See Table 9-8.
Physical Activity	Minimum goal: 30 minutes 3 or 4 times per week Assess risk with exercise test where appropriate to guide exercise prescription. Encourage 30–60 minutes of moderate intensity activity 3 or 4 times weekly (walking, jogging, cycling, or other aerobic activity). Advise medically supervised programs for moderate- to high-risk patients.
Weight Management	Start intensive diet and appropriate physical activity intervention in patients >120% of ideal weight for height. Emphasize need for weight loss in patients with hypertension, elevated triglycerides, or elevated glucose levels.
Blood-Pressure Control	Goal: <140/90 mmHg Initiate lifestyle modifications in all patients with blood pressure >140 mmHg systolic or 90 mmHg diastolic. Add medication if blood pressure is >140 mmHg systolic or 90 mmHg diastolic in 3 months *or* if initial blood pressure is >160 mmHg systolic or 100 mmHg diastolic.
Estrogens	Consider estrogen replacement in all postmenopausal women. Individualize consistent with other health risks.
Beta-Blockers	Start in high-risk post-MI patients (arrhythmia, left ventricular dysfunction, inducible ischemia) at 5–28 days. Continue 6 months minimum. Observe usual contraindications.
Antiplatelet Agents/Anticoagulants	Start aspirin 80–325 mg in all patients if not contraindicated. Begin warfarin (International Normalized Ratio 2–3.5) for post-MI patients unable to take aspirin.
ACE Inhibitors Post-MI	Start early in all high-risk patients post-MI (anterior wall MI, previous MI, CHF). Continue indefinitely in patients with left ventricular dysfunction (ejection fraction <40%) or symptoms of failure.

The postmenopausal woman is at increased risk for cardiovascular disease. ERT is generally believed to be of significant benefit. ERT confers a 50% reduction in the risk of developing CAD and an even greater risk reduction for subsequent coronary events among women with established CAD (Sullivan et al, 1990). Patients with severe coronary atherosclerosis by angiogram also demonstrate a marked reduction in CAD deaths with ERT. ERT should be considered in all postmenopausal women, and its use should be addressed on an individual basis. For women at risk of thromboembolic disease or those who have other associated risk factors (eg, hypertension, tobacco use, or a first-degree relative with breast cancer), ERT should be addressed in light of the potential risk/benefit ratio.

Finally, medical therapies aimed at reducing the rates of mortality and future coronary events should be initiated in all patients after MI unless specific contraindications exist. The use of aspirin, beta-blockers, and ACE inhibitors has documented benefit in the risk reduction of post-MI patients.

Cardiac Rehabilitation

It is the role of the primary care provider to initiate and coordinate rehabilitation for the patient who has sustained an MI. Rehabilitation begins in the hospital and is continued in a medically supervised progressive exercise program. The goal is to have the patient return to a maximal functional level. In-hospi-tal rehabilitation is most effectively achieved through a coordinated team approach that includes consultants, physical therapists, nurses, and other health professionals as well as access to community-based cardiac rehabilitative resources. The team approach also includes psychosocial support by the primary care provider as well as family, friends, and coworkers. Cardiac rehabilitation should be both comprehensive and individualized. Any program of rehabilitation must consider the severity of disease, medical and postsurgical risk factors, and the patient's physical condition, vocational status, and emotional state. In addition, the individualized exercise prescription is enhanced by dietary and pharmacologic modification and therapy as well as through lifestyle modifications.

The best available evidence indicates that physical activity is beneficial in both primary and secondary prevention. No single trial analyzing the effect of physical activity in patients with CAD has had enough power to demonstrate a risk reduction. However, intermediate endpoints (HDL cholesterol and blood pressure) are improved, and several meta-analyses have demonstrated a 20% to 30% reduction in CAD deaths with regular aerobic exercise (Haskell, 1994; O'Connor et al, 1989; Oldridge et al, 1988). The role of the primary care provider is to help set achievable goals and to provide encouragement and support. A minimum of 30 to 60 minutes of moderate-intensity activity should be encouraged three or four times weekly. Five sessions per week produces the maximal results and can be achieved in 4 to 6 weeks. All patients with known CAD should undergo treadmill testing before initiation of an exercise program, and patients at moderate to high risk should enter medically supervised programs.

COMMUNITY RESOURCES

Many hospitals sponsor support groups for their post-MI patients. These groups are often called "heart clubs" and are open to patients and their families. Also, the following national organizations provide resources and support for patients with coronary artery disease: the American Heart Association and the InterAmerican Heart Foundation, 7272 Greenville Ave., Dallas, TX 75231-4596 (1-800-AHA-USA1) and the Heart and Stroke Foundation of Canada, 160 George St., Suite 200, Ottawa, Ontario K1N 9M2 (613-241-4361). The following Internet sites also contain information relevant to CAD:

- Heart Home Page: www.hearthome.com
- American Heart Association: www.amhrt.org
- Merck Heart Diseases Information Page: www.merck.com
- Community Outreach Health Information Systems: www.bu.edu/COHIS/

REFERRAL POINTS AND CLINICAL WARNINGS

Early recognition and triage of patients with acute ischemia is a fundamental role of the primary care provider. Time to reperfusion is critical, and a rapid protocol should be instituted in the event that acute ischemia is diagnosed. Patients with anterior chest pain, dyspnea, diaphoresis, or a diagnostic 12-lead ECG in two or more contiguous leads do not provide a major diagnostic dilemma. These patients should undergo rapid referral to an emergency setting for immediate cardiac consultation and evaluation. Patients with known stable angina or those with multiple CAD risk factors who present acutely with gastrointestinal, esophageal, or other anginal equivalent symptoms should likewise undergo rapid referral and evaluation for evolving MI.

Patients may present with other signs and symptoms of myocardial ischemia in the absence of anginal pain that should prompt emergency referral. The acute onset of overt pulmonary vascular congestion or arterial oxygen desaturation may indicate ischemic left ventricular dysfunction. Arrhythmias, including new-onset atrial fibrillation, profound and prolonged sinus bradycardia, and second- or third-degree atrioventricular block, may also be signs of silent cardiac ischemia. The new appearance of a systolic murmur in the setting of pulmonary edema is an ominous sign for ischemic mitral valvular regurgitation.

Finally, the progression of stable angina to angina with minimal exertion or angina occurring at rest is a critical warning sign for the development of an unstable coronary syndrome. Such patients require urgent evaluation because this symptomatology frequently heralds the onset of acute coronary occlusion.

■ ■ ■ ■ CLINICAL PEARLS

- There are no clinical trails that indicate a decreased risk of coronary disease secondary only to an increase in HDL cholesterol.
- It has been suggested that HDL and triglycerides should not be considered separately when evaluating cardiac risk.

- Cigarette smoking adversely affects lipid profiles.
- While there is an increased incidence in the development of angina pectoris in those with the Type A personality, no subsequent increase in fatal cardiac events has been identified.
- It has been clearly established that esophageal pain and other syndromes may also respond to nitroglycerin.
- Physical examination of the patient's venous system can reveal previous coronary bypass grafting.
- Even cardioselective β1 blockers in high doses lose their selectivity and therefore are contraindicated in asthma and diabetes.
- Prophylactic postoperative β-blockade can reduce the incidence of atrial fibrillation and is routinely employed in patients without direct contraindications.
- Clinical signs of congestive heart failure, pulmonary edema, changes in mental status, arrhythmias, syncope, or stroke may also be the presenting manifestions of acute myocardial infarction.

EDITOR'S NOTE:
COMPLEMENTARY APPROACHES

A general discussion of complementary approaches can be found in Chapter 3. The following, while not an exhaustive list, are some complementary approaches being used for this condition. Additional information on these approaches, including precautions, can be found in Appendices A and B. Providers need to assess for the use of complementary approaches as part of the patient's history, as they may impact conventional therapies, and patients may not volunteer this information unless specifically asked. Efficacy of many complementary approaches is not as well documented as that of conventional therapies. Providers need to read the literature before suggesting these complementary approaches.

- Vitamins, minerals, herbs, supplements
  Carnitine
  Coenzyme Q10
  Fish oils
  Folate
  Garlic
  Magnesium
  Vitamin B_6
  Vitamin C
  Vitamin E
- Complementary Modalities
  Acupuncture
  Aromatherapy
  Biofeedback

References

Acute Infarction Ramipril Efficacy Study Investigators. (1993). Effect of ramipril on mortality and morbidity of survivors of acute myocardial infarction with clinical evidence of heart failure. *Lancet, 342,* 821–828.

Adams, J.E. III, Bodor, G.S., Davila-Roman, V.G., et al. (1993). Cardiac troponin I: A marker with high specificity for cardiac injury. *Circulation, 88,* 101–106.

Alderman, E.L., Bourassa, M.G., Cohen, L.S., et al. (1990). Ten-year follow-up of survival and myocardial infarction in the randomized Coronary Artery Surgery Study. *Circulation, 82,* 1629–1646.

Ambrosioni, E., Borghi, C., & Magnani, B., on behalf of the SMILE Study Investigators. (1994). Effects of the early administration of zofenopril on mortality and morbidity in patients with anterior myocardial infarction. Results of the Survival of Myocardial Infarction Long-Term Survival Trial. *N Engl J Med, 332*, 80–85.

American Diabetes Association. (1997). Clinical practice recommendations. *Diabetes Care, 20* (suppl), S1–70.

American Heart Association. (1991). *1991 heart and stroke facts.* Dallas: Author.

Antiplatelet Trialists' Collaboration. (1994). Collaborative overview of randomised trials of antiplatelet therapy: Prevention of death, myocardial infarction and stroke by prolonged antiplatelet therapy in various categories of patients. *British Medical Journal, 308*, 81–106.

Ardehali, A., Ports, T.A. (1990). Myocardial oxygen supply and demand. *Chest, 98*, 699–710.

Assman, G., & Schulte, H. (1992). Relation of high-density lipoprotein cholesterol and triglycerides to incidence of atherosclerotic coronary disease (the PROCAM experience). Prospective Cardiovascular Munster Study. *American Journal of Cardiology, 70*, 733–737.

Badimon, J.J., Fuster, V., Chesebro, J.H., & Badimon, L. (1993). Coronary atherosclerosis. A multifactorial disease. *Circulation, 87*(3 suppl), 113–116.

Barrett-Conner, E., & Bush, T.L. (1991). Estrogen and coronary heart disease in women. *JAMA, 265*, 1861–1867.

Barrett-Conner, E., & Bush, T.L. (1994). Estrogen and coronary heart disease. In: Pearson, T.A., Criqui, M.H., Luepker, R.V., Oberman, A., & Winston, M. (Eds.). *Primer in preventive cardiology.* Dallas, TX: American Heart Association.

Bassan, M.M. (1990). The daylong pattern of the antianginal effect of long-term three-times-daily administered isosorbide. *Journal of the American College of Cardiology, 16*, 936–945.

Berkman, L.F., Leo-Summers, L., & Horowitz, R.I. (1992). Emotional support and survival after myocardial infarction. A prospective, population-based study of the elderly. *Annals of Internal Medicine, 117*, 1003–1009.

Berliner, J.A., Navab, M., Fogelman, A.M., et al. (1995). Atherosclerosis: Basic mechanisms. Oxidation, inflammation and genetics. *Circulation, 91*, 2488–2496.

Bittl, J.A. (1997). Advances in coronary angioplasty. *N Engl J Med, 335*, 1290–1302.

Bush, T.L., Barrett-Conner, E., Cowan, L.D., et al. (1987). Cardiovascular mortality and noncontraceptive use of estrogen in women: Results from the Lipid Research Clinics Program Follow-up Study. *Circulation, 75*, 1102–1109.

Bush, T.L., & Korenman, S.G. (Eds.). (1990). Noncontraceptive estrogen use and risk of cardiovascular disease: An overview and critique of the literature. *Menopause: Biologic and clinical consequences of ovarian failure: Evaluation and management.* Norwell, MA: Serona Symposium.

Butler, W.J., Ostrander, L.D., Carman, W.J., & Lamphiear, D.E. (1985). Mortality from coronary heart disease in the Tecumseh study. Long-term effect of diabetes mellitus, glucose tolerance and other risk factors. *American Journal of Epidemiology, 121*, 541–547.

Bypass Angioplasty Revascularization Investigation (BARI) Investigators. (1996). Comparison of coronary bypass surgery with angioplasty in patients with multivessel disease. *N Engl J Med, 335*, 217–225.

Cates, C.U., Kronenberg, M.W., Collins, H.W., & Sandler, M.P. (1989). Dipyridamole radionuclide ventriculography: A test with high specificity for severe coronary disease. *Journal of the American College of Cardiology, 13*, 841–853.

Chaitman, B.R., Alderman, E.L., Sheffield, L.T., et al. (1983). Use of survival analysis to determine the clinical significance of new Q waves after coronary bypass surgery. *Circulation, 67*, 302–310.

Cohen, E.A., & Schwartz, L. (1996). Coronary artery stenting, indications and cost implications. *Progress in Cardiovascular Diseases, 39*, 83–110.

Cohn, P.E. (1996). Silent myocardial ischemia and infarction. *Cardiovascular Research and Reviews, 17*, 67–82.

Cohn, P.F., Maddox, D., Holman, B.L., Markis, J.E., Adam, D.F., & See, J.R. (1997). Effect of sublingually administered nitroglycerine on regional myocardial blood flow in patients with coronary artery disease. *American Journal of Cardiology, 39*, 672–678.

Collins, R., Peto, R., MacMahon, S., et al. (1990). Blood pressure, stroke, and coronary heart disease. Part 2, Short-term reductions in blood pressure: Overview of randomised drug trials in their epidemiological context. *Lancet, 335*, 827–838.

Cutler, J.A., Psalty, B.M., MacMahon, S., & Furberg, C.D. (1995). Public health issues in hypertension control: What has been learned from clinical trials. In: Laragh, J.H., & Brenner, B.M. (Eds.). *Hypertension: Pathophysiology, diagnosis, and management,* 2d ed. New York: Raven Press.

Dalen, J.E., & Hirsch, J. (1995). Fourth AACP Consensus Conference on Antithrombotic Therapy. *Chest, 108*, 380S–400S.

Deanfiels, J.E., Shea, M.J., Wilson, R.A., et al. (1986). Direct effects of smoking on the heart: Silent ischemic disturbances of coronary flow. *American Journal of Cardiology, 57*, 1005–1010.

de Bono, D. (1993). Complications of diagnostic cardiac catheterisation, results from 34,041 patients in the United Kingdom confidential enquiry into cardiac catheter complications. *British Heart Journal, 70*, 297–300.

Derrida, J.P., Sal, R., & Chiche, P. (1978). Favorable effects of prolonged nitroglycerin infusion in patients with acute myocardial infarction. *American Heart Journal, 96*, 833–840.

Diabetes Control and Complications Trial Research Group. (1993). The effect of intensive treatment of diabetes on the development and progression of long-term complications in insulin-dependent diabetes mellitus. *N Engl J Med, 329*, 977–986.

Eaker, E.D., Abbott, R.D., & Kannel, W.B. (1989). Frequency of uncomplicated angina pectoris in Type A compared with Type B persons. The Framingham Study. *American Journal of Cardiology, 63*, 1042–1056.

Ellis, S.G., Weintraub, W., Holmes, D., Shaw, R., Block, P.C., & King, S.B. (1997). Relation of operator volume and experience to procedural outcome of percutaneous coronary revascularization at hospitals with high interventional volume. *Circulation, 95*, 2467–2470.

English, J.P., Willus, F.A., & Berkson, J. (1940). Tobacco and coronary disease. *Journal of the American Medical Association, 13*, 1327–1329.

Farmer, J.A., & Gotto, A.M. (1997). In: Brauwald, E. (Ed.) *Heart disease: A textbook of cardiovascular medicine.* Philadelphia: W.B. Saunders.

Fibrinolytic Therapy Trialists' (FTT) Collaborative Group. (1994). Indications for fibrinolytic therapy in suspected acute myocardial infarction: Collaborative overview of early mortality and major morbidity results from all randomised trials of more than 1000 patients. *Lancet, 43*, 311–322.

Fischman, D.L., Leon, M.B., Baim, D.S., et al. (1994). A randomized comparison of coronary-stent placement and balloon angioplasty in the treatment of coronary artery disease. Stent Restenosis Study Investigators. *N Engl J Med, 331*, 496–501.

Franz, H., & Messerli, M.D. (1995). *Cardiovascular Drug Therapy,* 2d ed. Philadelphia: W.B. Sauders.

Freedman, D.S., Jacobsen, S.J., Barboriak, J.J., et al. (1990). Body fat distribution and male/female differences in lipids and lipoproteins. *Circulation, 81*, 1498–1506.

Friedlander, Y. (1994). Familial clustering of coronary heart disease: A review of its significance and role as a risk factor for disease. In: Goldbourt, U., de Faire, U., & Berg, K. (Eds.). *Genetic factors in coronary heart disease.* Hingham, MA: Kluwer Academic Publishers.

Garlin, R., & Sadock, K. (1994). Nitrates in the management of heart disease. *Clinical Cardiology, 21,* 4–6.

Gaziano, J.M., Buring, J.E., Breslow, J.L., et al. (1993). Moderate alcohol intake, increased levels of high-density lipoprotein and its subfractions, and decreased risk of myocardial infarction. *N Engl J Med, 329,* 1829–1834.

Gensini CG. (1975). *Coronary arteriography.* Mt. Kisco, N.Y.: Futura.

Getz, G.S. (1993). Report on the workshop on diabetes and mechanisms of atherogenesis, Sept. 17 and 18, 1992, Bethesda, Maryland. *Arteriosclerosis and Thrombosis, 13*(3), 459–464.

Gibbons, G.H., & Dzau, V.J. (1994). The emerging concept of vascular remodeling. *N Engl J Med, 330,* 1431–1438.

Gibbons, R.J., Balady, G.J., Beasley, J.W., et al. (1997). ACC/AHA guidelines for exercise testing: Executive summary. A report of the American College of Cardiology/American Heart Association Task Force on Practice Guidelines (committee on exercise testing). *Circulation, 96,* 345–354.

Goldstein, S. (1996). Beta-blockers in hypertensive and coronary heart disease. *Archives of Internal Medicine, 156,* 1267–1276.

Gordon, D.J., Probstfield, J.L., Garrison, R.J., et al. (1989). High-density lipoprotein cholesterol and cardiovascular disease. Four prospective American studies. *Circulation, 79,* 8–15.

Gould, K.L. (1989). How accurate is thallium exercise testing for the diagnosis of coronary disease ? *Journal of the American College of Cardiology, 14,* 1487–1497.

Graham, T.P., Jr., Corvell, J.W., Sonnenblick, E.H., et al. (1968). Control of myocardial oxygen consumption, relative influence of contractile state and tension development. *Journal of Clinical Investigation, 47,* 375–382.

Green, K.G. (1991). British MRC trial of treatment for mild hypertension—a more favorable interpretation. *American Journal of Hypertension, 338,* 1281–1285.

Green, M.S., Jucha, E., & Luz, Y. (1986). Blood pressure in smokers and non-smokers: Epidemiologic findings. *American Heart Journal, 111,* 932–941.

Grines, C.L., Browne, K.F., Marco, J., et al. (1993). A comparison of immediate angioplasty with thrombolytic therapy for acute myocardial infarction. The Primary Angioplasty in Myocardial Infarction Study Group. *N Engl J Med, 328,* 673–679.

GUSTO Investigators. (1993). An international randomized trial comparing four thrombolytic strategies for acute myocardial infarction. *N Engl J Med, 328,* 685–691.

Hammermeister, K.E., Burchfiel, C., Johnson, R., & Grover, F.L. (1990). Identification of patients at greatest risk for developing major complications at cardiac surgery. *Circulation, 82*(Suppl I), IV380–389.

Hamstn, A., & De Faire, U. (1987). Risk factors for coronary heart disease in families of young men with myocardial infarction. *American Journal of Cardiology, 59,* 14–19.

Haskell, W.L. (1994). Sedentary lifestyle as a risk factor for coronary heart disease. In: Pearson, T.A., Criqui, M.H., Luepker, R.V., Oberman, A., & Winston, M. (Eds.). *Primer in preventive cardiology.* Dallas: American Heart Association.

International Collaborative Study Group. (1984). Reduction of infarct size with the early use of timolol in acute myocardial infarction. *N Engl J Med, 310,* 9–15.

ISIS-1 (First International Study of Infarct Survival) Collaborative Group. (1986). Randomized trial of intravenous atenolol among 16,027 cases of suspected acute myocardial infarction. ISIS-1. *Lancet, 2,* 57–62.

ISIS-2 (Second International Study of Infarct Survival) Collaborative Group. (1988). Randomised trial of intravenous streptokinase, oral aspirin, or both, or neither among 17,187 cases of suspected acute myocardial infarction: ISIS-2. *Lancet, 2,* 349–360.

Joint National Committee (1993). The fifth report of the Joint National Committee on Detection, Evaluation, and Treatment of High Blood Pressure. *Archives of Internal Medicine, 153,* 154–183.

Jonas, M.A., Oates, J.A., Ockene, J.K., & Hennekens, C.H. (1992). Statement on smoking and cardiovascular disease for health care professionals. American Heart Association. *Circulation, 86,* 1664–1669.

Jugdutt, B.I., & Warnica, W. (1988) Intravenous nitroglycerin therapy to limit myocardial infarct size, expansion, and complications. Effect of timing, dosage, and infarct location. *Circulation, 78,* 906–919.

Kaplan, G.A., & Keil, J.E. (1993). Socioeconomic factors and cardiovascular disease: a review of the literature. *Circulation, 88,* 1973–1998.

Kirklin, J.W., Akins, C.W., Blackstone, E.H., et al. (1991). ACC/AHA guidelines and indications for coronary artery bypass graft surgery. A report of the American College of Cardiology/American Heart Association Task Force on assessment of diagnostic and therapeutic cardiovascular procedures. *Circulation, 83,* 1125–1140.

Kirklin, J.W., & Barratt-Boyes, B.G. (1993). *Cardiac surgery.* New York: Churchill-Livingstone.

Kleinman, J.C., Donahue, R.P., Harris, M.I., et al. (1988). Mortality among diabetics in a national health sample. *American Journal of Epidemiology, 128,* 389.

Kober, L., Torp-Pedersen, C., Carlsen, J.E., et al. (1995). A clinical trial of the angiotensin-converting-enzyme inhibitor trandolapril in patients with left ventricular dysfunction after myocardial infarction. Trandolapril Cardiac Evaluation (TRACE) Study Group. *N Engl J Med, 335,* 1670–1676.

Koss, J.H., Kobren, S.M., Grunwald, A.M., & Bodenheimer, M.M. (1987). Role of exercise thallium-201 myocardial perfusion scintigraphy in predicting prognosis in suspected coronary artery disease. *American Journal of Cardiology, 59,* 531–543.

Krieger, M. (1995). Lipoprotein receptors and atherosclerosis. In: Haber, E. (Ed.) *Scientific American molecular cardiovascular medicine.* New York: Scientific American.

Langford, H.G., Stamler, J., Wassertheil-Smoller, S., & Prineas, R.J. (1986). All-cause mortality in the Hypertension Detection and Follow-up Program. Findings for the whole cohort and for persons with less severe hypertension with and without other traits related to risk of mortality. *Progress in Cardiovascular Diseases, 29,* 29–37.

Leitch, J.W., Thomson, D., Baird, D.K., & Harris, P.J. (1990). The importance of age as a predictor of atrial fibrillation and flutter after coronary artery bypass grafting. *Journal of Thoracic and Cardiovascular Surgery, 100,* 338–347.

Lewis, H., Archibald, G., Steinke, W.E., et al. (1983). Protective effects of aspirin against myocardial infarction and death in men with unstable angina. *N Engl J Med, 309,* 396–403.

Lichtlen, P.R., Hugenholtz, P.G., Rafflenbeul, W., et al. (1990). Retardation of angiographic progression of coronary artery disease by nifedipine, results of the international nifedipine trial on antiatherosclerotic therapy (INTACT). *Lancet, 335,* 1109–1113.

Loscalzo, J. (1992). The relation between atherosclerosis and thrombosis. *Circulation, 86*(6 suppl), 1195–1199.

Macaya, C., Serruys, P.W., Ruygrok, P., et al. (1996). Continued benefit of coronary stenting versus balloon angioplasty: One year follow-up of Benestent trial. *Journal of the American College of Cardiology, 27,* 255–261.

MacMahon, S., Peto, R., Cutler, J., et al. (1990). Blood pressure, stroke, and coronary heart disease. Part 1, Prolonged differences in blood pressure: Prospective observational studies corrected for the regression dilution bias. *Lancet, 335*(8692), 765–774.

Manninen, V., Tenkanen, L., Koskinen, P., et al. (1992). Joint effects of serum triglyceride and LDL cholesterol and HDL cholesterol concentrations on coronary heart disease risk in the Helsinki Heart Study. Implications for treatment. *Circulation, 85,* 37–45.

Manson, J.E., Willet, W.C., Stampfer, M.J., et al. (1995). Body weight and mortality among women. *N Engl J Med, 333,* 677–685.

Mark, D.B., Califf, R.M., Morris, K.G., et al. (1984). Clinical characteristics and long-term survival of patients with variant angina. *Circulation, 66,* 588–600.

Mehta, J., Pepine, C.J., Day, M., et al. (1981). Short-term efficacy of oral verapamil in rest angina, a double-blind placebo-controlled trial in CCU patients. *American Journal of Medicine, 71,* 977–982.

MIAMI Trial Research Group. (1985). Metoprolol in acute myocardial infarction (MIAMI). A randomized placebo-controlled international trial. *European Heart Journal, 6,* 199–210.

Migas, O.D. (1988). The lipid effects of smoking. *American Heart Journal, 115,* 272–278.

Morris, D.L., Kritchevsky, S.B., & Davis, C.E. (1994). Serum carotenoids and coronary heart disease. The Lipid Research Clinics Coronary Primary Prevention Trial and Follow-up Study. *JAMA, 272,* 1439–1441.

Muller, D.W., Shamir, K.J., Ellis, S.G., & Topol, E.J. (1992). Peripheral vascular complications after conventional and complex percutaneous interventional procedures. *American Journal of Cardiology, 69,* 63–68.

Muller, D.W., & Topol, E.J. (1990) Selection of patients with acute myocardial infarction for thrombolytic therapy. *Ann Intern Med, 113,* 949–960.

National Institute of Health; National Heart, Lung and Blood Institute. (1994). *Morbidity and mortality chartbook on cardiovascular, lung, and blood disease.* Bethesda, MD: U.S. Government Printing Office.

Neaton, J.D., & Wentworth, D. (1992). Serum cholesterol, blood pressure, cigarette smoking, and death from coronary heart disease. Overall findings and differences by age for 316,099 white men. Multiple Risk Factor Intervention Trial Research Group. *Archives of Internal Medicine, 152,* 56–64.

NIH Consensus Development Panel on Triglyceride, HDL, and Coronary Heart Disease. (1993). Triglyceride, high-density lipoprotein, and coronary heart disease. *JAMA, 269,* 505–510.

Nygard, O., Nordrehaug, J.E., Refsum, H., Ueland, P.M., Farstad, M., & Vollset, S.E. (1997). Plasma homocysteine levels and mortality in patients with coronary artery disease. *N Engl J Med, 337,* 230–236.

O'Connor, G.T., Buring, J.E., Yusuf, S., et al. (1989). An overview of randomized trials of rehabilitation with exercise after myocardial infarction. *Circulation, 80,* 234–244.

O'Connor, N.J., Manson, J.E., O'Connor, G.T., & Buring, J.E. (1995). Psychosocial risk factors and non-fatal myocardial infarction. *Circulation, 92,* 1458–1464.

Oldridge, N.B., Guyatt, G.H., Fischer, M.E., & Rimm, A.A. (1988). Cardiac rehabilitation after myocardial infarction. Combined experience of randomized clinical trials. *JAMA, 260,* 945–950.

Olsson, G., Tuomilehto, J., Berglund, G., et al. (1991). Primary prevention of sudden cardiovascular death in hypertensive patients. Mortality results from the MAPHY Study. *American Journal of Hypertension, 4*(2 Pt 1), 151–158.

Parker, J.O., Amies, M.H., Hawkinson, R.W., et al. (1995). Intermittent transdermal nitroglycerin therapy in angina pectoris: Clinically effective without tolerance or rebound. The Minitran Efficacy Study. *Circulation, 91,* 1368–1374.

Passamani, E., Davis, K.B., Gillespie, M.J., Killip, T., CASS Principal Investigators. (1985). A randomized trial of coronary bypass surgery, survival in patients with a low ejection fraction. *N Engl J Med, 312,* 1665–1671.

Pepine, C.J., Cohn, P.F., Deedwania, P.C., et al. (1994a). Effects of treatment on outcome in mildly symptomatic patients with ischemia during daily life. The atenolol silent ischemia study (ASIST). *Circulation, 90,* 762–768.

Pepine, C.J., Cohn, P.F., & Ellenbogen, K.A. (1994b). Advisory Group reports on silent myocardial ischemia, coronary atherogenesis, and cardiac emergencies. Council for Myocardial Ischemia and Infarction. *American Journal of Cardiology, 73,* 39B–44B.

Pfeffer, M.A., Braunwald, E., Moye, L.E., et al. (1992). Effects of captopril on mortality and morbidity in patients with left ventricular dysfunction after myocardial infarction. *N Engl J Med, 327,* 669–677.

Pohost, G.M., & Johnson, L.L. (1992). Indications for thallium scanning. *Heart Disease and Stroke, Nov/Dec,* 348–356.

Reducing the health consequences of smoking: 25 years of progress. Washington DC: U.S. Government Printing Office, 1989.

Reichard, P., Nilsson, B.Y., Rosenqvist, U. (1993). The effect of long-term intensified insulin treatment on the development of microvascular complications of diabetes mellitus. *N Engl J Med, 329,* 304–309.

Rigotti, N.A., & Pasternak, R.C. (1996). Cigarette smoking and coronary artery disease: Risks and management. *Cardiology Clinics, 14,* 51–68.

RISC Group. (1990). Risk of myocardial infarction and death during treatment with low-dose aspirin and intravenous heparin in men with unstable coronary artery disease. *Lancet, 340,* 1421–1425.

Rissanen AM. (1979). Familial occurrence of coronary heart disease: Effect of age at diagnosis. *American Journal of Cardiology, 59,* 60–66.

Roberts, R., Croft, C., Gold, H.K., et al. (1984). Effect of propranolol on myocardial infarct size in a randomized blinded multicenter trial. *N Engl J Med, 311,* 218–225.

Rooke, G.A., & Fiegel, E.O. (1984). Work as a correlate of canine left ventricular oxygen consumption and the problem of catecholamine oxygen wasting. *Circulation Research, 55,* 734–741.

Ross, R. (1993). The pathogenesis of atherosclerosis, a perspective for the 1990s. *Nature, 362,* 801–808.

Ryan, T.J., Anderson, J.L., Antmann, E.M., et al. (1996). ACC/AHA guidelines for the management of patients with acute myocardial infarction: Executive summary. A report of the American College of Cardiology/American Heart Association task force on practice guidelines (Committee on Management of Acute Myocardial Infarction). *Circulation, 94,* 2341–2350.

Scandinavian Simvastatin Survival Study (4S). (1994). Randomised trial of cholesterol lowering in 4444 patients with coronary heart disease. *Lancet, 344,* 1383–1389.

Schwartz, C.J., Valente, A.J., Sprague, E.A., Kelley, J.L., Cayatte, A.J., & Rozek, M.M. (1992). Pathogenesis of the atherosclerotic lesion. Implications for diabetes mellitus. *Circulation, 15*(9), 1156–1157.

Schwartz, D.S., Ribakove, G.H., Grossi, E.A., et al. (1997). Single and multivessel port-access coronary artery bypass grafting with cardioplegic arrest: Technique and reproducibility. *Journal of Thoracic and Cardiovascular Surgery, 114,* 46–52.

Seiler, P., Corona, P., Audoin, P., et al. (1988). Influence of training on blood lipids and coagulation. *European Heart Journal, 9,* 32–41.

Serruys, P.W., de Jaegere, P., Kiemeneij, F., et al. (1994). A comparison of balloon-expandable-stent implantation with balloon angioplasty in patients with coronary artery disease. Benestent Study Group. *N Engl J Med, 331,* 489–495.

Serruys, P.W., Emanuelsson, H., van der Giessen, W.J., et al. (1996). Heparin-coated Palmaz-Schatz stents in human coronary arteries: Early outcome of the Benestent-II pilot study. *Circulation, 93,* 412–422.

Severi, S., & Michelassi, C. (1991) Prognostic impact of stress testing in coronary artery disease. *Circulation, 85*(suppl I), III82–88.

Shaper, A., Wannamethee, G., & Walker, M. (1988). Alcohol and mortality in British men: Explaining the u-shaped curve. *Lancet,* 1267–1273.

Shepherd, J. (1995). The West of Scotland Coronary Prevention Study: A trial of cholesterol reduction in Scottish men. *American Journal of Cardiology, 76*(9), 113C–117C.

Shepherd, J., Cobbe, S.M., Ford, I., et al. (1995). Prevention of coronary heart disease with pravastatin in men with hypercholesterolemia. *N Engl J Med, 333,* 1301–1306.

Silverman, N.A., Wright, R., & Levitsky, S. (1982). Efficacy of low-dose propranolol in preventing postoperative supraventricular tachyarrhythmias. A prospective randomized study. *Annals of Thoracic Surgery, 196,* 194–201.

Stamler, J. (1987). Epidemiology, established major risk factors, and the primary prevention of coronary heart disease. In: Parmley, W.W., & Chatterjee, K. (Eds.). *Cardiology.* Philadelphia: J.B. Lippincott.

Stamler, J., Dyer, A.R., Shekelle, R.B., Neaton, J., & Stamler, R. (1993a). Relationship of baseline major risk factors to coronary and all-cause mortality, and to longevity; findings from long-term follow-up of Chicago cohorts. *Cardiology, 82,* 191–222.

Stamler, J., Neaton, J., & Wentworth, D. (1993b). Blood pressure (systolic and diastolic) and risk of fatal coronary heart disease. *Hypertension, 13,* 2–12.

Subramanian, V.A. (1997). Less invasive arterial CABG on a beating heart. *Annals of Thoracic Surgery, 63*(6 Suppl), S68–71.

Sullivan, J.M., Vander Zwaag, R., Hughes, J.P., et al. (1990). Estrogen replacement therapy and coronary artery disease. Effect on survival in postmenopausal women. *Archives of Internal Medicine, 150,* 2557–2562.

Summary of the second report of the National Cholesterol Education Program (NCEP) Expert Panel on Detection, Evaluation and Treatment of High Blood Cholesterol in Adults (Adult Treatment Panel II). (1993). *JAMA, 269,* 3015–3023.

Swedberg, Held, P., Kjekshus, J., et al. (1992). Effects of the early administration of enalapril on mortality in patients with acute myocardial infarction. Results of the Cooperative New Scandinavian Enalapril Survival Study II (CONSENSUS II). *N Engl J Med, 327,* 678–684.

Tranchesi, B., Jr., Barbosa, V., de Albugueaque, C.P., et al. (1992). Diagonal earlobe crease as a marker of the presence and extent of coronary atherosclerosis. *American Journal of Cardiology, 70,* 1417–1425.

Varnauskas, E., & the European Coronary Surgery Study Group. (1988). Twelve-year follow-up of survival in the randomized European Coronary Surgery Study. *N Engl J Med, 319,* 332–337.

Veterans Administration Coronary Artery Bypass Surgery Cooperative Study Group. (1984). Eleven-year survival in the Veterans Administration randomized trial of coronary bypass surgery for stable angina. *N Engl J Med, 311,* 332–337.

Viscoli, C.M., Horwitz, R.I., & Singer, B.H. (1993). Beta-blockers after myocardial infarction: Influence of first-year clinical course on long-term effectiveness. *Annals of Internal Medicine, 118,* 99–105.

Viskin, S., Kitzis, I., Lev, E., et al. (1995). Treatment with beta-adrenergic blocking agents after myocardial infarction: From randomized trials to clinical practice. *Journal of the American College of Cardiology, 25,* 1327–1332.

Weiner, D.A. (1988). Calcium channel blockers. *Medical Clinics of North America, 72,* 83–115.

Weiner, D.A., Ryan, T.J., McCabe, C.H., et al. (1979). Exercise stress testing. Correlations among history of angina, ST-segment response and prevalence of coronary-artery disease in the coronary surgery study (CASS). *N Engl J Med, 301,* 230–343.

Wikstrand, J., Warnold, I., Olsson, G., Tuomilehto, J., Elmfeldt, D., & Berglund, G. (1992). Primary prevention with metoprolol in patients with hypertension. Mortality results from the MAPHY study. *Journal of the American Medical Association, 259,* 1976–1982.

Wilson, R.F., Marcus, M.L., Christensen, B.V., et al. (1991). Accuracy of exercise electrocardiography in detecting physiologically significant coronary arterial lesions. *Circulation, 83,* 412–420.

Winder, A.F. (1983). Relationship between corneal arcus and hyperlipidemia is clarified by studies in familial hypercholesterolemia. *British Journal of Ophthalmology, 67,* 789–794.

Yano, K., Rhoads, G., & Kagan, A. (1977). Coffee, alcohol and the risk of coronary heart disease among Japanese men living in Hawaii. *N Engl J Med, 297,* 405–409.

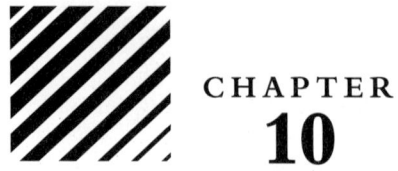

CHAPTER

10

Dyslipidemias

Joseph Reilly, PharmD, and Steven Richardson, MD

Coronary artery disease (CAD) is the leading cause of death for both men and women in the United States, and its incidence increases linearly with age. Large population studies demonstrate a clear relation between cholesterol levels and CAD risk, especially in subjects with cholesterol levels more than 200 to 240 mg/dL. Over the last two decades, overwhelming evidence has accumulated demonstrating this relation as well as the benefits of reducing serum cholesterol with a reduced risk of CAD. This bidirectional relation has led to the establishment of a National Cholesterol Education Program (NCEP) (Expert Panel, 1994). The approach of the NCEP is to identify and treat high-risk patients with elevated cholesterol levels and to encourage the general public to modify life habits to reduce cholesterol concentrations with other risk factors for CAD that have been identified (see Chap. 9) (Table 10-1).

Successful management of hyperlipidemic patients requires a thorough understanding of nonpharmacologic and pharmacologic therapies. Health care providers must also have an understanding of the multifactorial nature of the process of atherogenesis (see Chap. 9). Although the focus of this review is the role of hyperlipidemia in CAD and the current approaches to correcting hyperlipidemia, many patients who have CAD and suffer a myocardial infarction (MI) do not have high cholesterol levels.

ANATOMY, PHYSIOLOGY, AND PATHOLOGY

Lipid Metabolism and Pathophysiology

Cholesterol is a water-insoluble molecule that is essential for cell membrane formation and the synthesis of steroid hormones and bile acids. Cells derive cholesterol from intracellular synthesis or extraction from the systemic circulation. Daily cholesterol intake ranges from 250 to 500 mg, with approximately 50% being absorbed (Grundy et al, 1978). Body synthesis of cholesterol ranges from 500 to 1000 mg/dL (Grundy et al, 1966, 1969). Therefore, approximately 25% of the body's total cholesterol source is from dietary intake and 75% is synthesized *in vivo*. Cellular synthesis of cholesterol takes place through a series of biochemical steps involving a number of enzymes (Fig. 10-1). An important class of drugs, the hydroxymethylglutaryl coenzyme A (HMG CoA) reductase inhibitors, also referred to as the statins, disrupts this process; these drugs are commonly used in patients with elevated cholesterol levels.

Cholesterol and triglycerides in the diet enter into the exogenous pathway of lipid transport. Cholesterol in the intestine must be solubilized before it can be absorbed, and absorption is incomplete because cholesterol is highly insoluble in aqueous solutions (Grundy et al, 1996). In the intestine, cholesterol is in the unesterified (free) form and becomes esterified with a fatty acid when it enters the intestinal mucosa. Triglycerides are reformulated from absorbed fatty acids and monoglycerides and are incorporated with cholesterol esters into chylomicrons. These lipoproteins eventually reach the systemic circulation and undergo partial catabolism to chylomicron remnants carrying newly absorbed cholesterol into the liver (Grundy et al, 1996).

Hepatic cholesterol comes from newly absorbed cholesterol, from the uptake of serum lipoproteins, and via hepatic synthesis. In the liver, cholesterol can be incorporated into lipoproteins that are secreted into the plasma; their density is determined by their relative content of protein and lipid. Hepatic cholesterol synthesis (endogenous pathway) is regulated by the quantity of cholesterol in the liver. Bile acid synthesis is governed by the quantity of bile acids returning to the liver via enterohepatic circulation (Grundy et al, 1996). The primary route of cholesterol excretion is into the bile as cholesterol or as bile acids. About one third of the cholesterol synthesized or absorbed is converted into bile acids, which can be reabsorbed into the portal circulation and return to the liver (Grundy et al, 1966, 1969).

Lipid disorders can result from a dysfunction in any one of the numerous steps involved in the process of lipid metabolism. Table 10-2 categorizes the more common lipid disorders.

Lipoproteins

Lipids are present in the plasma as circulating lipoproteins that transport cholesterol and triglycerides. The basic structure of a typical lipoprotein is shown in Figure 10-2. These lipoproteins are divided into classes, typically based on their density and composition. The major lipoproteins include chylomicrons, very-low-density lipoproteins (VLDL), intermediate-density lipoproteins or remnant particles, low-density lipoproteins (LDL), and high-density lipoproteins (HDL) (Table 10-3). LDL accounts for approximately 60% to 70% of total serum cholesterol, HDL 20% to 30%, and VLDL about 10% to 15%. In addition, each lipoprotein particle contains proteins on its outer surface called apolipoproteins. These proteins have several functions, such as activating enzyme systems, providing structure to the lipoprotein, and binding with cell receptors.

Apolipoproteins

Four major classes of apolipoproteins exist: apo B, apo A, apo C, and apo E (Table 10-4). Patients with abnormal metabolism of apolipoproteins may be at an increased risk of atherosclerosis even if they have normal cholesterol levels. Therefore, many health care providers believe that apolipoprotein levels should be used to evaluate hyperlipidemic patients.

TABLE 10-1	Risk Factors for Coronary Heart Disease

POSITIVE RISK FACTORS

Sex/age (years)
    Male ≥45
    Female ≥55 or premature menopause without estrogen replacement therapy

Family history of premature coronary heart disease
    (Definite myocardial infarction or sudden death before 55 years of age in
    father or other first-degree male relative, or before 65 years of age in
    mother or other female first-degree relative)

Current cigarette smoking

Hypertension
    Blood pressure ≥140/90 mmHg or taking an antihypertensive medication)

Low high-density lipoprotein cholesterol level
    <35 mg/dL)

Diabetes mellitus

NEGATIVE RISK FACTORS

High high-density lipoprotein cholesterol level
    (≥60 mg/dL)

---

* If ≥60 mg/dL, subtract one positive risk factor because high levels of high-density lipoprotein decrease the risk of coronary heart disease.

Chylomicrons

Synthesized in the intestine, chylomicrons are large triglyceride-rich particles with apolipoproteins B-48, apo A, apo C, and apo E. In the peripheral circulation, chylomicrons interact with lipoprotein lipase on the vascular endothelium, which hydrolyzes the triglycerides into free fatty acids and monoglycerides, which are then absorbed by muscle and adipose tissues. The resultant product is a cholesterol-rich chylomicron remnant that is taken up by the liver. In patients with a lipoprotein lipase deficiency, this process is defective and hypertriglyceridemia results.

Newly absorbed cholesterol thus passes into the liver in chylomicron remnants. Fatty acids of chylomicron triglycerides are released into the peripheral circulation and can be used by muscle for energy, adipose tissue, and the liver. After a fatty meal, chylomicron levels are elevated, and therefore triglycerides are high. However, after a 12- to 24-hour fast, chylomicrons will have cleared from the blood. Fasting triglyceride concentrations reflect hepatic production and that which is carried by in VLDL and other remnant particles. For this reason, patients are required to fast before obtaining a lipoprotein profile.

Very-Low-Density Lipoproteins

Triglyceride-rich VLDL particles are produced by the liver and contain apo B-100 and apo E on their surface. The nascent VLDL particles circulate and acquire cholesterol esters and apolipoproteins (including apo C), developing into mature VLDLs. The B and E proteins are ligands for LDL receptors, and a defect in these receptors results in increased levels of cholesterol. Apolipoprotein C-II activates lipoprotein lipase, which interacts with VLDL as it does with chylomicrons. Fatty acids are released, producing remnant VLDL and intermediate-density lipoproteins. These remnants are eventually metabolized by the liver or converted to LDL. Most of the triglycerides are removed and replaced with cholesterol esters. Deficiencies of C-II apolipoproteins result in faulty triglyceride metabolism and hypertriglyceridemia.

Low-Density Lipoproteins

The LDLs are the major cholesterol transport lipoproteins in the plasma. They contain cholesterol ester in their core and only apolipoprotein B-100 on their surface. LDL is derived from VLDL catabolism and cellular synthesis. LDL is cleared by the liver and extrahepatic tissues, which recognize the apo B-100 and bind and internalize the particle, which is then degraded. Excess circulating LDL will result in deposition of cholesterol outside the cell, causing the formation of atherogenic plaques in the vascular endothelium. Because LDL contains 60% to 70% of the total blood cholesterol and there is a direct relation between the LDL concentration in the systemic circulation and atherosclerosis, LDL is the primary target of cholesterol-lowering therapies, in accordance with NCEP guidelines.

High-Density Lipoproteins

The smallest of the lipoprotein particles, HDL appears to transport cholesterol from peripheral cells to the liver. The liver and the gut secrete nascent HDL that consist of apo A and phospholipids. These particles acquire unesterified cholesterol that becomes esterified by lecithin–cholesterol acyltransferase, forming HDL-3 particles. HDL-3 acquires more cholesterol, forming HDL-2, which in turn may be converted back to HDL-3 by hepatic lipase and by transferring cholesterol esters to the liver, LDL, and VLDL. The transfer of cholesterol from HDL particles to lipoproteins is catalyzed by the enzyme cholesterol ester transfer protein. This complex HDL cycle is a critical part of the reverse cholesterol transport process, where cholesterol is returned to the liver for excretion.

In contrast to LDL, high HDL concentrations are desirable because they provide protective effects against the atherogenic process. Because HDL particles contain apo A-I, which activates lecithin–cholesterol acyltransferase, levels of apo A-I have a strong inverse correlation with CAD. Patients with abnormally low HDL levels (<35 mg/dL) are at an increased risk for CAD, presumably because of the decreased ability to remove

Acetyl CoA
↓
HMG CoA
      ↓ * HMG CoA reductase
(rate-limiting enzyme)
Mevalonate
↓
Mevalonate pyrophosphate
↓
Isopentenyl pyrophosphate
↓
Geranyl pyrophosphate
↓
Farnesyl pyrophosphate → ubiquinone, dolichol
↓
Squalene
↓
Lanosterol
↓
Cholesterol
↓↓↓
Bile acids, lipoproteins, steroid hormones

FIGURE 10-1 Biosynthetic Pathway for Cholesterol

TABLE 10-2	Common Lipid Disorders		
Disorder	Defect	Effect	
DEFECTIVE CLEARANCE			
Familial hypercholesterolemia (heterozygous)	LDL receptors	↑ LDL	
Dysbetalipoproteinemia (type III hyperlipidemia)	Apo E	↑ IDL, remnant VLDL	
Familial defective apo B-100	Apo B	↑ LDL	
Polygenic hypercholesterolemia	LDL receptor activity	↑ LDL	
INCREASED PRODUCTION			
Familial hyperapobetalipoproteinemia	↑ Apo B	↑ Apo B	
Familial combined hyperlipidemia	↑ Apo B and VLDL	↑ Cholesterol and/or ↑ triglycerides	
Hypoalphalipoproteinemia	↑ HDL catabolism (low HDL)	↓ HDL	

LDL, low-density lipoprotein; VLDL, very-low-density lipoprotein; IDL, intermediate-density lipoprotein.

TABLE 10-3	Classification of Major Lipoproteins		
Lipoprotein	Density (g/mL)	Primary Composition	Source
Chylomicron	0.98	Triglyceride-rich	Intestine
VLDL	0.98–1.006	Triglyceride-rich	Liver
IDL	1.006–1.019	Cholesterol esters & triglycerides	VLDL catabolism
LDL	1.019–1.063	Cholesterol-rich	IDL catabolism
HDL	1.063–1.21	Cholesterol-rich	Liver, intestine

(From the Expert Panel [1988] Report of the National Cholesterol Education Program Expert Panel on detection, evaluation and treatment of high blood cholesterol in adults. *Archives of Internal Medicine*, 148, 36–39. Chicago: American Medical Association.)

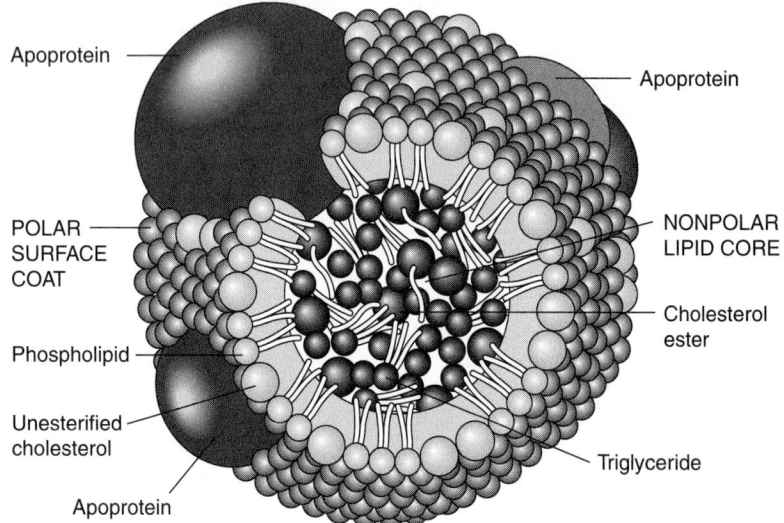

FIGURE 10-2 Basic structure of lipoproteins.

TABLE 10-4	Classification of Major Apolipoproteins	
Apolipoprotein	Lipoproteins	Sources
APOLIPOPROTEIN Bs		
B-48	Chylomicrons	Intestine
B-100	VLDL, LDL	Liver
APOLIPOPROTEIN As		
A-I	Chylomicrons, HDL	Liver, intestine
A-II	Chylomicrons, HDL	Liver
A-IV	Chylomicrons, HDL	Intestine
APOLIPOPROTEIN Cs		
C-I	Chylomicrons, VLDL, HDL	Liver
C-II	Chylomicrons, VLDL, HDL	Liver
C-III	Chylomicrons, VLDL, HDL	Liver
OTHER		
D	HDL	?
E2-E4	Chylomicrons, VLDL, HDL	Liver

(From the Expert Panel [1988] Report of the National Cholesterol Education Program Expert Panel on detection, evaluation and treatment of high blood cholesterol in adults. *Archives of Internal Medicine*, 148, 36–39. Chicago: American Medical Association.)

circulating cholesterol. In general, for every 1% decrease in HDL, there is a 2% to 3% increase in CAD (Gordon et al, 1989). In contrast, an elevated HDL level (≥60 mg/dL) is considered a negative risk factor for CAD.

Low-Density-Lipoprotein Receptors

Cholesterol uptake by hepatic and peripheral cells is accomplished by the binding of apolipoproteins found on circulating lipoproteins to LDL receptors on cell surfaces. LDL receptor synthesis occurs when there are low concentrations of intracellular cholesterol. These receptors are capable of binding with lipoproteins containing apolipoproteins E or B-100. Once bound, these lipoproteins are degraded. Drugs capable of reducing the intracellular synthesis of cholesterol can upregulate LDL receptors, thus enhancing removal of cholesterol from the systemic circulation.

ETIOLOGY OF HYPERLIPIDEMIA

The most severe forms of hyperlipidemia occur in patients with a defect in lipid metabolism or transport (see Table 10-2). Persons with these hereditary diseases or primary causes of hyperlipidemia typically require pharmacotherapy in conjunction

TABLE 10-5	Secondary Causes of Hyperlipidemia (Disease-Induced)
Acromegaly	Glycogen storage disease
Diabetes mellitus	Nephrotic syndrome
Hypothyroidism	Anorexia nervosa
Chronic renal failure	Lipodystrophy
Hepatic disease	Systemic lupus erythematosus

(From the Expert Panel [1988] Report of the National Cholesterol Education Program Expert Panel on detection, evaluation and treatment of high blood cholesterol in adults. *Archives of Internal Medicine*, 148, 36–39. Chicago: American Medical Association.)

TABLE 10-6	Secondary Causes of Hyperlipidemia (Drug-Induced)
Medication Class	Comments
Diuretics	Thiazides: ↑ cholesterol and triglycerides, with exception of indapamide, Loop: ↓ HDL
Beta-blockers	Selective and nonselective: ↑ triglycerides and ↓ HDL, with exception of those that are alpha-blocking or with ISA activity
Cyclosporine	↑ cholesterol
Anabolic steroids	↑ cholesterol
Isotretinoin	↑ cholesterol and triglycerides, ↓ HDL
Glucocorticoids	↑ cholesterol and triglycerides
Alcohol	↑ triglycerides
Oral contraceptives	↑ cholesterol and triglycerides, ↑ HDL: because of progestins; estrogen alone is protective; effects will vary between available formulations

with lifestyle modifications to correct or normalize their condition.

Secondary causes of hyperlipidemia can be attributed to lifestyle and underlying disease states (Table 10-5). In addition, many medications can have a negative effect on the lipid profile (Table 10-6). Many of these medications are used to treat comorbid disease states such as hypertension, congestive heart failure, and angina. Health care providers should evaluate the hyperlipidemic patient's current medications and identify the drugs that may be contributing to the dyslipidemic state. In some cases, a suspected medication can be replaced by one that has a neutral effect on lipids or one that has a beneficial effect. Angiotensin-converting enzyme (ACE) inhibitors and calcium channel blockers have a neutral effect on lipids; postsynaptic alpha-1 receptor blockers (eg, prazosin, terazosin, doxazosin) have favorable lipoprotein effects.

A person's dietary habits and lifestyle have a significant effect on the lipid profile and body weight, which can be positively correlated with LDL and triglyceride levels and negatively correlated with HDL levels. Patients who are overweight will benefit from weight loss, as seen by reduced LDL and triglyceride levels and an increased HDL level. Modifications in diet can result in weight loss and improvements in the lipoprotein profile. For these reasons, lifestyle modifications including dietary therapy are considered the foundation of therapy.

RATIONALE FOR THERAPY OF DYSLIPIDEMIA

Epidemiologic studies have greatly contributed to our understanding of CAD in patients with high blood cholesterol levels. A direct relation between total cholesterol and LDL levels in the blood and death and disability from coronary heart disease (CHD) has been demonstrated consistently. One of the most notable studies is the Framingham Heart Study (Kannel et al, 1971). In this ongoing study, the population of Framingham, Massachusetts, has been followed for more than 30 years, documenting that cardiovascular risk factors are related to CHD rates where serum cholesterol levels are correlated with CHD rates. In addition, long-term survival is inversely related to total cholesterol level at entry to the study (Anderson et al, 1987).

Another investigation, the Multiple Risk Factor Intervention Trial, involved more than 360,000 men in the United States (Stamler et al, 1986). The study participants were screened and followed for 6 years for CHD mortality. This trial showed a positive curvilinear correlation between initial cholesterol levels and subsequent CHD mortality, further emphasizing the relation between high cholesterol levels and CHD.

Individual lipoprotein fractions and CHD rates have similarly been established. The Framingham Heart Study (Kannel et al, 1979). revealed the association between risk factors and CHD: a high LDL level was found to be more predictive of CHD than the total cholesterol level. The significance of this relation is evident in the NCEP's recommendations, in which LDL is the primary target of therapy in patients with hyperlipidemia. This same study (Kannel et al, 1979; Cordon et al, 1977) has also provided valuable data about the negative relation between HDL level and CHD.

Serum triglyceride concentrations are also correlated with CHD risk (Austin, 1991). The Framingham Heart Study (Castelli, 1986) showed that the VLDL level (reflecting serum triglycerides) was a predictor of CHD. However, the specific relation between serum triglyceride levels and CAD was not very clear. Atherosclerotic plaques primarily contain cholesterol, not triglycerides. However, in patients with hypertriglyceridemia, there is often an accompanying increase in other atherogenic lipoproteins and a decreased HDL level. Therefore, an elevation in triglycerides may result in an increase of other lipoproteins that promote CAD. When serum triglycerides exceed 1000 mg/dL, the most immediate danger is acute pancreatitis. In patients with diabetes mellitus, reduction of glucose levels may significantly lower triglyceride levels.

The benefits of cholesterol-lowering therapies in patients with existing CHD (secondary prevention) and those without CHD (primary prevention) have been firmly established. The following is a brief review of the major primary and secondary prevention trials.

TEACHING AND SELF-CARE

Primary Prevention

The key primary prevention trials—those establishing the relation between blood cholesterol levels and CHD in patients without evidence of CHD—are summarized in Table 10-7. These studies evaluated the treatment of hyperlipidemic patients with diet and with and without pharmacotherapy. These trials justify the use of cholesterol-lowering therapies in asymptomatic patients to prevent CHD.

The Lipid Research Clinics Coronary Primary Prevention Trial (Lipid Research Clinics Program, 1984a, 1984b) involved more than 3800 hypercholesterolemic men, dividing them into placebo and cholestyramine treatment groups. After 7 years of treatment, the active treatment group had 19% fewer CHD events than the placebo group. Thus, patients receiving cholestyramine had significantly fewer CHD deaths and nonfatal MIs.

Another major drug trial was the Helsinki Heart Study, which compared gemfibrozil and placebo in more than 4000 Finnish men (Frick et al, 1987; Manninen et al, 1988). Over the 5-year period of the trial, the gemfibrozil group had a 34% reduction in major coronary events.

The West of Scotland Coronary Prevention Study (Shepherd et al, 1995) included more than 6500 men with hyperlipidemia. Patients were assigned to receive pravastatin 40 mg/day or placebo for approximately 5 years. Patients receiving the

pravastatin had a more than 30% reduction in CHD deaths, nonfatal MIs, and the need for revascularization procedures when compared to the placebo group. There was also a 22% reduction in total mortality in the pravastatin group, a clinically significant finding.

These clinical trials provide ample support for the identification and management of patients for primary prevention. More specifically, they demonstrated that for every 1 mg/dL reduction in cholesterol, the risk for CAD is reduced by 1%. However, most primary prevention trials have failed to show a decrease in the total mortality rate. This can be explained by a number of reasons, including study design and a lack of statistical power. In contrast, the pharmacologic agents used in these studies may have had deleterious side effects that offset their beneficial cholesterol-lowering properties. However, the abundance of data supporting cholesterol-lowering therapies justifies the treatment of patients without CAD and with elevated cholesterol levels.

Secondary Prevention

A number of secondary prevention trials, conducted in patients who have had MI or evidence of atherosclerotic vascular disease, have demonstrated the benefits of cholesterol-lowering interventions (see Table 10-7). The first study using an HMG CoA reductase inhibitor demonstrated the benefits of this potent class of drugs. In the Scandinavian Simvastatin Survival Study (4S, 1994), 4444 patients received simvastatin or placebo and were followed for more than 5 years. Patients in the simvastatin group had a 30% decrease in the total mortality rate, a 42% decrease in CHD deaths, a 37% decrease in revascularization procedures (eg, percutaneous transluminal coronary angioplasty or coronary artery bypass grafting), a 34% decrease in nonfatal MI or CHD death, and a 30% decrease in stroke. The difference between the treatment groups was evident by 2 years, after which the groups continued to diverge. Positive results were seen across all patient types, including women and the elderly. This landmark trial was the first to improve the overall mortality rate with a statin and therefore justified what many health care providers were already doing—using a statin as a first-line agent.

Since the 4S trial, another study involving pravastatin, the Cholesterol and Recurrent Events trial (Sacks et al, 1996), has provided more evidence for the use of statins in secondary prevention. This study involved more than 4100 patients with lower baseline cholesterol levels than those in the 4S trial. Study participants received either pravastatin or placebo, and the mean follow-up was 5 years. When compared to placebo, patients receiving pravastatin had a 24% reduction in CHD deaths and nonfatal MI, a 25% reduction in MI alone, and a 27% reduction in revascularization procedures.

From these secondary prevention trials, we have learned that the magnitude of LDL reduction was again correlated with the degree of benefit. It is clear from the results of these trials that aggressive LDL reduction in patients with high LDL levels has profound effects. There is still a benefit if the LDL is lower, but as expected it is not quite as great.

Angiographic Regression Trials

Another group of studies in patients with established CAD used angiography (see Table 10-7). The goal of these studies was to determine whether lipid-lowering interventions can retard

TABLE 10-7 Selected Major Lipid-Lowering Intervention Trials

Study	Treatment*	Outcome
PRIMARY PREVENTION TRIALS		
LRC-CPPT (Lipid Research Clinics 1984a, 1984b)	Cholestyramine	↓ CHD death and nonfatal MI
Helsinki Heart Study (Frick et al, 1987)	Gemfibrozil	↓ CHD death and nonfatal MI
WOSCOPS (Shepherd et al, 1995)	Pravastatin	↓ CHD death and nonfatal MI ↓ revascularizations ↓ total mortality
SECONDARY PREVENTION TRIALS		
Coronary Heart Project Coronary Drug Project, 1975; Canner et al, 1986)	Niacin	↓ nonfatal MI (at 6 years) ↓ total mortality (at 15 years)
Stockholm Heart Study (Carlson et al, 1988)	Clofibrate + niacin	↓ CHD mortality ↓ CHD death + nonfatal MI ↓ total mortality
4S Trial (Scandinavian Simvastatin Survival Study, 1991)	Simvastatin	↓ CHD mortality ↓ CHD death + nonfatal MI ↓ revascularizations ↓ total mortality ↓ stroke
CARE (Sacks et al, 1996)	Pravastatin	↓ CHD mortality ↓ CHD death + nonfatal MI ↓ revascularizations ↓ stroke
ANGIOGRAPHIC STUDIES		
CLAS (Blankenhorn et al, 1987)	BAS + niacin	↓ progression with Rx ↑ regression with Rx
FATS (Brown et al, 1990)	Statin and BAS	↓ progression with Rx ↑ regression with Rx
	Statin and niacin	↓ progression with Rx ↑ regression with Rx
Lifestyle (Ornish et al, 1990)	Diet + exercise	↓ progression with Rx ↑ regression with Rx
LCAS (?)	Statin +/− BAS	↓ progression with Rx ↑ regression with Rx

* Many of the trials also included concomitant dietary therapy.

BAS, bile acid sequestrant

progression and promote regression of coronary lesions. The findings of these trials indicate that by reducing cholesterol, the rate of coronary lesion progression was slowed, and in some cases regression was evident with changes in lumen size. An important benefit found was lesion stabilization and a decrease in CHD events. The lipid-lowering effects of an intervention are believed to reduce the lipid core of the unstable atherosclerotic lesion, rendering the lesion more stable and less likely to rupture and form a thrombus, producing an acute coronary event. These results support aggressive lipid-lowering interventions in patients with angiographic evidence of atherosclerosis to prevent CHD events.

DIAGNOSTIC CRITERIA

According to NCEP guidelines, serum total cholesterol and HDL levels should be measured in all adults age 20 and up at least once every 5 years in the nonfasting state. Two determinations, taken approximately 1 to 8 weeks apart, with the patient on a stable diet and in the absence of acute illness are recommended to decrease variability and obtain a reliable baseline.

If the two levels differ by more than 30 mg/dL, a third test should be taken, and the average of all three should be used to make an assessment. Patients should be thoroughly assessed with a complete evaluation (eg, complete history, physical examination, and basic laboratory tests) (see Chap. 9), and CHD risk factors should be identified. If a patient is found to have hyperlipidemia that cannot be explained by secondary causes, genetic factors may be the cause of the elevated lipids. In these

TABLE 10-8 Classification Based on Total Cholesterol Levels and HDL Levels

Level	Initial Classification
TOTAL CHOLESTEROL	
<200 mg/dL	Desirable
200–239 mg/dL	Borderline high
≥240 mg/dL	High
HDL	
<35 mg/dL	Low

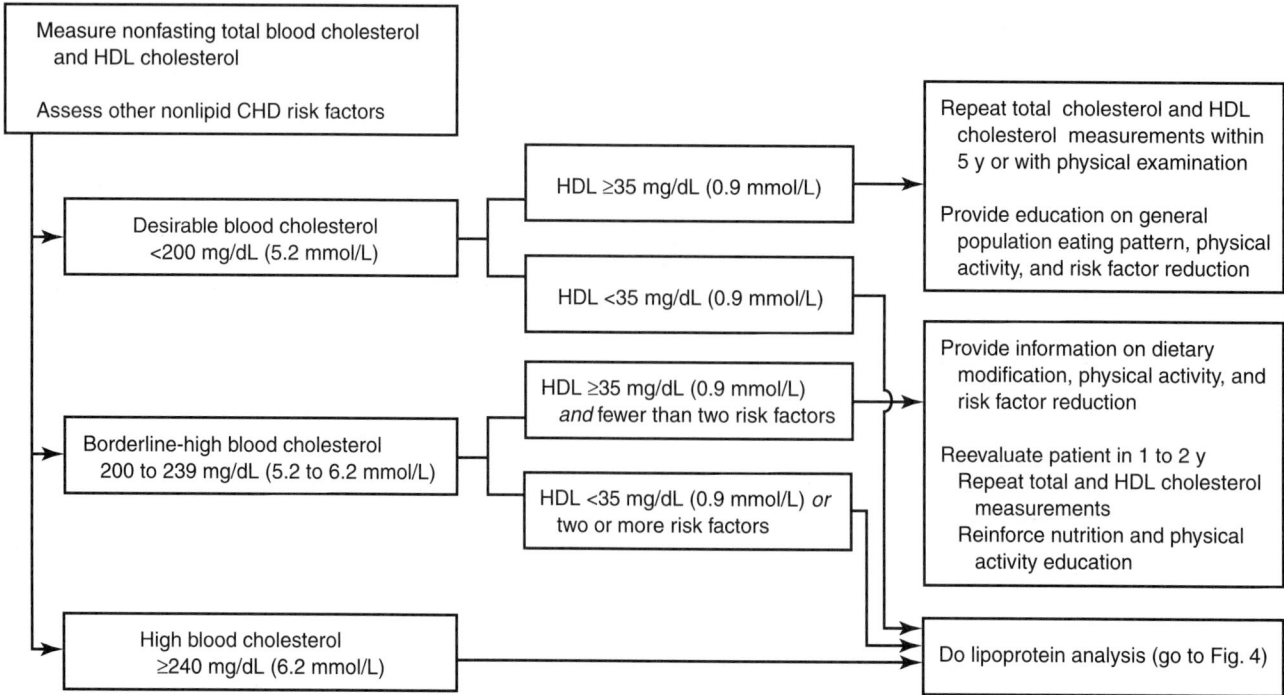

FIGURE 10-3 Primary prevention in adults without evidence of coronary heart disease (CHD). Initial classification is based on total cholesterol and high-density lipoprotein (HDL) cholesterol level.

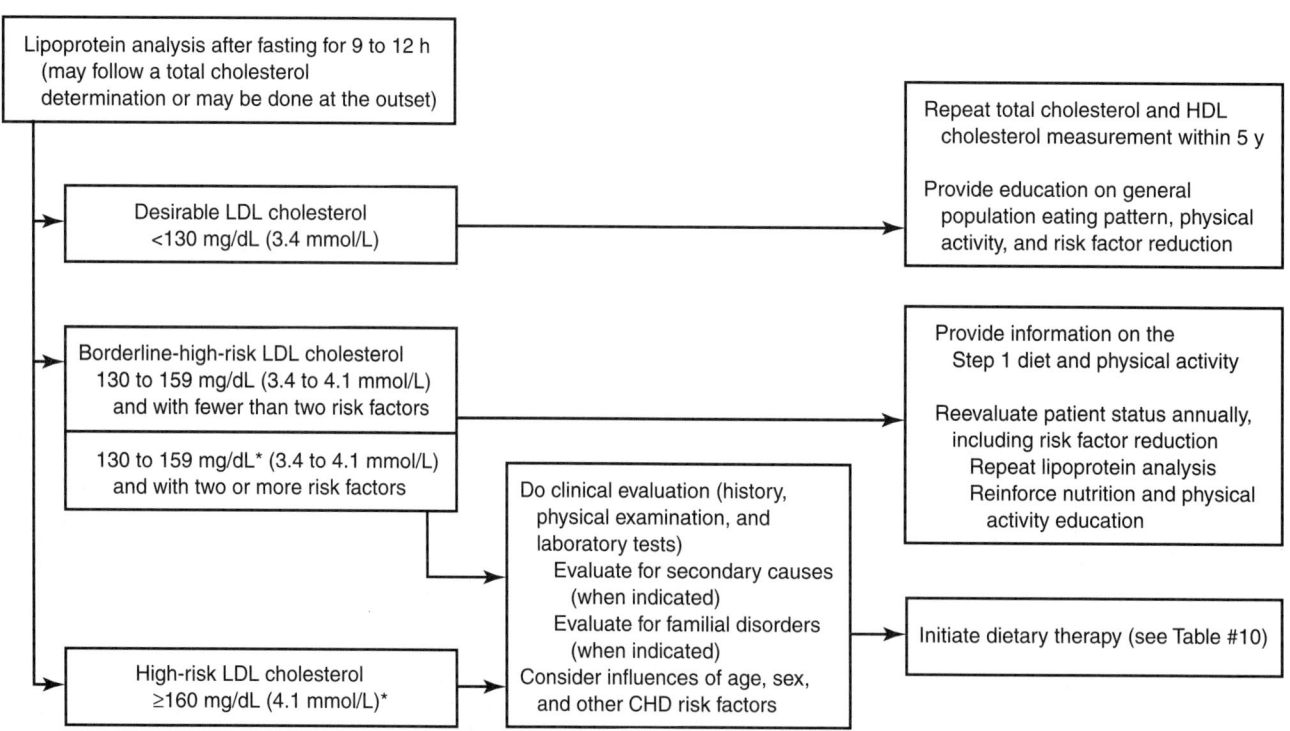

*On the basis of the average of two determinations. If the first two LDL-cholesterol test results differ by more than 30 mg/dL (0.7 mmol/L), a third test result should be obtained within 1 to 8 weeks and the average value of the three tests used.

FIGURE 10-4 Primary prevention in adults without evidence of coronary heart disease (CHD). Subsequent classification is based on low-density lipoprotein (LDL) cholesterol level.

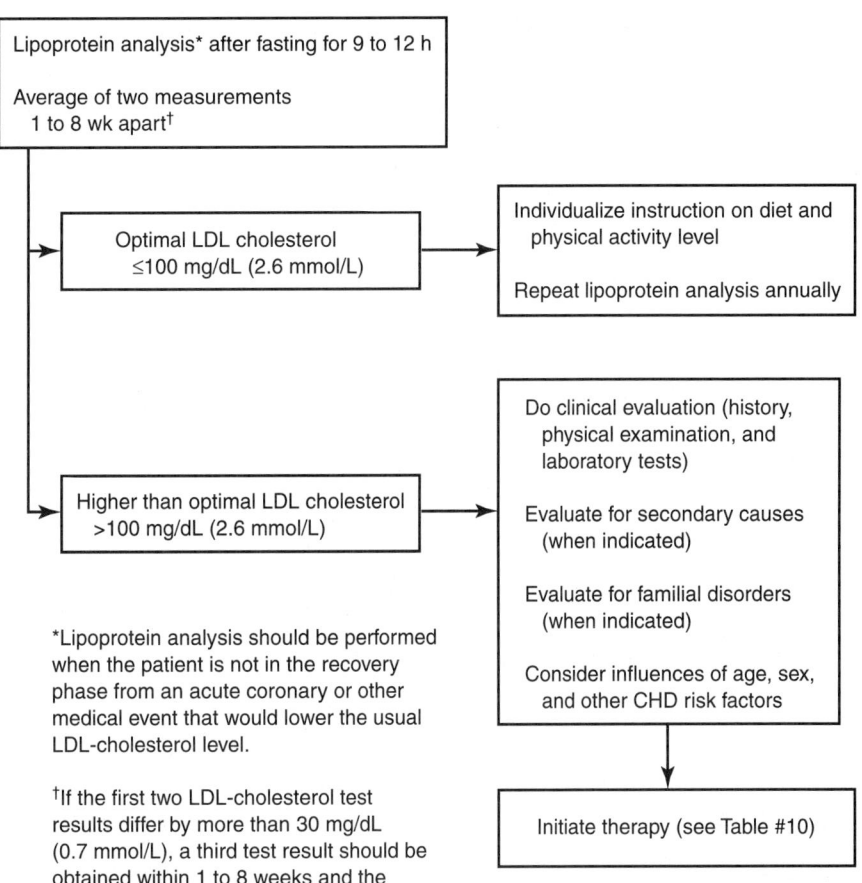

Lipoprotein analysis* after fasting for 9 to 12 h

Average of two measurements
1 to 8 wk apart†

Optimal LDL cholesterol
≤100 mg/dL (2.6 mmol/L)

Individualize instruction on diet and physical activity level

Repeat lipoprotein analysis annually

Higher than optimal LDL cholesterol
>100 mg/dL (2.6 mmol/L)

Do clinical evaluation (history, physical examination, and laboratory tests)

Evaluate for secondary causes (when indicated)

Evaluate for familial disorders (when indicated)

Consider influences of age, sex, and other CHD risk factors

Initiate therapy (see Table #10)

*Lipoprotein analysis should be performed when the patient is not in the recovery phase from an acute coronary or other medical event that would lower the usual LDL-cholesterol level.

†If the first two LDL-cholesterol test results differ by more than 30 mg/dL (0.7 mmol/L), a third test result should be obtained within 1 to 8 weeks and the average value of the three tests used.

FIGURE 10-5 Secondary prevention in adults with evidence of coronary heart disease (CHD). Classification is based on low-density lipoprotein (LDL) cholesterol level.

cases, lipid testing in first-degree relatives may be in order. This may help identify the type of hyperlipidemia as well as other family members requiring treatment.

In persons without CHD, total cholesterol levels can be categorized as desirable, borderline high, and high according to the classification in Table 10-8. The initial classification in this population is summarized in Figure 10-3. Subsequent classification can be made based on LDL levels: patients with high blood cholesterol levels, patients with borderline-high blood cholesterol levels with a low HDL or two or more risk factors, or patients with desirable blood cholesterol and low HDL levels. Figure 10-4 summarizes the classification of these patients.

Secondary prevention in adults requires a lipoprotein analysis and classification based on LDL levels (Fig. 10-5). Based on the lipoprotein analysis, the patient can be evaluated based on total cholesterol, LDL, and triglyceride levels (Table 10-9). The lipoprotein profile includes total serum cholesterol, total triglycerides, LDL, and HDL. The LDL can be estimated by using the following equation:

$$LDL = (total\ cholesterol) - (triglycerides/5) - HDL$$

In the above equation, the term "triglycerides/5" represents the VLDL. This equation is valid when triglyceride levels are below 400 mg/dL.

The decision to initiate therapy should be based on the previously stated patient classifications and the recommendations in Table 10-10. These patients should be treated with dietary therapy and if needed drug therapy. Often drug therapy can be delayed in young adult men (<35 years of age) and premenopausal women who have LDL levels below 220 mg/dL and are not otherwise at high risk. In developing a cholesterol-lowering program, many factors need to be considered, and treatment decisions should be individualized.

TABLE 10-9	Classifications and Lipoprotein Levels		
	Concentration (mg/dL)		
Lipoprotein	Desirable	Borderline	High
Cholesterol	<200	200–239	≥240
LDL	<130	130–159	>160
Triglycerides	<200	200–399	>400

TABLE 10-10	Treatment Guidelines Based on LDL Levels		
Patient Category	Goal LDL (mg/dL)	Dietary Therapy	Drug Therapy
Without CHD, <2 risk factors	<160	≥160	≥190
Without CHD, ≥2 risk factors	<130	≥130	≥160
With CHD	≤100	≥100	≥130

TREATMENT OPTIONS, EXPECTED OUTCOMES, AND COMPRENSIVE MANAGEMENT

Studies now provide a clear rationale for decreasing levels of cholesterol and LDL in patients with hyperlipidemia, with (secondary prevention) or without (primary prevention) established CHD. Despite the overwhelming evidence that hypercholesterolemia plays a role in CHD mortality and morbidity, most Americans who need treatment for high cholesterol levels are still not receiving it (Cohen et al, 1991; Giles et al, 1993; Nieto et al, 1995).

TEACHING AND SELF-CARE

Dietary Therapy and Lifestyle Modifications

Diet should be considered the cornerstone of therapy for most forms of hyperlipidemia. In many patients, dietary therapy alone is insufficient and pharmacologic therapy needs to be added. Health care providers must keep in mind that nondrug therapy is considered a lifestyle modification for the patient because it requires not only changes in diet but also changes in the patient's normal eating habits (eg, eating on the run, eating at restaurants, preparing meals).

The typical American diet consists of excessive fat and cholesterol intake for normal patients, not to mention those with lipid abnormalities. In fact, the step I NCEP diet (Table 10-11) is recommended for all Americans, whether or not they have elevated cholesterol levels. The rationale for dietary therapy is based on the overproduction of VLDL and LDL. Excessive cholesterol intake with saturated fatty acids results in decreased hepatic clearance of LDL and deposition in tissues (Dietschy et al, 1993).

The step I diet specifies that total fat intake be limited to 30% of daily calories; saturated fats and cholesterol are restricted to 8% to 10% and 300 mg/day, respectively. A low-fat diet should reduce total and LDL cholesterol and triglycerides. The estimated reduction in total serum cholesterol after an adequate trial of the step I diet is 3% to 14%; the average reduction is 5% to 7% in men with 13% to 14% of their calories as saturated fat. Because these reductions are modest at best, many providers may opt for drug therapy. Health care providers must remember that dietary therapy is essential even in conjunction with drug therapy if optimal reductions in cholesterol are expected.

Patients need to be thoroughly counseled and encouraged to participate in their treatment. Patient education for dietary therapy may best be implemented with the help of a dietitian, who can teach patients how to count calories and grams of fat, read food labels, and prepare meals and can provide general instruction on how to select low-fat foods (Table 10-12). Dietary therapy may provide benefits for the patient beyond the scope of hyperlipidemia, and simply treating laboratory values (total cholesterol, LDL) should be discouraged. Dietary therapy should decrease the patient's weight as well, especially in conjunction with exercise. Minor to moderate weight loss has been reported to double the LDL reductions achieved with a low-fat diet alone (Caggiula et al, 1981). Weight loss should also reduce triglyceride levels and raise HDL cholesterol levels, as well as reducing the risk of developing hypertension and diabetes (Wood et al, 1988). Exercise programs should be individualized for each patient. Aerobic exercise is most beneficial and ideally should be done at least 4 days weekly. Table 10-13 describes lifestyle interventions.

Progressing to the step II diet is advocated for patients who do not achieve control with the step I diet or those with CHD. The step II diet still restricts total fat to 30% of total calories, but it reduces saturated fats to below 7% and cholesterol to 200 mg/day. Because saturated fats elevate the LDL level, reducing their intake results in a greater decrease in total cholesterol than a simple restriction of total cholesterol intake (Blake et al, 1995). The step II diet should further reduce total cholesterol by about 3% to 7%. Some patients are more responsive to dietary therapy than others for a variety of reasons, so deviations from predicted reductions should be expected. The addition of 3 g/day of soluble fiber from oat products can further lower cholesterol (Rispin et al, 1992).

Unfortunately, patients may participate in dietary therapy for the short term only, as many Americans do not maintain diets to lose weight. Because these low-fat diets are often necessary indefinitely to sustain benefits, encouragement from all the patient's health care providers should be advocated. To achieve optimal and sustained cholesterol reductions from nondrug therapy, the patient may need positive reinforcement and education throughout treatment. The benefits of reducing cholesterol (eg, morbidity, mortality) should be emphasized.

It is important to assess the patient's current dietary habits before prescribing a therapeutic diet, because he or she may already be participating in the recommended diet. Depending on the response to initial dietary therapy, the patient should be maintained on the step I diet or advanced to the step II diet to reach the target levels of total cholesterol and LDL. Each phase of the diet should be maintained for 1 to 3 months before therapy is advanced, assessing lipids at 4 to 6 weeks and at 3 months. In primary prevention, patients should try dietary therapy for 6 months (3 months step I diet, 3 months step II diet) before instituting drug therapy. However, patients with severe forms of hyperlipidemia, those with two or more risk factors, or patients with established CHD are exceptions; treatment may be more aggressive and begin with the step II diet.

Dietary therapy works adjunctively with other risk factor interventions such as smoking cessation and treatment of hypertension. Also, if drug therapy is needed, the cholesterol lowering that is achieved from diet will be additive, therefore permitting the use of lower, less toxic, and less expensive doses of lipid-lowering agents. Assessment of dietary therapy can be done with a dietary assessment instrument described in the NCEP report.

For patients who have been treated with dietary therapy and whose LDL levels fall between their goal level and the threshold to initiate drug therapy, clinical judgment is required. Similarly,

TABLE 10-11	**Dietary Therapy for Hyperlipidemia**	
Nutrient	Step I Diet	Step II Diet
Total fat	≤30%	≤30%
Saturated fats	8–10%	<7%
Polyunsaturated fats	Up to 10%	Up to 10%
Monounsaturated fats	Up to 15%	Up to 15%
Carbohydrates	≥55%	≥55%
Cholesterol	<300 mg/day	<200 mg/day

TABLE 10-12	Recommended Diet Modifications to Lower Blood Cholesterol (The NCEP Step 1 Diet)	
Category	**Choose**	**Decrease**
Fish, chicken, turkey, and lean meats	Fish, poultry without skin, lean cuts of beef, lamb, pork or veal, shellfish	Fatty cuts of beef, lamb, pork, spare ribs, organ meats, regular cold cuts, sausage, hot dogs, bacon, sardines, roe
Skim and low-fat milk, cheese, yogurt, and dairy substitutes	Skim or 1% fat milk (liquid, powdered, evaporated), buttermilk	Whole milk (4% fat; regular, evaporated, condensed, cream, half-and-half, 2% milk, imitation milk products, most nondairy creamers, whipped toppings)
	Nonfat (0% fat) or low-fat yogurt	Whole-milk yogurt
	Low-fat cottage cheese (1% or 2% fat)	Whole-milk cottage cheese (4% fat)
	Low-fat cheeses, farmer or pot cheeses (all of these should be labeled no more than 2 to 6 g of fat per ounce)	All natural cheeses (eg, bleu, Roquefort, Camembert, cheddar, Swiss), low-fat or light cream cheese, low-fat or light sour cream, cream cheeses, sour cream
	Sherbet, sorbet	Ice cream
Eggs	Egg whites (2 egg whites equal 1 egg in recipes), cholesterol-free egg substitutes	Egg yolks
Fruits and vegetables	Fresh, frozen, canned, or dried fruits and vegetables	Vegetables prepared in butter, creams, or other sauces
Bread and cereals	Homemade baked goods using unsaturated oils sparingly, angel food cake, low-fat crackers, low-fat cookies	Commercial baked goods: pies, cakes, doughnuts, croissants, pastries, muffins, biscuits, high-fat crackers, high-fat cookies
	Rice, pasta	Egg noodles
	Whole-grain breads and cereals (oatmeal, whole wheat, rye, bran, multigrain, etc.)	Breads in which eggs are a major ingredient
Fats and oils	Baking cocoa	Chocolate
	Unsaturated vegetable oils: corn, olive, rapeseed (canola oil), safflower, sesame, soybean, sunflower	Butter, coconut oil, palm oil, lard, bacon fat
	Margarine or shortenings made from one of the unsaturated oils listed above, diet margarine	
	Mayonnaise, salad dressings made with unsaturated oils listed above, low-fat dressings	Dressings made with egg yolk
	Seeds and nuts	Coconut

(From the Expert Panel [1988] Report of the National Cholesterol Education Program Expert Panel on detection, evaluation and treatment of high blood cholesterol in adults. *Archives of Internal Medicine*, 148, 36–39. Chicago: American Medical Association.)

if the use of one medication lowers the LDL level into this range, clinical judgment is required as to whether to add a second drug. However, with the availability of the highly potent LDL-reducing statins, many patients can reach their goal with monotherapy.

Pharmacotherapy

Diet therapy alone, even in the most motivated persons, is frequently not sufficient to reduce cholesterol levels to recommended NCEP levels. Pharmacotherapy should be instituted after an adequate trial of diet therapy when the LDL level is 190 mg/dL or more in patients without CHD or two other risk factors. In patients without CHD but with two or more risk factors, drug therapy should be considered when the LDL level is 160 mg/dL or more. Patients who have CHD and LDL levels above 130 mg/dL should receive drug therapy after and in conjunction with dietary therapy (see Table 10-10).

The NCEP recognizes bile acid resins, niacin, and the HMG CoA reductase inhibitors (or statins) as the major drugs for cholesterol reduction. Although there are many efficacious agents from these major categories with varying cholesterol-reducing potencies, no single agent is effective for all lipoprotein disorders, and all are associated with adverse effects and limitations. Available agents, dosage ranges, expected effects, and comments are listed in Table 10-14.

Bile Acid Resins

Cholestyramine and colestipol, the bile acid resins, effectively lower LDL levels. They have a strong safety record and were associated with a reduced CHD risk in the Coronary Primary Prevention Trial (Lipid Research Clinics Program, 1984b; Criqui, 1991). The major actions of these anion exchange resins are to bind or sequester bile acids in the intestine, interrupt the enterohepatic circulation of bile acids, and increase the ex-

TABLE 10-13	Practical Aspects of CHD Lifestyle Interventions	
Clinical Quotes	Translation into Risk Factor Reduction	Translation into Specific Recommendation
Stay lean	■ Reduces total, VLDL, and LDL cholesterol levels ■ Reduces triglyceride levels, increases HDL levels ■ Reduces blood pressure ■ Increases exercise tolerance	■ Control portion sizes ■ Avoid "empty" calories from excess ■■■ ■ Avoid overconsumption of food—■■■ food" consumed in excess results in ■■■
Adopt a healthy diet	■ Reduces total, VLDL, and LDL cholesterol levels ■ Reduces triglyceride levels, increases HDL levels ■ Reduces blood pressure ■ Increases exercise tolerance	No more than 6 oz. lean meat per day ■ 2 or 3 servings low-fat dairy products daily ■ 4–6 servings fruit, vegetables daily ■ 8–10 servings grain products daily ■ This serving distribution not only ■■■ ronutrient content of the diet (protein, carbohydrates, fat), but also improves the ■■■ content of the diet (vitamins, minerals)
Exercise	■ Reduces resting blood pressure ■ Increases HDL cholesterol levels ■ Increases exercise tolerance	■ Regular program of exercise, 30 min per week ■ Take advantage of opportunities: ■ Stairs ■ Walk the dog ■ Park farther from the store

From Denke, M.A. (1994). Diet and lifestyle modification and its relationship to atherosclerosis. *Medical Clinics of North America*, *78*, 218.

TABLE 10-14	Drug Therapy in Hyperlipidemia	
Drug	Effect on Lipoproteins	Dosage Range
BILE ACID SEQUESTRANTS		
Cholestyramine	↓ LDL, ↑ VLDL	4–8 g, divided doses (24 g/day max)
Colestipol	↓ LDL, ↑ VLDL	Powder: 5–10 g divided doses Tabs: 4–8 g divided doses

Comments: Problems with patient acceptance; higher doses are difficult to tolerate because of side effects. May bind coadministered drugs. Dose titration recommended. Questran Light, Prevalite, and Flavored Colestid contain aspartame.

NIACIN		
Niacin	↓ LDL, ↓ VLDL, ↑ HDL	750–1500 mg b.i.d.

Comments: Problems with patient acceptance; higher doses are difficult to tolerate because of side effects. Dose titration required. Many cautions/contraindications. Must monitor liver enzymes. Coadminister with aspirin to reduce flushing.

STATINS		
Lovastatin	↓ LDL, ↓ VLDL, ↑ HDL	10–80 mg q.h.s. or b.i.d. if >20 mg
Pravastatin	to varying degrees	20–40 mg q.h.s.
Simvastatin		10–80 mg q.h.s.
Fluvastatin		20–80 mg q.h.s. or b.i.d. if >20 mg
Atorvastatin		10–80 mg q.d.

Comments: Must monitor liver enzymes. Lovastatin and fluvastatin may be more effective given b.i.d. if doses exceed 20 mg daily. Administer lovastatin with food to increase bioavailability. Higher doses may increase risk of hepatotoxicity and myopathy.

Gemfibrozil	↓ VLDL, ↓↑ LDL, ↑ HDL	600 mg b.i.d.

Comments: Toxicities may be less than clofibrate. Primarily reserved for patients with hypertriglyceridemia.

Probucol	↓ LDL, ↓ HDL	250–500 mg b.i.d.

Comments: Benefits and place in therapy unclear.

cretion of cholesterol in the feces. In turn, the liver is stimulated to convert hepatocellular cholesterol into bile acids, which are further sequestered. As a result, there is an upregulation of LDL receptor synthesis and uptake of LDL, thus decreasing serum cholesterol levels. An increase in hepatic cholesterol biosynthesis may be accompanied by an increase in hepatic VLDL production, which may result in increased triglyceride levels. Patients with homozygous familial hypercholesterolemia cannot increase synthesis of LDL receptors; therefore, bile acid resins are typically ineffective for those patients. However, these agents are effective for most patients when used alone, and combining a drug that reduces hepatocellular cholesterol biosynthesis (statins) with a resin is considered synergistic and can cause upregulation of LDL receptors with enhanced clearance of cholesterol, resulting in dramatic reductions of cholesterol (Expert Panel, 1994; Brown et al, 1986).

Resins reduce total and LDL cholesterol in a dose-dependent manner. LDL levels are reduced approximately 15% with a colestipol does of 5 g/day (equivalent to 4 g of cholestyramine), 23% with 10 g/day, and 27% with 15 g/day (Superko et al, 1992). However, side effects may also increase as the dose escalates. Resins are available in powder and tablet forms, and doses need to be titrated upward slowly. Patients should be started on a low dosage initially (one scoop or packet daily), with the dosage increased gradually and divided usually into four doses daily to minimize adverse effects. The patient should be instructed to mix the resin powder with a noncarbonated liquid or pulpy juice before administration; preparation of the whole daily dose can be done the night before and refrigerated to save time and increase palatability. Also, patients should mix the dose well and try to swallow it without engulfing air.

The major drawbacks of using the resins are the side effects, which often cause patients to discontinue therapy. Resin therapy frequently causes gastrointestinal complaints such as constipation, bloating, epigastric fullness, nausea, and flatulence (Lipid Research Clinics Program, 1984b). Patients may also complain that the resins have a gritty texture and are not easily administered. Because these agents have troublesome side effects and require frequent dosing and special preparation before administration, 40% of patients or more discontinue therapy within 1 year (Andrade et al, 1995). Patients should increase their fluid and fiber intake and may use stool softeners as needed to manage side effects. Other potential adverse effects include gastrointestinal obstruction and impaired absorption of fat-soluble vitamins A, D, E, and K. However, these occurrences are rare at typical doses used in the clinical setting and may occur only with high dosages (eg, 30 g/day cholestyramine). In addition, there are a number of potential drug interactions with resins: there is reduced absorption of medications such as warfarin, digitoxin, thiazide diuretics, and beta-blockers. Concurrent medications should be taken 1 hour before or 4 to 6 hours after the resin dose.

Niacin (Nicotinic Acid)

Niacin (vitamin B_6) is a water-soluble B vitamin that may also be used for primary hypercholesterolemia as monotherapy or in combination with other available agents. At high doses, niacin improves levels of all serum lipids; in contrast, its metabolite, nicotinamide, has no effect on cholesterol. Niacin produces its effects on cholesterol by reducing hepatic synthesis of VLDL, thus producing a reduced synthesis of LDL. Triglyceride levels are also decreased, and HDL catabolism is reduced, resulting in increased levels. Because of its effects on cholesterol and triglycerides, niacin is commonly used for mixed hyperlipidemias or hypertriglyceridemia. Niacin lowers LDL levels by approximately 15% to 30% and triglyceride levels by approximately 30% to 60% and increases HDL levels by approximately 20% to 35% (Coronary Drug Project Research Group, 1975; McKenney et al, 1994; Drood et al, 1991; Keenan, 1991). When niacin is used in combination with a resin, studies have revealed even more dramatic improvements in all serum lipids (Blankenhorn et al, 1987; Brown et al, 1990). Benefits of niacin monotherapy were seen in the Coronary Drug Project study, which demonstrated a reduced rate of MI and a decrease in the mortality rate.

Despite the beneficial effects of niacin, its over-the-counter availability, and its low cost, many providers are hesitant to prescribe niacin because of its frequent, bothersome side effects. Vasodilation, causing cutaneous flushing and itching, is common and appears to be prostaglandin-mediated. Flushing may be related to the rising serum concentrations of niacin; sustained-release preparations may alleviate these complaints (Kane et al, 1981). Patients can take niacin with meals and 325 mg of aspirin or 200 mg of ibuprofen 30 to 60 minutes before each dose to reduce these effects as well as reducing gastrointestinal symptoms (eg, dyspepsia, nausea, activation of peptic ulcer). Patients should avoid alcoholic beverages and hot drinks with niacin because they may contribute to vasodilation and flushing. Niacin can also cause elevation of uric acid levels, precipitating gout, and may cause glucose intolerance, which is problematic in persons with diabetes. Table 10-15 lists the contraindications to niacin therapy; however, some of the listed comorbid states can be considered relative contraindications.

Hepatotoxicity is a major concern with niacin therapy. This adverse effect seems to occur more with sustained-release niacin products and is likely to be dose-dependent, occurring at dosages above 1500 mg/day (McKenney et al, 1994). It may occur more often when there are abrupt increases in dose or when patients are switched from regular niacin to a sustained-release product without reducing the dose. Sustained-release niacin in about half the dose of regular niacin gives equivalent efficacy in reducing LDL levels (Brown, 1995). Hepatotoxicity is manifested by an elevation in liver transaminase enzymes and may be accompanied by fatigue, anorexia, and nausea. Patients' liver

TABLE 10-15	Contraindications to Niacin Therapy
Liver disease, jaundice	
Peptic ulcer disease	
Significant glucose intolerance, diabetes mellitus*	
Severe hypotension	
Hypersensitivity	
Gallbladder disease	
Inflammatory bowel disease	
Arterial hemorrhaging	
Hyperuricemia	

* Relative contraindication in cases of severe hypertriglyceridemia

Deke, MA. Diet and lifestyle modification and its relationship to atherosclerosis. *Medical Clinics of North America.* 78:218.

transaminase levels should be monitored before niacin therapy and every 6 to 8 weeks for the first year of therapy, after dose changes, and periodically thereafter. Patients who experience mild liver enzyme elevations can have their dose reduced or can temporarily discontinue the drug. Discontinuation of therapy is warranted when liver transaminase levels remain elevated to more than three times pretreatment levels. Sustained-release products are more expensive than regular niacin, and because they may be more likely to cause hepatitis, many providers think they should be reserved for patients who cannot tolerate crystalline niacin. However, if high doses of sustained-release niacin are avoided, and the product is titrated carefully, patients may be more satisfied, and the incidence of serious adverse reactions is no greater than with crystalline niacin (Brown, 1995).

CLINICAL WARNING: When niacin is used in combination with HMG CoA reductase inhibitors or gemfibrozil, there may be an increased incidence of myopathy.

Dosages of crystalline niacin should be started very low at approximately 100 mg twice daily and titrated every 3 to 7 days (eg, in increments of 200 to 300 mg up to 3000 mg) as tolerated. Patients will often need 2000 to 3000 mg/day for sufficient efficacy. Sustained-release niacin should also be titrated (eg, 250 mg twice daily up to 2000 mg). The authors recommend starting therapy at the beginning of a weekend so the patient may experience the effects of the first several doses at home rather than at work.

Similar to the bile acid sequestrants, patients need to be thoroughly educated about the anticipated side effects of niacin and the benefits of therapy. They should be encouraged to participate actively in their therapeutic plan.

HMG CoA Reductase Inhibitors (Statins)

Lovastatin, pravastatin, simvastatin, fluvastatin, and atorvastatin are enzyme inhibitors that interrupt the conversion of HMG CoA to mevalonate, the early rate-limiting step in the biosynthesis of cholesterol (see Fig. 10-1). Lovastatin was the first available product and therefore is the most studied. Pravastatin, simvastatin, fluvastatin, and atorvastatin have subsequently been approved for use in the United States. These agents significantly decrease cholesterol production and cause upregulation of LDL receptors, further enhancing the clearance of circulating LDL from the blood. Statins reduce triglycerides and increase HDL to varying degrees, depending on the agent and dose used. The ability of these medications to reduce LDL is dose-dependent and log-linear; low doses produce marked reductions and larger doses produce less dramatic reductions. Fluvastatin appears to be the least potent of the statins but still can allow many patients to reach their desired LDL goal as determined by NCEP guidelines. The newest statin, atorvastatin, is the most potent agent: the lowest dose of 10 mg can provide up to a 40% reduction in LDL. However, such large reductions may not be necessary for all patients. In addition, atorvastatin is effective in reducing triglyceride levels to a greater extent than the other statins. Differences in efficacy of the statins are summarized in Table 10-16.

The availability of statins has made control of hypercholesterolemia easier to achieve. Several trials have shown that statins can slow the progression of CAD or cause regression of atherosclerosis. Recent primary prevention and secondary prevention trials demonstrate that statins provide major benefits in patients, reducing the incidence of cardiac events and the mortality rate. It is unclear whether these benefits exist for all the HMG CoA reductase inhibitors.

Statins are well tolerated by most patients and seem to be the preferred cholesterol-lowering agent by many providers. Adverse effects are usually mild and include headache and gas-

TABLE 10-16	Comparison of the Available Statins			
Drug	Dosage	LDL (%)	HDL (%)	TG (%)
Lovastatin	20 mg Qpm	−24	+6.6	−10
Lovastatin	40 mg Qpm	−30	+7.2	−14
Lovastatin	20 mg b.i.d.	−34	+8.6	−16
Lovastatin	40 mg b.i.d.	−40	+9.5	−19
Pravastatin	10 mg Qpm	−22	+7	−15
Pravastatin	20 mg Qpm	−32	+2	−11
Pravastatin	40 mg Qpm	−34	+12	−24
Simvastatin	5 mg Qpm	−24	+7	−10
Simvastatin	10 mg Qpm	−33	+9	−10
Simvastatin	20 mg Qpm	−33	+11	−19
Simvastatin	40 mg Qpm	−40	+12	−19
Atorvastatin	10 mg q.d.	−39	+6	−19
Atorvastatin	20 mg q.d.	−43	+9	−26
Atorvastatin	40 mg q.d.	−50	+5	−29
Atorvastatin	80 mg q.d.	−60	+5	−37

TG, triglycerides.
(Kellick: *Hospital Formulary*.)

trointestinal symptoms. More serious side effects include hepatotoxicity and myopathy. An elevation in liver transaminase enzymes is a dose-dependent effect seen in approximately 1% to 2% of patients (Bradford et al, 1991). After discontinuation of the drug, liver enzymes return to normal, and rechallenge at a lower dose would be acceptable. As is the case with niacin therapy, liver enzymes need to be monitored in a similar fashion.

Myopathy, manifested by elevation of creatine kinase levels with or without symptoms (eg, muscle aches and weakness), has occurred with statin therapy. Creatine kinase levels may increase more than 10 times the upper limit of normal, and rhabdomyolysis has been reported.

CLINICAL WARNING: Rhabdomyolysis appears to occur more commonly when statin therapy is used in combination with other agents such as cyclosporine, erythromycin, gemfibrozil, and niacin. The exact mechanism for myopathy is not understood but may be related to the depletion of ubiquinone (coenzyme Q).

Fibric Acid Derivatives

Gemfibrozil and clofibrate are primarily used for their ability to lower triglyceride levels. In patients with dysbetalipoproteinemia or those at risk for pancreatitis with triglyceride levels above 1000 mg/dL, fibrates are considered first-line agents. Gemfibrozil, used in combination with dietary therapy, in the Helsinki Heart Study was associated with a reduction in CHD deaths and nonfatal MIs (Frick et al, 1987).

Fibrates exert their effects by increasing the activity of lipoprotein lipase, thus increasing VLDL catabolism. Fibrates also reduce the secretion of VLDL from the liver, reduce cholesterol biosynthesis, and promote cholesterol secretion into the bile (Saku et al, 1985; Grundy et al, 1987). Gemfibrozil lowers triglyceride levels by approximately 20% to 50% and raises HDL levels by 10% to 15% in patients with hypertriglyceridemia (Manttari et al, 1990; Rubins et al, 1992; Miller et al, 1993). In patients with mixed lipid elevations who are diabetic, gemfibrozil is particularly useful because niacin may worsen glucose intolerance. The LDL-lowering effect of fibrates may be limited to patients with isolated hypercholesterolemia (Manttari et al, 1990; Manninen et al, 1989; Hunninghake et al, 1987), but their role in this population is limited.

In general, gemfibrozil is well tolerated in patients and is associated with gastrointestinal side effects. Fibrate use may lead to the formation of cholesterol gallstones and myositis. Myopathy may occur with fibrate use, but does more frequently when a statin is used concurrently. Therefore, this combination of drugs should be used only when necessary. Creatine kinase elevations and accompanying muscle symptoms support the diagnosis.

Safety of the fibric acid derivatives has been a concern. Although gemfibrozil demonstrated some beneficial effects in the Helsinki Heart Study, it also increased the non-CHD mortality rate, so there was no net change in the total mortality rate. Clofibrate appears to be less effective in reducing VLDL production than gemfibrozil. Clofibrate also causes more adverse effects and was associated with an increase in the total mortality

rate in the World Health Organization trial; thus, it has fallen out of favor in the United States (Knodel et al, 1987; Committee of Principal Investigators, 1978). For these reasons, cautious use of fibrates is warranted. Triglyceride-lowering drugs should be considered in patients with moderate hypertriglyceridemia when other risk factors for CHD are present.

Probucol

The role of probucol in treating hyperlipidemic patients is unclear. It decreases LDL levels but also significantly reduces HDL levels as well. Similar to vitamins E and C and beta carotene, probucol has potent antioxidant properties (Baumstark et al, 1992; Kuzuya et al, 1993). Therefore, probucol may reduce or prevent the development of atherosclerosis (Parthasarathy et al, 1986; Kita et al, 1987) and has been shown to cause regression of xanthomas in patients with severe hypercholesterolemia (Yamamoto et al, 1986). Because probucol only modestly decreases LDL, has HDL-reducing properties, and can produce arrhythmias by prolonging the Q–T interval, clinical use is uncommon.

Fish Oils

The omega-3 fatty acids found in fish oils significantly lower triglyceride levels and may have some use in patients with hypertriglyceridemia. Their ability to decrease cholesterol levels is less clear, as is their role in the management of hyperlipidemia (see Chap. 9).

Hyperlipidemia in Women and Estrogen Replacement Therapy

CHD is the leading cause of death in women as well as men. In general, women, particularly premenopausal women, are at less of a risk for CHD than men of equivalent age. In premenopausal women, drug therapy for hyperlipidemia should generally be delayed if possible. However, the risk for CHD increases progressively after menopause. Postmenopausal women not taking hormone replacement therapy are at an increased risk for CHD. The use of estrogens in this particular population may obviate the need for standard cholesterol-lowering medications. Women who use estrogens may have up to a 50% lower CHD rate than those who do not (Stampfer et al, 1991; Barrett-Connor et al, 1991; Grady et al, 1992). Estrogens offer even greater benefits to women with established CHD (Grady et al, 1992; Gruchow et al, 1988). Estrogen replacement therapy (eg, 0.625 mg/day of conjugated estrogens) can decrease LDL levels by approximately 15% to 25% and raise HDL levels by 15% to 20%; thus, it can be used in this population instead of other antihyperlipidemics. However, increases in triglyceride levels commonly occur. The benefits of estrogen replacement also extend to its ability to reduce the incidence of osteoporosis and perimenopausal symptoms. See Chapters 9 and 67 for discussions on estrogen replacement.

COMMUNITY RESOURCES

- American Heart Association, 7272 Greenville Avenue, Dallas, TX 75231; 1-800-AHA-USA1; www.amhrt. org

- COHIS Diet and Nutrition Main Menu: www.bu.edu:80/COHIS/nutrition/nutri.hym
- Heart Point: wwww.heartpoint.com/cholesterol main.html

SUMMARY

The association between hypercholesterolemia and CHD has clearly been established. LDL is the primary target for lipid-lowering therapies. Patients with (secondary prevention) and without (primary prevention) CHD who have elevated cholesterol levels need to be identified and evaluated by health care providers to ensure appropriate treatment. Aggressive treatment of hypercholesterolemia results in fewer patients developing CAD, coronary events, and the need for revascularization procedures.

A multidisciplinary approach to treatment is required to provide a satisfactory outcome. Dietary therapy and lifestyle modifications are the initial therapy for patients with high blood cholesterol levels. Patients need to be counseled and given positive reinforcement if optimal outcomes are expected. Pharmacotherapy may be used if nonpharmacologic interventions do not produce the desired results. Bile acid sequestrants, niacin, and the HMG-CoA reductase inhibitors are considered the major lipid-lowering drugs. The majority of patients can be treated with these medications to attain desirable serum cholesterol levels. The decision to initiate pharmacologic agents should be patient-specific and should involve a complete analysis of each patient's history and clinical status.

■ ■ ■ ■ CLINICAL PEARLS

- Primary care providers should evaluate the hyperlipidemic patient's current medications and identify those drugs that may be contributing to the dyslipidemic state. When possible, these medications should be substituted for those that have a positive or neutral lipid effect.
- Dietary therapy may provide benefits to patients whose laboratory values may or may not reflect hyperlipidemia. The recommendation for dietary therapy, therefore, should not be based solely on the patient's laboratory values.
- It is important to assess the patient's current dietary habits, as they may already be participating in the recommended diet.
- Patients who experience flushing with niacin may reduce this effect by taking the niacin with meals and 325 mg of aspirin or 200 mg of ibuprofen 30–60 minutes prior to each dose.
- The primary care provider and patient should identify the best time to initiate niacin therapy to assure that the patient's life and work schedule will be best able to accommodate any discomfort the patient may experience.
- The LDL-lowering effects of fibrates may be limited to patients with isolated hypercholesterolemia.
- In premenopausal women with hyperlipidemia and no coexisting risk factors, drug therapy should be delayed.

EDITOR'S NOTE:

COMPLEMENTARY APPROACHES

A general discussion of complementary approaches can be found in Chapter 3. The following, while not an exhaustive list, are some complementary approaches being used for this condition. Additional information on these approaches, including precautions, can be found in Appendices A and B. Providers need to assess for the use of complementary approaches as part of the patient's history, as they may impact conventional therapies, and patients may not volunteer this information unless specifically asked. Efficacy of many complementary approaches is not as well documented as that of conventional therapies. Providers need to read the literature before suggesting these complementary approaches.

- Vitamins, minerals, herbs, supplements
  Carnitine
  Fish oils
  Garlic
  Niacin
- Complementary Modalities
  Acupuncture
  Aromatherapy

References

Anderson, K.M., et al. (1987). *JAMA, 257,* 2176.

Andrade, S.E., et al. (1995). *N Engl J Med, 332,* 1125–1131.

Austin, M.A. (1991). *Arteriosclerosis and Thrombosis, 11,* 2.

Barrett-Connor, E., et al. (1991). *JAMA, 265,* 1861–1867.

Baumstark, M.W., et al. (1992). *Clinical Biochemistry, 25,* 395–397.

Blake, G.H., et al. (1995). *American Family Physician, 51,* 1157–1156.

Blankenhorn, D.H., et al. (1987). *JAMA, 257*(23), 3233–3240.

Bradford, R.H., et al. (1991). *Archives of Internal Medicine, 151,* 43–49.

Brown, et al. (1986). *Science, 232,* 34–47.

Brown, et al. (1990). *N Engl J Med, 323*(19), 1289–1298.

Brown, V.W. (1995). *Postgraduate Medicine, 98,* .

Caggiula, A.W., et al. (1981). *Preventive Medicine, 10,* 443–475.

Canner, P.L., et al. (1986). *Journal of the American College of Cardiology, 8,* 1245–1255.

Carlson, L.A., et al. (1988). *Acta Medica Scandinavia, 223,* 405–418.

Castelli, W.P. (1986). *American Heart Journal, 112,* 432.

Cohen, et al. (1991). *Circulation, 83,* 1294–1304.

Committee of Principal Investigators. (1978). *British Heart Journal, 40,* 1069–1118.

Cordon, T., et al. (1977). *American Journal of Medicine, 62,* 707.

Coronary Drug Project Research Group. (1975). *JAMA, 231,* 360–381.

Criqui, M.H. (1991). *Annals of Internal Medicine, 115,* 973–976.

Dietschy, J.M., et al. (1993). *Journal of Lipid Research, 34,* 1637–1659.

Drood, J.M., et al. (1991). *Journal of Clinical Pharmacology, 31,* 641–650.

Expert Panel on Detection, Evaluation, and Treatment of High Blood Cholesterol in Adults (Adult Treatment Panel II). (1994). *Circulation, 89,* 1329.

Frick, M.H., et al. (1987). *N Engl J Med, 317,* 1237.

Giles, et al. (1993). *JAMA, 269*(9), 1133–1138.

Gordon, D.J., et al. (1989). *Circulation, 79,* 8–15.

Grady, D., et al. (1992). *Annals of Internal Medicine, 117,* 1016–1037.

Gruchow, H.W., et al. (1988). *American Heart Journal, 115*(5), 88–94.

Grundy, S.M. (1978). *Western Journal of Medicine, 128,* 13.

Grundy, S.M. (1996). In: *Etiology and treatment of hyperlipidemia.* Mosby-Wolfe Medical Communications.

Grundy, S.M., et al. (1966). *Journal of Clinical Investigation, 9,* 1503.

Grundy, S.M., et al. (1969). *Journal of Lipid Research, 10,* 91.

Grundy, S.M., et al. (1987). *American Journal of Medicine, 83,* 9–20.

Hunninghake, D.B., et al. (1987). *American Journal of Medicine, 83,* 44–49.

Kane, J.P., et al. (1981). *N Engl J Med, 304,* 251–258.

Kannel, W.B., et al. (1971). *Annals of Internal Medicine, 74,* 1.

Kannel, W.B., et al. (1979). *Annals of Internal Medicine, 90,* 85.

Keenan, J.M., et al. (1991). *Archives of Internal Medicine, 151*(7), 1424–1432.

Kita, T., et al. (1987). *Proceedings of the National Academy of Sciences of the USA, 84,* 5928–5931.

Knodel, L.C., et al. (1987). *Medical Toxicology, 2,* 10–32.

Kuzuya, M., et al. (1993). *Biological Medicine, 14,* 67–77.

LCAS

Lipid Research Clinics Program. (1984a). The Lipid Research Clinics Coronary Primary Prevention Trial results I. *JAMA, 251,* 351–364.

Lipid Research Clinics Program. (1984b). The Lipid Research Clinics Coronary Primary Prevention Trial results II. *JAMA, 251,* 365–374.

Manninen, V., et al. (1988). *JAMA, 260,*.

Manninen, V., et al. (1989). *American Journal of Cardiology, 63,* 42H–47H.

Manttari, M., et al. (1990). *Atherosclerosis, 81,* 11–17.

McKenney, J.M., et al. (1994). *JAMA, 271,* 672–677.

Miller, M., et al. (1993). *American Journal of Medicine, 94,* 7–12.

Nieto, et al. (1995). *Archives of Internal Medicine, 155,* 677–684.

Ornish, D., et al. (1990). *Lancet, 336,* 129–133.

Parthasarathy, S., et al. (1986). *Journal of Clinical Investigation, 77,* 641–644.

Rispin, C.M., et al. (1992). *JAMA, 267,* 3317–3325.

Rubins, H.B., et al. (1992). *Journal of Internal Medicine, 231,* 421–426.

Sacks, F.M., et al. (1996). *N Engl J Med, 335,* 1001–1009.

Saku, K., et al. (1985). *Journal of Clinical Investigation,* 1702–1712.

Shepherd, J., et al. (1995). *N Engl J Med, 333,* 1301–1307.

Scandinavian Simvastatin Survival Study Group. (1994). *Lancet, 344,* 1383.

Stamler, J., et al. (1986). *JAMA, 256,* 2823.

Stampfer, M.J., et al. (1991). *N Engl J Med, 325,* 756–762.

Superko, H.R., et al. (1992). *American Journal of Cardiology, 70,* 135–140.

Wood, P.D., et al. (1988). *N Engl J Med, 325,* 461–466.

Yamamoto, A., et al. (1986). *American Journal of Cardiology, 57,* 29H–35H.

CHAPTER
11

Heart Failure

Judy Cheng, PharmD, BCPS

Heart failure is a public health problem of enormous and growing significance. According to the NHANES III data (MMWR, 1994), heart failure affects approximately 4.7 million people in this country. As the population ages and the incidence of patients surviving other symptomatic cardiac diseases such as myocardial infarction continues to rise, the incidence of heart failure and its mortality rate will continue to increase. Heart failure is the only cardiovascular disease that is increasing in prevalence.

The management of heart failure has become one of the most challenging problems confronting our health care system today. Each year, the United States spends nearly $9 billion in managing patients with heart failure.

Treatment of heart failure is no longer confined to symptom relief. Because the underlying etiologies that contribute to ventricular dysfunction may progress independently from the development of symptoms, treatment to prevent and delay the progression of the disease is equally important. This chapter will discuss the pathophysiology, treatment, and social impact of heart failure, with emphasis on long-term management and patient education to prevent exacerbation and delay the disease progress to improve the patient's quality of life.

ANATOMY, PHYSIOLOGY, AND PATHOLOGY

Anatomy and Physiology of the Heart

FUNCTIONAL ANATOMY OF THE HEART

The heart is a four-chambered structure consisting of two atria and two ventricles. The atria are relatively thin-walled, low-pressure chambers that lie superior to the ventricles. Their primary function is to act as a reservoir, filling their respective ventricles. The ventricles are thick-walled chambers that function at higher pressures and pump blood from the heart into the respective great vessels. The atria and ventricles are more specifically identified as either right or left, according to their orientation in the chest. The right atrium and ventricle receive deoxygenated blood as it returns from the body. They then pump this blood to the lungs through the pulmonary artery. After the blood is oxygenated in the lungs, it returns via the pulmonary veins to the left atrium and is then pumped out to the rest of the body by the left ventricle via the aorta. The circulatory system thus consists of two circuits in series, the pulmonary and systemic, through which the blood sequentially flows.

The unidirectional blood flow is maintained by the four valves located in the heart. These valves allow the forward flow of blood and when closed prevent retrograde flow. The two atrioventricular valves, mitral and tricuspid, in the right and the left side of the heart respectively, separate the ventricles from their respective atria. The semilunar valves (aortic and pulmonic) divide the ventricles from their respective great vessel and artery. The left ventricle is separated from the aorta by the aortic valve; the right ventricle is separated from the pulmonary artery by the pulmonic valve.

CARDIAC PHYSIOLOGY AND HEMODYNAMICS

The primary physiologic function of the heart is to pump blood to supply oxygen and nutrients to the different body organ systems. Stroke volume is the volume of blood pumped per beat by each ventricle. Cardiac output is the volume of blood pumped per minute. Cardiac output and stroke volume are therefore related by the following equation:

$$\text{Cardiac output (mL/min)} = \text{stroke volume (mL/beat)} \times \text{heart rate (beats/min)}$$

Stroke volume is regulated by three variables: the end-diastolic volume, the mean aortic or arterial blood pressure, and the contractility of the ventricles. End-diastolic volume (EDV) is the amount of blood in the ventricles just before contraction. Because this is a workload imposed on the ventricles before contracting, it is clinically referred to as the preload. Arterial pressure represents an impedance to the ejection of blood from the ventricles, or an afterload imposed on the ventricles after contraction has begun. The stroke volume is directly proportional to the preload and contractility but inversely proportional to the afterload.

The portion of the EDV that is ejected (the ejection fraction) against a given afterload depends on the strength of ventricular contraction. The left ventricular ejection fraction is one of the most important objective criteria used in describing the severity of heart failure. Normally, contraction strength is sufficient to eject two thirds of the EDV with each heart beat. In a healthy heart, this fraction remains relatively constant, even with an increase in EDV. This implies that the strength of ventricular contraction must increase as the EDV increases in a normal heart. Such intrinsic control of contractile strength was first described by two physiologists, Frank and Starling, and thus is named the Frank-Starling law of the heart.

The other factor that controls cardiac output is the heart rate. Heart rate is regulated by the autonomic nervous system. Stimulation of the sympathetic nervous endings in the musculature of the atria and ventricles increases the strength of contraction (positive inotropic effect) and decreases slightly the time spent in systole. On the other hand, enhancing the effect of the parasympathetic nervous system decreases cardiac rate and contractility.

TABLE 11-1	Etiologies of Heart Failure

ISCHEMIC HEART DISEASE/MYOCARDIAL INFARCTION

Cardiomyopathy
    Idiopathic
    Infectious
    Toxic (eg, doxorubicin)

Hypertension

Aortic stenosis

Mitral regurgitation

Aortic regurgitation

Pericardial diseases
    Pericardial effusion
    Constrictive pericarditis

Arrhythmias
    Atrial fibrillation
    Ventricular tachycardia

Pathophysiology

PATHOPHYSIOLOGY OF HEART FAILURE

The pathophysiology of heart failure begins with myocardial cell damage caused by etiologies such as ischemic heart disease and hypertension. Table 11-1 details the causes of heart failure (Willerson & Cohn, 1995). As myocardial damage becomes significant, cardiac output decreases and intraventricular pressure increases to the point where body organ perfusion and functions are compromised. In the left ventricle, an increase in diastolic pressure leads to a rise in pressure in the pulmonary circulation. This causes pulmonary edema and prevents proper oxygenation of the blood, leading to dyspnea. In the right ventricle, an increase in diastolic pressure leads to an elevation of venous pressure, resulting in peripheral edema.

In the presence of a primary abnormality in myocardial contractility or excessive hemodynamic stresses, the heart relies on three major adaptive mechanisms in attempts to maintain cardiac output:

- The Frank-Starling mechanism, in which an increase in preload brought about in part by salt and water retention helps sustain cardiac performance (stroke volume is directly proportional to preload)

- Increased release of catecholamines by adrenergic cardiac nerves and the adrenal medulla activation of the renin–angiotensin–aldosterone system, and other neurohormonal adjustments that act to maintain arterial pressure and vital organ perfusion
- Myocyte hypertrophy with or without chamber dilatation, in which left ventricular mass is increased in an attempt to enhance contractility.

Figure 11-1 illustrates the interactions of the different compensatory mechanisms in heart failure.

Initially, these mechanisms can maintain cardiac output, arterial blood pressure, and organ perfusion, but they may also exert more stress on the already injured myocardium. Therefore, in the later phase of the disease, such compensatory mechanisms actually contribute to the worsening of symptoms. Table 11-2 illustrates the short-term and the long-term responses of the impaired myocardium to these compensatory mechanisms.

HEMODYNAMIC COMPENSATORY MECHANISMS IN HEART FAILURE

In the early phase of heart failure, activation of the sympathetic nervous system increases both the heart rate and the contractile force, thus increasing cardiac output. However, an important cardiac compensatory mechanism called myocardial remodeling, which occurs during myocardial injury and in a state of enhanced sympathetic nervous activities, may be both adaptive and maladaptive (Braunwald, 1992; Grossman et al, 1975; Patterson & Adams, 1996). Unlike skeletal muscle cells, myocardial cells cannot divide to increase their numbers, but they undergo remodeling by which they increase in length or volume (dilatation and hypertrophy). Early in heart failure, dilatation and hypertrophy may enhance contraction, but chronically they often worsen cardiac damage. In addition, dilatation of heart chambers leads to an increase in myocardial wall stress, which is one of the determinants of myocardial oxygen demand and supply imbalance. Hypertrophy, if severe and longstanding, leads to loss of contractile force.

NEUROHORMONAL COMPENSATORY MECHANISMS IN HEART FAILURE

One of the most significant compensatory mechanisms of heart failure is the activation of certain endogenous neurohormones.

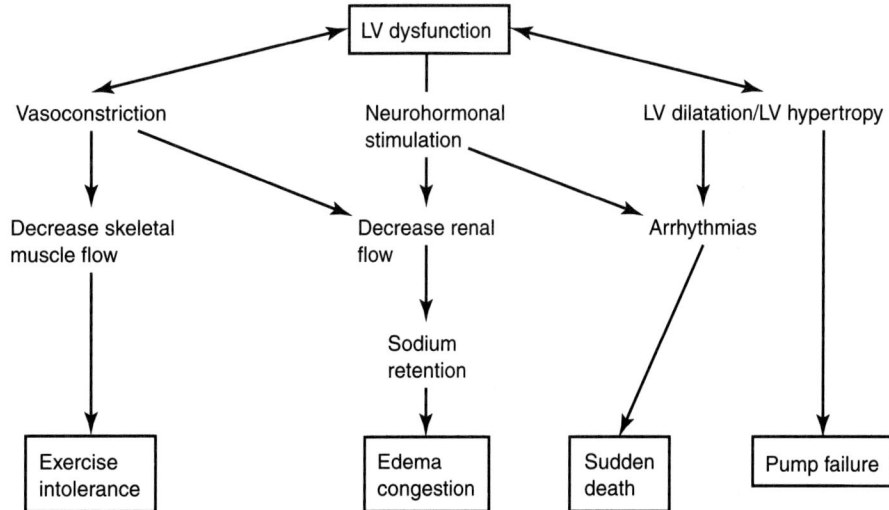

FIGURE 11-1 Pathophysiology of heart failure.

TABLE 11-2	Short-Term and Long-Term Responses of Impaired Myocardium to Different Compensatory Mechanisms	
	Short-Term Effects	**Long-Term Effects**
Frank Starling Mechanisms: Salt and water retention (renin–angiotensin activation)	Increases preload	Causes peripheral and pulmonary congestion
Sympathetic nervous stimulation	Maintains blood pressure and organ perfusion by vasoconstriction	Increases energy expenditure. Long-term stimulation also leads to desensitization of adrenergic receptors.
Myocardial hypertrophy		Deterioration and death of cardiac cells

Reduction of cardiac output stimulates other body systems to try to maintain normal blood pressure and organ perfusion. The major neurohormonal systems that regulate these compensatory mechanisms are the sympathetic, renin–angiotensin, and atrial natriuretic systems.

SYMPATHETIC NERVOUS SYSTEM

Plasma norepinephrine levels are increased in heart failure (Packer, 1988). With such activation of the sympathetic nervous system, there is an initial increase in cardiac contractility. Vasoconstriction also occurs and afterload increases. As mentioned, this is intended to enhance cardiac output and maintain vital organ perfusion. Chronically, however, this leads to an increase in systemic vascular resistance and adds to the strain of a failing heart. Increasing afterload leads to a decrease in blood perfusion to different organs, increasing preload (venous return to the heart). Vasoconstriction also leads to a reduction of blood flow to the kidneys, which stimulates the retention of sodium and water to compensate for the perceived lack of blood volume. Such retention of fluid and water does not improve stoke volume; rather, it contributes to the congestive symptoms of heart failure.

RENIN–ANGIOTENSIN SYSTEM

In states of low cardiac output, the renin–angiotensin–aldosterone axis is activated. This acts in concert with the activated adrenergic nervous–adrenal medullary system to maintain arterial pressure (Dzau, 1987). Renin is released by the kidneys in response to reduced blood flow. Renin converts angiotensinogen to angiotensin I in the circulation. Angiotensin I circulates to the lungs and other tissues, where angiotensin-converting enzymes (ACE) converts it to angiotensin II. Angiotensin II is a potent vasoconstrictor and therefore significantly increases afterload. Aldosterone production is also increased by angiotensin II. Aldosterone has potent sodium-retaining properties and contributes to the general volume overload state of heart failure. Finally, angiotensin II has an important role in the stimulation of the cell growth and development that leads to myocyte hypertrophy of the heart (Fig. 11-2).

Atrial natriuretic peptide (ANP) is a hormone produced by the atrial tissue of the heart. Its level is also increased in chronic heart failure (Packer, 1988). ANP is a counter-regulatory hormone that opposes the action of many of the vasoconstricting and salt- and water-retaining effects of the renin–angiotensin–aldosterone system. ANP acts as a vasodilating agent, suppresses the formation of renin, and enhances the excretion of salt and water. However, because of its relatively weak action and short duration of effect, it cannot totally reverse the detrimental effects of the renin–angiotensin system and the sympathetic systems. Investigational pharmacologic agents that mimic the action of ANP may have an important role in the management of heart failure.

EPIDEMIOLOGY

Each year, more than 2 million Americans suffer from heart failure, and approximately 400,000 new cases are diagnosed. Despite recent advances in the management of heart failure,

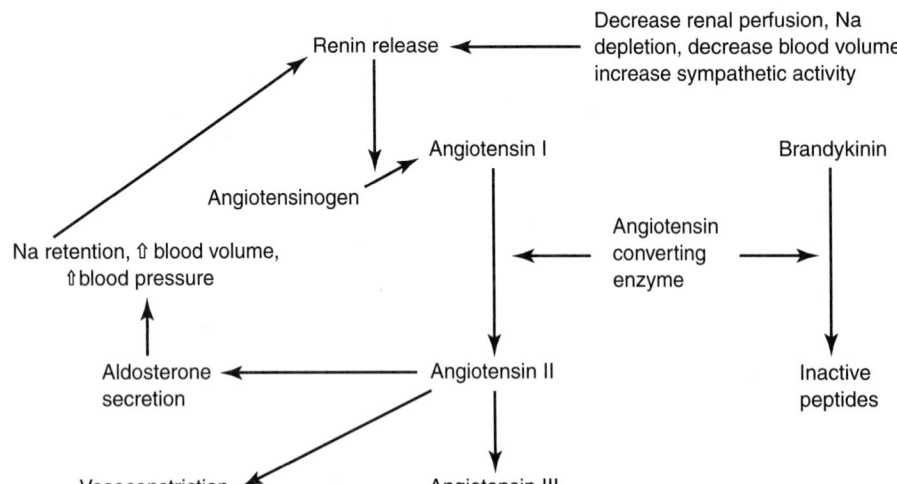

FIGURE 11-2 The Renin-angiotensin-aldosterone system.

both surgical and pharmacologic, the mortality rate of this disease remains high. The 5-year mortality rate is approximately 50%, and 92% of the deaths are in people older than 65. Potential causes of this phenomenon include the increasing average age of the American population and the longer survival of people with other symptomatic cardiac diseases who subsequently develop heart failure at an older age (Gillum, 1993). Race-specific death rates have also reflected a higher incidence for younger African Americans. This may suggest an earlier onset of disease and a greater severity of heart failure among African Americans (*MMWR*, 1994).

The management of heart failure patients exerts a heavy economic burden on society. Based on the information supplied by the Health Care Financing Administration, Medicare spends an average of $2.4 billion per year on patients admitted to the hospital with a primary diagnosis of heart failure (Konstam et al, 1994).

DIAGNOSTIC CRITERIA

Although the definition of heart failure remains unclear, the condition may be characterized by a pathophysiologic state in which the heart cannot provide adequate forward cardiac output to meet the perfusion and oxygenation requirements of the body organs and tissues. Although the etiologies of heart failure are numerous, the majority of cases can be classified as either systolic dysfunction, in which there is impaired cardiac contractility, or diastolic dysfunction, in which decreased compliance of the heart (manifesting as the heart's inability to relax) impairs ventricular filling. Distinguishing between these disorders is important clinically because they are treated very differently. Nevertheless, there is a common symptomatology, including fatigue, shortness of breath at rest, dyspnea on exertion, peripheral/pulmonary edema, and weight gain caused by fluid retention and congestion.

Systolic and diastolic heart failures are also commonly referred to in clinical situations as congestive heart failure. Systolic heart failure, which is the more common form, is characterized by a dilated ventricular chamber with a poorly contracting ventricle and usually a thinned ventricular wall, ultimately producing a reduced left ventricular ejection fraction (<45%) (Cohn, 1996). In most laboratories, an ejection fraction of >45% to 50% is considered normal. In patients with pure diastolic heart failure, the ventricular chamber size may not increase and the wall thickness is usually enhanced. The most important diagnostic criterion, which distinguishes systolic and diastolic heart failure, is the left ventricular ejection fraction. Patients with diastolic failure may have a normal or increased left ventricular ejection fraction. Many patients with heart failure have elements of both systolic and diastolic dysfunction. Table 11-3

summarizes the major characteristics and diagnostic criteria of systolic and diastolic heart failure.

HISTORY AND PHYSICAL EXAMINATION

Obtaining a complete medical history is extremely important in diagnosing heart failure. Symptoms suggestive of heart failure include:

- Paroxysmal nocturnal dyspnea
- Orthopnea
- Dyspnea on exertion
- Lower extremity edema
- Decreased exercise tolerance
- Unexplained confusion, altered mental status, or fatigue in an elderly patient
- Abdominal symptoms associated with ascites or hepatic engorgement (eg, nausea or abdominal pain).

Patients should be questioned about a previous history of angina or the equivalent (such as flash pulmonary edema), myocardial infarction, hypertension, other heart diseases, diabetes, and renal, pulmonary, thyroid, or gastrointestinal diseases. A complete medication history is also important to obtain. Table 11-4 lists some common medications that may cause or exacerbate heart failure symptoms. If symptoms of progressive dyspnea, orthopnea, or paroxysmal nocturnal dyspnea are present in conjunction with the above cardiac history, the likelihood that the patient has heart failure dramatically increases.

The physical examination can provide important information about the etiology of the patient's symptoms and the appropriate therapies. Physical signs suggesting heart failure include:

- Elevated jugular venous pressure or positive hepatojugular reflux
- Third heart sound (positive S_3)
- Laterally displaced apical impulse
- Bibasilar pulmonary rales that do not clear up with cough
- Peripheral edema not caused by venous insufficiency.

The most sensitive physical finding is the third heart sound (Mattleman et al, 1983). Jugular venous distention and peripheral edema appear to be the least sensitive signs (Harlan et al, 1977). Because physical signs may not be highly sensitive and specific indications of heart failure, and some patients with moderate to severe left ventricular dysfunction do not manifest any physical signs, patients with symptoms highly suggestive of heart failure should be referred for echocardiography or radionuclide ventriculography to measure ejection fraction.

TABLE 11-3	Diagnostic Criteria of Heart Failure	
	Systolic	**Diastolic**
Symptoms	Fatigue, shortness of breath, dyspnea on exertion, pulmonary or peripheral congestion, fluid retention	Similar to systolic heart failure
Left ventricular ejection fraction	<45%	≥45%–50%
Heart chamber size	Increased	Normal or increased
Wall thickness	Thinned	Typically enhanced

TABLE 11-4	Medications That May Induce or Exacerbate Heart Failure
Medications	**Effects**
Antiarrhythmic agents (eg, quinidine, procainamide, flecainide, propafenone, sotalol)	Most antiarrhythmic agents have negative inotropic effects and may induce heart failure when used in patients with other underlying heart diseases.
Calcium channel blockers (verapamil, diltiazem)	Most first-generation calcium channel blockers have negative inotropic effects and may induce heart failure when used in patients with other underlying heart diseases.
Beta-blockers (eg, atenolol, metoprolol, propranolol)	Negative inotropic effects can lead to heart failure when used in patients with other underlying heart diseases.
Heroin, cocaine, alcohol, amphetamines, doxorubicin, cyclophosphamide, sulfonamides, lead, arsenic, cobalt, phosphorus, ethylene glycol	Direct cardiac toxins

DIAGNOSTIC STUDIES

Recommended routine diagnostic studies for patients with suspected heart failure are listed in Table 11-5 (ACC/AHA, 1995). Many of these tests are recommended to rule out other diseases that have clinical symptoms similar to those of heart failure and to delineate the underlying causes of heart failure so they can be managed properly to reverse or prevent further progression of symptoms.

TREATMENT OPTIONS, EXPECTED OUTCOMES, COMPREHENSIVE MANAGEMENT

Systolic Heart Failure

The treatment of systolic heart failure includes general measures (eg, exercise and dietary changes), pharmacotherapy, and interventional or surgical therapy.

Medication Regimen

A pharmacotherapeutic plan includes (Cohn, 1996):

- Treating the underlying etiology whenever possible
- Relieving symptoms. This can be achieved by using pharmacologic agents that can improve the heart's pumping performance (eg, positive inotropic agents such as digoxin), reduce the heart's workload (eg, ACE inhibitors, vasodilators such as hydralazine, nitrates), relieve congestion (eg, diuretics), and reduce neurohormonal activation (eg, ACE inhibitors).
- Treating complications such as arrhythmia, cardiogenic shock, or thromboembolic events (stroke)
- Improving the mortality rate and prolonging survival (eg, ACE inhibitors).

Table 11-6 lists the pharmacotherapeutic options for managing systolic heart failure. Those that are used for the manage-

TABLE 11-5	Recommended Routine Diagnostic Studies for Patients With Suspected Heart Failure
Test	**Purpose**
Complete blood count	To rule out anemia, which decreases the blood's oxygen-carrying capacity, thus leading to or aggravating heart failure
Urinalysis	To rule out nephrotic syndrome or glomerulonephritis, which may cause a fluid overload state similar to heart failure
Serum electrolytes, urea nitrogen, creatinine, glucose, phosphorus, magnesium, calcium, and albumin	To determine fluid status and to rule out volume overload caused by renal failure or an increase in extravascular volume hypoalbuminemia
Thyroid-stimulating hormones	To check if the patient has atrial fibrillation and unexplained heart failure
Chest x-ray	To detect cardiomegaly and pulmonary congestion and to rule out other pulmonary causes of dyspnea such as pneumonia
Electrocardiogram	Abnormal changes such as ST-segment elevation/depression, T-wave inversion, and presence of Q waves may indicate ischemia or myocardial infarction, which if not managed promptly and appropriately may lead to heart failure
Transthoracic Doppler–two-dimensional echocardiography	To study myocardial wall motion and define ejection fraction
Exercise stress test, coronary angiography (in patients with coronary artery disease)	To optimize management of coronary artery disease, which ultimately prevents or retards the progression of heart failure

TABLE 11-6	Pharmacologic Therapy for Management of Systolic Heart Failure

FOR SYMPTOMATIC RELIEF

Positive inotropic agents: digoxin, intravenous/inotropes (dobutamine, dopamine, amrinone, milrinone)

Diuretics

Vasodilators (ACE inhibitors, nitrates, and hydralazine)

TREATMENT OF COMPLICATIONS

Antiarrhythmic agents (amiodarone)

Anticoagulants (warfarin)

Intravenous inotropic agents (for cardiogenic shock)

IMPROVE MORTALITY OR PROLONG SURVIVAL

ACE inhibitors

Nitrates and hydralazine

Amlodipine

Beta-blockers

ment of chronic heart failure will be discussed in more detail below.

Relieving Symptoms

POSITIVE INOTROPIC AGENTS

Digoxin is a positive inotropic agent that is used in systolic heart failure to improve myocardial contractility. The therapeutic efficacy of digoxin in patients with systolic heart failure and normal sinus rhythm has always been controversial. Digoxin can prevent clinical deterioration in systolic heart failure and improve patients' symptoms. However, there is no significant reduction of the mortality rate (Cohn, 1996; Packer et al, 1993). Digoxin should be used in patients with severe heart failure and should be added to the medical regimen of patients with mild to moderate left ventricular dysfunction who remain symptomatic after optimization of ACE inhibitor and diuretic therapy.

The usual dose of digoxin is 0.125 to 0.25 mg given orally once a day. A loading dose is not required unless the patient also has atrial fibrillation. Because digoxin has a vaguely defined but narrow therapeutic range, it is important to use doses that do not carry a risk of toxic effects. The Digitalis Investigation Group has put forward a simple rule in dosing digoxin (Cohn, 1996): for a patient weighing 50 to 70 kg, the dose is 0.25 mg/day for a creatinine clearance of >50 mL/min and 0.125 mg/day for a creatinine clearance of <50 mL/min.

If the patient is obese, add an extra 0.125 mg/day to the daily dose recommended. Serum digoxin levels are available in many laboratories and can be measured to ensure safety. The therapeutic range is generally defined as 0.8 to 2 ng/mL. However, the correlation between therapeutic levels and efficacy is not strong. Therefore, routine monitoring of digoxin levels is not necessary to ensure efficacy or safety. However, patients should be educated about the possible side effects of digoxin and if necessary a serum level can be obtained to confirm toxicity.

Adverse drug reactions of digoxin include nausea and vomiting (usually the first sign presented), diarrhea, abdominal pain, headache, fatigue, depression, yellow-green halos, and cardiac arrhythmias (Table 11-7).

CLINICAL WARNING: Elderly patients receiving digoxin who complain of anorexia or gastrointestinal disturbances should be assessed for digoxin toxicity. Hypokalemia may precipitate digoxin toxicity.

DIURETICS

Diuretics are used in heart failure to relieve circulatory congestion and peripheral edema. The role of diuretics in heart failure management is for symptomatic relief and should not be used if the patient has no signs of congestion. Table 11-8 lists common diuretics used in the management of heart failure. Thiazides are used to maintain a normal intravascular volume in mild states of congestion; more severe congestion usually requires the use of loop diuretics. If patients have persistent congestion, metolazone therapy may be added to loop diuretic therapy for a synergistic effect caused by their different sites of action at the renal tubule. Doses of diuretics are individualized based on the patient's condition. Patients receiving diuretic therapy should be monitored for electrolyte abnormalities, especially hypokalemia (except those receiving potassium-sparing diuretics). Hypokalemia may precipitate digoxin toxicity. Potassium supplements should be administered if necessary. Patients may also be advised to consume foods that are high in potassium, such as oranges and bananas. Potassium-sparing diuretics may be substituted to moderate the loss of potassium. However, potassium-sparing diuretics are not as potent a natriuretic agent as loop diuretics. Symptomatic hypotension and progressive elevation of the blood urea nitrogen concentration are signs of overdiuresis. Patients should be advised to weigh themselves daily to ensure efficacy and prevent overdiuresis.

VASODILATORS

Vasodilators can reduce preload, afterload, or both by relaxing the arterial and venous smooth muscle, reducing resistance to left ventricular ejection. This increases cardiac output, thus relieving congestion symptoms and improving exercise tolerance.

ACE inhibitors are the first choice of vasodilators used for systolic heart failure management because they not only relieve symptoms but also improve survival. ACE inhibitors reduce preload and afterload by inhibiting ACE, thus reducing the production of angiotensin II, which is a potent vasoconstrictor. Table 11-9 lists ACE inhibitors used in the management of heart failure. Therapy with ACE inhibitors should be initiated

TABLE 11-7	Adverse Effects of Digoxin

Nausea, vomiting (first sign presented)

Diarrhea

Abdominal pain

Headache

Fatigue

Depression

Yellow-green halo

Cardiac arrhythmia

TABLE 11-8	Use of Diuretics in the Management of Heart Failure		
Drugs	**Dose (mg)**	**Frequency**	**Common Adverse Effects**
THIAZIDE DIURETICS			
Hydrochlorothiazide	25–50	Daily	Hypokalemia, hyperglycemia, hyperuricemia, hypercholesterolemia
Chlorthalidone	25–100	Daily	
Metolazone	2.5–10	Once or twice daily	
LOOP DIURETICS			
Furosemide	20–200	Once or twice daily	Same as thiazide diuretics. High dose may also cause ototoxicity.
Bumetanide	0.5–4	Once or twice daily	
POTASSIUM-SPARING DIURETICS			
Spironolactone	25–100	Once or twice daily	Hyperkalemia, gynecomastia

at a low dose to avoid hypotension. Attempts should be made to achieve the target dosages, because survival benefits have been demonstrated at these dosages. Moderate asymptomatic hypotension and azotemia (serum creatinine <2.5 mg/dL) are acceptable side effects of ACE inhibitors, and reduction or discontinuation of therapy is not warranted. Reduction of diuretic doses may be adequate to correct these problems. However, symptomatic hypotension, progressive azotemia, or intolerable cough occasionally require discontinuation of ACE inhibitor therapy. Other side effects of ACE inhibitors include rash and angioedema.

For patients who cannot tolerate ACE inhibitors, other vasodilators can be substituted. Hydralazine (a direct arterial dilator that reduces afterload) and nitrate (a venous dilator that reduces preload) combinations have also been shown to improve hemodynamics as well as prolong survival. The target dosage of hydralazine is 75 mg three times a day. The target dosage of nitrates, given as isosorbide dinitrate, is 40 mg three times a day. Most patients cannot tolerate the target dose due to the development of headaches from the nitrate therapy. The need to take medications three times a day makes participation in the regimen difficult. Substituting long-acting nitrate formulations such as isosorbide mononitrate (administered once or twice daily) may help. An overnight interval of more than 10 hours between doses of isosorbide dinitrate is desirable to minimize the development of nitrate tolerance. Other side effects of this combination regimen include lupus syndrome from hydralazine, which is common at a daily dose of 200 mg or more.

Treating Complications

ANTIARRHYTHMICS
Ventricular arrhythmia is one of the two leading causes of death in patients with heart failure (the other being cardiogenic shock). It is not currently recommended that antiarrhythmic

agents be routinely administered to suppress ventricular arrhythmias, except in the event of sustained ventricular tachycardia or ventricular fibrillation. Patients with heart failure are also susceptible to developing atrial fibrillation because of the fluid stretch of the atrium during a fluid overload state. Conversion to normal sinus rhythm should be attempted because patients with heart failure do not tolerate symptoms of atrial fibrillation. Amiodarone is the most often used antiarrhythmic agent in patients with heart failure because of the low incidence of proarrhythmia and the lack of negative inotropic effect (Doval et al, 1994; Singh et al, 1995). Antiarrhythmic therapies have not been proven to prolong survival in patients with heart failure.

ANTICOAGULANTS
Thromboembolism is a potential complication in patients with heart failure. A poorly pumping heart promotes formation of blood clots (thrombi) in the ventricles. These thrombi may dislodge and eventually form emboli in the brain (stroke), the lung (pulmonary emboli), or the coronary artery (myocardial ischemia). Routine use of prophylactic anticoagulation is not recommended because of a lack of any prospective trial supporting its efficacy. However, patients who are at particularly high risk of developing thromboembolic events, such as those who have a history of atrial fibrillation or thromboembolic events or those with very low ejection fractions (<20% to 25%) should receive maintenance anticoagulation therapy. Warfarin is the drug of choice in this situation. When given, doses should be titrated to achieve an International Normalized Ratio (INR) of 2 to 3.

Improving the Mortality Rate and Prolonging Survival

ACE INHIBITORS
All patients with left ventricular dysfunction should be treated with ACE inhibitors unless contraindicated. Numerous studies on the use of ACE inhibitors in heart failure have demonstrated a reduction of the mortality rate in patients with moderate to severe heart failure (symptomatic or asymptomatic) and those in the early phase of recovery from myocardial infarction. Table 11-10 summarizes some of these important clinical trials. As previously mentioned, these drugs should be given at the dosages found in the clinical trials to increase survival. The various ACE inhibitors have not been directly compared by clinical trial. However, when initiating therapy, it is advisable to use a

TABLE 11-9	ACE Inhibitors Used in Systolic Heart Failure	
Drugs	**Initial Dose (mg)**	**Target Dose (mg)**
Captopril	6.25 3 times daily	50 3 times daily
Enalapril	2.5 twice daily	10 twice daily
Lisinopril	5 daily	20 daily
Quinapril	5 twice daily	20 twice daily

TABLE 11-10	Studies on the Use of ACE Inhibitors in Heart Failure	
Trial	**Therapy**	**Endpoints and Outcomes**
CONSENSUS I (1987)	Enalapril (PO) vs. placebo	Enalapril ↓ mortality 31% from heart failure, no difference in sudden cardiac death
CONSENSUS II (Swedberg et al, 1992)	Enalapril (IV) vs. placebo, given within 24 hours post-MI for 41–180 days	Terminated early at 6 months, trend toward ↑ mortality with enalapril (↑ heart failure and hypotension)
V-HeFT II (Cohn et al, 1995)	Enalapril vs. hydralazine + isosorbide dinitrate (Hyd/ISDN)	2-yr. mortality rate was 18% for enalapril and 25% Hyd/ISDN. 5-yr. mortality-rate was 48% for enalapril and 54% for Hyd/ISDN.
SOLVD (1992)	Enalapril (PO) vs. placebo	Enalapril significantly reduced the incidence of heart failure and hospital admission.
SAVE (Pfeffer et al, 1992)	Captopril vs. placebo, given 3–16 days post-MI for mean duration of 42 months	Captopril: ↓ mortality 19%, ↓ development of congestive heart failure 37%, ↓ recurrent MI 25%
AIRE (1993)	Ramipril vs. placebo given 2–9 days post-MI for mean duration of 15 months	Ramipril ↓ mortality 27%, ↓ development of congestive heart failure 29%
GISSI-3 (1994)	Lisinopril vs. IV/transderm NTG vs. combination vs. control given within 24 hours post-MI for 42 days	Lisinopril ↓ 6-week mortality 12%, IV/transderm NTG no effect, combination ↓ mortality 17%
ISIS-4 (1995)	Captopril vs. ISMO vs. combination vs. control given within 24 hours post-MI for 28 days	Captopril ↓ mortality 9%, ISMO no effect on mortality

CONSENSUS: **Co**operative **N**ew **S**candinavian **En**alapril **Sur**vival **S**tudy
V-HeFT: VA Cooperative Trial
SAVE: Survival and Ventricular Enlargement Trial
AIRE: The **A**cute **I**nfarction **R**amipril **E**fficacy Trial
GISSI: **G**ruppo **I**taliano per lo **S**tudio della **S**opravvivenza nell'**I**nfarto
ISIS: **I**nternational **S**tudy of **I**nfarct **S**urvival

short-acting agent such as captopril so that the dosage can be titrated delicately to prevent profound hypotension. Once the patient is stabilized, a longer-acting, once-daily agent should be given to help patients participate more easily in their suggested regimen.

HYDRALAZINE AND ISOSORBIDE DINITRATE

The combination of hydralazine and isosorbide dinitrate has been shown to improve the mortality rate in patients with congestive heart failure who were given digoxin and diuretic therapy (Cohn et al, 1991, 1986). In terms of survival benefit, this combination therapy did not compare as favorably as ACE inhibitors; however, it did provide a more favorable effect on left ventricular function and exercise capacity. This combination should be reserved for patients who cannot tolerate ACE inhibitors. It is important that both drugs be used at the same time to ensure mortality and hemodynamic benefits. Both of these drugs need to be taken three times daily.

BETA-ADRENERGIC BLOCKERS

The use of beta-blockers has been traditionally thought to be contraindicated for patients who have systolic heart failure because of their negative inotropic effects, which may further reduce myocardial contractility. A more recent understanding of the pathophysiology of heart failure has led to a redefinition of the role of beta-blockers. Because increases in sympathetic nervous activities and down-regulation of beta-receptors are believed to play an important role in the advanced stages of heart failure, beta-blockers may theoretically be able to resensitize the endogenous beta-receptors, thus changing the natural history of the disease. Clinical studies support this theory. Trials with metoprolol and bisoprolol have both provided evidence that beta-adrenergic antagonists may have a favorable effect on the course and prognosis of heart failure (Waagstein et al, 1993; CIBIS, 1994). Carvedilol, a second-generation beta-blocker with alpha-blockage activity and antioxidant properties, has shown a 48% reduction in mortality in patients with heart failure (Packer et al, 1996).

Despite these promising benefits, the optimal dosage of beta-blockers has yet to be defined. It is important to adjust the dose carefully to ensure maximum beneficial effects without severely decreasing myocardial contractility. Clinical trials are under way to answer this question. Until the results of these trials become available, use of beta-blockers should be considered only in patients who are not optimally controlled with digoxin, diuretics, and ACE inhibitors and are not in severe clinical heart failure. The dosage should be started low and titrated up slowly to the optimal response. Constant monitoring for worsening signs of heart failure is essential. Referral to a cardiologist is probably warranted.

CALCIUM CHANNEL BLOCKERS

Similar to beta-blockers, calcium channel blockers were traditionally believed to be contraindicated in systolic heart failure because of their negative inotropic effect. Second-generation calcium channel blockers, which have minimal negative inotropic effects, exert their actions more at the vascular wall than the heart. These agents are believed to be beneficial in systolic heart failure by decreasing preload and afterload. The administration of two such agents, amlodipine and felodipine, in systolic heart failure has been studied. Preliminary results suggested that there are no detrimental effects on long-term mortality rates (Packer et al, 1996; Cohn et al, 1995). Amlodipine is now routinely recommended for use in patients with systolic heart failure who require extra agents for blood-pressure control (after optimal doses of ACE inhibitors and diuretics are given) and for angina control. Amlodipine is given in a dosage of 5 to 10 mg daily. It is very well tolerated and side effects are minimal.

OTHER DRUG THERAPIES

Angiotensin II inhibitors (eg, losartan), drugs that inhibit neurohormonal activation (eg, neutral endopeptidase inhibitors), and other positive inotropic agents with antiarrhythmic action (eg, vesnarinone) are in various stages of evaluation as possible therapy for systolic heart failure. As the results of these trials become available, the treatment options for systolic heart failure may continue to expand.

Diastolic Heart Failure

The treatment of diastolic heart failure has both similarities to and differences from the treatment of systolic heart failure. Similar to systolic heart failure, any underlying causal or aggravating conditions need to be corrected, if possible. Recommendations regarding antiarrhythmics and anticoagulation therapy for systolic heart failure also apply to diastolic heart failure.

MEDICATION REGIMEN

The major differences between the treatment of systolic and diastolic function is that the goal of drug treatment in diastolic heart failure is to reduce symptoms by lowering the elevated filling pressures without significantly reducing cardiac output. This goal can be achieved with the judicious use of diuretics and nitrates, which decreases preload. Because adequate cardiac output depends on the elevated filling pressure, the dose of diuretics and nitrates has to be started low to prevent hypotension, to which patients with diastolic heart failure are prone. Calcium channel blockers and beta-blockers have been used to improve diastolic dysfunction by augmenting ventricular relaxation and compliance. ACE inhibitors are also frequently used, but studies demonstrating their efficacy in patients with diastolic function are limited. Because systolic function is generally normal, positive inotropic agents have little role in this situation.

Surgical Interventions

The decision to pursue interventional therapy for patients with heart failure is based on the underlying etiology of the disease. Revascularization is indicated for patients with evidence of viable but hypofunctional myocardium (Bonow, 1995). This may be accomplished by coronary angioplasty or coronary artery bypass graft surgery (CABG). Any underlying structural problems should be corrected. For instance, patients with aortic stenosis or severe valvular regurgitation should be considered for valve replacement.

Dual-chamber pacing may be useful for patients with severe first-degree or second- and third-degree heart block. Therapeutic ablation may be useful in patients with recurrent or refractory tachyarrhythmia that leads to congestive heart failure. Cardiomyoplasty is an experimental technique in which part of the latissimus dorsi muscle is released and wrapped around the heart. Survival benefits have not been proven.

Consideration should be given to cardiac transplantation in patients with severe limitation or repeated hospitalization because of heart failure despite aggressive medical therapy in whom other surgical interventions are unlikely to be beneficial.

Comprehensive Management

PRIMARY PREVENTION

Management of heart failure should focus on prevention and treatment of the underlying conditions associated with an increased risk of development of this disease. Table 1 lists the etiologies for heart failure development. Those that are modifiable include ischemic heart disease/myocardial infarction and hypertension.

To understand how to prevent ischemic heart disease/myocardial infarction and hypertension, one must first examine the risk factors for developing these conditions, discussed in the coronary artery disease chapter (Chap. 9).

To prevent heart failure, it is important to emphasize reduction in dietary fat or sodium consumption, weight maintenance, regular physical activity, and smoking cessation. In patients who already have a history of myocardial infarction, prevention of a second heart attack is also crucial. (Please refer to the chapters on hypercholesterolemia, coronary artery disease [9], hypertension [12], and diabetes [17] for further prevention strategies.)

Secondary Prevention

In heart failure, secondary prevention refers to the prevention of the appearance of clinical symptoms in asymptomatic patients. The prevention of clinically evident heart failure is one of the most important opportunities for decreasing the mortality and morbidity rates from this condition (Gould et al, 1971).

All patients with the following complaints should undergo evaluation for heart failure unless the history and physical examination clearly demonstrate otherwise:

- Paroxysmal nocturnal dyspnea
- Orthopnea
- New-onset dyspnea on exertion
- Lower extremity edema
- Decreased exercise tolerance
- Abdominal symptoms associated with ascites or hepatic engorgement
- Altered mental status, especially in the elderly.

This is especially applicable if the patient also has a history of other cardiac diseases.

Treatment to Prevent and Retard Disease Progression

Once the diagnosis of heart failure is made and the patient's condition has been stabilized, plans need to be implemented to prevent exacerbation and to slow the progression of the disease. In patients with moderate or severe left ventricular dysfunction (left ventricular ejection fraction <35% to 40%) and no clinical symptoms of congestive heart failure, ACE inhibitors should be given to reduce the chance of developing progressive clinical heart failure (Konstam et al, 1994). This recommendation is supported by the Survival and Ventricular Enlargement (SAVE) trial (Pfeffer et al, 1992) and the Studies of Left Ventricular Dysfunction (SOLVD) prevention trial (SOLVD, 1992). In the SAVE study, patients with a left ventricular ejection fraction ≤40% were randomized to receive either captopril titrated to 50 mg t.i.d. as tolerated or placebo. The proportion of patients who developed heart failure was 16% in the control group and 11% in the group receiving captopril. The proportion of patients requiring hospitalization for heart failure was 17% in the control group and 14% in the group receiving captopril. Similar to the SAVE study, patients in the SOLVD study receiving enalapril (titrated to 10 mg given orally b.i.d.) experienced reduced development of symptomatic heart failure (30% for the control group, 21% for the enalapril group).

Tertiary Prevention

REHABILITATION

Because heart failure is a lifelong disease, aggressive rehabilitation plans should be implemented to help patients live the fullest, least disabling life possible. Patients should be encouraged to perform regular exercise, such as walking or cycling (Konstam et al, 1994). Heart failure, when properly managed, should not prohibit patients from performing regular daily activities. Referral to supervised rehabilitation programs may also benefit patients who are anxious, are dyspneic at a low work level, or have angina, recent myocardial infarction, or coronary bypass surgery (Konstam et al, 1994).

Another important management strategy is dietary sodium restriction. Sodium consumption in patients with heart failure should be limited to 2 g/day if possible (definitely <3 g/day) (Konstam et al, 1994). A 3-g diet can be achieved fairly easily by not adding salt to foods and by avoiding salty foods. Many patients, especially the elderly, may find this unpalatable. Counseling and flexibility are required to promote participation and to ensure that patients do not become malnourished. Referral to a dietitian and involvement of the spouse, companion, or family members may be necessary to increase patient participation.

Patients with heart failure should also be advised to avoid excessive fluid intake. Strict restriction is not necessary unless the patient develops hyponatremia. Alcohol consumption should also be discouraged because acute ingestion of alcohol may depress myocardial contractility in patients with cardiac diseases.

Because pharmacologic agents used in the treatment of heart failure not only improve or eliminate symptoms but also prolong survival, good participation in a pharmacotherapeutic regimen becomes extremely important. However, this is sometimes difficult to achieve because patients with heart failure usually are receiving multiple medications for heart failure and other underlying disease states. To facilitate participation, long-acting formulations of medications that can be given once daily create a more convenient schedule for the patient. Providing patient and family education to improve their knowledge of the conditions and of the medications will also encourage patients to take a more active role in their medical management.

General Management Summary

The following is a summary of management recommendations for systolic and diastolic heart failure (Fig. 11-3).

- Mild to moderate exercise to tolerance, such as walking or biking, should be encouraged.
- Salt restriction (<3 g/day) should be recommended.
- Underlying etiologies should be treated whenever possible.
- Heart transplantation should be considered in patients with heart failure refractory to medical and surgical therapy.

SYSTOLIC HEART FAILURE

- ACE inhibitors should be administered to all patients with significantly reduced left ventricular ejection fraction (<45%) unless contraindicated.
- A combination of hydralazine and isosorbide dinitrate can be substituted if patients have contraindications to ACE inhibitors.
- Diuretic therapy should be administered to patients with fluid overload.
- Digoxin should be given to patients with systolic heart failure not adequately responsive to ACE inhibitors and diuretic therapy.
- Digoxin should also be given to patients with systolic heart failure and atrial fibrillation with rapid ventricular rates.
- Anticoagulation therapy with warfarin should be given to patients with atrial fibrillation, a previous history of systemic or pulmonary embolism, or a very low ejection fraction (<20% to 25%).
- Beta-blockers should be considered for patients who are not adequately responsive to digoxin, diuretics, and ACE inhibitors, but not in clinical heart failure.
- Second-generation calcium channel blockers (amlodipine or felodipine) may be considered if patients require additional blood-pressure or angina control.
- Antiarrhythmic agents (amiodarone) should be given to patients for sustained ventricular tachycardia or ventricular fibrillation or conversion to normal sinus rhythm from atrial fibrillation only.

DIASTOLIC HEART FAILURE

- Diuretics and nitrates are the drugs of choice for patients with congestive symptoms.
- Calcium channel blockers, beta-blockers, and ACE inhibitors may be beneficial.
- Agents with positive inotropic actions are not indicated if systolic function is normal.

TEACHING AND SELF-CARE

After the diagnosis of heart failure is made, patients and their families or caregivers should be counseled regarding the following aspects (Konstam et al, 1994):

- Nature of the disease: Explanation of heart failure, etiology, expected symptoms, and symptoms of worsening heart failure

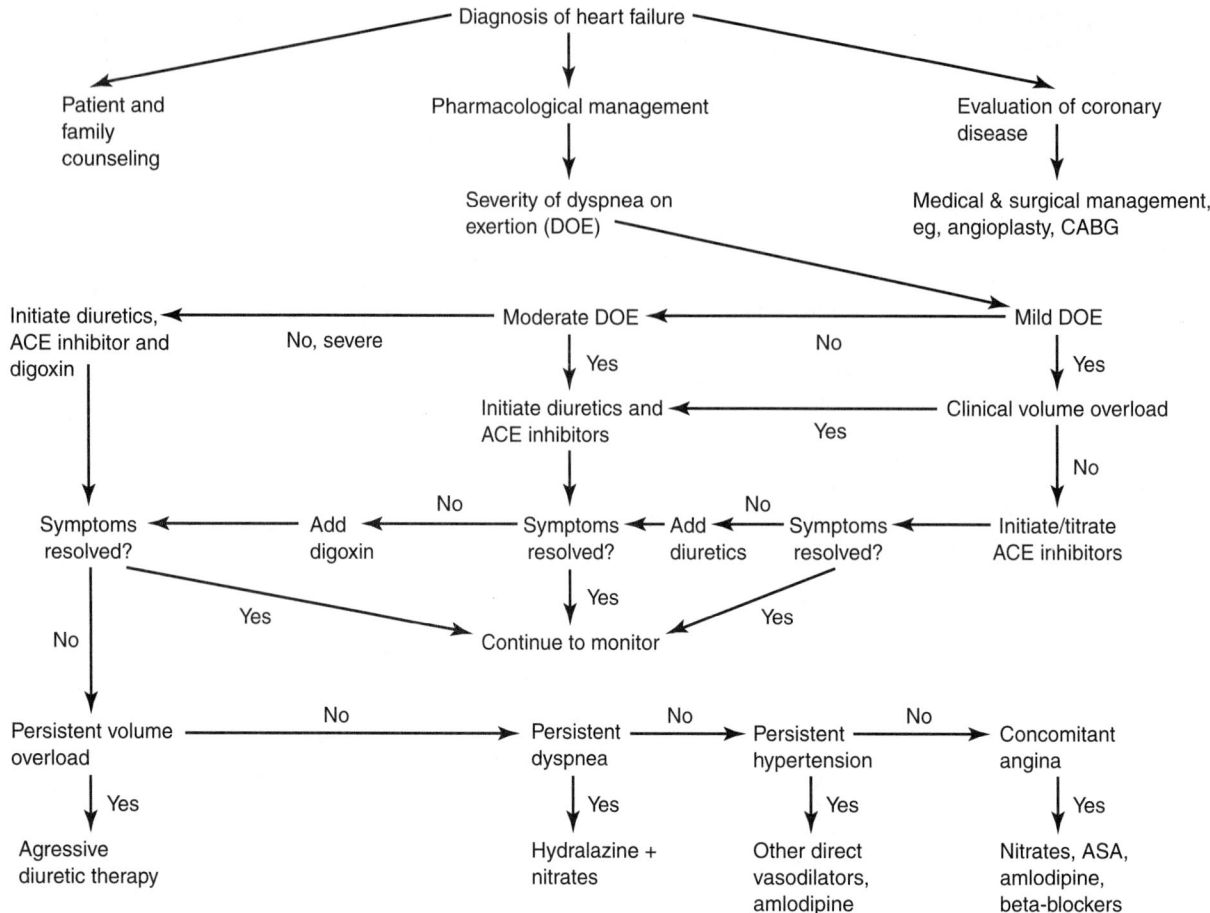

FIGURE 11-3 Management of heart failure.

- Prognosis: Life expectancy, advance directives, advice for family members in the event of sudden death
- Activity recommendations: Recreation, leisure and work activities, exercise, and sexual activity
- Dietary recommendations: Sodium restriction, avoidance of excessive fluid (or fluid restriction if necessary), alcohol restriction
- Medications: Effects of medication, dosing, side effects, financial assistance with medications
- Other treatment plans: Self-monitoring of daily weights, smoking and recreational drug use cessation, role of patients and family members in the treatment plan, availability of support groups, what to do when symptoms worsen, importance of obtaining vaccinations against influenza and pneumococcal disease
- Importance of active participation with the whole treatment/care plan.

Such education is most effectively provided by a multidisciplinary team involving different health care professionals, including primary care providers, nurses, pharmacists, physical therapists, dietitians, and social workers. Motivation and participation from patients themselves and their family members are also crucial.

COMMUNITY RESOURCES

In addition to professional counseling, there are numerous local support groups for patients with heart failure. These groups offer patients the chance to talk to others about their feelings and experiences dealing with the disease. Many support groups also offer educational programs about heart problems. For more information about support groups, patients can contact The Mended Hearts, Inc., 7272 Greenville Ave., Dallas, TX 75231 (214-706-1442) or The Coronary Club, Inc., 9500 Euclid Ave., E-37, Cleveland, OH 44195 (216-444-3690).

The following organizations also provide information, booklets, brochures, videotapes, and audiotapes about heart failure for patients: The American Heart Association, 7272 Greenville Ave., Dallas, TX 75231-4596 (1-800-AHA-USA1) or the National Heart, Lung, and Blood Institute Information Center, Public Health Service, P.O. Box 30105, Bethesda, MD 20824 (301-251-1222).

REFERRAL POINTS AND CLINICAL WARNINGS

Primary care providers should be aware of the appropriate indications for referral to cardiologists and hospitalization of patients with heart failure. Any of the findings listed in Table 11-11 usually signify a need for referral (Konstam et al, 1994).

TABLE 11-11	Clinical Findings Signifying the Need for Referral

1. Clinical or electrocardiographic changes that indicate acute myocardial ischemia

2. Pulmonary edema or severe respiratory distress

3. Markedly decreased oxygen saturation (<90% measured by arterial blood gas) not caused by pulmonary diseases

4. Anasarca

5. Symptomatic hypotension or syncope

6. Arrhythmia (severe symptomatic bradycardia, tachycardia, or atrial fibrillation)

7. Heart failure refractory to the optimal, patient-specific outpatient therapy

■ ■ ■ CLINICAL PEARLS

- While digoxin can prevent clinical deterioration in systolic heart failure and improve the patient's symptoms, there is no significant reduction in mortality.

- The correlation between digoxin's therapeutic levels and efficacy is not strong. Therefore, routine monitoring of digoxin levels is not necessary to ensure efficacy or safety.

- Nausea and vomiting are usually the first signs of digoxin toxicity. Any elderly patients on digoxin complaining of anorexia or gastrointestinal disturbance should be assessed for digoxin toxicity.

EDITOR'S NOTE:
COMPLEMENTARY APPROACHES

A general discussion of complementary approaches can be found in Chapter 3. The following, while not an exhaustive list, are some complementary approaches being used for this condition. Additional information on these approaches, including precautions, can be found in Appendices A and B. Providers need to assess for the use of complementary approaches as part of the patient's history, as they may impact conventional therapies, and patients may not volunteer this information unless specifically asked. Efficacy of many complementary approaches is not as well documented as that of conventional therapies. Providers need to read the literature before suggesting these complementary approaches.

- Vitamins, minerals, herbs, supplements
  Carnitine
  Coenzyme Q10
  Fish oils
  Hawthorne
  Taurine
- Complementary Modalities
  Acupuncture
  Aromatherapy

References

ACC/AHA Task Force on Practice Guidelines. (1995). Guidelines for evaluation and management of heart failure. *Journal of American College of Cardiology, 26*(5), 1376–1398.

Acute Infarction Ramipril Efficacy (AIRE) Study Investigators. (1993). Effect of ramipril on mortality and morbidity of survivors of acute myocardial infarction with clinical evidence of heart failure. *Lancet, 342,* 821–828.

Bonow, R. (1995). The hibernating myocardium: Implications for management of congestive heart failure. *American Journal of Cardiology, 75,* 17A–25A.

Braunwald, E. (1992). *A textbook of cardiovascular medicine.* Philadelphia: W.B. Saunders.

CIBIS Investigators and Committees. (1994). A randomized trial of beta-blockade in heart failure: the Cardiac Insufficiency Bisoprolol Study (CIBIS). *Circulation, 90,* 1765–1773.

Cohn, J. (1996). The management of chronic heart failure. *N Engl J Med, 335*(7), 490–498.

Cohn, J., Archibald, D., Ziesche, S., et al. (1986). Effect of vasodilator therapy on mortality in chronic congestive heart failure: Results of a Veterans Administration Cooperative Study. *N Engl J Med, 314,* 1547–1552.

Cohn, J., Johnson, G., Ziesche, S., et al. (1991). A comparison of enalapril with hydralazine-isosorbide dinitrate in the treatment of chronic congestive heart failure. *N Engl J Med, 325,* 303–310.

Cohn, J., Ziesche, S., Loss, L., Anderson, G., & V-HeFT Study Group. (1995). Effect of felodipine on short-term exercise and neurohormone and long-term mortality in heart failure: Results of V-HeFT III. *Circulation, 92* (suppl I) [abstract].

CONSENSUS trial study group. (1987). Effects of enalapril on mortality in severe congestive heart failure. *N Engl J Med, 316,* 1429–1435.

Doval, H., Nul, D., Grancelli, H., Perrone, S., Bortman, G., & Curiel, R. (1994). Randomized trial of low-dose amiodarone in severe congestive heart failure. *Lancet, 344,* 493–498.

Dzau, V. (1987). Renal and circulatory mechanisms in congestive heart failure. *Kidney International, 31,* 1402.

Gillum, R. (1993). Epidemiology of heart failure in the United States. *Am Heart J, 126,* 1042–1047.

GISSI-3. (1994). Effects of lisinopril and transdermal glyceryl trinitrate singly and together on 6-week mortality and ventricular function after acute myocardial infarction. *Lancet, 343,* 1115–1122.

Gould, L., Zahir, M., DeMartino, A., et al. (1971). Cardiac effects of a cocktail. *JAMA, 218,* 1799–1802.

Grossman, W., Jones, D., & McLaurin, P. (1975). Wall stress and patterns of hypertrophy in the human left ventricle. *Journal of Clinical Investigation, 56,* 56-64.

Harlan, E., Oberman, A., Grimm, R., et al. (1977) Chronic congestive heart failure in coronary artery disease: Clinical criteria. *Annals of Internal Medicine, 86,* 133–138.

ISIS-4. (1995). A randomized factorial trial assessing early oral captopril, oral mononitrate, and intravenous magnesium sulphate in 58,050 patients with suspected acute myocardial infarction. *Lancet, 345,* 669–685.

Konstam, M., Dracup, K., Baker, D., et al. (1994) *Heart failure: Evaluation and care of patients with left ventricular systolic dysfunction.* Rockville, MD: U.S. Department of Health and Human Services.

Mattleman, S., Tobin, J., Wassertheil-Smoller, D., et al. (1983). Reliability of bedside evaluation in determining left-ventricular function: Correlation with left ventricular ejection fraction determined by radionuclide ventriculography. *Journal of American College of Cardiology, 1,* 417–420.

MMWR. (1994). Mortality from congestive heart failure—United States, 1980–1990. *MMWR, 43*(5),77–81.

Packer, M. (1988). Neurohormonal interactions and adaptations in congestive heart failure. *Circulation, 77,* 721.

Packer, M., Bristow, M., Cohn, J., et al. (1996) The effect of carvedilol on morbidity and mortality in patients with chronic heart failure. *N Engl J Med, 334,* 1349–1355.

Packer, M., Gheorghiade, M., Young, J., et al. (1993). Withdrawal of digoxin from patients with chronic heart failure treated with angiotensin converting enzyme inhibitors. *N Engl J Med, 329,* 1–7.

Packer, M., O'Connor, C., Ghali, JK., et al. (1996). Effect of amlodipine on morbidity and mortality in severe chronic heart failure. *N Engl J Med, 335,* 1107–1114.

Patterson, H., & Adams, K. (1996). Pathophysiology of heart failure: Changing perceptions. *Pharmacotherapy, 16*(2), 26S–36S.

Pfeffer, M., Braunwald, E., Moye, L., et al. (1992). Effects of captopril on mortality and morbidity in patients with left-ventricular dysfunction after myocardial infarction: Results of the survival and ventricular enlargement trial. *N Engl J Med, 327,* 669–677.

Singh, S., Fletcher, R., Fisher, S., et al. (1995). Amiodarone in patients with congestive heart failure and asymptomatic ventricular arrhythmia. *N Engl J Med, 333,* 77–82.

SOLVD Investigators. (1992). Effect of enalapril on mortality and the development of heart failure in asymptomatic patients with reduced left-ventricular ejection fractions. *N Engl J Med, 327,* 685–691.

Swedberg, K., Held, P., Kjekshus, J., et al. (1992). Effects of the early administration of enalapril on mortality in patients with acute myocardial infarction. *N Engl J Med, 327,* 678–684.

Waagstein, F., Bristow, M., Swedberg, K., et al. (1993). Beneficial effects of metoprolol in idiopathic dilated cardiomyopathy. *Lancet, 342,* 1441–1446.

Willerson, J., & Cohn, J. (1995). *Cardiovascular medicine.* New York: Churchill-Livingstone.

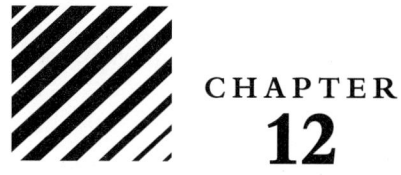

CHAPTER

12

Hypertension

Judy Cheng, PharmD, BCPS

Hypertension is one of the most common and most important risk factors in developing cardiovascular diseases such as coronary artery, cerebrovascular, and renal diseases. Prevention and proper control of hypertension can reduce the risk of developing such diseases. Since the inception of the National High Blood Pressure Education Program in 1972, remarkable progress has been made in detecting, treating, and controlling hypertension (Joint National Committee, 1997). Management of hypertension to date thus revolves around primary prevention via lifestyle modifications, early detection, and optimal treatment, with consideration of patients' other concurrent medical problems. This chapter will discuss the primary prevention strategy for hypertension as well as the proper therapeutic management once the diagnosis is established. Issues related to the implementation and dissemination of these approaches will be emphasized.

ANATOMY, PHYSIOLOGY, AND PATHOLOGY

Anatomy and Physiology

Arterial blood pressure is defined hemodynamically as the product of the cardiac output and the total peripheral resistance. It reaches its peak during cardiac systole (SBP) and its nadir at the end of diastole (DBP). The cardiac output is the major determinant of SBP, and total peripheral resistance determines DBP. Cardiac output, in turn, depends on stroke volume, heart rate, and venous capacitance. Factors that increase stroke volume and heart rates will increase cardiac output and subsequently SBP. Alternatively, venous capacitance affects the volume of venous blood (preload) that is returned to the heart. Venous dilatation increases venous capacitance and decreases preload, thus decreasing SBP. Total peripheral resistance is regulated by contraction and dilation of the arterioles. Other factors that may also affect intravascular resistance include the elasticity of arteries and blood viscosity.

The difference between SBP and DBP (pulse pressure) is an indicator of the tone of the vessel walls. The mean arterial pressure, which is defined as one third of the pulse pressure plus DBP, is the average pressure throughout the cardiac cycle.

Blood pressure can be regulated by the kidneys, which control blood volume, and the sympathomimetic nervous system. Increased sympathomimetic activity stimulates vasoconstriction of arterioles, thus raising total peripheral resistance, and increases cardiac output, thus elevating blood pressure. For blood pressure to remain within normal limits, specialized receptors (baroreceptors) are used. These stretch receptors are located in the aortic arch and in the carotid sinuses. An increase in blood pressure causes these receptors to stretch and stimulate the activity of the sensory nerve. Sensory nerve activity from the baroreceptors is transmitted via the vagus and glossopharyngeal nerves to the medulla oblongata, which directs the autonomic system to respond appropriately. An effective baroreceptor reflex helps to maintain adequate blood flow to the brain on standing.

Pathophysiology

The vast majority of patients who have hypertension have essential (primary) hypertension. Secondary hypertension makes up only about 10% of the hypertensive population (Joint National Committee, 1997). Some possible causes of secondary hypertension include kidney disease, pheochromocytoma, primary aldosteronism, hyperthyroidism, or drug-induced hypertension (eg, cyclosporine, erythropoietin, sympathomimetic agents). Primary hypertension, on the other hand, may be caused by multiple factors, including abnormal neural mechanisms, defects in peripheral autoregulation, disturbances in sodium, calcium, and natriuretic hormone levels, and malfunctions in either humoral or vasodepressor mechanisms.

Abnormal Neural Mechanisms

The central and the autonomic nervous systems are intricately involved in the maintenance of arterial blood pressure. Located in the presynaptic and postsynaptic nervous endings are alpha and beta receptors. Stimulation of presynaptic alpha and beta receptors will lead to inhibition and enhancement, respectively, of norepinephrine release; stimulation of postsynaptic alpha-1 receptors leads to vasoconstriction. Stimulation of postsynaptic beta-2 receptors leads to vasodilation. Stimulation of beta-1 receptors in the heart enhances cardiac contractility and increases heart rate. The major negative feedback system of the sympathetic nervous system is the baroreceptor reflex. A pathologic disturbance in any of these neural components could lead to sustained elevations of blood pressure.

PERIPHERAL AUTOREGULATION

A defect in renal adaptive mechanisms can lead to plasma volume expansion and increased blood flow to peripheral tissues, even when blood pressure is normal. To offset such increases in blood flow, local tissue autoregulatory processes would induce arteriolar constriction to raise the peripheral vascular resistance.

DISTURBANCES IN SODIUM, CALCIUM, AND NATRIURETIC HORMONE

Increased sodium intake, together with an inherited defect in the kidney's ability to excrete sodium, leads to an increase in the level of circulating natriuretic hormones. Natriuretic hormones inhibit intracellular sodium transport, causing increased vascular reactivity and a rise in blood pressure.

Calcium homeostasis also contributes to the pathogenesis of hypertension. Lack of calcium in the blood circulation leads to a relative elevation of calcium concentration intracellularly, which leads to altered vascular smooth muscle function and increased peripheral vascular resistance.

Potassium depletion may also cause an increase in peripheral vascular resistance, but its clinical impact is not clearly defined.

MALFUNCTION OF HUMORAL MECHANISM

The renin-angiotensin system's involvement in hypertension has been well described. Renin is synthesized in the kidney and stored in the juxtaglomerular cells. Decreases in perfusion pressure to the kidney and the flux of sodium and chloride across the renal tubule trigger renin release. In blood, renin catalyzes the conversion of angiotensinogen to angiotensin I, which is then converted by angiotensin-converting enzymes (ACE) to angiotensin II. Angiotensin II is a direct vasoconstrictor. It also stimulates catecholamine and aldosterone release from the adrenal gland. This neurohormone will lead to hypertension. Angiotensin is also produced by local tissues of different organs, such as the heart and the brain. Local angiotensin may interact with other humoral regulators and endothelium-derived growth factors to stimulate vascular smooth muscle growth. Components of the local angiotensin system may be responsible for long-term adaptation to hypertension (eg, left ventricular hypertrophy, smooth muscle hypertrophy of blood vessels, and glomerular hypertrophy) (see Chap. 11).

Other neurohormonal mechanisms involved in hypertension include hyperinsulinemia and insulin resistance. Elevation in the serum insulin concentration may induce renal sodium retention and enhanced sympathetic nervous system activity and may cause vascular smooth muscle hypertrophy. The vascular endothelium also plays an important role in blood vessel tone. Vasoactive substances produced by the endothelium, such as prostacyclin, bradykinin, endothelium-derived relaxing factor, and endothelin I, interact with each other to maintain normal vessel tone. Imbalances of these vasoactive substances may contribute to hypertension.

EPIDEMIOLOGY

The Third National Health and Nutritional Examination Survey (NHANES III), which reviewed data collected from 1988 through 1994, indicated that approximately 50 million (or one in every four) adults in the United States have hypertension (Joint National Committee, 1997). Hypertension is associated with an increased risk of developing coronary artery disease, stroke, congestive heart failure, renal insufficiency, and peripheral vascular disease. There is no gender discrimination for such risk throughout the entire adult age range. However, the prevalence of hypertension increases progressively with increasing age. The risk of morbidity and mortality from cardiovascular disease increases in a curvilinear fashion with progressively higher levels of SBP and DBP. Research over the years has helped in identifying environmental, cultural, and social factors that may contribute to the current hypertension pattern.

Cultural Factors

Research in animals and humans has identified the following factors as the most important contributors to age-related increases in blood pressure (Joint National Committee, 1997):

- High sodium intake (beyond human physiologic needs)
- Overweight
- Lack of physical activity
- Excessive alcohol consumption
- Smoking
- Excessive stress
- Inadequate potassium intake
- Positive family history
- Members of minority populations (eg, African Americans).

In a culture with a high level of stress, low physical activity, and excessive consumption of salt and alcohol, the prevalence of hypertension may increase.

Socioeconomic Factors

Socioeconomic status can also be a determinant of blood pressure. In economically developed countries, only a relatively small proportion of the general population has a blood pressure within the optimal range (<120/80 mmHg). This is, however, the norm in less developed societies, where age-related increases in blood pressure are uncommon (Carvalho et al, 1989; He et al, 1991). Reasons that may explain this phenomenon include differences in lifestyle (eg, activity level) and diet (eg, alcohol consumption) among different societies.

DIAGNOSTIC CRITERIA

Hypertension management begins with early detection. Primary care providers should measure a patient's blood pressure at every clinic visit. Table 12-1 provides the Sixth Report of the Joint National Committee (JNC VI) classification of adult blood pressure based on the risk of developing cardiovascular events (Joint National Committee, 1997). All stages of hypertension are associated with an elevated risk of cardiovascular events and renal disease, but the higher the blood pressure, the greater the risk.

Hypertension should never be diagnosed based on a single measurement because various factors, such as coffee consumption and the medical white coat, may affect a patient's blood pressure. An initial elevated reading should be confirmed on at least two subsequent visits over 1 to several weeks, except if SBP is above 180 mmHg, DBP is above 110 mmHg, or signs and symptoms of end organ damage are present. In these situations, patients need to be referred to emergency care immediately. An overall average SBP above 140 mmHg or a DBP above 90 mmHg will require further diagnosis and treatment. Table 12-1 illustrates the proper follow-up recommendations based on the initial screening blood pressure for patients older than age 18.

Because the risk of developing cardiovascular disease in patients with hypertension is determined not only by the level of blood pressure but also by the presence or absence of target organ damage or other risk factors (as listed below), the JNC VI guidelines recommend that treatment of hypertension be based on the patient's risk group (Table 12-2).

Risk factors for developing cardiovascular diseases (besides hypertension) are:

- Smoking
- Hyperlipidemia
- Diabetes mellitus

TABLE 12-1	Recommendations for Follow-Up Based on Initial Screening Blood Pressure of Patients >18 Years of Age		
	Initial Screening (mmHg)		
Category	*Systolic*	*Diastolic*	**Follow-Up Recommendation**
Optimal	<120	<80	Recheck in 2 years.
Normal	<130	<85	Recheck in 2 years.
High-normal	130–139	85–89	Recheck in 1 year.
Hypertension			
Stage 1	140–159	90–99	Confirm within 2 months.
Stage 2	160–179	100–109	Evaluate and refer for care within 1 month.
Stage 3	≥180	≥110	Evaluate and refer for care immediately or within 1 week, depending on clinical situation.

When SBP and DBP fall into different categories, the higher category should be used.

- Age above 60 years
- Male gender
- Family history of cardiovascular disease (women <65 or men <55).

HISTORY AND PHYSICAL EXAMINATION

A complete medical history and physical examination should be performed in all hypertensive patients during their initial evaluation. This examination should include:

- Family history of high blood pressure, premature coronary heart disease, stroke, cerebrovascular disease, diabetes, and hypercholesterolemia
- Patient history or symptoms of cardiovascular, cerebrovascular, or renal disease, diabetes, hypercholesterolemia, or gout
- Known duration and levels of elevated blood pressure
- History of weight gain, stress, physical activity, and smoking
- Dietary assessment, including sodium intake, alcohol use, and intake of cholesterol and saturated fat
- Complete medication history, including the use of over-the-counter products as well as the results and side effects of previous antihypertensive agents
- Symptoms suggesting secondary hypertension
- Psychosocial and environmental factors that may influence blood-pressure control (eg, family and employment situations, educational level)

- Verification of blood pressure by two or more blood-pressure measurements separated by 2 minutes with the patient either supine or seated and after standing for at least 2 minutes
- Verification of blood pressure in the contralateral arm (if different, the higher value should be used)
- Height, weight, and waist circumference
- Funduscopic examination for arteriolar narrowing, arteriovenous nicking, hemorrhages, exudates, or papilledema
- Examination of the neck for carotid bruits, distended veins, or an enlarged thyroid gland
- Examination of the heart for tachycardia, hypertrophy, pericardial heave, clicks, murmurs, arrhythmias, and third or fourth heart sound
- Abdominal examination for bruits, enlarged kidneys, masses, and abnormal aortic pulsation
- Examination of extremities for diminished or absent peripheral arterial pulsations, bruits, and edema
- Neurologic assessment.

DIAGNOSTIC STUDIES

Once hypertension is diagnosed, further evaluation of patients should be targeted at answering the following questions:

- Is the patient having primary hypertension versus secondary hypertension?
- Is target-organ disease present?

TABLE 12-2	Risk Stratifications of Patients With Hypertension		
Blood-Pressure Stages	**Risk Group A***	**Risk Group B†**	**Risk Group C‡**
High normal	Lifestyle modification	Lifestyle modification	Drug therapy
Stage 1	Lifestyle modification (up to 12 months)	Lifestyle modification (up to 6 months)§	Drug therapy
Stages 2 and 3	Drug therapy	Drug therapy	Drug therapy

* Risk group A: No risk factors, no target organ disease or clinical cardiovascular disease

† Risk group B: At least 1 risk factor (not including diabetes), no target organ disease or clinical cardiovascular disease

‡ Risk group C: Target organ damage and/or diabetes, with or without other risk factors

§ For patients with multiple risk factors, drug therapy plus lifestyle modification should be considered as initial therapy.

■ Are other cardiovascular risk factors present?

Any diagnostic studies that are required to rule out secondary causes should be performed. In addition, diagnostic tests required to rule out target-organ damage and other cardiovascular risk factors are also necessary. Several laboratory tests should be performed routinely before initiation of drug therapy. These include urinalysis; a complete blood count; measurement of blood glucose, electrolytes, serum creatinine, and uric acid; lipid profile; and electrocardiography.

TREATMENT OPTIONS, EXPECTED OUTCOMES, AND COMPREHENSIVE MANAGEMENT

Primary Prevention

Despite the fact that antihypertensive drug treatment reduces cardiovascular risk in hypertensive patients, it is far from the complete solution to the problem. Treatment requires an ongoing commitment to the task of identifying and treating incidental cases. This reduces the risks of development of secondary diseases but does not cure the problem. Furthermore, not everyone with hypertension receives early diagnosis. Many sustain vascular damage to their heart, brain, eyes, or kidneys before they come to the attention of primary care providers. In addition, treatment of hypertension can impose a social and economic burden on patients. Therefore, primary prevention of hypertension is part of the long-term solution to the problem. It provides opportunities to interrupt and reduce the continuing cost cycle of managing hypertension and its complications.

HEALTH PROMOTION AND SPECIFIC PROTECTION

Clinical trials have demonstrated that the following lifestyle modifications are efficacious in the primary prevention of hypertension.

The following are definitely efficacious:

■ Weight loss if overweight; regular aerobic exercise (30 to 40 minutes most days of the week)
■ Sodium intake less than 100 mmol/day (<2.4 g of sodium or <6 g of sodium chloride)
■ Alcohol consumption 1 oz/day or less of ethanol (24 oz of beer, 8 oz of wine, or 2 oz of 100-proof whiskey)
■ Smoking cessation
■ Reduction of dietary saturated fat and cholesterol intake for overall cardiovascular health (also good for weight reduction).

The following are possibly beneficial with limited efficacy:

■ Stress management
■ Adequate dietary potassium, calcium, and magnesium intake.

Weight reduction reduces blood pressure in a large population of hypertensive persons more than 10% above their ideal weight (Langford et al, 1991). All hypertensive patients who are above their ideal body weight should be placed on an individualized, monitored weight-reduction program involving caloric restriction and regular exercise to increase caloric expenditure. In stage 1 hypertensive patients, weight loss and exercise programs should be tried for at least 3 to 6 months before the

patients are considered candidates for pharmacologic antihypertensive therapy. Even if patients require antihypertensive pharmacotherapy, they should still participate in a weight-loss program.

Epidemiologic observation indicates that within a population, a **reduction of sodium intake** to 100 mmol/day was associated with an SBP reduction of 5 to 10 mmHg (Law et al, 1991; Intersalt, 1988). African Americans and older hypertensive patients are more sensitive to changes in dietary sodium (Grobbee, 1991). Patients should be advised to reduce their sodium consumption to less than 100 mmol/day.

Excessive **alcohol consumption** can lead to an elevation of blood pressure or resistance to antihypertensive therapy (Maheswaran et al, 1991). Patients should be encouraged to limit their daily intake to no more than 1 oz of ethanol. Significant elevations in blood pressure may develop during alcohol withdrawal in patients with heavy alcohol consumption, but such pressor effects of alcohol withdrawal are reversed several days after alcohol consumption is reduced.

Patients who continue to **smoke** despite proper control of blood pressure will not receive the full protection from developing coronary artery disease. Counseling and referral to effective smoking cessation programs are essential. The use of nicotine gum and nicotine patches in conjunction with patient counseling may assist the provider in promoting smoking cessation.

If necessary, drug therapy for **hypercholesterolemia** is an important adjunct to the antihypertensive regimen. This is discussed elsewhere in this text.

Although there is little literature support, **stress** can raise blood pressure acutely and may contribute to hypertension. Therefore, patients should be encouraged to relax and reduce stress.

There is an inverse relation between **potassium, calcium, and magnesium intake** and blood pressure (Linas, 1991; Hamet et al, 1991). Although supplementation of potassium, calcium, and magnesium has not been demonstrated to lower blood pressure, maintenance of adequate dietary intakes may help to prevent hypertension.

Secondary Prevention

EARLY DIAGNOSIS, PROMPT TREATMENT, AND DISABILITY LIMITATION

Hypertension management begins with early detection and continued surveillance. For accurate diagnosis, blood pressure should be measured in a manner such that the values obtained are representative of the patient's usual levels. Patients should be asked to sit with arms bared, supported, and at heart level. No caffeine or cigarettes should be consumed within 30 minutes of blood-pressure measurement. If possible, measurements should not be obtained until the patient has rested for at least 5 minutes. The appropriate cuff size should be used to ensure an accurate measurement. It is also advisable that two measurements be obtained 2 minutes apart if possible; if the two readings differ by more than 5 mmHg, additional readings should be obtained.

Once hypertension has been diagnosed, treatment plans need to be implemented to achieve the ultimate goal of improving morbidity and mortality rates. Therefore, it is equally important to maintain a normal blood pressure and to control other modifiable risk factors of cardiovascular disease. Lifestyle modification similar to those used for primary prevention (weight reduction, increased physical activity, and moderation of dietary sodium and alcohol consumption) are used as adjunctive or definitive therapies for hypertension.

Medication Regimen

There are numerous classes of antihypertensive agents from which to choose when initiating pharmacotherapy. Each possess their own advantages and disadvantages. Table 12-3 lists the different classes, some commonly prescribed antihypertensive agents available on the market, and precautions and special considerations in using these agents. Choosing an appropriate agent for each patient requires consideration of numerous factors. The following section will review the pharmacology of each class of antihypertensive agents and the general approach in initiating therapy and proper follow-up.

Diuretics work by initially decreasing plasma volume and extracellular fluid. Chronically, they decrease total peripheral resistance with a slight decrease in extracellular fluid. Side effects of diuretics include hypokalemia (except with potassium-sparing diuretics), hypomagnesemia, hyponatremia, hyperuricemia, hypercalcemia, hyperglycemia, hypercholesterolemia, hypertriglyceridemia, sexual dysfunction, and weakness. Diuretics are one of the two antihypertensive drug groups that have been demonstrated to improve long-term mortality and morbidity rates and are therefore recommended as first-line therapy, provided there are no contraindications (Joint National Committee, 1997).

Beta-blockers decrease blood pressure by decreasing cardiac output and baroreflex. They also decrease plasma renin activity. Beta-blockers can be divided into cardioselective agents (block beta-1 receptors only), noncardioselective agents (block both beta-1 and beta-2 receptors), and agents with intrinsic sympathomimetic activity (partial agonist). Side effects of beta-blockers include bronchospasm, exacerbation of symptoms of peripheral vascular disease, fatigue, insomnia, exacerbation of heart failure, masking symptoms of hypoglycemia, hypertriglyceridemia, decreased high-density lipoprotein levels (except agents with intrinsic sympathomimetic activity), sexual dysfunction, and reduced exercise tolerance. Beta-blockers are also one of the drug therapies that have been shown to improve long-term mortality and morbidity rates when used in the treatment of hypertension and are therefore a recommended first-line choice, provided no contraindications are present. To avoid rebound hypertension, beta-blockers should never be discontinued abruptly.

Calcium channel blockers block the inward movement of calcium ions across cell membranes and cause smooth muscle relaxation. Side effects of calcium channel blockers include headache, dizziness, peripheral edema (dihydropyridines), gingival hyperplasia (dihydropyridines), tachycardia (dihydropyridines), bradycardia (diltiazem and verapamil), and heart failure. Short-acting calcium channel blockers (specifically nifedipine) have also been associated with an increased incidence of myocardial infarction in a meta-analysis (Psaty et al, 1995; Alderman, 1992). It is believed that this phenomenon is caused by the fluctuations in neurohormonal and sympathetic activity caused by short-acting calcium channel blockers. Therefore, it is recommended that short-acting agents should be reserved for acute situations only; whenever possible, long-acting agents should be used.

ACE inhibitors block the formation of angiotensin II; this promotes vasodilation and decreases aldosterone production, which reduces salt and water retention. They also increase bradykinin levels and vasodilatory prostaglandins. Side effects of ACE inhibitors include cough, hyperkalemia, angioedema, rash, and elevation of serum creatinine levels.

Angiotensin II receptor antagonists bind to angiotensin II receptors in vascular smooth muscle to promote vasodilation. The side effect profile is similar to that of ACE inhibitors. However, because they bind directly to the angiotensin II receptors and have less effect on bradykinin production, they are believed to produce a lower incidence of side effects than ACE inhibitors.

Alpha-1 blockers produce vasodilation by blocking postsynaptic alpha-1 receptors. Side effects of alpha-1 blockers include orthostatic hypotension, headache, and palpitations.

Alpha-beta blockers exert their action by blocking both alpha- and beta-adrenergic receptors. Their side effect profiles are a combination of those of alpha- and beta-blockers.

Centrally acting agents exert their action by stimulating central alpha-2 receptors that inhibit efferent sympathetic activity. Side effects of these agents include drowsiness, sedation, dry mouth, fatigue, and orthostatic hypotension. To avoid rebound hypertension, short-acting clonidine should never be discontinued abruptly.

Direct vasodilators exert their action through direct smooth muscle (primary arteriolar) vasodilation. Side effects of direct vasodilators include headache, tachycardia, and fluid retention. Hydralazine can also cause lupus. Minoxidil can cause hypertrichosis.

Special Treatment Considerations

AGE AND GENDER CONSIDERATIONS

Beta-blockers, alpha-blockers, and ACE inhibitors are considered the drugs of choice for treatment of primary hypertension in middle-aged patients because these patients have a relatively higher sympathetic tone compared to older patients. Alternative agents recommended include centrally acting alpha-agonists such as clonidine.

In elderly patients, isolated systolic hypertension (in which DBP remains normal) is a commonly observed phenomenon. In a double-blind placebo-controlled trial, the Systolic Hypertension in the Elderly Program (SHEP) study (1991), active treatment of isolated systolic hypertension with chlorthalidone, a diuretic, significantly reduced the risk of stroke and the number of cardiovascular events. Diuretics should be the drugs of choice for elderly patients. Because elderly patients are more sensitive to volume depletion and sympathetic inhibition, antihypertensive medications should be initiated at a smaller-than-usual dose.

Women taking oral contraceptives, especially if they are also obese or more than 35 years old, have a higher risk of developing hypertension (Joint National Committee, 1997). In this case, it is strongly advisable to stop the use of oral contraceptives. If other contraceptive methods are not acceptable to the patient, then treatment of hypertension should be considered.

TABLE 12-3			Commonly Used Antihypertensive Agents	
Drugs	**Usual Dose (mg)**	**Frequency (times/day)**	**Precautions and Special Considerations**	**Remarks**
DIURETICS				
Thiazides				
Chlorthalidone	125–500	2	Except for indapamide and metolazone, ineffective in renal failure (CrCl <30 mL/min)	Hydrochlorothiazide and chlorthalidone generally preferred for hypertension. Loop diuretics generally reserved for fluid overload conditions such as congestive heart failure.
Hydrochlorothiazide	12.5–50	1		
Indapamide	2.5–5	1		
Metolazone	0.5–5	1		
Loop				
Bumetanide	0.5–5	1	Effective in chronic renal failure	
Furosemide	20–320	1–2		
Torsemide	5–100	1–2		
Potassium-Sparing				
Amiloride	5–10	1	Danger in patients who are prone to hyperkalemia (eg, taking ACE-I concurrently)	
Spironolactone	25–100	2–3		
Triamterene	50–150	1–2		
BETA-BLOCKERS				
Atenolol	25–100	1	Avoid in patients with asthma/COPD. Use with caution in patients with heart failure, heart block, diabetes, and peripheral vascular disease. Never stop abruptly to avoid rebound.	In higher doses, even selective beta-blockers may lose their selectivity.
Betaxolol	5–10	1		
Bisoprolol	2.5–10	1		
Carteolol	2.5–10	1		
Metoprolol	50–200	2		
Metoprolol long-acting	50–300	1		
Nadolol	40–320	1		
Penbutolol	10–20	1		
Propranolol	30–240	3–4		
Propranolol long-acting	60–240	1		
Timolol	20–60	2		
BETA-BLOCKERS WITH ISA				
Acebutolol	200–1200	2	Avoid in patients with coronary artery disease. Others similar to beta-blockers.	
Pindolol	10–60	2		
ALPHA-BETA BLOCKERS				
Carvedilol	12.5–50	2	Same as beta-blockers	
Labetalol	200–1200	2–3		
ALPHA-BLOCKERS				
Prazosin	1–20	2–3	Caution in elderly patients for orthostatic hypotension	Prazosin is generally used for hypertension. Terazosin is generally used for benign prostatic hypertrophy.
Terazosin	1–20	1		

(continued)

| TABLE 12-3 | Commonly Used Antihypertensive Agents *(Continued)* |

Drugs	Usual Dose (mg)	Frequency (times/day)	Precautions and Special Considerations	Remarks
ACE-I				
Benazepril	10–40	1–2	Hyperkalemia can develop, especially in patients with renal failure. Hypotension may develop with initiation of medications.	
Captopril	12.5–150	2–3		
Enalapril	2.5–40	1–2		
Fosinopril	5–40	1–2		
Lisinopril	5–40	1–2		
Moexipril	7.5–15	2		
Quinapril	5–80	1–2		
Ramipril	1.25–20	1–2		
Trandolapril	1–4	1		
CCB				
Diltiazem	90–360	3	Use with caution in patients with heart failure, heart block (except amlodipine, felodipine). Avoid short-acting agents because of the possible linkage between short-acting CCB and increased incidence of MI.	
Cardizem CD	120–360	1		
Amlodipine	2.5–10	1		
Felodipine	5–20	1		
Isradipine	2.5–10	2		
Mibefradil	50–100	1		
Nicardipine	60–120	3		
Nifedipine	30–120	3		
Nifedipine long-acting	30–120	1		
Verapamil	80–480	3		
Verapamil long-acting	120–480	1		
CENTRALLY ACTING ALPHA-2 ANTAGONISTS				
Clonidine	0.1–1.2	2–3	May cause rebound hypertension if discontinued abruptly	
Clonidine patch	0.1–0.3	1 weekly		
Methyldopa	250–2000			
DIRECT VASODILATORS				
Hydralazine	50–300	2–4	Hydralazine may induce lupus. Minoxidil may aggravate pleural and pericardial effusion.	Generally more difficult to tolerate. Tolerance may develop with long-term use of hydralazine. Usually reserved for patients with more severe hypertension, such as hypertension in patients with renal failure.
Minoxidil	2.5–80	1–2		
ANGIOTENSIN II RECEPTOR ANTAGONISTS				
Losartan	25–50	1–2	Similar to ACE-I (possibly lower incidence of occurrence)	
Valsartan	81–320	1		

ACE-I, angiotensin-converting enzyme inhibitors; CCB, calcium channel blockers; CrCl, creatinine clearance; ISA, intrinsic sympathetic activity; COPD, chronic obstructive pulmonary disease.

CULTURAL CONSIDERATIONS

Hypertension is a common problem in all races and cultures. However, African American populations seem to be affected at a disproportionately higher rate. African Americans also usually suffer from a more severe degree of hypertension. Because of the lower plasma renin level and the increased blood-pressure response to sodium and fluid overloading observed in this population, diuretic therapy should be used as the initial antihypertensive treatment, provided there are no contraindications. Calcium channel blockers have proven to be as efficacious as diuretics as first-line therapy. Beta-blockers and ACE inhibitors may not be as effective as diuretics and calcium channel blockers when used as monotherapy. If an adequate response is not attained with diuretics or calcium channel blockers, beta-blockers and ACE inhibitors can be added with favorable results (Joint National Committee, 1997; Hawkins et al, 1993).

QUALITY OF LIFE CONSIDERATIONS

Antihypertensive agents may cause certain side effects that will affect a patient's quality of life (see Table 12-3). Examples include impotence, impairment of mental acuity, and reduction of exercise tolerance.

ECONOMIC CONSIDERATIONS

The cost of antihypertensive medication may be a barrier to optimal control of hypertension because treating blood pressure usually means a commitment to life-long therapy. Working with patients to choose the most affordable therapy may help

TABLE 12-4	Individualized Antihypertensive Agents Based on Coexisting Diseases
Indication	**Drug Therapy**
COMPELLING INDICATIONS UNLESS CONTRAINDICATED	
Diabetes (type 1) with proteinuria	ACE-I
Systolic heart failure	ACE-I, diuretics
Isolated systolic hypertension (elderly)	Diuretics (preferred), CCB (long-acting dihydropyridine)
MI	Beta-blockers (non-ISA), ACE-I
MAY HAVE FAVORABLE EFFECTS ON CORMORBID CONDITIONS	
Angina	Beta-blockers, CCB
Atrial tachycardia and fibrillation	Beta-blockers, CCB (nondihydropyridine)
Diabetes (types 1 and 2) with proteinuria	ACE-I (preferred), CA
Dyslipidemia	Alpha-blockers
Essential tremor	Beta-blockers (noncardioselective)
Systolic heart failure	Amlodipine, carvedilol, losartan
Hyperthyroidism	Beta-blockers
Migraine	Beta-blockers (noncardioselective), CCB (nondihydropyridine)
MI	Diltiazem, verapamil
Osteoporosis	Thiazides
Preoperative hypertension	Beta-blockers
Prostatism (benign prostate hypertrophy)	Alpha-blockers
MAY HAVE UNFAVORABLE EFFECTS ON COMORBID CONDITIONS	
Asthma, COPD	Beta-blockers
Depression	Beta-blockers, central alpha-agonists, reserpine
Diabetes (type 1 and 2)	Beta-blockers, high-dose diuretics
Dyslipidemia	Beta-blockers (non-ISA), diuretics (high doses)
Gout	Diuretics
Second- and third-degree heart block	Beta-blockers, CCB (nondihydropyridine)
Systolic heart failure	Beta-blockers (except carvedilol), CCB (except amlodipine and felodipine)
Liver disease	Labetalol, methyldopa
Peripheral vascular disease	Beta-blockers
Pregnancy	ACE-I, angiotensin II receptor blockers

ACE-I, angiotensin-converting enzyme inhibitors; CCB, calcium channel blockers; COPD, chronic obstructive pulmonary disease; ISA, intrinsic sympathomimetic activity.

in improving their participation in a mutually acceptable therapeutic plan.

COEXISTING DISEASES CONSIDERATIONS

Antihypertensive agents, while improving high blood pressure, may worsen other disease states. For instance, beta-blockers may aggravate asthma, diabetes, and peripheral vascular disease. However, they have improved the mortality rate in myocardial infarction, certain arrhythmias, and certain heart failure conditions. Therefore, antihypertensive agents should always be selected bearing the patient's coexisting diseases in mind. Table 12-4 summarizes the specific agents of choice and the agents contraindicated in different disease states.

Initiation of Dosages and Follow-up

When the decision has been made to begin drug therapy, and the patient has no indications for another type of drug (see Table 12-4), a diuretic or beta-blocker should be chosen (Joint National Committee, 1997). Whenever initiating antihypertensive therapy, the lowest dosage should be selected to prevent unnecessary side effects and hypotension. Unless the patient experiences signs and symptoms of end organ damage, the lowest dose should be given for several weeks before it is increased to the next dosage level. During the initial titration of dosages, short-acting agents may be necessary to allow fine-tuning of doses. Once stabilized, long-acting agents (given once or twice daily) should be used whenever possible to improve patient participation in the therapeutic plan.

If after 1 to 2 months of the initial therapy, the response is still inadequate, the dosage of the initial agent can be increased up to the maximum, an alternative agent can be substituted, or a second agent from another antihypertensive class can be added. Combining different agents may allow smaller doses of each agent to be used, minimizing side effects. It may be more difficult for patients to maintain a regimen of multiple medications; therefore, risk/benefit ratios always have to be consid-

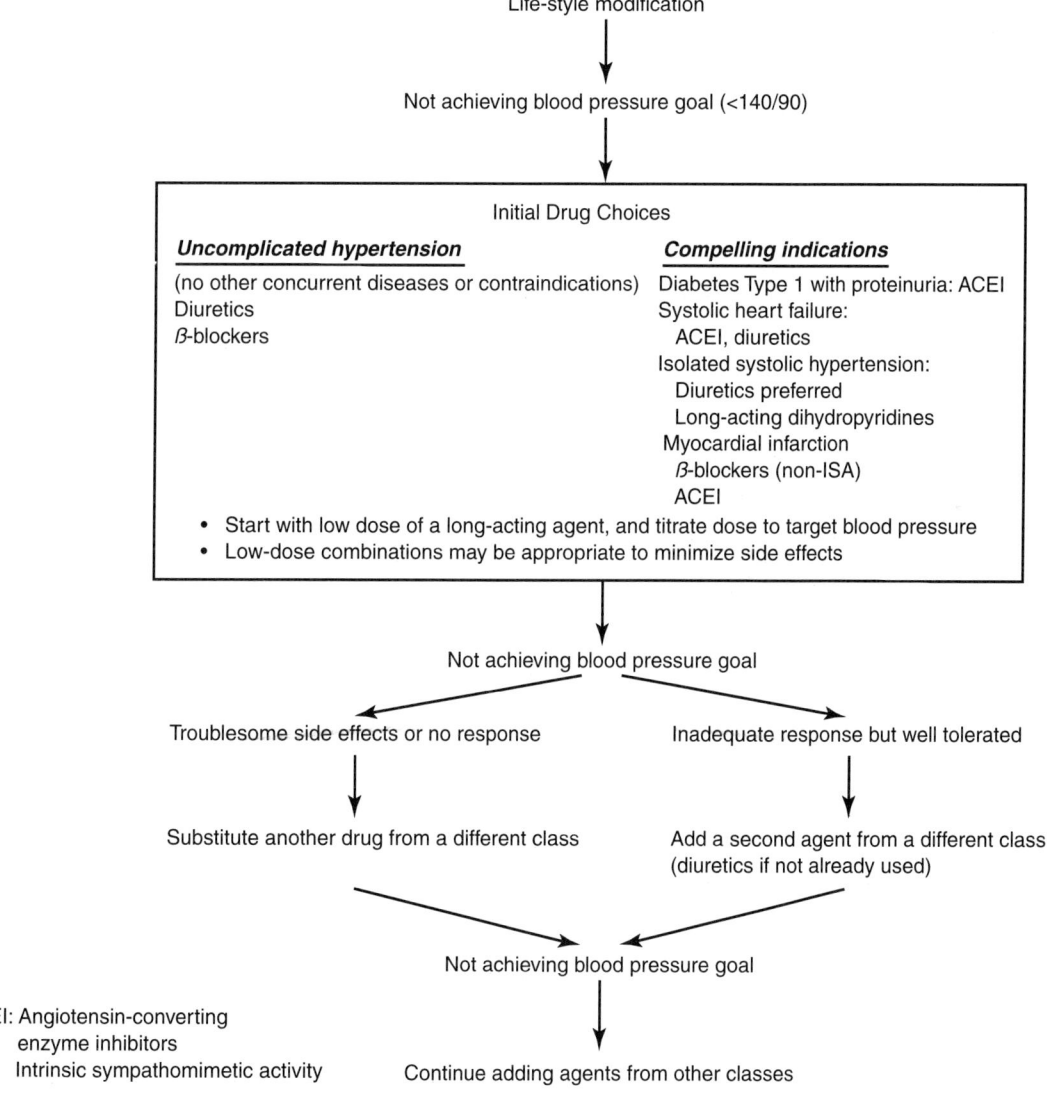

FIGURE 12-1 Treatment approach of essential hypertension.

ered. If a diuretic is not chosen as the initial agent, the addition of one usually enhances the effect of the other agents.

Achieving and maintaining the target blood pressure requires long-term follow-up. Once stabilized (optimal doses established), patients should be seen at 3- to 6-month intervals to ensure the blood pressure still remains normal.

STEP-DOWN THERAPY

Hypertension management should include attempts to decrease the dosage or number of antihypertensive drugs while maintaining lifestyle modifications. Although complete cessation of therapy is in general not indicated, after blood pressure has been controlled for 1 year, it may be possible to reduce antihypertensive therapy in a slow and progressive manner. Step-down therapy is especially successful in patients who are also participating in lifestyle modification programs. Patients who have drugs discontinued or reduced should have regular follow-up to detect recurrence of hypertension even after months or years, especially in the absence of sustained improvements in lifestyle.

Summary of Treatment

Treatment of hypertension should begin with aggressive lifestyle modifications. If this proves inadequate, antihypertensive agents should be initiated. Provided there are no contraindications or other concurrent disease states, diuretics and beta-blockers should be used as the drugs of choice because of their ability to improve long-term mortality and morbidity rates, as proven in controlled clinical trials. If the response is still inadequate, several approaches may be used. First, the dose of the initial agent may be increased and side effects monitored. Second, another agent may be substituted for the first. Third, a second agent from a different class may be added. Figure 12-1 summarizes the overall treatment approach to essential hypertension.

TEACHING AND SELF-CARE

Successful long-term control of hypertension requires intensive participation by patients. Therefore, proper patient education, patient self-care, and long-term support and follow-up are essential to ensure success. Strategies to improve participation in the therapeutic plan, and ultimately blood-pressure control, include:

- Use educational materials and programs stressing the importance of the primary prevention of hypertension and lifestyle modifications for long-term control of hypertension.
- Discuss with patients their concerns, and clarify any misunderstandings.
- Inform patients of their blood-pressure level. This gives patients a sense of control of their own disease.
- Involve patients in the decision-making process and in establishing the goals of treatment.
- Simplify the regimen as much as possible; this includes selecting the most cost-effective regimen.
- Incorporate the treatment into patient's daily lifestyle.
- Encourage blood-pressure monitoring by the patient; this may include home blood-pressure monitoring. Encour-

age discussion of side effects and concerns about the medication or diet regimen.
- Provide feedback regarding blood-pressure level.
- Provide positive encouragement for blood-pressure and behavioral improvement.
- Educate the patient's family members to be part of the blood-pressure control process and to provide positive reinforcement.
- Suggest small-group activities to enhance mutual support and motivation.
- Collaborate with other health care professionals to provide patients with more intensive counseling.

COMMUNITY RESOURCES

More information regarding the management of hypertension, epidemiologic data about hypertension, and community-based hypertension education programs can be obtained from the National High Blood Pressure Education Program, Office of Prevention, Education and Control, National Institutes of Health, P.O. Box 30105, Bethesda, MD 20892 (301-251-1222).

REFERRAL POINTS AND CLINICAL WARNINGS

Patients with the following signs and symptoms should be referred for further evaluation and management:

- SBP 180 mmHg or higher or DBP 120 mmHg or higher
- Signs and symptoms of target-organ damage, such as myocardial ischemia or congestive heart failure, stroke, absence of major pulses in extremities, proteinuria or significant elevation of serum creatinine level, and retinopathy
- Hypertension refractory to outpatient drug treatment
- Secondary hypertension that requires specialist consultation for the underlying cause (eg, pheochromocytoma)
- Hypertension in pregnancy.

■ ■ ■ CLINICAL PEARLS

- Even if patients require antihypertensive pharmacotherapy, they should still participate in a weight-loss program.
- African-Americans and older hypertensive patients are more sensitive to changes in dietary sodium.
- Short acting clonidine should never be discontinued abruptly, to avoid rebound hypertension.
- It is agreed that diuretics should be the drugs of choice for elderly patients.
- Antihypertensive agents, while improving high blood pressure, may worsen other disease states, i.e., beta-blockers may worsen asthma, diabetes, and peripheral vascular disease.
- During the initial titration of dosages, short acting agents may be necessary to allow fine tuning of doses. Once stabilized, long acting agents (given once or twice daily) should be used whenever possible to improve patient participation in the therapeutic plan.

EDITOR'S NOTE:

COMPLEMENTARY APPROACHES

A general discussion of complementary approaches can be found in Chapter 3. The following, while not an exhaustive list, are some complementary approaches being used for this condition. Additional information on these approaches, including precautions, can be found in Appendices A and B. Providers need to assess for the use of complementary approaches as part of the patient's history, as they may impact conventional therapies, and patients may not volunteer this information unless specifically asked. Efficacy of many complementary approaches is not as well documented as that of conventional therapies. Providers need to read the literature before suggesting these complementary approaches.

- Vitamins, minerals, herbs, supplements
  - Carnitine
  - Coenzyme Q10
  - Fish oils
  - Garlic
  - Magnesium
- Complementary Modalities
  - Acupuncture
  - Aromatherapy
  - Biofeedback
  - Massage therapy

References

Alderman, M. (1992). Which antihypertensive drugs first—and why? *JAMA, 267,* 2786–2787.

Carvalho, J., Baruzzi, R, Howard, P., et al. (1989). Blood pressure in four remote populations in the Intersalt study. *Hypertension, 14,* 238–246.

Despres, J., Moorjana, S., Lupien, P., Tramblay, A., Nadeau, A., & Bouchard, C. (1990). Regional distribution of body fat, plasma lipoproteins, and cardiovascular disease. *Arteriosclerosis, 10,* 497–511.

Grobbee, D. (1991). Methodology of sodium sensitivity assessment: The example of age and sex. *Hypertension, 17*(suppl I), I109–I114.

Hamet, P., Mongeau, E., Lambert, H., et al. (1991). Interactions among calcium, sodium, and alcohol intake as determinants of blood pressure. *Hypertension, 17*(suppl 1): I150–I154.

Hawkins, D., Bussey, H., & Prisant, M. (1993). Hypertension. In: *Pharmacotherapy: A pathophysiological approach.* Stamford, CT: Appleton & Lange.

He, J., Klag, M., Whelton, P., et al. (1991). Migration, blood pressure pattern, and hypertension: The Yi Migrant Study. *American Journal of Epidemiology, 134,* 185.

Intersalt Cooperative Research Group. (1988). Intersalt: An international study of electrolyte excretion and blood pressure. *British Medical Journal, 297,* 319–328.

Joint National Committee on detection, evaluation, and treatment of high blood pressure. (1997). *The sixth report.* NIH Publication No.98-4080.

Langford, H., Davis, B., Blaufox, M., et al. (1991). Effect of drug and diet treatment of mild hypertension on diastolic blood pressure. *Hypertension, 17,* 210–217.

Law, M., Frost, C., & Wald, N. (1991). By how much dose dietary salt reduction lower blood pressure? *British Medical Journal, 302,* 811–815.

Linas, S.L. (1991). The role of potassium in the pathogenesis and treatment of hypertension. *Kidney International, 39,* 771–786.

Maheswaran, R., Gill, J., Davies, P., & Beevers, D. (1991). High blood pressure due to alcohol: A rapidly reversible effect. *Hypertension, 17,* 787–792.

Psaty, B., Heckbert, S., Koepsell, T., et al. (1995). The risk of myocardial infarction associated with antihypertensive drug therapies. *JAMA, 274*(8), 620–625.

SHEP Cooperative Research Group. (1991). Prevention of stoke by antihypertensive drug treatment in older persons with isolated systolic hypertension. *JAMA, 265,* 3255–3264.

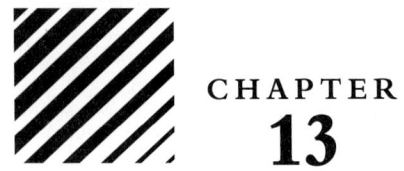

Peripheral Vascular Disease

Eileen M. Reilly, MS, RN, CS, FNP, Alice M. Arden, MA, RN, CS, ANP, and Harry L. Bush, Jr., MD

Peripheral vascular disease is a term used to describe a variety of disorders that affect the structure and function of the arterial, venous, and lymphatic systems. This chapter will discuss these disorders with regard to their clinical presentation, diagnostic criteria, and treatment options. It will also provide recommendations for patient education.

ARTERIAL INSUFFICIENCY

Arterial insufficiency is a progressively debilitating disease process caused by atherosclerotic plaque narrowing the lumen of the medium and long arteries. The innermost layer of the artery wall, the intima consists of endothelial cells that regulate the entry of substances from the blood into the artery wall. Atherosclerosis is a degenerative disease characterized by elevated plaques known as atheromas found within the intima. Atheromas narrow the vessels, resulting in stenosis or occlusion of the artery. Atherosclerosis impairs the ability of the endothelium to prevent platelet aggregation and cholesterol build-up. The distal vessels of the lower extremities are often the target for atherosclerotic plaque, usually found at the arterial branches in the regions of the intima. Patients with diabetes mellitus have an accelerated rate of atherosclerosis occurring at a relatively earlier age. Therefore, persons with diabetes have a greater risk for compromised circulation and the development of arterial ulcers (Auth, 1997).

Atherosclerosis is the leading cause of death in persons 65 years of age or older. It is suggested that more than 2 million people in the United States have arterial disease. Atherosclerosis in the arteries of the lower extremities is a strong indicator of atherosclerosis elsewhere in the body. Signs and symptoms of arterial insufficiency commonly develop in people between the ages of 50 and 70 (Saunders, 1997). Intermittent claudication is a common clinical condition that is estimated to affect at least 10% of the people over 70 years of age (Santilli et al, 1996).

The most common manifestation of lower extremity atherosclerosis is intermittent claudication (Olin, 1993). "Claudication" comes from the Latin word *claudicatio*, meaning "to limp" (Santilli et al, 1996). Intermittent claudication is a pain in the leg that is brought on by walking and relieved by rest. This pain, characteristic of peripheral arterial occlusion, results from diminished blood flow and the inability of the collateral circulation to meet the oxygen demand of the exercising muscles. Pain also occurs because the flow of blood is insufficient to remove metabolic wastes such as lactic acid, a byproduct of anaerobic metabolism. Development of this occlusive symptom indicates that the diameter of the affected vessel has been re-

duced by about 50% (Dumas, 1995). Pain often presents in the calf, thigh, or gluteal area (Auth, 1997).

Claudication develops in a muscle distal to the complete or partial obstruction of a main artery. Localization of symptoms depends on the anatomic pattern of the arterial occlusive disease. Pain is often felt in the muscle group below the level of the arterial obstruction. Aortoiliac occlusive disease may cause buttock and thigh claudication. This syndrome, known as Leriche's syndrome, causes atrophy and slow wound healing in the legs as well as an inability to maintain an erection. Iliofemoral occlusive disease results in thigh and calf claudication, and femoropopliteal occlusive disease results in calf claudication.

The most common site of peripheral arterial disease in both diabetic and nondiabetic patients is the superficial femoral artery. The second most common site is the aortoiliac segment. Tibial vessel disease, if present, may lead to critical ischemia of the leg, which is manifested by rest pain, nonhealing wounds, and gangrene (Santilli et al, 1996). Diseases affecting these vessels are more common in diabetic than nondiabetic patients (Krikorian & Vacek, 1995). Table 13-1 compares arterial and venous insufficiency.

A thorough patient history and physical assessment can help to distinguish ischemic ulcers caused by arterial disease from other types of ulcers (eg, venous, pressure, trauma, and vasculitis). The key to the diagnosis of arterial occlusive disease is the patient history (Auth, 1997). In taking the history, one must inquire about the onset and duration of symptoms and whether the leg pain is brought on by exercise and ceases with rest. How far can the patient walk before developing cramping pain? Which muscle groups are involved (calf, thigh, hips, buttock) (Uphold & Graham, 1994)? Does dangling the legs over the side of the bed relieve the pain? (This uses gravity to enhance circulation.) Males should be asked if impotence is present. Also, the provider should inquire about the patient's medical history of atherosclerosis, hypercholesterolemia, diabetes mellitus, and hypertension. A family history of arterial insufficiency should be elicited as well. The patient's social history (eg, smoking, sedentary lifestyle, and nutritional status) and a list of medications the patient is taking should be obtained.

The physical examination involves inspecting the patient's body for changes in appearance. Hair growth may be absent over the affected area. The nails may appear thick, yellow, and brittle. Motor function of the affected part may be impaired or absent. The muscles may also appear atrophied from severe nerve and skeletal muscle ischemia. Patients often complain of numbness and tingling in the extremity, as well as an inability to distinguish touch from pressure, pain, and temperature change.

The skin texture may also change with arterial insufficiency. The skin may appear shiny, taut and thin, or scaly and dry

TABLE 13-1	Comparison of Arterial and Venous Insufficiency	
Assessment	**Arterial**	**Venous**
Skin color	Extremely pale, pale when limb elevated, rubor when limb dependent	Brawny; brownish-red pigmentation, cyanotic when dependent
Skin texture	Thin, shiny, dry; hair loss on leg, ankle, and foot; thickened, rigid, yellow toenails	Stasis dermatitis, eczema, skin mottling, lipodermatosclerosis, thickened skin
Skin temperature	Cool	Warm
Edema	Absent or mild, usually unilateral	Present, usually foot to calf; may be unilateral or bilateral
Pain	Pain in the muscle of the buttocks, hip, thigh, or calf while walking that disappears at rest, worse while supine, disappears when dependent	Ache, dull, vague, localized on medial ankle; relieved with walking, leg elevation, and/or graduated compression stockings
Blood flow	Bruit may be present; pressure readings lower below stenosis	Normal
Pulses	Diminished or absent	Normal, although they may be difficult to feel through edema and thickened skin
Ulceration	Severely painful; involves toes or other bony prominences of foot, areas of trauma	Mildly painful; develops at medial malleolus
Ulcer characteristics	Well-demarcated edges Base: eschar or necrotic tissue common, punched-out appearance	Irregular edges, base: varies from granular to necrotic. Exudate varies from none to copious.
Impotence	May be present	Not present
Acute occlusion	Absent pulse, pale, cold, paralysis, and paresthesia present	Deep venous thrombosis: superficial phlebitis, redness, heat, calf tenderness, unilateral edema, acute dyspnea

from ischemia, or progress to a deep red when the feet are in a dependent position. To assess the degree of arterial insufficiency, a reactive hyperemia test may be performed. This involves raising the legs above the level of the heart for 5 minutes until the legs become a cadaveric pale color, followed by lowering the legs to a vertical position. If the leg remains red for longer than 15 seconds, the circulation is severely compromised.

The skin temperature may vary. It is usually cool from vascular occlusion or vasoconstriction, hindering the blood supply. The best way to assess the temperature is to palpate the extremity with the dorsum of the hand.

Breakdown of the skin may occur with severe ischemia, resulting in ulceration. These ulcers are often found over pressure points such as the heels, toes, bony prominences, the dorsum of the foot, or the metatarsal heads. Ulcers, which cause severe pain, are often symmetrical and without drainage. Mild edema may also be present. Patients experiencing pain at rest may have edema because they keep their legs in a dependent position for pain relief.

Palpating the patient's pulses provides information about the condition of the arteries. With arterial obstruction, the pulses may be absent or weak. Pulses should be assessed bilaterally for equality and strength using a Doppler stethoscope, if necessary. The physical examination should also include auscultation and evaluation of the blood flow. Normally, no sound is heard over a vessel that is patent. When blood flow becomes turbulent through an obstructed vessel, a blowing sound, or bruit, can be heard. Although the presence of a bruit is not always hemodynamically significant, it often indicates the start of chronic arterial occlusive disease long before symptoms such as cramps and pain appear (Bright & Georgi, 1992).

It is important in this patient population to check pulses in all regions of the body where major vessels are located, including the carotid, abdominal aorta, iliac, femoral, popliteal, posterior tibial, and dorsalis pedis. The clinical syndrome most difficult to distinguish from claudication is neurogenic claudication, more typically known as spinal stenosis. The pain characteristic of spinal stenosis is caused by a localized narrowing of the spinal canal caused by a structural abnormality that results in cauda equina compression. With spinal stenosis, the patient usually complains of pain in the lower back or buttock region as well as numbness and tingling in the feet with walking (Seller, 1996). Differentiation of claudication and spinal stenosis can be determined by the patient's response to exercise. Symptoms of intermittent claudication are brought on by exercise and relieved with rest. Onset at a given distance of walking can be predicted fairly accurately. Spinal stenosis may also be precipitated by walking, but the distance walked before symptoms appear will vary. Standing may cause discomfort in patients with spinal stenosis, whereas intermittent claudication relieves it (*Emergency Medicine*, July 1993).

Nocturnal muscle cramps may be another symptom that can mimic claudication. However, these cramps are a common complaint and have a tendency to occur in older persons. The cramps are not related to exercise. Tightness and pain in the calf after exercise can affect athletes with chronic compartment syndrome. This syndrome is usually found in young persons and presents after vigorous exercise and does not quickly subside with rest. Osteoarthritis of the hip may mimic thigh and buttock claudication. However, osteoarthritic pain occurs with variable amounts of exercise. It is relieved after long periods of rest and changes in severity from day to day (Santilli et al, 1996).

Acute arterial occlusion differs from intermittent claudication in terms of the presentation of pain. Claudication is a progressively debilitating symptom more chronic in nature. Acute arterial occlusion is abrupt in onset and is more severe. This excruciating, unrelenting pain may occur suddenly, and neither rest nor activity relieves it. With acute arterial occlusion, the progressive signs of arterial insufficiency (eg, dry skin, brittle nails, and hair loss) may not be present. Often the foot is white and cold (Bright & Georgi, 1992). The patient may experience muscle weakness, possible paralysis, and paresthesia. Because of the cessation of blood flow to the extremity, there will be loss of pulses distal to the occlusion (Saunders, 1997). This situation warrants immediate referral to a vascular surgeon.

Another differential diagnosis that can be included is Raynaud's disease. In Raynaud's disease, episodic vasospasm produces closure of the small arteries in the distal extremities. This may be elicited by exposure to cold, vibration, or emotional stimuli (Saunders, 1997). Refer to Chapter, where this is discussed in greater detail.

Intermittent claudication can be chronic in nature but may become more incapacitating. The body attempts to compensate for this ischemic state by developing collateral circulation. The collateral circulation may not be sufficient when oxygen demand exceeds supply. The patient may notice a decrease in endurance and tolerance with exercise, resulting in a decrease in the distance and amount of walking. The pain may begin to occur at night. This pain is often relieved by dangling the foot off the side of the bed. When arterial insufficiency has progressed to such a level that the pain is constant and severe, patients may be unable to function. At this point arterial ulcers may appear in conjunction with limb-threatening ischemia and ensuing gangrene, necessitating amputation (Bright & Georgi, 1992).

The diagnosis of peripheral vascular disease is based on patient history, physical examination, and noninvasive testing. A variety of diagnostic tests are used to diagnose vascular insufficiency. Doppler segmental pressures with an ankle/brachial index (ABI) provide information regarding the extent of the disease. Doppler segmental pressures are obtained by placing appropriately sized blood-pressure cuffs around the arm and at the proximal thigh, the distal thigh, the proximal calf, and the ankle of the affected leg. Normal values for Doppler segmental pressures show an increase of greater than 20 mmHg from the brachial artery to the proximal femoral artery. An increase of less than 20 mmHg signifies significant aortoiliac occlusive disease. A blood-pressure drop of more than 30 mmHg between any two successive blood-pressure cuffs in the leg signifies a significant arterial obstruction. The ABI is a ratio of the ankle blood pressure to the brachial blood pressure. An ABI of greater than 0.85 is considered normal, an ABI of 0.50 to 0.84 suggests arterial obstruction with claudication, and an ABI of less than 0.50 suggests significant arterial obstruction with critical ischemia (nonhealing wounds or rest pain). The sensitivity and specificity of Doppler segmental pressures and ABIs are in the range of 70% to 85%.

Occasionally, patients have normal ABIs and segmental pressures at rest, but their symptoms strongly suggest claudication. In these patients, segmental pressures and ABIs should be obtained before and after exercise. For this diagnostic test, the patient may walk or lift the heels repeatedly to elicit a pain response. Exercise may reveal the arterial obstruction, resulting in a significant change in the Doppler segmental pressures and the ABIs found at rest.

An angiogram is indicated after evaluation of Doppler segmental pressures and ABIs if a patient with claudication is to undergo surgical or endovascular treatment. Angiography helps to reveal the exact location of the arterial obstruction and provides a road map for operative reconstruction. Because of the low but significant risk of renal failure, hematoma formation, or arterial injury, angiography should be performed only in patients who are considering surgery (Santilli et al, 1996).

Magnetic resonance imaging (MRI) is a noninvasive, nonionic technique that produces cross-sectional images of the human anatomy through exposure to magnetic energy sources, without the use of radiation (Fischbach, 1996). MRI angiography provides both anatomic and hemodynamic information and is becoming a more common procedure to evaluate known vascular lesions. It may replace the gold standard of angiography, which requires the use of dye and the possible risk of renal failure.

There are several approaches to managing arterial insufficiency, beginning with risk factor modification. The single most important therapeutic intervention is smoking cessation. Hyperlipidemia should be controlled with dietary changes and if needed pharmacologic intervention. Dietary goals include a reduction of saturated fat intake and a reduction of cholesterol levels. For patients with diabetes, excellent glycemic control should be stressed. Blood pressure should be monitored and adequately controlled through mechanisms such as dietary changes, weight reduction, limitation of salt intake, stress reduction techniques, and pharmacologic management as needed. The patient should begin an exercise program that includes an aggressive walking program for approximately 30 minutes a day at a pace that elicits claudication. When claudication occurs, the patient should be instructed to walk a little further, stop, wait for the discomfort to pass, and then continue walking. A successful walking program can increase the distance to onset of claudication and help to develop collateral circulation (Olin, 1993).

Drug therapy for claudication enhances metabolic activity and increases blood flow to the affected muscles. Vasodilating agents have had little effect on patients with claudication. Antiplatelet agents and anticoagulants were thought to play a role in the treatment of claudication, but no data have been obtained to support their use in this condition. However, because of the high incidence of associated comorbidities in patients with claudication, consideration should be given to placing these patients on daily aspirin therapy.

Agents that decrease blood viscosity help promote blood flow to the extremities in patients with claudication. Pentoxifylline, a xanthine derivative, alters the structure of the red blood cell, decreases plasma viscosity, and decreases platelet aggrega-

TABLE 13-2	Patient Teaching Guidelines for Arterial Insufficiency

- Stop smoking
- Follow exercise plan
- Diet: low-fat, low-cholesterol
- Blood-pressure control
- Glucose control for the diabetic
- Hyperlipidemia control
- Avoid sitting or standing for prolonged periods
- Do not cross legs
- Inspect feet daily for ulceration, infection, redness, pressure points
- Protect bony prominences
- Wash, dry, moisturize feet well
- Protect feet from trauma or direct heat
- Keep feet and legs warm; report any numbness, tingling, pain
- Wear properly fitting shoes
- See podiatrist regularly

tion to enhance blood flow through the obstructed artery. Studies on the efficacy of pentoxifylline for claudication have produced conflicting results. This agent is the only medication approved by the U.S. Food and Drug Administration for the treatment of claudication. Pentoxifylline is given in a dose of 400 mg three times a day. Patients are usually given the drug for 1 to 3 months. If there is no change in the claudication after this time, the drug is discontinued. If the symptoms decrease, pentoxifylline therapy is continued. Reported symptomatic improvement rates vary from 10% to 20%. Five percent to 10% of patients cannot tolerate this drug because of gastrointestinal discomfort (Santilli et al, 1996).

Most patients with claudication respond to conservative therapy. Local infusion of a thrombolytic agent may be the next option before resorting to surgical revascularization in cases of acute limb-threatening ischemia (Elson, 1994). Before a decision is made to perform an invasive procedure, the risk of limb loss and the overall cardiovascular risk to the patient must be considered. Invasive procedures should be performed on patients who have failed to respond to optimal medical therapy such as risk factor modification, a progressive exercise program, and pharmacotherapy. These procedures should also be performed on patients who have symptoms so severe that they interfere with the quality of life, or on patients with progressive arterial occlusive disease with the manifestation of limb-threatening ischemia (pain at rest, nonhealing wounds, gangrene) (Santilli et al, 1996). Refer to Table 13-2 for patient teaching guidelines.

BUERGER'S DISEASE

Thromboangiitis obliterans, more commonly referred to as Buerger's disease, is a recurring inflammatory process affecting the small and medium-sized arteries and veins of the extremities. Buerger's disease is more commonly found in males than females between 35 and 50 years old. Risk factors include cigarette smoking and a family history. The cause is unknown.

Patients most often present with pain in either the feet or hands while at rest, numbness, and tingling, as well as color and

temperature changes. If any trauma to the affected extremity is experienced, ulceration may develop. Superficial thrombophlebitis manifested as erythema, warmth, and swelling often precipitates arterial signs and symptoms. Patients who develop ulceration are at great risk for infection, leading to possible amputation. Pulses in the extremities are either diminished or absent, and swelling is often noted in the feet. Angiography is indicated.

Patents should be taught to protect the extremities from trauma. Their hands and feet should be kept clean, dry, and moisturized. Patients may also promote circulation through exercise, such as the Buerger-Allen exercises. They should stop smoking. Pain can be controlled with analgesia or alternative therapies.

ANEURYSMS

An aneurysm is a defect in the anatomy of an artery resulting in weakness, stretching, and ballooning out of the arterial wall. The most commonly affected artery is the aorta; in 80% of cases the abdominal region is involved. There are three types of aneurysms: fusiform, saccular, and dissecting. Fusiform involves the ballooning of the entire circumference of the artery. Saccular involves only one side of the artery ballooning. A dissection occurs from a tear in the intima of the vessel, allowing blood to accumulate between the layers. A pseudoaneurysm is an accumulation of clot which forms outside an artery; it often occurs after trauma or an invasive procedure.

Aneurysms are more common in the population over 50 years of age, affecting men twice as often as women. Risk factors associated with aneurysmal dissection are hypertension, hyperlipidemia, atherosclerosis, smoking, diabetes, and a family history of aneurysm.

Most often aneurysms are asymptomatic and are discovered incidentally during ultrasound, computed tomographic (CT) scanning, or MRI. However, if a patient complains of symptoms such as chest, flank, or back pain, with any of the associated risk factors, an abdominal examination focusing on palpation and auscultation of the aorta should be performed. If suspicion of aortic aneurysmal disease arises, the patient should be referred to a vascular surgeon for consultation.

Aneurysms are diagnosed by ultrasound, CT scan, or MRI. Treatment, either surgical or monitoring every 4 to 6 months by imaging, should be implemented, along with risk factor modification. The primary care provider should also evaluate these patients for aneurysmal disease elsewhere in the body.

TEMPORAL ARTERITIS

Temporal arteritis, also known as giant cell arteritis, is a systemic condition characterized by chronic inflammatory changes of the aorta and its major branches. It occurs most commonly in Caucasian women over the age of 55. The onset of symptoms may be abrupt or insidious. The patient may present with headaches, often unilateral, and pain in both the pelvic and shoulder girdles (polymyalgia rheumatica). Visual disturbances, a particularly devastating complication of temporal arteritis, can also occur (Dean et al, 1995). Some atypical presentations include fever of unknown origin and weight loss.

On examination, the patient may have localized temporal artery tenderness, redness, decreased pulsation, induration, or in extreme cases scalp necrosis. Temporal arteries are normal in one third of the population. The patient may have ophthalmologic findings such as ophthalmoplegia and visual loss. On funduscopic examination, the patient may have pallor and swelling of the optic discs, an early sign of temporal arteritis; in the later stage of this disease, optic atrophy may exist. Systemic manifestations usually result from ischemia of affected arteries or inflammation. Bruits may be heard in the head and neck. The pulses in the upper extremities may be absent. Neurologic deficits, memory loss, delirium, dementia, or transient ischemic attacks may appear should this condition worsen.

If temporal arteritis is suspected, a temporal artery biopsy should be performed. However, a negative biopsy does not always rule out temporal arteritis. An erythrocyte sedimentation rate should be obtained; in temporal arteritis, it is almost always 50 mm/hour or more.

The treatment for temporal arteritis includes high-dose corticosteroids. These should be initiated promptly when the suspicion of temporal arteritis is high and when visual symptoms are present. Forty to sixty milligrams of prednisone daily is initially given. The initial doses can be given parenterally when there is a concern about visual compromise, but this must be started within the first 5 hours of visual impairment. Five days of high-dose parenteral methylprednisolone (1000 mg IV every 12 hours) is recommended by ophthalmologists. The steroid dose is titrated against symptoms and the sedimentation rate. This dose should be tapered after clinical and laboratory manifestations have normalized. Tapering to a dose of 20 to 30 mg/day within the first 2 months is a reasonable schedule. The goal is a maintenance dose of less than 10 mg/day. This may take over 1 year to achieve (Goroll et al, 1995).

FROSTBITE

Frostbite is a localized cold injury to the surface of the body. Its onset can be rapid or insidious. The traumatic effect of extreme cold on the skin and subcutaneous tissue is first recognized by the distinct pallor of exposed skin surfaces. Vasoconstriction and damage to blood vessels impair local circulation and result in anoxia, edema, vesiculation, and necrosis. Areas of the body at greatest risk from localized cold damage include the fingers, toes, hands, feet, nose, ears, and cheeks. Tissues that reach and maintain temperatures of −6° C. (21° F.) develop frostbite. This includes the epidermis, dermis, subcutaneous tissues, muscle, and bone, as well as nerves, lymphatics, and blood vessels.

The severity of the injury is difficult to determine on initial assessment of the patient with frostbite. In tissue that is damaged superficially, only the skin and subcutaneous tissues will be affected. Severe frostbite will penetrate deeper into muscles, nerves, and blood vessels and sometimes as deep as the bone. Frozen tissues will appear cold, white, bloodless, and hard on assessment. Generally, tissues that appear reddish or dusky blue have thawed, or thawed and refrozen. Tissue that is freshly thawed varies in appearance and in symptomatology. Even minor damage is frequently painful. The patient may describe a throbbing, stinging, stabbing, burning, or aching pain; the pain is caused by the return of blood flow to the affected area. On inspection, the skin may appear flushed and may develop clear yellowish or pink-tinged blisters over the first 24 hours after thawing. Deeper damage is evident if the patient feels no pain or sensation in the identified tissues. These tissues take on a ruddy-violet to purple-black dehydrated appearance. Areas that are damaged even further will become necrotic, taking on a black, desiccated appearance.

It is important to assess the patient frequently for any changes. These early observations of frostbite damage include frequent monitoring of circulation to the affected tissues. The patient should be queried about sensations, numbness, tingling, pain, pressure, or anesthesia. Patients may complain of an achiness or unpredictable spasms of piercing pain. Peripheral pulses should be assessed through palpation or by using a Doppler. Color, discoloration, texture, lines of demarcation, patterns, and the fullness and shape of the extremity should also be noted for comparison (Sullivan, 1993).

A potential complication that may develop is compartment syndrome, characterized by deep pain, decreased sensation, or tightness on the wound surface. A diminished pulse may also be present. Should this develop, the patient will require a fasciotomy to unburden the strangulating tissues.

When treating frostbite, it is important to remember not to rub or massage the affected extremity; the extremity should be protected from mechanical injury (Rakel, 1996). The initial treatment of frostbite is a thawing process. Before thawing is initiated, hypothermia, a more serious condition, must be ruled out (Sullivan, 1993). Hypothermia occurs when the body's core temperature drops below 35° C. (95° F.) and is considered severe when it falls below 28° C. (82.4° F.) (Jackson, 1995). If hypothermia exists, the patient should be admitted to an emergency department for closer monitoring and rapid rewarming. Thawing is performed by immersion in warm water baths and with the use of heating blankets. Warmed fluids enclosed in a container (such as an IV bag) can be placed under the arms and in the groin. Immersion is contraindicated if the patient's core temperature is less than 32° C. (90° F.). The affected part is immersed in a temperature-controlled whirlpool bath heated to 37.7° to 41.4° C. (100° to 106° F.), containing a solution of dilute (1:800) chlorhexidine gluconate. Frostbite on the ears is warmed with saline soaks. Thawing is complete when blood flow engorges the involved tissues, producing a pink or red flush. The tissue is then rinsed with a gentle stream of clean water with a temperature of about 35° C. (90° to 95° F.), gently patted dry or allowed to air-dry, and covered with a nonconstrictive protective barrier. Blisters should be left intact. If open wounds exist, a light application of silver sulfadiazine cream and sterile gauze is placed against the damaged tissues, then covered with a loose sterile bandage and a clean cotton mitt or bootie. Mupirocin ointment is applied to the ears.

Also, a diet high in protein, calories, vitamins, and minerals is recommended. Copious fluid intake is encouraged to replace pre-existing deficits and to provide a full reservoir to enhance circulation and repair. Caffeine intake and smoking are discouraged to minimize vasoconstriction.

Pharmacotherapy for frostbite may include enteric-coated aspirin (325 mg orally for 10 days) as an antiplatelet and analgesic agent. Additional analgesics may be given for very painful conditions. Phenoxybenzamine hydrochloride (10 mg/day for 10 days) may be given for its vasodilating effects. Antianxiety agents may be warranted because this is often a traumatic time for the patient. Medications that promote gastrointestinal stability, histamine antagonists, or proton pump inhibitors may also be warranted.

The patient should avoid acts that could disrupt circulation, risk infection, or traumatize fragile tissues. Affected extremities should be elevated to reduce edema. If the patient's arterial flow pattern is of concern, the affected extremity should be maintained in a neutral position.

Wound care consists of hydrotherapy twice daily. This allows the primary care provider to inspect the injuries and to prevent or manage infection. The hydrotherapy also helps to enhance circulation. The temperature of these gentle whirlpool baths should be 32° to 35° C. (90° to 95° F.), and again 1:800 chlorhexidine gluconate solution should be added to the water. These baths should last approximately 20 minutes. Unlike burn wounds, frostbite wounds are not actively debrided during these tubbings, or in the early weeks of care, because it is believed that these wounds are basically clean and that the trauma of debridement would contribute to an infection risk and might harm the already fragile blood flow. If eschar forms over healing tissues and begins to constrict underlying tissues, debridement is then cautiously attempted (Sullivan, 1993).

CLINICAL WARNING: Do not rub or massage the affected extremity. Protect the injured extremity from mechanical injury.

CHRONIC VENOUS INSUFFICIENCY

Chronic venous insufficiency can be a debilitating condition. It occurs predominantly in the elderly. This condition, which affects the lower extremities, develops when blood pools in the leg veins instead of returning to the heart. The normal anatomy of the venous system of the legs consists of three components: the deep venous system, the superficial venous system, and the perforator veins (Capeheart, 1996). The deep veins and arteries are located parallel to each other in the legs. The anterior and posterior tibial veins, the peroneal veins, the popliteal vein, the superficial and deep femoral veins, and the common femoral veins are included in this system. The superficial veins, consisting of two major veins (the greater and lesser saphenous veins), are located in the subcutaneous tissue. The greater saphenous vein extends from the dorsum of the foot up the medial aspect of the leg to the groin, where it empties into the common femoral vein. The lesser saphenous vein begins behind the lateral malleolus and enters the popliteal vein and the popliteal fossa. There are approximately 100 communicating or perforating veins in each leg. These veins are located medially and laterally in the lower leg and allow oblique blood flow from the superficial system through the fascia into the deep system. The most important communicating leg veins are located around the medial malleolus and, laterally, in the lower third of the leg (Lamont, 1991).

The venous system is a unique system consisting of valves that permit unidirectional flow of blood back to the heart. These delicate but very strong structures lie at the base of the segment of a vein that is expanded into a sinus. This arrangement permits the valves to open widely without coming into contact with the wall, thus allowing rapid closure when blood flow begins to reverse. There are fewer valves in the superficial veins. Approximately seven to nine valves exist in the greater and lesser saphenous veins. These valves allow blood flow to be directed centrally and prevent reflux. Perforating veins have valves that allow one-way flow of blood from the superficial system to the deep system. Competent valves are valves that ensure the unidirectional flow of blood to the heart.

For blood to return to the heart, the calf muscle must pump blood back into the central veins against gravity (Lovell et al, 1993). As the calf muscle contracts, it exerts pressure on the vein, thus setting the blood in motion. The pressure in the deep veins increases to 200 mmHg when the calf muscle contracts, pushing the blood flow toward the heart. The pressure in the superficial veins does not change during this contraction. As the calf muscle relaxes, the pressure in the deep veins decreases to between 0 and 10 mmHg, allowing the blood to flow into them through the perforator veins. At this point, the pressure in the superficial venous system decreases to 30 mmHg. The calf pump functions normally when foot vein pressure decreases from 90 to 30 mmHg during exercise of the calf muscle (Capeheart, 1996).

Venous disease occurs when there is an obstruction to or reduction of venous blood return to the heart. There are several different ways in which this happens, such as thrombus formation, incompetent valves, gravitational strain, and immobilization of the extremity. A thrombus or thrombophlebitis can obstruct a vein, producing acute pain or throbbing as a result of the inflammatory process. The valves in the veins can become incompetent, thereby causing a reduction in the venous blood flow. This in turn produces edema from the increased venous and capillary pressure, causing fluid to seep out into the surrounding tissues. The gravitational pressure of standing adds to the strain on veins because hydrostatic pressure increases venous pressure. Venous stasis occurs with immobilization or impairment of the pumping action of the calf muscles (Saunders, 1997). Calf pump failure occurs when the foot vein pressure is increased rather than reduced as the calf muscle relaxes. This failure is seen when there is an outflow obstruction (eg, intraluminal thrombosis, pelvic tumor), outflow tract regurgitation (eg, deep vein thrombosis, floppy valves), perforator vein incompetence (eg, congenital vein wall weakness), superficial vein regurgitation, or muscle failure (eg, paralysis) (Capeheart, 1996). Immobility, obesity, prolonged standing or sitting, and pregnancy are conditions that can cause venous stasis.

Conditions that produce hypercoagulability (ie, elevated platelet count, increased clotting factors, increased blood viscosity) can lead to the formation of thrombus that occludes venous circulation. These conditions include blood dyscrasias, the use of birth-control pills, malignant neoplasms, and pregnancy. Injury to the vein or vein wall can lead to decreased blood flow and can result from a variety of conditions, surgical and nonsurgical, including trauma, chemical sclerosing agents, and radiopaque dyes (Saunders, 1997).

The clinical manifestations of chronic venous insufficiency involve changes in the lower extremities. There are usually one or more visible cutaneous changes in the legs. These changes include edema, xerosis, brownish pigmentation (hemosiderin) deposition, eczema, ankle flare, and lipodermatosclerosis. They may be unilateral or bilateral.

Edema, an early sign of chronic circulatory insufficiency, is caused by the increase in venous pressure resulting from calf pump failure. When edema occurs, the capillary bed becomes distended. A brown or brownish-red pigmentation occurs as a result of extravasation of red blood cells, caused by venous hypertension, which distends the capillary walls and promotes leakage of the red blood cells through the endothelial cells in the surrounding tissues. This pigmentation, known as hemosiderin deposition, is noted on the skin, usually in the area superior to the medial malleolus in the gaiter area. Hemosiderin, an iron-containing pigment, is derived from hemoglobin as the red blood cell disintegrates. This pigmentation pattern may also be caused by melanin deposition.

Eczema is a condition that develops in response to xerosis, a chronic dryness, caused by the lack of oxygen and nutrients. It may present with erythema, scaling, pruritus, and occasional weeping. Ankle flare, a manifestation also called corona phlebectatica, is detected as dilated venules. These dilated venules are usually observed below the medial malleolus and extending onto the foot. The greater the number of capillaries noted in ankle flare, the greater the extent of venous disease.

Lipodermatosclerosis is the term used to describe the result of longstanding venous insufficiency. Fibrous tissue eventually replaces skin and subcutaneous tissue. The leg is no longer edematous; the lower third of the leg feels woody and has the appearance of an inverted champagne bottle or an inverted bowling pin. This dermal change, which may be mistaken for cellulitis, precedes and forebodes ulceration. The presence of lipodermatosclerosis, hemosiderin deposition, and epithelial scaling is referred to as venous dermatitis (Capeheart, 1996).

Chronic venous insufficiency of the legs is described throughout the literature as being among the most common medical problems. An estimated 7 million persons in the United States have chronic venous insufficiency; this accounts for an estimated 70% to 90% of all leg ulcers. Leg ulcers are thought to develop as a complication of chronic venous insufficiency three times more often among women as among men, especially in the population 65 years old and older (Capeheart, 1996).

The patient's health history is of utmost importance when assessing for venous insufficiency. To determine the significance of the symptoms of venous disease, it is important to inquire about any family history of venous disease and about any previous surgical history involving the affected extremity. Patients should be queried regarding other risk factors as described in Table 13-3.

The patient should identify and describe any areas of pain or heaviness in the limbs and rate the pain on a scale of 0 to 10, with 0 representing the least amount of pain and 10 being the worst amount of pain. It should be noted whether the patient has observed any changes in skin temperature or appearance, skin breakdown, or any history of ulcerations (Saunders, 1997).

The physical examination for the patient with venous insufficiency involves inspecting the skin for breakdown and noting

TABLE 13-3	**Pertinent History Questions**

- Recent hospitalization with prolonged bed rest (ie, surgery, illness, pregnancy)
- History of surgery or trauma to the leg
- Use of oral contraceptives
- History of superficial phlebitis or deep vein thrombosis
- History of prolonged sitting or standing
- Family history of venous disease

any scars from healed ulcers. The extremities should be inspected for edema, and if it is present they should be palpated for pitting edema. It is important to inspect and palpate the extremities for varicosities (tortuous or dilated veins). These are best seen in the standing position, when the gravitational pressure is greatest. The provider should also palpate for hard, cordlike segments along the veins. It is also important to palpate the feet and legs to detect any changes in the skin temperature and to assess all peripheral pulses. Any skin color changes, scaly skin, or open areas should be noted. Patients should be evaluated for a positive Homans' sign by dorsiflexing each foot and noting any pain (Saunders, 1997).

A common problem that arises from chronic venous insufficiency is the formation of a venous stasis ulcer. Unlike arterial ulcers, venous ulcers do not form at pressure points. Venous ulcers tend to be in the gaiter area, usually situated over the medial and lateral malleoli. Ulcer borders are usually shaggy and irregular. There may be brown-red hemosiderin pigmentation of the surrounding skin and eczematous changes around the ulcer with redness, scaling, and itching. Varicose veins may be present and ankle edema is common. In longstanding venous ulcers there may be a woody texture to the skin, as described earlier, which is known as lipodermatosclerosis. Chronic lymphedema may develop after repeated infections, and the ankle joint may eventually fuse because of prolonged immobility (Phillips, 1996). It is important to assess the patient's arterial circulation while treating venous disease, because they often coexist.

There are several diagnostic tests used to identify venous insufficiency. Doppler ultrasonography is used to establish the absence or presence of venous reflux and obstruction. Impedance plethysmography is used to assess venous outflow and measure variations in electrical impedance that accompany changes in blood volume. Photoplethysmography is used to measure vascular volume to provide an index of valvular competence. Duplex scanning with color-flow imaging is used to locate venous reflux in the superficial, deep, and perforator systems. Radionuclide venography is used to assess the venous system but does not allow for visualization of the tibial veins. Contrast venography provides radiographic pictures of the venous system.

The goals in the management of venous insufficiency are to prevent and eliminate infection. Here, the patient needs to be educated about meticulous skin care and the signs and symptoms of infection. Additional goals include stimulating the development of granulation tissue, implementing methods that promote venous return, and relieving pressure. Educating the patient is of prime importance in the management of venous disease. Patients need to be instructed in the areas of foot care, exercise, nutrition, leg elevation, activity, elastic support, nonsmoking, and medical follow-up.

Elastic compression stockings, which are applied from the toes to below the knee, aid in venous return by exerting a pressure greater at the foot and ankle area than at the calf area. These stockings should be put on as soon as the patient gets up in the morning. They should be worn all day and removed at night. Foot elevation is essential to promote venous return. This should be done several times daily with the feet elevated above the level of the heart. At night the foot of the bed should be elevated on 6″ blocks (Lovell et al, 1993). To enhance patient participation in elevation of the extremities, a "feet-up chart" can be used, as shown in the display (Capeheart, 1996).

FEET UP CHART
Patient log for foot elevation

DATE: _____

TIME: _____   LENGTH _____
morning

TIME: _____   LENGTH _____
afternoon

TIME: _____   LENGTH _____
evening

Meticulous skin care is imperative in ulcer prevention. Corticosteroids may be used to manage severe cases of dermatitis and pruritus. Xerosis is also known as winter itch because it is typically exacerbated during periods of low humidity and cold weather. It is prevalent on the lower extremities, and the patient may inadvertently cause the area to become inflamed through scratching because of the pruritic nature of the condition. Prevention measures include teaching the patient not to bathe every day, to use oils in the bath water, to use mild soaps or soapless cleansers, and to use a topical emollient to retard water loss from the epidermis. Patients should be instructed to buy emollients containing urea (10% to 20%) and lactic acid (5% or 12%). These ingredients assist in removing retained layers of stratum corneum and subsequently reduce the scaliness associated with xerosis. The patient should be educated to report any trauma sustained on the lower extremity or any signs of tissue breakdown (Capeheart, 1996).

Venous ulcers can be treated by several methods, including Unna's boot, hydrocolloid dressings, saline solution compresses, and leg compression and leg elevation. Various ointments and creams are also available and may be used in conjunction with dressings and elastic compression (Lovell et al, 1993).

The patient's nutritional status should be assessed through either blood tests or food diaries. In particular, deficits in vitamins C and A, zinc, and albumin should be identified. Low albumin levels may increase lower extremity edema by extending the distance between blood vessels and the dermal surface. Albumin levels lower than 3.5 g/dL warrant consideration for protein supplementation. In addition, patients with diabetes mellitus must be educated regarding the importance of keeping blood sugar levels under control, because hyperglycemia and ketosis may impair leukocyte function. Obese patients should be instructed about and placed on a weight reduction diet and encouraged to attend a weight loss support group, available through various senior centers, churches, or community centers.

Follow-up care should include a reassessment of the lower extremities at least every 6 months, or more frequently if indicated. A review of the patient's food diary and foot elevation record should occur at this time as well. This routine surveillance, feedback, and encouragement from the primary care provider can motivate the patient to participate actively in the prevention program (Capeheart, 1996) (Table 13-4).

TABLE 13-4	Education Tips for the Patient with Chronic Venous Insufficiency

THINGS YOU SHOULD DO

- Keep your legs elevated higher than your heart while sitting or lying down.
- Under the supervision of your primary care provider, begin a walking program.
- If you are on your feet for prolonged periods, wear graduated compression support hose.
- Maintain your ideal weight.
- Eat a balanced, nutritious diet.
- Inspect your legs and feet daily.
- Report any changes in your legs, feet, or existing ulcer, including color, size, temperature, itch, pain, odor.
- Keep legs and feet clean and well lubricated.
- Avoid bumping your legs.

THINGS YOU SHOULD NOT DO

- Stand or sit with legs in a dependent position for prolonged periods.
- Sit with your legs crossed.
- Wear constrictive clothing, such as girdles, nongraduated support hose, tight shoes, or high heels.
- Use heating pads, hot water bottles, heat lamps, ice packs.
- Take hot showers or hot baths or use a hot tub or whirlpool.
- Drink alcohol.
- Smoke.
- Scratch your legs.
- Use adhesive tape on your legs.

VARICOSE VEINS

Varicose veins are superficial veins, predominantly in the lower extremities, that have become dilated, tortuous, and elongated and are unable to function adequately, thus rendering them incompetent. It is unclear as to the exact cause of varicose veins, but certain risk factors or associations have been made (Table 13-5). Varicose veins are extremely common, effecting anywhere from 7% to 60% of the American adult population (Johnson, 1997). They are more common in women, possibly due to the hormonal changes encountered with pregnancy.

Varicose veins present as superficial purple or bluish bulging veins, usually in the thigh or calf region. Varicose veins appear to have a weakness in their walls that causes a dilation

TABLE 13-5	Risk Factors for Varicose Veins

- More common in women
- Overweight
- Pregnancy
- Family hisstory
- History of trauma
- History of venous insufficiency or superficial phlebitis
- Occupation requiring prolonged standing

of the lumen and valve incompetence. As time progresses these distended, tortuous veins become more and more visible. The patient may complain of heaviness, throbbing, and fatigue of the legs, at times accompanied with swelling that gets worse as the day progresses. The patient may also complain of itchiness and burning at the site of the varicosities, as well as leg cramps. Mild swelling is common, but a large amount may be caused by venous insufficiency affecting the deep vein system. As mentioned previously, this may progress to ulceration if left untreated. Varicose veins can also rupture as a result of some type of trauma, resulting in emergency department visits. Furthermore, of utmost concern is the development of superficial phlebitis, which occurs from the lack of smooth efficient transport of blood through the veins.

Conservative treatment of varicose veins starts with elevation of legs and avoidance of prolonged standing. It is best to elevate the legs above the level of the heart intermittently throughout the day. Additionally, the patient should wear compression stockings, usually with a 30 to 40 gradient. These stockings must be worn every day and put on first thing in the morning, when the legs become perpendicular and the pressure in the venous system rises. The third component is good local skin care to prevent breakdown or infection.

More aggressive approaches to treatment include sclerotherapy or laser or surgical repair. Sclerotherapy involves the injection of a sclerosing agent at the site of the varicosity, resulting in the complete fibrosis and collapse of the vein. Often more than one treatment is required. This is used for smaller varicosities. Laser treatment is a recent recommendation; however, it too involves multiple treatments and may lead to pigmentary and textural changes of the skin. This treatment is also reserved for smaller varicosities. Surgery, referred to as ligation and stripping, has become more refined, thus targeting only the more diseased area of the vein. As a result, the patient is left with several small stablike incisions. This procedure is more often performed on an ambulatory basis. Postsurgical care involves the application of Ace bandages to provide support and reduce the incidence of swelling. Patients are encouraged to ambulate, thus promoting circulation and preventing stasis of blood flow that may lead to superficial thrombophlebitis.

Venous thrombophlebitis is divided into two types: superficial and deep. This chapter will discuss superficial thrombophlebitis; refer to Chapter for a discussion of deep vein thrombosis. Superficial thrombophlebitis may arise from a source of trauma such as surgery, injury, or infection. It may also arise because of a lack of blood flow propelling forward (stasis) or a hypercoagulable state. The patient may complain of tenderness or pain over a specific region, swelling, redness, or warmth, or a palpable cordlike lesion. This usually occurs after plane or car travel with long hours of sitting, and dehydration.

The treatment involves warm compresses over the region, analgesics and anti-inflammatory agents, support stockings, and elevation. Patients must realize that this is a common complication that can arise again. Preventive measures the patient can take are to ambulate hourly if traveling for prolonged periods by car or plane. Patients should avoid prolonged periods of sitting, injuries, and dehydration. Superficial venous phlebitis is of minor concern. It resolves quickly and does not usually

travel to other areas of the body, as is the case with deep venous thrombosis.

LYMPHEDEMA

The lymph system is made up of lymphatic capillaries, ducts, and lymph nodes. This system is responsible for the movement of fluid and products (proteins, fat from the gastrointestinal tract, and certain hormones) from the interstitial spaces to the blood, as well as returning excess interstitial fluid to the blood in the prevention of edema (Lewis, 1996).

Lymph fluid is pale-yellow interstitial fluid that has diffused through lymphatic capillary walls. It circulates through its own vasculature system, much like blood moves through blood vessels. The formation of lymph fluid increases when the interstitial fluid pressure rises because there is more volume in the lymphatic system. When this interstitial pressure rises too high and interferes with the reabsorption of lymph, lymphedema develops (Lewis, 1996).

Lymphedema is a chronic swelling that results from the failure of the lymphatic system, causing accumulation of protein-rich interstitial fluid in the extremity. It affects one or more limbs and sometimes the adjacent quadrant of the trunk (Charge, 1995). The exact incidence of lymphatic disorders is not known, but it is estimated that the incidence of primary lymphedema is 1 per 10,000 persons. It affects most commonly women over age 40 (Saunders, 1997).

Lymphedemas are classified into two categories: primary and secondary. Primary lymphedemas are congenital or developmental in origin and occur worldwide. Secondary lymphedemas represent an acquired disruption in lymphatic flow, and their incidence varies geographically. Primary lymphedemas are caused by a poorly developed lymph system; secondary lymphedemas arise from an inflammatory process causing obstructions that impair the ability of the lymphatic channels to propel fluid forward to the vasculature (Wilson & Bilodeau, 1989). Secondary lymphedema may be caused by an infection, trauma, or a parasitic infiltrate known as filariae.

The pathophysiology of lymphedema is caused by an impaired lymphatic transport system that allows plasma proteins to accumulate in the interstitial fluid. This accumulation of fluid causes an increase in colloid osmotic pressure. The body attempts to compensate for this by reducing the elevated pressure and by drawing water into the interstitial areas. Consequently, the lymphatic channels dilate and lymphatic valves become incompetent. The extra fluid is no longer drained appropriately and accumulates in the tissues (Saunders, 1997).

The initial swelling caused by the leakage of fluid is known as the acute or latent stage of lymphedema. The patient presents with pitting edema without brawny skin changes. In the acute stage, the lymphedema may resolve during the night or with position changes during the day. Acute lymphedema can occur after a surgical procedure or trauma to an extremity and resolves within 2 weeks to 3 months. Long-term alteration in the size of the extremity does not usually result from this type of lymphedema.

Lymphedema present for at least 3 months is characterized as chronic and can occur after an acute episode of lymphedema. Skin changes are evident, with less pitting occurring in the acute form. The skin changes, which presumably are a result of the accumulation of fibroblasts and collagen, lead to brawny edema. Brawny edema is identified by a decrease in the tissue's ability to pit when pressure is applied. The capillaries and collecting vessels dilate, and the one-way valves become unable to function. Brawny edema is found with chronic lymphedema. Weakness, limited range of motion, stiffness, pain, and numbness of the extremity are associated with both acute and chronic lymphedema (Humble, 1995).

Permanent swelling involving only one of the lower extremities usually occurs. If bilateral swelling is present, it is asymmetric. A chronic, dull, heavy sensation develops in the affected extremity. Edema starts in the foot and progresses up the leg until the entire leg becomes edematous. In chronic peripheral lymphedema, it is the appearance that brings the patient for treatment. In the later stages of the disease, the affected limb loses its normal contour because of swelling, and the toes appear square (Saunders, 1997). The high protein concentration in the fluid changes the appearance of the extremity. These changes include deepened, enhanced natural skin creases and folds (hyperkeratosis). The tissue and skin become thick with less pitting and a positive Stemmer's sign, which is an ability to pick up a fold of skin at the base of the second digits. There is a distortion or exaggeration of the limb and an increased susceptibility to recurrent, acute inflammatory episodes such as cellulitis or fungal infections (Badger, 1996).

The diagnosis of lymphedema should be made only after a thorough history and physical examination are performed and the possibility of metastatic disease is ruled out. The onset of the swelling and any precipitating factors should be noted. A person with lymphedema will complain of heaviness or fullness of the extremity. Circumferential measurement of the extremity may be necessary to determine the degree of edema between extremities (Humble, 1995).

At the interview, the provider should inquire about the onset, location, duration, severity, and aggravating or alleviating factors as well as associated symptoms. The provider should also determine if there is an association with pain or changes regarding the time of day. The patient's use of other treatments for the condition should be noted. A thorough past medical history, including any coexisting medical problem, family history, and current pharmacotherapy, should also be obtained (Saunders, 1997).

The physical examination should include inspection for signs of inflammation or infection, such as a red streak extending along the course of the lymphatics as they drain. The provider should also palpate the lymph nodes for enlargement or tenderness and the lower extremities for edema. Edema should be classified as pitting or nonpitting; any pitting edema should be noted (Saunders, 1997). The extent of any edema can be measured by pinching folds of skin on both sides of the body. To promote maximal drainage from the limb, the adjacent quadrant of the trunk must be free of edema; thus, the degree of edema can be measured by comparing one limb to the other. The degree of edema will influence the choice of treatment as well as the hardness of the tissue. Signs of venous disease may include signs of venous hypertension on the arms and legs. Venous incompetence will tend to influence the outcome of treatment.

The provider should examine the condition of the skin, because this will also influence the choice of treatment. Signs of arterial insufficiency should be sought. The peripheral pulses should be assessed and the Doppler ultrasound probe used to measure the ABI (Badger, 1996).

On occasion, invasive testing may be necessary to establish the diagnosis of lymphedema. Use of MRI or CT can help to locate the area of obstruction caused by recurrent or metastatic disease. Lymphangiography, often considered the gold standard for lymphatic vessel imaging, involves the injection of a water-soluble contrast medium, followed by an x-ray to identify areas of insufficiency. This method is rarely used because of the potential side effects, such as lymphatic vessel injury and patient discomfort. Lymphoscintigraphy, another invasive procedure, uses a low-dose radioactive colloid and a gamma camera for scanning. This procedure can be used to detect the movement of fluid in the lymphatic system and collateral pathways and to confirm that the edema is of lymphatic origin (Humble, 1995). The colloid is injected into the distal subcutaneous tissue of the affected extremity, and the area is scanned 30 to 60 minutes later. Lymphedema is characterized by decreased or absent uptake of the radioactive isotope in the regional nodes (Saunders, 1997).

The treatment program for lymphedema should include external support, multilayer bandaging and compression stockings, skin care, exercise, and massage (Charge, 1995). The goals of therapy are to reduce the size of the swollen limb, to regain the original shape of the extremity, and to prevent recurrent acute inflammatory episodes (Badger, 1996). This may be achieved through an intensive treatment regimen followed by a maintenance treatment program. In the intensive phase, external compression with multilayer bandaging is used to reduce swelling. Manual lymph drainage promotes movement of the fluid out of the extremity and the adjacent quadrant of the trunk. Exercises to promote maximum lymph flow and to increase joint mobility are performed. Skin care instruction is given to preserve the integrity of the skin and prevent infection.

In the maintenance phase, strong external compression is applied, using hosiery to compress the drained tissue. Simple massage by the patient may be performed if the limb is still congested. Exercise should be continued to promote maximal lymphatic flow. Meticulous skin care is crucial to reduce the risk of infection (Badger, 1996).

Pharmacotherapy with appropriate antibiotics may be warranted to treat infections. Diuretic therapy is usually avoided in chronic therapy because it depletes the intravascular volume and produces metabolic abnormalities (Saunders, 1997).

If these methods do not control lymphedema, surgical intervention may be necessary. Failure may be caused by excessive swelling, uncontrollable persistent infection, or severe compromise of the patient's mobility. The two surgical options are a lymphatic-venous anastomosis and a total superficial lymphangiectomy (Wilson & Bilodeau, 1989).

For treatment of lymphedema to be successful, the patient needs to understand why the lymphedema occurs, what aggravates or enhances the swelling, and what helps lessen it. The patient must understand the reasons behind the treatment program that he or she will be encouraged to participate in; patients should know that the treatment should never be painful. No one component of the treatment program is effective on its own. For the treatment to work, all components of therapy must be considered. The patient should realize that good results depend on good participation and the avoidance of infection (Badger, 1996).

COMMUNITY RESOURCES

Because of the variety of peripheral vascular diseases, few community-based resources exist specific to a particular disease state. General information may be obtained from the American Heart Association. Additionally, patients who are encouraged to participate in weight reduction programs may find local support groups for this purpose.

CLINICAL WARNINGS AND REFERRAL POINTS

While evaluating and following patients with arterial and venous insufficiency, several situations may arise that warrant referral to a vascular surgeon. Any cessation of blood flow, as evidenced by a loss of pulse distal to an occlusion, should be immediately referred. The threat of gangrene is present when arterial insufficiency progresses to the point where pain is severe and persistent, with loss of function. Arterial ulcers may appear in conjunction with limb-threatening ischemia and warrant immediate referral. Also, any suspicion of aortic aneurysm should generate a consultation with a vascular surgeon. In patients with temporal arteritis, neurologic deficits may be present and should be evaluated by both a neurologist and a vascular surgeon. Patients with frostbite should have the extremity protected from rubbing or mechanical injury. If the frostbite is severe or hypothermia is present, the patient should be admitted to an emergency department. Consultation with a vascular surgeon may also be warranted for aggressive therapy of varicose veins and lymphedema.

■ ■ ■ ■   CLINICAL PEARLS

- Skin temperature of the extremity is best evaluated by palpating the extremity with the dorsum of the hand.
- Patients experiencing pain at rest may have edema because they keep their legs in a dependent position for pain relief.
- It is important in patients with peripheral vascular disease to check pulses in all regions of the body where major vessels are located, including the carotid, abdominal aorta, iliac, femoral, popliteal, posterior tibial and dorsalis pedis.
- Nocturnal muscle cramps, a symptom that mimics claudication, are a common complaint in older persons, and are not related to exercise.
- Vasodilating agents have had little effect on patients with claudication.
- If temporal arteritis is suspected it must be remembered that a negative biopsy does not always rule out temporal arteritis.
- In the patient with frostbite, deeper damage is evident if the patient feels no pain or sensation in the identified tissues.
- "Winter itch," in patients with venous insufficiency, also know as xerosis, is typically exacerbated during periods of low humidity and cold weather.
- In patients with lymphedema, permanent swelling involving only one of the lower extremities usually occurs. If bilateral swelling is present, it is asymmetric.
- Circumferential measurement of the patient with lymphedema may be necessary to determine the degree of edema between extremities.

> **EDITOR'S NOTE:**
> ## COMPLEMENTARY APPROACHES
>
> A general discussion of complementary approaches can be found in Chapter 3. The following, while not an exhaustive list, are some complementary approaches being used for this condition. Additional information on these approaches, including precautions, can be found in Appendices A and B. Providers need to assess for the use of complementary approaches as part of the patient's history, as they may impact conventional therapies, and patients may not volunteer this information unless specifically asked. Efficacy of many complementary approaches is not as well documented as that of conventional therapies. Providers need to read the literature before suggesting these complementary approaches.
>
> - Vitamins, minerals, herbs, supplements
>   Carnitine
>   Fish oils
> - Complementary Modalities
>   Acupuncture
>   Biofeedback

References

Auth, P.C. (1997). Assessment and treatment of arterial ulcers. *Physician Assistant, 21*(3), 64–79.

Badger, C. (1996). Treating lymphedema. *Nursing Times, 92*(11), 84–88.

Bright, L.D., & Georgi, S. (1992). Peripheral vascular disease: Is it arterial or venous? *American Journal of Nursing, 92*(9), 34–43.

Capeheart, J.K. (1996). Chronic venous insufficiency: A focus on prevention of venous ulceration. *Journal of Wound, Ostomy, and Continence Nursing, 23*(4), 227–234.

Charge, H. (1995). Treatment of lymphedema. *Nursing Times, 91*(30), 53–58.

Dean, R.H., Yao, J., & Brewster, D.C. (1995). *Current diagnosis and treatment in vascular surgery.* Norwalk, CT: Appleton & Lange.

Dumas, M.A.S. (1995). Clinical snapshot: Intermittent claudication. *American Journal of Nursing, 95*(12), 34–35.

Elson, J.D. (1994). Lower extremity ischemia. *Postgraduate Medicine, 95*(1), 103–107.

Fischbach, F. (1996). *A manual of laboratory and diagnostic tests,* 5th ed. Philadelphia: Lippincott-Raven.

Goroll, A., May, L., & Mulley, A. (1995). *Primary care medicine,* 3d ed. Philadelphia: J.B. Lippincott.

Humble, C.A. (1995). Lymphedema: Incidence, pathology, management, and nursing care. *Oncology Nursing Forum, 22*(10), 1503–1511.

Johnson, M.T. (1997). Treatment and prevention of varicose veins. *Journal of Vascular Nursing, 15*(3), 97–103.

Krikorian, R.K., & Vacek, J.L. (1995). Peripheral arterial disease: When to consider percutaneous revascularization. *Postgraduate Medicine, 90*(6), 109–116.

Lamont, L.J. (1991). Venous ulcers: A nursing challenge. *Journal of the American Academy of Nurse Practitioners, 3*(4), 158–165.

Lovell, M.B., Dixon, V., Harris, K.A., & Jamieson, W.G. (1993). The management of chronic venous disease. *Journal of Vascular Nursing, 11*(2), 43–47.

Olin, J.W. (1993). Lower extremity arterial disease: Tips on diagnosis and therapy. *Cleveland Clinic Journal of Medicine, 60*(1), 14–15.

Phillips, T.J. (1996). Leg ulcer management. *Dermatology Nursing, 8*(5), 333–341.

Rakel, R. (1996). *Saunders manual of medical practice.* Philadelphia: W.B. Saunders.

Santilli, J.D., Rodnick, J.E., & Santilli, S.M. (1996). Claudication: Diagnosis and treatment. *American Family Physician, 53*(4), 1245–1252.

(1997). *Saunders manual of nursing care.* Philadelphia: W.B. Saunders.

Seller, R. (1996). *Differential diagnosis of common complaints,* 3d ed. Philadelphia: W.B. Saunders.

Sullivan, S.A. (1993). Derm detective: How severe is this frostbite? *American Journal of Nursing,* ,59–64.

Uphold, C.R., & Graham, M.V. (1994). *Clinical guidelines in adult health.* Gainesville, FL: Barmarrae Books.

Wilson, C., & Bilodeau, M. (1989). Current management concepts for the patient with lymphedema. *Journal of Cardiovascular Nursing, 4*(1), 79–88.

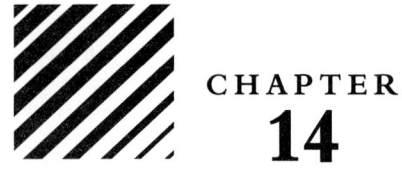

CHAPTER
14

Valvular Heart Disease

Jay A. Mazel, MD

The cardiac valves are designed to maximize the work performed by the heart. If the valves malfunction, a hemodynamic strain is placed on the heart. This strain is initially tolerated because the heart compensates by increasing in size or dimension. Over time, however, the hemodynamic burden leads to cardiac muscle dysfunction and congestive heart failure, and sometimes sudden death.

In the management of every case of valvular heart disease, the primary care provider must answer two major questions: Is the valvular disease severe enough to warrant mechanical intervention over medical therapy? If so, what is the best time to refer the patient for surgical intervention? This chapter will review these questions for the four major acquired left-sided valvular lesions: aortic stenosis, mitral stenosis, nonischemic mitral regurgitation, and aortic regurgitation.

ANATOMY, PHYSIOLOGY, AND PATHOLOGY

The compensatory mechanisms of the cardiovascular system depend on the type of hemodynamic strain imposed on the heart by the dysfunctional valve. If the valve is stenotic, the reduced valve area obstructs blood flow. To maintain an adequate cardiac output, more pressure must be generated to propel blood across the valve. Therefore, in stenosis, the heart undergoes hypertrophy to reduce the increasing wall tension. In contrast, if the valve is incompetent, forward stroke volume is reduced in proportion to the degree of regurgitation. To maintain the cardiac output, more volume must be generated to maintain forward flow. The heart dilates to accommodate the increasing volume. The hypertrophied or dilated heart decompensates when the pressure or volume creates excessive wall tension and overwhelms the ability of the heart to contract, resulting in a reduced cardiac output.

In valvular stenosis, the increased pressure and wall tension generated are dispersed proximal to the obstruction. In aortic stenosis, patients remain symptom-free for years because of the marked ability of the left ventricle to hypertrophy. Twice the baseline mass (105 to 275 g/m^2) is typical; however, even 10 times baseline mass has been reported (Passik et al, 1987). In contrast, in mitral stenosis the left atrium is in direct communication with the pulmonary vasculature and cannot adapt as easily. Thus, in mitral stenosis, increased atrial tension and pulmonary wall tension occur in the disease, manifested as dyspnea, orthopnea, and atrial arrhythmias.

Left ventricular dilatation occurs in both chronic aortic regurgitation and chronic mitral regurgitation. In aortic regurgitation, the increased volume is entirely ejected into the aorta. In contrast, in mitral regurgitation the regurgitant volume enters the left atrium. This is an important distinction because the increased stroke volume of aortic regurgitation increases pulse pressure, causing systolic hypertension. This imposes a significant increase in afterload on the left ventricle, as high as levels seen in aortic stenosis.

EPIDEMIOLOGY

Aortic Stenosis

Acquired aortic stenosis is usually an idiopathic disease resulting from degeneration and calcification of the aortic leaflets. When the disease is acquired in previously normal tricuspid aortic valves, stenosis develops in the sixth, seventh, and eighth decades. In persons born with a bicuspid aortic valve, stenosis is more likely to occur than in those with normal tricuspid valves. In these patients, stenosis typically develops earlier, in the fourth and fifth decades of life. It is unknown why aortic stenosis occurs in some people and not in others. Aortic stenosis does, however, share some of the same risk factors associated with coronary atherosclerosis, such as hypertension, hypercholesterolemia, calcification related to renal disease, and even infection with *Chlamydia pneumoniae* (Otto et al, 1994; Juvonen et al, 1997).

Mitral Stenosis

Mitral stenosis is usually a consequence of rheumatic heart disease, which primarily affects women. Although mitral valve involvement occurs in 40% of acute rheumatic fever cases, patients rarely recall having had rheumatic carditis. A history of rheumatic fever, therefore, is not helpful in establishing the presence or absence of mitral stenosis. In rheumatic heart disease, isolated mitral stenosis is the most common, followed by combined mitral stenosis and aortic stenosis. Isolated mitral regurgitation rarely occurs. The steady decline in the incidence of rheumatic fever has reduced the incidence of mitral stenosis in developed countries. In developing nations, however, both rheumatic fever and mitral stenosis remain common.

Regardless of the etiology, if aortic or mitral stenosis was not present at birth, the disease develops later in life from damage to the valve cusps. This causes abnormal flow patterns and predisposes the valve to fibrosis and calcification later in life. Because turbulent blood flow tends to persist, the stenosis can usually be expected to progress.

Mitral Regurgitation

The usual causes of mitral regurgitation are infective endocarditis, myxomatous degeneration of the mitral valve (eg, mitral valve prolapse), collagen vascular disease, spontaneous rupture of the chordae tendineae, rheumatic fever, and rarely eating disorders such as bulimia or anorexia.

Aortic Regurgitation

Aortic regurgitation results from disease of either the aortic leaflets or the aortic root that prevents coaptation of the leaflets. Leaflet abnormalities that result in aortic regurgitation can be secondary to infective endocarditis and rheumatic fever. Aortic root causes of aortic regurgitation include Marfan syndrome, aortic dissection, collagen vascular disease, syphilis, and annuloaortic ectasia.

HISTORY AND PHYSICAL EXAMINATION

Aortic Stenosis

The classic symptoms of aortic stenosis are angina, syncope, and the symptoms of congestive heart failure. Angina develops in aortic stenosis because of reduced coronary flow reserve and increased myocardial oxygen demand caused by high afterload. Exertional syncope results from either a vasodepressor response or an exercise-induced drop in total peripheral resistance that is uncompensated because the cardiac output is restricted by the stenotic valve. Heart failure in aortic stenosis results from diastolic dysfunction, systolic dysfunction, or both. Diastolic dysfunction results from increased left ventricular wall thickness and increased collagen content. Systolic dysfunction results from excess afterload, decreased contractility, or a combination of these factors.

A systolic ejection murmur radiating to the neck is the most common sign of aortic stenosis. It is usually heard best in the aortic area. It disappears over the sternum and then reappears in the apical area, mimicking mitral regurgitation (Gallivardin's phenomenon). In mild aortic stenosis, the murmur usually peaks early in systole. As the severity of stenosis increases, the murmur peaks progressively later in systole and may become softer as the cardiac output diminishes. The carotid upstrokes classically become diminished in amplitude and delayed in time (*parvus et tardus*). S_2 may become paradoxically split because of the delay in left ventricular emptying, or the second heart sound may become single because the aortic closing component is lost.

Mitral Stenosis

Patients with mitral stenosis usually have symptoms typical of left-sided heart failure: dyspnea on exertion, orthopnea, and paroxysmal nocturnal dyspnea. The increases in pulmonary vascular pressure can cause hemoptysis, hoarseness, and symptoms of right-sided heart failure. These symptoms are somewhat more specific for mitral stenosis but occur less frequently. Typically, patients first present with dyspnea or orthopnea when a cardiac stress such as pregnancy or atrial fibrillation occurs. The symptoms of mitral stenosis stem from increased left atrial pressure and reduced cardiac output, primarily caused by mechanical obstruction during filling of the left ventricle. Although the symptoms are those of left ventricular failure, the left ventricular function is usually normal in mitral stenosis. In some cases, however, the left ventricular ejection fraction is

reduced because of excessive afterload secondary to a reflexive increase in systemic vascular resistance. Because it is the right ventricle that ultimately propels blood through the mitral valve, right ventricular function is compromised, first by the afterload imposed on it by high left atrial pressure and then by the development of secondary pulmonary vasoconstriction.

During physical examination, mitral stenosis is suspected because of the presence of the classic diastolic rumble that follows an opening snap. S_1 is characteristically loud because the mitral valve is held open by the transmitral gradient until the force of ventricular systole closes the valve. A loud P_2, right ventricular lift, elevated neck veins, ascites, and edema indicate that pulmonary hypertension with right ventricular overload has developed. This is an ominous sign in the progression of the disease because pulmonary hypertension increases the risk associated with surgery.

Mitral Regurgitation

Chronic mitral regurgitation is compensated by the development of eccentric cardiac hypertrophy. Cardiac enlargement should therefore be manifest on physical examination. A holosystolic apical murmur heard on physical examination alerts the examiner that mitral regurgitation is present. An S_4 suggests that the disease is severe. An S_3 heard in mitral regurgitation, however, does not necessarily indicate the presence of congestive heart failure, because in this situation rapid filling of the left ventricle causes the sound by the large volume of blood stored in the left atrium in diastole.

Aortic Regurgitation

The large total stroke volume in aortic regurgitation increases pulse pressure, which produces a host of clinical signs. Although the typical diastolic blowing murmur heard along the left sternal border is the usual sign of aortic regurgitation, the peripheral signs of a hyperdynamic circulation indicate when the disease is severe. Table 14-1 is a partial list of these signs.

In addition to the typical murmur of aortic insufficiency, a diastolic rumble (Austin Flint murmur) may also be heard over the cardiac apex. Although its origin is debatable, the Austin Flint murmur is probably produced as the aortic jet impinges on the mitral valve, causing it to vibrate. Simultaneous diastolic filling of the left ventricle from the left atrium and aorta tends to close the mitral valve in diastole, producing physiologic stenosis.

The physical findings described above are summarized in Table 14-2.

TABLE 14-1	Findings in Aortic Regurgitation
Quincke's pulse:	Systolic engorgement and diastolic blanching in the nail bed when gentle pressure is placed on it
Corrigan's pulse:	A bounding, full carotid pulse with a rapid downstroke
Musset's sign:	Head bobbing
Hill's sign:	Systolic blood pressure in the leg at least 30 mmHg higher than that in the arm

TABLE 14-2	Physical Findings in Valvular Disease						
	Location	Radiation	Intensity/ Maneuvers	Pitch	Quality	Associated Signs	S_1 and S_2
SYSTOLIC							
Aortic stenosis	2nd right intercostal space	Neck, LSB, and apex	Variable, possible thrill	Medium	Harsh, musical at the apex	Thrusting apical impulse displaced inferolaterally, slow rising carotid impulse, narrow pulse pressure	Decreased S_1, possibly absent S_2
Mitral regurgitation	Apical area	Left axilla, possibly LSB and base	Often loud, possible apical thrill, does not increase with inspiration	High	Blowing	Enlarged sustained apical impulse, displaced inferolaterally	Decreased S_1, S_3
DIASTOLIC							
Aortic regurgitation	Mid-left sternal border	2nd intercostal space toward apex, possibly right sternal border	Faint, increased with leaning forward while exhaling	High	Blowing	Thrusting apical impulse displaced inferolaterally, systolic ejection murmor, apical diastolic murmur (Austin-Flint murmur), wide pulse pressure	S_3
Mitral stenosis	Apical area	Very little	Diminished, increased in left lateral position or exercise	Low	Rumbling	Increased RV impulse if pulmonary hypertension is present	Increased S_1, opening snap, increased P_2

LSB, left sternal border

(Dajani, A. et al. (1997). Prevention of bacterial endocarditis. Dallas: American Heart Association.)

DIAGNOSTIC STUDIES

Echocardiography is an excellent noninvasive diagnostic tool for assessing valvular disease. The degree of stenosis can accurately be determined with Doppler and planimetric calculation to obtain valve gradients and valve areas. For valvular regurgitation, color-flow jets and flow patterns provide only a rough estimate of severity. Echocardiography is also useful in assessing the extent of left ventricular hypertrophy or dilatation as well as estimating left ventricular ejection fraction.

Cardiac catheterization with ventriculography, aortography, or coronary angiography is the gold standard for assessing all valvular diseases. It is used only when surgery is being contemplated or the severity of the disease cannot be gauged accurately by noninvasive techniques. Catheterization is not suitable for longitudinal follow-up.

TREATMENT OPTIONS, EXPECTED OUTCOME, AND COMPREHENSIVE MANAGEMENT

Primary Prevention

All streptococcal infections should be diagnosed and treated to prevent acute rheumatic fever.

Secondary Prevention

Once valvular disease is diagnosed, most patients with valvular disease will require infective endocarditis prophylaxis for life before an invasive procedure is performed. Indications for anti-biotic prophylaxis are based on the type of valvular disease (Table 14-3) and the specific procedure anticipated (Table 14-4). Choice of antibiotics is based on the potential pathogenic organisms anticipated during a procedure (Tables 14-5 and 14-6). If the valve lesion in a child is rheumatic in origin, monthly prophylaxis for β-hemolytic streptococcal infection until adulthood is recommended.

Aerobic exercise should be encouraged in persons with mild asymptomatic valvular disease. In symptomatic aortic or mitral stenoses, vigorous exercise should be avoided altogether because it may precipitate serious symptoms, such as angina, syncope, and congestive heart failure (Schwartz et al, 1969). In aortic and mitral regurgitation, isometric exercise and physically strenuous occupations should be avoided because they can raise

TABLE 14-3	Valvular Conditions at Risk of Endocarditis

HIGH RISK

Prosthetic cardiac valves, including bioprosthetic and homograft valves

Previous bacterial endocarditis

MODERATE RISK

Acquired valvular dysfunction

Mitral valve prolapse with valvular regurgitation or thickened leaflets

(Dajani, A. et al. (1997). Prevention of bacterial endocarditis. Dallas: American Heart Association.)

TABLE 14-4	Prophylaxis	
Procedures	**Requiring Prophylaxis**	**Not Requiring Prophylaxis**
Dental	Procedures, including cleaning, where bleeding is anticipated Extractions Implants Periodontal procedures Endodontic instrumentation beyond the apex (root canal) Placement of orthodontic bands (not brackets) and subgingival antibiotic fibers or strips Intraligamentary local anesthetic injections	Restorative dentistry such as fillings or replacement of missing teeth Oral impressions, fluoride treatments, x-rays Shedding of primary teeth Intracanal endodontic treatment; post placement and build-up Prosthodontic or orthodontic appliance placement or adjustment Placement of rubber bands Suture removal Nonintraligamentary local anesthetic injections
Respiratory	Tonsillectomy Bronchoscopy with rigid bronchoscope Surgical operations that involve respiratory mucosa	Endotracheal intubation Bronchoscopy with flexible bronchoscope with or without biopsy Tympanostomy tube insertion
Gastrointestinal	Sclerotherapy for esophageal varices Esophageal stricture dilation Endoscopic retrograde cholangiography with biliary obstruction Biliary tract surgery Surgical operation that involves intestinal mucosa	Transesophageal echocardiography
Genitourinary	Prostatic surgery Cystoscopy Urethral dilation	Vaginal hysterectomy Vaginal delivery/cesarean section Uninfected: Urethral catheterization Uterine dilatation and curettage Therapeutic abortion Sterilization procedure Insertion and removal of IUD
Other		Cardiac catheterization, including percutaneous transluminal coronary angioplasty Implanted cardiac pacemakers, implanted defibrillators, and coronary stents Incision or biopsy of surgically scrubbed skin Circumcision

(Dajani, A. et al. (1997). Prevention of bacterial endocarditis. Dallas: American Heart Association.)

systemic blood pressure as high as 340 mmHg. The degree and type of exercise should be considered in choosing an occupation so that premature retirement will not be necessary.

Tertiary Prevention

MEDICAL THERAPY

Both aortic and mitral stenosis have no proven medical therapy. In aortic and mitral regurgitation, vasodilators such as angiotensin-converting enzyme inhibitors and dihydropyridine calcium channel antagonists are used to reduce afterload, increase forward output, and decrease left ventricular filling pressures. Because aortic regurgitation represents a state of excess afterload, it could be anticipated that reduction of afterload with vasodilators would improve left ventricular performance while simultaneously decreasing the amount of aortic regurgitation, thus reducing or delaying the need for surgery. The use of nifedipine in asymptomatic patients with severe aortic regurgi-

tation and normal left ventricular function has been shown to delay the need for surgery by 2 to 3 years (Scognamiglo et al, 1994). However, in mitral regurgitation, no long-term, large study has demonstrated that the use of vasodilators safely reduces or delays the need for surgery or improves outcome.

Atrial fibrillation commonly occurs in mitral stenosis and should be treated aggressively. Rate control with a beta-blocker, calcium channel blocker, or digoxin is important because a rapid heart rate further impairs left ventricular filling, further reducing the cardiac output and increasing left atrial pressure. Anticoagulation is extremely important because of the high risk of embolism.

SURGICAL THERAPY
Aortic Stenosis
The only effective relief of a mechanical obstruction to blood flow is valvular replacement. In aortic stenosis, a gradient of more than 50 mmHg or a valve area of less than 0.8 cm^2 indi-

TABLE 14-5	Prophylactic Regimen for Dental, Oral, and Esophageal Procedures	
Situation	**Agent**	**Regimen**
Standard general prophylaxis	Amoxicillin	2 g 1 hour before procedure
Unable to take oral medications	Ampicillin	2 g IM or IV ½ hour before procedure
Allergic to penicillin	Clindamycin *or*	600 mg 1 hour before procedure
	Cephalexin *or*	2 g 1 hour before procedure
	Cefadroxil *or* Azithromycin *or* Clarithromycin	500 mg 1 hour before procedure
Allergic to penicillin *and* unable to take oral medication	Clindamycin *or* Cefazolin	600 mg ½ hour before procedure 1 g ½ hour before procedure

No follow-up dose recommended

From: AHA/ACC guidelines, August 1997

cates critical stenosis that is capable of causing symptoms and death. The decision to replace the aortic valve is based primarily on the presence of classic symptoms of aortic stenosis rather than the severity of the stenotic valve. This is because until the onset of symptoms, the survival of patients with aortic stenosis is nearly normal. Once symptoms of angina, syncope, or heart failure develop, survival drops to 50% at 5, 3, or 2 years, respectively (Ross & Braunwald, 1968). Balloon aortic valvotomy is useful only for palliation of the disease in adult acquired aortic stenosis. The rate of serious complications, including death, stroke, aortic rupture, aortic regurgitation, and vascular injury, exceeds 10% (Berman et al, 1996). Furthermore, the mortality rate after this procedure is 60% at 18 months, a rate similar to that in an untreated population. The event-free survival rate at 2 years is only 20%, and many patients thought to be candidates only for balloon valvotomy eventually have a good outcome with aortic valve replacement (Lieberman et al, 1995).

Mitral Stenosis

When mild symptoms develop, diuretics are useful in lowering left atrial pressure and reducing symptoms. In mitral stenosis, symptoms usually occur at a mitral valve area less than 1 cm^2. If the symptoms are more than mild, or if there is evidence that pulmonary hypertension is beginning to develop, mechanical relief of the mitral stenosis is indicated because, as in aortic stenosis, further delay worsens the prognosis. Unlike valvotomy in aortic stenosis, balloon valvotomy for mitral stenosis provides excellent mechanical relief that usually results in prolonged benefit. Open commissurotomy, valve reconstruction, or mitral valve replacement is used when heavy valvular calcification, more than mild mitral regurgitation, or severe subvalvular distortion precludes against the use of balloon valvotomy (Carbello, 1991).

The symptoms of aortic and mitral regurgitation are those of left-sided heart failure (dyspnea, orthopnea, and fatigue) and occasionally angina. Unlike the stenotic lesions, regurgitant lesions may cause left ventricular damage before symptoms develop. Thus, valve surgery should be performed when asymptomatic left ventricular dysfunction has begun to develop and should be delayed until symptoms occur.

Mitral Regurgitation

In mitral regurgitation, preload is increased but afterload is normal or occasionally decreased; thus, the lesion itself facilitates left ventricular emptying. In the presence of normal muscle function, therefore, the ejection fraction should be supranormal in the patient with mitral regurgitation. Once the ejection fraction falls below 60%, the prognosis worsens. The end-systolic dimension is less dependent on preload than is the ejection fraction, and this can be used as another measure of left ventricular contractile function. When the end-systolic dimension exceeds 45 mm, the prognosis worsens.

Thus, patients should be referred for surgery if more than mild symptoms develop, or if the ejection fraction falls below 60% or the end-systolic dimension approaches 45 mm, even in the absence of symptoms (Crawford et al, 1990). Patients with a right ventricular ejection fraction of less than 30% are especially high risk (Hochreiter et al, 1986).

TABLE 14-6	Prophylactic Regimen for Genitourinary and Gastrointestinal (Excluding Esophageal) Procedures	
Situation	**Agent**	**Regimen**
High-risk patient	Ampicillin plus gentamicin	Ampicillin 2 g IM or IV plus gentamicin 1.5 mg/kg (not to exceed 120 mg) ½ hour before. Ampicillin 1 g IM or IV *or* amoxicillin 1 g PO 6 hours after procedure.
High risk, allergic to penicillin	Vancomycin plus gentamicin	Vancomycin 1 g over 1–2 hours plus gentamicin 1.5 mg/kg IV or IM; complete administration ½ hour before procedure
Moderate risk	Amoxicillin *or* ampicillin	2 g 1 hour before procedure 2 g IM or IV ½ hour before procedure
Moderate risk, allergic to penicillin	Vancomycin	1 g IV over 1–2 hours infused ½ hour before procedure

From: AHA/ACC guidelines, August 1997

Aortic Regurgitation

In general, aortic insufficiency should be surgically corrected before the ejection fraction falls below 55% or the end-systolic dimension exceeds 55 mm (the 55 rule), even in asymptomatic patients (Zile, 1991).

In contrast to mitral insufficiency, aortic insufficiency *increases* left ventricular afterload, in part because the high stroke volume produces a wide pulse pressure and systolic hypertension. After aortic valve replacement, afterload is reduced and the ejection fraction improves. Thus, it is not surprising that patients with aortic insufficiency can have a reduced ejection fraction and a larger end-systolic dimension than patients with mitral insufficiency but still have a good postoperative outcome.

■ ■ ■ CLINICAL PEARLS

Repair all valves *before* loss of systolic function. In stenotic disease, symptoms precede the loss of systolic function; therefore, operate primarily for symptoms. In regurgitant valve disease, systolic failure precedes diastolic failure. Therefore, serial noninvasive studies of systolic function should be performed and surgery undertaken at the first sign of systolic dysfunction.

SPECIAL DIAGNOSTIC AND TREATMENT CONSIDERATIONS

Age

Even though most patients with aortic stenosis are elderly, the prognosis with surgery, even in the elderly, is excellent in the absence of coexisting illnesses. The age-corrected survival after aortic valve replacement in patients older than 65 is not different from that in the general population. In mitral stenosis patients, however, patients over 75 years of age have a worse prognosis after surgery than younger patients do, especially if mitral valve replacement rather than repair has been performed or if coronary disease is present (Levinson et al, 1989).

Gender

Women with aortic stenosis are likely to have thicker ventricular walls, which reduces wall stress and causes higher ejection fractions.

■ ■ ■ CLINICAL PEARL

Preoperative recognition of these differences is important because postoperative management of low cardiac output requires volume expansion in women rather than the use of inotropic agents (Morris et al, 1994).

Coronary Artery Disease

The presence of coronary disease in patients with either mitral or aortic valve disease worsens the long-term prognosis. Although the operative risk may not be increased, the long-term prognosis in combined coronary and valvular heart disease is not as good as that in valvular disease alone, even when coronary bypass surgery is performed at the time of valve replacement. This is presumably a result of the progressive nature of coronary disease. Ischemic mitral regurgitation carries the worst prognosis: operative mortality is 10% to 20% and long-term survival is substantially lower than with nonischemic mitral regurgitation (Akins et al, 1994).

TEACHING AND SELF-CARE

The most important part of patient education is teaching the importance of endocarditis prophylaxis. The rationale for prophylaxis and the risks incurred if ignored should be clearly explained. Patients and families should be fully briefed on allowable activities and the early warning signs of worsening disease. Instructions should be reinforced at regular follow-up visits with the primary physician and consulting cardiologist to help involve the patient in his or her own care. Finally, the patient should be reminded of treatment options for his or her condition and the excellent prognosis when therapy is properly timed and applied.

COMMUNITY RESOURCES

Resources can be obtained from the American Heart Association, 7272 Greenville Ave., Dallas, TX 75231-4596 (1-800-AHA-4596; www.amhrt.org).

CLINICAL WARNINGS AND REFERRAL POINTS

The basic principle of repairing all valves before the loss of systolic function serves as the common referral point for all valvular heart diseases. In stenotic disease, symptoms precede loss of systolic function; referral for valvular surgery is indicated

TABLE 14-7	Critical Landmarks		
	Symptoms	**Findings**	
Aortic stenosis	Angina, congestive heart failure, syncope	Critical gradient ≥50 mmHg	Critical area ≤0.8 cm²
Mitral stenosis	Dyspnea, orthopnea, paroxysmal nocturnal dyspnea, fatigue	Critical gradient ≥20 mmHg*	Critical area ≤1.0 cm²*
Aortic regurgitation		End-diastolic dimension ≤55	Ejection fraction ≥55%
Mitral regurgitation		End-diastolic dimension ≤45	Ejection fraction ≥60%

* Because the lungs generally do not tolerate a pulmonary–capillary wedge pressure of >30 mmHg, the critical gradient and valve area are substantially reduced in mitral stenosis compared with aortic stenosis.

for symptoms. In regurgitant valve disease, systolic failure precedes diastolic failure; thus, serial noninvasive studies of systolic function should be performed and patients referred for surgery at the first sign of systolic dysfunction. Critical landmarks in the management (and surgical referral) of valvular disease are summarized in Table 14-7.

References

Akins, C.W., Hilgenberg, A.D., Buckley, M.J., et al. (1994). Mitral valve reconstruction versus replacement for degenerative or ischemic mitral regurgitation. *Annals of Thoracic Surgery, 58,* 668–675.

Berman, A.D., McKay, R.G., & Grossman, W. (1996). Balloon valvuloplasty. In: Baim, D.S., & Grossman, W. (Eds.). *Cardiac catheterization, angiography, and intervention,* 5th ed. Baltimore: Williams & Wilkins, pp. 659–687.

Carbello, B.A. (1991). Timing of surgery for mitral and aortic stenoses. *Cardiology Clinics, 9,* 229–238.

Crawford, M.H., Souchek, J., Oprian, C.A., et al. (1990). Determinants of survival and left ventricular performance after mitral valve replacement. *Circulation, 81,* 1173–1181.

Hochreiter, C., Niles, N., Devereux, R.B., Kligfield, P., & Borer, J.S. (1986). Mitral regurgitation. *Circulation, 73,* 900–912.

Juvonen, J., Laurila, A., Juvonen, T., et al. (1997). Detection of *Chlamydia pneumoniae* in human nonrheumatic stenotic aortic valves. *Journal of the American College of Cardiology, 29,* 1054.

Levinson, J.R., Akins, C.W., Buckley, M.J., et al. (1989). Octogenarians with aortic stenoses. *Circulation, 80*(suppl I), I49–I56.

Lieberman, E.B., Bashore, T.M., Hermiller, J.B., et al. (1995). Balloon aortic valvuloplasty in adults. *Journal of the American College of Cardiology, 26,* 1522–1528.

Morris, J.J., Schaff, H.V., Mullany, P.B., Frye, R.L., & Orszulak, T.A. (1994). Gender differences in the left ventricular functional response to aortic valve replacement. *Circulation, 80*(suppl II), II183–II189.

Otto, C.M., Kuusisto, J., Reichenbach, D.D., Gown, A.M., & O'Brien, K.D. (1994). Characterization of the early lesion of degenerative valvular aortic stenoses. *Circulation, 90,* 844–853.

Passik, C.S., Ackerman, D.M., Pluth, J.R., & Edwards, W.D. (1987). Temporal changes in the causes of aortic stenosis. *Mayo Clinic Proceedings, 62,* 119–123.

Ross, J., Jr., & Braunwald, E. (1968). Aortic stenoses. *Circulation, 38*(suppl V), V61–V67.

Schwartz, L.S., Goldfischer, J., Spraugue, G.J., & Schwartz, S.P. (1969). Syncope and sudden death in aortic stenoses. *American Journal of Cardiology, 23,* 647–658.

Scognamiglo, R., Rahimtoola, S.H., Fasoli, G., Nistri, S., & Dalla Volta, S. (1994). Nifedipine in asymptomatic patients with severe aortic regurgitation and normal left ventricular function. *N Engl J Med, 331,* 689–694.

Zile, M.R. (1991). Chronic aortic and mitral regurgitation. *Cardiology Clinics, 9,* 239–253.

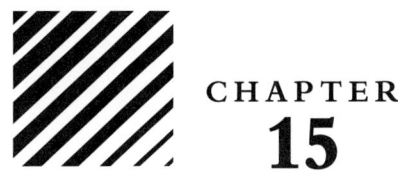

COMMON DERMATOLOGIC CONDITIONS

CHAPTER
15

Common Dermatologic Conditions

Goldie Gianoulis-Alissandratos, RN, MS, FNP, DNC

Of all the body organs that make up an individual, the skin is the largest and most visible. Information about a person can be revealed through mechanisms acting within the skin such as happiness, humor, anger, fear, embarrassment, health, and sickness. Age is revealed principally through changes in the pattern, fine structure, and mechanical properties of skin. Genetics also plays a role in determining the uniqueness of an individual at the level of the skin.

The skin plays a major role in maintaining the body's homeostasis. Through the maintenance of a constant body temperature, survival can be ensured. The skin serves as a barrier to prevent the loss of important body fluids and the entrance of possibly toxic environmental agents. The importance of the skin cannot be overlooked. Consider, for example, the color changes of the skin on a person in shock (pale, ashen) or a person with liver failure (yellow, jaundiced) or even a person with cardiac failure (blue, cyanotic). To the trained as well as the untrained eye, the skin may be an indicator of serious disease. The well-trained primary care provider, however, must be able to recognize the more subtle changes of the skin and distinguish between life-threatening diseases such as malignant melanoma and less serious, common skin conditions.

Patients present with skin lesions as an incidental finding or as the chief complaint. The role of the primary care provider in the diagnosis and treatment of common dermatologic conditions is increasingly important, because two thirds of these adult patients, who account for almost 10% of outpatient visits, will be seen by primary care providers. Furthermore, human suffering results from the disability, discomfort, and disfigurement that may be associated with various skin disorders. Through a relationship-centered approach, primary care providers may be able to assist their patients and help relieve their suffering.

Because of the nature of skin conditions, this chapter will include fundamental terms necessary to understand and describe skin lesions. Common skin diseases are then described in detail, including diagnosis and management.

ANATOMY, PHYSIOLOGY, AND PATHOLOGY

Skin Anatomy and physiology

The skin in composed of three layers: the epidermis, the dermis, and the subcutaneous tissues. Its outermost layer, the epidermis, is thin and devoid of blood vessels; therefore, it is dependent on the dermis for its nutrition. Melanin and keratin are formed in the epidermis. Well supplied with blood, the dermis

also contains connective tissue, sebaceous glands, and some hair follicles. The dermis merges below with the sucutaneous layer, which contains fat, sweat glands, and the remainder of the hair follicles. Hair, nails, mucous membranes, and sebaceous and sweat glands are considered to be appendages of the skin.

Major functions of the skin include:

- Protection from injurious external agents
- Maintenance of an internal environment by providing a barrier to water and electrolyte loss
- Regulation of body heat
- Self-maintenance by the eccrine and sebaceous glands of a buffered protective skin film
- Participation in Vitamin D production
- Delayed hypersensitivity reaction to foreign substances
- Sensation for touch, temperature, and pain.

Skin Disease Epidemiology

The true prevalence of skin disease is difficult to determine because many dermatologic studies have included only selected populations. Varying social and environmental factors also influence both the occurrence and the detection of skin disease. Persons whose occupation or hobbies require them to be outdoors may be more prone to the development of a skin cancer.

DIAGNOSTIC CRITERIA

The diagnosis and treatment of skin disease depend on the health care provider's familiarity with dermatology terms. Fitzpatrick and Bernhard (1993, p. 32) summed it up best when they said, "to read words, one must recognize letters; to read the skin, one must recognize the basic lesions." A barrier to communication among providers exists because of the lack of any standardization of basic dermatologic terminology. The International League of Dermatologic Societies has published a glossary of basic lesions in an attempt to standardize the definitions. To prevent confusion in the standard of measurement of lesions, a metric ruler is an essential tool for the provider to ensure accurate documentation of lesion size.

Primary Lesions

Primary lesions are the original lesions, whether they continue to full development or are modified by regression or trauma. These lesions assume a distinct characteristic (Table 15-1).

TABLE 15-1	Classification of Skin Lesions		
Type	**Appearance**	**Comments**	
PRIMARY LESIONS			
Macule	Flat, well-circumscribed area of any color change within the skin	Measures up to 1 cm in diameter. Area of pigment change is nonpalpable.	**A** Macule
Patch	Flat, well-circumscribed area of any color change within the skin	Measures greater than 1 cm in diameter. Area of pigment change is nonpalpable.	**B** Patch
Papule	Solid, raised, circumscribed	Measures less than 1 cm in diameter. Surface may be smooth or rough on palpation.	**C** Papule
Plaque	Solid, raised, circumscribed	Measures 1 or more cm in diameter. May develop as an individual lesion or a coalescence of papules. Color may range from normal skin color to any color of pigment change.	**D** Plaque
Nodule	Solid, palpable, possibly freely movable	Measures 1 to 2 in diameter. Extends deeper into the layers of the skin than do papules.	**E** Nodule
Tumor	Solid, palpable, possibly freely movable	Measures greater than 2 cm in diameter	**F** Tumor
Wheals	Elevated, flat-topped, edematous. White or usually pale red.	Also known as hives or urticaria. Vary in size. Fluid within the lesion is transitory. Lesions can develop within a few seconds and disappear slowly.	**G** Wheal
Vesicle	Circumscribed, elevated; contain fluid. Color may be clear, turbid, or hemorrhagic.	Also known as a blister. Measures up to 1 cm in diameter. Most often tense.	**H** Vesicle
Bullae	Circumscribed, elevated; contain fluid. Color may be clear, turbid, or hemorrhagic.	Measures greater than 1 cm in diameter. May be flaccid or tense.	**I** Bulla

(continued)

SECONDARY LESIONS

Pustules	Circumscribed elevations of the skin that contain pus	Also known as pimples. Pus is present as a result of the inflammatory nature of the lesion.	**J** Pustule
Scales	Increase in the formation of keratin cells	May vary in size from fine to coarse. Are produced when normal process of keratinization is interrupted. Papulosquamous is used to describe an eruption of scaling papules.	**K** Scales
Crust	Color may vary depending on the exudate. May be yellow, green to greenish-yellow, dark red, or brown.	Develops as a result of the opening and draining of a primary lesion	**L** Crust
Excoriation	Superficial lesions of the epidermis; may be linear or punctate	Commonly known as scratch marks	**M** Excoriation
Fissure	Linear crack that involves the epidermis and sometimes the dermis	Can vary in number and size. Frequently seen in conditions that cause dry skin. Flexural areas are commonly affected.	**N** Fissure
Erosion	Exudate may develop into a crust	Results from loss of viable epidermis. Usually heals with no scar.	**O** Erosion
Ulcer	Usually a rounded or irregularly shaped excavation	Results from loss of entire epidermis and some of the dermis. Can vary in diameter and depth. Scar likely to develop when ulcer heals.	**P** Ulcer
Scar	Caused by a deposition of fibrous tissue during the healing process. May become hypertrophic, keloidal, and even pruritic.	Size and shape determined by the preceding damage. Usually tend to become less obvious over time.	**Q** Scar
Atrophy	Appears as thin and somewhat transparent epidermis. Dermal atrophy manifests as a depression in the skin.	Loss of epidermis, dermis, or subcutaneous fat	**R** Atrophy

Art from: Smeltzer, S. and Bare, B. (1996). Brunner and Suddarth's Textbook of medical-surgical nursing, 8/e. Philadelphia: Lippincott-Raven Publishers.

Secondary Lesions

Secondary lesions are simply lesions that have undergone changes from their primary form (see Table 15-1).

HISTORY AND PHYSICAL EXAMINATION

The history of the present illness is critical in assessing a patient with a dermatologic concern. Along with the general medical history, a well-focused dermatologic history should be obtained. The history of a skin eruption should include:

- The onset, development, and progression of the skin lesion or lesions. Particular questions should focus on any relation of the skin eruption to the patient's occupation.
- An accurate medication history, including prescription and nonprescription medications, and use of recreational drugs
- Treatment obtained for any other ailment besides the skin eruption, including prescription and nonprescription medications
- The effect of the skin eruption on exposure to sunlight and seasonal variations
- Contact with animals, plants, chemicals, or metals
- The ingestion of certain foods and beverages may contribute to or even be the actual cause of a skin eruption; therefore, detailed dietary questioning is warranted.
- For the female patient, ask about any association of the skin eruption with menses or pregnancy.

In addition to the complete review of systems, constitutional symptoms that may indicate an acute illness syndrome or a chronic illness syndrome should be thoroughly investigated.

The physical examination must include the general appearance of the patient. A thorough head-to-toe examination of the skin should be conducted with proper lighting. Five major signs are assessed:

- Type of lesion
- Shape of lesion
- Arrangement of multiple lesions
- Color of lesion
- Distribution of the lesions.

DIAGNOSTIC STUDIES

Laboratory Tests and Diagnostic Tools

A hand lens magnifier is needed to examine the surface and detail of skin lesions. Oblique lighting of the skin surface may help to detect slight degrees of elevation or depression of the skin eruption. Low illumination of a room enhances the contrast between hypopigmented or hyperpigmented skin with normal skin. A Wood's lamp can be used to evaluate skin diseases that cause a loss or an increase in skin pigmentation; it should be used in a room that is completely dark. Diascopy is used to determine if a lesion is vascular. The examiner places a clear microscope slide or clear plastic ruler on the lesion while applying firm pressure. If the lesion turns white or fades as pressure is applied, the eruption is of vascular origin.

The dimple sign is a test used to aid in the differentiation of a benign lesion and a malignant melanoma. Lateral pressure is applied to the lesion with the thumb and index finger. If a dimpling occurs in the lesion, it is safe to assume that the lesion, which is most likely firm and pigmented, is not a melanoma.

Patch testing is used to aid in making the diagnosis and determining the causative agent of allergic contact dermatitis. Finn chambers are filled with specific allergens and usually placed on the patient's back. After 48 hours the patches are removed and the initial reading is done. A positive reaction to a specific chemical would be localized to the area that had direct contact with that chemical only. It may present as a faint macular erythema or it may become ulcerative. Another reading must be obtained after an additional 24 hours to document any delayed hypersensitivity reactions.

Microscopic examinations are used frequently in dermatology and include Gram stains, cultures (both bacterial and fungal), potassium hydroxide preparations, Tzanck tests, and hair pluck evaluation.

A serologic test for syphilis should always be considered for a patient with generalized erythematous and scaling eruptions.

Biopsy of the skin is a useful diagnostic tool. In most instances the clinical and histologic findings should be in agreement. If they are not, another biopsy should be obtained. Follow-up with the patient after a few days or a week is recommended. The most common technique for a skin biopsy involves the use of a tool called a punch (a small, sterile, disposable tubular knife) under local anesthesia. The site of the biopsy is very important and usually depends on the stage of the eruption.

Elliptical excisions and scalpel wedge excisions can also be performed and sent for examination. The excision method used should be based on the practitioner's experience and the laboratory's requirements for the requested tests.

ACNE

Pathology and Etiology

Acne vulgaris is a disease that affects the pilosebaceous unit and most commonly manifests on the chest, back, and face (Color Plate 1A–C). The pilosebaceous unit consists of sebaceous glands and hair follicles. These units are present on all skin surfaces except for the palms of the hands and soles of the feet.

Acne is a multifactorial disease that involves four principal factors in its pathogenesis: increased sebum production, abnormal keratinization of the follicular epithelium, proliferation of *Propionibacterium acnes* (*P. acnes*), and inflammation (Strauss, 1993).

INCREASED SEBUM PRODUCTION

Several factors influence sebum production, although the main influence is hormonal (Cunliffe & Gollnick, 1996). The secretory activity of the sebaceous gland is controlled by androgenic hormones (Leyden, 1995). Research has found that androgens are essential for the development of acne. No correlation, however, has been found between androgen levels and acne severity (Aizawa et al, 1995).

ABNORMAL KERATINIZATION OF THE FOLLICULAR EPITHELIUM

Abnormal or disordered shedding of the cells that line the sebaceous follicles is central to the pathogenesis of acne. This process is also known as follicular plugging (Arndt et al, 1995). The result of this abnormal shedding is comedo formation. If

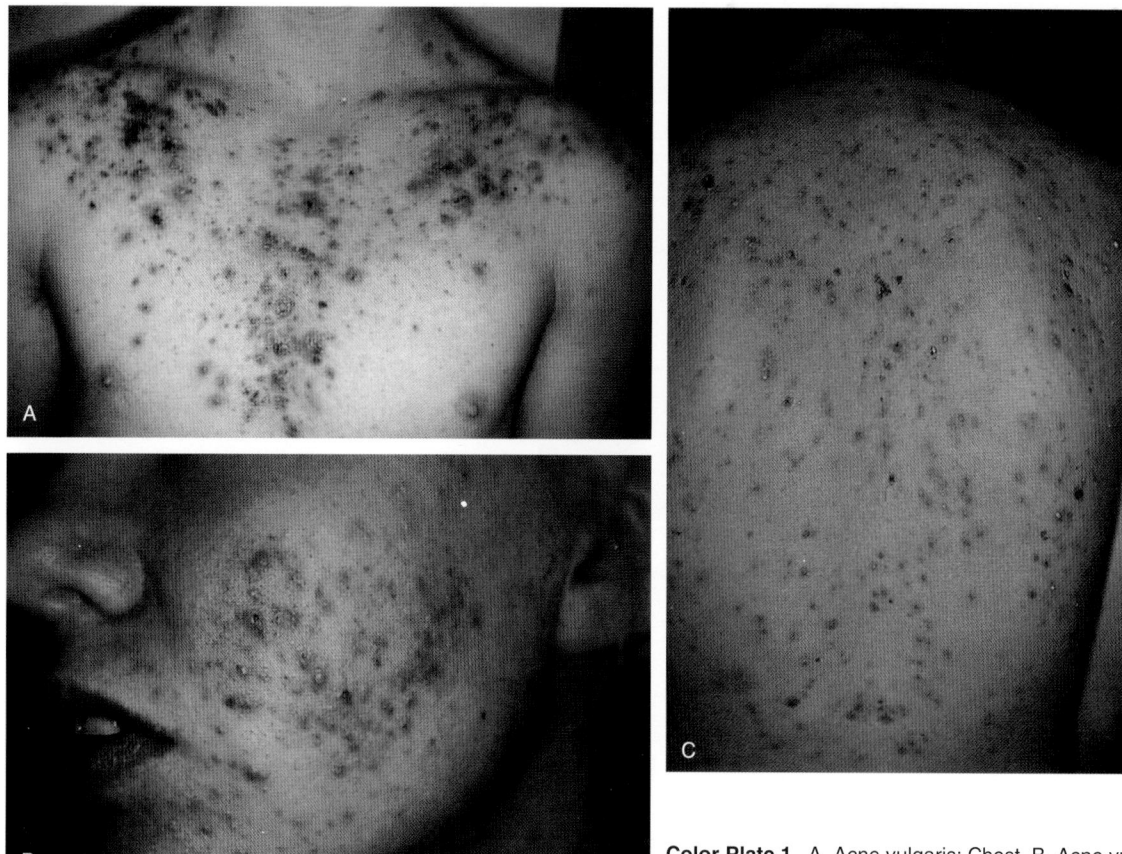

Color Plate 1. A. Acne vulgaris: Chest, B. Acne vulgaris: Face, C. Acne vulgaris: Back

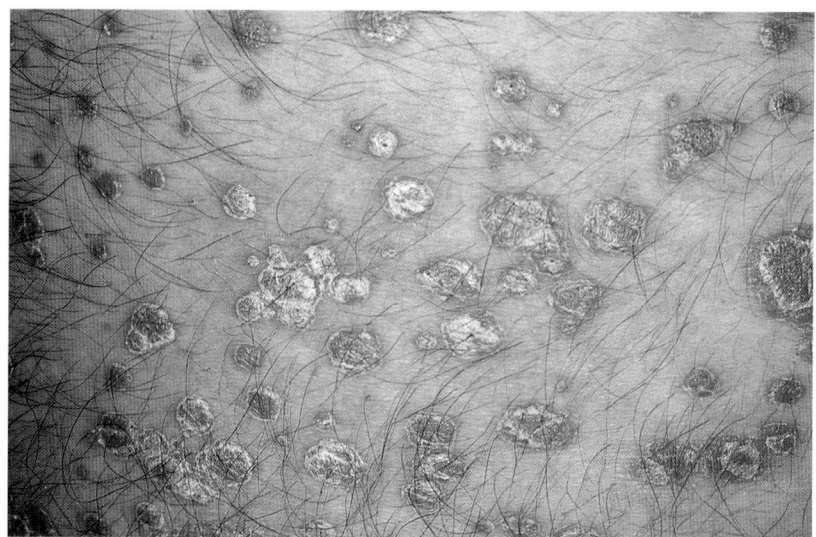

Color Plate 2. Psoriasis

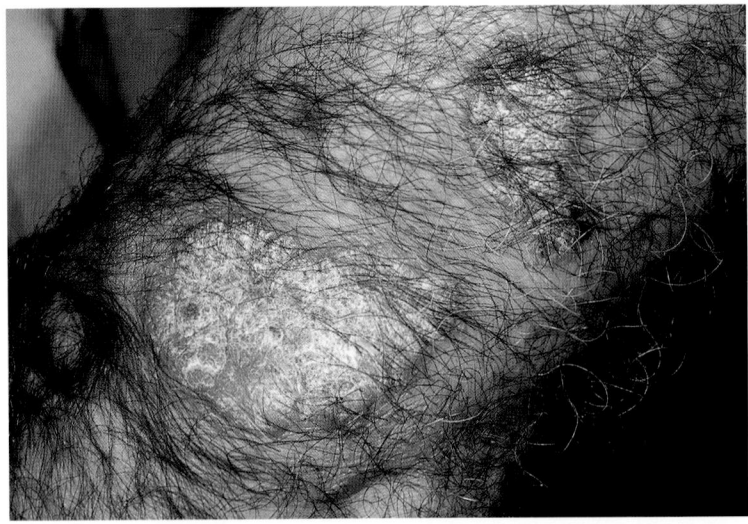

Color Plate 3. Plaque psoriasis

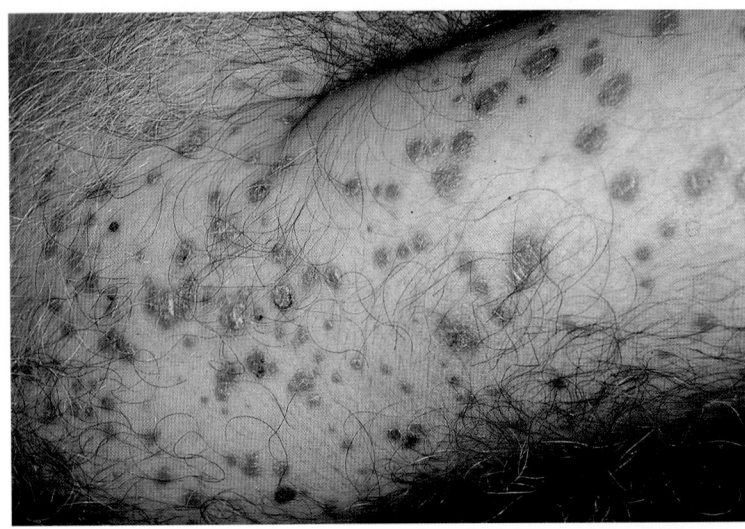

Color Plate 4. Guttate psoriasis

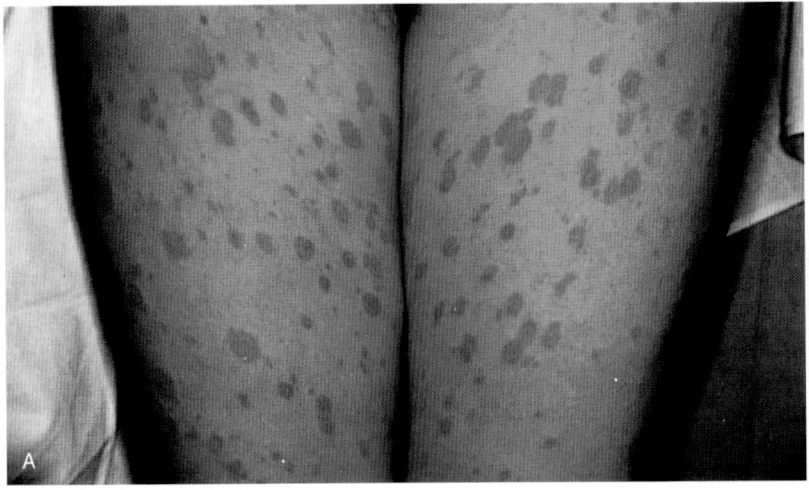

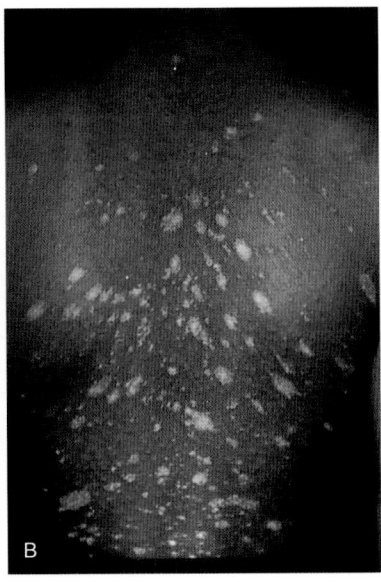

Color Plate 5. A. Pityriasis rosea: Thighs, B. Pityriasis rosea on the back of an African American male

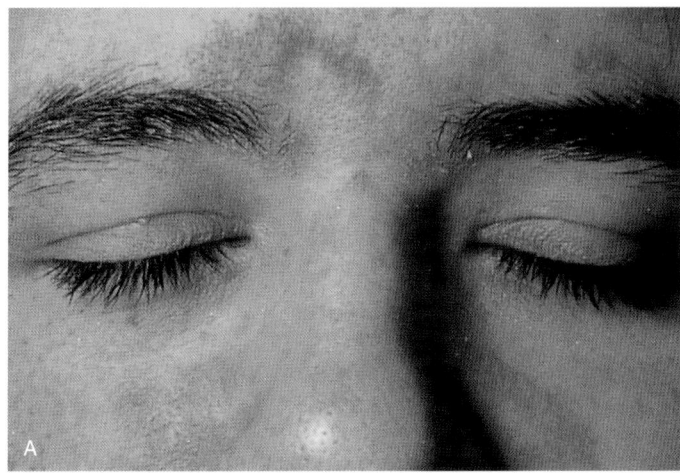 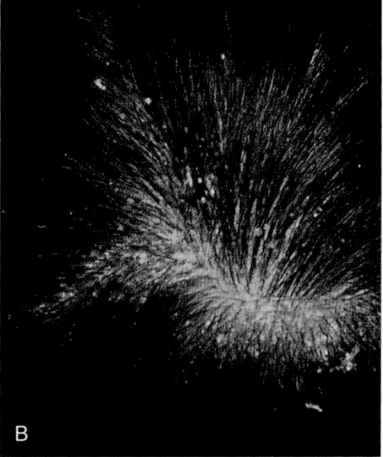

Color Plate 6. A. Seborrheic dermatitis: Eyes and nose, B. Seborrheic dermatitis

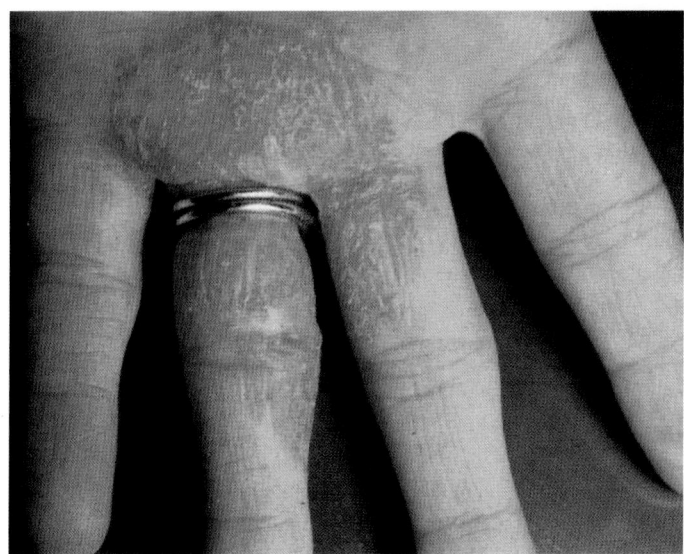

Color Plate 7. Contact dermatitis from soap under rings

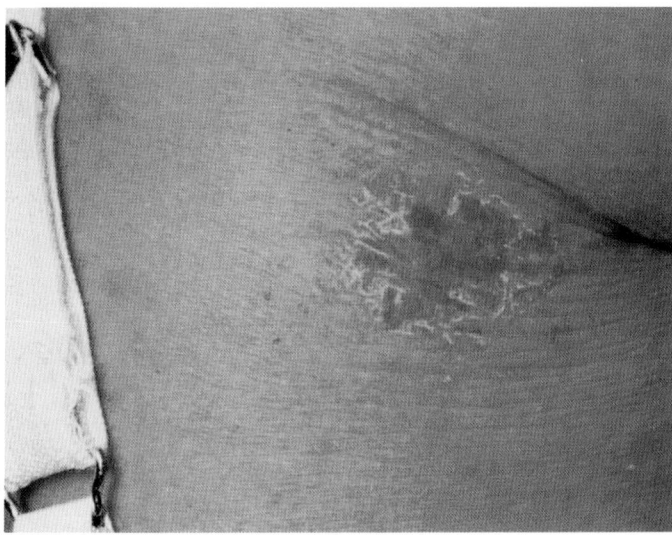

Color Plate 8. Contact dermatitis

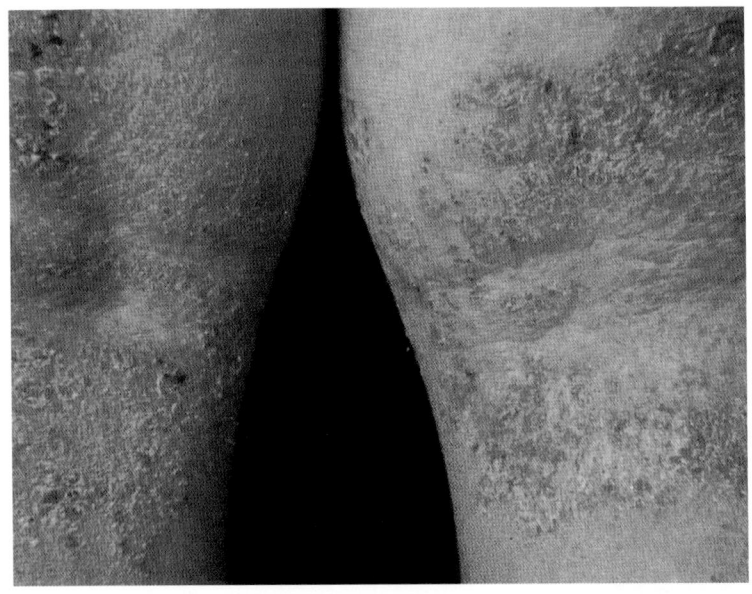

Color Plate 9. Atopic dermatitis

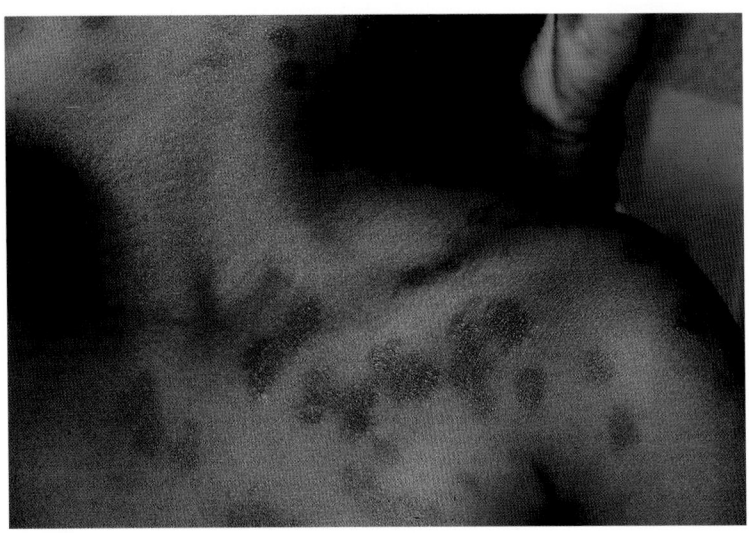

Color Plate 10. Tinea corporis

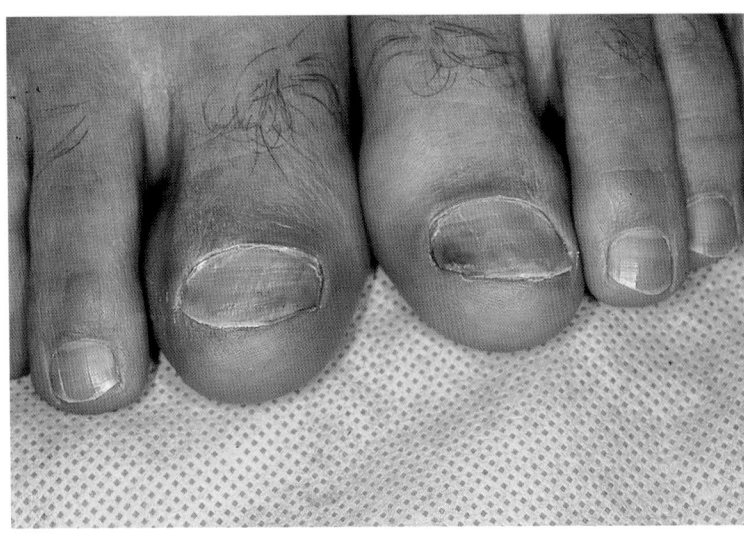

Color Plate 11. Tine ungium

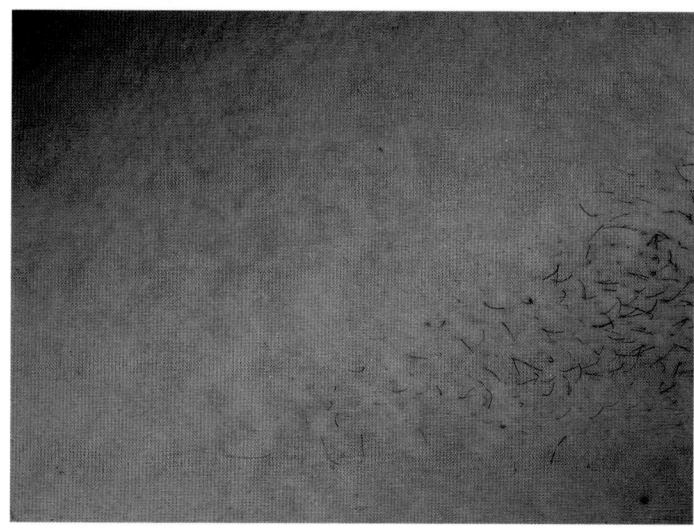

Color Plate 12. Tinea versicolor

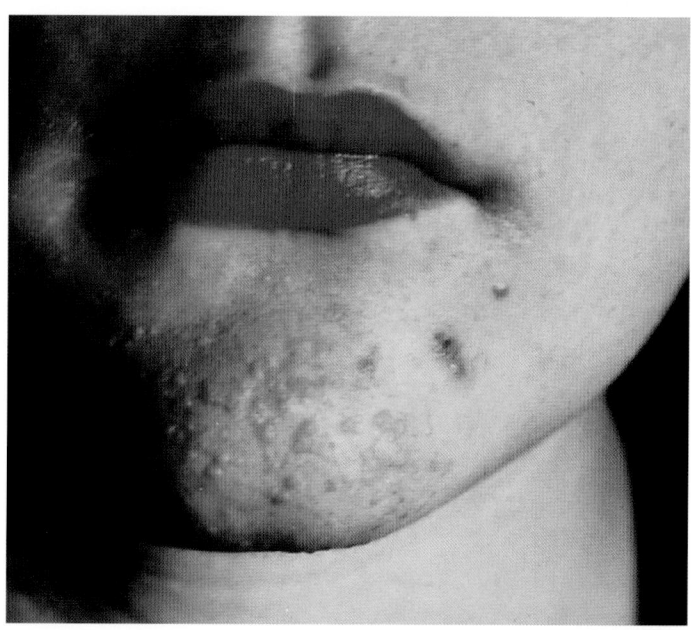

Color Plate 13. Herpes simplex

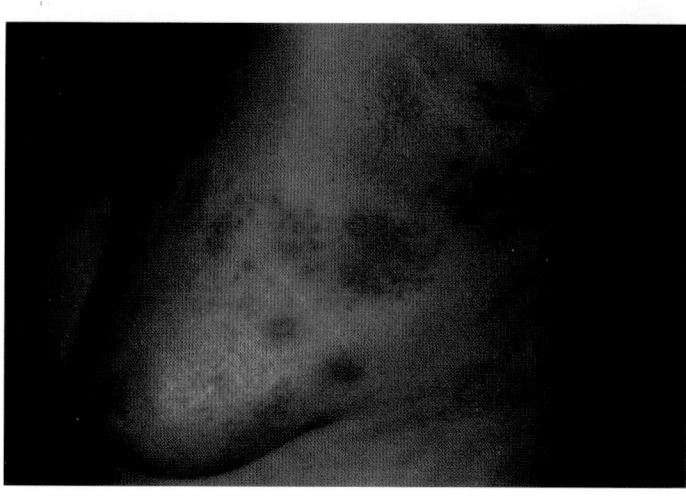

Color Plate 14. Herpes zoster

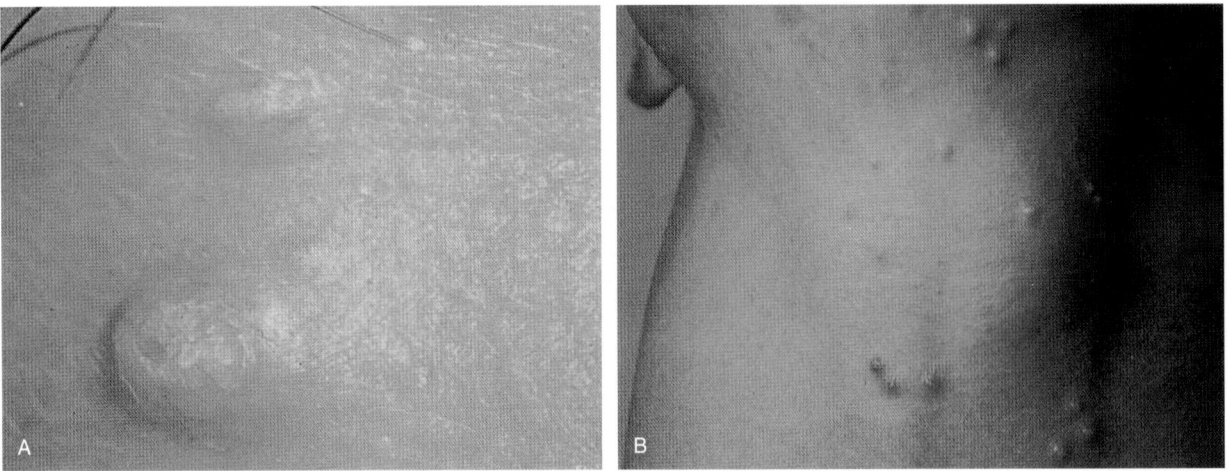

Color Plate 15. A. Molluscum contagiosum up close, B. Molluscum contagiosum: Neck

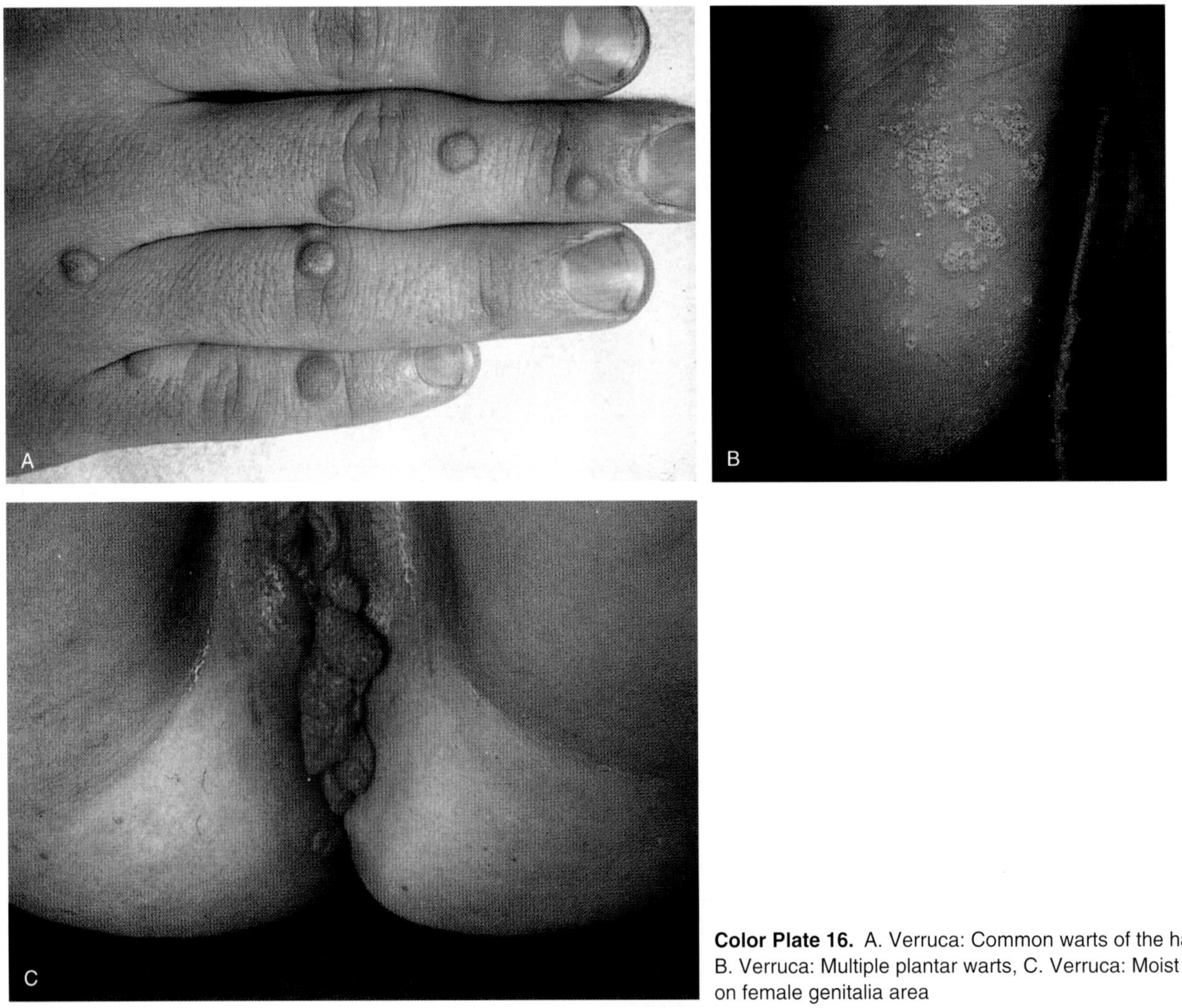

Color Plate 16. A. Verruca: Common warts of the hand, B. Verruca: Multiple plantar warts, C. Verruca: Moist warts on female genitalia area

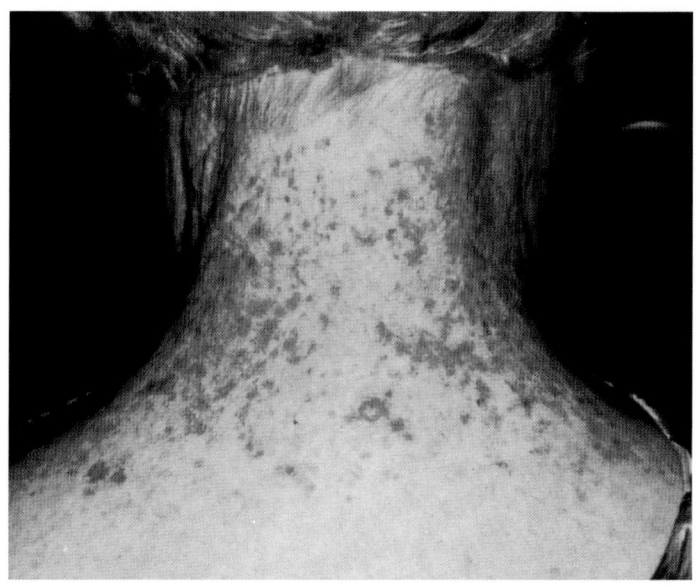

Color Plate 17. Actinic keratoses

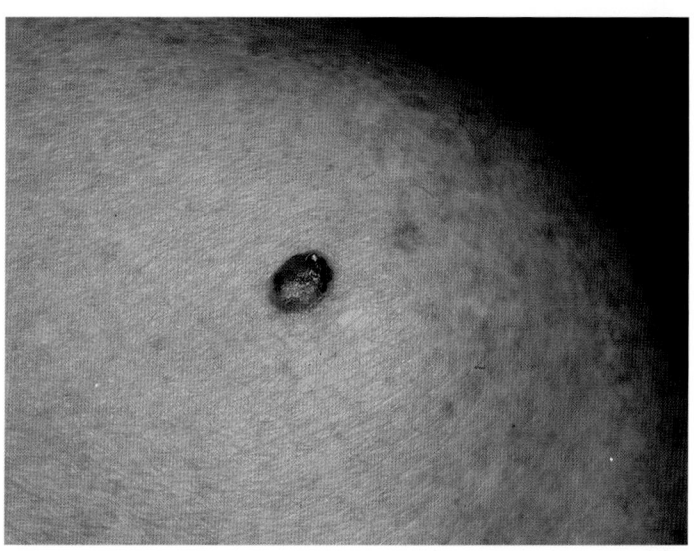

Color Plate 18. Basal cell carcinoma

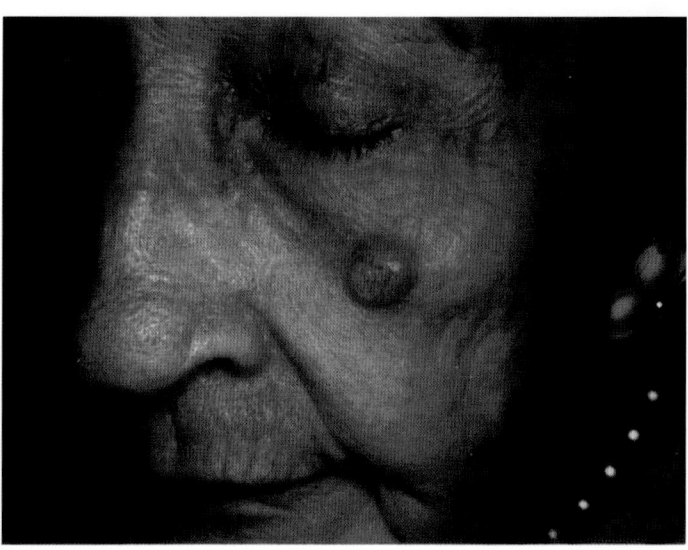

Color Plate 19. Squamous cell carcinoma on cheek

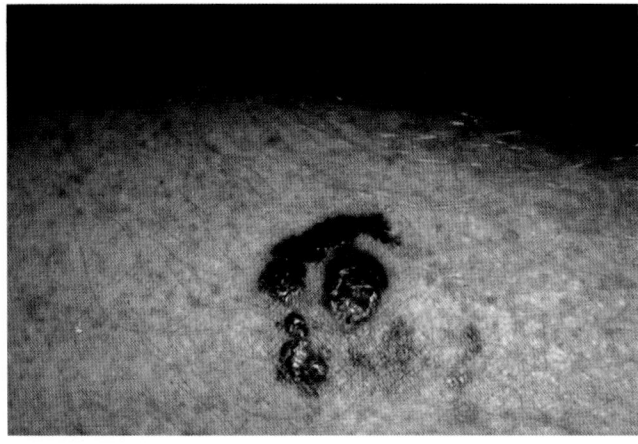

Color Plate 20. Malignant melanoma

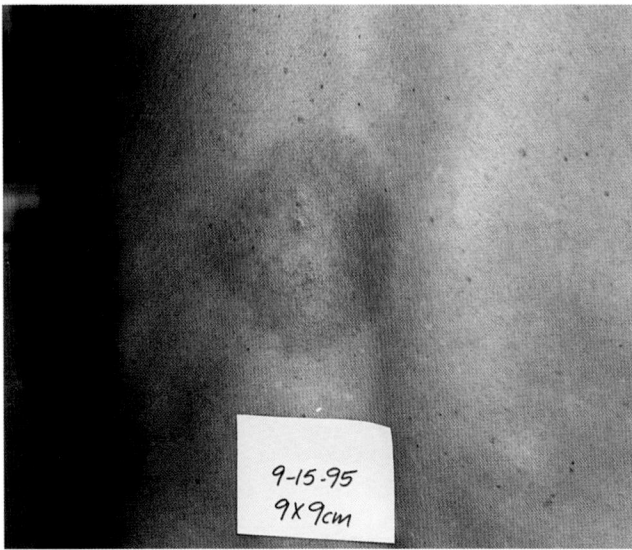

9-15-95
9×9cm

Color Plate 21. Classic erythema migrans rash

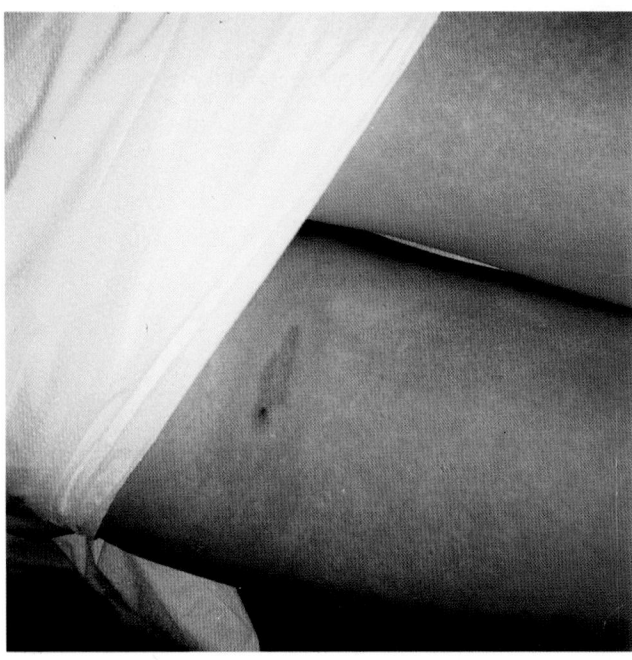

Color Plate 22. Brown recluse spider bite

the plug is formed within a dilated opening, it develops into a whitehead. If the comedonal mass protrudes from the sebaceous follicle, it develops into a blackhead. A whitehead is considered a closed comedo, whereas a blackhead is considered an open comedo (Leyden, 1995). These lesions, in and of themselves, are considered noninflammatory lesions of acne.

PROLIFERATION OF *P. ACNES* AND INFLAMMATION

P. acnes is an anaerobic diphtheroid that colonizes sebaceous follicles (Thiboutot, 1996). It is transported to the skin surface along with the production of sebum (Webster, 1995). Inflammatory acne lesions, described as papules, pustules, nodules, cysts, and abscesses, are produced when *P. acnes* proliferates and generates an inflammatory reaction. Most inflammatory acne lesions result from the intrafollicular rupture of a comedo as opposed to a visible rupture (Arndt et al, 1995). Clinically detectable inflammation results once the comedonal contents are exposed to the immune system. The severity of the response is variable. It may present as small, superficial papules or pustules, with or without cysts or deep nodules. Spontaneous fluctuations in the degree of involvement are the rule rather than the exception.

EPIDEMIOLOGY

Approximately 17 million people in the United States are afflicted with acne vulgaris (Kaminer & Gilchrest, 1995). In addition to disfigurement and scarring, acne may have an adverse effect on the victim's psychological development. Although often associated with adolescence, acne may be first diagnosed in patients who are in their 30s or 40s. Research has identified problems for some persons with this condition in terms of self-esteem, self-confidence, body image, social withdrawal, depression, and anger (Bergfeld, 1995).

OPTIONS, EXPECTED OUTCOMES, COMPREHENSIVE MANAGEMENT

Acne vulgaris is rarely misdiagnosed. It may, however, become confused with folliculitis, rosacea, or any other acneiform eruption. The diagnosis is usually based on the finding of comedones, pustules, papules, nodules, or cysts on the back, chest, or face.

There are many myths regarding factors that may aggravate or alleviate acne. The most common myth is that various foods such as shellfish, chocolate, and fatty foods aggravate acne. There is no evidence to support the value of eliminating these foods (Strauss, 1993). For patients who attribute their acne flare-ups to their dietary intake, it is best to encourage them to eliminate the foods they think produce the flare-up.

Several studies have shown that genetic factors may influence the susceptibility to acne (Ebling & Cunliffe, 1992). Stress can aggravate acne but it is not a primary cause (Cunliffe & Gollnick, 1996). Acne itself can cause stress and is certainly aggravated by picking at or popping the lesions.

Acne vulgaris has a very favorable prognosis. Management of acne should be directed toward a combination of the four factors associated with acne. Scarring, which can be minimized with proper treatment, is the only sequela of acne. Acne is considered a chronic disease that requires months, if not years,

of treatment. With the exception of isotretinoin, most therapies are prescribed on a long-term basis. Many treatment options are available, and treatment should be tailored to the patient based on the psychosocial impact the acne creates for the individual, as well as treatment costs.

TOPICAL THERAPY

Topical therapy is initially prescribed for patients with noninflammatory comedones. It may also be used for mild to moderate inflammatory acne. Topical therapies include comedolytic agents, antibiotics, and anti-inflammatory drugs.

COMEDOLYTIC AGENTS

The precursor of an acne lesion is the microcomedo. Therefore, therapy is initiated with a comedolytic agent.

Tretinoin

Tretinoin is an effective first-line comedolytic agent. It normalizes desquamation of the follicular epithelium and promotes drainage of pre-existing comedones. With continued use, normal shedding of follicular keratinocytes occurs within the lumen of the follicle (Thiboutot, 1996), preventing the development of new microcomedones.

There are various dosage forms and vehicle bases of tretinoin. It is usually applied once daily at bedtime after the face has been cleansed and adequate time allowed for it to dry. The mildest cream formulation should be prescribed first and the concentration increased depending on the clinical response. If the patient has excessively oily skin or lives in a humid climate, the gel formulation may be preferable. Dosage forms of tretinoin cream include 0.025%, 0.05%, and 0.1%. Gel formulation dosages include 0.01% and 0.025%. A 0.05% solution also exists. In terms of potency, the 0.05% cream and the 0.01% gel are roughly equivalent, as are the 0.1% cream and the 0.025% gel. The 0.05% solution is the most potent form of tretinoin.

Patients should always be informed of potential side effects, which include desquamation, burning, erythema, and exacerbation of inflammatory acne lesions. This irritation can be minimized by selecting the appropriate starting dose, applying the medication to dry skin, and increasing the concentration gradually. Tretinoin does not possess antimicrobial or anti-inflammatory activity. By reducing the number of microcomedones formed, a reduction in the number of inflammatory lesions can occur (Thiboutot, 1996).

Azelaic Acid Cream

Azelaic acid cream (20%) is a new topical therapy for acne that has recently become available in the United States. It is a naturally occurring compound that serves as an effective monotherapy in mild to moderate forms of acne (Graupe et al, 1996). The therapeutic benefits result from its ability to decrease the hyperproliferation of keratinocytes in the follicular infundibulum, an antibacterial effect against *P. acnes*, and direct anti-inflammatory properties. Azelaic acid cream has been found to have an overall efficacy comparable to that of 0.05% tretinoin, 5% benzoyl peroxide, and 2% topical erythromycin (Graupe et al, 1996). Significant advantages to the use of azelaic acid include excellent local tolerance and its favorable side effect profile: it is nonteratogenic, there are no photodynamic reactions, and it produces no induced resistance in *P. acnes* (Graupe et al, 1996). The proper application of azelaic acid cream is twice a day (morning and evening). It should be rubbed into the skin gently until it vanishes.

Anti-inflammatory Agents

P. acnes is the stimulus for inflammatory acne. Suppression of this organism will result in an improvement of inflammatory lesions. Topical antibiotics decrease the formation of *P. acnes* and possess intrinsic anti-inflammatory activity as well (Thiboutot, 1996). Antimicrobial agents, such as tetracycline and erythromycin, may also decrease the inflammatory potential of *P. acnes* (Webster, 1995).

Benzoyl peroxide is a potent bactericidal agent effective against *P. acnes*. It is considered a first-line choice of therapy in mild inflammatory acne (Thiboutot, 1996). Benzoyl peroxide is formulated as a wash, cream, lotion, or gel. It is available in concentrations of 2%, 5%, and 10%. It may be used once or twice daily. The more common side effects include erythema and dryness. It may also bleach clothing, which is an important consideration when the benzoyl peroxide is applied to the chest or back.

The more commonly used **topical antibiotics** include clindamycin, erythromycin, and sulfur. They are available in various formulations, including gels, lotions, solutions, and pads. In general, lotions are less drying to the skin than gels or pads; solutions tend to be more drying to the skin. The provider must always consider allergies that the patient may have and prescribe a topical antibiotic accordingly. Side effects include local irritation and the development of resistant bacteria. Topical antibiotics are effective for mild to moderate inflammatory acne, especially when used in combination with a comedolytic agent.

Topical clindamycin and erythromycin are available as solutions, lotions, pads, or gels. They may be used once or twice daily, depending on whether they are prescribed alone or with a comedolytic agent.

Topical sulfur is available as a lotion only. It can be used once or twice daily, depending on whether it is prescribed alone or in combination with a comedolytic agent. This particular lotion is also available in a tinted version, which would be a ideal choice for patients who would like to cover their acne lesions.

COMBINATION THERAPY

Studies have been done to test the efficacy and safety of various combinations. Tretinoin has been found to increase the penetration of other topical agents used in combination with it (Bearson & Shalita, 1995). It has also been found that when all lesion types are considered, the concurrent use of topical clindamycin and tretinoin, or clindamycin and benzoyl peroxide, is clinically superior to either of the agents used alone (Bearson & Shalita, 1995). These combinations also make the treatment better tolerated because the irritant effects of one agent are decreased with the addition of the other.

There has been a recent surge in the use of alpha-hydroxy acids in the treatment of both inflammatory and noninflammatory acne. The mechanism of action that has been proposed for these acids is their keratolytic activity. They are most effective when used as an adjunctive therapy, not alone (Bearson & Shalita, 1995).

SYSTEMIC THERAPY

Systemic drugs are usually added to the treatment regimen when inflammatory disease, whether mild, moderate, or severe, does not respond to topical combinations. The more commonly used oral antibiotics include tetracycline, erythromycin, and minocycline. The mechanism of action common among these antibiotics is their antibacterial effect against *P. acnes*. Many of them possess intrinsic anti-inflammatory activity as well as the ability to alter sebum production (Thiboutot, 1996).

Tetracyclines and Erythromycin

Tetracyclines are the mainstay of acne therapy. Tetracycline itself does not directly alter sebum production but it does decrease the concentration of free fatty acids, which has a direct effect on the secretion of other proinflammatory products (Strauss, 1993). Common side effects of tetracycline include gastrointestinal upset, vaginal candidiasis, phototoxicity, and decreased effectiveness of oral contraceptives. Because dairy products and iron can decrease the absorption of tetracycline, it should be taken on an empty stomach, preferably with a glass of water. Tetracyclines have the ability to mineralize tissues rapidly and are deposited in developing teeth; this may cause irreversible yellow-brown staining. Tetracyclines have also been reported to inhibit fetal skeletal growth (Strauss, 1993). Therefore, they should never be prescribed to pregnant women or to babies.

Minocycline, a tetracycline derivative, is commonly used in patients whose acne is unresponsive to tetracycline. It is a potent antibacterial agent with the ability to penetrate the sebaceous gland (Bearson & Shalita, 1995). It is less likely to cause gastrointestinal upset and phototoxic reactions, but these side effects may still occur. One common side effect associated with minocycline is vertigo-like symptoms. This can sometimes be avoided by gradually increasing the dose. Other potential side effects include slate-blue pigmentation (particularly in acne scars), headache, pseudotumor cerebri, and tooth discoloration, as with other tetracyclines.

Erythromycin is comparable to tetracycline in its efficacy (Thiboutot, 1996). However, the possibility of developing resistance is greater with erythromycin (Bearson & Shalita, 1995). It should be taken with food or milk to decrease the possibility of gastrointestinal upset. There is a theoretical risk of a decrease in the efficacy of oral contraceptives, but less than that with oral tetracyclines (Thiboutot, 1996). Erythromycin is a good alternative for photosensitive patients.

The dosages of tetracycline and erythromycin are usually 500 to 1000 mg/day. Minocycline is given at a dosage of 100 to 200 mg/day. The medications are usually taken twice daily in equally divided doses. It is important to inform patients that there is usually little improvement within the first month of therapy. As improvement of the acne condition is noted, the dosage of the oral antibiotic is decreased. Topical therapy should remain unchanged. Patients should always be informed of the possibility of restarting the oral antibiotic if an exacerbation occurs.

Isotretinoin

Isotretinoin is a synthetic oral retinoid. It is an analogue of vitamin A. The indication for isotretinoin is inflammatory acne or cystic acne that does not respond to conventional therapy. Isotretinoin is the only form of therapy that directly affects all four of the pathogenic factors of acne (Berson & Shalita, 1995). It has a direct influence on the abnormal keratinization of the follicle. A decrease in sebum production occurs as a result of sebaceous gland activity inhibition. Therefore, "the growth of *P. acnes* and its ability to generate proinflammatory mediators are diminished" (Bearson & Shalita, 1995, p. 37).

The minimal dosage for isotretinoin is 1 mg/kg/day for 20 weeks. Some providers initiate therapy at 1.5 mg/kg/day. Dosages as high as 2 mg/kg/day are indicated for patients with severe trunk involvement or resistant chest, back, and facial lesions (Strauss, 1993). Isotretinoin is an extremely effective drug (Berson & Shalita, 1995). Patients must be warned about the possibility of an acne flare-up during the initial 3 to 4 weeks of therapy. Maximum improvement continues for 6 to 8 weeks after the cessation of therapy (Strauss, 1993).

The use of isotretinoin must be carefully monitored. A complete blood count, serum chemistries, and levels of hepatic enzymes, cholesterol, and triglycerides should be obtained before initiating therapy and monthly thereafter. The greatest concern is the risk of the drug being administered during pregnancy. Isotretinoin is a teratogen (Berson & Shalita, 1995), making pregnancy an absolute contraindication. Women of childbearing age should be told to begin therapy on the second day of their menstrual cycle. A negative serum pregnancy test should be obtained within 2 weeks of initiation of therapy and monthly thereafter. Sexually active females should use two methods of birth control starting at least 1 month before therapy begins. These contraceptive methods should continue throughout the course of treatment and for 1 month after the cessation of treatment. No more than a 1-month prescription should be given to a female patient to reinforce her awareness of the hazards of pregnancy while taking this medication. Signed informed consent that the patient understands the risks and benefits of using this drug and becoming pregnant should be obtained.

Every patient taking isotretinoin will develop some degree of mucocutaneous side effects, which may be controlled with the use of emollients. Secondary infection of the skin with *Staphylococcus aureus* may complicate the mucocutaneous side effects. If this develops, a course of antibiotic therapy with either dicloxacillin or erythromycin is warranted. Benign intracranial hypertension, myalgia, arthralgia, and rarely diffuse interstitial skeletal hyperostosis are considered systemic side effects of isotretinoin (Cunliffe & Gollnick, 1996).

PSORIASIS

Psoriasis is one of the earliest skin diseases described. References date back to the Old Testament, where the general term *lepra* was used to describe various skin conditions, including psoriasis (Stern & Wu, 1996) (Color Plate 2).

Anatomy, Physiology, and Pathology

PATHOLOGY

Despite intensive research, little is known beyond the observation that psoriasis is characterized by an excessively rapid turnover of epidermal cells and inflammation (Christophers & Sterry, 1993). The generally accepted fundamental elements in the pathophysiologic mechanisms of psoriasis are accelerated proliferation of keratinocytes and disturbed maturation, altered

cyclic nucleotide levels, associated changes in polymorphonuclear leukocyte and prostaglandin biology, and dermal vascular abnormalities (Grizzard, 1991).

Epidemiology

For millions of people, "the heartbreak of psoriasis" is not just a familiar advertising slogan but an unfortunate fact of life. Psoriasis can wreak havoc not only on its victims' skin, but also on their lives. Dermatologists have always known that psoriasis increases the patient's stress and that increased stress exacerbates psoriasis. This is a vicious cycle, leading to discomfort and despair for both patient and provider alike.

Although rarely life-threatening, psoriasis has a social and economic impact that is frequently underestimated (Ginsburg, 1995). This skin disorder is a chronic, genetically influenced, remitting and relapsing, scaly inflammatory eruption affecting 1% to 3% of the population (Greaves & Weinstein, 1995). Control of this lifelong disease poses a great challenge to the patient, family, provider, and community. "Psoriasis is a disease that, in attacking the skin, attacks the very identity of the individual. Many patients have to deal on a daily basis with shame, guilt, anger, and fear of being thought dirty and infectious by others" (Ginsburg, 1995, p. 793).

Clinical Presentation

Because of the dynamic nature of psoriasis and the varied presentations of this disease, it is often confused with other dermatologic conditions. Psoriasis typically reveals itself in five different variations (Lowe, 1993):

- Plaque psoriasis
- Pustular psoriasis
- Guttate psoriasis
- Inverse psoriasis
- Erythrodermic psoriasis.

More than one pattern of psoriasis may be present at the same time. Each person with psoriasis is unique. A thorough skin examination is the crucial first step in diagnosing and managing patients with psoriasis.

PLAQUE PSORIASIS

The classical clinical appearance of plaque psoriasis is a well-demarcated, erythematous, scaling, and often raised lesion (Color Plate 3). These lesions account for the designation of psoriasis as a papulosquamous disorder. A plaque-type pattern of psoriasis occurs more frequently than any other (Stern & Wu, 1996). The scales, often silvery and thickened, may occur anywhere on the body and are usually relatively symmetrical. The most likely areas of involvement are the elbows, knees, scalp, and lower back. Usually plaque psoriasis has a gradual onset and chronic course. Complete spontaneous remission is unusual (Stern & Wu, 1996).

PUSTULAR PSORIASIS

Pustular psoriasis can be localized or generalized and is subtyped accordingly. It is often found on the palms or soles. Instead of thickened scaling plaques, this type of psoriasis presents as erythematous plaques studded with pustules. Some cases of pustular psoriasis may resolve spontaneously with supportive treatment only; in other cases, flare-ups and complications occur repeatedly.

GUTTATE PSORIASIS

The typical presentation of guttate psoriasis is an acute generalized eruption of erythematous, scaling, raindrop-like papules (Color Plate 4). These single lesions rarely become confluent. The palms and soles are often spared. The most affected area is usually the trunk. Acute guttate psoriasis predominantly occurs during the second or third decade of life and is often precipitated by streptococcal throat infections (Christophers & Kiene, 1995). Guttate psoriasis carries a better prognosis than plaque-type psoriasis. It responds rapidly to ultraviolet light therapy, and spontaneous remission may occur.

INVERSE PSORIASIS

Psoriasis that affects the intertriginous regions, which include the axilla, groin, intergluteal fold, navel, and submammary region, is termed **inverse psoriasis**. Most patients have psoriasis lesions elsewhere, but these specific areas of involvement can cause severe discomfort and can even disable the patient. Patches of inverse psoriasis may be cracked and fissured. Consequently, these moist, macerated areas often become colonized with yeast and bacteria, making inverse psoriasis difficult to treat. Because of the maceration and friction associated with these specific areas, the scales of psoriasis are often absent (Stern & Wu, 1996).

ERYTHRODERMIC PSORIASIS

When psoriasis completely covers the body, it is referred to as exfoliative, generalized, or **erythrodermic psoriasis**. This is a severe, life-threatening eruption that most often manifests as intense pruritus, generalized erythema, and scaling. Fever, chills, pruritus, malaise, difficulty in regulating body temperature, and fatigue are systemic symptoms associated with this condition. Fortunately, this type of psoriasis occurs in fewer than 10% of patients (Lowe, 1993). Erythroderma may be a complication associated with pustular or plaque psoriasis, or it may even be the initial manifestation of psoriasis. After the erythrodermic flare subsides, patients usually revert to their original pattern of disease (Stern & Wu, 1996).

PSORIATIC ARTHRITIS

Arthritis is a common systemic component of psoriasis and is estimated to occur in 6% to 10% of cases (Grizzard, 1991). It is an inflammatory arthritis that may cause stiffness, pain, and a decrease in range of motion. Oligoarticular and polyarticular involvement, affecting the hands, feet, knees, wrists, and ankles, is common (Stern & Wu, 1996). There is no single diagnostic laboratory finding in psoriatic arthritis. It is a seronegative arthritis, and therefore a negative test for rheumatoid factor may aid with the diagnosis. Bulbal et al (1995) have commented on important considerations that providers should not overlook when evaluating someone with arthritis:

- When considering psoriatic arthritis in the differential diagnosis, question the patient regarding any family history of psoriasis. A total body skin examination should also be performed in search of psoriatic lesions.

- Septic arthritis should always be ruled out, even in patients with an established diagnosis of psoriatic arthritis.
- Status of HIV infection should be considered in cases of fulminant disease.

Trigger Factors

A variety of stimuli, both local and systemic, have been reported to trigger the onset or exacerbation of psoriasis (Kadunce & Krueger, 1995). A genetic predisposition should always be taken into consideration. Pharmacologic triggers may include nonsteroidal anti-inflammatory drugs, beta-blockers, antimalarial agents, lithium, and systemic corticosteroids. Clinical studies have confirmed that stress exacerbates psoriasis (Weller, 1996). Other stimuli include infection by *Streptococcus pyogenes* and HIV, and pregnancy and the use of progesterone-containing birth-control pills (Stern & Wu, 1996). Cutaneous trauma, also referred to as the Koebner phenomenon, is seen mainly in unstable psoriasis, and is the development of psoriasis in response to cutaneous injury.

Treatment Options, Expected Outcomes, Comprehensive Management

Psoriasis follows an irregular, chronic course marked by exacerbations of unpredictable onset and duration, as well as spontaneous remissions. Patients with newly developed psoriasis often become disenchanted with their treatment; if they do not accept that there is no cure, they may switch providers in the hope of finding one. Although there is no cure, treatment usually offers significant temporary relief and sometimes clears the rash. Because psoriasis is a lifelong disorder, optimal therapy should be simple and inexpensive, whenever possible. The severity of the disease and its impact, as perceived by the patient and provider together, can serve as a guide in developing a rational treatment plan. Seriously considering the way psoriasis affects the patient physically, socially, and psychologically should increase the patient's participation in developing and maintaining the treatment plan. This in turn will be the best indicator of the effectiveness of the treatment plan.

The aim of treatment is to clear the skin and reverse inflammatory joint disease, if present. All too often, however, treatments that have kept the psoriasis in check will stop working. In cases where the condition becomes resistant, new therapeutic modalities are required.

There is a wide spectrum of treatments. Common treatments for psoriasis include topical therapy, phototherapy and photochemotherapy, combination therapies, and systemic therapies. Generally, treatment begins with topical medications, proceeds to phototherapy or photochemotherapy in combination with the topical therapy, and finally leads to systemic therapy. Emollients are a very important adjunctive agent with both topical and systemic therapies. They assist with hydration of the skin and soften and loosen the hyperkeratotic scales. They are safe and relatively inexpensive (Table 15-2).

TOPICAL THERAPIES
Topical Corticosteroids

Topical corticosteroids are frequently prescribed as the initial therapy for mild to moderate plaque psoriasis. Although the exact mechanism of action in psoriasis remains unknown, corti-

TABLE 15-2	Commonly Used Topical Steroids Ranked by Potency	

Brand Name	Generic Name
GROUP I (SUPER POTENT)	
Temovate cream 0.05%	Clobetasol propionate
Temovate ointment 0.05%	Clobetasol propionate
Diprolene cream 0.05%	Betamethasone dipropionate
Diprolene ointment 0.05%	Betamethasone dipropionate
Psorcon ointment 0.05%	Diflorasone diacetate
Ultravate ointment 0.05%	Halobetasol propionate
GROUP II (HIGH POTENCY)	
Elocon ointment 0.1%	Mometasone furoate
Florone ointment 0.05%	Diflorasone diacetate
Halog cream 0.1%	Halcinonide
Lidex cream 0.05%	Fluocinonide
Lidex gel 0.05%	Fluocinonide
Lidex ointment 0.05%	Fluocinonide
Topicort cream 0.25%	Desoximetasone
Topicort ointment 0.25%	Desoximetasone
GROUP III (HIGH POTENCY)	
Aristocort cream (HP) 0.5%	Triamcinolone acetonide
Diprosone cream 0.05%	Betamethasone dipropionate
Elocon ointment 0.1%	Mometasone furoate
Florone cream 0.05%	Diflorasone diacetate
Valisone ointment 0.1%	Betamethasone valerate
GROUP IV (MEDIUM POTENCY)	
Cutivate cream 0.05%	Fluticasone propionate
Elocon cream 0.1%	Mometasone furoate
Halog ointment 0.025%	Halcinonide
Kenalog cream 0.1%	Triamcinolone acetonide
Synalar cream 0.2%	Fluocinolone acetonide
Synalar ointment 0.025%	Fluocinolone acetonide
Westcort ointment 0.2%	Hydrocortisone valerate
GROUP V (MEDIUM POTENCY)	
Aclovate ointment 0.05%	Aclometasone dipropionate
Diprosone lotion 0.05%	Betamethasone dipropionate
Kenalog lotion 0.1%	Triamcinolone acetonide
Locoid cream 0.1%	Hydrocortisone butyrate
Synalar cream 0.025%	Fluocinolone acetonide
Valisone cream 0.1%	Betamethasone valerate
Westcort cream 0.2%	Hydrocortisone valerate
GROUP VI (MEDIUM POTENCY)	
Aristocort cream 0.1%	Triamcinolone acetonide
Synalar solution 0.05%	Fluocinolone acetonide
Synalar cream 0.01%	Fluocinolone acetonide
Valisone lotion 0.05%	Betamethasone valerate
GROUP VII (LOW POTENCY)	
Hytone cream 1%	Hydrocortisone

Adapted from Sloan, K., Araujo, O.E., & Flowers, F.P. In K.A. Arndt, P.E. Le Boit, J.K. Robinson, & B.U. Wintroub (Eds.). Cutaneous medicine and surgery, vol. 1 (p. 162). Philadelphia: W.B. Saunders.

costeroids have anti-inflammatory, antiproliferative, and antimitotic properties (Katz, 1995).

Topical corticosteroids are available in a variety of strengths and vehicles. They are categorized according to potency. Topical therapy is usually begun with a medium-strength agent. Higher-potency corticosteroids are most often reserved for plaques that are resistant to a weaker corticosteroid or are prescribed for short-term use in a patient with limited areas of involvement. Even with the high-potency agents, complete clearance occurs in only a minority of patients (Stern & Wu, 1996). Less potent steroids should be used for the face and intertriginous areas. By doing so, the risk of side effects is decreased.

Topical steroids are odorless, colorless, and relatively simple to use. The choice of vehicle is very important. Ointments are more potent than creams and provide the best delivery of the medication by acting as an occlusive agent. Ointments, however, have a greasy consistency and may be unpleasant. Creams are more tolerable but less effective. They are the vehicle of choice for intertriginous areas. Lotions penetrate less well but are more practical for hairy areas.

Topical steroids are generally applied twice a day. Use of ultrapotent steroids is limited to 2- to 3-week courses. Occlusive dressings enhance the delivery and increase the effectiveness of topical steroids. In general, however, occlusive dressings should not be used with high-potency steroids.

Side effects of topical steroids increase with the potency, amount, and length of treatment; the risk is also increased if they are used under occlusion. Local side effects, which may be seen after several weeks of treatment, include skin atrophy, telangiectasias, steroid acne, and a rebound worsening after discontinuing use. A rosacea-like syndrome may develop after long-term use of steroids on the face.

Anthralin

The mechanism of action of anthralin is unknown. Anthralin penetrates lesional skin more rapidly than normal skin (Stern & Wu, 1996). The irritation effect of anthralin causes a slight increase in the mitotic index in normal skin. In abnormal skin, continual use decreases proliferation gradually (Silverman et al, 1995). Anthralin should be used only to treat stable plaque psoriasis; the irritation it produces may aggravate erythrodermic and pustular psoriasis.

Anthralin is available in paste, cream, and ointment formulas. The paste allows the most precise application. The ointment and cream are easier to apply, but they may smear and therefore cause irritation of unaffected skin. A significant limitation to the use of anthralin is its staining properties. Staining of the skin and clothing is primarily caused by the oxidation of anthralin. Byproducts of oxidation bind to keratin, stain natural and synthetic fibers, and are increased by alkalis.

Tar Preparations

Tars are the products of the distillation of oil. The main type of tar used in psoriasis therapy is coal tar. Tar preparations have been used for many years as an adjunctive therapy with ultraviolet-B. They are messy and smelly; this limits their acceptability by patients. Tar has been reported to suppress epidermal hyperplasia in psoriasis (Silverman et al, 1995). Well-controlled trials, however, have failed to demonstrate substantial benefits when used as a monotherapy (Stern & Wu, 1996).

Vitamin D₃ Analogues

The identification of a high-affinity receptor in most skin cells for vitamin D has led to both oral and topical use of vitamin D analogues in the treatment of psoriasis. Epidermal keratinocytes produce vitamin D_3, metabolize it to its most active form, and respond with a decrease in proliferation and an increase in differentiation (Kragballe, 1995). Calcipotriene is currently the most promising analogues. The various clinical forms of psoriasis are not equally suitable for calcipotriol therapy. Calcipotriol is marketed for the treatment of plaque psoriasis. A cream and solution are also available. Even though calcipotriol usually decreases plaque thickness, some residual thickness often remains. Therefore, it may be necessary to supplement calcipotriol therapy with another antipsoriatic form of therapy. Skin irritation is the only local side effect noted with calcipotriol therapy. Skin atrophy and photosensitization have not been reported (Kragballe, 1995). Calcipotriol and the other topical vitamin D analogues are not teratogenic (Kragballe, 1995), but there are no data from clinical trials among pregnant women. It would be advisable to discontinue calcipotriol therapy if the patient becomes pregnant.

PHOTOTHERAPY AND PHOTOCHEMOTHERAPY

Phototherapy is the use of ultraviolet (UV) radiation to treat skin disorders. Light is absorbed by molecules in the skin, triggering a sequence of photochemical events that may alter the structure and function of the skin (Stern & Wu, 1996). Sunlight exposure has long been known to improve the symptoms of psoriasis. UVB may be used as a monotherapy or in combination with other therapies. UVA is used with topical or systemic photosensitizers. The use of exogenous photosensitizing agents to enhance the therapeutic effect of UV radiation is termed photochemotherapy.

UVB Phototherapy

The exact therapeutic mechanism of UVB in the treatment of psoriasis is unknown. Individual patient factors should govern the treatment schedules, although numerous protocols exist. Erythemogenic doses of UVB administered at least three times per week appear most effective (Stern & Wu, 1996). A hydrophobic emollient should be applied before each treatment to maximize UVB penetration. Treatments are continued until the lesions are cleared; 25 or more treatments are typically required. UVB maintenance therapy appears to prolong remission after clearing.

Photochemotherapy (PUVA)

PUVA is used to treat severe psoriasis. The mechanism of action is unknown. Treatment consists of oral ingestion of a potent photosensitizer at a constant dosage and variable doses of UVA, depending on the sensitivity of the patient. Treatments are given two or three times a week. In most patients, clearing occurs after 19 to 25 treatments (Christophers & Sterry, 1993). PUVA results in rapid pigmentation of the skin. To protect the eyes, UVA–blocking wraparound glasses should be worn while outdoors 24 hours after the ingestion of the photosensitizing agent. Ophthalmologic examinations should be performed before the initiation of PUVA and at yearly intervals thereafter. Long-term side effects make it necessary to restrict PUVA to patients with widespread and severe psoriasis. A major early side effect is pruritus. Late sequelae include long-term actinic skin damage (solar elastosis, dry and wrinkled skin) and hyper- and hypopigmentation. Skin cancers may also develop. All of these side effects are of considerable importance when deciding whether to begin PUVA therapy.

SYSTEMIC THERAPY

Systemic therapy can produce substantial to complete clearance of psoriatic lesions and psoriatic arthritis. Side effects of and contraindications to systemic therapy must be carefully considered before prescribing it. This type of therapy is most often reserved for refractory or severe cases of psoriasis.

Systemic Corticosteroids

The mechanism of action is thought to be anti-inflammatory. Dosages between 40 and 60 mg/day have resulted in improvement (Christophers & Sterry, 1993). Despite a transient relief of symptoms, systemic corticosteroid therapy is often followed by a severe flare of disease.

Methotrexate

Methotrexate is known to inhibit DNA synthesis and is thought to act directly on the rapidly dividing epidermal cells in psoriatic lesions (Christophers & Sterry, 1993). Because of the possible severe systemic side effects, methotrexate should not be given to anyone with significant renal or liver function abnormalities or to those who ingest excessive amounts of alcohol. Because of the risk of hepatotoxicity, a baseline liver biopsy should be obtained and repeated after each additional 1 g of medication. Methotrexate is given as a weekly oral, intravenous, or intramuscular dose or as a weekly divided dose over 24 hours (Stern & Wu, 1996). Salicylates and nonsteroidal anti-inflammatory agents interact with methotrexate by decreasing its renal excretion, and the result is an increase in methotrexate toxicity. Co-trimoxazole (Bactrim) should also be avoided while taking methotrexate because of an increased risk of myelosuppression and severe pancytopenia. The most common side effects of methotrexate therapy include malaise, headache, nausea, and anorexia. Stomatitis, diarrhea, and myelosuppression suggest acute toxicity to the rapidly proliferating cells of the gastrointestinal mucosa and bone marrow (Stern & Wu, 1996). Chronic hepatotoxicity is the most serious complication of long-term therapy and therefore warrants serial liver biopsies.

Retinoids

The retinoids are a group of compounds that include vitamin A and its derivatives. Etretinate and acitretin have been the focus of investigation in the treatment of psoriasis. The exact mechanism of action is unclear; however, etretinate suppresses DNA synthesis in psoriatic epidermis (Stern & Wu, 1996). Severe hyperlipidemia, active or recent hepatitis, pregnancy, and the inability or unwillingness to use long-term contraception are contraindications to retinoid therapy. A serum pregnancy test, lipid levels, and liver function tests should be obtained before initiation of therapy and monitored throughout. Side effects include cheilitis, generalized pruritus, dryness of the skin with erythema, and loss of the stratum corneum on the soles and palms, which leads to soreness in these areas (Christophers & Sterry, 1993). Continued therapy maintains the beneficial effect of etretinate; relapses usually occur when treatment is stopped (Christophers & Sterry, 1993).

COMBINATION THERAPIES

The goal of combination therapy is to maximize the efficacy and minimize the toxicity of the various therapies. Combination therapy is indicated for patients with severe recalcitrant psoriasis and should be prescribed with caution.

PITYRIASIS ROSEA

Pityriasis rosea is an acute inflammatory eruption of unknown etiology. It is self-limiting and often begins with a single isolated scaly plaque (referred to as the herald patch), followed by a generalized, usually symmetrical papulosquamous eruption (Color Plates 5a,b).

Pathology, Etiology, and Epidemiology

Although the etiology of pityriasis rosea is unknown, it has often been suggested, but never proven, that it is of viral origin. Women may have a slightly higher risk of developing the disease, but no racial or ethnic predisposition has been documented (Gonzalez, 1996).

Diagnosis and Clinical Presentation

Typical cases of pityriasis rosea can be recognized during the skin examination. Rarely is it necessary to confirm the diagnosis histologically. Ten medications have been proposed as causing pityriasis rosea-like eruptions:

- Captopril
- Arsenicals
- Bismuth
- Tripelennamine HCl
- Methoxypromazine
- Barbiturates
- Clonidine
- Metronidazole
- Gold
- Bacille Calmette-Guerin (BCG) vaccine.

The initial herald patch can appear anywhere on the body. It presents as a round, scaling, erythematous plaque. It may precede secondary lesions by 2 to 21 days (Gonzalez, 1996) and therefore is often not noticed by the patient.

Secondary lesions usually appear in crops on the trunk and proximal extremities. Typically they present as round or oval papular lesions of various sizes with a rim of fine scales (Arndt et al, 1995). The face, neck, and distal extremities are usually not affected. The long axes of the secondary lesions tend to parallel skin tension lines, producing a "Christmas tree" pattern of the rash (Emmons et al, 1997). By the time the patient is seen by a provider, it is common to see lesions in various stages.

Treatment Options, Expected Outcomes, Comprehensive Management

Most patients do not require any treatment. Spontaneous remission can occur with 6 to 10 weeks of the onset of the eruption. There are no permanent sequelae associated with pityriasis rosea.

Treatment is mainly symptomatic. Pruritus may be associated with this eruption but it is not a common feature. Antipruritic lotions (eg, Sarna lotion) and emollients can be used as often as necessary to help alleviate any pruritus. Oral antihistamines may even be prescribed. A medium-potency topical corticosteroid is useful to relieve the pruritus and to hasten any mild inflammation associated with the eruption.

Phototherapy has been proven effective in controlling the symptoms associated with this eruption, as well as inducing a faster remission (Gonzalez, 1996). It should, however, be reserved for patients with extensive or severe inflammatory variations.

A significant differential diagnostic consideration includes secondary syphilis. Therefore, a serologic test for syphilis should always be considered.

SEBORRHEIC DERMATITIS

Seborrheic dermatitis is an inflammatory disorder of unknown etiology that occurs primarily in areas of the skin rich in sebaceous glands. Initially, it appears as simple dandruff.

Anatomy, Physiology, Pathology

PATHOLOGY

The cause of seborrheic dermatitis remains unknown. However, a connection with *Pityrosporum ovale* (a lipophilic yeast) has been demonstrated by producing a favorable clinical response in certain lesions with topical antiyeast agents (Krenek & Gosen, 1996).

Epidemiology

Seborrheic dermatitis has a bimodal age distribution (Cropley, 1996): it is seen in early infancy and in adulthood. In infancy both boys and girls are affected equally; cradle cap is a form of seborrheic dermatitis. However, in adults, seborrheic dermatitis occurs more often in men than women. It is a common manifestation in persons with HIV infection or Parkinson's disease or other underlying central nervous system disorders (Krenek & Rosen, 1996). Exacerbations are common during the winter.

Diagnosis and Clinical Presentation

Seborrheic dermatitis is a papulosquamous disorder characterized by superficial white to yellow, greasy scales on an erythematous base (Color Plates 6a,b). Sebaceous gland-rich areas of the skin are typically affected (scalp, eyebrows, eyelids, nasolabial creases, ears, and sternum). The axillae, inframammary creases, umbilicus, groin, and gluteal creases may also be affected.

Pruritus of the scalp is a common manifestation of seborrheic dermatitis. Patients with facial or other areas of involvement may complain of an irritated or burning type of discomfort as opposed to pruritus (Cropley, 1996). Secondary impetigo caused by *S. aureus* or *Streptococcus* is common and will usually manifest with crusting or exudation. Severe cases of seborrheic dermatitis may be difficult to distinguish from psoriasis; therefore, the term sebopsoriasis is used.

Treatment Options, Expected Outcomes, Comprehensive Management

Treatment of seborrheic dermatitis is aimed at loosening and removing the scales with keratolytics and shampoos. Daily shampooing of the scalp, face, and other areas of involvement with one of the antidandruff shampoos containing salicylic acid and sulfur, selenium sulfide, zinc pyrithione, coal tar, or ketoconazole is recommended. For maximum effectiveness, the shampoo should be left in direct contact with the skin for at least 5 minutes. Alternating the use of two different types of shampoos may produce a more sustained result. Ketoconazole shampoo is available by prescription only, and therefore the cost may be offset if the patient has insurance.

Topical steroids are used to decrease the erythema, scaling, and pruritus associated with this condition. For the face, groin, and skinfold areas, a mild topical steroid cream or lotion is recommended. Higher-potency topical steroids are relatively safe for use on the trunk. Mid- to high-potency steroid solutions should be used for the scalp. The solution should first be applied onto the fingertips and then massaged directly into the affected areas of the scalp. All topical steroids are prescribed for twice-a-day use.

Topical antifungal agents such as ketoconazole 2% cream can be used to inhibit colonization by yeast at sites prone to steroid-induced side effects (face, groin, and skinfolds). Application should be twice a day in conjunction with topical steroid use or alone.

Systemic antibiotic therapy should be prescribed in cases of secondary infection. Before initiating the antibiotic therapy, a bacterial culture should be obtained. The patient should start taking the oral antibiotics while culture results are pending.

Patients must understand that all treatments available are used to control this chronic condition, not to cure it. Using topical antifungal medications alone should result in an improvement of the scaling, erythema, and pruritus, but it will be more gradual.

CONTACT DERMATITIS

Contact dermatitis is an inflammatory reaction in the skin arising from direct contact with an external agent. The causative agent is either a primary irritant or a contact allergen (Krenek & Rosen, 1996). Therefore, contact dermatitis can be divided into two categories: irritant contact dermatitis and allergic contact dermatitis (Color Plates 7, 8).

Irritant Contact Dermatitis

Acute irritant contact dermatitis results from direct exposure to an exogenous agent that has the ability to cause injury to the skin at the site of contact (Nethercott, 1996). The severity of the reaction is usually dependent on the integrity and thickness of the skin involved, as well as the concentration of the irritant. Previous exposure to an irritant is not necessary for a reaction to occur. Nonreactive chemicals may produce an injurious effect with adequate exposure over time (Krenek & Rosen, 1996). The onset of symptoms can occur anywhere from minutes to hours after exposure.

The reaction that the patient experiences can range from a well-demarcated erythema to erythematous scaling patches with indistinct borders and possibly some microvesiculation (Nethercott, 1996). Patients usually complain of itching, fissuring, and tenderness of the affected area. Simple handwashing may be enough to cause extreme discomfort.

Irritant contact dermatitis accounts for approximately 80% of all reported contact dermatitis cases (Emmons et al, 1997). Because the work environment is often a source of exposure, a patient's occupational history is of importance. Some of the substances that can cause irritant reactions include harsh chemicals such as soap, detergents, solvents, cleaning solutions, and insecticides.

Treatment of irritant contact dermatitis requires limiting exposure to the irritant. This may be accomplished by avoiding the irritant altogether or by using personal protective equipment such as gloves, aprons, and gauntlets (Nethercott, 1996). The use of emollient lotions (eg, Eucerin or Moisturel) may prevent skin damage from repeated contact with mild irritants. Topical steroid therapy serves a useful but limited role in treatment. Medium- to high-potency topical corticosteroid ointments prescribed for twice-daily application will help decrease local inflammation and pruritus and may serve as an emollient. However, chronic use of topical steroids may contribute to skin fragility, which in turn aggravates the irritant contact reaction. Mainstays of therapy include avoidance of contact with a known irritant, judicious use of topical steroids, and long-term use of emollients. Patients need to modify their skin care habits by avoiding exposure to irritants in general, both at work and at home.

Allergic Contact Dermatitis

Allergic contact dermatitis is an example of a delayed hypersensitivity reaction in which an allergen comes into contact with previously sensitized skin (Cruz, 1996). The patient may have been exposed to an allergen for many years before developing a reaction. Some of the more common causes of allergic contact dermatitis include nickel sulfate, thiomerosal, neomycin sulfate, formaldehyde, P-phenylenediamine, and toxicodendrons (Nethercott, 1996).

In allergic contact dermatitis, the patient presents with erythematous, edematous papules or plaques with distinct borders (Nethercott, 1996). Vesicles or bullae are also present. The skin manifestations are not caused by a direct injurious effect, as with irritant contact dermatitis; rather, they are the result of a delayed hypersensitivity reaction. Therefore, symptoms occur hours to days after exposure.

Nickel is the most common cause of an allergic metal dermatitis. It is commonly found in nickel-plated instruments or jewelry, including earrings, necklaces, bracelets, rings, wristwatches, clasps, and jeans buttons. Neomycin sulfate is a commonly used over-the-counter topical antibiotic. Formaldehyde is commonly found in permanent-press clothing. P-phenylenediamine is commonly found in semipermanent hair dyes.

Toxicodendron dermatitis results from contact with plants of the genus *Rhus* (poison ivy, poison oak, and poison sumac). The dermatitis is caused from contact with the plant oil. The rash generally appears within 24 to 48 hours after exposure to the allergen. Extreme pruritus may be the first sign, followed by the development of erythematous papules, vesicles, or bullae. The classic configuration of this type of reaction is linear, which most likely represents the brushing of the skin against the plant leaves or possibly the transfer of the allergen via the fingernails or clothing. It is important to inform patients that once the plant oil allergen has been washed off the body and clothing, there is usually no further spreading of the dermatitis. In addition, the fluid in the vesicles or bullae does not contain the allergen; therefore, new lesions will not develop if they rupture.

Treatment for allergic contact dermatitis should be based on the extent of involvement, severity of the reaction, and amount of discomfort the patient is experiencing. Mid- to high-potency topical steroids can be used with small, localized reactions. If large areas are involved or if new lesions continue to develop, a tapering dose of systemic corticosteroids is warranted.

Oral prednisone is usually given to adults at a dosage of 40 to 60 mg/day for at least 5 days. Once new lesions have stopped developing or the eruption has begun to regress, the prednisone should be tapered by 5 mg every other day. Inadequate duration or dosage of oral prednisone commonly results in a post-treatment flare of the allergic contact dermatitis (Krenek & Rosen, 1996). Patients should be advised to take the prednisone in the morning to decrease steroid-induced insomnia and to simulate endogenous glucocorticoid levels.

Oral antihistamines serve as an adjunct to relieve the pruritus associated with the eruption. Topical diphenhydramine preparations should be avoided because they may precipitate an allergic contact reaction (Krenek & Rosen, 1996). Adjunctive therapy includes open wet dressings with Burow's solution every 2 to 4 hours. Systemic oral antibiotics may be necessary for any evidence of infection.

The diagnosis of contact dermatitis (whether irritant or allergic) may be obvious in some cases and not so obvious in others. A detailed occupational and social history is important. Definitive diagnosis of an allergy to a certain chemical can be established through patch testing. This involves placing a series of suspect allergens in direct contact with the skin for approximately 48 hours. Patients should be referred to a specialist who is experienced with occupational skin disease and is equipped to perform the patch testing.

ATOPIC DERMATITIS

Atopic dermatitis, commonly referred to as eczema, is an intensely pruritic, chronic remitting and often relapsing eczematous dermatitis. It is probably the most common of the papulosquamous scaling disorders (Color Plate 9).

Epidemiology

Atopic dermatitis occurs primarily in infants and children with a personal or family history of allergic disease, which includes asthma, hay fever, or allergic rhinitis (Emmons et al, 1997). Although atopic dermatitis may disappear with time, studies have shown that 60% to 70% of patients will carry it into their adult life (Kristal & Clark, 1996).

Anatomy, Physiology, Pathology

PATHOLOGY

Controversy exists as to whether the inflammation associated with atopic dermatitis is a primary feature of the disorder or whether the histologic findings are produced by the rubbing and scratching associated with this condition. Stimulation of T cells by *S. aureus* has been implicated as one causative factor of the inflammatory response (Kemp & Campbell, 1996).

Clinical Presentation

Pruritus is the predominant symptom of atopic dermatitis. A persistent itch–scratch cycle develops and becomes so habitual that patients are unaware of their constant scratching, even at night (Krenek & Rosen, 1996).

The early changes seen in atopic dermatitis may be erythema and edema. These changes usually develop into scaling, vesiculation, oozing, and crusting. Once the condition becomes chronic, the skin thickens and becomes lichenified. From the inevitable rubbing and scratching, certain areas of skin involvement may become either hypopigmented or hyperpigmented.

Atopic dermatitis can be divided into acute, subacute, and chronic lesions. During the acute phase, the patient has intensely pruritic, erythematous papules or plaques and vesicles that have become excoriated, resulting in exudative drainage. Secondary staphylococcal infections commonly occur in these areas. In the subacute phase no vesicles or exudates are present. The affected skin usually has erythematous, scaling papules and plaques that have been excoriated.

Thickened skin with increased markings is described as lichenified. This typically defines the chronic lesions of atopic dermatitis. Lichenification results secondarily from repeated rubbing and scratching of the skin (Kristal & Clark, 1996).

Associated clinical findings may include dry skin, pigmentary changes (postinflammatory hyperpigmentation or hypopigmentation), Dennie-Morgan fold (a single or double fold in the lower eyelid), and elevated IgE levels (Kristal & Clark, 1996).

The infantile form of atopic dermatitis usually affects the face (including cheeks and forehead), scalp, and extensor surfaces of the extremities. Flexural involvement begins to develop around the age of 2 years, as does involvement of the posterior thighs and buttocks, chest, back, and abdomen (Kristal & Clark, 1996). Atopic dermatitis in adolescents and adults tends to occur in the neck, antecubital and popliteal fossae, ankles, back, and wrists (Kristal & Clark, 1996).

Complications of atopic dermatitis include secondary bacterial infection, increased susceptibility to viral and fungal infections, exfoliative erythroderma (a condition characterized by generalized scaling, erythema, lymphadenopathy, fever, and systemic toxicity), and mental and emotional dysfunction (Kristal & Clark, 1996).

Treatment Options, Expected Outcomes, Comprehensive Management

Therapy should be geared toward the management of acute, subacute, or chronic dermatitis. The goal of treatment is to restore hydration to the skin, recognize and eliminate any trigger factors, and decrease pruritus and inflammation (Kristal & Clark, 1996).

HYDRATION

Hydration is an essential element in the treatment of atopic dermatitis. This can be accomplished by soaking the affected areas (usually the entire body) in water for 15 to 20 minutes at least once per day. The temperature of the water should be comfortable but not too hot. Soap, fragrances, and oils should never be added to the water. A mild soap may be used during the last 2 minutes of the bath but should be applied only to the underarms, groin, buttocks, and feet. Excess water should be removed with a soft towel and the prescribed topical medication (usually a cortisone ointment) should be applied to the affected areas twice daily. White petrolatum or an emollient moisturizer should be applied to the uninvolved skin and can be used as often as desired. It is important to apply the prescribed topical medication to slightly dampened skin. Localized exudative lesions should be soaked in Burow's solution for 20 minutes at least four times per day.

TRIGGER FACTORS

The skin of patients with atopic dermatitis is already very dry and sensitive, thereby making it more susceptible to irritation from soaps, solvents, and fabrics (mostly wool and nylon). Soapless cleansers or mild, neutral pH soaps (eg, Dove, Purpose, Cetaphil) should be used when needed. A second rinse cycle may be necessary when doing laundry so that any residual detergent can be eliminated. Patients should modify their activities to avoid frequent handwashing and exposure to irritants. Surroundings where a constant temperature and humidity are maintained are optimal.

Patients with positive skin tests to environmental allergens should make every effort to avoid exposure to these allergens. Certain foods may cause a flare of dermatitis in some patients. Patients who know they have a sensitivity to certain foods will benefit by the avoidance of these foods. Diets that hasten the resolution of a patient's dermatitis, in conjunction with other therapies, do exist, but they are very restrictive. Patients should be informed of the strict self-discipline and commitment these diets require.

Bacterial, fungal, and viral infections commonly occur in patients with atopic dermatitis and may be a reason for recurrent flares (Kristal & Clark, 1996). *S. aureus* is the most common bacterial infection. A bacterial culture should be obtained from any weeping or crusted lesions to facilitate proper antibiotic therapy. Oral erythromycin, dicloxacillin, or a cephalosporin may be prescribed. Because *S. aureus* has been found to colonize in the nasal passages of patients with atopic dermatitis, topical mupirocin (Bactroban) ointment should be applied twice a day inside both nares (Nishijima et al, 1995).

Mild infections with herpes simplex may require no therapy. Burow's solution may be used to dry out vesicles. Systemic therapy with an antiviral drug should be used in cases of extensive local or widespread infection.

Topical antifungal medications, used twice daily, are usually all that is needed to treat any dermatophyte (fungal) infections. Recalcitrant infections may require oral therapy, and such patients should be referred to a specialist.

ANTIPRURITIC AGENTS

Oral antihistamines are the mainstay of therapy for pruritus, but used alone, without initiating hydration measures, they are of little benefit. However, they will suppress the pruritus by allaying anxiety and allowing the patient to sleep. Wearing loose-fitting cotton clothing may also help with the pruritus.

ANTI-INFLAMMATORY AGENTS

Topical corticosteroids are effective in decreasing the inflammation and pruritus associated with atopic dermatitis. With an acute flare, a mid- to high-potency topical steroid can be ap-

plied to affected areas on the trunk and extremities. A mild topical steroid should be applied to involved areas on the face and skinfolds. As the condition improves, the strength and frequency of application of the topical steroid should be decreased. Ointments and emollient creams provide more of an occlusive response. Whichever agent is used, it should be applied immediately after bathing to maximize the penetration through hydrated skin (Kristal & Clark, 1996). Patients should be monitored closely while using topical corticosteroids in an effort to prevent side effects such as atrophy and depigmentation.

Long-term systemic corticosteroid therapy is not encouraged for the treatment of atopic dermatitis. Short-term, tapering doses of oral prednisone or an intramuscular injection of triamcinolone may suppress an acute flare of atopic dermatitis. This method of treatment, however, should be left up to the discretion of a specialist.

Tar preparations also possess anti-inflammatory properties, but not to the same extent as topical cortisones. They are useful as an adjunctive therapy and may be alternated with the topical application of cortisone, may be applied at the same time to the affected skin, or may even be used in the bath water.

Because of its high content of gamma-linoleic acid, evening primrose oil has been shown to decrease the inflammation and pruritus associated with atopic dermatitis (Arndt et al, 1995). Oral doses of 6 g/day or more may be required.

Once the dermatitis is well controlled, hydration measures with the use of emollients (eg, petrolatum jelly, Aquaphor) should be used for routine skin care.

Both PUVA and UVB have been effective in the treatment of atopic dermatitis (Kristal & Clark, 1996). This type of treatment is usually reserved for patients with chronic and unresponsive disease. Patients must be referred to a specialist for this type of treatment. Acute side effects are phototoxicity; long-term side effects include an increased risk of developing skin cancers.

DERMATOPHYTE INFECTIONS

The majority of superficial fungal infections are caused by dermatophytes. The dematophytic fungi are a group of molds that invade keratinized tissue of the skin, hair, and nails. They are usually restricted to nonliving layers of the epidermis because of their inability to invade viable tissue in an immunocompetent host (Weitzman & Summerbell, 1995). Dermatophytes belong to three genera: *Epidermophyton, Microsporum,* and *Trichophyton.* Species of all three genera are similar in morphology, physiology, and pathogenicity (Elewski, 1996). Dermatophytoses (ringworm) are infections caused by dermatophytes. The classification of dermatophytic infections depends on the anatomic site involved. The word "tinea" is used with an adjective derived from Latin to designate the infected body. The classical lesion associated with tinea infections is a scaly annular patch.

Anatomy, Physiology, Pathology

PATHOLOGY AND ETIOLOGY

An important characteristic of dermatophyte pathogenesis is their ability to become dormant and survive within the environment for years before transmission (Elewski, 1996). Arthroconidia (spores) are the dormant form of dermatophytes. Because of their extracorporeal existence, dermatophytes are able to produce considerable morbidity. Some fungi produce an abundance of infective spores, constantly showering the environment with infected skin scales. Infective spores can be harbored in carpeting, furniture, shower stalls, and linen.

When infective spores come into contact with skin, various changes occur. The cutaneous changes that result from the growth of the fungal colony on the skin occur in three steps: adherence to the skin, invasion into the skin, and disease produced by host factors (Elewski, 1996). Adherence of the fungi and invasion into the keratinized tissue have not been thoroughly investigated.

ADHERENCE TO THE SKIN

Adherence of the fungi to the skin initiates the cascade of events that results in the clinical manifestation of the disease. Theoretically, the more readily the organism is able to adhere to the skin, the more likely it is that an infection will follow.

INVASION

For clinical dermatophytosis to ensue, invasion of the fungal organism into keratinized tissue must occur. "Unique among fungi, dermatophytes have the ability to produce keratinases and digest keratin *in vitro*, and this ability may be a virulence factor" (Elewski, 1996, p. 1050). The difference between dermatophyte hyphae and other common cutaneous fungal pathogens is that they may be able to squeeze between epidermal keratinocytes (Elewski, 1996).

HOST FACTORS

Clinical presentations of most cutaneous diseases are usually directly affected by host factors. After a dermatophyte has embedded itself in keratinized tissue, a variety of host factors determine the extent of the disease. Such host factors include the location of the infection, concomitant cutaneous disease, and the integrity of the epidermal surface of the skin. The integrity of the host immune system plays a significant role in restricting dermatophyte growth to keratinized surfaces. With impaired immune function, extensive cutaneous disease, subcutaneous abscesses, and even dissemination may result (Elewski, 1996).

Clinical Presentation

TINEA CAPITIS

Infection of the hair follicles of the scalp is termed tinea capitis. The organisms that have been isolated belong to the genera *Microsporum* and *Trichophyton*. *Trichophyton tonsurans* is the predominant pathogen in the United States (Elewski, 1996). Tinea capitis mostly affects children and is a rare event after puberty.

Three patterns of tinea capitis exist: ectothrix, endothrix, and favus. The location of spore invasion determines the classification. In ectothrix invasion, spores develop inside and outside the hair shaft with subsequent cuticle destruction. In endothrix invasion, the cuticle remains intact and spore formation occurs within the hair shaft. Favus occurs sporadically in Eastern Europe, North Africa, and the Middle East (Elewski, 1996). Scarring alopecia is a common sequela, and both children and adults can be infected.

In general, patchy hair loss, broken hairs, inflammation, and scaling are characteristic findings. A kerion may appear as a pustular folliculitis, causing a deep, boggy, and often painful area of purulence and swelling (Arndt et al, 1995).

TINEA CORPORIS

The trunk and extremities are the areas involved in tinea corporis. This term is also used to describe fungal infections of nonhairy skin. All species of dermatophytes can cause the infection. It is generally more prevalent in hot, humid climates, and the infection can be spread from human to human, animal to human, and soil to human (Elewski, 1996).

The classic lesions of tinea corporis start as erythematous macules or papules that spread outward and form annular scaling patches or plaques. The borders of the lesions are usually sharply circumscribed, scaling, and erythematous. As the lesions spread outward, a central clearing results. Tinea corporis may be mildly pruritic (Color Plate 10).

TINEA CRURIS

Often referred to as jock itch, tinea cruris is the term used for fungal infections involving the groin, including the suprapubic area, perineum, proximal medial thighs, buttocks, and gluteal cleft (Elewski, 1996). Predisposing factors include heat, maceration, and friction. It is more predominant in males and is thought to be associated with sports participation—hence the term jock itch. Pruritus is common and may be intense. Inflamed intertriginous areas rubbing together can cause discomfort, but many eruptions are asymptomatic.

TINEA PEDIS AND TINEA MANUUM

Tinea pedis, more commonly referred to as athlete's foot, is the most common of all fungal infections (Arndt et al, 1995). It is an infection of the plantar surface and toe webs. Dermatophytes that belong to the *Trichophyton* and *Epidermophyton* genera are the more common organisms. Pruritus is a very common symptom but is not always present. Interdigital scaling, crusting, and maceration can be seen predominantly in the fourth and fifth toe spaces. Moist, erosive, and malodorous infections may have a secondary bacterial or yeast component.

Tinea manuum is a fungal infection involving the palmar surfaces and interdigital spaces. Mild erythema with hyperkeratosis and scaling may be seen mainly over the palmar surfaces. Rarely is hand infection ever seen without foot involvement. The most common presentation is unilateral involvement of the hands and involvement of both feet—hence the name "one-hand, two-foot disease."

TINEA UNGUIUM (ONYCHOMYCOSIS)

Fungal infection involving the nail unit is termed tinea unguium or onychomycosis. This tinea is generally caused by dermatophytes that belong to the *Trichophyton* and *Epidermophyton* genera. Tinea unguium is more common in men, and the toenails are more often infected than the fingernails (Elewski, 1996) (Color Plate 11).

Invasion of the nail plate generally results from the nail bed. A white or yellow discoloration of the nail at the free margin or lateral borders is the beginning of the infection. As the infection progresses proximally, the nail may separate from the nail bed and become thickened and distorted, and an accumulation of subungual keratin and debris may result. The subungual keratin and debris may become a site for secondary bacterial infections (Emmons et al, 1997). Destruction of the nail can range from slight to very severe.

Diagnosis

A diagnosis of dermatophyte skin infection begins with a thorough examination of the skin and can be confirmed by direct microscopy or fungal cultures. Histologic diagnosis may be used to confirm unusual cases.

Examination of skin scales, nails, or hair using a microscope is performed by placing two drops of 20% potassium hydroxide, a keratin-clearing agent, directly onto scales, nail, or hair placed on a microscope slide. A cover slip is then applied. The slide should be viewed under low power first and then under high power. Definitive diagnosis is made by visualization of divided, nondistinct fungal hyphae and spores. Species identification is not possible.

In addition to microscopic examination, infection can be confirmed or identified by a fungal culture. Dermatophyte Test Medium is commonly used and contains phenol red, which changes the agar from yellow to bright red when its pH becomes alkaline from byproducts produced by dermatophyte fungi. Once the specimen is inoculated onto the medium, the cap should be loosely placed to provide air, which is required for fungal growth. A minimum of 2 weeks should be allowed for the culture to grow. It is safe to assume that if a color change does occur, it is the result of the presence of dermatophytes. Species identification is possible if the culture is sent to a laboratory for microscopic examination.

Regardless of the method used to confirm dermatophyte infection, the most appropriate site for specimen collection should be chosen. In patients with lesions that have advancing borders, the outer edge of the lesion should be sampled. In vesicular lesions, the roof of the blister generally has the most fungal particles. For nail clippings, the entire thickness of the discolored and thickened nail should be obtained. Debris in the nail bed as proximal as possible to the cuticle generally has the most viable fungi (Elewski, 1996).

Treatment Options, Expected Outcomes, Comprehensive Management

PROPHYLACTIC MEASURES

The development of fungal infections is increased by heat, moisture, and maceration. Intertriginous and interdigital areas should be thoroughly dried after bathing. Well-fitting, nonocclusive shoes are also important in the prevention of fungal infections. Plastic footwear should be avoided. Leather shoes or sandals are preferable. Patients with hyperhidrosis (excessive sweating) should be encouraged to wear absorbent cotton socks. Towels and clothing should be changed and laundered frequently.

SPECIAL CONSIDERATIONS

Most antifungal drugs' mode of action is to interrupt the integrity of the fungal cell membrane. Generally, topical therapy should be effective in the treatment of uncomplicated tinea pedis, tinea corporis, and tinea cruris. The medication prescribed should be applied twice a day and continued until the patient is clinically and mycologically clear of infection.

Systemic therapy is indicated for the treatment of tinea capitis and tinea unguium. Topical therapy may be used as an adjunct. Systemic therapy is also indicated for extensive dermatophytosis and in immunocompromised patients.

Terbinafine (Lamisil) is a fairly new antifungal drug and currently the only oral active fungicidal agent for dermatophytic infections. It has become the drug of choice in the treatment of fungal infections. This drug has an excellent safety profile, but screening blood work should be obtained before the initiation of therapy and again 6 to 12 weeks into therapy.

TINEA CAPITIS

The treatment of choice is ultramicronized griseofulvin (Gris-Peg). It is given twice a day at a dosage of 10 to 15 mg/kg/day for at least 6 weeks, or until cultures are negative. Alternate therapy includes ketoconazole (Nizoral) at a dosage of 200 mg/day for adults and 3.3 mg/kg/day for children. Because of the side effects associated with ketoconazole, it should be used for the treatment of tinea capitis in adults only. Adjunctive therapy includes selenium sulfide shampoo every other day.

TINEA CORPORIS AND TINEA CRURIS

When lesions are few in number and small in size, topical antifungal creams such as clotrimazole, miconazole, oxiconazole, sulconazole, ketoconazole, and terbinafine are usually effective. The cream should be applied twice a day to the affected areas until there is no more clinical evidence of infection. If the lesions are diffuse and cover a large percentage of the body, or if the infection is resistant to topical medication alone, a systemic antifungal drug should be given. A dosage of 250 mg/day of terbinafine for 2 weeks should be adequate. Because dermatophytes thrive in warm, moist, and humid environments, patients should apply a drying powder (eg, Zeasorb) once or twice a day to intertriginous areas.

TINEA MANUUM

Tinea manuum usually coexists with tinea pedis. Topical therapy alone is unlikely to be successful if tinea pedis is also associated. Topical therapy can be started with clotrimazole, miconazole, oxiconazole, sulconazole, ketoconazole, or terbinafine cream twice a day. If the infection does not improve within 2 weeks, oral terbinafine (250 mg/day) should be added to the regimen. Therapy should continue until there is no more clinical evidence of infection (3 to 6 weeks).

TINEA PEDIS

For tinea pedis without any nail involvement, topical therapy alone should suffice. Agents such as miconazole, oxiconazole, sulconazole, and terbinafine should be applied twice daily. Antifungal powders (eg, Tinactin, Zeasorb, or Desenex) may be used as an adjunct and will aid in keeping the interdigital areas dry.

TINEA UNGUIUM (ONYCHOMYCOSIS)

Topical antifungal medications are not effective in treating tinea unguium, but they may prevent the spread of infection (Emmons et al, 1997). If the goal of therapy is to cure the infection, then oral therapy is required. Traditionally, systemic therapy has been less than optimal. Griseofulvin was the first oral agent approved for the treatment of onychomycosis. Because of its poor bioavailability, it had to be given for at least 1 year to be effective. Subsequently, itraconazole and terbinafine have been approved.

Itraconazole can be given in one of two ways. Both regimens have a similar cure rate. The pulse dosage regimen is 400 mg/

day (200 mg b.i.d.) for 1 week per month for 3 or 4 months. The alternative regimen is 200 mg/day for 12 weeks. Because of possible hepatotoxicity, liver function tests are recommended before the initiation of therapy and monthly thereafter.

Since the approval of oral terbinafine, this drug seems to have become the drug of choice for the treatment of onychomycosis. The recommended therapy is 250 mg/day for 6 weeks with fingernail infections and 12 weeks for toenail infections. Patients should be monitored periodically while receiving therapy.

Tinea Versicolor

Tinea versicolor, also known as pityriasis versicolor, is a fungal infection affecting the superficial layers of the stratum corneum caused by the endogenous yeast *Malassezia furfur* (Elewski, 1996).

PATHOLOGY AND ETIOLOGY

M. furfur is a lipophilic yeast present on normal skin. Disease ensues when the fungus changes from the normal yeast form to the mycelial form. Conditions that favor growth and fungus transformation include warm, humid environments. Underlying conditions that may predispose people to infection include hyperhidrosis, systemic corticosteroid therapy, Cushing's syndrome, immunodeficiency, malnutrition, and pregnancy (Elewski, 1996). The presence of dicarbocyclic acids, which are cytotoxic for melanocytes, can explain the hypopigmentation.

Postpubertal healthy people can be afflicted with tinea versicolor. There is no gender or racial discrimination. Most people develop tinea versicolor in the summer.

CLINICAL DESCRIPTION

Patients generally have an asymptomatic rash on the upper trunk, arms, and neck. The lesions are slightly scaly, erythematous, hypopigmented or hyperpigmented patches (Color Plate 12). The face is rarely involved, except in young children. Involved areas do not usually tan in the summer and may become relatively darker in the winter.

DIAGNOSIS

The diagnosis is generally based on the cutaneous changes and confirmed by examination of scales under the microscope with potassium hydroxide. Microscopic examination should reveal numerous short hyphae and clusters of budding yeast cells. Wood's light examination magnifies the pigmentary changes and reveals the extent and margins of involvement more readily. Infected areas may fluoresce gold to orange.

TREATMENT

Topical therapy is generally used for treatment of tinea versicolor. For patients whose disease does not respond to topical therapy or who have severe or extensive involvement, systemic therapy should be considered.

Topical Therapy

The most economical therapy is selenium sulfide shampoo. The patient should apply the shampoo to wet skin from the earlobes to the knees and wrists with an abrasive type of sponge (eg, Buf-Puf) at bedtime to loosen the hyphae. The patient should sleep with it on overnight and in the morning should shower off. In addition, the scalp (and beard, if relevant) should be shampooed for 5 minutes with the selenium sulfide shampoo.

Topical antifungal medications effective against *M. furfur* include the azoles (eg, oxiconazole, sulconazole, ketoconazole). Terbinafine has also been effective when used topically (Elewski, 1996). For the highest cure rate, these medications should be applied twice daily to the entire trunk, upper extremities to the wrists, and lower extremities to the knees.

Patients should be made aware that evidence of the active infection (scaling) will resolve within several days. However, to ensure proper treatment and cure, therapy should be continued for several weeks. The pigmentary changes will resolve much more slowly.

Systemic Therapy

Tinea versicolor does not respond to griseofulvin or terbinafine. Several regimens exist for oral ketoconazole: 400 to 800 mg (each tablet is 200 mg) to be taken at once; 200 mg/day for 5 to 10 days (longer for severe infections); or a pulse dose of 400 mg initially, repeated in 7 days. Oral ketoconazole works best if the patient exercises to the point of sweating 20 to 30 minutes after taking the tablets. Itraconazole can be given at a dosage of 200 mg/day for 5 to 7 days. A single dose of fluconazole (400 mg) has been shown to be effective (Elewski, 1996).

Prophylactic Treatment

Prophylactic treatment may be necessary to avoid recurrent infections. Oral ketoconazole (200 mg) for 3 consecutive days every month or a monthly application of selenium sulfide shampoo has been proven effective.

VIRAL INFECTIONS

Herpes Simplex Virus

Herpes simplex virus (HSV) is a double-stranded DNA virus that affects only humans. There are two types of HSV: type 1, which is usually responsible for nongenital infections, and type 2, which is usually responsible for genital infections. HSV-1 is discussed in this chapter; refer to Chapter 69 for discussion of HSV-2. However, even though it is rare, HSV-1 may be found in genital infections and HSV-2 in nongenital infections.

Anatomy, Physiology, Pathology

PATHOLOGY

Cutaneous HSV infection assumes two distinct forms: the primary infection, which is often painful and disabling, and the recurrent infection, which is less painful and more bothersome and is also known as cold sores or fever blisters. Primary herpes infection develops with the first viral exposure in a seronegative person, most often as a result of direct mucocutaneous contact between infected and noninfected persons (Gulick, 1996). After primary infection, the virus remains latent in sensory ganglia. Recurrent infection develops from reactivation of the latent virus. The recurrent herpetic lesion develops as a consequence of viral conduction and replication via peripheral nerve fibers. Trigger factors associated with recurrent infection include emotional stress, sunburn, menses, fever, systemic infections, and physical trauma (Arndt et al, 1995). Patients with atopic dermatitis, whether the disease is active or not, risk the development of generalized herpes lesions. This condition is termed eczema herpeticum.

EPIDEMIOLOGY

HSV infection is one of the most common viral infections. By the age of 4, approximately 50% of the population has antibodies to HSV, which indicates prior exposure. By age 14 the percentage increases to 60% to 70% (Arndt et al, 1995). A disparity has been found between viral exposure and clinical manifestation of disease (Gulick, 1996). HSV-2 (genital herpes infection) recurs more frequently than HSV-1 (Arndt et al, 1995). Prior infection with one type of HSV does not provide immunity to subsequent infection from the other type.

CLINICAL PRESENTATION

Primary infection manifests approximately 3 to 12 days after exposure to an infected person. In general, it presents as a cluster of small vesicles on an erythematous base. A prodrome of burning, tingling, or pruritus may precede the development of the lesions. Over the course of a few days, the vesicles tend to rupture and a crust develops (Color Plate 13). It can take 1 to 3 weeks for the primary infection to resolve. Involvement ranges from subclinical to severe. Fever, pharyngitis, and lymphadenopathy may be present, along with painful vesicles that can develop into ulcers and may affect the face, lips, tongue, and oral mucosa.

Recurrent infections present in a manner similar to primary infections. Recurrent infections tend to be less severe and lesions heal more quickly (usually 7 to 10 days). Approximately 80% of patients with recurrent infections report a prodrome before the development of the lesions (Arndt et al, 1995).

DIAGNOSIS

Herpes should be suspected whenever a patient presents with vesicles or erosions on mucocutaneous skin. A Tzanck smear or a viral culture of the lesion may be performed to confirm the clinical diagnosis.

TREATMENT OPTIONS, EXPECTED OUTCOMES, COMPREHENSIVE MANAGEMENT

Acyclovir has been the treatment of choice for all forms of HSV infections. Rarely, acyclovir-resistant disease may result, especially in immunocompromised patients, in which case another antiviral drug should be used. Because of its specific uptake and viral enzyme inhibition, acyclovir remains a remarkably safe and active drug with low toxicity. A dosage of 200 mg five times per day for a total of 10 days has been established for the treatment of primary and recurrent HSV. Acyclovir is most effective when begun within 48 hours of prodromal symptoms. It decreases viral shedding and formation of new lesions and promotes more rapid healing. The use of topical acyclovir reduces viral shedding and possibly healing time. It is less effective than oral acyclovir and not recommended for routine primary or recurrent disease (Berger et al, 1990).

The more recently approved topical antiviral agent is penciclovir cream 1%. It should be used as an adjunct to oral therapy and is applied every 2 hours while awake to the affected area for a period of 4 days. The effects are similar to those of topical acyclovir.

Famciclovir (Famvir) and valacyclovir (Valtrex) are the more recently approved oral antiviral agents. Both are analogues of acyclovir intended to provide the same benefits. The advantage of prescribing one of these drugs over acyclovir is cost-effectiveness and ease of ingestion. For primary and recurrent HSV infection, famciclovir should be prescribed at 125 mg twice a day for 5 days, valacyclovir at 500 mg twice a day for 5 days.

For frequent recurrences (more than 6 to 12 per year), suppressive therapy with oral acyclovir is recommended. A dosage of 400 mg twice a day reduces recurrent episodes without significant toxicity over an indefinite period of time (Gulick, 1996). The use of drying agents (eg, benzoyl peroxide gel applied twice daily) for recurrent orofacial HSV may hasten the resolution of the eruption.

Herpes Zoster Virus

PATHOLOGY AND ETIOLOGY

Varicella zoster virus is a double-stranded DNA human herpes virus. The nasopharynx is the site of primary infection. Viremia results from viral replication in the upper respiratory tract. Primary varicella (chickenpox) results from subsequent dissemination to the skin and viscera (Gulick, 1996). During the primary viremia, sensory nerve ganglia become the site of latent varicella zoster virus infection. Secondary varicella zoster virus disease (herpes zoster or shingles) occurs as a result of reactivation of the latent virus.

EPIDEMIOLOGY

Herpes zoster can occur at all ages, but two thirds of patients are over 40 years old (Arndt et al, 1995). Postherpetic neuralgia is usually seen in patients over 60 years old and can be chronic and extremely painful. The interaction between viral and host immune factors plays a significant role in the reactivation of infection. Patients with malignancies have an increased incidence of zoster because of their altered immune system. A study, however, has demonstrated that patients with herpes zoster are no more likely to develop cancer (Gulick, 1996).

CLINICAL PRESENTATION

Zoster lesions are frequently preceded by a mild to severe pre-eruptive itch, tenderness, or pain. The pain may be generalized over an entire nerve segment, localized to part of it, or referred to some other internal organ. An average of 3 to 5 days elapses between the neurologic changes and the eruption. Lesions tend to appear posteriorly and progress anteriorly and peripherally along the dermatome involved. The eruption is almost always unilateral. Erythematous macules, papules, and plaques are the first lesions to appear. Plaques may be scattered irregularly along the dermatomal segment and may even become confluent. Grouped vesicles usually appear within 24 hours (Color Plate 14). In approximately 1 to 2 weeks the vesicles become purulent, crust, and fall off.

DIAGNOSIS

A diagnosis of herpes zoster is usually made from the history and physical examination. To confirm the clinical impression, a Tzanck smear or a viral culture of a vesicle may be performed.

TREATMENT OPTIONS, EXPECTED OUTCOMES, COMPREHENSIVE MANAGEMENT

Management of herpes zoster should include treatment for the acute eruption and any postherpetic neuralgia that may be a consequence.

Acute Management

Acyclovir has always been the gold standard of therapy. The recommended dosage is 800 mg orally five times per day for a total of 7 to 10 days. As with herpes simplex, famciclovir and valacyclovir have also been approved for the treatment of zoster. The advantage of choosing one of these two newer drugs is cost-effectiveness and their decreased dosing schedule, which helps patients maintain the regimen. The dosage for famciclovir is 500 mg orally every 8 hours for 7 days. The dosage for valacyclovir is 1000 mg orally every 8 hours for 7 days. None of the antiviral drugs has been approved for use as suppressive therapy in immunocompetent hosts.

General Measures

- Burow's solution applied four to six times per day may help speed drying of the lesions and removal of the crusts.
- An antibacterial sulfonamide cream (silver sulfadiazine 1%) applied two to four times per day can help prevent secondary bacterial infection and may even reduce discomfort.
- Patients with lesions around the eyes or on the nose should always be referred to an ophthalmologist, preferably within 24 hours.
- Patients should be advised to avoid contact with any immunosuppressed persons and persons who have not had chickenpox (varicella) until all the lesions have crusted over.

Postherpetic Neuralgia

The incidence of postherpetic neuralgia is directly related to age. Patients over 50 years of age are at a greater risk for postherpetic neuralgia (Berger et al, 1990). Various treatments may help relieve postherpetic neuralgia:

- Burow's solution soaks four to six times per day for 20 minutes each
- Capsaicin cream, 0.025%, applied three to five times daily
- An Ace wrap used to cover the area involved (easier with thoracic and extremity involvement)
- Acetaminophen and nonsteroidal anti-inflammatory agents may be adequate for pain relief; codeine may be added if the pain is not alleviated.
- Amitriptyline 25 to 75 mg at bedtime if the pain interrupts the patient's sleep or activities of daily living.

Patients should be referred to an anesthesiologist or a pain clinic for evaluation and treatment.

Molluscum Contagiosum

Molluscum contagiosum virus is an unclassified, common poxvirus that infects the skin and mucous membranes.

Anatomy, Physiology, Pathology

PATHOLOGY

The molluscum contagiosum virus has a propensity to infect follicular epithelium, with the most prominent feature of the lesions being umbilication (Groves, 1996). The disease is generally spread to other people through direct contact. Children with atopic dermatitis tend to be more susceptible to the infection. Genital lesions in adults are more than likely sexually transmitted, whereas children with genital lesions should be carefully evaluated for child abuse. The incubation period of the virus has been estimated to range from 2 weeks to 2 months.

EPIDEMIOLOGY

Molluscum contagiosum occurs throughout the world, and people of all ages are affected. Formerly, the majority of cases were seen in children, but the incidence among sexually active young adults has increased. The severity of the disease is increased in people who are immunocompromised; this is often an indicator of advanced disease.

CLINICAL PRESENTATION

Lesions can occur anywhere on the body and range in number from one to hundreds. Lesions have rarely been reported on the palms and soles (Gottlieb & Myskowski, 1994). The eruption begins with flesh-colored or pearly papules; as they progress they become centrally depressed or umbilicated (Groves, 1996). A white, curd-like core is usually present in the lesion. "Pearly umbilicated papules" is the hallmark description of this disease. Occasionally pruritus or inflammation may be associated with the lesions, but the eruption in general is asymptomatic (Color Plate 15a,b).

DIAGNOSIS

The clinical appearance of the eruption is usually characteristic of the disease. However, in cases of doubt, histologic examination should be used to confirm clinical suspicion. Warts are the lesions that are most often confused with molluscum.

TREATMENT OPTIONS, EXPECTED OUTCOMES, COMPREHENSIVE MANAGEMENT

The lesions of molluscum usually resolve spontaneously in immunocompetent hosts without any sequelae. If treatment is considered necessary, any of the following methods can be used alone or in combination:

- Cryotherapy with liquid nitrogen applied directly to the individual lesions using a cotton wool bud, for a total of 10 to 15 seconds or two 5-second freeze–thaw cycles
- Application of a vesicant such as cantharidin (Cantharone), alone or under occlusion with Blenderm tape, for 2 to 6 hours. This method may cause a severe inflammatory reaction; therefore, it is important to ensure the medication is dry to the touch before allowing the patient to move around or before occluding it with tape so that it does not spread to normal skin. Instruct the patient or parents to leave the medication on for no longer than 6 hours. If the patient is unable to tolerate the medication because of burning or irritation, then the medication should be washed off immediately. Lesions will usually crust and fall off. Cantharidin should not be used around the eyes.
- Pricking the surface of the lesion with a #11 blade or a large needle (18 gauge) and then manually expressing the core will almost guarantee resolution of that lesion. Manual expression can be performed using a comedo extractor or gentle but firm pressure with opposing fingers. A sharp curet may also be used to remove lesions. Anesthesia is generally not warranted.
- Topical b.i.d. applications of tretinoin (Retin-A) can be used in recurrent cases. The strongest dose that does not cause irritation to the patient should be used.

Adults with extensive lesions outside the genital area should be evaluated for immunosuppression. Patients should be advised that lesions are sexually transmissible and it is important for their sexual partner to be examined and treated, if necessary.

Because one treatment is usually inadequate, all patients should be seen biweekly until no more lesions are present. A final examination may be done 4 to 6 weeks after the last biweekly visit.

Verruca

Verruca, more commonly known as warts, are caused by infection with the human papillomavirus (HPV). There are four basic types of warts:

- Flat warts (verruca plana)
- Common warts (verruca vulgaris)
- Plantar warts
- Genital warts (condyloma acuminata) (see Chap. 69) (Color Plates 16a–c).

Anatomy, Physiology, Pathology

PATHOLOGY

A number of epithelial diseases are caused by the papillomaviruses. All papillomaviruses are made up of approximately 8000 deoxyribonucleotide bases on each of their two complementary strands of DNA (Androphy et al, 1996). DNA sequencing determines the order of nucleotides. The differences in the specific order of nucleotides are used to distinguish HPV types. HPV types 1, 2, 3, 4, and 7 are the dominant isolates from cutaneous warts.

Papillomaviruses gain access to a host through disruptions of the normal epithelial barrier. HPV infections are confined and therefore do not lead to systemic dissemination of the virus (Androphy et al, 1996). Warts can be spread via direct contact or by autoinoculation. A range of weeks to years can exist between the time of the initial infection to the time of clinically perceptible HPV infection.

EPIDEMIOLOGY

Warts are the most common clinical manifestation of HPV infection. They can occur in people of all ages but are more common between the ages of 12 and 16. Any cutaneous or mucosal epithelial surface can be affected, but the hands, face, feet, legs, and genitalia are the sites most often affected. Men and women are equally affected.

CLINICAL PRESENTATION

Warts are usually asymptomatic and often go unnoticed until they become large or ugly.

Common Warts

Common warts start out small and develop into large, raised hyperkeratotic papules with irregular, spiked scaly surfaces. Paring the lesion back may result in punctate bleeding points because of thrombosed capillaries.

Flat Warts

Flat warts are soft, small, 1- to 4-mm, slightly raised, discrete papules. They are often flesh-colored or tan.

Plantar Warts

Plantar warts are hyperkeratotic, firm, often raised lesions that interrupt the natural skin lines. Blue or black dots, representing thrombosed capillaries, may be apparent without having to pare back the lesion. A callus or corn can be differentiated from a wart because the former does not have the blue-black stippling, and the natural skin lines are not interrupted. The confluence of two or more lesions into one large lesion is called a mosaic wart.

DIAGNOSIS

The diagnosis of verruca is based on the clinical presentation. If there is any doubt, histologic confirmation may be used to substantiate the clinical assumption.

TREATMENT OPTIONS, EXPECTED OUTCOMES, COMPREHENSIVE MANAGEMENT

No ideal therapy exists for warts. They are benign cutaneous growths and therefore treatment should not present any hazards to the patient such as scarring or side effects, if possible. Warts should be treated to decrease any discomfort associated with them and to reduce the risk of transmission. The mainstay of therapy for nongenital warts is cryotherapy and keratolytics (Androphy et al, 1996).

Common Warts

Cryotherapy with liquid nitrogen includes two 5- to 10-second applications with a 30- to 45-second thaw time in between. The ice ball should extend 1 to 2 mm around the lesion. Premedicating with acetaminophen 30 minutes before the procedure improves patient tolerance. A blister should develop within 12 to 24 hours that may be filled with blood. This is not unusual, and the roof should be left intact. The fluid may be drained if the area becomes painful. Follow-up and additional treatment, if necessary, is indicated every 2 to 3 weeks, or when the blister roof falls off. All dead tissue should be pared back before retreating.

Application of keratolytics is a painless method of treatment. Single warts are more likely to be cured than are multiple warts. Use of this method is relatively slow and consistency of treatment is the major factor affecting the response rate. Most keratolytics contain salicylic acid and lactic acid in a flexible collodion (Duofilm, Occlusal) or transdermal system (Trans-Sal). This therapy may be combined with cryotherapy. However, keratolytics should not be applied to any lesions that have previously been treated with liquid nitrogen until all the inflammation has resolved. The proper application of keratolytics is as follows:

- Wash area with soap and water thoroughly. Soak warts in warm water for 5 minutes.
- Rub the surface of the wart gently using an emery board or pumice stone.
- Dry the surface and apply the medication.
- Once the liquid medication has dried, apply a Band-Aid for 24 hours.
- Repeat procedure for at least 6 weeks or until the warts have resolved.

A vesicant such as cantharidin (Cantharone or Verrusol) is a good method of treatment for patients who are unable to tolerate cryotherapy. Lesions are pared back, if necessary, and painted with the solution. Once dry to the touch, occlusive tape (Blenderm) is applied and left on for 24 hours or until the area begins to hurt. The tape is then removed and the area washed off. A blister should form and may be hemorrhagic in appearance. The blister will subsequently break, dry, and desquamate. Treatment may be repeated biweekly for refractory lesions.

Curettage surgery using local anesthesia may be necessary if other methods have not been of any benefit. Lidocaine without epinephrine should be used to anesthetize acral lesions of toes and fingers. Bleeding may be controlled using ferric subsulfate solution or 30% aluminum chloride.

Flat Warts

Flat warts almost universally resolve spontaneously, without treatment, over several months to years (Berger et al, 1990). If treatment is indicated, the following methods can be used:

- Cryotherapy with two 5-second freeze–thaw applications
- Very light and gentle curettage surgery
- Application of a keratolytic paint as described above. The surface of a flat wart does not need to be rubbed with an abrasive before the application.
- Retinoic acid (0.1% cream or 0.25% gel) applied twice daily should cause mild to moderate irritation with subsequent clearing.

Lesions on the face for men, and legs for women, pose a difficult problem because every time the patient shaves, the lesions can spread via autoinoculation. Use of an electric shaver may decrease the spread.

Plantar Warts

Plantar warts are the most difficult to treat. Overaggressive treatment should be avoided because it may result in permanent pain.

Mediplast (40% salicylic acid plaster) or another keratolytic therapy with salicylic and lactic acid, applied daily under occlusion, may lead to gradual resolution. Before the application, the wart should be soaked for 10 to 15 minutes and the surface rubbed with an abrasive device (emery board or pumice stone) to remove any dead tissue. The lesion should be dry before the application of the medication and again before occlusion.

Cryotherapy may produce good results, but not without discomfort during the procedure and subsequently as a result of blister formation. Treatment should be repeated at 2- to 3-week intervals. The lesion is pared back before retreating.

For one or a few lesions, curettage surgery may be the treatment of choice. Local anesthesia is given before the procedure. Aluminum chloride (30%) or ferric subsulfate can be used for hemostasis.

Recurrence of warts is common and does not necessitate a change of therapeutic modalities. However, patients with refractory, difficult, or extensive warts should be referred to a specialist. Therapeutic options may include intralesional DNA inhibitors (bleomycin) or laser ablation.

SKIN CANCER

At some point in their lifetime, approximately 20% of the population will be afflicted with some type of skin cancer (Marghoob, 1997). Screening for skin cancer should become part of the routine physical examination. Patients with any atypical or dysplastic-appearing nevi should be referred to a specialist. In general, three types of skin cancer exist: basal cell carcinoma, squamous cell carcinoma, and malignant melanoma. If caught early, most skin cancers can be easily treated and cured. Actinic keratoses are premalignant lesions caused by excessive sun exposure.

Assessment

The classic mnemonic used while evaluating moles is "the A, B, C, and Ds of moles and melanoma" (A, asymmetrical; B, border irregularity; C, color variation; and D, diameter). A standard of 5 mm has been used as the baseline guide for the normal diameter of a mole (the approximate size of a pencil eraser). However, a lesion should not be considered suspicious for skin cancer based on the diameter alone, unless the mole is extremely large.

Risk Factors

Most skin cancers are related to sun exposure. Other risk factors include:

- Exposure to ionizing radiation
- Exposure to inorganic arsenic
- Certain HPV subtypes
- Scars from old burns
- Chronic ulcerations or sinus tracts
- Impaired immune system
- Personal or family history of skin cancer
- Fair skin, light hair, and light color of eyes
- Sunburns or blistering burns as a child
- Occupational sun exposure.

Anatomy, Physiology, and Pathology

PATHOLOGY

Exposure to UV radiation is the single most predisposing factor in the development of skin cancer (Leshin & White, 1996). The exact mechanism is not clearly understood, but the use of sunscreens has become accepted as standard skin protection.

ACTINIC KERATOSES

Actinic keratoses develop in sun-damaged epidermis and if left untreated may progress from the clinically obvious keratosis to a squamous cell carcinoma.

BASAL CELL CARCINOMAS

Basal cell carcinomas tend to be slow-growing and have an extremely low rate of metastasis. They arise from cells located within the basal layer of the epidermis. There are three major subtypes of basal cell carcinoma: nodular, morpheaform, and superficial.

SQUAMOUS CELL CARCINOMAS

Squamous cell carcinomas tend to grow more rapidly than basal cells and also have a higher rate of metastasis. They arise from atypical epidermal keratinocytes.

MALIGNANT MELANOMA

Melanocytes are mostly located along the interface of the epidermis and dermis and are responsible for the production of pigment melanin. Cutaneous malignant melanoma is caused by malignant transformation of the melanocyte. There are four basic types of malignant melanoma: acral lentiginous, superficial spreading, nodular, and lentigo maligna.

Clinical Presentation

ACTINIC KERATOSES

Actinic keratoses are usually asymptomatic. They appear as flesh-colored or pink, flat or slightly raised, scaly lesions that are well demarcated (Color Plate 17). On palpation they feel rough like sandpaper.

BASAL CELL CARCINOMAS

Basal cell carcinomas usually start out as a nodule, ulcerate in the center, and develop a pearly or waxy border. There may be telangiectasias on the surface of the lesion. Other basal cell carcinomas may present as erythematous scaling plaques that resemble the plaques of psoriasis or eczema. However, these plaques are commonly found in areas of sun-damaged skin. An often-heard complaint during the history is a sore or pimple that won't heal (Color Plate 18).

SQUAMOUS CELL CARCINOMAS

An enlarging, scaling, dome-shaped nodule is the typical appearance of squamous cell tumors. They appear more rough, warty, crusty, and inflamed than do basal cell carcinomas. They may be tender to the touch because of their rapid growth and inflammatory reaction. Subsequent pain and dysesthesia may develop during the later stages of a squamous cell tumor because of local nerve invasion (Color plate 19).

MALIGNANT MELANOMA

Malignant melanoma may appear as a flat or slightly raised pigmented plaque or papule with irregular features. The color may vary from black to brown to blue-black; it may even lack pigment. The lesion may be slightly raised or cause the skin to pucker. Often the patient will report a new lesion or a change in a pre-existing mole. Itching, burning, or pain in a mole should arouse suspicion of possible malignant changes. Malignant melanomas are more friable (fragile and likely to bleed) than are basal cell and squamous cell carcinomas (Color Plate 20).

Diagnosis and Treatment Options

A mole that has changed in size, shape, or appearance, or any other suspicious lesions, should always be biopsied to confirm the diagnosis. Patients should be referred to a specialist for the histologic evaluation and subsequent treatment of any skin cancers. The choice of treatment by the specialist varies and is influenced by various factors, some of which include the histologic type of carcinoma, the diameter and location, and whether the tumor is a primary lesion or a recurrence of a previously treated skin cancer (Marghoob, 1997).

The treatment options include electrodesiccation and curettage, excision, topical fluorouracil (Efudex, Fluoroplex), radiation therapy, cryosurgery, and Mohs' surgery. Treatment should be individualized, with the ultimate goal being total tumor ablation with optimal cosmetic results. Prevention and early detection of skin cancer have the greatest impact on survival.

TEACHING AND SELF-CARE

Sunscreens

The causal relation between UV light and skin cancer has been documented. In addition, continual UVA or UVB exposure increases the rate of skin aging and early wrinkling. Sunscreen products have been developed to deter the harmful effects of the sun's rays. The development of nonmelanoma skin cancer is decreased with the application of UVB–blocking sunscreen (Friedlander & Lowe, 1996).

Sunscreen products may contain one or more chemical or physical protection agents. Chemical blocking agents include para-aminobenzoic acid (PABA), PABA derivatives, salicylates, cinnamates, benzophenones, and dibenzoylmethanes. Physical blocking agents include zinc oxide and titanium dioxide.

When choosing a sunscreen, it is important to select one that screens out both UVA and UVB rays and one in which the Sun Protection Factor (SPF) is adequate. The SPF is a numerical value of the ratio between the time required to produce minimal erythema using a sunscreen product and the time required to produce minimal erythema without using a sunscreen product. For example, if it takes 15 minutes of unprotected sun exposure to produce erythema on a person, then with use of an SPF 30 product it will take 30 times longer to obtain the same erythema (theoretically 450 minutes, or 7.5 hours).

"Water-resistant" implies that the sunscreen is able to maintain its original SPF after two 20-minute immersions. "Waterproof" implies that the sunscreen is able to maintain its original SPF after four 20-minute immersions.

Sunscreen should be applied on dry skin and allowed to dry thoroughly before the skin becomes wet. When perspiration, swimming, or rubbing of the skin occurs, the sunscreen should be reapplied every 2 to 4 hours. PABA-containing sunscreen may cause clothing to stain permanent yellow. Lip protector sunscreens should be included as part of the sun-protection routine (eg, PreSun, Neutrogena). The judicious use of sunscreen is important in preventing HSV-1 outbreaks.

Topical Corticosteroid Therapy

Topical corticosteroids are used to treat a variety of skin disorders ranging from mild to severe. When choosing a topical corticosteroid, it is important to consider the extent of skin involvement, the location of involvement, the nature and chronicity of the condition, and the duration of action desired.

Topical corticosteroids are available in five formulations: ointments, gels, creams, lotions, and solutions. Ointments provide the best occlusion, thereby enhancing penetration of the stratum corneum. They are best prescribed for conditions in which the skin is thick and lichenified, or for diseases that produce thick scales, such as psoriasis. A greasy feeling is the main disadvantage for patients. Creams are more cosmetically acceptable. They are best prescribed for areas of the skin that are sensitive, such as the face, groin, and intertriginous areas. They are less occlusive and more drying, making them an ideal choice for lesions that ooze. Gels, lotions, and solutions are preferred for hairy areas and may even be cooling to the skin.

All topical corticosteroids should be prescribed for twice-daily application and for no longer than 2 weeks (unless the disorder is one of a chronic nature). If long-term corticosteroid use is indicated, low- to medium-potency preparations should be used intermittently as opposed to continuously. High-potency preparations should be used in acute flares of chronic conditions and when the desired effect should be achieved in less than 2 weeks. Weaning patients from high- to lower-potency preparations is also recommended.

The amount of topical corticosteroid to be prescribed depends on the body surface area to be covered. Based on b.i.d. application for 2 weeks, the following amounts are appropriate:

- For face, hands, feet, and groin: 30 g
- For arms: 60 g
- For chest, back, and legs: 120 g
- For entire body: 480 g.

Solutions are usually dispensed in 60-mL amounts. When writing a prescription, it is important to include the name of the medication and the vehicle of choice to be used, the areas of the body the specific medication should be applied to and how often, the duration of application, and the amount to be dispensed with any refills, if necessary.

Despite the benefits that topical corticosteroids produce, there are side effects associated with their use, especially when used for chronic conditions. The most common side effects include atrophy, telangiectasias, striae, purpura, and rosacea. Less common side effects include hypopigmentation, hypertrichosis, steroid acne, and suppression of the hypothalamic–pituitary–adrenal axis. Systemic absorption, although rare, is the cause of such axis suppression. Generally, the higher-potency preparations tend to be responsible. When topical corticosteroids are prescribed and used judiciously, this side effect, as well as others, can generally be avoided.

COMMUNITY RESOURCES

- ACNENET (http://www.derm-infonet.com/acnenet/): General information, social impact of acne, acne treatment, interactive acne questions and answers, links to similar sites
- American Academy of Dermatology (http://www.aad .org): Patient education pamphlets on over 40 skin conditions; P.O. Box 4014, 930 N. Meacham Rd., Schaumburg, IL 60168-4014 (847-330-0230)
- American Society for Dermatologic Surgery (http://www.asds-net.org/index.html): Patient education on popular treatments, skin cancer fact sheet, links to other dermatologic sites; street address same as for the American Academy of Dermatology (847-330-9830 or 1-800-441-2737)
- Dermnet (http://www.dermnet.org.nz/index.html): Library of information on skin conditions; links to sites containing information on skin diseases and conditions, nail diseases, and hair disease; links to other dermatologic sites
- National Institute of Arthritis and Musculoskeletal and Skin Disease (http://www.nih.gov/niams/healthinfo/ psoriasis.html): Psoriasis facts
- National Psoriasis Foundation (http://www.psoriasis .org): General information, announcements, psoriasis therapies, services and publications, psoriasis research, links to similar sites; 6600 S.W. 92nd Ave., Suite 300, Portland, OR 97223 (503-244-7404; fax 503-245-0626)

- New Zealand Dermatology Society Skin Conditions Web Page (http://www.dermnet.org.nz/dnaza.html): Information on over 90 skin conditions.

CLINICAL WARNINGS AND REFERRAL POINTS

Any patient with a condition that does not improve with the recommended treatment within 6 to 8 weeks should be referred to a specialist. UV light therapy for psoriasis can be given only by a specialist. Follow-up with the specialist every 4 to 6 weeks is recommended. If abnormal side effects are reported with any type of treatment, the treatment should be discontinued immediately and the patient referred to a specialist if deemed necessary.

CLINICAL PEARLS

- Use of a well-lit examining room, a magnifying glass, and a pocket penlight will help with the complete examination of the skin. A pocket-sized ruler is also recommended to measure the size of lesions and moles.
- A pocket-sized topical steroid potency ranking table comes in handy when choosing which topical steroid to prescribe.
- Avoid use of ointment-based topical steroids on the face and intertriginous areas.
- Ointment-based topical steroids provide a better emollient effect than do creams, gels, or lotions.
- A thin film of water should be used with the application of cortisone ointments to minimize the amount of ointment used and maximize the area to be covered.
- Proper hydration measures with the use of emollients for routine skin care should be done at least once, if not twice, per day.

EDITOR'S NOTE:
COMPLEMENTARY APPROACHES

A general discussion of complementary approaches can be found in Chapter 3. The following, while not an exhaustive list, are some complementary approaches being used for this condition. Additional information on these approaches, including precautions, can be found in Appendices A and B. Providers need to assess for the use of complementary approaches as part of the patient's history, as they may impact conventional therapies, and patients may not volunteer this information unless specifically asked. Efficacy of many complementary approaches is not as well documented as that of conventional therapies. Providers need to read the literature before suggesting these complementary approaches.

- Vitamins, minerals, herbs, supplements
  Acne
    Zinc
  Dermatoses
    Garlic
    Fish oils
  Melanoma
    Melatonin
  Psoriasis
    Fish oils
- Complementary Modalities
  Psoriasis
    Acupuncture
  Aromatherapy

References

Aizawa, H., Nakada, Y., & Niimura, M. (1995). Androgen status in adolescent women with acne vulgaris. *The Journal of Dermatology, 22*(7), 530–532.

Androphy, E.J., Beutner, K., & Olbricht, S. (1996). Human papillomavirus infection. In K.A. Arndt, P.E. LeBoit, J.K. Robinson, & B.U. Wintroub (Eds.). *Cutaneous medicine and surgery,* vol. 2 (pp. 1100–1122). Philadelphia: W.B. Saunders.

Arndt, K.A. (Ed.). (1995). *Manual of dermatologic therapeutics,* 5th ed. Boston: Little Brown & Company.

Berger, T.G., Elias, P.M., & Wintroub, B.U. (1990). *Manual of therapy for skin diseases.* New York: Churchill Livingstone.

Bergfeld, W.F. (1995). The evaluation and management of acne: Economic considerations. *The Journal of the American Academy of Dermatology, 32*(Suppl. 3), 52–56.

Berson, D.S., & Shalita, A.R. (1995). The treatment of acne: The role of combination therapies. *The Journal of the American Academy of Dermatology, 32*(Suppl. 3), 31–41.

Bulbal, R., Williams, W.V., Schumacher, H.R. (1995). Psoriatic arthritis: Diverse and sometimes highly destructive. *Postgraduate Medicine, 97*(4), 97–108.

Christophers, E., & Kiene, P. (1995). Guttate and plaque psoriasis. In B.H. Thiers, M. Lebwohl, & M. Zanolli (Eds.). *Dermatologic clinics,* vol. 13 (pp. 751–756). Philadelphia: W.B. Saunders.

Christophers, E., & Sterry, W. (1993). Epidermis: Disorders of cell kinetics and differentiation. In T.B. Fitzpatrick, A.Z. Eisen, K. Wolff, I.M. Freedberg, & K.F. Austen (Eds.). *Dermatology in general medicine,* 4th ed., vol. 1 (pp. 489–514). New York: McGraw Hill.

Cropley, T.G. (1996). Seborrheic dermatitis. In K.A. Arndt, P.E. LeBoit, J.K. Robinson, & B.U. Wintroub (Eds.). *Cutaneous medicine and surgery,* vol. 1 (pp. 214–217). Philadelphia: W.B. Saunders.

Cruz, P.D. (1996). Allergic contact dermatitis: Cell-mediated immunity and Langerhans cell biology. In K.A. Arndt, P.E. LeBoit, J.K. Robinson, & B.U. Wintroub (Eds.). *Cutaneous medicine and surgery,* vol. 1 (pp. 167–173). Philadelphia: W.B. Saunders.

Cunliffe, W., & Gollnick, H. (1996). Acne: Sebaceous gland science, clinical description and therapies. In K.A. Arndt, P.E. LeBoit, J.K. Robinson, & B.U. Wintroub (Eds.). *Cutaneous medicine and surgery,* vol. 1 (pp. 461–473). Philadelphia: W.B. Saunders.

Ebling, F.J.C., & Cunliffe, W.J. (1992). Disorders of the sebaceous glands. In R.H. Champion, J.L. Burton, & F.J.C. Ebling (Eds.). *Textbook of dermatology,* 5th ed., vol. 3 (pp. 1699–1744). London: Blackwell Scientific Publications.

Elewski, B.E. (1996). The dermatophytoses. In K.A. Arndt, P.E. LeBoit, J.K. Robinson, & B.U. Wintroub (Eds.). *Cutaneous medicine and surgery,* vol. 2 (pp. 1043–1055). Philadelphia: W.B. Saunders.

Emmons, L., Callahan, P., Gorman, P., & Snyder, M. (1997). Primary care management of common dermatologic disorders in women. *The Journal of Nurse-Midwifery, 42*(3), 228–253.

Fitzpatrick, T.B., & Bernhard, J.D. (1993). The structure of skin lesions and fundamentals of diagnosis. In T.B. Fitzpatrick, A.Z. Eisen, K. Wolff, I.M. Freedberg, & K.F. Austen (Eds.). *Dermatology in general medicine,* 4th ed, vol. 1 (pp. 27–55). New York: McGraw-Hill.

Friedlander, J., & Lowe, N. (1996). Sunscreens. In K.A. Arndt, P.E. LeBoit, J.K. Robinson, & B.U. Wintroub (Eds.). *Cutaneous medicine and surgery,* vol. 1 (pp. 751–757). Philadelphia: W.B. Saunders.

Ginsburg, I.H. (1995). Psychological and psychophysiological aspects of psoriasis. In B.H. Thiers, M. Lebwohl, & M. Zanolli (Eds.). *Dermatologic clinics,* vol. 13 (pp. 793–804). Philadelphia: W.B. Saunders.

Gonzalez, E. (1996). Pityriasis rosea. In K.A. Arndt, P.E. LeBoit, J.K. Robinson, & B.U. Wintroub (Eds.). *Cutaneous medicine and surgery,* vol. 1 (pp. 218–221). Philadelphia: W.B. Saunders.

Gottlieb, S.L., & Myskowski, P.L. (1994). Molluscum contagiosum. *International Journal of Dermatology, 33*(7), 453–461.

Graupe, K., Cunliffe, W.J., Gollnick, H.P.M., & Zaumseil, R.P. (1996). Efficacy and safety of topical azelaic acid (20 percent cream): An overview of results from European clinical trials and experimental reports. *Cutis, 57*(Suppl. 1), 20–35.

Greaves, M.W., & Weinstein, G.D. (1995). Treatment of psoriasis. *N Engl J Med, 332,* 581–588.

Grizzard, D. (1991). Understanding the pathophysiology of psoriasis: A nursing perspective. *Dermatology Nursing, 3,* 305–311.

Groves, R.W. (1996). Poxvirus. In K.A. Arndt, P.E. LeBoit, J.K. Robinson, & B.U. Wintroub (Eds.). *Cutaneous medicine and surgery,* vol. 2 (pp. 1093–1099). Philadelphia: W.B. Saunders.

Gulick, R. (1996). Herpes virus infections. In K.A. Arndt, P.E. LeBoit, J.K. Robinson, & B.U. Wintroub (Eds.). *Cutaneous medicine and surgery,* vol. 2 (pp. 1074–1092). Philadelphia: W.B. Saunders.

Kadunce, D.P., & Krueger, G.G. (1995). Pathogenesis of psoriasis—current concepts. In B.H. Thiers, M. Lebwohl, & M. Zanolli (Eds.). *Dermatologic clinics,* vol. 13 (pp. 723–737). Philadelphia: W.B. Saunders.

Kaminer, M.S., & Gilchrest, B.A. (1995). The many faces of acne. *Journal of the American Academy of Dermatology, 32*(Suppl. 3), 6–14.

Katz, H.I. (1995). Topical corticosteroids. In B.H. Thiers, M. Lebwohl, & M. Zanolli (Eds.). *Dermatologic clinics,* vol. 13 (pp. 805–815). Philadelphia: W.B. Saunders.

Kemp, A.S., & Campbell, D.E. (1996). New perspectives on inflammation in atopic dermatitis. *Journal of Pediatric Child Health, 32*(1), 4–6.

Kragballe, K. (1995). Vitamin D-3 analogues. In B.H. Thiers, M. Lebwohl, & M. Zanolli (Eds.). *Dermatologic clinics,* vol. 13 (pp. 835–839). Philadelphia: W.B. Saunders.

Krenek, G., & Rosen, T. (1996). Eczema: The nuts and bolts of management. *Consultant, 36*(3), 486–506.

Kristal, L., & Clark, R.A.F. (1996). Atopic dermatitis. In K.A. Arndt, P.E. LeBoit, J.K. Robinson, & B.U. Wintroub (Eds.). *Cutaneous medicine and surgery,* vol. 1 (pp. 195–204). Philadelphia: W.B. Saunders.

Leshin, B., & White, L. (1996). Malignant neoplasms of keratinocytes. In K.A. Arndt, P.E. LeBoit, J.K. Robinson, & B.U. Wintroub (Eds.). *Cutaneous medicine and surgery,* vol. 2 (pp. 1378–1440). Philadelphia: W.B. Saunders.

Leyden, J.J. (1995). New understandings of the pathogenesis of acne. *Journal of the American Academy of Dermatology, 32*(Suppl. 3), 15–25.

Lowe, N.J. (Ed.). (1993). *Managing your psoriasis* (pp. 13–16). New York: Mastermedia Limited.

Marghoob, A.A. (1997). Basal and squamous cell carcinomas. *Postgraduate Medicine, 102*(2), 139–159.

Nethercott, J. (1996). Contact dermatitis and occupational dermatology. In K.A. Arndt, P.E. LeBoit, J.K. Robinson, & B.U. Wintroub (Eds.). *Cutaneous medicine and surgery,* vol. 1 (pp. 173–183). Philadelphia: W.B. Saunders.

Nishijima, S., Namura, S., Kawai, S., Hosokawa, H., & Asada, Y. (1995). *Staphylococcus aureus* on hand surface and nasal carriage in patients with atopic dermatitis. *Journal of the American Academy of Dermatology, 32*(4), 677–679.

Silverman, A., Menter, A., & Hairston, J. (1995). Tars and anthralins. In B.H. Thiers, M. Lebwohl, & M. Zanolli (Eds.). *Dermatologic clinics,* vol. 13 (pp. 817–833). Philadelphia: W.B. Saunders.

Stern, R., & Wu, J. (1996). Psoriasis. In K.A. Arndt, P.E. LeBoit, J.K. Robinson, & B.U. Wintroub (Eds.). *Cutaneous medicine and surgery,* vol. 1 (pp. 295–321). Philadelphia: W.B. Saunders.

Strauss, J.S. (1993). Acne vulgaris. In T.B. Fitzpatrick, A.Z. Eisen, K. Wolff, I.M. Freedberg, & K.F. Austen (Eds.). *Dermatology in general medicine,* 4th ed., vol. 1 (pp. 709–726). New York: McGraw-Hill.

Thiboutot, D.M. (1996). An overview of acne and its treatments. *Cutis, 57*(Suppl. 1), 8–12.

Webster, G.F. (1995). Inflammation in acne vulgaris. *Journal of the American Academy of Dermatology, 33*(Suppl. 1), 247–253.

Weitzman, I., & Summerbell, R.C. (1995). The dermatophytes. *Clinical Microbiology Review, 8*(2), 240–259.

Weller, P.A. (1996). Psoriasis. *Medical Journal of Australia, 165,* 216–221.

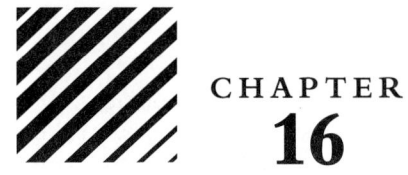

CHAPTER

16

Lyme Disease

Edwin J. Masters, MD

Lyme disease (also called Lyme borreliosis) is a multisystem illness caused by the spirochete *Borrelia burgdorferi*. It is the most prevalent tick-vectored illness in North America and Europe. The dermatologic and neurologic signs and symptoms were first described in Europe in the early 1900s. In the United States the first report of a case of erythema migrans (EM), the characteristic skin manifestation, occurred in Wisconsin in 1969. The broader clinical spectrum of the disease was recognized in the mid-1970s with the occurrence of a cluster of arthritis cases in the lower Connecticut River Valley town of Lyme, for which the disease was named.

Largely because this complex disease is newly recognized and incompletely studied, knowledge of it has had to be continually updated. This has created confusion and controversy. For example, it was first thought that the etiologic agent was a virus until the causative spirochete was discovered (Burgdorfer et al, 1982). Initially, the disease was termed Lyme arthritis, and "no arthritis, no Lyme" was a common dictum. The illness is now known to be more complex, and the name has been changed to Lyme disease. Arthritis is a common, but not necessary, component.

Patients who fulfill the diagnostic criteria are more numerous and geographically widespread than previously thought. Both seronegativity (Dattwyler et al, 1988; Liegner, 1993) and persistent infection after standard antibiotic therapy have been proven (Preac-Mursic et al, 1989). There has been a trend toward longer and more aggressive antibiotic therapy (Rakel, 1997). The *Ixodes dammini* deer tick as a separate tick species no longer exists and has been reclassified back to the more widespread *Ixodes scapularis* (Oliver et al, 1993). Increasing heterogeneity of the spirochetes is now known (Mathiesen et al, 1997), as is the ability of culture media to select or favor certain strains or genotypes (Norris et al, 1997). Failure to obtain a positive culture does not prove absence of infection.

The entire concept of Lyme disease in the lower Midwest and South challenges the prevailing paradigm (Oliver, 1996). Clinically the patients are similar (Masters et al., 1994; Masters & Donnell, 1995), but what to call the condition when the etiologic agent is found to be a related spirochete, but not *B. burgdorferi*, has not be determined. Regardless of the name, these Southern and Midwestern patients with clinical Lyme disease need to be treated (Masters & Donnell, 1996).

The primary care provider's role is paramount in the diagnosis and treatment of Lyme disease, as early diagnosis and treatment translate into better outcomes. The best opportunity for an accurate early diagnosis is the characteristic EM or bull's-eye rash stage (Fig. 16-1; Masters, 1995). The rash, however, may be transient, while the infection can persist and disseminate. Patients may get the rash, make an appointment that is

2 weeks away, and then have the rash fade. Believing they are getting well, patients might cancel the appointment, and an early therapeutic and diagnostic opportunity is missed. The rash is often relatively asymptomatic, and because tick bites on the hands and face are unusual, rarely are they found on a cosmetically sensitive body area. This adds to the lack of awareness by the patient of the seriousness of the condition. If patients with rashes or febrile illnesses after tick bites are not given prompt appointments, preferably within 2 or 3 days, the chances of dissemination, canceled appointments, and missed pathology are all increased.

Researchers and providers are still on the front end of the learning curve for this complicated disease, especially when it is in the late or disseminated phase. Providers can best serve their patients with education, early diagnosis, and effective treatment.

ANATOMY, PHYSIOLOGY, AND PATHOLOGY

Pathology

Lyme disease is transmitted by the bite of a tick infected with the causative spirochete, *B. burgdorferi*. *I. scapularis* ticks are the main vectors in North America. The tick itself may be as small as the period at the end of this sentence. Incubation time from tick attachment to disease onset can range from 1 to 31 days, with the average being about 1 week (Luft et al, 1996). The longer the tick is attached, the greater the likelihood of infection. Ticks that are removed within 24 hours are far less likely to transmit disease (Piesman et al, 1987). Just as most tick activity is in the summer, it is no surprise that June and July have the highest infection rates, although some new cases are reported year-round (CDC, 1997).

Lyme disease can usually be divided into three phases:

1. Early localized: EM rash only, with no other symptoms
2. Early disseminated: Rash plus evidence of spread (eg, fever, headache, lymphadenopathy)
3. Late: Infection has spread sufficiently to cause arthritis, carditis, neurologic involvement, or other late manifestations.

As with other spirochetal diseases, such as syphilis, Lyme borreliosis can have early and late phases and protean clinical manifestations that involve several organ systems. The EM rash involves the skin in about 60% of infected patients. A flu-like illness involving nausea and headache can also occur in the early phase. If untreated, or when treatment failure occurs, Lyme borreliosis can result in the spread of the bacteria to various areas of the body, including the skin, joints, eyes, heart, and

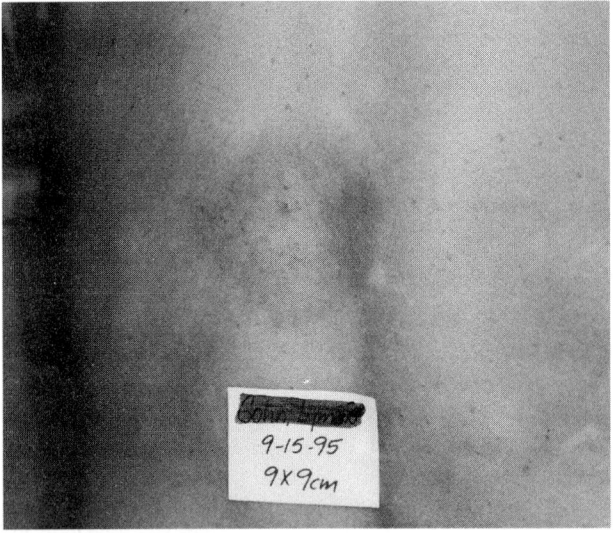

FIGURE 16-1 Classic erythema migrans rash (©Edwin J. Masters, MD).

the central and peripheral nervous systems. A migratory oligoarthritis is common, with the knee being the most common joint affected. The most prevalent neuropathy is a facial or seventh nerve palsy (Bell's palsy). Additional complications can include involvement of other peripheral nerves, radiculoneuropathy, lymphocytic meningitis, acute-onset high-grade (second- or third-degree) heart block, atrioventricular conduction defects, and myocarditis. Less common conditions range from myositis to keratitis.

EPIDEMIOLOGY

Most cases of Lyme disease occur in three generally recognized main endemic foci: the northeast, the north-central, and the far western regions. Hundreds of providers, however, in the Midwest and South have reported patients who fulfill both the surveillance and clinical criteria for diagnosis (CDC, 1997; Masters et al, 1998). Spirochetes have been observed in southern and midwestern ticks (Walker et al, 1996; Barbour et al, 1996; Feir et al, 1994). Studies to determine if these spirochetes are related to human clinical Lyme disease are underway. In the meantime, clinical Lyme disease in the South has been termed Lyme disease, Lyme-like disease (Masters & Donnell, 1995), erythema migrans rash disease (Walker et al, 1996), and Masters' disease (Telford et al, 1997). There is evidence that the clinical differences are negligible because the diagnosis, sequelae, and treatment are similar to those of Lyme disease elsewhere (Masters et al, 1994).

DIAGNOSTIC CRITERIA

Lyme disease is a clinical diagnosis that can be very difficult to confirm because the symptoms and signs may mimic those of other diseases. Great care should be taken to consider and rule out other illnesses. Laboratory tests for Lyme are supportive but are often inaccurate and can give both false-positive and false-negative results. Improved testing is a high research priority. The CDC has developed surveillance case definitions to be used for national reporting of Lyme disease (Table 16-1). These

TABLE 16-1	CDC Clinical Case Definition

CASE CLASSIFICATION

Confirmed: A case that meets one of the following clinical case definitions: Erythema migrans; *or* at least one late manifestation, as defined below, and laboratory confirmation of infection

LATE MANIFESTATIONS

This includes any of the following when an alternate explanation is not found.

Musculoskeletal system	■ Recurrent, brief attacks (weeks or months) of objective joint swelling in one or a few joints, sometimes followed by chronic arthritis in one or a few joints.
	■ Chronic progressive arthritis not preceded by brief attacks, and chronic symmetric polyarthritis, arthralgia, myalgia, or fibromyalgia alone is not a criterion for musculoskeletal involvement.
Nervous system	(any of the following, alone or in combination)
	■ Lymphocytic meningitis; cranial neuritis, particularly facial palsy (may be bilateral)
	■ Radiculoneuropathy; or rarely, encephalomyelitis (must be confirmed by showing antibody production against *B. burgdorferi* in the cerebral spinal fluid [CSF] demonstrated by a higher titer of antibody in CSF than in serum).
	■ Headache, fatigue, paresthesias, or mild stiff neck alone is not a criterion for neurologic involvement.
Cardiovascular system	■ Acute-onset, high-grade atrioventricular conduction defects that resolve in days to weeks and are sometimes associated with myocarditis. Palpitations, bradycardia, bundle branch block, or myocarditis alone is not a criterion for cardiovascular involvement.

LABORATORY CRITERIA FOR DIAGNOSIS

(any one is diagnostic)

■ Isolation of *B. burgdorferi* from clinical specimen

■ Demonstration of diagnostic levels of IgG antibody response to *B. burgdorferi* in paired acute- and convalescent-phase serum samples.

(Adapted from Wharton et al, 1990)

criteria are not designed for clinical diagnosis, but for surveillance. Patients whose disease meets these surveillance criteria should be reported by notifying the local or state health department. Lyme disease is reportable in all 50 states.

HISTORY AND PHYSICAL EXAMINATION

EM, when it is present, is the most specific clinical sign of Lyme disease infection. This rash was formerly called erythema chronicum migrans, but "chronicum" was deleted because the rash is not always chronic. Although the presentation can be variable, the EM rash typically appears as a centrifugally expanding, erythematous annular patch like a bull's eye. It may be accompanied by constitutional symptoms such as fever, headache, neck pain, myalgia, and nausea. Because the primary EM rash usually occurs within 1 to 31 days, with a median of 7 days, after a bite by a tick infected with *B. burgdorferi*, the rash offers an important opportunity for early diagnosis and treatment. The rash itself is minimally symptomatic and fades within a few weeks. In a minority of patients, multiple lesions may occur. In some 40% of cases, the EM rash is altogether absent. Despite this, many investigators consider the presence of the classic EM rash to be pathognomonic and, at a minimum, a marker for the disease. EM alone fulfills the CDC surveillance criteria for the diagnosis of Lyme disease.

Special care must be taken to differentiate Lyme disease from other conditions transmitted or caused by tick and spider bites. Allergic reactions to arthropod or insect bites can usually be differentiated by the early onset (often within hours) and intense itching. A history of similar reactions is also helpful. If patients with frequent tick exposure present with a nonpruritic rash occurring several days, usually a week, after a tick bite and say they have never had a tick bite react this way before, the provider should be suspicious regardless of the rash appearance. Atypical rashes are well documented. Although absent in 40% of cases, EM still offers clinicians the best opportunity for the early diagnosis and treatment of Lyme disease.

Five Diagnostic Steps for Erythema Migrans

1. Request the tick. Although testing of the tick may be difficult or even unnecessary in some geographic locations, it may be extremely helpful in areas where Lyme disease is not prevalent. If the tick has been saved, it can be sent for identification and testing, which are much easier if the tick is still alive. Keep in mind that many patients do not remember getting a tick bite (which is usually painless) and that the absence of a specific history of tick bite does not rule out a diagnosis of Lyme disease. Also, saving the tick might be useful in the event of a coinfection with another tick-borne illness such as ehrlichiosis or babesiosis. Put the tick in a small Ziploc bag with a blade of grass for moisture and save it for 31 days to cover the incubation times. If there is no fever or rash during that time, the probability of a tick-vectored illness is reduced to near zero. This follow-up can also decrease patient anxiety and will often lessen the pressure to treat asymptomatic tick bites prophylactically when the likelihood of infection is low.

2. Save frozen samples of blood and urine from the initial office visit. Do not order serologic testing for Lyme disease at the initial visit because the sensitivity of most tests is poor in the early stages of the disease. Better tests are on the way, however, and the ability to test for Lyme disease retrospectively might clarify a confusing clinical situation in the future. Therefore, take and store blood and urine specimens from each patient. A home freezer is not cold enough to store specimens indefinitely, but it should preserve enough antibodies to aid in a diagnosis for at least 2 years. If you do not have freezer space, give the samples to the patient to save, and note it in the chart. The availability of these specimens might be extremely useful in the future. Both our knowledge base and testing ability are continually changing.

3. Measure and photograph the rash. Good documentation of EM is more helpful in establishing the diagnosis than are any currently available serologic tests. The most potentially effective and convincing instrument used in documenting early Lyme disease at the rash stage is the camera. With a little practice, providers can become adept at photographing skin rashes. A simple 35-mm camera with an automatic zoom lens is satisfactory. For close-ups, covering about half of the flash will help avoid overexposure.

4. Obtain a culture, if possible. Culture of the causative organism is the irrefutable diagnostic procedure for Lyme disease. Specimens are usually obtained with a punch biopsy of the outside edge or advancing margin of the rash. Histologic examination by an experienced pathologist may identify changes consistent with EM.

5. Order serologic tests 4 to 6 weeks later. An ELISA or Western blot at 4 to 6 weeks can reinforce the diagnosis. With a convincing EM rash, serology is not necessary (Sigal, 1997). Remember that both false-positive and false-negative test results can occur. Negative serology, especially early in the disease, does not rule out Lyme borreliosis. Testing with an ELISA and using the Western blot as a second-line or confirmation test is a common and recommended practice (Verdon & Sigal, 1997).

Differentiating Loxoscelism From Lyme Disease

Cutaneous loxoscelism and Lyme disease are not only widespread in the United States, but they are also occurring in new, frequently overlapping geographic areas, raising the possibility of clinical confusion. Painful, necrotic bites from *Loxosceles* spiders, including *Loxosceles reclusa* (the brown recluse spider), are being reported across the country. This is the result of both increased clinical recognition and the spider's spread beyond the central and southern United States, its natural habitats. Both Lyme EM rashes (see Fig. 16-1) and early rashes from brown recluse spider bites (Fig. 16-2) have been described as sometimes having a bull's-eye appearance and have been confused by both patients and providers (Masters & King, 1994; Rosenstein & Kramer, 1987).

The following are distinguishing features of the brown recluse spider bite:

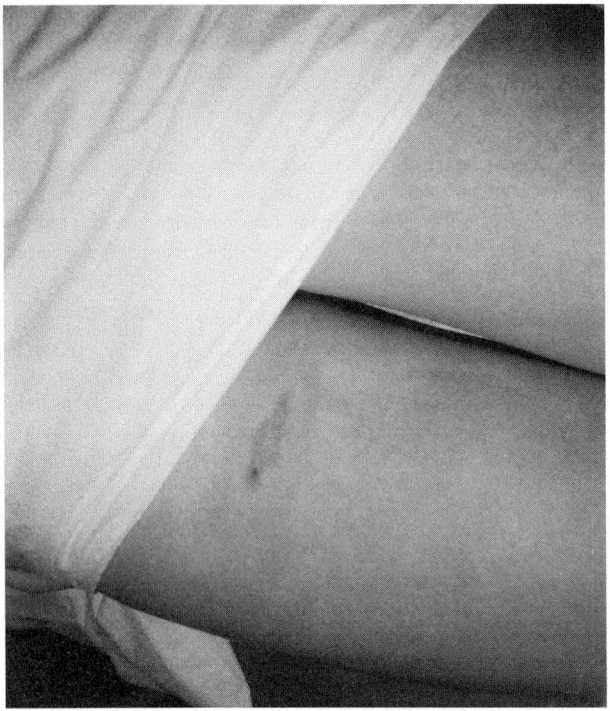

FIGURE 16-2 Brown recluse spider bite (©Edwin J. Masters, MD).

- Nonpruritic rashes appearing within 48 to 72 hours after a presumed arthropod bite are more likely to be caused by *Loxosceles* spiders than a tick. The tick-vectored EM rash usually has a more delayed onset, with an average incubation time of 6 or 7 days.
- The actual brown recluse spider bite site or punctum is usually off center or eccentric in relation to the remaining rash. Tick bite puncta, when visible, are usually at or near the center of the EM rash (see Fig. 16-2).
- Pain, often quite severe, within hours to a few days after the bite, strongly suggests the brown recluse spider. The EM rash of Lyme disease is seldom painful.
- The "red, white, and blue sign" generally appears 24 to 72 hours after a *Loxosceles* spider bite and is characterized by large areas of erythema, smaller areas of ischemia, and even smaller areas of skin necrosis.
- Intense inflammatory reactions from *Loxosceles* bites tend to extend downward from the site in a gravitationally dependent manner, often giving a "runny-egg" appearance.
- Tissue necrosis and prolonged healing are much more likely to be the result of *Loxosceles* envenomation than Lyme disease. Severe brown recluse bites may take weeks or even months to heal, whereas Lyme EM rashes usually

disappear in days or weeks, especially with antibiotic treatment.

Table 16-2 presents the distinguishing signs and symptoms of tick bite versus spider bite.

TREATMENT OPTIONS, EXPECTED OUTCOMES, COMPREHENSIVE MANAGEMENT

It is completely appropriate to treat EM solely on the basis of clinical findings. Various treatment regimens for early Lyme disease have been suggested. Even though early treatment failure occurs in only 5% to 10% of cases, disseminated disease is often devastating. All treatment guidelines for Lyme disease are based on limited data. Evidence of dissemination, dysesthesia, and multiple lesions may require more aggressive or longer therapy. Treatment for Lyme disease is presented in Table 16-3. Research has progressed to the point that Lyme vaccines are being tested.

Treatment of Late Lyme Disease

Clinical judgment is paramount in both diagnosing and treating late Lyme disease. Lyme serologic tests can result in both false-positive and false-negative results. Symptoms can persist even after treatment, and there is no current test of cure. Current treatment recommendations are published and can involve parenteral or intravenous antibiotic therapy. Ceftriaxone and cefotaxime are the most common choices, and the duration of therapy can range from 2 to 4 weeks (Verdon & Sigal, 1997) to 6 or more weeks (Rakel, 1997). The problem of chronic Lyme disease as a postinfectious syndrome, persistent infection, or autoimmune disorder is being studied. Without a consensus on the etiology of this debilitating condition, there is no agreement on treatment.

Teaching and Self-Care

Persons exposed to ticks should perform careful tick checks for early removal of ticks each day. Ticks can be more easily spotted and removed early. Only a very small percentage of ticks that are attached less than 24 hours actually transmit Lyme disease. The sooner a tick is removed, the less likely it is to cause an infection. Tick repellents work but have limitations and should be used carefully according to instructions. If possible, patients should avoid tick-infested endemic areas, especially in the peak months of May, June, and July. They should walk in the center of trails to avoid low vegetation that might harbor questing ticks. Tucking pant legs into socks or boots has also been shown to help. Removing leaves and tall grass from around houses can lower tick populations. Applying chemicals to kill ticks near

TABLE 16-2	Signs and Symptoms of Tick Bite Vs. Spider Bite	
Signs and Symptoms	**Tick Bite**	**Brown Recluse Bite**
Timing of rash	1–31 days (av. 7)	Hours to 3 days
Punctum location	Usually central	Usually eccentric
Pain	Rare	Common (may be severe)
Tissue necrosis	Rare	Common
Gravity-dependant erythema	No	Occasionally in severe cases

TABLE 16-3	Treatment of Lyme Disease

EARLY LOCALIZED PHASE

- Amoxicillin 1 g orally t.i.d., or 500 mg plus probenecid 500 mg orally t.i.d.; treat for ≥3 wk.
- Doxycycline 100 mg orally b.i.d. if <150 lb, t.i.d. if >150 lb; treat for ≥3 wk.
- Cefuroxime, 500 mg b.i.d.; treat for ≥3 wk.
- Azithromycin, 500 mg/day; treat for ≥10 days.

EARLY DISSEMINATED PHASE

- Treat longer with 6 wk of oral antibiotics.
- In severe cases, treat with IV antibiotics: ceftriazone, up to 2 g/day; or cefotaxime, 2 g t.i.d.; or penicillin G 20 M units every 4 hr for 2–6 wk, depending on response.

LATE PHASE

- Treat with IV antibiotics as above.
- IV antibiotics may be followed by 3–6 wk of oral antibiotics.
- Retreatment may be needed.

homes is being done, but again it should be done safely and strictly according to recommendations.

The manifestation of early disseminated and late Lyme disease can affect personal, professional, or social aspects of a patient's life regardless of response to treatment. Varying degrees of fatigue, malaise, memory loss, concentration difficulties, anxiety, and depression often accompany dissemination and neurologic involvement. The altered ability to perform daily activities, from simple tasks to work duties, because of the disease process or refractory infection can further compromise a patient's well-being. The primary care provider must recognize and address the possible complications of Lyme disease and their potential effects on the patient.

Management should be aimed at individualized and comprehensive care. A multidisciplinary approach may be indicated. Information on available support groups and psychological counseling if indicated should be provided. Patient education regarding the manifestations of the disease, along with continued reassurance that the symptoms are related to the disease process, is necessary. Patients should be encouraged to verbalize their concerns, maintain involvement in their care, and seek family support. Recommended self-care measures should include open communication and interaction with health care providers; adequate nutrition, exercise, and sleep; and stress management.

Tick Removal

Ticks should be removed as early as possible using a pair of tweezers or one of the commercially available tick-removal devices. Grasp the tick as close to the skin as possible and pull gently upward. Do not squeeze the body of the tick. Do not use a match, petroleum jelly, kerosene, or so forth; these methods are not effective in preventing spirochete transmission. Save the tick in a Ziploc bag with a blade of grass for 1 month. Having the tick might aid in the diagnosis should the person become ill.

COMMUNITY RESOURCES

- Lyme Disease Information Resource: http://www.sky.net/dporter/lyme1.html

- Lyme Disease Network: http://www.lymenet.org/Internet.
- American On Lyme: http://members.aol.com/ameronlyme/aolyme.htmlInternet.
- Lyme Disease Homepage, University of Connecticut: http://www.ycc.uconn.edu/wwwlymr/geninfo.html
- Lyme Disease Foundation, 1 Hartford Plaza, 18th Floor, Hartford, CT 06103 (1-860-525-2000)
- National Hotline Phone: 1-800-886-LYME
- American Lyme Disease Foundation, Inc., Mill Pond Offices, 293 Route 100, Suite 204, Somers, NY 10589 (914-277-6970, 1-800-886-LYME)

CLINICAL WARNINGS AND REFERRAL POINTS

- Treatment failure: Because this is a multisystem illness, depending on the host's immune response referral will be based on the most dominant presentation. Additional referrals may be necessary with subsequent system presentations.
- Complicating factors, such as pre-existing or coexisting conditions, also necessitate referral.

■ ■ ■ CLINICAL PEARLS

- EM, although absent in 40% of cases, offers the best opportunity for early diagnosis and treatment of Lyme disease. It is more helpful in establishing the diagnosis than any currently available serologic tests.
- The absence of a specific history of tick bite does not rule out a diagnosis of Lyme disease.
- If there is no fever or rash during the 30-day incubation period, the probability of a tick-vectored illness is reduced to near zero.
- The most effective and convincing instrument used in documenting early Lyme disease at the rash stage is the camera.
- It is completely appropriate to treat EM solely on the basis of clinical findings.

EDITOR'S NOTE:
COMPLEMENTARY APPROACHES

A general discussion of complementary approaches can be found in Chapter 3. The following, while not an exhaustive list, are some complementary approaches being used for this condition. Additional information on these approaches, including precautions, can be found in Appendices A and B. Providers need to assess for the use of complementary approaches as part of the patient's history, as they may impact conventional therapies, and patients may not volunteer this information unless specifically asked. Efficacy of many complementary approaches is not as well documented as that of conventional therapies. Providers need to read the literature before suggesting these complementary approaches.

- Complementary Modalities
    Massage Therapy

References

Barbour, A., Maupin, G., Teltow, G., et al. (1996). Identification of an uncultivable *Borrelia* species in the hard tick *Amblyomma americanum*: Possible agent of a Lyme disease-like illness. *Journal of Infectious Disease, 173*, 403–409.

Burgdorfer, W., Barbour, A., Hayes, S., Benach, J., Grunwaldt, E., & Davis, J. (1982). Lyme disease: A tick-borne spirochetosis? *Science, 216*, 1317–1319.

Centers for Disease Control. (1997). Lyme disease—United States, 1996. *MMWR, 46*(23), 531–535.

Dattwyler, R., Volkman, D., Luft, B., et al. (1988). Seronegative Lyme disease. *N Engl J Med, 319* (22), 1441–1446.

Feir, D., Santanello, C., Li, B., et al. (1994). Evidence supporting the presence of *Borrelia burgdorferi* in Missouri. *American Journal of Tropical Medicine and Hygiene, 51*, 475–482.

Liegner, K. (1993). Lyme disease: The sensible pursuit of answers [guest commentary]. *Journal of Clinical Microbiology, 31*(8), 1961–1963.

Luft, B., Dattwyler, R., Johnson, R., et al. (1996). Azithromycin compared with amoxicillin in the treatment of erythema migrans. *Annals of Internal Medicine, 124*, 785–791.

Masters, E. (1995). Erythema migrans rash as key to early diagnosis of Lyme disease. *Postgraduate Medicine, 94*, 133–142.

Masters, E., & Donnell, H. (1995). Lyme and/or Lyme-like disease in Missouri. *Missouri Medicine*, 345–353.

Masters, E., & Donnell, H. (1996). Epidemiologic and diagnostic studies of patients with suspected early Lyme disease, Missouri, 1990–1993 [letter]. *Journal of Infectious Disease, 173*, 1527–1528.

Masters, E., Donnell, H., & Fobbs, M. (1994). Missouri Lyme disease: 1989 through 1992. *Journal of Spirochetal and Tick-borne Disease, 1*, 12–17.

Masters, E., Granter, S., Duvay, P., et al. (1998). Physician-diagnosed erythema migrans and erythema migrans-like rashes following Lone Star tick bites. *Archives of Dermatology*, Vol. 134.

Masters, E., & King, L. (1994). Differentiating loxoscelism from Lyme disease. *Emergency Medicine, 26*(10), 46–49.

Mathiesen, D., Oliver, J., Kolbert, C. et al. (1997). Genetic heterogeneity of *Borrelia burgdorferi* in the United States. *Journal of Infectious Disease, 175*, 98–107.

Norris, D., Johnson, B., Piesman, J., et al. (1997). Culturing selects for specific genotypes of *Borrelia burgdorferi* in an enzootic cycle in Colorado. *Journal of Clinical Microbiology, 35*(9), 2359–2364.

Oliver, J. (1996). Lyme borreliosis in the southern United States: A review. *Journal of Parasitology, 82*(6), 926–935.

Oliver, J., Owsley, M., Hutcheson, J., et al. (1993). Conspecificity of the ticks *I. scapularis* and *I. dammini* (Acari: Ixodidae). *Journal of Medical Entomology, 30*(1), 54–63.

Piesman, J., Mather, T., Sinsky, R., & Spielman, A. (1987). Duration of tick attachment and *Borrelia burgdorferi* transmission. *Journal of Clinical Microbiology, 25*, 557–558.

Preac-Mursic, V., Weber, W., Pfister, W., et al. (1989). Survival of *Borrelia burgdorferi* in antibiotically treated patients with Lyme borreliosis. *Infection, 17*, 355–359.

Rakel, R. (1997). Lyme disease, method of J. Burrascano. In *Conn's current therapy*. Philadelphia: W.B. Saunders, pp. 140–143.

Rosenstein, E., & Kramer, N. (1987). Lyme disease misdiagnosed as a brown recluse spider bite [letter]. *Annals of Internal Medicine, 107*, 782.

Sigal, L. (1997). Myths and facts about Lyme disease. *Cleveland Clinic Journal of Medicine, 54*(4), 203–209.

Telford, S., Dawson, J., & Halupka, D. (1997). Emergence of tick-borne diseases. *Science and Medicine*, March/April, 24–33.

Verdon, M., & Sigal, L. (1997). Recognition and management of Lyme disease. *American Family Physician, 56*, 427–435.

Walker, D., Barbour. A., Oliver, J., et al. (1996). Emerging bacterial zoonotic and vector-borne diseases (special communication). *JAMA, 275*, 463–469.

Wharton, M., Chorba, T.L., Vogt, R.L., Morse, D.L., Buehler, J.W. (1990). Case definitions for public health surveillance. *MMWR Morb Mortal Wkly Rep* 39(RR-13):19-21.

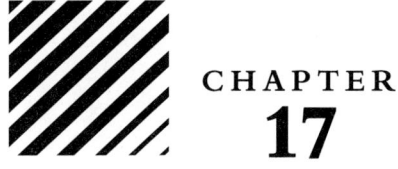

CHAPTER
17

Diabetes Mellitus

Carol Green-Hernandez, PhD, ANP/FNP-C

Diabetes mellitus is a disorder of endocrine function that affects metabolic and circulatory mechanisms. As a chronic disease, diabetes mellitus is characterized by glucose intolerance and distortions in fat metabolism, caused by either relative or absolute insulin deficiency. These two kinds of insulin deficiency are used to categorize the two primary variants of diabetes: type 1 (formerly called insulin-dependent diabetes [IDDM]) and type 2 (formerly called non-insulin-dependent diabetes [NIDDM]). This chapter will discuss each disease variant and current management strategies. Screening for and diagnosis of gestational diabetes is discussed within the context of type 2 disease; pregnancy management will not be covered, as it falls outside the parameters of this text. Screening, diagnosis, and management of other types of diabetes are also beyond the scope of this chapter, so their diagnosis and management will not be discussed. These include diabetes that occurs because of genetic defects of the beta cell; other genetic syndromes associated with diabetes (such as Down, Klinefelter, and Turner syndromes); immune-mediated diabetes; diseases of the exocrine pancreas secondary to pancreatic trauma, infection, or disease; and drug- or chemical-induced diabetes.

ANATOMY, PHYSIOLOGY, AND PATHOLOGY

Because type 1 differs so completely from type 2 diabetes, as well as from impaired glucose tolerance (IGT), the anatomy and physiology of each will be reviewed in turn. Maturity-onset diabetes of the young (MODY, or type 3) will also be presented.

Type 1 Diabetes

Type 1 diabetes is highly correlated with absence of insulin secretory reserve. This lack of a secretory reserve is derived from beta-cell destruction by glutamic acid decarboxylase antibodies. This is an autoimmune process; therefore, type 1 disease is classified as immune-mediated diabetes. It is one of two variants of type 1 disease. The second variant of type 1 diabetes is idiopathic, meaning that there are several forms whose etiologies are not all known. Idiopathic type 1 diabetes lacks an autoimmune cause of beta-cell destruction. Diabetes that results from cystic fibrosis exemplifies idiopathic type 1 diabetes. Like immune-mediated type 1, idiopathic diabetes also is characterized by absence of insulin secretory reserve. Patients with both variants of type 1 diabetes are prone to ketoacidosis (American Diabetes Association [ADA], Report of the Expert Committee, 1997).

Type 2 Diabetes

Type 2 diabetes is a polygenic disease characterized first by insulin resistance, leading to compensatory hyperinsulinemia (Service et al, 1997). At this time in the development of type 2 diabetes, the blood glucose level is normal, but high levels of insulin disrupt lipid metabolism. As the resistance increases, compensatory hyperinsulinemia cannot keep up, so the blood glucose level rises. At levels of 140 mg/dL or more, the glucose is toxic to the beta cell and to the sites where insulin works. Eventually, absolute hyperinsulinemia becomes relative hypoinsulinemia. Exogenous insulin administration cannot override the body's insulin resistance at this stage.

Abnormalities in hepatic glucose output are a secondary outcome rather than a primary cause of type 2 disease. Small amounts of insulin prevent hepatic glucose output. Much larger amounts of insulin are required to dispose of postprandial glucose loads. Although increased glucose output can complicate the course of type 2, abnormalities in hepatic glucose metabolism are reversible with adequate disease management (Olefsky, 1997).

This process can continue for some time, even several years, before the overt onset of type 2 disease. Persons at this stage of metabolic challenge may have normal glucose tolerance, or only IGT. This is an insulin-resistant state, but one for which there is metabolic compensation. Eventually, about 7% of persons with IGT develop type 2 diabetes in the United States every year. Who will develop this disease depends on several often interrelated factors, including genetic predisposition, ethnic heritage, overall health, and lifestyle. The onset of diabetes does not end its progression. If not diagnosed and adequately treated, type 2 diabetes will inexorably worsen, leading to complications and requiring more complex antidiabetic medication regimens. Some patients also see their disease progress through beta-cell destruction, thus bringing endogenous insulin secretion to a grinding, permanent halt.

Mouse research suggests that the genetic abnormalities seen in type 2 diabetes are themselves nondiabetogenic. Their coexistence in a person, however, can lead to the development of overt diabetes (Terauchi et al, 1997). Ongoing poor glycemic control places humans at risk for eventual diminishment of endogenous insulin secretory capacity. This problem is compounded by the concomitant decrease in beta-cell insulin content. The outcome is a marked decrease in insulin mRNA. This means that genetic transcription for insulin is suppressed in the chronically overstressed beta cells of type 2 if glycemic control

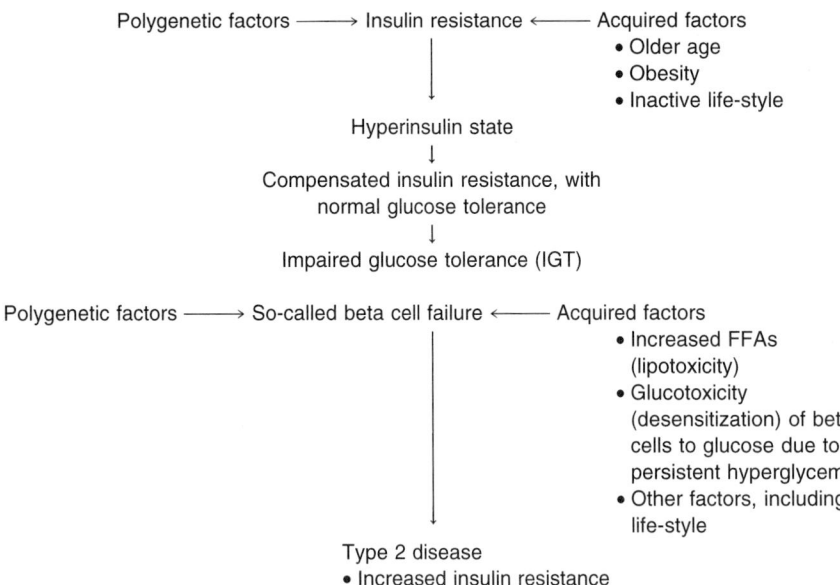

Polygenetic factors ——→ Insulin resistance ←—— Acquired factors
• Older age
• Obesity
• Inactive life-style

Hyperinsulin state

Compensated insulin resistance, with
normal glucose tolerance

Impaired glucose tolerance (IGT)

Polygenetic factors ——→ So-called beta cell failure ←—— Acquired factors
• Increased FFAs
(lipotoxicity)
• Glucotoxicity
(desensitization) of beta
cells to glucose due to
persistent hyperglycemia
• Other factors, including
life-style

Type 2 disease
• Increased insulin resistance
• Increased output of hepatic glucose
• Decreased secretion of insulin

FIGURE 17-1 From insulin resistance to Type 2 diabetes mellitus. (Adapted from Olefsky, J.M. [1997]. Pathophysiology of type 2 diabetes. Secaucus, NJ: Professional Postgraduate Services.)

is poor. Over time, the outcome may include glucose toxicity. Glucose toxicity is found in the type 2 beta cell when glycemic control is poor. Hyperglycemia is the outcome and leads to decreased sensitivity of the beta cells to normal glucose stimulation (Olefsky, 1997).

Yet another problem derived from poor glycemic control is lipogenesis. Lipogenesis includes elevation in levels of plasma free fatty acids, with attendant compromise in protein kinetics and overall cellular metabolism. The ultimate result is lipotoxicity, in which free fatty acid elevation progresses to beta-cell dysfunction. This process leads to a disruption in the glucose–insulin process, which is normally one of glucose stimulus followed by insulin response (Boden, 1997; Gougeon et al, 1997; Matsuoka et al, 1997; O'Rourke et al, 1997). Figure 17-1 illustrates the transition from insulin resistance to type 2 disease.

Human research suggests that the antecedents to insulin resistance in adulthood are not always the outcome of obesity or of aging. Lack of subcutaneous tissue at birth (ie, neonatal thinness) is associated with delayed activation of glycolysis as well as of glycogenolysis in adulthood. In exercising adults, it appears that this delay in providing for anaerobic metabolism results in an increase in muscle's reoxygenation rate. Only then can muscles anaerobically promote ATP synthesis. This process acts as a compensatory mechanism for the altered muscle microcirculation that developed because of neonatal thinness (Thompson et al, 1997).

■ ■ ■ CLINICAL PEARL

The outcome of delayed glycolysis and glycogenolysis in persons with very low birth weight (ie, lacking in subcutaneous tissue) means that they face increased risk of insulin resistance and, hence, type 2 disease in adulthood. Providers need to be cognizant of this risk in patients whose birth weight was very low and must apprise them of health-promoting activities that may help them to delay or avoid type 2 diabetes.

Impaired Glucose Tolerance

IGT defines impaired glucose homeostasis. This stage is not true type 2, but it is also not normal metabolism. IGT can actually be viewed as an early point on a continuum in the development of type 2 diabetes. When identified in a fasting specimen, IGT is comparable to impaired fasting glucose. Whether IGT or overt type 2 diabetes, glucose metabolism is a continuum that balances glycemic control with insulin response. Certainly, increased glucose levels are associated with microvascular complications such as retinopathy. Also, macrovascular (or large vessel) disease is the outcome of increased glucose as well as insulin levels (Sobel, 1997). Increased insulin response to glycemic loading in the nondiabetic state can serve to predict future type 2 and is clearly associated with macrovascular disease. Macrovascular complications include arteriosclerotic heart disease. Heart disease, hypertension, and coronary artery disease are seen in so-called syndrome X.

Syndrome X presents with significantly increased insulin levels that do not respond to the body's normal control mechanism of raising glucagon levels. Hyperinsulinemia is implicated in the disruption of normal fat metabolism, with elevation of total cholesterol levels, lowering of high-density lipoprotein cholesterol levels, undesirable elevation of low-density lipoprotein cholesterol levels, and elevation of serum triglyceride levels. Obesity and physical inactivity aggravate this process. Hyperinsulinemia also leads to blood vessel proliferation and, concomitantly, damage to vessel intimae. Atherosclerotic occlusion can be the end result of this process (Chaiken et al, 1993; DCCT Research Group, 1993b).

■ CLINICAL WARNING: In nondiabetics, both micro- and macrovascular diseases are seen as outcomes of increased serum glucose and insulin levels. These elevations commonly accompany normal aging, so their monitoring is the key to diabetes prevention in patients over age 55.

Maturity-Onset Diabetes of the Young

MODY, sometimes referred to as type 3 diabetes, is an autosomal dominant inherited disorder often mistakenly diagnosed as either type 1 or type 2. MODY is in fact neither purely type 1 nor type 2. It is a disorder of impaired insulin secretion without its absolute absence. Persons with MODY show no morphologic evidence of the glutamic acid decarboxylase antibodies characteristic of type 1. Nor is MODY characterized by any sign of the insulin resistance syndrome that is a hallmark of type 2 diabetes.

Providers can expect that further subphenotypic classification of diabetes variants will occur eventually (Lehto et al, 1997). That MODY's insulinemia may have a genetic underpinning is important information. This suggests that treatment methods will need to be better individualized if patients are to be supported in preventing or at least delaying complications of this disease.

Pregestational Diabetes

Pregestational diabetes is of concern to the woman with diabetes who is considering pregnancy, as well as to her primary care provider. Providers for fertile women with diabetes must inform them of the necessity for euglycemic control before becoming pregnant. This means encouraging such patients to keep blood sugar levels within the normal, nondiabetic range throughout the day. It has been demonstrated that abnormal blood sugar levels are teratogenic even before a woman knows that she is pregnant. If taking oral medication for her diabetes, any woman who plans to become pregnant should be managed on insulin to prevent possible fetal exposure to the chemicals in oral agents (Buchanan, 1997). Management of this variant is not a focus for this text.

Gestational Diabetes

Gestational diabetes also is not a focus for this text, although part of the provider's responsibility in primary care is to inform all fertile women of the importance of a healthy lifestyle before pregnancy. This lifestyle includes developing and maintaining well-rounded eating habits and active exercise patterns. These prevention activities will serve all women in good stead, including those who later decide to become pregnant.

Pathology of Complications Seen in Diabetes

OXIDATIVE STRESS AND ANTIOXIDANTS IN TYPE 2 DIABETES

Hyperglycemia sets cell walls up for disequilibrium, with the result that they undergo lipid peroxidation and accumulation of its end product, malondialdehyde. This process of lipid peroxidation is, simply, one of rancidification, wherein reactive oxygen species (ie, free radicals) are released at a rate that exceeds normal antioxidants' abilities to combat them. These free radicals ensure that the cell's metabolism will continue in chaos. Such chaos means that ATP formation and enzymatic pathway synthesis of proteins are compromised. Lipid peroxidation and its associated malondialdehyde accumulation also can turn on the protein glycation process.

Whether oxidative stress is a factor in type 2 diabetes is still being debated. There is a lack of reliable radical-trapping tools for assaying such stress. Research results are beginning to accrue, however, as testing methods for oxidative stress have become more reliable. Lowered antioxidant defenses of vitamins E and C in type 2 diabetes have been demonstrated in tissues, including those of the retina (Ceriello et al, 1997; Kowluru et al, 1997). Research has demonstrated that exogenous supplementation with vitamins C and E can block this process by inhibiting the formation of malondialdehyde, although specific dosage guidelines for vitamin E have not yet been established (Jin & Palmer, 1997; Kowluru et al, 1997). Chapter 5 provides guidelines for vitamin supplementation.

When euglycemia is restored in type 2 diabetes, reactive oxygen species production is reduced to normal. Research suggests that euglycemia not only protects against lipid peroxidation and its consequences, but can minimize or perhaps even mitigate against the clinical complications of diabetes as well (Kristal et al, 1997; Peuchant et al, 1997).

VASCULAR CHANGES

Flow-mediated dilation of blood vessels is impeded in the presence of hyperglycemia in type 2 disease. The reasons underlying this impedance were demonstrated by Jin and Bohlen (1997), who examined the intestinal mucosa in a rat model. Normally, blood flow is supported by the ongoing release of nitric oxide, which helps to maintain dilation and, thus, mucosal blood flow. In acute hyperglycemia, depressed acetylcholine release also decreases vasodilatory capacity, with the consequence that endothelial regulation is compromised. This compromise leads to an impairment of normal arteriole responsiveness to acetylcholine and a significant suppression in oxygen consumption.

RETINOPATHY

Glycemic control affects the incidence of microvascular retinopathies in type 1 disease as well as maculopathies in type 2 disease. Microvascular changes can in fact be found relatively early in the course of type 1 disease when glycemic control has been poor. Research suggests that the frequency and incidence of retinopathy can be reduced in type 1 disease with adequate glycemic control from the time of diagnosis (Klein et al, 1997). Specifics of pediatric control, especially for children under age 5, are outside the focus of this text.

Researchers examining the relation between anemia and retinopathy in diabetic subjects in Finland found that persons with diabetic retinopathy were at risk for severe retinopathy if they also had normocytic anemia. They then surmised that people who had diabetes and had normocytic anemia are at an increased risk of developing diabetic retinopathy, particularly of the severe type (Qiao et al, 1997).

EPIDEMIOLOGY

More than 16 million Americans have diabetes. No race, no ethnic group, and neither gender can claim exemption from this disease. Persons of all lifestyles—vegans or carnivores, smokers or not—are affected. Persons under 30 who become diabetic are more likely to develop type 1 diabetes or, to a lesser extent, MODY. People over age 30 are more likely to develop type 2 rather than type 1 disease. Less than 2% of people will develop type 2 diabetes before the age of 45. The prevalence increases at that point to 8% until age 54. Between age 55 and 64, the level rises to 12% and to 18% between 65 and 74 years.

Type 1 diabetes is more common in Caucasians of northern European heritage. Conversely, these persons have a lowered incidence of type 2 diabetes. Native North Americans have the highest level of type 2 disease; of these, members of the Southwestern desert tribes carry the greatest risk, particularly the Pima. Both lifestyle and ancestry seem to play an important role in diabetes onset in Native North Americans. Alaskan Native peoples, including the Inuit, report rates of 1% to 2%. Compare this relatively low incidence to that of the Pima of Arizona, whose reported prevalence rates stand at 50%. African Americans, Asian Americans, and Hispanic Americans have an incidence rate for type 2 disease 1.5 to 2 times that of whites of non-Hispanic European heritage. Further, the age at which diabetes occurs is lower in at-risk ethnic groups than for people of lesser ethnic predisposition (National Center for Health Statistics, 1993; Banerji et al., 1993a, b).

Overall, prevalence rates for type 2 diabetes have increased in the United States more than sevenfold what they were in the 1950s. This contrasts with the 50% to 80% increase in diagnosis of type 2 disease since the 1960s. Between 1991 and 1993, about 3% of the U.S. population stated they had diabetes (Harris, 1995). This figure represents only the tip of the iceberg, because screening data of a representative sample of people without known disease during this same period uncovered on average one unknown case for every diagnosed one, making 6% a more accurate figure. This translates to at least 1 in 17 people, or 15 million Americans—and half of this number are not diagnosed.

Ninety percent or more of diabetic cases are of the type 2 variant. The prevalence of diabetes is greatest after age 65, and people are now living long enough to develop type 2 disease (Kenny et al, 1995). This suggests that providers should actively add diabetes prevention to their management of nondiabetic patients.

The incidence of diabetes continues to rise in other Western countries as well, including among non-Western peoples. Lifestyle factors, including Western eating habits, obesity, sedentary occupational and recreational habits, and cigarette smoking, are likely culprits (Expert Committee, 1997; Harris et al, 1997; Ko et al, 1997; El-Kebbi et al, 1996; Hanson et al, 1996; Zaldivar & Smolowitz, 1994).

In the case of type 1 disease, infant exposure to bovine antigens and perhaps other environmental stimuli may account for its incidence in genetically susceptible children (Harris et al, 1997; Chaturvedi et al, 1996; Connolly & Kesson, 1996; Roshan et al, 1996; Schraer et al, 1996). In addition to the earlier-described risk factors, prenatal influences that lead to premature delivery or very low birth weight have been implicated in adult onset of type 2 diabetes (Thompson et al, 1997).

DIAGNOSTIC CRITERIA

A suspected diagnosis of diabetes mandates further investigation by the primary care provider. The provider should consider a diagnosis of diabetes when a patient presents with any of the findings outlined in Table 17-1.

TABLE 17-1	Diagnostic Criteria for Diabetes Mellitus

- Fasting plasma glucose (FPG, measured after > 8 hours of caloric fasting) elevation ≥ 126 mg/dL (7 mmol/L)
- Patients in the higher FPG ranges usually present with the classic symptoms of polydipsia, polyuria, and unexplained weight loss.
- Casual plasma glucose (ie, taken at any time of day, regardless of meal timing) ≥ 200 mg/dL (11.1 mmol/L) plus symptoms
- Oral glucose tolerance test (OGTT) is **not** recommended for routine use. If these data are obtained, then a level ≥ 200 mg/dL at 2 hours should be investigated using an equivalent 75-g anhydrous glucose/water load.
- Weight loss is common in type 1 but less so in type 2 disease, especially in persons with pre-existing obesity.
- A patient who presents with FPG between 110 and 126 mg/dL can be classified as having impaired glucose tolerance (IGT). The OGTT should not be routinely used in the average clinical setting. If this value is obtained, its level at 2 hours continues to be classified as IGT if it is between 140 and 200 mg/dL.
- FPG values:
  *FPG < 110 mg/dL = normal
  *FPG ≥ 110 and 126 mg/dL = IFG
  *FPG ≥ 126 = conditional diagnosis of diabetes

The above should be reconfirmed on a different day via repeat testing in any patient presenting without symptoms of hyperglycemia accompanied by acute metabolic decompensation.

Source: Expert Committee, 1997.

HISTORY AND PHYSICAL EXAMINATION

The primary care provider's history and physical examination should be thorough and careful if diabetes is to be diagnosed in a timely manner. History and physical data can alert the provider that a patient with other risk factors also risks glucose intolerance. Glucose intolerance can begin as impairment, but carries with it the risk of later overt diabetes. Table 17-2 presents questions specific to diabetes risk. Table 17-3 lists specific additional areas for physical examination that are indicated when screening for diabetes, as well as when providing ongoing care for the patient with diagnosed disease. It is important to note that 15% of patients already have evidence of complications at the time of diagnosis; these include retinopathy or neuropathy (DCCT Research Group, 1993b).

DIAGNOSTIC STUDIES

The means for diagnosing diabetes have been modified from previous recommendations (Expert Committee, 1997). These include preferred diagnosis by means of fasting plasma glucose (FPG), although other blood tests can also be used. Testing is not recommended for type 1 disease in patients who are healthy and who do not carry autoimmune risk. Patients age 45 and above should be screened for type 2 diabetes regardless of whether they are symptomatic. If the results of the screening FPG are normal, and in the absence of subsequent development of risk factors or diabetes symptoms, patients should continue to be screened at 3-year intervals, lifelong. More frequent testing should be considered in patients who are under 45 and who:

- Are obese (≥120% of desirable weight, or body mass index ≥27 kg/m²)
- Report a first-degree relative who had diabetes
- Are members of an ethnic group at high risk for diabetes (Native North American, African American, Asian American, or Hispanic American)

TABLE 17-2	History Questions in Screening for Diabetes (Age 18 and above)

- Family history of diabetes?
- If yes, then type 1 or type 2, and in whom?
- Classic symptoms (ie, polydipsia, polyphagia, unexplained weight loss)?
- Member of an ethnic group having a high incidence of diabetes (Native North American, African American, Asian, Hispanic)?
- Resident (past or present) of Sandy Lake, Ontario?
- Birth weight and, if known, approximate gestational age?
- History of gestational diabetes? Or of delivering an infant over 9 lb? Toxemia, stillbirth, polyhydramnios, or other complications associated with a pregnancy?
- Lifestyle stress?
- Recent stressful event (positive or negative)?
- Weight history (loss or gain)?
- Previous history of diabetes treatment? If yes, diet prescription, medications, self-management training? Glucose self-monitoring?
- History of complications, including ketoacidosis and hypoglycemia?
- Diet (including fluids) history for food types, amounts, and how prepared in a typical day. Include condiments and all snacks consumed.
- Aerobic as well as anaerobic exercise, noting type, amount of time, and frequency.
- Sleep–rest history (insomnia? nightmares?)
- Visual changes (blurring, diplopia, floaters)?
- Numbness, tingling, or burning in the hands or feet? This is a bilateral rather than unilateral neuropathy in diabetes and, although primarily sensory, motor nerve fibers may be involved. In more extreme cases, polyneuropathy may progress from severe pain to anesthesia, and with:
- Motor manifestations, including muscle weakness progressing to atrophy, with poor hand grasp or footdrop evident
- Unexplained indigestion or abdominal pain?
- Unexplained diarrhea?
- Infections, including urinary tract infections and candidiasis?
- Intertriginous infections/irritations (in skinfold areas of the obese; under the female breasts, crural areas in men)?
- Vaginitis?
- Impotence?
- History of chronic disease, including hypertension, endocrine, or autoimmune disease?
- Atherosclerosis risks, including diet, obesity, smoking, dyslipidemia, family history?
- Medications, prescribed and over-the-counter?
- Recreational drug use, including tobacco and alcohol (amounts and frequency)?
- Any other ethnic, psychosocial, socioeconomic, educational, or lifestyle considerations that could affect the provider and patient in their management of diabetes?

- Were diagnosed with gestational diabetes mellitus or delivered a baby over 9 lb
- Have high blood pressure (≥140/90 mmHg)
- Have a high-density lipoprotein cholesterol level of 35 mg/dL or less or a triglyceride level of 250 mg/dL or more
- Were found previously to have either IGT or impaired fasting glucose (ADA, 1996a, e, f).

Most case of diabetes can be diagnosed based on FPG, casual plasma glucose, or 2-hour plasma glucose. The oral glucose tolerance test (OGTT) can still prove useful in uncovering subclinical diabetes and, especially, insulin resistance in asymptomatic cases. The control exerted in the typical OGTT is not absolute; the test can be affected by a variety of factors, including smoking and stress. Still, the OGTT has value in uncovering patients otherwise at risk for subsequent diabetes and heart disease. This factor makes the OGTT a reasonable tool for the provider who questions the normalcy of a patient's overnight fasting or random blood work (McCance et al, 1994).

Table 17-4 presents specific laboratory tests to order when diabetes is suspected, as well as glycemic values for diagnosing the disease itself. Note that the FPG value (confirmed by re-

TABLE 17-3	Physical Examination for Diabetes (Age 18 and above)

- Height and weight
- Blood pressure (may need to obtain orthostatic measurements as well)
- Eyeground examination (preferably dilated, done by an ophthalmologist or licensed optometrist skilled in diabetes assessment) for signs of maculopathies and retinopathies. These can include:
  - retinal hemorrhages
  - scattered hard exudates
  - cotton-wool exudates (generally in concert with severe hypertension)
- Oral examination (eg, *Candida*)
- Thyroid auscultation and palpation
- Cardiac examination (eg, S₄)
- Abdominal examination (eg, hepatomegaly)
- Examination of pulses via palpation and auscultation
- Hand and finger examination
- Thorough skin examination (including insulin injection sites if applicable)
- Neurologic examination, including assessing for a positive Romberg sign (sometimes presents as swaying, destabilized pattern)
- Sensory stimulation changes (peripheral neuropathy and, if indicated by history, abdominal)
- Vibratory sense changes (peripheral neuropathy and, if indicated by history, abdominal)
- Foot examination, looking for evidence of foot ulcers or infection not otherwise explained
- Deep tendon reflex measurement (may be decreased, especially in presence of PN). Absence of ankle reflexes is an early sign.
- Gait analysis (may be unstable, especially in presence of peripheral neuropathy)
- If primary or differential diagnosis includes another endocrine disorder such as pheochromocytoma, Cushing syndrome, acromegaly, or hemochromatosis or pancreatic disease, be aware that secondary diabetes can occur in these patients (ADA, 1996e).

TABLE 17-4	Laboratory Evaluation and Criteria for Diagnosing Diabetes

- Fasting lipids (total cholesterol, high-density lipoprotein cholesterol, triglycerides, and low-density lipoprotein cholesterol)
- Serum creatinine
- Urinalysis for glucose, ketones, protein, and sediment
- Microalbuminuria (timed specimen, or the albumin/creatinine ratio)
- Urine culture if sediment or symptoms indicate need
- Thyroid function tests if indicated
- Electrocardiogram (establishing a baseline is important; obtain other measures if indicated)
- FPG at 8 or more hours of ≥126 mg/dL, or
- 2-hour plasma glucose ≥200 mg/dL during a 75-g OGTT, following WHO specifications. OGTT is not recommended for routine clinical analysis.

Unless in metabolic decompensation, repeat the glycemic measure used on a different day to confirm diagnosis.

Sources: Report of the Expert Committee, 1997; ADA, 1996a; ADA, 1996e.

peating the analysis) is the preferred testing method for diagnosis of diabetes mellitus as well as for impaired glucose homeostasis. The hemoglobin A_1c (HbA$_1$c) and any other glycosylated hemoglobins (GHBs) are not recommended for diagnostic testing. Because of the lack of standardization of these assays, GHBs are most reliably used as a measure to assess glucose deviations above normal over time.

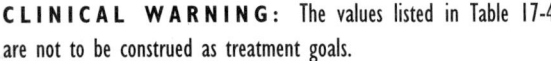

CLINICAL WARNING: The values listed in Table 17-4 are not to be construed as treatment goals.

As illustrated in Table 17-4, the provider who uncovers an FPG at about 126 mg/dL or greater on two different testings in a nonpregnant patient is advised to engage the patient in diabetes management. Although these guidelines seem more stringent than before, their strictness is supported by the presence of complications in 15% of those with FPG levels of 120 to 126 mg/dL (DCCT Research Group, 1993a, b).

Gestational Diabetes

The criterion for diagnosing gestational diabetes is considerably lower and, as recommended by Jovanovic-Peterson and Peterson in 1992, can be determined when the FPG on the OGTT is 90 mg/dL or higher after 100 g, not 75 g, of oral glucose. This recommendation is considerably more stringent than that currently advised by many obstetric sources, which stipulate that fasting rates that exceed 130 mg/dL should be considered as a reasonable screening criterion for gestational diabetes. The rationale for recommending the much lower range for screening of gestational diabetes comes from the latest research statistics, which indicate that fasting levels that exceed 90 mg/dL can have serious consequences for the developing fetus.

The new recommendations advise that screening be selective rather than universal for glucose intolerance in pregnancy. Women at low risk for such intolerance as well as for overt gestational diabetes include those who:

- Are under 25 years
- Are of normal weight
- Have no first-degree relatives with diabetes
- Are not a member of an ethnic group as previously identified (National Center for Health Statistics, 1993).

TREATMENT OPTIONS, EXPECTED OUTCOMES, AND COMPREHENSIVE MANAGEMENT

Treatment Options for Syndrome X

The clinical treatment of all factors seen in syndrome X, including hypertension, coronary artery disease, heart disease, and dyslipidemia, can be found in their respective chapters. The current discussion will focus on treating the diabetes component only.

Treating Diabetes

Whether type 1 or type 2, diabetes is characterized by consistent elevation of the blood glucose level and, in type 2, insulin resistance. Primary care management ideally leads to normalization of blood glucose and, if possible, improved glucose response to endogenous insulin in type 2 diabetes. The goal of treatment is not so much to control the disease but rather to prevent or decrease complications arising from the damaging effects of chronic hyperglycemia. Sound management plans arise from appropriate treatment options, and so lead to individualized plans of care that can maximize positive outcomes for a patient. For this reason, the following discussion will present various treatment options appropriate in different clinical circumstances. This discussion will be framed by appropriate management plans whose foci are optimal outcomes.

Matching Diagnosis to Treatment and Management

When symptoms of polydipsia, polyuria, and polyphagia present themselves, current diagnostic guidelines support making a clinical diagnosis of type 2 disease based on a single blood glucose measurement. This is true even in the absence of weight loss, which is more typical of type 1 than most variants of type 2 disease. The glucose need not be fasting. Specifics for each kind of glucose measurement should correspond with the values presented in Table 17-4 (ADA, 1997). If diabetes is not confirmed but is still suspected, then the provider can obtain an OGTT (ADA, 1997; Stolk et al, 1995).

When discussing treatment options with the patient, the effective primary care provider recognizes the importance of ethnic and cultural influences. This recognition begins before planning interventions. Food customs and eating rituals differ from family to family. Specific ethnic or lifestyle habits greatly influence diet and meal planning. Similarly, cultural beliefs and values surrounding the body and perceived self-harm will influence the patient's level of participation in self-monitoring and medical therapies. The primary care provider must inquire about and respect cultural influences, customs, beliefs, and values. This perspective is especially important when a patient's cultural, religious, or ethnic background, or even lifestyle, differs from that of the provider.

Developments in self-care education and pharmaceutical advances have revolutionized the potential for healthy outcomes for people with diabetes. The Diabetes Complications and Control Trial (1993a) provided firm evidence that optimal control of blood glucose, defined as HbA$_1$c of 7.4% or less, can delay or prevent long-term complications of diabetes. Further, any level of improved control will decrease complication rates.

The 1997 report from the Expert Committee on the Diagnosis and Classification of Diabetes Mellitus goes a step further, setting target goals of 80 to 120 mg/dL for FPG, bedtime glucose 100 to 140 mg/dL, and GHB (HbA$_1$c) of less than 7%. Newer pharmacologic interventions and insulin delivery systems can be combined to achieve these goals. Diabetes educators have developed curricula and teaching tools to help patients control their diabetes. Both patient and provider must continue to update their understanding of this disease.

The purpose of this section is to present the most current standards of practice in a clear and practical way. This information can be used to frame a plan of care that helps the patient with diabetes to obtain optimal metabolic control. Hyperglycemia must be eliminated to control the progression of diabetes as well as to delay or prevent complications, including micro- and macrovascular problems. These two problems will be discussed later in this chapter.

Goals of Diabetes Management

The immediate treatment goals in diabetes management include the achievement of optimal glycemic control based on HbA$_1$c of 7.4% or less and the absence of hypoglycemic episodes requiring assistance to treat. The overall goals of diabetic management are also two in number: correction of metabolic irregularities and prevention of micro- and macrovascular complications.

Achievement of these goals depends on maintaining the target blood glucose level. If frequent high and low blood sugar levels are encountered in the face of desirable HbA$_1$c, efforts must be made to smooth out glycemic control. Self-monitoring of blood glucose (SMBG) is critical to the success of this effort. SMBG and other components of diabetes management will be discussed after the following section, as lifestyle assessment is an important first step in managing blood glucose.

Lifestyle Assessment and Intervention

The importance of understanding the patient's activities of daily life cannot be overstated. Included in this assessment are meal planning, hours of sleep and activity, and variations in activities on a day-to-day, weekly, and seasonal basis. The provider also needs to assess the patient's educational level, employment, household, and potential for community support. Cultural and ethnic practices and religious beliefs may play an important role in health decisions, food choices, times for ritual fasting, and celebrations (Magnus, 1996). Family habits and customs also may affect the patient's self-management of diabetes. Ascertaining insurance status is important, as this often determines whether the patient has access to both primary care and specialty providers, support services, medication, and supplies.

It may prove helpful to have the patient complete a simple but thorough lifestyle assessment inventory. Appendix 1 presents a sample tool for lifestyle assessment. Ideally this intake could be reviewed by other office personnel, who could then assist the patient in completing written details if necessary. The

tool may also help assess the patient's literacy capabilities and visual acuity.

Lifestyle assessment can help the provider decide what to teach and how to teach it. Acting on these assessment data can help ensure that people with diabetes have sufficient and specific education to facilitate self-management. Providing diabetes education can be done effectively either in individual or group sessions (Arseneau et al, 1994; Hirsch et al, 1995).

A Certified Diabetes Educator (CDE) can assist the primary care provider in developing successful intervention strategies for patient teaching. The CDE is a nationally accredited role for professionals who have completed an extensive course of study through the American Diabetes Association. Most commonly, the CDE is a professional nurse (either BSN or MSN), a physician (MD or DO), a nutritionist (RD), or a social worker (MSW). The CDE has emerged as the recognized consultant for or provider of diabetes education. As a source of knowledge to the patient as well as the provider, CDEs are increasingly drawn into the patient–provider relationship. CDE services are often treated as reimbursable by third-party payers. Further information about CDEs as a resource is provided in the community resources section of this chapter.

Whether the sources of information and teaching are the provider, a CDE, or a combination of both professionals, it is important that information be given that will support the patient in managing his or her care in a systematic manner. This information includes but is not limited to:

- Understanding the rationale for GHB testing
- The relation of meal planning, food, and exercise control to glycemic control
- SMBG
- Mode of action and side effects of medications
- Sick-day management
- Signs and symptoms of hypo- and hyperglycemia and their management
- Possible acute and chronic complications.

Taken as a whole, this information constitutes the survival skills for the person with diabetes. The following discussion will focus on each of these content areas that providers and patients need to understand for successful management of diabetes.

Glycohemoglobin Testing

GHB testing helps the provider to determine a patient's blood glucose level for the 100 to 120 days before testing. A minor hemoglobin, GHB constitutes only 4% to 8% of the total hemoglobin. There are three components of GHB that are said to be glycosylated: A$_1$a, A$_1$b, and A$_1$c. A$_1$c is the most commonly measured GHB. If A$_1$a is measured, its value is computed at 2.4% higher than A$_1$c. GHB analysis is useful because this component of the red blood cell's hemoglobin combines with some of the blood stream's glucose load. This process is called glycosylation and is irreversible. In other words, how high a patient's GHB level is depends on how much glucose was available in the blood stream over the 100- to 120-day lifespan of the red blood cell. This determination is only an average of that glucose level, though, because red blood cells undergo a constant cycle of old cell destruction and new cell generation (Pagana & Pagana, 1997).

TABLE 17-5	Conditions That Interfere with GHB Determination

Low values can occur with:

- Sickle cell anemia
- Chronic renal failure
- Pregnancy

False elevations can occur whenever the lifespan of the red cell is lengthened, as in thalassemia.

Source: Pagana & Pagana, 1998.

Several assays exist for determination of GHB. Different assays may have different normal ranges. Providers must be aware of the assays available at a given practice site.

■ ■ ■ **CLINICAL PEARL**

The GHB should be assayed at least twice per year, although every 3 months is preferable (ADA, 1996d,e).

Refer to Table 17-5 for specific conditions that can affect GHB levels. GHB levels also can be increased or decreased by several conditions. Before making a final assessment of the GHB status of a patient, the provider should be aware of the coexistence of any of the states described in Table 17-6.

Meal Planning

Because "diet" is an emotionally charged and negative word, the concept of a meal plan is easier to accept and discuss. Many people plan their meals; people do not have to have a chronic disease to plan ahead for food. Meal planning is an important skill for patient learning. The provider must keep in mind that the primary goal of meal planning is control of blood sugar and lipid levels. Optimal glycemic control can be accomplished through planning meals. Planning includes meal composition, preparation methods, portion size, and condiments added. The provider should ask specific questions about favorite foods and about any food allergies or sensitivities, such as lactose intolerance.

TABLE 17-6	Conditions That Can Cause Increased or Decreased GHB Levels

INCREASED LEVELS

- New diabetes
- Poor diabetic control
- Chronic renal failure
- Hemodialysis
- Iron-deficiency anemia
- Splenectomy
- Pregnancy

DECREASED LEVELS

- Hemolytic anemia (due to increase in red cell turnover)

Source: Pagana & Pagana, 1998.

■ ■ ■ **CLINICAL PEARL**

Weight loss is a secondary target, and not easily sustained. In teaching meal planning, the provider should first aim at what can be done realistically to aid the patient in self-managing glycemic control. Very modest reductions in weight (3 to 10 lb) often yield dramatic improvements in glycemic control.

Details about composing a meal plan and measuring food intake are covered in Chapter 5. The provider should keep in mind that meal planning for the patient with diabetes includes 10% to 20% protein but not less than 0.8 g/kg/day, and no more than 10% saturated fats. Note that fat may need to be adjusted downward if the lipid profile indicates a cardiovascular risk. The rest of the day's calories should be derived from mono-unsaturated fats and complex carbohydrates. Both soluble and insoluble fibers should be consumed, and 20 to 35 g of soluble fiber should be eaten. Cholesterol intake should not exceed 300 mg/day (ADA, 1996c).

COMMON MYTHS IN DIABETIC MEAL PLANNING

There are at least three myths about food and diabetes management that must be dispelled (Dudley, 1998, personal communication; Norton, 1997, personal communication).

Myth 1 is, "Diabetes is a sugar disease. People with diabetes cannot eat sugar." In fact, diabetes is an insulin disease. Sugars such as sucrose, fructose, maltose, and so on are only foodstuffs that may affect the blood glucose level. As part of a balanced meal plan, different forms of sugar may be incorporated to provide variety in the diet (Dudley, 1998, personal communication).

Myth 2 is, "All persons with diabetes must have a bedtime snack." This myth is a holdover from the era when crude, long-acting insulins were used. These insulins exerted unpredictable peak actions; thus, it was deemed necessary to provide the patient with a hearty snack at bedtime. This myth pervades much of health care, contributing to fasting hyperglycemia both at home and in the hospital. Hepatic glucose output is maximal during the night, so additional caloric substrate is generally not required. Extra calories can lead to excessive weight gain.

■ ■ ■ **CLINICAL PEARLS**

- All patients on pharmacologic therapy should keep some form of sugar at the bedside in case of overnight hypoglycemic symptoms. Easily stored sugars include hard, easily chewed candies, or a tube of cake frosting.
- Bedtime snacks are indicated in persons who need extra calories to maintain weight or if glycogen storage is limited, as in liver disease. These patients are prone to overnight hypoglycemia and may require a snack containing some mixed nutrients (eg, 8 oz of 1% or skim milk and a slice of nonwhite bread toast with 0.5 oz of low-fat cheese).

■ **CLINICAL WARNING:** Juice and crackers are not recommended for bedtime consumption. Snacks containing only carbohydrate will provide only short-term fuel and, in fact, can potentiate higher blood glucose levels. Adding high-fat foods such as peanut butter may contribute to fasting hyperglycemia and general lipid excess in adults. Fats are not metabolized rapidly enough to prevent short-term hypoglycemia (Dudley, 1998, personal communication; Norton, 1997, personal communication).

Myth 3 is, " 'Unsweetened' and 'no added sugar' are the same as 'sugar-free'." All sugars, including fructose, can acutely elevate blood sugar levels. So-called "unsweetened" juice can deliver 20 to 30 g of carbohydrate in the form of fructose per 8-oz serving. This is nearly half the amount of a formal glucose tolerance test, which would raise the blood glucose of a person with diabetes to over 200 mg/dL. "Unsweetened" and "sugar-free" are not the same. Sugar-free foods provide few calories from carbohydrate (generally <4 calories per serving). Teach patients that any ingredient ending in "-ose" on a food label means that it contains a form of sugar (Norton, 1997, personal communication).

Activity and Exercise

Exercise can have positive effects on glucose control across the lifespan (Clark, 1997; Eriksson et al, 1997; Powell & Blair, 1994). Exercise is the missing link in the diabetes plan of care. Exercise can overcome or reverse many common mistakes in meal planning and eating patterns. Moving from the theoretical recognition of its importance to the daily practice of exercise is one of the most challenging tasks in clinical practice. Prochaska et al (1991, 1992, 1994) provide a model for understanding this barrier:

- Stage 1: Precontemplation. The person is uninterested in changing a behavior.
- Stage 2: Contemplation. The person is now interested in changing, but is not doing anything to act on this interest.
- Stage 3: Preparation. The person is now interested in change and is acting on this interest occasionally.
- Stage 4: Initial action. The person is now beginning a regular routine.

The primary care provider must be aware that the patient's participation in exercise (or lack thereof) may fit within the confines of this model. This awareness can prevent frustration for provider and patient alike and may help providers work with patients toward initiating and sustaining stage 4.

■ ■ ■   CLINICAL PEARL

Encourage a nonexercising or rarely exercising patient to approach exercise as a stepwise progression.

Walking is an excellent form of exercise that is low in cost and easy to initiate in patients without neuropathic impingement. Walking 45 to 60 minutes each day is optimal and should be undertaken 6 or 7 days a week (Zinman, 1997).

Meal planning must be linked to daily activities. Some persons require an altered meal plan or different doses of medications if their activities vary widely, such as the weekend athlete who sits in front of a computer Monday through Friday and is active on Saturday and Sunday.

All patients who take insulin (especially in type 1 diabetes) should take special care when exercising. SMBG is mandatory for determining the need for extra calories before an activity. If the blood glucose level is less than 100 mg/dL, then a pre-exercise snack should be eaten that contains 20 to 25 g of carbohydrate. This snack proportion should be repeated after 30 minutes of exercise. If the blood glucose level is 100 to 250 mg/dL, then exercise without snacking is probably safe. The patient should be instructed to check the urine for ketones if the blood glucose level exceeds 250 mg/dL. If the urine is positive for ketones, the patient should delay exercise. The rationale for this delay is that inadequate levels of insulin in an exercising person with diabetes will result in an increased blood glucose level.

■   CLINICAL WARNINGS:

- The provider needs to instruct the patient that exercise can alter the rate of insulin absorption. The patient should take care not to use any anatomic site for insulin injection that is used in exercising. For example, a runner or walker should avoid injecting the thigh before exercising. Because everyone responds differently to exercise, some patients may require insulin adjustments, whereas others may not.
- A cardiac stress test or cardiology evaluation should be done in nonexercisers over 40 years of age and in those with other cardiac risk factors. Refer to Chapter 9 for information about stress testing and exercise and cardiac disease.
- Patients who have neuropathy or retinopathy should be taught to be very selective in their exercise routines and other activities in which they participate. Those with peripheral neuropathy will be safer using a treadmill than walking or running outside, where the terrain may be uneven or fraught with potential foot hazards. Patients with preproliferative and proliferative retinopathy should avoid all activities that increase intraocular pressure. These include weight-lifting and arm wrestling. Activities of daily living such as lifting or moving objects (eg, grocery bags, furniture) also increase the risk of ophthalmic injury. Isometric exercise should be practiced only if the patient has had proper breath training.
- All patients who undertake an exercise program or activities should be advised of the importance of careful foot evaluation before and after the activity. They should also be encouraged to use proper equipment and footwear, and to replace them when needed.

Home Glucose Monitoring

The ADA (1996d) recommends that all patients who take insulin also self-monitor their blood glucose levels. This activity is especially important in all pregnant women who have diabetes, regardless of type. The provider should encourage SMBG in patients with unstable disease, those with a tendency toward hypoglycemia that occurs without forewarning, those with type 2 disease who are taking antidiabetic medication and whose glycemic control is tight, and in cases of ketoacidosis history. Whether type 1 or type 2, all patients who manage their disease via intensive insulin regimens must use SMBG as part of their therapy. This latter group includes those who use an insulin pump or who self-inject their insulin multiple times daily.

Any patient with a history of an abnormality in the renal glucose threshold should also be advised about the benefits of SMBG. This latter group includes all older patients who, as they approach their 60s and beyond, are also experiencing a decrease in the filtering capacity of their renal ultrastructure as well as overall renal weight. These normal changes of aging affect renal filtration of glucose, making renal measurement especially unreliable.

Caution should be used in teaching older patients how to perform SMBG, as normal changes of aging may make it a challenge to manipulate the SMBG process. These challenges can include decreased fine psychomotor skill in handling equipment, as well as a disturbance in blue-green color vision. Blue-green disturbance can lead to misinterpretation of SMBG results if the monitor's test pad relies on color changes (Young & Koda-Kimble, 1995). The provider can encourage the elderly patient using SMBG to purchase a device that provides a large-type readout on a screen.

There are many glucometers available. Package inserts provide excellent explanations on how to obtain a specimen and how to use the meter for its analysis and interpretation. Patients should be encouraged to bring their meters to the provider for one-on-one support and teaching about specimen collection and meter use. CDEs also are a good resource for up-to-date information related to meter choice and use.

Beginning Antidiabetic Medication

Achievement of optimal blood sugar control may require antidiabetic medication. The previous discussion on meal planning, exercise, and SMBG serves as the foundation to beginning a medication regimen. Food management and exercise may be enough for glycemic control in some patients with type 2 diabetes. But medications alone cannot create optimal blood sugar levels in diabetes. For those who also require medications, these modalities must be thought of as a threefold prescription. Together, they can assist the patient in maintaining the glucose profile at close to normal, or at least within optimal ranges at any given point in time.

Sound clinical judgment is the hallmark of providing safe and effective health care. The primary care provider must assess each patient on an individual, case-by-case basis. In organizing the patient's assessment and treatment plan, the provider should keep in mind the patient's stage of insulin resistance, glucose toxicity, and ability to produce insulin; these should be part of any decision in regard to treatment changes.

Others who require insulin include patients with beta-cell damage (if not complete destruction) secondary to surgery or exposure to some toxins, including certain medications. Patients who have blood glucose levels exceeding 200 mg/dL may also require temporary insulin therapy. Beta cells can shut down when they are exposed to prolonged high glucose levels. This process is referred to as glucose toxicity. It is important to remember that some patients with type 2 disease can become extremely ill, with or without hyperosmolar or diabetic ketoacidosis states. These patients usually present over a period of weeks to months, and are often over 30 years of age. They may have a history of obesity, though presenting with marked weight loss at times of prolonged hyperglycemia. Persons with type 2 disease of many years' duration can also experience dete-

rioration of beta-cell function, eventually requiring split and mixed regimens of insulin (eg, short- and long-acting) for optimal control (ADA, 1997).

CLINICAL WARNINGS:

- The patient with type 1 diabetes requires insulin at all times, and will have additional insulin requirements at times of illness and fasting. Withholding insulin in a person with type 1 disease who is vomiting can be a fatal mistake. Lack of insulin in type 1 disease allows the liver to produce ketones, precipitating illness and nausea and risking diabetic ketoacidosis.
- The patient with type 2 diabetes will require insulin when ill or if the blood sugar level is very high. Insulin absence in type 2 diabetes (for whatever reason) will prevent the movement of nutrients to tissues. This will precipitate metabolic acidosis. Metabolic acidosis results from a lack of insulin in the hepatocyte, which alters a metabolic pathway whose outcome is ketone production. Low doses of insulin are required to reverse this pathway. Increases in insulin dosage in persons taking insulin will be required at times of illness or fasting. Guidelines for these adjustments will be discussed under sick-day management later is this chapter.

Diabetic Therapies: How to Prescribe Insulin

The purpose of all diabetes therapies is to achieve glycemia as close to normal as possible without hypoglycemia. Insulin may be required for the maintenance of life or for the patient's level of wellness. Thus, insulin must be prescribed in a proactive manner that directly involves the patient in decision making and management. By anticipating peaks and troughs of blood glucose levels based on lifestyle assessments and, ideally, home glucose monitoring results, the provider can work with the patient to achieve smoother glycemic control. Insulin adjustments should be made after a pattern of insulin response is clear. Adjustments are made over a period of 3 or more days, within the context of a patient's diet, glucose levels, and exercise management. Once a dose is established, teaching, guidance, and support for self-administration of insulin must be provided. These activities can be done by a member of the health care team who is skilled in teaching this content.

When starting a patient on insulin, the provider should bear in mind that human insulin brings about a lesser antibody response than nonhuman insulin. Because of modern production methods, however, this response is considered slight and therefore of little true clinical significance (Young & Koda-Kimble, 1995). In any event, human insulin is less expensive than pork insulin.

Table 17-7 lists prescribing information for the insulins that are most widely available. Table 17-8 outlines methods for teaching insulin self-administration and injection site rotation. Table 17-9 describes how to draw up insulin.

■ ■ ■ ■ CLINICAL PEARLS

- Try to adjust only one insulin component at a time, unless all levels are consistently 200 mg/dL or greater.
- Because it is difficult to control and can affect the rest of the day's glycemic levels, start with the fasting glucose.
- Short-acting insulin delivered via inhaler is now in clinical trials. This delivery method should be available sometime after 2001.

TABLE 17-7	Types of Insulin				
Insulin Type	Source	Manufacturer/Brand Name	Onset and Peak Effectiveness	Usual Duration of Action	Notes
SHORT-ACTING					
Lispro	Insulin analogue	(Lilly) Humalog	2–15 min/30–90 min	2–4	Inject into abdomen to enhance rapid uptake. Consider individual response to site of injection. Dose time based on preprandial SMBG. If >200, then 20 min before meal If 150–200, then 10 min before If <150, then 5 min before meal. Because of hypoglycemia risk, advise SMBG 2–3 hours postmeal.
Standard	Beef/pork	(Lilly) Regular Iletin I	0.5–1.0 hour/ 2–4 hours	4–6 +	
Purified Pork	Pork	(Lilly) Regular Iletin II; also (Novo Nordisk)			
Human	Recombinant DNA	(Lilly) Humulin R; (Novo Nordisk) Novolin Rb,c			
INTERMEDIATE-ACTING					
Standard	Beef/pork	(Lilly) NPH or Lente Iletin I	1–2 hours/ 6–14 hours	16–24 +	
Purified	Pork	(Lilly) Pork NPH or Lente Iletin II; (Novo Nordisk) NPH Purified (N) or Lente (L)			
Human	Recombinant DNA	(Lilly) Humulin N or Humulin L; (Novo Nordisk) Humulin Nb or Humulin Lb			When given before meals, regular insulins should be injected depending on SMBG before injection, and, as for all insulins, site to be used for injection and individual patient responsiveness to regular insulin. Dose time based on preprandial SMBG: If >200, then approximately 1 hour before If 150–200, then 45 min before If <150, then 30 min before meal.
LONG-ACTING					
Ultralente	Recombinant DNA	(Lilly) Humulin U; Ultralente	4–6 hours/ 10–20 hours	24–28 +	
MIXTURES					
NPH/Regular (70/30%)	Recombinant DNA	(Lilly) Humulin 70/30; (Novo Nordisk) Novolin 70/30b,c	30 min	16–24	
NPH/Regular (50/50%)	Recombinant DNA	(Lilly) Humulin 50/50			

- Adjust the basic insulin dose 1 to 2 units at a time.
- If the patient has not taken insulin before, begin with a dose of synthetic U-100 human insulin in divided doses at 0.2 units/kg in the proportions outlined in Table 17-10.

Mixing Insulins

Mixing insulins is an important skill for all patients with type 1 and many with type 2 diabetes. Mixing insulins gives the patient and provider a truly individualized treatment plan. Should the provider need to prescribe an insulin plan that requires mixing, the patient needs to be taught how to draw up different insulin preparations in a single syringe. Table 17-11 provides information needed by the patient for mixing insulins.

Premixed insulins are available commercially. These insulins can be used in some cases because they are based on commonly occurring (but changeable) dose ratios. A frequently used combination ratio of NPH to regular is $\frac{2}{3}$ NPH and $\frac{1}{3}$ regular, or a ratio of 70:30. This provides 70 units of NPH and 30 units of regular per 100 units. For instance, the patient with a 70/30 prescription could take 9 units of a 70/30 preparation rather than mixing the breakfast dose of 6 units of NPH and 3 units of regular insulin (see Table 17-9).

Other ratios are available in many countries. Providers should familiarize themselves with what is available in their area.

TABLE 17-8	Teaching Insulin Self-Administration and Injection Site Rotation

- Use the smallest caliber needle available (currently 29- or 30-gauge), preferably silicon-coated.

- Use a low-dose syringe, with a dose indicator line gauged at 1 unit per line.

- 1-cc, ½-cc, ¼-cc, and ³/₁₀-cc syringes are available for U-100 insulin injection. ¼-cc or ³/₁₀-cc syringes are used for children and for insulin-sensitive adults taking small dosages.

- Needle sizes are ½″, 28- or 29-gauge and are silicon-coated.

- Assure the patient that the very small-gauged, silicon-coated needle will make insulin administration easier and virtually painless.

- Teach administration using a magnifying device if the patient requires help seeing the lines on the syringe. Encourage magnifier use at home for this patient.

- Select site and pinch tissue to be used.

- Hold the barrel straight up, like a pencil (or at a 45° angle if emaciated), and quickly thrust needle bevel side up into site.

- Check for blood by gently withdrawing plunger very slightly and, if none, inject insulin.

- Release the pinch and withdraw needle.

- Teach and encourage self-blood glucose monitoring.

- Teach injection site management to prevent alterations in insulin absorption, as well as lipohypertrophy. Sites should be chosen to ensure uniformity of insulin uptake, including exercise. Site rotation should be done within the same anatomic region. An ideal site is the abdomen, which is also one that is least affected by exercise.

Supplementary Doses

Sometimes supplementary insulin is needed to augment the once- or twice-daily doses of insulin. Regular insulin can be used to correct high premeal glucose concentrations. Planning how much supplemental insulin to prescribe depends on several factors, including the patient's sensitivity to insulin, meal planning, and exercise patterns.

■ ■ ■ ■ CLINICAL PEARLS

- Supplementation is generally made in the range of 1 to 2 units for every 50 mg/dL above the glycemic goal.

- When the FPG is 200 mg/dL or greater, consider either delaying the meal to occur 60 minutes after injection of regular insulin (rather than the more usual 20 to 30 minutes), or use lispro, whose onset of action is closer to 30 minutes than the approximately 56 minutes for regular insulin (see Table 17-7).

- If the preprandial glucose level is less than 60 to 70 mg/dL, decrease the premeal dose of regular insulin by 1 to 2 units, and give it immediately before eating. This meal needs to include 10 g of glucose if the SMBG was less than 50 mg/dL.

- If supplementation is required for 3 or more days, add 2 units of regular insulin to the prebreakfast insulin dose.

TABLE 17-9	How to Draw Up Insulin

- For all new, unused bottles of insulins **except** regular (R), agitate vigorously to loosen storage-induced sedimentation.

- Gently roll the bottle between the hands to avoid foaming.

- Keeping the bottle on a flat surface, wipe off the top of the bottle (unless brand new) with a clean alcohol wipe. Draw up air into the syringe in an amount that equals that of insulin to be withdrawn, put the needle into the bottle's diaphragm, and inject the air into the bottle.

- Keeping the needle in place, invert the bottle while supporting the syringe.

- Keeping the needle below the insulin's surface, pull back on the plunger to fill the syringe with insulin in the amount equal to the previously injected air.

- Carefully observe for air bubbles and, if seen, tap out. Gently pull back and forth on the plunger while moving the needle's bevel out of the insulin to push air out, and then moving it back under when pulling more insulin in. Alternate this with tapping, thus helping to dislodge stubborn bubbles.

INSULIN ANALOGUE (LISPRO)

Lispro is an insulin analogue that is structurally nearly identical to human insulin, except for reversal of amino acids lysine and proline in beta chain positions 28 and 29. Because of its very rapid peak onset and concomitant duration compared to regular insulin, dosage of intermediate-acting insulin may need readjustment.

Concentrations with abdominal injection are higher than those for deltoid or femoral area sites. It is recommended that this insulin be injected into the abdomen to enhance absorption and rapid uptake. Studies have shown that its absorption rate is consistently faster compared to regular, thus decreasing hypoglycemic risk between meals; however when it occurs, hypoglycemia may be more pronounced (Ter Braak et al, 1996; Tuominen et al, 1995). Mixing lispro with another insulin will blunt its rapid onset and may cause variability in that onset. If lispro is to be mixed with another insulin, care should be taken to draw it up first, before the other insulin, according to the following:

- When mixed with NPH, the time for lispro peak is increased, while absorption rate (but not bioavailability) is decreased. Blood glucose stabilization is delayed about 7 hours. Ives and Dunn (1997) report that mixing lispro with Ultralente does not produce this delay in absorption. For multiple combination dosing, Torlone et al. (1996) found that 20% to 40% NPH + 60% to 80% lispro before meals improved blood glucose stabilization to an average of 4 hours postprandial.

- If lispro is mixed with either NPH or Lente (human preparations), give within 5 minutes after mixing insulins and within 15 minutes premeal.

- Do not premix lispro with NPH ahead of time for storage, even if refrigerated, as its stability is not known.

■ **CLINICAL WARNING:** Consult with a diabetes specialty practice before prescribing lispro. Comanagement of the patient's insulinization may be necessary for patient safety. Hypoglycemia is less than for regular insulin. Therefore, advise 15 g rather than the normal 20 g of immediate-acting carbohydrate as treatment for hypoglycemic episode.

TABLE 17-10	A Plan for Prescribing Insulin for the First Time

- For a man weighing 76 kg, prescribe 16 units of synthetic insulin/day.

- To divide the dose, give two thirds in long-acting insulin (eg, NPH or Lente) and one third in short-acting regular. This would be 10 units of NPH and 6 units of regular for the man weighing 76 kg.

- This dose can now be divided over the day as follows: 3 units of regular + 6 units of NPH, administered ½ hour before breakfast, 3 units of regular taken ½ hour before dinner, and 4 units of NPH taken at bedtime.

- This total daily dose is usually small enough that the patient new to insulin therapy will be able to avoid hypoglycemia. Therefore, this dose will usually need to be adjusted upward.

- An alternative would be to give the NPH as described above, but give all the regular with the main meal of the day. This plan would delay the necessity for the patient to learn to mix insulins at the same time he or she learns basic insulin administration.

CLINICAL WARNING: The use of any short-acting insulin (such as regular) before bed is dangerous and generally should not be prescribed. Only clear consultation with a diabetes specialty practice can support the decision to add regular insulin at bedtime. In this instance, midsleep awakening for SMBG (3 AM) will be required for safeguarding against hypoglycemia.

CLINICAL WARNING: Hyperglycemia can cause transient or permanent visual blurring. Patients must be certain they are administering the correct dose. If the provider and patient determine that visual, special learning, or self-management needs exist, then a CDE or a provider from a diabetes specialty practice group should be consulted. Either of these professionals can provide information and teaching about possible alternative insulin delivery systems or assistive devices. These include information about syringe magnifiers for enlarging the calibration, and spring-loaded devices that can automatically insert an insulin needle with minimal hand pressure.

TABLE 17-11	How to Mix Insulins

Avoid contaminating a short-acting (regular [R]) insulin with an intermediate-acting insulin (N), which will obviously thus alter the ratio of R:N. The reverse risk of contaminating N with R is not problematic, as N's protamine can bind the R without altering N's efficacy. Mixing insulins mandates the following procedure:

- Gently roll the N bottle between the hands to disperse sediment.

- Cleanse the tops of both bottles, and then draw up and inject air into the N bottle in the amount to be given (eg, 12 U).

- Inject air into the R bottle in the amount that equals that of the insulin to be withdrawn (eg, 6 U).

- Leaving the syringe in place, invert the R bottle and draw up the desired amount (to the 6 U mark on the syringe).

- Withdraw the needle, and then carefully inject the needle into the N bottle, being careful not to push the plunger in.

- Invert the N and withdraw the desired amount (to the 18 U mark), taking care not to push the plunger into the N.

Anticipatory Insulin Doses

Because diet and exercise are connected to the need for insulin and its metabolic intake, the patient should be taught how to adjust the basic insulin dose to accommodate anticipated increased or decreased activity, exercise, and meal changes.

■ ■ ■ ■   **CLINICAL PEARL**

Increase the dose of regular insulin by 1 to 2 units for every additional 20 g of carbohydrate ingested (eg, birthday, holiday). Decrease the dose by 1 to 2 units if the meal is smaller than usual.

Exercise information related to glycemic monitoring, diet, and insulin prescription is provided in Table 17-12.

Intensive Insulin Therapy

Two methods for improving insulinization can be used in managing diabetes: insulin infusion via a pump, and the multiple injection technique. Providers interested in using the pump approach with a patient are advised to consult with a diabetes practice experienced in pump therapy.

Intensive insulin therapy using the multiple injection technique is best undertaken when patient, provider, and a consultant can work together to manage glycemic control. This regimen is designed to mimic the nondiabetic balance of meeting glycemic demand with insulinization. A total daily insulin dose is calculated, based on predicted calorie and exercise needs. The complexity of this approach requires careful attention to individual patient variances. This approach is best achieved with referral to a diabetes practice group familiar with calculating split-dosage regimens.

TABLE 17-12	Managing Metabolic Requirements, Medications, and Exercise

- SMBG before, during, and after exercise.

- If SMBG >240 to 300 mg/dL before, the patient should not exercise. Because high glycemic levels indicate severe low insulin bioavailability, the patient is at increased risk for hyperglycemia secondary to exercise.

- Inject R into abdomen 30 minutes before, to avoid increased absorption.

- If planning moderate exercise (eg, 30 to 45 minutes of bicycling or jogging), decrease the preceding R dose by 30% to 50%. Then if SBGM is normal or low just before activity, add a 10- to 15-g carbohydrate snack.

- Anyone whose glycogen stores may be low is at risk for hypoglycemia during and immediately after exercise. These patients include anyone who takes in 800 or less calories/day, those on a low-carbohydrate diet of <10 g/day, and alcoholics.

- Hypoglycemic risk is greater for patients on insulin than for those taking sulfonylureas. Diet-only therapy is generally not a risk for hypoglycemia from exercise.

- Postexercise hypoglycemia is a special risk after prolonged exercise, such as day-long hiking. Carbohydrate needs to be increased for that day. SMBG needs to be done during the night to monitor for postexercise nocturnal hypoglycemia, which can occur 8 to 15 hours later.

- Patients with severe proliferative retinopathy or retinal hemorrhage must avoid activities that will subject them to jarring, such as jogging, strenuous walking, horseback riding, skiing, bicycling, or aerobic dance. Any exercise that requires moving the head below waist level must also be avoided.

Oral Agents in Type 2 Diabetes

Oral antidiabetic agents can be very effective in the patient with type 2 disease who has some endogenous insulin capacity. These agents are prescribed when diet and exercise have not corrected hyperglycemia. Over the past 2 to 3 years, several new agents have become available that can control blood sugar with little or no risk of hypoglycemia. This has made it both reasonable and safe to achieve near-normal HbA$_1$c values in many patients who previously would have required insulin.

The choice of which oral agent to prescribe for a particular patient is based on many factors. Age, adiposity or leanness, lipid levels, blood pressure, and degree of hyperglycemia are some of the important considerations to bear in mind.

Sulfonylureas increase beta-cell insulin secretion through closure of ATP-sensitive potassium channels. They are usually well tolerated. Major side effects include hypoglycemia and, rarely, allergic reactions. Because they are highly protein-bound, sulfonylureas have relatively long durations of action. Sulfonylureas are appropriately used in leaner persons with moderate hyperglycemia (FPG < 140 mg/dL, HbA$_1$c < 8). Whether to use a first- or a second-generation agent depends on individual clinical factors. Second-generation sulfonylureas such as glipizide and glyburide are generally more potent on a milligram-per-milligram basis than first-generation drugs. Hypoglycemia is possible with all sulfonylureas but is less likely with the newer second-generation agents than with the first-generation drugs, such as tolbutamide or chlorpropamide. There are fewer side effects associated with second-generation sulfonylureas.

> **CLINICAL WARNING:** Patients with a known sulfa allergy should be carefully evaluated before beginning therapy to avoid an allergic response (Young & Koda-Kimble, 1995).

The primary mode of action of **biguanides** (metformin) is to decrease hepatic glucose production. This class of drugs also acts to increase intracellular glucose metabolism. To a lesser extent, biguanides also inhibit intestinal glucose absorption and may improve insulin sensitivity. Because of their efficacy in controlling glucose overproduction by the liver, biguanides are referred to as antihyperglycemics (as compared to other oral agents, which are referred to as hypoglycemics). There is virtually no risk of hypoglycemia when these agents are used as monotherapy. Metformin monotherapy, for example, does not promote weight gain and, in fact, may have favorable effects on lipid levels. This may be a good choice in obese patients with hyperlipidemia. Biguanides have been especially effective in interrupting the uncontrolled response of the liver to increased glucagon production. In rare cases, lactic acidosis has been reported in association with biguanide use. These instances include hypotension, hypoxemia, and any other condition that could place a patient at risk for lactic acidosis (Young & Koda-Kimble, 1995).

Alpha-glucosidase inhibitors (acarbose, miglitol) are a reasonable choice in mild hyperglycemia, especially in persons with a diet rich in carbohydrates. These drugs are helpful for patients whose FPGs are close to normal but whose postprandial glucose levels are elevated. Their primary mode of action is to decrease carbohydrate absorption from the gastrointestinal

tract. This means that there is a decrease in the normal postprandial glucose rise because glucose digestion is slowed. Because these agents do not enhance insulin secretion, they do not cause hypoglycemia if used as monotherapy, even if the patient is fasting. Their ability to enhance glycemic control is additive, making them a reasonable addition to an existing regimen, especially if postprandial glycemic control is refractory. Acarbose does not inhibit lactose; thus, lactose intolerance should not be seen with this agent.

> **CLINICAL WARNINGS:**
>
> - When used as monotherapy, an overdosage of metformin will not result in hypoglycemia. In this instance, the patient may experience gastrointestinal symptoms of relatively short duration.
> - When Metformin is used in combination therapy with other agents, hypoglycemia can occur.
> - Treatment of low blood sugar levels with alpha-glucosidase inhibition that has been combined with asulfonylurea or insulin requires the use of simple sugar, such as glucose tablets or gel. Table sugar, soda, and fruit juices all contain sucrose and will not be effective in treating this form of hypoglycemia.

When using combination therapy as outlined above, adding acarbose may prove helpful in lowering postprandial glucose levels as well as overall HbA$_1$c levels. As monotherapy, acarbose will not affect lipid levels, nor will it potentiate hypoglycemia. Hypoglycemia can occur when it is used in combination with other agents secondary to postprandial glucose reduction. As with metformin, significant gastrointestinal effects can be decreased through slow titration and diet management.

Troglitazone is a member of the **thiazolidinedione** class. Like metformin, it may prove to be effective as monotherapy in patients whose previous prescription was diet and exercise only. This agent is also indicated for patients whose HbA$_1$c level is consistently elevated at 8.5% or more, and whose poor glycemic control and insulin resistance remain refractory to intervention, including multiple insulin injections of more than 30 units/day (Raskin & Graveline, 1997). It is also a good choice for adding to the regimen of patients who are taking sulfonylurea and whose diabetes is not well controlled. Troglitazone works in a complementary manner with metformin. The combination was shown to lower both FPG and HbA$_1$c levels below baseline in a study examining their use in subjects with type 2 diabetes. These results suggest that the additive effect of these two agents is an important therapeutic option in the management of type 2 disease (Horton, 1997).

Thiazolidinediones are the newest class of drugs to be used in treatment of type 2 diabetes. Their primary mode of action is to increase insulin sensitivity of the liver, peripheral and adipose tissues, and skeletal muscle. They do not increase insulin secretion and are effective only in patients who are insulin-resistant. These patients include those who are obese, hyperinsulinized, hypertensive, or hyperlipidemic. Thiazolidinediones are also indicated for patients with high hip-to-waist ratios or large stores of abdominal fat, and for patients with an elevated serum creatinine level (1.5 in males and 1.4 in females) who are not able to take metformin. Troglitazone is the first thiazolidinedione

TABLE 17-13	Oral Agents			
Drug/Strength	Dose	Mean Half-Life (hours)	Duration (hours)	Notes
Chloropropamide 100 mg, 250 mg	0.1–0.5 g QD	35	24–72	Do not prescribe if risk of hyperglycemia is enhanced, as in renal failure, or in the case of decreased protein or energy stores. It has the highest frequency of side effects of sulfas. Should not be prescribed for elderly. Is associated with alcohol-induced flushing; warn about this side effect.
Acetohexamide 250 mg, 500 mg	0.25–1.5 g QD or in divided doses b.i.d.	6	12–18	Caution in elderly in renal disease
Tolazamide 100 mg, 250 mg, 500 mg	0.2–1 g QD or in divided doses b.i.d.	7	12–24	Renal failure may cause metabolites to accumulate.
Tolbutamide 250 mg, 500 mg	0.05–3 g in divided doses b.i.d. or t.i.d.	7	6–12	Shortest-acting of this class
Glipizide 5 mg, 10 mg	2.5–40 mg QD or in divided doses b.i.d.	3	12–24	Divide doses >15 mg. Take 30 min before meals. Adverse reactions range from dizziness to leukopenia, thrombocytopenia, mild anemia, hypoglycemia, dilutional hyponatremia, nausea, vomiting, urticaria, facial flushing, constipation, epigastric fullness, heartburn, weakness, and paresthesia. See package insert. May need to discontinue depending on severity of reaction(s).
Glipizide extended-release	5–20 mg QD or in divided doses b.i.d.	4–12	24	Same
Glyburide 1.25 mg, 2.5 mg, 5 mg	1.25–20 mg QD before breakfast or in divided doses b.i.d. before breakfast and supper	4–13	12–24	Initial dose with breakfast. Monitor closely for first week if substituting for chlorpropamide, due to prolonged retention of chlorpropamide. Refer to package insert for dosing information when changing from insulin to glyburide. Caution in elderly, renal failure, intestinal blockage; use with caution in patients tending to hypoglycemia. Adverse reactions resemble those for other sulfonylureas. Divide doses >10 mg to maximum 20 mg/d.
Micronized/glyburide 1.5 mg, 3 mg	1.0–12 mg QD	4	24	Same as for glyburide. Divide doses >6 mg.
Glimepiride	Initially 1–2 mg QD with breakfast or first main meal of day. Followed by gradual increases to a maximum of 8 mg QD. Most common maintenance dose ranges from 1 to 4 mg.	5	24	Dose increase after reaching initial 2-mg dose should be based on serum glucose response at no more than 1–2 mg at 1- to 2-week intervals. Is thought to cause less insulin secretion than others of this class due to different binding sites on cells, so potential for exacerbating insulin resistance may be less than for other second-generations, though clinical experience has not shown this. Adverse reactions resemble those for other sulfonylureas. Effective as monotherapy and, for those with type 2 in secondary beta cell failure (with FBG >150 mg/dL), has shown efficacy with insulin, decreasing insulin requirement. Encourage daily SMBG. In renal and hepatic insufficiency, start with 1 mg QD. No dosage adjustment needed in elderly, but recommended start with 1 mg and increase carefully.
Repaglinide	t.i.d., taken 15 min before meals	~1	~96	Works by producing insulin when needed (ie, at mealtime) should be available in 1999
Metaformin 500 mg, 850 mg	0.5–2.5 g in divided doses b.i.d. or t.i.d.	not know, but may be ½ to 3	6–12	Avoid in anyone lacking normal renal function, in hypotension, hypoxemia, or if predisposed to lactic acidosis (eg, ETOH). Discontinue before dye-cast studies or in dehydration. Expensive.

(continued)

| TABLE 17-13 | Oral Agents (Continued) |

Drug/Strength	Dose	Mean Half-Life (hours)	Duration (hours)	Notes
Acarbose 50 mg, 100 mg	Recommended initial dose is 25 mg (1.2 tablet) t.i.d., gradually titrate up to 50–100 mg t.i.d. chewed with first bite of meal. Alternatively, can start with 25 mg/day at largest meal (usually supper) for 1 week, then increase each week by 25 mg to a maximum of 100 mg t.i.d. chewed with first bite of each meal. This seems to decrease GI symptoms.	xx	~3	The major side effect is flatulence secondary to bacterial action in the colon on undigested carbohydrates. Base dosing changes on 1 hr postprandial blood sugar. Goal is to decrease this and bring HbA$_{1c}$ into therapeutic range. Benefits include no hypoglycemia or weight change effects, as well as decrease in postprandial insulin secretion and in triglyceride/cholesterol levels in FPGs. Contraindicated in bowel disease, ketoacidosis, any condition that may be worsened by gas formation. See package insert for other, less common adverse effects. Reinforce importance of preprandial SMBG to avoid periprandial hypoglycemia due to too high a dose.
Miglitol 25 mg (50 mg, 100 mg)	Recommended initial dose is 25 mg tid. Alternatively, can start at 25 mg once daily to minimize G1 symptoms and gradually increase to tid. Take orally tid with 1st bite of each main meal.	about 2		Should not cause hypoglycemia when used as monotherapy. Its effect is additive when used with a sulfonylurea. Contraindications same as for acarbose, as are side effects.
Troglitazone 200 mg, 400 mg, 600 mg	Continue the insulin dose when beginning this agent, at a dose of 200 mg/day. If FPG does not adequately respond within 2–4 weeks, increase dose. 400 mg is a typical daily dose; 600 mg is the maximum. Once FPG ranges less than 120 mg/dL, decrease daily insulin dose by 10% to 25%, using patient's response as a guide.	16–34		Obtain baseline liver panel before initiating, re-check serum transaminase monthly ×6 months, then q2 months for 1st year. Obtain liver function tests at 1st symptoms of hepatic dysfunction. Discontinue at 1st sign of jaundice and/or abnormal liver function tests. Bioavailability is increased if administered at breakfast. Dose adjustment is not needed for renal insufficiency. Use with caution in hepatic disease. Take with a meal. Does not induce hypoglycemia, but may need to adjust insulin downward to avoid hypoglycemia. Very expensive.

to be approved for use in the United States. It is expected that other agents will be marketed soon. Troglitazone is indicated in monotherapy in addition to diet and exercise, or in combination with insulin or sulfonylureas. The goal is improvement of glycemic control in type 2 diabetes.

CLINICAL WARNINGS:

- Drug interactions with troglitazone exist that include decreased efficacy of some oral contraceptives, resulting in loss of contraceptive protection. An alternative method for birth control may be needed.
- Do not give this agent to patients taking cholestyramine, as it interferes with troglitazone absorption by as much as 70%.
- Coadministration with terfenadine reduces the efficacy of the latter by 50% to 70%.

CLINICAL PEARL

Troglitazone is indicated in the treatment of type 2 diabetes if insulin in excess of 30 units per day in divided doses does not achieve an HbA$_1$c level of less than 8.5%, and for patients with documented insulin resistance.

Regardless of which agent is chosen for adding to a diabetic regimen, two principles must be kept in mind. FPG should be obtained 2 weeks after any dosage change. Continue to adjust the dosage at 2-week intervals until the FPG is in therapeutic range (80 to 120 mg/dL). If a single agent does not achieve the desired treatment goals, then a combination of oral agents can be used.

The major classes of oral agents and prescribing information are summarized in Table 17-13. This is not an exhaustive presentation of each agent. As with all medication, consult the package insert or a recent pharmacotherapeutics text for more detailed prescribing information.

Combining Oral Agents With Insulin

Just as not all patients with type 2 diabetes can be managed with diet and exercise alone, so too not all will be able to achieve adequate blood sugar control with the addition of oral agents. When all permutations of oral agents have been tried without success, it may be time to add insulin to the regimen. A variety of regimens are possible, including 10 to 15 units of NPH in a single bedtime dose added to metformin or sulfonylurea monotherapy, or to a combination of sulfonylurea, metformin, and acarbose. A single dose of 70/30 insulin just before the evening meal may also work well. The goal of this approach is to decrease the overnight production of hepatic glucose, thus supporting an FPG as close to normal as possible. Daytime glycemic control is managed with the oral agents (Horton, 1997). If glycemic goals are not achieved, adding troglitazone to this regimen may prove efficacious for patients who are insulin-resistant. Alternatively, switching to insulin therapy alone may be the best therapeutic option, especially in patients who are insulinopenic rather than insulin-resistant.

Insulin as Monotherapy in Type 2 Diabetes

Not all patients can tolerate combining oral agents, or maximal doses of certain oral agents. They may also be unable to tolerate combining such dosages with insulin, or their blood sugar levels may remain resistant to glycemic control despite these and dietary and exercise efforts. Further, some persons with type 2 diabetes may have progressed to the point where they no longer have sufficient beta-cell capability for endogenous insulin manufacture. In these instances, insulin as monotherapy may be tried.

NPH insulin can be prescribed b.i.d., with or without the addition of regular insulin, depending on glycemic control. Follow the same guidelines for insulin prescription as previously described.

Problems Associated With Insulin Therapy

WEIGHT GAIN, DAWN PHENOMENON, SOMOGYI EFFECT

Sometimes the foregoing plan all works so well that the patient with excellent glycemic control begins to gain weight. This weight gain may exceed desirable limits. Discern whether the patient is also experiencing some low blood sugar levels or a significantly increased appetite. This is the time to adjust some of the pharmacologic therapy.

Alternatively, some patients may experience variances in their glycemic control despite a strong management plan. Both the dawn phenomenon and the Somogyi effect can prove challenging to achieving glycemic control. The Somogyi effect is suspected when the patient's glycemic log shows bedtime normoglycemia, 3 AM hypoglycemia, and rebound prebreakfast hyperglycemia. Waning of the evening dose of NPH may in part contribute to this event. One third of the patients taking evening NPH experience asymptomatic nocturnal hypoglycemia, which rebounds into morning hyperglycemia in 10% (Young & Koda-Kimble, 1995). Elevated postbreakfast hyperglycemia that is refractory to treatment can also be a consequence of nocturnal hypoglycemia, and may be symptomatic of insulin resistance. Similarly, the dawn effect is suspected when the 3 AM SMBG is euglycemic, but hyperglycemia is then demonstrated between 4 and 8 AM.

■ ■ ■ CLINICAL PEARLS

■ Decrease the evening dose of NPH by 2 or 3 units. Monitor the 3 AM SMBG. Continue with the AM mixed-insulin dose, take only regular insulin for the evening (before supper) dose, and move the evening NPH dose to bedtime. Monitor the 3 AM SMBG until satisfied that this plan was successful. This realignment may be all that is needed to prevent nocturnal hypoglycemia and the hyperglycemic rebound in the morning, because NPH's peak effects are given full sway to cover the night and early morning period. This latter plan may also mitigate postbreakfast hyperglycemia as well as the dawn phenomenon.

■ Patients whose glycemic management proves challenging may benefit from referral to a diabetes specialty practice for consultation.
■ Doses of medications and even the medications themselves are rarely static in diabetes therapy.

CLINICAL WARNINGS:

■ The dawn phenomenon varies from one day to the next. To prevent asymptomatic nocturnal hypoglycemia and its attendant risks, patients who demonstrate nocturnal hypoglycemia should be encouraged to do SMBG at 3 AM a few or more times per week, depending on individual glycemic responses (Young & Koda-Kimble, 1995).
■ Short-acting insulin generally is not to be used at bedtime. Consult with a diabetes practice before embarking on using regular insulin at bedtime.
■ Whenever combination therapy is used, the risk of hypoglycemia is potentiated.
■ Sulfonylureas and troglitazone can all increase appetite, leading to weight gain and subsequently elevated blood glucose levels.

Special considerations for sick-day management for the patient taking diabetes medication are summarized in Table 17-14.

Diabetic ketoacidosis and hyperosmolar hyperglycemic nonketotic syndrome are complications of diabetes. Table 17-15 presents information on these two potentially fatal complications of diabetes.

HYPOGLYCEMIA

Prevention or timely management of hypoglycemia is important in controlling its dangerous effects as well as the metabolic disruptions that follow overcorrection. This is especially true should hypoglycemia become a management pattern. Hypoglycemia is defined as a blood glucose level of 50 mg/dL or less, regardless of whether the patient is symptomatic. Symptoms are generally reported when blood glucose levels drop below 40 mg/dL. Seizures and coma can be seen below 20 mg/dL. Frequent treatment to cover high or low blood sugar levels must be eliminated from diabetes management if the patient is to avoid or delay the complications of this disease. SMBG, meal planning, exercise, and pharmacologic agents are used together to maintain a glucose profile as close to normal as possible, or at least within optimal ranges at any given point in time. Table 17-16 provides information about hypoglycemia and its management.

Severe or Frequent Hypoglycemia

Severe hypoglycemia is generally defined as any hypoglycemic event that requires the patient to receive assistance to reverse the symptoms. Severe hypoglycemia generally occurs at blood glucose ranges of 50 mg/dL or less. Severe hypoglycemia is diagnosed when:

1. Symptoms of hypoglycemia occur
2. The blood sugar level is low when symptoms occur

3. Symptoms resolve with the administration of rapidly absorbed carbohydrate.

Frequent and recurrent hypoglycemia can lead to the development of long-term neurologic sequelae. Such sequelae could interfere with cognitive function and cause decreased perception of symptoms signaling a low blood sugar level. Obviously, the outcome of this complication is an increase in the frequency and severity of hypoglycemic events. Many patients (especially

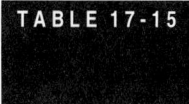

TABLE 17-14 | **Sick-Day Guidelines for Patients Taking Medication for Diabetes**

TYPE 1

- Avoid dehydration.

- Continue insulin.

- Check blood glucose every 2 hours.

- Give supplemental doses of regular insulin, using an individualized range developed in concert with diabetes specialist. Supplementation may, for example, be established as 1–2 units of R for every 30–50-mg/dL elevation above a prearranged glucose level (140 mg/dL).

- Check urine ketones every 4 hours or sooner if blood sugar > 240 mg/dL.

- Use a variety of clear fluids (some with sugar and some without) to maintain blood glucose level, especially if unable to eat. Strive for a caloric intake of 50 g of carbohydrate every 4 hours. Jello and popsicles (regular, not sugar-free), juices, regular soda, crackers, soups, and toast may be tolerated.

- Aim to drink 6–8 oz of clear fluids every hour. A sound protocol for vomiting or diarrhea could include replacing fluids and electrolytes with Pedialyte or similar solution.

CLINICAL WARNING: Patient should seek medical attention for:

- Continued vomiting or diarrhea, if SMBG exceeds 240 mg/dL, or if urine ketones continue elevated despite 2 or 3 supplemental doses of regular insulin if it is part of the patient's sick-day protocol, or if large amount of ketones or trace to small amounts in urine after 24 hours.

- Vomiting or diarrhea and temperature >101°F >24 hours.

- Signs of local infection (eg, urinary tract infection; open, purulent draining wound; cellulitis-like symptoms.)

- Signs of diabetic ketoacidosis, including extreme fatigue, abdominal cramping, and alterations in normal breathing pattern.

TYPE 2

- Avoid dehydration.

- If taking insulin, take ½ usual insulin dose if unable to eat as usual.

- If on oral agents and unable to eat, withhold agent for 1 hour. If able to eat after that time, take medication and some water. If unable to tolerate, notify provider.

- Monitor SMBG as above for type 1.

- Seek medical attention as above, or if illness is profound or protracted.

- Some patients will require insulin. Follow individualized protocol as above.

CLINICAL WARNING: If taking an alpha-glucosidase inhibitor or metformin, withhold dose if vomiting or diarrhea occurs. Do frequent SMBGs (every 2 hours or so), following guidelines as directed above. Resume medication when normal GI function returns.

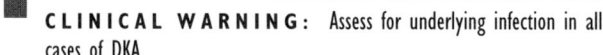

TABLE 17-15 | **Diagnosis and Deposition of Diabetic Ketoacidosis (DKA) and Nonketotic Hyperosmolar Syndrome (NKHS)**

DKA

- DKA is a medical emergency usually associated with type 1, but can (rarely) occur in type 2.

- Suspect DKA in adolescents and in any patient with type 1 who withholds insulin.

CLINICAL WARNING: Assess for underlying infection in all cases of DKA.

- Symptoms (most common): polyuria, polydipsia, vomiting (with or without abdominal pain and weakness)

- Laboratory tests may reveal hyperglycemia, though not always profoundly so, leukocytosis, hypertriglyceridemia, and anion gap acidosis. A serum pH of 7.25 or less and the presence of serum ketones are typical criteria for diagnosis of DKA.

NKHS

- NKHS occurs predominantly in patients with type 2 diabetes.

- NKHS is characterized by hyperglycemia (serum glucose levels often exceed 600 mg/dL), absence of serum ketones, and dehydration as evidenced by weight loss and, often, azotemia.

- Coma can occur in both DKA and NKHS.

- Mentation changes are common to both DKA and NKHS.

- Like DKA, underlying infection is common in NKHS.

- Intravenous insulin is usually required for treatment of profoundly dehydrated patients, as absorption from muscle and subcutaneous tissue is unpredictable.

- Lactic acidosis can compound either condition and increases the risk of death.

- Very mild DKA or early NKHS can sometimes be managed on an outpatient basis by an experienced primary care provider who is knowledgeable about diabetes.

CLINICAL WARNING: The general primary care provider should refer all suspected cases of DKA or NKHS for emergency room evaluation and treatment.

young people with type 1 diabetes) remain asymptomatic until the blood glucose level is profoundly low. Their first sign of metabolic distress may be changes in mentation or behavior.

CLINICAL ALERT

Patients at high risk for hypoglycemia include those with autonomic neuropathy, which predisposes them to hypoglycemic unawareness. Also at risk are patients who have undergone extensive gastrointestinal surgery or who have gastroparesis. Both of these situations can change the absorption of nutrients from the gut. Pancreatic damage from surgery interrupts insulin secretion in patients who maintain endogenous secretory capacity. Pancreatic damage also interferes with glucagon production, thus preventing the body's efforts at counterregulation in response to low blood sugar levels.

TABLE 17-16	Signs and Symptoms, Clinical Possibilities, and Management of Hypoglycemia

SIGNS AND SYMPTOMS

- Blurred vision, sweaty palms, slurred speech, hunger, confusion, shakiness, anxiety, combativeness; sometimes tingling and numbness around lips. Symptoms can be misinterpreted as signs of inebriation.

- Nocturnal signs and symptoms can include nightmares, disturbed sleep pattern, sweating, morning hangover. Reportedly up to 80% of patients have no symptoms.

CLINICAL POSSIBILITIES

- Last meal/snack eaten?
- Physical activity?
- Adverse sulfonylurea reaction (too much, or interaction with other medications)
- Other drug effects
- Delayed gastric emptying (gastroparesis)

MANAGEMENT

- 15–20 g simple, rapidly acting carbohydrate, depending on protocol. Symptoms and, if possible to obtain, SMBG guide amount to ingest. Repeat carbohydrate within 15 to 20 minutes if blood glucose continues under 60 mg/dL or if symptomatic. Eat a meal of complex carbohydrate and protein afterward.

- The preferred treatment is 3 or 4 B/D glucose tablets. If this is not possible, then some foods that contain 15 g of simple carbohydrate per serving include:
  ½ cup (4 oz) of orange juice
  6 oz of carbonated regular soft drink
  3 sugar cubes, or 3 tsp granulated sugar
  7 or 8 Lifesaver candies (quickly crunched—not tooth-friendly)

* The unconscious or seizing patient should be given:
  Glucose gel (comes in a tube. Squeeze into the inside of the patient's cheek), or
  Glucagon 1 mg SQ, IM, or IV (average response time 6.5 minutes), or
  Glucose 25 g IV (50 cc dextrose 50%). Average response time is 4 minutes.

* Follow-up hospitalization may be warranted.

Source: Young & Koda-Kimble, 1995.

CLINICAL WARNINGS:

- Hypoglycemia can be protracted in patients taking sulfonylureas or long-acting insulins. If these patients ingest alcohol, hypoglycemia can be both severe and prolonged. Also, these patients may again become hypoglycemic even after achieving normal blood glucose levels via intravenous dextrose. For safety, any patient in this situation should continue to be hospitalized after dextrose administration so that close professional supervision can be ensured.

- Tight control of blood sugar levels should be attempted with caution in patients who are at risk for severe hypoglycemia.

CLINICAL ADVICE

Along with their family members, patients with a history of severe hypoglycemia or established risk factors will need instruction in the use of glucagon, which is available by prescription. Glucagon can take up to 30 minutes to reverse the hypo-

glycemic episode. It is therefore important that the patient and the family members be able to use other, quicker oral methods for treating severe hypoglycemia. If the patient is conscious, a glass of orange juice with an added tablespoon of sugar can be quickly administered. A roll of hard candies can be easily kept in the bedside table for rapid access. At least seven or eight of these candies should be quickly crunched and swallowed. If the patient has lost consciousness, family or a friend who is trained to do so can administer glucose via glucagon injection or, if there is no danger of choking, by placing glucose gel in the patient's cheeks.

Patients should be instructed to keep a record whenever a hypoglycemic event occurs, including time of occurrence, relation to meals or snacks, exercise, sleep, and the last medication dosage and amount taken. Physical state immediately before the episode should also be noted. When next seen by the primary care provider, they can go over the record together. If any kind of pattern is seen to emerge in these episodes, a management plan can be developed that may help to alleviate the frequency or severity of these episodes.

OFFICE MANAGEMENT

The ADA (1996e) has published clear guidelines for the office management of diabetes and its complications. These standards will help the provider to give care that is current, organized, systematic, and scientifically based, and will serve as legal proof of diligent care. The goal should be to help the patient develop an individualized self-management plan. To the extent that the patient desires, the family should also be involved in this activity. The importance of actively involving the patient in developing problem-solving strategies cannot be overemphasized. Final acceptance of each component of the plan by provider and patient alike depends on understanding and acceptance by the patient.

The team approach used for management planning requires recognition of the shared expertise of all parties—patient, provider, nurse, nutritionist, social worker, psychologist, and often the family. Collaboration and trust are the keys to successful creation and implementation of a diabetes management plan. The team approach is important because no one professional has the time or skill needed to serve the patient in all areas. The diabetes team minimally includes one or more primary care providers who are committed to diabetes care, and a knowledgeable health care professional or CDE who will teach the patient about the disease, symptom monitoring, insulin management, and so on. Ideally, a social worker (MSW), a registered nutritionist (RD), and a licensed mental health professional are also available for team assignments when their expertise is needed. Table 17-17 summarizes the ADA's recommendations for office and lifestyle management.

Sometimes a patient has teaching or management needs that exceed the capabilities of this team. It is important that the patient then be referred to an endocrine specialist for medical needs specific to diabetes, or to a CDE for teaching and self-care needs. Sometimes patients are best served when they are referred for consultation with these professionals. In some instances, their continued comanagement of the patient is best.

TABLE 17-17	General Management Plan for All at Each Office Visit

- Patient's progress in self-management and in goal attainment for diabetes care
- Log of blood glucose levels. Ideally, the patient brings the control device to the office, where the stored glucose determinations can be downloaded. The printout serves two purposes: a valid and reliable record of patient's blood sugars since the last visit; and objective data for the patient's medical record.
- Diet and exercise regimens. These should be examined in tandem with the blood glucose record. Any episodes of hyper- or hypoglycemia should be closely correlated with these, with clarification of whether the patient was ill, had missed a meal, had eaten foods not normally consumed, etc. Look for patterns!
- Contraception (if indicated)
- Medications, including dosage and frequency
- Lifestyle changes since last visit? Biopsychosocial stress in general, and related to diabetes?
- Complications of diabetes
- Blood pressure control
- Dyslipidemia
- Were any referrals made at previous appointment? Check whether these were followed up. If not, work with patient to determine whether he or she can follow through on this aspect of the self-care plan.
- Specific knowledge related to diabetes self-care should be reviewed on an as-needed basis. Overall self-management knowledge related to medications, self-administration, diet, exercise, etc. should be reviewed annually.
- Encourage participation in support groups for diabetes, such as the local affiliate of the American Diabetes Association if available. Also encourage joining this organization's lay group. Patients receive *The Diabetes Forecast* as part of their membership. This excellent publication provides current information related to diabetes and its management. The address appears at the end of this chapter. Encourage patients to avail themselves of any continuing education programs on diabetes offered in their community.

Source: American Diabetes Association (1996e).

Table 17-17 summarizes the ADA's recommendations for office management, including those that pertain to lifestyle (ADA, 1996e). Table 17-18 suggests visit frequency and the continuing care activities that should occur at every office visit.

MANAGEMENT OF DIABETIC COMPLICATIONS

The Diabetes Complication and Control Trial in 1993 found that most diabetic complications are the result of prolonged hyperglycemia. High levels of glucose can cause proteins to bind together and form advanced glycation end products, which can interfere with multiple cellular activities (Brownlee, 1992).

Good glycemic control is the most powerful prevention for the complications of diabetes. At the very least, such control will delay or inhibit the development of micro- as well as macrovascular complications. Pimagedine, currently in clinical trials, may be of help in preventing or slowing the development of advanced glycation end products. This would mean that the progression of complications such as renal disease might be prevented by more than maintaining strict glycemic control only. In the meantime, the primary care provider must use a total approach to diabetes management that encompasses all metabolic deficits.

Dyslipidemia

Lipid abnormalities are associated with type 2 diabetes as well as type 1 (Sobel, 1997). These abnormalities can persist even with good glycemic control. The risk for dyslipidemia and its sequelae in diabetes is compounded in patients who have other major risk factors for coronary heart disease (ADA, 1996a). The provider needs to keep lipid management guidelines in mind for all patients with diabetes.

Triglyceride levels of 150 to 450 mg/dL are part of the insulin-resistant state in type 2 diabetes. Triglycerides frequently respond to good glycemic control through diet, exercise, and diabetic medications. Higher levels (450 to 900 mg/dL) may require separate medication schedules. Extreme hypertriglyceridemia (>1000 mg/dL), usually in the presence of chylomicronemia, is a serious metabolic illness and can lead to pancreatitis or death. In diabetes, such levels represent failure of the lipoprotein clearing enzyme, lipoprotein lipase, which is an insulin-dependent enzyme (Lahdenpera, et al., 1996). Even if the blood glucose level is not excessively high, these patients usually require insulin until their triglyceride levels return to less dangerous levels. Genfibvizal is most appropriate in these patients, with doses up to 2400 mg/day.

■ ■ ■ **CLINICAL PEARL**

Metformin and troglitazone have an effect on lipids.

For a more in-depth discussion of dyslipidemia, refer to Chapter 10.

Hypertension

Hypertension is strongly associated with diabetes and contributes significantly to the complications of retinopathy, coronary heart disease, and nephropathy (Sobel, 1997). Hypertension in people with type 2 diabetes may be of mixed etiology, with essential hypertension playing a larger role in this population. Hypertension that develops after the diagnosis of diabetes may be associated with accelerated nephropathy (Chaiken et al, 1995b). Patients with diabetes and hypertension should have a target blood pressure of less than 130/85 mmHg (ADA, 1996e, f). Diagnosis and management are discussed in Chapter 12; specifics of antihypertensive medications in relation to diabetes are discussed here.

ANTIHYPERTENSIVE MEDICATIONS

Antihypertensive medications can have metabolic effects that influence glycemic control and lipid levels. The provider must keep in mind that calcium channel blockers, angiotensin-converting enzyme (ACE) inhibitors, and direct angiotensin II blockers are metabolically neutral. Calcium channel blockers are particularly useful with coexisting coronary heart disease. ACE inhibitors have been shown to decrease proteinuria in type 1 diabetes. Clinical trials of direct angiotensin II blockers are underway to determine if these related compounds may also have renal-protective effects. Beta-blockers can be effective but should be used with caution. They can be used in patients newly diagnosed with diabetes, or when indicated after a myocardial infarction or in angina pectoris. However, beta-blockers may interfere with insulin secretion if nonselective agents are used.

TABLE 17-18	Visit Frequency				
Visit Frequency	Therapy Status	Ask	Examine	Plan	Phone or Office Follow-up
Every 3 months	All on insulin	Hypo or hyperglycemia episodes: cause, frequency, severity; glucose self-monitoring results; insulin and therapeutic regimen adjustments; problems with metabolic emergencies such as hypoglycemia requiring another's help; self-management of diet; exercise, etc. and other goals being met? Also, symptoms of complications, other illnesses; current medications; psychosocial or lifestyle issues	Height (if 18–20, pt is still growing); weight; B/P; any part of exam that was abnormal at last visit; fundi (preferably with dilation): refer stat to ophthalmologist or optometrist if new finding; if symptomatic feet, check sensation (using monofilament); check skin and nails	Refer to relevant specialist if findings suggest significant ischemia, infection, deformity, ulceration, etc. Reinforce diabetic teaching as well as foot care as needed.	Daily if new to insulin, and if major change in dose. May need daily visits as well until daily glucose controlled, hypoglycemia risk is low, and patient competent in implementing treatment. Hospitalization may be needed for some.
Every 3–6 months (depends on treatment goal achievement)	Oral hypoglycemics	As above	Any relevant system suggested by history	As above	May need to be seen or phoned weekly if new to treatment, until blood glucose range is reasonable or is able to manage regimen.
More frequent	All categories of diabetes	Self-management or medication problems. Acute complications or exacerbation, etc.	System relating to presented problem	As above	Phone or office follow-up needed when goals not being met; complications arise or worsen; also following metabolic emergencies such as hypoglycemia requiring another's help (if on medication); diabetic ketoacidosis; acute illness or appearance/exacerbation of chronic illness, including hypertension
Every 3–6 months (depends on treatment goal achievement)	Diet and exercise only	Self-management of diet, exercise, and other goals being met? Symptoms of complications; other illnesses, current medications; psychosocial or lifestyle issues	As above	As above	In-between phone follow-up as needed
Annually	All			Obtain laboratory data (see Table 17-4). Comprehensive visual and dilated eye exams by ophthalmologist or optometrist after 5 years of diabetes, and in all over age 30. Also, if reports visual/eye changes.	

■ **CLINICAL WARNING:** Beta-blockers can mute the adrenergic symptoms of hypoglycemia and decrease the movement of glycogen stores in muscle and liver in response to low blood sugar levels. This is especially true for patients taking insulin and for those with longstanding type I disease. In addition, response to counterregulatory hormones may be excessive because of the lack of alpha opposition of beta blockade. Patients with endogenous insulin capacity may be at risk for hyperosmolar nonketotic coma (Young & Koda-Kimble, 1995). Extreme caution should be used in persons with longstanding diabetes who may have hypoglycemic unawareness. Beta-blockers will further block normal awareness of and recovery from hypoglycemia because they mask symptoms such as tachycardia. The provider must carefully evaluate the risk for a fatal outcome of masked hypoglycemia when using beta-blockers.

Although they are the first step in medication management for hypertension, thiazide diuretics increase insulin resistance and decrease insulin production. They also can have adverse affects on lipids. All of these effects are generally dose-related. The use of thiazide in very low doses is often effective in lowering blood pressure, either alone or in combination with other antihypertensives. Thiazide is probably the least expensive of medications currently available.

CLINICAL WARNING: Avoid hypokalemia, as it can lead to decreased insulin secretion while worsening tissue resistance to insulin. Hypokalemia can also bring on arrhythmias. Therefore, endeavor to keep the dosage at 25 mg/day or less of hydrochlorothiazide, or 2.5 mg/dL of indapamide (Young & Koda-Kimble, 1995).

Selective alpha-blockers do not adversely affect insulin sensitivity. There is some evidence to suggest that they may actually improve levels of high-density lipoproteins and lower levels of low-density lipoproteins. These agents are particularly useful in persons with pulmonary problems, where beta-blockers are contraindicated. Selective alpha-blockers also can relieve urinary symptoms in men with benign prostatic hypertrophy (Young & Koda-Kimble, 1995).

Microvascular Disease

The major complications of microvascular disease in diabetes include nephropathy, proliferative retinopathy, including clinically significant macular edema, and neuropathy. Renal failure as an outcome of long-term nephropathy is seen less commonly in type 2 than in type 1 disease. This is quite possibly because patients with type 2 disease are more likely to die of cardiovascular disease, thus precluding the onset of renal failure. All of these complications can occur in both type 1 and type 2 diabetes. The news is not entirely grim, though, because all complications can be at least delayed and lessened, if not outright prevented, through sound glycemic control. This fact was well demonstrated by the Diabetes Control and Complications Trial (DCCT Research Group, 1993a, b). Given the poor outcomes for people with diabetes and end-stage renal disease (ESRD), the prudent primary care provider works with the patient to establish good control of blood pressure, blood sugar, and lipids. These controls can help to divert the otherwise inevitable downward course for the patient facing the complications of diabetes. The following discussion will cover each of the microvascular complications in turn.

NEPHROPATHY

Diabetes is one of the leading causes of ESRD. The 5-year survival rate for persons with diabetes and ESRD approaches only 20% (DCCT Research Group, 1993a). In patients with type 1 disease, renal disease commonly develops 10 to 20 years after the diagnosis of diabetes. The development of nephropathy is heralded by the onset of microalbuminuria several years before blood pressure or serum creatinine levels become abnormal (Gilbert et al., 1993). Only Caucasians with type 2 diabetes seem to be relatively spared excessive rates of nephropathy. Persons at greatest risk for nephropathy include those of Native

North American, Hispanic, Asian, African, and Pacific Island heritage (Chaiken et al., 1997). Kidney disease clusters in families. The incidence of diabetic nephropathy throughout a given practice area will vary considerably with the ethnic composition of the clinic and the family history of the patient.

The DCCT Research Group (1993a) showed that optimal control of blood glucose levels can prevent or delay progression of nephropathy in type 1 diabetes. Alzaid (1996) reported that in type 2 disease, higher levels of glucose and GHB are most strongly associated with microalbuminuria. Microalbuminuria is diagnosed when a urinary albumin/creatinine ratio of 30 to 300 mg/g creatinine is seen, or an albumin excretion range of 30 to 300 mg in a 24-hour urine sample (Pagana & Pagana, 1997). Microalbuminuria is often found in patients at the time of type 2 diagnosis. A urine screening for microalbuminuria via random urine for albumin/creatinine ratio should be done at that time, and annually thereafter. Alternatively, a 24-hour urine sample may be collected for the same purpose. Proteinuria and subsequent renal failure are long-term outcomes of poor glycemic control (Gilbert et al., 1994). Control of concomitant hypertension must be a goal in these patients to prevent, mitigate, or delay the progression of nephropathy.

ACE inhibitors are favored drugs in treating hypertension in diabetes (Perdneger et al, 1994; Kasiske et al, 1993). ACE inhibitors such as captopril have been shown to slow the progression of proteinuria in a population with type 1 diabetes (Lewis et al, 1993)

Ravid et al (1993) demonstrated that ACE inhibitors could decrease the excretion of urinary albumin in normotensive patients with type 2 diabetes. They also reported a slowing in the rate of decline in glomerular filtration. Clinical trials are continuing to examine the efficacy of ACE inhibitors in type 2 diabetes. What (if any) role ACE inhibitors have in delaying the onset of ESRD in type 2 populations thus is not yet established. Still, ACE inhibitors have been shown to decrease progression from microalbuminuria to clinical proteinuria in patients with hypertension and type 2 diabetes (Lebovitz et al, 1994).

Management of nephropathy may require the provider to consult with specialists in diabetes as well as in urology. Depending on the severity of the patient's needs, their continued presence in comanaging the patient's care may help both patient and provider. For more information in managing renal dysfunction and hypertension, the reader is referred to those respective chapters. The monitoring of kidney function in diabetes is presented in Table 17-19.

TABLE 17-19   **Monitoring Kidney Function in Diabetes**

- Yearly assessment of microalbuminuria, serum creatinine, and 24-hour urinary protein (begin yearly after first 5 years in type 1)

- Creatinine clearance determinations at time of type 2 diagnosis and every year thereafter. The use of albumin/creatinine (A/C) ratio on a spot urine specimen can help screen for early nephropathy. An A/C ratio of <20 mcg/g does not require confirmation by 24-hour or timed urinary collection. If creatinine clearance <100 mL/min/1.73 M^2, or if abnormal serum creatinine, then check more frequently.

- Consider nondiabetic causes of nephropathy if proteinuria occurs soon after diagnosis, or if creatinine rises with minimal proteinuria.

RETINOPATHY

Optimal control of the blood glucose level can reduce the incidence of retinopathy by 60% (DCCT Research Group, 1993b). However, 25% of patients with type 2 diabetes have some degree of retinopathy at the time of diagnosis. Diabetic retinopathy is the leading cause of new cases of adult blindness. Proliferative retinopathy that threatens vision is present in 25% of patients with type 1 diabetes of more than 15 years' duration. The timely use of laser photocoagulation can decrease the risk of visual loss by 50% to 60% (DCCT Research Group, 1993b).

The most common lesions seen on the retinas of persons with diabetes include hard exudates (a result of capillary leakage and macular edema) and proliferative changes caused by fragile new vessel formation. When they occur off the disc (which these vessels often do), there is a special risk for vision impairment (ADA, 1995). The reader is referred to the color plates that illustrate proliferative retinopathy, hard exudate formation, and macular edema. These pictures can be found in the color plates section of this text.

■ ■ ■ ■ CLINICAL PEARLS

- Annual eye examinations with pupillary dilation by an ophthalmologist or licensed optometrist skilled in retinopathic assessment are essential for all patients with type 2 diabetes. This should begin at the time of diagnosis. The provider is advised to document this advice in the patient's chart on an annual basis.

- Patients with type 1 diabetes should also have this dilation examination 5 years after the initial diagnosis and on an annual basis thereafter, lifelong. Document this advice.

- Any decrease in vision or onset of new floaters should be evaluated immediately by an ophthalmologist or licensed optometrist skilled in assessing diabetic retinas.

- Panretinal or scatter photocoagulation may be used on patients with high-risk characteristics, including proliferation of new vessels on the disc.

The primary care provider can support the patient with retinopathy to protect remaining vision. Besides achieving glycemic control, these supports may include hypertension and dyslipidemia management, assistance with smoking cessation, and provision of clinical advice (avoid isometric exercise, straining at stool [Valsalva maneuver], and hard sneezing or nose-blowing).

DIABETIC NEUROPATHY

Diabetic neuropathy is a painful, serious sequela of diabetes mellitus that affects patients and their families alike. Diabetic neuropathy is characterized by pain and associated symptoms of numbness and tingling in the hands and feet plus deep organ system neuropathy. Symptoms are difficult to diagnose and have potentially fatal consequences. When it occurs in its peripheral form, diabetic neuropathy is a generally bilateral rather than unilateral dysfunction. Its painful presentation can alternate with loss of sensory function, especially to the soles and palms. This loss can lead to patient confusion of where the feet are in relation to the physical environment, making walking difficult and, in extreme instances, impossible. Eventually the patient may report loss of all reasonable function in the affected extremities. Organ systems can also be affected. These include the ocular pupil, gastrointestinal tract, sweat glands, cardiovascular and adrenal medullary systems, and the bladder and sex organs. The primary care provider must thoroughly investigate any symptoms reported to discern systemic disease from diabetic neuropathy (Emanuele & Emanuele, 1997).

Allen et al (1997) reported that nerves die back in the presence of persistent hyperglycemia, with findings in both motor conduction and peripheral sensory pathways. Neuropathies occur in three major types, with overlapping clinical syndromes: distal symmetrical polyneuropathy, focal diabetic neuropathy, and autonomic neuropathy. The presentation and management of each of these three major types will be discussed in turn.

Distal symmetrical polyneuropathy is the most common type. Nearly 60% of patients will have this problem after 25 years of diabetes. Sometimes it is present at diagnosis (generally type 2 disease). The clinical syndrome associated with distal symmetrical polyneuropathy includes small-fiber neuropathy, large-fiber neuropathy, and acute painful neuropathy. Small-fiber neuropathy is characterized by distal loss of temperature sensation and of pinprick or pressure sensation. The use of monofilaments during the physical examination will help assess for small-fiber neuropathy. Large-fiber neuropathy is most strongly associated with neuropathic foot ulcers and joint deformities. It is characterized by impaired distal vibration sense and impaired proprioception. Ankle reflexes can be impaired, sometimes severely. Later findings can include alteration in gait and a positive Romberg sign. Acute painful neuropathy is relatively uncommon. Patients develop pain, in particular a severe burning sensation over the lower extremities. Numbness and tingling are also common. Acute painful neuropathy can be associated with the initiation of insulin therapy or with sudden weight loss (sometimes referred to as diabetic cachexia). Objective signs of neuropathy may be absent or minimal. Symptoms usually resolve over weeks to months of improved glycemic control. Relapses are rare.

Focal diabetic neuropathy, also called diabetic mononeuropathy, is characterized by sudden onset, asymmetrical distribution, and a self-limiting course to affected areas. Cranial nerves III and VI are most commonly affected in this kind of neuropathy. Recovery generally occurs over several weeks, and the disorder can take up to 18 months to resolve.

Autonomic neuropathies are associated with a wide range of pathologies and contribute significantly to the morbidity of diabetes. Autonomic neuropathies can complicate diabetic management to a significant degree. Autonomic neuropathies are generally seen in patients already found to have distal polyneuropathy. An autonomic neuropathy can be both uncomfortable and embarrassing for the patient. The treatment of autonomic dysfunction in primary care consists of patient support and, when indicated, referral to an appropriate specialist for symptom management. Examples of autonomic neuropathies include:

- Bladder dysfunction with incomplete emptying, resulting in frequent urinary tract infections (a common problem)
- Sexual dysfunctions
- Gastroparesis or impaired gastrointestinal motility, which can result in erratic glycemic control. Gastroparesis is characterized by early satiety, bloating, and decreased ap-

petite. Constipation and diabetic diarrhea often occur alternately. Diarrhea can last from hours to weeks and may be severe. Fecal incontinence can be a late manifestation.

■ Orthostatic hypotension, which can be associated with syncope, visual impairment, or postural dizziness.

Bladder Dysfunction

Patients complaining of frequency, dribbling, incomplete bladder emptying, or hesitancy should have their bladder function evaluated. The provider should augment careful history-taking with analysis of objective data. These data include examination of the glycemic record and vaginal and bladder muscle evaluation in women and prostate examination in men. The reader is referred to Chapters 67 and 68 for assessment and management strategies. *Referral Point:* If the appropriate glycemic control measures and vaginal, bladder, or prostate interventions are not effective, then referral to a urologic specialist may be in order. The specialist can assess the need for more specific bladder dysfunction interventions, including bethanechol chloride or, eventually, self-catheterization.

Sexual Dysfunction

Sexual dysfunction occurs in both men and women as a result of vascular and neurologic impairment.

Referral Point: Women may experience dyspareunia and vaginal dryness (see Chap. 67). Women whose dyspareunia does not respond to normal primary care interventions may require further evaluation by a gynecologic specialist.

■ ■ ▢ **CLINICAL PEARL**

Women who present with complaints of vaginal dryness or dyspareunia may respond well to Replens or a similar, nonmedicated product that improves mucosal moisture. Cooking oils may also prove effective; however, the patient will need to weigh their low-cost benefit against their propensity for staining any fabrics that come in contact with oils.

Men may become impotent. When associated with diabetes, impotence has a gradual onset. Alcohol and concomitant medication use may compound the problem. Initially, erections are decreased in frequency and rigidity, progressing to complete impotence. Before this occurs, other causes should be ruled out. If glycemic control is especially poor, improved control may restore function. *Referral Point:* Patients with impotency symptoms should be referred to a urologist who specializes in erectile dysfunction. This person can provide evaluation and management of these problems. Support can include use of a vacuum pump, intrapenile injections with prostaglandins, or a prosthesis (Genuth, 1997). There are a growing number of medical treatments, mechanical devices, and penile prostheses available. Many men can be successfully treated with sildenafil citrate taken prn 1 hour or so before intercourse. The provider is cautioned to carefully review prescribing materials related to this drug in concert with the patient's clinical record, including cardiac disease and medication history, before prescribing.

Gastroparesis

A referral should be given for gastroenterology consultation when a patient complains of gastrointestinal motility symptoms secondary to autonomic neuropathy. The patient may respond to pharmacologic intervention aimed at improving gastric motility. Some agents that the gastroenterologist may recommend to improve motility might include cisapride, erythromycin, or metoclopramide (Genuth, 1997). Diet can also assist in improving gastric motility. Interventions may include increasing soluble or insoluble fiber intake while making adjustments in the overall amount of fiber in the diet. The reader is referred to Chapter 5 for more information about sources and amounts of dietary fiber.

Orthostatic Hypotension

Vasoconstrictor medications may be indicated for the treatment of orthostatic hypotension in some patients, but referral to a diabetes specialist is usually prudent before embarking on pharmacologic treatment. The specialist can assist in discerning whether the management of a patient's orthostatic hypotension requires additional intake of salt and, perhaps, treatment with fludrocortisone.

■ ■ ▢ **CLINICAL PEARL**

Special waist-high support hose may benefit some patients.

■ **CLINICAL WARNING:** Autonomic neuropathies will certainly progress if blood glucose is not well controlled. Aggressive glycemic control also will help in improving the pain associated with distal symmetrical polyneuropathy and focal neuropathy. Glycemic control can prevent permanent nerve damage (DCCT Research Group, 1995). Prevention is key, because it is difficult to manage autonomic neuropathies (Genuth, 1997).

Peripheral Neuropathies

The pain associated with distal symmetrical polyneuropathy and focal neuropathy usually improves with optimal glucose control (DCCT Research Group, 1995). Supportive measures can include:

■ Tricyclic medication, which seems to give some pain relief
■ Serotonin reuptake inhibitors, which provide variable success; however, pain relief is not an approved use.
■ Vitamin B_6
■ Capsaicin cream 0.075% applied four times daily is often helpful and is approved for the pain associated with neuropathy. The cream depletes nerve fibers of their substance P, thus depriving them of the capacity to secrete this stimulus to pain.
■ Physical therapy can be helpful in improving function and flexibility and teaching the patient safe methods for movement when sensation is compromised.
■ Several aldose reductase inhibitors are in varying stages of clinical trial. These agents act by inhibiting sorbitol (created in the glucose metabolism pathway) from accumulating in peripheral nerves. When they become available, they will need to be taken lifelong. They should

assist in preventing complications of diabetes (Ives & Dunn, 1997).

See Chapter 56 for additional information.

Foot Care

The prevention of lower extremity amputations depends initially on identifying feet at risk. The results of the Seattle Prospective Diabetic Foot Study provided information key to primary care assessment of feet at risk for neuropathy (Adler et al, 1997). The study demonstrated that aggressive therapy decreased the risk for polyneuropathies in type 2 diabetes. This finding was echoed by Adler et al, who found that subjects with higher mean GHB values tested positive for foot neuropathy; their cohorts with normal GHB levels were free of neuropathy. A history of increased alcohol intake (whether overt or occult) was described as an important predictor for diabetic foot problems. Aging, duration of diabetes, and history of lower extremity ulceration were also found to be factors that preceded the clinical occurrence of foot neuropathy, as diagnosed by monofilament testing.

It is difficult to quantify the time frame for changes of aging. Preaging determinants of blood vessel and nerve integrity include genetic predisposition to problems, diet and exercise history, smoking and alcohol use, and the presence of other conditions such as coronary artery disease. The duration of diabetes is also difficult to pigeonhole, at least in type 2 disease. Patients typically deal with disruptions in fat and carbohydrate metabolism for several months or even years before they are formally diagnosed with diabetes. Thus, the primary care provider must use history of alcohol abuse (even if just suspected) as well as the presence of ulceration (current or in the past) in the neuropathy assessment.

One sign of vascular disease in the compromised foot is often hairlessness; the skin appears mottled and there may be a dependent rubor. Neuropathy assessment is done using the 5.07 monofilament. There is decreased pressure sensation as assessed by monofilament. This simple tool provides a pressure of 10 g and has demonstrated an ability to predict ulceration of the lower extremity (Mueller, 1996; Rith-Najarian et al, 1992) (a source for obtaining this tool is provided in the resources section at the end of this chapter). Decreased vibratory sense also is usually present.

■ ■ ■ ▫ **CLINICAL PEARL**

Tracking the neuropathic course is key to preventing complications. Therefore, the primary care provider should carefully examine and do monofilament testing on both feet at every visit. Record the results in the patient record at every visit. Vigilant daily foot examination and care are vital to preserving function (ADA, 1996b).

All persons with diabetes should wear comfortable shoes that do not rub against any portion of the feet. Patients with decreased sensation need to be especially vigilant. Anyone who has diabetes should avoid going barefoot and should be advised not to trim their own toenails. The primary care provider should teach the patient how to examine the feet, using a mirror

to examine hard-to-visualize spots, including the sole. This examination should be carried out nightly, after bathing. The feet should be dried thoroughly. The provider should encourage the patient to apply a rich emollient cream daily.

■ ■ ■ ▫ **CLINICAL PEARL**

Powders and creams may be used, except between the toes.

The goal of care is healthy foot maintenance and prevention of any unnoticed injury that might otherwise progress, perhaps with dangerous consequences. Foot care resources are listed at the end of this chapter.

Refer the patient to a podiatrist for an annual assessment and, if necessary, follow-up podiatric management. Document that this referral was made.

For more in-depth discussion of neuropathies and their management, consult Chapter 56.

Macrovascular Disease

Of the macrovascular complications of diabetes, coronary artery disease is the most prevalent. Its incidence is 55% in adults with type 2 disease, compared to 2% to 4% of persons without diabetes. The risk of death from coronary artery disease is sixfold greater in men with diabetes and fourfold greater in women with diabetes compared to the general population (Sobel, 1996). Diabetes in and of itself is a risk factor for subsequent cardiovascular disease.

Obesity, hypertension, and dyslipidemia are all covariates of diabetes. Their presence may potentiate the risk for cardiovascular complications in persons with diabetes. Patients who do not have diabetes are placed at increased risk for diabetes development should they have these covariates. Hyperinsulinemia and insulin resistance syndrome confer cardiovascular risk if the patient's type 2 diabetes is poorly controlled. Alterations in platelet function and increased aggregability, combined with disruptions in normal fibrinolysis, also may play a significant role in the development of macrovascular complications in diabetes. The reader is referred to the chapters dealing with each of these topics for a more detailed picture of their diagnosis and management.

Other Problems Seen in Diabetes

INCREASED SUSCEPTIBILITY TO INFECTION

All primary care providers are familiar with the problems associated with infection and its resolution in patients with diabetes. Neuropathy seems to be at least in part responsible for this situation, but it is also compounded by other physiologic variables. Specifically, leukocyte function is impaired in diabetes, with decreased complement activation seen as a sequela. This scenario is exacerbated by the compromise in vascular function, including basement membrane changes, which alter filtration functions in the blood vessel wall, as well as alterations in overall vessel function. Patients with vascular disease face even greater compromise in vascular function. When glycemic control is poor, leukocyte motility through the now-hyperosmolar serum is hindered. The outcome of such physiologic compromise is a propensity for infection that, especially when in the distal periphery, can lead to osteomyelitis.

SKIN CHANGES

There are several classic skin changes associated with diabetes mellitus:

- Acanthosis nigricans is a thickening and darkening of the skin at the back of the neck. This finding is associated with insulin resistance and so is most commonly found in patients with type 2 diabetes (Sauer & Hall, 1996).
- Glycation permits cross-linking of skin proteins, diminishing suppleness and limiting flexibility. The inability to place palms and fingers of each hand in direct contact with each other is sometimes seen in diabetes of long standing. This phenomenon is called the praying hands sign.
- Thickening of the skin is sometimes seen. This is referred to as scleredema and is generally found over the back of the arms.
- Lipodystrophy can occur at the site of multiple injections. Presenting with a lumpy, wasted appearance, lipodystrophy can sometimes be altered by deliberate injection to the site with insulin. It can generally be avoided if the patient is vigilant in rotating insulin therapy among multiple sites.
- Necrobiosis diabeticorum can occur in patients with longstanding diabetes. It typically presents with dark, dry, clustered patches overlying tight skin on the anterior surface of the lower leg. Although unattractive, this condition is benign.

Prevention of skin sores or ulcers is vital to health maintenance in diabetes. Like diabetic foot care, as previously described, the provider should emphasize the importance of careful washing and drying of skin, in concert with daily moisturizing with a rich emollient product. Daily skin inspection should round out this management plan.

TEACHING AND SELF-CARE

The best advice in diabetes self-management is healthy lifestyle. Antioxidants may prove helpful for reasons outlined in the pathology portion of this chapter. Vitamin E is an important antioxidant. Because vitamin E is fat-soluble, doses exceeding 400 IU/day are not generally recommended. Vitamin C is also a common antioxidant, and supplementation may be part of a healthy lifestyle. Anderson et al (1996) suggest that chromium picolinate improves glucose tolerance, but their findings are not definitive. The ADA (1996c) does not recommend that patients use chromium supplementation as part of their self-management plan.

See Tables 17-5, 17-6, 17-8, 17-9, 17-11, 17-12, 17-14, 17-15, and 17-16 for content specific to teaching self-care.

COMMUNITY RESOURCES

For general patient teaching strategies, provider and patient "cheat sheets" for diabetic foot inspection and foot care, as well as tips for provider documentation, **Ideabetes** provides ideas and equipment for teaching patients about the physiologic consequences of poor glycemic control. Foot care management packets, including assessment check-off sheets that the provider can use for examination and chart documentation, are wonderful. *Contact:* Mary Jo Dudley, BSN, RN, CDE, 38 Silver St., Dover, NH 03820; (603) 749-3899.

Monofilaments (10-g size) can be obtained from Gill Podiatry Supply and Equipment Co., 7803 Freeway Circle, Middleburg Heights, OH 44130; (800) 321-1148 or (216) 243-3700.

A list of CDEs in every state can be obtained from The American Association of Diabetes Educators, (800) TEAM-UP-4. A list of registered dietitians can be obtained from National Center for Nutrition and Dietetics of the American Dietetic Association, (800) 366-1655.

All patients with diabetes should be given access to **Diabetes Forecast**, a patient-focused publication of the American Diabetes Association. This magazine's approach to diabetes and its management is up to date and patient-empowering. It provides knowledge and support.

Internet sites for patient information on diabetes at http://www.niddk.nih.gov/diabetesdocs.html include:
Diabetes Control and Complications Trail
Diabetes Dictionary
Diabetes in America, 2nd Edition
Diabetes in African Americans
Diabetes in Hispanics Americans
Diabetes Overview
Diabetes Recipes and Cookbooks
Diabetes Statistics
Summary Fact Sheet for Diabetes Statistics
Diabetic Eye Disease
Diabetic Neuropathy: The Nerve Damage of Diabetes
End-stage Renal Disease
Feet Can Last a Lifetime
Hypoglycemia
Insuficiencia Renal Cronica Terminal: Eleccion del tratamiento que le conviene a usted (in Spanish)
End-Stage Renal Disease: Choosing a Treatment That's Right for You
Insulin-Dependent Diabetes
Kidney Disease of Diabetes
Other Diabetes Subjects
Questions to Ask Your Doctor about Blood Sugar Control
Understanding Gestational Diabetes
Diabetes Organizations, Professional and Voluntary . . . and many other topics
National organizations include:

- National Diabetes Information Clearinghouse, 1 Information Way, Bethesda, MD 20892-3560; (301) 654-3327; fax: (301) 907-8906; E-mail: ndic@aeri.com
- Weight-Control Information Network, 1 WIN Way, Bethesda, MD 20892-3665; (800) 946-8098 or (301) 570-2177; fax: (301) 570-2186; E-mail: WINNIDDK @aol.
com; home page: http://www.niddk.nih.gov
- National Center for Chronic Disease Prevention and Health Promotion, TISB Mail Stop K-13, 4770 Buford Highway NE, Atlanta, GA 30341-3724; (770) 488-5080; fax: (770) 488-5969
- Indian Health Service, Diabetes Program Headquarters West, 5300 Homestead Road NE, Albuquerque, NM 87110; (505) 837-4182; fax: (505) 837-4188

- American Association of Diabetes Educators, 444 N. Michigan Ave., Suite 1240, Chicago, IL 60611; (312) 644-2233 or (800) 338-3633; fax: (312) 644-4411; Diabetes Educator Access Line: (800) TEAM-UP-4 (800-832-6874); home page: http://www.aadenet.org
- American Diabetes Association, National Service Center, 1660 Duke St., Alexandria, VA 22314; (703) 549-1500 (National Service Center) or (800) 342-2383 (800-DIABETES) (reaches affiliate office in the state in which the call is placed); home page: http://www.diabetes.org
- American Dietetic Association, 216 W. Jackson Blvd., Suite 800, Chicago, IL 60606-6995; (312) 899-0040; fax: (800) 877-1600; home page: http://www.eatright.org

REFERRAL POINTS AND CLINICAL WARNINGS

The primary care provider should strive for timely diagnosis of type 2 diabetes, before complications have the opportunity to develop. Patient and provider can work together to develop, monitor, and adjust management strategies. Other health care providers, including the diabetologist, CDE, nutritionist, and psychologist, can all play important team roles in the comanagement of this potentially deadly disease. Tight glycemic control is the gold standard of management. Patients need to be referred to another provider if complications in management arise; these are noted throughout the chapter.

EDITOR'S NOTE:

COMPLEMENTARY APPROACHES

A general discussion of complementary approaches can be found in Chapter 3. The following, while not an exhaustive list, are some complementary approaches being used for this condition. Additional information on these approaches, including precautions, can be found in Appendices A and B. Providers need to assess for the use of complementary approaches as part of the patient's history, as they may impact conventional therapies, and patients may not volunteer this information unless specifically asked. Efficacy of many complementary approaches is not as well documented as that of conventional therapies. Providers need to read the literature before suggesting these complementary approaches.

- Complementary Modalities
   Acupuncture

References

Adler, A.I., Boyko, E.J., Ahroni, J.H., et al. (1997). Risk factors for diabetic peripheral sensory neuropathy. *Diabetes Care, 20*(7), 1162–1167.

Allen, C., Shen, G., Palta, B., et al. (1997). Long-term hyperglycemia is related to peripheral nerve changes at a diabetes duration of 4 years. *Diabetes Care, 20*(7), 1154–1158.

Alzaid, A.A. (1996). Microalbuminuria in patients with NIDDM: An overview. *Diabetes Care, 19,* 7-9-89.

American Diabetes Association. (1995). Screening for diabetic retinopathy (position statement). *Diabetes Care, 18*(Supp. 1), S21–23.

American Diabetes Association. (1996a). Detection and management of lipid disorders in diabetes (consensus statement). *Diabetes Care, 19*(Supp. 1), S96–102.

American Diabetes Association. (1996b). Foot care in patients with diabetes mellitus (position statement). *Diabetes Care, 19*(Supp. 1), S23–24.

American Diabetes Association. (1996c). Nutrition recommendations and principles for people with diabetes mellitus (position statement). *Diabetes Care, 19*(Supp. 1), S16–19.

American Diabetes Association. (1996d). Self-monitoring of blood glucose (consensus statement). *Diabetes Care, 19*(Supp. 1), S62–66.

American Diabetes Association. (1996e). Standards of medical care for patients with diabetes mellitus (position statement). *Diabetes Care, 19*(Supp. 1), S8–15.

American Diabetes Association. (1996f). Treatment of hypertension in diabetes. *Diabetes Care, 19*(Supp. 1), S107–113.

American Diabetes Association. (1997). Report of the Expert Committee. *Diabetes Care, 20*(7), 11.

Anderson, Cheng, & Bryden et al. (1997). Elevated intakes of supplemental chromium improve glucose and insulin variables in individuals with type 2 diabetes. *Diabetes, 46*(11), 1786–1791.

Arseneau, D.L., Mason, A.C., Wood, O.B., et al. (1994). A comparison of learning activity packages and classroom instruction for diet management of patients with non-insulin dependent diabetes mellitus. *Diabetes Educator, 20,* 509–514.

Banerji, M.A., Chaiken, R., Huey, H., et al. (1993a). Hybrid diabetes in African Americans: GAD antibody negative NIDDM in subjects with diabetic acidosis (DKA) who are positive for HLA DR3 and DR4. *Diabetes,* (Supp.), Abstract No. 195.

Banerji, M.A., Norin, R.L., & Lebovitz, H.E. (1993b). HLA-DQ associations distinguish insulin-resistant and insulin-sensitive variants of NIDDM in Black Americans. *Diabetes Care, 16,* 429–433.

Boden, G. (1997). Role of fatty acids in the pathogenesis of insulin resistance and NIDDM (review article). *Diabetes, 46*(1), 3–10.

Brownlee, M. (1992). Glycation products and the pathogenesis of diabetic complications. *Diabetes Care, 15,* 1835–1843.

Buchanan, T.A. (1997). Diabetes and pregnancy: A focus on type 2 and gestational diabetes. In J.M. Olefsky. (Ed.). *Current approaches to the management of type 2 diabetes.* Secaucus, N.J.: Professional Postgraduate Services.

Ceriello, A., Bortolotti, N., Fallete, E., et al. (1997). Total radical-trapping antioxidant parameter in NIDDM patients. *Diabetes Care, 20*(2), 194–197.

Chaiken, R.L., Banerji, M.A., Huey, H., & Lebovitz, H.E. (1993). Does Syndrome X exist in Black Americans? *Diabetes, 42,* 444–449.

Chaiken, R.L., Khawaja, R., Norton, M.E., Banerji, M.A., & Lebovitz, H.E. (1997). Utility of untimed urinary albumin measurements in assessing albuminuria in Black NIDDM subjects. *Diabetes Care, 20*(5) 709–713.

Chaiken, R.L., Norton, M.E., Pasmantier, R., et al. (1995a). Metabolic effects of dargliazone, an insulin sensitizer, in NIDDM subjects. *Diabetologia, 38,* 1307–12.

Chaiken, R.L., Palmisano, J., Norton, M.E., et al. (1995b). The interaction of hypertension and diabetes on renal function in Black NIDDM subjects: Cross-sectional data. *Kidney International, 47,* 1697–1702.

Chaturvedi, N., Fuller, J., Stephenson, J., & the EURODIAB IDDM Complications Study Group. (1996). The relationship between socioeconomic status and diabetes control and complications in the EURODIAB IDDM Complications Study. *Diabetes Care, 19*(5), 423–430.

Clark, D.O. (1997). Physical activity efficacy and effectiveness among older adults and minorities. *Diabetes Care, 20*(7), 1176–1182.

Connolly, V.M., & Kesson, C.M. (1996). Socioeconomic status and clustering of cardiovascular disease risk factors in diabetic patients. *Diabetes Care, 19*(5), 419–422.

Diabetes Control and Complications Trial (DCCT) Research Group. (1993a). The effect of intensive treatment of diabetes on the development and progression of long-term complication in insulin-dependent diabetes mellitus. *N Engl J Med, 329,* 977–986.

Diabetes Control and Complications Trial (DCCT) Research Group. (1993b). The relationship of glycemic exposure (HbA₁c) to the risk of development and progression of retinopathy in the Diabetes Control and Complications Trial. *Diabetes, 44,* 968–983.

Diabetes Control and Complications (DCCT) Research Group. (1995). The relationship of glycemic exposure (HbA₁c) to the risk of development and progression of retinopathy in the Diabetes Control and Complications trial. *Diabetes, 44,* 968–983.

Dudley, W.E. III. (January, 1998). Personal communication.

El-Kebbi, I.M., Bacha, G.A., Ziemer, D.C., et al. (1996). Diabetes in urban African Americans. Use of discussion groups to identify barriers to dietary therapy among low-income individuals with non-insulin-dependent diabetes mellitus. *Diabetes Educator, 22*(5), 488–492.

Emanuele, N.V., & Emanuele, M.A. (1997). Diabetic neuropathy: Therapies for peripheral and autonomic symptoms (a review). *Geriatrics, 52*(4), 40–9.

Eriksson, J., Taimela, S., & Koivisto, V.A. (1997). Exercise and the metabolic syndrome. *Diabetologia, 40,* 125–135.

Expert Committee. (1997). The report on the diagnosis and classification of diabetes mellitus. *Diabetes Care, 20*(7), 1883–1897.

Genuth, S.M. (1997). Complications of diabetes: Microvascular disease. In J.M. Olefsky (Ed.). *Current approaches to the management of type 2 diabetes.* Secaucus, N.J.: Professional Postgraduate Services.

Gilbert, R.E., Cooper, M.E., McNally, P.G., et al. (1994). Microalbuminuria: Prognostic and therapeutic implications in diabetes. *Diabetic Medicine, 11,* 636–645.

Gilbert, R.E., Tsalamandris, C., Bach, L.A., et al. (1993). Long-term glycemic control and the rate of progression of early diabetic kidney disease. *Kidney International, 44,* 855–859.

Gougeon, R., Pencharz, P.B., & Sigal, R.J. (1997). Effect of glycemic control on the kinetics of whole-body protein metabolism in obese subjects with non-insulin-diabetes mellitus during iso- and hypoenergetic feeding. *American Journal of Clinical Nutrition, 65,* 861–870.

Hanson, R.L., Jacobsson, L.T.H., McCance, D.R., et al. (1996). Weight fluctuation, mortality and vascular disease in Pima Indians. *International Journal of Obesity, 20,* 463–471.

Harris, M. (1995). *Diabetes in America.* Washington, D.C.: National Institutes of Health Publ. 95-1468.

Harris, S.B., Gittelsohn, J., Hanley, A., et al. (1997). The prevalence of NIDDM and associated risk factors in native Canadians. *Diabetes Care, 20*(2), 185–187.

Hirsch, S.R., Norton, M.E., & Harrington, P. (1995). Education increases rate of near-normoglycemic remission in newly diagnosed NIDDM. *Diabetes, 44,* 1995.

Horton, E.S. (1997). Therapeutic options for the treatment of type 2 diabetes. In J.M. Olefsky (Ed.). *Current approaches to the management of type 2 diabetes.* Secaucus, N.J.: Professional Postgraduate Services, 35–41.

Inzucchi, S.E., Maggs, D.G., & Spollett, G.R. (1997). Efficacy and metabolic effects of troglitazone and metformin in NIDDM. *Diabetes, 46*(Supp. 1), 34A.

Ives, T.J., & Dunn, P.F. (1997). The effect of oxygen radicals metabolites and vitamin E on glycosylation of proteins. *Free Radical Biology and Medicine, 22*(4), 593–596.

Jovanovic-Peterson, L., & Peterson, C.M. (1992). Pregnancy in the diabetic woman. *Endocrine and Metabolic Clinics of North America, 21,* 433.

Jin, J.S., & Bohlen, H.G. (1997). Non–insulin-dependent diabetes and hyperglycemia impair rat intestinal flow-mediated regulation. *American Journal of Physiology, 272* (2, Pt.2), H728–734.

Jin, S.K., & Palmer, M. (1997). Non-insulin-dependent diabetes and hyperglycemia impaired rat intestinal flow-mediated regulation. *American Journal of Physiology, 272*(2 Pt. 2), H728–734.

Kasiske, B.L., Kalil, R.S.N., Ma, J.Z., Liao, M., & Keane, W.F. (1993). Effect of antihypertensive therapy on the kidney in patients with diabetes. *Annals of Internal Medicine, 118,* 129–138.

Kenny, S.J., Aubert, R.E., & Geiss, L.S. (1995). Prevalence and incidence of non-insulin-dependent diabetes. In Harris, M. (1995). *Diabetes in America.* Washington, D.C.: National Institutes of Health Publ. 95-1468.

Klein, R., Palta, M., Allen, C., et al. (1997). Incidence of retinopathy and associated risk factors from time of diagnosis of insulin-dependent diabetes. *Archives of Ophthalmology, 115*(3), 351–356.

Ko, G.T, Chan, J.C., Lau, E., Woo, J., & Cockram, C.S. (1997). Fasting plasma glucose as a screening test for diabetes and its relationship with cardiovascular risk factors in Hong Kong Chinese. *Diabetes Care, 20*(2), 170–172.

Kowluru, T.A., Kern, T.S., & Engerman, R.L. (1997). Abnormalities of retinal metabolism in diabetes or experimental galactosemia. *Free Radical Biology and Medicine, 22*(4), 587–592.

Kristal, B.S., Jackson, C.T., Chung, H.Y., et al. (1997). Defects at center P underlie diabetes-associated mitochondrial dysfunction. *Free Radical Biology and Medicine, 22*(5), 823–833.

Lahdenpera, S., Syvanne, M., Kahri, J., & Taskinen, M-R. (1996). Regulation of low-density lipoprotein particle size distribution in NIDDM and coronary artery disease: Importance of serum triglycerides. *Diabetologia, 39,* 453–461.

Lebovitz, H.E., Weigmann, T.B., Cnaan, A., et al. (1994). Renal protective effects of enalapril in hypertensive NIDDM: Role of baseline albuminuria. *Kidney International, 45*(Supp. 45), S150–155.

Lehto, M., Tuomi, M.M., Widen, E., et al. (1997). Characteristics of the MODY3 phenotype. Early-onset diabetes caused by an insulin secretion defect. *Clinical Journal of Investigation, 99*(4), 582–591.

Lewis, E.J., Hunsicker, L.G., Bain, R.P., & Rhode, R.D. for The Collaborative Study Group. (1993). The effect of angiotensin-converting enzyme inhibition on diabetic nephropathy. *N Engl J Med, 329,* 1456–1462.

Magnus, M.H. (1996). Nutrition update: What's your IQ on cross-cultural nutrition counseling? *Diabetes Educator, 22*(1), 57–62.

Matsuoka, T., Kajimoto, U., Watada, H., et al. (1997). Glycation-dependent, reactive oxygen species-mediated suppression of the insulin gene promoter activity in HIT cells. *Journal of Clinical Investigation, 9*(1), 144–150.

McCance, D.R., Hanson, R.L., Charles, M.A., et al. (1994). Comparison of tests for glycated hemoglobin and fasting and two-hour plasma glucose concentrations as diagnostic methods for diabetes. *British Medical Journal, 308,* 1323–1328.

Mueller, M.J. (1996). Identifying patients with diabetes mellitus who are at risk for lower-extremity complications: Use of Semmes-Weinstein monofilaments. *Physical Therapy, 76,* 68–71.

National Center for Health Statistics. (1993). *Current estimates from the National Health Interview Surveys, 1992.* Vital and Health Statistics, Series 10(189).

Norton, M. (August, 1997). Personal communication.

Olefsky, J.M. (1997). Pathophysiology of type 2 diabetes. In J.M. Olefsky (Ed.). *Current approaches to the management of type 2 diabetes.* Secaucus, N.J.: Professional Postgraduate Services.

O'Rourke, C.M., Davis, J.A., Saltiel, A.R., & Cornicelli, J.A. (1997). Metabolic effects of troglitazone in the Goto-KaKizaki rat, a non-obese and normolipidemic rodent model of non-insulin-dependent diabetes mellitus. *Metabolism: Clinical and Experimental, 46*(2), 192–198.

Pagana, K.D., & Pagana, T.J. (1998). *Mosby's manual of diagnostic and laboratory test reference.* St. Louis: Mosby.

Perneger, T.V., Brancati, F.L., Whelton, P.K., & Klag, M.J. (1994). End-stage renal disease attributable to diabetes mellitus. *Annals of Internal Medicine, 121,* 912–918.

Peuchant, E., Delmas, M.C., Couchouron, A., et al. (1997). Short-term insulin therapy and normoglycemia. Effects on erythrocyte lipid peroxidation in NIDDM patients. *Diabetes Care, 20,* 202–207.

Powell, K.E., & Blair, S.N. (1994). The public health burdens of sedentary living habits: Theoretical but realistic estimates. *Medical Science and Sports Exercise, 26,* 851–856.

Prochaska, J.O. (1991). In search of how people change: Applications to addictive behaviors. *American Psychologist, 47*(9), 1102–1114.

Prochaska, J.O., Norcross, J.C., & DiClemente, C.C. (1994). *Changing for good.* New York: William Morrow.

Prochaska, J.O., Norcross, J.C., Fowler, J.L., Follick, M.J., & Abrams, D.B. (1992). Attendance and outcome in a worksite weight-control program: Processes and stages of changes as process and predictor variables. *Addictive Behaviors, 17*(1), 35–45.

Qiao, Q., Keinanen, S., & Laara, E. (1997). The relationship between hemoglobin levels and diabetic retinopathy. *Journal of Clinical Epidemiology, 50*(2), 153–158.

Rith-Najarian, S.J., Stolusku, T., & Gohdes, D.M. (1992). Identifying diabetic patients at high risk for lower-extremity amputation in a primary care setting. *Diabetes Care, 15,* 1386–1389.

Roshan, M., Burden, A., & Burden, M. (1996). Indo-Asians with diabetes: A special case, a different pattern of complications. *The Practitioner, 240*(2), 120–124.

Sauer, G.C.X., & Hall, J.C. (1996). *Manual of skin diseases.* Philadelphia: Lippincott-Raven.

Schraer, C.D., Ebbsson, S., Boyko, E., et al. (1996). Hypertension and diabetes among Siberian Yupik Eskimos of St. Lawrence Island, Alaska. *Public Health Reports, 111*(Supp. 2), 51–52.

Service, F.J., Rizza, R.A., Zimmerman, B.R., et al. (1997). The classification of diabetes by clinical and C-peptide criteria. A prospective-based study. *Diabetes Care, 20*(2), 198–201.

Sobel, B.E. (1996). Altered fibrinolysis and platelet function in the development of vascular complications of diabetes. *Current Opinion in Endocrinology and Metabolism, 3,* 355–360.

Sobel, B.E. (1997). Complications of diabetes: Macrovascular disease. In J.M. Olefsky (Ed.). *Current approaches to the management of type 2 diabetes.* Secaucus, N.J.: Professional Postgraduate Services.

Stolk, R.P., Orchard, T.J., & Grobbee, D.E. (1995). Why use the oral glucose tolerance test? *Diabetes Care, 18*(7), 1045–1049.

Terauchi, Y., Iwamoto, K., Taemoto, H., et al. (1997). Development of non-insulin-dependent diabetes mellitus in the double knockout mice with disruption of insulin receptor substrate-1 and beta cell glucokinase genes. Genetic reconstitution of diabetes as a polygenic disease. *Journal of Clinical Investigation, 99*(5), 861–866.

Ter Braak, E., Woodwroth, J.R., Bianchi, R., et al. (1996). Injection sites on the pharmacokinetics and glucodynamics of insulin lispro and regular insulin. *Diabetes Care, 19,* 1437–1440.

Thompson, C.H., Sanderman, D., Stein, C., et al. (1997). Fetal growth and insulin resistance in adult life: Role of skeletal muscle morphology. *Clinical Science, 92*(3), 291–296.

Torlone, E., Pampanelli, S., Lalli, C., et al. (1996). Effects of the short-acting insulin analog [Lys (B28), pro (B29)] on postprandial blood. *Diabetes Care, 19*(9), 945–952.

Tuominen, J.A., Karonen, S.L., Melamies, L., Bolli, G., & Koivisto, V.A. (1995). Exercise-induced hypoglycemia in NIDDM patients treated with a short-acting insulin analogue. *Diabetologia, 38,* 106–111.

Young, L.Y., & Koda-Kimble, M.A. (1995). *Applied therapeutics.* Vancouver, Wash.: Applied Therapeutics.

Zaldivar, A., & Smolowitz, J. (1994). Perceptions of the importance placed on religion and folk medicine by non-Mexican-American Hispanic adults with diabetes. *Diabetes Educator, 20*(4), 303–306.

Zinman, B. (1997). Guidelines for the management of type 2 diabetes. In J.M. Olefsky (Ed.). *Current approaches to the management of type 2 diabetes.* Secaucus, N.J.: Professional Postgraduate Services.

APPENDIX I-I

BACKGROUND QUESTIONS

Date of birth: _____   Age: _____   Zip Code: _____   Sex: ___ Male   ___ Female

In general, my overall health is: (please circle a number)

| 0 | 1 | 2 | 3 | 4 | 5 | 6 | 7 | 8 | 9 | 10 |

unhealthy/ill   very healthy

How far away in miles is your nearest emergency care? _____

Medication Status: Do you take any prescription or over-the-counter medication regularly? ___ yes   ___ no.
If yes, what is (are) the name(s) of the medication?

_____

_____

_____

_____

_____

HEALTH HABITS

Do you smoke cigarettes?   ___ yes   ___ no

If yes, how many cigarettes a day? _____   for how many years? _____

If no, did you ever smoke cigarettes?   ___ yes   ___ no

DIET/EXERCISE

What is your height? _____   What is your weight? _____

Are you on a special diet?   ___ yes   ___ no   If yes, please describe _____

Do you exercise regularly?   ___ yes   ___ no   If yes, please describe _____

SLEEP/REST

How many hours do you sleep per night? _____

Do you have problems with insomnia?   ___ yes   ___ no   Do you feel rested upon awakening?   ___ yes   ___ no

Do you use sleeping aids?   ___ yes   ___ no   If yes, please specify type and frequency _____

(Continued)

COGNITIVE/PERCEPTUAL

Do you have any hearing difficulty? ___ yes ___ no   If yes, please describe _____

Do you have any visual problems? ___ yes ___ no   If yes, please specify _____

Do you have any learning difficulties? ___ yes ___ no   If yes, please describe _____

Do you have trouble remembering events or people? ___ yes ___ no

If yes, how good is your memory _____

Are you ever confused? ___ yes ___ no   If yes, please describe

SELF/RELATIONSHIPS

Marital status: ___ married ___ single ___ living in a committed relationship ___ divorced ___ separated ___ widowed. (please check one)

Number of Children? _____   Ages: _____   How many at home? _____

How many people live in your household? _____   Do you have pets? ___ yes ___ no

My occupation is: _____ . I work _____ hours/week

Education level completed (please circle the appropriate number)

Grade School						High School					College					Graduate	
1	2	3	4	5	6	7	8	9	10	11	12	13	14	15	16	17	18+

Please check all roles that apply to you:

___ friend ___ child ___ parent ___ employer ___ employee ___ spouse ___ caretaker

___ community volunteer ___ other (specify: _____)

What resources do you have for emotional support? (check all that apply) ___ spouse ___ family ___ friends ___ religion/spiritual

___ other (specify: _____).

How satisfied are you with your sex life? ___ very satisfied ___ satisfied ___ dissatisfied

STRESS/COPING

Do you feel that you have an excessive amount of stress in your life? ___ yes ___ no

What is your perception of daily stressors which may interfere with your life? (Please circle the number of corresponding to each, 1 being no stress and 10 being the worst stress possible.)

Work:	1	2	3	4	5	6	7	8	9	10
Family:	1	2	3	4	5	6	7	8	9	10
Social:	1	2	3	4	5	6	7	8	9	10
Finances:	1	2	3	4	5	6	7	8	9	10
Health:	1	2	3	4	5	6	7	8	9	10

Other (please specify): _____

1 2 3 4 5 6 7 8 9 10

Do you meditate or practice a relaxation technique? ___ yes ___ no.

If yes, please check those that apply:

___ yoga ___ imagery ___ abdominal breathing ___ meditation ___ progressive muscle relaxation

___ Tai Chi ___ prayer ___ other: _____

Appendix 1 Lifestyle Assessment Inventory (Source: Patricia Winstead-Fry, PhD, The University of Vermont, Burlington, VT. Used with permission).

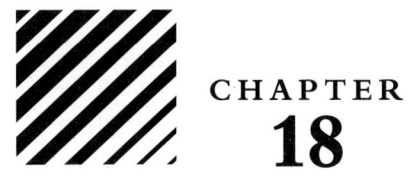

CHAPTER

18

Diseases of the Adrenal Glands

Muriel N. Nathan, PhD, MD

The adrenal glands, which sit on top of the kidneys, are very small organs with complex functions. The gland has a cortex that secretes glucocorticoids and mineralocorticoids. The medulla of the adrenal gland produces catecholamines, epinephrine, and norepinephrine. Each of these will be discussed in detail. Diseases of the adrenal glands can lead to syndromes of wasting, hypotension, and hypoglycemia if adrenal hormones are lacking, whereas diseases that increase the production of adrenal hormones can produce hypertension, weight gain, and virilization. The following chapter will give the primary care provider information needed for the diagnosis and management of several adrenal diseases: adrenal insufficiency, adrenal overactivity, hyperaldosteronism, hypoaldosteronism, and pheochromocytoma. Appropriate referral information will also be given.

ANATOMY, PHYSIOLOGY, AND PATHOLOGY

The adrenal glands are small pyramidal organs, measuring 3×6 cm and weighing about 2.5 to 5 g each, embedded in the retroperitoneal fat medial to the superior pole of the kidneys (Rittmaster & Arab, 1995). The blood supply branches off multiple sites; vascular sites drain from the suprarenal vein into the inferior vena cava on the right and the renal vein on the left. Autonomic innervation of the glands is extensive.

Histologically, the cortex is composed of three parts: the zona glomerulosa, which secretes mineralocorticoids, and the zona fasciculata and zona reticularis, which secrete glucocorticoids and androgens. The medulla arises from neural crest cells. It is very vascular and consists of chromaffin cells, arranged in a network, that secrete catecholamines (Rittmaster & Arab, 1995).

When adrenal loss is caused by autoimmune disease, the cortices of the adrenal glands are decreased in size and infiltrated by lymphocytes. Normal adrenal architecture is replaced by fibrosis. When adrenal failure is caused by tuberculosis or fungal infection, the glands are often large and calcified. Adrenal insufficiency can also occur secondary to hemorrhage within the gland, which has a plentiful arterial supply but limited venous drainage, increasing the risk of thrombosis (Rittmaster & Arab, 1995; Loriaux, 1995).

Synthesis of the steroid hormones is regulated by the hypothalamic–pituitary–adrenal axis (HPA) and, with the exception of aldosterone from the zona glomerulosa, is dependent on adrenocorticotrophic hormone (ACTH). ACTH is produced in the anterior pituitary. Its regulation is maintained by the feedback inhibition of cortisol. In addition, corticotropin-releasing hormone (CRH) stimulates ACTH release. Circadian rhythms and stress also influence the release of ACTH. Corti-

sol, when present in higher-than-physiologic levels, will inhibit ACTH secretion (negative feedback loop). ACTH and cortisol have a diurnal variation, with maximal secretion between 2 AM and 8 AM and nadir around midnight. ACTH secretion is also increased by fever, hypoglycemia, pregnancy, strenuous exercise, anorexia nervosa, and depression (White et al, 1995).

Corticotropin (ACTH) can stimulate aldosterone secretion, but its effect is short-lived. Aldosterone is instead regulated by the renin–angiotensin system and potassium. Receptors in the wall of the afferent arteriole of the kidney respond to hypovolemia and stimulate the release of renin from the juxtaglomerular cells. This cleaves angiotensinogen, a protein made by the liver and found in the plasma, to angiotensin I. Angiotensin-converting enzyme (ACE), elaborated by pulmonary endothelial cells, then cleaves angiotensin I, a decapeptide, to angiotensin II, an octapeptide. Angiotensin II binds to a membrane receptor on the zona glomerulosa cells that is in the family of G-protein-type receptors. Activated second messengers raise intracellular calcium concentrations, leading to aldosterone secretion. Potassium can also increase aldosterone secretion via depolarization of cell membranes, leading to calcium influx through voltage-gated channels (White, 1994).

The primary precursor of adrenal steroid hormones is cholesterol, which is stored in the adrenal cortex. Multiple enzymatic steps produce the steroid hormones along three pathways, producing mineralocorticoids, glucocorticoids, and androgens.

ADRENAL INSUFFICIENCY

Adrenal insufficiency results from a decreased concentration of glucocorticoids, such as cortisol. The most common cause is the withdrawal of exogenous steroids, often given to treat asthma or rheumatologic conditions. Primary adrenal insufficiency is caused by loss of the adrenal cortex; more than 90% of the cortex must be destroyed for adrenal insufficiency to occur (Loriaux, 1995). Secondary adrenal insufficiency is the loss of cortisol secretion because of loss of pituitary ACTH secretion (Oelkers, 1996). Causes of adrenal insufficiency are presented in Table 18-1.

Epidemiology

Primary adrenal insufficiency is caused by autoimmune destruction of the adrenal cortex in industrialized countries. About 70% of the cases of adrenal loss (40 to 60 per 1 million in North America) involve autoimmune adrenal insufficiency or Addison's disease. This can occur from age 17 to 72, but usually presents by age 40. It is three times more common in women

TABLE 18-1	**Causes of Adrenal Insufficiency**
Etiology	**Occurrence**
PRIMARY ADRENAL INSUFFICIENCY	
Autoimmune	70%
Tuberculosis	20%
Other	10%
Fungal infections	
Adrenal hemorrhage	
Congenital adrenal hyperplasia	
Sarcoidosis	
Amyloidosis	
AIDS	
Adrenoleukodystrophy	
Adrenomyeloneuropathy	
Metastatic disease	
SECONDARY ADRENAL INSUFFICIENCY	
Exogenous steroid use	Very common
After cure of Cushing's	Common
Pituitary and hypothalamic lesions	Uncommon

Source: White et al, 1995.

than men. Half of the patients with autoimmune adrenal insufficiency have other autoimmune illnesses, such as early gonadal failure, insulin-dependent diabetes mellitus, Hashimoto's hypothyroidism or Graves' hyperthyroidism, hypoparathyroidism, or pernicious anemia. Autoimmune adrenal insufficiency is called Addison's disease. Schmidt's syndrome is the combination of autoimmune adrenal insufficiency and diabetes with or without hypothyroidism. When more than two autoimmune diseases coexist, the syndrome is called polyglandular autoimmune syndrome, where antibodies to 21-hydroxylase (an enzyme involved in steroid synthesis) are found in the blood (Loriaux, 1995; Oelkers, 1996; Rao et al, 1989).

The second leading cause of adrenal insufficiency, found in 20% of those with adrenal loss, is cortical destruction from infectious diseases, such as tuberculosis or fungal infections. In developing countries, tuberculosis rather than autoimmune disease is the leading cause of adrenal insufficiency. Adrenal failure can be seen in up to 5% of patients with AIDS, usually late in the course of the disease and a result of cytomegalovirus infection (Loriaux, 1995).

Other causes of adrenal failure include hemorrhage in the adrenal gland (Loriaux, 1995; Oelkers, 1996; Rao et al, 1989). Unrecognized, this can lead to shock and death, which is then incorrectly attributed to sepsis or ischemia. This is seen in patients who have hypercoagulable states such as lupus, diabetes, or pregnancy, patients using anticoagulants, or patients in the postoperative period. This can also be seen during sepsis, particularly meningococcemia, pneumococcal pneumonia, or *Haemophilus influenzae* (Friedrich-Waterhouse syndrome). Patients with antiphospholipid syndrome, often associated with lupus, can also lose adrenal function because of arterial and venous thrombi (Oelkers, 1996).

Drugs that work by interfering with steroid synthesis or that accelerate steroid degradation can cause loss of adrenal function. These drugs include those used to treat excessive steroid production (ie, Cushing's syndrome) and adrenal carcinoma, such as aminoglutethimide, mitotane (o,p′-DDD, related to the insecticide DDT), and ketoconazole. The latter, for example, inhibits two enzymes in the glucocorticoid-synthetic pathway and binds to the glucocorticoid receptor. Drugs such as rifampin, phenytoin, and phenobarbital accelerate the catabolism of cortisone by stimulating hepatic microsomal enzymes. Their use causes adrenal insufficiency in patients with compromised adrenal function (Loriaux, 1995).

Rarer causes of adrenal cortical loss include metastatic disease, although adrenal failure is rare. This can occur in up to 58% of women with breast cancer, 42% of those with lung cancer, and 50% of those with malignant melanoma. Other infiltrating diseases, such as amyloidosis, sarcoidosis, or hemochromatosis, can lead to loss of adrenal cortical function. Familial disorders—X-linked or autosomal recessive metabolic disorders, adrenoleukodystrophy, and the milder adrenomyeloneuropathy—cause adrenal deficiency primarily in young men (Loriaux, 1995).

History and Physical Examination

Adrenal insufficiency can present as an insidious process or as an acute crisis (Loriaux, 1995; Oelkers, 1996). Patients complain of anorexia, weight loss, and weakness (Table 18-2). Fatigue, sweating, and loss of concentration can occur, especially as the loss of glucocorticoids enhances hypoglycemia. About half the patients have gastrointestinal complaints, usually nausea, vomiting, abdominal or loin pain, and diarrhea. In primary adrenal insufficiency, the patient notes darkening of the skin, caused by enhanced secretion of pro-opiomelanocortin-derived peptides. The increased pigmentation is found at the elbows, knees, creases of the palmar surface, gingival margin, or buccal mucosa. Vitiligo is also seen. Hypotension, with systolic readings under 110 mmHg, and orthostatic blood pressure changes are found. Women report hair thinning and irregular menses. Psychiatric symptoms are seen in 64% to 84% of patients with adrenal insufficiency. The most common findings are depression, apathy, or confusion, but there are reports of psychosis, paranoia, schizophrenia, and self-mutilation (Loriaux, 1995).

Adrenal hemorrhage with loss of adrenal function can be a complication of several illnesses, including sepsis, trauma with shock, coagulopathies, and ischemic disorders. The clinical signs can be vague, but usually patients have abdominal, flank, back, or chest pain with fever and hypotension. Anorexia, vomiting, psychiatric symptoms, and abdominal rigidity with rebound also occur (Loriaux, 1995; Rao et al, 1989).

Pituitary or hypothalamic disease can lead to secondary adrenal failure. Secondary adrenal failure is often associated with other secondary losses, such as hypothyroidism or hypogonadism (Loriaux, 1995; Oelkers, 1996). Thus, patients may present with fatigue, loss of menses, loss of libido, or difficulty getting

TABLE 18-2	**Symptoms and Signs of Adrenal Insufficiency**

ACUTE

Abdominal pain, postural hypotension, fever, confusion

CHRONIC

Weakness, fatigue, salt craving, anorexia, nausea, diarrhea, dizziness, and syncope; weight loss, orthostatic hypotension, vitiligo, pigmentation of skin and mucous membranes, and alopecia

erections. In secondary adrenal insufficiency, aldosterone secretion is preserved because aldosterone is regulated by the renin–angiotensin axis rather than ACTH (White, 1994).

Loss of aldosterone secretion can occur in isolation (hyperreninemic hypoaldosteronism) or as a result of diminished secretion of renin or angiotensin II (hyporeninemic hypoaldosteronism). Hyporeninemic hypoaldosteronism is commonly found in patients with mild renal insufficiency (eg, diabetes [50% of the patients]) or those with nephritis, but it can also be caused by use of nonsteroidal anti-inflammatory drugs (NSAIDs; see section on hypoaldosteronism). Hyperreninemic hypoaldosteronism is usually seen in critically ill patients and may be caused by hypotensive injury to the adrenal glands. It can also be seen in patients with diabetes or those taking heparin (Loriaux, 1995). These patients are usually asymptomatic but can have cardiac arrhythmias or muscle weakness because of hyperkalemia.

Diagnostic Studies

LABORATORY FINDINGS

Sixty-five percent of patients with primary adrenal insufficiency are hyperkalemic, and 90% are hyponatremic from renal salt wasting. In primary but not secondary adrenal insufficiency, mineralocorticoids (aldosterone) are lost along with the glucocorticoid secretion, causing intravascular volume depletion (hypotension) and elevated serum potassium levels. Primary adrenal insufficiency frequently causes hypoglycemia, hypercalcemia, and a mild normocytic anemia with lymphocytosis and mild eosinophilia (Loriaux, 1995; Oelkers, 1996).

In secondary adrenal insufficiency, hyponatremia but not hyperkalemia can occur, but from a different cause. The lack of ACTH leads to low cortisol levels, which increase vasopressin secretion and water retention (Loriaux, 1995; Oelkers, 1996). These patients also show evidence of other pituitary hormone abnormalities, such as elevated prolactin if there is a pituitary tumor, or low levels of thyroid-stimulating hormone, follicle-stimulating hormone, luteinizing hormone, and free thyroxine.

In adrenal hemorrhage, there is a precipitous drop in the hematocrit while the number of white blood cells increases (leukocytosis) (Loriaux, 1995). Hyponatremia and hyperkalemia with renal insufficiency (azotemia) and acidosis are also seen.

The definitive diagnosis of adrenal insufficiency is the lack of response of the adrenal gland to ACTH stimulation. Random cortisol levels may not distinguish patients with mild disease from the normal population, but morning cortisol levels greater than 25 mcg/dL (>525 nmol/L) are likely to indicate normal function, whereas patients with 8 to 9 AM cortisol levels under 4 mcg/dL (83 nmol/L) probably have adrenal insufficiency (Oelkers, 1996). The ACTH stimulation test can be done at any time and consists of giving 250 mcg of synthetic ACTH intravenously or intramuscularly (Oelkers, 1996). To differentiate primary from secondary disease, an ACTH level can be drawn before the synthetic ACTH is given: it will be high in primary disease (> 100 pg/mL or 22 pmol/L) and low in secondary disease (Oelkers, 1996). Alternatively, serum aldosterone could be measured; if low, it is indicative of primary disease, whereas its level is normal in secondary disease.

IMAGING STUDIES

In patients with primary adrenal insufficiency from autoimmune disease, imaging of the adrenal glands is not necessary. In other cases, computed tomography (CT) of the adrenal glands should be done to diagnose fungal disease or cancer (Loriaux, 1995; Oelkers, 1996). In patients with secondary disease from a pituitary or hypothalamic process, magnetic resonance imaging (MRI) of the pituitary and hypothalamic region is done.

Treatment Options, Expected Outcomes, and Comprehensive Management

The usual replacement is cortisone, 12 to 15 mg/m²/day, usually given as 25 mg in the morning and 12.5 mg in the evening to try to mimic the natural circadian rhythm of higher steroid production in the morning. British researchers have shown that there is no advantage to giving the greater dose of steroid in the morning, preferring to give 10 mg three times a day (Loriaux, 1995). If other steroids are used, dosages are adjusted according to the relative potency of the drug. For example, prednisone is about four times as potent as hydrocortisone, so replacement is given as 5 mg in the morning and 2.5 mg in the evening. Because steroids can cause gastritis, weight gain, and osteoporosis, the goal is to give the lowest dosage that relieves symptoms; this can be as low as 15 to 20 mg/day of hydrocortisone (Oelkers, 1996). The steroid replacement dose may be adjusted based on 24-hour measurements of urinary cortisol. Mineralocorticoids are necessary in 75% of patients with primary adrenal insufficiency; the dosage is usually 50 to 200 mcg 9-alpha-fludrocortisol (Florinef) given each morning with a liberal-salt diet. This aldosterone substitute can be adjusted by measuring blood pressure, potassium, and plasma renin activity (PRA), which should be in the upper end of the normal range (Oelkers, 1996).

Teaching and Self-Care

Concern about causing iatrogenic alterations in the pituitary–adrenal axis is widespread because of the common use of glucocorticoids to treat chronic diseases such as arthritis, inflammatory bowel disease, asthma, and emphysema.

CLINICAL WARNING: When the adrenal axis is suppressed from glucocorticoid use, abruptly decreasing or stopping the medication or missing a dose could precipitate an adrenal crisis (adrenal insufficiency) with symptoms of weakness, hypotension, and hypoglycemia.

The degree of suppression of the adrenal axis depends on many factors, such as the type of steroid used, the dosage, and the duration of treatment. Nonetheless, many studies show that suppression is not predictable in individual patients, and thus random cortisol levels are not helpful. Patients taking 20 mg or more of prednisone (or its equivalent) for more than 5 days should be suspected of having adrenal suppression, and thus are at risk for adrenal crisis if the medication is not appropriately weaned. Some patients have symptoms of adrenal insufficiency with normal cortisol and ACTH levels, probably from a sudden elevation in prostaglandin levels after steroid disuse (steroid withdrawal syndrome) (Schlaghecke et al, 1992).

Alternate-day therapy is an approach used by many providers to minimize adrenal axis suppression and decrease side effects from glucocorticoids while sustaining therapeutic effects (Schlaghecke et al, 1992). This use of a short-acting steroid (prednisone or methylprednisolone) every 48 hours should be the regimen of choice in patients facing more than a few weeks of glucocorticoid therapy for conditions other than adrenal insufficiency. Those lacking cortisol or ACTH secretion must take replacement daily.

During periods of stress such as febrile illness (temperature >100.4°F), gastroenteritis, or outpatient surgery (eg, tooth extraction), additional steroid coverage is given. The oral dose of steroid can be doubled for the first 2 or 3 days until the underlying fever or "24-hour bug" resolves. If patients are unable to take medications orally, they can be instructed to give glucocorticoid by subcutaneous injection or to use glucocorticoid suppositories for replacement (Oelkers, 1996). Patients may also make changes in their diet and lifestyle to manage symptoms of adrenal insufficiency. These include eating a healthy diet that contains ample fresh fruits and vegetables and is low in simple carbohydrates. Moderate exercise should be encouraged, both for overall good health as well as to aid in stress management. If the latter is a problem, patients may benefit from stress-management techniques that are individualized for them. Patients on steroid replacement should be encouraged to wear a Med-Alert bracelet or to carry a medical identification care stating that they use this medication.

Because steroid-related gastritis can be a problem, patients should be encouraged to avoid smoking and the use of aspirin and ibuprofen and to limit caffeine and alcohol intake. They should be advised to take their steroid with food. Some patients may find that eating small, frequent meals helps their tolerance of steroid medication.

Self-care for bone loss and osteoporosis is covered in Chapter 48.

Referral Points and Clinical Warnings

Chronic adrenal failure may persist for months or years before diagnosis, but acute adrenal insufficiency (adrenal crisis) must be promptly recognized and treated to avoid death, which is usually caused by the underlying illnesses (Loriaux, 1995; Oelkers, 1996; Rao et al, 1989). It can be difficult to diagnose acute adrenal crisis; it is often misdiagnosed as sepsis or an acute abdomen. Acute loss of cortical secretion leads to tachycardia, hypotension and vascular collapse, severe abdominal pain, nausea and vomiting, hyponatremia, and hyperkalemia.

■ ■ ■ **CLINICAL PEARL**

The provider should consider referring a patient with suspected adrenal insufficiency to an endocrine specialty practice for diagnosis and management planning.

■ **CLINICAL WARNING:** Acutely ill patients may be severely hypotensive. They may need emergency referral.

When a patient with known adrenal insufficiency must undergo emergency surgery, steroid coverage is increased and is given intravenously until oral medication can be reliably taken.

If patients have a history of steroid use, and the length of steroid treatment, the time since last use, or the dosage that was given is not clearly known, the safest and most practical clinical solution is to assume they may be adrenal-insufficient.

■ **CLINICAL WARNING:** It is recommended practice to give steroid coverage during emergency situations for any patient taking steroids over the past 12 months, even if the patient took alternate-day glucocorticoids (Schlaghecke et al, 1992).

ADRENAL OVERACTIVITY

Cushing's Disease and Cushing's Syndrome

Cushing's syndrome is a group of diseases characterized by excessive glucocorticoid secretion. The syndrome can be caused by increased ACTH secretion (pituitary or ectopic), or it can be ACTH-independent (adrenal disease). In Cushing's disease, a subset of the group, a pituitary lesion leads to increased ACTH secretion, which in turn leads to bilateral adrenal hyperplasia and increased glucocorticoid production.

EPIDEMIOLOGY

The most common cause of systemic illness from exposure to excessive glucocorticoid is iatrogenic, from the use of exogenous glucocorticoids (steroids) to treat inflammatory or respiratory diseases. Endogenous excessive glucocorticoid production causing Cushing's syndrome is most often ACTH-dependent. A pituitary tumor secreting excessive ACTH is the cause in 68% of all patients; this is called Cushing's disease. Ectopic production of ACTH from a cancer or islet cell tumor occurs in 12% of cases and is also ACTH-dependent. ACTH-independent disease is caused by autonomous adrenal activity (adrenal adenomas or carcinomas) in 19% of cases (Orth, 1995). Cushing's syndrome occurs at a rate of 10 cases per 1 million in the population.

HISTORY AND PHYSICAL EXAMINATION

Cushing's syndrome should be considered in patients who have a history of hyperglycemia, hypertension, osteoporosis, and a recent gain in weight without use of steroids (Orth, 1995; Tsigos & Chrousos, 1994). The presence of marked virilization in women increases the likelihood of adrenal carcinoma, whereas marked hypertension may indicate ectopic ACTH secretion (Orth, 1995). The symptoms and signs of hypercortisolism are caused by alterations in the metabolism of lipids, protein, and carbohydrates. Signs and symptoms include:

- Weight gain
- Hypertension
- Glucose intolerance or diabetes
- Facial rounding and plethora
- Filling in of supraclavicular fat pads and central obesity
- Loss of muscle strength and thinning of arms and legs
- Easy bruising
- Increased body hair
- Irregular menses in women; decreased libido and gynecomastia in men

- Peripheral edema
- Loss of height, back pain, and osteoporosis.

Fatigue, weakness, polyuria, polydipsia, and increased frequency of skin and urinary tract infections from hyperglycemia also are common complaints. Altered protein metabolism can lead to easy bruisability and striae wider than 1 cm on the abdomen or proximal extremities. Oligomenorrhea or amenorrhea occurs in premenopausal women; men report decreased libido (Orth, 1995). Depression and insomnia often occur; major depression is found in as many as 66% to 75% of patients (Orth, 1995; Tsigos & Chrousos, 1994; Gadde & Krishnan, 1994).

The typical cushingoid appearance is that of a patient with a round face (moon facies) with plethora (telangiectasias), fat pads that bulge above the supraclavicular fossae, and central obesity with spindle-like extremities. An increased prominence of the dorsal fat pad (buffalo hump) is less specific for Cushing's and can be found in patients with weight gain from any cause. There may be increased facial hair, thinning of the skin with petechiae and ecchymoses, and increased pigmentation of the skin, especially in the groin and palmar creases if the Cushing's syndrome is ACTH-dependent. There is proximal muscle wasting from protein catabolism, so the patient has difficulty rising from the seated position (Orth, 1995). There can also be osteoporosis or frank fractures with minimal trauma.

Pseudo-Cushing's syndrome is a diagnosis given to the disorder in which patients appear to have the physical signs of Cushing's syndrome, but the excess glucocorticoid is from secondary causes, such as alcoholism or depression. Patients with alcoholism have hormonal abnormalities that disappear during abstinence; the hormonal abnormalities are probably caused by increased CRH or impaired hepatic metabolism of cortisol. Major depression can also lead to abnormally regulated cortisol metabolism, although hypersecretion of cortisol is minimal. The hormonal defect disappears on remission of the depression (Tsigos & Chrousos, 1994; Gadde & Krishnan, 1994).

DIAGNOSTIC STUDIES
Laboratory Findings
Single cortisol values are not of value in diagnosing Cushing's syndrome. There is nonetheless a loss of the usual diurnal variation in cortisol secretion, and evening cortisol levels are equal to or higher than morning values (Oelkers, 1996; Orth, 1995). In a patient with the signs of Cushing's syndrome, low cortisol values may indicate the previously unsuspected use of exogenous steroids.

Screening tests for Cushing's syndrome involve either the collection of two or three 24-hour urine samples for free cortisol measurement, or the overnight dexamethasone suppression test. To verify the completeness of a 24-hour urine collection, urine creatinine is also measured in the sample, as its level should not vary by more than 10%. Both tests can have false-negative and false-positive results, but a morning serum cortisol greater than 5 mcg/dL after an 11 PM dose of 1 mg dexamethasone or a urine free cortisol value greater than 80 mcg/dL warrants referral for further investigation (Orth, 1995). Stress can lead to false-positive results. Testing is best done in the outpatient setting.

The ideal time to screen a patient for Cushing's syndrome is between midnight and 2 AM, when cortisol and ACTH levels are usually low because of circadian rhythms. For patient convenience, this can be done after 4 PM, and a ACTH level above 15 pg/mL (>3.3 pmol/L) in the face of a cortisol level above 15 mcg/dL (>415 nmol/L) suggests ACTH-dependent Cushing's, either Cushing's disease or ectopic ACTH syndrome. If ACTH levels are under 5 pg/mL (<1.1 pmol/L) with elevated cortisol levels, a primary adrenal lesion may be present (Orth, 1995).

The classic endocrine specialty workup for Cushing's syndrome involves looking at the endogenous steroid production after low- and high-dose steroids are given. The low-dose test consists of giving 0.5 mg dexamethasone every 6 hours for 48 hours. Because the classic 2-day low-dose and high-dose dexamethasone testing may be too complicated for patients to do in the outpatient setting, some endocrinologists do a more rapid high- and low-dose test. Patients can take increasing amounts of dexamethasone at night and have morning cortisol and ACTH levels measured. For the low-dose test, 2 mg dexamethasone is given, and for the high-dose test, 8 mg dexamethasone is given. Table 18-3 presents laboratory findings in pituitary-caused Cushing's versus those in adrenal and ectopic syndrome.

CRH has recently become available for clinical testing. CRH given IV induces a rise in ACTH and cortisol in normal subjects, while the increase is exaggerated in those with Cushing's disease. Those with ectopic production of ACTH often show no response to CRH.

In a minority of patients, the testing may give inconclusive or false-positive or false-negative results. Some patients may have episodic secretion of cortisol, or production of ectopic ACTH may not be uniform (Orth, 1995). There have been reports where the excessive steroid production is found only after eating.

TABLE 18-3	**Laboratory Findings in Pituitary-Caused Cushing's Disease Versus Findings in Adrenal and Ectopic Cushing's Syndrome**		
	Pituitary	**Ectopic**	**Adrenal**
BASELINE			
Cortisol	High	Very high	High
ACTH	High	Very high	Suppressed
RESPONSE TO DEXAMETHASONE			
Low dose	No change	No change	No change
High dose	Decreased >50%	No change	No change

Pseudo-Cushing's syndrome can be differentiated from Cushing's syndrome by checking evening cortisol levels (Orth, 1995). Cortisol concentrations in the blood have a diurnal rhythm, high in the morning and low between 10 PM and 2 AM. This evening nadir is preserved in pseudo-Cushing's syndrome and not in Cushing's syndrome, so patients with the former should demonstrate a low midnight cortisol value (<5 mcg/dL or 138 nmol/L).

Imaging Studies

Before the advent of MRI, pituitary tumors were identified in less than 50% of those with Cushing's disease, because Cushing's disease is often caused by a microadenoma (a lesion <1 cm). Now with MRI scanning, pituitary tumors can be identified in up to 75% of those with Cushing's disease. In some patients, there are signs that the defect originates in the hypothalamus rather than in the pituitary (Orth, 1995; Sonino et al, 1996).

Patients with adrenal adenomas have an equal chance of having benign or malignant tumors. MRI imaging, although it is more expensive than CT, can occasionally differentiate benign from malignant masses (Kloos et al, 1995). With the advent of better CT and MRI scanners, small adrenal lesions (<0.5 cm) are being identified that are nonfunctional; these are called adrenal incidentalomas. Seventy percent to 94% of adrenal masses found incidentally are nonsecretory and benign adenomas (Kloos et al, 1995). Tumors that are small and nonfunctional need not be removed. A cancerous lesion is suspected if the tumor is greater than 6 cm.

CLINICAL WARNING: Functioning adrenal masses that oversecrete hormone require surgical removal or medical therapy if the former is not possible. CT and MRI scanning cannot distinguish hormonally active from inactive lesions, and lesions that produce hormones can be clinically silent (Kloos et al, 1995). Most malignant tumors produce hormones, but they can be inefficient at making cortisol; thus, women with malignant adrenal tumors often appear virilized from overproduction of adrenal androgens, which would provide the clinical clue for further investigation (Orth, 1995).

If no pituitary tumor is seen on MRI and the patient has nonsuppressible cortisol secretion, bilateral inferior petrosal vein catheterization and sampling for ACTH during stimulation with CRH can differentiate pituitary from ectopic ACTH-dependent disease (Orth, 1995; Oldfield et al, 1991). This catheterization procedure is expensive and invasive and can produce dire complications, including brain stem damage; thus, it cannot be recommended as a routine procedure (Orth, 1995).

TREATMENT OPTIONS, EXPECTED OUTCOMES, AND COMPREHENSIVE MANAGEMENT

Surgical Treatment

The treatment of Cushing's syndrome depends on the cause. If Cushing's disease is found, the pituitary adenoma should be removed by transsphenoidal surgery. The surgery is curative in 60% to 90% of cases.

For larger tumors (macroadenomas), total hypophysectomy is required. If the symptoms of Cushing's syndrome are very pronounced, bilateral adrenalectomy may be preferred, as this stops the organ damage from hyperglycemia, hypertension, and protein catabolism. In up to 25% of patients treated in this fashion, there is a risk of developing Nelson's syndrome (a state created by the lack of feedback of exogenous steroid replacement on the pituitary tissue) (Sonino, 1996), because removal of the adrenal glands allows pituitary secretion of ACTH to increase. This is more likely to occur if the original pituitary lesion was an adenoma rather than hyperplasia, and if there was a high level of pretreatment urinary cortisol.

Radiation Therapy

Pituitary irradiation can be used, although the cure rate is not high (Orth, 1995). Relapse of Cushing's in adults is less likely when unsuccessful pituitary surgery is followed by radiation (Estrada, 1997).

Pharmacotherapy

In cases of Cushing's syndrome, where the tumor cannot be resected and radiation may take years to decrease cortisol production, drugs that inhibit steroid production can be used. These include aminoglutethimide and ketoconazole, and a drug that actually destroys adrenal cortical cells, mitotane (o,p'-DDD) (Orth, 1995). Ketoconazole is preferred because of its lack of side effects, but in men it can inhibit androgen secretion, leading to gynecomastia, and in women it can lead to hirsutism. Aminoglutethimide and mitotane can cause significant gastrointestinal side effects, particularly anorexia and vomiting. These drugs are less effective in the treatment of Cushing's disease than in other causes of Cushing's syndrome because the block in steroid synthesis actually increases ACTH secretion, which can ultimately overcome the drug's ability to block steroid synthesis.

TEACHING AND SELF-CARE

Patients with obesity often present to the primary care provider for evaluation of pituitary or adrenal function to determine if a hormonal imbalance has led to difficulty losing weight. The patient may know a friend or relative with Cushing's syndrome or may have seen information in the press, on television, or on the Internet about adrenal gland disorders. It can be difficult to separate patients with syndrome X, a genetic tendency for weight gain, hypertension, type 2 diabetes, gout, and in women hyperandrogenism (hirsutism), from those with early Cushing's syndrome, especially if the patients with syndrome X are depressed. Laboratory findings discussed previously and serial examinations can be helpful, realizing that Cushing's syndrome is rare and obesity, type 2 diabetes, hypertension, and depression are more common (Tsigos & Chrousos, 1994).

Hypersecretion of CRH can occur in depression, anorexia nervosa, excessive exercise, panic disorders, chronic alcoholism or drug withdrawal, diabetes mellitus with neuropathy, and central obesity. There may be higher levels of glucocorticoids in hyperthyroidism and premenstrual tension syndrome and in survivors of childhood sexual abuse (Tsigos & Chrousos, 1994). Lower levels of CRH or HPA axis dysregulation and "hypoarousal" may be found in patients with hypothyroidism and seasonal depression and chronic fatigue syndromes, including fibromyalgia (Tsigos & Chrousos, 1994). The weight gain, depression, and fatigue in Cushing's syndrome from chronic hypercortisolism might then be attributed to suppression of CRH secretion (Tsigos & Chrousos, 1994).

The primary care provider can assist the patient with Cushing's syndrome by encouraging regular exercise and stress management. Other healthy lifestyle choices have been previously discussed, including diet and tobacco, alcohol, and caffeine management. The provider should also discuss the benefits of limiting refined carbohydrates in the diet.

REFERRAL POINTS AND CLINICAL WARNINGS

Patients with adrenal tumors should at least be screened for pheochromocytoma, because 65% of these may have the signal intensity of adrenal metastases on MRI and appear bright. Percutaneous needle biopsy of an unsuspected pheochromocytoma could lead to release of catecholamines, causing hypertensive crisis, retroperitoneal bleeding, and death (Kloos et al, 1995).

■ ■ ■ CLINICAL PEARL

The use of female hormones can create a falsely elevated serum cortisol value. If results of screening tests for Cushing's are equivocal, consider whether the use of female hormones may have influenced free hormone levels. In this instance, measure free cortisol in the urine. Alternatively, birth-control pills or female hormones can be stopped for 6 to 8 weeks before testing.

INCREASED PRODUCTION OF MINERALOCORTICOIDS

Hyperaldosteronism

Excessive production of mineralocorticoids can occur as the result of primary disease (overproduction of aldosterone) or secondary disease from excessive stimulation by the renin–angiotensin system. In both these cases, glucocorticoid production is normal.

Primary hyperaldosteronism can be caused by an adrenal adenoma, bilateral adrenal hyperplasia (sometimes referred to as idiopathic hyperaldosteronism), or adrenal carcinoma (Gill, 1995). In bilateral hyperplasia, it is thought that the adrenals may be stimulated by a pituitary or hypothalamic factor, causing the overstimulation of aldosterone secretion (Gill, 1995).

EPIDEMIOLOGY

Primary aldosteronism is a rare cause of hypertension, accounting for 1% of patients with hypertension. In hypertensive patients with spontaneously occurring hypokalemia, the incidence of primary aldosteronism is increased to 50%. It affects women more often than men, and the peak age of diagnosis is between ages 30 and 50. More than 60% of the cases are caused by benign adenomas; 30% of patients have idiopathic hyperaldosteronism (White, 1994; Gill, 1995).

HISTORY AND PHYSICAL EXAMINATION

Patients with hyperaldosteronism may have no specific symptoms, but could have some complaints caused by mild hypokalemia; a low potassium level is found in up to 90% of patients. These complaints include polyuria, polydipsia, and muscle weakness. When the loss of potassium is severe, there may be paresis or tetany. The loss of potassium will also bring out glucose intolerance. Edema is not seen unless there is coexistent congestive heart disease or nephrotic syndrome (Gill, 1995). Hypertension (blood pressure >140/90 mmHg) is almost always seen in hyperaldosteronism, although there are some rare patients who are normotensive but have hypokalemic alkalosis caused by hyperaldosteronism.

OTHER CAUSES OF HYPERALDOSTERONISM

Some patients with hyperaldosteronism have hypokalemia but no hypertension; this is called Bartter's syndrome and is caused by excessive renin production from hyperplasia of the renal juxtaglomerular apparatus. There is also increased excretion of prostaglandins, and the hypokalemia responds to treatment with prostaglandin inhibitors such as indomethacin. Nonetheless, potassium supplementation is often used as the sole therapy because of the undesirable long-term side effects of NSAIDs (Gill, 1995).

Dexamethasone-suppressible hyperaldosteronism is an autosomal dominant disorder with features identical to those of primary aldosteronism, but the excessive aldosterone secretion can be eliminated by giving steroids such as dexamethasone (White, 1994; Gill, 1995).

Excessive ingestion of licorice can cause hypertension and laboratory findings of mineralocorticoid excess (Gill, 1995).

Secondary aldosteronism that also leads to hypokalemia is caused by elevated renin levels. Hyperreninemic hyperaldosteronism can occur in malignant hypertension, unilateral renal artery stenosis, and renin-secreting tumors of the kidney's juxtaglomerular apparatus (Gill, 1995).

DIAGNOSTIC STUDIES
Laboratory Findings

For an accurate evaluation of the renin–aldosterone axis, many patients have to discontinue drugs known to affect hormones in the pathway. Spironolactone and estrogens should be stopped for 6 weeks; prostaglandin inhibitors (NSAIDs), calcium channel blockers, ACE inhibitors, sympathomimetics, and adrenergic inhibitors should be withheld for 2 weeks (Gill, 1995). If patients experience hypertension after discontinuing these drugs, prazosin or other alpha-1 adrenergic inhibitors can be substituted during this period.

Laboratory testing in patients with hyperaldosteronism demonstrates a low potassium level (3 to 3.5 mEq/L) with alkalosis (Gill, 1995). The potassium value may be normal if the patient has been eating a low-sodium diet, so these tests should be done after 2 or 3 days of sodium loading (>200 mEq or 120 mM Na) (Gill, 1995). Primary aldosteronism is suspected if there are borderline or low potassium levels, low stimulated PRA, and high aldosterone levels. Aldosterone values are high in the serum (>14 ng/dL), and urinary aldosterone and potassium levels are also high (K > 30 mEq) (Gill, 1995). In secondary hyperaldosteronism, the major distinguishing feature is elevation of PRA. In contrast to secondary hyperaldosteronism, the PRA is suppressed in primary aldosteronism and does not increase in response to an upright position (standing for 4 hours) or volume depletion after a 40-mg dose of furosemide (Gill, 1995).

Many providers prefer to avoid salt loading in patients who are hypertensive and may be prone to congestive heart failure.

To look for hyperaldosteronism, they evaluate the plasma aldosterone level and the ratio of plasma aldosterone to PRA before and 90 minutes after administration of captopril (25 to 50 mg), an ACE inhibitor. This test does not require dietary preparation and does not expose the patient to salt loading. Those with secondary hyperaldosteronism, like normal patients, show a rise in PRA and a fall in aldosterone levels.

Single Adenoma Versus Bilteral Adrenal Hyperplasia

Once the diagnosis of primary aldosteronism is confirmed, it is important to then distinguish between causative factors—either a single adrenal adenoma or bilateral adrenal hyperplasia.

Imaging Studies

Imaging studies using CT or MRI scanning can distinguish adrenal hyperplasia from a benign adenoma. MRI is more expensive but in some circumstances can differentiate benign from malignant disease (Kloos et al, 1995).

Other Studies

Hypokalemia (K < 3 mEq/L) can be seen on electrocardiogram tracings as depression of the ST segment and inversion of the T wave. As potassium levels continue to fall, a prominent U wave is seen in the anterior leads.

TREATMENT OPTIONS, EXPECTED OUTCOMES, AND COMPREHENSIVE MANAGEMENT

In patients with a benign adenoma, surgical removal of the adrenal gland that contains the adenoma is curative in more than 70% of patients (Gill, 1995). Surgery is not indicated in idiopathic hyperaldosteronism (bilateral hyperplasia), which is treated with a potassium-sparing diuretic, ACE inhibitors, or calcium channel blockers, which inhibit aldosterone secretion.

Spironolactone (50 to 200 mg/day) is the most effective agent for hyperaldosteronism that cannot be treated surgically, as it is a competitive antagonist. It can create side effects because of its antiandrogen activity, leading to decreased libido, breast pain, and gynecomastia in more than 50% of men treated (Gill, 1995). In women, breast pain and irregular menstrual bleeding can occur. If spironolactone is not tolerated, calcium channel blockers with potassium-sparing diuretics can be used (Gill, 1995).

TEACHING AND SELF-CARE

Hyperaldosteronism is a rare cause of hypertension. Nonetheless, it should be considered as a diagnosis in patients with high blood pressure who have low potassium levels while not taking diuretics, or in those taking diuretics who appear to need greater potassium supplementation than usual.

Potassium can be replaced orally as a liquid or as a slow-release tablet, which is usually preferred because of the unpleasant taste of liquid potassium. The slow-release tablets must be taken with a copious amount of water to avoid gastric irritation. Most patients taking diuretics do not need routine potassium replacement. Patients who have potassium levels less than 3 mEq/L, those with coexistent cardiac disease (especially those who take cardiac glycosides [digoxin, digitalis]), those with chronic liver disease, and those at risk for diuretic-induced glucose intolerance (diabetes) should take oral potassium while taking commonly used diuretics.

Self-care management includes maintaining a healthy lifestyle. The provider can counsel the patient about diet, including sources of potassium. Exercise as well as stress-relieving activities can be important parts of the self-care plan. Balancing exercise and activities with adequate sleep and quiet recreation can round out a successful self-management regimen.

REFERRAL POINTS AND CLINICAL WARNINGS

Although many providers routinely evaluate outpatients for hyperaldosteronism by oral salt loading or short-term intravenous salt loading (2 L NS over 4 hours), these tests can lead to serious side effects, primarily congestive heart failure and severe hypertension. Normal patients have aldosterone values of 5 ng/dL or less after saline infusion; those with hyperaldosteronism have values greater than 10 ng/dL. Some authors advise never giving sodium to a hypokalemic patient in whom primary aldosteronism is suspected. Such loading will increase further potassium loss and trigger cardiac arrhythmias (Gill, 1995).

It is best to replace potassium orally, unless a life-threatening cardiac arrhythmia or vomiting makes this route unfeasible. It is also best to give the replacement slowly to avoid inducing hyperkalemia, ventricular fibrillation, and cardiac standstill.

Hypoaldosteronism

Hypoaldosteronism can also be a primary disease or can occur secondary to low renin levels. Usual causes of hypoaldosteronism include primary adrenal insufficiency, salt-wasting forms of congenital adrenal hyperplasia, or the use of drugs (White, 1994). Primary loss of aldosterone secretion can also be caused by genetic mutations of enzymes in the synthetic pathway for mineralocorticoids. Hyperreninemic hypoaldosteronism can also occur in critically ill patients as a likely response to chronic stress, ischemia in the zona glomerulosa, or a reaction to pyrogenic factors (eg, interleukin-1, tumor necrosis factor). Secondary hypoaldosteronism from low levels of renin (hyporeninemic hypoaldosteronism) is a common cause of hyperkalemia. It often occurs in patients with mild renal insufficiency, and most of these patients have diabetes mellitus. Drugs known to inhibit aldosterone secretion or interfere with its actions include heparin, cyclosporin A, calcium channel blockers, beta-blockers, NSAIDs, ACE inhibitors, spironolactone, and aminoglutethimide (Melby, 1995).

EPIDEMIOLOGY

Primary deficiency of aldosterone (hyperreninemic hypoaldosteronism) is usually caused by adrenal insufficiency and was described earlier. Secondary aldosterone deficiency caused by hyporeninemic hypoaldosteronism is also called type IV renal tubular acidosis. It most often occurs in middle-aged men, and chronic renal insufficiency is found in 80% of cases. Diabetes mellitus occurs in 50% of patients. Persons with diabetes are predisposed to hyperkalemia because of hyperglycemia and low insulin levels, which produce an extracellular flux of potassium. Autonomic neuropathy may also be a factor in the acquisition of the hyporeninemic state (Melby, 1995).

HISTORY AND PHYSICAL EXAMINATION

The clinical signs of hypoaldosteronism are caused by salt wasting and hyperkalemia. The hyperkalemia can lead to muscle weakness, muscle cramps, and cardiac arrhythmias (Melby,

1995). Salt wasting can cause orthostatic blood pressure changes and hyponatremia, which can lead to mental confusion.

DIAGNOSTIC STUDIES

Laboratory Findings

The diagnosis of hypoaldosteronism is made by measuring the PRA and the aldosterone level in the blood during a period of salt restriction (die with 10 to 20 mM Na) (Melby, 1995). If PRA is high, then hypoaldosteronism is an isolated defect; if PRA is low, hypoaldosteronism is secondary to the low renin level.

Other Studies

Hyperkalemia, when the potassium level is above 5.5 mEq/L, can be seen on the electrocardiogram as peaked T waves. With further increases in the plasma potassium level above 7 mEq/L, the P wave disappears, the ST segment is depressed, and the QRS complex widens, becoming sinusoidal. Untreated, patients with severe hyperkalemia present with ventricular fibrillation or cardiac standstill, unresponsive to electrical cardioversion, unless hypokalemia is corrected.

TREATMENT OPTIONS, EXPECTED OUTCOMES, AND COMPREHENSIVE MANAGEMENT

If hyperkalemia is mild, restriction of dietary potassium and avoidance of drugs that exacerbate hyperkalemia are useful. If dietary restrictions do not correct the hyperkalemia, mineralo-corticoid replacement with 100 to 200 mcg/day of 9-alpha-fludrocortisol (Florinef) is tried. This therapy may promote edema from sodium retention and coexisting congestive heart failure or renal failure, so a balance between salt retention and fluid overload must be individualized. If Florinef cannot be tolerated, kaliuresis can be promoted using appropriate diuretics, such as chlorthalidone or hydrochlorothiazide. Sodium polystyrene sulfonate (Kayexalate), a cation exchange resin, removes potassium, but it also increases the sodium load, is expensive, and is difficult to use in the outpatient setting (Melby, 1995).

Teaching and Self-Care

Patients with hypertension often consume products advertised as being low in sodium. Nonetheless, patients with hyperkalemia or mild renal insufficiency should avoid low-sodium foods because they often contain high amounts of potassium. A healthy lifestyle, as previously described, should be encouraged.

■ **CLINICAL WARNING:** Potassium restrictions need to be taught. This includes warning about specific medications, including over-the-counter drugs, as well as foods that are high in potassium. Potassium levels should be monitored (Melby, 1995).

REFERRAL POINTS AND CLINICAL WARNINGS

Patients with diabetes mellitus are at higher risk of becoming hyperkalemic because insulin transports glucose and potassium into cells. Patients with poorly controlled glucose levels, who are absolutely or relatively insulin-deficient, can experience cardiac arrhythmias and arrest from hyperkalemia. Therefore, after starting medications that inhibit aldosterone activity in patients with diabetes (eg, spironolactone, ACE inhibitors, NSAIDs), potassium levels should be monitored, looking for hyperkalemia.

Hyperkalemic crisis, where a high serum level of potassium (>7 mEq/L) causes electrocardiogram changes (T-wave peaking and arrhythmias), is treated emergently. Calcium gluconate (10 to 20 mL of a 10% solution) is given to counteract the effect of hyperkalemia on the heart. Then glucose and insulin (25 to 50 g/hour glucose and 5 units of regular insulin intravenously every 15 minutes) are used to drive potassium into cells. Hemodialysis can also be used once the acute crisis is reversed.

Pheochromocytoma

Catecholamine-secreting tumors of the adrenal medulla, and rarely from extra-adrenal sites, are called pheochromocytomas. Pheochromocytoma is a rare cause of hypertension. Most cases are sporadic, but some are associated with the familial syndromes of multiple endocrine neoplasia, where pheochromocytoma is found with hyperparathyroidism and medullary thyroid cancer. Pheochromocytomas can also be associated with neurofibromatosis and von Hippel-Lindau disease (Neumann et al, 1993).

ANATOMY, PHYSIOLOGY, AND PATHOLOGY

The medulla of the adrenal gland is formed from cells that migrate from the fetal neural crest; thus, they are related to the cells that form the sympathetic nervous system (Goldstein, 1995). These cells are called neuroendocrine cells and form catecholamines from the amino acid precursor tyrosine (Goldstein, 1995).

Because plasma catecholamines are labile, samples must be taken fasting, resting, and supine (with the needle placed 20 to 30 minutes before sample-taking) and processed rapidly. Urinary catecholamines are greater in magnitude and give a more integrated function over 24 hours, but use of certain drugs can give false-positive and false-negative results (Bouloux & Fakeeh, 1995). Methyldopa, terbutaline, and isoproterenol will give falsely elevated catecholamine values.

EPIDEMIOLOGY

Pheochromocytomas arise in the adrenal gland 90% of the time. They can be bilateral in 10%, especially in those with multiple endocrine neoplasia syndrome. When the tumor is located outside the adrenal gland, it is called a paraganglioma. Pheochromocytomas are the cause in less than 0.3% of patients with hypertension. When patients are hypertensive and have an adrenal mass or present with hypertension, episodic headaches, palpitations, and sweating, the yield increases to about 6%. Tumors are equally common in men and women and can occur at any age, although most are found in patients 30 to 40 years old. Many tumors are found on autopsy and are clinically silent during life (Kloos et al, 1995; Bouloux & Fakeeh, 1995; Keiser, 1995).

HISTORY AND PHYSICAL EXAMINATION

The main sign of pheochromocytoma is either sustained hypertension or paroxysmal hypertensive crises on a background of mild hypertension. Other signs and symptoms can include:

- Hypertension (> 95%)
- Headache (71%)
- Sweating (65%)
- Palpitations (65%).

In contrast, orthostatic hypotension may be the main finding when the tumor secretes mainly epinephrine (Goldstein, 1995; Insel, 1996). The hypertension of pheochromocytoma is characterized by earlier age of onset, increased severity, resistance to correction with standard antihypertensive drugs, and exacerbation by beta-adrenergic blockers. During hypertensive crises, patients may note throbbing headaches of short duration (<15 minutes), palpitations, anxiety, diaphoresis, tachycardia, abdominal pain, and nausea. Syncope, tremor, and facial blanching followed by flushing can occur (Bouloux & Fakeeh, 1995; Bravo & Gifford, 1993). The presence of all three symptoms—headaches with sweating and palpitations—in patients who are hypertensive at the times of these attacks increases the sensitivity of finding pheochromocytomas to 90% (Keiser, 1995). Episodes may be triggered by eating, defecation, urination, exercise, or induction of anesthesia. Norepinephrine secretion can lead to vasoconstriction, leading to hypovolemia, orthostatic postural changes, arrhythmias, and shock (Bouloux & Fakeeh, 1995).

DIAGNOSTIC STUDIES
Laboratory Findings
The diagnosis of pheochromocytoma is based on the finding of elevated catecholamine levels, usually measuring the urinary metabolites norepinephrine and normetanephrine in a 24-hour period. VMA levels can be elevated but are not as specific as normetanephrine levels (65% versus 84%) (Bouloux & Fakeeh, 1995; Keiser, 1995). In recent literature, where HPLC assays were used, collection of urinary free catecholamines was as sensitive as catecholamine metabolites such as normetanephrine, and may be more sensitive (>95%) for smaller lesions with rapid catecholamine turnover (Bouloux & Fakeeh, 1995).

The 24-hour collection of the urine is done in a jug containing acid, and creatinine should also be measured to ensure that the sample is adequate. Patients need not follow a special diet for detection of pheochromocytoma, but most antihypertensive medications should be stopped if possible. If the patient is severely hypertensive after discontinuing medication, hydralazine, minoxidil, calcium channel blockers, diuretics, or ACE inhibitors can be used. Drugs that are more apt to cause false elevations or to interfere with the collections are to be avoided, including:

- Amphetamines
- Catecholamines
- Clonidine withdrawal
- Ethanol
- Methyldopa, L-dopa
- Quinidine
- Theophylline
- Tetracycline
- Metyrosine
- Reserpine
- Guanethidine.

VMA collections can also be affected by monoamine oxidase inhibitors and clofibrate.

Plasma catecholamines are usually not collected as an initial screening test for two reasons: tumors can have episodic secretion that would be missed, and in some patients the stress of testing or pain during the procedure can lead to false-positive results. Nonetheless, plasma norepinephrine levels greater than 2000 pg/L are highly suggestive of a pheochromocytoma during a hypertensive crisis. The catabolic effects of excessive catecholamines and decreased tissue perfusion promote lactic acidosis, and a lactate level above 5 mmol/L should increase the suspicion of a pheochromocytoma (Keiser, 1995).

Giving clonidine (0.3 mg) orally can be useful in separating patients with baseline plasma catecholamine levels above normal into those likely to have a pheochromocytoma and those with elevations caused by stress. Pheochromocytoma is suspected when, 3 hours after clonidine dosing, the plasma catecholamine levels are greater than 500 ng/L (Keiser, 1995). Provocative testing can be done with glucagon, histamine, or metoclopramide but is not advised because these drugs can cause life-threatening cardiac responses in those with pheochromocytomas.

Special Laboratory Staining
Cells that produce catecholamines stain for neuron-specific enolase and chromogranin. In patients with pheochromocytoma, blood levels of chromogranin A are often elevated.

Imaging Studies
Most pheochromocytomas are found within the adrenal gland. Adrenal tumors can usually be seen by CT examination, but if there is concern that the iodine contrast material could trigger a hypertensive crisis or paroxysm, MRI also can be used (Kloos et al, 1995; Bouloux & Fakeeh, 1995; Keiser, 1995). MIBG (metaiodobenzylguanidine) is a nuclear tracer that can locate these tumors in 80% to 95% of patients, but it is not available at many sites (Kloos et al, 1995, Keiser, 1995). Isotope-labeled octreotide (Sandostatin) can also detect pheochromocytomas and is more widely available than MIBG, but it is expensive. Using MIBG or octreotide scanning, whole body images can be obtained, so that pheochromocytomas outside the adrenal area can be detected. If nuclear scanning to locate extra-adrenal sites of pheochromocytoma is not feasible, MRI scans of the chest, abdomen, and pelvis should be done to find those rarer tumor sites (eg, the bronchial tree, pancreatic tissue, bladder wall, or sympathetic-parasympathetic ganglia).

TREATMENT OPTIONS, EXPECTED OUTCOMES, AND COMPREHENSIVE MANAGEMENT
Surgical resection of the pheochromocytoma reverses the manifestations of the disease, although mild hypertension may persist in 25% of cases (Bouloux & Fakeeh, 1995). Some lesions can be multifocal or present at different times.

CLINICAL WARNING: Lifelong surveillance of pheochromocytoma is necessary. It can be difficult to discern malignant from benign lesions on cytology alone. Malignancy is found in up to 13% of tumors. It is more common when the pheochromocytoma is extra-adrenal. Malignant spread to lymph tissue, liver, and bone can be seen (Bouloux & Fakeeh, 1995).

Patients need preparation before surgery to avoid hypertensive crises and cardiac arrhythmias during anesthesia and hypotension on removal of the lesion. This preparation is ideally managed by an endocrine specialist. Hypertension lasting a month after surgery indicates multifocal disease or metastases or renal vasculature changes from the prior disease (Keiser, 1995). Discussion of surgical management is outside the bounds of this text.

Teaching and Self-Care

It may prove a diagnostic challenge to differentiate symptoms of a pheochromocytoma from those of thyrotoxicosis, drug withdrawal, anxiety disorders and panic attacks, carcinoid syndrome, paroxysmal tachycardia, mitral valve prolapse, migraine headaches, or hypoglycemia (Keiser, 1995). Many patients with pheochromocytomas are asymptomatic, but those with short episodes of throbbing headache, palpitations, and sweating are more likely to have these tumors than those with a history of long-lasting headaches and incapacitation.

■ ■ ■ ■ **CLINICAL PEARL**

Patients with pheochromocytoma may want to lie down during an attack, whereas those with panic and anxiety disorders tend to want to leave the site of an attack.

The body's ability to respond to stress involves the HPA and the efferent sympathetic nervous system (Tsigos & Chrousos, 1994). Women may experience irregular or missed menstruation during stress. Stress can cause alterations in thyroid hormones, such as euthyroid sick syndrome. Thus, stress management, relaxation techniques, and regular aerobic exercise can help reduce hormonal alterations and decrease symptoms and signs associated with excessive catecholamine release in the absence of a known adrenal tumor.

REFERRAL POINTS AND CLINICAL WARNINGS

The hypertensive crisis caused by a pheochromocytoma leads to symptoms that could be confused with stroke, myocardial infarction, or sepsis. Crisis can be precipitated by activity (bending over, urinating, or defecating) or by exposure to certain drugs (histamine, tyramine, glucagon, naloxone, metoclopramide, ACTH, tricyclics, and phenothiazines) (Bouloux & Fakeeh, 1995). Crisis can also occur spontaneously or from hemorrhage within the tumor. Patients present with severe hypertension, arrhythmias, and headache. There may be anxiety and confusion with hypertensive encephalopathy. Some patients can present with myocarditis, a dilated congestive cardiomyopathy that can be accompanied by pulmonary edema. If shock intervenes from arrhythmias or sudden vasodilation from epinephrine secretion, acute bowel obstruction could result from bowel ischemia (Bravo & Gifford, 1993).

COMMUNITY RESOURCES

- Addison News, 6142 Territorial, Pleasant Lake, MI 49272; (517) 769-6891; http://www2.dmci.net/users/hoffmanrj: Education and support for persons with Addison's disease

- National Cushing's Association, 4645 Van Nuys Blvd., Sherman Oaks, CA 91403; 818–788-9239: Education and support for persons with Cushing's disease
- Cushing's Support and Research Foundation, Inc., 65 East India Row, Suite 22B, Boston, MA 02110; http://world.std.com/csrf/: Information and support for persons with Cushing's disease
- Brain-Pituitary Foundation of America, 281 E. Moody Ave., Fresno, CA 93720-1524; 209–434-0610: Support for patients and families affected by adult pituitary tumors, including Cushing's disease
- Pituitary Tumor Network Association, 16350 Ventura Blvd., Suite 231, Encino, CA 91436; 818–499-9973: Support for patients, promotes medical and public awareness
- National Adrenal Diseases Foundation, 505 Northern Blvd., Great Neck, NY 11021; (516) 487-4992; http://medhlp.netusa.net/www.nadf.htm: Education and support for those with adrenal diseases and their families

---

EDITOR'S NOTE:

COMPLEMENTARY APPROACHES

A general discussion of complementary approaches can be found in Chapter 3. The following, while not an exhaustive list, are some complementary approaches being used for this condition. Additional information on these approaches, including precautions, can be found in Appendices A and B. Providers need to assess for the use of complementary approaches as part of the patient's history, as they may impact conventional therapies, and patients may not volunteer this information unless specifically asked. Efficacy of many complementary approaches is not as well documented as that of conventional therapies. Providers need to read the literature before suggesting these complementary approaches.

- Complementary Modalities
  Massage therapy

References

Bouloux, P., & Fakeeh, M. (1995). Investigation of phaeochromocytoma. *Clinical Endocrinology, 43,* 657–664.

Bravo, E.L., & Gifford, R.W. (1993). Pheochromocytoma. *Endocrinologic and Metabolic Clinics of North America, 22*(2), 329–343.

Estrada, J., Boronat, M., Mielgo, M., et al. (1997). The long-term outcome of pituitary irradiation after unsuccessful transsphenoidal surgery in Cushing's disease. *N Engl J Med, 336*(3), 172–177.

Gadde, K.M., & Krishnan, K.R.R. (1994). Endocrine factors in depression. *Psychiatric Annals, 24*(10), 521–524.

Gill, J.R. (1995) Hyperaldosteronism. In K.L. Becker (Ed.). *Principles and practice of endocrinology and metabolism,* 2d ed. Philadelphia: J.B. Lippincott, pp. 716–729.

Goldstein, D.S. Physiology of the adrenal medulla and the sympathetic nervous system. In K.L. Becker (Ed.). *Principles and practice of endocrinology and metabolism,* 2d ed. Philadelphia: J.B. Lippincott, pp. 753–762.

Insel, P.A. (1996). Adrenergic receptors—evolving concepts and clinical implications. *N Engl J Med, 334*(9), 580–585.

Keiser, H.R. (1995). Pheochromocytoma and other diseases of the sympathetic nervous system. In K.L. Becker (Ed.). *Principles and practice of endocrinology and metabolism*, 2d ed. Philadelphia: J.B. Lippincott, pp. 762–770.

Kloos, R.T., Gross, M.D., Francis, I.R., et al. (1995). Incidentally discovered adrenal masses. *Endocrine Review, 16*(4), 460–480.

Loriaux, D.L. (1995). Adrenocortical insufficiency. In K.L. Becker (Ed.). *Principles and practice of endocrinology and metabolism*, 2d ed. Philadelphia: J.B. Lippincott, pp. 682–686.

Melby, J.C. (1995). Hypoaldosteronism. In K.L. Becker (Ed.). *Principles and practice of endocrinology and metabolism*, 2d ed. Philadelphia: J.B. Lippincott, pp. 729–734.

Neumann, H.P.H., Berger, D., Sigmund, G., et al. (1993). Pheochromocytomas, multiple endocrine neoplasia type 2, and von Hippel-Lindau disease. *N Engl J Med, 329*(21), 1531–1538.

Oelkers, W. (1996). Adrenal insufficiency. *N Engl J Med, 335*(16), 1206–1212.

Oldfield, E.H., Doppman, J.L., Nieman, L.K., et al. (1991). Petrosal sinus sampling with and without corticotropin-releasing hormone for the differential diagnosis of Cushing's syndrome. *N Engl J Med, 325*(13), 897–905.

Orth, D.N. (1995). Cushing's syndrome. *N Engl J Med, 332*(12), 791–803.

Rao, R.H., Vagnucci, A.H., & Amico, J.A. (1989). Bilateral massive adrenal hemorrhage: Early recognition and treatment. *Annals of Internal Medicine, 110*, 227–235.

Rittmaster, R.S., & Arab, D.M. (1995). Morphology of the adrenal cortex and medulla. In K.L. Becker (Ed.). *Principles and practice of endocrinology and metabolism*, 2d ed. Philadelphia: J.B. Lippincott, pp. 640–647.

Schlaghecke, R., Kornely, E., Santen, R., & Ridderskamp, P. (1992). The effect of long-term glucocorticoid therapy on pituitary-adrenal responses to exogenous corticotropin-releasing hormone. *N Engl J Med, 326*(4), 226–230.

Sonino, N., Zielezny, M., Fava, G.A., et al. (1996). Risk factors and long-term outcome in pituitary-dependent Cushing's disease. *Clin Endocrinol Metab, 81*(7), 2647–2652.

Tsigos, C., & Chrousos, G.P. (1994). Physiology of the hypothalamic-pituitary-adrenal axis in health and dysregulation in psychiatric and autoimmune disorders. *Endocrinologic and Metabolic Clinics of North America, 23*(3), 451–470.

White, P.C. (1994). Disorders of aldosterone biosynthesis and action. *N Engl J Med, 331*(4), 250–258.

White, P.C., Pescovitz, O.H., & Cutler G.B. Jr. (1995). Synthesis and metabolism of corticosteroids. In K.L. Becker (Ed.). *Principles and practice of endocrinology and metabolism*, 2d ed. Philadelphia: J.B. Lippincott, pp. 647–682.

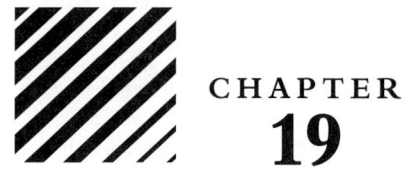

CHAPTER
19

Diseases of the Thyroid and Parathyroid Glands

Muriel N. Nathan, PhD, MD

This chapter will discuss thyroid and parathyroid diseases. Because of the complexity of this information, the chapter will be divided into several parts. First, hyperthyroidism, including Graves' disease, goiter, subacute thyroiditis, and thyroid storm, will be discussed. This will be followed by hypothyroidism, including chronic autoimmune thyroiditis, postpartum and treatment-related hypothyroid conditions, rarer forms of the disease, secondary hypothyroidism, and thyroid resistance syndromes. Thyroid cancer will be discussed. Hyperparathyroidism and the rarer state of hypoparathyroidism will follow. After a discussion of parathyroid diseases, community-based resources will be covered at the chapter's end.

THE THYROID GLAND

Thyroid disease is a common cause of outpatient visits to primary care providers. The size and texture of the gland can change. Goiter is a generalized enlargement of the thyroid gland, whereas a thyroid nodule is a focal enlargement. Symptoms can be caused by overactivity of the thyroid gland (hyperthyroidism) or underactivity (hypothyroidism). Autoimmune diseases can affect the function of the thyroid gland and can lead to hyperthyroidism (Graves' disease) or hypothyroidism (Hashimoto's thyroiditis). Lack of iodide in the diet or excessive iodine loading can lead to alterations in thyroid hormone synthesis.

HYPERTHYROIDISM

Anatomy, Physiology, and Pathology

The adult thyroid gland is composed of two lobes on each side of the trachea and a connecting isthmus. Some people have a pyramidal lobe, a remnant of the thyroglossal duct, that extends superiorly from the isthmus to the hyoid (Pintar, 1996). The normal gland weighs about 20 g, with each lobe about 5 cm long and 3 cm wide. It is palpable in most persons.

Connective tissue divides the thyroid into irregular portions. Thyroid hormone is synthesized by the follicular cells and stored in the colloid, where it can be taken up by the thyroid follicular cells for recycling or released into nearby capillaries. Thyroid tissue also contains vascular and nervous tissue elements and parafollicular cells that secrete calcitonin (Pintar, 1996).

The thyroid gland is diffusely enlarged in Graves' hyperthyroidism. Microscopic evaluation shows follicular hyperplasia, the colloid content is reduced, and the cells look activated, with more numerous mitochondria and increased microvilli at the cell surface (Pintar, 1996). In subacute thyroiditis, biopsy of the gland shows thyroid tissue infiltrated by granulocytes, monocytes, and giant cells. In some cases, lymphoid germinal centers are found (Lazarus, 1996).

Thyroid hormones are formed from two tyrosine molecules that are iodinated. Tetraiodothyronine or thyroxine (T_4) is produced only by the thyroid gland, whereas triiodothyronine (T_3) is produced by the thyroid and by conversion of T_4 at extrathyroidal sites. Thyroid hormone synthesis is dependent on the dietary intake of iodide and its subsequent transport to the follicular cells. To remain euthyroid, the minimal recommended intake of iodide is 150 mcg/day (Reed & Pangaro, 1995). In the United States, iodide is added to salt and flour, and dietary intake is usually 500 to 800 mcg/day (Reed & Pangaro, 1995). Daily production of T_4 is about 100 mcg/day, half of which is then converted to T_3 (Reed & Pangaro, 1995).

T_3 and T_4 travel in the bloodstream bound to serum proteins, particularly thyroxine-binding globulin, which binds T_4 more avidly than T_3. At the level of the cell, T_4 and T_3 dissociate from the binding proteins and enter as free hormones. Membranes within the cells contain receptors for T_4 and T_3, and at the nucleus receptors have a 10-fold increased avidity for T_3; there, the hormone stimulates mRNA production. Thyroid hormone ultimately stimulates thermogenesis by increased ATP use and promotes the synthesis of many structural proteins (Usala, 1995).

Thyroid hormone synthesis is regulated by the availability of intrathyroidal iodide and by thyrotropin or thyroid-stimulating hormone (TSH) (Scanlon & Toft, 1995). TSH is secreted by pituitary thyrotrophs. Its alpha subunit is identical to luteinizing hormone, follicle-stimulating hormone, and human chorionic gonadotropin, but its beta subunit is unique. As in all hormone systems, its secretion is pulsatile and its release is stimulated by thyrotropin-releasing hormone (TRH), which is made in the paraventricular nucleus of the hypothalamus. Low levels of free T_4 and free T_3 stimulate TRH and TSH release by negative feedback. Dopamine and somatostatin, on the other hand, inhibit TSH secretion (Scanlon & Toft, 1995).

Epidemiology

HYPERTHYROIDISM

Hyperthyroidism is a common disorder, occurring in about 19 per 1000 women and 1.6 per 1000 men in North America (Burman, 1995). The annual incidence rate is 3 per 1000 women (Burman, 1995). In Europe, the annual incidence rate is 25 per 100,000 people (Hay & Morris, 1996). Graves' disease is the most common cause of hyperthyroidism. It most commonly occurs in young women in the reproductive years, but it can occur in children and in men and women of any age. In the older patient (>40 years), hyperthyroidism is usually caused by a toxic multinodular goiter. The prevalence of toxic multinodular goiter appears to vary depending on the rate of endemic goiter. In areas of iodine deficiency (eg, Malmo, Sweden), toxic multinodular goiter is more common, occurring in 9% to 21% of the patients with thyrotoxicosis. In areas of iodine excess (eg, Great Britain), the rate of toxic nodular goiter is 3% (Hay & Morris, 1996).

Excessive exogenous thyroid ingestion is a common cause of mild hyperthyroidism (Burman, 1995; Nuovo, 1995). This ingestion could be prescribed or surreptitious, and can be found in many persons taking doses of 0.2 mcg or greater of L-thyroxine, 0.075 mg/day or more of L-triiodothyronine, or more than 180 mg/day (3 grains) of thyroid extract.

■ ■ ■ CLINICAL PEARL

Thyrotoxicosis is more likely to develop in persons with autonomous nodules or persons taking thyroid extract or combinations of T_3 and T_4, because the T_4 measurements in the serum underestimate the dose of thyroid hormone delivered (Burman, 1995; Hay & Morris, 1996). Although this hyperthyroidism is usually caused by ingestion of thyroid medication, there have been epidemics of hyperthyroidism caused by the ingestion of meat from neck strap muscles contaminated with thyroid gland (Burman, 1995).

Hyperthyroidism can also be caused by exposure to iodine in persons with a degree of thyroid autonomy (toxic nodules, multinodular goiter) (Burman, 1995; Hay & Morris, 1996). The hyperthyroidism can occur 3 to 8 weeks after an iodine load (eg, use of expectorant or intravenous contrast) and persists for several months. Likewise, use of amiodarone for cardiac arrhythmias can induce thyroiditis and cause hyperthyroidism, which is quite difficult to treat (Bartelena, 1996), because the iodine content of the drug is high (33%) and the half-life is prolonged (55 days). Radioactive iodine cannot be used in these cases, but antithyroid medication and steroids are helpful until the drug is eliminated and hyperthyroidism remits (Bartelena, 1996).

Rare cases of hyperthyroidism can be caused by excessive TSH secretion from a pituitary adenoma (Burman, 1995; Franklyn, 1994). These patients have goiter but no ophthalmopathy. Tumors of trophoblastic tissue (hydatidiform mole, choriocarcinoma) can also cause hyperthyroidism, because the human chorionic gonadotropin produced by such tumors has a weak thyroid-stimulating ability (Burman, 1995). Ectopic thyroid tissue within the ovary (struma ovarii, a dermoid tumor or teratoma of the ovary) can cause hyperthyroidism (Burman, 1995). Here, radioisotope scanning will show no uptake in the neck, but rather uptake in the pelvic area; this is diagnostic. In rare cases of thyroid cancer, patients will become hyperthyroid if they have a large amount of metastatic deposits of thyroid tissue (Burman, 1995).

GRAVES' DISEASE: PATHOPHYSIOLOGY

Graves' hyperthyroidism is an autoimmune disease caused by the production of antibodies that bind to the thyroid cell's TSH receptor, altering its function. It is believed that an intrinsic thyroidal cell defect changes immune cell function, activating a normally suppressed population of B lymphocytes (Burman, 1995). The B lymphocytes produce the autoantibody thyrotropin-binding inhibitory immunoglobulin, which mimics the action of TSH (Burman, 1995). This causes excessive production of thyroid hormone and growth of the thyroid gland. Many believe that autoimmune thyroid disease, Graves' and Hashimoto's thyroiditis (discussed under hypothyroidism), although not immunogenetically identical, represent opposite ends of a single illness. Both diseases have strong genetic components, involve lymphocytic infiltration of the gland, and elaborate autoantibodies (Burman, 1995).

Graves' hyperthyroidism appears to be an inherited disease because there is an increased frequency of certain genetic markers (histocompatibility complexes) in affected persons, especially HLA-B8 and DR3. In addition, there is a high concordance rate for the disease among monozygotic twins (Burman, 1995). Although autoantibodies cause the goiter and hyperthyroidism of Graves' disease in a genetically predisposed person, not all people with these genetic markers develop autoimmune thyroid disease. The development of disease may be linked to an environmental stimulus that permits expression of the gene or allows the thyroidal defect. At present this stimulus is unidentified, but it may involve viral infections, sex hormone levels, or stress, factors that could change immune cell function.

History and Physical Examination

Hyperthyroidism or thyrotoxicosis is the clinical syndrome that results when tissues are exposed to excessive thyroid hormone. Hyperthyroidism can have multiple causes and can vary in severity and length of illness. Its causes are presented in Table 19-1.

Symptoms are caused by the effects of excessive thyroid hormone on the various organ systems. Although different causes of hyperthyroidism may produce similar symptoms and signs of disease, it is important to differentiate the cause of the hyperthyroidism to devise the best treatment strategy.

Patients with hyperthyroidism display restlessness, anxiety, and emotional lability (Burman, 1995; Singer et al, 1995). Their ability to concentrate is diminished, as is their exercise tolerance because of proximal muscle weakness. They may notice a hand tremor, excessive perspiration, heat intolerance, and weight loss despite an increase in appetite. About 20% of patients gain weight. Increased gut motility leads to an increased frequency of bowel movements, but not true diarrhea.

■ **CLINICAL WARNING:** Hyperthyroidism can occasionally cause potassium wasting and loss of muscle tone, which results in episodes of localized or generalized weakness called periodic paralysis (Burman, 1995). Periodic paralysis is most often seen in patients who are Asian, and episodes of paralysis can be brought on by strenuous activity, consumption of carbohydrates or alcohol, or use of medications such as insulin.

TABLE 19-1	Causes of Hyperthyroidism
Disorder	**Comments**
Graves' disease	Elevated iodine uptake, eye findings, TSH rec. ABs
Toxic multinodular goiter	No eye findings, inhomogeneous scan, large goiter
Toxic nodule	No eye findings, usually T_3 toxicosis
Subacute thyroiditis	Fever, tender neck, iodine uptake low
TSH-secreting tumor	No eye signs, CNS signs, increased alpha-subunit
Interleukin-2 or interferon use	Causes thyroiditis and usually hypothyroidism

Patients usually seek care because of the thyroid enlargement, eye changes, cardiopulmonary symptoms, or difficulty at work or in their personal relationships. Table 19-2 presents additional symptoms and signs of hyperthyroidism.

Graves' disease has some unique signs and symptoms. The disease is characterized by a triad of findings: hyperthyroidism, diffuse thyroid enlargement (goiter), and infiltrative ophthalmopathy and dermopathy (pretibial myxedema) (Burman, 1995). Infiltrative ophthalmopathy is present in up to 50% of patients with Graves' disease, and it can develop before hyperthyroidism is evident (Burman, 1995; Prummel & Wiersinga, 1995). Ophthalmopathy is caused by the accumulation of glycosaminoglycans in the orbital fat, connective tissue, and muscle (Bahn & Heufelder, 1993). There is infiltration of the tissues by lymphocytes and plasma cells and edema (Bahn & Heufelder, 1993). Symptoms include:

- A sensation of grittiness in the eyes
- Blurred vision
- Photophobia
- Diplopia
- Increased lacrimation
- A feeling of increased orbital pressure (Burman, 1995; Bahn & Heufelder, 1993).

Signs of ophthalmopathy are:

- Bilateral proptosis, usually symmetrical
- Periorbital and conjunctival edema
- Limited ocular movement, especially upward gaze

- Increased intraocular pressure (Burman, 1995; Bahn & Heufelder, 1993; Franklyn, 1994).

■ ■ ■ CLINICAL PEARL

It is believed that both uncontrolled thyrotoxicosis and hypothyroidism worsen ophthalmopathy (Torring, 1996; Tallstedt, 1992).

Infiltrative dermopathy is a rare manifestation of Graves' disease, found in less than 10% (Burman, 1995). These nontender lesions are scaly plaques that are erythematous or hyperpigmented on the feet, ankles, or tibial region. Biopsy reveals epidermal atrophy, fibrosis, and mucinous edema of the dermis (Burman, 1995). Even rarer is thyroid acropachy, the clubbing of fingers and toes from subcutaneous fibrosis and periosteal bone formation involving the phalanges, metatarsals, and metacarpals (Burman, 1995).

On physical examination, the skin of a hyperthyroid patient is warm and smooth. Lid lag and lid retraction occur and can be found in hyperthryoidism of any cause (Burman, 1995). Infiltrative ophthalmopathy with protrusion of the eye and limited movement of the globe is most often caused by Graves' hyperthyroidism or autoimmune thyroid disease. Thyroid enlargement is generally found but can be absent in 20% of patients with Graves' (Burman, 1995). Because of increased blood flow to the hyperactive gland, a bruit or venous hum can be auscultated over the gland. Systolic hypertension, sinus

TABLE 19-2	Symptoms and Signs of Hyperthyroidism
System	**Effects**
General	Nervousness, insomnia, fatigue, heat intolerance, weight loss, tremulousness
Skin	Warm and moist, onycholysis, acropachy, pretibial myxedema, urticaria, pruritus, vitiligo
Eyes	Exophthalmos, chemosis, ophthalmoplegia, vision loss
Cardiovascular	Sinus tachycardia, shortness of breath and dyspnea on exertion, palpitations, atrial fibrillation, increased angina, congestive heart failure
GI	Hyperphagia, hyperdefecation, elevated liver function tests
Metabolic	Hypercalcemia, potassium wasting, increased alkaline phosphatase
Neuromuscular	Fine tremor of hands, proximal muscle weakness, loss of muscle tone, periodic paralysis
Osseous	Osteoporosis (if of long standing)
Neurologic	Fever, delirium, coma, choreoathetosis
Reproductive	Irregular menses, gynecomastia
Hematologic	Normochromic, normocytic anemia, lymphocytosis

Source: Burman, 1995.

tachycardia, and atrial fibrillation can be found. There is a fine hand tremor that is apparent when the hands are stretched out in front of the examiner (Burman, 1995; Singer et al, 1995).

TOXIC MULTINODULAR GOITER

Hyperthyroidism is also commonly the later stage of a multinodular goiter (Plummer's disease) (Hay & Morris, 1996; Singer et al, 1995; Franklyn, 1994). In toxic multinodular goiter, the gland is more irregular and nodular than in Graves' disease. Patients thus present with complaints of an enlarging neck mass or difficulty swallowing. Hyperthyroidism usually presents in an insidious manner and there is no infiltrative ophthalmopathy or dermopathy (Hay & Morris, 1996; Singer et al, 1995). In some cases, hyperthyroidism can follow exposure to drugs rich in iodine, such as intravenous contrast used in a computed tomography (CT) examination, the use of cough syrup with expectorants, or the use of amiodarone, an antiarrhythmic drug.

A few patients present with hyperthyroidism from a toxic (autonomous) nodule. This is found mostly in patients with a thyroid nodule that measures 3 cm or greater who are younger than 20 or older than 60 years (Hay & Morris, 1996).

SUBACUTE THYROIDITIS

Subacute thyroiditis (nonsuppurative thyroiditis, granulomatous thyroiditis, or De Quervain's disease) is an inflammatory disease of the thyroid gland that can cause overt hyperthyroidism. It is the most common cause of pain and tenderness of the thyroid gland (Lazarus, 1996). Its onset can be abrupt or gradual, and the pain is over the thyroid gland, with radiation to the jaw, throat, and ears. Many patients give a history of a recent upper respiratory infection, and they may give a history of fever, sore throat, and myalgias. The pain and hyperthyroidism are transient, subsiding in weeks to 2 to 3 months. Transient hypothyroidism may follow this period of hyperthyroidism because of leakage of stored hormone from the gland and a disruption of the biosynthesis of hormone. Permanent hypothyroidism is unusual (Lazarus, 1996).

Thyroid inflammatory disease can present in a silent or painless mode (Lazarus, 1996). This usually occurs in the postpartum period, and it can be difficult to differentiate painless thyroiditis from early Graves' disease. Nonetheless, postpartum thyroiditis is transient and does not lead to infiltrative ophthalmopathy. Women will report faster-than-expected weight loss after parturition, mood changes, anxiety, and palpitations that may all be erroneously attributed to the postpartum blues.

Diagnostic Studies

LABORATORY TESTING

Assays for Total T_4 and T_3

The concentrations of total T_4 and T_3 are measured in the blood using radioimmunoassay. Serum total T_4 and T_3 reflect hormonal production and also the serum concentration of thyroid hormone-binding proteins. When the level of serum thyroxine-binding globulin (thyroid hormone-binding protein) is increased, serum total T_4 and T_3 are increased, whereas the free hormones are not.

Estimation of Serum Free T_4 and T_3: Free Thyroxine Index

The amount of free T_4 can be estimated by separation of the free from the bound T_4 by a semipermeable membrane in equilibrium dialysis, a very expensive procedure, or by partition of tracer T_3 between serum proteins and a nonspecific solid-phase matrix (resin uptake). A serum free T_4 index can be calculated from the serum total T_4 and the thyroid hormone-binding ratio. Labeled T_3 is used because it is less tightly bound to proteins. The thyroid hormone-binding ratio or T_3 resin uptake estimates the number of unoccupied serum protein binding sites. Table 19-3 presents these values in hyperthyroidism and other states.

In hyperthyroidism, the TSH level is low or undetectable when using the ultrasensitive assays that are now available. The finding of a low TSH with elevated free thyroid hormones confirms the state of hyperthyroidism (Burman, 1995; Hay & Morris, 1996; Singer et al, 1995; Franklyn, 1994).

CLINICAL WARNING: Finding an elevated total T_4 may not indicate hyperthyroidism, because pregnancy or the use of conjugated estrogens increases the level of thyroxine-binding globulin (Burman, 1995). It is important in women with elevated total T_4 levels that hyperthyroidism is confirmed by the finding of a low TSH value.

There are some patients with a low TSH level who have high T_3 but not T_4 levels. T_3 thyrotoxicosis is more likely to occur in patients with a toxic thyroid nodule, but it can be seen in hyperthyroidism of any cause. Other patients have isolated elevations of T_4 and a low TSH level. In these cases, there is an intervening serious illness that inhibits T_4 to T_3 conversion (euthyroid sick syndrome) or the concomitant use of a drug, such as propranolol, that inhibits T_4 to T_3 conversion, so that T_3 levels are normal. Some persons show subclinical hyperthyroidism, in which TSH levels are low but free hormone levels are normal. This is often found in patients with autonomous thyroid function, such as euthyroid Graves', thyroid adenoma, or multinodular goiter (Burman, 1995; Hay & Morris, 1996; Singer et al, 1995).

Some patients on routine testing have low TSH values without clinically apparent disease. A low TSH level can be normal for that population, but free T_4 and total T_3 levels should be checked to look for thyrotoxicosis. Asymptomatic patients may

TABLE 19-3	Laboratory Values in Hyperthyroidism and Other States			
Disease	Total T_4	T_3RU	Free T_4	TSH
Hyperthyroidism	High	High	High	Low
Pregnancy Normal	High	Low	Normal	
Subclinical hyperthyroidism	Normal	Normal	Normal	Low

T_3 RU, T_3 resin uptake.

have apathetic hyperthyroidism, which is seen more frequently in the elderly, or thyroid autonomy (toxic nodule or toxic multinodular goiter) or sick euthyroidism.

TSH values are also low in secondary hypothyroidism, but the T_4 (free hormone) level is not elevated (see section on hypothyroidism). A normal or elevated TSH value in the presence of elevated free thyroid hormone levels indicates excessive pituitary secretion of TSH from a pituitary adenoma or thyroid resistance syndrome (Singer et al, 1995).

Thyroid antibodies are also found in the blood of patients with Graves' hyperthyroidism. The antibodies that are most specific are those that bind to TSH receptors, which include thyrotropin-binding inhibitor immunoglobulins or thyroid-stimulating immunoglobulins. Thyroid antibodies may be present during periods of remission, and their absence does not seem to be predictive for permanent remission (McIver, 1996). Antithyroid antibodies that bind to other cellular components are called antithyroglobulin and antimicrosomal, or thyroid peroxidase antibodies. These levels are also elevated, although titers are usually lower than those in patients with autoimmune thyroiditis (Burman, 1995) (see section on hypothyroidism).

Other laboratory abnormalities found in patients with hyperthyroidism include increased liver function tests, specifically aminotransferase and alkaline phosphatase; high calcium levels; glucose intolerance (patients with diabetes may note that their insulin requirements increase); and anemia with a relative decrease in granulocytes and an increase in lymphocytes. Patients with subacute thyroiditis have an elevated erythrocyte sedimentation rate (Lazarus, 1996; Burman, 1995; Franklyn, 1994). Thyroglobulin levels are increased, unless the hyperthyroidism is caused by exogenous intake of thyroid hormone.

RADIONUCLIDE IMAGING STUDIES

Most patients with hyperthyroidism have increased iodine uptake 24 hours after a tracer dose of radioactive iodine (^{131}I). The exceptions, showing low uptake during clinical hyperthyroidism, are patients with thyroiditis or patients who have taken thyroid hormone or received iodine loads (intravenous contrast or amiodarone) before the test. Uptakes are done to confirm the presence of hyperthyroidism and are not necessary for the diagnosis of classic cases of Graves' disease (Lazarus, 1996; Burman, 1995; Singer et al, 1995). Uptakes are also done to differentiate cases of thyroiditis from Graves' if clinical cues are inadequate to distinguish these causes of hyperthyroidism.

Thyroid scans that allow images of the gland to be generated are done with labelled iodine (^{123}I) or pertechnetate (technetium, ^{99}Tc). Both radioisotopes emit gamma particles that are detected by a gamma camera. ^{99}Tc is less expensive and has a shorter half-life, allowing less radiation exposure. In Graves' disease, the distribution of radionuclide within the thyroid is homogeneous, whereas toxic adenomas or toxic multinodular goiters are heterogeneous, showing some areas of increased uptake and other areas of decreased uptake (Burman, 1995; Hay & Morris, 1996). It is important that patients with areas of decreased uptake on thyroid scanning (cold nodules) are evaluated for thyroid cancer. Although most have multinodular goiters, some patients will harbor thyroid carcinoma in nonfunctioning tissue. Patients with hypothyroidism or thyroiditis demonstrate low or no uptake of radionuclide, and thyroid scans either cannot be generated or may look patchy (Lazarus, 1996).

COMPUTED TOMOGRAPHY AND MAGNETIC RESONANCE IMAGING

Graves' disease causes thickening of the eye muscles in more than 50% of patients; this can be detected by CT or magnetic resonance imaging (MRI) of the orbits. Orbital CT or MRI is particularly useful when the patient has euthyroid Graves' (normal thyroid function) or unilateral eye involvement, where the etiology of the proptosis may not be easily recognized. Although CT scanning does expose the lens to radiation, it is the preferred imaging modality because of its lower cost and its ability to provide bony anatomic detail.

Treatment Options, Expected Outcomes, and Comprehensive Management

Graves' disease is characterized by exacerbations, perhaps provoked by physical or emotional stress, and spontaneous remissions, where long periods of euthyroidism (normal thyroid function) can occur after the withdrawal of medical therapy. Remissions occur in about 25% of patients and are more likely with:

- Hyperthyroidism of recent onset
- Mild disease
- Modest thyroid enlargement
- Modestly elevated total T_3 levels (Burman, 1995; Singer et al, 1995; Franklyn, 1994).

Treatment strategies depend on the expected length of disease and its severity.

■ ■ ■ **CLINICAL PEARL**

Graves' disease has no one specific therapy, and it is difficult to predict who will go into remission and how long a remission will last. Thus, most patients are offered either antithyroid drug therapy or ablative treatment with radioactive iodine. The latter option is used most often in older patients with Graves'. Antithyroid drugs bring about euthyroidism more rapidly, do not cause permanent thyroid damage, and are inexpensive. Thus, antithyroid drugs are usually the initial treatment plan. If a side effect to medication occurs, or if hyperthyroidism is not controlled within a reasonable length of time, drug therapy can be withdrawn and radioactive iodine given. Radioactive iodine almost always results in hypothyroidism, which can occur any time after treatment (Burman, 1995; Franklyn, 1994; Torring, 1996).

■ **CLINICAL WARNING:** Radioactive iodine is contraindicated in pregnant women, and pregnancy should be deferred for at least 3 months after treatment.

DRUG THERAPY FOR HYPERTHYROIDISM

Antithyroid drugs that are available in the United States include propylthiouracil (PTU) and methimazole (Tapazole, MMI). Both work by inhibiting thyroid hormone synthesis, blocking iodine oxidation and iodotyrosine coupling. Both may inhibit antithyroid antibody production by inhibiting lymphocyte function. PTU also blocks, in a limited fashion, T_4 to T_3 conversion (Burman, 1995; Franklyn, 1994). Both drugs are absorbed from the gut rapidly, but MMI is better concentrated in the gland and metabolized slowly (Singer et al, 1995). MMI is usually given as 10 to 40 mg/day in two or three doses; per day PTU is given in two or three doses a day at 300 to 1200 mg. The larger the goiter, the larger the dose given.

There is biochemical improvement in 2 to 6 weeks and clinical improvement in 4 to 6 weeks (Burman, 1995; Franklyn, 1994; Torring, 1996). Most patients reach euthyroidism in 8 to 10 weeks, and the dose can be reduced by 25% to 50% (Burman, 1995). Initial therapy is to inhibit thyroid synthesis altogether until thyroid stores are depleted. Once euthyroidism is reached, the goal is partial inhibition, being careful to prevent hypothyroidism, which could aggravate thyroid enlargement or orbitopathy. Failure to control hyperthyroidism is often caused by noncompliance with therapy or inadequate doses of drug; often T_4 levels fall, but T_3 levels are still elevated, leading to persistent hyperthyroidism.

Patients are seen every 4 to 6 weeks until euthyroid on the medication and then every 3 months thereafter (Burman, 1995; Franklyn, 1994). Antithyroid medication is given for up to 24 months or longer to ensure remission; shorter periods of treatment usually lead to a recurrence of the hyperthyroidism within months of drug withdrawal. Franklyn (1994) states that one study that looked at patients 1 year after stopping treatment for Graves' disease found that 31% of patients who used antithyroid medication for 6 months were in remission, but 82% of patients on medication for 2 years were still euthyroid.

■ ■ ■ CLINICAL PEARL

There is no test that reliably predicts remission, although normal free hormone levels on low doses of medication and a dramatic decrease in the goiter size are good indicators (Franklyn, 1994).

An alternative treatment protocol for Graves' disease is to give high doses of antithyroid medication; when the patient responds, instead of decreasing the dose, thyroid supplement is added to prevent hypothyroidism. This dual therapy of "blockade and add back" allows higher doses of antithyroid drug to be given to suppress antithyroid antibody formation, supposedly increasing the rate of remission without causing hypothyroidism. The efficacy of this therapy has been shown in Japan and Europe. In a European study, medical therapy using antithyroid drug alone for 6 months and then with thyroxine for an additional 12 months was successful during a 4-year follow-up in 58% of young adults and 66% of adults over age 35 (Torring, 1996). This same therapy has not been as successful in North America, where the recurrence rate of hyperthyroidism (about 30%) was similar in patients given antithyroid medication and those given antithyroid medication followed by antithyroid medication plus thyroxine (McIver et al, 1996).

CLINICAL WARNING: All patients taking antithyroid medication should be warned to look for the minor and major side effects of the medication. A common minor reaction, especially to PTU, is an itchy skin rash. Often the rash improves with antihistamine use and as the hyperthyroidism is controlled, but bothersome skin eruptions

may mandate changing to MMI or stopping medication and using radioablation to reverse hyperthyroidism. More serious side effects, such as hepatitis, fever, and agranulocytosis (which occurs in 0.3%), require immediate cessation of medication and often hospitalization until blood tests improve. White blood counts should be obtained as a baseline because Graves' disease can produce mild leukopenia (Burman, 1995; Singer et al, 1995; Franklyn, 1994).

Inorganic iodine can decrease thyroid hormone levels by inhibiting the release of T_4 and T_3 by the thyroid gland (Burman, 1995; Franklyn, 1994). Iodide also blocks T_4 to T_3 conversion. This usually requires 5 to 10 mg of iodide daily. Escape from the antithyroid effects of iodide occurs within 7 to 14 days, but it is useful in patients with severe hyperthyroidism. Iodide is given several hours after starting antithyroid medication to avoid stimulating thyroid hormone synthesis. A saturation solution of potassium iodide (SSKI, 50 mg iodide/drop) or oral iodinated-contrast agents (Telepaque, 500 to 1000 mg b.i.d.) can be used (Burman, 1995).

Beta-adrenergic antagonists reverse many of the clinical symptoms and signs of hyperthyroidism. Propranolol is often used in a dosage of 40 to 160 mg/day to treat palpitations, tachycardia, nervousness, and hand tremors. Propranolol used alone does not reverse the catabolic effects of hyperthyroidism. It is the treatment of choice in thyroiditis and to control the symptoms of hyperthyroidism before ^{131}I therapy becomes effective (Lazarus, 1996; Burman, 1995; Singer et al, 1995; Franklyn, 1994).

RADIOIODINE ABLATION

Radioactive iodine (^{131}I) is an effective treatment for Graves' disease because it reduces the volume of functioning thyroid tissue. The advantages of using radioactive ablation over antithyroid medication are its lack of side effects and its efficacy. Nonetheless, hyperthyroidism may not be reversed for many months. Thus, severely ill patients may need to be pretreated with antithyroid medication until they are more stable (Burman, 1995; Franklyn, 1994; Torring, 1996). Before therapy, iodine-containing drugs and contrast agents must be avoided. The usual dose of ^{131}I is 8 to 12 mCi for Graves' disease, delivering 10,000 to 20,000 rad to the thyroid (Burman, 1995). Higher doses of ^{131}I (12 to 15 mCi) are given to patients who used antithyroid drugs before radioablation (Burch, 1994). Acute exacerbation of hyperthyroidism may occur within the first 2 weeks after treatment from radiation-induced thyroiditis (Franklyn, 1994). There may be some swelling of the goiter and neck pain, which responds to aspirin or steroids. Persistent hyperthyroidism may occur, especially if lower doses are used for treatment. Clinical and biochemical improvement occurs within 2 to 3 months; most patients are euthyroid or hypothyroid within 3 to 6 months. Hypothyroidism ensues in about 80% of treated persons within the following year, and 2% per year thereafter. Thyroidal underactivity is caused by radiation necrosis and the failure of the surviving cells to replicate.

CLINICAL WARNING: The primary care provider should refer any patient needing radioiodine ablation to a thyroid specialty practice for evaluation and treatment.

Concerns that ^{131}I can cause secondary thyroid cancers or other tumors has not been borne out in the literature (Burman, 1995; Franklyn, 1994). There may be a risk for gastric carcinoma in patients treated with ^{131}I for Graves' who have a family history of gastric cancer and pernicious anemia. Nonetheless, because of the concerns about potential gonadal radiation and leukemia, ^{131}I is not the preferred treatment for children and adolescents or women in their reproductive years. Adult men may not face the same risk after exposure to ^{131}I because the testicles are farther removed from the bladder than the ovaries and because the testicles manufacture new spermatocytes every 90 days.

CLINICAL WARNING: Pregnant women are not candidates for radioablation because the radioactive iodine can cross the placental barrier and destroy the fetal thyroid. Women who are fertile need to have a pregnancy test before treatment with ^{131}I.

SURGICAL ABLATION

Surgical treatment for hyperthyroidism is indicated for pregnant women who cannot tolerate antithyroid medication (Burman, 1995); patients with large goiters, especially those with compressive symptoms (Hay & Morris, 1996); patients intolerant of antithyroid medication who do not want radioactive iodine (Torring, 1996); and patients found to have coexistent suspicious nodules (Burman, 1995). Surgery can be preceded by short-term antithyroid medication, or in the nonpregnant patient iodide. Surgery is more expensive than treatment with radioiodine. Postoperative complications include vocal cord paralysis and transient or permanent hypocalcemia from hypoparathyroidism. Subtotal thyroidectomies, although safer in terms of less risk of vocal cord paralysis and hypoparathyroidism, may lead to recurrent hyperthyroidism because the thyroid remnant can be stimulated by remaining antithyroid antibodies. Many surgeons thus prefer to do near-total thyroidectomies (Burman, 1995) because it is difficult to reoperate in the neck. The recurrence rate for hyperthyroidism is about 3% to 8%; it tends to occur more than 5 years after surgery (Torring, 1996).

CLINICAL WARNING: All patients who undergo near-total thyroidectomies will be on lifelong thyroid hormone replacement and need to be followed for recurrence and adjustment of replacement by their primary care provider.

Surgical decompression is indicated if ophthalmopathy threatens vision.

CLINICAL PEARL

Periorbital edema from Graves' ophthalmopathy can be improved by using mild diuretics at night and sleeping with the head raised. Methylcellulose (0.5%) drops can also be used for eye irritation (Burman, 1995; Bahn & Heufelder, 1993). Ophthalmopathy that is more severe is treated with oral steroids or orbital irradiation.

The lesions of infiltrative dermopathy associated with Graves' disease usually require no therapy, but if extensive they can be treated with topical 0.5% fluocinolone covered with an occlusive dressing (Burman, 1995).

Follow-up for Graves' disease is lifelong to ensure that there is no recurrence of disease, to detect hypothyroidism after treatment, and to ensure that thyroid replacement therapy is adequate.

TREATMENT FOR TOXIC GOITER

Treatment for hyperthyroidism caused by multinodular thyroid disease is ablative, either with radioactive iodine or surgery (Hay & Morris, 1996). Despite the greater doses of radioiodine (15 to 29 mCi) used to treat multinodular goiter, hypothyroidism is less commonly seen after ablation than after Graves' because of the heterogeneous uptake. As hypertrophic areas of the nodular gland are destroyed, previously atrophic areas resume thyroid function. Antithyroid drugs can be taken until definitive therapy is undertaken (Hays & Morris, 1996; Franklyn, 1994). For large compressive goiters, surgery is curative, although for the elderly or those with concurrent heart disease who are not surgical candidates, large doses of radioactive iodine (>70 mCi) can be given (Huysmans, 1994). For younger patients with toxic nodules, which are usually follicular adenomas greater than 3 cm, surgical removal of the overactive nodule is the preferred treatment because this decreases the risk of persistent or recurrent hyperthyroidism and late-occurring hypothyroidism from the ^{131}I exposure.

TREATMENT FOR SUBACUTE THYROIDITIS

Treatment of subacute thyroiditis consists of relieving the pain and symptoms of hyperthyroidism. For pain relief, anti-inflammatory drugs (2.4 to 3.6 g salicylate or in more severe cases 30 to 40 mg prednisone) are used for 3 to 4 weeks and then tapered and withdrawn over 4 weeks (Lazarus, 1995; Burman, 1995; Franklyn, 1994). The neck pain usually totally resolves within 72 hours if prednisone is given; if pain persists, other diagnoses, including anaplastic thyroid cancer, should be considered. Propranolol or other beta-antagonists can be used for symptomatic palpitations or anxiety. It is essential to differentiate thyroiditis, where the hyperthyroid state lasts 4 to 8 weeks, from Graves' disease so that radioactive iodine and surgical remedies are avoided. Antithyroid medication is not given because of the transient nature of the hyperthyroidism. More importantly, because thyroiditis is a disease in which stored hormone is released and there is no increased synthesis of T_3 and T_4, PTU or MMI, which interfere with thyroid synthesis, have no beneficial effect (Lazarus, 1995).

Teaching and Self-Care

Stress may be a trigger for Graves' disease: more patients with Graves' disease report antecedent stress compared with controls in several studies. There are also reports of a higher incidence of Graves' disease among concentration camp survivors. Acute and chronic stress may induce a state of immune suppression (see Chap. 18) via the actions of corticotropin-releasing hormone and cortisol on immune cells.

Sex steroids also seem to play a role in the initiation of Graves' disease and other autoimmune diseases of the thyroid, because far more women have these diseases than men. Graves' disease is rare before puberty and during pregnancy; T- and B-cell function decrease, whereas the corticotropin-releasing hormone/cortisol axis is activated. Postpartum thyroiditis is caused by the rebound from this immunosuppression.

There is also a higher rate of disease persistence and ophthalmopathy in patients who smoke.

Referral Points and Clinical Warnings

Thyroid storm is a medical emergency and occurs in hyperthyroid patients who have an intercurrent illness or stress, such as an infection, motor vehicle accident, or heart attack (Burman, 1995; Franklyn, 1994; Burch & Wartofsky, 1993). It can also occur after stopping or missing doses of antithyroid medication, or rarely after ^{131}I therapy. Patients with thyroid storm have the same symptoms as those with thyrotoxicosis, but the symptoms and signs are more extreme:

- Fever (often >100.4°F)
- Nausea and vomiting
- Tachycardia and congestive heart failure
- Anxiety, confusion, or frank psychosis.

Thyroid storm is a clinical and not a biochemical diagnosis; these patients have elevated free thyroid hormone levels, but no more elevated than their less ill counterparts with hyperthyroidism. Thyroid storm has a fatality rate of 20% to 50% (Burch & Wartofsky, 1993), so treatment consists of hospitalization and aggressive reversal of thyrotoxicosis. Table 19-4 presents the treatment of thyroid storm. Serum T_4 and T_3 levels should improve within 48 hours.

To avoid thyroid storm, patients with hyperthyroidism should be told to contact their thyroid specialist or primary care team if they develop an intercurrent illness, and to avoid minor surgery, even dental procedures, until they are on adequate treatment for their thyrotoxicosis.

Hyperthyroidism can also be difficult to recognize and treat in the pregnant patient (Burman, 1995). This is because normal pregnancy may mimic some signs of hyperthyroidism. Hyperthyroidism should be suspected in pregnant women who have weight loss, severe nausea and vomiting, muscle weakness, marked tachycardia, and goiter; thyroid enlargement should not occur in pregnant women who have adequate iodide intake (Burman, 1995;, Singer et al, 1995; Franklyn, 1994). Hyperemesis gravidarum may be caused by occult hyperthyroidism; thus, free thyroid hormone levels and TSH should be obtained in pregnant women with intractable nausea and vomiting. Management of hyperthyroidism in pregnancy is outside the bounds of this text. Referral to a thyroid specialist for evaluation and guidance in the treatment plan is necessary.

In the postpartum period, hyperthyroidism is usually caused by recurrence of Graves' disease (Burman, 1995) or painless thyroiditis (Lazarus, 1996), which does not need aggressive therapy because of its transient nature. It is differentiated from Graves' by low uptake on iodine scanning.

Treatment of Graves' ophthalmopathy includes referral to the ophthalmologist and thyroid specialist, because achieving the euthyroid state (normal thyroid function) often improves diplopia and irritative symptoms. Swelling and edema of the orbital contents can cause optic nerve compression. Thus, patients complaining of loss of visual acuity or loss of color perception should be told to contact their ophthalmologist immediately to avoid sight loss.

HYPOTHYROIDISM

Hypothyroidism is the clinical and biochemical syndrome resulting from decreased thyroid hormone production. It may be caused by thyroid disease (primary hypothyroidism) or by diseases of the pituitary or hypothalamus (secondary hypothyroidism). Primary hypothyroidism is often caused by an autoimmune destruction of the thyroid follicular cells called chronic thyroiditis, but it can also be unrelated to autoimmune processes and thus idiopathic. Chronic thyroiditis can occur in an atrophic (nongoitrous) form or a goitrous form, often called Hashimoto's thyroiditis. Nonthyroidal illness can mimic hypothyroidism and must be distinguished from the latter because sick euthyroidism causes transient changes in the thyroid hormone production.

Causes of hypothyroidism include chronic autoimmune thyroiditis, history of treatment with radioactive iodine or external radiation to the head and neck, surgical removal of the thyroid gland, or thyroid gland dysgenesis. Causes of hypothyroidism are presented in Table 19-5.

Pathology

Chronic autoimmune thyroiditis can be subdivided into lymphocytic versus Hashimoto's thyroiditis. The former glands show thyroid tissue infiltrated by lymphocytes; the latter have areas of eosinophilic changes (Hurthle cells) and fibrosis (Dayan & Daniels, 1996). Glands from patients with the goitrous form of Hashimoto's thyroiditis reveal follicular hyperplasia and lymphoid germinal centers.

Epidemiology

The frequency of hypothyroidism varies with the population studied, increasing in women in the menopausal period. The incidence is about 5 to 10 per 1000, with overt hypothyroidism in up to 2% of the patients going for medical examinations

---

TABLE 19-4   **Treatment of Thyroid Storm**

BLOCK THYROID HORMONE SYNTHESIS

Loading dose 600–1000 mg propylthiouracil (PTU)

Followed by 200 mg PTU every 4–6 hours

PTU can be given orally, via nasogastric tube, or rectally.

BLOCK THYROID-ASSOCIATED CARDIAC ARRHYTHMIAS

Propranolol to control pulse (60–80 mg every 4–6 hours)

Can give propranolol intravenously, 0.5–1 mg/minute

BLOCK T_4 TO T_3 CONVERSION

Hydrocortisone is given (50 mg every 8 hours).

Iodine can also be used if treatment with radioactive iodine is not to be given in the next few days (SSKI 5 drops every 6 hours or Telepaque 500–1000 mg every 12 hours).

SUPPORTIVE MEASURES

Reduce fever.

Treat any underlying infection.

Give fluid (usually 3–5 L/day) and glucose.

TABLE 19-5	Causes of Hypothyroidism

PRIMARY HYPOTHYROIDISM

Destruction of thyroid tissue

Chronic autoimmune thyroiditis

Radiation (^{131}I, external for lymphoma, neck cancer)

Subtotal or total thyroidectomy

Infiltrative disease (amyloid, scleroderma)

Defective hormone synthesis

Iodine deficiency

Drugs that block synthesis (lithium, iodine)

CENTRAL HYPOTHYROIDISM

Pituitary disease

Hypothalamic disease

TRANSIENT HYPOTHYROIDISM

Silent thyroiditis (usually postpartum)

Subacute thyroiditis (usually viral)

Withdrawal of thyroid hormone therapy in a euthyroid patient

(Dayan & Daniels, 1996). Another 3% to 4% of all examined patients have subclinical hypothyroidism.

CHRONIC AUTOIMMUNE THYROIDITIS

Chronic autoimmune thyroiditis is the most common cause of hypothyroidism, occurring in 3% to 4.5% of the population. It occurs in children and adults but is more common in women. As many as 20% of perimenopausal women have antithyroid antibodies detected in their blood, although the disease may be clinically silent. As these women age, the frequency of finding antimicrosomal antibodies increases up to 33% after age 70 (Dayan & Daniels, 1996). Abnormal antibody production links this disease to Graves' hyperthyroidism. There are patients who develop Graves' after a bout of thyroiditis (Burman, 1995). In euthyroid patients with the nongoitrous, atrophic form of thyroiditis, overt hypothyroidism occurs in 5% to 25% per year. In patients with goiter, hypothyroidism seems to be more likely. The mean age of diagnosis is 59 years (Dayan & Daniels, 1996).

Up to 28% of patients with Down syndrome develop thyroid autoimmune thyroid disease. There may be a genetic link between damage to chromosome 21 and chronic thyroiditis. Women with Turner's syndrome, especially those who are XO, also have a high prevalence of chronic thyroiditis (up to 50%). Chronic thyroiditis is also associated with Addison's disease (20%) and polyglandular autoimmune syndrome type II (70%). Thus, there are probably several genetic sites related to autoimmune thyroid disease (Dayan & Daniels, 1996).

Similar to Graves' disease, chronic thyroiditis is an autoimmune disease with a strong genetic component, in which immunoglobulins are found in the serum of patients. There is an increased incidence of atrophic thyroiditis among persons positive for HLA-DR3, whereas HLA-DR5 positivity is associated with goitrous thyroiditis (Lazarus, 1996; Dayan & Daniels, 1996).

POSTPARTUM THYROIDITIS

Postpartum thyroiditis is a form of silent or painless thyroiditis and can also occur at other times. There may be a link between increased consumption of iodide in the diet and autoimmune thyroiditis. In areas that are not iodine-poor, postpartum thyroiditis can occur in up to 85% of pregnant women with positive antithyroid antibodies. In most populations of pregnant women, the prevalence of postpartum thyroiditis is about 9% (Lazarus, 1996; Dayan & Daniels, 1996).

HYPOTHYROIDISM AFTER CERVICAL RADIATION OR SURGERY

Hypothyroidism is an almost invariable consequence of ablative treatment with radioactive iodine for Graves' disease, and sometimes occurs after treatment for toxic multinodular goiter. External neck irradiation in doses of 2500 rad or more, as used to treat lymphoma or laryngeal cancer, can cause hypothyroidism after therapy. Hypothyroidism also follows surgical ablation of the gland, especially if near-total thyroidectomies are used to remedy Graves' disease or thyroid cancer.

RARER CAUSES OF HYPOTHYROIDISM: GENETIC MUTATIONS, NUTRITIONAL DEFICIENCIES, DRUG-INDUCED CHANGES

Normal thyroid hormone production depends on the availability of iodide and the ability of the gland to take up iodide and perform several biosynthetic steps. There are several nutritional and genetic causes of hypothyroidism. Penrod's syndrome is a genetically inherited goiter associated with sensorineural deafness. Dietary iodide deficiency leads to reduced thyroid hormone production, goiter, and hypothyroidism in children, called cretinism (Reed & Pangaro, 1995). Untreated, childhood hypothyroidism can lead to failure to thrive and developmental delays, which can result in lower IQs. Countries with a high prevalence of endemic goiter are now provided funding for equipment to iodinize salt, resulting in a dramatic decrease in goiter and cretinism.

■ ■ ■ ■ **CLINICAL PEARL**

Cabbage and broccoli are examples of natural goitrogens. These foods should be consumed in modest amounts by people with nodular disease or a family history of thyroid nodular disease. Certain drugs such as lithium, propylthiouracil, and amiodarone can cause hypothyroidism by interfering with iodine uptake or organification (Reed & Pangaro, 1995; Surks & Sievert, 1995).

SECONDARY HYPOTHYROIDISM (CENTRAL DEFECTS)

Secondary hypothyroidism is caused by decreased thyroid hormone production because of deficiencies of TSH or TRH. This type of hypothyroidism is much less common than primary hypothyroidism and is caused by the destruction of pituitary thyrotrophs from a pituitary lesion (macroadenoma) or by the loss of the pituitary function after irradiation, surgery, or infiltration of the pituitary by a neoplasm, granulomatous disease, or other infectious process (Reed & Pangaro, 1995).

THYROID RESISTANCE SYNDROMES

Thyroid enlargement and elevated TSH levels can also be found in generalized resistance to thyroid hormone syndrome. This is a rare disease where the total T_4 and T_3 levels are elevated but the TSH level is not suppressed. Some of these patients also have stippled epiphyses, deafness, and short stature, indicative of functional hypothyroidism since childhood. The resistance to the action of thyroid hormone is partial, because the higher T_4 and T_3 levels lead to normal peripheral thyroid hor-

TABLE 19-6	Symptoms and Signs of Hypothyroidism	
System	**Symptoms**	**Signs**
General	Cold intolerance, fatigue, mild weight gain	Hypothermia
Neuromuscular	Lethargy, memory deficits, personality change, weakness, muscle cramps	Somnolence, slowed speech, hoarseness, myxedema madness, ataxia, delayed relaxation of deep tendon reflexes, carpal tunnel
GI	Nausea, constipation	Large tongue, ascites
Cardiovascular	Inability to exercise	Bradycardia, mild hypertension, pericardial effusion
Reproductive	Irregular menses, decreased fertility	
Skin	Dry and rough, dry hair, hair loss, brittle nails	Nonpitting edema, facial pallor/swelling (myxedema), yellow skin (carotenemia), periorbital swelling

Source: Singer et al, 1995.

mone actions. The abnormality appears to be a postreceptor defect and may also be found in a minority of patients with attention deficit disorder (Surks & Sievert, 1995).

History and Physical Examination

The symptoms of hypothyroidism increase as the disease becomes more severe and of longer standing. Most symptoms are caused by the fact that thyroid hormone affects every major organ system (Table 19-6).

Macroglossia and laryngeal myxedema can lead to obstructive sleep apnea. Decreased gastrointestinal motility may result in nausea and abdominal distention. Complaints of angina may be less frequent because of reduction in the oxygen requirements of the myocardium. Women may note longer and heavier menstrual bleeding. There may be hoarseness, difficulty staying alert, depression, and arthralgias (Singer et al, 1995).

Physical examination reveals a symmetrically enlarged gland that is firm and nontender in patients with goitrous autoimmune thyroiditis; the gland may not be palpable in those with atrophic thyroiditis or in secondary hypothyroidism (Lazarus, 1006; Dayan & Daniels, 1996). Bradycardia, distant heart sounds, and pericardial effusion or cardiomyopathy are present (Singer et al, 1995). Neurologic examination reveals proximal muscle weakness, slowed speech, and delayed recovery of deep tendon reflexes.

Hypothyroidism can occur from the use of drugs that interfere with thyroid secretion (Surks & Sievert, 1995). These are listed in Table 19-7. Note that lithium causes goiter in 50% of users and overt hypothyroidism in 20%. It is believed that those prone to lithium-induced hypothyroidism have pre-existing thyroiditis (Surks & Sievert, 1995). Amiodarone is iodine-rich; it can cause hypothyroidism in those predisposed to thyroiditis (Surks & Sievert, 1995).

CLINICAL WARNING: In managing hypothyroidism, it is practical to continue lithium and amiodarone if their benefits outweigh the risks of concomitant use of thyroxine.

Diagnostic Studies

LABORATORY RESULTS

In primary hypothyroidism, the free T_4 level is low but the pituitary secretion of TSH is elevated. Laboratory test ranges are presented in Table 19-8. T_3 levels are generally maintained because the increased production of TSH results in preferential T_3 synthesis and an increase in T_4 to T_3 conversion. Thus, in hypothyroidism, it is generally unnecessary to check free or total T_3 levels. In secondary hypothyroidism, TSH levels are low, normal, or slightly increased, whereas synthesis of both

TABLE 19-7	Drugs That Influence Thyroid Functions or Thyroid Replacement
Action	**Drugs**
Increase total T_4	Estrogens, clofibrate, opiates
Decrease total T_4	Androgens, glucocorticoids, danazol
Inhibit binding to thyroxine-binding globulin	Salicylates, diphenylhydantoin, furosemide, sulfonylureas, diazepam, heparin
Inhibits thyroid function	Iodine, lithium, sulfonylureas, interleukin-2
Inhibits T_4 to T_3 Conversion	Glucocorticoids, ipodate, propranolol, amiodarone, propylthiouracil
Increases TSH	Iodine, lithium, dopamine antagonists, cimetidine
Decreases TSH	Glucocorticoids, dopamine agonists, somatostatin
Inhibits GI Absorption of hormone	Cholestyramine, colestipol, soybean flour, iron, sucralfate, cimetidine

TABLE 19-8	Laboratory Tests and Hypothyroidism			
Disease	Total T$_4$	T$_3$RU	Free T$_4$	TSH
Primary hypothyroidism	Low	Low	Low	High
Secondary hypothyroidism	Low	Low	Low	Low, normal
Subclinical hypothyroidism	Normal	Normal	Normal	High

T$_3$RU, T$_3$ resin uptake.

T$_3$ and T$_4$ is reduced. Subclinical hypothyroidism involves a slightly elevated TSH level (less than three times the upper range of the assay), with normal free T$_4$ levels. In nonthyroidal illness (sick euthyroidism), TSH levels can be low, normal, or elevated, depending on the phase of the illness during which the sample was taken (Singer et al, 1995).

Autoantibodies to thyroid antigens are found in the serum of patients with autoimmune hypothyroidism. Antibodies include those to thyroglobulin, the storage protein for thyroid hormone; microsomal (or thyroid peroxidase), the rate-limiting enzyme in thyroid biosynthesis; and TSH receptors. Both forms of thyroiditis lead to a high titer of antimicrosomal antibodies in the blood, whereas up to 20% have antithyrotropin receptor antibodies. In patients with diffuse goiter and hypothyroidism, antithyroid antibodies are positive in 95% of cases. Hypothyroidism results from the inhibition of thyroid function, blockade of the TSH receptor, or cellular damage from the cytotoxic activity, or a combination of factors (Lazarus, 1996; Dayan & Daniels, 1996).

Tests for thyroid peroxidase antibody are more sensitive than those for antimicrosomal antibody and are usually done by enzyme-linked immunoassay or radioimmunoassay. Titers of more than 1:6400 for antimicrosomal antibodies or more than 200 IU/mL for thyroid peroxidase antibodies are strongly suggestive of autoimmune thyroiditis (Dayan & Daniels, 1996).

In patients with secondary hypothyroidism, free thyroxine levels in the blood or free thyroxine index is measured. Other pituitary functions may also be measured, because secondary hypothyroidism is more often associated with panhypopituitarism than with an isolated loss of the thyrotrophs.

Other laboratory tests can be abnormal in hypothyroidism, including elevations in creatine phosphokinase, liver enzymes, cholesterol, and triglycerides (Singer et al, 1995). Sodium may be reduced because of water retention, whereas prolactin can be increased by elevated TRH secretion (Scanlon & Toft, 1996).

Often patients present for clinical evaluation who are taking thyroid supplements but for whom the initiating events for thyroid therapy are not well documented. In these cases, thyroid supplements should be stopped and thyroid functions rechecked in 4 to 6 weeks. The half-life of thyroxine is 6 days, and the serum thyroxine level should fall to the hypothyroid range in 2 weeks (Toft, 1994). It is necessary to delay blood tests for 4 to 6 weeks to allow recovery of the suppressed thyrotrophs. In normal persons, the pituitary should recover function and resume the manufacture of thyroid hormones. In truly hypothyroid patients, symptoms and laboratory evidence of hypothyroidism will remain at the end of that time.

IMAGING STUDIES

Imaging studies with radioactive iodine are usually not done because the underactive gland is not iodine-avid and uptake is reduced. Iodine uptake can be increased in rare cases of goitrous autoimmune thyroiditis. Iodine uptake can also be in-

creased in iodine deficiency and in inherited defects of thyroid hormone biosynthesis.

Severe primary hypothyroidism can cause pituitary enlargement and increased prolactin secretion because of stimulation of the thyrotrophs (TSH-producing cells) and lactotrophs (prolactin-producing cells) by the elevated TRH level (Scanlon & Toft, 1996). Pituitary imaging and surgery should be avoided in this instance of hyperprolactinemia. Correction of the hypothyroid state with thyroid replacement will resolve the pituitary enlargement and hypersecretion of prolactin.

Treatment Options, Expected Outcomes, and Comprehensive Management

MEDICATIONS: THYROXINE REPLACEMENT

Patients with elevated TSH values, usually three times the upper limit of the assay, should be treated with synthetic L-thyroxine (levothyroxine, T$_4$). Treatment for overt hypothyroidism is lifelong. The goal is to give enough thyroid supplement orally to result in normal free T$_4$ and TSH levels. Usual replacement doses are based on weight (1.7 mcg/kg) in adults. Elderly patients require less than 1 mcg/kg. Replacement for most women is 75 to 100 mcg/day. Elderly patients are started on 25 to 50 mcg/day to avoid inducing cardiac arrhythmias or precipitating angina or congestive heart failure (Toft, 1994). After 4 to 6 weeks, the TSH level can be rechecked and the dose adjusted. Patients usually note an improvement of symptoms within 2 weeks (eg, stabilizing of weight loss and facial puffiness), but it takes several months for all symptoms (eg, skin changes and anemia) to resolve. Elderly patients and patients with Graves' treated with radioactive iodine may need smaller doses of medication; the former have decreased clearance of the drug and the latter may have some stimulation of the thyroid remnant by thyroid-stimulating antibodies (Toft, 1994).

Some fluctuations in thyroid function may be noted while taking replacement because the bioavailability of the thyroid supplement may vary from company to company, and about 80% of the oral dose is absorbed (Singer et al, 1995; Toft, 1994). By either interfering with thyroxine absorption or increasing its elimination, some medications increase the amount of thyroxine needed for adequate replacement.

CLINICAL WARNING: Drugs known to decrease thyroxine absorption include resins (cholestyramine), aluminum-containing antacids, iron, sucralfate, and cimetidine (Surks & Sievert, 1995). Most antiseizure medications increase the hepatic metabolism of thyroxine, so patients need higher doses of thyroxine while taking these (Surks & Sievert, 1995). Smoking cigarettes may also increase thyroid replacement requirements. Adjustments in dose are made based on the TSH; if it is low, too much drug is being given; if it is high, the dose is increased.

There are reports documenting a change in serum thyroid hormone levels when one brand of thyroxine is replaced by a different brand or when a generic rather than a brand-name product is used (Toft, 1994). Experts in North America advise that patients should avoid generic thyroxine and should stick to one brand to avoid expensive testing and readjustment in doses. Toft (1994) states that the generic preparations are fine, because there is no proof of increased morbidity from these drugs and there is a substantial cost saving.

Patients with mild elevations of the TSH level or with subclinical hypothyroidism (normal free hormone levels) might benefit from T_4 replacement if there is goitrous enlargement of the gland (Dayan & Daniels, 1996; Toft, 1994; Oppenheimer, 1996). Most report a 30% reduction in goiter size after 6 months, but shrinkage is variable because of the presence of fibrosis in the gland.

■ ■ ■ **CLINICAL PEARL**

Thyroid replacement for subclinical hypothyroidism should be given in those who are without heart disease and are symptomatic, those with a TSH level above 10 mU/L, those with strongly positive antithyroid antibodies, those older than 45 years, and male patients (Dayan & Daniels, 1996).

In patients with subclinical hypothyroidism, the progression to overt hypothyroidism is slow. Many patients feel better on replacement. Unlike overt hypothyroidism, most patients with subclinical hypothyroidism do not show increased serum cholesterol levels, compared to the normal population, and starting thyroxine in this context does not change the low-density lipoprotein level (Toft, 1994). Furthermore, most patients do not lose weight while taking thyroid replacement unless they take a dose that renders them hyperthyroid.

Thyroid replacement is unnecessary during the transient period of hypothyroidism caused by subacute or painless thyroiditis (Lazarus, 1996). Full recovery is generally the rule, but there can be relapses.

Women with hypothyroidism from chronic thyroiditis may experience a remission (Toft, 1994) and can remain euthyroid after thyroxine replacement is withdrawn. Remission from the disease can be established only by stopping thyroxine replacement for 6 to 8 weeks.

■ **CLINICAL WARNING:** Withdrawal of thyroxine replacement should not be done routinely, because only 5% of women with autoimmune thyroiditis regain euthyroidism (Dayan & Daniels, 1996). This occurs more often if the thyroiditis occurred after the use of medications (eg, lithium, amiodarone), after parturition, or after a bout of viral thyroiditis.

Hypothyroidism during pregnancy increases the risk of fetal loss (Tallstedt, 1992). Three fourths of pregnant women need to have their thyroxine replacement increased, usually by more than 50 mcg/day, to avoid a rise in the TSH level (Reed & Pangaro, 1995; Singer et al, 1995; Toft, 1994). This increased need for thyroxine is caused by the estrogen-induced rise in thyroxine-binding globulin, lowering free hormone levels. In pregnancy, the TSH level should be measured each trimester.

USE OF THYROID SUPPLEMENTS OTHER THAN SYNTHETIC L-THYROXINE

Other thyroid hormone supplements are available but are not the treatment of choice (Singer et al, 1995; Toft, 1995; Oppenheimer, 1996). There are synthetic T_3 supplements (Cytomel) and combinations of synthetic T_3 and T_4 (Thyrolar) and desiccated thyroid (thyroid extract containing T_3 and T_4). Preparations containing T_3 lead to a supraphysiologic rise in serum T_3 levels several hours after ingestion and may cause cardiac arrhythmias and angina in older patients. Many providers do not recognize that the serum T_4 level should be in the lower part of the normal range when using combination preparations to avoid overtreatment (Toft, 1994). The main advantage of using synthetic thyroxine as replacement is that the serum T_3 level, formed by extrathyroidal conversion of the ingested thyroxine, is controlled physiologically; this is beneficial during illness and fasting, when the production of T_3 from T_4 is normally decreased (Toft, 1995; Oppenheimer, 1996).

Recently, more strengths of synthetic thyroxine have become available, and so-called tight replacement has been promoted, giving the strength of thyroxine that normalizes both free T_4 and TSH levels (Oppenheimer, 1996).

■ **CLINICAL WARNING:** There is concern that chronic overuse of thyroxine replacement increases the risk for osteoporosis and cardiac arrhythmias. It is not yet known whether chronically overreplaced patients are at risk for serious health problems. Most studies of patients taking thyroxine show that excessive use of thyroxine (>150 mcg/day or suppressed TSH values) leads to lower bone density, but bone loss was not found in menopausal women or in adolescent girls in recent studies (Oppenheimer, 1996; Saggessel, 1996; Langdahl, 1996).

Referral Points and Clinical Warnings

Concomitant illness, exposure to sedating drugs, or lack of treatment for a sustained time can lead to a medical emergency called myxedema coma, which carries a mortality rate of 20%. This coma usually develops gradually among older patients, especially those living in cold climates. It can happen more abruptly in persons with infection, gastrointestinal bleeding, or respiratory disease or those who use narcotics and analgesics. Overt hypothyroidism and mental obtundation develop before stupor and coma. Patients are pale and have periorbital edema. There is also macroglossia, dry skin, and lowered body temperature (Singer et al, 1995; Jordan, 1995).

Physical examination in this instance reveals distant heart sounds, bradycardia, and delayed relaxation of deep tendon reflexes. The patient may have hyponatremia, seizures, hypotension, and hypoglycemia. There is hypoventilation with respiratory acidosis, hypoxia, and retention of carbon dioxide (Singer et al, 1995; Jordan, 1995). The diagnosis is not based on a certain level of TSH, but is confirmed when the free thyroxine level is low and the TSH level is high. Diagnosis is more difficult if the T_4 level is low and the TSH level is low or normal, and the differential includes myxedema coma from secondary hypothyroidism or sick euthyroidism. It then may be helpful to get creatine phosphokinase levels, which are usually high in hypothyroidism because of type II muscle atrophy (Singer et al, 1995; Jordan, 1995).

Myxedema coma is a clinical diagnosis and is not based on the level of the total T_4 or TSH. When the criteria are met, including bradycardia, congestive heart failure, and hypothermia, T_4, TSH, and cortisol determinations should be done. Supportive measures must be initiated immediately, including aggressive replacement with T_4. Signs associated with poor outcome and death are advanced age, body temperature less than 93°F, persistent hypothermia beyond day 2, bradycardia of less than 44 beats/minute, sepsis, myocardial infarction, hypotension, and treatment with T_3 (Jordan, 1995).

NODULAR THYROID DISEASE

Patients who are clinically euthyroid can present with an enlarged thyroid. The enlargement can be diffuse or focal; there can be a smooth thyroid surface or a nodular gland. Evaluation for autoimmune thyroid disease, such as euthyroid Graves' or Hashimoto's, involves checking for high antithyroid antibody titers. More importantly, thyroid carcinoma must be ruled out in patients presenting with nodularity of the thyroid gland.

Pathology

On biopsy, multinodular glands have areas of focal hyperplasia. Some hyperplastic areas outgrow their blood supply and undergo hemorrhagic necrosis (become partly cystic) and fibrosis (Hay & Morris, 1996). Other areas accumulate large amounts of colloid.

Epidemiology

Thyroid nodules occur in 4% of the population. About half of affected persons have a single nodule. The incidence increases with increasing age (Mazzaferri, 1993). Women are more likely to have a thyroid nodule, and a history of radiation exposure or living in an area endemic for iodine deficiency also increases the incidence of thyroid nodularity. Ultrasound may increase the yield of finding thyroid nodules, and they may be present in up to 60% in the elderly. The main purpose of finding thyroid lesions is to identify those containing thyroid cancer. Thyroid cancer is rare, occurring in 4 per 100,000. Of nodules removed surgically, 20% to 50% contain cancer (Mazzaferri, 1993; Gharib & Goellner, 1993). Risk factors for thyroid cancer include:

- Previous head and neck irradiation
- Family history of thyroid cancer, such as multiple neoplasia (MEN) syndrome
- Gardner's syndrome (familial polyposis)
- Young age or elderly
- Male gender (Mazzaferri, 1993).

The two most common types of thyroid cancer are papillary and follicular. Papillary thyroid cancer, the more common form, is slow-growing and asymptomatic. The cancer can be multicentric within the thyroid gland and can spread to the local cervical structures, including the cervical lymph nodes,

musculature, trachea, and esophagus (Mazzaferri & Jhiang, 1994).

> **CLINICAL WARNING:** Young patients with enlarged cervical lymph nodes should be evaluated for papillary thyroid cancer. Follicular cancer is usually encapsulated and metastasizes to lung and bone via blood vessel invasion (DeGroot, 1995).

Medullary thyroid cancer is a tumor of the parafollicular cells of the thyroid gland and can occur sporadically or in families with genetic mutations (MEN syndrome or familial medullary thyroid cancer) (Eng, 1996; Moers et al, 1996). When a genetic mutation is present, medullary thyroid cancer develops in childhood (as early as 2 years) or early adulthood. Although those with MEN 2A fare best in terms of survival with this disease (85% >10 years), this syndrome can lead to hyperparathyroidism and bilateral adrenal pheochromocytomas that can be life-threatening (Eng, 1996). Patients with sporadic medullary thyroid cancer have the disease in about the sixth decade. Sixty percent of these patients die from the disease over 10 years. The worst prognosis is for those with MEN 2B syndrome, where there is a marfanoid habitus, pheochromocytomas, and neuromas of the lips, tongue, and gastrointestinal tract (Eng, 1996).

Anaplastic thyroid cancer usually appears in the sixth decade, is very aggressive, and often appears in a nontoxic multinodular goiter as a hard, rapidly enlarging mass that causes pain and hoarseness (Hay & Morris, 1996).

Lymphoma of the thyroid gland can develop in patients with goitrous (Hashimoto's) thyroiditis. It should be sought in patients who have a rapidly expanding nodule and autoimmune thyroid disease (Dayan & Daniels, 1996).

History and Physical Examination

Nodular thyroid glands often cause no symptoms, but they can lead to compression of the trachea, esophagus, and jugular venous blood flow (Hay & Morris, 1996; Dayan & Daniels, 1996). Thyroid enlargement can cause difficulty swallowing and neck discomfort. The natural history is slow growth, increased nodularity, and increasing hyperthyroidism.

Most nodules containing cancer are asymptomatic and are found on physical examination. Symptoms and signs suggestive of cancer include rapid growth, neck pain, hoarseness, and dysphagia. Other signs of more ominous disease, papillary or anaplastic thyroid cancer, include fixation of the nodule, hard consistency, and lymphadenopathy in the cervical region (Mazzaferri, 1993; Gharib & Goellner, 1993). Thyroid nodularity can be part of a multinodular goiter, but it is often caused by a thyroid adenoma or cyst. It can also be a sign of thyroiditis or ectopic parathyroid gland.

Diagnostic Studies

LABORATORY TESTING

Most patients with nodular thyroid disease are euthyroid, with normal levels of TSH and free hormones. Some may have an area of thyroid autonomy (toxic nodule or multinodular goiter) and show a low TSH level with normal free hormone levels (Hay & Morris, 1996). As the nodular disease progresses, the patient may show more signs and symptoms of hyperthyroidism and become overtly thyrotoxic, with elevated free hormone levels. Autoimmune thyroid disease causing nodular disease should be evaluated by checking the TSH and thyroid antibodies. Almost all patients with thyroid cancer are euthyroid, unless they have coexistent Graves' disease or Hashimoto's thyroiditis.

CLINICAL WARNING: Patients with thyroid nodules should have thyroid functions measured and in some cases calcitonin levels if there is a family history suggestive of MEN, multiple nodules, or a history of pheochromocytoma or hyperparathyroidism (Eng, 1996).

CLINICAL PEARL

Genetic testing is available for persons having a family history of MEN syndrome. This is done via RET proto-oncogene screening (Eng, 1996).

IMAGING STUDIES

Thyroid ultrasound allows the detection of lesions as small as 2 to 3 mm, but the disadvantage of this method is that its use may identify lesions (<1.5 cm) that are unlikely to cause clinical disease. The workup for these small lesions can create needless expense and patient anxiety (Tan & Gharib, 1997). Many times, patients with solitary thyroid nodules found clinically are found to have multinodular disease using ultrasonography (Mazzaferri, 1993).

CLINICAL WARNING: All nodules greater than 1 to 1.5 cm should be evaluated by a thyroid specialist to rule out the presence of thyroid carcinoma (Tan & Gharib, 1997). Thyroid ultrasound can reveal whether lesions are cystic or solid, but again many lesions are mixed and could represent degenerating benign adenomas or cystic papillary thyroid cancers (Mazzaferri, 1993).

Thyroid scans with iodine (^{123}I) or pertechnetate (^{99}Tc) reveal that most nodules (85%) are hypofunctioning (cold) while the remainder are normal or hyperfunctioning (hot). Of the cold lesions, about 20% are cancer (Gharib & Goellner, 1993). Thus, scanning does not reveal whether a nodule is cancer, because most nodules are hypofunctioning. Although the images of thyroid glands are similar during iodine and pertechnetate scanning, there are instances where nodules that appear hot by ^{99}Tc are cold by ^{123}I, and thus more worrisome for cancer (Reed & Pangaro, 1995).

The most direct evaluation of a palpable thyroid nodule is fine-needle aspiration. This is done by a specialist in the outpatient clinic. An important cause of false-negative reports is an inadequate sample of too few cells. The provider can avoid this problem by referring the patient to a specialist who does the procedure 20 to 35 times a year (Mazzaferri, 1993).

Treatment Options, Expected Outcomes, and Comprehensive Management

THYROID CYSTS

Thyroid cysts may be drained by aspiration. Cystic fluid from a thyroid nodule does not guarantee that the lesion is benign; the fluid should be examined because walls of cystic lesions can contain papillary thyroid cancer. The use of thyroid supplements does not decrease the likelihood of fluid reappearance (Mazzaferri, 1993). Cysts can be reaspirated, but if the fluid reaccumulates rapidly after aspiration or the size is large, patients may prefer to have the cystic area surgically removed. Recently, ethanol has been instilled into benign cysts or small thyroid adenomas, leading to shrinkage of the lesion.

HOT NODULES

Hyperfunctioning follicular adenomas (large hot nodules) are more common in young adults and can cause hyperthyroidism in those with thyroid nodules 3 cm or greater (Burman, 1995; Mazzaferri, 1993). Treatment of these nodules includes radioactive iodine ablation. Surgical ablation is preferred in the young. Surgery will prevent recurrence or subsequent hypothyroidism from exposure of the normal gland to radioactive iodine.

COLD NODULES

Hypofunctioning (cold) nodules contain cancer in 20%, so for most patients, cold nodules are benign follicular adenomas or colloid adenomatous nodules within a multinodular goiter (Hay & Morris, 1996; Mazzaferri, 1993). Thyroid suppression may shrink the nodules in some patients; studies show that there can be a 30% reduction in nodule size. Thyroid supplements do not change nodule size for many patients. This is because of the presence of fibrous tissue. More importantly, thyroid supplements do not prevent the formation of new nodules (Toft, 1994; Oppenheimer, 1996). Thyroid supplementation may lead to subclinical hyperthyroidism in a patient with a multinodular gland.

CLINICAL WARNING: Suppressed TSH is a risk factor in older patients for cardiac arrhythmias and osteoporosis, although the rate of bone fracture is probably not increased (Singer et al, 1995; Oppenheimer, 1996). For most patients, observation is the treatment of choice for a euthyroid multinodular goiter. The provider should watch for signs or symptoms of hyperthyroidism or for the development of suspicious nodules. If the gland becomes cosmetically unacceptable or causes dysphagia, surgical extirpation must be planned. Radioactive iodine can reverse hyperthyroidism and shrink the gland for some patients with toxic nodular goiter. For patients with very fibrotic or large goiters, only surgery will reduce the size of the gland.

Thyroid lobectomy is the treatment of choice for benign nodules that are cosmetically unacceptable or that are causing symptoms of tracheal compression. Euthyroid patients cannot be treated with radioactive iodine, and thyroid lobectomy is unlikely to result in hypoparathyroidism. In young adults with small nodules that contain thyroid cancer (<1 cm), thyroid

absorption (sprue), and alcoholism and those exposed to certain drugs, such as amphotericin, aminoglycosides, and cisplatin. Table 19-11 presents the target tissues affected in hypoparathyroidism.

ELECTROCARDIOGRAM FINDINGS AND IMAGING STUDIES

Hypocalcemia causes the QT interval to be prolonged, which can increase the risk of ventricular arrhythmias and sudden death. Longstanding hypocalcemia can cause calcification of the basal ganglia, apparent on skull x-ray or CT (Streeten & Levine, 1995).

Treatment Options, Expected Outcomes, and Comprehensive Management

Treatment of hypoparathyroidism depends on the severity of the defect. Mild cases are treated with calcium supplements. Most patients with more severe disease are treated with calcitriol (1,25-dihydroxy-vitamin D) because its half-life is short and use is less likely to result in toxicity than with ergocalciferol, the more traditional treatment of vitamin D and calcium (Streeten & Levine, 1995).

Teaching and Self-Care

Creating a healthy lifestyle is important in parathyroid diseases. Striking the right balance between diet and exercise and balancing the need for adequate rest with job, home, and recreation are challenging even when health is optimal. Parathyroid diseases require greater emphasis on these entities if adequate calcium management is to ensue. The stakes are high, for calcium is key to cell function and overall tissue health. The primary care provider should give extra emphasis to working with the patient to develop or improve lifestyle plans that enhance wellness. Referral to a registered nutritionist may prove helpful in dietary management.

A moderate exercise program should be agreed on. Stress management should be discussed, and concrete plans for stress control should be mapped out. Patients taking medication should be encouraged to wear a Med-Alert item. Local pharmacies generally carry pamphlets and applications for the purchase of these nominally priced articles.

Referral Points and Clinical Warnings

Patients taking vitamin D supplements are at an increased risk for renal stone disease. Vitamin D increases calcium absorption from the gut, causing hypercalciuria. Patients with hypocal-

TABLE 19-11	Effects of Hypoparathyroidism on PTH Target Tissues

- Decreased intestinal absorption of calcium
- Decreased bone resorption and turnover
- Decreased renal reabsorption of calcium
- Decreased phosphate excretion
- Calcium levels 5–8 mg/dL range
- High phosphate levels
- Low 1,25-dihydroxy-vitamin D levels

TABLE 19-12	Drugs That Cause Changes in Serum Calcium

- Thiazide diuretics can create hypercalcemia.
- Loop diuretics such as furosemide can worsen hypocalcemia.
- Glucocorticoids or antiseizure medications can block the actions or increase the clearance of vitamin D supplements.

cemia are corrected to low-normal values to avoid presenting higher calcium loads to the kidney (Streeten & Levine, 1995). Vitamin D toxicity can occur suddenly in patients if they become dehydrated and is manifested by nausea and vomiting. It is essential to monitor calcium levels frequently for patients on replacement and to monitor urine calcium levels as well to avoid renal stones. The concomitant use of other drugs can also increase or decrease vitamin D requirements, as shown in Table 19-12.

CLINICAL WARNING: Hypocalcemic crisis can occur in patients with intercurrent illnesses if they are unable or unwilling to take their supplements or if they add medications that block or inhibit vitamin D activity. Crisis is rarely the initial manifestation of the disease. Signs of crisis include severe tetany, laryngospasm, and convulsions.

Hypocalcemia can be a transient phenomenon after thyroidectomy or parathyroid surgery (Burman, 1995; Streeten & Levine, 1995). Another cause of hypocalcemia after surgery is "hungry bone syndrome," in which previous thyrotoxicosis (of long standing) or hyperparathyroidism leads to calcium depletion of the bones. When caused by hungry bone syndrome, transient hypocalcemia usually leads to low calcium and phosphorus levels, whereas postsurgical hypoparathyroidism leads to low calcium levels with high phosphorus levels (Streeten & Levine, 1995). Levels of PTH and calcium usually recover within the week of surgery.

Resistance to PTH is rare but is called pseudohypoparathyroidism because these patients have low calcium levels with high levels of intact PTH. One subtype of this disease, type Ia, produces phenotypic changes and bony changes that include short stature, round facies, and shortened fourth and fifth metacarpals (Albright's hereditary osteodystrophy). This disease is identified around age 8, and the hypocalcemia is milder than that of hypoparathyroidism. The peripheral resistance to PTH is caused by a defect in the regulatory subunit (Gs) of adenylate cyclase, the second messenger through which PTH activates its target organ activities. Other subtypes of the disease do not display these phenotypic features and may not have the defect in Gs (Streeten & Levine, 1995). Patients with the Gs defect may display resistance to other peptide hormones, TSH, follicle-stimulating hormone, and luteinizing hormone.

COMMUNITY RESOURCES

- The American Thyroid Association, Inc., Montefiore Medical Center, 111 E. 210th St., Bronx, NY 10467; 800-542-6687; fax: 718-882-6085; E-mail: admin@thyroid.org; Web page: www.thyroid.org. This is a good resource for patient brochures about thyroid disease. Informative pamphlets are available at no charge. Leave your name and address on the 800 number to receive information on the thyroid gland and thyroid disease appropriate for both providers and the general public.

- National Graves' Disease Foundation, c/o Dr. Nancy Patterson, 320 Arlington Rd., Jacksonville, FL 32211; 904-724-0770; E-mail: ndgf@citcom.net; Web page: www.ndgf.org/. Provides information on support groups and information on Graves' disease. Membership is $25, which includes the quarterly newsletter and six health bulletins, most written by doctors. Information on specific problems is available. Referrals to other members in the geographic area are available. The information is appropriate for providers and the general public.

- The Thyroid Foundation of America, Inc., Ruth Sleeper Hall, RSL 350, 40 Parkman St., Boston, MA 02114-2698; 800-832-8321; fax: 617-726-4136; Web page: www.clark.net/pub/tfa/. Staff members field calls and answer general thyroid disorder questions. To receive information by mail, send a self-addressed business-size envelope with first-class postage. Information available is for both physicians and the general public. An optional membership fee of $25 includes a quarterly newsletter, one free book, and five free articles or brochures (discounted rate of $15 for students and seniors). Referrals to specialists in the geographic area are available, as is a complete publication list.

- The Thyroid Foundation of Canada, 1040 Gardiners Rd., Suite C, Kingston, Ontario K7P 1R7; 800-267-8822; Fax: 613-634-3482; E-mail: thyroid@io.org; Web page: http://home.ican.net/thyroid/ Canada.html. Up-to-date information on thyroid diseases for patients and families. Membership is $25 for family, $15 for seniors and students; a quarterly newsletter is included. There are 21 chapters across Canada. Their goal is to provide support and education. Information is offered on public meetings, telephone help-line, and community education. Information is appropriate for providers and the general public.

- The Thyroid Society for Education and Research, 7515 S. Main St., Suite 545, Houston, TX 77030; 800-THYROID or 713-799-9909; E-mail: help@the-thyroid-society.org; Web page: www.houston-interweb.com/thyroid/thyroid.html. Staff members field calls and answer thyroid questions as well as help explain test results. Information available includes a complete thyroid information packet, specific topics, such as Graves' disease, specialized providers in the geographic area, recommended readings, and referrals to organizations. Members ($20) receive the quarterly newsletter. This information is appropriate for both providers and the general public.

- The Thyroid Home Page: www.thyroid.com. This offers information for providers and the general public. Support group information is available, as well as "Ask the Doc" via e-mail. General information is free.

References

Bahn, R.S., & Heufelder, A.E. (1993). Pathogenesis of Graves' ophthalmopathy. *New England Journal of Medicine, 329*(20), 1468–1475.

Bartelena, L. (1996). Treatment of amiodarone-induced thyrotoxicosis, a difficult challenge: Results of a prospective study. *Journal of Clinical Endocrinology and Metabolism, 81*(8), 2930–2933.

Bartley, G.B. (1995). The incidence of Graves' ophthalmopathy in Olmsted County, Minnesota. *American Journal of Ophthalmology, 120*(4), 511–517.

Burch, H.B. (1994). Discontinuing antithyroid drug therapy before ablation with radioiodine in Graves' disease. *Annals of Internal Medicine, 121*(8), 553–559.

Burch, H.B., & Wartofsky, L. (1993). Life-threatening thyrotoxicosis: Thyroid storm. *Endocrinologic and Metabolic Clinics of North America, 22*(2), 263–277.

Burman, K.D. (1995). Hyperthyroidism. In K.L. Becker (Ed.). *Principles and practice of endocrinology and metabolism*, 2d ed. Philadelphia: J.B. Lippincott, pp. 367–385.

Burtis, W.J. (1995). Nonparathyroid hypercalcemia. In K.L. Becker (Ed.). *Principles and practice of endocrinology and metabolism*, 2d ed. Philadelphia: J.B. Lippincott, pp. 520–532.

Dayan, C.M., & Daniels, G.H. (1996). Chronic autoimmune thyroiditis. *New England Journal of Medicine, 335*(2), 99–107.

DeGroot, L.J., Kaplan, E.L., Shukla, M.S. et al. (1995). Morbidity and mortality in follicular thyroid cancer. *Journal of Clinical Endocrinology and Metabolism, 80*, 2946–2953.

Eng, C. (1996). The RET proto-oncogene in multiple endocrine neoplasia type 2 and Hirschsprung's disease. *New England Journal of Medicine, 335*(13), 943–951.

Franklyn, J.A. (1994). The management of hyperthyroidism. *N Engl J Med, 330*(24), 1731–1739.

Gharib, H., & Goellner, J.R. (1993). Fine-needle aspiration biopsy of the thyroid: An appraisal. *Annals of Internal Medicine, 118*, 282–229.

Goltzman, D., & Hendy, G.N. (1995). Parathyroid hormone. In K.L. Becker (Ed.). *Principles and practice of endocrinology and metabolism*, 2d ed. Philadelphia: J.B. Lippincott, pp. 455–467.

Hay, I.D., & Morris, J.C. (1996). Toxic adenoma and toxic multinodular goiter. In L.E. Braverman & R.D. Utiger (Eds.). *Werner and Ingbar's The thyroid: A fundamental and clinical text*, 7th ed. Philadelphia: J.B. Lippincott, pp. 566–572.

Hermann, M. (1994). Thyroid surgery in untreated severe hyperthyroidism: Perioperative kinetics of free thyroid hormones in the glandular venous effluent and peripheral blood. *Surgery, 115*, 240–245.

Huysmans, D.A.K.C. (1994). Large, compressive goiters treated with radioiodine. *Annals of Internal Medicine, 121*(10), 757–762.

Jordan, R.M. (1995). Myxedema coma: Pathophysiology, therapy and factors affecting prognosis. *Medical Clinics of North America, 79*(1), 185–194.

Langdahl, B.L. (1996). Bone mass, bone turnover and body composition in former hypothyroid patients receiving replacement therapy. *European Journal of Endocrinology, 134*(6), 702–709.

Lazarus, J.H. (1996). Silent thyroiditis and subacute thyroiditis. In L.E. Braverman & R.D. Utiger (Eds.). *Werner and Ingbar's The thyroid: A fundamental and clinical text*, 7th ed. Philadelphia: J.B. Lippincott, pp. 577–591.

Livolsi, V.A. (1995). Morphology of the parathyroid glands. In K.L. Becker (Ed.). *Principles and practice of endocrinology and metabolism*, 2d ed. Philadelphia: J.B. Lippincott, pp. 432–436.

Mazzaferri, E.L. (1993). Management of a solitary thyroid nodule. *New England Journal of Medicine, 328*(8), 553–539.

Mazzaferri, E.L., & Jhiang, S.M. (1994). Long-term impact of initial surgical and medical therapy on papillary and follicular thyroid cancer. *American Journal of Medicine, 97*, 418.

McIver, B., Rae, P., Beckett, G. et al. (1996). Lack of effect of thyroxine in patients with Graves' hyperthyroidism who are treated with an antithyroid drug. *N Engl J Med, 334*(4), 220–224.

Moers, A.M., Landsvater, R.M., Schaap, C. et al. (1996). Familial medullary thyroid carcinoma: Not a distinct entity? Genotype–phenotype correlation in a large family. *American Journal of Medicine, 101*, 635–641.

Nuovo, J. (1995). Excessive thyroid hormone replacement therapy. *Journal of the American Board of Family Practice, 8*(6), 435–439.

Nussbaum, S.R. (1993). Pathophysiology and management of severe hypercalcemia. *Endocrinology and Metabolism Clinics of North America, 22*(2), 343–362.

Oppenheimer, J.H. (1996). A therapeutic controversy: Thyroid hormone treatment: When and what? *Journal of Clinical Endocrinology and Metabolism, 80*(10), 2973–2978.

Pearce, S., & Brown, E.M. (1996). The genetic basis of endocrine disease: Disorders of calcium ion sensing. *Journal of Clinical Endocrinology and Metabolism, 81*(6), 2030–2035.

Pintar, J.E. (1996). Normal development of the hypothalamic-pituitary-thyroid axis. In L.E. Braverman & R.D. Utiger (Eds.). *Werner and Ingbar's The thyroid: A fundamental and clinical text,* 7th ed. Philadelphia: J.B. Lippincott, pp. 9–14.

Prummel, M.F., & Wiersinga, W.M. (1995). Medical management of Graves' ophthalmopathy. *Thyroid, 5*(3), 231–234.

Reed, L., & Pangaro, L.N. (1995). Physiology of the thyroid gland I: Synthesis and release, iodine metabolism and binding and transport. In K.L. Becker (Ed.). *Principles and practice of endocrinology and metabolism,* 2d ed. Philadelphia: J.B. Lippincott, pp. 285–291.

Saggessel, G. (1996). Bone mineral density in adolescent females treated with L-thyroxine: A longitudinal study. *European Journal of Pediatrics, 155*(6), 452–457.

Scanlon, M.F., & Toft, A.D. (1996). Regulation of thyrotropin secretion. In L.E. Braverman & R.D. Utiger (Eds.). *Werner and Ingbar's The thyroid: A fundamental and clinical text,* 7th ed. Philadelphia: J.B. Lippincott, pp. 220–240.

Silverberg, J., & Bilezikian, J.P. (1996). Extensive personal experience: Evaluation and management of primary hyperparathyroidism. *Journal of Clinical Endocrinology and Metabolism, 81*(6), 2036–2040.

Silverberg, S.I. (1995). Primary hyperparathyroidism. In K.L. Becker (Ed.). *Principles and practice of endocrinology and metabolism,* 2d ed. Philadelphia: J.B. Lippincott, pp. 512–520.

Singer, P.A., Levy, E.G., Ladenson, P.W. et al. (1995). Treatment guidelines for patients with hyperthyroidism and hypothyroidism. *JAMA, 273*(10), 808–812.

Sofferman, R.A. (1996). Preoperative technetium-Tc-99m-sestimibi imaging: Paving the way to minimal-access parathyroid surgery. *Archives of Otolaryngology Head and Neck Surgery, 122,* 369–374.

Sofferman, R.A. (November 1997). Personal communication.

Streeten, E.A., & Levine, M.A. (1995). Hypoparathyroidism and other causes of hypocalcemia. In K.L. Becker (Ed.). *Principles and practice of endocrinology and metabolism,* 2d ed. Philadelphia: J.B. Lippincott, pp. 532–546.

Surks, M.I., & Sievert, R. (1995). Drugs and thyroid function. *New England Journal of Medicine, 335*(25), 1688–1694.

Taillefer, R., Boucher, Y., Potrin, C. et al. (1992). Detection and localization of parathyroid adenomas in patients with hyperparathyroidism using a single radionuclide imaging procedure with technetium-99m-sestimibi (double-phase study). *Journal of Nuclear Medicine, 33,* 1801–1807.

Tallstedt, L., Lundell, G., Torring, O. et al. (1992). Occurrence of ophthalmopathy after treatment for Graves' hyperthyroidism. *New England Journal of Medicine, 326*(26), 1733–1738.

Tan, G.H., & Gharib, H. (1997). Thyroid incidentalomas: Management approaches to nonpalpable nodules discovered incidentally on thyroid imaging. *Annals of Internal Medicine, 126*(3), 226–231.

Toft, A.D. (1994). Thyroxine therapy. *New England Journal of Medicine, 331*(3), 174–181.

Torring, O. (1996). Graves' hyperthyroidism: Treatment with antithyroid drugs, surgery or radioiodine—a prospective, randomized study. *Journal of Clinical Endocrinology and Metabolism, 81,* 2986–2993.

Tunbridge, W.M. (1977). The spectrum of thyroid disease in a community: The Whickham survey. *Clinical Endocrinology, 7,* 481–493.

Tuttle, R.M. (1995). Treatment with propylthiouracil before radioactive iodine therapy is associated with a higher treatment failure rate than therapy with radioactive iodine alone in Graves' disease. *Thyroid, 5*(4), 243–247.

Usala, S.J. (1995). Physiology of the thyroid gland II: Receptors, postreceptor events and hormone resistance syndromes. In K.L. Becker (Ed.). *Principles and practice of endocrinology and metabolism,* 2d ed. Philadelphia: J.B. Lippincott, pp. 292–299.

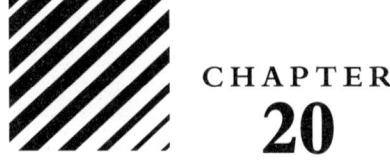

CHAPTER
20

Bowel Obstruction

Paul Cohen, MD

Bowel obstruction refers to a blockage in either the small or the large bowel (colon). When a patient presents with symptoms suggestive of obstruction, it is important to determine the location of the obstruction. Based on the location, certain etiologies will be more likely. Both the history and the physical examination play essential roles in helping to determine both the location and the cause of a bowel obstruction.

ANATOMY, PHYSIOLOGY, AND PATHOLOGY

Adhesions form as a result of previous surgery and can form from days to years after the surgery. They occasionally occur in the "virgin" abdomen (with no previous history of surgery) because of peritonitis. Adhesions cause obstruction in the following manner. Two external walls of bowel adhere to each other, and a loop of bowel wraps around or becomes lodged between the adhesion(s). There is a compromise in blood supply to that segment of intestine, with resultant ischemia and necrosis.

External hernias and *internal hernias* are the second most common causes of small bowel obstruction and less commonly colonic obstruction. Common examples of an external hernia are inguinal, paraumbilical, and ventral hernias. Internal herniation is rare by comparison. These occur within the abdominal cavity and are often symptomatically intermittent, obstructing and reducing spontaneously. Between episodes, when patients are often asymptomatic, it is difficult to make the proper diagnosis (Turley, 1979). Incarceration of a hernia is caused when the bowel becomes trapped in a hole in the muscle wall or in a foramen. Delay in diagnosing the obstruction leads to ischemic changes in the bowel wall (strangulation). Necrosis (death) of the small bowel, secondary to either external or internal hernias, will result if the ischemic changes are not reversed. The mortality rate associated with necrosis of the bowel, small or large, is very high and increases in patients with multiple medical problems (Sachs et al, 1981; Marston, 1989).

Volvulus occurs most often in the large bowel and is associated with a redundant portion of bowel, most often in the sigmoid colon and much less often in the cecum (Ballantyne, 1981; Frizelle & Wolff, 1996). Chronic constipation and laxative abuse have been suggested as causes of the redundant sigmoid colon. A volvulus is a twist in the colon, much like a twist in a pretzel, resulting in a compromise in the blood flow and ischemia. Patients usually present with abdominal distention and inability to pass flatus or have a bowel movement; they may or may not have abdominal pain.

Inflammatory conditions such as *diverticulitis* commonly cause bowel obstruction, usually in the sigmoid colon (Sleisenger, 1993). Occlusion of a diverticulum from fecoliths, peanuts, or any object small enough to enter and lodge within the diverticulum can result in diverticulitis. Microperforation of the diverticulum can occur as a complication of diverticulitis and can result in a peridiverticular abscess. The intense inflammatory response to this microperforation results in edematous changes and subsequent obstruction. This form of obstruction is usually not difficult to diagnose because it usually occurs in the left lower quadrant and is accompanied by fever, leukocytosis, and focal rebound tenderness.

The *inflammatory bowel diseases*, Crohn's disease and ulcerative colitis, can also cause bowel obstruction. The most common site of obstruction in Crohn's disease is the ileocecal region because it is the narrowest segment in the entire gastrointestinal tract. The mechanism for obstruction with inflammatory bowel disease initially involves inflammation and then stricture formation. In ulcerative colitis, which involves only the large bowel, chronic inflammation can lead to stricture formation with resultant obstruction (see Chap. 27).

Malignant causes of intestinal obstruction are due to mechanical obstruction secondary to the bulkiness of the tumor within the lumen of the intestine. Larger tumors are needed to cause obstruction in the cecum and other areas with a larger diameter. The descending colon has a narrower lumen, and malignancy in this part of the colon may present as an obstruction (see Chap. 24).

Occasionally a tumor can cause an obstruction by initiating an *intussusception*. This is most commonly seen in the small bowel and can be caused by both malignant and benign lesions. At the site of intussusception, the tumor acts as an initiator, and one portion of bowel "telescopes" over the adjacent piece of intestine. This causes edema and obstruction as well as a decrease in blood flow to the loops of intestine involved, with resultant ischemia.

Paralytic ileus must always be considered when a patient presents with evidence of an obstruction. With paralytic ileus, the peristaltic function of the small and large bowel is disrupted, and the intestine dilates. Patients who present with histories suggestive of sepsis more than likely have a paralytic ileus rather than an obstructive process. Other causes of a paralytic ileus include perforation, peritonitis, and electrolyte abnormalities. Peptic ulcer disease, blunt trauma to the abdomen, and cancers with resultant perforations all can result in the development of a paralytic ileus. Another common cause for a paralytic ileus is abdominal surgery. All patients undergoing a laparotomy will have a postoperative ileus for a short period of time. This is expected and should not cause alarm. The bowel function usually returns to normal within a few days.

EPIDEMIOLOGY

The most common benign causes of small bowel obstruction include adhesions and external and internal hernias. Adhesions can occur in anyone who has ever had abdominopelvic surgery. Volvulus is a less common cause of obstruction, occurring mostly in the elderly or institutionalized patients. Diverticular disease with obstruction also occurs most commonly in the elderly (Painter & Burkitt, 1975). Approximately 10% to 20% of patients with a history of diverticulosis will develop diverticulitis during their lifetime (Almy & Howell, 1980). Intussusception is an uncommon cause of obstruction in adults, accounting for approximately 5% of all obstructions (Azar & Berger, 1997). In adults, a causative factor can be found in up to 90% of cases of intussusception (Agha, 1986).

Malignant causes of bowel obstruction usually occur in the colorectal region and are most commonly secondary to adenocarcinomas. Less common causes of malignant obstruction include carcinoid tumors in the distal ileum, lymphoma (more commonly in the distal small bowel), and adenocarcinoma in the proximal small bowel.

DIAGNOSTIC CRITERIA

A diagnosis of obstruction is made clinically. It is based on the history and physical examination. The diagnosis can be supported by objective findings, such as those on x-rays. In all cases of obstruction, it is necessary to diagnose the obstruction and identify the etiology.

HISTORY AND PHYSICAL EXAMINATION

The typical history from a patient presenting with an obstruction includes abdominal distention, nausea, vomiting, and a sudden onset of constipation or obstipation. The patient may or may not have abdominal pain. Other symptoms include loss of appetite, weakness, and general discomfort. Although obvious after a diagnosis is made, obstruction is often not considered when a patient presents with these symptoms. If a patient has a history of abdominopelvic surgery or an external hernia, obstruction must always be strongly considered. When obstruction is secondary to the other causes mentioned (namely, volvulus, intussusception, or an intestinal malignancy), making the correct diagnosis from the history alone becomes more difficult.

The timing of vomiting in relation to meals and the content of the vomitus are significant factors in helping to determine the location of the obstruction. Patients with a small bowel obstruction will often present with delayed vomiting (>1 hour after eating), and the vomitus is bilious. Bilious content is present when the level of obstruction is below the second portion of the duodenum. A similar presentation can also occur with a colonic obstruction. Thus, bilious vomitus helps to identify only if the obstruction is above or below the second portion of the duodenum.

Physical examination usually reveals a grossly distended abdomen, increased bowel sounds, diffuse tenderness without rebound tenderness (unless the bowel has perforated), and increased tympany. If the patient is thin, peristalsis can occasionally be observed on the abdominal wall. If diverticulitis is the cause of the obstruction, localized rebound tenderness, usually in the left lower quadrant, may be present. This is especially true in the presence of a peridiverticular abscess.

Unlike patients with mechanical obstruction, patients with a paralytic ileus will often lack bowel sounds. They do, however, have abdominal distention and increased tympany, as in mechanical obstruction. Some patients may appear septic (as seen in peritonitis), and others may appear relatively comfortable (as seen in postlaparotomy patients).

DIAGNOSTIC STUDIES

Flat plate and upright abdominal x-rays are usually the first diagnostic studies obtained when obstruction is suspected (Gonzalez et al, 1982). If an obstruction is present, the level of the obstruction can often be suggested by these studies. Proximal to the obstruction there are dilated loops of bowel and often air–fluid levels. The air–fluid level is an interface between air and the fluid in a loop of bowel. On x-ray this appears as a straight line and is usually found in multiple areas throughout the abdomen. Distal to the obstruction, the bowel is often flaccid from a lack of air or intestinal fluid. Air–fluid levels are also noted when an ileus is present.

Other radiologic modalities, such as duplex Doppler ultrasonography, are likely to play an increasing role in the initial evaluation of patients who present with an obstructive process (Gimondo & LaBella, 1995). By evaluating the different degrees of signal intensity and frequency, a sonographer may be able to distinguish a mechanical obstruction from a paralytic ileus, as well as locating the level of obstruction.

If a colonic obstruction is suspected, a barium enema can be obtained to help assess both the level of obstruction and possible etiologies. This is usually considered safe.

Colonoscopy is also a useful tool in helping to assess a colonic obstruction. It is arguably the procedure of choice after an x-ray of the abdomen because the level of obstruction can be reached and biopsies taken if appropriate. Colonoscopy, however, is an invasive procedure and perforation is a major risk. In addition, sedatives and analgesics are often administered for colonoscopies, and these pose a risk as well. Barium studies are noninvasive and pose a lesser risk of perforation. However, if performed under higher pressures (as with air-contrast studies), perforation also remains a concern.

Laboratory Studies

There are no serologic studies considered pathognomonic for bowel obstruction. Early in the course of an obstruction, all blood test results are usually normal. As time elapses and the condition worsens, the white blood cell count may be increased because of stress, inflammation, or infection. Measuring electrolytes, blood urea nitrogen, and creatinine are helpful in assessing hydration status. Dehydration occurs when the patient has repeated vomiting because of the obstruction. Lactic acidosis occurs once ischemia and necrosis develop. In addition to the lactic acidosis, other enzyme elevations can be seen in the presence of ischemia or necrosis. Serum amylase, aspartate aminotransferase, alanine aminotransferase, and alkaline phosphatase levels may be elevated.

TREATMENT OPTIONS, EXPECTED OUTCOMES, AND COMPREHENSIVE MANAGEMENT

Self-Care and Prevention

Obstruction of the bowel is an emergent situation requiring hospitalization and often surgical intervention. Patients with previous surgeries and patients with hernias should be aware of potential complications, and if they suspect obstruction, they should seek immediate attention. Patients with inguinal hernias or large ventral hernias may opt for surgical repair and reduce their risk of obstruction. Because the recurrence rate of a sigmoid volvulus is quite high, patients with a history of volvulus may agree to have a resection of the redundant bowel. Patients with diverticular disease should be instructed about dietary restrictions, including avoidance of nuts and seeds. These difficult-to-digest foods can lodge in the diverticula and cause ischemia and eventually necrosis.

Inpatient Treatment

The hydration status and electrolyte balance must be addressed immediately. Once the cause of obstruction has been determined, definitive therapy can be instituted. If there is evidence of bowel necrosis or perforation, emergency surgery must be done (Fig. 20-1).

A nasogastric tube attached to intermittent suction is placed in all patients with suspected obstruction in an attempt to decompress the distended bowel and to remove secretions. Often a Cantor tube is placed via the nasogastric route and allowed to "float" down the gastrointestinal tract with peristaltic activity. Cantor tubes are attached to suction and work by decompressing the distended proximal bowel, with the goal of relieving the edema in the entrapped loop of bowel. They also help decrease the amount of vomiting by removing intestinal secretions.

Surgery remains the mainstay of treatment for most obstructions. If the obstruction is secondary to adhesions, adhesiolysis is performed. If the bowel remains viable, resection is not necessary, and separating the bowel is all that is done. If the bowel is necrotic, it must be removed. Incarcerated and strangulated hernias are also treated surgically. If the obstruction is secondary to a malignancy, resection of the involved portion of bowel is performed. Intussusception also requires surgical intervention, both to treat the situation and to search for the etiology of the intussusception.

If diverticulitis is suspected as the cause of obstruction and there is no evidence of perforation, treatment with intravenous antibiotics is indicated. However, if there is a peridiverticular abscess, surgery is usually required. Laparoscopic surgery is being done with increased frequency for the treatment of diverticular abscesses (Bruce et al, 1996). In Crohn's disease, treatment of the obstruction with intravenous steroid therapy is often effective (see Chap. 27).

Obstruction secondary to a volvulus can be treated initially via colonoscopic decompression. Unfortunately, because the cause of a volvulus is redundancy of the colon, the recurrence rate after decompression is high (Bok & Boley, 1986). Surgical resection of the redundant bowel is definitive therapy.

Treatment of a paralytic ileus depends heavily on the treatment of the underlying cause. Treatment of sepsis with antibiotics, surgical repair of a perforation, and simply waiting for the expected postoperative ileus to resolve are some of the usual ways to treat an ileus. Supportive measures such as placement of a nasogastric tube for suction and keeping the patient without any oral intake (NPO) are essential in managing these patients and preventing the nausea and vomiting that would otherwise inevitably result.

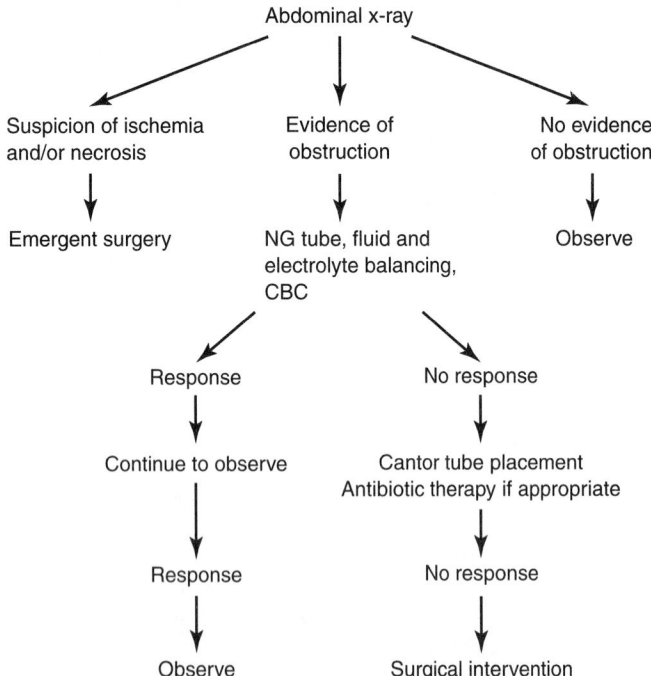

FIGURE 20-1 Treatment approach to suspected obstruction.

REFERRAL POINTS

Obstruction is an emergency. Patients with signs of obstruction need immediate referral to the emergency room or the hospital. Consultation with a gastroenterologist or gastrointestinal surgeon is usually necessary.

▮ ▮ ▮ CLINICAL PEARLS

- A lack of abdominal pain does not rule out obstruction.
- A lack of bowel sounds does not rule out obstruction. After a certain amount of time, the increased bowel sounds from an obstruction often subside.
- Peritonitis can be localized (as with diverticulitis).
- Immediate attention is essential when dealing with obstruction. Delay often results in ischemic changes and necrosis.

EDITOR'S NOTE:
COMPLEMENTARY APPROACHES

A general discussion of complementary approaches can be found in Chapter 3. The following, while not an exhaustive list, are some complementary approaches being used for this condition. Additional information on these approaches, including precautions, can be found in Appendices A and B. Providers need to assess for the use of complementary approaches as part of the patient's history, as they may impact conventional therapies, and patients may not volunteer this information unless specifically asked. Efficacy of many complementary approaches is not as well documented as that of conventional therapies. Providers need to read the literature before suggesting these complementary approaches.

- Complementary Modalities
  Aromatherapy

References

Agha, F.P. (1986). Intussusception in adults. *American Journal of Roentgenology, 146*, 527.

Almy, T.P., & Howell, D.A. (1980). Diverticular disease of the colon. *N Engl J Med, 302*, 324.

Azar, T., & Berger, D.L. (1997). Adult intussusception. *Annals of Surgery, 226*(2), 134–138.

Ballantyne, G.H. (1981). Volvulus of the splenic flexure: Report of a case and review of the literature. *Diseases of the Colon and Rectum, 24*, 630.

Bok, M.D., & Boley, S.J. (1986). Sigmoid volvulus in elderly patients. *American Journal of Surgery, 151*, 71.

Bruce, C.J., Coller, J.A., Murray, J.J., Schoetz, D.J. Jr., Roberts, P.L., & Rusin, L.C. (1996). Laparoscopic resection of diverticular disease. *Diseases of the Colon and Rectum, 39*(10 suppl), S1–6.

Frizelle, E.A., & Wolff, B.G. (1996). Colonic volvulus. *Advances in Surgery, 29*, 131–139.

Gimondo, P., & LaBella, A. (1995). Experimental use of duplex Doppler ultrasonography in the evaluation of intestinal motility in occlusive syndromes. *Radiologic Medicine (Torino), 89*(3), 264–269.

Gonzalez, R., Siskind, B.N., & Burrell, M.I. (1982). The role of radiology in the evaluation of intestinal obstruction. In Fielding, L.P., Welch, J.P., & Moore, F.D. (Eds.). *Intestinal obstruction.* Edinburgh: Churchill-Livingstone, p. 28.

Marston, A.M. (1989). Vascular occlusion. In Marston, A.M., Bulkley, G.B., Fiddian-Green, R.G., & Haglund, U.H. (Eds.). *Splanchnic ischemia and multiple organ failure.* London: Edward Arnold, p. 51.

Painter, N.S., & Burkitt, D.P. (1975). Diverticular disease of the colon, a 20th century problem. *Clinical Gastroenterology, 4*, 3.

Sachs, S.M., Morton, J.H., & Schwartz, S.I. (1982). Acute mesenteric ischemia. *Surgery, 92*, 646.

Sleisenger, M. & Fordtran, J. (1993). *Gastrointestinal disease*, 5th ed., Ch. 30, Sect. IV. Philadelphia: WB Saunders, 591.

Turley, K. (1979). Right paraduodenal hernia. A source of chronic abdominal pain in the adult. *Archives of Surgery, 114*, 1072.

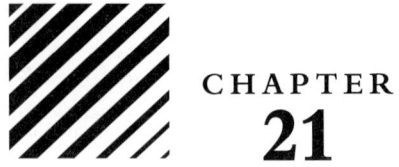

CHAPTER
21

Cirrhosis of the Liver

Rosalinda Margulies, BSN, MPH, RNC and Albert D. Min, MD

Cirrhosis of the liver is defined as the destruction of normal hepatic architecture through fibrosis and nodular regeneration. It is the seventh leading cause of death in the United States, and thus it is important for the primary care provider to formulate a comprehensive, collaborative plan to provide high-quality care in a cost-effective and efficient manner. This chapter will focus on the comprehensive approach used by the primary care provider in caring for patients with cirrhosis.

ANATOMY, PHYSIOLOGY, AND PATHOLOGY

The liver weighs approximately 1500 g. There are two anatomic lobes, the right one about six times the size of the left. The liver participates in multiple functions essential to life, including storage and metabolism of carbohydrates and detoxification of toxins. The clinical sequelae of cirrhosis result from necrosis and regeneration of liver cells, followed by an increase in fibrous tissue formation. The normal structure of the hepatic lobules is distorted, leading to impaired hepatocellular function, obstruction of bile flow through the liver, and alterations in hepatic blood flow. In cirrhosis, regardless of the etiology or clinical status, the triad of parenchymal necrosis, regeneration, and scarring is present (Conn & Atterbury, 1993).

Although the mechanism of cirrhosis is unknown, its etiology is diverse and extensive. It may be classified into two major categories, hepatocellular and cholestatic liver diseases (Min & Bodenheimer, 1996). This is illustrated in Table 21-1.

EPIDEMIOLOGY

Cirrhosis is the fourth leading cause of death in Caucasian American men between 25 and 64 years of age living in an urban setting (Bureau of Health Statistics, 1986). Alcoholic liver disease is a major clinical problem for primary care providers because early diagnosis is sometimes difficult and definitive treatment for alcoholism remains elusive. Alcoholism is the most common cause of chronic liver disease in Western societies, and approximately 18 million Americans abuse alcohol (Crabb & Lumeng, 1995). The peak prevalence of alcoholic liver disease occurs between 40 to 55 years of age. Incidence is disproportionately high in African Americans, Hispanics, and native Americans (Bureau of Health Statistics, 1986). In addition, cirrhosis accounts for 75% of all medical deaths among alcoholics. The male:female ratio in alcoholic liver disease is about 3:1 (Crabb & Lumeng, 1995).

Hepatitis B has a worldwide distribution and is the most common cause of chronic viral disease, cirrhosis, and hepatocellular carcinoma. End-stage liver disease from hepatitis C cirrhosis is responsible for 8000 to 10,000 deaths annually, and it is now the leading indication for liver transplantation in the United States (NIH, 1997).

Biliary cirrhosis is found in all races and occurs worldwide. It accounts for 0.6% to 2% of deaths from cirrhosis throughout the world (Kaplan, 1996).

DIAGNOSTIC CRITERIA

A definite diagnosis of cirrhosis and its etiology can be usually made by a liver biopsy demonstrating characteristic histologic changes in conjunction with serologic tests and viral markers. Various serologic tests are useful as initial diagnostic measures, especially in patients with chronic hepatitis. A liver biopsy is often required to assess the degree of hepatocellular injury, in addition to pointing toward the etiology. Noninvasive radiologic imaging studies such as abdominal ultrasound with Doppler, computed tomography scanning, or magnetic resonance imaging do not have an important role in making the diagnosis of cirrhosis. Although either a nodular surface or an enlarged caudate lobe seen on these imaging studies may be suggestive of underlying cirrhosis, such findings are usually seen in advanced cirrhosis (Dodd, 1996). However, these studies are helpful and are often used to assess the size of the liver and the patency of hepatic vessels and to detect concomitant hepatic lesions.

HISTORY AND PHYSICAL EXAMINATION

History

Patients with cirrhosis range from the asymptomatic, otherwise healthy patient to the patient presenting acutely with hepatocellular failure. However, more typical is the patient presenting with symptoms of fatigue, anorexia, insomnia, or pruritus of varying degrees. A detailed history is essential because it may point toward the etiology of the cirrhosis. Specific questions must be asked regarding risk factors for acquiring viral hepatitis, such as transfusion of blood products, history of intravenous drug abuse, sexual behavior, occupational hazards (eg, health care worker), and birthplace or travel in endemic areas. A family history of liver diseases is helpful in diseases such as hemochromatosis and Wilson's disease. Obtaining a past medical or surgical history is warranted because associated extrahepatic diseases can often tip the possibility of a liver disease. The presence of inflammatory bowel disease in patients with abnormal liver chemistry results can lead to investigation of possible primary sclerosing cholangitis. Patients with decompensated liver diseases may have insomnia, abdominal discomfort, or a history of gastrointestinal bleeding.

Physical Examination

The physical examination is invaluable in establishing a diagnosis of cirrhosis. There may be evidence of temporal muscle wasting in a decompensated cirrhotic patient. Scleral icterus is usu-

| **TABLE 21-1** | **Classification and Etiologies of Cirrhosis** |

HEPATOCELLULAR DISEASES

Alcohol

Hepatotropic viruses
  Hepatitis B
  Hepatitis C
  Hepatitis D

Drugs and toxins

Autoimmune hepatitis

Right-sided heart failure

Nonalcoholic steatohepatitis

Hemochromatosis

Alpha-1-antitrypsin deficiency

Wilson's disease

Cryptogenic

CHOLESTATIC DISEASES

Primary biliary cirrhosis

Primary sclerosing cholangitis

ally detected at total bilirubin levels above 3 to 4 mg/dL. Spider angiomas—visible small arterioles—are common, particularly on the upper arms and chest.

Several findings are noted on examination of the hand. Palmar erythema is characterized by redness of the ball of the palm with the thenar and hypothenar eminences. Dupuytren's contracture may be a nonspecific finding but is often seen in alcoholic liver disease; it involves the fourth and fifth fingers because of thickening of the palmar fascia. White nails and clubbing are often present. Asterixis (flapping tremor) can also be noted in decompensated patients with hepatic encephalopathy.

Gynecomastia, testicular atrophy, and pectoral alopecia are also commonly present. Xanthelasma, xanthomas, and calcinosis can be seen in patients with biliary cirrhosis. Xanthelasmas usually occur below the inner canthal fold of the eye and the eyelid. Xanthomas are most commonly found in the creases of the hands, arms, and legs. Calcinoses typically occur at pressure points such as elbow and the ulnar surface of the forearm. Ascites, peripheral edema, splenomegaly, umbilical hernia, and caput medusae are seen in patients with advanced cirrhosis.

Disease Course

Patients with cirrhosis may live productive lives, but their disease may cause complications and death. Complications of cirrhosis include portal hypertension, often associated with the development of esophageal varices and ascites, hepatic encephalopathy, and spontaneous bacterial peritonitis. Further, cirrhosis often leads to the development of hepatocellular carcinoma, especially in the setting of cirrhosis stemming from hepatitis B and C. Once a cirrhotic patient experiences a complication of portal hypertension with evidence of decreased hepatic synthetic function, the overall prognosis is very poor, and the patient should be evaluated for liver transplantation.

DIAGNOSTIC STUDIES

The evaluation, diagnosis, and treatment of patients with cirrhosis are expensive endeavors. Duplicate workups, such as performing a liver and spleen nuclear scan in a patient scheduled

for a liver biopsy, add little to the diagnosis and should be minimized. However, much of the costs are incurred during evaluation and symptomatic treatment of various complications of chronic liver disease, and optimal therapy without unnecessary costs can be obtained only with accurate diagnosis and evaluation.

Laboratory Tests

Routine laboratory tests play a crucial role in recognizing chronic liver disease and subsequently delineating the etiology, particularly in healthy, asymptomatic persons. Rather than a single specific test, the combination of several tests assessing different aspects of hepatic physiology, measured over a period of time, can lead to the diagnosis.

Serum aminotransferase levels are a sensitive indicator of liver cell injury and hepatocellular necrosis. Alanine aminotransferase (ALT, SGPT) and aspartate aminotransferase (AST, SGOT) are two such enzymes commonly measured in the routine assessment of liver dysfunction. ALT is thought to be more sensitive and specific for liver injury because it is present in highest concentration there, whereas AST is found in the liver, cardiac and skeletal muscles, the kidneys, the brain, and elsewhere. Aminotransferase levels are usually elevated in all liver disorders. However, in cirrhosis the degree of elevation is less than in acute hepatitis and rarely rises above eight times the upper limit of normal except during flare-ups of chronic viral and autoimmune hepatitis. The AST : ALT ratio is of little diagnostic value except in the recognition of alcoholic liver disease, in which the AST : ALT ratio is often greater than 2.

Enzymes that detect cholestasis include alkaline phosphatase and gamma-glutamyl transpeptidase (GGTP). Alkaline phosphatase is a group of enzymes that catalyze the hydrolysis of organic phosphate esters at an alkaline pH and are mainly found in the bile canalicular surface of the hepatocytes and biliary epithelium and bone. Hepatobiliary alkaline phosphatase elevations may be differentiated from other sources of alkaline phosphatase elevations either by measuring isoenzymes or by evaluating the serum activity of another "hepatic" enzyme, such as GGTP. Elevation of serum GGTP is found predominantly in hepatobiliary disease. About three quarters of patients with cholestatic liver disease have alkaline phosphatase values at least three times the upper limit of normal, with a minimal rise in the aminotransferases. However, these elevations do not distinguish between the intrahepatic and extrahepatic bile duct abnormalities.

The serum bilirubin level depends on a balance between the rate of production and removal from the liver. Unconjugated (indirect) hyperbilirubinemia results from overproduction (eg, hemolysis) or impaired hepatic uptake or conjugation, as in Gilbert's syndrome, which is a benign hereditary condition of mildly increased levels of serum unconjugated bilirubin. Conjugated (direct) hyperbilirubinemia results from decreased hepatic excretion or leakage of the conjugated bilirubin from diffuse liver injury or damaged bile ducts. Detection of bilirubin on a routine urinalysis indicates the presence of hepatobiliary disease because the unconjugated bilirubin is not excreted by the kidney.

The biosynthetic capacity of the liver is assessed by serum albumin and prothrombin time. Albumin is synthesized exclusively by the liver, and hypoalbuminemia is common in cirrhosis. A serum albumin level below 3 g/dL usually reflects severe liver damage. The liver is the most important site of synthesis for most blood coagulation proteins, and various components of the clotting cascade may be abnormal in cirrhosis. The prothrombin time is a most useful test in predicting the severity of hepatocellular damage. On a complete blood count, thrombocytopenia or leukopenia may be found (from hypersplenism secondary to portal hypertension), and microcytic anemia (from chronic gastrointestinal blood loss) or macrocytic anemia (eg, alcoholic liver disease) is commonly present.

Although not a routine study, a liver biopsy is often necessary to diagnose cirrhosis and confirm the etiology. The biopsy, usually done via a percutaneous approach in an outpatient setting, should be done only after clotting factors are assessed and a complete blood count, including platelet count, is done. The results are not always conclusive, and further testing may need to be done.

Specific Findings

Detection of hepatitis B surface antigen in cirrhotic patients typically establishes the diagnosis of hepatitis B cirrhosis, whereas hepatitis C virus (HCV) infection is diagnosed by testing for anti-HCV antibody. If a test for anti-HCV by second-generation Enzyme Linked Immunosorbent Assay (ELISA) is positive, a recombinant inmmunoblot assay or HCV RNA by polymerase chain reaction is performed to confirm the true HCV infection. Furthermore, HCV RNA by quantitative polymerase chain reaction is now used to measure the viral load, with a significant role in antiviral therapy.

Autoimmune hepatitis is characteristically associated with hyperglobulinemia and circulating autoantibodies such as antinuclear and anti-smooth muscle antibodies. Often, one clue to its diagnosis is the coexistence of other diseases with immune or autoimmune features, such as thyroiditis (Krawitt, 1996). The diagnosis of primary biliary cirrhosis is made by a combination of positive antimitochondrial antibodies and increased immunoglobulin M on immune protein electrophoresis, in addition to characteristic histologic findings on liver biopsy (Kaplan, 1996). Primary sclerosing cholangitis is diagnosed when endoscopic retrograde cholangiopancreatography demonstrates the characteristic beaded bile duct appearance.

Hemochromatosis is an autosomal recessive metabolic disorder in which there is increased iron absorption over many years. Elevated serum ferritin levels and an increased percentage of transferrin saturation are typical biochemical findings. However, the best method of confirming the diagnosis is to measure quantitative hepatic iron content through liver biopsy. Alpha-1-antitrypsin deficiency is an inherited condition in which early-onset emphysema and a variable spectrum of liver disease can be found. About 1% of adult patients with cirrhosis are homozygous deficient. An adult with diagnosis of cryptogenic cirrhosis should be evaluated for this disease, and serum alpha-1-antitrypsin level should be measured and Pi typing carried out.

Another hereditary condition, Wilson's disease, is an autosomal recessive disorder resulting in abnormalities in copper metabolism. Deficiency of the plasma copper protein ceruloplasmin, because of its impaired synthesis, is seen in more than 95% of these homozygote patients.

Nonalcoholic steatohepatitis or fatty liver may be caused by various conditions, including diabetes, obesity, and jejunoileal bypass. Because the liver biopsy shows steatosis, portal mononuclear inflammation, and Mallory bodies, alcohol abuse must be excluded before making this diagnosis.

TREATMENT OPTIONS, EXPECTED OUTCOMES, AND COMPREHENSIVE MANAGEMENT

Comprehensive Management

Treatment of patients with cirrhosis is entirely dependent on the etiology of their liver disease and whether they have compensated or decompensated cirrhosis. Management of patients with decompensated cirrhosis involves symptomatic treatment of the complications of portal hypertension. The extent and timing of follow-up visits are thus dependent on the therapy instituted, the clinical condition, and the severity of the liver injury. All patients with cirrhosis, especially those with viral hepatitis, should be routinely screened for development of hepatocellular carcinoma with abdominal ultrasound and serum alpha-fetoprotein measurement once or twice a year.

Teaching and Self-Care

The management of cirrhosis by the primary care provider must take into account not only the history, physical examination, and blood and diagnostic tests but also the patient's and family's ability to understand their role in this process. Assessment of the nutritional (see Chap. 5) and rehabilitative needs on a regular basis is essential in managing the patient. Hepatic decompensation may occur gradually, and initial clinical manifestation may include weight loss and changes in daily activities. Therefore, to ensure early and timely intervention, patient education is essential so that the patient can monitor for weight gain or loss, signs of early satiety (eg, feelings of bloating and fullness), and manifestations that may interfere with ambulation (eg, shortness of breath, increased ankle swelling). This collaboration between the patient and the primary care provider will help to maintain an optimal level of functioning.

Self-care and preventive measures for cirrhosis vary in effectiveness, depending on the underlying liver disease. Encouraging abstinence in a patient with alcoholism may prevent the progression of liver disease to cirrhosis. The immunization of all newborns and vaccination of persons at increased risk with hepatitis B vaccines are effective for the prevention of hepatitis B virus acquisition and its subsequent clinical sequelae (Lemon & Thomas, 1997). Unfortunately, there is no HCV vaccine thus far. Patients need to be educated about the sexual transmission of hepatitis B virus (approximately 30%) and HCV (4%) and protective measures, such as using condoms.

Patients and providers may also teach family members about their risk for cirrhosis. In addition to the transmissability of hepatitis B virus and HCV (noted above), screening for early hemochromatosis in first-degree relatives is crucial, particularly in brothers of the patient with hemochromatosis. Affected siblings may also be identified by comparing their human leukocyte antigen (HLA) serotypes with that of the patient. Those treated in the precirrhotic stage, before tissue damage has ensued, have a normal life expectancy.

Treatment

In considering the therapeutic options, the primary care provider should consider three factors: etiology, duration of disease, and complications of underlying cirrhosis. For chronic viral hepatitis B and C, alpha-interferon is the only treatment approved by the Food and Drug Administration. Patients with chronic hepatitis B and cirrhosis who have evidence of replicating virus with positive hepatitis B e antigen and hepatitis B virus DNA and an elevated aminotransferase level should be considered for alpha-interferon therapy. Similarly, patients with hepatitis C with evidence of viremia and an elevated ALT level should be considered for antiviral therapy. The details of such treatments are outlined in Chapter 26. By changing from an active replicative viral state to a dormant state in patients with hepatitis B and by decreasing the viral load in patients with hepatitis C, such antiviral therapy may prevent or delay the progression of the underlying liver disease.

For a patient with autoimmune hepatitis, a daily combination of 10-mg prednisone and 50-mg azathioprine is the optimal therapeutic regimen that minimizes the side effects while achieving the desired clinical, biochemical, and histologic improvement. In patients who cannot take or tolerate azathioprine, 20 mg/day prednisone is a suitable alternative therapy. In autoimmune hepatitis, the superiority of treatment with prednisone alone or in combination with azathioprine over nontreatment is well established. Patients with decompensated cirrhosis or those with a subfulminant picture who do not immediately respond to immunosuppressive therapy should be evaluated for liver transplantation.

Although various medical therapies to increase serum levels of alpha-1-antitrypsin have been attempted with variable success in adult patients with emphysema, it is unclear that any medical therapy alters the course of this deficiency-associated liver disease. However, liver transplantation cures this genetic disorder, including improvement or correction of pulmonary complications.

The therapy in Wilson's disease is aimed at removing the excess copper from the liver and other organs as much as possible, and medical therapy includes use of D-penicillamine or trientine. Liver transplantation is indicated for progressive hepatic insufficiency refractory to drugs in Wilson's disease.

Treatments for hemochromatosis include phlebotomy and chelation therapy with deferoxamine mesylate. After histologic assessment with a liver biopsy, the patient with primary biliary cirrhosis should be started on ursodeoxycholic acid, which improves biochemical tests of cholestasis and hepatic inflammation and may slow the progression of the liver damage (Combes, 1997). In contrast, ursodeoxycholic acid has recently shown to be ineffective in patients with primary sclerosing cholangitis (Lindor, 1997).

If a patient develops decompensated cirrhosis associated with hepatic synthetic dysfunction, therapy is aimed at alleviating the symptoms, such as sodium restriction and diuretics for ascites, band ligation or sclerotherapy for esophageal variceal bleeding, and lactulose, neomycin, or both for hepatic encephalopathy. The hepatic synthesis of factors II, VII, IX, and X requires vitamin K, the deficiency of which can be seen in obstructive jaundice. However, a prolonged prothrombin time (>4 seconds from control values or INR of 1.5 to 2) that is not corrected by vitamin K injection suggests severe parenchymal disease. Patients with severe portal hypertension despite normal hepatic synthetic function should be considered for a portal decompressive procedure such as portosystemic shunt, whereas liver transplantation is indicated, regardless of the etiology of cirrhosis, for patients with complications of portal hypertension and poor hepatic synthetic function.

The primary care provider must collaborate with the patient, family, and other health care members to avoid delays in instituting appropriate therapy, such as a liver transplant. Continuity of care by the primary care provider is also important after the transplant in managing some of the medical complications of immunosuppressive therapy, such as steroid-induced diabetes mellitus and hyperlipidemia.

COMMUNITY RESOURCES

Dealing with a chronic, perhaps life-threatening, disease is difficult. Even if the patient has the most supportive family possible, talking with someone who was or is in the same situation can be very helpful. Therefore, the primary provider must have information readily available regarding such community resources for the patient. Such resources are noted at the end of the unit on gastrointestinal disorders.

REFERRAL POINTS AND CLINICAL WARNINGS

In general, once the primary care provider suspects chronic liver disease, routine blood and serologic testing should be ordered to delineate the underlying etiology. When a definite diagnosis is not obvious by laboratory tests or a specific therapy is being considered, a referral to a gastroenterologist or hepatologist is recommended for further diagnostic and possibly invasive tests.

Once patients develop the signs and symptoms of decompensated cirrhosis, such as esophagogastric variceal bleeding, hepatic encephalopathy, ascites, or spontaneous bacterial peritonitis, in addition to evidence of decreased hepatic synthetic function, they should be referred to a liver transplant program as early as possible, as outlined in Figure 21-1. After the referral to a transplant center is made, the challenge for the primary care provider is to maintain collaboration with the transplant team to ensure patient cooperation and to continue managing and monitoring the patient's clinical condition closely to detect any further sign of decompensation and to alert the transplant team about a need for urgent transplant. Thus, the primary care provider must maintain a continuing and cooperative relationship with the transplant team.

Although liver transplantation itself is not a remedy for eradicating hepatitis viruses from cirrhotic patients, nearly 40% of liver transplants are performed because of end-stage liver diseases from viral hepatitis B, C, or D. In fact, hepatitis C cirrhosis is the leading underlying liver disease in transplant patients, accounting for approximately 35% of all liver transplants in the United States.

■ ■ ■   **CLINICAL PEARLS**

- Patients with cirrhosis may present with classical findings on the physical examination or may be completely asymptomatic, with only abnormal liver function testing raising the suspicion.
- Establishing the etiology of cirrhosis is essential in planning a treatment strategy.
- All patients with cirrhosis, especially those with viral hepatitis, should be routinely screened for the development of hepatocellular carcinoma with abdominal ultrasound and alpha-fetoprotein measurement once or twice a year.

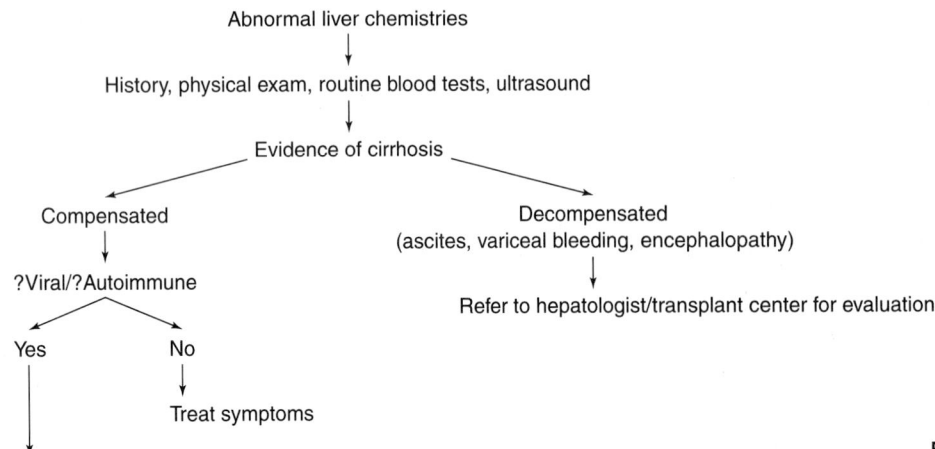

FIGURE 21-1 Comprehensive management of patients with cirrhosis.

- Liver transplantation is often necessary in cases of decompensated cirrhosis. Patients need to be educated about this, and the primary care provider must collaborate with the gastroenterologist and the transplant team to coordinate this effort.

EDITOR'S NOTE:

COMPLEMENTARY APPROACHES

A general discussion of complementary approaches can be found in Chapter 3. The following, while not an exhaustive list, are some complementary approaches being used for this condition. Additional information on these approaches, including precautions, can be found in Appendices A and B. Providers need to assess for the use of complementary approaches as part of the patient's history, as they may impact conventional therapies, and patients may not volunteer this information unless specifically asked. Efficacy of many complementary approaches is not as well documented as that of conventional therapies. Providers need to read the literature before suggesting these complementary approaches.

- Vitamins, minerals, herbs, supplements
  Milk thistle
- Complementary Modalities
  Aromatherapy

References

Bureau of Health Statistics and Analysis. (1986). *Summary of vital statistics and analysis.* New York: Centers for Disease Control and Prevention.

Combes, B. (1997). Ursodeoxycholic acid in primary biliary cirrhosis. *Seminars in Liver Disease, 17,* 125–128.

Conn, H.O., & Atterbury, C. (1993). Cirrhosis. In L. Schiff & E.R. Schiff (Eds.). *Diseases of the liver,* vol. 2, 7th ed., pp. 875–943. Philadelphia: J.B. Lippincott.

Crabb, D., & Lumeng, L. (1995). *Alcoholic liver disease,* vol. 3, 5th ed., pp. 2215–2240. Philadelphia: W.B. Saunders.

Dodd, G.D.,(1996). Imaging in cirrhosis. In P.C. Freeny (Ed.). *Radiology of the liver, biliary tree and pancreas,* pp. 65–69. Reston, Va.: American Roentgen Ray Society.

Kaplan, M.M. (1996). Primary biliary cirrhosis. *N Engl J Med, 3*(35), 1570–1580.

Krawitt, E.L. (1996). Autoimmune hepatitis. *N Engl J Med, 3*(34), 897–903.

Lemon, S.M., & Thomas, D.L. (1997). Vaccines to prevent viral hepatitis. *N Engl J Med, 3*(36), 196–204.

Linder, K.D. (1997). Ursodiol for primary sclerosing cholangitis. *N Engl J Med, 336*(70), 691–695.

Min, A.M., & Bodenheimer, H.C. Jr. (1996). Evaluation of patients with chronic liver disease. In J.W. Hurst (Ed.). *Medicine for the practicing physician,* 4th ed., pp. 1734–1736. Norwalk, Conn.: Appleton & Lange.

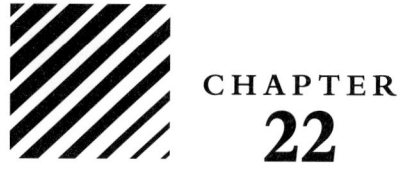

CHAPTER
22

Gallbladder

Charles Berk, MD

The problems of the gallbladder related to gallstones present along a broad clinical spectrum. Most patients with gallstones remain clinically silent. Symptoms in many patients are mild and may be evaluated and treated in the outpatient setting and on an elective basis. However, gallstones can cause a variety of complications requiring hospitalization and rapid intervention. Previously, surgical removal of gallstones and the gallbladder from symptomatic patients was the only viable treatment option for most patients. However, now there are medical and endoscopic options aimed only at the treatment of the stones themselves that may be appropriate for selected patients. Further, laparoscopic cholecystectomy has largely replaced open cholecystectomy as the surgical procedure of choice for patients with gallstones. Appropriate management, especially with emergencies, requires a multidisciplinary team.

ANATOMY, PHYSIOLOGY, AND PATHOLOGY

The anatomy of the gallbladder is described in Chapter 24. Biliary pain results from impaction of the cystic duct by a gallstone, causing distention of the gallbladder (Giurgiu & Roslyn, 1996). In acute cholecystitis, occlusion of the cystic duct is accompanied by inflammation of the gallbladder. Bacteria can sometimes be cultured from the bile of patients with acute cholecystitis, but this is currently thought to represent an incidental and not a causal relation (Somberg et al, 1993).

Choledocholithiasis is associated with stones obstructing the common duct. Cholangitis is an infectious complication related to bile duct obstruction. The increased intraluminal pressure results in the reflux of bacteria into the hepatic veins and through the lymphatics into the systemic circulation. The commonly cultured organisms in cholangitis are *Escherichia coli*, *Klebsiella*, *Pseudomonas*, enterococci, and *Proteus*. Anaerobes are found in approximately 15% of infections, but these are usually present simultaneously with aerobic species. Common anaerobic bacterial infections in cholangitis are *Bacteroides fragilis* and *Clostridium perfringens* (Giurgiu & Roslyn, 1996; Somberg et al, 1993).

Gallstone Formation

There are three types of gallstones: cholesterol stones and two types of pigmented stones, brown and black. In the developed world, 70% to 80% of stones are the pure cholesterol type, or mixed cholesterol with calcium (Goldschmid & Brady, 1993). Brown stones are more common in developing countries. They develop as a result of parasitic infections leading to biliary stasis and secondary chronic anaerobic infection. Brown stones usually form in the intrahepatic bile duct rather than the gallbladder (Carey, 1993). Black stones form in sterile bile and are associated with conditions producing chronic hemolysis, such as sickle cell disease.

CHOLESTEROL GALLSTONES

There are three contributory factors identified in the current model of cholesterol stone formation: supersaturation of the bile with cholesterol, accelerated nucleation, and gallbladder hypomotility. All three of these factors must be present for the formation of gallstones to occur, although each factor may predominate under different clinical circumstances.

Cholesterol is itself insoluble in aqueous solutions such as bile. However, with the addition of bile salts and lecithin, the three components come together to produce a soluble structure known as a micelle. Either hypersecretion of cholesterol or insufficient quantities of bile salts can result in a situation where the ability of cholesterol to be held in suspension in the bile is exceeded. Supersaturated bile is considered to be lithogenic. Increased cholesterol secretion is much more commonly implicated in stone formation, but decreased bile salts have been found as a risk factor in some indigenous populations in the American Southwest (Johnston & Kaplan, 1993).

Nucleation is the second step in stone formation. Studies done comparing the bile from patients with stones to patients without stones have shown that for any given concentration of cholesterol, crystal formation occurs more readily in patients with gallstones. Initially the cholesterol crystals are small and trapped in a mucin gel. This thick substance is referred to as biliary sludge and has been associated with pancreatitis. The mucoproteins in sludge are thought to be at least one of the pronucleating factors contributing to gallstone formation. The cholesterol microcrystals coalesce and grow into gallstones (Johnston & Kaplan, 1993).

Gallbladder stasis contributes to gallstone formation by interfering with the process by which sludge and microscopic crystals would normally be emptied from the gallbladder and by promoting prolonged contact between bile and pronucleating factors (Johnston & Kaplan, 1993; O'Donnell & Fairclough, 1993). Hypomotility is a prominent risk factor in pregnant patients, patients receiving total parenteral nutrition, patients with diabetes mellitus, and patients with spinal cord injuries.

EPIDEMIOLOGY

In the United States the incidence of gallstones is approximately 10% to 15% of the adult population (NIH, 1983). The incidence is greater in women, but increases in both men and women with age. Women and men in their 70s have an incidence of 40% to 50% and 16%, respectively. Past the age of 90, the incidence increases to over 80% among men and women (Watkins et al, 1993).

TABLE 22-1	Risk Factors for Gallstones

HYPERSECRETION OF BILIARY CHOLESTEROL
Women
Exogenous estrogen
Rapid weight loss
Obesity
Hypertriglyceridemia
Increasing age
Pregnancy
Clofibrate
Gemfibrozil

HYPOMOTILITY
Total parenteral nutrition
Vagotomy
Pregnancy
Spinal cord injury

PIGMENTED STONES
Hemolytic anemia
Biliary infection
Cirrhosis

DECREASED BILE ACID POOL
Disease of the terminal ileum
Resection of the terminal ileum

The development of symptomatic gallstone disease occurs at the rate of 1% to 4% a year in persons with gallstones (Gracie & Ransohoff, 1982). In 1991 about 600,000 cholecystectomies were performed in the United States. Gallstone disease is the most common cause of hospitalization for digestive disorders (Bowen, 1993; Ghiloni, 1993). Table 22-1 lists risk factors for gallstones.

DIAGNOSTIC CRITERIA

Diagnostic criteria are listed in Table 22-2.

HISTORY AND PHYSICAL EXAMINATION

Most cases of cholelithiasis are asymptomatic, and most patients will not proceed to the development of symptoms. Once patients develop clinical stone-related disease, the hallmark complaint is abdominal pain. The characteristics, however, are nonspecific, and biliary pain has a broad differential diagnosis, including gastritis, peptic ulcer disease, reflux esophagitis, pancreatitis, renal disease, diverticulitis, radicular pain, and angina (Giurgiu & Roslyn, 1996; Moscati, 1996). Because asymptomatic gallstones are common, the identification of stones in the gallbladder should not preclude a complete evaluation of patients whose symptoms suggest other diagnoses.

Biliary pain has previously been referred to as biliary colic, but most authors agree that the term colic, which implies a spasmodic type of pain, does not accurately describe the pain of patients with gallstones. The pain of cholecystitis usually comes on suddenly and builds to a plateau quickly. It lasts several hours, with gradual resolution (Ghiloni, 1993). Uncomplicated biliary pain usually lasts less than 3 hours but may last as long as 24 hours. An episode of pain lasting more than 6 hours is suggestive of acute cholecystitis rather than chronic cholecystitis (Moscati, 1996; Somberg et al, 1993). The most common location for biliary pain is the epigastrium. The right costal margin is actually the second most likely location in which patients describe their pain (Doran, 1967). Patients may have pain that is localized or that radiates to the right scapula

TABLE 22-2	Gallstone-Related Conditions: Presentation and Evaluation			
Disease	**Symptoms**	**Physical Exam Findings**	**Labs**	**Imaging**
Asymptomatic cholelithiasis	Absent	Normal	Normal	+ Ultrasound
Chronic cholelithiasis	Recurrent biliary pain usually <3 hrs	Normal	Normal or slight abnormalities similar to acute cholecystitis	+ Ultrasound + Cholecystogram
Acute cholecystitis	Biliary pain usually >6 hrs	Fever Murphy's sign	↑ WBC ↑ Bilirubin (usually <4 mg/dL) ↑ Alkaline phosphatase ↑ AST	+ Ultrasound + Cholescintigraphy
Choledocholithiasis	Biliary pain	Fever Jaundice	↑ WBC ↑ Bilirubin ↑ Alkaline phosphatase ↑ AST/ALT	+ ERCP + Endoscopic ultrasound + Intraoperative cholangiogram
Cholangitis	Biliary pain	Fever Jaundice	↑ WBC ↑ Bilirubin ↑ Alkaline phosphatase ↑ AST/ALT + Blood culture	+ ERCP

and shoulder. Atypical symptoms such as fullness, bloating, belching, heartburn, and early satiety are extremely common, especially in the elderly (Watkins et al, 1993). Restlessness, nausea, vomiting, diaphoresis, and low-grade fever are findings frequently associated with biliary pain. The older teaching that pain is precipitated by the ingestion of foods and especially fats is mistaken. Many patients have no such association, and many patients have their symptoms at night (Moscati, 1996).

Patients with chronic cholecystitis, characterized by recurrent bouts of biliary pain, usually have no fever, no abdominal tenderness, and no jaundice. Once patients begin to have symptoms from chronic cholecystitis, the episodes tend to recur with increasing frequency and severity. They usually have no fever, no abdominal tenderness, and no jaundice and have normal laboratory evaluations for white blood cell counts and bilirubin, liver enzyme, and alkaline phosphatase levels.

Patients with acute cholecystitis usually have biliary pain and may have fever. About 20% present with jaundice. Abdominal tenderness is common and a positive Murphy's sign (eliciting pain when palpating the right upper quadrant as the patient takes a deep inspiration) is a classic finding. The white blood cell count is usually elevated, but to less than $15,000/mm^3$. The serum bilirubin value may be elevated but is usually less than 4 mg/dL. Transaminase and alkaline phosphatase levels may also be elevated (Ghiloni, 1993; Somberg et al, 1993).

Choledocholithiasis and cholangitis are difficult to distinguish from each other on clinical grounds. Choledocholithiasis is caused by the presence of a gallstone in the common duct. Cholangitis is an infection of an obstructed bile duct and is usually found in association with choledocholithiasis. Both sets of patients may present with abdominal pain, jaundice, and fever. This combination of symptoms is known as Charcot's triad and is generally associated with cholangitis, but the same description may apply to patients with choledocholithiasis (Somberg et al, 1993).

Complications of acute cholecystitis include perforation, Mirizzi's syndrome, and emphysematous cholecystitis. Perforation may take three forms: localization by abscess formation; free spillage into the peritoneum; or erosion into an adjacent viscus, giving rise to fistula formation. Mirizzi's syndrome is a phenomenon in which extrinsic compression by surrounding inflammation leads to obstruction of the common hepatic duct or the common bile duct. Certain infections are associated with the production of gas in the gallbladder, the gallbladder wall, the bile ducts, or the pericholecystic area; this is referred to as emphysematous cholecystitis.

DIAGNOSTIC STUDIES

Screening asymptomatic patients for gallstones is currently not justified (NIH, 1983). The laboratory tests that are suggestive of biliary obstruction, as in choledocholithiasis and cholangitis, are elevations of the hepatic transaminases (AST and ALT), bilirubin (usually >4 mg/dL), GGT, and alkaline phosphatase (Wallach, 1992). Leukocytosis is also usually present. Blood cultures are usually positive in cholangitis.

In acute cholecystitis, the white count is usually elevated, and in 20% of patients the bilirubin level is also elevated, but less so than when obstruction is present. An elevated AST level is found in 75% of patients with acute cholecystitis. Patients with chronic cholecystitis have normal or mildly elevated laboratory values compared with patients with acute cholecystitis.

Ultrasonography

Ultrasonography is the most important diagnostic tool for identifying gallstones in the gallbladder. It is accurate, quick, readily available, and noninvasive and requires no special preparation. Useful information that may be obtained by ultrasound includes identifying a thickened gallbladder wall, which suggests chronic cholecystitis; assessing the number and size of stones, which can help determine if a patient qualifies for nonsurgical treatment; and identifying a dilated biliary tree, which may mean obstruction of the common duct and choledocholithiasis (Giurgiu & Roslyn, 1996; Watkins et al, 1993; Somberg et al, 1993).

Endoscopic ultrasonography is a more recent diagnostic approach. Its accuracy at detecting choledocholithiasis rivals that of endoscopic retrograde cholangiopancreatography (ERCP), and it carries no risk of pancreatitis. It may be particularly useful at ruling out choledocholithiasis in patients who have contraindications to ERCP or whose risk for choledocholithiasis is low.

Radiography

Plain x-rays are of limited value in assessing gallstones because most gallstones are radiolucent. Only 10% to 25% of stones are rendered radiopaque by the presence of calcium (Carey, 1993). The x-ray finding on plain abdominal films that suggests the presence of a gallstone is an incomplete ringed density in the right upper quadrant. Although it is not the method of choice for locating gallstones, information regarding calcium content is essential in evaluating patients for dissolution therapy because only pure cholesterol stones, which are radiolucent, are amenable to this treatment (Watkins et al, 1993).

Cholecystography

Oral cholecystography is a second-line test after ultrasound in diagnosing chronic cholecystitis. This study should be considered if ultrasonography fails to identify the gallbladder or if the ultrasound is negative for stones but gallstone disease is still a diagnostic consideration. A halogenated contrast medium is given to the patient orally. The contrast material is secreted into the bile and concentrated in the gallbladder, thus rendering it radiopaque. Gallstones are represented by filling defects within the contrast material. Two thirds of patients whose gallbladders do not visualize after the first dose of contrast material will respond to a second dose. Visualization of the gallbladder via cholecystography requires a patent cystic duct. This is an inclusion criteria for both lithotripsy and oral dissolution therapy. Additionally, oral dissolution therapy is more likely to succeed when stones are noted to float in halogenated bile (Goldschmid & Brady, 1993).

Cholescintigraphy

Cholescintigraphy is a nuclear medicine study that is useful in diagnosing acute cholecystitis. Radioactive-labeled iminodiacetic acid derivatives given intravenously are quickly excreted into the bile. Scans done at 30 to 60 minutes normally show radioactivity in the gallbladder, the common bile duct, and the small bowel. Nonvisualization of the gallbladder because of obstruction of the cystic duct is consistent with acute cholecystitis. Failure to see dye in the small intestine is suggestive of choledocholithiasis (Somberg et al, 1993; Watkins et al, 1993).

Endoscopic Retrograde Cholangiopancreatography

ERCP involves injecting contrast dye directly into the biliary tree. Stones may be identified in patients with abdominal pain in whom no other diagnosis can be made and in whom sonograms and cholecystograms are negative. However, its main use in gallstone disease is in diagnosing choledocholithiasis and cholangitis. Ultrasonography, as stated above, is not very sensitive for identifying common duct stones. Although certain clinical and laboratory findings may suggest these conditions, no set of findings is specific for these diagnoses. When the presence of ductal stones is suspected and when stones cannot be identified in the gallbladder or no common duct dilatation is noted on ultrasound, ERCP may be the method of choice for identifying common duct stones (Somberg et al, 1993; Watkins et al, 1993).

TREATMENT OPTIONS, EXPECTED OUTCOMES, AND COMPREHENSIVE MANAGEMENT

Prophylactic treatment of asymptomatic gallstones is not recommended (NIH, 1983). Few patients progress from asymptomatic to symptomatic disease, and in most cases the progression of symptoms is gradual. Also, few patients will develop serious complications from their disease (Thistle et al, 1984). This recommendation also applies to persons with diabetes and represents a recent change in thinking (Ransohoff et al, 1987). However, because morbidity and mortality rates are increased in patients with diabetes undergoing emergency cholecystectomies, they should be treated quickly once symptoms occur and the diagnosis of gallstone disease is made (Aucott et al, 1993).

Teaching and Self-Care

Primary prevention aimed at decreasing the incidence of asymptomatic gallstones is currently not recommended. The only available medical modality would be to treat patients with oral dissolution therapy; this would treat 90% of patients unnecessarily and would be prohibitively expensive. Lifestyle modifications that may theoretically decrease the risk of gallstones include weight loss (but avoiding dieting for rapid weight loss), increased exercise, high-calcium diets, frequent meals, and high-fiber diets, but there is no evidence that these interventions are effective (Hoffman, 1993).

Surgical Therapy

OPEN CHOLECYSTECTOMY

Until recently, open cholecystectomy was the surgical procedure of choice for cholecystitis. Mortality rates are very low, ranging from 0.1% to 1.3%, although for patients over 70 the mortality rate may be as high as 5% (Giurgiu & Roslyn, 1996). The morbidity rate is less than 5%, and complications include bleeding, infection, rupture of viscus, and complications related to anesthesia (Doran, 1967; Gholson et al, 1994). The average

hospital stay is 6 days. Postoperative convalescent time is 4 to 5 weeks. The main contraindication to surgery is inability to tolerate general anesthesia (Ghiloni, 1993; NIH, 1983).

An open cholecystectomy may be preferred in patients with generalized peritonitis, septic shock from cholangitis, severe acute pancreatitis, end-stage cirrhosis with portal hypertension, severe coagulopathy, cancer of the gallbladder, and known cholecystoenteric Fistules.

LAPAROSCOPIC CHOLECYSTECTOMY

Laparoscopic cholecystectomy has largely replaced open surgery as the procedure of choice for removal of the gallbladder. The advantages of the procedure include decreased postoperative pain, shorter hospital stays (1 to 2 days), and a convalescent time of only 1 to 2 weeks (NIH, 1983). The time under general anesthesia is slightly increased compared with open cholecystectomy, and there is a slightly greater risk of damage to the common cystic duct (Ponsky, 1991). These risks, however, are usually not great enough to alter the preference for this procedure. About 5% of laparoscopic procedures need to be converted to open cholecystectomies. Although the cost of a laparoscopic procedure is higher than that of an open cholecystectomy, this cost is offset by savings from decreased days of hospitalization and more rapid return to work.

The contraindications to laparoscopic cholecystectomy are similar to those for open cholecystectomy. Inability to tolerate general anesthesia is an absolute contraindication. Patients with choledocholithiasis can be treated with laparoscopic cholecystectomy, but they may require additional procedures to remove their ductal stones. ERCP with sphincterotomy is the procedure of choice for the management of patients with bile duct stones who have had a cholecystectomy. Preoperative ERCP to remove stones is more controversial and requires a higher level of technical skill. Therefore, the decision to manage patients with ERCP followed by laparoscopic cholecystectomy should depend on the expertise of the operator (Gholson et al, 1994; Sivak, 1989).

Nonsurgical Treatments

Several nonsurgical modalities have been developed for the treatment of gallstones. Unfortunately, many patients do not meet the criteria that would predict a good response to any of these treatments. Also, the recurrence of gallstone formation is high in all of them. At the same time, laparoscopic cholecystectomy has gained popularity both with providers and with patients because it offers the advantages of a surgical procedure with significantly fewer problems related to pain and convalescence.

ORAL DISSOLUTION THERAPY

Two agents are available for oral dissolution therapy. Chenodeoxycholic acid was available first, but its use was limited by side effects of diarrhea, elevated liver transaminase levels, and increased plasma cholesterol levels (Goldschmid & Brady, 1993; Price & Hartranft, 1995). Ursodeoxycholic acid is better tolerated, but it can promote the development of calcified gallstones, which would not be amenable to dissolution therapy. The dose of ursodeoxycholic acid is 8 to 10 mg/kg/day divided into two or three doses per day, or the entire dose may be given once at bedtime. Six to 12 months of treatment may be necessary, and regular ultrasound examination is recommended at 6-month intervals. Treatment should be continued for 3 months after complete dissolution as determined by ultrasound (Goldschmid & Brady, 1993). Recurrence rates are high and peak at 50% 5 years after discontinuation of therapy (Ghiloni, 1993; Lanzini & Northfield, 1994).

Patients who are poor surgical risks or who refuse surgery should be evaluated for nonsurgical treatment. Small cholesterol stones may respond well to oral dissolution therapy. Larger stones and multiple stones may be better treated with direct dissolution therapy or lithotripsy.

After successful medical treatment for gallstones, patients should be monitored annually with ultrasound. Oral dissolution therapy should be continued for 3 months after dissolution of stones is noted by ultrasound, but there is no recommendation for chronic prophylactic treatment of patients who have had their stones treated medically.

Table 22-3 lists the criteria for oral dissolution therapy.

CONTACT DISSOLUTION THERAPY

Methyl tertbutyl ether can be introduced via percutaneous transhepatic gallbladder puncture. Noncalcified cholesterol gallstones can be dissolved in about 7 hours in 90% of cases. Disadvantages to the procedure include the fact that the solvent is flammable and potentially explosive and the administration technique is cumbersome. Complications can arise from catheter insertion or from the solvent. Painful jaundice has been reported to occur in some patients. Like other nonsurgical treatments, its use is currently limited to patients with severe symptoms and noncalcified gallstones who are either poor surgical candidates or refuse surgery. The benefit of this treatment is that it is not limited by the number or size of the stones, as long as they are noncalcified (Goldschmid & Brady, 1993).

EXTRACORPOREAL SHOCKWAVE LITHOTRIPSY

Extracorporeal shockwave lithotripsy is still an experimental treatment. Shockwaves are generated underwater by various means and focused on the gallbladder. The best results are in patients with a single noncalcified stone that is less than 20 mm in a functioning gallbladder. The success rate in these patients is 95% (Bowen, 1993). In patients with a single stone 20 to 30 mm or with three stones, the success rate is 65%. Calcified or partially calcified stones can also be fragmented, but clearance of the fragments from the gallbladder is poor (Goldschmid &

TABLE 22-3	Criteria for Oral Dissolution Therapy
Comorbid condition that precludes safe operation	
Refusing therapy	
Cholesterol stones*	
Radiolucent stones†	
Functioning gallbladder*	
Floating gallstones†	
Stones <1.5 to 2 cm in diameter†	
Not pregnant	
No renal or hepatic disease	

* Required for oral dissolution therapy to work
† Predictors of better outcomes

Brady, 1993). Oral dissolution therapy is also used after lithotripsy to dissolve residual stone fragments (Lanzini & Northfield, 1994).

Choledocholithiasis

Common duct stones can be treated in a variety of ways. Common duct stones discovered during open cholecystectomy may be treated by open or laparoscopic duct exploration. Stones discovered during laparoscopic cholecystectomy may be treated by endoscopic sphincterotomy or conversion to an open procedure (Ponsky, 1991). Stones that are discovered or that develop after cholecystectomy can probably be treated by sphincterotomy via ERCP (Cameron, 1989).

Cholangitis

Mild to moderate cases of cholangitis should respond to a single-antibiotic regimen. Cefoxitin is recommended. In more severe cases, triple therapy with ampicillin, gentamicin, and metronidazole is more appropriate. Drainage of the biliary system is recommended in severe cases and in milder cases that do not respond to antibiotics alone. Associated common duct stones must be treated once the patient is stabilized.

Special Considerations

Older patients and patients with diabetes mellitus are at increased risk for complications related to symptomatic gallstone disease. Patients with diabetes, once diagnosed, should be treated promptly and definitively. Older patients present with more atypical symptoms and have a high incidence of gallstones. Providers should maintain a high level of suspicion for gallstones when confronted with symptoms such as dyspepsia, fullness, bloating, tightness, nausea, and heartburn. Diagnostic studies that further help make the diagnosis have already been reviewed. Surgery can be recommended for healthier older adults. The mortality rate for nonemergent cholecystectomy in older patients is less than 4%.

COMMUNITY RESOURCES

Community resources, national organizations, and Internet web sites are noted at the end of the unit on gastrointestinal disorders.

REFERRAL POINTS AND CLINICAL WARNINGS

Acutely and severely ill patients require the immediate involvement of at least a surgeon, but a multidisciplinary approach is likely to be required depending on the clinical presentation of the patient and the expertise available to perform laparoscopic and endoscopic procedures. The team may include a gastroenterologist and a radiologist. Any patient who presents with fever, jaundice, or a positive Murphy's sign, or who has leukocytosis and elevated liver function tests, should be referred for immediate evaluation and probable hospitalization.

Patients with a history suggestive of symptomatic gallstones but who are not acutely ill can be referred for noninvasive imaging studies. The initial follow-up evaluation can be with the primary provider. Surgical referral will be the best option for most patients. If surgery is contraindicated or if the patient

> **EDITOR'S NOTE:**
> ## COMPLEMENTARY APPROACHES
>
> A general discussion of complementary approaches can be found in Chapter 3. The following, while not an exhaustive list, are some complementary approaches being used for this condition. Additional information on these approaches, including precautions, can be found in Appendices A and B. Providers need to assess for the use of complementary approaches as part of the patient's history, as they may impact conventional therapies, and patients may not volunteer this information unless specifically asked. Efficacy of many complementary approaches is not as well documented as that of conventional therapies. Providers need to read the literature before suggesting these complementary approaches.
>
> ■ Complementary Modalities
>   Acupuncture
>   Aromatherapy

prefers a trial of dissolution therapy, a referral to a gastroenterologist should be considered.

References

Aucott, J., Cooper, G.S., Bloon, A.D., & David, C. (1993). Management of gallstones in diabetic patients. *Archives of Internal Medicine, 153,* 1053–1058.

Bowen, J.C. (1993). Gallstone disease: Current treatment. *Seminars in Ultrasound, CT, and MRI, 14*(5), 321–324.

Cameron, J.L. (1989). Retained and recurrent bile duct stones: Operative management. *American Journal of Surgery, 158,* 218–221.

Carey, M.C. (1993). Pathogenesis of gallstones. *American Journal of Surgery, 165,* 410–419.

Doran, F.S.A. (1967). The sites to which pain is referred from the common bile-duct in man and its implication for the theory of referred pain. *British Journal of Surgery, 54*(7), 599–606.

Ghiloni, B.W. (1993). Cholelithiasis: Current treatment options. *American Family Physician, 48*(5), 762–768.

Gholson, C.F., Sittig, K., & McDonald, J.C. (1994). Recent advances in the management of gallstones. *American Journal of Medical Sciences, 307*(4), 293–304.

Giurgiu, D.I.N., & Roslyn, J.J. (1996). Treatment of gallstones in the 1990s. *Primary Care, 23*(3), 497–513.

Goldschmid, S., & Brady, P.G. (1993). Approaches to the management of cholelithiasis for the medical consultant. *Medical Clinics of North America, 77*(2), 413–426.

Gracie, W.A., & Ransohoff, D.F. (1982). The natural history of silent gallstones: The innocent gallstone is not a myth. *N Engl J Med, 307*(13), 798–800.

Hoffman, A.F. (1993). Primary and secondary prevention of gallstone disease: Implications for patient management and research priorities. *American Journal of Surgery, 165,* 541–548.

Johnston, D.E., & Kaplan, M.M. (1993). Pathogenesis and treatment of gallstones. *N Engl J Med, 328*(6), 412–421.

Lanzini, A., & Northfield, T.C. (1994). Pharmacological treatment of gallstones. *Drugs, 47*(3), 458–470.

Moscati, R.M. (1996). Cholelithiasis and cholecystitis, and pancreatitis. *Emergency Medical Clinics of North America, 14*(4), 719–729.

National Institute of Health. (1983). Gallstones and laparoscopic cholecystectomy. *JAMA, 269*(8), 1018–1024.

O'Donnell, L.J.D., & Fairclough, P.D. (1993). Gallstones and gallbladder motility. *Gut, 34,* 440–443.

Ponsky, J.L. (1991). Complications of laparoscopic cholecystectomy. *American Journal of Surgery, 161,* 393–395.

Price, P., & Hartranft, T.H. (1995). New trends in the treatment of calculous disease of the biliary tract. *Journal of the American Board of Family Practice, 8*(1), 22–28.

Ransohoff, D.F., Miller, G.L., Forsythe, S.B., & Herman, R.E. (1987). Outcome of acute cholecystitis in patients with diabetes mellitus. *Annals of Internal Medicine, 106*(6), 829–832.

Sivak, M.V. (1989). Endoscopic management of bile duct stones. *American Journal of Surgery, 158,* 228–240.

Somberg, K.A., Way, L.W., & Sleisenger, M.H. (1993). Complications of gallstone disease. In M.H. Sleisenger & J. Fordtran (Eds.). *Gastrointestinal disease: Pathophysiology, diagnosis, management*, Philadelphia: W.B. Saunders, pp. 1805–1836).

Thistle, J.L., Cleary, P.A., Lachin, J.M., Tyor, M., & Hersh, T. (1984). The natural history of cholelithiasis: The National Cooperative Gallstone Study. *Annals of Internal Medicine, 101*(2), 171–175.

Wallach, J. (1992). *Interpretation of diagnostic tests*, Boston: Little, Brown & Company, pp. 205–206.

Watkins, J.L., Blatt, C.F., & Layden, T.J. (1993). Gallstones: Choosing the right therapy despite vague clinical clues. *Geriatrics, 48*(8), 48–54.

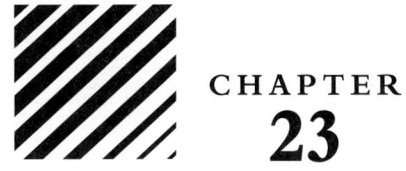

CHAPTER
23

Gastroesophageal Reflux Disease

Paul Cohen, MD

Gastroesophageal reflux disease (GERD) is such a common problem that it affects more than 1 out of 10 people on a daily basis. The presence or absence of a hiatal hernia often helps determine the severity of GERD and the ease or difficulty with which it can be treated. Several treatment options are available, but in addition to medications, use of self-care techniques is paramount.

ANATOMY, PHYSIOLOGY, AND PATHOLOGY

GERD occurs for various reasons, ranging from dietary factors to disruption of the antireflux barrier, allowing gastric content to reflux into the esophagus. In addition to these reasons, the lower esophageal sphincter (LES) normally relaxes approximately four times per hour (Mittal & McCallum, 1987; Holloway et al, 1995), and gastric juices may reflux during these times.

The antireflux barrier is composed of the crura diaphragm, the phrenoesophageal ligament, the acute angle of His, and the LES. These components physically block the reflux of gastric juices into the esophagus. The crura diaphragm wraps around the esophagus and helps create this barrier. The acute angle of His is the angle created when the esophagus passes through the diaphragm and empties into the stomach.

The LES is perhaps the most important component of this antireflux barrier. The intrinsic pressure of the LES keeps it closed until swallowing occurs. Once a bolus of food is swallowed, the LES receives a signal to relax and allows the bolus to pass into the stomach. The normal relaxation of the LES is believed to occur as part of digestion, perhaps to allow accumulating gases to escape. This relaxation is believed to play a major role in the etiology of reflux disease. Seasoned foods, cigarette smoking, alcohol ingestion, and caffeine are all well-known causes of LES relaxation with resultant reflux. Progesterone has also been found to decrease the LES pressure (Baron & Richter, 1992).

Hiatal Hernias

A hiatal hernia disrupts the antireflux barrier. Although the LES still functions normally, by allowing the LES to be displaced upward and separated from the other components of the antireflux barrier, the barrier is not as effective. The sliding hiatal hernia is the most common form of hiatal hernia. This type of hiatal hernia slides back and forth through the diaphragmatic hiatus. Because of this sliding back and forth, hiatal hernias, especially when small, may seem to appear and disappear on various diagnostic studies.

Paraesophageal hiatal hernias are more dangerous and far less common than sliding hiatal hernias. With paraesophageal hernias, GERD is not a complication, because the LES is not displaced. Rather, a distal portion of the stomach actually migrates upward and becomes trapped between the diaphragm and the esophagus. This can lead to ischemic changes and eventually necrosis of the stomach, with catastrophic consequences.

Histologic Changes

Histologic changes can be found in GERD, especially in patients with chronic GERD. The repetitive insult of the gastric juices causes metaplastic changes in the esophagus. Barrett's esophagus represents the replacement of the squamous epithelia of the esophagus with columnar epithelia normally found in the stomach or small bowel. Barrett's esophagus is a premalignant condition that occurs in 10% to 20% of patients with GERD (Spechler & Goyal, 1985; Reid et al, 1988). The incidence of adenocarcinoma in the presence of Barrett's esophagus varies, but studies suggest an initial prevalence of approximately 8% (Cameron et al, 1985).

Knowing the type of metaplastic change helps to determine the risk of developing adenocarcinoma. Intestinal metaplasia has a much greater malignant potential than gastric metaplasia (Chalasani et al, 1987). These adenocarcinomas often begin as flat lesions that can be missed on diagnostic studies. Therefore, any suspicious lesion should be biopsied at endoscopy and evaluated for dysplastic changes or a malignant focus.

EPIDEMIOLOGY

The incidence and prevalence of reflux disease are based more on estimates than actual data because there is no accepted gold standard for recognizing or excluding GERD (Wienbeck & Barnert, 1989). However, a study done by questionnaire (Isolauri & Laippala, 1995) found that 10.3% of the participants experienced gastroesophageal reflux on a daily basis. The group with the highest incidence of daily heartburn is pregnant women (48% to 79% in European studies; Bainbridge, 1983; Baron & Richter, 1992).

DIAGNOSTIC CRITERIA

A diagnosis of GERD is often made by history alone. A definitive diagnosis, however, can be made by endoscopy or, with more advanced inflammation, a barium swallow, or by pH probe monitoring.

HISTORY AND PHYSICAL EXAMINATION

Patients with GERD often have some degree of symptomatology, but the degree of symptoms and the objective findings on diagnostic studies do not always correlate. All too often, patients with GERD are evaluated via a barium swallow that is interpreted as normal, and patients are told nothing was found—therefore, nothing is wrong. In reality, they may have only mild inflammation, which is not detected by barium studies but nevertheless causes a great deal of discomfort.

The patient's description of the pain is usually burning and substernal, although often patients describe it as a dull ache. Other common features of the pain are that onset of symptoms occurs when the patient is supine or after meals; temporary relief is provided by antacids; and intermittent dysphagia occurs.

When obtaining the history, it is prudent to determine the duration of symptoms, the timing of symptoms (day or night), whether there has been a significant change in symptoms, and relieving or aggravating factors. Nocturnal symptoms are common because of the supine position at bedtime. When supine, gravity causes layering of gastric juices, which results in cephalad flow toward the distal esophagus.

Less typical presenting manifestations are cough and hoarseness. The cough is usually nocturnal and must be differentiated from other causes, such as asthma, postnasal drip, or congestive heart failure. GERD is sometimes diagnosed by the otolaryngologist when persistent hoarseness, secondary to inflammation of the vocal cords, is caused by acid reflux.

Water brash, another manifestation of GERD, is described as excess saliva ("water") in the mouth. Typically it has a bitter or sour taste and is caused by the reflux of gastric juices. Water brash occurs mostly at night and represents a more severe form of GERD.

Benign peptic strictures causing dysphagia may be a presenting manifestation of GERD. However, the provider can never be certain whether the stricture is benign or malignant by history alone. Clues in the history that suggest benignity include a prolonged history of reflux with a recent decrease in reflux symptoms. This is caused by the presence of the stricture.

DIAGNOSTIC STUDIES

Esophogastroduodenoscopy (EGD) remains the gold standard for diagnosing all degrees of GERD and its complications (Table 23-1), except for perforation. If a perforation is suspected, a chest radiograph and computed tomography scan of the chest to find free air in the mediastinum are the first studies performed. EGD is contraindicated in patients with suspected perforation because of the likelihood of further spillage into the mediastinum, with resultant severe mediastinal infection. EGD enables the provider to evaluate the esophagus for the degree of inflammation, erosive changes, Barrett's metaplasia, stricture formation, and hiatal hernia.

A barium swallow is also a popular method of evaluating the esophagus. The advantages of the barium swallow include its noninvasive nature; it is easily tolerated and safer for evaluating patients with dysphagia. In patients with dysphagia, it is sometimes difficult for the patient to locate the exact point at which the food tends to "stick." A barium swallow safely identifies the area of narrowing, which may be in the proximal, middle, or distal esophagus.

Few other laboratory studies are needed when diagnosing or treating GERD. If a patient has hemorrhaged, the hemoglobin/hematocrit becomes important. Another diagnosis to consider in patients with difficult-to-treat GERD is Zollinger-Ellison syndrome. A fasting serum gastrin level and, if indicated, a secretin stimulation test can be obtained (see Chap. 29 for a description of the secretin stimulation test).

TREATMENT OPTIONS, EXPECTED OUTCOMES, AND COMPREHENSIVE MANAGEMENT

Self-Care

Dietary therapy remains an essential part in both the initial treatment of GERD and in attempts to prevent relapse after completion of therapy (Fig. 23-1). Medical therapy is an adjunct to dietary therapy, and medical therapy should never be used in place of dietary therapy. Certain foods are commonly associated with worsening symptoms (Table 23-2) and should be avoided. These foods and beverages cause the LES pressure to decrease.

Other self-care measures must be stressed. Avoiding large meals 2 hours before bedtime and elevating the head while supine (with either an extra pillow or by elevating the head of the bed with wooden blocks) are usually helpful. Smoking cessation must be stressed, as should avoidance of alcohol.

Medication Therapy

Because reflux disease is such a common problem, patients have often attempted to treat themselves with either antacids or, more recently, over-the-counter H-2 blockers. When the patient presents, the provider must explore which remedies were tried and their effectiveness. If the patient's symptoms are of recent onset, empiric therapy with either proton pump inhibitors or high-dose H-2 blockers is reasonable. However, if the patient has had these symptoms for numerous months or years, Barrett's esophagus may be present, and further investigation should be considered.

Assuming that reflux esophagitis is diagnosed and Barrett's esophagitis is not present, aggressive acid suppression should be the next step. Proton pump inhibitors remain the gold standard for treatment of established esophagitis (Porro et al, 1992; Heudebert et al, 1997). Treatment for 10 to 12 weeks (Table 23-3) is now recommended to ensure 90% to 95% healing (Schulman & Orlando, 1995; Klinkenberg-Knol & Meuwissen, 1992), although patients will often note marked relief within days of initiating therapy.

H-2 blockers are much less effective at doses used to treat peptic ulcer disease (Marks & Richter, 1991). For years, patients with reflux disease were treated with the same twice-daily doses of H-2 blockers that were prescribed for ulcer disease. Not surprisingly, these patients often had temporary relief of symptoms but had recurrence of symptoms once off the H-2 blockers. Higher doses of H-2 blockers are more effective in treating GERD.

TABLE 23-1   Complications of GERD

- Perforation: a surgical emergency
- Peptic stricture: a benign condition, but malignant causes for strictures (ie, esophageal carcinoma) should always be excluded.
- Bleeding: occurs when mucosal damage extends to the underlying blood vessels

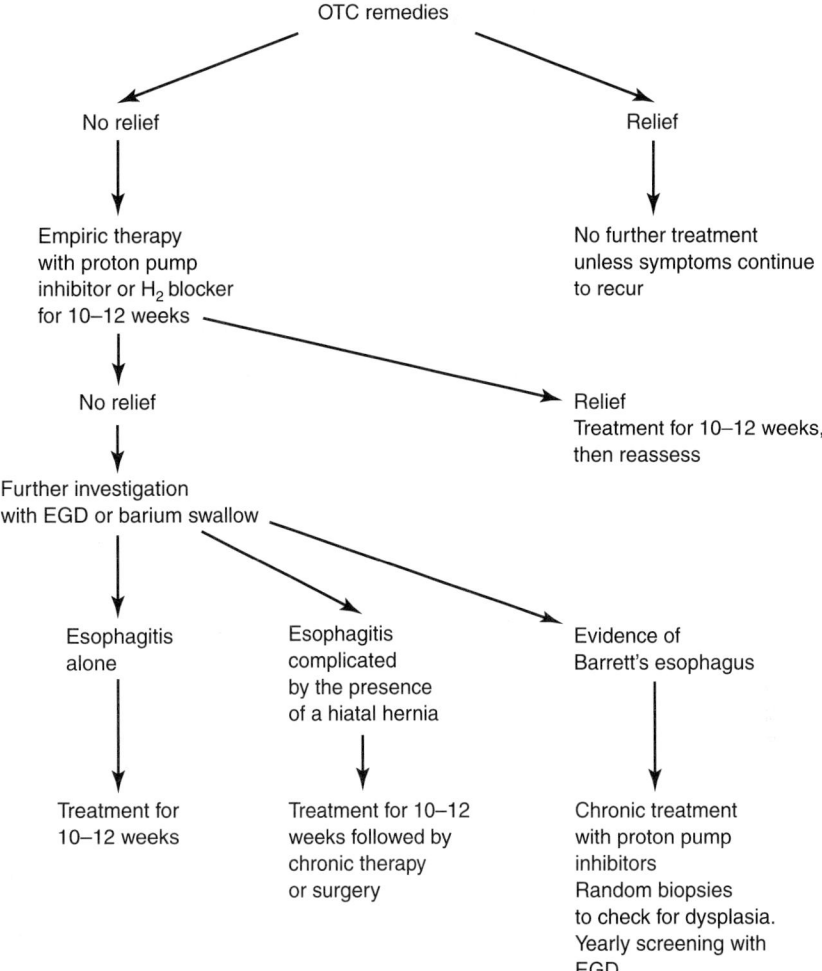

FIGURE 23-1 Treatment approach to patients with GERD.

After a full course of therapy (approximately 10 to 12 weeks), patients often require a lesser degree of acid suppression to remain symptom-free. Either low-dose proton pump inhibitors or H-2 blockers usually suffice. However, because no medication should be used indefinitely if possible, self-care measures should continue.

Cisapride is also used in the treatment of GERD. Its mechanism of action is multifactorial. Cisapride increases the LES pressure, increases the strength of esophageal peristalsis, and improves gastric emptying. This allows less reflux with greater gastric emptying.

TABLE 23-2	Foods Commonly Associated With GERD

- Chocolate
- Caffeine
- Alcohol
- Spearmint
- Spicy foods
- Fatty foods
- Acidic foods (eg, orange juice)

Surgical Treatment

When a patient's GERD is caused by the presence of a large hiatal hernia, chronic acid suppression is often required. Surgical repair remains a viable option for these patients. It would obviate the need for chronic acid suppression and is the most definitive way to approach GERD. However, as with any surgery, the risks and benefits of both anesthesia and the surgery itself must always be considered.

COMMUNITY RESOURCES

A list of community resources is located at the end of the unit on gastrointestinal disorders.

REFERRAL POINTS

In the following cases the patient should be referred to a gastroenterologist:

- Progressive dysphagia
- Intermittent dysphagia
- Persistent GERD despite treatment
- Weight loss associated with GERD
- Chronic GERD (>6 months)
- Evidence of a large hiatal hernia on barium studies.

TABLE 23-3	Treatment Regimens for GERD	
Medication	**Dosage**	**Duration (wk)**
Omeprazole (Prilosec)	20–40 mg/day	10–12
Lansoprazole (Prevacid)	30–60 mg/day	10–12
Ranitidine (Zantac)	300–600 mg/day	10–12
Nizatidine (Axid)	300–600 mg/day	10–12
Cimetidine (Tagamet)	800–1600 mg/day	10–12
Famotidine (Pepcid)	40–80 mg/day	10–12
Cisapride (Propulsid)	10 mg 15 minutes before meals and at bedtime	To be determined for each patient

■ ■ ■ CLINICAL PEARLS

- Cigarette smoking is a major cause of GERD.
- Chest pain often thought to be cardiac in origin may very well be secondary to GERD.
- If GERD symptoms improve and then dysphagia develops, consider a peptic stricture.
- Intermittent dysphagia in the presence of GERD is secondary to dysmotility induced by the inflamed esophagus. The dysphagia will resolve with aggressive treatment of the GERD.
- Nocturnal cough may be the only manifestation.

References

Bainbridge, E.T. (1983). Symptomatic gastroesophageal reflux in pregnancy. A comparative study of white Europeans and Asians in Birmingham. *British Journal of Clinical Practice, 37,* 53.

Baron, T.W., & Richter, J.E. (1992). Gastroesophageal reflux disease in pregnancy. *Gastroenterology Clinics of North America, 21*(4), 777–791.

Cameron, A.J., Ott, B.J., & Payne, W.S. (1985). The incidence of adenocarcinoma in columnar-lined (Barrett's) esophagus. *N Engl J Med, 313,* 857.

Chalasani, N, Wo, J.M., Hunter, J.G., & Waring J.P. (1997). Significance of intestinal metaplasia in different areas of esophagus including esophagogastric junction. *Digestive Disease Science, 42*(3), 603–607.

Heudebert, G.R., Marks, R., Wilcox, C.M., & Centor, R.M. (1997). Choice of long-term strategy for the management of patients with severe esophagitis: A cost-utility analysis. *Gastroenterology, 112,* 1078–1086.

Holloway, R.H., Penagini, R., & Ireland, A.C. (1995). Criteria for objective definition of transient lower esophageal sphincter relaxation. *American Journal of Physiology, 268*(1 Pt 1), G128–133.

Isolauri, J., & Laippala, P. (1995). Prevalence of symptoms suggestive of gastro-oesophageal reflux disease in an adult population. *Annals of Medicine, 27*(1), 67–70.

Klinkenberg-Knol, E.C., & Meuwissen, S.G.M. (1992). Medical therapy of patients with reflux oesophagitis poorly responsive to H$_2$-receptor antagonist therapy. *Digestion, 51*(suppl. 11), 44–48.

Marks, R.D., & Richter, J.E. (1991). Gastroesophageal reflux disease. In D. Zikim & A.J. Dannenberg (Eds.). *Peptic ulcer disease and other acid-related disorders.* New York: Academic Research Associates, pp. 247–314.

Mittal, R.K., & McCallum, R.W. (1987). Characteristics of transient lower esophageal sphincter relaxation in humans. *American Journal of Physiology, 252,* G636.

Porro, G.B., Pace, F., Peraccha, A., et al. (1992). Short-term treatment of refractory reflux esophagitis with different doses of omeprazole or ranitidine. *Journal of Clinical Gastroenterology, 1,* 72–75.

Reid, B.J., Haggitt, R.C., & Rubin, C.E. (1988). *Barrett's esophagus. Medical and surgical management.* Philadelphia: W.B. Saunders.

Schulman, M.I., & Orlando, R.C. (1995). Treatment of gastroesophageal reflux. The role of proton pump inhibitors. In R.W. Schrier, J.D. Baxter, F. Abboud F, et al (Eds.). *Advances in Internal Medicine.* St. Louis: Mosby, pp. 273–302.

Spechler, S.J., & Goyal, R.K. (1985). *Barrett's esophagus. Pathophysiology, diagnosis and management.* New York: Elsevier.

Wienbeck, M., & Barnert, J. (1989). Epidemiology of reflux disease and reflux esophagitis. *Scandinavian Journal of Gastroenterology, 24*(suppl. 156), 7.

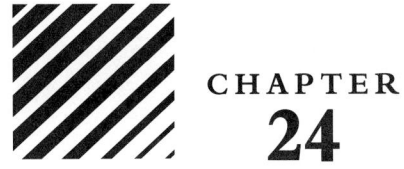

CHAPTER
24
Gastroenterologic Cancers

ESOPHAGEAL CANCER
Richard W. Golub, MD, FACS, and Nuria Lawson, MD

Cancer of the esophagus is a rare but aggressive malignancy, the etiology of which remains uncertain. Most patients present with locally advanced disease and have a poor overall survival rate and diminished quality of life. Approximately 95% of patients who have esophageal cancer will die from it, and 75% of patients will die within 1 year of diagnosis. Efforts to lower mortality rates in the United States have so far been disappointing. Despite many new and innovative approaches to the treatment of esophageal cancer, the 5-year survival rate has shown only modest improvement. Screening the population at large for early and perhaps treatable esophageal cancer is difficult and impractical. Nevertheless, epidemiologic data suggest that the incidence of esophageal cancer can be greatly reduced if environmental risk factors are controlled. In addition, identifying patients at risk for this disease increases the likelihood that patients will present with earlier, more favorably staged disease.

ANATOMY, PHYSIOLOGY, AND PATHOLOGY

The esophagus is a muscular tube, approximately 18 to 26 cm long, that extends from the level of the 6th cervical to the 11th thoracic vertebra. It has no significant secretory or absorptive functions and works solely to transport swallowed material from the pharynx to the stomach. In its mediastinal course, the esophagus is closely related to the trachea, bronchus, pulmonary veins, pericardium, and left atrium anteriorly, the pleura and lungs laterally, and the vertebral column and thoracic aorta posteriorly. Separating the esophagus from the vertebral column are the thoracic duct, azygos and hemiazygos veins, and posterior intercostal arteries. Unlike the remainder of the gastrointestinal tract, the esophagus has no serosa. It is separated from adjacent structures by only a loose connective tissue that provides little barrier to the local spread of tumor.

For convenience, the esophagus is often divided into upper, middle, and lower thirds. The upper third extends to the aortic arch, the middle third to the inferior pulmonary vein, and the lower third to the esophagogastric junction.

Cancer of the esophagus has a propensity for rapid invasion of the esophageal wall and easy, widespread dissemination by way of a rich lymphatic supply. In general, lymphatic metastases involve the regional nodes closest to the site of primary tumor. However, because of the rich anastomoses of intramural lymphatic channels, nodal involvement may occur at substantial distances from the primary lesion.

Distant metastases can be found anywhere throughout the body. The liver, lungs, pleura, and kidneys are the most common sites, but the adrenal glands, bone, brain, heart, and peritoneum can be involved. Occasionally, the tumor may extend directly into mediastinal structures before distant metastasis is evident.

PATHOLOGY
Squamous Cell Carcinoma

Squamous cell carcinoma is the most common tumor of the esophagus, accounting for approximately 95% of esophageal cancers worldwide and 60% of esophageal cancers in the United States. Unless detected in its earliest stages, it is usually fatal in less than 5 years. Histologically, the tumor is composed of sheets of polygonal or polyhedral cells with varying degrees of differentiation. Well-differentiated tumors contain features such as keratin pearls and intercellular bridges, whereas poorly differentiated tumors have marked nuclear and cellular pleomorphism. The majority of tumors, however, are moderately differentiated. Macroscopically, 60% of these lesions are fungating intraluminal growths, 25% are ulcerative lesions associated with extensive infiltration of the adjacent esophageal wall, and 15% are infiltrating. Approximately 8% of tumors occur in the cervical esophagus, 55% in the upper and midthoracic segments, and 37% in the lower thoracic segment (Orringer, 1997).

Adenocarcinoma

Adenocarcinomas can arise at any level but are located most often at or near the gastroesophageal junction. Histologically, various degrees of glandular differentiation are noted, but well-differentiated tumors predominate. Esophageal adenocarcinoma is typically flat or ulcerated, although about one third of lesions are polypoid or fungating.

Other Malignancies

Several other rare types of esophageal malignant tumors occur, and all have a poor prognosis. Anaplastic small cell (oat cell) carcinoma accounts for fewer than 2% of esophageal cancers. Like their pulmonary counterparts, they arise from the APUD cell system and demonstrate neurosecretory granules on electron microscopy. Malignant melanoma is exceedingly rare and constitutes less than 0.1% of esophageal malignancies. The tumor is more common in men and is clinically indistinguishable from other esophageal neoplasms. Adenoid cystic carcinoma typically occurs as a middle-third esophageal tumor and is usually discovered late in its course. Carcinosarcoma of the esophagus (also known as pseudosarcoma, spindle cell carcinoma, or polypoid carcinoma) is a tumor with histologic features of both squamous cell carcinoma and malignant spindle

277

cell sarcoma. Found primarily in the distal two thirds of the esophagus, it can grow large (10 to 15 cm) (Xu et al, 1984, Orringer, 1997). Sarcomas of the esophagus are rare, but a number of variants have been described. These include leiomyosarcoma, fibrosarcoma, rhabdomyosarcoma, liposarcoma, and malignant mesenchymoma. Primary malignant lymphoma is also infrequent but is occasionally reported in patients with AIDS (Moses et al, 1995). Finally, involvement of the esophagus by another primary tumor, either by direct extension or metastatic spread, has been reported with cancers of the breast, lung, liver, kidney, prostate, and stomach (Kadakia et al, 1992; Vansant & Davis, 1971; Nussbaum & Grossman, 1976).

EPIDEMIOLOGY

There is wide variation in the incidence of esophageal carcinoma throughout the world. Although the disease is uncommon in most of Western Europe and the United States, clusters of high incidence occur in certain parts of Asia and Africa. Esophageal cancer is of epidemic proportion in northeastern Iran, the Transkei of South Africa, Linxian County in the Henan province in northern China, certain areas of southern Russia, India, the Middle East, Singapore, southern Uruguay, and sporadic areas in Europe such as northern France and Italy (Duranceau, 1988). According to the World Health Organization, mortality rates are highest in China, Puerto Rico, and Singapore (Roth et al, 1997). This variation, which cannot be explained by differences in reporting, indicates a great geographic range in etiologic factors for this cancer.

By comparison, esophageal cancer is relatively uncommon in North America, Australia, and most European countries, where the reported incidence is 3 to 10 cases per 100,000 population. The peak incidence is between the fifth and seventh decades, and men predominate by six- to eightfold. The incidence among African American men (16.8/100,000) is higher than that of any other ethnic group. For both African American men and women, the death rate is approximately three times the rate in the white population (Duranceau, 1988).

Since the mid-1970s, tumor registry data obtained from the Surveillance, Epidemiology and End Results (SEER) program have shown a decrease in the incidence of squamous cell carcinoma of the esophagus and an increase in adenocarcinoma of 5% to 10% per year (Blot et al, 1991). This increase exceeded that of any other cancer during this period. In fact, nearly half of all newly diagnosed cases of esophageal cancer in the United States are adenocarcinomas, and white men account for the majority of these cases (Blot et al, 1991; Blot et al, 1993; Daly et al, 1996). Most of these tumors arise in the lower third of the esophagus in the sixth decade of life and have a male/female ratio of 3:1.

ETIOLOGY AND RISK FACTORS

The etiology of esophageal carcinoma remains unknown, but a number of factors, such as environmental exposure, dietary habits, chronic mucosal irritation, infection, cultural influences, and genetic predisposition, have been implicated (Table 24-1). A complex interaction among these risk factors probably exists, and their effects may be additive or even synergistic.

TABLE 24-1	**Risk Factors Associated With Esophageal Cancer**

DIETARY
N-nitroso compounds
Alcohol (liquor > beer)
Hot tea
Tannins
Vitamin deficiency (A, E, and C, niacin, zinc)
Retinol-containing foods

CHRONIC IRRITATION
Tobacco
Betel nut chewing
Esophagitis (GERD, hiatal hernia, radiation)
Strictures (lye, radiation)
Injection sclerotherapy
Barrett's esophagus

CHRONIC INFECTION
Fungal
Viral (HPV)

MISCELLANEOUS
Previous head and neck malignancy
Achalasia
Plummer-Vinson syndrome
Tylosis
Celiac disease
Previous gastrectomy
Esophageal diverticula

Several epidemiologic studies implicate tobacco use and alcohol consumption as predisposing factors in the development of squamous cell carcinoma of the esophagus, especially in the United States and Western Europe (Schoenberg et al, 1971; Pottern et al, 1981). The risk from alcohol is directly related to the quantity and the type of alcohol ingested, hard liquor posing a greater threat than wine or beer (Pottern et al, 1981).

Although cigarettes have received the most attention, tobacco can be carcinogenic in any form. Pipe tobacco, cigars, snuff, and chewing tobacco all increase the risk (Rogot & Murray, 1980; Doll & Peto, 1976; Mimic et al, 1988; Altorki et al, 1992). The precise mechanism of tobacco carcinogenesis has not been fully characterized, but smoke constituents such as nitrosamines presumably play a role. In general, smokers run a risk four times greater than nonsmokers of developing esophageal cancer (Krevsky, 1995).

Multiple risk factors for the development of adenocarcinoma of the esophagus have been proposed. Unlike squamous cell carcinoma, there is no evidence that tobacco, alcohol, or diet plays a major pathogenic role in the development of esophageal adenocarcinoma. The only known predisposing factor is Barrett's mucosa (metaplastic columnar epithelium), with severe dysplasia developing from chronic gastroesophageal reflux. Patients with a columnar-lined lower esophagus (Barrett's metaplasia) are 40 times more likely to develop adenocarcinoma than the general population (Cameron et al, 1985; Orringer, 1997).

TABLE 24-2	American Joint Committee on Cancer Staging of Esophageal Cancer

PRIMARY TUMOR (T)

TX	Primary tumor cannot be assessed
T0	No evidence of primary tumor
Tis	Carcinoma *in situ*
T1	Tumor invades lamina propria or submucosa
T2	Tumor invades muscularis propria
T3	Tumor invades adventitia
T4	Tumor invades adjacent structures

REGIONAL LYMPH NODES (N)

NX	Regional lymph nodes cannot be assessed
N0	No regional lymph node metastasis
N1	Regional lymph node metastasis

DISTANT METASTASIS (M)

MX	Distant metastasis cannot be assessed
M0	No distant metastasis
M1	Distant metastasis

TUMORS OF THE LOWER THORACIC ESOPHAGUS:

M1a	Metastasis in celiac lymph nodes
M1b	Other distant metastasis

TUMORS OF THE MIDTHORACIC ESOPHAGUS:

M1a	Not applicable
M1b	Nonregional lymph nodes or other distant metastasis

TUMORS OF THE UPPER THORACIC ESOPHAGUS:

M1a	Metastasis in cervical nodes
M1b	Other distant metastasis

STAGE GROUPING

0	Tis	N0	M0
I	T1	N0	M0
IIA	T2	N0	M0
	T3	N0	M0
IIB	T1	N1	M0
	T2	N1	M0
III	T3	N1	M0
	T4	Any N M0	
IV	Any T	Any N M1	
IVA	Any T	Any N M1a	
IVB	Any T	Any N M1b	

American Joint Committee on Cancer. (1998). AJCC Cancer Staging Manual, 5/e. Chicago: The American College of Surgeons.

DIAGNOSTIC CRITERIA

After a histologic diagnosis is made, patients with esophageal carcinoma are best staged by the Tumor–Node–Metastasis (TNM) system developed jointly by the American Joint Committee on Cancer and the International Union Against Cancer. In this system the esophagus is divided into four regions:

- Cervical, from the lower border of the cricoid cartilage to the thoracic inlet, approximately 18 cm from the upper incisor teeth
- Upper thoracic, from the thoracic inlet to the tracheal bifurcation at approximately 24 cm
- Midthoracic, from the tracheal bifurcation to half the distance to the esophagogastric junction at 32 cm
- Lower thoracic, extending to 40 cm and including the intra-abdominal portion of the esophagus and the esophagogastric junction (AJCC, 1997).

The most recent TNM classification and stage grouping is presented in Table 24-2.

In addition to stage, several aspects of tumor biology are associated with a poor prognosis. These include a poor histopathologic grade, DNA ploidy status, and a high score on the argyrophilic nucleolar organizer regions test (AgNOR number) (Haskell, 1995). Anatomic location has also been found to have prognostic significance, with upper and midthoracic lesions having a less favorable outcome than other sites (AJCC, 1997).

HISTORY AND PHYSICAL EXAMINATION

History

Dysphagia and weight loss are the initial symptoms of carcinoma of the esophagus in 90% of patients (Table 24-3). Unfortunately, these are late symptoms in the natural history of the disease. Because of its distensibility, difficulty in swallowing does not occur until at least half the circumference of the esophagus has been infiltrated by cancer (Skinner, 1976). By this time, the tumor may have grown to a significant size, with local invasion or metastases. Occasionally, the onset of dysphagia is sudden, but most patients complain of an ill-defined retrosternal discomfort or a vague difficulty in swallowing for the preceding 3 to 6 months. Although most patients can localize the site of obstruction, this does not always correlate with the actual location of the tumor. Odynophagia (painful swallowing) occurs in more than 20% of patients and may be the only presenting symptom. Weight loss is common, but severe weight loss and cachexia are infrequently seen and are usually indicative of locally advanced or widespread disease. Patients may also experience regurgitation of undigested food, epigastric pain, or aspiration pneumonia.

TABLE 24-3	Presenting Signs and Symptoms of Esophageal Cancer

Dysphagia
Regurgitation
Vomiting
Weight loss
Cough
Pain
Cachexia
Hoarseness
Dyspnea
Neck mass
Hemoptysis
Hematemesis
Tracheoesophageal fistula

American Joint Committee on Cancer. (1997). AJCC Cancer Staging Manual, 5/e. Chicago: The American College of Surgeons.

Advanced lesions may present with a variety of symptoms such as hematemesis, melena, superior vena cava syndrome, cough from a bronchoesophageal or tracheoesophageal fistula, hemoptysis, or problems related to nerve involvement (ie, Horner's syndrome or paralysis of the recurrent laryngeal or phrenic nerve) (Akiyama, 1990; Roth et al, 1997). Aortoesophageal fistula is a rare but lethal complication. Other signs of unresectable malignant disease may be found with malignant pleural effusion or malignant ascites.

Physical Examination

Apart from features of recent weight loss, the physical examination is often unremarkable, and the diagnosis of esophageal cancer will depend on radiographic or endoscopic data. However, the physical examination should encompass a thorough search for evidence of metastases. Supraclavicular or cervical lymph nodes should be sought and samples taken for biopsy if palpable. Enlargement of the left gastric, celiac, and retropancreatic nodes may be palpable in thin or cachectic patients, and there may be hepatomegaly in patients with liver metastases. Other evidence of intra-abdominal disease includes the presence of an epigastric mass, ascites, enlarged ovaries (Krukenberg tumors), or a Blumer's shelf on rectal examination (Fok & Wong, 1996). Documentation of metastatic disease establishes the presence of a stage IV tumor.

Disease Course

Squamous cell carcinoma of the esophagus is an aggressive tumor. It tends to infiltrate locally, involving adjacent lymph nodes and metastasizing widely by lymphatic or hematogenous routes. Lack of an esophageal serosal layer tends to favor local tumor extension into such structures as the pericardium, aorta, tracheobronchial tree, diaphragm, and left recurrent laryngeal nerve. Lymph node metastases are present in at least 75% of patients at the time of diagnosis. Distant spread to the liver and lung is common. The overall prognosis of invasive squamous cell carcinoma is poor, with only 5% to 12% of patients surviving 5 years. Extraesophageal tumor extension is present in 70% of cases at the time of diagnosis, and the 5-year survival rate is only 3% when lymph node metastases are present, compared with 42% when there is no lymph node spread (Orringer, 1997).

As is the case with squamous cell carcinoma, adenocarcinoma of the esophagus exhibits aggressive behavior, with frequent transmural invasion and lymph node metastases. Distant spread is common, with the liver and lung most frequently involved. The 5-year survival rate for esophageal adenocarcinoma is only 0% to 7%, with the presence of lymph node metastases significantly decreasing survival (Orringer, 1997).

DIAGNOSTIC STUDIES

Laboratory abnormalities are often nonspecific in patients with esophageal cancer, but they may reflect the disease stage and assist clinicians in deciding on appropriate therapy. Bleeding may result in microcytic anemia. Malnutrition may reduce the serum albumin and cholesterol levels and the white blood cell count. Elevated liver enzyme levels may be an indication of hepatic metastases. Hypercalcemia, which has been associated with a poor prognosis, has been reported in 16% to 28% of patients (Kuwano et al, 1989; Axelrad & Fleischer, 1998). The role of serum tumor markers, such as carcinoembryonic antigen, CA 19-9, CA-50, and T-4, is uncertain. Although their levels are elevated in many patients, there is still no good evidence for their use in diagnosis or screening for esophageal cancer. Pulmonary function testing and arterial blood gas measurements are helpful to quantify the extent of chronic obstructive pulmonary disease. Patients with underlying coronary artery disease should have an echocardiogram to assess left ventricular function and a stress test to assess the extent of ischemic heart disease.

A plain chest x-ray provides limited information in patients with esophageal cancer. Possible abnormalities include an air–fluid level secondary to an obstructed esophagus, infiltrates suggesting aspiration pneumonia, tracheal deviation, pulmonary nodules, pleural effusion, and mediastinal widening from lymphadenopathy. The chest film, however, may be deceptively normal, even with advanced disease.

Because dysphagia is the presenting complaint in 80% to 90% of patients with esophageal carcinoma, any patient who complains of progressive dysphagia warrants both a barium esophagram and esophagoscopy to rule out carcinoma. Barium swallow is usually the first procedure that identifies the lesion and should precede esophagoscopy whenever possible. The location of the tumor, its length, its gross pathologic characteristics, and its relation to adjacent structures may all be assessed by this study. The typical esophageal carcinoma presents with an irregular, ragged mucosal pattern with luminal narrowing. Irregular filling defects may represent polypoid or fungating lesions, and advanced tumors may present with complete luminal occlusion or demonstration of a tracheoesophageal fistula.

Regardless of how suspicious a lesion appears on contrast swallow, esophagoscopy with biopsy is mandatory to establish the diagnosis. This is especially true if cancer is suspected and the barium esophagogram is normal. Flexible fiberoptic or video endoscopy permits the direct visualization of the esophageal tumor, its anatomic extent, and associated or secondary lesions.

Accurate tissue specimens can be obtained easily under direct visual control using endoscopic instruments. Multiple biopsy specimens provide a positive yield of 85%, and in combination with brush cytology, accuracies of 90% to 100% should be readily attainable (Winawer et al, 1976).

Upper endoscopy should also include direct visualization of the oropharynx, hypopharynx, epiglottis, vocal cords, and the stomach and duodenum. The ability to inspect these regions permits the detection of synchronous lesions and allows assessment of the suitability of the stomach and duodenum for esophageal replacement.

Clinical Staging

Once the diagnosis of esophageal carcinoma has been established histologically, staging of the tumor is the next critical step in determining which therapeutic option is appropriate.

Computed tomography (CT) of the chest and upper abdomen is now the standard noninvasive technique for staging esophageal carcinoma. It may be of value in determining surgical resectability or planning for radiation therapy or endoscopic palliation. CT scanning permits evaluation of esophageal wall thickness, mediastinal invasion, and the presence of regional or distant metastases. It is particularly useful in assessing local extension of disease and its relation to adjacent structures, especially when oral contrast medium is used. It is less accurate in assessing the degree of periesophageal lymph node involvement and often underestimates the length of the esophageal lesion.

Experience with magnetic resonance imaging (MRI) seems to indicate that it does not have any particular advantage over CT and shares many of its limitations. A major problem with MRI is lack of a suitable intraluminal contrast agent. A direct comparison of CT and MRI found a comparable accuracy in predicting resectability, with both sensitivity and specificity of 85% (Takashima et al, 1991; Krevsky, 1995).

Endoscopic ultrasound (EUS) can define the depth of tumor wall invasion and associated paraesophageal lymph nodes. The use of EUS may be limited if there is an obstructing tumor that cannot be traversed by the ultrasound probe. In patients in whom the probe can be positioned within the esophageal lumen involved by tumor, however, this procedure has an 86% accuracy in defining involved mediastinal lymph nodes (Orringer, 1997).

Depending on the location of the tumor, some patients may require additional staging modalities such as mediastinoscopy, bronchoscopy, laparoscopy, thoracotomy, or thoracoscopy. Bronchoscopy may be useful in patients with carcinomas of the upper and middle third of the esophagus to evaluate for airway invasion. Endoscopic evidence of invasion to the tracheobronchial tree precludes a safe esophagectomy. Similarly, laparoscopic and thoracoscopic staging of esophageal cancer has been found to be advantageous. Preliminary results indicate that with its use, correct staging of esophageal tumors approaches 90%.

TREATMENT OPTIONS, EXPECTED OUTCOMES, AND COMPREHENSIVE MANAGEMENT

Operative Management

Surgical resection is the primary treatment modality for patients with carcinoma of the esophagus in the absence of known metastatic disease or medical contraindications to surgery. It is the only proven curative single-treatment modality for esophageal cancer and remains the gold standard by which all other therapeutic modalities are measured. Unfortunately, only half of patients have resectable disease at the time of presentation. The goal of surgical resection is the eradication of all disease, including regional lymph nodes, while relieving dysphagia and maintaining gastrointestinal continuity. Esophageal resection with lymphadenectomy offers the best chance for long-term survival in these patients, with many achieving 20% 5-year survival rates (Lee & Miller, 1997).

There are a variety of operative procedures used for the resection of esophageal cancers and subsequent reconstruction of the alimentary tract. The choice of procedure depends on many factors, including the preference of the surgeon, the location of the tumor, the patient's age and physiologic fitness, and the extent of disease on EUS and intraoperative staging. Of these, location of the tumor and the surgeon's preference are probably the two most important.

The most radical procedure is the *en bloc* resection. If preoperative staging is favorable, this procedure is undertaken with curative intent. The objective of *en bloc* resection is complete removal of the tumor with wide margins, together with most of the esophagus, adjacent connective tissue, and lymph nodes. Reconstruction of the gastrointestinal tract is usually accomplished with a gastric pull-up, but small bowel or colon can be substituted if necessary.

Regardless of the procedure used, surgical resection can be a formidable undertaking. Morbidity and mortality rates can be significant and are mainly caused by cardiopulmonary complications. A well-rehearsed team of experienced surgeons, anesthesiologists, intensivists, and support staff is critical for a successful outcome.

Radiation Therapy

Although squamous cell carcinoma is generally believed to be radiosensitive, radiation therapy as a single modality of treatment seldom achieves cure in patients with carcinoma of the esophagus. The 5-year survival rate is only 6% (Earlam & Cunha-Melo, 1980). Locoregional failure has been the main limitation and can be expected in 60% to 80% of patients (Axelrad & Fleischer, 1998). Despite these results, radiation is an important method of nonoperative palliation and provides relief of dysphagia in approximately 80% of patients, one half of whom will remain free of dysphagia until the time of death (DeMeester, 1997).

Endoluminal radiation therapy (brachytherapy) works by implanting a radioactive source directly at the tumor bed. Delivery of radiation by this means theoretically provides maximal effect to the tumor itself, with minimal risk to surrounding tissues. A complete or partial response has been seen in more than 90% of patients, and more than 90% experience significant relief of dysphagia (DeMeester, 1997). Unfortunately, nearly half of patients experience moderate to severe complications that require further therapy. Additional evaluation is therefore required to determine the ultimate role of this modality in the treatment of esophageal cancer.

Chemotherapy

Unlike surgery and radiation therapy, systemic chemotherapy has a theoretical advantage in treating esophageal cancer because most patients present with widespread systemic disease. Several drugs have been used against esophageal carcinoma, but when administered as single agents the responses are usually partial and short-lived. This has prompted an evaluation of combination chemotherapy; most protocols include cisplatin in combination with 5-fluorouracil, bleomycin, methotrexate, and vindesine. Unfortunately, with the exception of the potential to improve resectability, none of these regimens has proven effective in providing local control or improving survival.

Multimodal Therapy

Since the late 1970s, esophageal cancer trials have focused on adding chemotherapy to radiation therapy or surgical resection. The rationale is to control distant disease while dealing directly with the locoregional tumor. There is also the suggestion that certain chemotherapeutic agents may act as radiation sensitizers, thereby enhancing the efficacy of radiation therapy. At present, several ongoing studies are evaluating this form of therapy. Although surgical resectability has been improved, a clear survival advantage has not been seen. Most authors also report significant morbidity and mortality rates. Hence, there is no role for this form of therapy outside of a formal protocol.

Nonoperative Options

Because most patients with esophageal cancer present with advanced disease, curative treatment is generally not possible and palliation is the primary goal. Palliative options include surgery, radiation therapy, chemotherapy, endoscopic therapy, or supportive management only.

Mechanical dilatation is a simple and inexpensive modality that can afford relief of dysphagia in up to 70% of patients. Maloney (mercury-filled rubber) bougies or Eder-Puestow (metal olives) or Savary-Gilliard (tapered plastic) dilators have all been used successfully. Unfortunately, the procedure has a 15% failure rate and relief of dysphagia is short-lived. Complications, such as perforation and bleeding, occur in 2% to 10% of patients (DeMeester, 1997). Dilatation is useful, however, as the initial step in several alternative nonoperative palliative techniques.

Transoral intubation with a prosthesis is the most popular worldwide method for palliating advanced esophageal cancer. Advantages include simplicity, short hospitalization, and immediate improvement in dysphagia. The overall reported mortality rate ranges from 3% to 15%, and a 20% to 60% complication rate has been reported (DeMeester, 1997; Orringer, 1997). Although most patients have improved swallowing, only 10% to 50% can eat solid food. The average length of survival after palliative intubation for esophageal carcinoma is less than 6 months (Orringer, 1997). Recently, self-expanding metallic stents have been introduced in an effort to improve the ease of insertion and to lessen the complications of the standard prosthesis.

Endoscopic laser therapy is most commonly performed with a Nd-Yag (neodymium-yttrium-aluminum-garnet) laser because of its deep tissue penetration and reliable hemostatic property. Relief of dysphagia occurs in 70% to 85% of patients, but multiple treatments are usually required. The dysphagia-free period is only 6 to 8 weeks.

Photodynamic therapy has recently emerged as a more selective form of laser treatment. This involves injecting a hematoporphyrin derivative, which is selectively retained by neoplastic and reticuloendothelial tissues. Argon dye lasers or gold vapor lasers are typically used to activate the hematoporphyrin derivative, leading to release of free oxygen radicals and cell death. Limited experience with photodynamic therapy is available for esophageal cancer. Although potentially curative for early tumors, possible complications, such as stricture, hemorrhage, and perforation, have not been adequately assessed (Krevsky, 1995; Likier et al, 1991).

Injection therapy has been performed with a variety of agents, such as absolute alcohol and sodium morrhuate (Payne-James et al, 1990). The technique involves passing an endoscope beyond the tumor and injecting 0.5- or 1-mL aliquots of sclerosant directly into the tumor. Tumor necrosis and restoration of luminal patency have been achieved. The experience,

however, has not been extensive, and long-term results are inconclusive.

REFERRAL POINTS AND CLINICAL WARNINGS

Multiple treatment options and combinations have been used in the treatment of esophageal carcinoma. Because there is no standard regimen, joint assessment and management planning by a team including the primary care provider, gastroenterologist, surgeon, oncologist, and radiation therapist is often valuable. Generally, the goal of palliation is relief of dysphagia and prolongation of life, but it may also include pain management, nutritional support, or attention to the psychosocial and spiritual well-being of the patient and family.

■ ■ ■   **CLINICAL PEARLS**

- Most patients with esophageal carcinoma have widespread disease at the time of diagnosis.
- The physical examination should focus on identifying metastatic disease and comorbid factors.
- Cure is rarely achieved.
- The goals of palliation are relief of dysphagia and prolongation of life.
- The risk of developing esophageal cancer can be reduced by dietary and lifestyle modification.

References

Akiyama, H. (1990). *Surgery for cancer of the esophagus.* Baltimore: Williams & Wilkins; 10.

Altorki, N.K., Lightdale, C.J., & Skinner, D.B. (1992). Tumors of the esophagus. In S.J. Winawer (Ed.). *Management of gastrointestinal disease.* New York: Gower Medical Publishing; 1992, 24.1–24.31.

American Joint Committee on Cancer. (1997). Esophagus. In I.D. Fleming, J.S. Cooper, D.E. Henson, et al. (Eds.). *AJCC cancer staging manual,* 5th ed. Philadelphia: Lippincott-Raven; 1997, 65–69.

Axelrad, A.M., & Fleischer, D.E. (1998). Esophageal tumors. In M. Feldman, B.F. Scharschmidt, M.H. Sleisenger (Eds.). *Sleisenger & Fordtran's gastrointestinal and liver disease,* 6th ed. Philadelphia: W.B. Saunders; 540–554.

Blot, W.J., Devesa, S.S., & Fraumeni, J.F., Jr. (1993). Continuing climb in rates of esophageal adenocarcinoma: An update. *JAMA, 270,* 1320.

Blot, W.J., Devesa, S.S., Kneller, R.W., et al. (1991). Rising incidence of adenocarcinoma of the esophagus and gastric cardia. *JAMA, 265,* 1287–1289.

Cameron, A.J., Ott, B.J., & Payne, W.S. (1985). The incidence of adenocarcinoma in columnar-lined (Barrett's) esophagus. *N Engl J Med, 313,* 857.

Daly, J.M., Karnell, L.H., & Menck, H.R. (1996). National cancer data base report on esophageal carcinoma. *Cancer, 78,* 1820–1828.

DeMeester, T.R. (1997). Esophageal carcinoma: Current controversies. *Seminars in Surgical Oncology, 13,* 217–233.

Doll, R., & Peto, R. (1976). Mortality in relation to smoking: 20 years' observation on male British doctors. *British Medical Journal, 2,* 1525–1536.

Duranceau, A. (1988). Epidemiologic trends and etiologic factors of esophageal carcinoma. In N.C. Delarue, E.W. Wilkins Jr., J. Wong (Eds.). *International trends in general thoracic surgery,* vol. 4: Esophageal cancer. St. Louis: C.V. Mosby; 3–10.

Earlam, R., & Cunha-Melo, J.R. (1980). Oesophageal squamous cell carcinoma: II. A critical review of radiotherapy. *British Journal of Surgery, 67,* 457–461.

Fok, M., & Wong, J. (1996). Oesophagus. In T.G. Allen-Mersh (Ed.). *Surgical oncology.* London: Chapman & Hall; 127–138.

Haskell, C.M., Lavey, R.S., Ramming, K.P. (1995). Esophagus. In Haskell (ed.) *Cancer treatment,* 4th ed. Philadelphia: W.B. Saunders, 439–451.

Kadakia, S.C., Parker, A., & Canales, L. (1992). Metastatic tumors to the upper gastrointestinal tract: Endoscopic experience. *American Journal of Gastroenterology, 87,* 1418.

Krevsky, B. (1995). Tumors of the esophagus. In W.S. Haubrich, F. Schaffner, J.E. Berk (Eds.). *Bockus Gastroenterology,* 5th ed. Philadelphia: W.B. Saunders; 534–557.

Kuwano, H., Baba, H., Matsuda, H., et al. (1989). Hypercalcemia related to the poor prognosis of patients with squamous cell carcinoma of the esophagus. *Journal of Surgical Oncology, 42,* 229.

Lee, R.B., & Miller J.I. (1997). Esophagectomy for cancer. *Surgical Clinics of North America, 77,* 1169–1196.

Likier, H.M., Levine, J.G., & Lightdale, C.J. (1991). Photodynamic therapy for completely obstructing esophageal carcinoma. *Gastrointestinal Endoscopy, 37,* 75–78.

Mimic, Y., Garabrant, D.H., Peters, J.M., et al. (1988). Tobacco, alcohol, diet, occupation and cancer of the esophagus. *Cancer Research, 48,* 3843–3848.

Moses, A.E., Rahav, G., Bloom, A.I., et al. (1995). Primary lymphoma of the esophagus in a patient with AIDS. *Journal of Clinical Gastroenterology, 21,* 327.

Nussbaum, M., & Grossman, M. (1976). Metastases to the esophagus causing gastrointestinal bleeding. *American Journal of Gastroenterology, 66,* 467–472.

Orringer, M.B. (1997). Tumors, injuries, and miscellaneous conditions of the esophagus. In L.J. Greenfield, M.W. Mulholland, K.T. Oldham et al (Eds.). *Surgery: Scientific principles and practice,* 2d ed. Philadelphia: Lippincott-Raven; 694–735.

Payne-James, J.J., Spiller, R.C., Misiewicz, J.J., & Silk, D.B.A. (1990). Use of ethanol-induced tumor necrosis to palliate dysphagia in patients with esophagogastric cancer. *Gastrointestinal Endoscopy, 36,* 42–43.

Pottern, L.M., Morris, L.E., Blot, W.J., et al. (1981). Esophageal cancer among black men in Washington DC: I. Alcohol, tobacco, and other risk factors. *Journal of the National Cancer Institute, 67,* 777–783.

Rogot, E., & Murray, J.L. (1980). Smoking and causes of death among U.S. veterans: 16 years of observation. *Public Health Reports, 95,* 213–222.

Roth, J.A., Putnam, J.B., Jr., Rich, T.A., & Forastiere, A.A. (1997). Cancer of the esophagus. In J.T. DeVita, Jr., S. Hellman, S.A. Rosenberg (Eds.). *Cancer: Principles & practice of oncology,* 5th ed. Philadelphia: Lippincott-Raven; 980–1021.

Schoenberg, B.S., Bailar, J.C., & Fraumeni, J.R. (1971). Certain mortality patterns of esophageal cancer in the United States. *Journal of the National Cancer Institute, 46,* 1930.

Skinner, D.B. (1976). Esophageal malignancies: Experience with 110 cases. *Surgical Clinics of North America, 56,* 137–147.

Takashima, S., Takeuchi, N., Shiozaki, H., et al. (1991). Carcinoma of the esophagus: CT vs. MR imaging in determining resectability. *American Journal of Roentgenology, 156,* 297–302.

Vansant, J.H., & Davis, R.K. (1971). Esophageal obstruction secondary to mediastinal metastases from breast carcinoma. *Chest, 60,* 93–95.

Winawer, S.J., Melamed, M., & Sherlock, P. (1976). Potential of endoscopy, biopsy, and cytology in the diagnosis and management of patients with cancer. *Clinical Gastroenterology, 5,* 575–595.

Xu, L., Sun, C., Wu, L., et al. (1984). Clinical and pathological characteristics of carcinosarcoma of the esophagus: Report of four cases. *Annals of Thoracic Surgery, 37,* 197.

GASTRIC CANCER

Francis Cannizzo, Jr., MD, PhD,
and Richard W. Golub, MD, FACS

Cancer of the stomach is a disease with an almost uniformly poor prognosis. This, combined with its global distribution, makes gastric cancer a major worldwide public health concern. Research into the basic biology, prevention, diagnosis, and treatment of this disease has accrued over the past century. In that time, though, the greatest reduction in overall morbidity and mortality rates has been realized through primary prevention via public health initiatives and tertiary treatment by the introduction and refinement of new surgical techniques.

ANATOMY, PHYSIOLOGY, AND PATHOLOGY

Gastric Carcinoma

The vast majority of gastric malignancies are carcinomas. The incidence of gastric carcinoma increases with age. The current view is that carcinomas of the stomach have a long latency period that is often associated with recognizable precancerous lesions. Gastric acid inhibits the growth of bacteria within the stomach. Bacteria have been demonstrated to generate carcinogenic nitrosamine compounds from salivary and dietary nitrates. Conditions that lead to gastric achlorhydria may therefore predispose to gastric cancer. Intestinal metaplasia and chronic atrophic gastritis are two conditions associated with achlorhydria that have been linked with gastric cancer in correlation studies. Both chronic atrophic gastritis and intestinal metaplasia are more prevalent in areas with high rates of gastric cancer (Dobrilla et al, 1994).

Helicobacter pylori is a recently discovered microaerophilic, gram-negative, spiral-shaped bacterium that commonly has been found in patients with acute and chronic inflammation of the gastric antrum. Because of the known association between gastritis and gastric cancer, there has been speculation about the role of *H. pylori* in the causation of gastric cancer, and several large cohort studies have confirmed this suspicion. However, *H. pylori* infection is common in the general population, and most persons with *H. pylori* will not develop cancer (Mera, 1995; Graham et al, 1995).

One reason for the lack of success in indicting a particular agent or sequence as the definitive cause of gastric carcinoma is the large number of strongly associated factors that have been studied. The sharp fall in gastric cancer in this country began in 1930, shortly after the passage and enforcement of the Pure Food and Drug Act of 1927. This realization contributed to a search for a nutritional cause of gastric cancer that began in the 1950s and continues today. In the course of that work, it has been found that diets rich in smoked or pickled foods containing preformed N-nitroso compounds or nitrites, respectively, (Neugut et al, 1996) or high consumption of salted foods or alcohol (Francheschi & LaVecchia, 1994) are closely correlated with an increased lifetime risk of developing gastric carcinoma. Conversely, diets high in raw fruits and vegetables and antioxidants such as vitamins C, E, and beta-carotene (Correa, 1995; Hwang et al, 1994) are strongly correlated with a reduction in the risk of gastric carcinoma (Correa, 1995).

Two histologically distinct types of gastric carcinoma have been described (Lauren, 1965). The distinction between intestinal and diffuse types of carcinoma continues to have relevance today, not only as a descriptive device but because the two types are thought to have different origins, risk factors, population distributions, and prognoses (see the section on epidemiology).

Intestinal-type gastric tumors are true adenocarcinomas. They are characterized by a proliferation of atypical glandular elements containing large numbers of mucin-containing goblet cells. There is commonly a loss of polarization with a varying amount of nuclear atypia in the cells lining these glandular formations. Histologically, the diffuse type of gastric carcinoma largely lacks recognizable glandular elements and consists predominately of stromal tissue. The hallmark of this type of tumor is the large number of signet-ring cells with deeply staining basophilic nuclei. Grossly, either of these tumors may be raised, flat, or ulcerated on endoscopic examination; in addition, intestinal-type tumors may be polypoid. The gross appearance of the lesion has little association with the true depth of invasion.

Noncarcinoma Gastric Malignancies

Although 92% to 98% of all gastric malignancies are adenocarcinomas, there are also three relatively uncommon tumors. The first of these is the primary gastric lymphoma. This represents 3% to 4% of all gastric malignancies and is predominately of the non-Hodgkin's type. Gastric lymphomas arise from the mucosal-associated lymphoid tissue. The majority of these tumors are composed of B-lymphocytes and have long growth cycles, tending to remain within the stomach (Isaacson & Spencer, 1996). Primary T-cell lymphomas are much less common and tend to be more aggressive in their growth and spread. Finally, although histiocytic lymphomas and true Hodgkin's disease of the stomach have been reported in the literature, the incidence of these tumors is vanishingly small. Like lymphoma at most other sites in the body, gastric lymphomas tend to be highly responsive to radiation and chemotherapy. Nonetheless, surgical excision, where possible, remains an important part of the therapeutic regimen.

Prognosis for all of these tumors is related to the stage of the disease at diagnosis and the histologic type of tumor. Early B-cell lymphomas are reported to have a 75% 5-year survival rate and late-stage T-cell lymphomas as low as a 32% 5-year survival rate (Aozasa et al, 1988).

Gastric leiomyosarcomas constitute approximately 1% to 2% of all gastric malignancies. These smooth muscle tumors can grow to large size, protruding primarily into the peritoneal cavity rather than into the lumen of the stomach. They are usually slow-growing tumors and it can be challenging to distinguish them from benign leiomyomas. Often the definitive diagnosis of malignancy can be made only after surgical resection, when the entire specimen is available for examination. In most cases, though, size is a good indicator of malignancy: tumors less than 4 cm are likely to be benign, those exceeding 6 cm malignant. Five-year survival rates after surgical excision have been reported to be as high as 55% for patients with smaller tumors but 30% for those with tumors greater than 8 cm.

The third major noncarcinoma tumor is the gastric carcinoid tumor. These endocrine tumors have been estimated to represent 3% of all gastric tumors. Although histologically similar, the gastric carcinoids are divided into two classes based on the prevailing gastric mucosa (Bordi, 1995). The first class is the classic carcinoid tumor, which is strongly associated with chronic atrophic gastritis and Zollinger-Ellison syndrome. The hypersecretion of gastrin seen in these patients is thought to cause hyperplasia of enterochromaffin cells, resulting in carcinoid tumors. The second class of carcinoid-type tumors arises in histologically normal gastric mucosa without detectable antecedent endocrine abnormalities. These spontaneous or sporadic carcinoids are, in fact, true neuroendocrine carcinomas.

The gastritis-associated class of gastric carcinoid tumors is usually confined to the mucosa. Small tumors of this class are amenable to repeated endoscopic fulguration and treatment of the underlying gastric pathology, whereas larger tumors require surgical excision. The sporadic class is often poorly differentiated and more likely to metastasize to regional lymph nodes and distant sites. These tumors are rarely suitable for surgical intervention and have a markedly poor prognosis (Akerstrom, 1996).

EPIDEMIOLOGY

In the early part of this century, gastric cancer was the most common cancer in the United States. At that time it accounted for 35% of cancers in men and 22% of cancers in women (exceeded only by uterine cancer). Beginning around 1930, and continuing until the middle of the last decade, the incidence of stomach cancer in the United States fell to its currently stable rate of 3 per 100,000 women and 6 per 100,000 men (Boring et al, 1994). In 1994, 24,000 new cases of stomach cancer were reported. In that same year, there were 14,000 deaths attributed directly to it. The worldwide incidence of stomach cancer for men ranges from 35 per 100,000 in Japan to 6 per 100,000 in the United States, with the incidence for women averaging approximately half that of men. Within populations, rates for both sexes are higher among lower socioeconomic groups.

As the total incidence of gastric cancer declines worldwide, two apparently discrete populations of adenocarcinomas are becoming evident. The intestinal type (named for its histologic appearance) appears to be responsible for the majority of the decline. This is also the type that seems to be affected by environmental and dietary factors, because the risk of this type is reduced if a person moves from an area of high prevalence to one of low prevalence (Correa & Chen, 1994). The other type of tumor is called diffuse because of its predilection toward widespread involvement of the stomach. There is evidence linking this type of gastric cancer to genetic factors because its incidence has not been found to be associated with specific environmental factors (Elder, 1995). The incidence of diffuse-type gastric carcinoma has not changed significantly since its identification in 1965.

DIAGNOSTIC CRITERIA

There have been several systems proposed to stage gastric carcinomas throughout the years. Currently, the system most commonly used by providers in the United States is the TNM system adopted by the American Joint Commission on Cancer (AJCC; Table 24-4). This staging system is useful in standardizing communications about cancers by grouping them by extent and severity, which roughly correlates with prognosis.

The single most important property of the primary tumor in determining prognosis is the depth of invasion. Thus, the

TABLE 24-4	AJCC Staging System for Gastric Cancer

PRIMARY TUMOR

T0	No primary tumor detected
TX	Primary tumor unable to be assessed
Tis	Primary confined to the mucosa (carcinoma *in situ*)
T1	Primary involving the submucosa
T2	Primary involving the muscularis propria
T3	Primary involving the serosa
T4	Primary invading through the serosa and involving contiguous structures

LYMPH NODES

N0	No regional lymph node involvement
NX	Lymph node involvement unable to be assessed
N1	Involvement of 1 to 6 regional lymph nodes
N2	Involvement of 7 to 15 regional lymph nodes
N3	Involvement of more than 15 regional lymph nodes

DISTANT METASTASIS

M0	No distant metastasis
MX	Presence of distant metastasis unable to be assessed
M1	Distant metastasis present

STAGING

0	Tis	N0	M0
1A	T1	N0	M0
1B	T1	N1	M0
	T2	N0	M0
II	T1	N2	M0
	T2	N1	M0
	T3	N0	M0
IIIA	T2	N2	M0
	T3	N1	M0
	T4	N0	M0
IIIB	T3	N2	M0
IV	T1	N3	M0
	T2	N3	M0
	T3	N3	M0
	T4	Any N	M0
	Any T	Any N	M1

American Joint Committee on Cancer. (1997). AJCC Cancer Staging Manual, 5/e. Chicago: The American College of Surgeons.

AJCC system classifies primaries as limited to the mucosa, extending to the serosa, or extending through the serosa (with or without involvement of contiguous structures). Regional lymph node involvement is divided into three groups corresponding to the number of regional lymph nodes found to be involved with tumor (see Table 24-4). Formerly classified as regional lymph nodes, the para-aortic, hepatoduodenal, pancreatic, and mesenteric lymph nodes are now classified as distant metastases.

HISTORY AND PHYSICAL EXAMINATION

History and Physical Examination

Gastric cancer is characteristically silent in its early stages. This contributes to the late stage at which most gastric cancers are diagnosed. Characteristic symptoms of gastric tumors such as early satiety, pain, and obstruction appear late in the course of the disease. These symptoms herald extensive involvement of the gastric body or pylorus. Occasionally, large extraluminal tumors may be palpable through the abdominal wall. Linitis plastica (leather-bottle stomach) is a classic sign associated with tumor infiltration throughout the stomach. It manifests as extremely early satiety resulting from a dramatic decrease in gastric distensibility and can often be palpated through the abdominal wall in the right upper quadrant.

Disease Course and Prognosis

Although advanced gastric cancer continues to have a uniformly poor prognosis, when gastric cancer is found and treated early, survival rates can be quite high. In 1993, Wanebo et al reviewed the American experience with gastric cancer from 1982 to 1992. The results of this study found that 5-year survival rates after surgical resection with curative intent depended on stage. Patients with stage I tumors had a 50% 5-year survival, with stages II, III, and IV carrying survival rates of 29%, 13%, and 3%, respectively. An important point revealed by this study was that more than two thirds of these patients had advanced disease (stage III or IV) at the time of diagnosis. Further, most of these patients did not receive radical lymph node dissection. Local recurrence occurred in 40% of patients and distant disease in 60%.

Reports on the long-term survival of patients undergoing resection for cure and intraoperative radiotherapy are becoming available for review from many centers. The 5-year survival rate was improved in patients with stage II, III, and IV disease from 62%, 37%, and 0%, respectively, to 83%, 62%, and 14%, respectively, using mid- to high-dose radiation (28 to 36 Gy) in selected patients (Abe et al, 1987).

DIAGNOSTIC STUDIES

The association between gastric cancer and chronic gastritis should alert providers to be on the lookout for neoplasia in patients with this condition. Routine upper gastrointestinal endoscopy with biopsy of suspicious areas has been shown to be of value in increasing early detection of gastric tumors. Recently a resurgence in the use of the upper gastrointestinal series has shown that double-contrast (barium and gas) radiographic examinations may be equivalent to endoscopy in distinguishing lesions with clearly malignant or clearly benign hallmarks, with follow-up endoscopic biopsy reserved for equivocal lesions (Halvorsen et al, 1996).

These findings have led to the use of mass screening programs as an adjunct to the identification of populations at high risk for the development of gastric cancer. Such programs have been successful in Japan, where the incidence of gastric cancer is many times higher than in most places in the West. Nationwide Japanese screening programs have succeeded in increasing the proportion of gastric cancers diagnosed in early stage (before extragastric spread) to approximately 30% in recent years (Sugimachi, 1993). To reproduce these results in the United States would require enormous resources, and because of the relatively low incidence of the disease the actual outcome might still be marginal.

The workup for newly identified gastric lesions should include computed tomography (CT) or magnetic resonance imaging (MRI). Currently, CT is the preferred mode of abdominal imaging in these cases. CT is relatively sensitive in detecting gastric wall infiltration, regional and distant lymph node abnormalities, and liver and spleen extension or metastases. However, like MRI, it lacks specificity, and both are unable to distinguish tumor involvement in normal-sized lymph nodes.

A relatively new technology is currently under evaluation for its value in examining gastric cancer. Endoscopic ultrasonic (EUS) probes can be applied to the mucosal surface of the stomach to determine the depth of tumor wall invasion. In certain cases even the regional lymph nodes can be examined with much higher accuracy than conventional transabdominal techniques. The widespread use of EUS, however, is limited by several factors. The EUS-equipped endoscopes are substantially larger than standard endoscopes, preventing their passage in patients already sensitive to upper endoscopy as well as patients with esophageal narrowing. Second, accurate interpretation of data from EUS equipment requires experience, which should improve as the technology matures and research data are disseminated (Miller et al, 1997).

TREATMENT OPTIONS, EXPECTED OUTCOMES, AND COMPREHENSIVE MANAGEMENT

Because gastric cancer is commonly diagnosed late in its course, often at a stage beyond which it can be successfully excised, and because of its historically poor response to chemotherapy and radiation treatment, research into prevention, mass screening, and identification of populations at risk for earlier detection and multimodal treatment regimens has intensified in recent decades (Patino, 1994).

Surgical Treatment

The first-line treatment of newly diagnosed gastric cancer continues to be surgical excision. In most cases, total gastrectomy with attempts to remove all involved tissues back to microscopically clean margins is the ultimate goal. Such an operation is currently not possible for the majority of patients presenting with locally advanced or metastatic cancers (Dalton & Eisenberg, 1994). The standard surgical treatment in Japan has differed from that in Western countries. Japanese surgeons are generally more aggressive, making use of systemic or radical lymph node dissection. The results of such surgery have yielded significant improvements in long-term survival rates in Japanese populations. Attempts to reproduce these results in Europe and the United States have not been as successful. At first, this was attributed to lack of familiarity with the surgical technique, but with increasing Western experience with radical gastrectomy, it seems that at least a portion of the Japanese success may be related to differences in the pathophysiologic variants of gastric cancer between Japan and Western countries (Maruyama et al, 1996). These differences may render the Japanese variant more susceptible to surgical excision.

The radical nature of surgical gastrectomy for gastric cancer (whether Japanese or Western) is fraught with intra- and postoperative dangers. These are often long procedures associated with massive intra- and extracellular fluid shifts. Patients are frequently malnourished and compromised by pulmonary or cardiac abnormalities. In addition, many of these operations involve removal of the pylorus or pancreas, leaving the patient prone to dumping syndrome or postoperative diabetes (Averbach & Jacquet, 1996). Clearly, such treatment requires detailed preoperative discussion to ensure that the patient understands both the nature of the disease process and the risks of the surgical resection.

Radiochemotherapeutics

To date, no chemotherapeutic agent, either alone or in combination, has proven effective as the sole treatment for gastric cancer. As a consequence, recent research has turned toward the use of chemotherapy in conjunction with surgery. Adjuvant combination chemotherapy has shown some efficacy after curative resection, but an overall survival advantage has yet to be demonstrated (Schipper & Wagener, 1996), and toxicity can be significant. These agents affect all rapidly proliferating cell populations. This includes bone marrow suppression, with its immunocompromising effect; gastrointestinal mucosal sloughing, with concomitant malabsorption; and impairments in wound healing and regeneration of skin appendages, resulting in, among other things, hair loss.

Another strategy under study is the use of neoadjuvant therapy before surgical resection (Fink et al, 1995). Downstaging of tumor preoperatively may make curative resection more feasible. Initial studies have indicated improved tumor-free survival after neoadjuvant chemotherapy and primary resection with lymphadenectomy versus resection and lymphadenectomy alone (Nakajima, 1995). Further studies in this area are required to define which patients will benefit from this technique.

Finally, true multimodal therapy for gastric cancer is under study at various centers (Jessup et al, 1993). This approach makes use of neoadjuvant chemotherapy to shrink the tumor, followed by resection and lymphadenectomy with intraoperative radiotherapy. Although this therapy is promising, long-term survival data are not yet available and are eagerly awaited.

TEACHING AND SELF-CARE

The importance of including the patient and family in the decision-making process cannot be overstated. The goal should always be for each team member to develop a comprehensive plan that includes all available options as well as recommendations. This plan is then communicated to the other team members, including the patient, preferably at interval multidisciplinary meetings. In this way, patients can make informed decisions and assume ultimate control over their disease. For further information on self-care, refer to the section at the end of this chapter.

Complementary Therapies

Early in the history of gastric cancer research, a link was identified between certain dietary components (eg, smoked meats, salted foods, alcohol) and an increased incidence of gastric carcinoma. More recently, an association between common dietary antioxidants and a decreased risk of gastric cancer has been studied. Experimental and epidemiologic data to this effect suggest that vitamin C and carotenoids may be of value in preventing gastric cancer when taken consistently in adequate amounts. The evidence in favor of vitamin E and selenium is not as strong (Kono & Hirohata, 1996). These data support the recommendation of a diet high in fresh fruits and vegetables, consistent with current FDA recommendations. There is little

TABLE 24-8	AJCC Staging of Liver Carcinoma

PRIMARY TUMOR

TX	Primary tumor cannot be assessed
T0	No evidence of primary tumor
T1	Solitary tumor ≤2 cm without vascular invasion
T2	Solitary tumor ≤2 cm with vascular invasion; or multiple tumors limited to one lobe, none >2 cm without vascular invasion; or solitary tumor >2 without vascular invasion.
T3	Solitary tumor >2 cm with vascular invasion; or multiple tumors limited to one lobe, each <2 cm with vascular invasion; or multiple tumors limited to one lobe any >2 cm with or without vascular invasion.
T4	Multiple tumors in more than one lobe, or tumor(s) involving a major branch of the portal or hepatic vein(s)

REGIONAL LYMPH NODES

NX	Regional lymph nodes cannot be assessed
N0	No regional lymph node metastasis
N1	Regional lymph node metastasis

DISTANT METASTASIS

MX	Presence of distant metastasis cannot be assessed
M0	No distant metastasis
M1	Distant metastasis

STAGING

I	T1	N0	M0
II	T2	N0	M0
III	T1	N1	M0
	T2	N1	M0
	T3	N0	M0
	T3	N1	M0
IVA	T4	Any N	M0
IVB	Any T	Any N	M1

(American Joint Committee on Cancer. (1997). AJCC Cancer Staging Manual, 5/e. Chicago: The American College of Surgeons.)

HISTORY AND PHYSICAL EXAMINATION

The diagnosis of primary liver cancer should be suspected if a patient presents with weight loss, weakness, anorexia, malaise, right upper quadrant abdominal pain, jaundice, abdominal mass, and ascites or other evidence of portal hypertension (Keller et al, 1993). On the physical examination, firm nodular hepatomegaly, an hepatic rub, or an arterial bruit in the right upper quadrant may be found. Five percent of patients present with pulmonary metastasis, which is the most common site of metastatic disease, and many patients have metastatic disease at the time of diagnosis. HCC should be considered when patients with known cirrhosis develop signs such as unexplained clinical deterioration accompanied by changes in liver enzymes, pain, or fever.

DIAGNOSTIC STUDIES

Liver function tests evaluate liver activity by assessing the degree of functional impairment. They are not definitive diagnostic tools but can alert the clinician to a possible tumor or other liver disease. Occasionally, liver function tests may produce normal results despite the presence of significant lesions. Alkaline

phosphatase, aspartate aminotransferase (SGOT), and aspartate alanine transferase (SGPT) are three enzymes whose levels are abnormal in hepatic disease. SGOT is present in the liver, myocardium, skeletal muscles, kidney, and pancreas, and levels can be elevated if injury to any of these organs is present. SGPT is more significantly applicable to evaluation of liver disease because of its high hepatic content. Elevated levels of SGPT and lactic dehydrogenase can be indicative of hepatocellular damage and should prompt further studies. Bilirubin is an orange bile pigment produced by the breakdown of hemoglobin and excreted by liver cells. Failure of liver cells to excrete bile or bile duct obstruction can cause an increased amount of bilirubin in body fluids and thus lead to obstructive jaundice. In late liver disease, coagulopathies may occur from decreased synthesis of prothrombin.

Serum alkaline phosphatase is present in many tissues, and levels may be increased in many conditions not associated with liver disease. Levels are increased in bile duct obstruction, parenchymal disease, and liver mass lesions. Gamma-glutamyl transpeptidase (GGTP) increases in serum with hepatobiliary disease and also after myocardial infarction, in neuromuscular disease, and during ingestion of ethanol. GGTP may be useful to identify the source of an alkaline phosphatase increase but offers no clear advantage over the other available tests (Ockner, 1988). The plasma membrane 5'-nucleotidase may also help identify the source of elevated serum alkaline phosphatase activity (Ockner, 1988).

If HCC is suspected, alpha-fetoprotein (AFP) is a useful marker, especially if the patient has a cirrhotic liver or hepatitis B. Although no screening tests are routinely performed in the United States, in high-risk populations ultrasound and AFP are useful to detect liver tumors. Although AFP levels are not specific for HCC, they are elevated in 50% to 70% of those with HCC, and the increase is frequently proportional to the size or rapidity of growth of the tumor. A transient increase in AFP may also occur in benign chronic liver diseases such as cirrhosis. Ultrasound can detect small lesions and is a valuable screening tool in regions with high incidence rates of HCC.

Hepatic arteriography is helpful to confirm a liver lesion and to determine the extent of disease, particularly portal or arterial involvement. Computed tomography (CT) with intravenous contrast can define the tumor, assess the presence of extrahepatic disease, and detect lesions as small as 1 cm. CT can also differentiate among fatty, cystic, and solid lesions. Magnetic resonance imaging is useful to detect vascular lesions such as hemangioma (hemangiomas are benign vascular tumors that need no further intervention unless they bleed or cause a mass effect). Ultrasound-guided percutaneous needle biopsy can provide a histologic verification of diagnosis in patients without coagulopathy (Frogge, 1990). If hemangioma is suspected, a needle biopsy is contraindicated (Schwartz, 1994).

CT with arterial portography is the best method to study liver lesions. Contrast is injected into the superior mesenteric artery or the splenic artery, and when it has entered the portal system, delayed images are taken. The sensitivity of this test is reported to be as high as 97%. A chest x-ray should be performed to exclude pulmonary metastases.

The use of all the above liver imaging studies and laboratory tests does not increase the accuracy of diagnosis and can needlessly increase the expense associated with diagnosis (Schwartz, 1994). Consideration for radiologic studies should be based on cost-effective, appropriate clinical judgment.

As previously stated, metastatic liver disease from another primary is more common than primary liver cancer. It is critical to ascertain if the lesion is a primary liver tumor or a metastasis from another primary site. Histologic diagnosis is the key to planning treatment.

TREATMENT OPTIONS, EXPECTED OUTCOMES, AND COMPREHENSIVE MANAGEMENT

Early diagnosis, prompt treatment, optimizing quality of life, and limiting disability are the goals for patients with HCC. The tumor is difficult to detect and proliferates rapidly; although treatment options are improving, they remain suboptimal. Surgical excision is the only known curative treatment. Tumor location and size, histologic type, metastatic disease, and the general physical health of the patient must be considered when planning surgical intervention. Criteria that preclude surgery are listed in Table 24-9. If the primary tumor is a solitary mass without evidence of regional lymph node or distant metastases, or cirrhosis, surgery may be an option. The major complications of hepatic resection include hemorrhage, sepsis, biliary fistula, subphrenic abscess, pneumonia, portal hypertension, and coagulopathy (Frogge, 1990). Anemia, fluid and electrolyte status, and coagulation status should be corrected or optimized before surgery. Obviously, a total hepatectomy can be done only in the setting of liver transplant.

Cryosurgery—destruction of tumor cells by application of extreme cold—has been identified as a safe and feasible option for palliation in patients with cirrhosis (Wren et al, 1997). With this technique, liquid nitrogen is injected through the tumor using a metal probe, and one or more lesions may be treated. Anesthesia and laparotomy are necessary, and the 5-year survival rate for this procedure is about 10% (Yahanda, 1995).

Because of its multifocal nature, association with chronic liver disease, and frequent postresectional recurrence incidence, nonsurgical modalities are important in the management of these patients. Many patients with primary liver cancer are not candidates for surgery, and chemotherapy is the treatment of choice to offer symptomatic relief by arresting tumor growth. Systemic chemotherapy has provided poor results in patients with HCC. Intra-arterial (via the hepatic artery) infusions of cytotoxic drugs can deliver highly concentrated agents directly into the tumor. Studies have compared the use of single or multiple chemotherapeutic agents. Intra-arterial doxorubicin, alone or in conjunction with other agents, has produced the best response rates (Yahanda, 1995). Technical complications can arise with placement of these catheters, and complication rates vary depending on the expertise of the surgical team and arterial anatomy (Campbell et al, 1993). Angiography of the liver vasculature greatly assists the proper placement of these catheters. Percutaneous injection of ethanol and arterial chemoembolization offer a 3-year survival rate of approximately 55% to 70% and 20%, respectively (Liu & Fan, 1997).

Combined chemotherapy and external beam radiation therapy have been administered to patients with unresectable disease, rendering resectable status (Sitzmann & Abrams, 1993). The primary intra-arterial agents studied include doxorubicin, 5-fluorouracil, mitomycin C, and cisplatin. The use of effective antiemetics in conjunction with relaxation therapy can enhance the comfort of patients receiving emetogenic chemotherapy.

The role of radiation therapy alone is limited but can facilitate pain relief in some patients as a palliative measure. Distraction techniques, rhythmic breathing exercises, or imagery with appropriate analgesics may reduce pain perception (Devolder-McCray & Hogan, 1991). Jaundice is prevalent among patients with liver disease, and efforts should be made to reduce pruritus by avoiding the use of deodorant or perfumed soaps and detergents. Antihistamines can be administered to help reduce itching, but the most effective way to control the itching is by resolving the jaundice by improved liver function (if possible), resolution of ductal obstruction, or diversion of bile by stenting. These are the only methods to resolve persistent jaundice but often are not possible.

The 5-year survival rate for all stages of HCC is about 6% (Ravikumar, 1996). After treatment, surveillance by complete history and physical examination should be done at a minimum of 3-month intervals. Patients should be asked about jaundice, itching, nausea, vomiting, pain (abdominal or bone), urine color, bleeding, dyspnea, cough, and bowel function. The abdomen should be assessed for mass, organomegaly, and ascites. The lungs should also be assessed. Alkaline phosphate and bilirubin levels and a complete blood count should be obtained every 3 months (sooner if the patient is symptomatic) because biliary obstruction may indicate recurrence. A CT scan of the chest and abdomen and AFP assessment should be added at 6-month intervals.

TEACHING AND SELF-CARE

Primary care providers should be alert for patients who are at risk for HCC and should encourage health-promotion lifestyles, based on realistic goals for each patient. A reduction in the number of patients contracting hepatitis B and C will reduce the number of persons who will develop HCC. Hepatitis B vaccination should be encouraged in high-risk populations (see Chap. 26). Immigrants from countries where hepatitis B is endemic should be tested and vaccinated when appropriate. Alcohol intake should be assessed in all patients, and efforts made to teach patients about the constellation of medical issues that can evolve from chronic abuse of alcohol. If the efforts of the primary care provider fail, patients should be offered psychosocial counseling. Alcoholics Anonymous can provide support to patients who are willing to participate.

If HCC is detected early, when a lesion is localized and surgically resectable, patients have an improved prognosis. Quality of life should be considered when contemplating treatment options. Patients and their significant others should be supported to perceive some enjoyment in life despite adversity and to participate in treatment decisions. The stress of diagnosis and treatment can significantly affect a person's outlook and minimize quality of life. A psychological consultation, possibly

TABLE 24-9	**Criteria for Unresectability of Liver Carcinoma**

- Lung, bone, or lymph node metastases
- Multiple tumor nodules in both lobes of liver
- Ascites with tumor cell seeding in the peritoneum or cirrhosis
- Tumor extension or obstruction of the common bile duct
- Inferior vena cava involvement or retrograde intraluminal growth to the portal vein bifurcation

in conjunction with the use of antidepressants or mood elevators, should be considered. Manifestations of sadness, impending doom, and depression should be addressed and not dismissed as natural manifestations of the diagnosis of cancer. The best approach to treatment, surveillance, and tertiary care is a multidisciplinary one, using conventional medical therapies as well as other approaches such as guided imagery, relaxation, and hypnosis. For further information on self-care in patients with malignancy, see the self-care section at the end of this chapter.

COMMUNITY RESOURCES

Information on community resources, national organizations, and Internet sites for liver cancer is listed at the end of the unit on gastrointestinal disorders.

REFERRAL POINTS AND CLINICAL WARNINGS

On suspicion or diagnosis of HCC, appropriate referrals may include an oncologist, a surgical oncologist, a gastroenterologist, a radiation oncologist, and an interventional radiologist. Other health care workers who may need to be contacted include those who provide psychological support and the pain management team.

As participants in their care, patients and their significant others should be consulted about their wishes for management of this disease. The integrity of a person's existence is affected and multiple issues arise from the impact of cancer diagnosis and treatment. This is especially applicable to those with HCC because of its poor prognosis and insidious course.

References

American Joint Committee on Cancer. (1992). Liver (including intrahepatic bile ducts). In O.H. Beahrs, D.E. Henson, R.V. Hutter, & B.J. Kennedy (Eds.). *Manual For staging of cancer*, 4th ed. Philadelphia: J.B. Lippincott; 89–91.

Campbell, K.A., Burns, R.C., Sitzmann, J.V., Lipsett, P.A., Grochow, L.B., & Niederhuber, J.E. (1993). Regional chemotherapy devices: Effect of experience and anatomy on complications. *Journal of Clinical Oncology, 11*, 822–826.

Devolder-McCray, N., & Hogan, C. (1991). Psychosocial issues. In S.E. Otto (Ed.). *Oncology nursing*. St. Louis: Mosby Year Book; 452–467.

Frogge, M.H. (1990). Gastrointestinal cancer: Esophagus, stomach, liver, and pancreas. In S.L. Groenwald, M.H. Frogge, M. Goodman, & C.H. Yarbro (Eds.). *Cancer nursing: Principles and practice*, 2d ed. Boston: Jones and Bartlett; 806–844.

Keller, J.W., Peacock, J.L., & Smith, J.L. (1993). Cancer of the major digestive glands: Pancreas, liver, bile ducts, gallbladder. In P. Rubin (Ed.). *Clinical oncology: A multidisciplinary approach for physicians and students*, 7th ed. Philadelphia: W.B. Saunders; 597–615.

Liu, C.L., & Fan, S.T. (1997). Nonresectional therapies for hepatocellular carcinoma. *American Journal of Surgery, 173*, 358–365.

Niederhuber, J.E. (1995). Tumors of the liver. In G.P. Murphy, W. Lawrence, R.E. Lenhard (Eds.). *American Cancer Society textbook of clinical oncology*, 2d ed. Atlanta: American Cancer Society; 269–280.

Ockner, R.E. (1988). Laboratory tests in liver disease. In J.B. Wyngaarden & L.H. Smith, Jr. (Eds.). *Cecil textbook of medicine*, 18th ed. Philadelphia: W.B. Saunders; 814–817.

Parker, S.L., Tong, T., Bolden, S., & Wingo, P.A. (1997). Cancer statistics, 1997. *CA Cancer Journal for Clinicians, 47*, 5–27.

Ravikumar, T. (1996). Primary liver cancer and intrahepatic bile duct cancer. In D.S. Fischer (Ed.). *Follow-up of cancer: A handbook for physicians*. Philadelphia: Lippincott-Raven; 38–39.

Ries, L.A.G., Miller, B.A., Hankey, B.F., Kosary, C.L., Harras, A., Edwards, B.K. (Eds.). (1994). *SEER cancer statistics review, 1973–1991*. Bethesda, MD: National Cancer Institute. NIH Pub. No. 94-2789.

Saurin, J.C., Taniere, P., Mion, F., et al. (1997). Primary hepatocellular carcinoma in workers exposed to vinyl chloride, a report of two cases. *Cancer, 79*, 1671–1677.

Schwartz, S.I. (1994). Liver. In S.I. Schwartz, G.T. Shires, & F.C. Spencer (Eds.). *Principles of surgery*, 6th ed. New York: McGraw-Hill; 1319–1366.

Sitzmann, J.V., & Abrams, R. (1993). Improved survival for hepatocellular cancer with combination surgery and multimodality treatment. *Annals of Surgery, 217*, 149–154.

Wren, S.M., Coburn, M.M., Tan, M., et al. (1997). Is cryosurgical ablation appropriate for treating hepatocellular cancer? *Archives of Surgery, 132*, 599–603.

Yahanda, A.M. (1995). Hepatobiliary cancers. In D.H. Berger, B.W. Feig, & G.M. Fuhrman (Eds.). *The M.D. Anderson surgical oncology handbook*. Boston: Little, Brown & Co.; 194–223.

PANCREATIC CANCER

Wanda J. Cennerazzo

The American Cancer Society estimates that there were 27,600 new cases of pancreatic cancer and 28,100 deaths from pancreatic cancer in the United States in 1997 (Parker et al, 1997). It is the 10th most common type of cancer but the 5th most common cause of death from cancer. The 5-year survival rate for all stages is 3.3% (Caspar, 1996). Pancreatic cancer is difficult to detect and diagnose because of the anatomic location of the pancreas, the lack of screening tests, and the absence of symptoms until late in the course of the disease. As a result more than half of the cases are diagnosed at a late stage, with distant metastases already present. Fewer than 20% of patients survive 1 year after diagnosis (Lillemoe & Pitt, 1996). The overall prognosis for a patient with pancreatic cancer is poor because early detection is rare, treatment strategies are suboptimal, and the tumor is inherently aggressive.

ANATOMY, PHYSIOLOGY, AND PATHOLOGY

The anatomy of the pancreas is described in Chapter 28. Most (95%) pancreatic tumors develop in exocrine parenchyma as ductal adenocarcinoma (Evans et al, 1997). Usually ductal adenocarcinoma occurs in the head of the pancreas, but it may arise throughout the organ. Rarely (5%) islet cell carcinoma develops as a functioning insulinoma or as a nonfunctioning carcinoma. Other rare pancreatic tumors include cystadenocarcinoma (mucinous), adenosquamous carcinoma, and solid microglandular carcinoma.

EPIDEMIOLOGY

According to Surveillance, Epidemiology, and End Results (SEER) cancer statistics, white and African American men have a 1.12% and 1.08% lifetime risk, respectively, of being diagnosed and a 1.09% and 1.05% risk of dying from pancreatic cancer. White and African American women have a 1.21% and 1.4% lifetime risk, respectively, of being diagnosed and a 1.17% and 1.28% risk of dying from pancreatic cancer (Ries et al, 1994). Pancreatic cancer occurs at all ages, but the peak incidence is between 60 and 70 years of age. It is rare before age 40. Recently, the incidence of pancreas cancer has been increasing by 300 to 500 new cases per year without a clear explanation. Ethnicity may play a role in disease incidence. Japanese immigrants to the United States are slightly more likely to develop pancreatic cancer than native whites (Beazley & Cohn, 1995).

Relatively few causal effects are known for pancreatic cancer. Cigarette smoking is the most firmly established risk factor. High fat and meat intake is implicated, whereas a low-fat diet rich in fruit and vegetables seems to reduce the risk (Evans et al, 1997). There is limited evidence that alcohol abuse, coffee intake, diabetes, chronic pancreatitis, and lower socioeconomic status are associated with the incidence of pancreatic cancer, but none of these associations has been identified as conclusively causal.

DIAGNOSTIC CRITERIA

The diagnosis of pancreatic cancer is made histologically. However, the main triad of presenting symptoms comprises pain, jaundice, and weight loss. A high level of suspicion should be maintained in patients older than 40 who present with any of the clinical manifestations (Moosa, 1980) listed in Table 24-10. If the patient is a heavy smoker, the level of suspicion should be doubled (Moosa, 1980). Staging of pancreatic cancer is listed in Table 24-11.

HISTORY AND PHYSICAL EXAMINATION

The diagnosis of pancreatic cancer is usually made late in the course of the disease because there are usually no signs and symptoms until then; when present, the symptoms are often vague. Several weeks or months may pass before a diagnosis is established. Physical signs may include jaundice, abdominal mass, epigastric tenderness, palpable gallbladder, and hepatomegaly (Keller et al, 1993). About half of the patients lack physical findings except weight loss and an insidious onset of abdominal or back pain. A sudden onset of atypical diabetes with a rapid progression to insulin dependence could be a clue to the possibility of a pancreatic lesion (Noy & Bilezikian, 1994). Other signs that indicate progression of pancreatic cancer include abdominal or back pain that is aggravated by lying flat and worse at night, dark urine, clay-colored stool, fatigue, and depression.

TABLE 24-10	Clinical Manifestations of Pancreatic Cancer

- Obstructive jaundice
- Unexplained weight loss, >10% of body weight
- Recent unexplained upper abdominal or lumbar back pain, worse at night
- Recent vague, unexplained dyspepsia, with a normal upper gastrointestinal investigation
- Sudden onset of steatorrhea
- Attack of idiopathic pancreatitis

TABLE 24-11	AJCC Staging of Pancreatic Carcinoma

PRIMARY TUMOR (T)

TX	Primary tumor cannot be assessed
T0	No evidence of primary tumor
T1	Tumor limited to the pancreas
	T1a Tumor ≤ 2 cm
	T1b Tumor > 2 cm
T2	Tumor extends to duodenum, bile duct, or peripancreatic tissues
T3	Tumor extends to stomach, spleen, colon, or adjacent large vessels

REGIONAL LYMPH NODES (N)

NX	Regional lymph nodes cannot be assessed
N0	No regional lymph node metastases
N1	Regional lymph node metastases

DISTANT METASTASIS (M)

MX	Presence of distant metastasis cannot be assessed
M0	No distant metastasis
M1	Distant metastasis

STAGING

I	T1	N0	M0
	T2	N0	M0
II	T3	N0	M0
III	Any T	N1	M0
IV	Any T	Any N	M1

American Joint Committee on Cancer. (1997). *AJCC Cancer Staging Manual*, 5/e. Chicago: The American College of Surgeons.

DIAGNOSTIC STUDIES

Once the suspicion of pancreatic cancer is raised, confirmation should be attempted by abdominal ultrasound to evaluate extrahepatic biliary ductal dilatation and to assess the pancreatic head and liver. Abdominal ultrasound is relatively inexpensive, readily available, and useful for diagnosing obstructive jaundice. Thin-section, contrast-enhanced computed tomography (CT) is the study of choice to assess the extent of disease and to determine if the tumor is considered operable (Fuhrman et al, 1995). A CT scan is less costly than magnetic resonance imaging (MRI), and the usefulness of MRI for pancreatic cancer is uncertain. With appropriate use of CT scanning, ultrasound, and endoscopic retrograde cholangiopancreatography, it should be possible to diagnose pancreatic cancer in more than 90% of patients with the disease (Bell, 1993). Essential laboratory tests include a complete blood cell count with differential and platelet count; liver function tests; amylase, glucose, and electrolyte measurements; and coagulation tests (Table 24-12).

While obtaining diagnostic studies, the patient should be referred to a surgical oncologist and gastroenterologist. A gastroenterologist may perform an endoscopic retrograde cholangiopancreatography or an endoscopic ultrasound in a jaundiced patient to visualize the duodenum and ampulla of Vater, to localize the site of obstruction in the pancreatic and bile ducts, and to obtain a biopsy. Endoscopic ultrasound, the most recent addition to the diagnostic armamentarium, can help define the extent of the mass and guide biopsies. The surgeon may perform a laparotomy or laparoscopy to obtain a tissue diagnosis and determine resectability. However, ideally the laparotomy

TABLE 24-12	Common Abnormal Laboratory Results With Pancreatic Carcinoma

Test	Result
Hematocrit	↓
Hemoglobin	↓
Alk phos	↑
Bilirubin	↑
Glucose	↑
SGOT/SGPT	↑
LDH	↑
Albumin	↓
PT/PTT	↑

should be therapeutic, not diagnostic, and resectability should be determined preoperatively by use of the procedures noted above. A CT-guided percutaneous fine-needle aspiration can be performed for cytologic confirmation of malignancy in patients with locally advanced disease.

TREATMENT OPTIONS, EXPECTED OUTCOMES, AND COMPREHENSIVE MANAGEMENT

A multidisciplinary approach to treatment of pancreatic cancer is essential. Surgery is the only known curative modality, but cure is rare. Lesions in the head of the pancreas have the greatest likelihood of surgical cure, possibly because onset of jaundice occurs relatively quickly from ductal obstruction. A Whipple procedure (pancreaticoduodenectomy), first described by A.O. Whipple in 1935, is the standard for lesions in the head of the pancreas. This operation is appropriate only for patients with localized, potentially resectable lesions with a reasonable opportunity for cure. A Whipple procedure involves resection of the duodenum, head of the pancreas, common bile duct, gallbladder, and distal stomach. The remaining gastric pouch is anastomosed to the jejunum, and the common duct and pancreatic duct are joined to the jejunum proximal to the gastrojejunostomy. A pylorus-sparing pancreaticoduodenectomy preserves blood supply to the duodenum and reduces the postoperative incidence of dumping and diarrhea. Traditionally, these procedures have carried a high operative mortality rate (5% to 20%, depending on the expertise of the operative team; Bell, 1993), and they should be considered only if the prospects for cure outweigh the risks. Complications include sepsis, bleeding, and biliary or pancreatic fistula. In recent years, the operative mortality rate has been reported at less than 2% (Yeo et al, 1995). Reports of prognosis vary after a Whipple resection, with the 5-year survival rate ranging from about 5% (Bell, 1993) to about 20% (Cameron, 1995).

If a lesion is unresectable (Table 24-13), a palliative bilioenteric bypass to relieve jaundice and gastroenteric bypass to correct or obviate gastric outlet obstruction may be performed (Evans et al, 1997). Patients with ascites or liver metastases have a median survival of less than 6 months. In these patients, an endoscopic biliary stent placement may be preferred over surgical biliary bypass to eliminate unnecessary surgery (Evans et al, 1997), although gastrointestinal bypass is still required

in some patients (Wanebo & Vezeridis, 1996). About 20% to 30% of patients with biliary stents develop ascending cholangitis or technical problems associated with the stent (Beazley & Cohn, 1995). If a biliary stent is placed, patients and their caregivers require adequate instruction about its management, including collection, measurement, and documentation of drainage. Fever, change in quality or quantity of drainage, erythema or pus around the catheter site, increasing pain, or bloody drainage should be reported.

There is no known, standard, curative therapy available for patients with advanced, unresectable pancreatic cancer (Lionetto et al, 1995). The role of adjuvant radiation therapy to improve local control and adjuvant chemotherapy to control systemic recurrence is being investigated. The Gastrointestinal Tumor Study Group (1987) demonstrated an improved survival (20 months for the treatment group versus 11 months for the controls) using adjuvant 5-fluorouracil and radiation therapy after Whipple resection. Hoffman et al (1996) postulated that preoperative chemotherapy and radiation may offer benefit for localized pancreatic cancer. The use of chemotherapy alone has been disappointing for patients whose lesions are unresectable. Continued development of new approaches is essential to improve the treatment and survival of these patients.

Palliative care includes symptom management, nutritional support, and attempts at providing optimal quality of life. Pancreatic cancer is often associated with severe, unrelenting abdominal and back pain. A variety of approaches should be considered when addressing pain management. Pharmacologic and nonpharmacologic modalities have been shown to be effective, including percutaneous celiac nerve block and alterations in drug administration approaches (Caraceni & Portenoy, 1996). Narcotics, used to control pain, should be given on scheduled doses with rescues as needed, and laxatives should be administered judiciously to avoid constipation. Antidepressants and amphetamines may also be useful. Massage, therapeutic touch, relaxation techniques, proper positioning, and biofeedback may complement conventional modalities. Radiation therapy can provide pain relief when administered for localized bone pain.

TEACHING AND SELF-CARE

In terms of primary prevention, smoking cessation should be encouraged in all patients because it is linked as a contributing factor to numerous ailments. A high-fiber, low-salt, low-fat diet rich in fruits and vegetables remains the gold standard for health promotion.

TABLE 24-13	Criteria for Unresectability and Metastatic Sites in Pancreatic Carcinoma

■ Locally advanced disease—extension of tumor in the retroperitoneum along the superior mesenteric artery

■ Metastases to regional lymph nodes

■ Metastases to liver

■ Metastases to the visceral peritoneum of the small bowel mesentery

Pancreatic insufficiency may ultimately develop in some long-term survivors, and protein and fat malabsorption and vitamin deficiencies may result. Vitamin and mineral supplementation and pancreatic enzymes administered with meals are important components of nutritional management. Surgery involving the head of the pancreas can alter the secretion of insulin and the production of glucagon, and insulin therapy may be indicated. Patients and their families should be advised to recognize and report signs of pancreatic functional abnormalities such as steatorrhea, hyperglycemia and hypoglycemia, stupor, and lethargy.

The course of pancreatic cancer is insidious and rapid, and patients and their families need support through this process. All possible means for comfort should be explored and provided to minimize the incapacitating manifestations of the disease. For further information, see the self-care section at the end of this chapter.

Follow-up Care

Pertinent follow-up during and after treatment includes history and physical examination, complete blood count, and biochemical profile monthly or as needed for a patient with locally advanced tumor who opts for treatment (Casper, 1996). A chest x-ray and abdominal CT scan should be obtained at 6- to 12-month intervals, or sooner if symptoms develop. Nutritional status, including serum albumin level, also should be assessed during follow-up. Carcinoembryonic antigen and CA 19-9 have poor sensitivity and specificity and have limited value in follow-up care or screening for pancreatic cancer. In patients who choose comfort measures only, there is no rationale for repeated blood testing or radiologic studies, and care should be directed exclusively at symptom management.

COMMUNITY RESOURCES

With the advent of Internet searches and literature directed at keeping patients abreast of breakthroughs in medical research and treatment options, many patients investigate their disease and are able to participate in treatment decisions. In addition, national and local organizations provide a plethora of teaching materials suitable for providers and patients, as well as support groups. Such Websites and organizations are noted at the end of this unit.

REFERRAL POINTS AND CLINICAL WARNINGS

The primary care provider should oversee an interdisciplinary team to address the constellation of problems faced by these unfortunate patients. Appropriate referrals include surgeon, oncologist, gastroenterologist, radiation oncologist, nutritionist, social worker, oncology nurse, and anesthesia/pain management team. For some patients, hospice or home hospice is a viable and beneficial option. However, patients at all stages of this disease are living with a sword of Damocles over their heads, and the provider is in the position to calm their fear and anxiety by being available, by providing simple and appropriate information with symptom control, and by making proper referrals. An honest, direct approach should be taken when discussing the progression of the disease, but a fine balance is required to prevent patients and their loved ones from losing hope. Impending feelings of doom can be soothed by clergy or other spiritual support.

References

American Joint Committee on Cancer. (1992). Exocrine pancreas. In O.H. Beahrs, D.E. Henson, R.V. Hutter, & B.J. Kennedy (Eds.). *Manual for staging of cancer*, 4th ed. Philadelphia: J.B. Lippincott; 109–110.

Beazley, R.M., & Cohn, I. (1995). Tumors of the pancreas, gallbladder, and extrahepatic bile ducts. In G.P. Murphy, W. Lawrence, & R.E. Lenhard (Eds.). *American Cancer Society textbook of clinical oncology*, 2d ed. Atlanta: American Cancer Society; 251–268.

Bell, R.H. (1993). Neoplasms of the exocrine pancreas. In L.J. Greenfield, M.W. Mulholland, K.T. Oldham, & G.B. Zelenock (Eds.). *Surgery: Scientific principles and practice*. Philadelphia: J.B. Lippincott; 816–833.

Cameron, J.L. (1995). Long-term survival following pancreaticoduodenectomy for adenocarcinoma of the head of the pancreas. *Surgery Clinics of North America, 75*, 939–951.

Caraceni, A., & Portenoy, R. K. (1996). Pain management in patients with pancreatic carcinoma. *Cancer, 78 (3 Suppl)*, 639–653.

Caspar, E.S. (1996). Pancreatic cancer. In D.S. Fischer (Ed.). *Follow-up of cancer: A handbook for physicians*. Philadelphia: Lippincott-Raven; 44–45.

Evans, D.B., Abbruzzese, J.L., Rich, T.A. (1997). Cancer of the pancreas. In V.T. DeVita, S. Hellman, & S.A. Rosenberg (Eds.). *Cancer: Principles and practice of oncology*, 5th ed. Philadelphia: Lippincott-Raven; 1054–1087.

Fuhrman, G.M., Berger, D.H., & Feig, B.W. (1995). Pancreatic adenocarcinoma. In D.H. Berger, B.W. Feig, & G.M. Fuhrman (Eds.). *The M.D. Anderson surgical oncology handbook*. Boston: Little, Brown & Co.; 224–238.

Gastrointestinal Tumor Study Group. (1987). Further evidence of effective adjuvant combined radiation and chemotherapy following curative resection of pancreatic cancer. *Cancer, 59*, 2006–2020.

Hoffman, J.P., O'Dwyer, P., Agarwal, P., Salazar, H., & Ahmad, N. (1996). Preoperative chemoradiotherapy for localized pancreatic carcinoma. A perspective. *Cancer, 78 (3 Suppl)*, 592–597.

Keller, J.W., Peacock, J.L., & Smith, J.L. (1993). Cancer of the major digestive glands: Pancreas, liver, bile ducts, gallbladder. In P. Rubin (Ed.). *Clinical oncology: A multidisciplinary approach for physicians and students*, 7th ed. Philadelphia: W.B. Saunders; 597–615.

Lillemoe, K.D., & Pitt, H.A. (1996). Palliation, surgical and otherwise. *Cancer, 78 (3 Suppl)*, 605–614.

Lionetto, R., Pugliese, V., Bruzzi, P., & Rosso, R. (1995). No standard treatment is available for advanced pancreatic cancer. *European Journal of Cancer, 31A(6)* 882–887.

Moosa, A.R. (1980). *Tumors of the pancreas*. Baltimore: Williams & Wilkins; 433.

Noy, A., & Bilezikian, J.P. (1994). Diabetes and pancreatic cancer: Clues to the early diagnosis of pancreatic malignancy. *Journal of Clinical Endocrinology & Metabolism, 79(5)*, 1223–1231.

Parker, S.L., Tong, T., Bolden, S., & Wingo, P.A. (1997). Cancer statistics, 1997. *CA Cancer Journal for Clinicians, 47*, 5–27.

Ries, L.A.G., Miller, B.A., Hankey, B.F., Kosary, C.L., Harras, A., & Edwards, B.K. (Eds.). (1994). *SEER Cancer Statistics Review, 1973–1991*. Bethesda, MD: National Cancer Institute. NIH Pub. No. 94–2789.

Wanebo, H.J., & Vezeridis, M.P. (1996). Pancreatic carcinoma in perspective. A continuing challenge. *Cancer, 78 (3 Suppl)*, 580–591.

Yeo, C.J., Cameron, J.L., Lillemoe, K.D., et al. (1995). Pancreaticoduodenectomy for cancer of the head of the pancreas: 201 patients. *Annals of Surgery, 221,* 721–731.

COLORECTAL CARCINOMA

Michael T. Harris, MD

Colorectal carcinoma is the fourth most common cancer and the second most common cause of cancer deaths in the United States, with more than 130,000 new cases and 55,000 deaths annually (Parker et al, 1997). The real tragedy is that colorectal cancer can be prevented with effective screening and identification of high-risk patient groups. Prevention and management of this disease form a cornerstone of primary care and depend greatly on satisfactory communication between primary care providers and their patients.

ANATOMY, PHYSIOLOGY, AND PATHOLOGY

Anatomy

The colon is about 4 feet long and extends from the ileocecal valve in the right lower abdominal quadrant to the anus. It travels in a question-mark shape, essentially appearing in any and all areas of the abdomen (Fig. 24-1). The cecum, the most proximal portion of the colon, is approximately 7 to 8 cm in diameter and has the most distensible wall, which is why many right-sided colon carcinomas do not cause symptoms until they have grown quite large. The diameter decreases throughout the rest of the colon until it reaches the narrowest and least distensible portion, the sigmoid colon (where obstructive symptoms can occur fairly early in the course of a carcinoma). The rectal ampulla is again larger and more distensible, reflecting its function as a reservoir for stored stool. The anus, best defined as the canal extending from the pelvic floor to the anal verge, is surrounded by two highly specialized extensions of the muscular walls of the colorectum and the pelvic floor, known as the internal and external anal sphincters, respectively. These structures are of supreme concern when planning treatment for distal colorectal carcinomas.

Histologically, the colonic wall has four distinct layers: serosa, muscularis, submucosa, and mucosa. The serosal layer ends at the level of the upper rectum, which allows for early and extensive local and regional spread of some rectal tumors. The muscularis consists of an outer longitudinal and an inner circular muscle layer. This inner circular layer of muscularis becomes the internal anal sphincter below the level of the pelvic floor. The mucosal layer of the colon is columnar epithelium, which extends to the upper part of the anus. In the anal canal, there is a transition to cuboidal and then squamous epithelium (anoderm). The dentate line is a visible mucocutaneous junction within the anal canal. Colorectal carcinomas arise from the columnar mucosal layer. Tumors arising in the transition zone or below are uncommon and are best considered anal cancers.

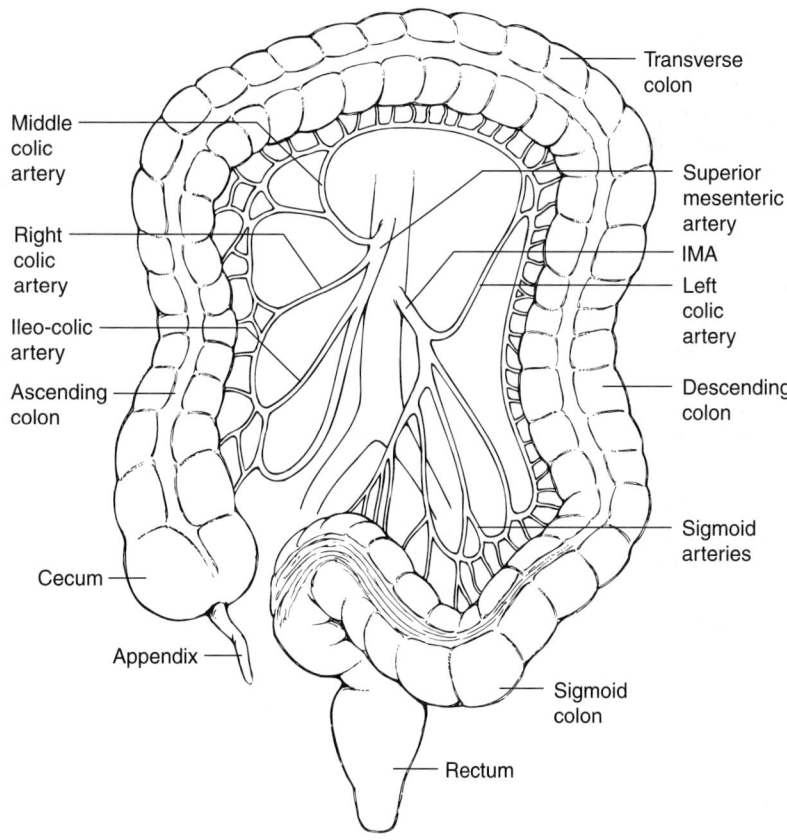

FIGURE 24-1 Anatomy of the colon.

Physiology

The colorectum can be considered as having essentially two physiologic functions: water and electrolyte balance and waste storage and elimination. Sodium and chloride are actively absorbed via the colonic mucosa in exchange for potassium and bicarbonate, respectively. Water passively follows the flow of sodium and chloride. Approximately 1500 mL of fluid enters the colon each day via the ileocecal valve, of which only approximately 100 to 150 mL is excreted in the form of stool. About 90% of the water volume is absorbed by the colonic mucosa.

Stool is stored in the left colon until a complex series of voluntary and involuntary reflex arcs are initiated, allowing movement of stool distally, relaxation of the anal sphincters and pelvic floor, and evacuation of feces in a socially acceptable situation.

Pathology

Colorectal neoplasms have been used as the prototypical model for the study of the biology of carcinomas, in large part because of the observed stages of development. It is widely believed that colorectal neoplasms generally progress from normal mucosa to adenomatous polyps to invasive carcinomas.

EARLY DISEASE

The adenomatous polyp is a benign colorectal neoplasm that is considered to be a premalignant lesion. Histopathologically, it represents a well-circumscribed area of unrestricted cell division within the colonic mucosa. Two essential forms of adenoma are described, based on visual appearance. The pedunculated polyp has a distinct body attached to the colon wall by a stalk or pedicle, often causing a mushroom-like appearance. Sessile polyps are flat, without stalks. The microscopic structure of either form of polyp can range from highly branched, tubular glands (tubular adenoma), to finger-like villous formation (villous adenoma), to a combination of the two (tubulovillous adenoma). Tubular adenomas are far more common and are less likely to harbor an occult malignancy than are villous tumors.

As the polyp matures, mucosal elements may undergo a series of changes leading to the development of cellular atypia or dysplasia, and ultimately progression to frank invasive carcinoma. This process is thought to occur over the course of approximately 10 years. Recently, it has been shown that a predictable sequence of genetic mutations frequently occurs during this transformation (Jessup et al, 1994).

LATE DISEASE

The end result of the sequence described above is the loss of regulation of cell division and growth, with ultimate invasion through the mucosal barrier into the deeper layers of the colon wall. As the tumor continues to progress, the depth of invasion into (and even through) the outer layers of the colon wall increases. In addition, invasion of tumor cells into the neurovascular and lymphatic structures can occur, leading to local, regional, and distant metastatic spread. The two most common sites of metastatic spread from colorectal cancer are the liver and the lungs. Occasionally, the ovaries, brain, or bone marrow becomes involved.

EPIDEMIOLOGY

Prevalence

Colorectal carcinoma is a very common disease entity in the Western world, with approximately 130,000 new cases and 55,000 deaths annually in the United States alone. It ranks fourth in the United States in new cancer cases and second in cancer deaths. Although the majority of new cases are sporadic occurrences, there is an increasing body of evidence to support the strong genetic nature of the disease (Jessup et al, 1997). The implication is that early identification of people at risk for developing colorectal carcinomas may affect outcomes in this disease.

Age

Sporadic colorectal carcinomas have a peak incidence in the seventh and eighth decades of life. Autopsy series have reported the incidence of adenomas to be approximately 17% in people younger than 50, 35% in those 50 to 59, 56% of those in their sixties, and 63% in people over 70 (Rickert et al, 1979). Age of disease onset appears to be important: younger patients have been shown to present with later stages of disease when compared with older patients (Polissar et al, 1981; D'Onofrio & Tan, 1985; Adkins et al, 1987; Smith & Butler, 1989; Taylor et al, 1988). Patients with genetic predispositions or premalignant disease states tend to present with more aggressive disease and at earlier ages.

Gender

Men and women have roughly the same incidence of colorectal adenomas and carcinomas at any age. Women tend to have more right-sided lesions than men (Kodner et al., 1994).

Ethnicity

Although the incidence of colorectal carcinoma is higher in whites than in African Americans, the frequency of stage I and II tumors at the time of diagnosis is significantly lower in African Americans (48%) than in whites (55%) (Jessup et al, 1996). In fact, although the cancer-specific death rate has declined over the past 30 years for white men and women, it has increased by 47% for African American men and 16% for African American women (Boring et al, 1992). This discrepancy may be attributable in part to limited access to health care, but this trend appears across all socioeconomic strata. Hispanics and Asians have rates similar to those of non-Hispanic whites.

Cultural Factors

Dietary patterns of different cultural groups have proven to be a significant etiologic factor in the development of colorectal carcinoma. Diets high in unsaturated animal fats and highly saturated vegetable oils are associated with a markedly increased incidence of colorectal carcinoma (Giovannucci et al, 1992). Other elements in the diet may be protective against the development of colonic neoplasia. Oxygen free-radical scavengers such as selenium and carotenoids are theorized to act at the colonic mucosal surface, preventing free-radical injury and tumorigenesis (Buring & Hennekens, 1993). Populations that eat high-fiber diets, such as some African populations, have a significantly reduced incidence of cancer, perhaps because of decreased transit time and bulk dilution of potential carcinogens. Many studies have demonstrated a definitive relation between fiber and colorectal carcinoma (Shankar & Lanza, 1991; Howe et al, 1992). Further evidence that diet does play a role in the pathogenesis of this disease is found in the fact that emigration from countries of low incidence, such as Japan, to countries of high incidence, such as the United States or the United Kingdom, causes an increase in colorectal carcinoma incidence to the level of the new country.

Genetic Predisposition

Several polyposis and nonpolyposis cancer syndromes have been identified, with delineation of clear-cut genetic inheritance patterns (Jessup et al, 1997). The most famous of these is familial adenomatous polyposis, which itself includes a spectrum of syndromes defined by various extraintestinal manifestations. The most common of these is Gardner's syndrome, characterized by polyposis of the small bowel, stomach, and colorectum; desmoid tumors; osteomas; and epidermoid cysts. The inheritance is autosomal dominant, with all patients containing the gene showing expression. The genetic defect, a mutation of the APC gene, has been identified on chromosome 5. If left untreated, 100% of patients with familial adenomatous polyposis will develop carcinoma.

Premalignant Diseases

Chronic ulcerative colitis has long been known to be a risk factor for colorectal carcinoma, but the mechanism is as yet unclear. The incidence of carcinoma is related to the duration of disease, with a rate of 5% to 8% after 8 years of disease, increasing 0.5% to 1% per year after that. Cancer risk is not correlated with disease activity. Ulcerative colitis is primarily a disease diagnosed in teenagers and young adults, so most patients will be affected for decades, carrying an enormous risk into middle and old age.

Crohn's disease most commonly involves the small intestine but can also affect the colon and rectum. It had long been thought that one of the primary differences between chronic ulcerative colitis and Crohn's colitis was the relative risk of developing colon cancer: Crohn's was not thought to be a significant risk factor for colorectal carcinoma. More recently,

however, it has become apparent that the risk of developing cancer in Crohn's colitis is actually identical to that in chronic ulcerative colitis (Lennard-Jones et al, 1990; Rubin et al, 1988).

DIAGNOSTIC CRITERIA

Definitive diagnosis of colorectal carcinoma depends largely on visualization of the colonic lumen or pathologic confirmation of tissue obtained on biopsy. Endoluminal evaluation may be obtained with either contrast enema (usually barium) or colonoscopy, both discussed below. Staging of colorectal carcinoma, like other cancers, is based on local tumor criteria, regional lymph node status, and the presence or absence of distant metastases. The two commonly used staging systems, TNM and Dukes', are summarized in Table 24-14.

HISTORY AND PHYSICAL EXAMINATION

History

Colorectal carcinomas may take years or even decades to develop, so it is not surprising that symptoms may be absent or minimal at the time of diagnosis. Patients with significant symptoms may already have advanced disease. Symptoms, when they occur, may be referable to the gastrointestinal tract, may be extracolonic, or may be constitutional in nature. Unfortunately, all of these symptom complexes are nonspecific and therefore often generate a large differential diagnosis.

SYMPTOMS REFERABLE TO THE GASTROINTESTINAL TRACT

Abdominal pain is one of the two common presenting complaints, occurring in 22% to 65% of patients. It is much more likely in patients with colon rather than rectal neoplasms (Weiss & Itzkowitz, 1995). Pain is generally vague and cannot be localized. Indeed, up to one third of these patients will undergo initial evaluation of the upper gastrointestinal tract because of upper abdominal discomfort (Speights et al, 1991).

Rectal bleeding as the initial complaint also occurs in approximately half of the patients with colorectal carcinoma (34% to 60%) (Weiss & Itzkowitz, 1995). Bleeding may be manifest across a large spectrum, from specks of blood in the bowel or on the toilet tissue to massive hematochezia. Small amounts of bright-red blood outside the stool or on the paper may reflect a distal lesion, whereas dark blood or maroon stool are more consistent with right-sided colon carcinomas. Frank rectal

TABLE 24-14	Comparison of TNM with Dukes' Staging of Colorectal Carcinoma			
TNM Stage	Depth of Tumor	Regional Lymph Nodes	Distant Metastasis	Dukes' Stage
0	*In situ*	Negative	Negative	A
I	Muscularis propria	Negative	Negative	B1
II	Full thickness	Negative	Negative	B2
III	Any	Positive	Negative	C1 or C2*
IV	Any	Positive or negative	Positive	D

* Depends on tumor thickness.

bleeding, particularly in the older age group, should not be assumed to reflect benign disease; approximately 10% of patients with rectal bleeding prove to have colorectal neoplasms (Goulston et al, 1986).

The third common gastrointestinal symptom is a change in bowel habits, occurring in 22% to 58% of cancer patients (Weiss & Itzkowitz, 1995). Diarrhea is as common as constipation. Patients may suffer alterations in stool caliber (ribbon stools), incontinence, incomplete evacuation, or tenesmus. These symptoms may be subtle or embarrassing, and therefore are often elicited only by careful, specific questioning. Symptoms of small or large bowel obstruction may occur in patients with right- or left-sided colon tumors, respectively, that occupy 75% or more of the colonic lumen.

CONSTITUTIONAL SYMPTOMS

Weakness, fatigue, and weight loss are common presenting symptoms of colorectal malignancies and are usually related to the iron-deficiency anemia of occult gastrointestinal bleeding. Colorectal carcinoma was found to be present in 6% to 11% of patients with iron-deficiency anemia, whose average ages were 60 to 63 (McIntyre & Long, 1993; Rockey & Cello, 1993). Iron deficiency in men or postmenopausal women should be assumed to be from a gastrointestinal neoplasm until proven otherwise. Even in the absence of gastrointestinal blood loss, advanced carcinomas themselves may cause fatigue and weight loss.

EXTRACOLONIC SYMPTOMS

Rarely, colorectal carcinomas may grow so large as to cause initial symptomatology from an adjacent or distant organ. Colovesical fistulas from colorectal carcinoma may initially present as recurrent or multiorganism urinary tract infections; indeed, multiorganism urinary tract infections mandate a colorectal workup. Rectovaginal fistulas may occur, particularly in the setting of previous hysterectomy. Even more rare, but almost pathognomonic of colorectal carcinoma, is the culture of *Streptococcus bovis* from the blood or cerebrospinal fluid.

Physical Examination

A complete physical examination is essential in any patient with suspected colorectal carcinoma. This must include a careful evaluation of the abdomen for evidence of a mass or of intestinal obstruction (eg, distention, tympany). A careful digital rectal examination is mandatory, including fecal occult blood testing. A bimanual pelvic examination in women is also indicated. Some centers even consider rigid sigmoidoscopy to be part of the physical examination.

In patients with palpable rectal lesions, the digital examination gives much useful information. The size of the tumor should be noted, as well as the degree of circumferential involvement. Fixation to the pelvic side wall suggests a locally advanced lesion.

Patients with late-stage disease may present with cachexia and temporal wasting. Firm periumbilical or left supraclavicular lymph nodes (Sister Mary Joseph's and Virchow's nodes, respectively) are evidence of widespread lymphatic obstruction with tumor and are ominous findings.

TABLE 24-15	Survival of Colorectal Carcinoma by Dukes' Stage
Dukes' Stage	**5-Year Survival Rate (%)**
A	93–100
B1	67–85
B2	54–63
C1	43–55
C2	23–28
D	0–6

Source: Kodner et al, 1994.

Disease Course and Prognosis

Long-term survival rates of patients treated for colorectal carcinoma are summarized in Table 24-15. Patients with late-stage disease (Dukes' C or D) should be strongly encouraged to consider preparing a living will and assigning a health care proxy. Family support and involvement should be sought at all stages of disease.

DIAGNOSTIC STUDIES

Laboratory Tests

Patients with known or suspected colorectal carcinoma should undergo routine blood work. Specific tests of interest are the complete blood count, with particular attention to red cell morphology. Microchromic, microcytic anemia is indicative of iron deficiency from chronic gastrointestinal blood loss. Alkaline phosphatase levels should be obtained because elevations may be an early sign of hepatic metastasis. Carcinoembryonic antigen (CEA) levels should be obtained in patients with known colorectal carcinoma as a baseline for later measurements.

Radiologic Studies and Endoscopic Evaluation

Although either colonoscopy or barium enema may be adequate to confirm the presence of a colorectal neoplasm, colonoscopy has several distinct advantages. First, the specificity and sensitivity of endoscopy have been shown repeatedly to be superior to those of contrast enema (Hixson et al, 1990; Anderson et al, 1991). Second, colonoscopic biopsy provides tissue for microscopic evaluation. In addition, the ability to perform complete polypectomy through the endoscope allows for the possibility of definitive therapy for some neoplasms.

Two prospective studies compared the combination of flexible sigmoidoscopy and barium enema versus colonoscopy alone in the evaluation of patients with lower gastrointestinal bleeding (Irvine et al, 1988; Rex et al, 1990). In one, the overall sensitivity of colonoscopy in detecting neoplasm was 100%, versus 83% with the combination examination. Specificity was also significantly greater with colonoscopy alone. In the second study, 32% of patients who underwent sigmoidoscopy and barium enema required colonoscopy for biopsy or polypectomy, or for an inadequate barium study.

Computed tomography (CT) has been widely used in the evaluation of patients with colorectal neoplasms. As a primary diagnostic test, its sensitivity and specificity pale in comparison with either barium enema or colonoscopy, and the cost is much greater. Although it has a definite role in the evaluation of extracolonic disease (particularly in rectal cancers), CT has been greatly overused in this disease.

Endorectal Ultrasound

Endoluminal ultrasound is becoming an important modality in the staging of mid- and distal rectal carcinomas. Detailed information regarding depth of invasion and local nodal status may be obtained. Tumor staging is significantly more accurate than that of CT scanning or any other preoperative staging modality (Solomon & McLeod, 1993).

TREATMENT OPTIONS, EXPECTED OUTCOMES, AND COMPREHENSIVE MANAGEMENT

Prevention

Diet has long been postulated to play an important epidemiologic role in the development of colorectal neoplasms. To date, most of the evidence to support this has been obtained from population studies. Although it has been shown that emigration has altered the incidence of colon cancers, dietary intervention has not yet been shown to alter cancer rates. Several prospective studies have recently been initiated to determine whether specific dietary interventions might prevent colon cancer (Table 24-16).

Patients taking aspirin and nonsteroidal anti-inflammatory drugs for long periods of time have been found to develop colorectal carcinomas less often than matched controls. Patients in one large study showed significantly less aspirin consumption than age- and sex-matched controls (Kune et al, 1988). Several other studies have confirmed the protective effect of both aspirin and nonsteroidal anti-inflammatories, both in cancer risk and in the development and recurrence of colorectal adenomas

(Suh et al, 1993; Peleg et al, 1994; Logan et al, 1993; Rosenberg et al, 1991; Thun et al, 1991; Thun et al, 1993).

Screening

Screening for colon carcinoma with fecal occult blood testing is simple and inexpensive. However, the sensitivity of guaiac-based tests ranges from only 50% to 70% in studies of known colorectal carcinomas, and only 10% to 20% for patients with known adenomas (Ahlquist et al, 1993; Lance et al, 1992; Winauer et al, 1991). The positive predictive value ranges from 22% to 58%. These same studies show that patients who undergo fecal occult blood screening for colorectal cancer have an earlier stage of disease at the time of diagnosis than patients who are not screened. Further, a 19% decrease in the mortality rate was seen in groups undergoing annual fecal occult blood screening (Towler et al, 1994).

Case-control studies show up to a 70% decrease in cancer-related deaths from tumors within reach of the sigmoidoscope (Selby et al, 1992; Newcomb et al, 1992; Gilbertson, 1974; Atkin et al, 1992). The greater reach of the flexible instrument (60 cm versus 25 cm) suggests its superiority over the rigid scope. These studies, although dramatic, do not demonstrate survival improvement for tumors beyond the reach of the endoscope. However, the high cost, increased risks, and need for expertise have thus far prevented widespread use of screening colonoscopy. As risk factors and genetic markers for colorectal carcinoma become clearer, the use of colonoscopy as a screening instrument for high-risk groups is likely to become more prevalent. New guidelines from the Centers for Disease Control and Prevention for colorectal cancer screening include routine full colonoscopy for patients over age 50 (Table 24-17).

Treatment of Colorectal Neoplasms

ENDOSCOPIC POLYPECTOMY
Endoscopic removal of an adenomatous polyp can be viewed as an essentially curative resection of a premalignant colorectal neoplasm. This viewpoint is justified by the National Polyp

TABLE 24-16	Ongoing Trials of Dietary Intervention for Colorectal Neoplasia		
Investigator	**Location**	**Intervention**	**Sample Size**
MacLennan	Australia	<25% calories from fat Wheat bran (25 g/d) Beta-carotene (20 mg/d)	424
Ritenbaugh	U.S.	Wheat bran supplement (13.5 g/d)	1,400
Decosse	U.S.	High-fiber supplement Vitamins C and E	62
McKeown-Eyssen	Canada	20% calories from fat 50 g fiber	201
Schatzkin	U.S.	20% calories from fat Dietary fiber (18 g/1000 kcal/d) Fruits & vegetables (5–8 servings/d)	2,079
Women's Health Initiative	U.S.	Hormones, calcium, vitamin D	48,000
Hill	Israel, Europe	Low-fat diet Fiber, calcium	800

Source: Weiss & Itzkowitz, 1995.

TABLE 24-17	Screening Guidelines for Colorectal Carcinoma		
Symptoms	Family History	Age to Begin Tests	Evaluation
Absent	None	50	Digital rectal exam Stool guaiac Colonoscopy: if neg, repeat in 3–5 yrs; if pos, repeat in 1 yr
Absent	First-degree relative	40	As above
Absent	Familial polyposis (FAP)	10	Digital rectal exam Colonoscopy: if neg, repeat in 3 yrs; if pos, repeat annually
Absent	Hereditary Nonpolyposis colorectal carcinoma (Lynch syndrome)	Late teens	As for FAP
Present	None	25	Digital rectal exam Stool guaiac Colonoscopy: if neg, repeat in 3–5 yrs; if pos, repeat in 1 yr

Source: Jessup et al, 1997.

Study, which found that clearing the colon of adenomatous polyps reduced the incidence of developing subsequent colorectal cancer by 80% to 90% (Winauer et al, 1993).

SURGERY

For invasive colorectal cancers, surgical resection offers the only chance for cure. The choice of procedure depends on the location of the lesion in the colon. In all resections, the tumor is removed with a wide margin of normal colon on either side and with all the draining lymph nodes for that segment. Cecal and ascending colon tumors are treated with right hemicolectomy and ileotransverse colon anastomosis. Left-sided lesions are best treated by left hemicolectomy with colocolonic anastomosis. Upper rectal cancers are treated by anterior resection with colorectal anastomosis. With the popularity of surgical staplers, the development of newer sphincter-sparing techniques, and the reduction of local recurrences with adjuvant therapies, more mid- and lower rectal cancers (down to 4 cm from the anal verge) are being resected without the sacrifice of intestinal continuity (Hansen et al, 1996; Williams, 1984).

Controversy exists regarding the performance of incidental oophorectomy in conjunction with colon resection for carcinoma in postmenopausal women. Although some colorectal tumors can secondarily involve the ovaries via direct extension or metastatic spread, far more common is the incidence of coexisting primary ovarian cancer (about 1%). The ease with which oophorectomy is performed has prompted many surgeons to recommend bilateral oophorectomy in any postmenopausal woman undergoing a laparotomy.

CHEMOTHERAPY

The use of levamisole in combination with 5-fluorouracil after complete resection of colon carcinoma resulted in a 41% reduction in tumor recurrence and a 33% reduction in the 3-year mortality rate for patients with stage III disease (Laurie et al, 1989). Other studies, using leucovorin and 5-FU, have confirmed these findings, particularly in those with more advanced disease (O'Connell et al, 1993; Wolmark et al, 1993; Erlichman et al, 1994). Although there is conflicting evidence regarding the advantages of various regimens on various stages of disease,

postoperative adjuvant chemotherapy is widely regarded as absolutely indicated for patients with Dukes' stage C disease, and possibly indicated for patients with Dukes' stage B2 disease (Table 24-18).

RADIATION THERAPY

External beam radiation therapy (XRT) is reserved for patients with rectal carcinomas distal to the peritoneal reflection (mid- and distal rectal lesions). Most studies of surgery and adjuvant XRT have demonstrated clear-cut reductions in local recurrence, but survival advantages have proven elusive (GTSG, 1985; Fisher et al, 1988; Willett et al, 1992). The great current controversy involves the use of preoperative versus postoperative versus "sandwich" therapy (pre- and postoperative XRT). The National Institutes of Health Consensus Conference on Rectal Cancer (1990) declared combined postoperative treatment of rectal carcinoma to be the standard of care for this disease. Newer studies are underway evaluating the additive effects of XRT and chemotherapy and the use of neoadjuvant (preoperative) chemoradiation protocols.

Surveillance of Patients Treated for Colorectal Carcinoma

Controversy exists over the necessary level of aggressiveness in surveying patients for recurrent or metachronous (new pri-

TABLE 24-18	Indications for Adjuvant Chemotherapy for Colorectal Carcinoma	
Dukes' Stage	TNM Stage	Indication for Chemotherapy
A	0	No
B1	I	No
B2	II	Unproven
C1, C2	III	Yes
D	IV	Unproven

mary) colorectal carcinoma. Although the pessimism of many providers may be justified with regard to survival after treatment of recurrent colorectal carcinoma, the high incidence of metachronous lesions (up to 6.3%), which act similarly to primary cases, seems to support regular follow-up (Cochrane et al, 1980; Vassilopoulos et al, 1982; Cali et al, 1993).

The mainstay of surveillance after potentially curative treatment of colorectal cancer is the measurement of serum levels of CEA. This has gained popularity because the assay is inexpensive and widely available, and because several reports have found clinically undetectable recurrences diagnosed by rising CEA counts (McCall et al, 1994; Moertel et al, 1993; Bruinuels et al, 1994). These reports, however, failed to demonstrate a survival advantage in patients with recurrences detected by CEA levels. Very high levels have been shown to be associated with lesions with a particularly poor prognosis. Although there is not universal acceptance, most clinicians follow patients with CEA levels every 3 months for the first 2 years after potentially curative treatment of colorectal cancer (when most recurrences will be detected), and every 6 months after that.

TEACHING AND SELF-CARE

Particular attention should be paid to diet in the initial postoperative period. A low-residue diet, avoiding uncooked fruits and vegetables, green vegetables, and nuts, will allow for relative rest of the distal bowel. Roughage can gradually be resumed 2 to 3 weeks after surgery. Ultimately, no restrictions on diet should be placed.

Feelings of depression, weakness, and loss of appetite are common during the first 6 to 12 weeks after surgery. Patients should be warned that even after several days of feeling energetic and "up," they may experience relapses. Chemotherapy, XRT, or both may prolong the recovery period extensively.

Because of the now-established genetic nature of colorectal carcinoma, patients should be encouraged to discuss their disease with family members. First-degree relatives are at increased risk of developing colon cancer and should be placed in a high-risk primary prevention program. For more information about self-care, refer to the section at the end of this chapter.

Rehabilitation

Recovery from treatment of colorectal carcinoma is similar to that from any major abdominal surgery. Patients should be encouraged to walk as much as possible because ambulation prevents both pulmonary and gastrointestinal complications. Stairs and hills are permissible. Strenuous exercise, particularly that which places a strain on the abdominal wall musculature, may predispose toward incisional hernias and should be avoided for 6 weeks after surgery. At this time, the tensile strength of the body wall closure has reached at least 80% of its maximum. Driving is prohibited for at least 2 weeks. Patients may shower as little as 48 hours after surgery.

STOMA CARE

Patients with ileostomies or colostomies benefit greatly from a program of teaching and self-care. Stoma care teaching is best begun preoperatively by a specially trained enterostomal therapist. The most common problems that occur with stoma care are related to stoma placement. These are also the most difficult to manage, because simple appliance manipulation frequently cannot compensate for a poorly placed stoma. Unfortunately, preoperative evaluation of stoma siting is frequently overlooked. Patients and providers are often overwhelmed by discussions of the cancer issues and body-image concerns that invariably dominate preoperative discussions.

Postoperatively, the therapist should resume teaching sessions as soon as the patient is able to concentrate (usually on the second or third postoperative day). The focus should be on the patient's ability to empty, clean, and change the appliance. Skin care is also a major concern and should be addressed early. After discharge, several home visits should be arranged for follow-up teaching.

PERISTOMAL IRRITATION

Skin problems are frequently encountered in patients with ostomies. Dermatoses are caused by prolonged contact with stoma effluent; this occurs with ill-fitting appliances or poorly placed stomas. Prevention and treatment are essentially the same. Meticulous care must be taken to ensure an air-tight and water-tight seal of the skin barrier. Patients should be instructed to change the appliance frequently (every 2 days or so) and to avoid soaps and detergents when washing the area. Persistent problems should be referred to a qualified enterostomal therapist. *Candida albicans* infection is very common in the peristomal skin and is usually easily managed with the use of nystatin powder and frequent appliance changes. With good teaching and meticulous self-care, these problems are largely avoidable.

COMMUNITY RESOURCES

For information on patient education, teaching materials, national organizations, and community resources on colon cancer, refer to the section on community resources at the end of this unit.

REFERRAL POINTS AND CLINICAL WARNINGS

Effective prevention and treatment of colorectal carcinoma require a true interdisciplinary team approach. The primary care provider must coordinate the efforts of the gastroenterologist, gastrointestinal surgeon, oncologist, dietitian, and social work services to provide the most effective and the most personal treatment.

■ ■ ■ **CLINICAL PEARLS**

■ Colorectal cancer is a preventable disease. Screening for asymptomatic patients significantly reduces the mortality rate. High-risk patients should be identified and educated in disease prevention.

■ In all patients except the very young, rectal bleeding should be assumed to arise from a gastrointestinal neoplasm until proven otherwise. Prompt evaluation is warranted.

■ Iron-deficiency anemia in men or postmenopausal women requires prompt evaluation.

EDITOR'S NOTE:

COMPLEMENTARY APPROACHES

A general discussion of complementary approaches can be found in Chapter 3. The following, while not an exhaustive list, are some complementary approaches being used for this condition. Additional information on these approaches, including precautions, can be found in Appendices A and B. Providers need to assess for the use of complementary approaches as part of the patient's history, as they may impact conventional therapies, and patients may not volunteer this information unless specifically asked. Efficacy of many complementary approaches is not as well documented as that of conventional therapies. Providers need to read the literature before suggesting these complementary approaches.

- Vitamins, minerals, herbs, supplements
  - Esophageal
    - Beta carotene
  - Stomach
    - Garlic
  - Colorectal
    - Vitamin E
- Complementary Modalities
  - Aromatherapy
  - Massage therapy

References

Adkins, R.B., Jr., DeLozier, J.B., McKnight, W.G., & Waterhouse, G. (1987). Carcinoma of the colon in patients 35 years of age and younger. *American Surgeon, 53,* 141–145.

Ahlquist, D.A., Wieand, H.S., Moertel, C.G., et al (1993). Accuracy of fecal occult blood screening for colorectal neoplasia: A prospective study using Hemoccult and HemoQuant tests. *JAMA, 269,* 1262–1267.

Anderson, N., Bramwell-Cook, H., & Coates, R. (1991). Colonoscopically detected cancer missed on barium enema. *Gastrointestinal Radiology, 16,* 123–127.

Atkin, W.S., Morson, B.C., & Cuzick J. (1992). Long-term risk of colorectal cancer after excision of rectosigmoid adenomas. *N Engl J Med, 326,* 658–662.

Boring, C.C., Squires, T.S., & Heath, C.W., Jr. (1992). Cancer statistics for African Americans. *CA Cancer Journal for Clinicians, 42,* 7–17.

Bruinvels, D.J., Stiggelbout, A.M., Kievit, J., et al (1994). Follow-up of patients with colorectal cancer, a meta-analysis. *Annals of Surgery, 219,* 174–182.

Buring, J.E., & Hennekens, C.H. (1993). Retinoids and carotenoids. In V.T. DeVita, S. Hellman, & S.A. Rosenberg (Eds.). *Principles and practice of oncology.* New York: Lippincott; 464–470.

Cali, R.L., Pitsch, R.M., Thorson, A.G., et al (1993). Cumulative incidence of metachronous colorectal cancer. *Diseases of the Colon & Rectum, 36,* 388–393.

Cochrane, J.P., Williams, J.T., Faber, R.G., & Slack, W.W. (1980). Value of outpatient follow-up after curative surgery for carcinoma of the large bowel. *British Medical Journal, 280*(6214), 593–595.

Devroede, G.J., Taylor, W.F., Sauer, W.G., et al (1971). Cancer risk and life expectancy of children with ulcerative colitis. *N Engl J Med, 285,* 17–21.

D'Onofrio, G.M.D., & Tan, E.G.C. (1985). Is colorectal carcinoma in the young a more deadly disease? *Australian & New Zealand Journal of Surgery, 55,* 537–540.

Erlichman, C., Marsoni, S., Seitz, J., et al (1994). Event-free and overall survival is increased by FUFA in resected B and C colon cancer, a prospective pooled analysis of 3 randomized trials [abstract]. *Proceedings of the American Society of Clinical Oncologists, 13,* 194.

Fisher, B., Wolmark, N., Rockette, H., et al (1988). Postoperative adjuvant chemotherapy or radiation therapy for rectal cancer: Results from NSABP protocol R-01. *Journal of the National Cancer Institute, 80,* 21–29.

Gastrointestinal Tumor Study Group. (1985). Prolongation of the disease-free interval in surgically treated rectal carcinoma. *N Engl J Med, 312,* 1465–1472.

Gilbertson, V.A. (1974). Proctosigmoidoscopy and polypectomy in reducing the incidence of rectal cancer. *Cancer, 34,* 936–939.

Giovannucci, E., Stampfer, M.J., Colditz, G., et al (1992). Relationship of diet to risk of colorectal adenoma in men. *Journal of the National Cancer Institute, 84,* 91–98.

Goulston, K.J., Cook, I., & Dent, O.F. (1986). How important is rectal bleeding in the diagnosis of bowel cancer and polyps? *Lancet, 2,* 261–263.

Hansen, O., Schwenck, W., Hucke, H.P., & Stock, W. (1996). Colorectal stapled anastomoses. Experience and results. *Diseases of the Colon & Rectum, 39,* 30–36.

Hixson, L.J., Fennerty, M.B., Sampliner, R.E., McGee, D., & Garewal, H. (1990). Prospective study of the frequency and size distribution of polyps missed by colonoscopy. *Journal of the National Cancer Institute, 82,* 1769–1772.

Howe, G.R., Benito, E., & Castelleto, R. (1992). Dietary intake of fiber and decreased risks of cancer of the colon and rectum: evidence from the combined analysis of 13 case-control studies. *Journal of the National Cancer Institute, 84,* 1887–1896.

Irvine, E.J., O'Connor, J., Frost, R.A., et al (1988). Prospective comparison of double contrast barium enema vs. colonoscopy in rectal bleeding. *Gut, 29,* 1188–1193.

Jessup, J.M., McGinnis, L.S., Steele, G., Jr., et al (1996). Colon cancer: Report from the National Cancer Data Base. *Cancer, 78,* 918–926.

Jessup, J.M., Menck, H.R., Fremgen, A., & Winchester, D.P. Diagnosing colorectal carcinoma: Clinical and molecular approaches. *CA Cancer Journal for Clinicians, 47,* 70–92.

Jessup, J.M., Steele, G., Jr., Thomas, P., et al (1994). Molecular biology of neoplastic transformation of the large bowel, Identification of two etiologic pathways. *Surgical Oncology Clinics of North America, 3,* 449–477.

Kodner, I.J., Fry, R.D., Fleshman, J.W., & Birnbaum, E.H. (1994). Colon, rectum, and anus. In S.I. Schwartz, G.T. Shires, & F.T. Spencer (Eds.). *Principles of surgery.* New York: McGraw-Hill; 1191–1306.

Kune, G.A., Kune, S., & Watson, L.F. (1988). Colorectal cancer risk, chronic illness, operations and medications, case control results from the Melbourne colorectal cancer study. *Cancer Research, 48,* 4399–4404.

Lance, P., Grossman, S., Marshall, J. (1992). Screening for colorectal cancer. *Seminars in Gastrointestinal Diseases, 3,* 22–32.

Laurie, J.A., Moertel, C.G., & Fleming, T.R. (1989). Surgical adjuvant therapy of large bowel carcinoma, an evaluation of levamisole and the combination of levamisole and fluorouracil. *Journal of Clinical Oncology, 7,* 1447–1456.

Lennard-Jones, J.E., Melville, D.M., Morson, B.C., et al (1990). Precancer and cancer in extensive ulcerative colitis, findings among 401 patients over 22 years. *Gut, 31,* 800–806.

Logan, R.F.A., Little, J., Hawkin, P., & Hardcastle, J.D. (1993). Aspirin and nonsteroidal anti-inflammatory drug (NSAID) use and the risk of asymptomatic colorectal cancer, a case control study of subjects participating in the Nottingham faecal occult blood (FOB) screening trial. *Gastroenterology, 104,* A422.

McCall, J.M., Black, R.B., Rich, C.A., et al (1994). The value of serum carcinoembryonic antigen in predicting recurrent disease following curative resection of colorectal cancer. *Diseases of the Colon & Rectum, 37,* 875–881.

McIntyre, A.S., & Long, R.G. (1993). Prospective survey of investigations in outpatients referred with iron deficiency anemia. *Gut, 34,* 1102–1107.

Moertel, C.G., Fleming, T.R., Macdonald, J., et al (1993). An evaluation of the carcinoembryonic antigen (CEA) test for monitoring patients with resected colon cancer. *JAMA, 270,* 943–947.

Newcomb, P.A., Norfleet, R.G., Storer, B.D., Surawicz, T.S., & Marcus, P.M. (1992). Screening sigmoidoscopy and colorectal cancer mortality. *Journal of the National Cancer Institute, 84,* 1572–1575.

NIH Consensus Conference (1990). Adjuvant therapy for patients with colon and rectal cancer. *JAMA, 284,* 1444–1450.

O'Connell, M., Maillard, J., Macdonald, J., et al (1993). An intergroup trial of intensive course 5-FU and low-dose leucovorin as surgical adjuvant therapy for high-risk colon cancer [abstract]. *Proceedings of the American Society of Clinical Oncologists, 12,* 190.

Parker, S.L., Tong, T., Bolden, S., & Wingo, P.A. (1997). Cancer statistics. *CA Cancer Journal for Clinicians, 47,* 5–27.

Peleg, I.I., Maibach, H.T., Brown, S., & Wilcox, C.M. (1994). Aspirin and nonsteroidal anti-inflammatory drug use and the risk of subsequent colorectal cancer. *Archives of Internal Medicine, 154,* 394–399.

Polissar, L., Sim, D., Phil, M., & Francis, A. (1981). Survival of colorectal cancer patients in relation to duration of symptoms and other prognostic factors. *Diseases of the Colon & Rectum, 24,* 364–369.

Rex, D., Weddle, R., Lehman, G., Pound, D., et al (1990). Flexible sigmoidoscopy versus colonoscopy for suspected lower gastrointestinal bleeding. *Gastroenterology, 98,* 855–861.

Rickert, R.R., Auerbach, O., Garfinkel, L., et al (1979). Adenomatous lesions of the large bowel, an autopsy study. *Cancer, 43,* 1847–1857.

Rockey, D.C., & Cello, J.P. (1993). Evaluation of the gastrointestinal tract in patients with iron deficiency anemia. *N Engl J Med, 329,* 1691–1695.

Rosenberg, L., Palmer, J.R., Zauber, A.G., Warshauer, M.E., Stolley, P.D., & Shapiro, S. (1991). A hypothesis, nonsteroidal anti-inflammatory drugs reduce the incidence of large bowel cancer. *Journal of the National Cancer Institute, 85,* 355–358.

Rubin, P.H., Chapman, M.L., Cortes, J.L., Harpaz, N., Bodian, C., & Present, D.H. (1998). Dysplasia and cancer in chronic Crohn's colitis, a 7-year experience with screening and surveillance colonoscopy. Presented at Digestive Disease Week, San Francisco.

Selby, J.V., Friedman, G.D., Quesenberry, C.P., Jr., Weiss, N.S. (1992). A case-control study of screening sigmoidoscopy and mortality from colorectal cancer. *N Engl J Med, 326,* 653–657.

Shankar, S., & Lanza, E. (1991). Dietary fiber and cancer protection. *Hematology & Oncology Clinics of North America, 5,* 25–41.

Smith, C., & Butler, J.A. (1989). Colorectal cancer in patients younger than 40 years of age. *Diseases of the Colon & Rectum, 32,* 843–846.

Solomon, M.J., & McLeod, R.S. (1993). Endoluminal transrectal ultrasonography: Accuracy, reliability, and validity. *Diseases of the Colon & Rectum, 36,* 200–205.

Speights, M.O., Johnson, M..W, Stoltenberg, P.H., Rappaport, E.S., Helbert, B., & Riggs, M. (1991). Colorectal cancer, current trends in initial clinical manifestations. *Southern Medical Journal, 84,* 575–578.

Suh, O., Petrelli, N.J., & Mettlin, C. (1993). Aspirin use, cancer and polyps of the large bowel. *Cancer, 72,* 1171–1177.

Taylor, M.C., Pounder, D., Ali-Ridha, N.H., et al (1988). Prognostic factors in colorectal carcinoma of young adults. *Canadian Journal of Surgery, 31,* 150–153.

Thun, M.J., Namboodiri, M.M., Calle, E.E., Flanders, W.D., & Heath, C.W., Jr. (1993). Aspirin use and risk of fatal cancer. *Cancer Research, 53,* 1322–1327.

Thun, M.J., Namboodiri, M.M., Heath, C.W., Jr. (1991). Aspirin use and reduced risk of fatal colon cancer. *N Engl J Med, 325,* 1593–1596.

Towler, B., Irwig, L., Glasziou, P., et al (1995). The potential benefits and harms of screening for colorectal cancer. *Australian Journal of Public Health, 19,* 24–28.

Vassilopoulos, P.P., Yoon, J.M., Ledesma, E.J., & Mittelman, A. (1982). Treatment of recurrence of adenocarcinoma of the colon and rectum at the anastomotic site. *Surgery Gynecology & Obstetrics, 152,* 777–780.

Weiss, A.A., & Itzkowitz, S.H. (1995). Clinical aspects of colorectal cancer. In A.K. Rustgi (Ed.). *Gastrointestinal cancers: Biology, diagnosis, and therapy.* Philadelphia: Lippincott-Raven; 353–365.

Willett, C.G., Tepper, J.E., Kaufman, D.S., et al (1992). Adjuvant postoperative radiation therapy for rectal adenocarcinoma. *American Journal of Clinical Oncology, 15,* 371–375.

Williams, N.S. (1984). The rationale of preservation of the anal sphincter in patients with low rectal cancer. *British Journal of Surgery, 71,* 575–581.

Winauer, S.J., Schottenfeld, D., & Flehinger, B.J. (1991). Colorectal cancer screening. *Journal of the National Cancer Institute, 83,* 243–253.

Winauer, S.J., Zauber, A.G., Ho, M.N., et al (1993). Prevention of colorectal cancer by colonoscopic polypectomy. *N Engl J Med, 329,* 1977–1981.

Wolmark, N., Rockette, H., Fisher, B., et al (1993). The benefit of leucovorin-modulated fluorouracil as postoperative adjuvant therapy for primary colon cancer. Results from National Surgical Adjuvant Breast and Bowel Project protocol C-03. *Journal of Clinical Oncology, 11,* 1879–1887.

TEACHING AND SELF-CARE FOR PATIENTS WITH GASTROINTESTINAL MALIGNANCIES

Quality of life for the patient with advanced malignant disease hinges on control of symptoms. Factors to be considered include pain, jaundice, pruritus, nausea and vomiting, constipation or diarrhea, intestinal obstruction, anorexia, cachexia, and dyspnea. Pain, in particular, can be a challenging problem and should be managed aggressively. Although not all cancer patients experience pain, those with advanced disease often require a multidisciplinary approach, using the expertise of a wide range of health care professionals. In this setting, a pain management team can be invaluable. In the great majority of patients, pain can be controlled using simple pharmacologic methods, but other concurrent interventions may be required. The goal of pain therapy is to allow patients to function at a level they choose, to lead as normal a life as possible, and to die free of pain.

Education on pain management should include continuous dosing, with as-needed dosing for breakthrough pain, and teaching about the side effects, such as constipation and nausea, that often occur with narcotic use. Use of a mild laxative or stool softener is helpful in preventing constipation.

Dietary considerations should be reviewed with all patients. In general, patients should be taught to follow a low-residue diet for the first 1 to 2 weeks after bowel resection, and then to resume roughage gradually. Patients with pancreatic cancer or pancreatectomy should be taught the signs and symptoms of hyperglycemia. They should also realize that diarrhea can be expected after a Whipple procedure or secondary to malabsorption. If an ostomy is present, careful attention should be given to care of the ostomy as well as local skin care (see the section on self-care in colon cancer for more information on ostomy and skin care).

Malnutrition is common and is frequently referred to as cancer cachexia. Although supplemental nutrition is often advocated by providers or sought by relatives and patients, there is little evidence that nutritional strategies can maintain or reverse malnutrition in the patient with advanced malignancy. Indeed, the issue of nutrition in patients with cancer poses far more questions than answers. Nevertheless, many health care providers continue to use nutritional support aggressively under specific circumstances. In general, supplemental nutrition, either enteral or parenteral, should be instituted only after very careful consideration of the likely benefit to the patient.

Finally, sexuality issues should not be overlooked in patient teaching. The psychological impact of cancer, as well as body image changes from weight loss, alopecia, jaundice, and ostomy surgery, can all affect the patient's sexuality. In general, once patients are cleared to drive, they can be cleared to resume sexual activity. However, fatigue and pain may preclude the resumption of usual activity. Open discussion with the partner should be encouraged.

The successful management of the cancer patient, with or without persistent or recurrent disease, requires the full range of medical skills of the primary care provider. Providers must remember that in patients with cancer, not all findings arise from the cancer; other treatable medical and surgical diseases can and do occur. The provider must carefully reassess and re-evaluate the patient throughout the course of the illness. Also necessary is an approach to management that incorporates the family as the unit of care. By fostering interaction among and participation by all those significantly involved in the patient's well-being, and by attending to the psychosocial and spiritual concerns of the family, the health care provider can have an indispensable role in meeting the needs of the cancer patient.

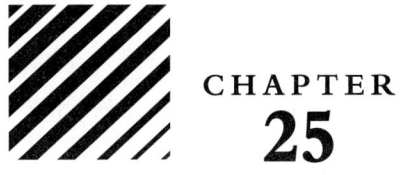

CHAPTER
25

Hemorrhoids

Steven Lowy, MD

Hemorrhoids (sometimes referred to as piles) are tumors made up of enlarged rectal and anal veins along with reactive tissue surrounding those veins. Although a common condition and one that causes significant patient discomfort and concern, hemorrhoids most often can be managed conservatively with good result, especially early in their course. Correct diagnosis is paramount, though, because hemorrhoids can coexist with other, more serious disease entities that cause similar symptoms.

ANATOMY, PHYSIOLOGY, AND PATHOLOGY

There are two sets of hemorrhoidal veins: the superior hemorrhoidal plexus, which gives rise to internal hemorrhoids, and the inferior plexus, which gives rise to external hemorrhoids. The superior plexus is connected to the relatively high venous pressure of the portal system, lies above the dentate line in its normal position, and is covered by rectal mucosa. The inferior plexus has little connection to intra-abdominal venous pressure, lies below the dentate line, and is covered by perianal skin.

Factors associated with the formation of hemorrhoids include the following:

- Genetic predisposition
- Increased venous pressure from various causes (eg, overlong sitting on the toilet seat, straining at constipated stool, prolonged standing, heavy lifting, coughing, pregnancy or other pelvic masses, and portal hypertension)
- Diarrhea
- Rectal tumors and causes for incomplete evacuation of stool from the rectum that cause excessive straining to empty the rectum.

Whatever the cause, formation of an internal hemorrhoid begins with swelling of a venous structure of the superior plexus, usually as a slow and gradual process. As the vein enlarges it pushes its covering mucosa into the lumen of the rectum. Once in the lumen it is subject to the expelling forces of defecation and gradually enlarges as peristalsis and fecal flow push it toward the anus.

As it stretches, the vein becomes attenuated and prone to bleeding, which is often the first symptom of a hemorrhoid. Although bleeding from a hemorrhoid is usually described as bright-red drops of blood in the toilet bowl or on the toilet tissue after defecation, it may be so slight as to go unnoticed or, in contrast, may have the quality of an arterial bleed, leading to hypotension and shock. Eventually, the hemorrhoidal mass can become large and long enough to extend below the dentate line and beyond the anal verge: at this point it becomes a prolapsed hemorrhoid.

EPIDEMIOLOGY

Exact epidemiologic data are difficult to determine because hemorrhoids are so common and are often not reported. Typical Western diets consisting of highly refined foods and little roughage cause firm, dry stools that are difficult to pass and lead to excessive straining at defecation. In poorer parts of the world, where food is less processed, hemorrhoids are less common.

DIAGNOSTIC CRITERIA

Diagnosis is made on the basis of history and a thorough examination. It is essential not to reach a diagnosis of hemorrhoids too quickly. Although hemorrhoids are the most common cause of many of the noted symptoms, other, more ominous processes, particularly rectal carcinoma, can cause these same symptoms. Benign conditions such as anal fissures and condylomata can also cause similar symptoms, but they require different treatment. A thorough digital examination and colonoscopy with particular attention to the rectosigmoid should be part of every diagnostic workup.

HISTORY AND PHYSICAL EXAMINATION

Bleeding and rectal discomfort are the most common complaints voiced about hemorrhoids. Essentials of the history are noted in Table 25-1. When the hemorrhoid prolapses, the following symptoms may appear, even if the prolapse is fully reducible manually or reduces spontaneously:

- A sense of incomplete evacuation and rectal tenesmus
- Irritation and itching
- Mucosal ulceration (another cause of bleeding)
- Acute onset of severe pain and swelling secondary to thrombosis.

Physical findings for internal hemorrhoids are one or more intrarectal masses, usually soft and sometimes tender, with or without the presence of bright-red blood. Characteristically, the bleeding of hemorrhoids coats the stool, whereas the stool itself is negative for occult blood; the finding of stool that is positive for occult blood should reinforce the need for a complete diagnostic workup of the gastrointestinal tract.

If internal hemorrhoids are large, they may be seen prolapsing through the anus or may prolapse as the finger is removed from the rectum. Thrombosed hemorrhoids can be firm, although not nearly so hard as a carcinoma, and are quite tender early in their course; there may be significant anal sphincter spasm. A prolapsed and thrombosed hemorrhoid presents as a

TABLE 25-1	**Essentials in the History of Hemorrhoids**

- Specifics concerning diet, especially the amount of roughage consumed
- Characteristics and degree of pain, itching, burning
- Degree of incapacitation caused by symptoms
- Character of bleeding—whether on toilet paper, in bowl, or mixed with stool
- Severity of bleeding, as best the patient can ascertain
- Symptoms not specific to hemorrhoids: mucus in stool, obstipation, diarrhea, tenesmus, character of stool

swollen, firm mass protruding through the anus with mucus and possibly ulceration. With resolution, there may remain only redundant tissue in the rectum, because the resultant fibrosis after thrombosis may actually cure the patient of that particular internal hemorrhoid. Chronic internal hemorrhoids may result in the formation of anal skin tags.

External hemorrhoids do not cause bleeding, itching, and tenesmus; pain is their singular symptom and occurs with thrombosis. The history usually will be one of sudden onset of intense pain with mild to minimal antecedent symptomatology. There is often no discernible precipitating cause for thrombosis of an external hemorrhoid, and its pathogenesis is unclear. On physical examination, external hemorrhoids are seen as asymptomatic to minimally tender bluish discolorations just distal to the anal verge.

TREATMENT OPTIONS, EXPECTED OUTCOMES, AND COMPREHENSIVE MANAGEMENT

Teaching and Self-Care

Many patients will self-administer treatment for hemorrhoids, either on their own or with guidance from their primary care provider. Proper bowel habits and eating habits are the best preventive measure. The frequent use of the toilet as a place to catch up on one's reading is a major contributor to the high incidence of hemorrhoids. Attention to these factors is also important in the treatment of early hemorrhoids. Use of bulk laxatives or a high-fiber diet, stool softeners, and lubricants such as mineral oil, as well as proper toilet habits, will resolve many, if not most, cases of early hemorrhoids.

For hemorrhoids that do not respond to the above regimens but are not yet severely prolapsed, the common astringent agents available over the counter work well in both cream and suppository forms. Still more acute cases often respond to warm sitz baths and iced witch hazel. These should be alternated hourly, as often as the patient's lifestyle allows. Witch hazel (Tucks) pads are commonly used but are much less effective than the full-strength witch hazel found in most pharmacies.

Medications

Commercial over-the-counter products such as Anusol suppositories and creams can be added to the above regimen, using them every 4 to 6 hours and skipping the sitz baths and witch hazel for that hour. The suppositories are particularly effective for smaller hemorrhoids that do not protrude through the anus but still cause pain, irritation, and an annoying sense of rectal fullness.

Itching that does not respond to the above regimen can be treated with any hydrocortisone cream or foam product. It is used directly on the perianal skin four times a day for up to 3 or 4 days. The patient should notice improvement in pain and spasm in 2 to 4 days, although severe cases may require a week for inflammation to resolve sufficiently that symptoms abate. Itching, if caused by the hemorrhoidal irritation, should resolve quickly with local care.

Follow-Up Care

If the patient's symptoms are not considerably improved within 4 to 7 days, if severe bleeding occurs, or if constipation is an unrelenting problem, the patient should be referred to a specialist.

Once the acute episode is resolved, recurrence can be minimized by adherence to good bowel habits and increasing stool bulk. Bulk is best ensured by having the patient increase dietary fiber intake from vegetable and fruit sources. If adequate stool bulk is not achieved with diet, a psyllium seed fiber product such as Metamucil may be intermittently added to the regimen as needed.

Definitive Treatment

A patient whose pain and discomfort do not resolve with conservative therapy should also be referred to a specialist for treatment. The specialist can perform several relatively noninvasive procedures for hemorrhoid removal, including injection with sclerosing solutions, rubber-band ligation, cryosurgery, and infrared or electric cauterization. Severe cases may require surgical resection. Although primary care providers do not perform resection, they should be aware of the contraindications to this surgery. Concomitant conditions that predispose to operative and postoperative hemorrhage, including portal hypertension, clotting disorders, and inflammatory diseases of the rectum, are contraindications to hemorrhoid surgery. Inflammatory rectal disease also predisposes to poor postoperative healing and possible fistula formation.

Complementary Therapies

Recent evidence has shown oral Daflon 500 mg to shorten significantly the resolution time for acutely thrombosed hemorrhoids (Cospite, 1994; Godeberge, 1994). Daflon is a combination of flavonoids that have beneficial effects on the integrity of veins and improve lymphatic circulation.

DMSO (dimethylsulfoxide) has been reported to be effective in the treatment of inflamed and thrombosed hemorrhoids (*Alternatives*, 1996). However, DMSO is not approved by the Food and Drug Administration for this use and is sold in health-food stores solely as a solvent.

During the acute attack, constipation may be ameliorated with mineral oil, either orally or by enema. One tablespoon of the oil by mouth two or three times daily is usually sufficient. Administration should be decreased or discontinued if stools become excessively oily. Aspiration of mineral oil can cause lipoid pneumonia, and oral mineral oil should be avoided in obtunded or debilitated patients. The oil is not recommended for long-term use, but solely for the passage of hard stool during the acute episode.

COMMUNITY RESOURCES

Community resources, patient education materials, and provider information are available from several organizations noted at the end of the unit on gastrointestinal disorders.

REFERRAL POINTS AND CLINICAL WARNINGS

Reasons for referral to a specialist include bleeding, thrombosis, and intractable symptoms. Treatment of bleeding requires, first and foremost, a full diagnostic workup to rule out a carcinoma. The patient with bleeding that is hemodynamically significant or does not cease with the use of the noninvasive methods outlined should be referred to a specialist.

Proper treatment of thrombosed hemorrhoids requires definitive differentiation of whether the affected hemorrhoid is internal or external. Although it is normally simple enough to determine if a hemorrhoid originates above or below the dentate line, that may not be true early in the thrombotic process. It is completely safe to incise and evacuate a low-pressure thrombosed external hemorrhoid in the office, but surgical evacuation or excision of an internal hemorrhoid is risky, with the potential for massive bleeding. These patients need a referral to an experienced specialist.

■ ■ ■ ■   CLINICAL PEARLS

- Rectal bleeding, tenesmus, mucus, or pain should not be quickly dismissed as hemorrhoidal in etiology once hemorrhoids are found. A complete history and physical examination, including proctosigmoidoscopy, is essential to avoid overlooking more serious pathology, especially rectal neoplasms.
- Before considering therapy, especially incision and evacuation of clot, the provider must be completely certain that the source of the symptoms is an external hemorrhoid, not an internal one. An error here can result in dangerous, even fatal, hemorrhage.

- When using psyllium fiber, the patient should be cautioned to take the psyllium fiber mixed in at least 8 ounces of liquid, because thicker preparations may swell and cause dangerous esophageal and airway problems.
- Excessive bleeding may be significant enough to cause shock and death.

EDITOR'S NOTE:
COMPLEMENTARY APPROACHES

A general discussion of complementary approaches can be found in Chapter 3. The following, while not an exhaustive list, are some complementary approaches being used for this condition. Additional information on these approaches, including precautions, can be found in Appendices A and B. Providers need to assess for the use of complementary approaches as part of the patient's history, as they may impact conventional therapies, and patients may not volunteer this information unless specifically asked. Efficacy of many complementary approaches is not as well documented as that of conventional therapies. Providers need to read the literature before suggesting these complementary approaches.

- Complementary Modalities
    Acupuncture
    Aromatherapy

References

Alternatives for the health-conscious individual. (Dec. 1996) Mountain Home Publishing, 6(18), p. 140.

Cospite, M. (1994). Double-blind, placebo-controlled evaluation of clinical activity and safety of Daflon 500 mg in the treatment of acute hemorrhoids. *Angiology, 45*(6 Pt 2), 566–573.

Godeberge, P. (1994). Daflon 500 mg in the treatment of hemorrhoidal disease: A demonstrated efficacy in comparison with placebo. *Angiology, 45*(6 Pt 2), 574–578.

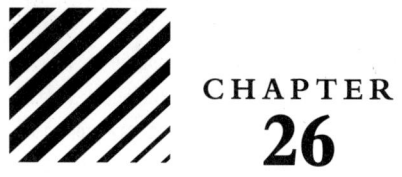

Hepatitis

Charlotte C. Cabello, MSN, RN

At present, there are at least five well-known hepatotropic viruses: hepatitis A, B, C, D, and E. A new hepatotropic virus, hepatitis G, has also been identified. These viruses can cause inflammation of the liver with hepatocellular damage ranging from mild to severe to potentially fatal. The type of hepatitis virus and the degree of liver damage will determine the medical intervention needed. Patients with acute hepatitis should be monitored until liver function tests become normal. Cases of known exposure to hepatitis A and E should resolve quickly and spontaneously. Known exposure to hepatitis B and C viruses may require ongoing monitoring to detect and manage chronic disease. The goal is to maximize the level of functioning by minimizing the severity of the liver failure.

Other viruses can also cause inflammation of the liver, such as Epstein-Barr virus, cytomegalovirus, rubella, herpes simplex, and varicella. For purposes of this chapter, the hepatotropic viruses will be reviewed (Table 26-1). Primary care providers must identify the virus causing liver damage, care for patients with these viral infections, and protect the community as well as themselves from exposure to these viruses.

HEPATITIS A (INFECTIOUS HEPATITIS)

Anatomy, Physiology, and Pathology

Hepatitis A is a single-stranded RNA virus of the enterovirus group. It is caused by the hepatitis A virus (HAV) and is primarily transmitted by the fecal–oral route. Transmission is facilitated by poor sanitation, intimate contact (household or sexual), and poor personal hygiene. Every year, outbreaks from water or food contaminated by infected food handlers are reported.

Epidemiology

The Centers for Disease Control reports that there are 75,000 to 100,000 cases of hepatitis A annually (Long & Kyllonen, 1997). Hepatitis A is a worldwide infection. It is nearly universal in childhood in overcrowded developing countries. It is thought that by adulthood, up to 50% of persons in the United States have been infected with HAV (Marx, 1993). Risk factors for infection with HAV include employment at day-care centers, international travel, intravenous drug use, and exposure to contaminated food or water.

History and Physical Examination

Symptoms consist of flu-like complaints. Jaundice may or may not appear. Other signs and symptoms of hepatitis can be found in Box 26-1. HAV is acute, self-limited, and rarely fulminant.

Hepatic failure occurs in approximately 0.1% of cases (Marx, 1993), with a mortality rate of 0.6%. There is no carrier state, and initial exposure confers lifelong immunity.

Approximately 42% of persons who acquire the infection have no identifiable risk factor (Long & Kyllonen, 1997). Persons infected with hepatitis A may be asymptomatic and still have the potential to transmit disease. The incubation period is about 2 to 6 weeks (average 28 to 30 days), with the highest concentration of HAV found during the 2 weeks before jaundice appears. It is during this period that the person is highly infectious. Although rare, HAV can be transmitted by blood transfusions if the donation is made in the prodromal phase of the infection.

Diagnostic Studies

Liver enzyme elevations, specifically alanine aminotransferase (ALT), are indicative of hepatocellular damage. HAV is confirmed by finding anti-HAV IgM (specific antibody to the hepatitis A virus) in serum during the acute or early convalescent phase of illness. This antibody to HAV usually lasts 6 to 12 months. IgG (immunoglobulin G) remains detectable in the serum for a lifetime and denotes a convalescent infection.

Prophylaxis

Recently, a vaccine for hepatitis A has been developed. Immune globulin administered before exposure or during the incubation period of hepatitis A is protective against clinical illness. Its efficacy is greatest (80% to 90%) when given within 2 weeks of exposure (Jackson & McPherson, 1991). Anyone with a known exposure to hepatitis A should be tested for hepatitis A infection and if not immune should receive the vaccine as well as prophylactic immune globulin. Known IgG to hepatitis A means that the person has immunity to this infection and needs no prophylaxis. In cases of known exposure to hepatitis A, close family members of the infected person should also be offered the hepatitis A vaccine, as well as immune globulin as prophylaxis after they are tested for hepatitis A antibodies. For travelers to endemic countries, prophylactic administration of the hepatitis A vaccine plus a course of immune globulin before exposure is recommended.

Treatment Options, Expected Outcomes, and Comprehensive Management

Prevention of hepatitis A is enhanced by a clean water supply. This includes handwashing in restaurants and day-care centers. Use of cloth diapers would minimize the introduction of fecal

TABLE 26-1	Types of Hepatitis				
Virus Type	**A**	**B**	**C**	**D**	**E**
Other names	Infectious	Serum	Parenteral non-A, non-B	Delta	Enteric non-A, non-B
Route of transmission	Fecal–oral Water supply Infected food handlers	Parenteral Blood/blood products Sexual exposure Maternal–Fetal	Parenteral Blood/blood products	Coinfection with hepatitis B via parenteral route Travel to endemic areas	Fecal–oral Water supply
Incubation period	2–6 weeks (28–30 days)	4 weeks–6 months (avg. 60 days)	5–12 weeks	15–60 days	2–7 weeks
Diagnostic criteria	IgM anti-HAV (acute state) IgG anti-HAV (convalescent state)	HBsAg (acute state) HBeAg (high infectivity) HBV DNA Anti-HBS (immunity to Hepatitis B)	Anti-HCV— confirmed by HCV (polymerase chain reaction) Confirmed by biopsy	Anti-HDV IgM anti-HBc (coinfection) Confirmed by biopsy	Anti-HEV IgM (acute state) Anti-HEV IgG (convalescence)
Prophylaxis	Hepatitis A vaccine	Hepatitis B vaccine Adults >50 yrs old may need 4 injections	No vaccine	Hepatitis B vaccine	No vaccine
Treatment	Immune globulin (IgG) prophylaxis best within 2 weeks of exposure	Hepatitis B immune globulin Interferon therapy Transplantation (if cirrhosis and end-stage liver disease develop)	Alpha-interferon injections Transplantation (if cirrhosis and end-stage liver disease develop)	Hepatitis B immune globulin for postexposure prophylaxis	None
Prognosis	No chronic state Lifelong immunity Rarely fatal (0.6% mortality)	Chronic carrier state Can become immune Chronic hepatitis B associated with hepatocellular carcinoma	Chronic carrier state Chronic hepatitis C associated with hepatocellular carcinoma (20%)	Chronic carrier state Immunity to B gives immunity to D	No chronic state 20% mortality in pregnant women in third trimester

---

SIGNS AND SYMPTOMS OF HEPATITIS

During acute phases of any hepatitis infection, the patient may experience any or all of the following symptoms:

- Loss of appetite
- Nausea and vomiting
- Low-grade fever
- Malaise
- Jaundice
- Change in color of urine or stool
- Right upper quadrant pain
- Liver enlargement.

If these symptoms are vague in nature (eg, fatigue, loss of appetite), they may not be sufficient to alert the patient to visit the primary care provider.

---

matter into landfills from disposable diapers. Universal enteric precautions are recommended for health care providers as they can care for potentially infectious asymptomatic patients. Outbreaks among health care workers show that inadequate handwashing and lack of appropriate glove use for handling stool result in exposure of health care workers to this virus.

Hepatitis A is a self-limiting disease. There currently is no treatment recommended for the disease itself, but symptomatic and supportive treatment should be given. These measures are discussed below in the section on self-care.

HEPATITIS B (SERUM HEPATITIS)

Anatomy, Physiology, and Pathology

Hepatitis B virus (HBV) is a DNA virus of the hepadnavirus family. It is transmitted parenterally, by sexual exposure, by contact with infected blood and tissues, and by maternal–fetal spread. HBV codes for a variety of proteins. There are three distinct antigens: surface antigen (HBsAg), core antigen (HBcAg), and the e antigen (HBeAg). These three antigens have antibodies that may appear during the infectious phase.

Epidemiology

There are 1 to 1.25 million hepatitis B carriers in the United States. Hepatitis B is a major cause of death in the Far East and Africa (Bodenheimer et al, 1995). There are about 15,000 new cases of hepatitis B each year in the United States (Bodenheimer et al, 1995). HBV is prevalent in people born in endemic countries as well as their descendants. Most HBV-infected persons in the United States are intravenous drug users, homosexual men, and men and women with multiple sexual partners. Other at-risk groups are prison inmates, household contacts of HBV carriers, infants born to HBV-infected mothers, and hemodialysis recipients. Parenteral transmission can also occur from shared needles and tattooing. Health care workers are at risk through contact with blood and blood products and tissue. The worldwide immunization of newborns and infants with the hepatitis B vaccine should markedly decrease the incidence of hepatitis B in the future.

History and Physical Examination

The incubation period of hepatitis B is 4 weeks to 6 months, with an average of 60 days (Jackson & McPherson, 1991; Lisanti & Talotta, 1994). During the acute phase, symptoms may last about 4 months. Typically, patients with acute hepatitis B infection present with nonspecific complaints such as fatigue and anorexia. Jaundice may appear as the conjugated bilirubin level rises, and the patient may notice dark urine and clay-colored stool. Other signs and symptoms are noted in Box 26-1.

There is a 10% likelihood that persons who become infected with hepatitis B in adulthood will become chronic carriers (Vail, 1997). However, persons infected with hepatitis B in infancy have a 90% likelihood of becoming chronic carriers in adulthood (Vail, 1997). The risk of being a hepatitis B carrier is twofold: first, one can transmit the infection to others; second, one is at increased risk for the development of cirrhosis, liver failure, and primary liver cancer. Some chronic carriers are asymptomatic, whereas others experience symptoms that require intervention.

Diagnostic Studies

Nonspecific liver enzyme elevations (serum transaminase with alanine aminotransferase) may be the first indication that a patient has hepatitis. Clinical evidence of liver disease of at least 6 months' duration, elevated serum aminotransferase levels with a liver biopsy showing an unresolved hepatic inflammation, and confirming serologic markers indicate chronic hepatitis B. HBsAg appears in the blood about 1 month after exposure and may remain for up to 6 months. Persistence of HBsAg for more than 6 months indicates a carrier or chronic state. The presence of hepatitis B core antibody (anti-HBc) occurs 2 weeks after HBsAg appears. The period between the disappearance of HBsAg and the appearance of hepatitis surface antibody (anti-HBs) is known as the window period. During the window period, the only serologic marker indicative of an acute

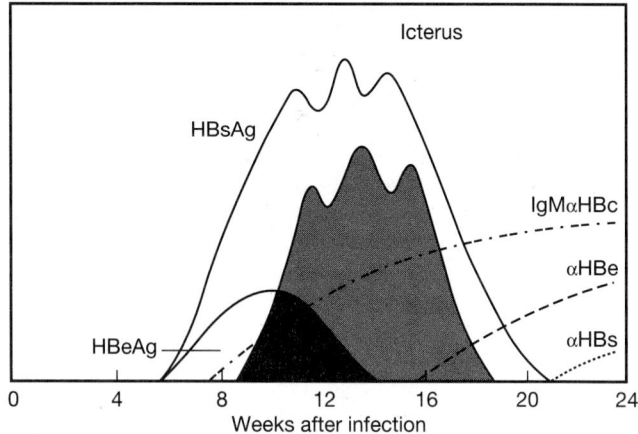

FIGURE 26-1 The course of acute type B hepatitis. HBsAg = hepatitis B surface antigen, HBeAg = hepatitis Be antigen, AST = aspartate transaminase, IgM αHBc = IgM antibody against hepatitis B core antigen, αHBe = antibody against hepatitis e antigen, αHBs = antibody against hepatitis B surface antigen. (Sherlock, S. & Dooley, J. (1997). *Disease of the liver and biliary system*, 9th ed. Boston: Blackwell Sciences)

hepatitis B infection is the presence of hepatitis B core IgM. The presence of anti-HBs indicates immunity to hepatitis B (Fig. 26-1).

Prophylaxis

There is a vaccine for hepatitis B that is 85% to 95% effective. It is a series of three injections, with the second dose given 1 month after the first and the third dose given 6 months thereafter. In adults older than age 50 who have low anti-HBs levels after three vaccine injections, a fourth injection is well tolerated and results in an improved immunogenic response (Bennett et al, 1996).

Recent changes in the Occupational Safety and Health Administration (OSHA) mandates for health care workers have resulted in prophylactic vaccination of health care workers. This step, in combination with barrier protections, should minimize the risk of hepatitis B transmission to health care workers. There is controversy over the beneficial effects of immune globulin administration after needle stick exposure or contact with blood or blood products in cases of hepatitis B or C.

In the United States and worldwide, vaccination programs for all newborns and persons at high risk for contracting hepatitis B are underway in an attempt to decrease the morbidity and mortality rates from HBV. Family members of persons with acute hepatitis B should be treated with the hepatitis B vaccine as well as hepatitis B immune globulin.

Treatment Options, Expected Outcomes, and Comprehensive Management

There is no specific treatment for an acute hepatitis B infection. Rather, supportive care must be provided based on the symptoms. The section on self-care at the end of this chapter outlines supportive care measures.

Chronic hepatitis B carriers with active viral replication and well-compensated liver disease are good candidates for interferon therapy (Davis et al, 1995). Recommended treatment is

5 million units of interferon daily for 6 to 12 months (Schluger, 1997). The most common side effects of interferon therapy are neutropenia, which requires monitoring, and flu-like symptoms, which are transient and usually diminish with continued treatment. The success rate for interferon therapy is these cases is 25% to 50% (Vail, 1997).

The recurrence of hepatitis B after liver transplantation has resulted in significant morbidity and mortality rates. Almost 85% of patients with elevated HBV DNA and HBeAg levels in serum will suffer a relapse of clinical hepatitis within 2 years after transplantation (Bodenheimer et al, 1995), and the 1-year survival rate after transplantation has only been 50% to 60% (Davis et al, 1995). Some transplant centers are treating patients with hepatitis B immune globulin after the transplant to improve survival rates and decrease the incidence of disease recurrence. This has had varying degrees of success. Much work still needs to be done to prevent reinfection, because the value of retransplantation for hepatitis B is questionable.

HEPATITIS C (PARENTERALLY TRANSMITTED NON-A, NON-B HEPATITIS)

Anatomy and Physiology

The hepatitis C virus (HCV) was identified in 1989 as the causative agent in most cases of non-A, non-B hepatitis. HCV is a small, single-stranded RNA virus of approximately 10,000 nucleotides and is most closely related to viruses of the *Flaviviridae* family (Terrault, 1995). There are at least six HCV genotypes based on the 5′ terminal region and nucleotide (NS5) sequence analysis. The main route of transmission is parenteral via contaminated blood and blood products.

Epidemiology

HCV is the most prevalent of the hepatotropic viruses leading to chronic liver disease in the United States. Each year, 150,000 new cases of hepatitis C infection occur in the United States (Jackson & McPherson, 1991; Brown et al, 1994). HCV is encountered worldwide, with a relatively high prevalence in Japan, the southern United States, and the Mediterranean countries of Europe, Africa, and the Middle East, where 0.5% to 1.5% of the blood donors are anti-HCV positive (van der Poel et al, 1994). Most HCV-infected persons are either intravenous drug users (46%) or recipients of blood products not screened for anti-HCV (6%) (Brown et al, 1994; Herreid, 1995). Other parenteral risk factors include tattoos and needle stick injuries among health care workers. HCV infection is common among dialysis patients from the procedure itself as well as from blood transfusions. Transmission of HCV to household contacts of people with HCV infection is low. However, mother-to-child transmission has been documented through HCV RNA detection as a marker of infection in infants.

History and Physical Examination

Classic findings of hepatitis such as abdominal pain and jaundice may be noted, but often the infection is subclinical and manifests years later in a chronic form. Other signs and symptoms of acute hepatitis are noted in Box 26-1. As mentioned above, once viral hepatitis is suspected, serologic assays can identify the specific cause. See Figure 26-1 for the serologic assays available to identify the type of viral hepatitis.

The incubation period of HCV is 5 to 12 weeks during the initial infection. Infection with hepatitis C is asymptomatic in 70% to 80% of people with HCV antibody (Najm, 1997; MacDonald et al, 1996). Chronic infection with HCV develops into chronic liver disease (70%), cirrhosis (20%), or hepatocellular carcinoma (20%) (MacDonald et al, 1996). Once cirrhosis has developed, screening for hepatocellular carcinoma with abdominal sonograms and measuring serum alpha-fetoproteins is essential. The number of deaths attributed each year to HCV is approximately 1% to 2% (Najm, 1997).

Diagnostic Studies

Hepatitis C infection is diagnosed by persistent elevation of serum transaminases, positive anti-HCV antibodies (confirmed by HCV polymerase chain reaction), and the presence of hepatitis on a liver biopsy. It may take as long as 6 months after primary infection for an anti-HCV antibody response to develop. HCV infection can produce fluctuations in serum transaminase levels; thus, serial testing (at 3 months and 6 months) may be required to detect a rise in the ALT.

Infection can be diagnosed by tests that detect the presence of specific antibody to HCV and by tests that detect the presence of HCV RNA itself. EIA2 is the most frequently used serologic test for diagnosing HCV infection. It is an enzyme-linked immunoassay that detects antibody to the C-100-3 antigen located in the NS4 region. Seroconversion occurs within a range of 15 days to 9 months after the onset of hepatitis in 85% of patients (Herreid, 1995).

The recombinant immunoblot assay (RIBA2) detects antibodies directed against the C-100-3 antigen and is a supplementary or confirmatory assay, with 90% accuracy. The polymerase chain reaction detects viral RNA within the first week of infection and when antibody production is impaired, providing increased sensitivity. HCV RNA is currently the best marker of viremia and infectivity.

Prophylaxis

There is no vaccine for hepatitis C. An exposed person should have a liver function panel and baseline testing for anti-HCV. Both these tests should be repeated at 3 and 6 months. Currently, all blood administered in the United States is screened for hepatitis C before transfusion.

Treatment Options, Expected Outcomes, and Comprehensive Management

Because a small percentage of people develop acute hepatitis, primary care providers are focusing their attention on preventing chronic disease and educating patients about risk factors for contracting HCV. With an acute infection, supportive measures, such as those noted in the section on self-care at the end of the chapter, may be implemented. The risk of fulminant hepatitis is 1%, with the mortality rate reaching 91% for this complication (Herreid, 1995). Corticosteroids are of no value because they increase viremia in anti-HCV-positive, autoantibody-positive patients with chronic hepatitis (Magrin, 1994).

Alpha-interferon, an antiviral agent, was first studied by Hoofnagle in 1986. Patients who responded showed normalization of ALT concentrations over a 1-year period. Renewed HCV RNA positivity may be a more sensitive indicator of relapse after interferon therapy than an increase in ALT. Alpha-interferon is used to treat both active and chronic infections, although studies report that 40% to 50% of patients still show viremia after treatment (Najm, 1997). Because it is not known why some patients respond and others do not, it is difficult to determine criteria for patient selection, predictors of response, and cost of treatment.

Antiviral agents are also being used to treat acute and chronic hepatitis C. Ribavirin, an orally administered guanosine analogue, normalizes ALT levels, but HCV RNA remains detectable during and after therapy. Combination therapy (interferon and ribavirin) is under study and may be effective in clearing viremia.

Liver transplantation has been done in patients with HCV. Nearly 95% of patients who had hepatitis C before the transplant became viremic after the transplant (Terrault, 1995). Some transplant centers are using alpha-interferon to treat hepatitis C after transplant, with varying success.

HEPATITIS D (DELTA HEPATITIS)

Anatomy, Physiology, and Pathology

The hepatitis D virus (HDV) was recognized as a new virus in 1977. Hepatitis D is a defective RNA virus and as an incomplete virus requires the presence or helper function of the HBsAg of HBV to survive and replicate. Therefore, it can infect only persons who are HBsAg positive. The hepatitis D infection that occurs simultaneously with HBV infection is self-limiting in 95% of patients (Gurevich, 1993b).

Epidemiology

Hepatitis D is endemic in the Mediterranean area, the Middle East, and South America. In the United States, it is thought that HDV accounts for 2% of all cases of acute viral hepatitis (Najm, 1997). HDV has been reported to cause outbreaks of both fulminant and chronic hepatitis in the northern part of South America but is virtually absent in areas of the continent with similar or higher HBV endemicity rates (Torres & Machado, 1994; Poss, 1989). High-risk groups such as intravenous drug users, hemophiliacs, and recipients of multiple blood transfusions have had an impact on endemic regions. This, coupled with poor sanitary conditions, has increased the prevalence of HDV in Latin America.

History and Physical Examination

Hepatitis D is a coinfection with HBV, so signs and symptoms specifically associated with HDV are indistinguishable from symptoms of other types of hepatitis. Signs and symptoms of hepatitis are noted above and in Box 26-1.

The incubation period for hepatitis D ranges from 15 to 60 days. The most common form of HDV infection occurs in the chronic HBsAg carrier who develops an acute episode of delta hepatitis (Najm, 1997; Torres & Machado, 1994). This is known as a superinfection. It can also occur as a coinfection, which means that hepatitis B and D infect the host simultaneously.

Diagnostic Studies

In coinfection with hepatitis B, aminotransferase levels become elevated, along with the appearance of clinical symptoms and jaundice. Acute coinfection can be identified by simultaneous detection of IgM anti-HBc, which along with HBsAg establishes acute HBV infection. In chronic hepatitis D, serodiagnosis depends on the presence of persistent HBsAg and antidelta antibodies. Liver biopsies can confirm the presence of the delta virus antigen.

Treatment Options, Expected Outcomes, and Comprehensive Management

Prevention of HBV infection will prevent delta hepatitis (see section on HBV). There is no known treatment for hepatitis D, although there have been trials using interferon therapy. The risk to health care workers is low and preventable with hepatitis B vaccination.

Sixty-seventy percent of patients with chronic delta hepatitis will develop cirrhosis over 2 to 15 years (Najm, 1997). However, the HDV superinfection does not accelerate the development of hepatocellular carcinoma (Huo, 1996). The development of hepatocellular carcinoma in hepatitis D patients does not produce worse disease outcomes than it does in hepatitis B patients, as long as the carcinoma is diagnosed early and actively treated.

HEPATITIS E (ENTERICALLY TRANSMITTED NON-A, NON-B HEPATITIS)

Anatomy, Physiology, and Pathology

The hepatitis E virus (HEV) is a nonenveloped, single-stranded RNA. Hepatitis E is similar to hepatitis A, with transmission through the fecal–oral route. Most outbreaks are associated with contaminated drinking water or tainted food. Direct contamination is rare, but there appears to be some vertical transmission from mother to infant that can be fatal.

Epidemiology

HEV is prevalent in regions with poor sanitation systems, where inadequate sewage disposal or communal bathing is practiced. Although rare in the United States, HEV infections have been documented in new immigrants and visitors from endemic areas such as Mexico, Asia, and West and North Africa. As such, HEV does not pose a major health threat in the United States. The best way to prevent infection is to avoid food or water that may be contaminated in endemic areas.

History and Physical Examination

HEV is an acute, self-limiting, icteric disease that does not produce chronic disease. Jaundice may be accompanied by malaise, anorexia, abdominal discomfort, nausea, vomiting, or liver enlargement. Other signs and symptoms are noted in Box 26-1.

The incubation period ranges from 2 to 7 weeks. As with hepatitis A, symptoms resolve in 4 to 8 weeks. There is a high mortality rate among pregnant women (20%), especially in the third trimester (Brown et al, 1994).

Diagnostic Studies

Serologic tests for hepatitis E have been developed but are not available commercially in the United States. It is an enzyme-linked immunosorbent assay for anti-HEV IgM, which is diagnostic of acute hepatitis E infection. Convalescence is confirmed by the presence of anti-HEV IgG.

Treatment Options, Expected Outcomes, and Comprehensive Management

There is no vaccine for HEV, although one is being developed. The best way to prevent transmission of HEV is through hand-washing and maintaining a clean water supply to reduce the number of cases in areas where the virus is endemic. OSHA mandates for universal precautions remain the best preventive method for health care workers (the use of gloves, goggles, and gowns as needed for contact with blood, blood products, and items contaminated with these fluids). Supportive treatment for acute infections is described below in the section on self-care.

HEPATITIS G

A new hepatotropic virus has recently been identified by reverse transcriptase–polymerase chain reaction using the NS5 region of the hepatitis G virus (HGV) genome. It is thought to be a non-A through non-E hepatitis virus. It is a single-stranded RNA genome and has the structure of a *Flaviviri-dae*-like virus. There appear to be two strains of the same virus, identified as GBV-C and HGV. It is thought to be transmitted parenterally.

The literature is inconclusive as to whether HGV has a causative role in acute and chronic hepatitis. However, some recent studies indicate that it has minimal clinical significance in causing chronic liver diseases such as cirrhosis or hepatocellular carcinoma (Zanetti, 1997; Colombatto, 1997; Kitamoto, 1997). In patients with chronic hepatitis C, it has been reported that interferon therapy had some effect on HGV RNA becoming negative (Baba, 1997).

TEACHING AND SELF-CARE

The patient's understanding of the disease and cooperation with management are essential. Patients must be educated about the importance of handwashing, using condoms, adhering to dietary restrictions, keeping appointments, and so forth. Patients must be able to recognize the symptoms that may indicate a worsening of their condition (eg, fatigue, anorexia, weight loss). Early in the disease process, the patient should be educated about appropriate dietary modifications and physical activity. Some primary care providers may insist on bed rest and a diet high in carbohydrates and low in fat. However, recommending small, frequent meals for those who report loss of appetite is a good strategy. Alcohol consumption should be avoided. A referral to a dietitian or physical therapist may be

appropriate. Return to work must be discussed and determined after an acute infection.

Family members of patients infected with hepatitis A and E need to be taught to wash their hands after contact with the patient and not to eat food prepared by the patient. Family members should be tested for the hepatitis virus.

A patient with a hepatitis B or C infection transmitted by intravenous drug use or shared needles should also be screened for HIV. Sexual contacts of hepatitis B-infected persons must be contacted and offered hepatitis B vaccine and hepatitis B immune globulin. Follow-up of those infected with hepatitis B is no longer needed when serologies reveal a negative HBsAg and the presence of anti-HBS, because this means that immunity to hepatitis B has developed.

For those who become chronic carriers of hepatitis B or C, education includes ways of preventing the spread of the disease:

- Condom use during sexual intercourse
- Avoiding sexual intercourse while menstruating
- Eliminate intravenous drug use
- No donating of blood
- No shared needle use.

A chronic hepatitis B carrier who becomes pregnant should be told that her newborn will be given hepatitis B immune globulin and the hepatitis B vaccine to avoid infection.

COMMUNITY RESOURCES

A list of community resources, national organizations, and Web sites about hepatitis is located at the end of the unit on gastrointestinal disorders.

REFERRAL POINTS AND CLINICAL WARNINGS

Referral to a gastroenterologist or hepatologist is recommended when the etiology of hepatitis is uncertain. As noted, there are many causes for hepatitis (eg, viruses, medications), and care of the patient depends on the etiology. If the etiology is presumed to be self-limiting but the hepatitis persists, this too is a reason for referral.

With the discovery of new viruses and treatments, patients who have chronic hepatitis B or C should be evaluated as candidates for treatment with alpha-interferon or other agents. This often requires a referral to a specialist.

Patients who are hepatitis B carriers are also at risk for the development of hepatocellular carcinoma. Whether caused by hepatitis B or C, if the lesion is small and without metastases or vascular invasion, potential treatment options include a liver resection or referral for liver transplant.

Hepatic failure resulting from end-stage liver disease caused by hepatitis B or C is an important indication for liver transplantation. Patients who develop chronic hepatitis B may eventually present with muscle wasting, ascites, and variceal bleeding. Cases of fulminant hepatic failure in the presence of HBsAg, accompanied by worsening liver function tests, a prolonged prothrombin time, and encephalopathy require immediate evaluation. In both of these cases, referral to a hepatologist and a liver transplant service for evaluation is indicated.

Patients diagnosed with acute hepatitis A, B, and C may be reported to the public health department for epidemiologic purposes.

EDITOR'S NOTE:

COMPLEMENTARY APPROACHES

A general discussion of complementary approaches can be found in Chapter 3. The following, while not an exhaustive list, are some complementary approaches being used for this condition. Additional information on these approaches, including precautions, can be found in Appendices A and B. Providers need to assess for the use of complementary approaches as part of the patient's history, as they may impact conventional therapies, and patients may not volunteer this information unless specifically asked. Efficacy of many complementary approaches is not as well documented as that of conventional therapies. Providers need to read the literature before suggesting these complementary approaches.

- Vitamins, minerals, herbs, supplements
  Milk thistle
- Complementary Modalities
  Aromatherapy

References

Baba, T., Makind, R., Shibata, M., et al. (1997). Interferon treatment for hepatitis G virus infection in patients with chronic hepatitis C. *Nippon-Rinsho, 55*(3); 625–630.

Bennett, R.G., Powers, D.C., Reemsburg, R.E., Scheve, A., & Clements, M.L. (1996). Hepatitis B virus vaccination for older adults. *Journal of the American Geriatrics Society, 44*(6), 699–703.

Bodenheimer, H.C. Jr., Schluger, L.K., & Sheiner, P. (1995). Viral hepatitis in liver transplant recipients. *Clinical Transplantation, 9,* 211–214.

Brown, E.A., Kawanishi, H., & Schiff, E.R. (1994). Hepatitis C and E: How much of a threat? *Patient Care, 28*(9), 105–117.

Davis, C.L., Gretch, D.R., & Carithers, R.L. (1995). Hepatitis B and transplantation. *Infectious Disease Clinics of North America, 9*(4), 925–941.

Gurevich, I. (1993b). Hepatitis part II. Viral hepatitis: B, C, and D. *Heart & Lung, 22*(5), 450–458.

Herreid, J. (1995). Hepatitis C: Past, present and future. *MedSurg Nursing, 4*(3), 179–187.

Huo, T., Wu, J.C., Lai, C., et al. (1996). Comparison of clinico-pathological features in hepatitis B virus-associated hepatocellular carcinoma with or without hepatitis D virus superinfection. *Journal of Hepatology, 25*(4), 439–444.

Jackson, M.M., & McPherson, D.C. (1991). Hepatitis A through E—Current and future trends. *Today's O.R. Nurse, 13*(10), 7–12.

Kitamoto, M., Moriya, T., Sasaki, F., et al. (1997). Detection of GBV-C RNA among non-B non-C hepatocellular carcinoma patients. *Nippon-Rinsho, 55*(3), 583–586.

Lisanti, P., & Talotta, D. (1994). An overview of viral hepatitis: A through E. *Journal of the American Operating Room Nurse, 59*(5), 997–1005.

Long, J., & Kyllonen, K. (1997). Adult vaccinations: A short review. *Cleveland Clinic Journal of Medicine, 64*(6), 311–316.

MacDonald, M., Crofts, N., & Kaldor, J. (1996). Transmission of Hepatitis C virus: Rates, routes, and cofactors. *Epidemiological Reviews, 18*(2), 137–148.

Magrin, S., Craxi, A., Fabiano, C., et al. (1994). Hepatitis C viremia in chronic liver disease: Relationship to interferon or corticosteroid treatment. *Hepatology, 19,* 280–285.

Marx, J.F. (1993). Viral hepatitis: Unscrambling the alphabet. *Nursing, 93,* 34–41.

Najm, W. (1997). Viral hepatitis: How to manage type C and D infections. *Geriatrics, 52*(5), 28–37.

Poss, J.E. (1989). Hepatitis D virus infection. *Nurse Practitioner, 14*(8), 13–15.

Terrault, N.A., Wright, T.L., & Pereira, B.J.G. (1995). Hepatitis C in the transplant recipient. *Infectious Disease Clinics of North America, 9*(4), 943–964.

Torres, J.R., & Machado, I.V. (1994). Special aspects of hepatitis B virus and delta virus infection in Latin America. *Infectious Disease Clinics of North America, 8*(1), 13–27.

Vail, B.A. (1997). Management of chronic viral hepatitis. *American Family Physician, 55*(8), 2749–2755.

Van der Poel, C.L., Cuypers, T.H., & Reesink, H.W. (1994). Hepatitis C virus: Six years on. *Lancet, 344,* 1475–1479.

Zanetti, A.R., Tanzi, E., Romano, L. et al. (1997). GBV-C/HGV: A new human hepatitis-related virus. *Respiratory Virology, 148*(2): 119–122.

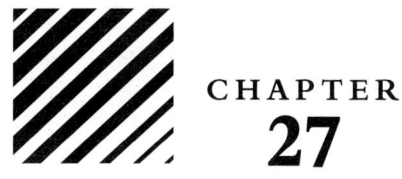

CHAPTER
27

Inflammatory Bowel Disease

James F. Marion, MD, and Catherine M. Concert, MS, RN, CS, FNP

Ulcerative colitis (UC) and Crohn's disease are chronic inflammatory diseases of the bowel and share many demographic, epidemiologic, and clinical features. Because UC and Crohn's disease lack any unique distinguishing features and can resemble many other diseases, there is considerable potential for misdiagnosis. The essential nature and etiology of these inflammatory bowel diseases are unknown; however, our understanding of the clinical patterns, immune dysfunction, environmental factors, and genetic predisposition underlying these conditions has increased considerably and has spurred the development of new therapies. The early recognition of these diseases and appropriate management can spare patients hospitalization and surgery. Primary care providers are invaluable members of the team caring for patients with inflammatory bowel disease (IBD) and can claim a leading role in early disease recognition and diagnosis, coordination of management among multiple specialties, prevention of disease recurrence, and cancer screening.

ANATOMY, PHYSIOLOGY, AND PATHOLOGY

Intensive investigation over the last 60 years has failed to produce a simple explanation of the pathophysiology of IBD. An infectious agent has eluded investigators, and searches for multiple candidate parasites, mycobacteria, viruses, and bacteria have proved futile.

There is strong evidence that immune cell dysfunction, especially T-cell activation, plays an important role in UC and Crohn's disease. Activated T lymphocytes produce IL-2 (an inflammatory cytokine), which may play a role in the inflammatory cascade in which the activation of other T cells, B cells, and macrophages occurs. Macrophages, the first line of defense, present luminal antigens to the sensitized T cells and release a host of proinflammatory cytokines. The cytokines produced in the cascade amplify the inflammatory response by recruiting neutrophils and monocytes. The subsequent release of oxygen metabolites, proteases, and other inflammatory cytokines then produces macroscopic mucosal injury (Pullman & Doe, 1992). Tumor necrosis factor alpha (TNF-α) and other cytokines then perpetuate the inflammatory response. The enteric nervous system and neuropeptides such as somatostatin may also play a role in regulating or perpetuating the inflammatory cascade. Platelet dysfunction and coagulation abnormalities, in close consort with the inflammatory cascade, are likely to contribute to the injury of the bowel.

Crohn's Disease

Crohn's disease is characterized by transmural granulomatous inflammation. It can involve any part of the gastrointestinal tract from the mouth to the anus but most commonly involves the terminal ileum (Crohn et al, 1932). Crohn's disease can also be called regional enteritis, and when it involves the colon, granulomatous colitis. Inflammation tends to be patchy and noncontiguous; a mucosal biopsy taken during endoscopy may miss submucosal involvement. Colonic involvement typically spares the rectum.

Early in the inflammatory process, edema, hyperemia, and aphthous ulceration of the mucosa predominate. As the disease progresses, these aphthae can enlarge and coalesce to form deep, serpiginous ulcerations with nodular swelling of the intervening inflamed mucosal lining, producing the classic cobblestone appearance seen on contrast radiography. The bowel can then become thickened, fibrotic, and narrowed. The surrounding mesentery can also become edematous and fatty and can even encase the involved bowel segment, producing a phlegmon. A phlegmon or abscess can produce an abdominal mass palpable on physical examination. Fistulas, the result of transmural inflammation and fissuring, can penetrate the bowel wall, producing local perforation and abscess formation. These fistulas can communicate with adjacent bowel, organs (eg, urinary bladder), or even skin.

Ulcerative Colitis

The inflammatory process of UC involves only the colonic mucosa. The inflammation can involve the rectum and sigmoid colon or the entire colon. UC is usually symmetrical and continuous and involves the colon from the anal verge. Some patients present with isolated proctitis that can progress to involve the proximal colon. If the disease involves the entire colon (also called universal colitis) and the inflammation is severe, indirect injury of the terminal ileum, called backwash ileitis, can occur. Otherwise, any proximal gut or small bowel involvement implies Crohn's disease.

Early inflammation can produce hyperemia, edema, and friability. As the inflammatory process progresses, spontaneous hemorrhage and superficial ulcerations of the mucosa develop. These can become diffuse and coalesce, forming deep, confluent ulcerations. With chronic recurrent injury, fibrosis can develop. Pseudopolyps, the result of chronic inflammation and healing, can protrude into the colonic lumen and cause obstruction. Longstanding inflammation can cause stricture formation, which can be a harbinger of underlying adenocarcinoma in patients with UC.

Severe inflammation causes thinning and dilation of the bowel wall and denudement of the mucosal lining, compromising the protective mucosal barrier. Toxic dilation, also called megacolon, can occur and possibly lead to perforation. Small rectovaginal or perirectal fistulas are rare but can occur in UC.

These distinguishing features of Crohn's disease and UC become less reliable with chronic or severe disease and after successful treatment. Healing of UC can be uneven or patchy. Use of rectal or topical medications can produce rectal sparing similar to Crohn's colitis.

PATHOLOGY

The traditional histologic, pathognomonic feature of Crohn's disease, the noncaseating epithelioid granuloma, is found in only 10% to 28% of endoscopic biopsies and only half of surgical specimens. As disease severity increases, and with multiple biopsies, this yield is greater (Surawica et al, 1981). The inflammatory process can traverse all four layers of the bowel, up to and including the serosal layer.

The typical histologic feature of UC is the crypt abscess with proliferation of neutrophils in the lamina propria. Distortion or atrophy of the crypts with a villous or irregular mucosal surface can also be seen. These histologic changes can even be seen in endoscopically normal-appearing mucosa (Spiliadis & Lennard-Jones, 1987).

EPIDEMIOLOGY

The incidence of Crohn's disease has been increasing over the last 50 years, whereas that of UC has remained stable (Whelan, 1990). UC is more prevalent than Crohn's disease. UC has an incidence of approximately 6 to 8 cases per 100,000 population. The prevalence rate ranges from approximately 39 to 117 per 100,000 population. The incidence of Crohn's disease is approximately 2 cases per 100,000 population. The prevalence rate is approximately 28 to 106 per 100,000 population.

Both are diseases of young people, and a diagnosis of IBD is most likely to be made in patients in their teens and 20s. Men and women are roughly equally affected. Although these diseases can occur in any age group, a second peak of incidence has been documented in the seventh and eighth decades of life (Lashner et al, 1986; Sedlack et al, 1980). This second peak may be attributable to confusion of diverticulitis or mesenteric ischemia with IBD or, more likely, a result of more intense evaluation of elderly patients suspected of having IBD.

There is considerable geographic variation in the incidence of IBD. The incidence in developed countries increases in direct proportion to the distance from the equator, with Scandinavia, the United Kingdom, and North America having the highest incidence. In the Southern Hemisphere, Australia and South Africa have an increased incidence. Whites are more likely to have IBD than patients of Asian or African descent. IBD is more common among patients of Jewish heritage. The geographic variability in incidence among Jewish populations appears to mirror that of the general population. Migrants to areas of higher incidence subsequently exhibit a higher rate of IBD. Studies that have indicated a higher incidence among urban residents or among members of certain occupations are probably undermined by referral bias.

Genetic Factors

A genetic component is suspected in IBD. Although the concordance between monozygotic twins is significantly less than 100%, siblings of patients with IBD are 17 to 35 times more likely to have IBD than the general population. Investigators have begun to focus on HLA alleles on chromosome 6, which may be associated with genes involved in the production of the inflammatory cytokine TNF-α. An "IBD gene" has not been discovered, and any heritable component to IBD is likely to involve multiple genes.

Environmental Factors

Certain environmental factors contribute to the pathogenesis of IBD. Smoking is positively associated with Crohn's disease, but in UC a negative association has been observed. An increased risk for IBD among users of oral contraceptives has not been confirmed.

Diet would seem a logical focus of investigation, but numerous studies examining diet and IBD have failed to demonstrate any dietary risk factors. Increased sugar intake among patients with Crohn's disease is more likely a result than a cause. There is no consistent evidence that prenatal vitamin supplements, tonsillectomy, childhood vaccinations, early childhood hygiene, toothpaste use, psychosocial factors, and breast-feeding or bottle-feeding play any role in the etiology of IBD (Sachar et al, 1980).

DIAGNOSTIC CRITERIA AND DIFFERENTIAL DIAGNOSIS

There are no set diagnostic criteria for IBD. The diagnosis of Crohn's disease is based on the history and clinical profile and supporting radiographic, histologic, or endoscopic data. Most patients will give a history of at least 6 weeks of symptoms, thus excluding most acute infectious enterocolitides. Several conditions can act as impostors of Crohn's disease, including tuberculosis, *Yersinia* enteritis, *Entamoeba histolytica*, and chlamydia. Appendicitis, intestinal lymphoma or carcinoma, carcinoid tumor of the small bowel, celiac sprue, and diverticulitis often can be mistaken for Crohn's disease.

UC can be mistaken for several conditions that produce inflammation and ulceration of the colonic mucosa and bloody diarrhea: *Escherichia coli*, *Salmonella*, *Shigella*, *Campylobacter*, *E. histolytica*, and cytomegalovirus. Other impostors include diverticulitis, cancer of the colon, ischemic colitis, nonsteroidal anti-inflammatory drug colopathy, radiation injury to the rectum, pseudomembranous or antibiotic-associated colitis, and solitary rectal ulcer syndrome (Marion et al, 1998).

HISTORY AND PHYSICAL EXAMINATION

Patients with IBD can present with multiple, often confusing, symptoms. Certain patterns in the history of these patients allow the provider to distinguish IBD from other gastrointestinal diseases and between UC and Crohn's disease (Table 27-1).

Crohn's Disease

The patient with Crohn's disease commonly presents with systemic symptoms, including malaise, fever, night sweats, and weight loss. Most commonly, patients complain of right lower

TABLE 27-1	Clinical Features Differentiating UC from Crohn's Disease	
	UC	**Crohn's Disease**
Gross blood in stool	Almost always	Occasionally
Mucus	Almost always	Occasionally
Systemic symptoms	Occasionally	Frequently
Pain	Occasionally	Frequently
Abdominal mass	Rarely	Frequently
Significant perineal disease	No	Frequently
Abdominal mass	Rarely	Frequently
Fistulas	No	Frequently
Abscess	No	Occasionally
Intestinal obstruction	Rarely	Frequently
Response to antibiotics	Occasionally	Frequently
Recurrence after surgery	No	Frequently
Current smoker	Rarely	Frequently
Former smoker	Frequently	Rarely
Previous appendectomy	Rarely	Occasionally ("missed")

Source: Alstrad et al, 1990.

quadrant pain indicative of distal ileal involvement. Involvement of the stomach and duodenum can produce pain similar to that of peptic ulcer disease. As the disease progresses, chronic scarring can cause gastric outlet or duodenal obstruction.

In the teenage patient, a history of developmental delay resulting from malabsorption may be elicited. Patients will often give a history of increased borborygmi. Nocturnal abdominal pain, severe enough to interrupt a sound sleep, or nocturnal bowel movements help to distinguish IBD from functional syndromes of the bowel. Gross rectal bleeding can be seen but is unusual. Most patients complain of frequent, loose, nonbloody stools and right lower quadrant pain.

Symptoms of intermittent small intestinal obstruction or a frank perforation may suggest underlying Crohn's disease. Fistulas can penetrate adjoining abdominal or perineal structures such as the urinary bladder, producing pyuria, fecaluria, or pneumaturia. Penetration of the skin or vagina may present with passage of air, stool, or mucus. Complications, including toxic megacolon and colonic perforation, associated with UC can also be seen in Crohn's disease. Patients may give a history of "missed" appendectomy—that is, ileitis that was mistaken for appendicitis.

Ulcerative Colitis

UC patients most often present with bloody stools accompanied by mucus and diarrhea. If only the rectum is inflamed, patients may complain of constipation with a sense of urgency and passage of bloody mucus. The passage of gross blood is the cardinal feature of UC. Disease limited to the distal or left colon is usually not accompanied by constitutional symptoms, whereas universal or more severe disease can produce symptoms of malaise, nausea, and diffuse abdominal pain. UC has a strong tendency toward recurrence, and patients may give a previous history of hospitalization for severe disease or toxic megacolon. A history of recent discontinuation of tobacco may also be elicited.

The primary provider may be faced with making the diagnosis of IBD in the pediatric patient. A child may present with severe, overt symptoms similar to those seen in adults, but often the provider is faced with a more subtle constellation of complaints, including unexplained fever, arthralgias, and growth retardation.

Extraintestinal manifestations occur in both UC an Crohn's disease (Table 27-2). The arthritis affects the larger joints. Some manifestations may precede the bowel symptoms, and diagnosing IBD may be difficult. Other manifestations (eg, ankylosing spondylitis) are not related to the severity of the disease, and treatment is challenging.

Cancer Prevention

The risk of colorectal cancer in patients with extensive UC and Crohn's colitis is considerably higher than in the general population. A patient with universal UC has a lifetime risk of

TABLE 27-2	Extraintestinal Manifestations of IBD

MORE LIKELY TO BE SEEN IN PATIENTS WITH UC
Primary sclerosing cholangitis, pericholangitis
Pyoderma gangrenosum

MORE LIKELY TO BE SEEN IN PATIENTS WITH CROHN'S DISEASE
Erythema nodosum
Aphthous stomatitis
Amyloidosis
Iritis and episcleritis

CAN BE SEEN IN EITHER CROHN'S DISEASE OR UC
Ankylosing spondylitis
Peripheral arthritis
Hypercoagulability (deep vein thrombosis, cerebrovascular accident, pulmonary embolus)

colorectal cancer of approximately 6%. The risk increases with the duration and extent of disease. A patient with extensive UC of 7 years' duration should be enrolled in a surveillance program of yearly colonoscopy. Patients with extensive Crohn's colitis should also be enrolled in a similar surveillance program (Gillen et al, 1994). Patients with UC limited to the rectosigmoid should be reassured that their risk of colorectal carcinoma is similar to that of the general population.

Considerations of Fertility and Pregnancy

Fertility is usually not altered in IBD. Patients with inactive IBD have roughly the same risks of miscarriage and prematurity as matched controls (Mayberry & Weterman, 1986). Active disease in the mother increases the risk of miscarriage, low birth weight, and prematurity (Khosla et al, 1984). In general, women should be counseled to postpone attempts at conceiving until they are in remission. Men taking sulfasalazine must be switched to a 5-ASA compound because of the reversible, adverse effect of sulfasalazine on sperm count, morphology, and motility.

It is inadvisable to discontinue medications if a patient with IBD becomes pregnant. A flare in disease activity from withdrawal of medicines is more likely to harm the fetus than any medicines currently in use. Use of 5-ASA, sulfasalazine, and corticosteroids appears to be safe throughout pregnancy. Increasingly, the safety of immunomodulators (6-mercaptopurine and azathioprine) is becoming apparent (Alstead et al, 1990; Dayan et al, 1996). Use of prednisone, 5-ASA, and sulfasalazine should not preclude breast-feeding. Data regarding breast-feeding and immunomodulator therapies are lacking, and mothers should be counseled against breast-feeding while taking these medicines.

DIAGNOSTIC STUDIES

Laboratory Tests

IBD can produce many abnormalities in routine screening laboratory tests. Anemia, leukocytosis, and elevated platelet counts may be noted on the complete blood count. Patients with UC are more likely to have a microcytic anemia, whereas those with Crohn's disease of the small bowel usually have macrocytic anemia from malabsorption of cobalamin (vitamin B_{12}) or folic acid. The erythrocyte sedimentation rate and the C-reactive protein level, both nonspecific indicators of inflammation, can be elevated in both forms of IBD. Abnormal liver function tests, including levels of alkaline phosphatase and transaminases, may be seen in IBD because of reactive hepatitis or primary sclerosing cholangitis.

Low serum protein and albumin levels can be seen in IBD and can indicate chronicity and severity. Electrolyte abnormalities, including hypokalemia, hypomagnesemia, and hypocalcemia, can be documented in many IBD patients, especially those taking steroids.

Serologic blood tests to help distinguish between UC and Crohn's disease are available but have yet to be evaluated prospectively. The presence of perinuclear antineutrophil antibodies suggests UC, whereas the presence of anti-*Saccharomyces cervisiae* antibodies suggests Crohn's disease. However, 10% of patients with IBD may not be categorized by these assays.

Radiography

Once a diagnosis of IBD is suspected, contrast radiography is a useful tool in making the diagnosis of IBD but not in determining clinical activity.

Crohn's disease most often affects the distal ileum and produces a characteristic appearance on a barium small bowel series. Stricturing, thickening of the bowel loops, fistulas, and aphthous ulceration can be detected in a small bowel series in a patient with Crohn's disease. A normal small bowel series is usually seen in UC. Barium enema is useful in evaluating the extent of disease in UC and the presence of fistula in Crohn's disease. It does not, however, correlate with disease severity and is not useful in screening for precancerous changes. Computed tomography (CT) is useful in the evaluation of an abdominal mass of Crohn's disease if an abscess is suspected. CT-guided needle aspiration of an intra-abdominal abscess associated with Crohn's disease rarely prevents surgery. Ultrasonography can detect hydronephrosis associated with Crohn's disease but overall plays a lesser role in the evaluation and management of IBD.

Endoscopy

Flexible sigmoidoscopy or even proctoscopy, especially when used in conjunction with a small bowel series, may be used to confirm a diagnosis of IBD. These modalities are particularly useful in the patient with severe, active colitis, where colonoscopy should be avoided. Colonoscopy is useful when the diagnosis is in question, the colitis is more quiescent, or surveillance colonoscopy is needed. The rectal mucosa is almost always involved in UC, whereas in Crohn's disease the rectum is often spared.

Stricture formation in Crohn's disease or UC can complicate the course of the disease and confound efforts at colonoscopic surveillance. Stricture formation in patients with IBD is associated with a high risk of carcinoma, particularly in patients with UC. Strictures encountered in patients with Crohn's disease, on the other hand, are typically benign. Endoscopic dilation of strictures in Crohn's disease can produce symptomatic relief in about 60% of patients, but multiple dilations are usually required and the risk of perforation is about 10%. Only endoscopists experienced with these procedures should be consulted (Marion et al, 1997).

TREATMENT OPTIONS, EXPECTED OUTCOMES, AND COMPREHENSIVE TREATMENT

The medical therapies used in the management of IBD control the inflammatory process and should be tailored to the severity, location, and type of IBD (Table 27-3). These medicines are used to treat active disease and, in most cases, maintain a remission once the acute attack has been controlled. Many patients will be managed with a combination of these drugs, and the importance of maintaining the medical regimen once remission has been achieved must be stressed. A consistent rule of medical therapy of IBD is that it is easier to maintain a remission with medicines once it is achieved than to regain a remission after it is lost. Prevention of a flare-up of IBD is essential.

Aminosalicylates

Aminosalicylates are effective for both UC and Crohn's disease and can be used in patients with mild to moderate disease. Sulfasalazine has been used for many years and is effective for

TABLE 27-3	Current Medical Therapies for IBD
Aminosalicylates	Azathioprine
Sulfasalazine	Methotrexate
Mesalamine	Cyclosporine
Olsalazine	FK-506
Antibiotics	Antidiarrheals
Metronidazole	Loperamide
Ciprofloxacin	Codeine
Clarithromycin	Deodorized tincture of opium
Ampicillin	Antispasmodics
Corticosteroids	Hyoscyamine
Hydrocortisone	Dicyclomine
Prednisone (oral)	Nutritional
Cortifoam (rectal)	Ensure, Sustacal, Resource
Cortisone enemas	supplements
Budesonide	Elemental diet
Immunomodulators	Low-residue diet
6-mercaptopurine	TPN

Crohn's disease and UC (Dissanyake & Truelove, 1973; Summers et al, 1979; Van Hess et al, 1981). Newer 5-ASA drugs, including mesalamine, have a theoretical advantage over sulfasalazine because of controlled release throughout the bowel and fewer side effects. None of the 5-ASA agents, however, has been shown to be more effective than sulfasalazine. Topical 5-ASA, either in suppository or enema form, is useful in treating ulcerative proctosigmoiditis.

Antibiotics

Antibiotics are effective in Crohn's disease and are a useful adjunct to 5-ASA therapy in mild to moderate disease. These drugs decrease the luminal antigenic load, treat suppurative and fistulizing complications, and may have an indirect immunomodulating effect. Metronidazole has been studied more extensively than other antibiotics and is most useful for perineal disease and colonic disease. Side effects, including nausea, dyspepsia, a metallic taste, and a furry tongue, are dose-related and reversible. Paresthesias related to the drug can persist for months after discontinuation. Other antibiotics, including ciprofloxacin and clarithromycin, have been studied in uncontrolled trials and may be useful. The role of antibiotics in treating UC has yet to be defined, and clinical controlled trials are ongoing.

Corticosteroids

Corticosteroids should be reserved for patients whose disease has failed to respond to 5-ASA agents or antibiotic therapy. The initial dose should be high (eg, prednisone 60 mg/day orally or hydrocortisone 300 mg/day intravenously) and should halt the inflammatory process. In severely ill patients, intravenous infusions of corticosteroids can bring about a remission. These medicines should be used only in acute exacerbations: they are not effective for long-term maintenance and should be tapered rapidly to avoid side effects such as osteoporosis, acne, striae, cataracts, glucose intolerance, weight gain, or infection.

The need to avoid long-term side effects of corticosteroids has driven the search for more rapidly metabolized steroids. However, budesonide, the newest, is less effective than prednisolone for active Crohn's disease, and at high doses produces the adrenal suppression and systemic side effects seen in other steroid preparations (Rutgeerts et al, 1994). Topical steroid preparations in suppository, foam, or enema formulations are useful adjuncts to oral medications in patients with distal colitis.

Immunomodulatory Therapy

Patients who become dependent on corticosteroids or whose disease fails to respond may respond to immunomodulatory agents such as 6-mercaptopurine and azathioprine. These medicines have a considerable steroid-sparing benefit and reduce clinical symptoms in two thirds of patients with Crohn's disease or UC (Present et al, 1980; George et al, 1996). Concerns about short- and long-term toxicity appear unwarranted (Pearson et al, 1995). Methotrexate has been shown to be effective in Crohn's disease in reducing the need for steroids and improving symptoms (Kozarek et al, 1989). Cyclosporine A, a potent immunosuppressant used for organ transplant patients, has been shown to be effective in patients with UC that has failed to respond to intravenous steroid therapy. Patients whose disease has failed to respond to 7 to 10 days of intravenous steroid therapy should be offered cyclosporine therapy, and a surgeon should be consulted to evaluate the patient for possible colectomy. More than 80% of these patients treated with cyclosporine can be spared colectomy, and long-term remission can be maintained with 6-mercaptopurine (Lichtiger et al, 1994; Marion & Present, 1997). If a patient's disease fails to respond to cyclosporine in 7 to 10 days, colectomy is indicated.

Nutritional Therapies

Nutrition can play an important adjunctive role in the management of IBD. Patients with Crohn's disease are often malnourished or exhibit signs and symptoms of malabsorption. Elemental diets have been demonstrated to be as effective as steroids in the induction of remission and can correct growth failure in the malnourished pediatric patient (Saverymuttu et al, 1985). Total parenteral nutrition (TPN) is also of value in nutritionally depleted patients who cannot tolerate oral intake. Patients who have had multiple ileal resections totaling more than 100 cm of small bowel can develop short bowel syndrome. Malabsorption and diarrhea can be severe in these patients, and TPN may be helpful. The risk of line infection with TPN precludes its routine use in the absence of severe disease.

Repletion of cobalamin (vitamin B_{12}) because of distal ileal malabsorption or folic acid because of proximal gut malabsorption or sulfasalazine therapy is important in patients with Crohn's disease. Patients with fibrostenotic Crohn's disease with stricturing are advised to remain on a low-residue diet to avoid mechanical obstruction.

Nutritional therapy for UC is more limited. Bowel rest is of no use in UC. These patients, even those with severe disease (but not those with toxic megacolon), should follow a low-residue diet with multivitamin supplementation. Fish oil supplements may help to reduce steroid requirements but produce an unacceptable odor in most patients. Short-chain fatty acid enemas have not been shown to be effective for UC.

Symptomatic Therapies

Patients with IBD often suffer debilitating symptoms of diarrhea and cramps. The slow onset of action of many of the medicines used to treat these illnesses often requires the use of symptomatic medicines such as antidiarrheals (eg, loperamide), antispasmodics (eg, hyoscyamine), and bile salt resins. These medicines can make an enormous difference in the quality of the patient's life. Caution should be observed in patients with severe or extensive colitis because antidiarrheals and anticholinergic medicines can precipitate toxic dilation of the colon. Bile salt resins (eg, cholestyramine) are particularly useful in patients who have recently had an ileal or ileocolic resection and are having symptoms of bile salt catharsis.

New Therapies

There are several new therapies, now in clinical trials, that will soon be used. The most promising biologic therapies to date are the monoclonal antibodies to TNF-α, which appear to block TNF and halt the inflammatory process. When available, these medicines will play an important role in the management of Crohn's disease (Stack et al, 1997; Targan et al, 1997). Studies using other anti-inflammatory cytokines are also in progress. Heparin has shown some promise for treating severe UC in uncontrolled studies but should not be used outside of a controlled trial. Nicotine therapy may be of use for mild UC, but more data are needed.

Surgery

CROHN'S DISEASE

Many patients with IBD face surgery in the course of their disease. Approximately 60% to 70% of all patients with Crohn's disease will undergo a bowel resection in their lifetimes. Indications for surgery include failure to respond to medical therapy, perforation, abscess formation, hemorrhage, and cancer. Symptoms that persist despite maximal medical therapy or reliance on steroids despite steroid-sparing therapy warrants surgical management. The most common surgical procedure for patients with Crohn's disease is an ileal or ileocolic resection of the diseased portion of bowel.

One of the most frustrating aspects of Crohn's disease for the patient and the provider is the incurability of the condition. Patients with Crohn's disease who require surgery almost always suffer a recurrence. The disease typically recurs proximal to the anastomosis in patients with ileitis. No risk factors for postoperative recurrence have been identified. Mesalamine given within 8 weeks of a resection can decrease the likelihood of clinical recurrence (McLeod et al, 1995).

ULCERATIVE COLITIS

Approximately 30% to 40% of patients with UC will require surgical intervention in their lifetimes because of failure to respond to medical therapy, perforation, toxic dilation, hemorrhage, stricture, dysplasia, or cancer. The standard Brooke ileostomy and total proctocolectomy remains the only reliable "cure" for UC but is unacceptable to many patients for cosmetic and emotional reasons. The ileal pouch anastomosis has become a popular choice, particularly among younger patients. In this surgery, the colon is removed and the distal small bowel is converted into a reservoir that is then attached to the anal musculature. This allows for rectal continence and does not require an external ileostomy appliance. Although the procedure is very appealing to patients for cosmetic reasons, the provider should not offer ileal pouch anal anastomosis as a "cure" for UC.

Psychological Aspects

The most common psychological complaints in patients with IBD are anxiety and occasionally depression. IBD is not caused by stress or psychopathology or personality disorders. There is no recognized "IBD personality." A careful psychological review of symptoms should be taken when IBD patients are seen. Appropriate referral for psychotherapy or psychopharmacologic intervention may be needed. The primary care provider must be aware of iatrogenic causes of psychological symptoms, such as corticosteroid or narcotic medications.

Teaching and Self-Care

The approach to treatment of IBD depends on the patient's current clinical status. The chief goal of treatment is to achieve and maintain a clinical remission. Patients should be encouraged to participate in their management and to gain a sense of control. Educating the patient and the family helps ensure their understanding of the frustrating elements of the disease. They should be familiar with the disease course, the prognosis, and the clinical warnings as to when urgent attention is warranted.

Part of the educational process is helping the patient understand not only what to do, but what not to do. Changing medications indiscriminately may cause an exacerbation. Regaining a remission is more difficult than maintaining a remission. When patients feel the need to change the medication regimen, whether it is because they feel well or poor, they should discuss any changes with the provider. This amplifies the need for ongoing communication between the patient and the provider.

Over-the-counter medicines should be used with caution. Even common medications, such as ibuprofen, may be toxic in patients with IBD. Often "cold and flu" preparations contain ingredients that may be harmful. Before using any over-the-counter medicine, the patient should be completely familiar with it and discuss its use with the provider.

COMMUNITY RESOURCES

Because patient education is an essential part of the treatment for IBD, community resources are invaluable. Several sources are listed in the section on community resources at the end of this unit.

REFERRAL POINTS AND CLINICAL WARNINGS

The primary care provider is a key member of the team caring for the patients with IBD. A gastroenterologist will be needed for severe disease, endoscopic intervention or surveillance, and the initiation of immunosuppressant therapies. A surgeon should be called for patients who develop intra-abdominal abscess, massive bleeding, stricture, intestinal obstruction, or perforation of the bowel. A nutritionist may be needed when a patient manifests severe weight loss, malnutrition, or vitamin and mineral deficiencies.

Extraintestinal manifestations, particularly arthritis, may warrant referral to a rheumatologist. Referral to a dermatologist may be needed to confirm skin manifestations such as erythema nodosum or pyoderma gangrenosum. An ophthalmologist may be needed for patients whose IBD is complicated by uveitis, iritis, or episcleritis.

Hospitalization of a patient with IBD is indicated for dehydration, inability to tolerate oral intake, failure of oral or topical therapy, or any indication for intravenous therapy or surgery. Additionally, abdominal pain may be severe enough to mimic an acute abdomen. Patients with complications such as toxic megacolon require emergent consultation.

■ ■ ■ CLINICAL PEARLS

- UC almost always has rectal mucosa involvement; Crohn's disease almost always affects the terminal ileum.
- Extra-intestinal manifestations may precede overt bowel disease.
- Strictures in patients with UC are more likely to be malignant than strictures in patients with Crohn's disease.
- Caution must be used when planning colonoscopic or contrast radiographic procedures on the acutely ill patient with severe colitis. These procedures and the bowel-cleansing preparations administered before the procedure can exacerbate the disease or precipitate toxic dilation of the colon (megacolon).
- Patients with UC of more than 7 years' duration and patients with severe Crohn's colitis should have yearly surveillance colonoscopy.
- Patients with Crohn's disease who require surgery will usually suffer recurrence.

References

Alstead, E.M., Ritchie, J.K., Lennard-Jones, J.E., et al. (1990). Safety of azathioprine in pregnancy in inflammatory bowel disease. *Gastroenterology, 99*, 443.

Crohn, B.B., Ginsburg, L., & Oppenheimer, G.D. (1932). Regional enteritis. *JAMA, 99*, 1323–1329.

Dayan, A., Rubin, P., Chapman, M., et al. (1996). 6-mercaptopurine in inflammatory bowel disease patients of childbearing years. *Gastroenterology, 100*, A824.

Dissanyake, A.S., & Truelove, S.C. (1973). A controlled therapeutic trial of long-term maintenance treatment of ulcerative colitis with sulphasalazine. *Gut, 14*, 923.

George, J., Present, D.H., Pou, R., et al. (1996). 6-mercaptopurine for the treatment of ulcerative colitis. *American Journal of Gastroenterology, 91*, 1711.

Gillen, C.D., Walmsley, R.S., Prior, P., et al. (1994). Ulcerative colitis and Crohn's disease. *Gut, 35*, 1590.

Khosla, R., Wiloughby, C.P., & Jewell, D.P. (1984). Pregnancy in Crohn's disease. *Gut, 25*, 52.

Kozarek, R.A., Patterson, D.J., Gelfand, M.D., et al. (1989). Methotrexate induces clinical and histologic remission in patients with refractory inflammatory bowel disease. *Annals of Internal Medicine, 110*, 353.

Lashner, B.A., Evans, A.A., Kirsner, J.B., et al. (1986). Prevalence and incidence of inflammatory bowel disease in family members. *Gastroenterology, 91*, 1395.

Lichtiger, S., Present, D.H., Kornbluth, A., et al. (1994). Cyclosporine in severe ulcerative colitis refractory to steroid therapy. *N Engl J Med, 330*, 1841.

Marion, J.F., George, J., & Waye, J. (1997). Crohn's disease. In A.J. Dimarino & S.B. Benjamin (Eds.). *Gastrointestinal disease, an endoscopic approach.* London: Blackwell, p. 511.

Marion, J.F., & Present, D.H. (1997). The modern medical management of severe ulcerative colitis. *European Journal of Gastroenterology and Hepatology, 9*, 831.

Marion, J.F., Rubin, P.H., & Present, D.H. (1998). Differential diagnosis of chronic ulcerative and Crohn's colitis. In J. Kirsner (Ed.). *Inflammatory bowel diseases.* Philadelphia-WB Saunders.

Mayberry, J.F., & Weterman, I.T. (1986). European survey of fertility and pregnancy in women with Crohn's disease. *Gut, 27*, 821.

McLeod, R.S., Wolf, B.G., Steinhart, A.H., et al. (1995). Prophylactic mesalamine treatment decreases postoperative recurrence of Crohn's disease. *Gastroenterology, 109*, 404.

Pearson, D.C., May, G.R., Fick, G.H., et al. (1995). Azathioprine and 6-mercaptopurine in Crohn's disease. *Annals of Internal Medicine, 122*, 132.

Present, D.H., Korelitz, B.I., Wisch, N., et al. (1980). Treatment of Crohn's disease with 6-mercaptopurine. *N Engl J Med, 320*, 981.

Pullman, W.E., & Doe, W.F. (1992). IL-2 production by intestinal lamina propria cells in inflamed and cancer-bearing colons. *Clinical and Experimental Immunology, 88*, 132.

Rutgeerts, P.R., Lofberg, R., Malchow, H., et al. (1994). A comparison of budesonide with prednisolone for active Crohn's disease. *N Engl J Med, 331*, 842.

Sachar, D.B., Auslander, M.O., & Walfish, J.S. (1980). Etiological theories of inflammatory bowel disease. *Clinical Gastroenterology, 9*, 231.

Saverymuttu, S., Hodgson, H.J., & Chadwick, V.F. (1985). Controlled trial comparing prednisolone with an elemental diet plus nonabsorbable antibiotics in active Crohn's disease. *Gut, 26*, 994.

Sedlack, R.E., Whisnant, J., Elveback, L.R., et al. (1980). Incidence of Crohn's disease in Olmstead County, Minn., 1935–1975. *American Journal of Epidemiology*, 759.

Spiliadis, C.A., & Lennard-Jones, J.E. (1987). Ulcerative colitis with relative rectal sparing. *Diseases of the Colon and Rectum, 30*, 334.

Stack, W.A., Mann, S.D., Roy, A.J., et al. (1997). Randomised controlled trial of CDP571 antibody to tumour-necrosis factor in Crohn's disease. *Lancet, 349*, 521.

Summers, R.W., Switz, D.M., Sessions, D.T., et al. (1979). National cooperative Crohn's disease study. *Gastroenterology, 77*, 847.

Surawicz, S.M., Meisel, J.L., Ylvisaker, T., et al. (1981). Rectal biopsy in the diagnosis of Crohn's disease. *Gastroenterology, 81*, 66.

Targan, S.R., Hanauer, S.B., van Deventer, S.J., et al. (1997). A short-term study of chimeric monoclonal antibody cA2 to tumor-necrosis factor-alpha for Crohn's disease. *N Engl J Med, 337*, 1029.

Van Hess, P.A., Van Lier, H.J.J., van Elteren, P.H., et al. (1981). Effect of sulfasalazine in patients with active Crohn's disease. *Gut, 22*, 404.

Whelan, G. (1990). Epidemiology of inflammatory bowel disease. *Gastroenterology Clinics of North America, 19*, 1.

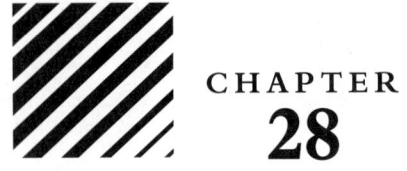

CHAPTER

28

Pancreatitis: Acute and Chronic

Gwyneth Davis, MD

Pancreatitis, an inflammatory disease of the pancreas, may be classified as acute or chronic. Most cases of acute pancreatitis are caused by either alcohol intake or gallstones. The clinical course may be mild, subsiding within 48 to 72 hours with conservative therapy, or may progress to necrosis and rapid deterioration to respiratory and other organ failure, sepsis, and death. Treatment is largely supportive, with intravenous hydration and parenteral analgesics. Treatment failure mandates a search for complications such as abscesses or pseudocysts.

The etiology of chronic pancreatitis is similar, with alcoholism as the predominant factor. Recurrent cholelithiasis or rarely hereditary factors or malnutrition (Sarner, 1995) may play a part in its pathogenesis. Continuing inflammation of the gland leads to fibrosis and a loss of exocrine and endocrine parenchyma. Pain is the predominant symptom until acinar tissue is completely effaced, at which point steatorrhea becomes the main problem (Braganza, 1996).

ANATOMY, PHYSIOLOGY, AND PATHOLOGY

The pancreas is a retort-shaped gland of soft consistency. It is more than 6″ long and has a finely lobulated surface. It lies somewhat obliquely, immediately behind the peritoneum of the posterior abdominal wall, and slopes from a large head, up through a neck and body, toward a narrow tail. The head lies in the C curve of the duodenum, and part of its posterior surface is prolonged and wedge-shaped, forming the uncinate process. The main pancreatic duct (Wirsung) is continuous from the tail to the head and joins the common bile duct at the ampulla of Vater, which then opens into the duodenum. The accessory pancreatic duct (Santorini) drains the uncinate process and lower part of the head and also opens into the duodenum separately from the main duct, although the two ducts often communicate. The blood supply is from the splenic and pancreaticoduodenal arteries; the corresponding veins drain into the portal system.

The pancreas has both endocrine (internal) and exocrine (external) secretory properties. The endocrine component of the pancreas consists of the islets of Langerhans. These produce insulin, glucagon, and somatostatin, which play a major role in the metabolism of food. Most endocrine tissue is contained in the tail and distal body of the pancreas. The exocrine pancreas consists of glandular, secretory units, the acinar cells. These produce and secrete pancreatic juice, which has two important components: bicarbonate (to neutralize stomach acid) and digestive enzymes, which are secreted into the duodenum via the main pancreatic duct.

ACUTE PANCREATITIS
Epidemiology and Etiology

An inflammatory process of the pancreas may subsequently involve other regional tissues or remote organ systems. The process can be mild or severe, mild being associated with minimal organ disruption and an uneventful recovery, and severe sometimes progressing to cell necrosis and death. Seventy-five percent of cases of acute pancreatitis fall into this mild category. The incidence of acute pancreatitis ranges from 54 to 238 episodes per 1 million per year (Levelle-Jones & Neoptolemos, 1990). About half the patients with acute pancreatitis are older than 60 years, and among them there is a slightly higher prevalence in women, probably caused by a higher incidence of gallstone-associated pancreatitis (Gullo et al, 1994). Histologically, acute pancreatitis is characterized by a wide spectrum of lesions, including edema, fatty necrosis, parenchymal necrosis, and hemorrhage.

There are many causes of acute pancreatitis (Table 28-1), but more than 80% of cases are caused by alcohol or gallstones. Another 10% of cases are idiopathic but might be related to the presence of biliary sludge (Lee et al, 1992). Other, rarer causes make up the final 10%.

History and Physical Examination

Clinically, abdominal pain and raised serum concentration of pancreatic enzymes are the most common features (Gullo et al, 1994). Signs and symptoms typically include sudden epigastric pain radiating to the back, associated with nausea and vomiting. The pain is severe and is aggravated by food and alleviated by leaning forward. The patient often moves about constantly in search of a comfortable position. There is often a history of alcohol excess, and the degree of alcohol consumption must be explored if there is no suggestion of cholelithiasis.

Physical findings of acute pancreatitis include fever, tachycardia, epigastric tenderness with guarding, and rebound tenderness, if severe. Bowel sounds are often diminished; absence of bowel sounds indicates paralytic ileus. Hypotension and tachypnea are indicative of severe pancreatitis, as are decreased breath sounds from pleural effusion. Rarely, there are ecchymoses on the flanks (Grey-Turner sign) or on the periumbilical region (Cullen's sign).

Approximately half the patients with acute pancreatitis recover spontaneously, as the disease has a self-limiting nature. There is a 10% mortality rate, with death usually occurring during the initial or second episode rather than subsequent ones. The more severe forms, however, are characterized by

TABLE 28-1	Causes of Acute Pancreatitis
Alcoholism	Idiopathic
Cholelithiasis	Infections
Drugs	Pancreas divisum
Hypercalcemia	Trauma
Hypertriglyceridemia	ERCP

pancreatic necrosis, and the mortality rate increases to 20% or 30% (Kusske et al, 1996). Prognostic criteria for acute pancreatitis were developed by Ranson et al (1974) and are shown in Table 28-2.

Complications of acute pancreatitis include those common to the pancreas itself, to adjacent organs, or to various systems within the body. Pseudocysts, abscesses, and hemorrhage into the pancreas are the most common complications. They require immediate surgical intervention, except for small cysts, which can be observed over a period of time. The first organ system to be affected is often respiratory, with adult respiratory distress syndrome developing early in severe acute pancreatitis. Pancreatitis can cause massive sequestration of fluid into the third space, causing severe hypotension and hypovolemic shock. Pleural effusion and atelectasis can occur, as well as renal failure. Electrolyte abnormalities are also common, and electrolytes must be constantly monitored.

Severe acute pancreatitis can lead to pancreatic infection and generalized sepsis as a result of bacterial translocation from the gut, which permits colonization of the necrotic tissue. Common bacteria implicated in such infection include *Escherichia coli* and other enteric aerobes. Anaerobes rarely cause pancreatic infections.

Diagnostic Studies

LABORATORY TESTS

Serum amylase is most frequently used to detect pancreatitis. However, elevated amylase levels occur only in acute exacerbations, so the usefulness of this test is limited. Serum amylase is

TABLE 28-2	Prognostic Criteria for Acute Pancreatitis

AT ADMISSION

Age >55 years

White count >16,000/mm^3

Blood glucose >200 mg/dL (>11 mmol/L)

Serum LDH >350 IU/L

AST (SGOT) > 250/L

DURING INITIAL 48 HOURS

Hematocrit drop >10 percentage pts.

BUN rise >5 mg/dL (>1.8 mmol/L)

Arterial Po$_2$ <60 mmHg

Base deficit >4 mEq/L

Serum calcium <8 mg/dL (<2 mmol/L)

Estimated fluid sequestration >6 L

If 3 or fewer of these signs are present, the mortality rate approaches 1%, and few patients are seriously ill. If 4 or more signs are present, the mortality rate can reach 25%, and about 50% of patients are seriously ill.

also found in saliva, so isoenzyme measurement may need to be done to determine its origin. Elevation of the serum lipase level is more specific but less sensitive than serum amylase analysis.

A complete blood count should be done and serum calcium, glucose, triglycerides, electrolytes, lactate dehydrogenase and alanine amino transferase (ALT), bilirubin, and alkaline phosphatase levels should all be checked. The hematocrit increases because of hemoconcentration as serum is lost into peritoneal and retroperitoneal spaces. The white cell count is usually elevated. The serum calcium level is decreased, possibly because of failure of homeostatic mechanisms. The serum glucose level is elevated because of decreased insulin or increased glucagon levels. Increased bilirubin and alkaline phosphatase values are evidence of cholestasis from compression of the common bile duct. Triglyceride levels are generally elevated, but a level above 1000 mg/dL would implicate an underlying hyperlipidemic disorder, usually a type V lipid profile. Mildly elevated levels of transaminases and alkaline phosphatase are also common. Hypokalemia and hypomagnesemia are the two most frequent electrolyte abnormalities, aside from hypocalcemia.

IMAGING STUDIES

A flat plate of the abdomen may reveal calculi in the gallbladder or sentinel loops (localized gas collections in loops of bowel overlying the pancreas) in a few cases. It will also rule out the presence of free air under the diaphragm, which would signify a perforation of a hollow viscus. Diffuse stippled calcification is seen in about 30% of patients with chronic pancreatitis.

Ultrasonography is limited mostly to evaluation of patients with possible gallstone disease. It can also be used to differentiate between a phlegmon (a solid inflamed mass of pancreatic tissue that subsides spontaneously) and a pseudocyst (a cystic collection of fluid and necrotic debris without a definitive formed wall).

Computed tomography of the abdomen may show calculi, pseudocyst, abscess, or ductal abnormalities. It may be normal in mild pancreatitis, or it may show focal or diffuse enlargement (Gupta & Al-Kawas, 1995). The presence of necrosis is an indicator of more severe disease.

Treatment Options, Expected Outcomes, and Comprehensive Management

Hospitalization is necessary for acute pancreatitis. Treatment is largely supportive and symptomatic, consisting of intravenous and parenteral analgesics. Pain can be controlled with narcotics or other injectable nonsteroidal anti-inflammatory agents such as ketorolac (Toradol). Hydration should be vigorous because there is sequestration of large quantities of fluid into extravascular spaces. Urine output should be monitored as an indicator of the adequacy of hydration. The patient should not have any oral intake (NPO) to avoid stimulation of pancreatic juices, although a nasogastric tube need not be placed unless there is vomiting or an ileus ensues. If acute pancreatitis is caused by gallstones, an endoscopic retrograde cholangiopancreatography (ERCP) with sphincterotomy and stone extraction should be done. Otherwise, ERCP exacerbates acute pancreatitis and should be avoided.

SELF-CARE

Patients need to be educated about what increases their risk for developing acute pancreatitis. Risk factors must be reviewed extensively, and all risk factors must be addressed. Because alcohol is such a common cause of pancreatitis, the use and abuse of alcohol need to be explored. Hypertriglyceridemia is often a cause for pancreatitis. One of the best methods to decrease triglyceride levels is to eat a low-fat, low-cholesterol diet; only when this dietary therapy is insufficient should further therapies be instituted. If the cause for pancreatitis is cholelithiasis, discussing the possibility of a cholecystectomy, after the acute episode subsides, may be warranted.

COMPLEMENTARY THERAPIES

Several modalities have been used in controlling pain, including transcutaneous electrical nerve stimulator (TENS), acupuncture, and biofeedback. Because the pain is severe, these modalities are used more with chronic pancreatitis than with acute pancreatitis. In the acute, hospital setting, opioid medications or potent nonsteroidal anti-inflammatories are usually administered.

Referral Points and Clinical Warnings

Although acute pancreatitis may subside spontaneously, it is a potentially life-threatening disorder and should be treated as such. Patients with suspected cases should be evaluated urgently for admission to the hospital. A gastroenterologist and possibly a surgeon may need to be consulted. In addition, social workers, dietitians, and possibly psychologists need to be involved, depending on the risk factors for pancreatitis and the severity of the disease.

CHRONIC PANCREATITIS

Epidemiology and Etiology

In the general population of Western countries, the incidence of chronic pancreatitis is 5 to 10 cases per 100,000 per year (Gullo et al, 1994). Clinical onset is usually between 30 and 40 years of age and the male : female ratio is about 8 : 2. Alcohol abuse is the most common cause in the United States, although in some parts of the world protein-calorie malnutrition predominates. There is a long latent period (on average 18 years) before the first symptom in men who drink more than 150 g of ethanol daily, demonstrating that alcohol is itself a weak etiologic factor (Braganza, 1996). The disease is idiopathic in many patients and may be genetically linked.

History and Physical Examination

Clinically, pancreatitis is chronic if the patient has persistent pain or a decrease in pancreatic secretion, whether exocrine or endocrine, after the initial attack. This is different from acute pancreatitis, where recovery is complete. Recurrent epigastric or left upper quadrant abdominal pain, radiating to the back, characterizes chronic pancreatitis. Pain is excruciating and constant and may be felt in almost any area of the abdomen. It is accompanied by steatorrhea (foul-smelling greasy stools), weight loss, and late in the course of the disease diabetes mellitus.

Diagnostic Studies

The history and physical findings of chronic abdominal pain and steatorrhea, in the presence of a past history of acute pancreatitis, are virtually pathognomonic for the disease. Fecal fat determination will both diagnose steatorrhea and monitor the efficacy of oral pancreatic supplements. Amylase levels are not as elevated as in acute disease, except during acute exacerbations. An abdominal x-ray shows diffuse calcification of the gland in about 30% of cases. Sonography or computed tomography scanning of the abdomen may be useful to confirm the diagnosis by demonstrating calcifications or to rule out the differential diagnosis of pancreatic carcinoma. ERCP may show a dilated main pancreatic duct with strictures and other intraductal filling defects and prominent side branches, consistent with chronic pancreatitis.

Treatment Options, Expected Outcomes, and Comprehensive Management

Therapy is directed predominantly at pain relief, control of diabetes, and correction of malabsorption. Pain is often initiated by an alcoholic binge, so cessation of alcohol forms an important part of treatment. Avoidance of narcotic analgesics as much as possible is suggested because the potential for addiction is strong, and it becomes very difficult to wean patients off these drugs. The initial drugs used should be salicylates and aspirin. Pancreatic enzymes may be helpful in some patients. If pain is resistant to analgesics, a celiac plexus block is the procedure of choice (Gullo et al, 1994). As the disease progresses, the pain becomes less intense and more manageable.

A variety of surgical procedures exist for the management of failed medical therapy. The choice of procedure is generally based on the state of the pancreatic duct and the residual function of the pancreas. For patients with narrow pancreatic ducts and impaired function, total pancreatectomy may be necessary (Fleming & Williamson, 1995). Although the disease is diffuse, localized accentuation of the pathologic process, usually in the head of the organ, has been used as an argument for localized resection, although some favor total pancreatectomy in all patients.

Teaching and Self-Care

Much of the self-care necessary for chronic pancreatitis is noted in the section on acute pancreatitis. The focus is on the exacerbating factors and how to control and eliminate them. In addition to reducing the pain and addressing the cause of the pancreatitis, patients may use supplements of pancreatic enzymes to help reduce some of the malabsorption and complications associated with pancreatitis. Enzyme replacement drugs usually contain amylase, protease, and lipase in varying amounts, depending on the manufacturer.

COMPLEMENTARY TREATMENTS

Some complementary therapies for pain management are noted above in the section on acute pancreatitis. The replacement of pancreatic enzymes is also described above. In addition to avoiding causative agents, some have theorized that antioxidants, such as organic selenium, beta-carotene, vitamin C, vitamin E, and methionine, may help reduce the recurrence of pancreatitis.

Referral Points and Clinical Warnings

Unlike acute pancreatitis, patients with chronic pancreatitis do not always require admission to the hospital. However, these patients are at extremely high risk for developing an "acute on chronic" situation, which raises their risk of morbidity and death. Patients with chronic pancreatitis may be able to be managed on oral, outpatient analgesics, but this alone is not enough. Risk factors, as noted in acute pancreatitis, must be identified and addressed by the appropriate providers on the health care team.

COMMUNITY RESOURCES

The etiology of acute and chronic pancreatitis should be sought. If alcohol is implicated, many local and regional self-help groups are available for rehabilitation purposes, as well as national organizations such as Alcoholics Anonymous. For further detail on alcohol abuse, see Chapter 64. Organizations and Web sites that focus on pancreatitis and digestive diseases are listed at the end of the unit on gastrointestinal disorders.

■ ■ ■ CLINICAL PEARLS

- Use the Ranson criteria to help assess the severity of disease, but do not forget to look at the overall clinical picture.
- The etiology of pancreatitis is usually alcoholism or gallstones. These possibilities must always be sought.

- Hospitalization is often required with acute pancreatitis but may or may not be necessary with chronic pancreatitis.
- Persons who are addicted to alcohol and have built up tolerance may also have built up tolerance to analgesic medications. Assessment and monitoring of liver function may be necessary with administration of analgesic medication.

References

Braganza, J.M. (1996). The pathogenesis of chronic pancreatitis *QJM,* *89,* 243–250

Fleming, W.R., & Williamson, R.C.N. (1995). Role of total pancreatectomy in the treatment of patients with end-stage chronic pancreatitis. *British Journal of Surgery, 82,* 1409–1412.

Gullo, L., Sipahi, H., & Pezzilli, R. (1994). Pancreatitis in the elderly. *Journal of Clinical Gastroenterology, 19*(1), 64–68.

Gupta, P.K., & Al-Kawas, F.H. (1995). Acute pancreatitis: Diagnosis and management. *American Family Physician, 52*(2), 435–443.

Kusske, A., Rongione, A., & Reber, H. (1996). Cytokines and acute pancreatitis. *Gastroenterology, 110*(2), 639–641.

Lee, S.P., Nicholls, J.F., & Park, H.Z. (1992). Biliary sludge as a cause of acute pancreatitis. *N Engl J Med, 326,* 589–593.

Levelle-Jones, M., & Neoptolemos, J.P. (1990). Recent advances in the treatment of acute pancreatitis. *Surgery Annual, 22,* 235–261.

Ranson, J.H., Rifkind, K.M., Roses, D.F., et al. (1974). Prognostic signs and the role of operative management in acute pancreatitis. *Surgery, Gynecology & Obstetrics, 139,* 69–81.

Sarner, M. (1995). Pancreatic inflammatory disease. *Gut, 37,* 455–456.

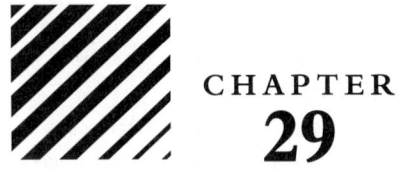

CHAPTER
29

Peptic Ulcer Disease

Paul Cohen, MD

Approaches to peptic ulcer disease (PUD) have changed throughout the years. The etiology of PUD is multifactorial. Initially thought of as a disease associated with excess acid production or a lack of protective mechanisms, or both, it is now known to have an infectious etiology as well. The yearly incidence is estimated at 15 to 30 cases per 1000 people. Obtaining an accurate history is very important in ascertaining these various causative factors. As with most diseases, knowing the cause of an ulcer remains the most important factor in deciding the treatment course and determining the prognosis.

ETIOLOGY, ANATOMY, PHYSIOLOGY, AND PATHOLOGY

The reason why one patient will develop a peptic ulcer and another will not is still unclear. Acid must be present for PUD to occur. The usual pH of the stomach is approximately 1. If an ulcer develops in a patient who is known to be achlorhydric, a gastric malignancy is the likely cause for the ulceration.

There are several protective mechanisms that play a role in preventing PUD. Disruption in any of these factors may result in ulcer formation. The gastric mucosal barrier is the main defense mechanism of the stomach. Another protective mechanism is cytoprotection. Tight junctions between mucosal cells help prevent leakage of acid into the gastric lining. There is always a small degree of leakage of hydrogen ions into these mucosal cells, but the rich vascular supply of the stomach helps sweep away these hydrogen ions. A third factor is the secretion of protective mucus and bicarbonate by the gastric mucosa.

Reversible culprits that can reduce the effectiveness of these protective factors include smoking, the presence of *Helicobacter pylori*, and the use of nonsteroidal anti-inflammatory agents (NSAIDs).

There are several proposed mechanisms by which cigarette smoking can cause PUD. Smoking may alter blood flow, with resultant hypoxic damage to the mucosa and ulcer formation. Smoking also increases basal and maximal acid secretion and has been reported to decrease gastric mucosal prostaglandin production (Endoh & Leung, 1994).

Recently, the eradication of *H. pylori* in PUD became a standard of care. *H. pylori* is a gram-negative rod found in the antrum of the stomach. It is also found in the duodenal bulb, where islands of gastric mucosa are commonly found. Originally called *Campylobacter pylori*, this organism's ability to survive in the acidic environment of the stomach comes from its ability to secrete urease and other enzymes into the mucous layer of the mucosa. This damages the protective barrier and allows ulcer formation. *H. pylori* is associated with 65% to 70% of gastric ulcers and 90% to 95% of duodenal ulcers (Tytgat &

Rauws, 1990; Hojgaard et al, 1996). The incidence of *H. pylori* increases in frequency with age: at age 50 years, it is found in about 50% of the general population, increasing by approximately 10% each decade thereafter.

The use of NSAIDs is strongly associated with PUD. NSAIDs are mainly associated with gastric ulcers; approximately 70% of ulcers caused by these agents occur in the stomach. NSAIDs work by inhibiting mucosal prostaglandin production. This results in an interference in mucous secretion, reduced gastric mucosal blood flow, and decreased bicarbonate secretion (Selling, 1987). Aspirin (acetylsalicylic acid) is the prototype NSAID and therefore damages the gastric mucosa as described above. It is also a weak acid, and in the potent acid environment of the stomach, it becomes un-ionized and penetrates the gastric mucosal cells, causing further damage.

EPIDEMIOLOGY

There are marked differences in the incidence of gastric and duodenal ulcers. Duodenal ulcers have a lifetime prevalence, in both men and women, of approximately 10% (Bernersen et al, 1990), whereas gastric ulcers occur much less frequently. However, the incidence of gastric ulcers rises sharply when NSAIDs are involved. PUD used to occur mainly in men; now it occurs almost equally in both sexes (Kurata et al, 1985). The increase in smoking, one of the contributors to PUD, among young women may help explain this increase.

DIAGNOSTIC CRITERIA

Often the diagnosis of "ulcer disease" is made on clinical grounds. The patient presents with a classical history of PUD, a therapeutic trial of appropriate agents is started, and if the patient improves, the diagnosis is considered validated. This is often the clinical scenario. However, a definitive diagnosis of PUD can be made only by radiologic studies or endoscopy.

HISTORY AND PHYSICAL EXAMINATION

Although the history of a patient with PUD may vary from no symptoms at all to severe crushing chest pains mimicking a myocardial infarction, PUD is classically described as a burning or gnawing epigastric pain. Ulcer disease can cause early morning awakening (typically 2 to 4 AM), believed to be secondary to the circadian changes in acid secretion (Sleisenger & Fordtran,). Although acid secretion is low in the early morning, there is typically no food in the stomach to buffer the acid; thus, even low levels of acid secretion may aggravate ulcer disease. Epigastric pain occurs in both duodenal and gastric ulcer disease, but radiation of the pain to the back is more common in duodenal ulcer disease, especially that found on the posterior wall of the duodenal bulb. The association of food with pain should be established. Eating often helps alleviate symptoms of duodenal ulcers but may exacerbate the pain of gastric ulcers.

In addition to the patient's abdominal complaints, the provider must also focus on exacerbating factors. Asking the patient about alcohol consumption (which may aggravate ulcer disease but is not a direct cause of ulcer disease) and smoking is essential. Inquiring about use of NSAIDs and steroids is also necessary. Often direct questioning needs to be done to elicit NSAID use because many patients do not consider over-the-counter medications to be "medicines." Identifying these culprits will help in both treatment and prevention of recurrent PUD.

The physical examination of patients with PUD may be unrevealing. It should focus on identifying complications of PUD. Vital signs and orthostatic pressures should be obtained to help identify blood loss secondary to gastrointestinal (GI) bleeding. Pain-free GI bleeding occurs most frequently in the elderly, especially when NSAIDs are involved. A thorough abdominal examination must be done, noting any masses and any signs of an acute abdomen (eg, rigidity and lack of bowel sounds), which occur with perforation of an ulcer and resultant peritonitis. A rectal examination should be done to reveal any occult blood or frank bleeding.

Although PUD is a common, usually benign, disease, complications of PUD may be fatal. Complications include perforation of the ulcer with resultant peritonitis; penetration of the ulcer into the pancreas, which can result in pancreatitis; excessive edema around the ulcer, causing an outlet obstruction; and bleeding significant enough to cause death.

DIAGNOSTIC STUDIES

Esophagogastroduodenoscopy (EGD) is considered the gold standard for evaluating the upper GI tract. It has several advantages over barium studies, including the ability to diagnose subtle mucosal lesions, to take samples of lesions for biopsy, and to perform therapeutic measures (eg, cauterization or injection therapy of bleeding ulcers). Endoscopy tends to take less time to perform than barium studies and is more appropriate in an acute setting. Disadvantages of EGD include the need for sedation, discomfort, and the invasiveness of the procedure, with the accompanying risk of tears and perforation. Patients with respiratory difficulties tend to have more difficulty with the procedure because they fear the endoscope will obstruct their airway. EGD may also be contraindicated in patients with recent myocardial infarctions. Endoscopy tends to cause excessive catecholamine release, possibly leading to arrhythmias. In addition, the rubbing of the endoscope as it passes next to the right atrium (while in the esophagus) may also cause arrhythmias.

Barium studies (an upper GI series) remain a useful tool in diagnosing various types of pathology in the upper GI tract, especially when EGD is contraindicated. They are also useful when community resources and access to an endoscopist are limited.

EGD or barium studies may be done when the patient presents initially, but they must be done if the disease does not respond to the treatment plan. Ulcers are often described as active, chronic, or healed or old. Active and chronic ulcers must

be addressed with appropriate medications and lifestyle changes. Healed or old ulcers with scarring do not necessarily require medications, but lifestyle modifications (described below) should begin.

Testing for *H. pylori* is often done when the diagnosis of PUD is made. However, a diagnosis of PUD cannot be made by the presence or absence of *H. pylori*. There are several methods of testing. Serologic testing for antibodies to *H. pylori* may reveal exposure to *H. pylori* but may not indicate active infection. Titers often remain positive after eradication of the organism (Cutler, 1996). Endoscopy with biopsy of the prepyloric area and placement of the tissue in a rapid urease test kit is another method to detect the organism. The advantages of this method are its high sensitivity and specificity (93% and 92%, respectively). The disadvantage is the need to perform an invasive procedure to obtain the tissue. A newer method is the urease breath test, which tests for the presence of urease in expelled air and avoids the need for endoscopy.

Testing for Zollinger-Ellison syndrome should be done when a patient presents with multiple ulcers in the upper GI tract or ulcers refractory to the usual treatment modalities. This is done by measuring the fasting serum gastrin level. An elevated level (800 to 1200 pg/mL) strongly suggests Zollinger-Ellison syndrome. The next step to help confirm the diagnosis is the secretin stimulation test. If a gastrinoma is present (usually located in the head of the pancreas or the second portion of the duodenum), the serum gastrin levels will rise rapidly in the presence of secretin. After a bolus of secretin is given intravenously, multiple venous blood samples are obtained at predetermined intervals, and the gastrin levels are then measured in each sample. If there is a rise of more than 200 pg/mL in any of the samples after the secretin is given, compared to the gastrin level before the secretin, a diagnosis of Zollinger-Ellison syndrome can be made.

Biopsy samples for PUD should be obtained based on the location of the ulcer. Samples should be taken for biopsy from all gastric ulcers and re-evaluated by endoscopy after 4 to 6 weeks of treatment. Duodenal ulcers do not need to be evaluated by biopsy. A biopsy sample must be taken in any ulcer in which healing cannot be documented.

TREATMENT OPTIONS, EXPECTED OUTCOMES, AND COMPREHENSIVE MANAGEMENT

Teaching and Self-Care

Patients may recognize some of the foods that seem to exacerbate their symptoms, but they should be educated about all offending agents. Smoking cessation cannot be overemphasized. Use of acetaminophen for analgesia, fever, or headaches may be preferable. Alcohol should be avoided because it may exacerbate ulcers already present.

Self-care is often started before the patient sees the health care provider. The patient may have already tried over-the-counter histamine antagonists or antacids or a friend's medication. Such use should be explored before recommending any treatment. "On demand" therapy (treatment when the patient is symptomatic only) has been advocated (Korman, 1995).

Medication Regimens

With a relatively benign presentation, several diagnostic and treatment paths can be followed (Fig. 29-1). An empiric trial of antisecretory medications (histamine blockers, proton pump

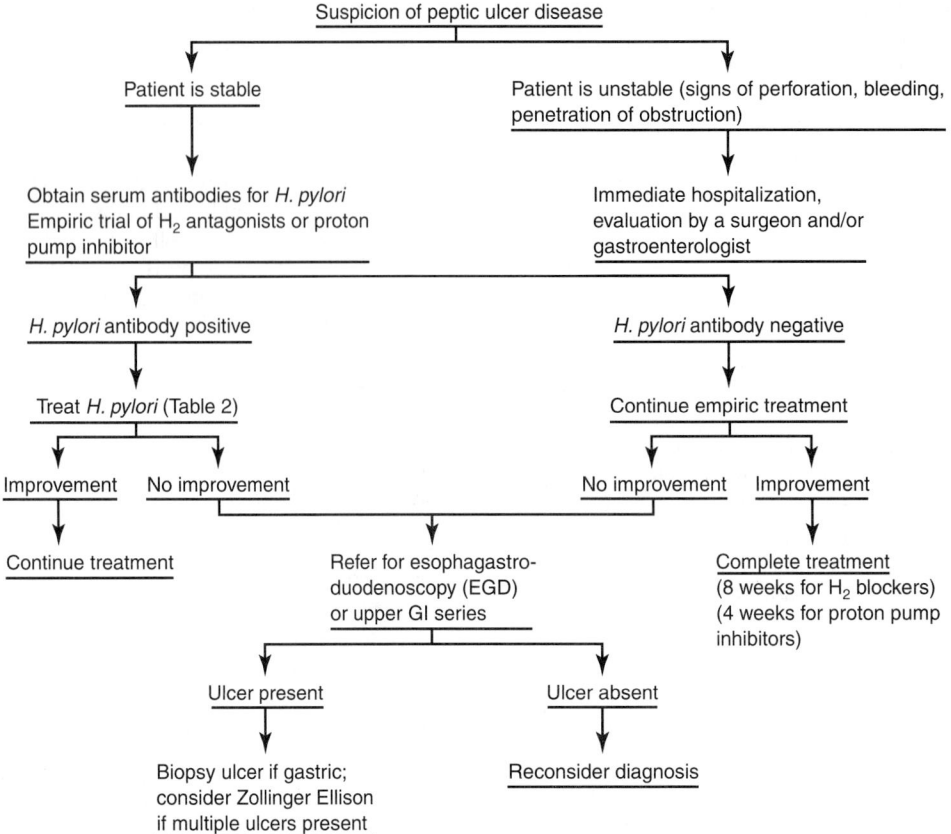

FIGURE 29-1 Treatment approaches for patients with peptic ulcer disease.

inhibitors) or sucralfate (Table 29-1) may be prescribed and the patient's course carefully monitored. Antacids can also be used to treat PUD. The appropriate dose to ensure healing is approximately 30 mL of liquid antacid every 4 to 6 hours; however, this much antacid often results in diarrhea, decreasing the likelihood of cooperation with treatment. Over-the-counter histamine blockers are now available in half-strength tablets

(compared to prescription strength; see Table 29-1). It is uncertain if the over-the-counter recommended doses are sufficient to heal ulcers. Active ulcers generally need 6 to 8 weeks of treatment with histamine blockers or sucralfate or 4 weeks of treatment with proton pump inhibitors.

Proton pump inhibitors require a shorter duration of therapy, healing 80% to 100% of duodenal ulcers in 4 weeks

TABLE 29-1	Pharmacologic Treatment of Peptic Ulcer		
	Dosing	**Duration**	**Maintenance Doses**
HISTAMINE BLOCKERS			
Ranitidine (Zantac)	150 mg b.i.d.	6–8 weeks	150 mg/day
	300 mg nightly	Same	
Cimetidine (Tagamet)	400 mg b.i.d.	6–8 weeks	400 mg/day
	800 mg nightly	Same	
Famotidine (Pepcid)	20 mg b.i.d.	6–8 weeks	20 mg/day
	40 mg nightly	Same	
Nizatidine (Axid)	150 mg b.i.d.	6–8 weeks	150 mg/day
	300 mg nightly	Same	
PROTON PUMP INHIBITORS			
Omeprazole (Prilosec)	20 mg/day	4 weeks	10 mg/day
Lansoprazole (Prevacid)	30 mg/day	4 weeks	15 mg/day
BARRIER PROTECTION			
Sucralfate (Carafate)	1 g q.i.d.	6–8 weeks	1 g b.i.d.
PROSTAGLANDIN THERAPY			
Misoprostol (Cytotec)	200 mcg q.i.d. to be taken for the duration of NSAID therapy		
	(100 mcg q.i.d. if diarrhea occurs with 200 mcg)		

(Maton, 1991). Some providers prefer proton pump inhibitors as first-line therapy in all patients who bleed from an ulcer. This is because the ulcers heal more rapidly and rebleeding may be avoided.

In addition to prescribing antisecretory drugs in the treatment of ulcers, *H. pylori,* if present, must be eradicated. Table 29-2 presents treatment options for the eradication of this organism. All these options are effective, with an eradication rate of approximately 70% to 85% (Labenz et al, 1993). These treatment options apply to duodenal ulcers as well as gastric ulcers. The recommended duration of combination therapy is usually 2 weeks, although shorter courses, such as 1 week and even 1 day (Kimura et al, 1995), have been described. The 2-week course involves both the antibiotic and the antisecretory medication. Once the 2-week course is over, the antisecretory medication should be continued because it often takes a longer duration of acid suppression to ensure healing of either duodenal or gastric ulcers. In other words, once the *H. pylori* has been eradicated, the patient must remain on an antisecretory medication for the full recommended course to ensure healing of the ulcer.

Sucralfate is also used to treat PUD. It works as a barrier protector and does not inhibit the secretion of acid. Dosing recommendations are noted in Table 29-1.

After completion of therapy, further evaluation of duodenal ulcers is not indicated. These ulcers respond very well to medical therapy, and the likelihood of duodenal malignancy is extraordinarily low. Duodenal carcinoma is rare, but 7% of gastric ulcers are secondary to malignancy (Gear et al, 1969; Wenger et al, 1971). As mentioned above, biopsy samples need to be taken from all gastric ulcers and healing must be closely monitored. Endoscopy should be repeated after 4 to 6 weeks of treatment for gastric ulcers. A biopsy sample must be taken from any ulcer that is not healing. However, even ulcers secondary to malignancy may heal, so caution and early biopsies must be practiced.

Misoprostol (Cytotec) is a synthetic prostaglandin E_1 analogue recommended for patients taking NSAIDs. This medica-

tion helps to protect the gastric mucosa, which is damaged by the NSAIDs because of their inhibition of prostaglandin formation. These prostaglandins act by increasing bicarbonate secretion, increasing mucous secretion, and inhibiting acid secretion from the parietal cells. These three mechanisms help to prevent ulcer formation in patients exposed to NSAIDs.

Approximately 25% of elderly persons taking NSAIDs develop ulcers. This number can be halved if misoprostol is taken at recommended doses (Soll et al, 1991; see Table 29-1).

Surgery may be necessary in cases of complicated PUD. Since the advent of histamine blockers and interventional endoscopy, the need for surgery has decreased markedly. However, if bleeding cannot be controlled via endoscopy or if perforation has occurred, surgery is often the last chance the patient has for survival. Surgery is also recommended for refractory ulcers (those that do not respond to prolonged therapy with histamine blockers, sucralfate, or proton pump inhibitors) and ulcers where malignancy is either strongly suspected or documented.

Complementary Therapies

Alternative approaches to treatment of PUD have included eating foods thought to buffer the acidic environment of the stomach and avoiding offending agents. Alcohol, spicy foods, or acidic foods may provoke symptoms in a particular patient. Avoidance of cigarettes is an essential part of PUD therapy.

COMMUNITY RESOURCES

A list of community-based resources can be found at the end of this unit.

REFERRAL POINTS AND CLINICAL WARNINGS

In the following cases the patient should be referred to a gastroenterologist or a GI surgeon:

- Gastric ulcers, so that an endoscopic biopsy may be obtained
- PUD that does not respond to conventional treatment and eradication of *H. pylori*
- Complicated PUD, including gastric outlet obstruction, penetration of the ulcer into the pancreas, perforation of the ulcer, and GI bleeding
- Clinical suspicion of Zollinger-Ellison syndrome.

TABLE 29-2	FDA-Approved Treatment Options for *Helicobacter pylori*

Omeprazole 40 mg/day *plus* clarithromycin 500 mg t.i.d. × 2 weeks, then omeprazole 20 mg/day × 2 weeks
OR

Ranitidine bismuth citrate 400 mg b.i.d. *plus* clarithromycin 500 mg t.i.d. × 2 weeks, then ranitidine bismuth citrate 400 mg b.i.d. × 2 weeks
OR

Bismuth subsalicylate (Pepto-Bismol) 525 mg q.i.d. *plus* metronidazole 250 mg q.i.d. *plus* tetracycline 500 mg q.i.d.* × 2 weeks *plus* histamine receptor antagonist therapy as directed × 4 weeks
OR

Lansoprazole 30 mg b.i.d. *plus* amoxicillin 1 g b.i.d. *plus* clarithromycin 500 mg b.i.d. × 2 weeks
OR

Lansoprazole 30 mg t.i.d. *plus* amoxicillin 1 g t.i.d. × 2 weeks.†

* Although not FDA-approved, amoxicillin has been substituted for tetracycline in patients in whom tetracycline is not recommended.

† This dual therapy regimen has restrictive labeling. It is indicated for patients who are either allergic or intolerant to clarithromycin or for infections with known or suspected resistance to clarithromycin.

■ ■ ■ **CLINICAL PEARLS**

- Always consider a history of black stools significant until proven otherwise.
- Always ask about the use of Pepto-Bismol or iron supplements in the patient who presents with black stools.
- Always suspect NSAIDs as a possible cause of ulcers because of the frequency of use in all age groups and their ready availability.
- Alcohol does not cause ulcers, but it may exacerbate them.
- In patients who are vomiting blood, distinguishing so-called bright-red blood from dark blood does not help determine the source of the bleeding.
- Do not combine sucralfate with histamine blockers or proton pump inhibitors. There is no synergistic activity.

EDITOR'S NOTE:

COMPLEMENTARY APPROACHES

A general discussion of complementary approaches can be found in Chapter 3. The following, while not an exhaustive list, are some complementary approaches being used for this condition. Additional information on these approaches, including precautions, can be found in Appendices A and B. Providers need to assess for the use of complementary approaches as part of the patient's history, as they may impact conventional therapies, and patients may not volunteer this information unless specifically asked. Efficacy of many complementary approaches is not as well documented as that of conventional therapies. Providers need to read the literature before suggesting these complementary approaches.

- Vitamins, minerals, herbs, supplements
  Garlic
  Glutamine (cabbage juice)
  Licorice
  Vitamin C
- Complementary Modalities
  Aromatherapy
  Massage therapy

References

Bernersen, B., Johnsen, P., Straume, B., et al. (1990). Towards a true Prevalence of peptic ulcer disease: The Sorreisa Gastrointestinal Disorder Study. *Gut, 31*, 989.

Cutler, A.F. & Prasad, V.M. (1996). Long-term follow-up of helicobacter pylori serology after successful eradication. *American Journal of Gastroenterology, 91*(January): 85–87.

Endoh, K., & Leung, F.W. (1994). Effects of smoking and nicotine on the gastric mucosa: A review of clinical and experimental evidence. *Gastroenterology, 107*(3), 864–878.

Gear, M.W.L., Truelove, S.C., Williams, D.G., Massarella, G.R., & Boddington, M.M. (1969). Gastric cancer simulating benign gastric ulcer. *British Journal of Surgery, 56*, 739.

Hojgaard, L., Mertz, A., Nielsen, A., & Rune, SJ. (1996). Peptic ulcer pathophysiology: Acid, bicarbonate and mucosal function. *Scandinavian Journal of Gastroenterology, 216*(suppl), 10–15.

Kimura, K. Ido, K., et al. (1995). Therapy for the treatment of helicobacter pylori infection. *American Journal of Gastroenterology, 90*, 60–63.

Korman, M.G. (1995). Influence of initial therapy on outcome of peptic ulcer disease. *Scandinavian Journal of Gastroenterology, 208*(suppl), 21–23.

Kurata, J.H., Haile, B.M., & Elashoff, J.D. (1985). Sex differences in peptic ulcer disease. *Gastroenterology, 88*, 96.

Labenz, J., Gyenes, E., Ruhl, G.H., et al. (1992). Two weeks treatment with amoxicillin/omeprazole for eradication of helicobacter pylori. *Gastroenterology, 30*(11), 776–778.

Maton, P.N. (1991). Omeprazole. *N Engl J Med, 324*, 965.

Selling, J.A., Hogan, D.L., Aly, A., et al. (1987). Indomethacin inhibits duodenal mucosal bicarbonate secretion and endogeneous prostaglandsin E2 output in humans. *Annals of Internal Medicine, 106*: 368.

Sleisenger, & Fordtran, (Eds.). *Gastrointestinal disease,* 5th ed., p. 591.

Soll, A.H., Weinstein, W.M., Kurata, J., & McCarthy, D. (1991). Nonsteroidal anti-inflammatory drugs and peptic ulcer disease. *Annals of Internal Medicine, 114*, 307.

Tytgat, G.N.J., & Rauws, E.A.J. (1990). *Campylobacter pylori* and its role in peptic ulcer disease. *Gastroenterology Clinics of North American, 19*, 183.

Wenger, J., Brandborg, L., & Spellman, F. (1971). Cancer Part I. Clinical aspects. *Gastroenterology, 61*, 598.

APPENDIX 29

COMMUNITY RESOURCES FOR GASTROINTESTINAL DISORDERS

There are many national organizations available for different gastrointestinal disorders. Some of the organizations are disease-specific and others are more general. Some are easily accessible by phone, others via the Internet. They offer patient teaching, classes, provider education, brochures, videos, and support groups and serve as a referral source. Each organization serves different functions, and providers are encouraged to familiarize themselves with each to know which will best serve the patient.

Acute and Chronic Pancreatitis

- Pancreatitis Supporter Network, 15 Mayfield Court, 59 Mayfield Road, Moseley, Birmingham B13 9HS, United Kingdom, 1-800-424-2923; http://ourworld.compuserve.com/homepages/psnjimarmour/: General pancreatitis information, traditional and alternative treatment options, newsletters
- NIDDK (National Institute of Diabetic and Digestive and Kidney Diseases) National Digestive Diseases Clearinghouse: http://www.niddk.nih.gov/Pancrea/Pancrea.htm: Extensive overview of pancreatitis
- American College of Gastroenterology, 4900-B S. 31st St., Arlington, VA 22206, 703-820-4400; http://www.acg.gi.org/acghome.html
- Healthtouch Online: http://www.healthtouch.com/level1/leaflets/105190/105237.htm: Overview of acute and chronic pancreatitis
- The Virtual Hospital, University of Iowa: http://www.vh.org/Providers/ClinRef/FPHandbook/Chapter04/11-4.html: Extensive overview of acute pancreatitis, family practice handbook

Cirrhosis

- American Liver Foundation, 1425 Pompton Ave., Cedar Grove, NJ 00709, 1-800-GO LIVER (465-4837); http://sadieo.ucsf.edu/ALF/ALFfinal/homepagealf.html: General information on cirrhosis, epidemiology, symptoms and treatment; links to similar Websites
- NIDDK Home Page (National Digestive Disease Clearinghouse), 2 Information Way, Bethesda, MD 20892-3570; http://www.niddk.nih.gov/DigestiveDocs.html: General information on cirrhosis
- American Association for the Study of Liver Disease (AASLD), 1200 19th St., NW, Suite 300, Washington D.C. 20036, 1-202-429-5179; http://hepar-sfgh.ucsf.edu: Links to liver-related sites, general information about AASLD
- Liver Disease Homepage-Cirrhosis: http://www.gastro.com/liverpg/livdz.htm: General information on liver disease
- American Gastroenterological Association, 7910 Woodmont Ave., 7th Floor, Bethesda, MD 20814, 301-654-2055
- Wilson's Disease Association, 4 Navcho Dr., Brookfield, CT, 1-800-399-0266
- Transplant Recipient International Organization (TRIO), 1000 16th St., NW, Suite 602, Washington D.C. 20035, 1-800-TRIO-386, 202-293-0980

- International Liver Transplantation Society: www.livertransplantation.org.

Gallbladder

- American Liver Foundation (address above; see cirrhosis resources): General information on gallbladder disease, epidemiology, symptoms and treatment; links to similar Websites
- NIDDK Home Page (address above; see cirrhosis resources): General information on gallstones
- American Association for the Study of Liver Disease (address above; see cirrhosis resources): Links to liver-related sites, general information about AASLD
- Health Resource Directory: http://www.stayhealthy.com /hrdfiles/hrd00346.html: Gallbladder, gallstones, laparoscopic cholecystectomy

Gastroesophageal Reflux Disease

- NIDDK (address above; see cirrhosis resources); GERD Page: http://www.niddk.nih.gov/Heartburn/Heartburn. html: Overview, treatment and home management, complications, recommended readings
- American College of Gastroenterologists: http://www. acg.gi.org/acghome.html: Understanding GERD, free video, extensive overview
- Healthtouch: http://www.healthtouch.com/level1/leaflets /105190/105206.htm: Overview of heartburn and GERD
- GERD Information Resource Center: http://www.gerd. com/: Overview of GERD
- American Gastroenterological Association (address above; see cirrhosis resources)
- American College of Gastroenterology (address above; see pancreatitis resources)

Gastrointestinal Cancers

- American Cancer Society, 1599 Clifton Rd., N.E., Atlanta, GA 30329 and local chapters in all 50 states; 1-800-ACS-2345; http://www.cancer.org: Information, newsletters and support grops for all types of cancers
- National Cancer Institutes, Office of Cancer Communication, 31 Center Dr., MSC 2580, Bethesda, MD 20892-2580, 1-800-422-6237
- http://cancernet.nci.nih.gov/clinpdq/pif/Colon—cancer —Patient.html
- http://cancernet.nci.nih.gov/clinpdq/pif/Extrahepatic—bile —duct—cancer—Patient.html
- http://cancernet.nci.nih.gov/clinpdq/pif/Gallbladder —cancer —Patient.html
- http://cancernet.nci.nih.gov/clinpdq/pif/Gastric—cancer —Patient.html
- http://cancernet.nci.nih.gov/clinpdq/pif/Gastrointestinal —carcinoid—tumor—Patient.html
- http://cancernet.nci.nih.gov/clinpdq/pif/Rectal—cancer —Patient.html
- http://cancernet.nci.nih.gov/clinpdq/pif/Small—intestine —cancer—Patient.html
- Healthtouch Online: http://www.healthtouch.com/level1/ leaflets/109207/109759.htm: Pancreatic and liver cancer information
- American Liver Foundation (address above; see cirrhosis resources): Information on benign and malignant tumors of the liver

- Aetna U.S. Healthcare Colorectal Info Page: http: //www.aetnaushc.com/topics/colorectal.html: General overview of colorectal cancer
- United Ostomy Association, 26 Executive Park, Suite 120, Irvine, CA 92714, 1-800-826-0826

Hemorrhoids

- American Association of Family Physicians: http: //www.aafp.org/patientinfo/hemorroh.html
- MedicineNet Power Points: http://www.medicinenet.com/ mainmenu/encyclop/article/art—h/ he morrd.htm
- NIDDK (address above; see cirrhosis resources)
- NIH Hemorrhoids Information Page: http://www .niddk.nih.gov/Hemorrhoids/Hemorrhoids.html
- American Gastroenterological Association (address above; see cirrhosis resources)

Hepatitis

- Hepatitis Weekly: http://www.newsfile.com/1h.htm
- Hepatitis Network: http://www.hepnet.com: General information, publications, Websites, and news reports about hepatitis A, B, C, D, and G; current news and events update; information for providers and patients
- American Liver Foundation (address above; see cirrhosis resources): Information on hepatitis A, B, C, D, E, and G, epidemiology, symptoms, and treatment; links to similar Websites
- NIDDK Home Page (address above; see cirrhosis resources): General information on hepatitis
- American Association for the Study of Liver Disease (address above; see cirrhosis resources): Links to liver-related sites

Inflammatory Bowel Disease

- Crohn's and Colitis Foundation of Canada, 21 St. Clair Ave. EasE, Suite 301, Toronto, Ontario M4T 1L9, 1-800-387-1479; http://www.ccfc.ca/html: Facts about Crohn's and ulcerative colitis
- Crohn's information page: http://web.bu.edu:80/COHIS/ help/find/catgry/gi.htm
- American College of Gastroenterology (address above; see pancreatitis resources)
- NIDDK (address above; see cirrhosis resources)

Peptic Ulcer Disease

- Aetna U.S. Health Care Peptic Ulcer Page: http: //www.aetnaushc.com/topics/peptic.html: Overview, signs and symptoms, diagnosis, and treatment
- Stomach and Duodenal Ulcers Page: http://www .gastro.com/ulcers.htm: Causes, diagnosis, and treatment; recommended readings; points to remember
- Healthtouch: http://www.healthtouch.com/level1/leaflets/ 105190/105206.htm: Overview of stomach ulcers
- Mayo Health Oasis: http://www.mayohealth.org/mayo/ askphys/qa970402.htm: Questions and answers, new treatments, ulcers and diet
- National Digestive Diseases Information Clearinghouse (address above; see cirrhosis resources)
- American Gastroenterological Association (address above; see cirrhosis resources)
- American College of Gastroenterology (address above; see pancreatitis resources)

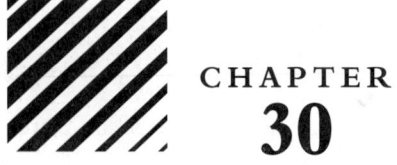

CHAPTER
30

Acute Renal Failure

Gail A. Breen, PharmD, BCPS

Acute renal failure (ARF) is a deterioration of renal function, over a period of hours to days, resulting in failure of the kidney to perform its necessary processes, which include the elimination of nitrogenous waste products, homeostasis of fluid and electrolytes, and acid–base balance. An elevation in nitrogenous wastes is referred to as azotemia. Uremia is the clinical manifestation of azotemia and consists of nausea and vomiting, altered sensorium, pruritus, asterixis, decreased appetite, and pericarditis.

ARF is commonly defined as an increase in the serum creatinine concentration of 0.5 mg/dL when the baseline creatinine is less than 3 mg/dL, or an increase in serum creatinine of 1 mg/dL if the baseline creatinine exceeds 3 mg/dL (Rose, 1987). However, the serum creatinine level does not always rise in proportion to renal damage. Therefore, ARF can be more broadly defined as a time when the body cannot maintain adequate acid–base balance and volume status or accumulates nitrogenous wastes.

ARF is divided into three categories: prerenal (resulting from renal hypoperfusion), intrarenal (resulting from direct damage to the kidney), and postrenal (resulting from a urine flow obstruction). It is important to identify which type of renal failure a patient has, because treatment approaches vary depending on the etiology.

Risk factors for developing ARF have been defined for different patient populations and will be discussed in this chapter. Identification of patients with such risk factors is important in the prevention of ARF. Early detection and intervention is important in minimizing permanent damage to the kidneys. Despite recent advances in the medical care of these patients, the treatment of ARF continues to pose a serious dilemma for the primary care provider.

ANATOMY, PHYSIOLOGY, AND PATHOLOGY

Anatomy and Physiology

Normally, people have two kidneys measuring 10 to 13 cm. Each kidney consists of approximately 2.5 million nephrons, the functional units of the kidney. The nephrons are responsible for production of an ultrafiltrate; reabsorption of electrolytes, bicarbonate, glucose, and essential amino acids; and secretion of electrolytes, medications, and other constituents of the blood that are not necessary for homeostasis.

Blood flows to each kidney via the renal artery, which divides into two branches before arriving at the kidneys. Each branch divides into approximately five segmental branches, providing blood flow to their respective portions of the kidney. Each segmental branch further breaks down into smaller arteries and arterioles. Each nephron consists of a glomerulus (a vascular tuft that joins the efferent and afferent arterioles) and the collecting tubules, which consists of the proximal tubule, the loop of Henle, and the distal tubule. In the proximal tubule, 60% to 70% of the filtered load of water and solute is reabsorbed, including amino acids, glucose, and bicarbonate. Reabsorption of calcium, potassium, and magnesium occurs at the loop of Henle, as well as maintenance of an osmotic gradient necessary for the concentration of urinary solutes. The distal tubules are responsible for acid–base balance, secretion of potassium, and reabsorption of water. Figure 30-1 illustrates the anatomy of the kidney.

Pathology

Prerenal failure results from decreased renal perfusion, with or without systemic hypotension. Under normal conditions, renal blood flow is approximately 25% of the cardiac output. In states of volume depletion or major bleeding, there is a decrease in blood volume and consequently a decrease in renal perfusion. In cases of congestive heart failure and shock, there is not a decrease in blood volume but there is a decrease in blood flow to the kidneys, which also results in renal hypoperfusion. An obstruction of the renal arteries bilaterally (or unilaterally in a solitary kidney) will also decrease renal perfusion (Brenner et al, 1987). The kidney is capable of maintaining an adequate glomerular and renal blood flow in the presence of moderate reductions in renal perfusion by autoregulation. Prerenal failure results when autoregulation fails to maintain the glomerular filtration rate.

Acute intrinsic renal failure results from damage to any part of the kidney, including the small blood vessels, glomerulus, renal tubule, and interstitium. Damage to the small blood vessels may result from cholesterol emboli deposition or malignant hypertension. Damage to the glomerulus can be caused by a number of diseases, including systemic lupus erythematosus, and Goodpasture's syndrome. Injury to the renal tubules may result from severe renal hypoperfusion or direct toxicity from exogenous and endogenous substances. Examples of exogenous nephrotoxic substances include radiocontrast dyes, aminoglycosides, and amphotericin B. Contrast nephropathy is a relatively common cause of ARF. Most contrast dyes are vasoconstrictive, and the decrease in renal blood flow can cause ischemic nephropathy. Myoglobin, a potential endogenous nephrotoxin, is released in rhabdomyolysis and may cause acute damage to the renal tubules. Nonselective backleak of filtrate across damaged renal tubules may also result in acute tubular necrosis (ATN). Damage to the interstitium may result from infections, such as HIV and streptococci, and many drugs, including penicillin and cephalosporin antibiotics, ciprofloxacin, sulfonamides, phenytoin, and nonsteroidal anti-inflammatory agents (NSAIDs). In the case of acute interstitial nephritis, eosinophils are usually present in the blood and urine; however, eosinophils are not found in interstitial nephritis caused by NSAIDs. Symptoms of acute interstitial nephritis include fever, rashes, eosinophilia, and eosinophiluria.

Postrenal obstruction is characterized by an acute onset of anuria. The incidence of postrenal failure is low: it accounts for less than 10% of all cases of ARF (Balsov & Jorgensen, 1963). It must occur in both kidneys to cause ARF, or in one kidney if the patient has a solitary kidney. Crystal deposition from oxalate or drugs such as acyclovir or sulfonamides may cause a urinary obstruction. Malignancy, atonic bladder, or urethral stricture can cause obstruction. Benign prostatic hypertrophy, a progressive enlargement of the prostate, is a common cause of acute postrenal failure, particularly in men older than age 50 (Wood & Bosley, 1991).

ARF can also be classified based on urine output. In the absence of obstruction, urine output directly correlates with the glomerular filtration rate in patients with ARF. Anuria is

TABLE 30-1	Causes of Acute Renal Failure
PRERENAL	
Decreased intravascular volume	Multiple myeloma
Bleeding	Pyelonephritis
Dehydration	Vascular
Decreased renal blood flow	Wegener's granulomatosis
Congestive heart failure	Polyarteritis nodosa
Shock	Thrombotic thrombocytopenic purpura
Sepsis	Pre-eclampsia
Vasodilating drugs	Scleroderma
INTRINSIC	Arterial embolization
Glomerular	Hemolytic uremic syndrome
IgA nephropathy	**POSTRENAL**
Systemic lupus erythematosus	Prostatic hypertrophy
Goodpasture's syndrome	Tumor
Postinfectious	Stones
Tubulointerstitial	
Acute tubular necrosis	Emboli
Acute interstitial nephritis	Crystals

defined as a 24-hour urine production of less than 50 mL. Oliguria is defined as a 24-hour urine output of 50 to 400 mL. Nonoliguria is defined as a 24-hour urine output of greater than 400 mL. Patients with nonoliguric ARF have a better prognosis than those with oliguric renal failure, probably because of the decreased severity of the insult (Corwin et al, 1987). Tables 30-1 and 30-2 outline the causes of ARF.

EPIDEMIOLOGY

ARF is more common in the hospital setting than in the community setting. For example, the incidence of ARF is 1% at the time of admission to the hospital (Kaufman et al, 1991), increases to 2% to 5% during hospitalization (Maher et al, 1989; Shusterman et al, 1987), and rises to 4% to 15% after cardiopulmonary bypass (Zanasrdo et al, 1994). However, because of the difficulty in defining and ultimately diagnosing ARF, the exact incidence is unknown.

There are a number of risk factors for ARF, including sepsis, bleeding, volume depletion, surgery, chronic liver disease, and nephrotoxic drugs. There appears to be a direct relation between the number of failed organ systems and the death rate associated with ARF (Maher et al, 1989). The mortality rate increases two- to eightfold as the number of failed organ systems increases from zero to three (Maher et al, 1989).

The mortality rate associated with ARF has improved in recent years, probably because of more aggressive nutritional therapy and earlier and improved renal replacement therapies. Before the development of dialytic therapies, the most common causes of death in patients with ARF were uremia, hyperkalemia, and volume overload. With the improvement of dialytic techniques, the most common causes of death now are sepsis, cardiovascular and pulmonary dysfunction, and the withdrawal of life-support measures (Turney, 1990; Woodrow & Turney, 1991).

DIAGNOSTIC CRITERIA

The first step in the diagnostic process is to determine whether the ARF is the result of a prerenal, postrenal, or intrinsic renal event. Prerenal failure and intrinsic renal failure from ischemia

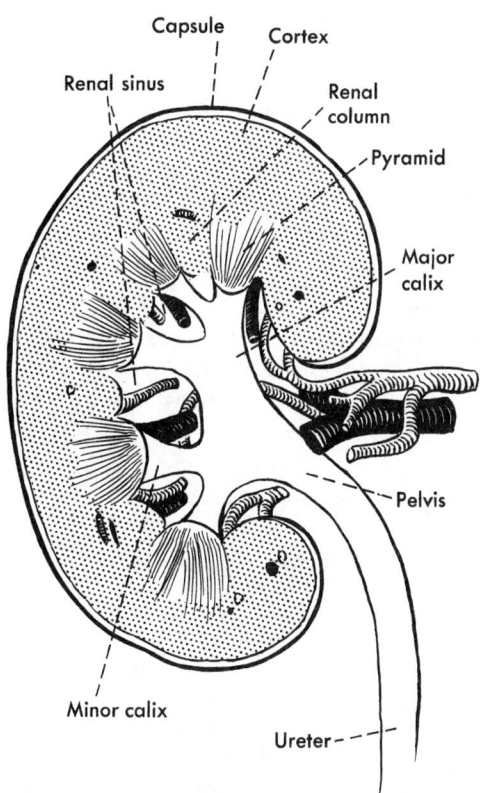

FIGURE 30-1 The kidney. The renal vessels anterior to the renal pelvis have been cut in removing the anterior half of the kidney; the fat in the renal sinus has also been removed. (From Rosse, C. & Gaddum-Rosse, P. (1997). *Hollinshead's Textbook of Anatomy*, 5/e. Philadelphia: Lippincott-Raven Publishers.)

TABLE 30-2	Drugs Associated With Acute Renal Failure
Mechanism	**Drug**
Allergic interstitial nephritis	Penicillins, NSAIDs, cephalosporins, sulfonamides, rifampin, allopurinol, cimetidine, phenytoin, vancomycin, ciprofloxacin
Decreased renal perfusion	Angiotensin-converting enzyme inhibitors, NSAIDs, radiocontrast agents, cyclosporine
Direct tubular toxicity	Aminoglycosides, amphotericin B, cisplatin, cyclosporine, foscarnet, pentamidine, heavy metals
Rhabdomyolysis	Cocaine, lovastatin*
Tubular obstruction	Acyclovir, sulfonamides, chemotherapeutic agents†
Hemolytic-uremic syndrome	Cyclosporine, cocaine, quinine

* Rhabdomyolysis has been reported with lovastatin when combined with cyclosporine.

† Uric acid crystals form as a result of tumor lysis.

Adapted from Thadhani et al, 1996.

or nephrotoxins are responsible for most episodes of ARF (Thadhani et al, 1996). Diagnostic tests that may help with the diagnosis of ARF are listed in Tables 30-3, 30-4, and 30-5.

Blood tests that help in the diagnosis and workup of ARF include serum creatinine and blood urea nitrogen (BUN); levels of both are usually elevated. The rise in creatinine may lag behind the rise in BUN and may not be detected until some time after the renal insult. The ratio between BUN and creatinine can be used to help pinpoint the cause of kidney dysfunction. The BUN/creatinine ratio is usually 10:1, but it varies depending on the etiology of ARF. An increase in creatinine kinase levels in association with a traumatic event or prolonged ischemia may be indicative of rhabdomyolysis (Kurokawa, 1983). Hypercalcemia and hyperuricemia may indicate a malignant cause; eosinophilia may point to an allergic interstitial nephritis. Tests for immunologic substances such as serum complement 3 and 4 would suggest glomerulonephritis and alert the provider to a systemic cause, such as lupus nephritis.

An extensive examination of the urinalysis is crucial to the diagnosis. Proteinuria and hematuria indicate a glomerular injury; glucosuria suggests a tubular injury. Microscopic examination of the urine is also important. Examples of diagnostic findings on the microscopic urinalysis include pigmented, muddy-brown granular casts, which are characteristic of tubular necrosis; red blood cell casts, which are suggestive of a glomerular injury; and white cell casts, which are indicative of interstitial nephritis.

Urine indices, including urine osmolality, urine sodium concentration, and fractional excretion of sodium, help differen-

tiate between prerenal azotemia and ATN (Rose, 1987). The equation for calculating the fractional excretion of sodium is (Thadhani et al, 1996):

$$(U_{Na} \times P_{Cr} \times 100)/U_{Cr} \times P_{Na}$$

In prerenal conditions, the concentration ability of the kidneys and the reabsorptive function of the tubules are usually intact, whereas in ATN these processes are usually lost or impaired. Because the ability of the kidneys to concentrate the urine is diminished in the setting of ATN, urine osmolality is decreased, and the urinary fractional excretion of sodium (and hence the urine sodium concentration) is increased. However, the guidelines for urine indices are not rigid. For example, early in ATN secondary to contrast nephropathy, urinary excretion of sodium is low. Concomitant diuretic administration may limit the usefulness of the fractional excretion of sodium by increasing sodium excretion (Rose, 1987).

Prerenal azotemia and ATN together account for 70% to 75% of cases of ARF in the hospital setting (Miller et al, 1978). Prerenal azotemia and ATN are often difficult to differentiate, because prerenal failure may lead to ATN. Treatment options differ between these two causes; therefore, every effort must be made to distinguish the cause. Aggressive fluid administration would be the primary treatment modality of prerenal azotemia but may be detrimental in ATN. Laboratory data, as mentioned previously and in Table 30-1, will aid in the correct diagnosis.

HISTORY AND PHYSICAL EXAM

A careful history is crucial in the initial evaluation. A history of concomitant disease states, family medical history, and medication use are all pertinent in the diagnosis. A recent history of an exacerbation of congestive heart failure, volume depletion secondary to a traumatic injury, or angiography may suggest the diagnosis of ARF.

A thorough physical exam is a necessary part in the workup of ARF. Clinical findings of thirst and orthostatic dizziness and physical findings of orthostatic hypotension, tachycardia, and dry skin turgor suggest prerenal failure secondary to volume depletion. A rash may suggest allergic interstitial nephritis. Flank pain may indicate a renal artery or vein occlusion. Digital ischemia may suggest atheroembolization.

TABLE 30-3	Utility of Diagnostic Tests
Test	**Utility**
Renal ultrasound	Will help differentiate if renal insult is acute or chronic by assessing the number and size of the kidneys; will indicate whether an obstruction is present
Pyleography Renal angiography	Diagnostic for renal artery obstruction
Renal biopsy	Primary etiology is suspected; pre- and postrenal ARF have been ruled out

TABLE 30-4	Diagnostic Parameters for the Differentiation of Acute Renal Failure		
	Prerenal	**Intrinsic**	**Postrenal**
Urinalysis	Hyaline casts	Proteinuria, WBC, RBC, casts	Frequently normal; hematuria
Urinary sodium concentration (mEq/L)	<10	>10	Acute: <10 Chronic: >10
Urine osmolality (mOsm/kg)	>500	<300	Variable
Fractional sodium excretion (%)	<1	>1	Acute: <1 Chronic: >1
BUN/plasma Cr	>20	15	15

WBC, white blood cell; RBC, red blood cell; BUN, blood urea nitrogen; Cr, creatinine.

TABLE 30-5	Diagnostic Parameters for the Differentiation of Intrinsic Acute Renal Failure		
Area of Kidney Affected	**Suggestive Clinical Features**	**Urinalysis**	**Confirmatory Tests**
LARGE RENAL VESSELS			
Renal artery thrombosis	h/o a.fib or recent MI	Proteinuria, red cells	Renal arteriogram
Atheroembolism	Age>50, recent manipulation of aorta, HTN	Often normal, eosinophiluria, rarely casts	Eosinophilia
Renal vein thrombosis	Pulmonary embolism, flank pain	Proteinuria, hematuria	Inferior vena cavagram and renal venogram
SMALL VESSELS AND GLOMERULI			
Glomerulonephritis vasculitis	Clinical history (infection)	Red cell or granular casts, red and white cells, mild proteinuria	Renal biopsy, blood cultures
Hemolytic-uremic syndrome	History (GI infection, CSA use)	May be normal, red cells, mild proteinuria, rarely red cell or granular casts	Anemia, thrombocytopenia, increased LDH renal biopsy
Malignant hypertension	Severe HTN with headaches, retinopathy	Red cells, red cell casts, proteinuria	Resolution of ARF with control of BP
ACUTE TUBULAR NECROSIS			
Ischemia	Recent hemorrhage hypotension	Muddy-brown granular or tubular epithelial cell casts	Clinical assessment and U/A usually sufficient for diagnosis
Exogenous toxins	Recent nephrotoxic substance	Muddy-brown granular or tubular epithelial cell casts	Clinical assessment and U/A usually sufficient for diagnosis
Endogenous toxins	Rhabdomyolysis (seizure, ethanol), hemolysis, tumor lysis (chemotherapy)	Urine supernatant positive for heme	↑ K, ↑ PO_4, ↑ uric acid, rhabdo: also ↑ CK, ↑ LDH ↑ AST/↑ ALT
TUBULOINTERSTITIUM			
Allergic interstitial nephritis	Recent ingestion of drug, rash, fever, arthralgias	White cell casts, white cells, eosinophiluria, red cells, rarely red cell casts, proteinuria	Systemic eosinophilia, skin biopsy of rash
Bilateral pyelonephritis	Flank pain and tenderness, febrile	Leukocytes, proteinuria, red cells, bacteria	Urine and blood cultures

Adapted from Brady, H.R., et al. (1996). In *The Kidney,* 5th ed., Brenner, B.M. (ed.). Philadelphia: WB Saunders.

TREATMENT OPTIONS, EXPECTED OUTCOMES, AND COMPREHENSIVE MANAGEMENT

ARF is commonly a result of iatrogenic causes, so emphasis must be placed on prevention. Risk factors for the development of ARF secondary to a number of causes have been defined, and their identification is the first step in prevention. Once risk factors are identified, different measures can be taken to avoid ARF. For example, if a patient is at risk for aminoglycoside nephrotoxicity, a different antibiotic may be used, such as a cephalosporin antibiotic with gram-negative coverage. If a patient is at risk for postoperative ARF, medical treatment may be employed, or surgery may be delayed until an underlying risk is corrected. If a patient is at risk for contrast-associated nephrotoxicity, adequate hydration and volume expansion should be implemented. Risk factors for the development of ARF are outlined in Table 30-6.

Patients at risk for the development of ARF should receive preventive therapy. This includes maintaining adequate hydration before a potentially nephrotoxic event, sodium loading, and the use of pharmacologic agents.

Ensuring adequate hydration with 0.9% or 0.45% normal saline is essential in the prevention of ARF. Renal perfusion is improved with proper hydration, and the workload of the tubules is reduced. Providing adequate hydration also dilutes the nephrotoxic substance and reduces the concentration of the substance in the tubule (Conger, 1995). On the other hand, administering intravenous fluids to patients who are volume-overloaded would be detrimental. These patients must be treated differently to prevent respiratory failure and pulmonary edema. Patients must be examined daily for evidence of volume overload or pericardial friction rubs. Hemodynamic parameters should be monitored frequently (specifically, pulmonary capillary wedge pressure, systolic and diastolic pulmonary artery pressures, central venous pressure, cardiac output, cardiac index, and systemic vascular resistance). Fluid intake and output assessments must include insensible losses. Patients should be weighed daily. In states of volume accumulation, approximately 1 L of fluid is equal to 1 kg of body weight gain. Patients with ARF are in a hypercatabolic state and therefore would be expected to lose weight, so a small weight gain may indicate an actually higher gain in water weight. Monitoring the serum sodium level also helps in the assessment of fluid balance. In states of volume overload, a dilutional hyponatremia occurs. The choice of intravenous solution and the amount to be administered for fluid replacement must be individualized.

Examples of clinical situations where hydration is beneficial in the prevention of ARF include rhabdomyolysis and tumor

TABLE 30-6	Risk Factors for the Development of Acute Renal Failure
Etiology	**Risk Factors**
Aminoglycoside	Advanced age, high cumulative dose of the aminoglycoside, renal hypoperfusion, concomitant nephrotoxic drugs, hypokalemia
Contrast media	Ionic contrast agents, advanced age, diabetes, concomitant use of nephrotoxic drugs, liver disease, renal impairment
Postoperative	Advanced age, male sex, pre-existing renal insufficiency, left ventricular dysfunction, hypotension, hypertension

lysis syndrome. In both instances, tubular-toxic substances (phosphate and nucleic and uric acids) are released in the body; aggressive hydration dilutes these toxic substances, decreasing the contact with the renal tubules.

Sodium loading is another preventive strategy in ARF. Sodium loading enhances the tubular glomerular reflex. The reflex works as follows. The kidney senses a high sodium concentration, and subsequently there is a decrease in renal blood flow and the glomerular filtration rate and ultimately a conservation of solutes and fluid. This decrease in renal blood flow results also in a reduction of the amount of nephrotoxic substance that passes through the tubules. Sodium loading is routinely used before amphotericin B administration in hopes of preventing nephrotoxicity (Solomon et al, 1994).

Conversion of oligoanuric to nonoliguric ARF is associated with an increased survival rate and reduced complications (Dixon & Anderson, 1985). Several agents, including mannitol, furosemide, and dopamine, alone and in combination, have been investigated for their role in ARF, with controversial results. Studies addressing these issues are difficult to evaluate: a number of these studies incorporated small numbers of patients, were uncontrolled, and included a variety of patient populations.

Mannitol is used as a prophylactic and therapeutic agent in ARF. Mannitol increases solute excretion, decreases cell swelling, inhibits tubular obstruction, and enhances vasodilation (Teschan & Lawson, 1966; Flores et al, 1972; Burke et al, 1983; Hanley & Davidson, 1981; Slekurt, 1945; Morris et al, 1972). If initial therapy with mannitol is not effective, subsequent doses should not be administered, because high doses of mannitol aggravate ARF. Fluid and electrolyte status, as well as the osmolar gap, must be monitored closely. Prolonged use of mannitol in severely oliguric patients should be avoided. Overdiuresis with mannitol may result in hypernatremia and a hyperosmolar state, and accumulation of mannitol may result in excessive extracellular volume expansion (Gubern et al, 1988; Dorman et al, 1990). Acute convulsions, coma, and death have been reported with the use of mannitol.

A small number of case reports have advocated the use of diuretic therapy and have claimed benefit in retrospective settings; therefore, many providers continue to use diuretic therapy in this setting (Cantarovich et al, 1973; Minuth et al, 1973; Karayannopoulos, 1974; Fries et al, 1971). The beneficial effect of loop diuretics may result from renal vasodilation, decreased tubular obstruction, suppressed tubuloglomerular feedback, or more than one of these (Cantarovich et al, 1973; Minuth et al, 1973). Furosemide increases urine output, hastens the time of oliguria or anuria, and reduces the need for dialysis; however, it does not appear to alter the mortality rate (Conger, 1995). Loop diuretics may be used alone, but in the setting of ARF high doses are needed, and often diuretic resistance is encountered (Mueller, 1997). Diuretic resistance can be a result of decreased oral bioavailability, excessive sodium intake, reduced delivery of diuretic to its site of action, and increased sodium reabsorption, specifically in congestive heart failure and cirrhosis (Mueller, 1997). Risks of high-dose loop diuretics include reversible ototoxicity, which is associated with rapid administration (furosemide administered intravenously at a rate >4 mg/min), and volume depletion (Conger, 1995).

Loop diuretics may be used in conjunction with a diuretic that has a different site of action in the kidney. Thiazide di-

TABLE 30-7	Pharmacologic Agents Used in the Treatment of Acute Renal Failure	
Agent	**Dosage Regimen**	**Selected Considerations**
Mannitol (20%)	12.5–25 g IV over 3–5 min, may repeat in 1 hour if no response; if urine output follows, give mannitol 20% 20 mL/hr with furosemide	Monitor fluid status, urine output, serum electrolytes, serum osmolality
Furosemide	100 mg IV; if no response within 1 hr, give 250 mg IV; if urine output follows, give 500–2000 mg/d in divided doses or continuous infusion 5–50 mg/hr	Monitor urine output and serum electrolytes
Dopamine	0.5–3 ug/kg/min IV infusion	Monitor urine output

Adapted from Mueller, 1997.

uretics, specifically metolazone, are commonly combined for their synergistic action in this setting.

Dopamine administered at low doses (0.5 to 3 μg/kg/min) may also be used in the prevention and treatment of ARF by increasing renal blood flow secondary to dopamine-induced renal vasodilation (McDonald et al, 1964; Szerlip, 1991). There is little clinical evidence that dopamine is effective in this setting, and in some cases it has proven to be detrimental. Adverse effects that may be associated with dopamine include pulmonary shunting, tachyarrhythmias, and gastrointestinal or digital necrosis (Thompson & Cockrill, 1994).

Calcium channel blockers may prevent ARF by their dilatory effect on the afferent arteriole of the kidney and subsequent increase in the glomerular filtration rate (Neumayer et al, 1992). Also, in states of reduced oxygen supply, calcium channel blockers may inhibit cell death, which is thought to be a result of calcium in the mitochondria and renal tubules. The protective effect of calcium channel blockers on the kidney is not definitive and still in the experimental stages. Research with these agents has been mostly in the prevention of radiocontrast-induced nephropathy, cyclosporine-induced vasoconstriction nephropathy, and post-transplant ATN (Ruggenenti et al, 1991; Neumayer et al, 1989).

Other agents that have been investigated in the prevention of ARF include antiendothelin, renal growth factors, and atrial natriuretic peptide (Rahman et al, 1994; Kon et al, 1989; Fine et al, 1992).

Guidelines on the order in which mannitol, furosemide, and dopamine should be used are not available. When using these agents, it is important to monitor electrolytes and volume status closely (see Table 30-4). Patients may become overhydrated, or conversely may be overdiuresed and dehydrated, which could exacerbate existing damage to the kidneys. Maintenance of adequate circulation volume and oxygen delivery to the kidneys at all times provides the best proven protection against ARF. The response to a therapeutic maneuver depends on the phase of ARF in which the intervention is initiated. A therapeutic maneuver initiated in the first 24 hours of ARF may elicit a different response than if it is initiated later (>48 hours). Table 30-7 outlines the agents used in ARF.

The approach to nutritional support in patients with ARF is controversial and the target of recent research. Patients with ARF are in a hypercatabolic state, which may lead to muscle wasting, a compromised immunologic state, and impaired wound healing. Protein administration in the patient with ARF leads to azotemia; therefore, historically protein administration was limited in this setting and conditioned by the type of renal replacement therapy available. Research has found that although amino acid administration may cause azotemia in the patient with ARF, if the patient is adequately dialyzed, azotemia can be avoided and nitrogen balance maintained (Kopple, 1996). The current thought is that aggressive protein administration is safe and easily achieved when continuous renal replacement therapy is used, because these therapies remove more fluid and nitrogenous wastes in the hemodynamically unstable patient (Kopple, 1996). Aggressive protein administration coupled with adequate dialysis results in a detectable improvement in daily nitrogen balance when compared with standard approaches, without inducing uncontrolled azotemia (Sponsel & Conger, 1995).

Dosage regimens of drugs that are renally eliminated must be modified, and potential toxicities must be monitored closely. The use of standard formulas to calculate creatinine clearance cannot be used in this setting, because these formulas are useful only when renal function is stable; renal function may be overestimated when using standard formulas. Most antibiotics are renally eliminated; this is of particular concern because infection is a common complication in ARF. Examples of antibiotics that are renally eliminated are aminoglycosides, vancomycin, many penicillin and cephalosporin antibiotics, ciprofloxacin, and sulfonamides.

Hyperkalemia is a common and potentially life-threatening complication in ARF. It results not only from decreased renal excretion of potassium but also from increased release of potassium from damaged tissue and release of intracellular potassium because of acidosis. Hyperkalemia can be aggravated in this setting by the administration of exogenous substances (Table 30-8). Potassium concentrations, in conjunction with an elec-

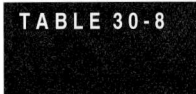

TABLE 30-8	Exogenous Substances That Aggravate Hyperkalemia in the Setting of Acute Renal Failure
Potassium salts	
Penicillin G potassium salts	
Digoxin	
Beta-blockers	
Angiotensin-converting enzyme (ACE) inhibitors	
Nonsteroidal anti-inflammatory drugs	
Heparin	
Trimethoprim	
Blood transfusions	

trocardiogram, should be used to monitor severity. Severe hyperkalemia (serum potassium concentration >6 mEq/L) in the presence of electrocardiogram changes (peaked T waves, shortened Q-T interval, lengthening of the PR interval and QRS complex) is a clinical emergency and must be treated immediately. Table 30-9 outlines the treatment regimens for hyperkalemia.

Severe metabolic acidosis (arterial pH <7.2, serum bicarbonate concentration <15 mmol/L) is another life-threatening complication of ARF and requires immediate treatment. Sodium bicarbonate may be administered orally or intravenously for metabolic acidosis. However, because of volume overload secondary to the large amount of sodium bicarbonate needed to correct the acidosis, dialysis is usually needed for correction of volume overload and pulmonary edema.

Anemia, another complication of ARF, is a result of a combination of processes, including multiple blood collections, decreased production of erythropoietin by the kidneys, and uremia-induced shortened red blood cell survival. Red blood cell transfusions are indicated in the acute setting (hemoglobin <8 g/dL), especially in patients who have compromised cardiovascular systems, such as those with unstable angina. Erythropoietin may also be used, but because it takes 1 to 2 weeks to have an initial effect, it is usually reserved for patients with chronic renal failure or those with prolonged ARF.

Uremia hinders the function of platelets by decreasing their aggregation ability. Patients should be closely monitored for signs of bleeding. Bleeding may be prevented by using saline flushes in place of heparin flushes and administering vitamin K daily (Olivero, 1994). If bleeding occurs, it can be treated with packed red blood cell transfusions, vasopressin analogues such as desmopressin (DDAVP; 0.3 μg/kg/day intravenously), conjugated estrogens (0.6 mg/kg/day intravenously), and dialysis, with varying effects (Peterson, 1985). DDAVP is also used prophylactically in the setting of ARF before any procedure that carries a risk of bleeding.

Infection is a common complication and is the leading cause of death associated with ARF. Patients with ARF are more susceptible to infection because of their abnormal host-defense mechanisms caused by impaired leukocyte function and depressed cell-mediated immunity. Indwelling catheters are a potential site for infection; therefore, intermittent catheterization should be used whenever possible. Intravascular catheters used to monitor hemodynamic parameters are another source of infection. Catheters should be examined frequently for infection and changed or removed as needed. Respiratory infections are also common, so patient mobilization and respiratory therapy should be initiated early to reduce the risk of infection. If an infection is suspected, aggressive antibiotic therapy should be initiated.

Gastrointestinal complications may also be encountered. Nausea and vomiting may occur from a buildup of uremic toxins; this responds well to dialysis. Stress ulcers leading to gastrointestinal bleeding are common. Patients should receive stress ulcer prophylaxis with histamine antagonists or antacids (Dickson & Hillman, 1991). Sucralfate may interfere with diagnostic tests involved in the workup of gastrointestinal bleeding; therefore, antacids or histamine antagonists may be preferred. Dosage regimens of histamine antagonists must be adjusted in settings of renal failure. Table 30-10 outlines the complications of ARF.

Hyperphosphatemia may occur in ARF because of the decreased ability of the kidneys to excrete phosphorus. Excess phosphorus in the body binds to calcium and causes hypocalcemia. Hypocalcemia may also occur because of the inability to absorb calcium in the gastrointestinal tract secondary to a failure of the kidneys to produce the active form of vitamin D (1,25-dihydroxy-vitamin D_3); however, this is more common in chronic renal failure. Muscle twitching and convulsions may occur as a result of hypocalcemia. Hyperphosphatemia may be treated with phosphate binders such as calcium carbonate and calcium acetate, which should also help correct hypocalcemia. Aluminum binders may be used in the acute setting; however, if the patient develops chronic renal failure, another binder should be used to avoid the long-term side effects of aluminum (microcytic anemia, encephalopathy, bone disease). Magne-

TABLE 30-9	Treatment Modalities for Hyperkalemia		
Agent	**Adult Dosage**	**Onset**	**Special Considerations**
Calcium Gluconate (10%)	10–30 mL IV at 1 mL/min	Immediate	Monitor EKG. Calcium and bicarbonate are incompatible.
Sodium bicarbonate (8.4%)	50 mL IV over 1–5 min	30–60 min	Sodium and alkaline load. Be cautious in patients with congestive heart failure.
Glucose/insulin	50 mL $D_{50}W$ with 10 U insulin IV or 1000 mL $D_{10}W$ with 25–50 U insulin at 350–500 mL/hr	30–60 min	Monitor glucose control.
Albuterol	10–20 mg nebulized or 0.5 mg IV over 15 min	10–30 min	Monitor pulse.
Kayexalate	25–50 PO or as a retention enema	2–3 hr	Monitor for GI disturbances. Avoid in the early postsurgical setting. Many preparations contain sorbitol.
Dialysis	—	Hours	Requires vascular access and nursing expertise

Adapted from Mueller, 1997.

TABLE 30-10	Complications of Acute Renal Failure
Cardiovascular	Sepsis
Arrhythmias	Urinary tract infection
Hypertension	Metabolic
Myocardial infarction	Acidosis
Pericarditis	Hyperkalemia
Pulmonary edema	Hyperphosphatemia
Gastrointestinal	Hyperuricemia
Gastrointestinal bleeding	Hypocalcemia
Nausea	Hyponatremia
Vomiting	Malnutrition
Hematologic	Neurologic
Anemia	Asterixis
Bleeding tendency	Coma
Immunologic	Mental status changes
Pneumonia	Seizures

sium binders are not very effective binders of phosphorus, may accumulate in renal failure, and are associated with diarrhea; therefore, they should be avoided.

In addition to medical treatment, dialysis is also used. Traditionally, most patients who required treatment of ARF in the intensive care setting were managed with intermittent hemodialysis or peritoneal dialysis. There are, however, complications of hemodialysis, such as severe hypotension and oxygen desaturation. Contraindications to peritoneal dialysis include diaphragmatic splinting, causing problems with mechanical ventilation. Peritoneal dialysis in the highly catabolic setting is not as efficient as hemodialysis. Problems associated with traditional methods of dialysis have led to the development of continuous forms of treatment, which can provide similar clearance of waste products from the blood in a slower, controlled manner, avoiding such problems. Continuous renal replacement therapy refers to any treatment that can provide a continuous form of dialysis for patients in ARF. There are different forms of continuous dialysis, including continuous arteriovenous hemofiltration and hemodiafiltration and continuous venovenous hemofiltration and hemodiafiltration (Dickson & Hillman, 1991). The choice of renal replacement therapy is principally a medical one, based on the availability of equipment and resources, nursing knowledge and expertise, vascular access, and hemodynamic stability. Complications of continuous renal replacement therapy include dehydration and hypovolemia if overdiuresed, and fluid overload and pulmonary edema if underdiuresed. These patients need continuous anticoagulation; therefore, both over- and undercoagulation are potential complications.

Patients receiving any type of dialysis should have their blood pressure monitored frequently because hypotension associated with dialysis may slow recovery from renal failure. If hypotension occurs, dopamine, albumin, or normal saline may be administered. In edematous patients with hypoalbuminuria, albumin may be the preferred agent.

Recovery of the kidney usually takes 10 to 14 days, although this may be prolonged for as long as 8 weeks (Haglund, 1994). Survival rates for patients with ARF are largely dependent on its original cause and whether other major organ failure is involved. The average mortality rate for intensive care unit patients with ARF exceeds 60%, although for those who do survive, renal function returns to within 80% of normal within 1

year (Haglund, 1994). Approximately 5% of patients do not fully recover from an episode of ARF go on to develop chronic failure, requiring maintenance dialysis or renal transplantation.

COMMUNITY RESOURCES

- National Kidney Foundation, 30 E. 33d St., New York, NY 10016
- Acute renal failure: www.healthanswers.com/database/ami/converted/000501.html

REFERRAL POINTS AND CLINICAL WARNINGS

Hyperkalemia, metabolic acidosis, and fluid overload (pulmonary edema) are acute, life-threatening complications of ARF. Treatment, whether dialysis or pharmacologic agents, must be initiated immediately to prevent detrimental effects and possible death.

CLINICAL PEARLS

- Patients with ARF are in a catabolic state and are expected to lose weight; even modest weight gain can reflect a higher gain in water weight. These patients should be weighed daily to monitor states of fluid accumulation. Each kilogram of weight gain is approximately equal to 1 L of fluid.
- To prevent nephrotoxicity with amphotericin B use, patients may receive sodium loading.
- Maintenance of adequate circulation volume and oxygen delivery to the kidneys at all times provides the best proven protection against ARF.
- Standard formulas for calculating creatinine clearance cannot be used in the setting of ARF; these formulas are accurate only when renal function is stable.
- To prevent bleeding, saline flushes should be used instead of heparin flushes when maintaining intravenous catheters.
- Patients with ARF should receive stress ulcer prophylaxis but should not receive sucralfate, which may interfere with diagnostic testing.

References

Balsov, J.T., & Jorgensen, H.E. (1963). A survey of 499 patients with acute renal insufficiency. *American Journal of Medicine, 34,* 753–764.

Brenner, B.M., Coe, F.L., & Rector, F.C. (Eds.). (1987). Acute renal failure. In: *Clinical nephrology.* Philadelphia: W.B. Saunders, pp. 36–72.

Burke, T.J., Arnold, P.E., & Schrier, R.W. (1983). Prevention of ischemic acute renal failure with impermeant solutes. *American Journal of Physiology, 244,* F646–F649.

Cantarovich, F., Galli, C., Benedetti, L., et al. (1973). High-dose furosemide in established acute renal failure. *British Medical Journal, 24,* 449–455.

Conger, J.D. (1995). Interventions in clinical acute renal failure: What are the data? *American Journal of Kidney Disease, 26,* 565–576.

Corwin, H.L., Teplick, R.S., Schreiver, M.J., Fang, L.S., Bonventre, J.V., & Coggins, C.H. (1987). Prediction of outcome in acute renal failure. *American Journal of Nephrology, 7,* 8–12.

Dickson, D.M., & Hillman, K.M. (1991). Continuous renal replacement therapies versus intermittent hemodialysis in acute renal failure: What do we know? *American Journal of Kidney Disease, 28,* S90–S96.

Dixon, B.S., & Anderson, R.J. (1985). Nonoliguric acute renal failure. *American Journal of Kidney Disease, 6,* 71–80.

Dorman, H.R., Sondheimer, J.H., & Cadnapaphornchai, P. (1990). Mannitol-induced acute renal failure. *Medicine, 69,* 159.

Fine, L.G., Hammernan, M.R., & Abboud, H.E. (1992). Evolving role of growth factors in the renal response to acute and chronic disease. *Journal of the American Society of Nephrology, 2,* 1163–1170.

Flores, J., DiBona, D.R., Beck, C.H., et al. (1972). The role of cell swelling in ischemic renal damage and the protective effect of hypertonic solute. *Journal of Clinical Investigation, 51,* 118–126.

Fries, O., Pozet, N., Dubois, N., et al. (1971). The use of large doses of furosemide in acute renal failure. *Postgraduate Medicine, 47,* 18.

Gubern, J.M., Sancho, J.J., Simo, J., & Sitges-Serra, A. (1988). A randomized trial on the effect of mannitol on postoperative renal function in patients with obstructive jaundice. *Surgery, 103,* 39–44.

Haglund, M. (1994). Making sense of continuous renal replacement therapy. *Nursing Times, 90,* 37–38.

Hanley, M.J., & Davidson, K. (1981). Prior mannitol and furosemide infusion in a model of ischemic acute renal failure. *American Journal of Physiology, 241,* F556–F564.

Karayannopoulos, S. (1974). High-dose furosemide in renal failure. *British Medical Journal, 2,* 278–279.

Kaufman, J., Khakal, M., Patel, B., & Hamburger, R. (1991). Community-acquired acute renal failure. *American Journal of Kidney Disease, 17,* 191–198.

Kon, V., Yoshioka, T., Fogo, A., & Ichikawa, I. (1989). Glomerular actions of endothelin in vivo. *Journal of Clinical Investigation, 83,* 1762–1767.

Kopple, J.D. (1996). The nutrition management of the patient with acute renal failure. *Journal of Parenteral and Enteral Nutrition, 20,* 3–12.

Kurokawa, K. (1983). Acute renal failure and rhabdomyolysis. *Kidney International, 23,* 888–898.

Maher, E.R., Robinson, K.N., Scoble, J.E., et al. (1989). Prognosis of critically ill patients with acute renal failure. APACHE II score and other predictive factors. *Quarterly Journal of Medicine, 72,* 857–866.

McDonald, R.H., Goldverg, L.I., Mcnay, J.L., & Tuttle, E.P. Jr. (1964). Effects of dopamine in man: Augmentation of sodium excretion, glomerular filtration rate, and renal plasma flow. *Journal of Clinical Investigation, 43,* 1116–24.

Miller, T.R., Anderson, R.J., Linas, S.L., et al. (1978). Urinary diagnostic indices in acute renal failure: A prospective study. *Annals of Internal Medicine, 89,* 47–50.

Minuth, A.N., Terrell, J.B., & Suki, W.N. (1973). Acute renal failure: A study of the course and prognosis of 104 patients and of the role of furosemide. *American Journal of Medical Sciences, 271,* 317–324.

Morris, C.R., Alexander, E.A., Bruns, F.J., et al. (1972). Restoration and maintenance of glomerular filtration by mannitol during hypoperfusion of the kidney. *Journal of Clinical Investigation, 51,* 1555–1564.

Mueller, B.A. Acute renal failure. In Dipiro, J.T., Talbert, R.L., Yee, G.C. et al. (eds). *Pharmacotherapy, A pathophysiological approach,* 3rd ed., Stamford, CT: Appleton & Lange, 887–912.

Neumayer, H.H., Junge, W., Kufner, A., & Wenning, A. (1989). Prevention of radiocontrast-media-induced nephrotoxicity by the calcium channel blocker nitrendipine: A prospective randomized clinical trial. *Nephrology Dialysis & Transplantation, 4,* 1030–1036.

Neumayer, H.H., Kunzenforf, U., & Schreiver, M. (1992). Protective effects of calcium antagonists in human renal transplantation. *Kidney International, (Suppl)36,* S87–S93.

Olivero, J.J. (1994). Postsurgical acute renal failure: Which patients are at greatest risk? *Journal of Critical Illness, 9,* 673–685.

Peterson, W.L., & Richardson, C.T. (1985). Sustained fasting achlorhydria: A comparison of medical regimens. *Gastroenterology, 88,* 666.

Rahman, S.N., Kim, G.E., Mathew, A.S., et al. (1994). Effects of atrial natriuretic peptide in clinical acute renal failure. *Kidney International, 45,* 1731–1738.

Rose, B.D. (Ed.). (1987). Acute renal failure: Prerenal disease versus acute tubular necrosis. In: *Pathophysiology of renal disease.* New York: McGraw-Hill, pp. 63–112.

Ruggenenti, P., Perico, N., Mosconi, L., et al. (1991). Calcium channel blockers protect transplant patients from cyclosporine-induced daily renal hypoperfusion. *Kidney International, 43,* 706–711.

Shusterman, N., Strom, B.L., Murray, T.G., Morrison, G., West, S.L., & Maislin, G. (1987). Risk factors and outcome of hospital-acquired acute renal failure: Clinical epidemiologic study. *American Journal of Medicine, 83,* 65–71.

Slekurt, E. (1945). Changes in renal clearance following complete ischemia of the kidney. *American Journal of Physiology, 144,* 395.

Solomon, R., Werner, C., Mann, D., D'Elia, J., & Silva, P. (1994). Effects of saline, mannitol, and furosemide on acute decreases in renal function induced by radiocontrast agents. *N Engl J Med, 331,* 1416–1420.

Sponsel, H., & Conger, J.D. (1995). Is parenteral nutrition of value in acute renal failure patients? *American Journal of Kidney Disease, 25,* 96–102.

Szerlip, H.M. (1991). Renal-dose dopamine: Fact and fiction. *Annals of Internal Medicine, 115,* 153–154.

Teschan, P.E., & Lawson, N.L. (1966). Studies in acute renal failure. Prevention by osmotic diuresis and observations on the effect of plasma and extracellular volume expansion. *Nephron, 3,* 1.

Thadhani, R., Pascual, M., & Bonventre, J.V. (1996). Acute renal failure. *N Engl J Med, 334,* 1448–1460.

Thompson, B.T., & Cockrill, B.A. (1994). Renal-dose dopamine: A siren song? *Lancet, 344,* 7–8.

Turney, J.H. (1990). Why is mortality persistently high in acute renal failure? *Lancet, 35,* 971.

Wood, J.M., & Bosley, C.L. (1991). BPH: Treating older men's most common problem. *RN, 54,* 32–38.

Woodrow, G.G., & Turney, J.H. (1991). Cause of death in acute renal failure. *Nephrology Dialysis & Transplantation, 7,* 230–234.

Zanasrdo, G., Micheilon, P., Paccagnella, A., et al. (1994). Acute renal failure in the patient undergoing cardiac operation: Prevalence, mortality rate, and main risk factors. *Journal of Thoracic and Cardiovascular Surgery, 107,* 1489–1495.

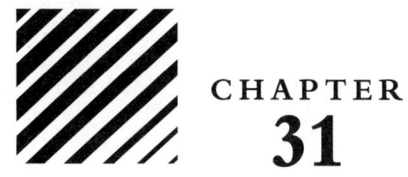

CHAPTER
31

Chronic Renal Failure

Richard MacDougall, RPA-C

The kidney has many important regulatory functions, such as body fluid volume, solute dilution and concentration, acid–base balance, and excretion of waste products. The kidney also secretes hormones that regulate red blood cell production, blood pressure, and calcium metabolism. Progressive loss of renal function—chronic renal failure (CRF)—regardless of cause affects these vital processes, with changes seen throughout all organ systems. The kidneys exhibit remarkable adaptive abilities, and symptomatic changes usually do not become apparent until the glomerular filtration rate (GFR) declines to less than 25% of normal.

When dealing with CRF, watchful waiting is the key phrase. The progression of the disease is slow, and the presenting symptoms are nonemergent. Baseline laboratory values are obtained. If hypertension is present, it is pharmacologically managed. The class of drug chosen depends on the etiology of the renal failure. Once the blood pressure is stabilized and any other presenting symptoms are dealt with, it becomes a matter of time. The creatinine level does not rise quickly, as it does in acute renal failure. In 1 year's time, the creatinine level might rise one tenth of a point; the next year it may rise three tenths of a point. As long as the patient is hemodynamically stable, intervention is unnecessary.

While monitoring the patient's renal function, the process that brought the patient to this stage must be understood. The goal here is to slow the progression toward dialysis or renal transplant. For this to happen, it is important to become familiar with the anatomy and physiology of the kidney, as well as the most common causes of CRF.

ANATOMY, PHYSIOLOGY, AND PATHOLOGY

Anatomy

The kidneys are paired organs located on the posterior abdominal wall, outside the peritoneal cavity. They lie on either side of the vertebral column, with upper and lower poles extending from the 12th thoracic to the 3rd lumbar vertebrae. Each kidney is approximately 11 cm long, 5 to 6 cm wide, and 3 to 4 cm thick. The right kidney is displaced downward by the overlaying liver and thus is lower than the left kidney. Each kidney is surrounded by the tightly adhering renal capsule and embedded in a mass of fat. The capsule and fatty layer are covered with a double layer of renal fascia, a fibrous tissue that attaches the kidney to the posterior abdominal wall. The medial indentation, called the hilus, serves as the entry and exit site for the renal blood vessels, nerves, lymphatic vessels, and ureters (see Fig. 30-1).

The major components of the kidney are the renal cortex and the renal medulla. The renal cortex contains all the glomer-uli and portions of the tubules. The renal medulla contains a series of wedges called the renal pyramids. These pyramids are divided into outer and inner zones. The renal columns extend from the renal cortex down between the pyramids. The apex, which is the point of the renal pyramid, extends down into the minor calyx (a cup-shaped cavity) and joins with other minor calyxes to form the major calyx. The major calyxes join to form the renal pelvis, an extension of the upper end of the ureter.

INTERNAL STRUCTURE

The nephron is the functional unit of the kidney (Fig. 31-1). There are approximately 1.2 million nephrons per kidney. The nephron is a tubular structure made up of many subunits. The glomerulus is the tuft of capillaries that loop into a circular space called the Bowman's capsule. The space within the capsule, known as Bowman's space, descends toward the renal medulla. Bowman's capsule then merges into the proximal convoluted tubule. The proximal convoluted tubule is made up of two segments. The initial convoluted segment is the pars convoluta. The straight separate segment is the pars recta, which descends to the renal medulla, forming the loop of Henle. As the loop of Henle emerges from the renal medulla, it becomes the distal convoluted tubule. The distal tubule is formed by straight and convoluted segments and extends from the macula densa to the collecting ducts. These ducts are large tubules that descend down the renal cortex and through the renal pyramids of the inner and outer medulla into a minor calyx. The glomerulus is lined with epithelial cells. Mesangial cells lie between the capillaries of the glomeruli and hold them together, forming Bowman's capsule.

There are two kinds of nephrons. First are the cortical nephrons, which extend only partially into the renal medulla. They originate close to the surface of the renal cortex. The juxtamedullary nephrons, the second type, extend deep into the medulla. They are important for concentration of urine. The juxtamedullary nephrons are located deep inside the renal cortex, close to the renal medulla. There are structural differences between the two types of nephrons. The cortical nephrons have a short loop, so they may not extend into the renal medulla. The juxtamedullary nephrons have a loop that may extend the whole length of the medulla (40 mm); these represent approximately 12% of all nephrons.

The walls of the glomerular capillaries act as a filtration membrane and comprise three layers. The first is the inner capillary endothelium, which is composed of cells in continuous contact with the basement membrane. It is perforated by many small openings called fenestrae. The second layer is the middle basement membrane, a selectively permeable network of glycoproteins and mucopolysaccharides. The third layer is the epithe-

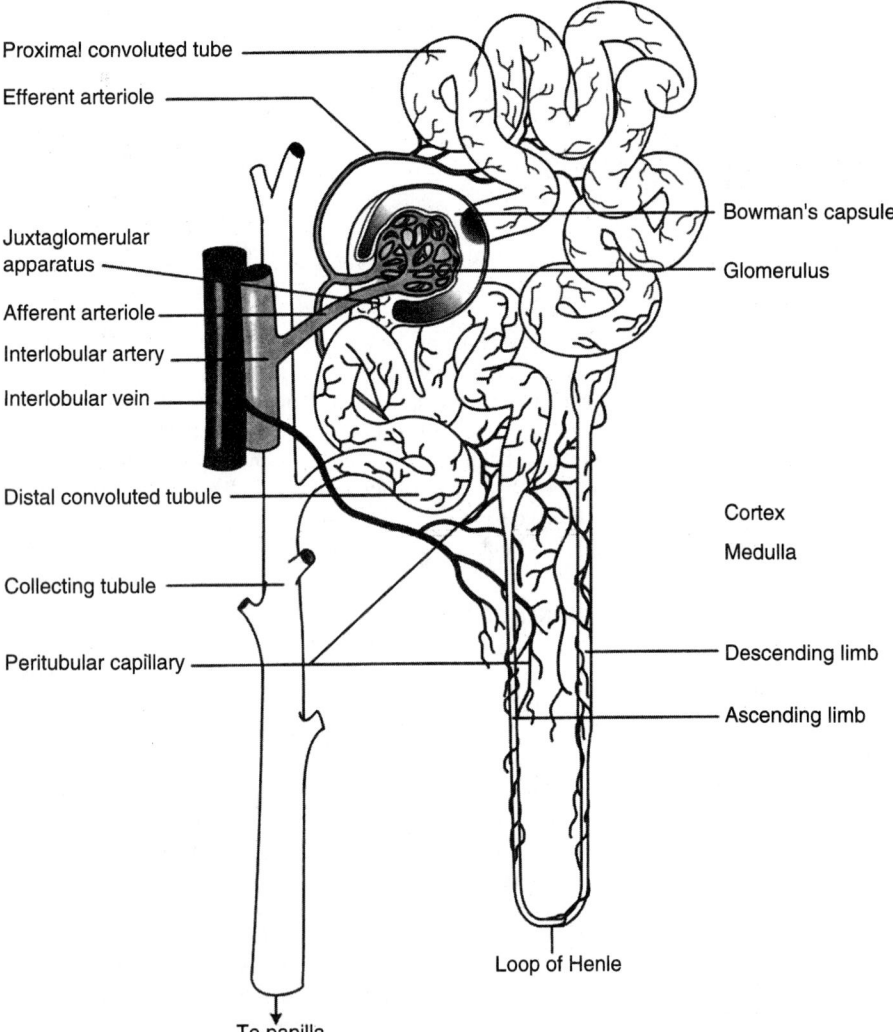

Proximal convoluted tube

Efferent arteriole

Juxtaglomerular apparatus

Afferent arteriole

Interlobular artery

Interlobular vein

Distal convoluted tubule

Collecting tubule

Peritubular capillary

Bowman's capsule

Glomerulus

Cortex

Medulla

Descending limb

Ascending limb

Loop of Henle

To papilla

FIGURE 31-1 Nephron, showing the glomerular and tubular structures along with the blood supply. (From Porth, Carol M. (1998). *Pathophysiology, 5/e.* Philadelphia: Lippincott-Raven Publishers.)

lium. This layer has specialized cells called podocytes, footlike structures that radiate from the epithelium and adhere to the basement membrane. The pedicle of one podocyte interlocks with the pedicle of an adjacent podocyte, forming an elaborate network of intercellular clefts called filtration slits. The glomerular filtration membrane separates the blood of the glomerular capillaries from the fluid in Bowman's space. The glomerular filtrate passes through the three layers of the glomerular membrane and forms the primary urine.

As the glomerular filtrate leaves Bowman's capsule, it enters the proximal tubular lumen, which consists of one layer of cells. This is the only surface inside the nephron that contains microvilli (a brush border). The microvilli create an expanded surface area inside the tubule, enhancing its reabsorptive function. The glomerular filtrate that is not reabsorbed in the proximal tubule then enters the loop of Henle. The loop is composed of two separate segments: a thin segment, composed of thin squamous cells with no active transport, and a thick segment. This area, constructed of cuboidal cells, actively transports several solutes out of the filtrate.

Toward the end of the loop of Henle, at its ascending loop, a transitional segment is formed. This is known as the macula densa. Here the distal tubule coming off the ascending loop

passes between and contacts the afferent and efferent arterioles at their point of attachment to the macula densa and glomerulus. This linkage forms the juxtaglomerular apparatus. The juxtaglomerular apparatus has the important function of controlling renal blood flow, glomerular filtration, and renin secretion. Specialized cells in the walls of afferent and efferent arterioles secrete the hormone renin, which contributes to the control of arterial blood pressure.

BLOOD VESSELS

The renal arteries arise from the fifth branch of the abdominal aorta. As the renal artery enters the kidney at the renal hilus, it divides into anterior and posterior branches. These branches further divide into lobar arteries. The lobar arteries supply blood to the lower, middle, and upper thirds of the kidney. The interlobar arteries are further subdivisions of the lobar arteries that travel down between the renal columns and between the renal pyramids. At the corticomedullary junction, the interlobar arteries branch into the arcuate arteries. These vessels arch over the base of the renal pyramids and run parallel to the surface of the kidney. These further branch into the interlobular arteries, which extend through the renal cortex toward the periphery and form the afferent arterioles. These arterioles subdivide into fistlike structures of four to eight glomerular capillaries. The blood supply proceeds through the glomerular capillaries and empties into the efferent arterioles, conveying blood into a second capillary bed, the peritubular capillaries. This is the only place in the body where an arteriole is positioned between two capillary beds. The positioning of the peritubular capillaries is important for glomerular filtration. The capillaries surround the convoluted portions of the proximal and distal tubules of the loop of Henle. There are two types of peritubular capillaries. The first type supplies the cortical nephrons. These capillaries are similar to the capillaries of other tissues. The second are the capillaries that supply the juxtamedullary nephrons. These capillaries, called vasa recta, form loops and closely follow the loop of Henle. The peritubular capillaries of the vasa recta are the capillaries that influence the osmolar concentration of the medullary extracellular fluid, which is important to the formation of a concentrated urine. These capillaries are the only blood supply to the renal medulla.

All capillaries then drain into the venous system. The renal veins follow the same path as the renal arteries, only in the reverse direction.

Physiology

The kidney is a highly vascular organ, receiving approximately 20% to 25% of the cardiac output (1000 to 1200 mL blood/min). Approximately 20% of the plasma is filtered (120 to 140 mL/min) at the glomerulus and passes into Bowman's capsule. The GFR is the filtration of plasma per unit of time. The GFR is directly related to the perfusion pressure in the glomerular capillaries. The rest of the plasma (80%) flows through the efferent arterioles to the peritubular capillaries. The ratio of glomerular filtration to renal plasma flow per minute is called the filtration fraction. All but 1 to 2 mL of the glomerular filtrate is normally reabsorbed and returned to the circulation by the peritubular capillaries.

The GFR is directly related to renal blood flow. This is regulated by three factors. Intrinsic autoregulatory mechanisms help keep the GFR stable and constant over changing arterial pressures (80 to 180 mmHg). Renal blood flow and GFR are constant; thus, solute and water excretion are constant. The second factor affecting renal blood flow is neural regulation. Neural regulation results in interruption of renal blood flow by the autonomic nervous system through sympathetic fibers that can cause vasoconstriction. Hormonal regulation is the third factor affecting renal blood flow. The renin angiotensin system produces an enzyme formed and stored in the cells of the arterioles of the juxtaglomerular apparatus. Numerous factors stimulate the release of renin, including:

- Decreased plasma sodium
- Decreased plasma potassium
- Decreased blood pressure in the afferent arterioles (this reduces the stretch of the juxtaglomerular cells)
- Sympathetic stimulation of the beta-adrenergic receptors on the juxtaglomerular cells.

The release of renin cleaves an alpha-globulin molecule (angiotensinogen) in the plasma to form angiotensin I. In the presence of a converting enzyme, angiotensin I is converted to angiotensin II and III. Angiotensin II stimulates the secretion of aldosterone by the adrenal cortex; this is a potent vasopressor and in turn inhibits renin release (a biofeedback mechanism).

Kidney Function

The function of the nephron is to form a filtrate of protein-free plasma. This process, known as ultrafiltration, occurs across the glomerular capillaries. The nephron then regulates the filtrate to help maintain body fluid volume and electrolyte composition within narrow limits. This fluid regulation happens through two processes. The first, tubular reabsorption, consists of movement of fluids and solutes from the proximal convoluted lumen into the peritubular capillary plasma. The second process, tubular secretion, is the active and passive transfer of substances from the plasma of the peritubular capillary into the lumen of the proximal convoluted tubule.

GLOMERULAR FILTRATION

The total volume filtered by the kidney in 24 hours is approximately 180 L. Changes in the GFR can occur with changes to the arterioles. For instance, constriction of the afferent arteriole will decrease the amount of blood entering Bowman's capsule, thereby decreasing the GFR. On the other hand, constriction of the efferent arteriole will cause an increase in the pressure in the capillaries inside Bowman's capsule, causing an increase in GFR. An endpoint to this is an increase in urinary excretion. By the time the filtrate travels to the end of the proximal tubule, 60% to 70% of the filtered sodium and water and 50% of the urea has been reabsorbed. In addition, 90% of the potassium, glucose, bicarbonate, calcium, phosphate, and uric acid have also been reabsorbed. All this is done by active transport. In the proximal tubule, active reabsorption of sodium is the primary function. Cotransported with the sodium are water, most electrolytes, and other organic substances.

At the loop of Henle, concentration or dilution of urine occurs, with additional concentration or dilution at the collecting ducts. When the process occurs at the loop of Henle, the strength of the concentrated filtrate is related to the length of the loop and the depth of penetration the loop has into the renal medulla. The primary function of the loop is to establish a hyperosmotic state within the medullary interstitial fluid. Each portion of the loop of Henle is permeable to different aspects of the filtrate. The thin descending segment is highly permeable to water and moderately permeable to sodium, urea, and other solutes. The thin ascending segment is more permeable to sodium but almost impermeable to water. The thick ascending portions of the loop of Henle are highly permeable to sodium, potassium, and chloride and less so to urea and water. The convoluted portion of the distal tubule is poorly permeable to water but readily absorbs ions and contributes to the dilution of the tubular fluid. Finally, the straight segment of the distal tubule and the collecting duct are permeable to water and sodium. The absorption rate of the water is controlled by antidiuretic hormone (ADH). Sodium is readily absorbed by the distal tubule and collecting duct under the regulation of the hormone aldosterone.

■ ■ ■   **CLINICAL PEARL**

When the GFR increases or decreases, the renal tubules, primarily the proximal tubules, automatically adjust their rate of reabsorption of sodium and water to balance the change in GFR.

URINE

Urea is an end product of protein metabolism and is the major constituent of urine, along with water. The glomerulus freely filters urea, and tubular reabsorption of urea depends on the urine flow rate. There is less reabsorption at higher flow rates. About 50% of the urea is excreted in the urine; the other 50% is recycled within the kidney. The recycling of urea from the tubules and collecting ducts contributes to an osmotic gradient in the renal medulla and is necessary for the concentration and dilution of urine. Because urea is an end product of protein metabolism, persons with protein deprivation will not be able to concentrate their urine maximally.

The final concentration of urine is controlled by ADH. ADH increases the permeability of water in the last segment of the distal tubule and along the entire length of the collecting ducts. The collecting ducts pass through the inner and outer zones of the renal medulla.

In the presence of ADH, water reabsorption is high. Most of the water is reabsorbed in the medullary collecting ducts because of the high osmotic gradient in the medullary interstitium. The water diffuses into the ascending limb of the vasa recta and returns to the systemic circulation. Excreted urine can have a high osmotic concentration (up to 1400 mOsm). The volume is normally reduced to about 1% of what is filtered at the glomerulus.

ADH secretion is one cause of oliguria (urine excretion of less than 30 mL/hr or 400 mL/day). In the absence of ADH, water diuresis takes place. The distal tubule and collecting ducts become impermeable to water. The water remains in the tubular lumen and is excreted as a diluted and large volume of urine. ADH has no effect on sodium reabsorption; it continues to be transported actively from the distal tubule and back into the renal vasculature.

RENAL HORMONES

Vitamin D is a hormone that can be obtained from the diet or synthesized by the action of ultraviolet light or cholesterol in the skin. These forms of vitamin D_3 (cholecalciferol), from the diet or skin, are inactive and require two hydroxylations, one hepatic and one renal, to establish a metabolically active form, 1,25-dihydroxycholecalciferol (OH_2D_3). Vitamin D is necessary for the absorption of calcium and phosphate by the small intestine. The renal hydroxylation step is stimulated by the parathyroid hormone. A decreased calcium level (less than 10 mL/dL) stimulates the secretion of parathyroid hormone.

Serum phosphate fluctuation can also influence the renal hydroxylation of vitamin D. Decreased serum levels of phosphate stimulate active $1,25\text{-}OH_2D_3$ formation. Increased phosphorus levels inhibit formation of $1,25\text{-}OH_2D_3$. This results in compensatory phosphate absorption from the bone and intestine. The clinical significance of the role of the kidney in calcium and phosphate metabolism is evident in renal disease: patients with renal disease have a deficiency of $1,25\text{-}OH_2D_3$ and manifest symptoms of disturbed calcium and phosphate balance.

Erythropoietin is a renal hormone that stimulates the bone marrow to produce red blood cells in response to perceived tissue hypoxia. The stimulus for increased erythropoietin release is a lowered oxygen delivery to the kidneys. The anemia of chronic disease produced by CRF may be caused by nonfunctional kidney cells and the lack of this hormone.

Natriuretic hormone is also referred to as atrial natriuretic peptide (ANP). Although not a renal hormone, it is a hormone that can affect the loss of sodium and water and the regulation of fluid balance. When the extracellular fluid volume is expanded, ANP secretion is increased and sodium reabsorption is depressed. This causes increased amounts of sodium and water to be excreted in the urine. ANP is released from cardiocyte granules located in the atria of the heart in response to the increased atrial stretch.

EPIDEMIOLOGY

Data on the incidence and prevalence of end-stage renal disease (ESRD) are available from the U.S. Renal Data System (USRDS, 1997). Based on these data, 68,870 patients developed ESRD in 1995, and 257,266 ESRD patients were alive in the continental United States. The incidence and prevalence of ESRD have grown each year; however, the growth rates may be decreasing. The incidence and prevalence of ESRD increase with increasing age, peaking in the eighth decade, with the mean age around 60 to 64 years. ESRD is more common in men than women and is highest in the African American population.

Diabetes, hypertension, and primary glomerulonephritis are the three most common attributed causes of ESRD. The incidence of diabetic, hypertensive, and glomerulonephritic ESRD from 1993 to 1995 was 94, 70, and 27 per million persons for each year, respectively; the prevalence was 274, 233, and 167 per million persons for each year. The difference between the diagnosis-specific prevalence and incidence rates indicates variations in average survival, with smaller differences suggesting higher mortality rates.

Primary glomerulonephritis and cystic, hereditary, and congenital diseases are the most common causes of ESRD among patients younger than age 20. Diabetes predominates in persons age 20 to 64. Hypertension is the largest attributed cause of ESRD in those older than 65. Primary glomerulonephritis and hypertension are more common in men than women; diabetic ESRD is more common in women than men. African Americans have a higher incidence of hypertensive ESRD than other ethnic groups. Asians have a higher incidence of primary glomerulonephritis, and Native Americans have the highest incidence of diabetic ESRD, with a relatively low incidence of hypertensive ESRD.

DIAGNOSTIC CRITERIA

Renal insufficiency refers to a decline in renal function to about 25% of normal kidney filtration, or a GFR of 25 to 30 mL/min. Serum chemistries show the mildly elevated levels of serum creatinine and blood urea nitrogen (BUN). A significant loss of renal function (approximately 10% to 25%) is termed renal failure. When less than 10% of renal function remains, this is termed end-stage renal failure (ESRF). Renal failure can be chronic, with progression to ESRF over a period of months to years.

Uremia is a syndrome of renal failure that includes elevated BUN and creatinine levels, accompanied by fatigue, anorexia, nausea, vomiting, pruritus, and neurologic changes. Electrolyte disorders and retention of toxic waste can also accompany this syndrome. Azotemia is a term sometimes used interchangeably with uremia. Both azotemia and uremia indicate an accumulation of nitrogenous waste products in the blood.

The common feature of CRF and uremic syndrome is the diminishing numbers of functioning nephrons that operate normally, except for increased excretion of the solute. Known as the intact nephron hypothesis, this theory proposes that the loss of nephron mass with progressive kidney damage causes the remaining nephrons to sustain normal kidney function. These nephrons are capable of a compensatory expansion in their state of reabsorption and secretion. They also can maintain a constant rate of excretion in the presence of a declining GFR. The increased workload is achieved primarily by hypertrophy of the remaining nephrons. Another theory proposes an adaptive response by the nephrons. This adaptive response depends on the location of kidney damage. For example, with tubular interstitial disease, damage occurring primarily in the tubular or medullary parts of the nephron produces problems such as renal tubular acidosis, salt-wasting, and difficulty with dilution and concentration of the urine. Conversely, when there is primarily vascular or glomerular damage, persistent hematuria and nephrotic syndrome are more prominent. This theory is useful for planning treatment in the early stages of renal failure, when symptomatic differences in renal diseases may be distinct.

The intact nephron hypothesis explains the adaptive changes in solute and water regulation that occur with advancing renal failure. Although the urine of a patient with CRF may contain abnormal amounts of red and white blood cells and casts, the major end products of excretion are similar to those of normally functioning kidneys. There is no significant alteration to the urine until advanced stages of renal failure, when there is a significant reduction of functioning nephrons.

Urinary excretion of potassium is primarily related to distal tubular secretion, which is mediated by aldosterone and sodium-potassium ATPase. In renal failure, there are adaptions by the distal tubules and large intestine to the effects of aldosterone and other factors to enhance the secretion of potassium. This provides effective regulation of potassium until the onset of oliguria. The symptoms of hyperkalemia are usually not evident in CRF until the GFR falls below 5 mL/min. When the GFR is greater and clinical symptoms are present, endogenous sources of increased serum potassium, trauma, infection, or hemolysis should be investigated. Volume depletion, as well as the use of beta-blockers, angiotensin-converting enzyme (ACE) inhibitors, and potassium-sparing diuretics (eg, spironolactone) may also precipitate an increase in the potassium level. The use of the antirejection medication cyclosporine can also elevate potassium levels. With the progression of the disease to ESRF, total serum potassium can increase to life-threatening levels and must be controlled by dialysis.

Acid–Base Balance

The normal diet produces 50 to 100 mEq of hydrogen per day. These ions are secreted in the renal tubules and excreted in the urine, combined with phosphate and ammonia buffers. In the early stages of renal insufficiency, individual nephrons maintain normal pH by increasing the rate of acid excretion and bicarbonate absorption. Metabolic acidosis begins when the GFR falls below 30% to 40%, occurring primarily because of the decreased ammonia synthesis and decreased bicarbonate reabsorption at each nephron. Phosphate buffers remain effec-

tive until very late in the process. When ESRF develops, serum bicarbonate levels stabilize at 15 to 20 mEq/L, partly because the excess hydrogen ions are buffered by anions in skeletal bone. Patients with ESRF can develop metabolic acidosis, which may be severe enough to require dialysis.

The metabolism of calcium and phosphate is mediated by parathyroid hormone (PTH) and vitamin D. Changes in the acid–base balance also influence the status of calcium and phosphate. The major disorders associated with CRF are reduced renal phosphate excretion, decreased synthesis of 1,25-OH_2D_3, and hypocalcemia. In the early stages of CRF, as the GFR falls, urinary excretion of phosphate falls and the plasma phosphate concentration rises. This causes a binding with calcium, which causes hypocalcemia. Decreased serum calcium causes increased PTH secretion. The PTH stimulates the release of calcium from the bone and enhanced phosphate excretion. This adaptive effect is a cause of secondary hyperparathyroidism.

With each incremental decrease in the GFR, the effectiveness of PTH in maintaining phosphate balance decreases. When the GFR is less than 25%, PTH is no longer effective in maintaining serum phosphate levels. The persistently decreased GFR and secondary hyperparathyroidism cause progressive hyperphosphatemia, hypocalcemia, and dissolution of skeletal bone. Hypocalcemia and bone disease are accelerated by the impaired synthesis of 1,25-OH_2D_3. When the loss of functioning nephrons is significant and the GFR is less than 25%, the lack of active forms of vitamin D can cause reduced intestinal absorption of calcium. This impairs the effectiveness of calcium and phosphate resorption from the bone by PTH. The toxicity of uremia may also suppress vitamin D action in the intestines. The development of uremia can also precipitate the development of uremic osteodystrophy, a bone disease caused by the loss of calcium from the bone as a result of increased serum phosphorus levels. This depletion can be treated with vitamin D supplementation. A negative calcium balance also occurs when acidosis is present, which is common in CRF.

HISTORY AND PHYSICAL EXAM

The history and physical exam involve a series of diagnostic tests, described below.

DIAGNOSTIC STUDIES

Renal clearance techniques determine how much of a substance can be cleared from the blood by the kidneys per a given unit of time. The application of this principle permits an indirect measure of GFR, tubular secretion, tubular reabsorption, and renal blood flow.

GFR provides the best estimate of the amount of functioning renal tissue. Loss of, or damage to nephrons leads to a corresponding decrease in GFR. The GFR is calculated by multiplying the urinary creatinine value by the amount of urine produced for a given duration, usually 24 hours. This value is divided by the plasma creatinine value. Normal values are 130 ± 20 mL/min in males and 120 ± 15 mL/min in females.

Creatinine is a natural substance produced by the muscle; it is released into the blood at a relatively constant rate, and this is a commonly used clinical indicator. It is freely filtered at the glomerulus, but a small amount is released by the renal tubules. Therefore, creatinine clearance overestimates the GFR, but within tolerable limits. Creatinine clearance provides a good measure of GFR because only one blood sample is required, in addition to the volume of urine. Creatinine clearance may be estimated by the formula: ([140 − age]/serum creatinine) × (ideal body weight/72).

The clearance of urea is similar to that of creatinine. Because urea is both filtered and reabsorbed, and the level varies with the state of hydration and diet, urea clearance is less than the GFR. If protein intake and metabolism are constant, plasma levels will increase as the GFR declines. Adaptation by the tubules does not modify urea levels because urea is excreted primarily by glomerular filtration.

A chronic decline in the GFR over weeks or months is reflected in the plasma creatinine concentration; normal values are 0.7 to 1.2 mg/dL. The plasma creatinine concentration is stable when the GFR is stable because creatinine has a constant rate of production as a product of muscle metabolism. The amount filtered is about equal to the amount excreted. When GFR decreases, the plasma creatinine level increases proportionately. Thus, the GFR and plasma creatinine are inversely related. If GFR decreases by 50%, the filtration and excretion of creatinine would be decreased by 50%, and creatinine would accumulate in plasma to twice the normal value. Therefore, an elevated plasma creatinine volume represents a decrease in the GFR.

This test is helpful for monitoring progressive changes in renal function. It is most valuable for monitoring the progress of CRF rather than acute renal disease because it takes 7 to 10 days for the plasma creatinine level to stabilize when the GFR declines. Plasma creatinine levels become elevated during trauma or breakdown of muscle tissue.

The concentration of urea nitrogen in the blood (BUN) reflects glomerular filtration and the urine-collecting capacity of the kidney. Because urea is filtered at the glomerulus, BUN levels rise as the GFR decreases. Because urea is reabsorbed by the blood through the permeable tubules, BUN rises in states of dehydration. There is also a rise of BUN with acute and chronic renal failure when passage of the glomerular filtrate through the tubules is slowed. Altered protein intake and protein catabolism can also alter BUN. Normal values of BUN in an adult are 10 to 20 mg/dL.

Urinalysis

During urinalysis, the color, turbidity, protein, pH, specific gravity, sediment, and supernatant are evaluated. Color is normally light yellow. When formed substances (crystals, blood cells or casts) are in the urine, it appears turbid. Protein in the urine creates foam when shaken, and bile pigment makes the urine foam yellow.

Urine pH ranges from 5 to 6.5, but it can vary from 4 to 8. Urine is more alkaline postprandially and then acidifies before the next meal. Because sleep is accompanied by intermittent hypoventilation, a person produces more acidic urine after awakening.

Specific gravity is an estimated measure of the solute concentration of the urine. This value is compared to the same amount of volume as distilled water. Although specific gravity is not a true measure of the number or concentration of particles in the urine, it correlates well with osmolality. The normal values are 1.016 to 1.022.

Urine osmolality is primarily a function of ADH, which controls water reabsorption in the collecting ducts. If the kidneys cannot concentrate a dilute urine with a given stimulus, the cause is usually a malfunction of the renal tubules or inappropriate ADH secretion by the posterior pituitary gland. Hydration status also affects the urine specific gravity, so hydration status should be evaluated before making a diagnosis. This determination is helpful for differentiating oliguria caused by intrinsic renal disease from hypovolemia as a result of dehydration.

Urinary sediment can represent cells, casts, crystals, and bacteria. Epithelial cells may be seen; they are shed naturally throughout the urinary tract. Normal urine contains few or no red blood cells (RBCs). Hematuria is the term used when large numbers of RBCs are present in the urine. The sediment may be red when hematuria is present. An alkaline or hypotonic urine causes lysis of the red blood cells, so the cells will not be seen. When RBCs are present, the urine will be positive for hemoglobin and the specific gravity will be elevated.

Casts are accumulations of cellular precipitates. They originate in the renal tubules (from which they take their shape). They are cylindric and have distinct borders. All casts arise primarily from the ascending limb of the distal tubule. RBC casts indicate bleeding into the tubule. White cell casts are associated with an inflammatory process. Epithelial cell casts indicate degeneration of the tubular lumen or necrosis of the renal tubules.

Crystals are composed of cystine, uric acid, calcium oxalate, or phosphate. They tend to form in a concentrated acidic or alkaline urine. They are generally not clinically significant. Diagnostically, they indicate an inflammation, infection, or metabolic disorder.

TREATMENT OPTIONS, EXPECTED OUTCOMES, AND COMPREHENSIVE MANAGEMENT

The eight most common causes of CRF are:

- Chronic glomerulonephritis
- Nephrotic syndrome
- Hypertensive nephropathy
- Diabetic nephropathy
- Polycystic kidney disease
- Systemic lupus erythematosus
- Polyarteritis nodosa
- Interstitial nephritis.

Nephritis and nephrotic syndromes are described in Chapter 32. Hypertensive and diabetic nephropathy and polycystic kidney disease are described here.

Regardless of category, all are slowly progressive, with the end result being the failure of the organ. Treatment is aimed at arresting the progressive deterioration of organ function. Almost all forms of renal insufficiency have hypertension as a hallmark symptom. Also, uncontrolled hypertension advances the stage of the disease. The mainstay of therapy is to keep the blood pressure controlled.

If there is volume overload, diuretics are used to maintain the proper fluid balance. Diuretics enhance the flow of urine. Clinically, diuretics interfere with renal sodium reabsorption and reduce extracellular fluid volume. They are commonly used to treat hypertension, edema associated with congestive heart failure, nephrotic syndrome, and ascites from cirrhosis of the liver. Diuretics affect the tubular reabsorption at different sites, depending on their type. The four general types are:

- Osmotic diuretics
- Carbonic anhydrase inhibitors
- Inhibitors of loop sodium chloride transport
- Aldosterone antagonists.

Common side effects of diuretics are alterations of the acid–base balance and electrolyte balance.

■ ■ ■ CLINICAL PEARL

If the patient has diabetes, use of an ACE inhibitor will lower the GFR and keep the blood pressure controlled.

Hypertensive Nephropathy

Whether the hypertension is "essential" or of another etiology, persistent exposure to elevated blood pressure results in increased renal circulation. The increased renal circulation leads to elevated intraluminal pressure, which in turn results in intrinsic lesions of the renal arterioles (hyaline arteriolosclerosis). This eventually leads to loss of nephron function (nephrosclerosis).

There are two types of nephrosclerosis. The benign type is seen in patients who are hypertensive for an extended period of time, with the blood pressure above 150/90 mmHg. The increased blood pressure is found on a routine exam, and the patient complains of nonspecific symptoms (headaches, palpitations). The kidneys are normal to reduced in size, with a loss to the cortical mass. This leads to a fine granularity, shown by renal biopsy under microscopy. Characteristic pathology shows a thickening of the afferent arteriole walls as a result of the deposition of homogenous eosinophilic material (hyaline arteriolosclerosis). This is composed of plasma proteins and fats deposited in the arterial wall, secondary to injury to the endothelium. The narrowing of the vascular lumen results from consequent ischemic injury to the glomeruli and tubules. The renal disease caused by benign nephrosclerosis may manifest as mild to moderate elevation of the serum creatinine level, microscopic hematuria, or mild proteinuria. Clinical evaluation does not reveal any abnormalities. Patients with benign nephrosclerosis maintain a near-normal GFR despite a reduction in renal blood flow.

The second type of nephrosclerosis, malignant arteriolar nephrosclerosis, occurs in patients with previous benign nephrosclerosis or in patients with no previous history of hypertension. It is defined as the sudden elevation of blood pressure (more than 130 mmHg diastolic), accompanied by papilledema and central nervous system manifestations (altered state of consciousness, focal or generalized seizures). There is also cardiac decompensation and acute progressive deterioration of renal function. With this nephrosclerosis, the kidneys appear flea-bitten secondary to hemorrhages in the surface capillaries. Two distinct lesions occur: fibrinoid necrosis (infiltration of the arteriolar wall with eosinophilic material, including fibrin) with associated thickening of the vessel wall, and a lesion involving the interlobular arteries. Concentric hyperplastic proliferation

of the cellular elements of the vascular wall with deposition of collagen to form hyperplastic arterioles. Malignant hypertension is likely to develop in patients with a previous history of hypertension. This usually occurs in the third to fourth decade of life, with a higher incidence among African American men (Harrison's, 1991). Renal abnormalities include an increased serum creatinine level, hematuria, and proteinuria. In the urinary sediment, red and white cells may be present.

Control of the blood pressure is the principal goal of therapy for both forms of nephrosclerosis. Untreated, most patients die from the extrarenal complications of hypertension. Whereas patients with malignant hypertension have a true medical emergency, the natural course of this disease has a death rate of 80% to 90% in the first year after diagnosis, secondary to uremia (Harrison's, 1991).

Increasing evidence indicates that some classes of antihypertensive agents offer greater protection against renal insufficiency, even though they produce similar blood-pressure control as other antihypertensive agents. Epstein (1998) describes the benefits of calcium channel antagonists and ACE inhibitors in this population. The apparent benefits include a retardation of renal disease progression by protecting the kidney from hemodynamically mediated glomerular damage. The calcium channel antagonists may also offer protective effects independent of their renal microvasculatory effects. Woittiez et al (1998) have studied differences among the calcium channel antagonists as related to renal protective effects. In their clinical study population of CRF patients with mild to moderate hypertension, those who received mibefradil had a significantly better response in their blood pressure than did those who received sustained-release nifedipine: more mibefradil-treated patients achieved normalization of blood pressure within 12 weeks. In this study, renal function parameters and adverse events were similar between the groups. More studies may be forthcoming.

Diabetic Nephropathy

The natural history of diabetic nephropathy occurs at the onset of the diabetes. The kidneys are usually enlarged from the increased glomerular and tubule size. When glycemic control is poor, the GFR is high. Microproteinuria (less than 550 mg/24 hours) includes mainly albumin of glomerular origin and can be seen in the patient with poor control. With intensive insulin therapy, the proteinuria clears within 72 hours. The glomerular size, however, remains above normal even after glycemic control has been achieved. The reversibility is attributed to the combination of hemodynamic abnormalities and the loss of charge selectivity of the glomerular membranes. In the absence of macroproteinuria (more than 550 mg/24 hours), end-stage diabetic nephropathy rarely develops. Renal hyperfunction continues until macroproteinuria develops. Persistent macroproteinuria indicates glomerular basement disease and may predict future renal failure. Once macroproteinuria develops, the GFR decreases by about 11 mL/min/yr, and renal failure is inevitable. Hypertension accelerate this process (William's, 1992).

In the type 1 diabetic, proteinuria at the time of diagnosis is rare. Its incidence begins to increase 6 to 8 years after the diagnosis, with its peak incidence 16 years after diagnosis. This figure then decreases to about 1% per year after 30 years of diabetes (Davidson, 1991). Male diabetics are at an increased risk of developing proteinuria. After 16 years, incidence of proteinuria is 50% greater in men, a pattern that persists even after 40 years of diabetes. In addition, passage through puberty by members of either sex seems to increase the incidence of proteinuria (Davidson, 1991). Because it is difficult to establish the exact time that hyperglycemia develops in the type 2 diabetic, nearly 15% of all type 2 patients have proteinuria at the time of diagnosis (Davidson, 1991) (Table 31-1).

Diabetic nephropathy with proteinuria is the initial presentation in most patients, although some diabetics present with hypertension. Diabetic nephrosclerosis is one of the most significant of the diabetic renal lesions and one of the most frequent causes of ESRF in diabetics. Renal disease is first observed as episodic, asymptomatic proteinuria. Once proteinuria develops and the GFR decreases, the remaining nephrons attempt to compensate for the loss of function in the damaged glomeruli. This compensation is accomplished by increasing blood flow (hyperperfusion) to the healthy glomeruli, with a concomitant increase in the intraglomerular pressure (Davidson, 1991). Eventually, progression to a fixed, moderate to heavy proteinuria occurs rapidly, about 1 to 2 years after the onset of proteinuria. Once proteinuria occurs, a rapid fall in the GFR follows. ESRF usually occurs within 5 years (Harrison's, 1991). The occurrence of hypertension usually parallels that of proteinuria. Monitoring for microalbuminuria is the accepted method for identifying early nephropathy (Fig. 31-2).

Aiello (1998) reinforces the need for primary care providers to be aware of current screening guidelines, managing patients with tight glycemic control, risk factor modification, and ACE inhibitor administration. With these early interventions, the progression of renal disease can be deterred.

Diabetic retinopathy is usually seen along with diabetic nephropathy. The appearance of nephrotic syndrome in a patient with diabetic nephropathy of less than 10 years' duration, or in the absence of retinopathy, should alert the provider to consider a nondiabetic etiology of the renal disease.

The classic (pathognomonic) lesion of diabetic nephropathy is nodular diabetic glomerular sclerosis, frequently termed the Kimmelstiel-Wilson lesion. The lesion consists of nodular enlargement of the mesangial compartment of the glomerulus (Stein, 1994). Diffuse glomerular sclerosis is more commonly seen, especially when heavy proteinuria is present. Associated with this pathology is atherosclerosis of the afferent and efferent arterioles. Basement membrane thickening and interstitial atrophy can be seen. Early in the disease, the GFR is 20% to 30% above normal. Control of the blood pressure can slow the rate of renal insufficiency.

ACE inhibitors are used to treat this condition. Various studies have shown that they slow the progression of ESRF by reducing early manifestations such as hyperfiltration and microalbuminuria, and they may be particularly effective in reducing intraglomerular pressure. It is believed that these agents have a selective effect on the afferent arteriole of the glomerulus, causing a reduction in arteriolar resistance. Allen et al (1997) demonstrated that these beneficial effects are related to the blockade of angiotensin II, not bradykinin. These researchers also found similar beneficial effects of administering angiotensin II receptor antagonists versus ACE inhibitors for renoprotection.

■ ■ ■ **CLINICAL PEARLS**

■ These agents can cause hyperkalemia. In patients with associated renal artery stenosis, these agents may induce reversible acute renal failure. Therefore, creatinine and potassium levels should be monitored during therapy (Stein, 1994).

■ Patients with chronic renal insufficiency and diabetes are also at a higher-than-average risk for congestive heart failure. The choice of therapy in these patients can be complicated by the need to manage lipids, glucose control, and blood pressure. DiGregorio (1998) reviewed this combination of problems and recommended ACE inhibitors as the treatment of choice in these patients.

Polycystic Kidney Disease

Polycystic kidney disease (PKD), the most significant renal cystic kidney disease, is a process in which cysts are diffusely scattered throughout the renal cortex and medulla. Autosomal dominant disease is usually recognized in the third to forth decade of life. This is a familial disease, with the trait inherited as an autosomal dominant trait. The gene has been linked to chromosome 16. Virtually all who have this trait have some cystic changes, but not all affected persons will progress to renal failure. By age 50, about 25% of those affected will have ESRF. This percentage increases to 50% at age 70 (Stein, 1994). PKD is found worldwide and in all races. Approximately 6000 new cases are diagnosed in the United States each year (Stein, 1994).

Cysts are the most common structural abnormality encountered in the adult kidney. Nearly all renal cysts are derived from nephrons or collecting duct elements. They begin as hair-sized

TABLE 31-1	Typical Clinical Course of Diabetic Neuropathy
Years After Onset of Diabetes (approximate)	**Clinical Course**
0	Enlarged kidneys, supernormal function, microalbuminuria reversed by meticulous insulin treatment
2	Thickening of glomular basement membrane and increase in mesangial matrix
10–15	Silent period: no overt proteinura; microalbuminuria may be present, especially after exercise (.30 μg/m indicative of future protenuria)
10–20	Proteinuric period intermittent at first, then persistent (0.5g/24 h); this means that a relentless decline in glomular function has begun
<15	Azotemic period begins in average 17 y after onset
20	Uremic period: diabetic retinopathy, hypertension, and nephrotic syndrome may be present

(From: Wilson, J.D. & Foster, Daniel W. (eds.) (1992). *William's Textbook of Endocrinology*, 8th ed., Philadelphia: WB Saunders)

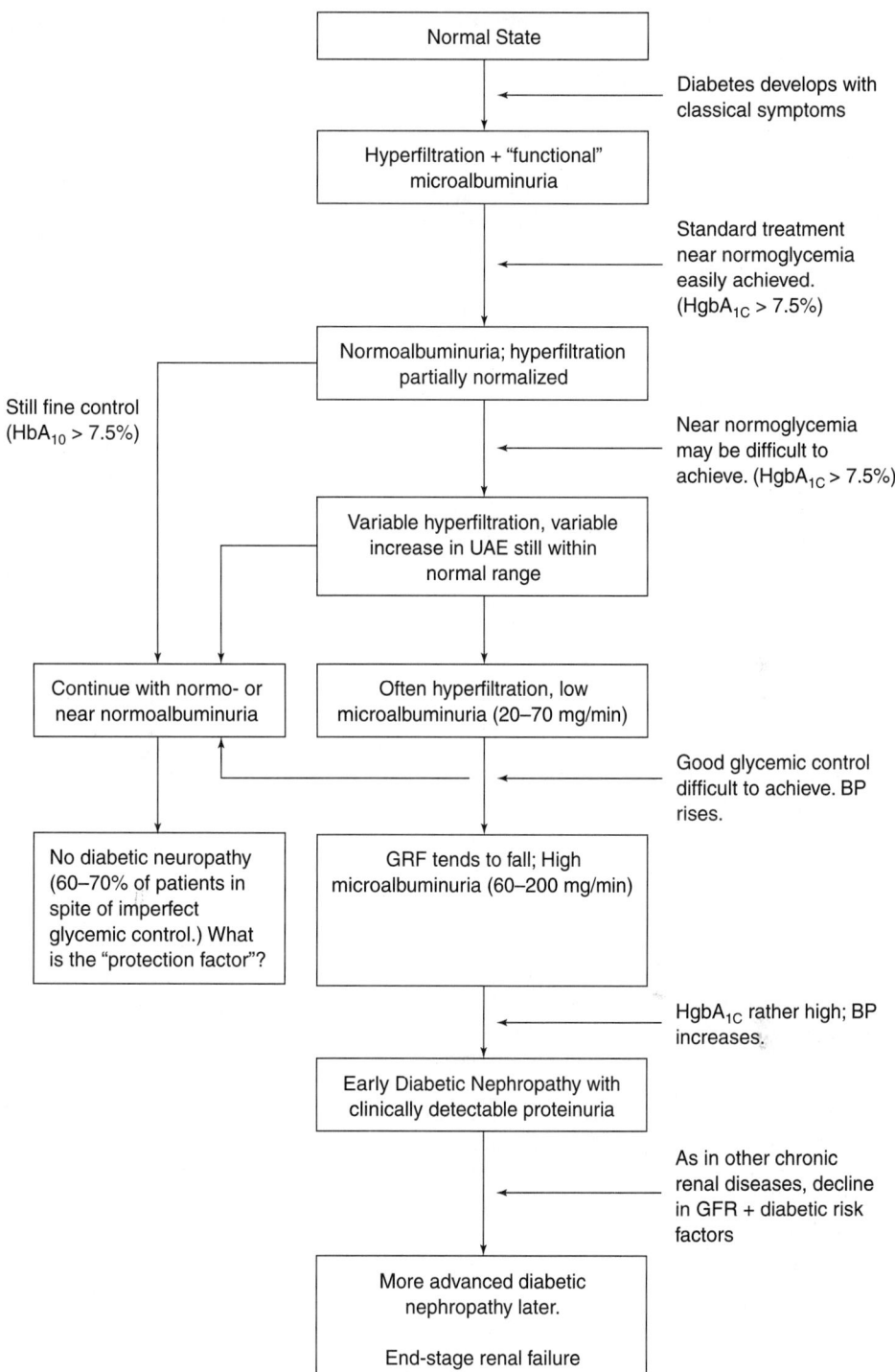

FIGURE 31-2 Natural history of neuropathy in untreated diabetes mellitus. UAE: urinary albumin excretion; BP: blood pressure; GFR: Glomular filtration rate; HgbA$_{1C}$: hemoglobin A, C. (Mogensten, C.E. (1988). Therapeutic interventions in neuropathy of IDDM. *Diabetes Care 11* [Suppl. 1]:10)

structures, enlarging to several centimeters in diameter and containing several hundred milliliters of fluid. Generalized cystic diseases are characterized by cysts spread throughout the renal cortex and renal medulla of one of both kidneys. In PKD, cysts are scattered, bilaterally, throughout the kidney and vary in size from several millimeters to several centimeters. Most cysts are filled with straw-yellow fluid resembling urine. Blood is also found in some cysts. The cysts originate in all segments

of the nephron (Bowman's capsule, proximal tubule, loop of Henle, distal tubule, collecting tubule, and the papillary collecting duct) and are lined with single-cell epithelium.

The liver also contains cysts in 40% to 60% of patients with autosomal dominant PKD (Stein, 1994). Women have greater enlargement of the liver than do men. In some cases, the cysts can grow so large that they cause portal hypertension or obstruction of the common bile duct. Arterial aneurysms of the circle of Willis are found in 10% of patients with autosomal dominant PKD (Stein, 1994). There is also an increased incidence of aortic aneurysm, abnormalities of the mitral valve, and inguinal hernia. Diverticulosis is also seen more frequently in patients with this disease.

Clinical symptoms of hematuria, polyuria, hypertension, and abdominal pain rarely occur in persons younger than 20 to 25. Nonspecific, dull lumbar pain is usually the most frequent symptom. This usually occurs when the kidneys are large enough to be palpable on the abdominal exam. Sharp localized pain can occur from cystic rupture. By urine dipstick, microhematuria without RBC casts can be noted. Hypertension usually occurs at an early stage of PKD. Nocturia is present at diagnosis, and most patients show impaired salt conservation. Urinary tract infections and pyelonephritis are common complications. CRF usually occurs in the fifth to sixth decade of life. As the cystic nephrons increase in size, there is atrophy and fibrosis of the associated kidney tissue. It is thought that the cyst fluid is derived from glomerular filtrate and transepithelial fluid secretion.

Abdominal pain and hematuria are common presenting symptoms. Infected renal cysts secondary to urinary tract infections are also common. Fifty percent of patients have associated hypertension, and this side effect usually precedes the disease (Stein, 1994). There are no specific laboratory values for the diagnosis.

Ultrasound is the preferred method for screening. If more than five cysts per kidney are found, and there is a family history of PKD, then the diagnosis is made. If the ultrasound is equivocal, then a computed tomography scan of the kidney is recommended for a definitive diagnosis.

Diagnosis can also be made with intravenous pyelography and renal ultrasound, which will show lucent cysts surrounded by attenuated strands of functional renal tissue. A patient cannot be judged free of the disease until after age 30 to 35. An adolescent is at high risk for the disease if a morning urine osmolality after an overnight water fast exceeds 800 mOsm/kg.

Therapy is directed at control of the hypertension and prevention of early urinary tract infections and renal stones. Nephrectomy is sometimes indicated for persistent gross hematuria.

Patients should be told that this is an autosomal dominant disease and that there is a 50% chance that their children will inherit the defective gene (Stein, 1994).

COMMUNITY RESOURCES

- American Kidney Fund, 6110 Executive Boulevard, Rockville, MD 20852
- National Kidney Foundation, 30 E. 33d St., New York, NY, 10016
- National Kidney and Urologic Disease Information Clearinghouse (NKUDIC), 3 Information Way, Bethesda, MD 20892
- Chronic Renal Failure, www.healthanswers.com/data base/ami/converted/00047.html
- The Virtual Medical Center, Chronic Renal Failure Educational Material, www.mediconsult.com/noframes/renal/shareware/content.html

REFERRAL POINTS AND CLINICAL WARNINGS

Many of these patients will be comanaged by a primary care provider and a nephrologist. Most providers are comfortable managing a patient until a creatinine level of 2 to 2.5 mg/dL is reached; at that point, a visit with the subspecialist is considered.

REFERENCES

Aiello, J.H. (1998). Preventing diabetic nephropathy: the role of primary care. *Nurse Practitioner, 23(2)*, 12–24.

Allen, T.J., Cao, Z., Youssef, S., Hulthen, U.L., & Cooper, M.E. (1997). Role of angiotensin II and bradykinin in experimental diabetic nephropathy; functional and structural studies. *Diabetes, 46*, 1612–1618.

Davidson, J.K. (1991). *Clinical diabetes mellitus,* 2d ed. Thieme.

DiGregorio, R. (1998). Managing heart failure in diabetic patients. *US Pharmacist, 23(6)*, 101–112.

Epstein, M. (1998). Calcium antagonists and the progression of chronic renal failure. *Current Opinion in Nephrology & Hypertension, 7(2)*, 171–176.

Stein, J.H. (1994). *Internal medicine,* 4th ed. St. Louis: Mosby.

USRDS. (1997). Incidence and prevalence of ESRD. *American Journal of Kidney Diseases, 30*(2 suppl 1):S40–53.

Wilson, J.D., Braunwald, E., Isselbacher, K.J., et al. (eds.) (1991). *Harrison's principles of internal medicine,* 12th ed. New York: McGraw-Hill.

Wilson, J.D. & Foster, D.W. (eds.) (1992). *William's textbook of endocrinology,* 8th ed. Philadelphia: W.B. Saunders.

Woittiez, A.J., Jobrin, I., Villa, G., et al. (1998). A comparison of the safety and efficacy of mibefradil and nifedipine SR in patients with renal disease and hypertension. *Clinical Nephrology, 49(3)*, 160–166.

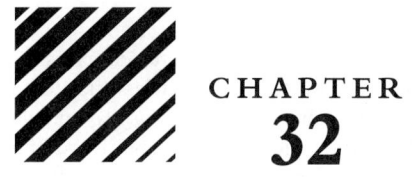

CHAPTER

32

Nephrotic and Nephritic Renal Disease

Hillary Wall, Pharm.D., Joseph A. Grillo, Pharm.D., and Eva Fischer, M.D.

Glomerular disease is the third largest cause of chronic renal insufficiency in the United States. The U.S. Renal Data System estimates that 12.6% of cases of end-stage renal failure are the result of glomerular nephritis (National Institute of Diabetes, 1994). Glomerular diseases are similar in that they are all related to abnormalities within the glomerulus. However, the glomerulopathies comprise a somewhat diverse group of disorders in terms of prevention, presentation, prognosis, and treatment (Glassock et al, 1995; Adler et al, 1995; Glassock & Cohen, 1996). Although glomerular diseases often ultimately require renal biopsy for diagnosis, careful evaluation of a patient's history, physical exam, urinalysis, and age may allow the provider to narrow the diagnosis significantly. This chapter is intended to give an overview of glomerular disease. Patient referral to a specialist in nephrology would be prudent.

ANATOMY, PHYSIOLOGY, AND PATHOLOGY

A comprehensive review of the anatomy and physiology of the kidney are discussed in the chapters on chronic and acute renal disease (Chaps. 30 and 31).

The glomerulopathies are often confusing in that they may be grouped according to their histology, cause, presentation, type of urinary sediment, or some combination of all of the above (Glassock, 1991; Shayman, 1995). Glomerulopathies are categorized as primary or secondary. Primary glomerulopathies originate in the glomeruli of the kidney. Secondary glomerulopathies are a consequence or complication of a systemic disease (Table 32-1). The strong association of primary glomerulopathies with certain diseases suggest that some are in fact systemic diseases that are limited to the kidney. Histologically, the patterns observed in the kidney cannot be differentiated based on primary or secondary glomerulopathies (Glassock, 1991). Glomerular disease may also be divided into a nephrotic or nephritic (ie, focal or diffuse) category based primarily on urinary findings. Some of the more common causes (both primary and secondary) of nephrotic and nephritic glomerular disease will be discussed.

Nephrotic Diseases

MINIMAL CHANGE DISEASE (NIL DISEASE)

Minimal change disease accounts for about 15% to 25% of all cases of glomerulonephritis seen in adults (Pontcelli & Patrizia, 1994). Light microscopy reveals normal or minimal (hence the name) changes in the mesangial cell proliferation. Most of the cases are idiopathic in origin. Some occurrences are attributed to drugs, including nonsteroidal anti-inflammatory drugs (in particular fenoprofen), lithium, tiopronin, ampicillin, rifampin,

and interferon (Glassock & Cohen, 1996; Glassock, 1991). Malignancy, in particular Hodgkin's lymphoma, has also been associated with minimal change disease (Meyrier et al, 1992). The tumor is thought to produce cytokines that are lethal to the glomerular epithelial cells. Secondary minimal change disease responds well to removal of the cause or treatment of the underlying disease.

Usually patients with minimal change disease present with edema and proteinuria in the nephrotic range. Many patients improve with corticosteroids; other therapies have also been tried (Pontcelli & Passerini, 1994; Fujimoto et al, 1991; Glassock, 1993). Overall, the prognosis for patients with minimal change disease is good. Progression to end-stage renal disease is unusual (Nalasco et al, 1986).

MEMBRANOUS GLOMERULONEPHRITIS (OR NEPHROPATHY)

Membranous nephropathy is the most common cause of nephrotic syndrome in adults. The majority of the cases diagnosed are idiopathic, although cases associated with hepatitis B infections, malignancy, systemic lupus erythematosus, and drugs (penicillamine and gold) have been reported (Glassock et al, 1995; Glassock, 1991; Pontcelli & Patrizia, 1994). Membranous nephropathy is more prevalent in patients in their 40s and 50s. Clinically, most patients present with edema and nephrotic-range proteinuria. Hematuria is seen in about half of the patients. Hypertension is noted in less than 40% of the patients. Increased plasma creatinine concentrations are seen in patients with advanced disease, and these patients are more likely to have hypertension (Glassock et al, 1995; Glassock & Cohen, 1996; Pontcelli & Passerini, 1994).

The natural history of membranous nephropathy is variable. Some reports estimate that as many as half the patients presenting with nephrotic syndrome will develop end-stage renal disease within 10 years from diagnosis (Pontcelli & Patrizia, 1994). Other patients have a very benign course, with spontaneous remissions. As with most of the glomerulopathies, long-term studies on outcome and progression to renal disease are limited. The variability in the natural course of the disease makes the evaluation and selection of therapy quite difficult and controversial (Schieppati et al, 1993; Hebert, 1995; Imperiale et al, 1995; Piccoli et al, 1994; Remuzzi et al, 1994). Factors that are associated with increased risk of progression to end-stage renal disease include male gender, age greater than 50 years, heavy proteinuria, abnormal plasma creatinine concentrations, interstitial fibrosis on biopsy, and hypertension (Glassock et al, 1995; Glassock & Cohen, 1996; Schieppati et al, 1993; Hebert, 1995; Imperiale et al, 1995; Piccoli et al, 1994; Remuzzi et al, 1994).

TABLE 32-1	Systemic Diseases Associated With Secondary Glomerular Nephropathies
Endocrine	Wegener's granulomatosis
Diabetes	Scleroderma
Oncology	Mixed connective tissue
Multiple myeloma	disease
Lymphoma	Henoch-Schönlein purpura
Leukemias	Behçcet's
Carcinomas	Sjögren's syndrome
Hematologic	Infectious
Sickle cell disease	Poststreptococcal
Thrombotic thrombocytopenia purpura	Hepatitis B and C
	Endocarditis
Connective Tissue	Other
Systemic lupus	HIV
Polyarteritis	Drugs

FOCAL SEGMENTAL GLOMERULOSCLEROSIS

Focal segmental glomerulosclerosis is notable for scarring or sclerosing of the glomeruli. "Focal" refers to the fact that not all the glomeruli are involved. It is more common in young adults less than 40 years of age. It is one of the primary glomerulopathies, so the majority of the cases are thought to be idiopathic. However, as is typical, systemic disease is associated with focal segmental glomerulosclerosis, most notably HIV disease. HIV nephropathy appears to produce a more rapid deterioration of renal function than focal segmental glomerulosclerosis from idiopathic causes (Glassock & Cohen, 1996; Glassock, 1991; Pontcelli & Passerini, 1994).

Patients with focal segmental glomerulosclerosis usually present with proteinuria in the nephrotic range, impaired renal function, and hypertension; red cells and red cell casts can be observed in the urine sediment. Many patients progress to end-stage renal disease. Some think that focal segmental glomerulosclerosis may be a degenerative change from minimal change disease (Glassock & Cohen, 1996).

DIABETIC NEPHROPATHY (DIFFUSE AND NODULAR GLOMERULOSCLEROSIS)

Diabetic nephropathy causes renal failure in almost a third of patients with type I diabetes and about 5% of type II patients (Perneger et al, 1994). Diabetic glomerular disease is the most common cause of end-stage renal disease requiring dialysis (Markett & Freidman, 1992). Diabetic nephropathy is described as a diffuse and nodular glomerulosclerosis. Diffuse thickening in the glomerular basement membrane is observed with the light or electron microscope in patients with diabetic nephropathy. Kimmelstiel-Wilson lesions are nodules that can be seen in more advanced stages of diabetic renal disease (Glassock, 1991). The exact mechanism of diabetes glomerular disease is not clearly understood. One theory is that advanced glycosylation end products (produced by the glycosylation of proteins) accumulate and alter the mesangial matrix (Makita et al, 1991). Persons with diabetes are noted to have an increase in glomerular filtration (hyperfiltration) before they develop microalbuminuria. This hyperfiltration may be damaging to the glomerulus (Rudbert et al, 1992). Additionally, increased glucose concentrations may contribute to increased pressures within the glomerulus, which are detrimental (Glassock, 1991).

Clinically, patients with diabetic nephropathy may initially present with microalbuminuria (not detectable on the routine urine protein dipstick), then proteinuria, which can be in the nephrotic range. In patients with type I diabetes, progression to end-stage renal disease occurs 15 to 20 years after the onset of microalbuminuria.

AMYLOIDOSIS

Patients with renal amyloidosis usually present with severe proteinuria, severe edema, and low albumin concentrations. Patients may also present with hepatosplenomegaly, congestive heart failure, and carpal tunnel syndrome. The plasma creatinine concentration may be normal or moderately elevated. Amyloidosis can be primary or secondary. Secondary disease is usually associated with multiple myeloma, tuberculosis, rheumatoid arthritis, infection, or chronic inflammation. The majority of patients have primary amyloidosis. Primary amyloidosis is usually seen in adults older than 40 years. The prognosis and treatment options for primary amyloidosis are limited. Treatment of the cause of secondary amyloidosis (eg, infection) may lead to resolution of the amyloidosis and as such a more favorable outcome (Adler et al, 1995; Glassock, 1991).

Nephritic Glomerular Diseases

IgA (BERGER'S)

IgA, or Berger's disease, is the most common glomerulopathy. Granular IgA deposits observed under immunofluorescence are diagnostic for Berger's disease (Glassock et al, 1995; Glassock & Cohen, 1996; Glassock, 1991). Approximately half of the patients with IgA nephropathy have high plasma IgA concentrations. IgA typically presents with intermittent gross hematuria and flank pain. Often the diagnosis is made when mild proteinuria and microscopic hematuria are noted on a urinalysis. IgA has been observed to present about 5 days after the onset of an upper respiratory tract infection. The majority of cases of IgA are thought to be idiopathic; other causes include cirrhosis, gluten enteropathy, nil disease, oat cell carcinoma, disseminated tuberculosis, and HIV infection (Galla, 1995). IgA is considered to have a better outcome than some of the other glomerulopathies, although end-stage renal disease may develop in 20% of patients within 20 years of diagnosis. Factors that have been suggested to increase the chance of developing end-stage renal disease are increased in plasma creatinine concentration, hypertension, urinary protein excretion greater than 1 g/day, or morphologically glomerular scarring, crescent formation, or tubulointerstitial changes. The natural history of IgA is generally favorable, taking 10 to 20 years to develop into end-stage renal disease, if it occurs (Glassock et al, 1995; Glassock, 1991; Galla, 1995).

HEREDITARY NEPHRITIS

Hereditary nephritis, or Alport's syndrome, is an X-linked disorder associated with hearing loss and lenticular opacities. Men generally progress to end-stage renal disease; women tend to have a more benign course. Histologically, thinning of the glomerular basement membrane is observed early in the disease course. Later, splitting or laminating of the basement membrane is more diagnostic of Alport's syndrome. Asymptomatic hematuria and proteinuria or gross intermittent hematuria is the typical early presentation. Family history of deafness would favor the diagnosis of Alport's over IgA nephropathy; the presentation of the disease may be quite similar in other respects (Glassock et al, 1995; Glassock & Cohen, 1996; Glassock, 1991; Bodziak, 1994).

POSTINFECTIOUS GLOMERULONEPHRITIS

A proliferative type of glomerulonephritis can be observed as a complication of infection, particularly of the throat and skin. Most cases involve only mild renal disease that may not even be identified. The most common infections associated with postinfectious glomerulonephritis are certain strains of streptococci. Clinically, poststreptococcal glomerulonephritis presents 1 to 3 weeks after pharyngitis or impetigo infections, respectively (Glassock, 1991). Patients may present with severe hematuria, bilateral flank pain, a decrease in glomerular filtration rate, and oliguria. Nephritic urine sediment is typical, although white blood cells may be observed. The majority of patients have low plasma C_3 concentrations, whereas antistreptolysin O values are elevated. Spontaneous resolution occurs in most patients, although some patients develop acute renal failure. Endocarditis is also associated with postinfectious glomerulonephritis (Adler et al, 1995; Glassock, 1991; Montseny et al, 1995).

RAPIDLY PROGRESSING GLOMERULONEPHRITIS

Rapidly progressing glomerulonephritis is the clinical presentation of a disorder noted for red blood cells of variable size and shape, proteinuria (usually not in the nephrotic range), and rapid deterioration in renal function. Untreated, it may progress to end-stage renal disease within months. Renal insufficiency tends to be severe because pathologically, rapidly progressing glomerulonephritis is associated with crescent formation in almost all the glomeruli. Crescent formation is not diagnostic, however; it can occur in almost any type of proliferative glomerulonephritis. Thus, the term "crescentic glomerulonephritis" should not be used as a synonym for rapidly progressing glomerulonephritis (Glassock et al, 1995; Glassock & Cohen, 1996). Rapidly progressing glomerulonephritis is the result of primary and secondary causes. The primary causes are classified as types I to V. In type I, also known as antiglomerular basement membrane antibody disease, antibodies are directed against antigens in the glomerular basement membrane. These patients have antibodies that can be detected in the serum. Secondary causes are often grouped into infectious (endocarditis, hepatitis), systemic (lupus, malignancy), or drug-related (allopurinol, hydralazine), and as complications of other primary glomerulopathies (membranous nephropathy, IgA nephropathy) (Glassock,; Merkel et al, 1994). Treatment depends on the cause and if primary the particular subtype (Glassock et al, 1995; Adler et al, 1995; Glassock & Cohen, 1996; Glassock,).

LUPUS NEPHRITIS

Renal disease probably occurs in some form or another in the majority of patients with systemic lupus erythematosus (Boumpas et al, 1995). Ninety percent have renal abnormalities identified from renal biopsy even if they do not have clinical evidence of disease (Leehey et al, 1982). Immune complex glomerular

diseases are the most common type of renal disease in patients with lupus, but nonglomerular renal disorders also occur. The types of lupus glomerular disease are mesangioproliferative, focal proliferative, diffuse proliferative, and membranous glomerulonephritis (Appel et al, 1978). Diffuse proliferative glomerulonephritis is the most common type of glomerular disease; it also has the worst renal prognosis, with progression to end-stage renal disease if untreated (Glassock, 1991). Mesangioproliferative glomerulonephropathy occurs in less than 20% of patients with lupus nephritis and has an excellent prognosis. Lupus glomerular disorders can be identified on electron microscopy by the tubuloreticular structures in the glomerular endothelial cells. Patients may convert from one form of glomerular disease to another, which may confuse the natural history of the particular type of disease (Glassock, 1991).

DIAGNOSTIC CRITERIA

Proper diagnosis of the subtype, cause, and stage of glomerular diseases is crucial to appropriate treatment, preventing or decreasing the risk of progression. An important consideration is the risk of progressive renal insufficiency leading to end-stage renal disease. The utility of treatments to prevent these renal syndromes is most extensively studied in the diabetic population.

Urinalysis is necessary in all patients with suspected glomerular disease. The urine sample should be evaluated within 30 to 60 minutes of voiding. Correct interpretation of urinalysis data (Table 32-2) is key to placing a patient into one of the classifications of glomerular disease (focal nephritic, diffuse nephritic, or nephrotic). The information obtained from urinalysis, combined with the patient's age and comorbid state, may help determine the diagnosis. Many patients with glomerular disease are asymptomatic, with evidence of renal disease found only by abnormalities seen on a routine urinalysis. The two symptoms that often alert the provider to the possibility of glomerular disease are hematuria and proteinuria. Evidence of decreased glomerular filtration rate, hypertension, and edema suggest severe disease. Other nonglomerular causes of hematuria such as infection, coagulation defects, renal tumors, renal cysts, renal stones, and trauma should be ruled out.

HISTORY AND PHYSICAL EXAM

A thorough history and physical exam are essential in the diagnosis of a patient with suspected glomerular disease. History of other diseases such as diabetes, lupus, or chronic active hepatitis may help predict the abnormal renal histology; for example, malignancy is associated with membranous glomerulonephritis. A detailed family history is also important because a history of kidney disease or deafness might suggest hereditary nephritis. Lastly, a medication history, including illicit drug use, is essential: intravenous heroin use is associated with the development of focal glomerulosclerosis (Glassock, 1991).

Hypertension and edema are clinical manifestations that are commonly associated with glomerular disease and are usually detectable on the physical exam. In addition to a routine physical exam, evaluation of the kidneys is essential: this may identify large or abnormally shaped kidneys that are suggestive of renal cell carcinoma or polycystic kidney disease. Patients should be

TABLE 32-2	Characteristic Patterns of Urinary Sediment and Causes of Glomerular Disease	
	Nephritic	
Nephrotic	*Focal*	*Diffuse*
COMMON URINALYSIS FINDINGS		
▪ Proteinuria (>3 g/d)	▪ Red blood cell casts	▪ Proteinuria (usually mild, <1.5g/d)
▪ Fatty casts	▪ Red blood cells (variable size and shape)	▪ Hematuria
▪ Oval fat bodies		▪ Broad waxy casts
▪ Free fat droplets	▪ White cells	▪ Granular casts
▪ Hematuria (variable)	▪ Proteinuria (mild, <1.5g/d)	
▪ Few cells or casts		
MAJOR CAUSES		
▪ Focal glomerulosclerosis	▪ IgA nephropathy	▪ Lupus
▪ Minimal change disease	▪ Lupus	▪ Hereditary nephritis
▪ Benign nephrosclerosis	▪ Henoch-Schönlein purpura	▪ Membranous proliferative glomerulonephritis
▪ Pre-eclampsia	▪ Postinfectious glomerulonephritis (mild)	▪ Postinfectious glomerulonephritis
▪ Membranous nephropathy	▪ Hereditary nephritis	▪ Rapidly progressing glomerulonephritis
▪ Diabetic nephropathy		
▪ Primary amyloidosis		
▪ Postinfectious glomerulonephritis (late)		

evaluated for the presence of a malar rash: this might suggest lupus as the cause of glomerular disease.

DIAGNOSTIC STUDIES

Urine Dipstick for Protein

The urine dipstick for protein is a semiquantitative test for protein in urine. The scale is negative, trace, 1+, 2+, and 3+; these are equal to none, less than 10 mg/dL, 10 mg/dL, 100 mg/dL, and greater than 500 mg/dL, respectively (Shayman, 1995). These represent concentrations of protein in the urine. Diagnostic criteria are based on 24-hour urine protein excretion. Normal protein excretion in adults is less than 150 mg per 24 hours, so even trace protein on the urine dipstick (10 mg/dL) can represent an abnormal amount of protein excretion. The urine dipstick tests primarily for albumin. Other urinary proteins, such as those seen in multiple myeloma, may not be detected on a urine dipstick. The sulfosalicylic acid test may be done to determine the presence of other proteins (Shayman, 1995; Hrick & Smith, 1986).

24-Hour Urine Protein Concentration

A 24-hour timed urine collection for protein is used to determine the amount of protein excreted within a 24-hour period. Before beginning the collection, the patient voids. This urine is discarded, and the specimen collection is begun from that time forward. All urine for the entire study period must be collected. Twenty-four hours after the collection has begun, the patient must void one final time (this urine is included in the collection). The total urine volume is noted, and one 10-mL aliquot is analyzed. Nephrotic-range proteinuria is usually considered greater than 3.5 g of protein per day.

A common problem with 24-hour collections is incomplete samples. Measurement of urine creatinine concurrently can as-

sist in determining if a sample is complete. Knowing that males usually excrete 20 to 25 mg/kg/day of creatinine and females 15 to 20 mg/kg/day, the total amount of creatinine from the 24-hour urine collection can be compared to the average 24-hour creatinine excretion. If the sample urinary creatinine is less than expected, it may indicate an inadequate urine collection (Shayman, 1995).

Urine Protein/Creatinine Ratio

Another method to quantify urine protein excretion is the urine protein/creatinine ratio (Ginsberg et al, 1983). This is calculated by dividing the urine protein concentration by the urine creatinine concentration. The ratio is equal to the number of grams of protein excreted per day per 1.73 m². A protein/creatinine ratio of less than 0.2 is normal. A ratio of greater than 3.5 correlates with the nephrotic range of proteinuria in average-sized adult (1.73 m²).

Urinalysis

A fresh, first-morning, properly obtained midstream urine specimen should be evaluated for blood, specific gravity, pH, and protein and should undergo microscopic evaluation for cellular elements and casts (red blood cell casts, white blood cell casts, oval fat bodies, red and white cells, granular casts, fatty casts). The diagnostic criteria outlined in Table 32-2 will help with interpretation of the urinary sediment seen in the various glomerular diseases.

Red cell casts in the urine are essentially diagnostic of some types of glomerular disease as the cause of bleeding. If proteinuria is also noted with the hematuria, it implies a glomerular cause. Hematuria can be the result of many nonglomerular disorders. Abnormally shaped (dysmorphic) red blood cells are seen in glomerular disease; the damage is though to occur as they pass through the glomerular basement membrane. More normal-appearing red blood cells suggest a lower tract source of hematuria (Glassock et al, 1995; Adler et al, 1995; Glassock & Cohen, 1996; Glassock, 1991; Shayman, 1995).

URINE PROTEIN ELECTROPHORESIS

This allows the identification of proteins: albumin, alpha₁-antitrypsin, alpha₂-macroglobulin, haptoglobulin, transferrin, C3 complement, and immunoglobulins. A urine protein electrophoresis in proteinuria from a glomerular source has albumin, alpha₁-antitrypsin, and transferrin bands. Light chain monoclonal proteins are often observed in patients with multiple myeloma. Beta-2 microglobulin suggests a tubular cause of the proteinuria (Shayman, 1995).

URINE IMMUNOELECTROPHORESIS

Proteins in urine are separated and identified against a series of antigens to potential human immunoglobulins known to cause pathology. Immunoelectrophoresis can test for the presence of IgG, IgM, IgA, anti-kappa, anti-lambda, and antipolyvalent (Shayman, 1995).

Serologic Studies

Some of the glomerular disorders have specific serologic data that are helpful in diagnosing the type or cause of the injury. This is particularly true for the secondary causes of glomerular diseases. For example, levels of antistreptolysin O antibodies are elevated in postinfectious glomerulonephritis; levels of antiglomerular basement membrane antibodies are increased in antiglomerular basement membrane antibody disease; levels of antineutrophil cytoplasmic antibodies are high in Wegener's granulomatosis; and levels of antinuclear antibodies are elevated in lupus. These studies are noninvasive and often allow the practitioner to avoid or delay renal biopsy.

Renal Biopsy

Percutaneous renal biopsy is the gold standard for identifying the specific type of glomerular disease. The precise type of glomerular disease is determined by evaluating the tissue samples by light, immunofluorescence, and electron microscopy.

Not all patients with glomerular renal injury evidenced by the physical exam, medical history, and urinary and plasma laboratory determinations will require renal biopsy. Patients with nephrotic syndrome from an obvious cause (eg, diabetic nephropathy) generally do not require a biopsy. Patients with concurrent lupus usually require a biopsy to identify the type of glomerular disease. Biopsy may be helpful in some patients to assess the severity of disease.

Contraindications to percutaneous renal biopsy include single kidney, large renal cysts, bleeding diathesis, renal carcinoma, and acute pyelonephritis. Percutaneous renal biopsy in relatively safe. Complications include pain at the site of biopsy, hematuria, and hematoma. The mortality rate is about 0.1% (Radford et al, 1994).

TREATMENT OPTIONS, EXPECTED OUTCOMES, AND COMPREHENSIVE MANAGEMENT

The therapy for each glomerular disease varies. Some are more amenable to therapy than others. Therapeutic guidelines have not been established for all the glomerular diseases. For example, considerable controversy exists regarding treatment of membranous glomerulopathy. If the glomerular disease is secondary to a systemic disease or another medical disorder or drug, removing the offending agent or treating the underlying problem tends to be the most effective treatment.

Primary Glomerular Disease

Corticosteroids are considered the mainstay of therapy for some of these diseases, such as minimal change disease. Minimal change disease can be treated with oral prednisone at a dose of 1 mg/kg/day (as a single dose), to a maximum of 80 mg/day (Glassock & Cohen, 1996; Fujimoto et al, 1991; Glassock, 1993). Optimal dose and duration have not been established. This course is continued for 8 to 16 weeks, although some patients may require 16 to 20 weeks before responding. Poncelli and Passerini (1994) suggested using the same starting dose until a response is observed (but at least 6 weeks), then changing to alternate-day therapy at 1.6 mg/kg/48 hours and decreasing the dose by 0.2 to 0.4 mg/kg/48 hours every month. Adults do not respond as well or as quickly to treatment as children: only 50% to 60% respond by 8 weeks, and 25% of patients take 12 to 16 weeks to respond. Relapse of minimal change disease occurs in about a third of patients; another third are considered steroid-dependent (Fujimoto et al, 1991). First relapses are usually treated with a repeat course of corticosteroids. Cyclophosphamide, chlorambucil, and cyclosporine have been used in patients with frequent relapses or steroid dependence (Glassock et al, 1995; Glassock & Cohen, 1996; Glassock, 1993).

In the management of Berger's disease, corticosteroids are generally not thought to be helpful unless the patient presents with rapidly progressing or crescentic IgA (Galla, 1995). Essential fatty acid deficiencies in patients with IgA nephropathy have prompted trials with fish oils (Donadio et al, 1994). Angiotensin-converting enzyme (ACE) inhibitors have also been evaluated in IgA (Cattran et al, 1994).

Treatment for antiglomerular basement membrane antibody disease may include plasmapheresis to remove antibodies and immunosuppressive therapy to reduce new antibody formation. Chronic dialysis is usually necessary in patients who present with a serum creatinine level greater than 6 mg/dL. Drug therapy for this group may be less effective and too risky. Treatment of secondary causes of rapidly progressing glomerulonephritis are usually directed at the underlying cause. Treatment must be started immediately, and renal biopsy is usually required to identify the precise type of disease for appropriate treatment (Glassock et al, 1995; Glassock & Cohen, 1996; Glassock, 1991; Merkel et al, 1994).

The utility of drug therapy depends on the exact subtype of disease, its cause, and the stage of diagnosis. For example, in other variants of glomerular disease, corticosteroids may either be ineffective or worsen the natural course of the disease. An important consideration with these syndromes is the risk of progressive renal insufficiency leading to end-stage renal disease.

Secondary Glomerular Disease

Secondary glomerular diseases are a consequence or complication of a systemic disease. Prevention and treatment of the underlying cause is the most effective therapy. For example, treatment of postinfectious glomerulonephritis is directed at using appropriate antibiotic therapy to treat the underlying infectious process.

Prevention of glomerulopathies is poorly understood. Most reports focus on the prevention of diabetic nephropathy. The exact mechanism of how diabetes leads to glomerular disease is not completely understood, but the impact of glycemic control on its incidence and progression are clear. The Diabetes Control and Complications Trial (DCCT, 1993 & 1995) confirmed that strict glucose control in patients with type I diabetes decreased the development and progression of diabetic nephropathy. Blood-pressure control is also imperative in the management of diabetic nephropathy (Vijan et al, 1997). Antihypertensive therapy to lower blood pressure to 130/85 mmHg is recommended (Sixth Report, 1997). ACE inhibitors should be considered as first-line therapy (unless comorbidities or intolerance contraindicate their use). ACE inhibitors appear to have beneficial effects on preserving renal function, in addition to the benefits of reducing blood pressure on kidney function. These effects are thought to be related to their effect on decreasing urinary protein excretion and decreasing intraglomerular pressures. Even in normotensive patients, there are benefits to initiating ACE inhibitor therapy with evidence of microalbuminuria or proteinuria (Ravid et al, 1993; Ravid et al, 1996; Bennett et al, 1995). Early detection and prevention are the keys in helping to avoid or slow the progression of

diabetic nephropathy. Screening for proteinuria and microalbuminuria should be done at least annually (Vijan et al, 1997; Bennet et al, 1995). Proteinuria can be detected with urine dipstick. If negative, patients should be tested for microalbuminuria. Strict glycemic control is also essential. Patient education on the disease, potential complications, and the benefit of preventive therapies is crucial in total management of this disease.

Management of Clinical Manifestations of Nephrotic Syndrome Associated With Both Primary and Secondary Glomerular Disease

An overall approach to the treatment of clinical manifestations (edema, hypertension, hyperlipidemia, hypercoagulablity, hypoalbuminemia, and infection) associated with glomerular diseases that cause nephrotic syndrome is shown in Figure 32-1.

EDEMA
Edema resulting from nephrotic syndrome is particularly difficult to manage. Dietary modification is essential. Sodium intake should be restricted to approximately 2 g/day. At the same time, potent diuretic therapy (eg, loop diuretics) should be initiated. Patients with nephrotic syndrome are generally resistant to loop diuretic therapy (ie, furosemide, bumetanide, torsemide) to some degree (Keller et al, 1982) for two reasons.

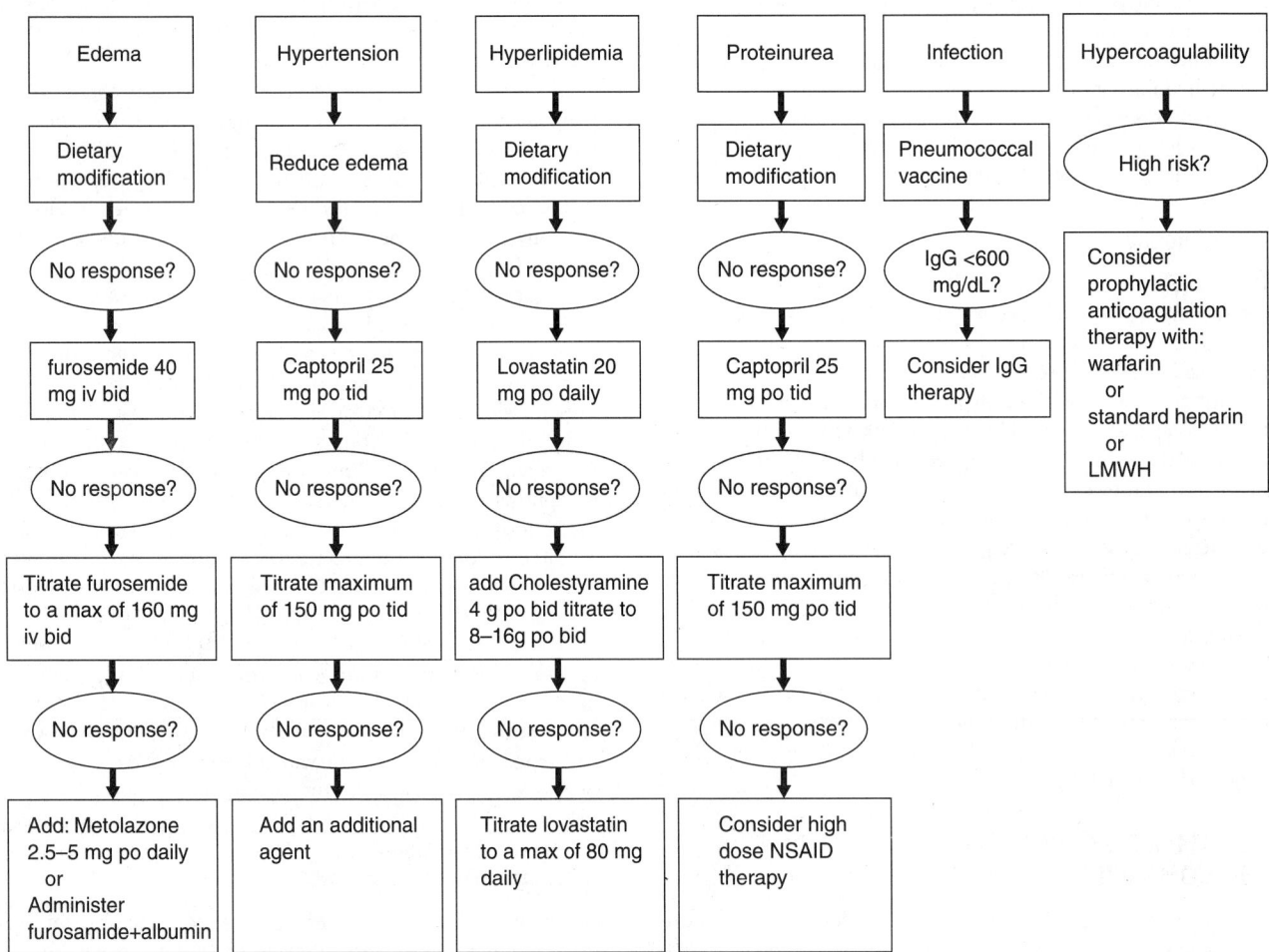

FIGURE 32-1 Overall management of clinical manifestations of nephrotic syndrome.

The reason for this observed "resistance" is two-fold. The diuresis elicited by this class of drugs is caused by inhibition of the $Na^+/K^+/Cl^-$ cotransporter at the ascending loop of Henle. This site of action is reached intraluminally, after the loop diuretic is excreted by the proximal tubule. Because all commercially available loop diuretics are highly bound to plasma proteins (eg, albumin) in the plasma, a major portion of a dose remains in the vascular tree under normal conditions. This would allow more drug to be available for transport to the site of action. Hypoalbuminemia secondary to nephrotic syndrome may reduce the rate of delivery of the loop diuretic secondary to increased extravascular distribution (Keller et al, 1982; Smith et al, 1985). In addition, loop diuretics that reach the kidney and enter the renal tubular lumen can become bound to abnormally filtered albumin in the tubule and rendered inactive (Kirchner et al, 1991; Kirchner et al, 1990).

Furosemide is the most widely studied and economical loop diuretic for this indication. Treatment is generally begun at an intravenous dose of 40 mg administered twice daily. This dose can be doubled and even tripled if required. Patients requiring greater than 160 mg of furosemide twice daily should be started on a second diuretic that effects urinary sodium loss in a different manner. A thiazide diuretic such as metolazone is a common choice. Another therapeutic manipulation in the setting of diuretic resistance secondary to hypoalbuminemia is to administer 40 to 80 mg of furosemide added to a 50-mL vial of 25% albumin. The theory is that the additional albumin will force more furosemide to remain intravascularly, thereby increasing the rate to drug delivery to the kidney. One study reports a three- to fivefold increase in sodium excretion with this method of delivery (Inoue et al, 1987). A follow-up study failed to corroborate these findings, however (Akcicek et al, 1995). This therapy is still considered controversial and should only be used as a last resort. Other measures, such as bed rest and supportive stockings, should also be incorporated into the overall management plan.

HYPERTENSION

Hypertension is a common complication of nephrotic syndrome. One study noted that 78% of adult patients with minimal change disease were hypertensive during the edematous phase before steroid therapy (Kuster et al, 1990). Blood-pressure control is key because systemic hypertension increases the loss of protein in the urine and may accelerate the progression of glomerular disease. Systemic hypertension associated with nephrotic syndrome is generally considered to be the result of volume expansion secondary to renal sodium retention (Abrass, 1997). As a result, plasma renin activity is usually low (Rodriguez-Iturbe et al, 1981).

Initial therapy is aimed at removing edema, as discussed in the previous section. The goal is to maintain an average blood pressure of 125/75 mmHg. In most cases, patients respond to this intervention alone (Abrass, 1997). However, patients who are hypertensive in the absence of significant edema generally have a high plasma renin activity and respond well to the addition of an ACE inhibitor (Stockigt et al, 1979). In addition, ACE inhibitors slow the progression of the glomerulopathy and also provide an antiproteinuric effect independent of their antihypertensive effect (Abrass, 1997; Keilani et al, 1993). Other antihypertensive agents such as dihydropyridine calcium channel blockers (eg, nifedipine), hydralazine, and minoxidil

should be used with caution in this population because they may worsen peripheral edema.

HYPERLIPIDEMIA

Hyperlipidemia secondary to nephrotic syndrome usually correlates with the degree of proteinuria (Abrass, 1997). A combination of dietary modification and pharmacologic intervention is the cornerstone of management, although the outcome is highly variable. D'Amico and Gentile (1991) reported that a vegetarian soy diet (ie, low fat, moderately low protein, and high polyunsaturated fats) can reduce serum lipid concentrations by as much as 30% in patients with nephrotic syndrome-induced hyperlipidemia.

In addition to dietary modification, most patients require a pharmacologic agent. The most successful agents for this condition are the HMG-CoA reductase inhibitors (eg, lovastatin 20 mg/day) and the bile acid sequestrants (eg, cholestyramine starting at 4 g once or twice daily, titrated to a maintenance dose of 8 to 16 g/day in two divided doses) (Kean, 1994; Valeri et al, 1986; Rabelink et al, 1988; Golper et al, 1989). These agents, used alone or in combination, can lower plasma cholesterol and triglyceride concentrations by as much as 45% (Rabelink et al, 1988; Golper et al, 1989). Fibric acid agents (eg, gemfibrozil) can reduce total cholesterol by as much as 30% in this population but are generally contraindicated because they will accumulate in the setting of renal dysfunction, resulting in an increase in the incidence of serious adverse events associated with this class (ie, myopathy, gallstones, and gastrointestinal disorders) (Groggel et al, 1989).

Reduction in the degree of proteinuria alone will also reduce levels of total and low-density lipoprotein cholesterol by as much as 15%. Adjunctive therapy with ACE inhibitors, as described above, can reduce proteinuria and further reduce hyperlipidemia associated with nephrotic syndrome (Keilani et al, 1993).

HYPERCOAGULABILITY

Thromboembolism is one of the most serious complications of the nephrotic syndrome and has an overall incidence of 20% (Llach et al, 1985). The routine use of prophylactic anticoagulation is controversial; it is usually reserved for patients who are at high risk (ie, membranous nephropathy and a plasma albumin level <2 g/dL). Warfarin therapy is extremely difficult to optimize in this population because of inconsistent absorption and fluctuating synthesis of hepatic coagulation factors (Ganeval et al, 1986). Unfractionated heparin is also an option; however, it requires frequent monitoring and is difficult to administer on an outpatient basis. Low-molecular-weight heparin is a better alternative in this population because it can easily be administered at home and no significant monitoring is required. Rostoker et al (1995) reported that enoxapirin, a low-molecular-weight heparin, is safe and effective in patients with severe nephrotic syndrome. Treatment of a thromboembolic event generally involves the initial use of heparin therapy, followed by chronic warfarin therapy for the duration of time the patient is nephrotic. The benefit of low-molecular-weight heparin in the treatment of an acute thromboembolic event has not been elucidated.

PROTEINURIA AND HYPOALBUMINEMIA

Proteinuria secondary to nephrotic syndrome can be somewhat reduced through dietary modification and drug therapy (eg, ACE inhibitors). Protein intake should be restricted to 0.8 to

1 g/kg/day. Pharmacotherapy can include ACE inhibitors and high-dose nonsteroidal anti-inflammatory agents. The latter are approximately 30% effective in reducing proteinuria through a reduction in the glomerular filtration rate (Abrass, 1997). All of these interventions are temporary, with the goal of reducing other sequelae until remission can be achieved with appropriate therapy for the type of glomerular disease.

INFECTION

Patients with nephrotic syndrome are more susceptible to infection than the normal population, primarily because of their reduced serum immunoglobulin concentrations, reduced cell-mediated immunity, and malnutrition (Heslan et al, 1982). Adults with severely depressed immunoglobulin levels should receive the pneumococcal vaccine (Bodziak et al, 1994). Unfortunately, one study suggested that 50% of patients fail to maintain adequate antibody concentrations within 1 year of vaccination (Spika et al, 1986).

Intravenous immunoglobulin therapy is generally restricted to nephrotic patients with severely depressed serum immunoglobulin concentrations (ie, <600 mg/dL). Although this treatment is still controversial, one study suggested treatment with 10 to 15 g of intravenous IgG per month in this population. The authors reported a return to an infection rate similar to that of the normal population with this regimen (Ogi et al, 1994). The method of admixture and the rate of administration differ significantly depending on the immunoglobulin product used.

COMMUNITY RESOURCES

- American Society of Nephrology, 1200 19th St. NW, Washington D.C. 20036
- National Kidney Foundation, 30 E. 33d St., New York City, NY 10016
- National Kidney and Urological Disease Information Clearinghouse, 3 Information Way, Bethesda, MD 20892

■ ■ ■ CLINICAL PEARLS

- Clinically, patients with diabetic nephropathy may initially present with microalbuminuria (not detectable on the routine urine protein dipstick), then proteinuria, which can be in the nephrotic range.
- A detailed family history is also important, because a history of kidney disease or deafness might suggest hereditary nephritis.
- The urine dipstick primarily tests for albumin. Other urinary proteins, as seen in multiple myeloma, may not be detected on a urine dipstick.
- Some of the glomerular disorders have specific serologic data that are helpful in diagnosing the type or cause of the injury. Studies of antistreptolysin antibodies, antiglomerular basement membrane antibodies, antineutrophil cytoplasmic antibodies, and antinuclear antibodies are noninvasive and often allow the provider to avoid or delay renal biopsy.
- Patients with nephrotic syndrome from an obvious cause (eg, diabetic nephropathy) generally do not require a biopsy.
- Optimal glucose and blood pressure control are imperative in the management of diabetic nephropathy.

- Patients requiring more than 160 mg of furosemide twice daily should be started on a second diuretic that effects sodium loss in a different manner.
- Warfarin therapy is difficult to optimize in nephrotic and nephritic syndrome because of inconsistent absorption and fluctuating synthesis of coagulation factors.

References

Abrass, C. (1997). Clinical spectrum and complications of the nephrotic syndrome. *Journal of Investigative Medicine, 45,* 143.

Adler, S.G., Cohen, A.H., & Glassock, R.J. (1995). Secondary glomerular diseases. In B. Brenner (Ed.). *The kidney,* 5th ed. Philadelphia: W.B. Saunders, pp. 1498–1596.

Akcicek, F., Yalniz T, Basci A, et al. (1995). Diuretic effect of furosemide in patients with nephrotic syndrome: Is it potentiated by intravenous albumin? *British Medical Journal, 310,* 162.

Appel, G., Silva F.G, Pirani C.L, et al. (1978). Renal involvement in systemic lupus erythematosus: A study of 56 patients emphasizing histologic classification. *Medicine, 57*(5):371–410.

Bennet, P.H., Haffner S, Kasiske B.L, et al. (1995). Diabetic renal disease recommendations. *American Journal of Kidney Disease, 25,* 107–112.

Bodziak, K., Hammond, W., & Molitoris, B. (1994). Inherited diseases of the glomerular basement membrane. *American Journal of Kidney Disease, 23,* 605.

Boumpas D, Austin H.A 3rd, Fessler B.J, et al. (1995). Systemic lupus erythematosus: Emerging concepts. *Annals of Internal Medicine, 122*(12):940–950.

Cattran, D., Greenwood, C., & Ritchie, S. (1994). Long-term benefits of angiotensin-converting enzyme inhibitor therapy in patients with severe immunoglobulins A nephropathy: A comparison to patients receiving treatment with other antihypertensive agents and to patients receiving no therapy. *American Journal of Kidney Disease, 23*(2):247–254.

D'Amico, G., & Gentile, M.G. (1991). Pharmacologic and dietary treatment of lipid abnormalities in nephrotic patients. *Kidney International, 39*(suppl 31), S65.

Diabetes Control and Complications Trials Research Group. (1993). The effect of intensive treatment of diabetes on the development and progression of long-term complications in insulin-dependent diabetes mellitus. *N Engl J Med, 329*(14):977–986.

Diabetes Control and Complications Trial Research Group. (1995). Effect of intensive therapy on the development and progression of diabetic nephropathy in the Diabetes Control and Complications Trial. *Kidney International, 47*(6):1703–1720.

Donadio, J., Bergstralh E.J, Offord K.P, et al. (1994). A controlled trial of fish oil in IgA nephropathy. *N Engl J Med, 331*(18):1194–1199.

Fujimoto, S., Yamaoto Y, Hisanaga S, et al. (1991). Minimal change nephrotic syndrome in adults: Response to corticosteroid therapy and frequency of relapse. *American Journal of Kidney Disease, 17*(6):687–692.

Galla, J. (1995). IgA nephropathy. *Kidney International, 47*(2): 377–387.

Ganeval, D., Fischer, A.M., Barre, J., et al. (1986). Pharmacokinetics of warfarin in the nephrotic syndrome and effect on vitamin K-dependent clotting factors. *Clinical Nephrology, 25,* 75.

Ginsberg, J.M., Chang B.S, Matarese R.A, et al. (1983). Use of a single voided urine sample to estimate quantitative proteinuria. *N Engl J Med, 309*(25):1543–1546.

Glassock, R.J. (1993). Therapy of idiopathic nephrotic syndrome in adults. *American Journal of Nephrology, 13*(5):422–428.

Glassock, R.J. (1991). The glomerulopathies. In R.W. Schrier (Ed.). *Renal and electrolyte disorders,* 4th ed. Boston: Little, Brown & Co.

Glassock, R.J., & Cohen, A.H. (1996). The primary glomerulopathies. *Dis Mon, 42*(6), 329–383.

Glassock, R.J., Cohen, A.H., & Adler, S.G. (1995). Primary glomerular diseases. In B. Brenner (Ed.). *The kidney*, 5th ed. Philadelphia: W.B. Saunders, pp. 1392–1497.

Golper, T., Illingworth D.R, Morris C.D, et al. (1989). Lovastatin in the treatment of multifactorial hyperlipidemia associated with proteinuria. *American Journal of Kidney Disease, 13*(4):312–320.

Groggel, G., Cheung A.K, Ellis-Benigni K, et al. (1989). Treatment of nephrotic hyperlipoproteinemia with gemfibrozil. *Kidney International, 36*(2):266–271.

Hebert, L.A. (1995). Therapy of membranous nephropathy. *Journal of the American Society of Nephrology, 5,* 1543–1545.

Heslan, J.M., Lautie, J.P., Intrator, L., et al. (1982). Impaired IgG synthesis in patients with nephrotic syndrome. *Clinical Nephrology, 18*(3):144–147.

Hrick, D.E., & Smith, M.C. (1986). *Proteinuria and the nephrotic syndrome.* Chicago: Year Book.

Imperiale, T.F., Goldfarb, S., & Berns, J.S. (1995). Are cytotoxic agents beneficial in idiopathic membranous nephropathy? A meta-analysis of the controlled trials. *Journal of the American Society of Nephrology, 5,* 1553–1558.

Inoue, M., Okajima K, Itoh K, et al. (1987). Mechanism of furosemide resistance in analbunemic rats and analbuminemic patients. *Kidney International, 32*(2):198–203.

Kean, W. (1994). Lipids and the kidney. *Kidney International, 46*(3): 910–920.

Keilani, T., Schlueter W.A, Levin M.L, et al. (1993). Improvement of lipid abnormalities associated with proteinuria using fosinopril, an angiotensin-converting enzyme inhibitor. *Annals of Internal Medicine, 188*(4):246–254.

Keller, E., Hoppe-Seyler, G., & Schollmeyer, P. (1982). Disposition and diuretic effect of furosemide in the nephrotic syndrome. *Clin Pharmacol Ther, 32*(4):442–449.

Kirchner, K., Voelker, J., & Brater, D. (1990). Intratubular albumin blunts the response to furosemide: A mechanism for diuretic resistance in the nephrotic syndrome. *Journal of Pharmacology and Experimental Therapy, 252*(3):1097–1101.

Kirchner, K., Voelker, J., & Brater, D. (1991). Binding inhibitors restore furosemide potency in tubule fluid containing albumin. *Kidney International, 40*(3):418–424.

Kuster, S., Mehls, O., Seidel, C., & Ritz, E. (1990). Blood pressure in minimal change and other types of nephrotic syndrome. *American Journal of Nephrology, 10*(suppl 1), 76.

Leehey, D., Katz A.I., Azaran A.H., et al. (1982). Silent diffuse lupus nephritis: Long-term follow-up. *American Journal of Kidney Disease, 2*(suppl 1):188–196.

Llach, F., Papper, S., & Massry, S.G. (1985). Hypercoagulability: Renal vein thrombosis and other complications of the nephrotic syndrome. *Kidney International, 28,* 429.

Makita, Z., Radoff S, Rayfield E.J., et al. (1991). Advanced glycosylation end products in patients with diabetic nephropathy. *N Engl J Med, 325*(12):836–842.

Markell, M., & Freidman, E.A. (1992). Diabetic nephropathy: Management of the end-stage patient. *Diabetes Care, 15,* 1226.

Merkel, F., et al. (1994). Course and prognosis of anti-basement membrane mediated disease. *Nephrology Dialysis & Transplantation, 9*(4):372–376.

Meyrier, A., Delahousse M, Callard P, et al. (1992). Minimal change nephrotic syndrome revealing solid tumors. *Nephron, 61*(2): 220–223.

Montseny, J.J., Meyrier A, Kleinknecht D, et al. (1995). The current spectrum of infectious glomerulonephritis. *Medicine, 74*(2):63–73.

National Institute of Diabetes and Digestive and Kidney Disease, The National Institutes of Health. (1994). *USRDS 1994 Annual Data Report.* Bethesda, Md.

Nolasco, F., Cameron J.S., Heywood E.F., et al. (1986). Adult-onset minimal change nephrotic syndrome: A long-term follow-up. *Kidney International, 29*(6):1215–1223.

Ogi, M., Yokoyama, H., Tomosugi, N., et al. Risk factors for infection and immunoglobulin replacement therapy in adult nephrotic syndrome. *American Journal of Kidney Disease, 24*(3):427–436.

Perneger, T.V., Brancati, F.L., Whelton, P.K., et al. (1994). End-stage renal disease attributable to diabetes mellitus. *Annals of Internal Medicine, 121*(12):912–918.

Piccoli, A., Pillon, L., Passerini P., et al. (1994). Therapy for idiopathic membranous nephropathy: Tailoring the choice by decision analysis. *Kidney International, 45,* 1193–1202.

Pontcelli, C., & Passerini, P. (1994). Treatment of the nephrotic syndrome associated with primary glomerulonephritis. *Kindery International, 46,* 595.

Rabelink, A., Hene, R.J., Erkelens, D.W., et al. (1988). Effect of simvastatin and cholestyramine on lipoprotein profile in hyperlipidaemia of nephrotic syndrome. *Lancet, 2*(8624):1335–1338.

Radford, M.G., Donadio, J.V., Holley, K.E., et al. (1994). Renal biopsy in clinical practice. *Mayo Clinic Proceedings, 69,* 983–984.

Ravid, M., Savin, H., Jutrin, I., et al. (1993). Long-term stabilizing effect of angiotensin-converting enzyme inhibitors on plasma creatinine and proteinuria in normotensive type II diabetic patients. *Annals of Internal Medicine, 118,* 577.

Ravid, M., Land, R., Rachmani, R., et al. (1996). Long-term renoprotective effects of angiotensin-converting enzyme inhibition in non-insulin dependent diabetes mellitus: A 7-year follow-up study. *Archives of Internal Medicine, 156,* 286–289.

Remuzzi, G., Schiepatti, A., & Garattini. (1994). Treatment of idiopathic membranous glomerulopathy. *Current Opinion in Nephrology and Hypertension, 3,* 155–163.

Rodriguez-Iturbe, B., Baggio, B., Colina-Chourio, J., et al. (1981). Studies on the renin-aldosterone system in the acute nephritic syndrome. *Kidney International, 19*(3):445–453.

Rostoker, G., Durand-Zaleski, I., Petit-Phar, M., et al. (1995). Prevention of thrombotic complications of the nephrotic syndrome by low-molecular-weight heparin enoxapirin. *Nephron, 69*(1):20–28.

Rudberg, S., Perrson, B., & Dahlquist, G. (1992). Increased glomerular filtration rate as a predictor of diabetic nephropathy: An eight-year prospective study. *Kidney International, 41,* 822–828.

Schiepatti, A., Mosconi, L., Perna, A., et al. (1993). Prognosis of untreated patients with idiopathic membranous nephropathy. *N Engl J Med, 329*(2):85–89.

Shayman, J.A. (1995). *Renal pathophysiology.* Philadelphia: J.B. Lippincott, pp. 93–116.

Sixth Report on the Joint Committee on Detection, Evaluation and Treatment of High Blood Pressure (JNC VI). (1997). National Institute of Health Publication Number 98-4080.

Smith, D., Hyneck, M.L., Berardi, R.R., et al. (19985). Urinary protein binding kinetics and dynamics of furosemide in nephrotic patients. *Journal of Pharmacy Science, 74*(6):603–607.

Spika, J.S., Halsey, N.A., Le, C.T., et al. (1986). Decline of vaccine-induced antipneumococcal antibody in children with nephrotic syndrome. *American Journal of Kidney Disease, 7*(6):466–470.

Stockigt, J., Topliss, D., & Hewett, M. (1979). High-renin hypertension in necrotizing vasculitis. *N Engl J Med, 300,* 1218.

Valeri, A., Gelfand, J., Blum, C., et al. (1986). Treatment of hyperlipidemia of the nephrotic syndrome: A controlled trial. *American Journal of Kidney Disease, 8*(6):388–396.

Vijan, S., Stevens, D.L., Herman, W.H., et al. (1997). Screening, prevention, counseling, and treatment for the complications of type II diabetes mellitus: Putting evidence into practice. *Journal of General Internal Medicine, 12*(9):567–580.

33

Renal Tumors

B. Mayer Grob, MD

Benign and malignant renal tumors are often diagnosed in the workup of hematuria. In addition, incidental renal masses are frequently seen in the evaluation of nonurologic abnormalities on sonograms, computed tomography (CT) scanning, and magnetic resonance imaging (MRI). The primary care provider should be acquainted with the appropriate evaluation and treatment of the common renal neoplasms. Working together with the urologist, these problems can usually be managed successfully.

OVERVIEW OF RENAL TUMORS

Diagnostic Criteria

Although the number of renal masses detected incidentally is increasing, many are still found in the workup of hematuria. The definition of hematuria is not completely clear. Excretion rates of red blood cells (RBC) for normal persons is 500,000 to 1 million per 12 hours. The semiquantitative method of counting the number of cells per high-power field of urine sediment has been shown to correlate well with the 12-hour excretion rates. Ninety percent of normal persons have less than 1 RBC per high-power field, and 97% have less than 5 RBCs per high-power field of urine sediment (Larcom, 1948). There is no universally accepted standard amount of microscopic hematuria that should prompt a full evaluation. Some providers believe that 1 RBC per high-power field is abnormal enough to initiate a workup, but almost all would agree that a urinalysis showing more than 5 RBCs should be evaluated further. Hematuria in the presence of significant proteinuria, however, is often attributable to glomerular disease, and a urologic evaluation is not usually necessary. It may be more reasonable to refer the patient to a nephrologist.

History and Physical Exam

A complete history and physical exam are part of any hematuria workup. The precise nature of the hematuria should be elucidated. Hematuria accompanied by pain, either in the flank or the pelvis, may be an indication of stone disease. Pain from stone disease is often colicky and of sudden onset compared to pain from a slowly growing mass. Fever may be an indication of an infection, possibly pyelonephritis. Pyuria is significant in almost all cases, and hematuria, without pyuria, should not be attributed to infection. The passage of blood clots can sometimes help to localize the site of bleeding to the upper tracts—long and string-like versus more clumped (bladder). Recent trauma may be readily apparent in some patients, but hematuria secondary to apparently trivial trauma may indicate a condition such as a ureteropelvic junction obstruction. Recent

strenuous physical exercise is sometimes associated with hematuria as well. A past history of urologic conditions or procedures is obviously important. A family history of urologic disease may be crucial because some cases of renal cell carcinoma (RCC) are familial, with and without von Hippel-Lindau (VHL) disease. Occupational exposures to the rubber and dye industry are particularly relevant to transitional cell carcinoma (TCC), and a social history, including cigarette use, is important.

A thorough exam of the flank, abdomen, and genitalia should be included in the physical. Any unusual mass should be carefully characterized. Adenopathy is an ominous sign.

Diagnostic Studies

Urinary exfoliative cytology is also important in the workup of hematuria. TCC, whether of the bladder or upper urinary tract, has a loosely coherent outer layer. These are the cells that are often identified on a urinary cytology. Bladder cancers are much more common than renal tumors. Although a negative result on cytology does not rule out bladder cancer, a positive cytology result often helps direct the course of therapy. In addition, because some renal TCCs are difficult to distinguish from RCC, a positive cytology result can shift the treatment plan for renal tumors; as will be described later, the surgical approach for renal TCC is different from that for RCC.

Two new urine tests have recently become available in the evaluation of hematuria. The Bard BTA-stat (bladder tumor-associated analyte) and the Matritech NMP22 (nuclear matrix protein) (Sarosdy, 1995; Soloway, 1996) urine tests identify unique markers in the urine of patients with bladder cancer. Although their role has not clearly been defined, these tests may be particularly helpful in following patients with bladder cancer. They are mentioned here for completeness in the diagnostic criteria for hematuria. Whether either will play a role in the evaluation of upper tract TCC is not known at the time of this writing.

Intravenous urography (IVU) remains the initial imaging study of choice for most patients in the workup of hematuria. Ultrasonography (US) is an excellent test to differentiate solid from cystic lesions of the kidney; however, US alone is not sensitive enough to identify most urothelial tumors, specifically TCC of the renal pelvis or ureter. Masses seen on US that meet the strict criteria for a simple cyst need no further evaluation. These criteria include a fluid-filled mass with a distinct posterior wall and acoustic enhancement, without calcification, septation, or nodularity. In some cases, US may not confirm the existence of a mass seen initially on IVU; a CT scan should then be obtained with and without contrast to take advantage of the vascular nature of most RCCs. In patients allergic to contrast media and unwilling to accept intravenous contrast after steroid preparation, and in patients with marginal renal function, an MRI with gadolinium is also an excellent test in the evaluation of renal masses. Renal angiography is seldom necessary today, although in the past it was often used to clarify an abnormal IVU. Angiography is sometimes helpful in preparation for a partial nephrectomy, especially in a patient with a solitary kidney or multiple renal masses.

Imaging studies provide information about the kidneys and ureters but cannot adequately assess the bladder. Large bladder tumors are sometimes seen on an IVU or CT scan, but smaller tumors and carcinoma in situ are not reliably detected on any imaging test. Cystoscopy is necessary to complete the hematuria workup. This can often be performed in the urologist's office or an ambulatory surgery center. If the result of the urine cytology is positive, or if an abnormality is detected on upper tract imaging studies, the cystoscopy may be performed with anesthesia. This allows samples to be taken for bladder biopsy or ureteropyelography to be accomplished without patient discomfort.

SPECIFIC RENAL TUMORS

Benign Renal Neoplasms

RENAL ADENOMA

Anatomy, Physiology, and Pathology

The classification "renal adenoma" is controversial. It may be possible to distinguish an RCC from a renal adenoma based on nuclear and cytoplasmic criteria, but there are no reliable gross, microscopic, or ultrastructural differences between the two lesions. Previously, size alone was the standard criteria. This was based on the autopsy study by Bell (1950), demonstrating that renal lesions smaller than 3 cm rarely metastasized, whereas almost 70% of lesions greater than 3 cm had metastasized. There are, however, several reports of lesions as small as 5 mm with metastases. Small, solid renal masses that enhance with intravenous contrast are probably small RCCs.

One recent study of several thousand autopsy and surgical specimens described two distinct histologic types of adenomas (Faria, 1994). Adenomas with a papillary or tubulopapillary pattern are more common, are smaller, are frequently multiple, and probably are not precursors of RCC. They are usually composed of basophilic or oncocytic cells. Adenomas with a solid or papillary pattern are frequently solitary, are larger, and may be a morphologic precursor of RCC. They are often composed of clear cells.

Epidemiology

In autopsy series, renal adenomas have been found in about 20% of cases (Bonsib, 1985). In large screening ultrasound series, however, the clinical detection rate is much less than 1%. The male/female ratio is 3:1. Certain diseases have a significantly higher incidence of adenomas. Patients with VHL disease have a tendency to develop renal cysts and solid renal tumors. Some of these may be adenomas, but there is an association with potentially lethal RCC as well. Patients with acquired renal cystic disease on dialysis for end-stage renal disease are also prone to develop small but potentially metastatic renal tumors. These have historically been labeled adenomas but are probably small RCCs.

Treatment Options, Expected Outcomes, and Comprehensive Management

Most small adenomas are asymptomatic. They are detected incidentally on CT or US during the workup for an unrelated medical problem. Rarely, they can present as a source of bleeding. Even larger adenomas are usually discovered incidentally, but they are more likely to present with symptoms referable to the urinary tract. Flank pain and hematuria have been associated with larger adenomas.

Renal adenomas appear as solid masses on IVU. They cannot be distinguished from RCC by imaging techniques, and most urologists think these tumors should be treated as if they were RCCs. How should these small RCCs or renal adenomas be managed? Although the standard therapeutic approach for RCC remains radical nephrectomy, there is growing interest in the use of partial nephrectomy, especially for incidentally discovered lesions. In select cases, it may even be reasonable to observe small tumors. A recent report by Bosniak et al (1995) showed that for lesions less than 3 cm at diagnosis, and followed for at least 2 years, no metastases were clinically detectable. The majority of patients eventually went on to have surgery, and none developed metastases. This "watchful waiting" approach may be acceptable for an elderly patient with other significant medical problems, but it should be undertaken in consultation with a urologist. It is certainly not to be suggested in the young and otherwise healthy patient, because small renal tumors do grow and do have the capacity to metastasize.

RENAL ONCOCYTOMA

Anatomy, Physiology, and Pathology

Grossly, oncocytomas are well-circumscribed tumors with a characteristic mahogany color. A large stellate central scar is often seen. Hemorrhage and necrosis are typically absent. Microscopically, the tumor is composed of large well-differentiated cells with intensely eosinophilic cytoplasm. These oncocytes rarely exhibit mitoses.

Epidemiology

Oncocytomas account for 3% to 14% of all renal tumors. The male/female ratio is 2:1. They are usually solitary, and the peak age of incidence is 55 years. They are occasionally found in the same kidney with RCC, on rare occasions within the same lesion.

Treatment Options, Expected Outcomes, and Comprehensive Management

Approximately 70% of oncocytomas are detected incidentally. The remainder present with complaints referable to the genitourinary system. Hematuria, flank pain, and a flank mass are the typical symptoms. Oncocytomas appear as solid masses on IVU or US. They cannot be distinguished from RCC on radiologic grounds. A central scar seen on CT or a "spoke-wheel" appearance on angiography may suggest an oncocytoma, but there is simply no reliable method to rule out RCC preoperatively.

Pure oncocytomas are benign lesions. However, because there is no reliable clinical method to differentiate oncocytomas from RCCs, they are usually treated as RCCs and managed with nephrectomy. As is the case for renal adenomas, small incidentally discovered lesions suggestive of oncocytoma may be treated successfully with a partial nephrectomy. This scenario is not an indication for a percutaneous renal biopsy. Because of the occasional occurrence of oncocytoma and RCC in the same lesion, and because some RCCs have oncocytic features, the diagnosis of oncocytoma cannot be made with a small sampling of tissue.

ANGIOMYOLIPOMA

Anatomy, Physiology, and Pathology

The gross appearance is determined by the relative amounts of the various cellular components. If the lesion is composed predominantly of fat, it will have a homogeneous yellowish appearance, but all three cell types must be present to establish the diagnosis. The lesion will be more heterogeneous if there is an even distribution of fat, muscle, and vessels. Calcification and necrosis are rare, but hemorrhage is frequent.

Epidemiology

Hamartomas are neoplastic masses of disorganized cells or tissue normally seen in a particular organ. The most familiar renal hamartoma is the angiomyolipoma, named for the three components observed in this lesion: blood vessels, smooth muscle, and fat. These tumors are particularly interesting because they are the only benign renal masses that can be reliably diagnosed radiographically.

Angiomyolipomas are seen in two distinct clinical settings: sporadic and in association with tuberous sclerosis. The sporadic form accounts for more than 80% of cases. It is more common in women, with a ratio of 4:1, and the mean age is 43 years. Tuberous sclerosis is a congenital and familial disorder characterized by brain gliosis, mental retardation, epilepsy, adenoma sebaceum, and hamartomas of the retina, lungs, liver, pancreas, bone, and kidneys. Angiomyolipomas associated with tuberous sclerosis present as larger lesions, at a younger age, and are more likely to be symptomatic and require surgical intervention.

Treatment Options, Expected Outcome, and Comprehensive Management

Plain radiographs occasionally show lucent areas within large angiomyolipomas, suggesting the diagnosis, but typically the IVU demonstrates an expansile mass that cannot be distinguished from RCC. On US, they are usually more echogenic than surrounding parenchyma. They share this feature with about one third of RCCs, however. With the development of high-quality CT scanning, it was realized that the detection of fat within a renal lesion allows confident preoperative diagnosis and the potential to avoid surgery in most cases that are not symptomatic (Fig. 33-1).

The most common presentation is incidental discovery during imaging for other medical conditions. Patients may present with acute flank pain with or without spontaneous hemorrhage. Occasionally, the onset of symptoms is preceded by seemingly trivial trauma. The blood vessels of angiomyolipoma lack a complete elastic layer, predisposing these lesions to aneurysm formation and bleeding. Steiner et al demonstrated that lesions less than 4 cm rarely become symptomatic, whereas lesions greater than 4 cm require surgical intervention in about half the cases for bleeding (Steiner, 1993).

When the CT scan is unequivocal and the patient is asymptomatic, no intervention is required for small angiomyolipomas. In cases where the diagnosis is in question, exploration and partial or radical nephrectomy may be necessary. Symptomatic

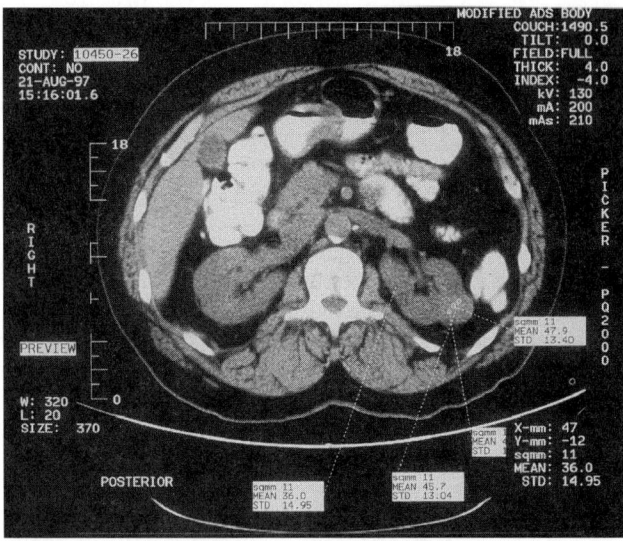

A

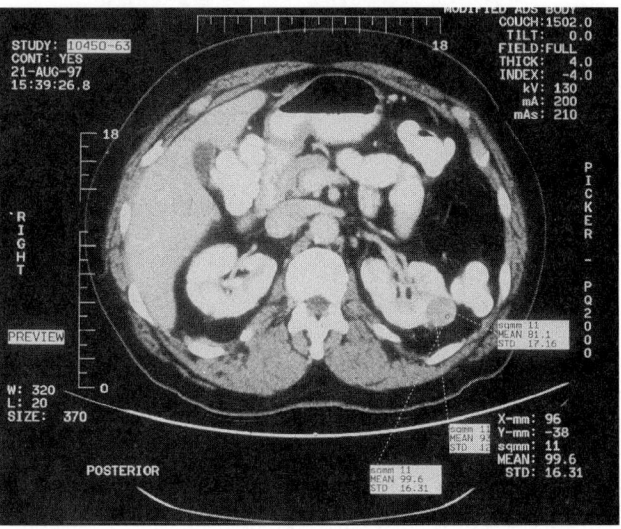

B

FIGURE 33-1 Pre- and post-contrast injection CT scan demonstrating increased enhancement measured in Hounsfield units of hypervascular renal mass. A partial nephroctomy was performed, revealing renal cell carcinoma.

patients with angiomyolipomas can often be treated successfully with percutaneous angioinfarction (Table 33-1).

Malignant Renal Neoplasms

RENAL CELL CARCINOMA

Anatomy, Physiology, and Pathology

The origin of RCC is the renal cortex. Grossly, the tumors are often yellow or orange because of the abundance of fat seen in the clear cell variant. The clear cytoplasm observed by light microscopy of the clear cell variety is caused by removal of glycogen and lipids during histologic processing. The granular type is usually more white to gray. The sarcomatoid cell type is less frequently seen. Usually there is a mixed picture. As RCC grows, it compresses the normal parenchyma, forming a pseudocapsule. RCC has a propensity for invasion into vascular

TABLE 33-1	Benign Renal Neoplasms		
Tumor Type	**Epidemiology**	**X-Ray Criteria**	**Noteworthy**
Renal adenoma	M:F = 3:1; von Hippel-Lindau association	Small, enhancing, solid mass	Probably a small RCC
Oncocytoma	M:F = 2:1	Central scar, spoke-wheel appearance	Cannot be distinguished from RCC clinically
Angiomyolipoma	F:M = 4:1; tuberous sclerosis association	Fat density on CT is diagnostic	>4 cm usually require surgery

spaces, including the renal vein, inferior vena cava, and occasionally even the right atrium.

Histologic grading of RCC cells has been used with variable success to predict the clinical behavior of these tumors. Compared to pathologic stage, no additional prognostic information has been consistently obtained. Nuclear grade has recently become a more accepted prognostic factor. At the time of this writing, a new grading system is being evaluated by a multi-institutional panel of pathologists and will be available soon to assist in prognosis.

Epidemiology

RCC accounts for 85% of all renal parenchymal cancers and represents 2% to 3% of all adult malignancies. RCC has been designated by many terms, including hypernephroma, Grawitz' tumor, and nephrocarcinoma. There were approximately 30,000 new cases in 1996, resulting in 12,000 deaths (Franklin, 1996). It occurs most commonly in the fifth to sixth decade, although it has been reported in children and young adults. The male/female ratio is 2:1. Recent advances in imaging have led to increased incidental detection of RCC and improved prognosis of patients with such tumors.

Most cases of RCC are sporadic in nature. However, it has been shown that in rare familial cases and in RCC associated with VHL disease, loss of tumor suppressor gene activity, particularly at the VHL locus on chromosome 3p, may be responsible for tumorigenesis (Franklin, 1996).

No clear understanding of how environmental and genetic factors interact in the pathogenesis of RCC has been determined. Two strong cases for environmental exposure are cigarette smoking and phenacetin-containing analgesic abuse. There is a dose-related risk of developing RCC in cigarette smokers (approximately a twofold increase). An increased risk has also been reported in shoe workers, leather tanners, and workers exposed to cadmium, petroleum products, and asbestos.

Treatment Options, Expected Outcomes, and Comprehensive Management

The classic triad of hematuria, pain, and palpable flank mass occurs in only 10% of cases. More commonly, a patient will present with one or two of these symptoms. Other symptoms may be associated with paraneoplastic syndromes from elaboration of various humoral factors. Stauffer's syndrome (abnormal liver enzymes), hypercalcemia, polycythemia, and hypertension are the best known of these. These findings do not imply metastatic disease.

The most common test to evaluate extent of disease is the CT scan. RCC is seen as a solid lesion that enhances after intravenous contrast administration. An increase in Hounsfield units of at least 20 is considered positive enhancement. Ten to 20 units of enhancement are considered intermediate and inconclusive. Approximately 10% of RCCs are hypovascular, however, and will not enhance with intravenous contrast (Gillenwater, 1996).

When involvement of the vena cava by tumor thrombus is in question, an MRI is often helpful. Occasionally, a cavogram or transesophageal US is necessary to determine the exact location of a tumor thrombus in the vena cava. Knowledge of the superior extent of the thrombus is crucial for planning the surgical approach. Even patients with tumor in the right atrium can be cured of RCC with a radical nephrectomy and thrombectomy, although the potential morbidity and mortality rates of the procedure are certainly higher in this setting.

Tumor stage is recognized as the most important prognostic factor in RCC (Table 33-2). The two systems in use are the Robson and the TNM classification. The Robson system includes renal vein, vena cava, and lymphatic involvement in stage III. The key difference in the TNM system of the International Union Against Cancer (UICC) is the attention paid to the size of the primary and the separate designation for lymphatic involvement. The 2.5-cm cutoff for stage II tumors is controversial, however, and was revised in 1997. The new cutoff is 7 cm.

Surgical excision remains the standard therapy for clinically organ-confined RCC. Radical nephrectomy entails en bloc removal of the kidney and its enveloping fascia (Gerota's). The classic radical nephrectomy includes the ipsilateral adrenal gland as well. However, recent studies have shown a very low involvement of the adrenal. Thus, adrenalectomy has fallen out of favor for all but large upper pole lesions, which may be more likely to involve the adrenal by direct extension. Regional lymphadenectomy is often performed, but there are no controlled studies that demonstrate improved survival with this additional procedure. The main value of removing the lymph nodes may be in more accurate staging, which can lead to participation in appropriate clinical trials.

Partial nephrectomy or nephron-sparing surgery implies removal of the tumor while leaving enough functional parenchyma to support life without dialysis in the event that the other kidney is already absent or lost in the future. A partial nephrectomy is often performed in a patient with impaired renal function or a patient with bilateral renal tumors. The size and location of the tumor are crucial determinants of whether a partial nephrectomy can be attempted. Because of the increase in the number of smaller, incidentally discovered renal masses, interest has grown in the use of partial nephrectomy even in patients with normal renal function and a normal contralateral kidney. Early results using this approach in a series by Herr

TABLE 33-2	Comparison of the TNM Staging System With the Robson System for RCC

ROBSON

Stage 1	Confined to the kidney
Stage 2	Perirenal fat or adrenal involvement but confined to Gerota's fascia
Stage 3	A. Renal vein or inferior vena cava involvement B. Lymphatic involvement C. Vascular and lymphatic involvement
Stage 4	A. Adjacent organs B. Distant metastases

TNM

Primary Tumor (T)

TX	Primary tumor cannot be assessed
T0	No evidence of primary tumor
T1	Tumor ≤7 cm in greatest diameter and confined to kidney
T2	Tumor >7 cm in greatest diameter and confined to kidney
T3a	Tumor invades adrenal or perirenal fat, but confined to Gerota's fascia
T3b	Tumor grossly involves renal vein or subdiaphragmatic inferior vena cava
T3c	Tumor involves inferior vena cava above the diaphragm
T4	Tumor invades beyond Gerota's fascia

Lymph Node (N)

NX	Regional lymph node status cannot be assessed
N0	No regional lymph node involvement
N1	Metastasis in a single node, ≤2 cm in greatest dimension
N2	Metastasis in a single node, >2 cm but ≤5 cm in greatest dimension, or multiple nodes ≤5 cm in greatest dimension
N3	Metastasis in node(s) >5 cm in greatest dimension

Distant Metastasis (M)

MX	Status of distant metastasis cannot be assessed
M0	No distant metastasis
M1	Distant metastasis present

(1994) are excellent, with survival of about 95% and acceptable local recurrence rates of about 2%.

About 30% of patients with RCC show distant metastases at the time of diagnosis (Franklin, 1996). There is a great need for effective systemic therapy for these patients, but currently such treatment is lacking. Cytotoxic chemotherapy with agents such as vinblastine shows an objective response rate of up to 15%, but durable responses are rare. Some RCCs are hormonally responsive, but objective remissions are seen in less than 5% of cases.

Immunotherapy with biologic response modifiers has been the most promising approach in the last 5 to 10 years. The three agents that have shown the most efficacy are interferon (IFN), interleukin-2 (IL-2), and lymphokine-activated killer (LAK) cells. The first IFN to show efficacy against metastatic RCC was IFN-alpha. On average, the various studies show a remission rate of about 14%, but the range of responses varies widely, from 0% to almost 40% (Wirth, 1993). This variability is most likely caused by patient selection. The other IFNs have shown a similar range of responses. IFN-alpha has occasionally been combined with the most effective cytotoxic agent vinblas-

tine, but the results were not significantly better than with IFN-alpha alone, and the side effects were substantially increased. IL-2 has also been studied extensively in RCC. Early results as a single agent were promising, but the most recent data show somewhat less efficacy than IFN-alpha as monotherapy. IL-2 has been combined with other agents. Lymphocytes isolated from peripheral blood and incubated in vitro with IL-2 are stimulated to become LAK cells. These LAK cells can destroy human tumor cells. When given in combination with IL-2, objective response rates of 30% have been obtained. This treatment is associated with significant side effects, however. Because follow-up studies have not confirmed the initial results, other effective treatments are still needed.

The issue of nephrectomy before immunotherapy for metastatic RCC is a controversial one. Several studies have reported improved survival rates in patients who undergo preimmunotherapy nephrectomy to reduce the tumor burden. However, there is no way to account for selection bias in these series. It is likely that patients who were thought to have a better chance to survive surgery, because of a better performance status, were offered nephrectomy, whereas those in poor medical condition were not. A randomized study is necessary to prove the benefit of a debulking nephrectomy before immunotherapy. Such a trial in the Southwest Oncology Group is nearing completion.

Resection of all metastatic disease in conjunction with nephrectomy has also been shown to be associated with prolonged survival in patients with widespread disease. Once again, it is difficult to account for selection bias and the natural history of the disease.

CARCINOMA OF THE RENAL COLLECTING SYSTEM AND PELVIS
Anatomy, Physiology, and Pathology
More than 90% of upper tract urothelial tumors are TCC. Most of these are papillary in configuration. Papillomas of the upper tract are single, delicately branching, fern-like tumors. They are covered by cytologically benign epithelium resembling normal urothelium and are not thought to have the capacity to invade or metastasize. Papillary carcinomas are usually broad-based and the urothelium is hyperplastic. The epithelial cells have lost their orientation and uniformity. The outer layers are only loosely coherent, which explains the increased likelihood of a positive result on urinary cytology. Squamous carcinoma of the renal urothelium accounts for 5% to 10% of cases and is usually associated with chronic inflammation secondary to indwelling catheters or stone disease (Melamed, 1993). Grossly, squamous carcinoma is nonpapillary, poorly circumscribed, and infiltrating. The tumors typically have areas of keratinization. They are highly aggressive tumors and are usually detected at a late stage. Adenocarcinomas are rare, accounting for 1% or less of tumors of the upper tract. Metastatic carcinoma must be ruled out before accepting this diagnosis. These tumors are also found at higher stages, and these patients have a uniformly poor prognosis.

Epidemiology
Cancer of the urothelium of the upper urinary tract accounts for 5% to 10% of all renal tumors but only about 5% of all urothelial tumors (Melamed, 1993). Bladder cancer is much more common, representing 90% of such lesions. Renal urothelial tumors have a peak incidence in the sixth to seventh decade and occur three times more commonly in men than women.

The etiology of upper tract urothelial cancer is unknown but is probably similar to that of bladder cancer. Environmental factors thought to be significant include cigarette smoking and exposure to chemicals used in the rubber and textile industries. Long-term exposure to phenacetin has been implicated in some cases of urothelial cancer of the renal pelvis. Chronic urinary tract infections over many years and urolithiasis may play a role, particularly in the etiology of the squamous cell variety. Inhabitants of the Balkan countries (Bulgaria, Greece, Rumania, and the former Yugoslavia) are at risk for developing a particular type of nephropathy that is associated with cancers of the renal pelvis. This Balkan nephropathy accounts for more than 40% of the renal cancers in these countries. These tumors are often bilateral and less biologically aggressive (Gillenwater, 1996).

Upper tract urothelial tumors can occur in patients with a prior history of bladder carcinoma, although the reverse is much more common. Among all patients with prior TCC of the bladder, 2% to 4% will develop malignancies of the kidney or ureter. Bladder cancer patients who have required intravesical chemotherapy or immunotherapy, such as bacillus Calmette-Guerin, are at much higher risk, however, with as many as 15% to 20% developing upper tract TCC. Roughly 40% of patients with initial upper tract tumors will subsequently develop bladder cancer.

Treatment Options, Expected Outcomes, and Comprehensive Management

There are no characteristic clinical features of renal urothelial cancer. Microscopic or gross hematuria occurs in 60% to 75% of cases. Flank pain occurs in roughly one third of patients and is usually a dull ache; with the passage of clots, however, it can be acute and more intense.

Cystoscopy is particularly helpful during active bleeding to localize the site and to rule out a synchronous bladder cancer. Often blood and clots can be seen effluxing from one of the ureteral orifices. IVU demonstrates an abnormal filling defect in 50% to 75% of cases (Gillenwater, 1996). Filling defects may also be seen with stones, fungus balls, blood clots, and sloughed papillae.

Often an IVU will not completely clarify the issue, and a retrograde ureteropyelogram will be performed. This requires the use of contrast media, which is injected up the ureter from the ureteral orifice cystoscopically. With the recent improvements in optics and working instruments, direct vision of the lesion can usually be accomplished with either rigid or flexible ureteroscopy. Then a biopsy or brushing cytology sample can be obtained. With all these recent advances, it may still be impossible to make a pathologic diagnosis preoperatively. Based on the judgment of the urologist, the kidney may have to be removed.

Tumor stage is the single most important prognostic factor for carcinoma of the renal urothelium. The prognosis of patients with invasive tumors that have not penetrated the wall of the pelvis is excellent. Extension into perirenal or peripelvic soft tissue carries a dismal prognosis. The UICC staging system for renal pelvic tumors is closely modeled after the system for bladder cancer. The system proposed by Grabstald and others has largely been replaced by the UICC system (Table 33-3).

The standard treatment for TCC of the renal pelvis and ureter is nephroureterectomy. The kidney and the entire length

TABLE 33-3	Comparison of Grabstald and TNM Staging Systems for Renal Pelvic Tumors
GRABSTALD	
Stage O	Noninvasive
Stage A	Superficially invasive
Stage B	Deeply invasive but not though kidney or renal pelvis
Stage C	Invasion into perirenal or peripelvic tissue
TNM	
Primary Tumor (T)	
TX	Primary tumor cannot be assessed
T0	No evidence of primary tumor
Tis	Carcinoma in situ
Ta	Noninvasive papillary tumor
T1	Tumor invades lamina propria
T2	Tumor invades muscularis propria
T3	Tumor invades renal parenchyma or peripelvic fat
T4	Tumor invades into perinephric fat
Lymph Node (N)	
NX	Regional lymph node status cannot be assessed
N0	No regional lymph node involvement
N1	Metastasis in a single node ≤2 cm in greatest dimension
N2	Metastasis in a single node >2 cm but ≤5 cm in greatest dimension or multiple nodes ≤5 cm
N3	Metastasis in node(s) >5 cm in greatest dimension
Distant Metastasis (M)	
MX	Distant metastasis cannot be assessed
M0	No distant metastasis
M1	Distant metastasis present

of ureter are removed. A separate incision is often required to open the bladder and excise the intramural portion of the ureter with a cuff of normal bladder tissue. In a radical nephrectomy for RCC, only the proximal portion of the ureter is removed. A regional lymphadenectomy is often performed, mainly to assist in staging. If the tumor has spread to regional nodes, adjuvant chemotherapy is often recommended, although there are little data to support its use in this setting. In a patient with a solitary kidney or renal insufficiency, a more conservative approach may be warranted, especially for lesions that appear to be of low stage and low grade. Tumors can be resected ureteroscopically or ablated with a laser fiber through either a rigid or flexible ureteroscope. Percutaneous approaches have also been used, but these carry a risk of seeding the tract. Conservative measures are gaining acceptance even for patients with normal renal function, but the standard treatment for upper tract TCC remains nephroureterectomy.

Patients with metastatic TCC from the renal urothelium have a poor prognosis. Protocols originally designed for advanced bladder carcinoma are often used in upper tract TCC. The most successful regimen against advanced TCC of the bladder combines methotrexate, vinblastine, doxorubicin (Adriamycin), and cisplatin (M-VAC). Some protocols do not use doxorubicin. Combined partial and complete response rates are about 50% in bladder carcinoma, but the durable complete responses are uncommon. New agents are desperately needed for these patients. Ifosfamide, gallium nitrate, and paclitaxel (Taxol) are currently under investigation, either alone or in combination, and offer the most promise.

RENAL SARCOMA
Epidemiology
Primary sarcoma of the kidney is a rare entity, representing 1% of all renal malignant tumors.

Treatment Options, Expected Outcome, and Comprehensive Management
The treatment of renal sarcoma is nephrectomy with a wide margin of normal tissue. Complete surgical resection is recognized as an important prognostic factor, and resection of adjacent organs is often required. Tumor grade is also an important prognostic factor. Patients with high-grade lesions tend to have a more unfavorable disease-free survival than those with lower-grade tumors. Although tumor size has been thought to be important in other sites, the average renal sarcoma is greater than 10 cm, so size is less of a factor. Renal sarcomas have a poorer prognosis than sarcomas at other sites not in the retroperitoneum, probably because of the space for growth of the tumor and lack of symptoms until late in the course. The use of adjuvant irradiation therapy or chemotherapy in the treatment of renal sarcomas remains unproved.

Pain and palpable mass are the most common presenting symptoms, but diagnosis is often delayed until the tumors are quite large. Gross hematuria is variably present. There are no distinguishing characteristics, making the distinction between sarcoma and RCC difficult preoperatively. The most common histologic tumor type is leiomyosarcoma, followed by liposarcoma, hemangiopericytoma, rhabdomyosarcoma, and osteogenic sarcoma, in descending order of frequency.

ADULT WILMS' TUMOR
Anatomy, Physiology, and Pathology
Wilms' tumor or nephroblastoma is the most common renal malignancy of childhood. Seventy-five percent of cases are seen before age 5. However, this lesion can be seen in adolescents and adults.

Epidemiology
Patients typically present with abdominal masses, flank pain, or hematuria. On IVU, a focal renal mass may be observed, or the affected kidney may not visualize because of renal vein occlusion, ureteral obstruction, or replacement of the parenchyma by the tumor. Calcification is common. CT is often helpful in determining the local extent of the tumor. Wilms' tumor in adults is usually hypovascular, but there are no radiologic criteria to distinguish adult Wilms' from a hypovascular RCC. Therefore, the diagnosis is rarely made before surgery.

Treatment Options, Expected Outcome, and Comprehensive Management
Although survival in children has increased to about 90%, the prognosis in adults remains less favorable. This is true even when the disease is compared on a stage-for-stage basis (Hentrich, 1995). Because adult Wilms' tumor is so rare, randomized trials cannot be performed. There is no standard treatment as there is in children. In children, after nephrectomy, adjuvant

chemotherapy alone is recommended for low-stage lesions and favorable histology. Irradiation therapy is added for patients with higher-stage tumors or poor histology. Many authors argue that multimodal treatment is necessary for adults regardless of stage. All adult cases of Wilms' tumor should be reported to the National Wilms' Tumor Study.

Tumors of hematologic origin often involve the kidney, but they infrequently cause symptoms indicating their presence. Renal involvement is most commonly a manifestation of systemic disease. In rare cases, no other site of disease is identified and the lymphoma, leukemia, or multiple myeloma appears to originate in the kidney. Suspicion of a primary hematologic malignancy involving the kidney is one of the rare instances when a percutaneous renal biopsy is warranted. More often the diagnosis of renal involvement is made in the setting of clinically apparent advanced hematologic disease, obviating the need for renal biopsy.

In older autopsy series, leukemia was found to infiltrate the kidney secondarily in nearly 70% of cases (Gillenwater, 1996). Involvement is usually bilateral and diffuse in the renal cortex. Focal accumulations of leukemic cells may also occur. Although IVU and CT scans may show diffuse renal enlargement, radiologic evidence of leukemic involvement may be lacking. Treatment is directed at the primary disease process and usually entails chemotherapy and occasionally irradiation therapy.

Involvement of the kidney with lymphoma has been reported in 36% of patients before effective chemotherapy (Colevas, 1996). The incidence is higher in patients with non-Hodgkin's lymphoma than in those with Hodgkin's disease. Involvement may occur as multiple nodules, diffuse infiltration, extension from lymphatics, or rarely as a solitary mass. Extranodal lymphoma limited to the kidney is so rare as a presenting diagnosis that some have challenged the existence of such an entity. CT is probably the most accurate method of assessment, although MRI is also useful. The mainstay of treatment is systemic multidrug chemotherapy. Irradiation therapy is sometimes used, especially in cases of bulky disease with a high risk of relapse.

Plasma cell infiltration of the kidneys is seen occasionally in patients with multiple myeloma, but solitary plasmacytomas without other evidence of disease are exceedingly rare. If there are no abnormal blood or urine findings, distinction from RCC is usually not possible. More commonly, myeloma causes renal disease secondary to tubular precipitation of myeloma proteins. Chemotherapy is the standard treatment.

SECONDARY MALIGNANCIES
Epidemiology
Renal metastases occur more frequently than primary renal neoplasms in autopsy series. These lesions rarely become symptomatic because of their small size and the brief survival of most of these patients. With the increased use of CT scanning to stage other primary malignancies, renal metastases are being diagnosed more commonly. Lung, breast, and pancreas are the most common primary tumors that produce renal metastases.

Anatomy, Physiology, and Pathology
Metastatic lesions are not typically vascular; therefore, significant contrast enhancement is not often encountered on CT. Large lesions may show irregular, diminished attenuation cen-

TABLE 33-4	Malignant Renal Neoplasms		
Tumor Type	Epidemiology	X-Ray Criteria	Noteworthy
RCC	M:F = 2:1	Enhancing, solid renal mass	Surgery is only effective curative treatment
TCC	M:F = 3:1	Filling defect on IVU	Surgery is primary; some respond to chemo
Sarcoma	Rare, <1% renal malignancies	Difficult to distinguish from RCC	Resection of adjacent organs often required
Adult Wilms' tumor	Rare	Usually hypovascular	Poor prognosis, unlike pediatric Wilms'
Renal lymphoma	Rarely, if ever, primary in the kidney	Usually infiltrative, not a solid mass	Chemo is primary
Metastatic tumor	Lung, breast, and pancreas are most common primaries	Usually hypovascular with areas of necrosis	May be a rare indication for a percutaneous biopsy

trally, suggestive of necrosis. The presence of multiple renal masses in the setting of a known primary with other metastatic sites strongly suggests metastatic disease. Even a solitary renal mass in a patient with known metastatic disease from another primary can be assumed to be metastasis, and pathologic proof is rarely needed. The treatment of a patient with a solitary renal mass and a history of cancer with no known metastasis is more controversial. If the lesion is radiologically suspicious for RCC, it should probably be treated as such. If the CT shows areas of necrosis often seen in metastatic disease, without contrast enhancement, a biopsy may be useful to establish the diagnosis with certainty before surgical exploration (Table 33-4).

TEACHING AND SELF-CARE

Educating patients about renal masses is similar to educating patients about any oncologic diagnosis. Patients should be informed of the prognosis and treatment options for the specific type of tumor diagnosed. Patients should also participate in a discussion regarding the tolerability of the available chemotherapeutic agents and testing procedures before they are instituted.

COMMUNITY RESOURCES

- National Kidney Foundation, 30 E. 33d St., New York City, NY 10016, 800-622-9010
- American Kidney Fund, 6110 Executive Blvd., Rockville, MD 20852, 800-638-8299
- University of Pennsylvania Cancer Center, 3451 Walnut St., Philadelphia, PA 19104, 800-789-PENN
- www.healthtouch.com/level1/leaflets/
- www.ncifcrf.gov/kidney/
- oncolink.upenn.edu/disease/kidney/

■ CLINICAL WARNINGS:

- Hematuria, whether microscopic or gross, is a significant abnormality, even if it occurs only once. RBCs in the urine, in the absence of white blood cells, should not be attributed to a urinary tract infection, thereby delaying timely evaluation. Instead, after a full history and physical exam, urine should be sent for cytologic evaluation and

appropriate imaging studies should be performed. Urologic evaluation should then ensue.
- Once a renal mass has been detected, indications for a percutaneous needle biopsy are rare. This is generally a safe procedure, but there is a low but definite risk of morbidity. There is a small risk of seeding the tract, especially in TCC. More importantly, because of the significant chance of sampling error, the negative predictive value is unacceptably low. Therefore, there are only very select cases when a biopsy is indicated. These have been reviewed, but urologic consultation before needle biopsy of a suspicious renal mass is always warranted.

■ ■ ■ ■ CLINICAL PEARLS

- Although some providers believe that 1 RBC per high-power field is abnormal enough to initiate a workup, almost all would agree that a urinalysis showing more than 5 RBCs should be evaluated further.
- Small, solid renal masses that enhance with intravenous contrast are probably small RCCs.
- Although conservative measures are gaining acceptance even for patients with normal renal function, the standard treatment for upper tract TCC remains nephroureterectomy.
- Wilms' tumor in adults is usually hypovascular, but there are no radiologic criteria to distinguish adult Wilms' from a hypovascular RCC. Therefore, the diagnosis is rarely made before surgery.
- Tumors of hematologic origin often involve the kidney, but they infrequently cause symptoms indicating their presence. Renal involvement is most commonly a manifestation of systemic disease.
- Extranodal lymphoma limited to the kidney is so rare as a presenting diagnosis that some have challenged the existence of such an entity.
- Metastatic lesions are not typically vascular; therefore, significant contrast enhancement is not often encountered on CT.
- Even a solitary renal mass in a patient with known metastatic disease from another primary can be assumed to be metastasis, and pathologic proof is rarely needed.

References

Amin, M., Crotty, T., Tickoo, S., & Farrow, G. (1997). Renal oncocytoma: A reappraisal of morphologic features with clinicopathologic findings in 80 cases. *American Journal of Surgical Pathology, 21*(1), 1–12.

Bell, E. (1950). *Renal diseases.* Philadelphia: Lea & Febiger, p. 435.

Bonsib, S. (1985). Renal parenchymal tumors: A. Pathologic features. In *Genitourinary Oncology.* Philadelphia: Lea and Febiger, 185.

Bosniak, M. (1995). Observation of small incidentally detected renal masses. *Seminars in Urologic Oncology, 13*(4), 267–272.

Colevas, A., Kantoff, P., DeWolf, W., & Canellos, G. (1996). Malignant lymphoma of the genitourinary tract. In *Comprehensive textbook of genitourinary oncology.* Baltimore: Williams & Wilkins, pp. 1140–1151.

Faria, V., Reis, M., & Trigueiros, D. (1994). Renal adenoma: Identification of two histologic types. *European Urology, 26,* 170–175.

Franklin, J., Figlin, R., & Belldegrun, A. (1996). Renal cell carcinoma: Basic biology and clinical behavior. *Seminars in Urologic Oncology, 14*(4), 208–215.

Gillenwater, J., Grayhack, J., Howards, S., & Duckett, J. (Eds.). (1996). *Adult and pediatric urology.* Chicago: Year Book Medical Publishers.

Gold, P., Feter, A., & Thompson, J. (1996). Paraneoplastic manifestations of renal cell carcinoma. *Seminars in Urologic Oncology 14*(4), 216–222.

Guinan, P., Saffrin, R., Stuhldreher, D., Frank, W., & Rubenstein, M. (1995). Renal cell carcinoma: Comparison of the TNM and Robson stage groupings. *Journal of Surgical Oncology, 59,* 186–189.

Hentrich, M., Meister, P., Brack, N., Lutz, L., & Hartenstein, R. (1995). Adult Wilms' tumor: Report of two cases and review of the literature. *Cancer, 75*(2), 545–551.

Herr, H. (1994). Partial nephrectomy for incidental renal cell carcinoma. *British Journal of Urology, 74,* 431–433.

Larcom, R. & Carter G. (1948). Erythrocytes in urinary sediment: Identification and normal limits. *Journal of Laboratory and Clinical Medicine, 33,* 875.

Licht, M. (1995). Renal adenoma and oncocytoma. *Seminars in Urologic Oncology, 13*(4), 262–266.

Melamed, M., & Reuter, V. (1993). Pathology and staging of urothelial tumors of the kidney and ureter. *Urologic Clinics of North America, 20*(2), 333–347.

Pollack, E. (Ed.). (1990). *Clinical urography.* Philadelphia: W.B. Saunders.

Robey, E. & Schillhammer, P. (1986). The adrenal gland and renal cell carcinoma: Is ipsilateral adrenalectomy a necessary component of radical nephrectomy? *Journal of Urology, 135,* 453.

Sarosdy, M., DeVere White, R., Soloway, M., et al. (1995). Results of a multicenter trial using the BTA test to monitor for and diagnose recurrent bladder cancer. *Journal of Urology, 154,* 379–384.

Soloway, M., Briggman, J., Carpinito, G., et al. (1996). Use of a new tumor marker, urinary NMP22, in the detection of occult or rapidly recurring transitional cell carcinoma of the urinary tract following surgical treatment. *Journal of Urology, 156,* 363–367.

Spellman, J., Driscoll, D., & Huben, R. (1995). Primary renal sarcoma. *The American Surgeon, 61,* 456–459.

Steiner, M., Goldman S., Fishman, E., & Marshall F. (1993). The natural history of renal angiomyolipoma. *The Journal of Urology, 150,* 1782–6.

Wagner, B., Wong-You-Cheong, J., & Davis, Jr., C. (1997). Adult renal hamartomas. *Radiographics, 17,* 155–169.

Wirth, M. (1993). Immunotherapy for metastatic renal cell carcinoma. *Urologic Clinics of North America, 20*(2), 283–295.

CHAPTER
34

Urinary Incontinence

Elena M. Umland, Pharm.D.

Urinary incontinence (UI) is the involuntary loss of urine. It is not a disease, but rather a symptom of an underlying process. It is a symptom that may be significantly improved or cured in approximately 80% of affected patients (Maloney, 1995). Additionally, UI is not only a physical problem, but may also be debilitating psychosocially. It is associated with medical problems such as rashes, skin infections, pressure sores, and urinary tract infections. Psychosocial issues including depression, embarrassment, restricted social interaction, reduced activities outside the home, reduced sexual activity, and sleep disturbances may ensue (*MMWR*, 1995). Patients perceive UI as a very disturbing problem that restricts their activities, and the majority of these patients believe that UI could be treated (McDowell et al, 1996). Given this patient belief, in conjunction with effective treatment options, primary care providers are compelled to identify UI in their patients. This is a difficult task, because patients may not volunteer such information to their health care provider. The provider must be aware of UI and make a more concerted effort to identify its existence and its classification to make appropriate treatment choices.

UI may be classified as either transient or chronic. Transient causes of UI include elements that form the mnemonic DIAPPERS: delirium, infection (urinary), atrophic urethritis, pharmacologic agents, psychological elements (eg, depression), excessive urine output, restricted mobility, and stool impaction (Resnick, 1996). Chronic or established UI is characterized as stress, urge, overflow, or functional (Table 34-1).

ANATOMY, PHYSIOLOGY, AND PATHOLOGY

Male and female urinary systems are similar in that both consist of the following elements: the bladder, surrounded by the detrusor muscle; an internal sphincter muscle; and an external sphincter muscle. The major differences include the prostate gland and a longer urethra in males. Figure 34-1 illustrates the similarities and differences. Knowledge of the anatomy and physiology of the male and female urinary systems provides a clear understanding of the potential areas where urinary continence can be affected.

The detrusor muscle, responsible for the propulsive force in bladder emptying, is under parasympathetic autonomic control through the pelvic nerves (Isselbacher et al, 1995). Bladder contraction results from cholinergic stimulation. The internal and external sphincter muscles, located in the bladder outlet area, are responsible for maintaining urethral pressure. Comparably, the internal sphincter is innervated by the alpha-adrenergic pathway. Alpha-stimulation results in muscle contraction, preventing urine flow (Young & Koda-Kimble, 1995). The

external sphincter is composed of striated muscle that is under voluntary control.

In the female, estrogen receptors are located in both the internal and external sphincters. Estrogen receptor stimulation, then, contributes to sphincter competence. In the absence of estrogen, as in postmenopausal women, the internal and external sphincters may not resist urine passage in situations of increased stress (eg, coughing, sneezing, climbing stairs, and other physical activities), resulting in small amounts of urine leakage. This is secondary to the lack of estrogen-stimulated competence of these sphincters.

Stress incontinence in males may result after prostate surgery in which damage to the external sphincter has occurred. Transurethral resection of the prostate may result in damage to both the internal and external sphincters such that mechanical incontinence ensues (Isselbacher et al, 1995).

Overflow incontinence may result from obstruction of the bladder neck or urethra or from neurologic damage such as spinal cord injury. Bladder outlet obstruction often occurs in men with benign prostatic hypertrophy. When enlarged, the prostate gland, which surrounds the urethra, impedes urinary outflow from the bladder. This results in symptoms such as nocturia, reduced size and force of the urinary stream, straining to void, and terminal dribbling. Detrusor instability leads to uncontrollable bladder contractions and may arise from central nervous system diseases such as cerebrovascular accidents, dementia, neoplasia, and perhaps normal-pressure hydrocephalus (Isselbacher et al, 1995).

EPIDEMIOLOGY

Although UI is not exclusive to the elderly population, it does occur most frequently in this group of patients, with 15% to 30% affected (*MMWR*, 1995; Barker et al, 1995; Rosenthal & McMurty, 1995). This number rises to 35% of patients in the acute-care hospital setting and up to 60% of nursing home residents (Rosenthal & McMurty, 1995). As much as 70% of cases of UI in the elderly may be attributed to detrusor instability (Isselbacher et al, 1995).

Established risk factors in UI include age, gender, and parity (Rosenthal & McMurty, 1995; Wilson & Herbison, 1995). Based on these risks, women are affected more often than men. Involuntary loss of urine secondary to activity has been reported by 50% of nulliparous women 18 to 25 years of age (Lemcke et al, 1995). Additionally, 26% of women aged 30 to 59 years have experienced UI at some time in their adult life, and often perceive it as a social or hygienic problem (Diokno, 1995).

Other potential risk factors that have not been thoroughly studied include urinary tract infection, obesity, menopause,

TABLE 34-1	Types of UI
Classification	**Description**
Stress incontinence	Involuntary loss of urine during coughing, sneezing, laughing, lifting, or other physical activity. Caused by sphincter insufficiency. Occurs when urethra pressure falls below bladder pressure.
Urge incontinence	The inability of a patient to suppress the sensation of bladder fullness, resulting in loss of urine. The detrusor muscle is unstable. Patient experiences an abrupt and strong desire to void.
Overflow incontinence	Occurs when there is inadequate detrusor function, inadequate sensory perception within the bladder wall, or significant outlet obstruction.
Functional incontinence	Incontinence secondary to impaired mobility. The voiding mechanism is adequate. However, involuntary urine loss occurs secondary to a patient's inability to get to a toilet.

genitourinary surgery, lack of postpartum pelvic floor strengthening exercise, cigarette smoking, chronic illness, and certain pharmacologic agents (Rosenthal & McMurty, 1995; Wilson & Herbison, 1995). Such agents include, but are not limited to, diuretics, anticholinergics, sedatives, neuroleptics, calcium channel blockers, alcohol, and alpha-adrenergic agonists and antagonists (Resnick, 1996; Barker et al, 1995).

As previously noted, UI has both medical and psychosocial consequences. The overall cost of health care is increased for patients with UI, and the morbidity and perhaps mortality rates of these patients may also be affected. UI is not a disease, but rather a symptom of an underlying problem. Once that process has been identified, successful treatment may be chosen to improve or cure UI.

DIAGNOSTIC CRITERIA

Definitive criteria have not been clearly established, and diagnosis is largely based on symptomatology gathered in the history and physical exam. In the case of overflow incontinence,

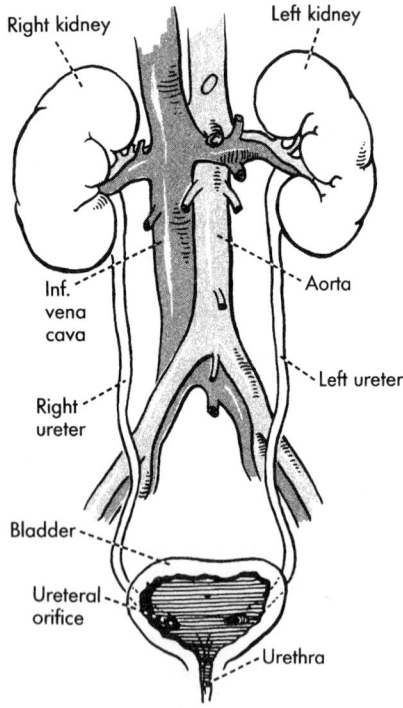

FIGURE 34-1 Bladder and urinary system anatomy. (From Rosse, C. & Gaddum-Rosse, P. (1997). *Hollinshead's Textbook of Anatomy, 5/e.* Philadelphia: Lippincott-Raven Publishers.)

however, measuring postvoid residual urine volume may be of aid. Urine volume of greater than 100 mL may be indicative of overflow incontinence; concern rises as the volume exceeds 200 mL (Barker et al, 1995).

HISTORY AND PHYSICAL EXAM

The evaluation of UI begins with the identification of its presence. If a reversible cause such as drug therapy or urinary tract infection cannot be identified, further workup for chronic UI begins. The first step is gathering a complete patient history (Table 34-2).

After the history, a physical exam helps classify the type of UI. Key aspects include urinalysis, palpation of the bladder, a neurologic exam, exams of the rectum and pelvic areas (appropriate to gender), and catheterization of the bladder (Chutka et al, 1996). Urinalysis may be performed to identify the presence of leukocytes, blood, or nitrites, which may be indicative of infection, a cause of reversible UI if appropriately treated. A palpable bladder is suggestive of overflow incontinence. The neurologic exam of the perineal area provides information regarding a potential neurologic cause for the UI. While doing this exam, the provider assesses sensation in the perineal area using fine touch and also observes the presence of voluntary anal sphincter tone (Barker et al, 1995). The rectal exam can identify fecal impaction and, in men, prostatism. The pelvic exam in women may help to identify atrophic vaginitis. Additionally, with the pelvic exam, the presence of urinary sphincter insufficiency may be observed. Catheterization is performed after the patient has completely emptied the bladder. This measures the postvoid residual volume in the bladder (Rosenthal & McMurty, 1995).

TABLE 34-2	Information Collected in the Patient History

- Frequency of urinating in a toilet vs. small leaking accidents vs. large accidents
- Description of the accidents, regarding their association with:
  Inability to suppress the urge to void that results in large-volume losses
  Occurrence of coughing or sneezing that results in increased abdominal pressure, contributing to small-volume losses
- Presence of neurologic symptoms, including paresthesias and gait disturbances
- Symptoms of prostatism
- Patient or family history of metabolic diseases such as diabetes
- Presence of urinary tract infection symptoms such as dysuria, urinary frequency, urinary urgency

DIAGNOSTIC STUDIES

Age and Gender Considerations

Given that the highest prevalence of UI is in the elderly, with women more commonly affected, specific age and gender considerations must be taken into account in diagnosing and treating UI. One example of a special diagnostic consideration, outside the realm of the elderly, occurs in the younger woman. In this situation, it is important to distinguish incontinence from a gynecologic source. A history of chronic dampness in the absence of activity or urge suggests this or perhaps a vesicovaginal or ureterovaginal fistula or ectopic ureter. Use of pharmacologic agents that discolor the urine, such as phenazopyridine or methylene blue, may help in distinguishing between these two potential sources (Lemcke et al, 1995).

The focused diagnostic exam, including urinalysis, palpation of the bladder, and neurologic evaluation, is similar regardless of sex. The same questions are posed and similar medical and laboratory tests are performed. A major point of difference exists, however, regarding anatomy: in the male patient, prostatism must be evaluated as a contributing factor to UI.

TREATMENT OPTIONS, EXPECTED OUTCOMES, AND COMPREHENSIVE MANAGEMENT

There are a number of treatment options for UI. These include not only behavioral modification and related techniques, but also medical management and potentially surgery. In any of these instances, the expected outcome is the same: the improvement of incontinence by reduction or complete discontinuation of incontinent episodes. As a result, morbidity is reduced and overall medical, psychosocial, and monetary costs are also reduced. The overall care of a patient with UI, after appropriate diagnosis, entails education about the therapeutic regimen chosen and alternatives that may exist. Figure 34-2 illustrates, ac-

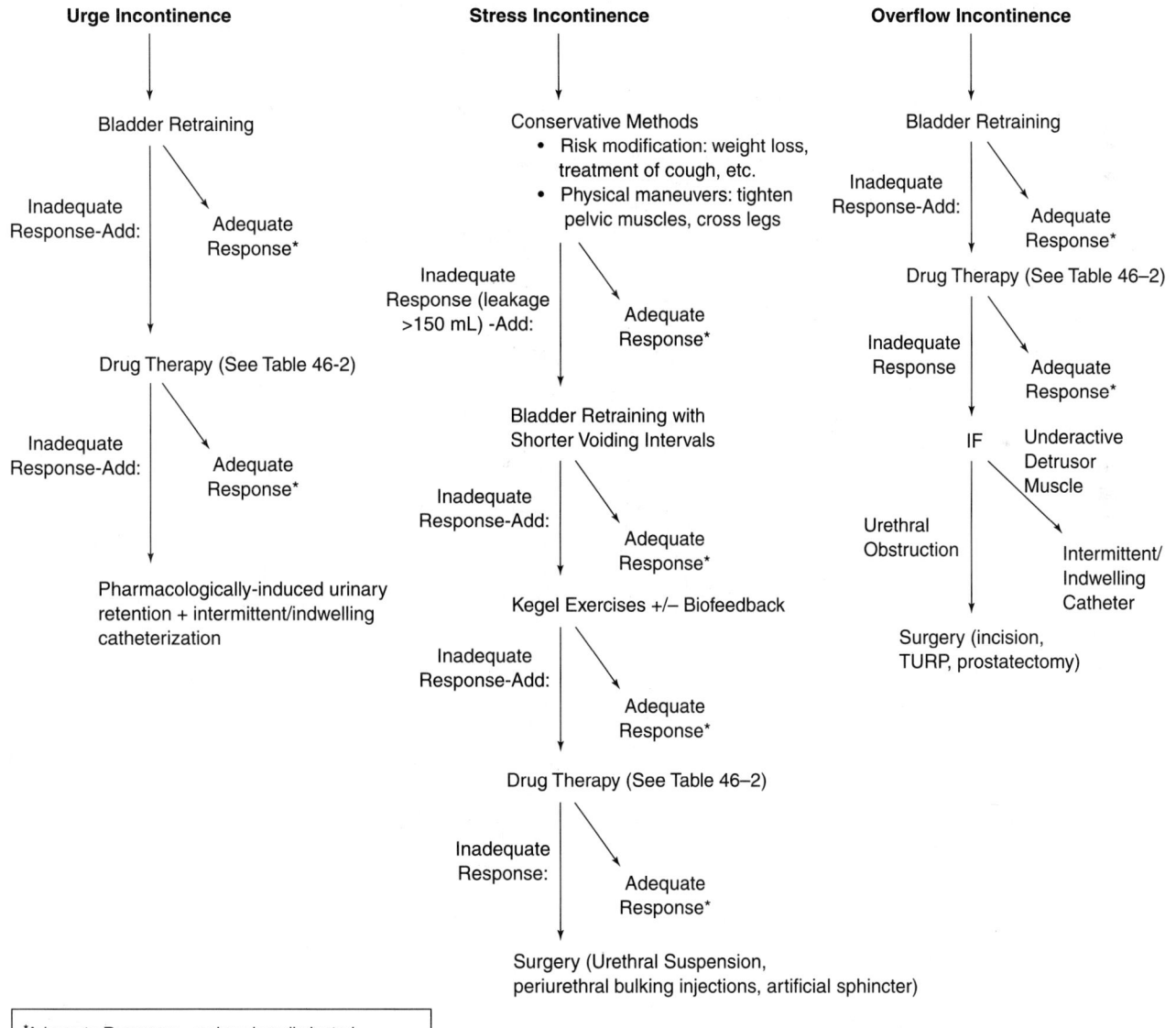

FIGURE 34-2 UI comprehensive management.

cording to UI classification, the therapeutic management steps to be taken.

Behavior Modification

Behavioral interventions for the treatment of UI include but are not limited to timed-voiding bladder training and pelvic floor exercises (Kegel exercises). Other interventions include biofeedback and electrical stimulation. Timed-voiding bladder training is most effective for patients who have detrusor instability. However, it may also be effective for stress and urge incontinence. In this form of therapy, patients void at regular intervals (every 1 to 2 hours). If the urge to void occurs within this time frame, the patient is instructed not to void, even at the expense of incontinence. Every 1 to 2 weeks, the interval is increased by 15 to 60 minutes. Success occurs when the interval is 3 to 4 hours, the patient remains continent, and symptoms (eg, urgency, frequency) are minimal (Weinberger, 1995; Beckman, 1995).

Pelvic floor exercises, also known as Kegel exercises, are especially effective in genuine stress incontinence and may also be used to treat urge incontinence. Repetitive voluntary contractions of the pelvic muscles may stabilize the proximal urethra such that urethral pressure will be less likely to fall below bladder pressure. These muscles may be described as the muscles contracted when trying to stop the urine stream (Weinberger, 1995; Beckman, 1995). A woman can be taught to perform these exercises during a gynecologic exam as the provider assesses the strength of the musculature. A man may be taught to perform these exercises during a rectal examination by having him squeeze the anal sphincter around the examiner's finger. This is effective because the anal and urethral sphincters are almost identically innervated (Barker et al, 1995).

Biofeedback, which uses visual feedback to teach the patient to control various muscle groups affecting continence, may be highly effective. It is especially beneficial in elderly patients who have sphincter insufficiency (Barker et al, 1995). Electrical stimulation may be used in conjunction with biofeedback or alone. Patients with stress incontinence, detrusor instability, and sensory urgency have benefited from its use (Wilson & Herbison, 1995). This treatment involves low-dose electrical stimulation of the perianal and vaginal bladder inhibitory reflexes (Barker et al, 1995).

Drug Therapy

The pharmacologic agents used in the treatment of UI are chosen based on the classification of UI (stress, urge, or overflow). Table 34-3 lists the medications, usual doses, and expected side effects according to the specific category of UI. Drug therapy is not always the first treatment choice for UI. The therapeutic option chosen, whether drugs, behavioral therapy, or surgery, depends on the nature and severity of the UI.

Surgery

According to the 1992 U.S. Agency for Health Care Policy and Research guidelines regarding the management of UI, the first choice of treatment should be that which is the least invasive and least dangerous. Therefore, in the great majority of cases, the surgical option is chosen only after treatment failure

with behavioral or drug therapy. Many of the cases requiring surgery are those in which the primary problem is outlet obstruction. Prostate enlargement and urethral stricture are examples of situations where surgery may be undertaken.

Prevention

Because UI is a symptom, pure prevention is not entirely realistic. However, raising the awareness of primary care providers to the previously noted risk factors and the potential pharmacologic agents that may contribute to UI may allow for earlier identification of this problem. With heightened awareness, primary care providers should be better prepared to identify at-risk patients and make it a point to question them regarding the presence of UI.

Measures that may be helpful in preventing UI, but that have not been proven beneficial, include modification of certain risk factors, such as weight reduction and smoking cessation (Wilson & Herbison, 1995). Improved stress incontinence has been observed after weight loss because of lower increases in abdominal pressure with physical stress. In smokers, presumably secondary to more frequent and violent coughing, early development of stress incontinence ensues; the number of cigarettes smoked positively correlates with this. Smoking cessation and reduced numbers of women smokers have been thought to have a great effect on the declining prevalence of stress incontinence in women (Wilson & Herbison, 1995).

TEACHING AND SELF-CARE

The cornerstone of patient education regarding UI is to identify the type of UI and explain it briefly to the patient. Then the possible interventions can be discussed, including risk factor modification. Weight loss and smoking cessation may help in improving UI as well as the patient's overall health status. Other educational issues to be considered include explaining how and why to keep a bladder record. This record illustrates all times when the patient willingly voided throughout the day and whenever involuntary urine loss occurred. Involuntary voiding is further described in the record as excessive or small amounts dribbled, and the impetus for this (eg, a sneeze, cough, laughing, or inability to suppress the urge) is noted. This record provides information that is important in the diagnosis of UI.

Bladder retraining, as previously described, also requires explanation by the primary care provider. When used in conjunction with the bladder record, the patient and the primary care provider can easily evaluate its efficacy. The provider should explain the role of Kegel exercises and how to perform them, as well as evaluating the role of biofeedback and electrical stimulation of the pelvic floor.

Primary care providers have a major role in teaching patients with UI. In addition to providing reassurance that UI can be improved or possibly cured, they can also provide tips to patients (eg, avoid drinking large amounts of fluid before going on a trip or if access to a toilet may be limited; make it a point to be aware of the location of toilets). The primary care provider is a good source of information and support for patients with UI.

COMMUNITY RESOURCES

The provider is encouraged to identify community-based resources for patients with UI, such as:

TABLE 34-3   Common Drug Therapy for UI

Type of UI	Drug Therapy	Dose	Adverse Effects
Stress Incontinence	1. Alpha-sympathomimetic agonists (ephedrine, pseudoephedrine, phenylpropanolamine) 2. Imipramine 3. Estrogen cream (women) 4. Oral estrogen (women)	1. Ephedrine - 25 mg TID—50 mg QID; pseudoephedrine—15 mg BID—60 mg QID; phenylpropanolamine—25 mg BID—75 mg QID immediate release 2. 10 mg BID—75 mg BID 3. Initial: ½–1 applicator 3×/week; maintenance: ⅓–½ applicator 1–2×/week 4. 0.625 mg conjugated estrogens/day	1. Excitation, tremulousness, insomnia, palpitation, vertigo, dryness of the nose and throat, acute urinary retention (occasionally) 2. Orthostatic hypotension, tachycardia, confusional states (especially elderly), dry mouth, blurred vision, constipation, urinary retention/delayed micturition **3. Vaginal irritation 4. GI upset, vaginal bleeding, headache, increased risk of endometrial hyperplasia***
Urge Incontinence	1. Oxybutynin 2. Dicyclomine 3. Flavoxate 4. Propantheline 5. Imipramine	1. 2.5–5 mg TID–QID 2. 10–20 mg TID–QID 3. 100–200 mg TID–QID 4. 7.5–15 mg QID 5. As above	1. Palpitations, tachycardia, constipation, dry mouth/eyes, urinary hesitation/retention, asthenia, dizziness, drowsiness 2. See oxybutynin 3. Nausea, vomiting, dry mouth/eyes, drowsiness, tachycardia, palpitation, increased ocular pressure 4. Drying of salivary secretions, blurred vision, urinary hesitancy/retention, constipation, drowsiness 5. See above
Overflow Incontinence	1. Alpha-adrenergic blockers (prazosin, terazosin, doxazosin) 2. Bethanechol 3. Finasteride (men)	*1. Prazosin—1–5 mg BID–TID; terazosin—1–5 mg QD–BID; doxazosin—1–8 mg QHS 2. 10–25 mg TID–QID 3. 5 mg QD	1. Dizziness, headache, drowsiness, lack of energy, weakness, palpitations, nausea 2. Malaise, abdominal discomfort, diarrhea, nausea/belching, urinary urgency, hypotension 3. Impotence, decreased libido, decreased ejaculate volume, breast tenderness/enlargement

* Alpha-adrenergic blockers are initiated at the lowest possible dose HS due to orthostatic hypotension

** Up to 25% of a dose of vaginal estrogen cream may be absorbed, contributing to systemic side effects

*** Risk greatly reduced, to that normally seen in the usual population, by the addition of progesterone

- Help for Incontinent People, P.O. Box 544R, Union, SC 29379
- The Simon Foundation, P.O. Box 835, Wilmette, IL 60091
- United Ostomy Association, 2001 W. Beverly Blvd., Los Angeles, CA 90057
- Bladder Health Council, 300 W. Pratt St., Suite 401, Baltimore, MD 21201
- www.medaccess.com.seniors/agepg/ap38.htm
- www.uib.no/isf/people/inkter.htm

These resources can provide information regarding local support groups and offer videos, brochures, or newsletters that may be helpful to the patient (Umlauf et al, 1996).

REFERRAL POINTS AND CLINICAL WARNINGS

Referral to a subspecialist, usually a urologist, is straightforward. The following criteria indicate the need for such action (Maloney, 1995; Barker et al, 1995; Rosenthal & McMurty, 1995):

- Recurrent urinary tract infection
- Postvoid residual bladder volume of more than 200 mL

without infection, with suspicion of renal impairment, or with bladder outlet obstruction

- Suspected overflow incontinence secondary to outlet obstruction or atonic bladder
- Marked pelvic prolapse or significant stress incontinence
- Suspicion of prostate cancer
- Presence of hematuria

After a referral, with the help of the subspecialist, a decision about the most appropriate therapy is made.

■ ■ ■ CLINICAL PEARLS

- A history of chronic dampness in the absence of activity or urge may suggest either incontinence or a vesicovaginal or ureterovaginal fistula or ectopic ureter. Use of pharmacologic agents that discolor the urine (eg, phenazopyridine or methylene blue) may help in distinguishing these two potential sources.
- A man may be taught to perform Kegel exercises during a rectal examination by having him squeeze the anal sphincter around the examiner's finger. This is effective because the anal and urethral sphincters are almost identically innervated.

EDITOR'S NOTE:

COMPLEMENTARY APPROACHES

A general discussion of complementary approaches can be found in Chapter 3. The following, while not an exhaustive list, are some complementary approaches being used for this condition. Additional information on these approaches, including precautions, can be found in Appendices A and B. Providers need to assess for the use of complementary approaches as part of the patient's history, as they may impact conventional therapies, and patients may not volunteer this information unless specifically asked. Efficacy of many complementary approaches is not as well documented as that of conventional therapies. Providers need to read the literature before suggesting these complementary approaches.

- Complementary Modalities
  Biofeedback

References

Barker, L.R., Burton, J.R., & Zieve, P.D. (1995). *Principles of ambulatory medicine.* Baltimore: Williams & Wilkins.

Beckman, N.J. (1995). An overview of urinary incontinence in adults: Assessments and behavioral interventions. *Clinical Nurse Specialist, 9*(5), 241–247.

Chutka, D.S., Fleming, K.C., Evans, M.P., et al. (1996). Urinary incontinence in the elderly population. *Mayo Clinic Proceedings, 71*(January), 93–101.

Diokno, A.C. (1995). Epidemiology and psychosocial aspects of incontinence. *Urologic Clinics of North America, 22*(3), 481–485.

Isselbacher, K.J., Braunwald, E., Wilson, J.D., et al. (1995). *Harrison's principles of internal medicine.* New York: McGraw-Hill.

Lemcke, D.P., Pattison, J., Marshall, L.A., & Cowley, D.S. (1995). *Primary care of women.* Norwalk, CT: Appleton & Lange.

Maloney, C. (1995). Evaluation and treatment of urinary incontinence: A primary care approach. *Nurse Practitioner, 20*(2), 74–75.

McDowell, B.J., Engberg, S.J., Rodriguez, E., et al. (1996). Characteristics of urinary incontinence in homebound older adults. *Journal of the American Geriatrics Society, 44*(8), 963–968.

MMWR. (1995). Knowledge, attitudes, and practices of physicians regarding urinary incontinence in persons aged ≥65 years—Massachusetts and Oklahoma, 1993. *MMWR, 44*(4), 747–749.

Mold, J.W. (1996). Pharmacotherapy of urinary incontinence. *American Family Physician, 54*(2), 673–680.

Resnick, N.M. (1996). Geriatric incontinence. *Urologic Clinics of North America, 23*(1), 55–74.

Rosenthal, A.J., & McMurty, C.T. (1995). Urinary incontinence in the elderly. *Postgraduate Medicine, 97*(5), 109–121.

Umlauf, M.G., Goode, P.S., & Burgio, K.L. (1996). Psychosocial issues in geriatric urology. *Urologic Clinics of North America, 23*(1), 127–136.

U.S. Agency for Health Care Policy and Research. (1992). *Urinary incontinence in adults: A patient's guide.* Rockville, MD: Dept of Health and Human Services, Public Health Service, Agency for Health Care Policy and Research, 1992; DHHS publication No. (AHCPR)92-0040.

Weinberger, M.W. (1995). Conservative treatment of urinary incontinence. *Clinical Obstetrics and Gynecology, 38*(1), 175–188.

Wilson, D., & Herbison, P. (1995). Conservative management of incontinence. *Current Opinion in Obstetrics and Gynecology, 7,* 386–392.

Young, L.Y., & Koda-Kimble, M.A. (1995). *Applied therapeutics: The clinical use of drugs.* Vancouver, WA: Applied Therapeutics.

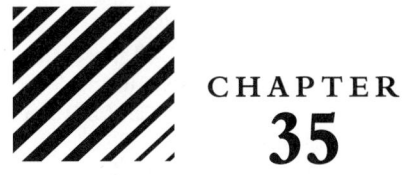

CHAPTER
35

Urinary Tract Infection

Tracy N. Offerdahl, Pharm.D., Elena M. Umland, Pharm.D.

Urinary tract infections (UTIs) are common and may range in severity from uncomplicated cystitis to severe pyelonephritis. These infections result in millions of visits to health care providers each year and may also become an unexpected complication of a hospital admission. Both men and women experience UTIs, but the incidence in females far exceeds that of males until the age of 50. UTIs may also become complications of pregnancy, paralysis, diabetes mellitus, renal transplantation, and many renal diseases (Kunin, 1994a; Young & Koda-Kimble, 1995).

UTIs may be classified according to where the infection occurs or by the frequency of infection. For instance, cystitis or urethritis are both considered lower tract infections because they usually involve the bladder and urethra. In contrast, pyelonephritis is considered an upper tract infection because it involves inflammation of the renal parenchyma. Patients may also experience an acute UTI, or they may experience chronic exacerbations of infection from either relapse or reinfection (Young & Koda-Kimble, 1995; DiPiro et al, 1997; Perdue & Plaisance, 1995).

UTIs can further be classified as uncomplicated or complicated—no structural or neurologic abnormalities versus a predisposing lesion of the urinary tract. Other patient factors that may be associated with a complicated UTI include pregnancy, diabetes mellitus, and immunosuppression (Young & Koda-Kimble, 1995; DiPiro et al, 1997; Perdue & Plaisance, 1995).

Additionally, patients may present with nephrolithiasis (kidney stones) of infectious origin. Patients may have symptoms of a UTI, such as bacteriuria or dysuria, without actually having a UTI (Young & Koda-Kimble, 1995; DiPiro et al, 1997; Perdue & Plaisance, 1995).

ANATOMY, PHYSIOLOGY, AND PATHOLOGY

Bacteria enter and spread throughout the urinary tract in three ways: the ascending route, the hematogeneous route, and the lymphatic route. The ascending route is the most common (Young & Koda-Kimble, 1995; Stamm & Hooton, 1993; Hatton et al, 1994; Mandell et al, 1995).

In comparing the female and male anatomies, the urethra in the female is shorter and in close proximity to the rectal area, making it an easy target for fecal contamination. Once bacteria have colonized the urethral area, they multiply, leading to retrograde infection of the bladder (Young & Koda-Kimble, 1995; Stamm & Hooton, 1993; Hatton et al, 1994; Mandell et al, 1995).

Although both urine elements and bladder mucosal elements have protective properties against infection, certain risk factors may predispose patients to infection. These will be discussed later in the chapter. Bacteria can further move to involve the bladder (upper tract infection), especially in patients with decreased urethral peristalsis, such as in pregnancy, urethral obstruction, urethral massage, self-catheterization, diaphragm use, or virulent gram-negative bacterial infections (Young & Koda-Kimble, 1995; Stamm & Hooton, 1993; Hatton et al, 1994; Mandell et al, 1995).

The hematogenous route of bacterial entry involves bloodborne pathogens that infect the renal parenchyma. The lymphatic route has been examined in animals, where a lymphatic connection was found between the ureters and the kidneys. This, however, seems to be a relatively unimportant route of infection in humans (Young & Koda-Kimble, 1995; Stamm & Hooton, 1993; Hatton et al, 1994; Mandell et al, 1995).

Nephrolithiasis

In addition to UTI development, other disorders of the urinary tract exist. One of these disorders is renal stone disease, or nephrolithiasis. The pathophysiology of nephrolithiasis is multifaceted. Renal stones may contain calcium, uric acid, struvite, cystine, and other substances, but calcium-containing stones account for a large number of recovered renal stones in cases of noninfectious nephrolithiasis (Mandell et al, 1995).

For a renal stone to develop, three requirements have been identified: the formation of a nidus, retainment of the nidus within the urinary tract, and growth of the nidus. Risk factors that contribute to stone formation are many. Hypercalciuria is a common finding in stone formers. Idiopathically it has been found to occur in 40% to 60% of these patients (Mandell et al, 1995). Other contributing factors to the formation of renal stones include dietary factors, level of patient activity, primary hyperparathyroidism, renal tubular acidosis, and hyperoxaluria (Mandell et al, 1995).

Pathology

Patients with structural abnormalities (eg, vesicoureteral reflux, neurogenic bladder, neoplasm, stricture) may experience complicated UTIs from less virulent strains of bacteria. Patients who are wheelchair-bound because of paralysis often experience these problems. These patients are categorized as having complicated UTIs, regardless of the location of the infection (Mandell et al, 1995; Lipsky, 1989; Kunin, 1994b).

EPIDEMIOLOGY

UTIs: Acute, Chronic, Pyelonephritis

UTIs are among the most frequently observed infections in clinical medicine. Primary complaints of painful urination, frequency, and urgency or actual UTI account for an estimated 6.2 million annual health care visits in the United States (Mandell et al, 1995). In more than 95% of these infections, a single bacterial species was responsible (Kunin, 1994b).

UTIs occur in both men and women at any age, independent of race. However, the risk of acquiring a UTI (Table 35-1) and the subsequent actual incidence varies according to age and gender. Between the ages of 1 and 50 years, UTIs predominantly affect females. Women in young adulthood are 30 times more likely to develop a UTI compared to males in this age group (Stamm & Hooton, 1993; Kunin, 1994b). It is estimated that 10% to 20% of the female population will experience a symptomatic UTI in their lifetime (Kunin, 1994a; Kunin, 1994b; Lemcke et al, 1995). Additionally, about half of school-aged girls found to have significant bacteriuria will develop symptomatic infection about the time they become sexually active (Perdue & Plaisance, 1995).

Gender Factors

FEMALE GENDER

Women, particularly those of childbearing age, experience UTIs at a much higher rate than do their male counterparts. About 20% of young women with an initial episode will have recurrent infections. Greater than 90% of these will be reinfections, occurring months apart. Recurrence has been associated with diaphragm use and the use of spermicides, because spermicides induce *Escherichia coli* colonization of the vagina (DiPiro et al, 1997). Generally, frequency of sexual intercourse, diaphragm use, and lack of urination after intercourse are risk factors for UTIs in women (Kunin, 1994b).

TABLE 35-1	UTI Risk Factors

GENERAL RISK FACTORS
- Extremes in age
- History of recent UTI
- Neurologic dysfunction: spinal cord injury, stroke, atherosclerosis, diabetes mellitus
- Renal disease
- Sexual intercourse
- Urinary tract instrumentation (eg, catheterization)
- Urinary tract obstruction

FEMALE RISK FACTORS
- Delayed postcoital micturition
- Contraceptive methods (eg, diaphragms, spermicides)
- Female gender
- Pregnancy

MALE RISK FACTORS
- Lack of circumcision
- Sexual practices (anal intercourse)
- Female sexual partner with vaginal colonization
- Obstructive uropathy from prostate and loss of bactericidal prostatic secretions

Pregnancy is an independent risk factor for UTI. Bacteriuria occurs in 4% to 10% of pregnant women, double the incidence in nonpregnant women of similar age. Hormones and anatomic changes have been suggested as causes (Kunin, 1994a).

Twenty-five to 30% of postpartum women have bacteriuria (Stamm & Hooton, 1993; Hatton et al, 1994). After age 65 years, approximately 20% of women have bacteriuria. Women older than 80 years of age have a 20% to 50% incidence of bacteriuria (Stamm & Hooton, 1993; Hatton et al, 1994; Warren, 1992). This incidence is highest in nursing-home residents, women with incomplete bladder emptying, those with fecal incontinence, and those requiring intermittent bladder catheterization. Postmenopausal estrogen deficiency has been implicated in contributing to increased vaginal pH, thus altering the vaginal flora and possibly contributing to bacteriuria and increased UTI occurrence in this population (Stamm & Hooton, 1993; Warren, 1992).

MALE GENDER

In general, uncomplicated UTI is rare in school-aged boys and men 20 to 50 years of age. However, by age 65 the incidence of UTI in men is comparable to that observed in women. Potential causes for this increased incidence in older men include obstructive uropathy from the prostate, fecal incontinence, and increased instrumentation and bladder catheter usage (Kunin, 1994b).

In older men, the presence of benign prostatic hypertrophy can greatly increase the incidence of UTIs. This may occur because of urethral obstruction from the size of the prostate, as well as a decrease in the bactericidal activity of the prostatic secretions. The major concern here is that bacteria may infect the prostate gland, causing bacterial prostatitis (Hatton et al, 1994; Mandell et al, 1995; Lipsky, 1989).

UTI is rare in men younger than 50 years of age, and if present it may be considered indicative of an underlying abnormality of the urologic system. In other cases, risk factors play some role. These factors include anal intercourse without a condom, in which exposure to *E. coli* has been noted; lack of circumcision, associated with enhanced *E. coli* colonization of the glans and prepuce; and sex with a partner who is vaginally colonized with uropathogens (DiPiro et al, 1997; Lipsky, 1989).

Nephrolithiasis

Nephrolithiasis affects approximately 12% of the population. It has an annual incidence in the United States of 1.6 per 1000 population (Mandell et al, 1995).

DIAGNOSTIC CRITERIA

Diagnosis of a UTI is based on patient signs and symptoms as well as laboratory testing. Another important point to consider is whether this is a first UTI or a recurrent UTI, because females with recurrent UTIs may need to be evaluated for interstitial cystitis. Symptomatic female patients with lower tract infection may complain of the following (Young & Koda-Kimble, 1995; Stamm & Hooton, 1993):

- Abrupt or gradual onset of dysuria
- Increased frequency of urination
- Urgency of urination

- Difficulty in urinating
- Suprapubic or lower back pain.

Signs and symptoms of an upper tract infection may include any of the above and also the following (Young & Koda-Kimble, 1995; Stamm & Hooton, 1993):

- Fever
- Chills
- Nausea or vomiting
- Headache
- Malaise
- Hematuria
- Flank pain.

Differentiating between a lower tract infection and an upper tract infection may be difficult, however, based on symptoms alone. Some patients with upper tract infections fail to present with the typical upper tract symptoms. Therefore, a urinalysis is important to identify any other components of infection (Young & Koda-Kimble, 1995; Stamm & Hooton, 1993).

Men with acute or chronic prostatitis may experience a variety of signs and symptoms, but many men with chronic prostatitis are totally asymptomatic. Symptoms may be similar to the typical ones experienced by patients with acute cystitis (eg, frequency of urination, difficulty on urination, and painful urination). Other signs and symptoms may include the following (Stamm & Hooton, 1993; Hatton et al, 1994; Mandell et al, 1995; Lipsky, 1989):

- Fever
- Chills
- Perineal pain
- Tender or swollen prostate gland that is warm to the touch on exam.

Nephrolithiasis

Although renal stones may form in patients of any age, the highest incidence is in patients between the ages of 20 and 40. Idiopathic hypercalciuria is the primary cause in most cases. In the elderly, primary hyperparathyroidism and drug-induced etiologies should be considered (Mandell et al, 1995).

Microbiology

In the large majority of uncomplicated cases, a single bacterial species is responsible for causing a UTI. *E. coli* is by far the most common pathogen isolated in acute cases of uncomplicated cystitis. Urine samples that contain multiple organisms are seen in patients with complicated UTIs or in contaminated specimens. Organisms that may indicate a contaminated specimen include *Staphylococcus epidermidis*, diphtheroids, lactobacilli, and anaerobes. These are normally found on the skin and urethra. Additional organisms frequently found to cause UTIs include other enteric (found in the gastrointestinal tract) gram-negative organisms such as *Klebsiella* spp., *Proteus* spp., *Enterobacter* spp., *Staphylococcus* spp., and *Enterococcus* spp. These organisms, along with *Pseudomonas* spp. and *Acinetobacter* spp., are more likely to be a problem in patients with recurrent or complicated UTIs, as well as in hospitalized patients. Hospitalized patients experience infection more frequently with resistant strains of these organisms (Young & Koda-Kimble, 1995; Stamm & Hooton, 1993; Hatton et al, 1994; Mandell et al, 1995).

Men with acute or chronic prostatitis may be infected with a variety of organisms, including *E. coli*, *Pseudomonas* spp., *Enterococcus* spp., *Klebsiella* spp., *Enterobacter* spp., and *Proteus* spp. (Hatton et al, 1994; Mandell et al, 1995; Lipsky, 1989).

Patients with indwelling genitourinary catheters or those receiving antimicrobial therapy may also experience UTIs caused by fungi such as *Candida* spp. Organisms such as *Chlamydia trachomatis*, *Neisseria gonorrhoeae*, and herpes simplex virus have been isolated in cases of sexually transmitted urethritis. These infections should be ruled out, especially in sexually active patients (Young & Koda-Kimble, 1995; Stamm & Hooton, 1993; Hatton et al, 1994; Mandell et al, 1995).

Patients with infection-induced stones, or nephrolithiasis, usually have struvite stones, which form in the presence of urease-producing bacteria that cause alkaline urine (pH $\geq$ 7). Many bacteria are capable of producing urease enzyme; examples include *Proteus* spp. and *Ureaplasma urealyticum* (Young & Koda-Kimble, 1995; DiPiro et al, 1997; Mandell et al, 1995) (see Table 35-1).

HISTORY AND PHYSICAL EXAM

Specific signs and symptoms are mentioned above.

DIAGNOSTIC STUDIES

Urinalysis is performed in virtually all patients suspected of having a UTI or prostatitis. It can give a quick laboratory diagnosis of infection. The midstream clean-catch method of urine collection is one of three acceptable methods of urine collection for analysis. It is the most common method for routine exam. Once the urethral area has been cleaned appropriately, patients are instructed to void and discard a small amount of urine. The rest of the midstream urine is then collected for analysis (Young & Koda-Kimble, 1995; DiPiro et al, 1997; Stamm & Hooton, 1993; Hatton et al, 1994). The two other methods of urine collection are catheterization and suprapubic aspiration, and these will be discussed later in the chapter. Regardless of the method of collection, problems with sterility and contamination of urine specimens may affect the results of the urinalysis. These problems are mainly caused by poor or inconsistent collection methods or failure to take the specimen to the laboratory immediately (or failure to refrigerate the specimen). Therefore, bacteriuria alone is not diagnostic of a UTI (Young & Koda-Kimble, 1995; DiPiro et al, 1997; Stamm & Hooton, 1993; Hatton et al, 1994).

The urinalysis includes both macroscopic and microscopic evaluation of the urine specimen. The macroscopic analysis is done by the dipstick method and consists of measuring or analyzing the urine color, specific gravity, pH, glucose, protein, ketone, blood, and bilirubin. Often the macroscopic evaluation and the dipstick portion of the urinalysis are the only parts evaluated in the laboratory. Another quick but indirect method to detect the presence of bacteria in the urine is the nitrite test: bacteria in the urine break down urinary nitrate into nitrite, resulting in a positive test (Young & Koda-Kimble, 1995; DiPiro et al, 1997; Stamm & Hooton, 1993; Hatton et al, 1994; Kunin, 1994b).

Microscopic examination is performed on the urine sample once it has been centrifuged; the sediment is then examined under a microscope. The presence and the quantity of white blood cells, or leukocytes (pyuria), erythrocytes, and bacteria is determined. Also examined in the microscopic analysis of urine is the presence of epithelial cells, crystals, and casts. The presence of white blood cell casts on the microscopic exam may be an indication of upper tract involvement; however, the absence of such casts does not rule out upper tract involvement. Table 35-2 lists normal and abnormal levels for these components of the urinalysis (Young & Koda-Kimble, 1995; DiPiro et al, 1997; Stamm & Hooton, 1993; Hatton et al, 1994; Kunin, 1994b; Traub, 1992).

A more reliable method than urinalysis for diagnosis is the urine culture. This may be warranted in certain patients, such as patients with recurrent UTIs, pregnant patients, or patients suspected of having pyelonephritis. Because urine is normally sterile, and assuming that an acceptable method of urine collection has been used (the midstream clean-catch method) and the sample has been analyzed immediately, the quantity of bacteria can be estimated. The presence of more than 10^5 bacteria/mL of urine in an asymptomatic patient is considered diagnostic of a UTI. Comparably, in a symptomatic patient, more than 10^2 or 10^3 bacteria/mL is indicative of infection (Young & Koda-Kimble, 1995; DiPiro et al, 1997; Perdue & Plaisance, 1995; Stamm & Hooton, 1993; Hatton et al, 1994).

Age and Gender Considerations

As in any disease state, the diagnosis and treatment of very old and pregnant patients require a degree of caution beyond that observed in other patient populations (Perdue & Plaisance,

1995). The diagnosis of an upper tract UTI in the elderly may be clouded because the presentation is often atypical. These patients may present with mental status changes; they may be afebrile and have respiratory or gastrointestinal complaints, such as a decrease in appetite. Therefore, UTI should be included in the differential diagnosis for any elderly patient. Alternatively, asymptomatic bacteriuria is often encountered in elderly patients. Although it rarely leads to progressive renal damage in the absence of urinary tract obstruction, it has been associated with an increased mortality rate in this select subpopulation of the elderly (Kunin, 1994a; Stamm & Hooton, 1993; Hatton et al, 1994).

Bacterial prostatitis, either acute or chronic, is a potential concern in any male experiencing a UTI. Acute and chronic prostatitis present very differently, and one infection does not usually precede the other—in other words, acute prostatitis does not usually result in chronic prostatitis. In general, these infections are of particular concern because they are more difficult to treat. The anti-infective agent must reach high prostatic levels to be effective, and therefore patients must be treated for longer periods of time (Hatton et al, 1994; Mandell et al, 1995; Lipsky, 1989).

Occupational Hazards

Certain occupational hazards may predispose patients to the development of UTIs:

- People with multiple sex partners, such as prostitutes
- Jobs that do not allow for adequate hydration and toilet breaks.

TREATMENT OPTIONS, EXPECTED OUTCOMES, AND COMPREHENSIVE MANAGEMENT

Surgical Intervention

Surgical management for UTIs is usually performed to remove obstructive lesions or calculi, to repair any ureter or bladder malformations, or to remove stones, as in nephrolithiasis. Any active UTI should be treated with antimicrobial therapy before surgery to decrease the possibility of bacteremia. With nephrolithiasis, surgical management to remove stones may be a primary therapeutic intervention. Another option is the use of lithotripsy, where the goal is to remove all traces of stone fragments. Surgical intervention to remove kidney stones seems to be relatively successful, with cure in approximately 60% of patients (Young & Koda-Kimble, 1995; Hatton et al, 1994; Mandell et al, 1995).

Medication Regimens

Once a patient has been evaluated, appropriate antimicrobial therapy and follow-up must be initiated to ensure eradication of the infecting organism and cure of the infection. Because most UTIs are acute, uncomplicated cases in young women, the cure rate is quite high when the patient is treated with appropriate antimicrobial therapy to which the likely infecting organism is sensitive. Specific management considerations are listed in Table 35-3 (DiPiro et al, 1997; Bailey, 1993).

TABLE 35-2	Urinalysis in Urinary Tract Infections	
	UTI Values	Normal Values
MACROSCOPIC EXAM AND DIPSTICK		
Color	clear to cloudy[a]	Clear to amber
Specific gravity	normal[b]	1.010–1.020
pH	normal to alkaline	4.5–8.0[c]
Glucose	0 to trace	0 to trace
Protein	0 to +2	0 to +1
Ketone	0 to trace	0 to trace
Blood	0 to +3	0 to trace
Leukocytes	0 to +3	0 to trace
Bilirubin	0 to trace	0 to trace
MICROSCOPIC EXAM		
Bacteria	>10^3 or 10^5/mL	None
White blood cells	8/mm^3 or 2–5/HPF[d]	0 or 1/HPF
Red blood cells	normal or >2–3/HPF	2 or 3/HPF
Epithelial cells	0 or 1/HPF	0 or 1/HPF
Casts	0 to many[e]	0 to trace

[a] Urine may be clear or cloudy because of bacteria or leukocytes; it may also be red or orange because of blood in the urine (hematuria).

[b] Specific gravity may be abnormally high or low in UTIs from other causes.

[c] Average pH = 6.0

[d] HPF = high-power field

[e] Casts may be helpful in diagnosing upper tract infection (pyelonephritis).

TABLE 35-3	UTI Management Considerations

INITIAL EVALUATION OF PATIENT

Severity of illness (Any gastrointestinal symptoms or dehydration? Is the infection uncomplicated or complicated?)

Site of infection (lower tract versus upper tract; prostate)

PATIENT-RELATED FACTORS

Allergies

Concomitant disease states

Renal function or hepatic function[a]

PHARMACOLOGIC FACTORS

Antimicrobial concentration in urine

Antimicrobial spectrum of activity

Side effect profile of antimicrobial agent

Cost of antimicrobial agent

[a] Depending on antimicrobial agent chosen, may need to adjust dose based on renal or hepatic function

CHOICE OF ANTIMICROBIAL AGENT

Many of the important decisions involved in choosing an antimicrobial agent to treat a UTI are identified in Table 35-3 under management considerations. First, medications chosen should have activity against any known or suspected organisms. These agents should also be well tolerated by patients: medications with many side effects actually result in treatment failure because patients do not want to take them. If two agents are equally effective in eradicating the most likely organism, the agent with fewer side effects should be chosen. Antimicrobial agents chosen for treatment of a UTI should achieve high urinary or prostatic concentrations (in the case of prostatitis). Many antimicrobial agents fulfill all of these characteristics, so a wide variety of treatments are available. Classes of agents will be discussed in general. For specific information regarding dosing, adverse effects, precautions, and contraindications, a more thorough review of these agents is available in any pharmacotherapeutics textbook (DiPiro et al, 1997; Stamm & Hooton, 1993; Hatton et al, 1994; Mandell et al, 1995, Kunin, 1994b; Norrby, 1994; Bailey, 1993).

Folate antagonists such as trimethoprim-sulfamethoxazole (TMP/SMX) have been the mainstay of therapy in the treatment of UTIs. This agent has high renal tissue concentrations, has good activity against most organisms implicated in UTIs, and is generally well tolerated. Adverse effects associated with this agent include nausea, vomiting, anorexia, some hematologic abnormalities, and allergic skin rash. TMP/SMX should be discontinued at the first appearance of any adverse effect. This agent should also be used with caution in patients with renal or hepatic impairment. It is generally contraindicated in pregnant patients and nursing mothers and therefore should be used only in situations where the benefits definitely outweigh the risks. This agent should never be used in the third trimester of pregnancy because of the risk that the fetus will develop kernicterus. Patients with a known allergy to sulfa agents should avoid this product (DiPiro et al, 1997; Stamm & Hooton, 1993; PDR, 1997).

Patients taking TMP/SMX should be advised to take this medication on an empty stomach and to drink plenty of fluid because of the risk of crystalluria or stone formation. They should also be instructed to avoid sun exposure because of the photosensitivity associated with this agent. Tablets are available in regular or double-strength, and the double-strength agent is usually used in the treatment of UTIs. TMP is also sometimes used alone for treatment of UTIs (DiPiro et al, 1997; Stamm & Hooton, 1993; PDR, 1997).

Fluoroquinolone antibiotics such as ciprofloxacin, norfloxacin, or ofloxacin have become important treatment options in the last several years for both complicated and uncomplicated UTIs. They also achieve excellent concentrations in the entire genitourinary system, exhibit excellent activity against all potential pathogens that cause UTIs, and are generally well tolerated. Adverse effects associated with these agents include diarrhea, nausea, vomiting, anorexia, abdominal discomfort, dizziness, headache, central nervous system stimulation, and hypersensitivity reactions. These agents are not recommended for use in pregnant or nursing women and should be used only when the benefits clearly outweigh the risks. Fluoroquinolones should also be avoided in patients less than 18 years of age because of the risk of arthropathy. Patients should be advised to avoid overexposure to the sun because of the risk of photosensitivity, and should also be warned against the concomitant use of antacids or any di- or trivalent cations (eg, iron, multivitamins) because of a significant decrease in the absorption of the fluoroquinolone. Fluoroquinolones also have drug interactions with other agents, such as theophylline and warfarin; therefore, close attention must be paid to a patient's concomitant medication regimen (DiPiro et al, 1997; Bailey, 1993; Reeves, 1994; von Rosenstiel & Adam, 1994).

Beta-lactam antibiotics such as ampicillin, amoxicillin, amoxicillin plus clavulanic acid, and cephalosporins are also used in the treatment of UTIs. Problems with ampicillin and amoxicillin include potential gram-negative resistance (a fair number of E. coli isolates are now resistant to amoxicillin), as well as the potential for adverse effects such as skin rash, hives, and diarrhea. Amoxicillin and ampicillin should be avoided in patients with penicillin allergy. Patients should be advised to take ampicillin on an empty stomach and amoxicillin/clavulanic acid with food to decrease some of the gastrointestinal symptoms (DiPiro et al, 1997; Perdue & Plaisance, 1995; PDR, 1997).

Cephalosporins may be used as alternatives for patients who are allergic to penicillin, although cross-allergenicity may occur. Adverse effects associated with these agents include rash, nausea, vomiting, and diarrhea, although they are generally well tolerated. Second- and third-generation cephalosporin antibiotics should be reserved for patients who are infected with an organism that is resistant to first-generation cephalosporins (DiPiro et al, 1997; Perdue & Plaisance, 1995; PDR, 1997).

Nitrofurantoin is another highly effective agent against most strains of E. coli, and organisms previously sensitive to this agent rarely develop resistance. However, other organisms that may be associated with the development of UTIs, such as Proteus spp. and Klebsiella spp., are generally resistant to nitrofurantoin. Adverse effects associated with this agent include a high incidence of gastrointestinal complaints, including flatulence and nausea. It is therefore recommended that this agent be taken with food. Other possible side effects include pulmonary reactions and peripheral neuropathy. This drug is contraindicated in patients with anuria, oliguria, or renal impairment (estimated creatinine clearance <60 mL/min) because of the possibility of toxicity resulting from impaired excretion. This drug is also contraindicated at term in pregnancy and in mothers nursing infants less than 1 month of age because of the possibility of hemolytic anemia. Nursing mothers should be warned of this potential effect (Young & Koda-Kimble, 1995; DiPiro et al, 1997; Perdue & Plaisance, 1995).

Patients should be advised that these agents may cause the urine to become dark yellow or rusty brown. Nitrofurantoin is available in macrocrystal or microcrystal formulations; some evidence suggests that there may be fewer adverse effects associated with the macrocrystalline product (Young & Koda-Kimble, 1995; DiPiro et al, 1997; Bailey, 1993).

Nalidixic acid is also used in the treatment of UTIs and is effective against a wide variety of gram-negative organisms. However, this agent has no activity against *Staphylococcus* spp. Adverse effects associated with this agent are many, so the use of nalidixic acid has been superseded by the development of newer, better-tolerated agents such as the fluoroquinolones (Young & Koda-Kimble, 1995; DiPiro et al, 1997; Perdue & Plaisance, 1995).

Fosfomycin tromethamine (Monurol) is an agent recently approved as a one-dose antibiotic for the treatment of uncomplicated UTIs, such as acute cystitis. It appears to be generally well tolerated. Adverse effects from clinical trials include diarrhea, vaginitis, nausea, and headache. Fosfomycin tromethamine is supplied in a sachet containing 3 g of orange-flavored powder to be mixed with water, according to the manufacturer's instructions (Lowers, 1997).

Other antimicrobial agents such as the aminoglycosides, imipenem/cilastatin, and aztreonam are reserved for the treatment of serious UTIs caused by resistant organisms in hospitalized patients. A thorough discussion of these agents is beyond the scope of this chapter.

DURATION OF TREATMENT

Therapy can be separated into single-dose treatment, 3-day treatment, and longer durations of treatment. Single-dose treatment has been shown to be effective in females with acute, uncomplicated UTIs. Advantages of this type of regimen include decreased cost, enhanced participation in the regimen, and decreased adverse drug effects because only one dose is administered. One drawback of the single-dose regimen is the potential for recurrence of the UTI. Candidates for single-dose therapy include young women (nonpregnant) with a first or isolated episode of acute, uncomplicated cystitis, early onset (presentation within a couple of days), or patients with catheter-acquired bacteriuria. Specific single-dose regimens are listed in Table 35-4. Antimicrobial agents chosen for single-dose therapy must achieve high urinary concentrations for at least 12 hours. Patients whose disease fails to respond to a single-dose regimen should receive a longer duration of therapy of

TABLE 35-4	Single-Dose Regimens for Treatment of UTIs

- Trimethoprim-sulfamethoxazole DS 2 tabs
- Norfloxacin 400–800 mg
- Ciprofloxacin 250–500 mg
- Trimethoprim 400–600 mg
- Fosfomycin tromethamine 3 g
- Amoxicillin 3 g

TABLE 35-5	Three-Day Courses of Therapy for UTIs

- Trimethoprim-sulfamethoxazole DS every 12 hours
- Trimethoprim 100 mg every 12 hours
- Ciprofloxacin 250 mg every 12 hours
- Norfloxacin 400 mg every 12 hours
- Nitrofurantoin 100 mg every 6 hours
- Nalidixic acid 500 mg every 8 hours
- Amoxicillin 250 mg every 8 hours
- Amoxicillin/clavulanic acid 500 mg (amox.) every 12 hours

approximately 10 to 14 days (Young & Koda-Kimble, 1995; Hatton et al, 1994; Mandell et al, 1995 Kunin, 1994b).

Three-day courses of therapy are the current mainstays of treatment for acute, uncomplicated UTIs in females and are usually preferred over single-dose therapy. The one exception may be the single-dose administration of fosfomycin tromethamine, which produces tissue concentrations in excess of 3 days. It is difficult to predict, however, what this new agent's role will be. In general, 3-day courses of therapy are as effective as traditional longer courses of therapy and may be more effective than single-dose treatment. Three-day treatment regimens have advantages similar to single-dose therapy, such as enhanced participation in completing the regimen, decreased cost, and decreased adverse drug effects as compared to longer durations of therapy. Specific regimens are listed in Table 35-5. This abbreviated regimen is again reserved for female patients with acute, uncomplicated UTIs (Young & Koda-Kimble, 1995; Hatton et al, 1994; Mandell et al, 1995; Kunin, 1994b).

Although the traditional 7- to 14-day regimen for treatment of UTIs is considered excessive in many patient populations currently, some patients may still be reasonable candidates. Patients in this group include but are not limited to pregnant women, patients with pyelonephritis, and males. Patients with diabetes mellitus or prostatitis and those who relapse may need even longer courses of therapy (up to 4 to 6 weeks). Specific regimens are listed in Table 35-6 (Young & Koda-Kimble,

TABLE 35-6	Longer Treatment Regimens for UTIs

7- to 14-day treatment regimens may be used in any of the following patient populations:

Pregnant patients

Male patients

Patients with pyelonephritis

Patients with other complicated UTIs, such as prostatitis (may require 2–6 weeks of therapy)

Potential regimens are similar to 3-day treatment regimens and include:

Trimethoprim-sulfamethoxazole DS every 12 hours

Trimethoprim 100 mg every 12 hours

Ciprofloxacin 250 mg every 12 hours

Norfloxacin 400 mg every 12 hours

Nitrofurantoin 100 mg every 6 hours

Nalidixic acid 500 mg every 8 hours

Amoxicillin 250 mg every 8 hours

Amoxicillin/clavulanic acid 500 mg (amox.) every 12 hours

1995; Mandell et al, 1995; Lipsky, 1989; Kunin, 1994b; Norrby, 1994).

ROUTE OF ANTIMICROBIAL ADMINISTRATION

Oral antimicrobial therapy is usually sufficient to treat patients with a lower tract UTI. The route of administration may become an issue, however, in the treatment of upper tract infections such as pyelonephritis. The decision here is whether a patient requires oral or parenteral therapy. Patients with mild pyelonephritis without gastrointestinal symptoms (nausea, vomiting) or dehydration are also reasonable candidates for outpatient oral antimicrobial therapy. Inpatient, parenteral antimicrobial therapy is recommended, at least initially, in patients with severe pyelonephritis with gastrointestinal complaints and dehydration. These patients can usually be switched to an oral antimicrobial agent within a few days to complete the course of therapy (Young & Koda-Kimble, 1995; Kunin, 1994b).

AGE AND GENDER CONSIDERATIONS

Treatment of elderly patients with asymptomatic bacteriuria may not result in cure, and relapse is common, requiring continued treatment or chronic prophylaxis. Therefore, many practitioners choose not to treat asymptomatic bacteriuria in the elderly on the basis of cost, side effects, and potential complications of drug therapy. When drug therapy is used (eg, in the case of symptomatic bacteriuria or UTI), certain issues should be kept in mind when choosing the appropriate drug therapy. In the event of compromised renal function, drug dosages may need to be reduced accordingly. Elderly patients may be more sensitive to the adverse effects of the drugs used in the management of UTIs. The cephalosporins are a relatively common cause of *Clostridium difficile*-associated diarrhea. This should be considered in the treatment of elderly patients. The central nervous system side effects (ie, difficulty sleeping, nightmares, hallucinations, and other altered mental states) observed with the fluoroquinolones should be monitored when these agents are prescribed for this older patient population. In the elderly, given the presence of polypharmacy, the potential for drug interactions also exists. For example, the effects of warfarin and phenytoin may be potentiated by the use of TMP-SMX (Kunin, 1994a; Stamm & Hooton, 1993; Hatton et al, 1994).

SPECIFIC ANTIMICROBIAL REGIMENS

See Tables 35-4, 35-5, and 35-6.

PATIENT MONITORING AND FOLLOW-UP

In most cases of uncomplicated UTI, a patient's response to therapy can be evaluated clinically, with resolution of signs and symptoms as the major therapeutic goal. Patients should see relatively rapid resolution of these symptoms, usually within 48 to 72 hours after initiation of antimicrobial therapy (Perdue & Plaisance, 1995; Hatton et al, 1994; Mandell et al, 1995).

Microbiology follow-up would ideally consist of a return visit 10 to 14 days after drug treatment for a second urine specimen evaluation. Thorough patient follow-up classifies patients into one of four categories: cure, persistence of UTI, relapse, or reinfection. A patient defined as cured is one with negative urine cultures during drug therapy as well as 10 to 14 days after drug therapy (Perdue & Plaisance, 1995; Hatton et al, 1994; Mandell et al, 1995). Persistence of a UTI is defined as significant bacteria in the urine after 48 hours of antimicrobial

therapy, or the continued presence of the actual infecting organism in low numbers after 48 hours of antimicrobial therapy. Reasons for persistence include the presence of a resistant organism, subtherapeutic antimicrobial levels in the urine (because the patient took the medication inappropriately or missed doses, or there was insufficient dosing or absorption of the antimicrobial agent), or the presence of bacteria in soft tissue or renal calculi. The majority of these patients experience a relapse of the UTI (Hatton et al, 1994; Mandell et al, 1995).

RECURRENCE, RELAPSE, AND REINFECTIONS

Recurrent UTIs are subdivided into relapse or reinfection, with the large majority caused by reinfection. Relapse in female patients usually occurs from infection with the same organism causing the initial UTI, and these cases usually occur within 7 to 14 days after completion of the initial medication regimen. Another point of evaluation in patients with frequent recurrences is whether a correct diagnosis has been made, as in the case of interstitial nephritis. In general, patients with a relapsed UTI respond to a longer duration of treatment, ranging from 2 to 6 weeks (Perdue & Plaisance, 1995; Stamm & Hooton, 1993; Mandell et al, 1995; Kunin, 1994b).

Some female patients have frequent UTIs from reinfection. Reinfection is usually defined as a UTI caused by a different organism, such as a change in bacterial species, and can occur at any time during or after treatment with an antimicrobial agent. Risk factors in women that may be associated with frequent reinfection include sexual intercourse or diaphragm use. Antibiotic prophylaxis may be an option for many of these women, and this subject will be discussed in the next section (Young & Koda-Kimble, 1995; Perdue & Plaisance, 1995; Stamm & Hooton, 1993; Hatton et al, 1994; Lemcke et al, 1995).

Male patients may also experience recurrent UTIs, usually within 1 month of antimicrobial therapy, and frequently from relapse with the same microorganism causing the initial infection. Recurrent infection in males may be caused by persistence of bacteria in the prostate gland or a structural or anatomic abnormality of the urinary tract. In general, these male patients should be treated with a longer duration of antimicrobial therapy (about 1 month) (Lipsky, 1989).

ANTIBIOTIC PROPHYLAXIS

Chronic UTIs may be managed in a number of ways, including treatment of each recurrence with a short duration of therapy, treatment of each recurrence with a longer duration of therapy, or the administration of prophylactic antibiotic therapy. The frequency of recurrence usually determines whether a patient is a candidate for antibiotic prophylaxis. Patients with more than two or three UTIs per year are reasonable candidates for antibiotic prophylaxis. Other patients who may be reasonable candidates are elderly patients with chronic colonization with potential pathogenic organisms, patients with vesicoureteral reflux, and patients with long-term indwelling catheters (Kunin, 1994a; Young & Koda-Kimble, 1995; Perdue & Plaisance, 1995; Stamm & Hooton, 1993; Hatton et al, 1994).

Antibiotic prophylaxis regimens consist of the administration of low-dose antimicrobial agents for several months, with the goal being to prevent bacterial colonization of the urinary tract. Antimicrobial agents are given either daily or every other day (three times weekly) for several months. The duration of

TABLE 35-7	Antibiotic Prophylaxis for UTIs

Low-dose, chronic prophylaxis regimens, usually given daily or 3 times a week (every other day):

Trimethoprim-sulfamethoxazole SS[a] ½ to 1 tab

Trimethoprim 100 mg

Nitrofurantoin 50–100 mg

Cephalexin 125–250 mg

Norfloxacin 200 mg

[a] SS = single-strength tablets

antibiotic prophylaxis should be individualized for each patient; however, regimens longer than 6 months may increase the possibility of antimicrobial resistance. Specific regimens are listed in Table 35-7 (Kunin, 1994a; Young & Koda-Kimble, 1995; Perdue & Plaisance, 1995; Stamm & Hooton, 1993; Hatton et al, 1994).

In women with recurrent UTIs associated with sexual intercourse or contraceptive use, single-dose treatment should be taken either immediately before or after intercourse. This type of regimen is beneficial because of its efficacy, low cost, good patient acceptance and participation in completing the regimen, and decreased incidence of adverse drug reactions because of the administration of only one dose. Specific regimens are listed in Table 35-8 (Kunin, 1994a; Young & Koda-Kimble, 1995; Perdue & Plaisance, 1995).

Another option is for women with frequent UTI recurrences to initiate therapy themselves when symptoms occur. These regimens consist of therapy with either a single dose or a 3-day regimen. Women who are not candidates for this regimen because of patient acceptance and reliability issues or for other reasons should be considered for chronic, low-dose antibiotic prophylaxis (Kunin, 1994a; Young & Koda-Kimble, 1995; Perdue & Plaisance, 1995).

In all of these cases, the risk of using these antibiotics (eg, the development of resistance) needs to be weighed against the benefits of using such a regimen.

Nonmedication Regimens

Nonpharmacologic therapies also play a role in the management of UTIs. These include hydration, urinary acidification, and the use of analgesics. Hydration is theorized to be of importance in diluting out bacteria in the urine, which are then excreted. This practice is controversial, and patients should be counseled to drink according to the specific directions given by their primary care provider or pharmacist; any medications that may require more fluid should be noted (Perdue & Plaisance, 1995; Mandell et al, 1995).

TABLE 35-8	Postcoital Prophylaxis Regimens

Regimens to be taken immediately before or after sexual intercourse:

Trimethoprim-sulfamethoxazole SS[a] ½ to 1 tab

Cephalexin 250 mg

Nitrofurantoin 50–100 mg

[a] SS = single-strength tablet

Keeping the urine acidic allows more antibacterial activity to be exerted by the urine. However, urinary acidification is also somewhat controversial; a better intervention may be to try to eliminate items from the diet that cause urinary alkalinization (eg, antacids, milk, and sodium bicarbonate). Overall, urinary acidification is rarely warranted for long-term antimicrobial therapy (Perdue & Plaisance, 1995; Mandell et al, 1995).

Controversy exists regarding the use of cranberry juice in the prevention of UTIs. It was once thought that cranberry juice exerted its effect through urinary acidification, although some of this thinking is changing. There may be some antibacterial activity associated with the ingestion of cranberry juice in volumes as little as 300 mL/day or the use of cranberry tablets, and it is thought to be caused by the hippuric acid from the berry. Although the use of cranberry juice and cranberry tablets may be an easy preventive measure, absolute recommendations regarding its use remain controversial (Perdue & Plaisance, 1995; Mandell et al, 1995).

Urinary analgesics such as phenazopyridine hydrochloride may play a small role in the short-term management of dysuria associated with an acute, uncomplicated UTI. These symptoms, however, usually respond relatively rapidly to antimicrobial therapy, so urinary analgesics may not be needed at all. Systemic analgesics may be helpful in patients with severe dysuria or flank pain (eg, acetaminophen, aspirin, or ibuprofen) (Perdue & Plaisance, 1995; Mandell et al, 1995).

Comprehensive Management Recommendations

The following regimens are for empiric treatment of UTIs; therapy should always be individualized for each patient. If urine cultures are performed, therapy may need to be changed based on the results of the culture and sensitivity.

ACUTE, UNCOMPLICATED, LOWER TRACT UTI

For nonpregnant females with no complications, initiate therapy with a 3- or 7-day course of oral TMP-SMX or fluoroquinolone antimicrobial agent, assuming there are no contraindications. Some patients may be candidates for single-dose therapy. For specific regimens, see Tables 35-4, 35-5, and 35-6 (Young & Koda-Kimble, 1995; Stamm & Hooton, 1993; Hatton et al, 1994; Kunin, 1994b; Lemcke et al, 1995).

For men with no complications, initiate therapy with a 7- to 14-day course of oral TMP-SMX or fluoroquinolone antimicrobial agent, assuming there are no contraindications. Male patients should not be considered candidates for abbreviated therapeutic regimens because of concern about the development of bacterial prostatitis. For specific regimens, see Table 35-6 (Stamm & Hooton, 1993; Hatton et al, 1994; Lipsky, 1989).

UPPER TRACT INFECTIONS IN FEMALES

For mild to moderate pyelonephritis without severe gastrointestinal symptoms or dehydration, initiate therapy with a 10- to 14-day course of an oral antimicrobial agent such as TMP-SMX or fluoroquinolone, assuming there are no contraindications. For specific regimens, see Table 35-6 (Young & Koda-Kimble, 1995; Kunin, 1994b).

RECURRENT UTI

For postcoital prophylaxis, initiate therapy with a single oral dose of cephalexin, nitrofurantoin, or TMP-SMX, assuming no contraindications are present. For specific regimens, see Table 35-8 (Perdue & Plaisance, 1995; Stamm & Hooton, 1993; Hatton et al, 1994).

For continuous prophylaxis, initiate therapy either daily or every other day (three times weekly) with an oral antimicrobial agent such as cephalexin, TMP-SMX, nitrofurantoin, or a fluoroquinolone. The duration should be individualized, ranging from 6 weeks to 6 months of continuous therapy. Once the course is completed, patients should be re-evaluated. For specific regimens, see Table 35-7 (Young & Koda-Kimble, 1995; Perdue & Plaisance, 1995; Stamm & Hooton, 1993; Hatton et al, 1994).

ASYMPTOMATIC BACTERIURIA

In elderly patients, the management of asymptomatic bacteriuria is controversial. Either no therapy or a 3-day course of an oral antimicrobial agent is appropriate (Young & Koda-Kimble, 1995; Mandell et al, 1995; Lemcke et al, 1995). In patients with catheters, the management of asymptomatic bacteriuria is controversial. If the patient is asymptomatic, treatment is not generally recommended.

DYSURIA AND STERILE PYURIA ON URINALYSIS

These patients (males and females) need to be evaluated for other possible causes of dysuria, such as a chlamydial or gonococcal infection.

NEPHROLITHIASIS

Once stones have been removed, postoperative stone solvent irrigations may be warranted to remove any microscopic fragments. Examples of such solutions include Suby's G solution or hemiacidrin. An in-depth discussion of this therapy is beyond the scope of this chapter (Mandell et al, 1995).

Antibiotics are used as adjunctive therapy in the management of infection-induced nephrolithiasis and should be chosen based on the results of culture and sensitivity. Long-term use of antimicrobial agents may be warranted in specific patient populations (Mandell et al, 1995).

Prevention

PRIMARY PREVENTION

Knowledge of the risk factors for UTIs, and taking action to alter these factors, may help reduce the incidence of UTIs. In general, these alterations include improved sexual hygiene and use of improved, more sterile techniques for urinary catheterization.

Health Promotion and Specific Protection

Because the highest incidence of UTIs occurs in women of childbearing age, it is important that specific steps be taken to reduce their UTI risk. Women should empty their bladders completely after sexual intercourse. Because frequency of sexual intercourse has been suggested as a UTI risk factor, education about and alteration of this practice may lower the risk of UTI.

In postmenopausal women, estrogen deficiency has been suggested as a contributing factor to the increased incidence of UTIs. It has been suggested that estrogen supplementation,

TABLE 35-9	Self-Initiated Prophylaxis for UTIs

Candidates for self-initiated treatment:

- Women willing to participate in pharmacotherapy
- Women who have frequent or recurrent UTIs

Therapeutic regimens consist of either a single dose or a 3-day regimen as listed in Tables 35-4 and 35-5.

either orally or via estrogen vaginal cream, may help to reduce this incidence, but evidence is lacking (Stamm & Hooton, 1993; Lemcke et al, 1995).

UTI risk can be lowered in women of all ages by modifying the periurethral wiping technique used. Front-to-back wiping, as opposed to back-to-front wiping, can help minimize urethral exposure to uropathogens such as *E. coli*, which may be colonized in the anal area.

UTIs attributed to *E. coli* obtained through anal intercourse have been observed. The use of condoms during this sexual practice may help reduce a man's risk of contracting a UTI in this manner.

Cases of catheter-associated UTI exceed 1 million annually in the United States; therefore, lowering this risk is imperative. Strategies used to reduce rates of morbidity and mortality and costs of catheter-related infection include sterile insertion and care of the catheter, prompt catheter removal, and the use of a closed collecting system (DiPiro et al, 1997; Hatton et al, 1994; Mandell et al, 1995). Additionally, lower rates of bacteriuria have been observed with intermittent versus long-term indwelling catheterization (DiPiro et al, 1997).

Secondary Prevention

Early Diagnosis, Prompt Treatment, and Disability Limitation

As previously mentioned, a fair number of patients experience recurrent UTIs. Effective prophylactic measures prevent such recurrences in susceptible females and males with a prostatic focus. In addition to the primary prevention modalities mentioned, medical prophylaxis is often used in patients with recurrent UTIs.

TERTIARY PREVENTION

See Table 35-9.

TEACHING AND SELF-CARE

Patients with UTIs and nephrolithiasis must recognize the signs and symptoms of these disorders and then take the appropriate action. Whether this action includes presentation to a primary care provider or immediate self-treatment with a pre-prescribed supply of antibiotics is a conclusion to be reached jointly by the provider and the patient. The appropriate treatment plan chosen is very patient-specific.

Dispelling and clarifying the myths surrounding the treatment of these conditions is also of great importance. Two such myths previously discussed include increased hydration and the use of cranberry juice (Hatton et al, 1994; Mandell et al, 1995; Kunin, 1994b; von Rosenstiel & Adam, 1994).

TABLE 35-10	Self-Care: Ways to Reduce UTI Risk

GENERAL SUGGESTIONS

- Good perineal hygiene (eg, front-to-back wiping)

SUGGESTIONS RELATIVE TO SEXUAL ACTIVITY

- Complete postcoital voiding of the bladder
- Good postcoital hygiene (eg, appropriate cleansing of perineal area after coitus and after the use of diaphragm or spermicidal jelly)

SUGGESTIONS RELATIVE TO CATHETER USE

- Use of sterile technique with insertion and care of catheter (eg, in intermittent catheterization, wash hands before catheter insertion and properly sterilize the catheters if they are reused)
- Prompt catheter removal
- Use of a closed collecting system when chronic catheterization, internal or external, is used
- Use of intermittent catheterization whenever possible versus long-term, indwelling catheterization

General considerations regarding the self-care of UTI and nephrolithiasis include awareness of the presenting signs and symptoms, which may differ among various patient populations. A healthy young woman will have different presenting symptoms than a paraplegic patient who requires intermittent catheterization. In addition to increased awareness is the importance of keeping the lines of communication open between the patient and the primary care provider. Following these general guidelines should help to reduce the morbidity associated with UTIs and nephrolithiasis. Specific suggestions that patients can follow to help reduce their risk of developing UTIs and nephrolithiasis can be found in Table 35-10.

COMMUNITY RESOURCES

- American Board of Urology, 2216 Ivy Rd., Suite 210, Charlottesville, VA 22903
- American Foundation of Urologic Disease, 300 W. Pratt St., Suite 401, Baltimore, MD 21201
- National Institute of Diabetes and Digestive and Kidney Disease—Urinary Tract Infections in Adults: www.niddk.nih.gov.UrinaryTractInfections.html
- University Health Service—Urinary Tract Information: www.rochester.edu/student-srvcs/UHS/urinary.html

REFERRAL POINTS AND CLINICAL WARNINGS

Although many patients contact their primary care provider with classic UTI symptomatology, leading to appropriate diagnosis and timely treatment, others present with symptoms well beyond those of the classic lower UTI. The need for further referral or perhaps hospitalization in these situations depends on a number of factors, including:

- Symptomatology
- Social situation
- Ability of the patient to maintain adequate fluid intake
- Tolerance of oral medications
- Excessive recurrence of UTIs despite appropriate prophylactic therapy

- Complicated UTIs
- Suspected or diagnosed pyelonephritis
- Relapsing UTIs
- Resistant UTIs.

Symptomatology indicative of bacteremia (eg, fever and rigors) or symptoms of endotoxemia, including hypotension, signal the need for hospitalization and treatment with intravenous antibiotics. These symptoms are also frequently accompanied by an inability to tolerate oral medications or hydration. Particularly in patients with diabetes, hospitalization is important because acute pyelonephritis may predispose such a patient to diabetic ketoacidosis.

Referral may also be important in the patient with recurrent UTIs. In the case of relapsing UTIs, in which an organism persists despite appropriate antimicrobial therapy, an increased duration of therapy may be warranted. If such a treatment duration is unsuccessful, referral for anatomic and functional evaluation of the urinary tract should be made (Perdue & Plaisance, 1995).

■ ■ ■ CLINICAL PEARLS

- UTI recurrence has been associated with diaphragm use and the use of spermicides, because spermicides induce *E. coli* colonization of the vagina.
- Problems with sterility and contamination of urine specimens may affect the results of the urinalysis. These problems are mainly caused by poor or inconsistent collection methods or failure to take the specimen to the laboratory immediately (or failure to refrigerate the specimen). Therefore, bacteriuria alone is not diagnostic of a UTI.
- Many agents used as antibiotics for UTIs may cause photosensitivity. Patients should be warned about this potential effect and should use sunscreens while taking these antibiotics.
- Elderly patients may be more sensitive to the adverse effects of the drugs used in the management of UTIs.
- There may be some antibacterial activity associated with the ingestion of cranberry juice in volumes as little as 300 mL/day or the use of cranberry tablets, and it is thought to be caused by the hippuric acid from the berry.

EDITOR'S NOTE:

COMPLEMENTARY APPROACHES

A general discussion of complementary approaches can be found in Chapter 3. The following, while not an exhaustive list, are some complementary approaches being used for this condition. Additional information on these approaches, including precautions, can be found in Appendices A and B. Providers need to assess for the use of complementary approaches as part of the patient's history, as they may impact conventional therapies, and patients may not volunteer this information unless specifically asked. Efficacy of many complementary approaches is not as well documented as that of conventional therapies. Providers need to read the literature before suggesting these complementary approaches.

- Complementary Modalities
  Aromatherapy

References

Bailey, R.R. (1993). Management of lower urinary tract infections. *Drugs, 45*(Suppl 3), 139–144.

DiPiro, J.T., Talbert, R.L., Yee, G.C., Matzke, G.R., Wells, B.G., & Posey, L.M. (1997). *Pharmacotherapy: A pathophysiologic approach.* Stamford, CT: Appleton & Lange.

Hatton, J., Hughes, M., & Raymond, C.H. (1994). Management of bacterial urinary tract infections in adults. *Annals of Pharmacotherapy, 28*(November), 1264–1272.

Kunin, C.M. (1994a). Chemoprophylaxis and suppressive therapy in the management of urinary tract infections. *Journal of Antimicrobial Chemotherapy, 33*(Suppl A), 51–62.

Kunin, C.M. (1994b). Urinary tract infections in females. *Clinical Infectious Diseases, 18*(January), 1–10.

Lemcke, D.P., Pattison, J., Marshall, L.A., & Cowley, D.S. (1995). *Primary care of women.* Norwalk, CT: Appleton & Lange.

Lipsky, B.A. (1989). Urinary tract infections in men: Epidemiology, pathophysiology, diagnosis, and treatment. *Annals of Internal Medicine, 110*(2), 138–150.

Lowers, J. (1997). First single-dose therapy approved for treating UTIs. *Pharmacy Today, 3* (2), 14.

Mandell, G.L., Bennett, J.E., & Dolin, R. (1995). *Principles and practice of infectious disease.* New York: Churchill-Livingstone.

Norrby, S.R. (1994). Evaluation of antibiotics for treatment of urinary tract infections. *Journal of Antimicrobial Chemotherapy, 33*(Suppl A), 43–50.

Perdue, B.E., & Plaisance, K.I. (1995). Treatment of community-acquired urinary tract infections. *American Pharmacy, NS35*(12), 37–45.

Physicians' desk reference. (1997) Montvale, NJ: Medical Economics.

Reeves, D.S. (1994). A perspective on the safety of antibacterials used to treat urinary tract infections. *Journal of Antimicrobial Chemotherapy, 33*(Suppl A), 111–120.

Stamm, W.E., & Hooton, T.M. (1993). Management of urinary tract infections in adults. *N Engl J Med, 329*(18), 1328–1334.

Traub, S.L. (1992). *Basic skills in interpreting laboratory data.* Bethesda, MD: American Society of Health-System Pharmacists.

von Rosenstiel, N., & Adam, D. (1994). Quinolone antibacterials: An update on their pharmacology and therapeutic use. *Drugs, 47* (6), 872–901.

Warren, J.W. (1992). Catheter-associated bacteriuria. *Clinics in Geriatric Medicine, 8*(4), 805–819.

Young, L.Y., & Koda-Kimble, M.A. (1995). *Applied therapeutics: The clinical use of drugs.* Vancouver, WA: Applied Therapeutics.

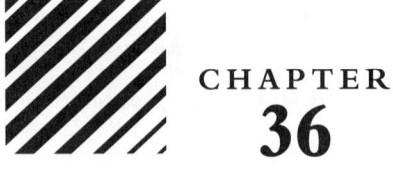

CHAPTER
36

Anemia

Duke Kasprisin, M.D.

The term "anemia" literally means "without blood" and is often used as if it were a disease, rather than a manifestation of an underlying disease process. Anemia is a condition of a decrease in the volume of blood, the number of erythrocytes, or the quantity of hemoglobin. Tissue hypoxia caused by the loss of oxygen is the principal defect caused by anemia.

Because of the numerous etiologies of anemia, they are frequently subdivided into their distinguishing characteristics, such as morphology, red cell size (microcytic, normocytic, macrocytic), or laboratory screening tests. An often-used method to categorize anemias is to describe them as decreased production, increased destruction (hemolysis), or bleeding. In reality, such clear distinctions are artificial. For example, a patient with chronic blood loss may have iron deficiency with a decrease in production. Still, these subdivisions are useful in making anemia more understandable.

ANATOMY, PHYSIOLOGY, AND PATHOLOGY

The most important function of erythrocytes is to transport oxygen to the tissues through hemoglobin. Hemoglobin accounts for 95% of erythrocyte protein (with most of the rest as enzymes, which provides energy for oxygen transfer and protection from oxidation and denaturation). Hemoglobin consists of a complex iron containing a porphyrin molecule called heme and a protein, globin.

The globin protein consists of two pairs of different polypeptides forming four intertwining chains. These chains are called alpha (α), beta (β), gamma (γ), and delta (δ). The type of polypeptide chain varies with age. The combination of globin chains determines the name of the hemoglobin.

In later fetal development, α and γ chains form fetal hemoglobin, (Hb F or $\alpha_2\gamma_2$), which is the first hemoglobin to exist postnatally. Hb F is the predominant hemoglobin of fetal life and decreases rapidly after birth. In adults, the majority of hemoglobin consists of two α chains and two β chains, named hemoglobin A (Hb A or $\alpha_2\beta_2$). Synthesis of this hemoglobin increases rapidly after birth and becomes the dominant form by the first few months of life. In addition to Hb A and the small remaining Hb F, an adult has minimal Hb A_2, which consists of $\alpha_2\delta_2$. The heme portion of hemoglobin is consistent throughout life and does not vary.

Both the percentage of erythroid precursors and bone marrow cellularity decrease shortly after birth, returning to normal adult level at 1 to 3 months of age. During the decrease in erythrocyte production in this postnatal period, insults cannot be compensated for by increasing red cell production. Therefore, this period of life is an especially vulnerable time.

In adults, replication and maturation of erythrocytes occur in the bone marrow. As the erythrocyte matures, it accumulates hemoglobin, loses its nucleus, and develops its final appearance of a biconcave disc. A critical characteristic of erythrocytes is deformability, which allows for negotiation through the capillary channels of the microcirculation.

As the erythrocyte ages, the cell begins to fragment and progressively loses its deformability. Changes in the biophysical characteristics cause the erythrocyte to become phagocytised by the macrophages in the spleen, liver, and bone marrow. The hemoglobin is degraded, the iron is reused or stored, and the protein portion of hemoglobin is metabolized to bile pigments, biliverdin and bilirubin. When these pigments are overproduced, the patient appears jaundiced.

The life span of erythrocytes is approximately 120 days. One percent of new cells are released each day to compensate for an equal number being destroyed. If this equilibrium is not maintained, tissue hypoxia results. Hypoxia is the primary stimulus for erythrocyte production through the release of erythropoietin. Erythropoietin is a hormone produced in the kidneys and to a lesser extent in the liver. Erythropoietin is the most important regulatory factor for erythropoiesis and is responsible for the proliferation and differentiation of erythroid progenitor cells. In the presence of anemia, erythropoietin production increases and stimulates a six- to eightfold increase of red cell production in the bone marrow.

TYPES OF ANEMIA

The subdivision of anemia by etiology is useful but does not account for the multiple mechanisms often present. For instance, chronic renal failure causes a loss of erythropoietin production, but hemolysis and coagulopathy can be components as well. Therefore, the etiology of anemia will be categorized by the principal mode of action, understanding these limitations.

Decreased Production

Effective erythropoiesis requires a functional marrow, adequate erythropoietin stimulation, and a sufficient quantity and proper assimilation of nutrients. Any problem maintaining effective erythropoiesis leads to a decrease in red cell production.

Some of the more common causes of anemia caused by decreased production are listed in Table 36-1.

TABLE 36-1	Anemias Caused by Decreased Erythropoiesis

Bone marrow depression or inhibition
    Aplastic anemia, congenital or acquired
    Pure red cell aplasia

Marrow replacement
    Leukemia
    Malignancy
    Others (myelofibrosis, osteopetrosis)

Myelodysplastic syndromes

Abnormalities in metabolism or deficiencies of substances needed for hemoglobin or red cell formation
    Erythropoietin
    Iron, B_{12}, folic acid, protein, others

Others—anemia of chronic disease, endocrine disorders

MYELOPHTHISIC ANEMIA

Myelophthisic anemia or marrow failure is a consequence of the infiltration of nonhematopoietic-producing cells. This can be caused by the abnormal proliferation of marrow components, as in the leukemias and multiple myeloma, or by metastasis from cancers, such as breast or prostate cancer or neuroblastoma, or from noncancerous cells' crowding normal marrow components, as in the osteopetroses (marble bone disease), the lipid storage diseases, and myelofibrosis.

Myelofibrosis, the replacement of the bone marrow by fibrosis, can be primary (idiopathic) or secondary to other diseases, such as myeloproliferative disorders (eg, chronic myelogenous leukemia). Myelofibrosis is often associated with myeloid metaplasia that is extramedullary.

The myelophthisic anemias produce a normocytic, normochromic anemia. If the infiltration of the bone marrow is extensive, there is considerable variation of red cell shapes and immature red cells and granulocytes in the peripheral smear (leukoerythroblastosis) (Table 36-2).

MYELODYSPLASTIC SYNDROME

This syndrome is characterized by a clonal hematopoietic stem cell anomaly with abnormal maturation and ineffective hematopoiesis. The bone marrow can be either hypercellular or normocellular. Red cells are macrocytic but not as large as in megaloblastic anemia; they are occasionally normocytic.

In the past, this syndrome was identified as preleukemia, refractory anemia, or sideroachrestic anemia. The French-American-British classification system includes refractory anemia, refractory anemia with sideroblasts, refractory anemia with

TABLE 36-2	Specific Appearance of Red Blood Cells
Sickle cells	Sickle cell disease, sickle–thalassemia
Spherocytes	Hereditary spherocytosis, some immune hemolytic anemias
Elliptocytes	Hereditary elliptocytosis
Target cells	Thalassemia, Hb C and other hemoglobinopathies, iron deficiency, postsplenectomy, liver disease
Premature red cells in peripheral smear	Myelophthisic anemias, severe hemolysis, thalassemia major, postsplenectomy, some infections

excess blasts, chronic myelomonocytic leukemia, and refractory anemia with excess blasts in transformation (Kouides & Bennett, 1996). The distinction between these categories is based on morphology and the number of blasts seen. The abnormal clone of cells is not stable and can gradually degenerate into a less favorable classification, including acute nonlymphocytic leukemia.

Treatment is controversial. Early therapy does not appear to affect the progression of the disease.

Marrow failure can also result from an acquired absence of erythrocyte precursors (pure red cell aplasia) or of hematopoietic cells in general (aplastic anemia). Drugs are a frequent cause of marrow failure, including cancer chemotherapeutic drugs, resulting in a usually reversible marrow aplasia. Chloramphenicol has been associated with a rare idiosyncratic aplastic anemia.

CONGENITAL PURE RED CELL APLASIA

Congenital pure red cell aplasia (congenital hypoplastic anemia, Blackfan-Diamond syndrome) has multiple etiologies. Acquired pure red cell aplasia often is autoimmune, with the autoantibody directed against erythroid precursors or erythropoietin. Many adult cases are associated with thymoma. Other causes include drugs, toxins, riboflavin deficiency, infection, renal failure, malnutrition, and leukemia. The anemia is normochromic and normocytic or less commonly macrocytic. The reticulocyte count is reduced and the bone marrow shows an absence of red cell precursors, although precursors to other hematopoietic cell lines are abundant.

APLASTIC ANEMIA

The aplastic or hypoplastic anemias are characterized by a hypocellular bone marrow with fatty replacement as well as thrombocytopenia and leukopenia, leaving patients at risk for hemorrhage and infection. The best-known congenital or constitutional aplastic anemia is Fanconi's anemia, an autosomal recessive disorder associated with pancytopenia and skeletal anomalies, mostly of the hands and forearms. Other signs include café-au-lait spots, short stature, renal anomalies, microcephaly, and other central nervous system disease. Acquired aplastic anemias are most often idiopathic (50%), although drugs, toxins, radiation, paroxysmal nocturnal hemoglobinuria, and infections such as hepatitis can all play a role.

INEFFECTIVE ERYTHROPOIESIS

Ineffective erythropoiesis occurs in renal failure from lack of erythropoietin production. Lack of an adequate quantity or assimilation of nutrients is another common cause of this anemia.

Iron Deficiency Anemia

Iron deficiency anemia is the most common type of anemia. Anemia caused by dietary deficiency of iron is most often seen in infants and children and during pregnancy, when rapid growth requires increased amounts of iron. Dietary iron deficiency anemia in adults is uncommon in this country, although not in nations with severely inadequate diets. However, iron deficiency without anemia is extremely common in the United States.

In this country, iron deficiency anemia in adults is more often related to chronic blood loss. Many women are iron-deficient secondary to menstrual bleeding or pregnancy. Adolescent girls are particularly prone to iron deficiency anemia because of menstruation combined with a diet lacking adequate iron content.

In men, iron deficiency anemia is usually pathologic and often the first sign of colon cancer. Intestinal parasites are a major cause of iron loss in some areas of the world. Deficient iron ingestion may also be seen in the elderly or in alcoholics, and inadequate absorption can be seen in severe inflammatory bowel disease.

Iron deficiency can be associated with pica, the craving to ingest nonfood items; this is most common in children and pregnant women. Ice-eating (pagophagia) and dirt-eating (geophagia) are two of the most common, but a great variety of objects may be ingested.

Iron-Related Anemias

Other iron-related anemias include defects in the iron transfer to red cell precursors. In atransferrinemia, the protein transferrin, which transports iron from storage sites to the erythrocyte precursors, is either absent or abnormal. Total iron-binding capacity is low, in contrast to iron deficiency anemia, in which it is high.

In the sideroblastic anemias, iron is not properly used for hemoglobin synthesis. Iron stores are increased, with erythroid hyperplasia in the bone marrow. Using special stains to detect iron, ringed sideroblasts or iron deposits on developing erythrocytes can be seen. This anemia is primary, idiopathic, or secondary to drugs, toxins, alcohol, and other diseases. Some of the hereditary forms of this disease respond to pyridoxine therapy.

Other Nutritional Anemias—B_{12} and the Macrocytic Anemias

Vitamin B_{12} and folic acid deficiencies lead to megaloblastic anemia or large red cells and disordered maturation. Dietary deficiencies of these two vitamins are uncommon in this country. The liver can store large quantities of B_{12}, so prolonged periods of deficiency would be required to deplete these stores before the patient became symptomatic.

The most common form of anemia related to B_{12} is pernicious anemia. These patients lack a protein, intrinsic factor, which is secreted by the parietal cells of the gastric mucosa. Intrinsic factor binds B_{12} and allows absorption by the intestinal mucosa. Pernicious anemia is associated with atrophic gastric mucosa and hypochlorhydria. Some types are congenital; others are autoimmune, because autoantibodies to the gastric parietal cell or intrinsic factor are frequently observed, as well as endocrine deficiencies, particularly of the thyroid and adrenal glands. Other conditions that affect B_{12} include fish tapeworms, blind loop syndrome, intestinal inflammatory diseases, and gastric resections where changes in intestinal flora result.

Folic acid, which is abundant in green leafy vegetables, liver, mushrooms, and yeast, is easily destroyed by overcooking. Because the body cannot store as much folic acid as B_{12}, it is easier to develop folic acid deficiency. However, folic acid deficiency is more commonly associated with alcoholism, malabsorption syndromes, dialysis, and drugs (eg, methotrexate and other folic acid antagonists, some anticonvulsants, and drugs that affect DNA metabolism).

There are increased requirements for folic acid in pregnancy, infancy, malignancy, some hyperhematopoiesis conditions (eg,

sickle cell disease and thalassemia), and hypermetabolic conditions (eg, hyperthyroidism). In patients with megaloblastic anemia, it is important to rule out B_{12} deficiency, because treatment with folic acid will help the anemia but the neurologic defects will progress.

OTHER ANEMIAS CAUSED BY DECREASED PRODUCTION

Endocrine deficiencies, especially hypothyroidism, frequently result in anemia. Pituitary dysfunction, especially when thyroid-stimulating hormone is involved, produces a hypoproliferative anemia. Adrenocortical deficiency (Addison's disease) is also associated with anemia. Loss of androgen production in males causes a decrease in hematocrit to female levels. Anemia is reversed by hormonal replacement in endocrine diseases.

ANEMIA OF CHRONIC DISEASE

Anemia secondary to infection, inflammation (eg, rheumatoid arthritis), and neoplasm is common, although anemia of chronic disease does not have to be associated with a chronic disease. These normochromic, normocytic anemias are usually mild but difficult to resolve. Besides decreased production of red cells, there is also a slight decrease in red cell survival in this anemia.

Anemia of chronic disease results from an abnormality of iron reuse, causing a failure in erythroid hyperplastic compensation. A decrease in erythropoietin may also be a factor.

Increased Destruction

Table 36-3 lists some of the more common causes of anemia caused by increased destruction or hemolysis. The hemolytic anemias are usually divided into those whose etiology is intrinsic to the red cell (corpuscular) and those that are extrinsic to the red cell (extracorpuscular). Intrinsic red cell defects can be caused by abnormalities in the red cell membrane, the enzyme systems that enable the red cell to function, and hemoglobinopathies. Extrinsic defects are immune or nonimmune.

INTRINSIC RED CELL DEFECTS
Membrane Defects—Hereditary Spherocytosis
Many of the intrinsic red cell defects are genetic in nature and manifest as alterations in structural proteins. The most common is hereditary spherocytosis (Hassoun & Palek, 1996). This disease is autosomal dominant, and the red cells take on a sphero-

TABLE 36-3	**Anemias Due to Increased Destruction**

Defects intrinsic to the red cell
    Membrane (eg, hereditary spherocytosis)
    Enzyme (eg, G6PD deficiency)
    Hemoglobinopathies (eg, sickle cell, thalassemia)
Defects extrinsic to the red cell
    Mechanical
        Vascular (eg, microangiopathic hemolysis)
        Hypersplenism
        Iatrogenic (eg, artificial heart valves, extracorporeal oxygenation)
        Other (eg, infections, malignancies)
    Immune
        Isoimmune
        Autoimmune

cytic shape instead of the normal biconcave disc, increasing the osmotic fragility of the cell. The abnormal shape impedes red cell flexibility and ability to navigate the microcirculation of the spleen, resulting in increased phagocytization by the macrophages. The spleen enlarges and traps still more spherocytes, resulting in severe anemia and congestive heart failure if untreated. If the hemolysis is brisk, the patient appears jaundiced. Cholelithiasis is common because the rapid destruction of cells results in bilirubin stones in the gallbladder.

A family history of multiple members with anemia, jaundice, splenomegaly, or gallstones is common. However, because of incomplete penetrance of the gene, generations may be skipped, or both mild and severe symptoms may appear in the same family.

Patients with concurrent infections may go into aplastic crises. Severe hemolytic anemia accompanied by decreased red cell production can be life-threatening. Splenectomy is the only treatment that resolves the anemia. The spherocytosis is unaffected by splenectomy, but the rate of red cell production in the bone marrow is able to compensate for the loss by hemolysis once the major site of destruction has been removed. However, the immunologic risks of splenectomy include increased susceptibility to pneumococci and other encapsulated bacteria, particularly in children.

Red Cell Enzyme Defects—Glucose-6-Phosphate Dehydrogenase

As the red cell matures, it loses its nucleus, mitochondria, and microsomes, leaving very limited metabolic capacity. To maintain the energy necessary to function and transport oxygen, the primary source of energy for red cells is glucose. Glucose is metabolized via one of two pathways: the Embden-Meyerhof (glycolytic) or the hexose monophosphate shunt. Numerous enzymes can be affected by hereditary defects in these two pathways, resulting in clinical disorders, including hemolytic anemias. The most common of these enzyme defects involves an enzyme in the hexose monophosphate shunt pathway, glucose-6-phosphate dehydrogenase (G6PD). The gene for this enzyme is present on the X chromosome. More than 350 variants of this protein have been identified. Although some are capable of causing disease, others are protective. For instance, many variants of red cell enzymes and hemoglobins have evolved because they impart a partial resistance to *Plasmodium falciparum* malaria. Malaria, one of the most lethal infectious diseases in the world, reproduces in red cells. Severe G6PD deficiency impedes the survival of erythrocytes to these parasites.

The predominant form of this enzyme is Gd^B, G6PD B, or G-6-PD^B. The most common variant is Gd^A, which functions 80% to 90% as well as Gd^B. Gd^B differs from Gd^A by a single amino acid, the substitution of aspartic acid for asparagine. The variant Gd^{A-}, which is frequently seen in African Americans, has markedly decreased enzyme activity and can cause hemolysis. Males with this variant and females homozygous for this gene usually have no symptoms but can develop a severe hemolysis when their red cells are stressed (eg, infection, certain drugs, diabetic acidosis). A reaction to primaquine, an antimalarial, first identified this enzyme deficiency.

Another variant, $Gd^{Mediterranean}$, has even less enzyme activity than Gd^{A-}. Caucasians, especially Italians, Greeks, Arabs, and Sephardic Jews, are affected with this gene. This disease results in an even more severe hemolysis than Gd^{A-}.

Because the gene for G6PD is on the X chromosome, all males who inherit this gene are affected. Women with one affected gene are usually normal, but abnormal G6PD genes are so common that homozygous females are often seen. In females, only one of the two X chromosomes is active in any cell (Lyon hypothesis). Therefore, males and females with normal variants of G6PD have equal enzyme levels. If a woman is heterozygous for one of the deficient genes, she will have approximately half the normal level of enzyme. However, women with severely deficient genes may have normal enzyme levels. This is because red cells that inactivate X chromosomes containing affected genes are quickly destroyed. The only red cells that survive have the normal gene.

In patients with the most severe deficiency of G6PD, jaundice, hemoglobinuria (with resulting dark urine), renal failure, and severe, symptomatic anemia usually result within 1 to 3 days of the causative stress. In patients with less severe hemolysis, there is a moderate decline in hemoglobin. These episodes can easily be missed unless the diagnosis is considered.

Screening tests for this disease can detect the abnormality only if sufficient red cells are affected. Unfortunately, after a hemolytic episode, the oldest cells, with the lowest enzyme activity, are destroyed. The remaining younger cells have greater G6PD levels, and because these are the only ones that can be measured, false-negative results may occur. Because younger red cells contain more G6PD, the Gd^{A-} variant is usually self-limiting once the older cells are destroyed.

Drugs that cause hemolytic episodes include antimalarials (primaquine, quinacrine), antibiotics (sulfonamides, nitrofurantoin), and analgesics (acetylsalicylic acid). A G6PD-deficient patient treated with certain antibiotics and analgesics becomes a prime candidate for a hemolytic episode. Drugs that cause hemolysis in G6PD-deficient patients are listed in Table 36-4.

TABLE 36-4	Drugs Commonly Leading to Hemolysis in G6PD Deficiency	
ANTIMALARIALS		**ANALGESICS**
Primaquine		Acetanilid
Quinacrine (Atabrine)		Acetylsalicylic acid*
		Acetophenetidin (phenacetin)*
SULFONAMIDES		**SULFONES**
Sulfanilamide		Diaminodiphenyl sulfone (Dapsone)
Salicylazosulfapyridine (Azulfidine)		
Sulfisoxazole (Gantrisin)*		
OTHER ANTIBACTERIALS		**MISCELLANEOUS**
Nitrofurantoin (Furadantin)		Dimercaprol (BAL)
Nitrofurazone (Furacin)		Naphthalene (mothballs)
Chloramphenicol*		Methylene blue*
Para-aminosalicylic acid		Vitamin K (water-soluble analogues)*
Nalidixic acid		Ascorbic acid*

A more comprehensive list of drugs that have been implicated in oxidant-induced hemolysis appears in Beutler, E. (1969). *Pharmacology Review*, 21, 73.

* Hemolysis is infrequent and generally requires high concentrations of the drug. Probably a risk in Gd^{A-} but not in $Gd^{Mediterranean}$ or Gd^{Canton}.

Source: Beck, W.S., & Tepper, R.I. (1991). Hemolytic anemias. IV. Metabolic disorders. In W.S. Beck (Ed.). *Hematology*. Cambridge, MA: The MIT Press, p. 294.

Hemoglobinopathies

Other common causes of hemolysis are abnormalities in hemoglobin (hemoglobinopathies) or in hemoglobin synthesis (thalassemias). For oxygen to be bound in the lung and released in tissue, a very defined structure of hemoglobin is required. Variations can cause increased or decreased oxygen affinity, resulting in hemoglobin that either does not bind or does not release oxygen. Other variations may affect red cell shape and cause rapid destruction of cells and anemia.

Sickle Cell Disease

Sickle hemoglobin, the most common hemoglobinopathy, is caused by the replacement of a glutamic acid by valine at position 6 of β chain and is written Hb S or $\alpha_2\beta_2^S$ or $\alpha_2\beta_2^{6Glu \rightarrow val}$. The α chains are normal in Hb S. There is a one-in-four chance that two persons with sickle trait will have a child with sickle cell disease.

Patients with sickle cell disease produce mostly sickle hemoglobin, variable amounts of Hb F, and normal but small amounts of Hb A$_2$. The morphology of the red cells in sickle cell trait is normal. In sickle cell disease, however, the peripheral smear is markedly abnormal, with many bizarre-looking cells, especially the hallmark of the disease: red cells in the shape of sickles. The sickle cells are rigid, occlude small blood vessels, and damage tissue. The abnormally shaped cells quickly hemolyze, leading to the severe anemia that is classic in this disease.

The predominant form of hemoglobin in the newborn is Hb F, which contains no β chains. As a result, patients with sickle cell disease are rarely symptomatic as newborns. When β-chain production increases, sickle cells begin to appear and patients begin to have myriad symptoms. Almost every body system is eventually involved. Morbidity is caused by severe anemia and vaso-occlusive problems.

Patients with sickle cell disease usually have hematocrits between the high teens and low 30s. The anemia can be exaggerated by marrow failure caused by infection (particularly parvovirus B19), folic acid deficiency caused by increased erythrocyte production as a response to the anemia, and splenomegaly from increased entrapment and destruction of red cells.

Symptoms begin in infancy, often with acute and painful swelling of the hands and feet. Growth and maturation are hindered. Anemia develops quickly and can progress to congestive heart failure. The vaso-occlusive nature of the disease causes severe painful crises, often triggered by infection. Although these painful episodes can occur almost anywhere, they frequently occur in the abdomen, chest, and joints. It is often difficult to distinguish painful crises from other pathology because of the numerous systems that can be involved in this disease.

The clinical manifestations of sickle cell disease are listed in Table 36-5. Many symptoms can present a diagnostic dilemma. The development of gallstones and cholecystitis is often difficult to differentiate from abdominal pain crises. Bony changes mimic osteomyelitis on x-ray.

Other manifestations cause treatment difficulties as well. The kidneys lose their ability to concentrate the urine, so patients can dehydrate easily. Recurring strokes may require chronic transfusion to prevent further vaso-occlusive episodes, but transfusions add to the possibility of further complications.

TABLE 36-5	Sickle Cell Disease Clinical Manifestations
Organ	**Clinical Manifestations**
Constitutional signs	Impaired growth and development, failure to thrive; painful crisis, most commonly in the abdomen and extremities
Hematologic	Severe anemia, complicated by folic acid deficiency; cardiopulmonary symptoms
Immunologic	Spleen autoinfarcts; increased risk of infection and sepsis, particularly *Pneumococcus, Haemophilus,* and salmonella
Hepatobiliary	Jaundice, gallstones, impaired liver function, infarcts
Skeletal system	Bone infarcts with characteristic fish-mouth appearance on x-ray; aseptic necrosis of femoral head; osteomyelitis
Genitourinary	Isosthenuria; hematuria; priapism; complications with pregnancy
Pulmonary	Impaired pulmonary function, hypoxemia
Skin	Skin ulcers, especially on the lower extremities
Ocular	Retinal infarcts; AV anomalies, vitreous hemorrhage, retinitis proliferans, retinal detachment
Neurologic	Strokes, hemiplegia, coma, convulsions

The spleen infarcts early in life and the patient suffers all the immunologic risks of asplenia. Autosplenectomy is usually complete by age 8. Because of the increased risk of infection with *Pneumococcus, Haemophilus,* and salmonella, patients should be seen quickly if infection is a concern. Pneumococcal sepsis can progress from an asymptomatic state to death within a few hours. Therefore, pneumococcal vaccine is routinely given to these patients. Neurologic symptoms are common and recurring strokes usually require chronic transfusions to prevent further vaso-occlusive episodes.

In general, persons with sickle cell trait are completely asymptomatic. However, on occasion they may experience hematuria, splenic infarcts when exposed to severe hypoxia, problems concentrating urine, and crises that may proceed to death with extreme exercise, especially at high altitudes. Anesthesiologists must be particularly careful to avoid hypoxia in any patient with sickle hemoglobin.

Hemoglobin C Disease

The second most common hemoglobinopathy caused by a single amino acid substitution is hemoglobin C. Hemoglobin C consists of two normal α chains and β chains with a replacement of a glutamic acid by lysine at position 6, and is written Hb C or $\alpha_2\beta_2^C$ or $\alpha_2\beta_2^{6Glu \rightarrow lys}$. Persons who inherit the Hb C gene from only one parent and Hb A from the other have Hb C trait, with 60% to 75% Hb A and 25% to 40% Hb C. The gene occurs in approximately 2% of African Americans.

Heterozygous persons are asymptomatic, but their peripheral blood smears contain numerous target cells, which look like little bull's-eyes. Persons with homozygous Hb C have a mild anemia and splenomegaly. The peripheral smear demonstrates numerous target cells and intracellular crystals of hemoglobin. Recurrent arthralgias and abdominal pain are the predominant symptoms. Jaundice may be present.

Thalassemia

The thalassemias are inherited disorders with absence or diminished synthesis of one or more of the globin chains. Any chain can be involved. Like many of the abnormal hemoglobins, thalassemia parallels the malaria belt. The severity of the thalassemia depends on the chain involved and the degree to which synthesis is decreased. For example, because δ chains represent only a small proportion of hemoglobin chain synthesis, complete absence of δ-chain synthesis exists but is not a clinically significant entity.

The lack of balanced synthesis among hemoglobin chains in thalassemia leads to deficient production of one chain, with decreased hemoglobin and hypochromic, microcytic cells. There is an abundance of a second chain, which precipitates in the red cell, causing cell membrane damage. Thalassemia is a mixture of ineffective erythropoiesis and hemolysis.

Most populations have two genes for α chains on each chromosome for a total of four genes. If all four genes fail to produce α chains, a condition termed hydrops fetalis results. The patient becomes severely anemic and edematous and dies in utero or shortly after birth. If only one α gene is functional, the patient has Hb H disease, named because the excess β chains form a tetramer β_4 called Hb H. These patients suffer a moderate anemia (thalassemia intermedia).

If two α genes are functional, the severity may vary depending on whether the two genes are on the same chromosome (cis) or there is one on each chromosome (trans). Cis appears to be more severe, but both cause only mild anemias. A single affected gene cannot be clinically discerned and is usually diagnosed only by studying families with the more severe forms of the disease.

There appears to be only one gene for β-chain production on each chromosome 11. The β-thalassemia gene may produce a decreased number of β chains; this is referred to as a β^+ gene. When there are no β chains produced by the gene, it is termed β^0. When a person inherits only one thalassemia gene of either type, a mild microcytic, hypochromic anemia termed thalassemia minor results. The measurement of cell size is disproportionately low for the degree of anemia, which helps distinguish this from iron deficiency.

If both genes are involved with either β^+ or β^0, a severe anemia termed thalassemia major results. Milder β-thalassemia variants, sometimes termed silent carriers, also exist. When this gene is inherited with one of the severe β-thalassemia genes, an anemia of intermediate severity occurs, called thalassemia intermedia. Persons have varying degrees of residual Hb F production, which gives some protection against thalassemia. Numerous other thalassemia genes cause disease of variable severity, but they are not as common.

In β-thalassemia major, the patient is normal in the first months of life, when β-chain synthesis is normally limited. As the anemia progresses, hepatosplenomegaly develops, as well as cardiovascular changes related to congestive heart failure. Without transfusion, the thalassemic child usually dies within the first year of life from anemia and heart failure.

Combined Hemoglobinopathies

Because hemoglobinopathies are so common, combinations of abnormal hemoglobins are routinely encountered. The most common are Hb SC, S-β-thalassemia, and SS-α-thalassemia, although many other combinations have been reported.

Hb SC produces a much milder anemia than sickle cell disease. On peripheral smear, there may be sickle forms, or cells partially sickled with a central bulge of Hb C. There are many target cells, classic of Hb C. Hemoglobin electrophoresis demonstrates approximately equal amounts of Hb S and Hb C but no Hb A. The spleen remains palpable, and recurrent pain crises are usually less severe and more easily managed. Priapism and stroke may also occur. Other problems commonly encountered include hematuria, aseptic necrosis of the femoral head, ocular disease, and complications during pregnancy.

S-β-thalassemia exhibits more variability than other thalassemias, although this is dependent on the variant of β-thalassemia inherited. Microcytic cells, sickle forms, and target cells are seen on peripheral smear. The mean corpuscular volume (MCV) is low. Hemoglobin electrophoresis reveals Hb S and less or no Hb A. In S-β^0-thalassemia, there is more Hb A_2. On hemoglobin electrophoresis, mild forms of S-β-thalassemia can be distinguished from sickle trait, because sickle trait shows more Hb A than Hb S. Patients with S-β^0-thalassemia often have disease as severe as sickle cell anemia. Those with milder β-chain anomalies usually have less severe anemia and symptoms.

SS-α-thalassemia patients have two sickle cell genes and one α-thalassemia gene. Because these patients generally have milder symptoms and anemia, the primary care provider should be suspicious of this entity when a homozygous sickle cell patient has a low MCV. Family studies can identify this syndrome. Ocular disease and osteonecrosis are more commonly seen in these patients.

EXTRINSIC RED CELL DEFECTS

There are numerous causes of hemolysis related to factors extrinsic to the red cell. For example, mechanical damage to the red cell membrane can be caused by extracorporeal oxygenation during surgery, or by artificial heart valves. Strenuous exercise can lead to red cell injury within the blood vessels and can cause hemolysis and hemoglobinuria (march hemoglobinuria). Extensive burns may traumatize the red cell membranes, also leading to hemolysis. The passage of erythrocytes through damaged small blood vessels causes mechanical injury of the cell with fragmentation. Microangiopathic hemolytic anemia of this type is seen in disorders such as thrombotic thrombocytopenic purpura, hemolytic-uremic syndrome, and disseminated intravascular coagulopathy.

Antibody-Mediated Anemias—Isoimmune

Antibody-mediated anemia can be isoimmune or autoimmune. Maternal–fetal red cell incompatibility is caused by a fetal red cell antigen that is not shared by the mother. Hemolytic disease of the fetus and newborn occurs when the mother produces an antibody directed against this red cell antigen. The antibody must be able to cross the placenta (IgG can, IgM cannot). Death in utero results if a large quantity of antibody develops early in pregnancy. In live births, morbidity and mortality rates depend on the severity of the anemia and the quantity of bilirubin.

In the past, Rh incompatibility was the most common cause of severe disease. With the advent of Rh_O immune globulin, the incidence of hemolytic disease of the newborn caused by Rh_O has decreased dramatically. Rh_O immune globulin is given to Rh-negative women at 28 weeks' gestation and again shortly after birth.

In the rare case of Rh$_O$ immune globulin failure, or in cases caused by other red cell antigens, measurement of the level of maternal antibody titers may be indicative of fetal problems. Amniocentesis can predict the degree of anemia and the presence of symptoms in the fetus and newborn. Treatment of severe cases includes intrauterine transfusion or exchange transfusion once the baby is delivered.

Patients who develop antibodies against transfused red cells will coat these cells with antibody, and they may be destroyed. The rate of destruction determines the degree of symptoms. The presence of antibodies or complement on the red cells can be detected by a direct antiglobulin test (direct Coombs'), and antibodies directed against red cell antigens can be discovered with an indirect antiglobulin test (indirect Coombs'). The correlation between the degree of positivity and the potential for hemolysis may be poor. However, this test frequently yields significant information when a patient with hemolysis has an immune etiology.

Autoimmune Hemolytic Anemias

The development of autoantibodies directed against red cell antigens can be symptomatic or asymptomatic. When hemolysis occurs in the presence of autoantibodies, the anemia is termed autoimmune hemolytic anemia. Autoimmune hemolytic anemia can be divided into two main categories, warm and cold.

Warm autoimmune hemolytic anemia is the more common disorder. Autoantibody can be identified by a positive direct antiglobulin test at 37°C. In this disease, either IgG or complement can be found on the surface of the red cell. Sometimes IgM or IgA is the causative agent. The etiology of autoimmune hemolytic anemia caused by warm reactive antibodies is idiopathic in more than half of the cases. It is also associated with drugs such as α-methyldopa and penicillin, lymphoproliferative disorders, and other maladies, such as lupus erythematosus.

Autoimmune hemolytic anemia caused by cold-reacting antibodies (cold-agglutinin disease) is caused by autoantibodies that react best at temperatures less than 37°C. Patients may have symptoms of vaso-occlusion in the distal extremities. Hemolysis, when present, is usually mild but is occasionally severe, particularly after cold exposure. Surgery requiring the body to be cooled can be a problem for persons with this disorder. Transient disease occurs in younger patients after infection with *Mycoplasma pneumoniae* and less often infectious mononucleosis. In older patients, cold-agglutinin disease is more commonly idiopathic or associated with lymphoproliferative disorders. The causative antibody is usually IgM, more rarely IgG. IgA can cause acrocyanosis but not hemolysis.

Paroxysmal cold hemoglobinuria is now a rare cause of intravascular hemolysis after cold exposure. It was commonly associated with congenital or acquired syphilis but also occurs with viral illnesses.

Bleeding

Hemorrhage as a cause of anemia can be subdivided into acute and chronic bleeding. Symptoms from rapid blood loss secondary to trauma, surgery, hemostatic failure, or rupture of a large blood vessel depend on the volume of blood lost and the speed with which it is lost.

The initial problems associated with sudden, massive blood loss are related to volume depletion and cardiovascular collapse.

Most healthy persons can withstand a 15% to 20% loss of blood volume without serious complication. As the volume loss approaches 20% to 30%, cardiovascular distress occurs. More than 30% loss leads to shock, and 40% or more is acutely life-threatening. Fluid replacement is critical to maintain blood volume and pressure. Fluid resuscitation and the emergency management of acute blood loss are complex and the focus of emergency medical practice (Fakhry & Sheldon, 1994).

Initially, the hematocrit and other indices are misleading in acute blood loss. Until fluids enter the circulation and hemodilute the remaining red cells, the hematocrit appears higher than it actually is. It may take a few hours before the significance of the drop in hematocrit can be fully appreciated. The resulting anemia is normocytic and normochromic. As red cell production increases, the patient becomes microcytic and hypochromic if there are inadequate iron stores. In chronic blood loss, the patient usually demonstrates a microcytic, hypochromic anemia as progressive iron deficiency occurs.

EPIDEMIOLOGY

The epidemiology of anemia is frequently genetic. The other etiologies tend to be secondary to primary diseases, and therefore patients are not at independent risk of acquiring those diseases. Myelodysplastic syndrome is a group of diseases that are more likely to occur in patients older than 50, but younger patients and children are also at risk. Congenital pure red cell aplasia can be genetic, and some types are associated with skeletal and other congenital anomalies.

In G6PD deficiency, 20% of African Americans have the common variant Gd^A and 11% have the hemolytic type Gd^{A-}. The frequency of the sickle cell gene parallels the incidence of *P. falciparum* malaria. Approximately 8% of African Americans are heterozygous for sickle hemoglobin, and 1 in 400 African Americans has sickle cell disease. The gene is also seen in Greeks, Italians, Arabs, and Asian Indians.

Anomalies of β-chain synthesis, β-thalassemia or Cooley's anemia, are most commonly seen in Mediterranean populations (eg, Italians, Greeks). α-thalassemia is most common in Asian populations and among Africans and African Americans.

Although α-thalassemia appears in many populations, the severe forms involving three or four genes appear almost exclusively in Asian populations. This may be caused by a higher incidence of two affected genes per chromosome (cis); other populations are more likely to have only one affected gene per chromosome (trans).

DIAGNOSTIC CRITERIA

A decreased hemoglobin or hematocrit is the laboratory definition of anemia. Normal values, however, vary with age, geographic location, and especially gender. Androgens stimulate erythropoiesis, and estrogen does not. Therefore, normal hemoglobin levels for men are higher than for women, which becomes apparent at puberty. Normal hemoglobin levels are 14 to 16 g/dL for men and 12 to 14 g/dL for women. The hematocrit is approximately three times the level of hemoglobin, so the normal hematocrit for men is 48 and for women 42.

A reduction in the oxygen content of air at high altitudes leads to a compensatory increase in red cell mass (polycythemia). Polycythemia can also result from tissue hypoxia in such conditions as congenital heart disease with right-to-left shunt or some chronic pulmonary diseases.

HISTORY AND PHYSICAL EXAM

The history in anemia varies with the age of onset and whether the anemia is acute or chronic. Family history can reveal hereditary forms of anemia. Questions regarding a family history of anemia or anemia treatment, bleeding disorders, splenomegaly, cholelithiasis, jaundice, transfusions, or drug sensitivities should be asked.

A history of bleeding, including abnormal bleeding from recent surgery, should be elicited. Recent infection and drug ingestion may identify drug-induced anemia or secondary marrow failure. Recent travel, toxin exposure, radiation, and parasite infestations should be explored.

Symptoms depend on the severity and duration of the anemia and may affect multiple organ systems. Weakness, fatigue, and drowsiness are common, as are central nervous symptoms such as headache, dizziness, vertigo, irritability, and behavioral changes. Cardiovascular and pulmonary compensatory responses include increases in heart rate and cardiac output. Heart murmurs are a manifestation of increased output and are common in severe anemia. Heart failure results if the demand on the heart exceeds its compensatory capacity. Other symptoms include amenorrhea, loss of libido, and gastrointestinal complaints.

The underlying cause of the anemia may lead to additional signs and symptoms. An acute and severe blood loss will lead to shock, but chronic blood loss leading to the same degree of anemia may be accommodated by increased red cell production. Severe hemolysis may cause jaundice and splenomegaly. Petechiae may indicate a platelet deficiency secondary to leukemia. Neoplastic replacement of the marrow will result in anemia as well as thrombocytopenia and leukopenia.

Concave or spoon-shaped fingernails (koilonychia) are seen with iron deficiency anemia. Iron-deficient patients may also lose red cells, proteins, and minerals through the intestines, leading to edema and guaiac-positive stools. Poor temperature regulation is also associated with iron deficiency anemia, as are atrophic glossitis, dysphagia, esophageal webs, and atrophic gastritis.

B_{12} deficiency is associated with a variety of symptoms, but neurologic problems are classic. These symptoms are particularly difficult to diagnose because they may occur even in the absence of anemia. Neurologic deficits become permanent if the B_{12} deficiency is not corrected in a timely manner.

DIAGNOSTIC STUDIES

Reticulocyte Count

Reticulocytes are red cell precursors that have lost their nuclei but still maintain ribosomes and mitochondria and retain the ability to synthesize heme and globin. On the peripheral smear they appear larger than red cells and bluish (basophilic), which is termed polychromatophilia, allowing special stains to be used to quantify them.

In the presence of anemia, an elevated reticulocyte count (reticulocytosis) implies a functioning bone marrow; therefore, the red cell loss is caused by hemolysis or hemorrhage. A low reticulocyte count (reticulocytopenia) suggests marrow failure, as in pure red cell aplasia or aplastic anemia. It can also be seen in an occupied marrow as in leukemia, or a malfunctioning marrow caused by a deficiency state such as iron deficiency or renal disease.

Normally, reticulocytes are produced at 1% per day. The lack of older red cells caused by bleeding or hemolysis will produce an artificially elevated reticulocyte count. This can be corrected mathematically by calculating the reticulocyte index ([patient's hematocrit/normal hematocrit] × reticulocyte percentage).

If the bone marrow is functional, it will take a few days for an elevated reticulocyte response to follow an acute blood loss.

Red Cell Morphology

Red cell size and the presence of abnormal cells help identify the pathologic mechanism causing the anemia. Sometimes the presence of abnormal morphology yields a definitive diagnosis, as in sickle cell disease.

On most automated blood counts, a quantitative evaluation of cell size is included with the hemoglobin, hematocrit, and red cell count. The MCV, the mean corpuscular hemoglobin (MCH), and the mean corpuscular hemoglobin concentration (MCHC) are usually included on the blood count. A reticulocyte count, a microscopic viewing of the peripheral smear, a platelet count, and a white cell differential are part of some routine screenings or can be ordered separately (Gulati & Huyn, 1994).

Table 36-6 describes the initial laboratory screening that can be used to distinguish the major causes of anemia. The reticulocyte count separates anemia into the three major pathophysiologic mechanisms (decreased production, increased destruction, and hemorrhage). The MCV separates the microcytic (low MCV) and hypochromic (low MCHC) anemias from the normocytic (normal MCV), normochromic (normal MCHC), and macrocytic (high MCV) anemias.

The peripheral smear can reveal signs of specific anemias. Sickle cells are seen in sickle cell disease and some other hemoglobinopathies combined with the sickle gene (eg, sickle–thalassemia). Spherocytes are observed in hereditary spherocytosis and in immune hemolytic anemias. Target cells are common in Hb C disease and thalassemia. Basophilic stippling is often present in lead poisoning (Gulati & Huyn, 1994).

An absolute decrease in platelets and white cells or the appearance of reduced numbers of these cells on the peripheral smear may indicate a marrow failure of all cell lines.

The serum haptoglobin is a good screening test for hemolysis. Haptoglobin is a protein formed in the liver that binds free hemoglobin released by the lysis of red cells. Low levels of haptoglobin suggest the presence of hemolysis. Haptoglobin levels are also low in severe hepatic disease.

The heme component of hemoglobin metabolizes to bilirubin. Bilirubin is not very soluble in water and is excreted by the liver and through the feces. This type of bilirubin is termed unconjugated or indirect bilirubin. Some of the excreted bilirubin is absorbed through the gut and transported to the liver, where it is joined with glucuronic acid to form conjugated (direct) bilirubin. Conjugated bilirubin is water-soluble and is excreted by the kidney. An elevated indirect bilirubin level is a

TABLE 36-6	Laboratory Management of Anemia		
Initial			
Reticulocytosis		Reticulocytopenia	
Hemolysis or chronic hemorrhage		Marrow failure or replacement	
MCV/MCH and Peripheral Smear			
Hypochromic			
Microcytic	Macrocytic	Normochromic	
Iron deficiency Nutritional	B_{12} deficiency	Acute blood loss	
	Folate deficiency	Marrow failure Aplastic/red cell aplasia Renal disease Chronic illness	
Iron deficiency Chronic blood loss	Folic acid antagonists		
Sideroachrestic anemias	Other megaloblastic anemias	Myelophthisic anemias	
Thalassemia		Corpuscular hemolytic anemias Membrane Enzyme Some hemoglobinopathies	
Lead poisoning		Extracorpuscular hemolytic anemias Immune Nonimmune	

measure of hemolysis or defects in bilirubin metabolism. Direct bilirubin is elevated most commonly by hepatitis, liver, and gallbladder disease and by certain drugs. Total bilirubin levels are a combination of both direct and indirect forms. Bilirubin is an unreliable test for hemolysis but can be used to confirm the clinical suspicion of jaundice.

More specific tests can confirm the diagnoses of anemia. In hemolytic anemia, a Coombs' test may distinguish an immune anemia in the absence of characteristic cells in the peripheral smear. In a microcytic, hypochromic anemia, tests for iron deficiency and for blood loss, such as testing stool for occult blood, would follow. Hemoglobin electrophoresis may be indicated if iron deficiency is ruled out. A bone marrow aspiration will identify aplastic anemia, pure red cell aplasia, marrow invasion, and a variety of other causes for anemia (Hyun et al, 1994). Tests for specific systemic disease are indicated if it appears the anemia is secondary.

Populations at risk for hemoglobinopathies, G6PD, and other hereditary forms of anemia can be screened to detect carrier status for abnormal genes. Genetic counseling allows couples to make informed decisions concerning the transmission of a hereditary disease to their offspring. The hemoglobinopathies, thalassemias, and other hereditary anemias can be diagnosed prenatally by studying fetal DNA from amniotic fluid cells, chorionic villi, or fetal blood samples.

Laboratory Diagnosis of Iron Deficiency

Multiple laboratory tests are used to diagnose iron deficiency because of the lack of one specific diagnostic tool. Laboratory diagnosis is made initially in the presence of a microcytic, hypochromic anemia. Serum iron levels are decreased, and the total iron-binding capacity is increased. The serum iron multiplied by 100 and divided by the iron-binding capacity value is the percent transferrin saturation and is markedly depressed. Serum ferritin levels measure iron stores and are typically low. Ferritin levels can be falsely normal in the presence of other diseases such as infection and neoplasms.

Protoporphyrin, the prophyrin that combines with iron to form heme, accumulates when there is an inadequate iron supply. Free erythrocyte protoporphyrin measures conditions interfering with heme synthesis and is elevated in iron deficiency and other diseases, such as lead poisoning, where it is markedly elevated. Iron staining of the bone marrow can be diagnostic but is usually not necessary.

Laboratory Studies of Hemoglobinopathies

Sickle cell disease is suspected when a patient has a positive family history and a personal history, physical exam, and peripheral blood smear consistent with the disease. The definitive diagnosis is made by hemoglobin electrophoresis. Those with sickle cell trait usually have about 60% Hb A and 40% Hb S.

The peripheral blood smear in thalassemia major is very characteristic with small, pale-red cells, target cells, and nucleated red cells. The MCV is very low. Unlike in iron deficiency, the bilirubin level is usually elevated, and iron levels are high. Hemoglobin electrophoresis can identify the common variants of both α-thalassemia, such as Hb H disease, and β-thalassemia. Hb F and Hb A_2 are elevated unless the patient has a variant of $\beta\delta$-thalassemia, where Hb A_2 levels may be decreased and the Hb F level is elevated. Recombinant DNA technology, such as polymerase chain reaction, can be used to diagnosis thalassemias in utero, even when there is little Hb A production.

TREATMENT OPTIONS, EXPECTED OUTCOMES, AND COMPREHENSIVE MANAGEMENT

Treatment of anemia depends on the underlying cause. In congenital pure red cell aplasia, many patients respond to corticosteroids, which yield the best results when started early. Immunosuppressive therapy and bone marrow transplantation have helped some patients. Patients often respond to steroids and other immunosuppressive therapies or thymectomy if a thymoma is present.

Aplastic Anemia

Treatment of this disease is beyond the scope of the primary care provider. For example, common treatment modalities include bone marrow transplantation for nontransient forms of this disease and immunosuppressive therapy (eg, antithymocyte globulin and cyclosporine) for immune etiologies and even for those whose disease failed to respond to allogeneic bone marrow transplantation. The response to therapeutic measures helps to clarify the pathophysiology of acquired aplastic anemia (Young & Maciejewski, 1997).

Aplastic anemia can also degenerate into hematologic malignancy. Androgens and hematopoietic growth factors have been used, particularly in Fanconi's disease. Supportive therapy of the bleeding and infectious complications is critical. Transfusions are often needed, but paradoxically they may have an adverse affect on the success of bone marrow transplantation if that becomes necessary.

Pernicious Anemia

■ ■ ■ CLINICAL PEARL

In B$_{12}$ deficiency, replacement must be administered intramuscularly, because oral B$_{12}$ is not effective in pernicious anemia.

Anemia of Chronic Disease

Treatment or management of the underlying disease is the most effective therapy, although erythropoietin is being studied as a potential treatment for this condition.

Sickle Cell Disease

Therapy depends on the degree and type of symptoms. Pain management is critical. Painful crises need prompt treatment with hydration and analgesics. Infections need to be detected early and aggressively treated. Because folic acid deficiency is common and aggravates the anemia, folic acid supplementation is routinely administered.

Red cell transfusions are limited to circumstances that cannot be managed medically or for specific problems (eg, providing a temporizing solution for patients with severe pneumonia or other infection, reducing the risk of surgery, and reducing the recurrence of strokes). Caution must be exercised when transfusing these patients, because increasing the viscosity of blood by transfusion can trigger a sickling crisis. Rapid transfusion can precipitate congestive heart failure. Therefore, transfusions are given slowly or exchange transfusion is used, removing and replacing blood in small increments.

Recent studies have shown the benefit of trying to increase the amount of Hb F in sickle patients by the use of hydroxyurea (Steinberg et al, 1997). Hydroxyurea may help decrease the incidence of pain crises (Charache et al, 1996). Bone marrow transplant has also been attempted in this disease, and initial results are promising (Walters et al, 1996).

Thalassemia

Maintaining the hemoglobin level at more than 10 g/dL by transfusion has been shown to be an effective way to avoid the complications of this anemia. These "hypertransfusion" programs, which necessitate a transfusion every 3 weeks, suppress erythropoiesis and the signs that accompany it (eg, anemic symptoms, growth retardation, and disfiguring bony changes). Some clinical investigators advocate maintaining the hemoglobin at even higher levels, but this is controversial. Recently, a more moderate transfusion program has been tried, maintaining the hemoglobin level at 9 to 10 g/dL. This regimen appears to suppress erythropoiesis while reducing the number of transfusions and the resultant problems with overabundant iron stores (Cazzola et al, 1997).

The problems associated with iron overload (hemochromatosis) from the breakdown of transfused red cells have complicated the benefits from transfusion, especially the greatly improved life expectancy and quality of life for many patients with anemia. These patients normally have an increased absorption of dietary iron, which is suppressed in part by transfusion. However, each unit of red cells contains approximately 200 to 250 mg of iron, and the body does not have an effective way to excrete the accumulating iron. The iron from the transfusions is engulfed by the reticuloendothelial system. As it becomes saturated, the iron deposits in other tissues. The skin color becomes bronze to slate gray. Liver failure ensues, gallstones are common, and diabetes mellitus develops when the pancreas is damaged. Iron deposition in the heart leads to arrhythmias and congestive heart failure. Further, patients develop an increased risk of infection, particularly by infectious agents that are more virulent in the presence of large iron stores. Some patients with hemoglobinopathies have enlarged spleens that trap and destroy red cells, increasing the transfusion requirement and perpetuating the cycle. Splenectomy can be helpful, but it further increases the infectious risks.

Deferoxamine is the only iron-chelating drug approved for clinical use, although several potential agents are in clinical trials. Deferoxamine binds iron, which can then be excreted through the stool and urine. Iron in hemoglobin and in the cytochromes is too securely bound to be dislodged by this drug. Life expectancy has increased dramatically with the use of this medication (Zurlo et al, 1989). To be maximally effective, chelation therapy must be aggressive and start soon after the transfusion therapy begins. Deferoxamine must be given parenterally by intravenous or subcutaneous infusion for 8 to 12 hours by pump. This complex therapy presents difficulty for many patients; catheter complications, expense, and drug toxicity are additional problems. Risks with this drug include visual and hearing loss.

Ascorbic acid deficiency commonly occurs in patients with iron overload, but it is the correction by ascorbic acid supplementation that increases the urinary excretion of iron by deferoxamine.

■ CLINICAL WARNING: The primary care provider must be very careful when ascorbic acid is used in patients with iron overload, because it can lead to a rapid cardiac decompensation. Therefore, ascorbic acid therapy should not be given until chelation therapy is well established.

Because of the complexity and expense of chelation therapy, the problems of patient participation, and the risks of transfusion therapy, bone marrow transplantation is becoming more common, particularly now that a National Bone Marrow Registry exists. This registry helps to identify a compatible donor when none can be found among family members (Lucarelli et al, 1995).

An oral iron-chelating agent, deferiprone, has been approved in India and is being tested elsewhere (Hoffbrand, 1996). This advance could greatly affect the therapy of thalassemia in the future.

Treating liver disease has been more complicated. In addition to the hepatic damage caused by iron overload, chronically transfused patients are constantly exposed to the risk of transfusion-associated hepatitis. However, with the addition of hepatitis C antibody testing and surrogate testing for hepatitis, the risk of transfusion has declined dramatically.

A final complication is that patients who are chronically transfused develop antibodies against donor erythrocytes and leukocytes. This makes the search for compatible donors progressively more difficult.

Autoimmune Hemolytic Anemia

Treating the warm variety of this disease can be extremely difficult. Transfusions should be avoided, but if they are necessary, they should be infused slowly with close monitoring. Frequently, the autoantibody reacts with all red cells in the bloodstream, including transfused cells. However, when a patient requires transfusion and compatible blood cannot be found, it is possible to use blood that is less compatible, because it may not be as reactive with the antibody as the patient's own red cells.

Most patients with warm autoimmune hemolytic anemia respond to corticosteroids, or to immunosuppressive drugs and splenectomy if steroids fail. Splenectomy rarely works unless the patient has splenomegaly and accrues red cells in the spleen (which can be diagnosed by radiolabeling red cells). Other therapies include intravenous gamma globulin, danazol, a modified androgen, and plasmapheresis.

Therapy for the cold type of this disease includes avoidance of cold exposure and treatment of any underlying disease. Generally, only the IgG variety of the disease responds to corticosteroids and splenectomy, although immunosuppressive therapy can be more widely beneficial. Blood should be warmed with a blood warmer when transfusion is necessary. Some investigators have studied the removal of antibodies by plasmapheresis before inducing hypothermia during surgery.

Transfusions

When disease-specific treatments are not available and the patient's symptoms secondary to the anemia require intervention, transfusion may be warranted. However, there are numerous risks associated with transfusion. Some of the more common or more dangerous include the following:

- *Hemolytic transfusion reactions* are most commonly caused by blood group incompatibility, with ABO the most dangerous. Shortness of breath, nausea, vomiting, pain (often at the site of infusion or in the chest or back), hypotension, shock, acute renal failure, and death are all possible. Hemolytic reactions during surgery may lead to

uncontrollable bleeding. A common problem in chronically transfused patients is the development of antibodies against red cell antigens. Patients who develop clinically significant antibodies require red cells that do not contain that antigen for subsequent transfusions.

- *Nonhemolytic immune transfusion reactions* include febrile reactions caused by antibodies against donor leukocytes and allergy to donor plasma proteins. Febrile reactions can usually be prevented by filtration of red cells as they are transfused. Allergic reactions are usually mild and consist of urticaria. However, anaphylaxis can occur, particularly in IgA-deficient patients who have developed an anti-IgA antibody.

- *Disease transmission*: The risk of AIDS has been greatly reduced in the past few years. Present estimates for transmission of HIV by transfusion are 1 in 450,000 to 660,000 (Lackritz et al, 1995; Schrieber et al, 1996). The risk has again been lowered by the implementation of HIV p24 antigen testing to reduce the HIV window. Hepatitis is another significant infectious risk. The risk for hepatitis B is estimated at 1 in 63,000 (Schrieber et al, 1996), and for hepatitis C 1 in 103,000 donors. Cytomegalovirus is a major risk to premature neonates or severely immunocompromised patients (eg, bone marrow transplant patients). Other infectious agents possibly transmitted through transfusion include Chagas' disease, *Yersinia enterocolitica*, bacterial contaminants, and rarely malaria (Klein et al, 1997). All units of blood are tested for HIV-1/HIV-2 antibodies, HIV p24 antigen, hepatitis B surface antigen, antibodies to hepatitis B core antigen, alanine aminotransferase, syphilis serology, antibodies to human T-lymphotropic virus types I and II, and antibodies to hepatitis C. Albumin, plasma protein fraction, and intramuscular gamma globulin preparations do not appear to carry a risk of spreading viral or bacterial infections.

- *Metabolic complications* are physiologic changes resulting from stored blood. Hypothermia from infusing cold blood can cause arrhythmias and cardiac arrest. Commercial blood warmers are available if patients need to be transfused rapidly. Hyperkalemia is caused by the lysis of aging red cells, although it is rarely a problem except in patients receiving massive transfusions or exchange transfusions or those with renal failure. Citrate toxicity caused by the anticoagulants can be a problem in patients with liver disease. Massive transfusions carry the risk of hemodilution of the clotting factors, miniclots or microaggregates in the stored blood, and decreases in red cell 2,3-diphosphoglycerate (2,3-DPG), which increases oxygen affinity and slows the release of oxygen to the tissues.

- *Other complications* include iron overload, air embolism, and circulatory overload. Graft-versus-host disease is caused when donor lymphocytes, live and immunologically competent, precipitate a rejection reaction in the recipient. Immune competency may also be affected by transfusion; this may explain why survival of patients with colorectal cancer is lower in patients who have been transfused.

The risks of transfusion have encouraged attempts to create a safer alternative. The two major areas of research have been with perfluorocarbon solutions and hemoglobin solutions. Perfluorocarbons are organic molecules similar to the refrigerant freon. Hemoglobin solutions involve polymerization of the hemoglobin molecule or attachment of hemoglobin to larger molecules to prevent rapid loss in the urine (Gould et al, 1994).

Erythropoietin was originally approved for treating the anemia of chronic renal failure. It is now used for treatment of anemia in HIV-infected patients receiving zidovudine treatment and for cancer patients undergoing chemotherapy. It is being actively investigated in the treatment of anemia of chronic disease, bone marrow transplant, anemia of prematurity, myelodysplastic syndromes, and sickle cell disease. Erythropoietin can increase the number of autologous units a patient can donate for surgical purposes, an issue especially important to Jehovah's Witnesses. It can also be used to prepare for surgery patients who cannot donate autologous units because of their health, size, or anemia or those who are alloimmunized (Goodnough, 1994; Goodnough et al, 1997).

Cultural Considerations

Each culture and religion has traditions that affect their beliefs about illness and therapy. Primary care providers must be attentive to these culturally derived attitudes toward health. Assessing a patient's viewpoint and practices concerning nutrition, breast feeding, nontraditional remedies, and pain can prevent obstacles to effective therapy.

A lack of awareness of the genetic nature of many anemias, especially in high-risk racial and ethnic groups, has led some primary care providers to underdiagnose and mistreat these diseases. For example, the development of severe anemia after medical treatment often goes unrecognized in patients with G6PD deficiency. Patients with sickle cell disease may be given inadequate pain management if the frequency and severity of pain crises are mistaken for an appeal for addictive drugs.

Attitudes toward treatment should be considered as well. Personal and religious opinions regarding transfusion can be very strong. The media's coverage of AIDS has created concern about blood safety. Many patients respond to the fear of getting AIDS from a transfusion by wanting to chose their donors, a process termed directed donations. Requests for directed donors are often for blood products from persons with racial, socioeconomic, or geographic features similar to those of the patient. However, scientific studies have not shown directed donors to be any safer than the regular volunteer donor population.

Additional problems with transfusion include the development of red cell antibodies (alloimmunization) from frequent exposure to the red cells of other people. This is exaggerated by the fact that the racial background of the donor population is often different from that of patients with chronic anemia. Nationally, most donors are white, and many of the anemias requiring transfusion are genetically transmitted among people of African descent. There is also a difference in frequency of some of the less common red cell antigens among racial groups. Therefore, when multiple antibodies do develop, it is often necessary to seek donors among the rare-blood donor files. These donors are likely to be persons whose racial background is similar to that of the patient. It is important for the primary care provider to explain these facts to patients without inadvertently playing into any prejudices they may have concerning the donor population or receiving blood from a different racial group from their own.

Religious attitudes are also critical. Jehovah's Witnesses oppose the use of blood transfusions, regardless of the circumstance. Persons of other religions, such as Christian Scientists, do not believe in medical treatment of any sort.

> ■ ■ ■ **CLINICAL PEARL**
>
> Helping patients negotiate the complexities of their treatment is crucial if their religious beliefs conflict with medical therapy.

Socioeconomic Factors

The economic impact of anemia can be overwhelming, especially for patients with hereditary anemias, which can cause lifelong illness, and for those with anemia secondary to other chronic diseases. It has been estimated that the cost of chelation therapy for a disease such as thalassemia can be $30,000 to 60,000 a year. Even more modestly priced therapies may be beyond the economic capability of the affected family. Health and life insurance can be difficult or impossible to obtain. Even when the direct costs are covered by insurance or Medicare or Medicaid, lost time from work caused by illness or caring for an affected family member can take an economic toll. In some cases, treatment that would be covered by third-party payers is not sought or obtained by the patient because of the expense of travel or lack of affordable child care.

Newer, more experimental therapies, such as bone marrow transplantation, are not covered by many third-party payers, and most families cannot afford this expensive option without aid. The dangers associated with transplantation and the difficulty of finding compatible donors limits the potential of this therapy, but the chief problem is that this important treatment is simply too expensive for most patients and too costly for some third-party payers, especially if they cover a population with large numbers of patients with hereditary anemias.

Prevention

Patients with hereditary anemia can often be diagnosed in utero. Genetic counseling helps the family understand the inheritance patterns and statistical risks in each pregnancy and the medical options that are available. To offer appropriate advice, the provider must understand the patient's religious and social beliefs toward these options and having children.

Patients with an increased erythrocyte turnover, as in sickle cell anemia, thalassemia, and hereditary spherocytosis, are prone to folic acid deficiency. Prophylactic folic acid prevents some of the complications of these diseases. In addition, autosplenectomy in sickle cell disease or surgical splenectomy for hereditary spherocytosis places these patients at great risk of sepsis. Pneumococcal vaccine and judicious use of antibiotics when infection is first suspected are important therapeutic interventions to prevent the complications of splenectomy.

TEACHING AND SELF-CARE

Iron deficiency is the most common cause of anemia in the United States. Typically, patients include multiparous women, infants on a prolonged milk diet with no iron supplementation, and patients who are bleeding from the gastrointestinal tract or from a neoplasm. Adolescent girls are also at risk because of menstruation combined with weight-loss diets that have little nutritional value.

Treatment for iron deficiency anemia depends on the cause and the severity of the anemia and should combine a pharmacologic and nonpharmacologic approach. Patients are encouraged to augment their diet with foods high in iron, as well as taking supplemental iron tablets. Foods that are high in iron include red meats, pinto beans, and dried fruits such as apricots, prunes, and raisins. Foods that have lesser amounts of iron include spinach, peas, beans, carrots, sweet potatoes, and peaches.

If the patient is prescribed a supplemental oral iron, the least expensive form of iron is ferrous sulfate, containing 60 mg of elemental iron per tablet. Patients should brush their teeth after each dose to avoid iron stains. Treatment will continue for at least 3 months. Ferrous sulfate should be taken with meals to decrease gastrointestinal upset. Some foods help in iron absorption, such as citrus fruits, but others, such as tea, inhibit absorption. Common side effects of ferrous sulfate include nausea, indigestion, diarrhea, abdominal cramping, and constipation. Constipation and black stools are perhaps the most common side effects, and patients should be warned about these in advance. The provider should consider prescribing a mild anticonstipation agent, such as Colace or Metamucil.

If ferrous sulfate is not tolerated, ferrous gluconate can be considered: it produces less constipation than ferrous sulfate. In patients with reduced oral iron absorption or those who cannot tolerate oral iron, parenteral iron can be used.

■ ■ ■ CLINICAL PEARL

To maintain adequate hydration, it is not sufficient to "push fluids." Quantitative guidelines and a description of potentially good sources of fluids should be given, based on what the patient is most likely to accept.

COMMUNITY RESOURCES

Numerous associations have been created to help patients with anemia and their families. Some offer support services to patients; others have programs that increase public awareness, disseminate educational materials, promote research, or provide other services. Many of these organizations have local chapters.

- Community Outreach Health Information System (COHIS): http://web.bu.edu/COHIS/cardvasc/cvd.htm: What is anemia, causes, diagnosis, treatment, types of anemia, nutritional topics
- Aplastic Anemia Answer Book: http://medic.med.uth.tmc.edu/ptnt/00001038.htm: General information, diagnosis, initial treatment, bone marrow transplantation, drug therapy
- Aplastic Anemia Foundation of America, Inc.: http://www.teleport.com/nonprofit/aafa/
- Fanconi Anemia Handbook: http://www2.cybernex.net/jj/fa/fabook.html
- Sickle Cell Information Center: http://www.emory.edu/PEDS/SICKLE/

- RxMed—Anemia during Pregnancy: http://www.rxmed.com/illnesses/anemia during pregnancy.html: General information, causes, prevention, diagnosis and treatment, possible complications
- RxMed—Pernicious Anemia: http://www.rxmed.com/illnesses/anemia, pernicious.html: General information, causes, diagnosis and treatment, risk factors and prevention
- National Association for Sickle Cell Anemia, 3345 Wilshire Blvd., Suite 1106, Los Angeles, CA 90010, 800-421-8453
- National Sickle Cell Disease Program, National Heart, Lung, and Blood Institute, Bldg. 31, Room 4A-21, Rockville Pike, Bethesda, MD 20205, 301-496-4236
- Aplastic Anemia Foundation of America, Inc., P.O. Box 613, Annapolis, MD 21404, 800-747-2820; fax 410-867-0240; aafacenter@aol.com
- Sickle Cell Information Center, P.O. Box 109, Grady Memorial Hospital, 80 Butler St., Atlanta, GA 30335; 404-616-3572; aplatt@emory.edu
- Cooley's Anemia Foundation, 129-09 26th Ave., Flushing, NY 11354, 800-522-7222
- The Hemochromatosis Research Foundation, Inc., P.O. Box 8569, Albany, NY 12208, 518-489-0972

REFERRAL POINTS AND CLINICAL WARNINGS

The management of anemia and the underlying conditions is complex, and many of the treatments are fraught with risks and hazards.

- Massive blood loss needs immediate attention to avoid cardiovascular compromise, shock, and death.
- Sickle cell disease patients can deteriorate rapidly because of marrow shutdown after infections, hyperhemolytic episodes, strokes, and sepsis. They are at increased danger from anesthesia and hypoxia when undergoing surgery.
- Patients with splenectomies face septic risks.
- Immediate hemolytic transfusion reactions can lead to renal failure and death and must be quickly recognized and treated.

Pregnancy needs to be carefully monitored in patients with sickle cell disease thalassemia, and other anemias (Rust & Perry, Koshy, 1995).

Management of anemia requires a comprehensive understanding of its pathophysiology and treatments and the cooperation of specialists to help ensure that the patient receives timely and appropriate therapy.

References

Cazzola, M., Borgna-Pignatti, C., Ocatelli, F., Ponchio, L., Beguin, Y., & De Stefano, P. (1997). A moderate transfusion regimen may reduce iron loading in β-thalassemia major without producing excessive expansion of erythropoiesis. *Transfusion, 37,* 135–140.

Charache, S., Barton, F.B., Moore, R.D., et al. (1996). Hydroxyurea and sickle cell anemia. *Medicine, 75,* 300–326.

Fakhry, S.M., & Sheldon, G.F. (1994). Massive transfusion in the surgical patient. In L.C. Jeffries & M.E. Brecher (Eds.). *Massive transfusion.* Bethesda, MD: American Association of Blood Banks, pp. 17–42.

Goodnough, L.T. (1994). Reducing the need to transfuse: Applications of hematopoietic growth factors. In J.P. Aubuchon & L.A. Issitt (Eds.). *Limiting donor exposure in hemotherapy.* Bethesda, MD: American Association of Blood Banks, pp. 1–15.

Goodnough, L.T., Monk, T.G., & Andriole, G.L. (1997). Erythropoietin therapy. *N Engl J Med, 336,* 933–938.

Gould, S.A., Sehgal, L.R., Sehgal, H.R., & Moss, G.S. (1994). The role of hemoglobin solutions in massive transfusion. In L.C. Jeffries & M.E. Brecher (Eds.). *Massive transfusion.* Bethesda, MD: American Association of Blood Banks, pp. 43–64.

Gulati, G.L., & Hyun, B.H. (1994a). The automated CBC: A current perspective. *Hematology/Oncology Clinics of North America, 8,* 593–603.

Gulati, G.L., & Hyun, B.H. (1994b). Blood smear examination. *Hematology/Oncology Clinics of North America, 8,* 631–650.

Hassoun, H., & Palek, J. (1996). Hereditary spherocytosis: A review of the clinical and molecular aspects of the disease. *Blood Reviews, 10,* 129–147.

Hoffbrand, A.V. (1996). Oral iron chelation. *Seminars in Hematology, 33,* 1–8.

Hyun, B.H., Stevenson, A.T., & Hanau, C.A. (1994). Fundamentals of bone marrow examination. *Hematology/Oncology Clinics of North America, 8,* 651–663.

Jeffries, L.C., & Brecher, M.E. (Eds.). (1994). *Massive transfusions.* Bethesda, MD: American Association of Blood Banks.

Klein, H.G., Dodd, R.Y., Ness, P.M., Fratantoni, J.A., & Nemo, G.J. (1997). Current status of microbial contamination of blood components: Summary of a conference. *Transfusion, 37,* 95–101.

Koshy, M. (1995). Sickle cell disease and pregnancy. *Blood Reviews, 9,* 157–164.

Kouides, P.A., & Bennett, J.M. (1996). Morphology and classification of the myelodysplastic syndromes and their pathologic variants. *Seminars in Hematology 33,* 95–110.

Lackritz, E.M., Satten, G.A., Aberle-Grasse, J., et al. (1995). Estimated risk of transmission of the human immunodeficiency virus by screened blood in the United States. *N Engl J Med, 333,* 1721–1725.

Lucarelli, G., Giardini, C., & Baronciani, D. (1995). Bone marrow transplantation in thalassemia. *Seminars in Hematology 32,* 297–303.

Rust, O.A., & Perry, K.G. (1995). Pregnancy complicated by sickle hemoglobinopathy. *Clinical Obstetrics & Gynecology, 38,* 472–484.

Schrieber, G.B., Busch, M.P., Kleinman, S.H., & Korelitz, J.J. (1996). The risk of transfusion-transmitted viral infections. *N Engl J Med, 334,* 1685–1690.

Steinberg, M.H., Lu, Z.H., Barton, F.B., Terrin, M.L., Charache, S., & Dover, G.J. (1997). Fetal hemoglobin in sickle cell anemia: Determinants of response to hydroxyurea. Multicenter Study of hydroxyurea. *Blood, 89,* 1078–1088.

Walters, M.C., Patience, M., Leisenring, W., et al. (1996). Bone marrow transplantation for sickle cell disease. *N Engl J Med, 335,* 369–376.

Young, N.S., & Maciejewski, J. (1997). The pathophysiology of acquired aplastic anemia. *N Engl J Med, 336,* 1365–1372.

Zurlo, M.G., DeStefano, P., Borgna-Pignatti, C., et al. (1989). Survival and causes of death in thalassemia major. *Lancet, 2,* 27–30.

Bibliography

Beutler, E., Williams, W.J., Lichtman, M.A., Coller, B.S., & Kipps, T.J. (Eds.). (1995). *Williams' hematology,* 5th ed. New York: McGraw-Hill.

Hackel, E., Westphal, R.G., & Wilson, S.M. (Eds.) (1992). *Transfusion management of some common heritable blood disorders.* Bethesda, MD: American Association of Blood Banks.

Jaffe, M.S., & McVan, B.F. *Davis's laboratory and diagnostic test handbook.* Philadelphia: F.A. Davis.

Kasprisin, D.O., & Luban, N.C. (Eds.). (1987). *Pediatric transfusion medicine,* Vol. I & II. Boca Raton, FL: CRC Press

Lee, G.R., Bithell, T.C., Foerster, J., Athens, J.W., & Lukens, J.N. (Eds.). (1993). *Wintrobe's clinical hematology,* 9th ed. Philadelphia: Lea & Febiger.

Massa, J. (1995). *Manual of clinical hematology,* 2d ed. Boston: Little, Brown & Co.

Mollison, P.L., Engelfriet, C.P., & Contreras, M. (Eds.). (1993). *Blood transfusion in clinical medicine,* 9th ed. Oxford: Blackwell.

Petz, L.D., Swisher, S.N., Kleinman, S., Spence, R.K., & Strauss, R.G. (Eds.). (1996). *Clinical practice of transfusion medicine,* 3d ed. New York: Churchill-Livingstone.

Rossi, E.C., Simon, T.L., Moss, G.S., & Gould, S.A. (Eds.). (1996). *Principles of transfusion medicine,* 2d ed. Baltimore: Williams & Wilkins.

Winslow, R.M. (1992). *Hemoglobin-based red cell substitutes.* Baltimore: The Johns Hopkins University Press.

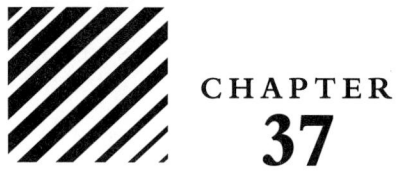

CHAPTER
37

Coagulopathies

Ian Rabinowitz, M.D.

Coagulopathies, include hemorrhage, thrombosis, and embolism and represent common clinical manifestations of hematologic disease. Normally, bleeding is controlled by clot formation, which results from the interaction of platelets, plasma proteins, and the vessel wall. The clot ultimately is dissolved through clot lysis. A derangement of any of these components may result in a bleeding disorder. Individual disease states will be examined under the broad headings of coagulation factor deficiencies, disorders of platelets, and mixed disorders. Thrombotic states will also be examined (Table 37-1).

ANATOMY, PHYSIOLOGY, AND PATHOLOGY

Blood Coagulation

Coagulation is initiated after blood vessels are damaged, enabling the interaction of blood with tissue factor, a protein present beneath the endothelium (Fig. 37-1). Small amounts of factor VII present in plasma bind to tissue factor, and this tissue factor–factor VII complex activates factor X. Activated factor X, in the presence of factor V, activates prothrombin (II) to thrombin (IIa), which subsequently cleaves fibrinogen to fibrin. The fibrin polymerizes into an insoluble gel. This is stabilized by the action of factor XIII. This process constitutes the extrinsic pathway.

Coagulation is consolidated by the intrinsic pathway. Factor XI is activated (possibly by thrombin generated in the extrinsic pathway), resulting in the activation of factor IX, which then activates factor X in the presence of factor VIII. Activated factor X produces a fibrin clot, as outlined above in the extrinsic pathway. Decreased levels of clotting factors may be caused by defective synthesis, excessive use, circulating inhibitors of clotting factors, or excessive proteolysis by the fibrinolytic system.

The coagulation pathway is controlled by a number of mechanisms. Protein C is a plasma protein that inhibits factors V and VIII, thus inhibiting the activity of factors IX and X, respectively. This inhibition is catalyzed by protein S. Antithrombin III (AT III) primarily inhibits the activity of thrombin and factor X, and this inhibition is greatly enhanced by heparin. Loss of function of these proteins would result in uninhibited coagulation and hence a predisposition to spontaneous thrombosis.

Fibrinolysis is a mechanism for dissolving fibrin clots. Plasmin, the activated form of plasminogen, cleaves fibrin to produce soluble fragments. Fibrinolytics such as tissue plasminogen activator and urokinase activate plasminogen, resulting in dissolution of a fibrin clot.

CLASSES OF BLEEDING DISORDERS

Vascular Defects

Vascular defects usually cause bleeding only into the skin and mucous membranes. Congenital causes include Osler-Weber-Rendu syndrome and Ehlers-Danlos disease. Acquired causes of vascular purpura include infections, drugs, uremia, connective tissue disorders, and dysproteinemias. Treatment is directed to the primary illness.

Inherited Coagulation Disorders

Deficiencies of any of the known coagulation factors are present from birth and may be inherited or result from a spontaneous disruption in the associated coagulation factor gene. Only deficiencies of factors VIII and IX, and von Willebrand's disease (vWD) will be discussed in more detail, because the other disorders are rare.

HEMOPHILIA

Hemophilia is an X-linked recessive disorder associated with a congenital deficiency of factor VIII or IX (hemophilia A or B, respectively). Hemophilia is suspected in any male who has excessive bleeding after trauma, or spontaneous bleeding into joints or soft tissues. Patients with severe hemophilia (factor level <1%) are at risk for spontaneous hemarthrosis and soft-tissue bleeding. Patients who have moderate disease (factor level 1% to 4%) or mild hemophilia (factor level 5% to 25%) are at a reduced risk of spontaneous hemorrhage, but may bleed excessively after trauma or surgery.

VON WILLEBRAND'S DISEASE

von Willebrand factor (vWF) is a plasma protein that is required for the adhesion of platelets to sites of vascular damage. Deficiency of vWF is called type I; qualitative abnormality of vWF is called type II. vWD is an autosomally inherited hemostatic disorder of variable severity, characterized by mucosal and cutaneous bleeding, similar to patients with platelet disorders. Patients may have a prolonged bleeding time and a prolonged activated partial thromboplastin time (aPTT).

Mixed Coagulation Disorders

Mixed coagulation disorders are a group of acquired diseases. They usually involve multiple elements of the hemostatic system and are often associated with a particular disease or clinical syndrome.

TABLE 37-1	Overview of Coagulopathies						
Disorder	Clotting/ Bleeding	Labs	History	Assoc. Factors	Rx	Information for Patients	Intervention
Hemophilia A	B	↑ PTT ↓ factor VIII	Lifelong bleeding, joints, soft tissue	Males	Factor replacement DDAVP	Genetic counseling Support groups	Prophylactic factor replacement Avoid aspirin, NSAIDs
Hemophilia B	B	↑ PTT ↓ factor IX	As above	Males	As above	As above	As above
vWD	B	↑ bleeding time ↓ Ristocetin cofactor activity ↓ vWF Ag.	Lifelong bleeding, mucosal epistaxis		Cryoprecipitate DDAVP	Genetic counseling	As above
DIC	B	↑ PTT, ↑ FDP ↓ platelets ↓ fibrinogen		Sepsis, retained placenta	Treat underlying cause	N/A	N/A
Liver disease	B	↑ PT ↓ Fibrinogen (↑ PTT)	Mucosal and GI bleeding	Liver disease	FFP, platelets	N/A	Avoid alcohol and other hepatotoxic drugs
Vitamin K deficiency	B	↑ PT	Bruising, visceral bleeding	Obstructive liver disease coumadin	Vit. K	N/A	Treat cause
ITP	B	↓ plts.	Petechiae, epistaxis	SLE, HIV, lymphoproliferative disorders	Prednisone IVIgG	Possibility of chronicity	Monitor platelets, long-term
TTP	B	↓ plts, ↓ HB, ↑ retic, ↑ BUN/ creat ⊕ Schistocytes	Petechiae, epistaxis	Chemotherapy, HIV	Plasma pheresis and FFP	Possibility of relapse	Monitor platelets, retic, LDH long-term
Protein C deficiency	C	↓ protein C	Thrombosis <40 years Recurrent DVT family history		Anticoagulation (see text)	Genetic defect Possible family member affected	Avoid oral contraceptives Prophylaxis before surgery Prophylaxis during pregnancy
Protein S deficiency	C	↓ protein S	As above		As above	As above	As above
AT III deficiency	C	↓ AT III	As above		As above	As above	As above
Lupus anticoagulant	C	↑ PTT, ⊕ anticordio ab ⊕ dilute RVVT			As above	As above	As above
Hyperhomocysteinemia	C	↑ homocystein	As above		As above	As above	As above
APC resistance	C	DNA test APC resistance assay	As above		As above	As above	As above

DISSEMINATED INTRAVASCULAR COAGULATION

Disseminated intravascular coagulation (DIC) can be caused by the activation of either the coagulation or fibrinolytic system and therefore can result in bleeding or thrombosis. Conditions associated with DIC include infections such as gram-negative sepsis, meningococcemia, Rocky Mountain spotted fever, and typhoid fever; obstetric complications (abruptio placentae, eclampsia, retained dead fetus); massive trauma; surgery; shock; and certain malignancies.

LIVER DISEASE

Coagulation disorders are common in patients with liver disease. These may arise from malabsorption of vitamin K, decreased synthesis of clotting proteins, or synthesis of abnormal proteins. Fibrin degradation products may be elevated because of poor hepatic clearance, resulting in impaired coagulation resembling DIC. Liver disease associated with hypersplenism may result in thrombocytopenia.

VITAMIN K DEFICIENCY

Factors II, VII, IX, and X are vitamin K-dependent coagulation factors that are synthesized in the liver. Vitamin K is naturally synthesized by intestinal bacteria. It is a fat-soluble vitamin and is absorbed only in the presence of bile salts. Depletion of vitamin K-dependent factors may occur in patients receiving antibiotics; in obstructive jaundice, malabsorptive states, or hepatic parenchymal disease; and in patients receiving warfarin therapy. Patients have an increased, international normalization ratio (INR).

Platelet Disorders

Platelet disorders include thrombocytopenia, which may be caused by diminished platelet production, enhanced platelet destruction, or sequestration of platelets (Table 37-2). Qualitative platelet disorders may be congenital or acquired. Congenital disorders may affect platelet adhesion, aggregation, or platelet secretion, and are rare. Acquired qualitative platelet disorders are secondary to uremia, myeloproliferative disorders, drugs, and dysproteinemias.

IMMUNE THROMBOCYTOPENIC PURPURA

Immune thrombocytopenic purpura (ITP), the autoimmune destruction of platelets, usually presents as ecchymoses, petechiae, or bleeding. The differential diagnosis includes aplastic

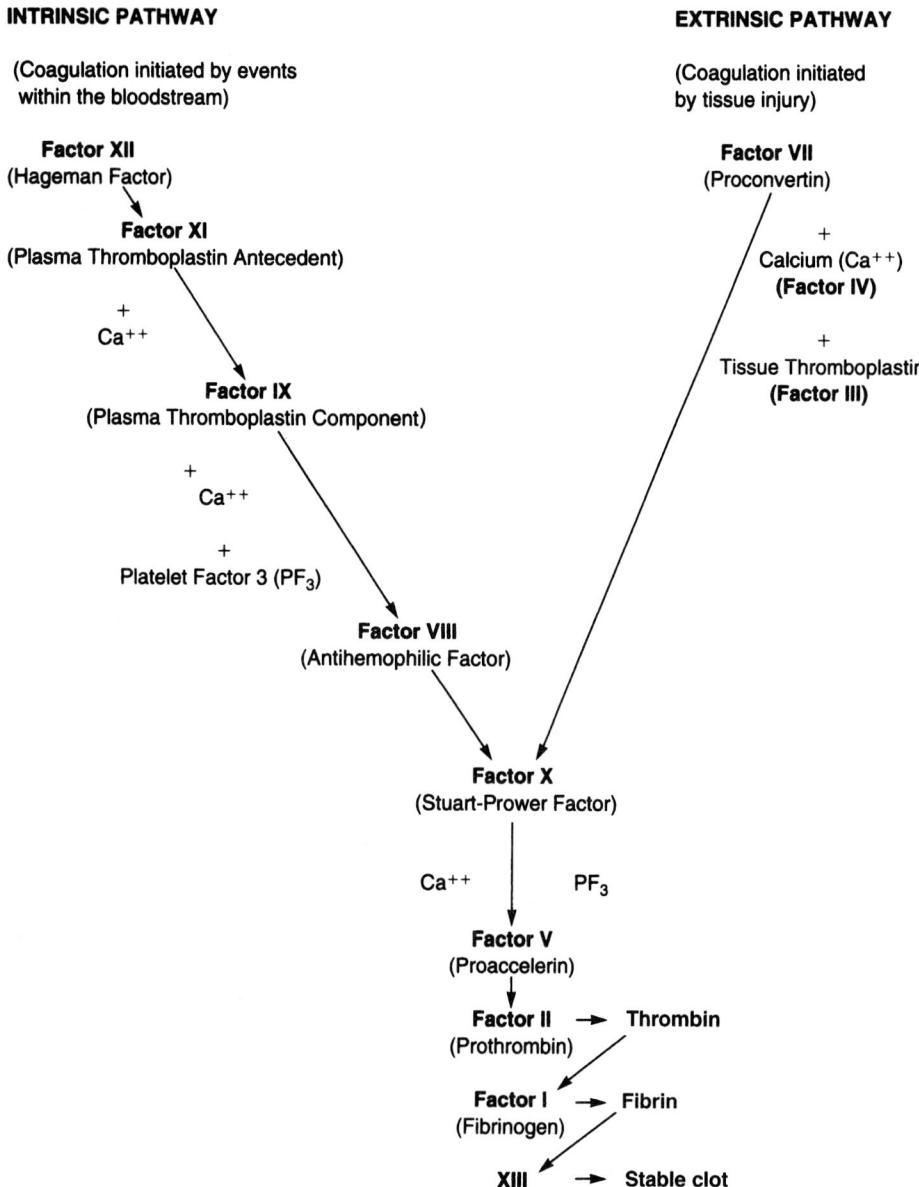

INTRINSIC PATHWAY

(Coagulation initiated by events
within the bloodstream)

Factor XII
(Hageman Factor)

Factor XI
(Plasma Thromboplastin Antecedent)

+
Ca++

Factor IX
(Plasma Thromboplastin Component)

+
Ca++

+
Platelet Factor 3 (PF$_3$)

Factor VIII
(Antihemophilic Factor)

EXTRINSIC PATHWAY

(Coagulation initiated
by tissue injury)

Factor VII
(Proconvertin)

+
Calcium (Ca++)
(Factor IV)

+
Tissue Thromboplastin
(Factor III)

Factor X
(Stuart-Prower Factor)

Ca++   PF$_3$

Factor V
(Proaccelerin)

Factor II → **Thrombin**
(Prothrombin)

Factor I → **Fibrin**
(Fibrinogen)

XIII → **Stable clot**
(Fibrin stabilizing factor)

FIGURE 37-1 The coagulation cascade is initiated by the "extrinsic pathway" and consolidated by the "intrinsic pathway." Coagulation is controlled by the inhibition of factors VIII and V by APC, and by AT III inhibition of II and X.

anemia, sepsis, DIC, acute leukemia, drug-induced thrombocytopenia, and infiltrative bone marrow disorders. The diagnosis is made by excluding other causes of thrombocytopenia, after a careful history, physical exam, and peripheral smear. Patients with risk factors for HIV should be tested for the HIV antibody. Bone marrow aspiration may be indicated in elderly patients or patients with atypical findings.

Chronic ITP usually occurs in adults, with a 3:1 ratio of females to males. It is common in patients between the ages of 20 and 50 years. ITP may also be associated with HIV infection, systemic lupus erythematosus, lymphoproliferative disorders, ulcerative colitis, and carcinoma. The thrombocytopenia is often chronic and unremitting, requiring definitive therapy. Acute ITP occurs primarily in children.

DRUG-INDUCED THROMBOCYTOPENIA

Drug-induced thrombocytopenia is diagnosed after excluding other causes, and by noting a temporal relation between the onset of thrombocytopenia and the administration of the drug, as well as resolution on discontinuation of the drug. Although any drug can be implicated, alcohol, thiazide diuretics, quinine, quinidine, penicillins, gold, sulfa, and heparin are more commonly associated with drug-induced thrombocytopenia. Myelosuppressive drugs used to treat malignancies and other disorders can produce thrombocytopenia by suppressing platelet production.

Heparin-induced thrombocytopenia is associated with an early nonimmune clinical syndrome and a later immune-mediated thrombocytopenia that occurs 5 to 7 days after the initiation of heparin. This type of thrombocytopenia may be associated with paradoxical thrombosis instead of bleeding.

In all cases, the offending drug should be discontinued if possible.

THROMBOTIC THROMBOCYTOPENIC PURPURA

Thrombotic thrombocytopenic purpura (TTP) is a complex clinical syndrome characterized by a clinical pentad of neurologic dysfunction, which may range from headaches or blurred

TABLE 37-2	Causes of Thrombocytopenia

Diminished platelet production
    Marrow infiltration with tumor, fibrosis, infection
    Aplastic/hypoplastic anemia
    Ionizing radiation
    Nutritional deficiencies (B_{12}, folate)
    Viral infections
    Drugs (thiazides, alcohol, myelosuppressive agents)
    Paroxysmal nocturnal hemoglobinemia

Splenic sequestration
    Lymphoproliferative disorders
    Portal hypertension
    Myeloproliferative disorders
    Infections (bacterial, viral, parasitic)

Increased platelet destruction
    Nonimmune
        Vascular prosthesis
        DIC
        Sepsis/infection
        TTP
    Immune
        Drug-induced antibodies
        ITP

vision to seizures or profound coma; purpura and petechiae from thrombocytopenia; jaundice and pallor from a microangiopathic hemolytic anemia; fever; and renal dysfunction. The cause of TTP is unknown, although this disease has been associated with certain drugs and HIV infection.

Laboratory findings include anemia, thrombocytopenia, fragmented red blood cells seen on peripheral smear, elevated blood urea nitrogen and creatinine levels, proteinuria, hematuria, and an elevated level of lactic dehydrogenase. The INR and aPTT are usually normal.

Thrombophilia

Thrombophilia refers to a tendency to have recurrent venous thromboembolism. Acquired causes of thrombosis such as malignancy, myeloproliferative disorders, systemic lupus erythematosus, and the antiphospholipid syndrome should be excluded. Thrombophilia should be considered in patients who have venous thrombosis and who are less than 45 years old, have a family history of venous thromboembolism, have recurrent spontaneous episodes of venous thromboembolism, have thrombosis in an unusual site (eg, mesenteric vein, cerebral vein), or have recurrent fetal loss. Patients who demonstrate thrombophilia should be evaluated for evidence of deficiencies of protein C, protein S, and AT III, as well as activated protein C resistance (APC resistance), hyperhomocysteinemia, and the lupus anticoagulant. The frequency of inherited thrombophilia in patients with recurrent venous thrombosis is about 5% for AT III, protein C, and protein S deficiencies. Hyperhomocysteinemia is found in 10% and APC resistance in about 25% to 50% of such patients (De Stefano, 1996).

Because protein C and protein S are vitamin K-dependent factors, assays of these factors as well as APC resistance should be performed when the patient is not receiving warfarin. Similarly, patients who are receiving heparin may have decreased levels of AT III.

The lupus anticoagulant is an acquired disorder characterized by an antibody that interferes with and prolongs the aPTT and less commonly increases the INR. Despite the prolonged aPTT, this disorder is not associated with bleeding, but it may be associated with thrombosis. The diagnosis is confirmed by performing the dilute Russell viper venom time and an anticardiolipin antibody assay.

EPIDEMIOLOGY

The incidence of hemophilia is 1 case per 10,000 live male births (hemophilia A) and 1 case per 50,000 live male births (hemophilia B). vWD has a prevalence of about 1% in the general population. The majority of patients (80%) have type I vWD.

DIAGNOSTIC CRITERIA

Basic tests to diagnose a bleeding disorder includes a bleeding time, which tests quantitative and qualitative platelet disorders; an INR, which examines the extrinsic pathway of the coagulation cascade (ie, a deficiency or inhibition of factors VII, X, V, II, I); an aPTT, which examines the intrinsic pathway of the coagulation cascade (ie, a deficiency or inhibition of prekallikrein, high-molecular-weight kininogen, and factors XII, XI, IX, VIII, X, V, II, I); and the thrombin time, which tests for deficiencies or inhibitors of thrombin and fibrinogen. A complete blood count will determine if there is a quantitative platelet deficiency.

HISTORY AND PHYSICAL EXAM

Any recurrent bleeding, especially if it begins in early childhood or includes a family history of bleeding, is suggestive of an inherited bleeding diathesis. Spontaneous hemarthroses or hematomas are associated with severe hemophilia A or B but may be observed with other severe coagulopathies. Abnormal bruising and mucosal bleeding, including epistaxis, gum bleeding, and menorrhagia, are typical of abnormalities of platelets or vascular endothelium. Neonatal umbilical cord bleeding and defective wound healing may indicate factor XIII deficiency, afibrinogenemia, or rarely dysfibrinogenemia.

A patient of European Jewish descent with postsurgical and mucosal bleeding may have a deficiency of factor XI, which occurs predominantly in this population. Deficiencies of the intrinsic contact factors (factor XII, prekallikrein, or high-molecular-weight kininogen) do not produce abnormal bleeding.

A detailed drug history (notably aspirin, nonsteroidal anti-inflammatories, anticoagulants, and antibiotics) and an evaluation for underlying medical conditions such as liver disease, cancer, uremia, or collagen vascular disorders are essential. A careful history of every previous surgical, dental, or traumatic event should be taken, noting the amount of blood loss and measures needed to control the bleeding.

DIAGNOSTIC TESTS

If a patient with a bleeding history has an increased INR or a prolonged aPTT, then a mixing study should be performed using a 50:50 mix of patient plasma and control plasma (Fig. 37-2). The INR or aPTT would correct to normal with a coagulation factor deficiency, whereas plasma with an inhibitory antibody would not correct in mixing studies.

In a patient with a bleeding history and normal screening tests, one should suspect vWD. Repeated determinations of the bleeding time and activity of vWF may be necessary to establish the diagnosis. The laboratory workup may include the func-

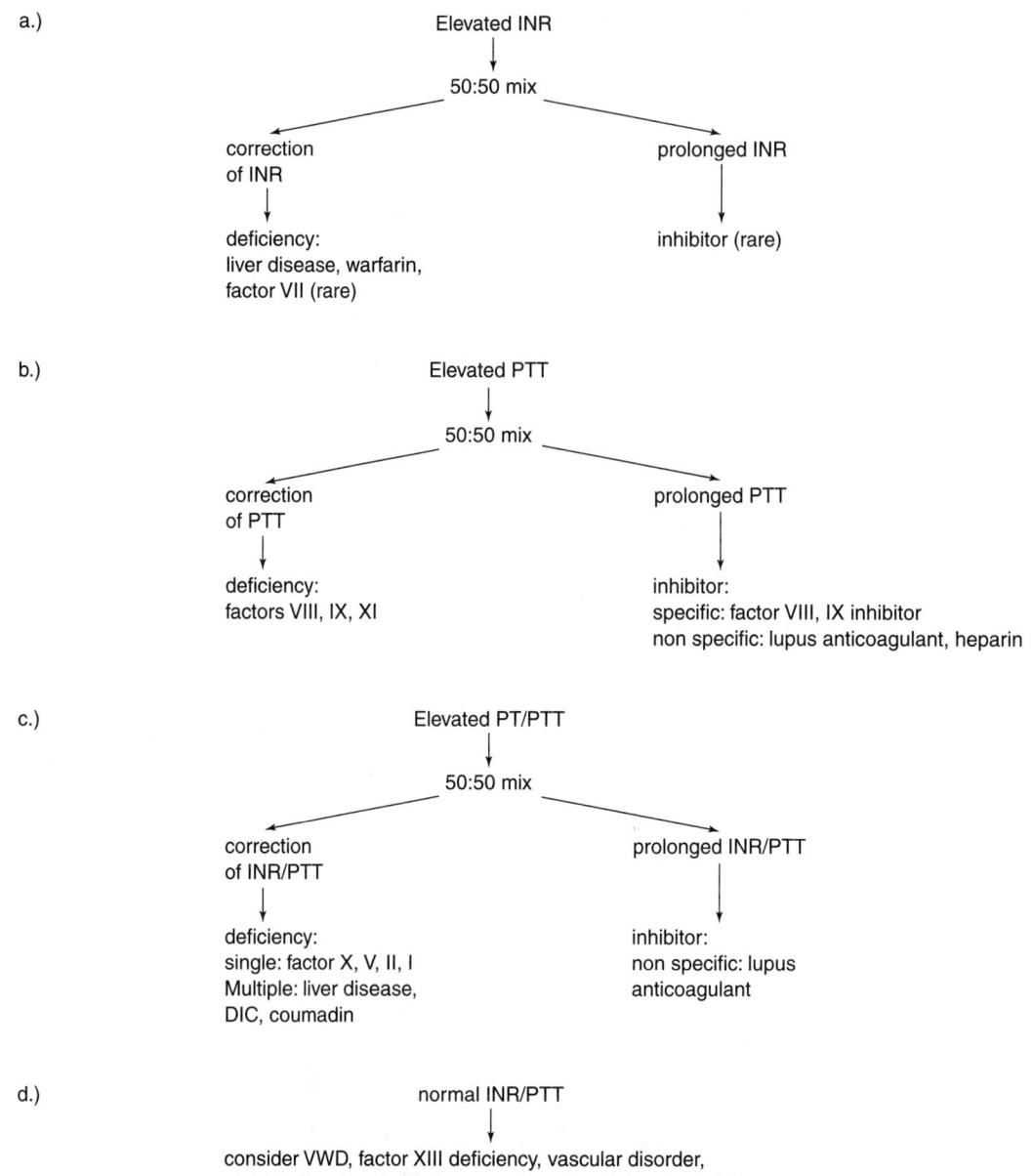

FIGURE 37-2 An algorithm for the evaluation of a bleeding patient.

tional ristocetin cofactor assay to determine the plasma level of vWF, and characterization of the multimeric structure of the vWF molecule by gel electrophoresis.

If these tests are normal in a patient with a bleeding history, testing for factor XIII should be performed by testing for increased solubility of the fibrin clot in urea. Further testing should rule out deficiencies of plasminogen activator inhibitor, or α2 antiplasmin. These latter tests are seldom necessary unless a positive history of bleeding and negative screening laboratory tests indicate a high probability of such disorders.

Platelet function can be evaluated in vitro by platelet aggregation studies, in which light transmission through turbid platelet-rich plasma increases as platelets aggregate after the addition of an agonist. Laboratory findings in DIC include thrombocytopenia, an increased INR, prolonged aPTT and thrombin time, increased levels of fibrin degradation products, and hypofibrinogenemia.

Laboratory abnormalities in hemophilia include a variable prolongation of the aPTT and reduced factor activity. Inhibitory antibodies are present in about 10% of patients with hemophilia A and 2% of patients with hemophilia B. Inhibitory antibodies in hemophiliacs should be suspected when mixing studies with normal plasma fail to normalize the factor level in vitro.

TREATMENT OPTIONS, EXPECTED OUTCOMES, AND COMPREHENSIVE MANAGEMENT

Hemophilia

In patients with mild hemophilia A, desmopressin (DDAVP), which stimulates the release of both factor VIII and vWF, can be used for the control of bleeding and as prophylaxis before some surgical procedures. DDAVP should not be used as therapy in patients with life-threatening bleeding or in patients with severe deficiencies of factor VIII. DDAVP is administered as an intravenous infusion (0.3 mg/kg) and can be repeated every 8 to 12 hours. Prolonged administration of DDAVP may result in tachyphylaxis.

In patients undergoing a dental procedure, epsilon-aminocaproic acid (EACA), an inhibitor of fibrinolysis, can be used to control bleeding. One regimen is to administer EACA on the day before the dental procedure and for 5 to 7 days afterward, along with a single 50% factor replacement dose immediately before the procedure.

Severe hemophilia A is treated with factor VIII concentrates. Hemophilia B is usually treated with high-purity factor IX concentrate. Minor cuts and abrasions for all types usually require no therapy.

Uncomplicated hemarthrosis and symptomatic hematomas in noncritical locations can be managed by administering factor VIII or IX intravenously to achieve levels of about 50% of normal for 2 to 4 days. A single dose administered by the patient at home at the onset of symptoms is often sufficient therapy for a hemarthrosis. Prompt initiation of therapy can minimize bleeding and subsequent joint deformity. Immobilization of the joint for 2 to 3 days is important. Needle aspiration of blood from the joint space is performed only if severe pain and swelling are present. Life-threatening hemorrhage, hematomas in critical locations, and major surgery require achievement of factor levels of 100% and longer courses of therapy. Therapy is monitored by assaying factor VIII or IX activity after a replacement dose.

With replacement therapy, the average life expectancy now exceeds 60 years. Unfortunately, 70% to 90% of patients treated with factor concentrates before 1985 were infected with the AIDS and hepatitis viruses. Since 1985, heat and other treatments have been used to inactivate these viruses.

von Willebrand Disease

All types of vWD are responsive to replacement therapy with cryoprecipitate or intermediate-purity factor VIII concentrates containing functional vWF. However, these products carry the risk of transmitting viral diseases such as HIV and hepatitis. Thus, these therapies are reserved for patients with severe type I disease and the majority of type II vWD patients.

DDAVP, administered at 0.3 mg/kg by intravenous infusion, can elevate vWF activity for 6 to 8 hours in most cases of type I vWD. The response to DDAVP in type II vWD is variable and in some cases potentially harmful. Some authorities recommend testing certain type II vWD patients with DDAVP well in advance of surgery to assess if they will respond. The concomitant use of antifibrinolytics such as EACA is recommended, particularly for dental procedures and minor mucosal bleeding.

Disseminated Intravascular Coagulation

The treatment of DIC is aimed primarily at the underlying disease process and secondarily at the coagulopathy that results in the thrombotic or hemorrhagic manifestation. In patients with severe bleeding, fresh-frozen plasma (FFP), cryoprecipitate, or platelets can be used. In patients with thrombosis, hepa-rin may be useful, usually at lower-than-normal doses, to reduce the risk of bleeding (eg, 500 units/hour intravenous infusion). However, unless the thrombotic or hemorrhagic complications are serious, specific therapy for DIC is probably of no benefit.

Liver Disease

Patients with liver disease and a prolonged INR should empirically be given vitamin K 10 mg/day subcutaneously for 3 days, although only a minority of patients will respond. Patients who are actively bleeding may be given FFP, which may temporarily replace the deficient coagulation factors. Usually 2 to 4 units of FFP are administered every 4 to 6 hours. Care needs to be taken to avoid fluid overload with this therapy.

Vitamin K Deficiency

Treatment with vitamin K 10 mg/day subcutaneously for 3 days will replace the vitamin K stores and reverse the coagulopathy. In patients with severe hemorrhage, immediate replacement of coagulation factors can be achieved by the administration of FFP, 2 to 4 units every 4 to 6 hours.

Thrombocytopenia

In general, patients who are bleeding with thrombocytopenia associated with platelet counts of less than 50,000/mL should be treated with platelet transfusions. Asymptomatic patients with a platelet count less than 10,000/mL should receive similar prophylaxis.

Patients with thrombocytopenia from platelet destruction rarely benefit from platelet transfusions, and treatment is directed at the cause of the thrombocytopenia. Patients with thrombocytopenia from platelet sequestration may require far greater quantities of platelets than normal. Occasionally a splenectomy may be indicated to correct the thrombocytopenia.

Acquired qualitative platelet disorders are generally treated with platelet transfusions. Uremic bleeding associated with qualitative platelet abnormalities can be treated with DDAVP or dialysis, however.

Treatment for chronic ITP includes prednisone, 1 to 2 mg/kg daily. Splenectomy should be considered for patients who need an excessively high dose of prednisone to maintain an adequate platelet count, or for patients whose disease does not respond to steroid treatment. Splenectomy normalizes the platelet count in about 70% of patients (George et al, 1996).

Intravenous immune globulin, 400 mg/kg daily for 5 days, usually increases the platelet count more rapidly than steroids alone and can be used in actively bleeding patients. Transfused platelets are cleared rapidly and are therefore rarely beneficial. Patients who suffer relapses after splenectomy may be treated with a variety of drugs, including cyclophosphamide, azathioprine, vincristine, or danazol, with variable success.

Patients with HIV-associated thrombocytopenia requiring treatment may be given zidovudine (AZT) 600 mg/day. Because the response to AZT may be slow, other interim therapies such as steroids or intravenous immune globulin may be necessary in patients with severe symptomatic thrombocytopenia with a platelet count less than 10,000/mL.

Without appropriate treatment, TTP is almost universally fatal. However, 70% of patients will survive with expediently administered exchange transfusions with FFP (3 to 4 L/day). Many authorities also recommend the administration of prednisone, 1 to 2 mg/kg daily. Plasma exchange is continued until the clinical status has improved and the platelet count and level of lactic dehydrogenase are normal for several consecutive days.

The cryosupernatant fraction of plasma may be used in patients whose disease does not initially respond to plasma exchange with FFP. Approximately 20% of patients whose disease initially responds suffer a relapse and require retreatment. Splenectomy, azathioprine, cyclophosphamide, and vincristine are also used as salvage therapies for patients with refractory disease or relapse. Platelet transfusions should be withheld in patients with TTP, except for patients with severe hemorrhage.

Prevention

Patients with severe thrombocytopenia should be warned against taking aspirin or nonsteroidal anti-inflammatories, which interfere with platelet function and could increase the risk of bleeding.

Prenatal testing for both hemophilia A and B can be performed via chorionic villous sampling on women who are carriers of the gene and who are pregnant with a male fetus. As with any postconception screening, moral and emotional issues may make this diagnostic tool unacceptable for some people. Excellent genetic counseling should be given to persons considering this test.

Lifelong prophylaxis should not be considered for asymptomatic persons with inherited thrombophilia who are not exposed to thrombotic risk factors. However, prophylactic measures should be implemented when the patient is exposed to thrombotic risk (eg, surgery, prolonged immobilization, pregnancy and the postpartum period).

CLINICAL WARNING: Patients with thrombophilia should be counseled about the high risk of venous thrombosis associated with oral contraceptive use. Because pregnancy and the 4 weeks after delivery are times associated with high thrombotic risk, the administration of unfractionated heparin, 5000 units three times a day, is recommended.

Before and after surgery, patients should receive subcutaneous unfractionated heparin, 5000 units three times a day. When the risk is exceptionally high, as in certain orthopedic procedures, transfusion of AT III or protein C concentrates may be considered as additional therapy for patients with AT III or protein C deficiency, respectively.

Patients with documented venous thromboembolism and no previous venous thrombosis or history of thrombophilia should receive 3 to 6 months of oral anticoagulation therapy. If the patient has a transient clinical risk factor (eg, orthopedic surgery), oral anticoagulation for 4 to 6 weeks is appropriate, provided the patient is mobile at that time.

The true incidence of recurrence in patients with thrombophilia who discontinue anticoagulant therapy after a single episode of venous thrombosis is unknown. Thus, the risks and benefits of lifelong anticoagulation should be individualized. Most authorities would offer lifelong anticoagulation to thrombophilic patients who have had more than one episode of venous thrombosis. Usually lifelong anticoagulant therapy is not offered after the first thrombotic episode, especially if it developed in association with surgery, pregnancy, or other circumstances associated with a high risk of thrombosis.

If the first thrombotic event was life-threatening or if there are multiple inherited genetic defects, lifelong oral anticoagulant therapy may be considered. Patients with thrombophilia and a first episode of venous thrombosis are treated with standard heparin therapy, followed by oral anticoagulation for 3 to 6 months. In addition, patients with hyperhomocysteinemia associated with thrombosis should receive lifelong folate 1 mg/day, pyridoxine 100 mg/day, and cobalamin 0.4 mg/day, all of which reduce the level of serum homocysteine.

TEACHING AND SELF-CARE

Patient and family education focuses on the particular features of the bleeding disorder in question. General guidelines for counseling include the following:

- Physical exercise that is safe and aerobic in nature is strongly encouraged. Being in good physical condition can reduce the number and minimize the damage of bleeding complications. The physical regimen should be planned to reduce the chance of potential bleeding from trauma; contact sports are discouraged.
- All patients should be taught to detect warning signs and to seek immediate treatment should they occur. This is especially important for the patient with thrombocytopenia. Bruising, nose bleeds, oral bleeding, or petechiae may indicate danger.
- Bleeding disorders can be treated with blood transfusions. Patients with bleeding disorders who have not been exposed to hepatitis B should receive the hepatitis B vaccine series.
- Genetic counseling is important for patients with inherited diatheses.

COMMUNITY RESOURCES

- Healthtouch Online—Immune Thrombocytopenia Purpura: http://www.healthtouch.com/level1/leaflets/nhlbi/nhlbi025.htm: General overview

- Lupus Foundation of America—Blood Disorders in SLE: http://www.lupus.org/lupus/topics/blood.html#3
- NIH Publication, Facts About Immune Thrombocytopenic Purpura: gopher://fido.nhlbi.nih.gov:70/00/educprog/other/gppubs/itpfs.txt: General overview
- Community Outreach Health System: http://web.bu.edu/COHIS/cardvasc/cdv.htm: What is coagulation, platelet disease information
- National Heart, Lung, and Blood Institute Information Center, P.O. Box 30105, Bethesda, MD 20824-0105, 301-251-1222

REFERRAL POINTS AND CLINICAL WARNINGS

The care of patients with severe bleeding diatheses should be supervised by a hematologist experienced in hemostatic disorders. Referrals should be made to a hematologist for such patients before surgical procedures and in the event of significant hemorrhagic episodes. Hemophiliacs with inhibitory antibodies are especially difficult to treat and should be evaluated by a hematologist. Patients with thrombocytopenia should be evaluated by a hematologist, especially if the cause is not immediately evident, if the platelet count is less than 50,000/mL, or if the patient is actively bleeding.

References

De Stefano, V., Finazzi, G., & Mannucci, P.M. (1996). Inherited thrombophilia: Pathogenesis, clinical syndromes, and management. *Blood, 87*(9), 3531–3544.

Furie, B., Limentani, S.A., & Rosenfield, C.G. (1994). A practical guide to the evaluation and treatment of hemophilia. *Blood, 84*(1), 3–9.

George, J.N., Woolf, S.H., Raskob, G.E., et al. (1996). Idiopathic thrombocytopenic purpura: A practice guideline developed by explicit methods for the American Society of Hematology. *Blood, 88*(1), 3–40.

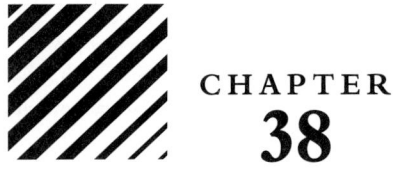

Lymphoma

Candis Morrison, Ph.D., C.R.N.P.

Hodgkin's and non-Hodgkin's lymphoma are neoplasms of lymphocytes that affect the lymph nodes, the spleen, and the hematopoietic system. These cancers may spread to other tissues and structures, including the gastrointestinal tract, bone marrow, and liver. They are often referred to as immunologic cancers because of the immunologic function of the lymphocyte (Carson, 1996).

Although the clinical presentation and diagnostic evaluation of these two diseases are similar, the pathologic identification of marker cells distinguishes the two types of lymphoma. The diagnostic category determines both treatment and prognosis, despite the fact that the staging systems overlap.

The development of less toxic therapies and growth factors have lessened the complication of severe cytopenia, enabling many patients with lymphoma to be treated as outpatients. Primary providers participating in the care of these patients must understand the disease entities, the treatment modalities and their side effects, and complications. A multidisciplinary team approach is optimal to help decrease the morbidity and mortality rates associated with these hematologic malignancies.

ANATOMY, PHYSIOLOGY, AND PATHOLOGY

The intricate interrelation between the hematologic and the immunologic systems protects the body from foreign invaders, such as pathogens and toxins. There are three primary components of the immune system. The first is phagocytosis, in which invading substances are ingested and destroyed by individual immune cells. Mononuclear phagocytes recognize invaders, engulf foreign particles, and activate specific immunity. The second component is inflammation, in which cells and proteins defend the body against infection and repair tissue damage. The third component is cellular and humoral immunity. In cellular immunity, T lymphocytes initiate the response; in humoral immunity, the trigger is serum antibodies. Phagocytosis and inflammation are predominantly nonspecific immune responses, whereas humoral and cellular responses are characteristic of specific immunity (Post-White, 1996).

The primary cells of the immune system are lymphocytes and mononuclear phagocytes. Lymphocytes are formed from pluripotent stem cells, found primarily in the bone marrow. These cells differentiate into all of the recognized mature cell lines produced by the various hematopoietic cytokines, or growth factors (Lowry, 1996). Figure 38-1 illustrates normal hematopoiesis, and Table 38-1 describes the clinically relevant cytokines (Hoffman & Williams, 1994).

More than 1 billion lymphocytes are produced in the marrow daily. There are two functional classes of lymphocytes—the T lymphocytes, which regulate antibody synthesis and cellular immune processes, and the B lymphocytes, which contribute to the humoral response of antigen sensitization. The lymphoid stem cell is programmed by the bone marrow to develop into either a T-cell or a B-cell precursor. B-cell maturation occurs in the follicles of the lymph nodes after exposure to an antigen (Paradiso, 1995).

Lymphocytes are the only immunocompetent cells able to recognize antigens. T cells are produced in the marrow, mature in the thymus, and then are released to secondary lymphoid organs, such as the lymph nodes, the spleen, the tonsils, and Peyer's patches in the ileum, as well as throughout all the connective and epithelial tissues of the body. Lymphocytes continuously circulate through the lymphatic network and vascular channels throughout the body and within nodes, which are densely clustered in the neck, axillae, abdomen, and pelvis (David, 1994).

Surface markers and receptors, which are macromolecules with a binding affinity for a specific antigen, appear on the immune cell during maturation. They signal each other to recognize, bind, and kill antigens. Surface markers differentiate between lymphocyte subsets and are recognized by monoclonal antibodies. These groups of lymphocytes, surface markers, and monoclonal antibodies are called "clusters of differentiation" (CD). The most commonly known surface markers are CD4 and CD8. CD4 defines the helper function of T cells, CD8 the suppressor or cytotoxic function (Post-White, 1996).

When B lymphocytes are activated by a signal from T lymphocytes, they differentiate into one of the five classes of immunoglobulins (Ig); IgM, IgG, IgD, IgE, and IgA. In the primary immune response, there is a latent period in which B cells make contact with the antigen, proliferate, differentiate, and secrete antibody. Because resting B cells express only IgM and IgD, and IgD is rarely secreted, IgM is the dominant antibody secreted in the primary immune response. Other isotypes, including IgG, IgA, and IgE, appear with second exposure to the same antigen. The secondary antibody response is more rapid than the primary because of the added ability of memory. This complicated host response is distorted by malfunctions in hematopoiesis, especially the proliferation of abnormal cells.

Hodgkin's Disease

Hodgkin's disease (HD) is a unifocal disease that usually spreads in a contiguous manner. Early in the course of the disease, only the lymph nodes are affected, making diagnosis difficult until multiple nodes are involved. The disease spreads predictably from the original site to lymph nodes in adjacent areas. This orderly pattern of contiguous spread is most evident in nodular sclerosing HD.

Some lesions that originate in the mediastinum spread to nodes in the lower neck and then to the upper retroperitoneal area. Other histologic types may skip the mediastinum and

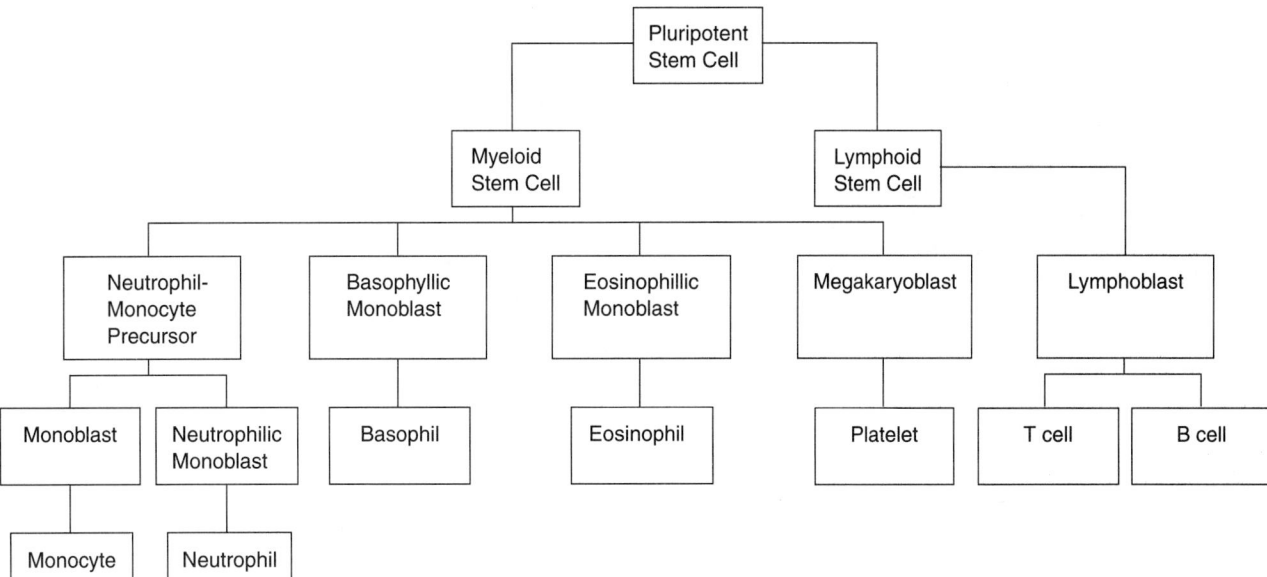

FIGURE 38-1 New blood cells are constantly produced by the body. In healthy adults, an estimated 100 billion red cells and 400 million white cells are produced each hour. The life span of mature blood cells is short, only a few days or months. 95% of the body's blood cell production takes place in the bone marrow, with the remaining 5% occurring in the spleen. While most blood cells produced in the bone marrow are discharged directly into the bloodstream, T cells first travel to the thymus gland, where they receive further programming before being released. Here they also acquire new functions and surface antigens and then emigrate to peripheral tissues. Development of the various cell lines proceeds through many steps and phases. A simplified diagram of the process is presented above.

spread to the retroperitoneal nodes without ever causing intrathoracic disease. Disease spreads to extranodal areas by direct extension and then invades the vasculature, resulting in hematologic dissemination. The spleen is the final lymph node area of involvement before hematologous dissemination occurs.

■ ■ ■ **CLINICAL PEARL**

The absence of splenic disease is a positive prognostic indicator for HD.

Non-Hodgkin's Lymphoma

Normally, the early lymphocyte matures in a predictable manner into a mature immunocompetent cell. However, in non-Hodgkin's lymphoma (NHL), an abnormal proliferation of monoclonal cells occurs. Instead of progressing to the next developmental phase, the cells fix at one phase of development and continue to proliferate.

The neoplastic cell population is cloned from a single neoplastic hematopoietic stem cell and ultimately proliferates into

TABLE 38-1	Clinically Useful Hematopoietic Growth Factors and Interleukins
Growth Factor	**Functions**
Interleukin-1 (IL-1)	Radioprotective agent (decreases degree of granulocytopenia/thrombocytopenia) Antitumor activity against renal cell carcinoma and melanoma with or without lymphokine activated killer cells
Interleukin-2 (IL-2)	Stimulates T cells, B cells, natural killer cells, and monocytes Aids in differentiation and maturation of B cells
Interleukin-3 (IL-3)	Lessens degree of granulocytopenia/thrombocytopenia after chemotherapy or bone marrow transplantation (BMT)
Interleukin-6 (IL-6)	Stimulates platelet production Lessens degree of granulocytopenia/thrombocytopenia after chemotherapy or BMT
Granulocyte-macrophage colony-stimulating factor (GM-CSF)	Lessens degree of granulocytopenia after chemotherapy or BMT Used to treat chronic neutropenic disorders
Granulocyte colony-stimulating factor (G-CSF)	Lessens degree of granulocytopenia after chemotherapy or BMT Used to treat chronic neutropenic disorders
Macrophage colony-stimulating factor (M-CSF)	Adjunctive therapy for fungal infections after chemotherapy or BMT Antitumor therapy when administered with monoclonal antibodies
Erythropoietin	Treatment of anemias of chronic renal disease, chronic inflammation, cancer, and HIV infection

Adapted from Hoffman & Williams, 1994, and Schrier, 1994.

lymphoma. Surface markers and immunoglobulins are formed after the proliferation of neoplastic cells and designate the cell type of lymphoma. This progression of events has important implications for the prognosis and treatment of this disease.

Seventy percent of lymphomas are B cell. B cells can be divided into four cytologic types: small cleaved, large cleaved, small noncleaved, and large noncleaved. It is possible to predict some of the clinical manifestations of NHL based on the characteristics of the predominant cell type. Neoplastic cells often retain the surface of their cells of origin, so it is also possible to group them according to the phenotypic properties of their surface markers.

The two major classes of NHL are indolent and aggressive. Indolent NHL is a generalized disease usually diagnosed late (stage III or IV in 70% to 90% of cases). Indolent NHL spreads noncontiguously, and bone marrow involvement is evident most of the time. Spread to the central nervous system is rare, and systemic symptoms are present in only 15% to 20% of cases. Aggressive NHL is often diagnosed early (stage I or II in 30% to 40% of cases). Mediastinal involvement is rare; the bone marrow is affected only 10% to 30% of the time. Ten percent to 15% of patients have central nervous system disease, and 20% to 30% have systemic symptoms (Sunderland & Coltman, 1993).

EPIDEMIOLOGY

With an incidence in excess of 61,000 cases a year, the malignant lymphomas collectively represent the sixth most common cause of cancer in the United States (ACS, 1998). Approximately 85% of patients with malignant lymphomas have NHL, and the remaining 15% have HD.

Hodgkin's Disease

There are 7000 to 8000 cases of HD diagnosed in the United States each year. The incidence follows a bimodal curve. The first peak occurs between ages 20 and 25, followed by a plateau lasting until age 55. There is a second peak in the seventh decade (Klitz et al, 1994). HD is uncommon in children, with only 10% to 15% of cases occurring in patients younger than 16 (Weinstein & Tarbell, 1997). HD is more common in males than in females for all age groups, and half as common among African Americans as whites.

The etiology of HD is unknown. Evidence suggests that impaired growth factor genes, viruses, genetic alterations, and immune defects all contribute to tumorigenesis in HD (Durkop et al, 1992). Certain HLA phenotypes are associated with increased susceptibility, and there are several examples of multiple family occurrences. Siblings of patients with HD have a five- to ninefold increased risk of developing the disease, and that risk may be even higher in same-sex siblings (Sunderland & Coltman, 1993). It occurs more frequently in first-born children and in those from small families.

Patients with a higher standard of living or who are better educated are also at increased risk. One hypothesis suggests that exposure to common environmental pathogens is protective against HD, and this exposure is reduced in wealthier young people. In older patients, social class characteristics play a less significant role (Sunderland & Coltman, 1993).

An association between Epstein-Barr virus infection and HD has been postulated as a result of an increased incidence of HD in persons with a history of infectious mononucleosis. Prospective studies have also shown elevated Epstein-Barr virus titers in patients before the diagnosis of HD.

Non-Hodgkin's Lymphoma

More than 53,600 cases of NHL are diagnosed each year. It is the sixth most common cause of cancer-related death in the United States, accounting for more than 23,800 deaths yearly (ACS, 1998). This is approximately three times the number of HD cases (Carson, 1996). Males outnumber females by 10:7. Because of the young average age of lymphoma patients (42 years) and the resulting number of years of life lost to these diseases, NHLs rank fourth in economic impact among cancers in the United States (Shipp et al, 1997).

There has been a 50% increase in the incidence of NHL in the past 15 years, one of the largest increases for any cancer group. Certain highly aggressive NHLs occur in the setting of AIDS, accounting for the biggest increase in overall incidence. Indolent lymphomas have also significantly increased in recent years (Shipp et al, 1997).

In the United States, the incidence of NHL shows a steady age-dependent increase from childhood through the eighth decade of life. Certain subcategories are more likely to occur in specific age groups. Diffuse large B-cell, lymphoblastic, and Burkitt's lymphoma are the most common lymphomas in children. Aggressive lymphomas are the most common lymphoid neoplasms in young adults. Indolent lymphomas affect adults averaging age 56 years. Because the incidence of both indolent and aggressive lymphomas increases with age, they are the most common lymphoid malignancies in patients over 60 years of age (Shipp et al, 1997).

NHLs are more common in males than females and in whites than African Americans. Although NHLs are reported worldwide, specific subtypes occur more frequently in particular locales. Follicular lymphomas are rare in Latin America. Burkitt's lymphoma occurs more frequently in tropical Africa, and adult T-cell lymphoma is more common in southwest Japan and the Caribbean (Shipp et al, 1997).

Some lymphomas have been associated with chromosome translocations and rearrangement of proto-oncogenes such as bcl-2 and c-myc. These changes may be important to the etiology and progression of the disease. Genetic abnormalities of chromosome 14 are recognized in many follicular lymphomas as well as in Burkitt's lymphoma (Carson, 1996).

Some research suggests that exposure to certain herbicides, industrial solvents, or vinyl chloride may increase a person's risk. Other possible risk factors include exposure to excessive amounts of radiation or treatment with high-dose chemotherapy for cancer, or with immunosuppressive agents such as those used after solid organ transplant (ACS, 1998). NHL is 45 to 100 times more likely among renal transplant patients receiving immunosuppressive therapy, with lymphomas accounting for 29% of cancers in these patients. Other patients predisposed to NHL are those with autoimmune diseases such as rheumatoid arthritis and systemic lupus erythematosus.

Certain viral etiologies have been implicated in NHL, including Epstein-Barr (particularly in the immunocompromised host), *Helicobacter pylori*, HTLV-1, and Kaposi Sarcoma herpesvirus. Burkitt's lymphoma is associated with the presence of the Epstein-Barr virus. The HTLV-1 virus has been implicated in some adult T-cell lymphomas, especially in those occurring in the Caribbean, parts of South Africa, and southwestern Japan. The HTLV-1 infection has also been detected in AIDS patients who develop lymphomas.

DIAGNOSTIC CRITERIA

Lymphomas are diagnosed and categorized by the histologic exam of an excised lymph node. Both HD and NHL are staged via the Ann Arbor system (Table 38-2). This classification does not account for changes in histology, bulky disease, or extranodal involvement, all of which are important prognostic indicators in NHL. The Cotswold additions, which address bulk and site of disease, make this system much more useful for staging NHL.

Lymphomas are classified by cell type. NHL classifications are presented in Table 38-3. This new system includes lymphomas that have been reclassified or newly recognized. There is currently a version of lymphoma classification under development.

When diagnosing lymphomas, needle biopsy specimens are not adequate: the cell architecture must be preserved to make an accurate diagnosis. Lymphomas without accessible lymph nodes may be diagnosed on the basis of bone marrow or peripheral blood smears using special stains and cytogenetics.

The histologic diagnosis of HD is based on recognition of Reed-Sternberg (RS) cells in the appropriate cellular and architectural setting. The RS cell is large, with two or more nuclei, each containing a single prominent nucleolus (Fig. 38-2). A clear zone surrounding the nucleolus is a distinctive feature. However, cells similar to RS cells can be detected in other lymphomas and solid tumors, infectious mononucleosis, and lymphoid hyperplasia associated with phenytoin therapy. Therefore, the presence of RS cells can be a confusing finding (Horner, 1996).

In HD, the lymph node architecture is effaced by a cellular infiltrate composed of normal lymphocytes, eosinophils, histiocytes, and plasma cells, with RS cells scattered throughout this background of inflammatory cells. The accompanying lymphocytes are primarily host response and polyclonal T and B cells. Most of the T-cell population belongs to the T-helper subset.

The Rye system classifies HD into four histopathologic categories: lymphocyte-predominant, mixed cellularity, lymphocyte-depleted, and nodular sclerosis. The first three categories differ primarily in their relative proportion of RS cells, mononuclear variants, and reactive lymphocytes. The fourth category, nodular sclerosis, has broad collagen bands that divide lymphoid tissue into circumscribed nodules. Nodular sclerosis HD also has distinctive clinical features: it is the only HD subtype more common in women than in men, and it has a propensity to involve lower cervical, supraclavicular, and mediastinal lymph nodes.

In lymphocyte-predominant HD, two variants, diffuse and nodular, are recognized. The diffuse form is associated with a good prognosis; however, patients with the nodal variant have an increased risk of relapse after completion of therapy. This form may be related to the B-cell malignancies of NHL. Further, the prevalence of histologic subtypes of HD varies widely by age. In patients younger than age 35, the majority (70%)

TABLE 38-2	Staging System for Lymphoma	
Stage	Ann Arbor Staging System	Cotswold Modification
I	Involvement of a single lymph node region (I) or of a single extralymphatic organ or site (I$_E$)	Involvement of a single lymph node region or lymphoid structure
II	Involvement of two or more lymph node regions on the same side of the diaphragm alone (II) or with involvement of limited, contiguous extralymphatic organ or tissue (II$_E$)	Involvement of two or more lymph node regions on the same side of the diaphragm (the mediastinum is considered a single site, whereas the hilar lymph nodes are considered bilaterally); the number of anatomic sides should be indicated by a subscript (eg, II$_3$).
III	Involvement of lymph node regions on both sides of the diaphragm (III), which may include the spleen (III$_S$), a limited, contiguous extralymphatic organ or side (III$_E$), or both (III$_{ES}$)	Involvement of lymph node regions on both sides of the diaphragm: III$_1$ (with or without involvement of splenic, hilar, celiac, or portal nodes) and III$_2$ (with involvement of para-aortic, iliac, and mesenteric nodes)
IV	Multiple or disseminated foci of involvement of one or more extralymphatic organs or tissues, with or without lymphatic involvement	Involvement of one or more extranodal sites in addition to a site for which the designation E has been used

All cases are subclassified to indicate the absence or presence of the systemic symptoms of significant fever (>38°C), night sweats, and unexplained weight loss exceeding 10% of normal body weight within the previous 6 months. The clinical stage denotes the stage as determined by all diagnostic examinations and a single diagnostic biopsy. In the Ann Arbor classification, the term "pathologic stage" is used if a second biopsy of any kind has been obtained, whether negative or positive. In the Cotswold modification, the pathologic stage is determined by laparotomy; X designates bulky disease (widening of the mediastinum by more than one third or the presence of a nodal mass >10 cm), and E designates involvement of a single extranodal site that is contiguous or proximal to the known nodal site.

TABLE 38-3		Characteristics of Non-Hodgkin's Lymphoma Classifications	
Neoplasm	**B or T Cell**	**Usual Course**	**Other Disease Characteristics**
Small lymphocyte lymphoma/Chronic lymphocytic leukemia	B	Indolent	Common disorder, representing approximately 90% of chronic lymphoid leukemias. Most patients are older adults with both marrow and peripheral blood involvement at diagnosis. They present with generalized lymphadenopathy, hepatosplenomegaly, and extranodal infiltrates. Extent of disease at time of diagnosis is the best predictor of survival. Patients may have hypogammaglobulinemia, which is associated with infectious complications, and autoimmune phenomena such as hemolytic anemia or thrombocytopenia. Death is usually a result of infectious complications in patients whose disease has become refractory to treatment.
Lymphoplasmacytic lymphoma Waldenstrom's macroglobulinemia	B	Course is indolent but more aggressive than CLL Disseminated	Much less common; about 5% to 10% of indolent disseminated lymphomas. Patients are usually older adults with bone marrow involvement and a monoclonal serum paparotein (IGM type). If associated with hyperviscosity, is labeled Waldenstrom's. Lymph node or splenic involvement may occur.
Splenic marginal zone lymphoma (with or without villous lymphocytes)	B	Extremely indolent Disseminated	Rare, accounting for 1% to 2% of chronic lymphoid malignancies identified in bone marrow. Patients typically have bone marrow involvement and may have a small M component; peripheral lymphadenopathy is uncommon. Tumor may be resistant to chemotherapy. Splenectomy may be followed by prolonged remission.
Extranodal marginal zone (MALT)	B	Indolent Extranodal	Extranodal MALT lymphoma constitutes most of low-grade gastric lymphomas, up to 40% of orbital lymphomas, and most indolent pulmonary, thyroid, and salivary gland lymphomas. Most patients present with localized disease and are older adults. A slight female predominance has been reported. Patients may have a history of autoimmune disease such as Sjögren's syndrome or Hashimoto's thyroiditis. In gastric MALT lymphoma, a strong association with *Helicobacter* gastritis has been discovered.
Nodal marginal zone lymphoma	B	Indolent nodal	Rare disorder. Patients present with isolated or generalized nodal disease and bone marrow and rarely peripheral blood involvement. The clinical course is similar to other indolent B-cell lymphomas.
Follicle center (follicular) lymphoma	B	Indolent nodal	Most common adult lymphoma in U.S., representing 35% to 40% of all NHLs. Affects predominantly older adults, with an equal gender incidence. Most patients have widespread nodal disease at diagnosis, with additional involvement of the spleen and bone marrow. There is occasional involvement of peripheral blood and extranodal sites.
Mantle cell lymphoma	B	Indolent nodal (actually has moderately aggressive course)	Approximately 5% of adult NHLs in U.S. Usually occurs in older adults. Marked male predominance. Patients usually have widespread disease at diagnosis. Involved sites include lymph nodes, spleen, Waldeyer's ring, and often bone marrow, blood, and extranodal sites such as the GI tract. Median survival is only 3 years.
Diffuse large B-cell lymphoma	B	Aggressive	Constitutes 30% to 45% of adult NHL cases. Median age at diagnosis is in the 6th decade, but the range is broad and these tumors may be seen in children. Patients present with single or multiple rapidly enlarging, symptomatic masses in nodal or extranodal sites. Up to 40% of these are extranodal. The most common extranodal site is the stomach, although most primary lymphomas of the CNS, bone, kidney, and testes are also diffuse large B-cell lymphomas. These tumors are aggressive but potentially curable with intensive therapy. They may result from transformation from an indolent NHL.
Primary mediastinal (thymic) large B-cell lymphoma	B	Aggressive	Unknown incidence. Female predominance with median age in the fourth decade. Patients present with a locally invasive anterior mediastinal mass originating in the thymus. Frequently, airway compromise and superior vena cava syndrome complicate care. Relapses are usually extranodal.
Anaplastic large cell lymphoma	T	Aggressive	Unknown incidence. Disease has bimodal age distribution but has been recognized in all age groups. May arise as a high-grade transformation of an indolent extranodal T-cell lymphoma such as mycosis fungoides. Either presents as a systemic disease involving lymph nodes or extranodal sites, or as a primary cutaneous form without extracutaneous spread.
Peripheral T-cell lymphomas, unspecified	T	Aggressive	Less than 15% of NHL cases in U.S.; more common in other parts of the world. Patients are usually adults with generalized disease. Occasionally eosinophilia, pruritus, or hemophagocytic syndromes are demonstrated. Lymph nodes, skin or subcutus, liver, spleen, and other viscera may be involved. These diseases are potentially curable, but relapses are more common than in B-cell lymphomas of similar histology grades.

(continued)

	B or T		
TABLE 38-3	**Characteristics of Non-Hodgkin's Lymphoma Classifications** *(Continued)*		
Neoplasm	**B or T Cell**	**Usual Course**	**Other Disease Characteristics**
Angioimmunoblastic T-cell lymphoma	T, specific variant	Moderately aggressive with some spontaneous remissions	One of most common peripheral T-cell lymphomas encountered in Western countries but still rare. Accounts for 20% of T-cell lymphomas and about 4% of all NHL cases. Patients typically have generalized lymphadenopathy, fever, weight loss, skin rash, and polyclonal hypergammaglobulinemia. They have increased susceptibility to infections.
Nasal/nasal-type T/NK-cell lymphoma	T	Indolent or aggressive	Rare disorder in U.S. May affect children or adults. Extranodal sites are involved, including nose, palate, upper airway, GI tract, and skin.
Intestinal T-cell lymphoma	T	Aggressive	Occurs in adults who often have a history of gluten-sensitive enteropathy. Uncommon in most areas of U.S. Patients present with abdominal pain, often associated with jejunal perforation. Stomach and colon are affected less often. Death usually occurs from multifocal intestinal perforation caused by refractory malignant ulcers.
Hepatosplenic T-cell lymphoma	T	Very aggressive	Rare condition, incidence unknown. Patients are predominantly adolescent or young adult males. They present with marked hepatosplenomegaly and circulating neoplastic cells, and subtle bone marrow involvement may be present. They may respond to chemotherapy initially, but relapse and death are common.
Adult T-cell lymphoma/leukemia	T	Indolent to very aggressive	The majority of patients are adults who have antibodies to HTLV-1. Most cases occur in Japan. Acute form is most common in patients presenting with a high white cell count, hepatosplenomegaly, hypercalcemia, and lytic bone lesions; survival only a few months. A chronic form (with less marked lymphocytosis, no hypercalcemia or hepatosplenomegaly) has a slightly longer survival. Both forms produce skin rashes.
Precursor B lymphoblastic leukemia/lymphoma	T	Aggressive	Constitutes 40% of childhood lymphomas and 15% of acute lymphoblastic leukemias. Patients are predominantly adolescent or young adult males, but older adults may be affected. They typically have mediastinal (thymic masses) or peripheral lymphadenopathy, or both. CNS involvement is common. Untreated disease is rapidly fatal.
Burkitt's lymphoma	T	Aggressive	Most common in children (30% of non-African pediatric lymphomas); rare adult cases (only 1% to 2%) of NHL often associated with immunodeficiency, particularly AIDS. The male/female ratio is 2 to 3:1. In African (endemic) cases, the jaws and other facial bones are often involved. In non-African (nonendemic) cases, most present in the abdomen, often involving the distal ileum, cecum, or mesentery; ovaries, kidneys, and breasts may also be involved.

Adapted from DeVita, Hellman & Rosenberg, 1997.

have nodular sclerosis HD and less than 20% have the mixed cellularity form. For older patients, 20% have nodular sclerosis and 40% mixed cellularity (Horner, 1996). The proportion of patients with early-stage disease is highest in lymphocyte-predominant disease and progressively decreases through nodular sclerosis, mixed cellularity, and lymphocyte-depleted subtypes.

Patients are classified, or staged, by the extent of lymph node involvement for stages I, II, and III. Stage IV includes patients with disease disseminated outside the lymph system. Patients are further classified with either "A" or "B" on the presence or absence of constitutional symptoms. The occurrence of "B" symptoms correlates with stage. Fewer than 10% of stage I patients are symptomatic at diagnosis, whereas over 80% of those with stage IV disease have one or more "B" symptoms. The subscript "E" denotes direct extension outside a lymph nodal area and the subscript "S" the involvement of the spleen.

Approximately 60% of patients with HD in the United States are stages I and II at the time of diagnosis. The percentage of patients with stages III and IV is generally higher in developing countries and in lower socioeconomic groups. This reflects the predominance of mixed cellularity and lymphocyte-depleted subtypes in these populations (Aisenberg, 1995).

HISTORY AND PHYSICAL EXAM

Hodgkin's Disease

The most common presenting feature of HD is a single or multiple, painless lymph node enlargement above the diaphragm. Mediastinal adenopathy is especially common among

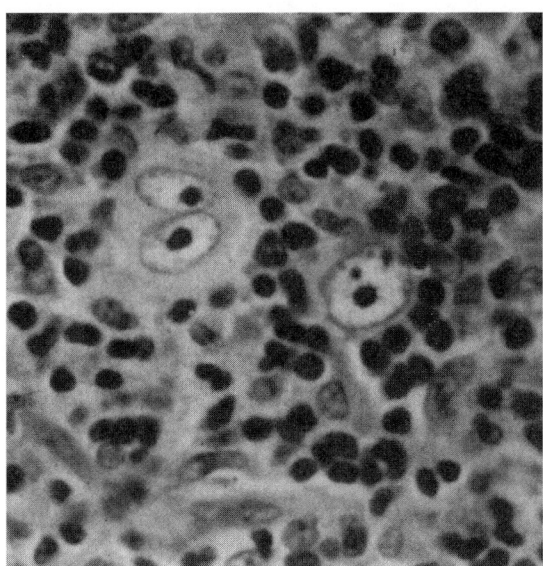

FIGURE 38-2 Reed-Sternberg cell. (DeVita et al, 1993)

patients between 15 and 35 years of age who have the nodular sclerosis subtype. Constitutional symptoms of fever, night sweats, and weight loss, termed "B" symptoms, may be present and debilitating in up to 40% of patients. For some patients, the fever is cyclic, with febrile episodes lasting several days to weeks and alternating with periods of normal temperature. Occasionally the "B" symptoms are the sole manifestations of this disease, and adenopathy is minimal or occult. This presentation is more common among older men with the histologic type of mixed cellularity or lymphocyte-depleted.

Severe generalized pruritus of unknown etiology is another presenting symptom in some patients. Patients may complain of pain in lymphoid tissue shortly after consuming alcohol; the mechanism for this phenomenon is not clear. Subdiaphragmatic involvement is less common. Although HD occasionally presents with cough, chest discomfort, or superior vena cava syndrome, most patients do not experience symptoms from enlarged lymph nodes.

The physical exam should include careful assessment of all lymph node regions to judge the extent of peripheral adenopathy. HD nodes are nontender and rubbery and are located in the neck region in 60% to 80% of cases (DeVita et al, 1997). Evaluation of the chest wall, palpation of the vertebral column to elicit tenderness, and a careful abdominal examination to detect hepatosplenomegaly are essential.

Non-Hodgkin's Lymphoma

The clinical presentation of NHL is similar to that of HD. Differential diagnosis is dependent on the size, shape, and location of lymph nodes. The most frequent clinical presentation is painless superficial adenopathy. Systemic symptoms occur in 15% to 20% of indolent cases and 20% to 30% of aggressive cases. Noncontinuous adenopathy is common, and NHL frequently involves sites such as epitrochlear nodes and Waldeyer's ring. Adenopathy of these nodes may wax and wane over a period of time. Extranodal involvement may occur, and multiple organ systems may be affected (eg, gastrointestinal tract, central nervous system, skeleton). Symptoms depend on whether the organ is invaded or obstructed. Characteristics of HD and indolent and aggressive NHL are presented in Table 38-4.

DIAGNOSTIC STUDIES

Indolent lymphomas are often diagnosed incidentally by leukocytosis on a routine complete blood count or adenopathy on a routine physical exam. Once a histopathologic diagnosis is established by lymph node biopsy, further evaluation is required for staging each patient. This staging process is necessary to determine the prognosis and extent and sites of disease, to direct therapeutic modalities, and to establish parameters to follow the patient's response. Routine laboratory tests include a complete blood count with differential and sedimentation rate, serum alkaline phosphatase and calcium levels, urinalysis, and liver and renal function tests.

The most common hematologic abnormality is normocytic, normochromic anemia, which is often associated with symptomatic, extensive disease. Rarely, cytopenias secondary to hypersplenism or bone marrow disease are noted. The erythrocyte sedimentation rate is commonly elevated in HD, and several studies have demonstrated that the degree of elevation has prognostic significance in patients with limited disease (DeVita, 1997).

Routine chemistries, including calcium and uric acid, can be used to screen for hypercalcemia, hyperuricemia, acidosis,

TABLE 38-4	Characteristics of Hodgkin's Disease and Non-Hodgkin's Lymphoma		
Characteristic	**Hodgkin's Disease**	**Indolent NHL**	**Intermediate to Aggressive NHL**
Extent of disease	Often localized	Rarely localized	Often localized in early stages
Site of origin	Nodal	Extranodal in 10%	Extranodal in 25%–40%
Stage I or II at diagnosis	60%	10%–25%	30%–40%
Nodes	Contiguous spread	Noncontiguous spread	Noncontiguous spread
Mediastinal involvement	>50% of cases	<20% of cases	Rare except in lymphoblastic lymphoma
Bone marrow involvement	<10%	70%–90%	10%–30%
CNS involvement	Rare	Rare	10%–15%
Hepatic involvement	Uncommon	Common	May or may not be associated
Extranodal involvement	Uncommon	More common involvement of GI tract, testes, bone marrow	May or may not be associated
Systemic symptoms	Common (30%–40%)	Uncommon (15%–20%)	20%–30%

Adapted from Sunderland, M.C. & Coltman, C.A. (1993). Lymphomas. In G.R. Weiss *Clinical Oncology,* Norwalk, CT: Appleton & Lange, p 285.

and electrolyte abnormalities, all of which may reflect the extent and complications of lymphoma. Modest elevations of alkaline phosphatase can occur in patients with limited disease; higher levels are associated with hepatic, osseous, or marrow involvement. Hypercalcemia is a rare paraneoplastic manifestation.

After a positive lymph node biopsy, radiologic assessment is a very important aspect of diagnosis and staging. A screening chest x-ray may demonstrate mediastinal, hilar, and paratracheal lymphadenopathy as well as parenchymal involvement. It is usually performed early in the diagnostic workup. Computed tomography (CT) of the chest can detect smaller lymphadenopathy, parenchymal disease, and mediastinal masses and is required for patients with abnormal chest x-rays. CT scans of the abdomen and pelvis are also a component of staging; they assess nodes in the celiac, para-aortic, retroperitoneal, mesenteric, and inguinal nodal areas and visualize tumor nodules in the liver and spleen.

Bone marrow aspirate and core biopsies are required. Marrow involvement denotes stage IV disease, and the aspirated material can be used for flow cytometry, which can detect disease in just a small number of cells. Additional special stains for surface markers, immunophenotyping, and cytogenetics may be needed for difficult diagnoses.

Several additional diagnostic procedures have been used to evaluate selected cases. Intravenous pyelography may be performed in patients with renal abnormalities demonstrated on CT. However, contrast dye is contraindicated in the presence of a paraproteinemia or renal failure from hypercalcemia or hyperuricemia.

Nuclear medicine studies, such as gallium scans, can complement CT scans in determining response to treatment. Gallium, which is avidly taken up by involved tissue in HD, is useful in the assessment of treatment response. Gallium is most sensitive for lymphomas above the diaphragm. Several studies suggest that the failure to convert from a positive to a negative gallium scan after therapy indicates a high likelihood of persistent HD (DeVita, 1997). Others studies include scans of the liver, spleen, or bone. These tests provide a guide for the surgeon if a staging laparotomy is to be performed. Staging laparotomy, although occasionally used in HD, is not performed in NHL.

Lumbar punctures with cytology are indicated in cases of diffuse histiocytic lymphoma that have demonstrated marrow involvement, lymphoblastic lymphoma, and undifferentiated lymphoma. Any lymphoma patient presenting with unexplained neurologic symptoms or an alteration in mental status requires evaluation of the cerebrospinal fluid.

Lymphangiograms are used infrequently, although they are indicated in stages I and II HD, after all other noninvasive evaluations have been negative. They provide a more accurate evaluation of lower abdominal involvement, such as the lower aortic, iliac, and retroperitoneal lymph nodes. This confirms early disease that has the potential for cure with radiation treatment. However, lymphangiograms are not performed in many medical centers because they are invasive, time-consuming for the patient, and more expensive than CT (Aisenberg, 1995).

A major problem with all radiologic techniques is the inability to diagnose splenic involvement. Exploratory laparotomy is the only diagnostic tool that can assess the extent of subdiaphragmatic disease in HD. It remains the definite method for detecting occult nodal, splenic, and hepatic disease. However, it is used only for patients who plan to undergo radiotherapy

and is currently not indicated for patients who will receive only chemotherapy. The procedure involves splenectomy and sampling and removal of celiac, splenic hilar, portahepatic, and para-aortic nodes. Sampling of the liver by wedge and needle biopsy under direct vision and open iliac crest bone marrow biopsy are also involved in staging laparotomies.

TREATMENT OPTIONS, EXPECTED OUTCOMES, AND COMPREHENSIVE MANAGEMENT

Treatment

HODGKIN'S DISEASE

The initial treatment of HD is based on the extent of disease. Those with a favorable stage and prognosis are candidates for radiotherapy, which is likely to cure the disease. If the presentation is unfavorable, chemotherapy is required.

Radiation therapy is generally offered to patients with a nonbulky, supradiaphragmatic presentation with no extranodal involvement, or involvement of only one extranodal site in an otherwise asymptomatic patient. Because HD spreads in an orderly fashion, through adjacent lymph node groups, localized high-dose radiation that is directed at affected lymph nodes and contiguous uninvolved lymph node regions can produce a high rate of relapse-free survival. Megavoltage radiation therapy is administered in daily dosages of 180 to 200 cGy to a total of 3500 to 4400 cGy. Relapse-free survival results in 75% to 80% of pathologically staged patients.

Combination chemotherapy is the treatment of choice for many patients with stage IIB disease and all patients with stage III and IV disease. Stage IIIA is highly curable with a number of chemotherapy regimens. With current therapy, a 65% to 70% relapse-free survival rate can be achieved even in patients with the least favorable presentations. Because of the vesicant nature of chemotherapeutic agents used to treat HD and the frequency of treatments (every 2 weeks for 6 months), central lines are usually surgically installed.

A variety of factors determine the prognosis for patients with HD. Age is the most significant, with younger patients achieving better cure rates. Poor outcome in older patients is attributable to both a less favorable response to treatment and inadequate therapy (Table 38-5). Both of the regimens in Table 38-5 are administered every 28 days. ABVD is currently favored in most centers because of its comparable effectiveness in clinical trials and its lower incidence and severity of toxicities.

CLINICAL WARNING: Patients successfully treated for HD suffer a number of late effects, including an increased risk of leukemia and sterility after some types of chemotherapy and an increased risk of solid tumors and cardiac disease after radiotherapy. New treatments have been designed to maintain the high cure rates while reducing acute and chronic toxicities.

NON-HODGKIN'S LYMPHOMA

Since the 1970s, NHLs have been treated with combination regimens. The use of combination chemotherapy regimens containing cyclophosphamide (CHOP), doxorubicin, vincristine, and prednisone yield very high cure rates, in excess of 75%

TABLE 38-5	Chemotherapy Regimens for HD	
Regimen	**Agents**	**Adverse Effects**
ABVD	Adriamycin (doxorubicin)	Nausea, vomiting
	Bleomycin	Alopecia
	Vinblastine	Bleomycin-related lung disease
	Dacarbazine	Potentiation of radiation-related cardiopulmonary disease
MOPP	Mechlorethamine	Nausea, vomiting
	Oncovin (vincristine)	Myelosuppression
	Procarbazine	Neuropathy
	Prednisone	Sterility
		Increased risk of acute leukemia

in patients with stage I and nonbulky stage II diffuse aggressive NHL. CHOP remains one of the most frequently used regimens and is considered a first-generation protocol. Second-generation combinations include agents such as methotrexate, bleomycin, dexamethasone, leucovorin, etoposide, and cytarabine.

The most important factor affecting outcome is dose intensity (Armitage, 1995). The intensity of treatment can be increased by the use of hematopoietic growth factors to allow an increased dose or shortened treatment intervals. Patient selection for these regimens is based on favorable disease characteristics and patient tolerance. Age appears to be a limiting factor because drug toxicity escalates in patients over age 50 (Carson, 1996).

Although indolent lymphomas are highly sensitive to a wide range of chemotherapies, the duration of remissions is typically short, usually less than 24 months. These conditions are considered incurable, except in some cases when bone marrow transplantation is successful. Therefore, many providers advocate observation and initiate therapy only to provide symptomatic relief of fevers, night sweats, or weight loss or to reverse severe cytopenia. Using this policy of "watchful waiting," treatment can be avoided in 50% of patients for 1 to 3 years and in 10% for 5 years, and approximately 30% will have partial spontaneous regression. This regression may be prolonged but is usually not permanent. Some trials have shown that early treatment may result in longer remission, but long-term survival is unchanged (Carson, 1996).

Once the decision to treat indolent lymphoma is made, there are many options, although whether to palliate symptoms or attempt complete remission remains controversial. For the less than 10% of patients with stage I or II disease, field radiation therapy is the treatment of choice because they have a 50% to 80% chance of disease-free survival exceeding 10 to 20 years. For stage III and IV disease, chemotherapy with single alkylating agents such as chlorambucil or cyclophosphamide or one of several combination regimens is used. Combination regimens yield slightly higher complete remission rates than single agents, but there is no regimen that stands out as the most efficacious. Newer drugs such as purine analogues, fludarabine, and CdA have shown promising results. Other classes such as topoisomerase I inhibitors (campathotecin-11, topotecan) and the taxanes (Taxol, Taxotere) are also being studied (Cheson, 1993).

Combination chemotherapy has dramatically improved the prognosis for aggressive lymphomas, which were formerly fatal within 1 year. Although these tumors grow rapidly, they respond better to chemotherapy and therefore present a greater potential for cure than most low-grade, indolent NHLs. In diffuse aggressive NHL, complete remission can be achieved in 60% to 80% of adults and long-term disease-free survival can be expected in 30% to 50% (Roncadin et al, 1994).

Health Promotion and Specific Protection

The most important new risk factor for lymphoma is the association of AIDS with aggressive NHLs. The rate of new cases has grown 65% since the 1970s, largely because of the increased incidence of AIDS among young men (ACS, 1998). Preventing the spread of HIV disease through safe sex practices and precautions against bloodborne pathogens could prevent these lymphomas.

Rehabilitation

Patients live longer because of improved treatment strategies, although problems arise associated with survivorship. Studies of patients with HD and NHL have identified several physiologic and psychological difficulties of long-term survival. Long-term comprehensive care will help to ensure the quality as well as the quantity of life.

Fatigue, lack of energy, or tiredness is a common complaint, often accompanied by depression. It may take 12 to 18 months after treatment for energy to return. Similarly, loss of libido and problems with infertility secondary to chemotherapy may cause major physical, mental health, and lifestyle complications for survivors of HD. Impairment of memory may be a short- or long-term effect. Anxiety and the fear of relapse and further treatment are common problems but decrease the longer the patient remains disease-free. The failure of some patients to return to work or to resume normal activities years after treatment is a cause for intervention. However, those returning to work may experience job discrimination or difficulties at work, in part stemming from career interruptions while they completed their treatment. Insurance-related problems are common (Kornblith, 1992). Increased divorce rates and marital difficulties have been attributed to role changes, the stress of treatment, and anger at the well spouse. Educating the patient about potential psychosocial difficulties during treatment and recovery will decrease the impact of these difficulties and may prevent many of them.

Age and Gender Considerations

The cure rate for children with all stages of HD is approximately 85% to 90%. Younger patients are generally better able to tolerate more intensive chemotherapy. In most cases, there is little use for radiation in these patients because it appears to add toxicity without improving outcome (Engelkrug & Hummard, 1996). Because the central nervous system is the initial site of relapse in almost one third of cases of childhood NHL, central nervous system prophylaxis with intrathecal chemotherapy is warranted in most patients (Armitage, 1995).

NHL is an increasingly common problem in the elderly. The response rate in older patients is worse and median survival is shorter, probably because of poor initial response to therapy and increased treatment-related toxicity (Armitage, 1993). However, even aggressive NHL can be cured in some elderly patients with standard chemotherapeutic regimens. For elderly patients with low-grade lymphomas, treatment my be deferred until symptoms or functional compromise occurs. Treatment options that are well tolerated by elderly patients include a combination of alkylating agents (cyclophosphamide or chlorambucil) and glucocorticoids (prednisone). Patients with high blood pressure, congestive heart failure, diabetes, or osteoporosis need extremely close supervision when receiving steroids.

TEACHING AND SELF-CARE

To achieve optimal results, patients must understand their disease process, its course, and the treatment options available to them. The timing of teaching is important and is determined by the readiness to learn. The stress of receiving a diagnosis of cancer may inhibit a patient's ability to assimilate new information, and it is often necessary to repeat information several times. Materials such as pamphlets, books, or tapes may help. Many patients are currently retrieving vast amounts of information from the Internet, but they often need help deciphering it.

Patients need to be aware of the effects of both the disease and the modalities used to threat their lymphoma. The treatment regimens for aggressive lymphomas result in potentially severe side effects and toxicities. Patients need education regarding the specific toxicities of the chemotherapeutic agents in their regimen. For example, bleomycin causes pulmonary fibrosis, vincristine causes peripheral neuropathies, and doxorubicin can be cardiotoxic. Patients should be familiar with signs and symptoms to report and the diagnostic testing schedule conducted to monitor for them. Because chemotherapy attacks rapidly growing cells, temporary alopecia is associated with many regimens, particularly those containing doxorubicin and cyclophosphamide. Wigs, hats, and scarves can make this transition less traumatic.

Complications of radiotherapy include loss of taste, dry mouth, dysphagia, nausea, vomiting, diarrhea, anorexia, malaise, and bone marrow depression, depending on the amount delivered. Mucositis is a continual problem because many patients remain neutropenic throughout treatment. Nausea and vomiting can be minimized or even eliminated with proper administration of antiemetics. Instruction in proper dental hygiene is important because of the increased risk of dental caries caused by dry mouth. Late reactions may include radiation pneumonitis, transient aspermia in men, and artificial menopause in women who have not had an oophoropexy or shielding of the ovaries.

As a compromised host, the lymphoma patient is at risk for developing infections as the result of altered or deficient defense mechanisms (Dean et al, 1996). In addition to marrow replacement by tumor, chemotherapy and radiotherapy both suppress the immune system. The best predictor of infection is neutropenia, defined as an absolute neutrophil count of less than $1000/cells/mm^3$. Patients need to monitor their temperatures two or three times per day and report elevations of 100.5°F or higher. They should understand the different blood parameters that are being monitored and record their counts. Calendars with treatments, counts, temperatures, and symptoms are very useful. Hospitalization and intravenous antibiotics are indicated if the patient becomes febrile in the neutropenic state.

Proper rest and nutrition affect the immune system and should be encouraged. Immunocompromised patients should avoid persons who have recently been given live vaccines. Fungal infections are an additional threat, and neutropenic patients should avoid construction and landscaping projects, where fungal spores, such as *Aspergillus*, may be unearthed.

COMMUNITY RESOURCES

As more lymphoma management moves into outpatient venues, the community will meet the needs of patients who were once on inpatient units. Home care now assists with the administration of intravenous antibiotics. Cancer centers often have free-standing satellite clinics to provide chemotherapy and blood products in a more convenient and less costly environment.

In the past decades, organizations have been formed, ranging from professional societies to community and service organizations, with the goal of supporting cancer patients. In 1993, the American Cancer Society celebrated 80 years of service, and the Leukemia Society of America dates back to 1949 (Ades, 1996). These organizations provide information and support for professionals, patients, and families.

- The American Cancer Society, 1699 Clifton Rd., NE, Atlanta, GA 30329-4251, 1-800-ACS-2345, 404-320-3333; http://www.cancer.org: A community-based voluntary health organization that supports research, education, advocacy, and service. It offers programs to educate the public and provides programs and services to patients and families.
- Leukemia Society of America, National Headquarters, 600 Third Ave., New York, NY 10016, 1-800-955-4LSA, 212-573-8484: A volunteer organization dedicated to the cure of hematologic cancers and to improving the quality of life of patients and their families through research, patient aid, public and professional education, and community service. Their Web site, http://www.leukemia.org, provides information on leukemia, lymphoma, myeloma, and Hodgkin's disease.
- National Coalition for Cancer Survivorship (NCCS), 1010 Wayne Ave., Fifth Floor, Silver Spring, MD 20910, 301-650-8868: A network of people, organizations, and treatment centers working in the area of cancer survivorship and support to generate awareness of survivorship. As a peer support group, it facilitates communication, promotes peer support, serves as an information clearinghouse, advocates for the interests of survivors, and encourages the study of survivorship.

- National Cancer Institute/Cancer Information Service, Public Inquiry Section, Office of Cancer Communications, Building 31, Room 10A24, Bethesda, MD 20892, 1-800-4-CANCER: Government agency-sponsored nationwide telephone service for cancer patients and their families, as well as health care professionals. CIS specialists are trained to provide current and understandable information about all types of cancer.
- Lymphoma Research Foundation of America, Inc., 8800 Venice Boulevard, Suite 207, Los Angeles, CA 90034, 310-204-7040, 310-204-7043; http://www.lympho ma.org: Links to similar sites and resources, support groups, lymphoma overview, LRFA resources
- National Association of Hospital Hospitality Houses, Inc., 1-800-542-9730: An association of more than 100 nonprofit organizations throughout the United States that provides lodging and support services to persons receiving medical treatment away from home.

REFERRAL POINTS AND CLINICAL WARNINGS

Patients with progressive lymphoma are at risk for a number of oncologic emergencies, including problems that are obstructive, metabolic, infiltrative, and infective. Patients with lymphomas on the right side of the superior mediastinum are at risk for superior vena cava syndrome, in which the mass obstructs the blood return to the heart. This produces a characteristic syndrome of edema of the upper body and requires emergent treatment with radiation and chemotherapy. Bowel obstructions, particularly large bowel obstructions in the case of lymphomas, are a potential emergency, as is third space syndrome. The latter is caused by the shift in fluid from the vascular to the interstitial space secondary to lowered plasma proteins, increased capillary permeability, or lymphatic blockage from disease (Miaskowski, 1996). Patients with gastric lymphomas, particularly those with bulky disease, have a high incidence of perforation.

Metabolic emergencies include syndrome of inappropriate antidiuretic hormone, hypercalcemia, septic shock, and disseminated intravascular coagulation (DIC). These are often life-threatening and require immediate intensive care admission. Syndrome of inappropriate antidiuretic hormone presents with signs and symptoms of water intoxication. Tumor lysis syndrome, as a result of the rapid breakdown of cells from aggressive chemotherapy, contributes to metabolic derangements and can produce life-threatening elevations of uric acid. Hypercalcemia can present with neuromuscular symptoms, gastrointestinal dysfunction, or cardiovascular effects. Septic shock, produced by the release of endotoxin and subsequent dilation of arteries and veins, results in a series of signs and symptoms, including mental confusion, chills, fever, flushed and warm skin, tachycardia, tachypnea, and decreased Po_2. Untreated, this progresses to cold shock, in which the patient has cold skin, peripheral edema, tachycardia, hypotension, tachypnea, pulmonary congestion, hypoxemia, oliguria, and metabolic acidosis.

DIC results from an alteration in the normal clotting mechanisms that manifests as diffuse clotting occurring simultaneously with hemorrhage. In cancer patients, DIC has been seen with intravascular hemolysis from transfusion reaction, overwhelming viral or bacterial sepsis and shock, particularly from gram-negative sepsis, and release of thrombin from malignant cells (Carson, 1996).

Infiltrative emergencies include cardiac tamponade and spinal cord compression. Spinal cord compression is commonly seen in progressive lymphoma. It develops rapidly, with signs and symptoms of weakness of the lower extremities, increased deep tendon reflexes, a positive Babinski's sign, and development of sensory loss. Early diagnosis and intervention are crucial in preventing neurologic impairment and paralysis. Complaints of leg weakness or bowel or bladder dysfunction, especially in patients with back pain, require immediate diagnostic and therapeutic intervention. Patients with central nervous system involvement are at risk for increased intracranial pressure, which also requires immediate intervention to circumvent associated sequelae.

Bone marrow depression—from the disease itself or from the therapies used to treat it—can produce life-threatening cytopenias. Transfusion support is often required. Febrile neutropenia requires hospitalization with intravenous antibiotics because sepsis may ensue.

Because of the high tumor load characteristic of many lymphomas, these complications have the potential to occur with increased frequency. Early recognition and intervention can diminish associated morbidity and mortality rates.

References

A.C.S. (1988). Cancer 1998 statistics. In CH, *A Cancer Journal for Clinicians, 48*(16), 10–29.

Ades, T. (1996). Cancer organizations. In R. McCorkle, M. Grant, M. Frank-Stromberg, & S.B. Band. (Eds.). *Cancer nursing*, 2d ed. Philadelphia: W.B. Saunders, pp. 1425–1429.

Aisenberg, A.C. (1995). Hodgkin's disease. In R.I. Handen, T.P. Stossell, & S.E. Lux (Eds.). *Principles and practice of hematology*. Philadelphia: J.B. Lippincott, pp. 813–850.

Armitage, J.O. (1995). Non-Hodgkin's lymphoma. In R.I. Handen, T.P. Stossell, & S.E. Lux (Eds.). *Principles and practice of hematology*. Philadelphia: J.B. Lippincott, pp. 851–884.

Armitage, J.O. (1993). Treatment of non-Hodgkin's lymphoma. *N Engl J Med, 328*, 1023–1030.

Carson, C. (1996). Hodgkin's disease and non-Hodgkin's lymphomas. In R. McCorkle, M. Grant, M. Frank-Stromberg, & S.B. Band (Eds.). *Cancer nursing*, 2d ed. Philadelphia: W.B. Saunders, pp. 729–751.

Cheson, B.D. (1993). New chemotherapeutic agents for the treatment of low-grade non-Hodgkin's lymphomas. *Seminars in Oncology, 20*(Suppl. 5), 96–110.

David, J. (1994). Organs and cells of the immune system. In D.C. Dale & Federman, D.D. *Scientific American Medicine*, Vol. 2. New York: Scientific American, pp. 1–17.

Dean, G.E., Haeuber, D., & Rivera, L.M. (1996). Infection. In R. McCorkle, M. Grant, M. Frank-Stromberg, & S.B. Band. (Eds). *Cancer nursing*, 2d ed. Philadelphia: W.B. Saunders, pp. 963–977.

DeVita, V.T., Hellman, S. & Jaffe, E. (1993). Hodgkin's disease. In V.T. DeVita, S. Hellman & S.A. Rosenberg (Eds.). *Cancer Principles and Practice of Oncology*, 4th ed. Philadelphia: J.B. Lippincott, p. 821.

DeVita, V.T., Mauch, P.M., & Harris, N.L. (1997). Hodgkin's disease. In V.T. DeVita, S. Hellman & S.A. Rosenberg (Eds.). *Cancer Principles and Practice of Oncology*, 5th ed. Philadelphia: J.B. Lippincott-Raven, pp. 2242–2283.

Durkup, H., Latza, V. Hummel et al. (1992). Molecular cloning and expression of a new member of the nerve growth factor receptor family that is characteristic for Hodgkin's disease. *Cell, 68*, 422.

Engelking, C., & Hummard, S.M. (1996). Current issues and controversies in the management of non-Hodgkin's lymphoma. Educational monograph. New York: Triclinica Communications.

Fisher, R.I. (1994). Treatment of aggressive non-Hodgkin's lymphomas. Lessons from the past 10 years. *Cancer, 74,* 2657–2661.

Hoffman, R., & Williams, D.A. (1994). Molecular and cellular biology of hematopoiesis. In J.H. Stein (Ed.). *Internal Medicine,* 4th ed. St. Louis: Mosby, pp. 684–690.

Klitz, W., Aldrich, C.L., Eildes, V et al. (1994). Localization of predisposition to HD in the HLA class II region. *American Journal of Human Genetics, 54,* 497.

Kornblith, A.B., Anderson, J., & Celia D.F. (1992). Hodgkin's disease survivors at increased risk for problems with psychosocial adaptation. *Cancer, 70,* 2214.

Lowry, P.A. (1996). Nonmalignant white cell disorders. In J. Noble (Ed.). *Textbook of primary care medicine,* 2d ed. St. Louis: Mosby, pp. 734–736

Miaskowski, C. (1996). Oncologic emergencies. In McCorkle, Frant, Farnk-Stromberg, & Band. *Cancer Nursing,* 2nd ed. Philadelphia: W.B. Saunders, 1183–1192.

Paradiso, C. (1995). *Pathophysiology.* Philadelphia: J.B. Lippincott, pp. 383–413.

Post-White, J. (1996). Principles of immunity. In R. McCorkle, M. Grant, M. Frank-Stromberg, & S.B. Band. (Eds.). *Cancer nursing,* 2d ed. Philadelphia: W.B. Saunders, pp. 171–189.

Rabkin, C., Devesa, S.S., Zahm, S.H., & Gail, M.H. (1993). Increasing incidence of non-Hodgkin's lymphoma. *Seminars in Hematology, 30,* 286.

Roncadin, M., et al. (1994). Total body irradiation and predmustine in chronic lymphocytic leukemia and low-grade non-Hodgkin's lymphomas. *Cancer, 74,* 978–984.

Schrier, S.L. (1994). Hematopoiesis and red blood cell function. In D.C. Dale & D.D. Federman. *Scientific American Medicine,* Vol. 2. New York: Scientific American, pp. 5–11.

Shipp, M.A., Mauch, P.A., & Harris, N.L. (1997). Non-Hodgkin's lymphomas. In V.T. Devita, S. Hellman, & S.A. Rosenberg (Eds.). *Cancer: Principles and practice of oncology,* 5th ed. Philadelphia: Lippincott-Raven, pp. 2165–2220.

Shipp, M.A. (1994). Prognostic factors in aggressive non-Hodgkin's lymphoma: Who has "high-risk" disease? *Blood, 83,* 1165.

Weinstein, H.J., & Tarbell, N.J. (1997). Leukemias and lymphomas of childhood. In V.T. Devita, S. Hellman, & S.A. Rosenberg (Eds.). *Cancer: Principles and practice of oncology,* 5th ed. Philadelphia: Lippincott-Raven, pp. 2145–2165.

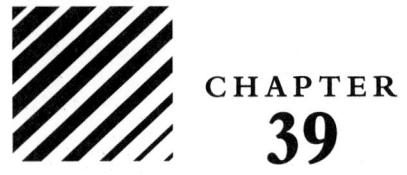

CHAPTER
39

Myeloproliferative Diseases

Elaine B. Owen, R.N.C.S., M.S.N., A.O.C.N.

Myeloproliferative disorders are characterized by a malfunction of the bone marrow. Both preleukemic dysfunction and acute leukemia can present with symptoms found in a primary care setting. The increased incidence, because of an aging population, and the chronic nature of these diseases mean that many more primary care providers are likely to have patients in their practices with bone marrow disorders.

Chronic leukemia and acute leukemia are malignant disorders, whereas nonmalignant disorders, characterized by various cytopenias and dysplastic cell features, include diseases such as myelodysplastic syndrome and myelofibrosis. Some consider myelodysplastic syndrome a malignant condition because long-term survival data are sparse. All of these disorders involve the hematopoietic system and lead to disruption of normal hematopoiesis. They can be characterized by autonomous proliferation of poorly differentiated cells or, in the case of the chronic leukemias, by uncontrolled expansion of mature cells. The more common problems associated with these diseases will be discussed.

ANATOMY, PHYSIOLOGY, AND PATHOLOGY

Anatomy and Physiology

Hematopoiesis is the process of making blood cells. All the cellular components of blood come from a single cell line progenitor called stem cells. Stem cells reside in the bone marrow, but they also circulate in peripheral blood. They can be harvested from the peripheral blood, obviating the need to extract bone marrow for use in transplant situations. The potential for plurality of these stem cells has led them to be labeled pluripotent progenitor cells.

Stem cells have the ability to self-replicate or differentiate into one of several cell-specific progenitors. Self-replication ensures replenishment of the cell line. Differentiation of stem cells commits cells to a path of distinct function. A pluripotent stem cell can be committed to become, for instance, either a leukocyte or an erythrocyte. Thus, hematopoiesis is the process of proliferation and differentiation of these self-renewing, pluripotent progenitor cells.

Figure 39-1 illustrates the hematopoietic cascade (Shoemaker, 1993). When a stem cell divides, the daughter cells may in turn self-replicate or further differentiate. This succession of stem cells (progenitors) and their daughter cells is called a lineage.

Not all the factors that cause a stem cell to differentiate are known. It is known that as each tributary of the pathway branches or differentiates, there is an increasingly restrictive capacity to renew itself. The first major branching of the pathway divides into myeloid and lymphoid precursor cells. The myeloid cells are called colony-forming unit/granulocyte-erythrocyte-monocyte-megakaryocyte (CFU-GEMM); the lymphoid precursors are called simply lymphoid. The committed cells cannot be distinguished at this stage of hematopoiesis. Subsequent divisions and differentiations are necessary for these precursor cells to be recognizable.

The first recognizable cells in the CFU-GEMM line are myeloblasts (precursors of granulocytes and monocytes) and erythroblasts (precursors of red blood cells). Normally immature blast cells are not present in peripheral blood. A relatively small number of these immature cells are contained in the bone marrow and constitute less than 5% of the bone marrow space.

The cycle of blood cell reproduction, growth, maintenance, and destruction is a highly efficient and orderly process, tightly controlled by growth factors and suppressors. Abnormal proliferation and defective cell production of any cell line disrupt the delicate blood cell balance necessary to sustain the body's good state of health.

Pathology

The adult leukemias constitute about 10% of all cancers. They are a heterogeneous group of diseases, with myeloid and lymphoid subclasses, and are broadly divided into acute and chronic disorders. The acute leukemias are characterized by autonomous proliferation of undifferentiated cells, whereas the chronic leukemias are distinguished by uncontrolled expansion of mature cells. Cellular proliferation genes and tumor suppressor genes are responsible for regulation of cellular growth. There are genes that also regulate apoptosis or programmed cell death. Bone marrow dysfunction may result from aberrant regulation of this homeostasis.

CHRONIC LEUKEMIA AND RELATED DISORDERS

Two types of chronic conditions affect the myeloid cell lineage, which consists of granulocytes, red cells, and platelets. Myeloproliferative disorders, the first type, are characterized by an efficient abnormal proliferation, resulting in an overproduction of mature cells. They include chronic myelocytic leukemia, polycythemia vera, essential thrombocythemia, and chronic myelofibrosis. Myelodysplastic syndromes (MDS), the second type, involve inefficient abnormal proliferation, resulting in an underproduction of mature, normal blood cells. MDS patients have a cellular marrow but low blood counts.

Myelofibrosis

Myelofibrosis, or fibrosis of the bone marrow, can be seen with malignant conditions such as the leukemias, lymphomas, and solid tumors, as well as nonmalignant conditions such as Paget's disease, osteoporosis, lupus erythematosus, and chemical expo-

HEMATOPOIESIS

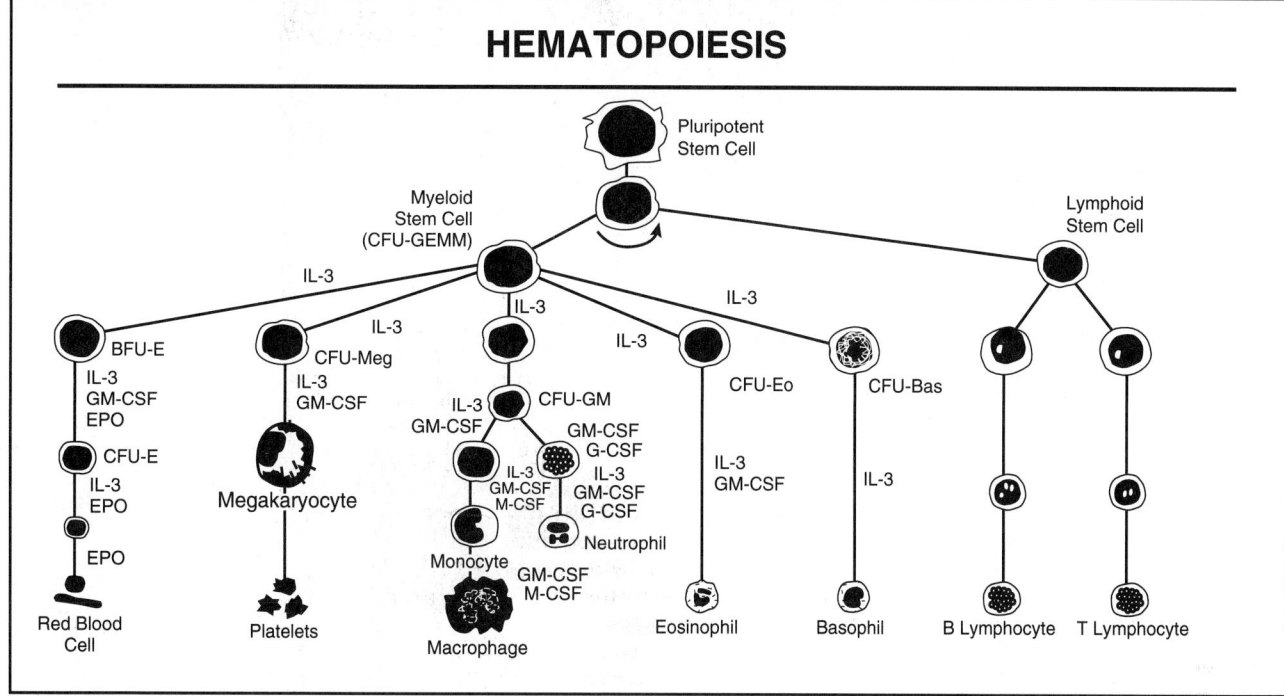

FIGURE 39-1 Hematopoietic Cascade. CFU-GEMM = colony-forming unit, granulocyte-erythrocyte-monocyte-megacaryocyte; IL-3 = interleukin-3; BFU-E = burst-forming unity, erythroid; CFU-Meg = CFU, megacaryocyte; CFU-GM = CFU, granulocyte-macrophage; CFU-Ec = CFU, eosinophil; CFU-Bas = CFU, basophil; GM-CSF = granulocyte-macrophage colony-stimulating factor; EPO = erythroprotein; M-CSF = macrophage CEF; G-CSF = granulocyte CSF. (Shoemaker, 1993) (McCall, R.E. & Tankersley, C.M. (1998). *Phlebotomy essentials, 2/e.* Philadelphia: Lippincott-Raven Publishers)

sures. Agnogenic myeloid metaplasia is another term used to describe myelofibrosis. Myelofibrosis is considered a neoplastic disorder because of chromosomal and genetic abnormalities, the presence of certain enzyme and cell defects, and its chronic progressive nature.

In most presentations of myelofibrosis, an underlying disease state is the causative agent. Myelofibrosis also may occur de novo, in which extramedullary hematopoiesis is a prominent feature (Athens, 1993). Extramedullary hematopoiesis, or blood formation outside the marrow space, most commonly occurs in the spleen, although the liver, lymph nodes, skin, thymus, or other organs can be affected.

Chronic Myelogenous Leukemia

Chronic myelogenous leukemia (CML) is characterized by a proliferation of granulocytes, especially neutrophils, and the hallmark Philadelphia chromosome. This chromosome is the G group chromosome 22 missing a portion of the long arm, which has been translocated to the long arm of chromosome 9. The translocation activates a gene that produces a protein. This protein stimulates growth factor receptors, inducing uncontrolled growth of the cell line (Ellerhorst-Ryan, 1997). CML has three distinct phases: the chronic phase with minimal physical symptoms, an accelerated phase with erratic cytopenias, and a phase marked by excessive myeloblasts, known as a blast crisis.

Chronic Lymphocytic Leukemia

The chronic leukemia that affects the lymphoid cell line is known as chronic lymphocytic leukemia (CLL). It is characterized by the accumulation of mature-appearing lymphocytes in

the peripheral blood associated with infiltration of the bone marrow, spleen, and lymph nodes. It is important to distinguish early CLL from reactive lymphocytosis in asymptomatic patients. In reactive lymphocytosis, the cells are polyclonal and predominantly T lymphocytes, whereas in CLL they are usually B cells.

ACUTE LEUKEMIA

The acute leukemias are also a heterogeneous group of disorders. Acute myelogenous leukemia, also known as acute nonlymphocytic leukemia, arises from the myeloid stem cell. The term "acute myelogenous leukemia" is often used nonspecifically to encompass all the subgroups. In contrast, acute lymphocytic leukemia (ALL) arises from the lymphoid stem cells.

Leukemic subtypes are defined by the hematopoietic stage that was interrupted by the disease. Leukemia is not "hyperproliferative" because the mitotic rate of leukemic cells is not greater than normal white blood cells. Rather, leukemia results from an overabundance of nonfunctional white blood cells, which proliferate until there are so few normal white blood cells that the patient is overcome, often by infection, and dies.

CYTOGENETICS

Cytogenetic abnormalities, or the rearrangement, translocation, and deletion of chromosomes, take many forms. A cytogenetic evaluation at the time of diagnosis of a myeloproliferative disease enables the evaluator to classify the tissue submitted for review and enables the provider to form a prognosis. For example, in MDS, the 5q minus (chromosome 5 missing part of its longer arm) is associated with a disease course longer than 5 years. Alternatively, if chromosome 7 is missing in MDS, the prognosis is worse, and patients tend to develop leukemia within the year (Sensenbrenner, 1995). Unfortunately, except for the presence of the Philadelphia chromosome in CML, it is difficult to judge whether a particular genetic event is associated with malignant transformation. This is because of the heterogeneous nature of chromosomal abnormalities and the apparent lack of such features in many of the people diagnosed with these disorders (Brock, 1993).

EPIDEMIOLOGY

There were approximately 27,600 new cases of leukemia diagnosed in 1996, about equally divided between acute and chronic leukemia (American Cancer Society, 1996). Each year in the United States there are approximately 3000 new cases of MDS diagnosed (Castro-Malaspina, 1995). The incidence for these disorders combined is 9 of every 100,000 people. Leukemia is the sixth most common type of cancer in both men and women. In children, however, leukemia is the leading cause of death from disease (Sandler, 1992). Although leukemia is often thought of as a childhood cancer, it is much more common in adults: 10 times more adults than children are affected by leukemia. This seems to be an age-related phenomenon, and the incidence rises sharply for every decade after age 40 (American Cancer Society, 1996).

A few risk factors have been clearly identified in the development of myeloproliferative diseases, including chemical toxins (industrial, environmental, and iatrogenic), radiation, viruses, and congenital disorders. Table 39-1 outlines known leukemogenic pathogens.

Socioeconomic Factors

Socioeconomic factors play a role in the risk of developing leukemia: a higher standard of living has a greater association with the disease. Industrialized countries have higher rates of leuke-

TABLE 39-1	Pathogenesis of Myeloproliferative Disorders

I. Toxins
  A. Radiation
    1. Ionizing
    2. Medical
  B. Chemical
    1. Occupational (benzene, solvents)
    2. Medical (alkylating agents, phenylbutazone)
II. Congenital disorders
  A. Down syndrome
  B. Fanconi's syndrome
  C. Klinefelter's syndrome
  D. Turner's syndrome
  E. Bloom syndrome
  F. Wiskott-Aldrich syndrome
III. Acquired disorders
  A. Malignancies
  B. Myeloproliferative
    1. Polycythemia vera
    2. Primary thrombocytosis
    3. Agnogenic myeloid metaplasia
  C. Myelodysplastic syndromes
  D. Paroxysmal nocturnal hemoglobinuria (PNH)

(Williams, W., Beutler, E., Ersler, AJ, et al (eds.) (1990). *Hematology.* Edina, MN: McGraw-Hill)

mia than nonindustrialized countries, and international studies concur that ALL occurs more frequently among more affluent persons in urban areas. However, the lack of controlled data collection or epidemiologic trials looking specifically at individual socioeconomics may play a role in these conclusions.

Cultural Factors

Leukemia is a disease with worldwide incidence, but some national groups are at higher risk than others. Persons in India, Japan, and China do not experience the rapid increase in incidence with age that we do in North America. Asians who have emigrated to the United States may have higher rates, however, depending on their degree of cultural assimilation. The Japanese and Chinese populations of San Francisco continue to have a low incidence of lymphoid leukemia, but the rate of myeloid leukemia approaches that of persons of Northern European origin. Otherwise, race is not a predisposing factor in the United States.

DIAGNOSTIC CRITERIA

Historically, disorders of the hematopoietic system were classified morphologically, which often led to a lack of clarity in the classification of a disorder. More recent studies such as Southern blot techniques and molecular abnormalities identified through polymerase chain reaction, cytogenetics, and fluorescence studies for bone marrow or peripheral blood samples are more precise. Differentiation and maturation are a continuum, and cells may not always fit neatly into scientific conceptions.

Sullivan (1993) has organized a classification scheme that outlines neoplastic diseases of the hematopoietic system according to blood cell differentiation and the location in the pathway where the malfunction probably occurred. Classifying bone marrow disorders has been likened to a Chinese puzzle:

A piece that will not fit always seems to be left over. For example, the distinction between lymphoid leukemia and lymphoma cannot be justified on the basis of lineage alone. Although patients with lymphoma typically present with the bulk of their disease confined to the lymphoid organs, the disease often progresses to a leukemic phase. Also, the cells of the lymphoid system, with few exceptions, do not undergo the dramatic shape change and organelle failure characteristic of the myeloid derivatives. Thus, this scheme retains the standard morphologic divisions, but has incorporated evidence obtained from biochemical, immunohistochemical and cytogenetic methods. We must acknowledge, however, that any classification is tentative and reflects the perceptions, comprehension and prejudice of its user. (Sullivan, 1993)

HISTORY AND PHYSICAL EXAM

The symptoms and disease course for the myeloproliferative disorders vary with subtype and are closely related to two main factors: the severity of cytopenia and the number of myeloblasts. In general, the signs and symptoms of acute leukemia are present for a few days to a few weeks (Table 39-2).

Symptoms are mild and nonspecific early in the course of all the myeloproliferative disorders. Complaints include malaise, fatigue, decreased exercise tolerance, weight loss, low-grade fever, night sweats, early satiety, left upper quadrant discomfort

TABLE 39-2	Clinical Features of Acute Leukemia Related to Pathophysiology		
Symptoms	**Signs**	**Laboratory Abnormalities**	**Cause**
Fatigue, weakness	Pallor, lethargy, weakness	Anemia, hypocalcemia, hypercalcemia, hypomagnesemia	Marrow failure, release of cellular ions and metabolite
Weight loss	Weight loss		Reduced food intake, anemia, hepatosplenomegaly, increased catabolism
Bleeding in skin, mucous membranes, gums, gastrointestinal and genitourinary tracts	Purpura, gum oozing or hypertrophy, hematuria, melena	Thrombocytopenia; hypofibrinogenemia; reduced factors V, VIII; increased fibrin split products	Marrow failure, disseminated intravascular coagulation
Infection of skin, throat, gums, respiratory or urinary tracts	Fever, chills, tissue infiltrates, pyoderma gangrenosum	Granulocytopenia, x-ray evidence of pneumonia, sinusitis, etc., positive cultures	Marrow failure, granulocytopenia, immunodeficiency
Headache, nausea, vomiting, blurred vision, cranial nerve dysfunction	Papilledema, cranial nerve palsy, meningeal irritation	Spinal fluid pleocytosis, reduced CSF sugar, increased CSF protein	Meningeal, CNS, or nerve infiltration or compression
Bone pain and tenderness	Increased bone tenderness	Periosteal elevation, bone destruction by x-ray, abnormal bone marrow pressure, fibrosis	Local leukemic infiltration
Abdominal fullness, anorexia	Hepatosplenomegaly, abdominal tenderness	Hyperfibrinogenemia; elevated SGOT, SGPT; alkaline phosphatase	Infiltration of abdominal viscera, effusion
Enlarged lymph nodes or tumor masses	Enlarged lymph nodes, masses in node areas, skin, breast, testes	Abnormal biopsy, liver, spleen, and bone scans	Local tumor growth or infiltration
Oliguria	Oliguria	Concentrated urine, elevated BUN, elevated uric acid	Dehydration, uric acid nephropathy, disseminated intravascular coagulation
Obstipation	Abdominal fullness, tenderness	Abnormal scans or x-ray contrast studies	Local infiltration, obstruction, calcium/magnesium imbalance

(Holleb, A. Fink, D., Murphy, G. (eds). *American Cancer Society Textbook of Clinical Oncology.* Atlanta: The American Cancer Society)

or fullness, bone pain, and easy bruising. In more advanced stages, symptoms may include weakness, shortness of breath, bleeding, edema, headache, nausea, or vomiting.

Physical findings in patients with myeloproliferative disorders often include fever, pallor, ecchymoses, purpura, and petechiae. Sinusitis, pneumonia, perirectal cellulitis, and skin abscesses are common localized infections. Gingival hyperplasia,

skin infiltrates, lymphadenopathy, splenomegaly, and pleural effusions may also be present.

Acute leukemia is a lethal disease with an untreated median survival of 2 months. In contrast, the chronic leukemias are often discovered incidentally. This is especially true of CLL, where more than 25% of patients are diagnosed as a result of office visits for other complaints, such as gastritis. Table 39-3

TABLE 39-3	Rai Staging of CLL	
Stage	**Findings**	**Survival***
0	Lymphocytosis alone**	>150
I	Lymphocytosis and adenopathy	101
II	Lymphocytosis with splenomegaly and/or hepatomegaly	71
III	Lymphocytosis with anemia (Hb <11 g/dL)**	19
IV	Lymphocytosis with thrombocytopenia (plt <100,000/mm)***	19

* Median survival from diagnosis in months

** Peripheral blood >15,000/mm^3, bone marrow >40%

*** May occur on a hypoproliferative or immune basis
(Holleb, A. Fink, D., Murphy, G. (eds). *American Cancer Society Textbook of Clinical Oncology.* Atlanta: The American Cancer Society)

outlines the physical findings and survival rates for CLL according to Rai (1990).

Many patients die from the complications associated with this problem or the measures taken to treat it. For instance, patients who are transfusion-dependent may develop hemochromatosis from the accumulation of excess iron contained in transfused red cells.

DIAGNOSTIC STUDIES

A bone marrow biopsy and aspirate are required to make the diagnosis of any myeloproliferative disorder, with the exception of CLL, which can be diagnosed by a peripheral blood smear. Biopsy, however, is required to stage the extent of bone marrow involvement. Smears of the bone marrow aspirate are stained to define subtypes of myeloproliferative disorders. When leukemias are suspected, the aspirate is heparinized and sent for cytogenetic analysis, fluorescence-activated cell sorting, and polymerase chain reaction.

Because stem cells and mature white cells can infiltrate any body tissue, a host of symptoms can result. A chemistry panel, coagulation studies, HLA typing, urinalysis, and chest x-ray make up an initial evaluation for suspected disease. If neurologic symptoms are present, an examination of the cerebrospinal fluid may be included.

TREATMENT OPTIONS, EXPECTED OUTCOMES, AND COMPREHENSIVE MANAGEMENT

Rehabilitation

Rehabilitation, or a return to a preillness state of health, is often impossible with myeloproliferative disorders because of the disease itself or the long-lasting side effects of the treatment. This can have a devastating effect, impairing functional status, decreasing independence, and affecting overall quality of life (Ferrel et al, 1996).

Fatigue has been identified as the most common side effect of cancer treatment (Nail & Jones, 1995). A natural response to feeling fatigued or depressed is to decrease physical activity. Further, when patients complain of being fatigued, health care providers often recommend additional rest and decreased activity. Over time, this leads to reduced functional capacity and a decreased ability to tolerate exercise and normal activity.

During stable periods, an optimal level of functioning can be expected. Exercise is one of the few tested interventions that has reliably decreased fatigue in patients receiving treatment for cancer (Mock et al, 1997). A moderate, self-paced walking program for women undergoing radiation therapy demonstrated good physical and psychosocial benefits.

Treatment Options and Expected Outcomes

Treatment options for people with myeloproliferative disease are based on the particular diagnosis. High-dose chemotherapy with or without peripheral stem cell or bone marrow transplantation (BMT) may be indicated in a number of cases. The goal of therapy for these regimens is to cure the disease.

BMT has evolved over the last 30 years from an experimental procedure to a relatively common treatment for many carefully selected patients. There are three types of BMT: syngeneic transplant, when the donor is an identical twin and therefore a perfect HLA match; allogeneic transplantation by a phenotypically identical donor, either a family member or a stranger who is HLA-compatible; and autologous transplant, when a patient's own marrow is removed and then replaced after chemotherapy is administered. This last type is used if ablative chemotherapy is needed but no HLA match is found, or an allogeneic transplant is unnecessary. With any of the transplant procedures, radiation therapy may or may not be used.

Complications of BMT depend on the type of procedure. Allogeneic transplants require the most supportive care as a consequence of the chemotherapy treatment regimens and the possibility of graft-versus-host disease (Whedon & Wujcik, 1997).

Because technology has improved, it is not always necessary to harvest blood precursors from bone marrow. Currently, peripheral blood progenitor cells can be used to reconstitute bone marrow after ablative therapy. Rapid reconstitution of hematopoiesis has made peripheral blood progenitor cell transplants a valuable clinical tool (Chao et al, 1993).

Many patients diagnosed with myeloproliferative disorders are not candidates for ablative therapy or allogeneic BMT. For these persons, low- to moderate-dose chemotherapy or other drug therapies may be used.

Supportive Care

For many people with myeloproliferative disorders, transplantation is not indicated. Transfusion to control cytopenia may be indicated for those not in blast crisis, those who have early-stage disease, or those in the midst of a long chronic phase. The frequency of red blood cell or platelet transfusions is highly individual. A hematologist or oncologist will transfuse a patient because of the degree of symptoms, anemia, or thrombocytopenia. The current guideline is that a patient with a hemoglobin level less than 8 to 9 g/dL should be transfused with packed red cells. Patients with a platelet count less than 10,000 to 20,000 mm^3/dL are often transfused, although controversy exists if transfusion should be ordered prophylactically in the absence of bleeding (Stehling et al, 1994; Walker et al, 1993). All transplant patients should receive irradiated blood products, and all hematology/oncology patients should receive leukocyte-filtered products.

Hematopoietic growth factors may be used to minimize or eliminate the need for transfusions. In patients with MDS, growth factors have been used with varying degrees of success. Interleukin, erythropoietin, granulocyte-colony-stimulating factor, granulocyte-macrophage-stimulating factor, and thrombopoietin have all been used to increase the production of red blood cells, white blood cells, and platelets. These hormones stimulate the marrow to produce blood cells (Gobel, 1997; Castro-Malaspina, 1995).

Nontraditional therapies have been tried to decrease the severity of acquired bone marrow disorders. Vitamin therapy aimed at correcting deficiencies that can worsen pancytopenia is useful in some people. Hormone manipulation through the use of steroids, androgens, danazol, and other preparations has also helped small numbers of patients.

Immunosuppression therapy with agents such as antithymocytic globulin and cyclosporine has had limited success. Low-dose chemotherapy with agents such as cytosine arabinoside (Ara-C) and azacytidine has been used in an attempt to induce differentiation or to suppress the abnormal clone in the hope that the bone marrow repopulates with normal clones.

Infectious Complications

Patients with chronic illness are at very high risk for developing infections. The relation among malignancy, immunocompromised status, and infection is well known.

CLINICAL WARNING: Neutropenia signals the need for prompt identification and treatment of possible infection.

Opportunistic infections are common. The primary care provider must be familiar with the infectious agents most common among patients with immunocompromise and the medications used to treat them.

Comprehensive Management Recommendations

The many issues that need to be addressed in patients with myeloproliferative disorders are not unlike those of other chronic and catastrophic illnesses. Specialists are apt to focus on the apparent issues of disease management and assume that other important issues are being addressed elsewhere. It is vital to the patient's well-being that primary care providers not only manage physical symptomatology but also address nutritional, psychosocial, spiritual, and end-of-life concerns.

TEACHING AND SELF-CARE

A hematologic problem is not as easy to understand as the concept of a solid tumor. Describing the basic physiology of the bone marrow, beginning with "marrow is a place in the center of the bones where blood is formed" is a good start (Wujcik, 1997). Figure 39-2 is a teaching sheet that can be used as an aid in the early management of serious problems.

Patients with acute leukemia and other bone marrow disorders are concerned with infection and bleeding. Self-care is aimed at prevention through good nutrition, good hygiene, and protective measures. Patients should be taught that even though the white blood cell count is often high, the cells may be immature or dysfunctional and unable to fight infection. Patients and close contacts should be taught the following infection precautions:

- Wash hands frequently with antibacterial soap.
- Use meticulous hygiene.
- Brush teeth frequently with a soft toothbrush (or sponge swab if gums are bleeding), rinse with mild mouthwash, and receive dental care as needed.
- Keep the home environment clean.

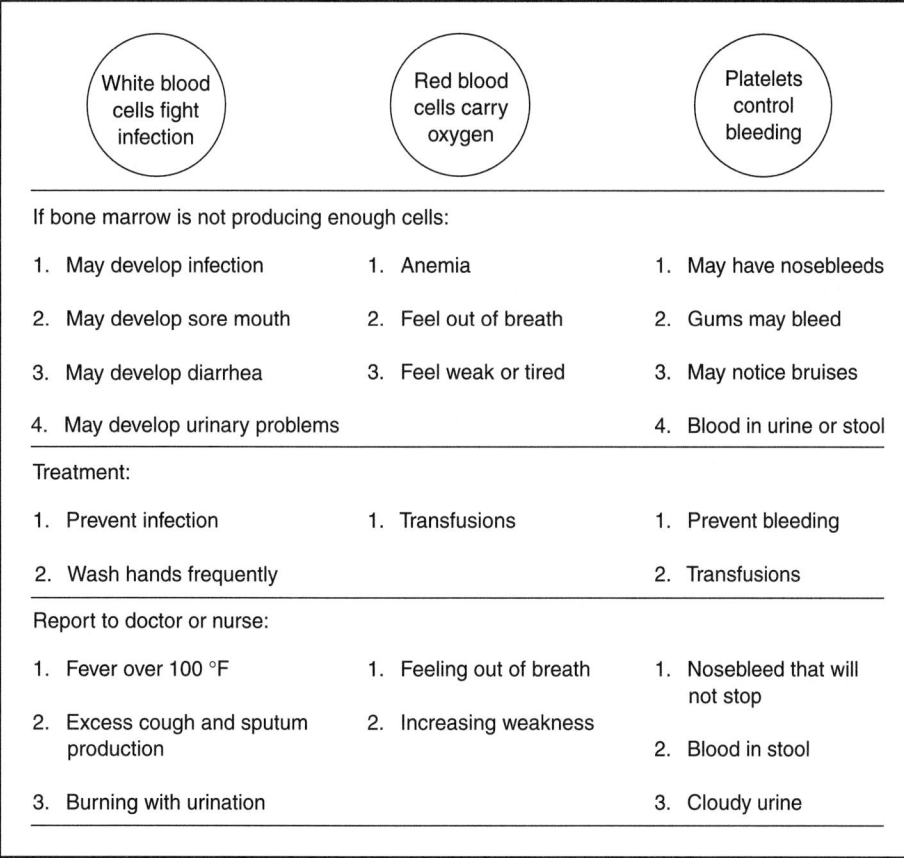

FIGURE 39-2 Teaching sheet. (Groenwald, S., Frogge, M. Goodmen, S. et al (eds). (1997). *Cancer Nursing Principles and Practice, 4/e.* Audbury, MA: Jones & Bartlett)

- Avoid contact with crowds and persons with colds and flu.
- Avoid stagnant water, improperly prepared foods, or spoiled foods.
- Clean the perianal area after each bowel movement.

Patients should also be taught to recognize signs and symptoms of infection and to notify a provider immediately if they occur. These may include fever; malaise; chills; anorexia; red, warm, tender, and inflamed patches of skin; sore throat; inflamed perianal area; mouth lesions; shortness of breath and cough; restlessness; irritability; confusion; or headache.

Small, frequent feedings and nutritional supplements are necessary to help prevent emaciation. The skin should be protected to prevent breakdown, which may act as a portal of infection. Patients should also be reminded to return for periodic blood counts.

The primary care provider should also discuss the risk of bleeding. Platelet counts may be elevated or decreased, but clotting function may be abnormal. The patient should watch for signs of abnormal bleeding such as petechiae formation, excessive bruising, conjunctival hemorrhage, severe nose bleeds, gum bleeding, vaginal spotting or unusually heavy menses, and oozing from skin puncture sites. In addition, the patient and caretakers should be taught the symptoms of internal bleeding, such as headache with change in responsiveness, possible blurred vision, hemoptysis, hematemesis, melena, change in level of consciousness, dizziness, and tachycardia.

The patient must be cautioned to prevent injury by using only a soft or sponge toothbrush, using an electric razor, preventing constipation, avoiding the use of knives or sharp objects, not taking products that contain aspirin or nonsteroidal anti-inflammatory agents, and restricting activity when the platelet count is low. Minor bleeding should be controlled by applying direct pressure followed by ice.

Patients with polycythemia are at risk for bleeding as well as thrombosis and heart failure. They should be encouraged to ambulate regularly and avoid long periods of bed rest. They should be alert for signs of thromboembolism, such as painful extremity, swelling, redness, painful joint, chest pain, and shortness of breath. Signs of heart failure should be taught, including exertional fatigue and dyspnea, dry cough, orthopnea, and restlessness.

COMMUNITY RESOURCES

- American Cancer Society, 1599 Clifton Rd., NE, Atlanta, GA 30329-4251, 404-320-3333, 800-ACS-2345
- Aplastic Anemia Foundation of America, P.O. Box 22689, Baltimore, MD 21203, 410-955-2803
- Cancer Care Inc., 1180 Avenue of the Americas, New York, NY 10036, 212-221-3300, 800-813-HOPE
- Cancer Information Service, National Cancer Institute—Office of Cancer Communications, Bldg. 31, Room 10A16, Bethesda, MD, 800-4-CANCER, 800-422-6237
- National Cancer Institute—Myeloproliferative disorders: http://cancernet.nci.nih.gov/clinpdq/soa/MyeloproliferativedisordersPhysician.html:

Prognosis, stage information, treatment option overview, general information
- Corporate Angel Network, Inc., Westchester County Airport, Bldg. 1, White Plains, NY 10604, 914-328-1313
- Hospice Education Institute, 190 Westbrook Rd., Essex, CT 06426-1511, 860-767-1620, 800-331-1620
- Leukemia Society of America, National Headquarters, 600 Third Ave., New York, NY 10016, 212-573-8484; 800-955-4LSA
- National Cancer Care Foundation, 1180 Avenue of the Americas, 2d Floor, New York, NY 10036, 212-221-3300
- National Leukemia Research Association, Inc., 585 Stewart Ave., Suite 536, Garden City, NY 11530, 516-222-1944
- National Marrow Donor Program, Coordinating Center, 3433 Broadway St., NE, Minneapolis, MN 55413, 612-627-5844; potential donor 800-MARROW-2
- Myeloproliferative Disorders: http://www.acor.org/diseases/hematology/MPD/: Medical resources, support groups, glossary

REFERRAL POINTS AND CLINICAL WARNINGS

There are key times to consult a hematologist/oncologist:

- Infections not responsive to first-line management. These can be a serious problem for immunocompromised patients. There are seven common sites of infection for patients with myeloproliferative disease. Infection in one of these sites could mean danger.
- Acceleration of disease, signified by a change in circulating blast count. For example, a patient who has a circulating blast count that has been stable at 5% comes in for follow-up, and the blast count is 10%; this patient may need to be restaged, and this implies that a new treatment strategy may be warranted.

References

American Cancer Society. (1996). *Cancer facts and figures, 1996.* Atlanta, GA: American Cancer Society.

Athens, J. (1993). Myelofibrosis. In R. Lee, T. Bithell, J. Foerster et al. (Eds.). *Wintrobe's clinical hematology*, 9th ed. Philadelphia: Lea & Febiger.

Brock, D.J. (1993). Molecular genetics for the clinician. Cambridge, England: Cambridge University Press.

Castro-Malaspina, H. (1995). *Myelodysplastic syndromes answer book.* Annapolis, MD: Aplastic Anemia Foundation of America.

Chao, N., Schriger, J., Grimes, K., et al. (1993), Granulocyte colony-stimulating factor mobilized peripheral blood progenitor cells accelerate granulocyte and platelet recovery after high-dose chemotherapy. *Blood, 81*, 2031.

Ellerhorst-Ryan, . (1997). The nature of cancer. In C. Varricchio. (Ed.). *A cancer source book for nurses*, 7th ed. Atlanta, GA: American Cancer Society.

Ferrel, B., Grant, M., et al. (1996). Quality of life in breast cancer. *Cancer Practice, 4*, 331.

Gobel, B. (1997). Bleeding disorders. In S. Groenwald, M. Frogge, M. Goodman, & C. Yarbro. (Eds.). *Cancer nursing: Practice and principles.* Boston: Jones & Bartlett.

Mock, V., Dow, K., et al. (1997). Effects of exercise on fatigue, physical functioning, and emotional distress during radiation therapy for breast cancer. *Oncology Nursing Forum, 24,* 991.

Nail, L., & Jones, S. (1995). Fatigue as a side effect of cancer treatment: Impact on quality of life. *Quality of Life, 4,* 8.

Rai, K.R. & Han, T. (1990). Prognostic factors and clinical staging in chronic lymphocytic leukemia. *Hematology Clinics of North America,* 4:447.

Sandler, O.(1992). Epidemiology and etiology of acute leukemias: An update. *Leukemia, 6,* 3–5.

Sensenbrenner, L. (1995). *Myelodysplastic syndromes.* Published oral presentation, Annapolis, MD: Aplastic Anemia Foundation of America.

Shoemaker, D. (1993). *Hematopoiesis and the impact of cancer therapy.* New York: Triclinica Communications.

Stehling, L., Luban, N., Anderson, K., et al. (1994). Guidelines for blood utilization review. *Transfusion, 34,* 438.

Sullivan, A. (1993). Classification, pathogenesis, and etiology of neoplastic diseases of the hematopoietic system. R. Lee, et al. (Eds.). *Wintrobe's clinical hematology,* 9th ed. Philadelphia: Lea & Febiger.

Walker, R., Branch, D., Dzik, W., et al. (1993). *Technical manual of the American Association of Blood Banks,* 11th ed. Bethesda, MD: AABB.

Whedon, M. & Wujcik, D. (1997). *Stem cell and marrow transplantation: Principles, practice and nursing insight,* 2d ed. Boston: Jones & Bartlett.

Wujcik, D. (1997). Leukemia. In S. Groenwald, M. Frogge, M. Goodman, & C. Yarbro. (Eds.). *Cancer nursing: Principles and practice,* 4th ed. Boston: Jones & Bartlett.

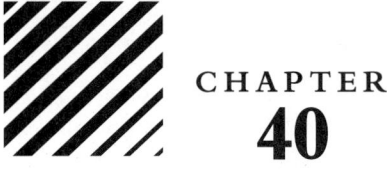

CHAPTER
40

Connective Tissue Disorders

Naomi Schlesinger, M.D.

The connective tissue diseases, also called collagen vascular diseases, are a group of multisystemic diseases. They include but are not limited to systemic lupus erythematosus (SLE), Sjögren's syndrome, systemic sclerosis, rheumatoid arthritis, Raynaud's phenomenon, and the vasculitides. These diseases are characterized by pathologic changes in the blood vessels and connective tissues. The connective tissue diseases are autoimmune diseases. The basic cause of the defective immunity is uncertain but most likely involves an interaction between genetic factors and environmental agents.

Diagnosing these diseases definitively is often difficult because many patients fulfill only part of the diagnostic criteria. Further, many of these diseases overlap, making diagnosis difficult. However, in many of the connective tissue disorders, the affected target organs may be different. In scleroderma, typical skin findings may be noted, whereas in Sjögren's, the lacrimal glands and salivary glands are the prime targets. Most have musculoskeletal involvement as an important feature of the disease.

Inflammatory connective tissue diseases respond to corticosteroids and other immunosuppressive medications. Although clinical response to corticosteroids is usually the rule in SLE or the vasculitides, it is not so with scleroderma. Through knowledge of the common and the unique clinical features, immunologic mechanisms, organ involvement, and the response to treatment, providers can have a better understanding of the connective tissue diseases.

The provider–patient relationship is essential with any disease. Given the multisystemic nature of the connective tissue disorders, almost any organ may be affected. Providers need to treat the disease, but they must also understand the impact of the disease on the patient and the family as a whole. Patients need to be educated about sequelae and prognosis. Depending on the severity of the disease, connective tissue disorders affect every aspect of life, including planning a family, raising a family, employment, and even ability to perform daily activities. Continual counseling must occur, and often it is the primary provider who does this.

Systemic Lupus Erythematosus

SLE is the most common of the connective tissue diseases. It is a multisystemic disease with a wide variety of clinical manifestations, ranging from a benign, easily treated disease with a rash and arthritis to a life-threatening illness with progressive nephritis or central nervous system damage. SLE is characterized by exacerbations and remissions.

ANATOMY, PHYSIOLOGY, AND PATHOLOGY

SLE is characterized by excessive autoantibody production, immune complex formation, and immunologically mediated tissue injury. The pathologic findings of SLE occur throughout the body and are manifested by inflammation and blood vessel abnormalities. This is noted as bland vasculopathy and vasculitis as well as immune complex deposition.

Hematoxylin bodies, also known as LE bodies, containing both DNA and immunoglobulin are highly suggestive of SLE (Godman & Deitch, 1957). They can be found in any organ but are more commonly found in glomeruli and the endocardium. LE cells are phagocytes that engulf these bodies.

Different organs have various histologic findings in SLE. Some findings are pathognomonic for SLE, whereas others are not specific at all. The pathology of the kidney has been studied extensively because renal biopsies are commonly performed to assess the disease activity. The kidney in SLE displays varying degrees of inflammation, increased mesangial cells and matrix, cellular proliferation, basement membrane abnormalities, and immune complex deposition. Skin lesions in SLE show inflammation and degeneration at the dermal–epidermal junction. Complement components and immunoglobulins can be demonstrated in a band-like pattern by immunofluorescence microscopy. Concentric periarterial fibrosis or onion-skin changes in the spleen are considered pathognomonic for SLE.

EPIDEMIOLOGY

The prevalence of SLE varies throughout the world. Its prevalence in the United States has been estimated in the range of 15 to 50 per 100,000. It is more prevalent in women (female/male ratio of 9 : 1), particularly those in their reproductive years. The disease may affect as many as 1 in 1000 young women. Initial presentation is usually between the first and fourth decade. Approximately 10% of SLE patients present after the age of 60. The prognosis for men (Miller et al, 1983) and children (Barron et al, 1993) with SLE is less favorable than it is for women. SLE that begins after the age of 60 (in both sexes) tends to have a more benign course; arthritis, pleurisy, rash, and anemia are the major manifestations (Baker et al, 1979).

TABLE 40-1	American College of Rheumatology Revised Criteria for SLE*
Criterion	**Definition**
Malar rash	Fixed erythema over the malar eminences
Discoid rash	Erythematous raised patches with adherent keratotic scaling and follicular plugging. Atrophic scarring may occur in older lesions.
Photosensitivity	Skin rash secondary to sunlight
Oral ulcers	Usually not painful
Arthritis	Nonerosive arthritis involving two or more peripheral joints
Serositis	Pleuritis or pericarditis
Renal disorder	Persistent proteinuria >0.5 g/day or cellular casts
Neurologic disorder	Seizures or psychosis in the absence of offending drugs or a known metabolic impairment
Hematologic disorder	Hemolytic anemia or leukopenia or lymphopenia or thrombocytopenia
Immunologic	Positive LE cell preparation or anti-DNA or anti Sm, or false-positive test for syphilis
Antinuclear antibody	Titer 1/80 or more

* Four or more of the criteria need to be met for diagnosis.
(Tan, E, Cohen, A.S. et al (1982). The 1982 Revised criteria for the classification of systemic erythematosus. *Arthritis and Rheumatism, 25*(11):1271–1277.)

In the United States, SLE is more common among African Americans and Hispanics than whites. The average incidence in the United States is 25.5 per 1 million population for white females and 75.4 per 1 million for African American females. African American patients with SLE have also been shown to have anti-Smith antibody and antiribonucleoprotein antibody, discoid skin lesions, cellular casts, and serositis more commonly (Ward & Studenski, 1990). They have also been considered to have a poorer prognosis than white patients (Reveille et al, 1990). Patients with a lower education level, which may reflect a lower socioeconomic status, do less well than those with a higher education level (Callahan & Pincus, 1990).

DIAGNOSTIC CRITERIA

Table 40-1 lists the manifestations of SLE (Tan et al, 1982). Signs and symptoms of almost all the organ systems are included, in addition to distinct laboratory findings. The presence of four or more of these manifestations is the American College of Rheumatology (ACR) criteria for diagnosing SLE. The ACR criteria help distinguish patients with SLE from patients with other connective tissue diseases but are not helpful in assessing the severity or prognosis of the disease. Further, there may be times when not all the diagnostic criteria are met, but clinical suspicion for SLE remains high.

HISTORY AND PHYSICAL EXAM

The most important part of the examination of the patient suspected of having SLE is the history. The patient must be asked about systemic symptoms such as fever, malaise, and weight loss; musculoskeletal complaints such as arthritis and arthralgia, myalgias; cardiopulmonary complaints such as chest pain and shortness of breath; cutaneous lesions including alopecia, rash, photosensitivity, and oral or nasal ulcers; and nervous system complaints such as headaches and migraines, psychosis, depression, and seizures. The family history is very important because 10% to 15% of patients have a first-degree relative with

SLE and 18% to 22% of patients have a relative with SLE (Pistiner et al, 1990; Hull, 1975).

The exam of the patient should not be limited to the skin or the musculoskeletal system; attention should be paid to all the other organ systems that may be involved. The exam should begin with vital signs, including temperature, respirations, pulse, blood pressure, and weight. Weight loss is often noted through serial evaluations. The skin (including mucosal surfaces), hair, and scalp are usually examined first. A thorough pulmonary and cardiac exam is required, as is a careful neurologic exam.

- Musculoskeletal features: Arthralgia or arthritis is a presenting manifestation of 95% of patients with SLE (Cronin, 1988). The acute arthritis may involve any joint but typically involves the small joints of the hands, wrists, and knees. It is characteristically episodic, oligoarticular, and migratory; unlike rheumatoid arthritis, it is not destructive. Radiographic findings, therefore, are usually minimal. Myalgia and generalized muscle tenderness occur frequently during exacerbations of the disease: they are observed in up to 80% of patients. Tendinitis is also common and can result in tendon rupture (Furie & Chartash, 1988).
- Cutaneous manifestations: Skin lesions seen can be divided into acute lesions, subacute cutaneous lupus erythematosus, and chronic lupus. The classic "butterfly" malar rash over the cheeks and the bridge of the nose is the acute lesion. It is present from days to weeks and is often pruritic or painful. Commonly precipitated by sunlight, it occurs in only one third of SLE patients. A patchy rash on the upper trunk and sun-exposed areas (photosensitivity) is more common (Callan, 1988). Subcutaneous lupus erythematosus refers to a cutaneous lesion that is nonscaring, is papulosquamous or annular (or both), and has LE-specific histopathology. It is present on the trunk, limbs, face, and palms. Most patients with this type of rash have antibodies to the Ro (SS-A) antigen. Discoid lesions are chronic lesions. Patients with skin lesions of discoid lupus

may or may not have evidence of SLE. In general, when other features of SLE are present, the course tends to be more indolent in patients with discoid lupus (Prystowsky et al, 1976). In addition, the oropharyngeal and nasal mucosa may reveal painless ulcerations.

■ Renal disease: Specific symptoms are not voiced by patients until they have advanced nephrotic syndrome or renal failure. Clinically, renal disease is reported in about 50% of patients during the first year of the clinical diagnosis of SLE. The prevalence seems to increase in subsequent years. Although most patients have some renal lesions (Bennett et al, 1977), severe renal disease that leads to death or the need for renal transplant occurs in only a small percentage (15% to 20%) of patients. A renal biopsy provides the most reliable information about the type and severity of renal involvement. In general, the more severe the glomerular inflammation, the worse the prognosis. The major indications for a renal biopsy are to determine whether irreversible renal disease is present, to investigate atypical renal failure, and to document the subtype and stage of nephritis for study purposes.

■ Neuropsychiatric manifestations: Neurologic manifestations of SLE (CNS lupus) are present in most SLE patients at some point during the course of their disease. The neurologic manifestations of the disease can affect any part of the central nervous system. Symptoms may include headaches, migraine headaches (Brandt & Lessel, 1978), seizures, strokes, frank psychosis, cognitive dysfunction, and dementia. Up to two thirds of patients with SLE show some cognitive impairment or other signs of CNS lupus. However, it is sometimes difficult to determine if these manifestations are secondary to lupus, treatments for lupus (eg, steroids), or concomitant disease.

■ Cardiopulmonary manifestations: Although pericarditis is clinically present in up to 45% of patients, pericardial lesions are found in 60% to 80% of the cases at autopsy. The physical exam may reveal a pericardial friction rub, and an electrocardiogram may reveal ST elevations in the precordial leads. Pleuritis, secondary to a pleural effusion, is present in up to 60% of lupus patients during the course of their disease. Attacks of pleuritic pain often last for days to weeks. The pleural effusion generally occurs on the side of the chest pain, and during the physical exam there may be crackles or a decrease in breath sounds over the area of the effusion. When an infiltrate is seen on the chest x-ray, the most common cause is an infection. Lupus pneumonitis is uncommon.

DIAGNOSTIC STUDIES

Antinuclear antibodies (ANAs) is a general term used to describe any autoantibodies directed against a component of the nucleus. The detection of an ANA is a sensitive screening test for SLE but is not very specific. ANAs occur in 95% of SLE patients (Hochberg, 1990). The degree of positivity of the ANAs is diagnostically important. The positive predictive value of the test increases with higher titers.

ANAs include antibodies to each of the following: dsDNA (anti-double-stranded DNA), ssDNA (anti-single-stranded DNA), Sm (anti-Smith), RNP (antiribonucleoprotein), SS-A (Ro), SS-B (La), Scl-70, centromere, Jo-1, PM-Scl, histones, enzymes, tRNAs, and structural proteins.

SS-A (anti-Ro) and SS-B (anti-La) antibodies are found in just less than half and nearly a fifth of lupus patients, respectively. SS-A is associated with photosensitive skin rash, interstitial pneumonitis, thrombocytopenia, and nephritis. SS-B is associated with absence of nephritis in SLE. The presence of SS-A and SS-B is associated with congenital heart block, Sjögren's syndrome, subacute cutaneous lupus, and neonatal lupus dermatitis. Although levels of these antibodies may change, monitoring levels of SS-A or SS-B is not warranted because the relevance to disease expression is not known (Harley & Reichlin, 1993).

Antibodies to double-stranded DNA (found in 30% of patients with inactive disease and in 60% with active disease) and to Smith, a ribonucleoprotein antigen (found in 30% of SLE patients), are more specific than other ANAs for the diagnosis of SLE. The titer of the antibody is a useful measure of disease activity (Ter Borg et al, 1990).

Patients with clinically active SLE have depressed complement levels. Evaluation of the complement system can serve as an indirect measure of the presence of immune complexes. The total hemolytic complement level (CH50) represents the sum of all the components of the system. Separate complement components (C3, C4, and C1q) should also be measured. SLE patients with renal disease tend to have lower mean levels of CH50, C1q, C4, and C3 than those without renal disease (Schur, 1993). Normal C3 and anti-DNA levels usually correlate with improvement in disease activity (Schur, 1993). Following CH50, C3, C4, C1q, and anti-dsDNA antibody levels appears to be most useful in predicting exacerbations of disease and in following therapy.

Antiphospholipid antibodies and anticardiolipin antibodies are found in increased frequency in patients with SLE. They should be sought in patients who have increased thromboembolic events, venous thrombosis, and recurrent spontaneous abortions.

Routine screening of chemistries, complete blood count, and urinalysis need to be included as part of a regular evaluation. Anemia, leukopenia, and thrombocytopenia are often present. The erythrocyte sedimentation rate, although nonspecific, is usually elevated in SLE. Patients with worsening disease may need to be seen weekly, but patients with stable SLE need less frequent evaluations.

The principal tests used to follow lupus nephritis are blood urea nitrogen, creatinine, creatinine clearance, 24-hour urine for protein, urinary sediment, C3, and anti-dsDNA antibody. Serum creatinine or creatinine clearance reflects the level of renal function but reveals little about disease activity. Nearly all patients with clinically important renal disease have microscopic urine findings. The appearance of five or more red blood cells in a clean midstream urine specimen, especially with at least a trace of albumin, suggests active nephritis.

TREATMENT OPTIONS, EXPECTED OUTCOMES, AND COMPREHENSIVE MANAGEMENT

Self-Care and Complementary Therapies

Although it is impossible to prevent the onset of SLE, prevention of exacerbations may be possible. Avoidance of exacerbating factors may help reduce the number and severity of flare-ups. These include sun exposure, injuries, insufficient rest, emotional crises, and medication cessation. Abruptly stopping medications, particularly large doses of corticosteroids, may even be fatal. Patients must be counseled about these factors. Several authors have implicated stress as a factor that can induce or exacerbate SLE. Different techniques such as biofeedback, visual imagery, stress reduction maneuvers, and acupuncture could be considered.

General therapeutic considerations must always include rest and exercise. Rest is important in the treatment of fatigue secondary to SLE. It is essential during the early stages of the disease. These rest periods can be abolished when the patient feels better. Exercises that strengthen muscles and improve endurance while avoiding undue stress on the affected joints are recommended. Aquatic therapy is ideal.

The impact of the disease on the family needs to be discussed. Patients are often young adults who have children and other family members at home. Frequent office visits, hospitalizations, and even transplants will obviously affect each member of the family. Provisions for care of the other family members must be addressed. Other issues include women who want their own biologic children but are unable to maintain a pregnancy because of recurrent spontaneous abortions or the side effects of the medications.

Patients need to understand their disease and participate in their care. In addition to avoiding the exacerbating factors (see above), they must be reminded that SLE is multisystemic. All health providers, including dentists, should be told about their disease. All patients with SLE should receive antimicrobial prophylaxis before and during surgery, including dental procedures (Klippel, 1997). Patients may learn more about SLE from the Arthritis Foundation (see the list of resources at the end of this chapter).

Before initiating treatment, the following questions should be answered:

1. Does the patient fulfill the ACR criteria for SLE (see Table 40-1)?
2. If the patient has lupus, is life-threatening organ involvement present, or does the patient have mild disease?
3. Does a particular aspect of the patient's disease require specific treatment (eg, seizures, Raynaud's phenomenon, or cognitive dysfunction)?

Medication Regimen

Nonsteroidal anti-inflammatory drugs (NSAIDs) are mainstays in the therapy of non-organ-threatening lupus. Eighty percent of lupus patients are given NSAIDs. The NSAIDs are useful in treating fever, arthralgia, headaches, pleuritis, and pericarditis. However, complications of NSAID use are more common in SLE patients than in patients with nonrheumatic diseases.

Antimalarial drugs such as chloroquine and hydroxychloroquine are effective nonsteroidal drugs for some patients with non-organ-threatening lupus. These drugs are most effective for the treatment of cutaneous lesions, arthritis and arthralgia, fatigue, and serositis. Chloroquine tends to be more effective than hydroxychloroquine. Atabrine is most effective for cutaneous lesions and fatigue. The chloroquines and atabrine are effective in 1 to 2 months and may be used synergistically. Generalized gastrointestinal and musculoskeletal complaints may occur, but they are reversible and often minor. The chloroquines can cause retinal damage; however, retinal damage has not been reported in patients taking recommended doses who undergo ophthalmologic exams every 6 months.

Corticosteroids are potent anti-inflammatory and immunosuppressive medications. They are used in the active lupus patient who has heart, kidney, hematologic, or central nervous system involvement. They are also used in small doses in patients with fever, arthritis, mild serositis, rash, and fatigue whose disease did not respond to NSAIDs or antimalarial drugs. Daily oral dosing is used in most patients with active disease. With severe disease, such as severe nephritis, high-dose intravenous pulse therapy may be warranted. The most commonly used corticosteroid preparations are prednisone and methylprednisolone. However, side effects such as hyperglycemia, hypertension, edema, premature cataracts, osteoporosis, depression and psychosis, gastric irritation, and predisposition to infections limit their use.

The use of cytotoxic or immunosuppressive drugs such as cyclophosphamide and azathioprine is limited by their common and potentially life-threatening side effects. They are used only in patients with organ-threatening disease or patients whose disease fails to respond to corticosteroid treatment, or when the benefits of a steroid-sparing agent outweigh the risks of administering these medications.

Controlled trials have demonstrated the superiority of using cytotoxic drugs plus corticosteroids over the use of corticosteroids alone. These studies include well-designed controlled trials in lupus nephritis and chronic active "lupoid" hepatitis.

REFERRAL POINTS AND CLINICAL WARNINGS

Early warnings that may indicate a flare-up of SLE include chills, fatigue, fever, or any of the symptoms listed in Table 40-1. The provider should be notified if any new symptom occurs. If a patient is still having flare-ups while taking oral corticosteroid therapy, a consultation with a specialist is recommended. Because SLE is potentially fatal, whenever the diagnosis is questioned, treatment seems ineffective, or uncertainty about the prognosis or sequelae exists, a referral is warranted.

■ ■ ■ **CLINICAL PEARLS**

- A positive test for ANA does not necessarily mean the patient has SLE. The frequency of ANA positivity increases with age. Twenty-five percent of persons over age 60 have a positive ANA test.
- A negative test for ANA makes the diagnosis of SLE unlikely.
- The symptoms of SLE may be vague. At times, constitutional symptoms, arthralgia, and a rash may be the only manifestations. Whenever more than one organ system is involved, think connective tissue disorder.
- SLE may be fatal. When in doubt about any aspect of the disease, diagnosis, or treatment, request a consultation.
- SLE is multisystemic. Remember to examine all organs (on physical exam and with laboratory testing) for possible involvement.

Sjögren's Syndrome

Sjögren's syndrome (sicca syndrome) is a slowly progressive inflammatory autoimmune disease affecting primarily the salivary and lacrimal glands. In the absence of other autoimmune diseases, the syndrome is classified as primary Sjögren's syndrome. Secondary Sjögren's syndrome accompanies other connective tissue diseases such as rheumatoid arthritis, systemic lupus erythematosus, and systemic sclerosis.

ANATOMY, PHYSIOLOGY, AND PATHOLOGY

The histopathologic hallmark of Sjögren's syndrome is focal lymphocytic infiltration of the salivary glands, lacrimal glands, or extraglandular organs without structural destruction. These foci range from small foci to diffuse lesions. The extent of inflammation in a biopsy specimen is established by a focus score; a focus is defined as an aggregate of 50 or more cells. At least 2 foci/4 mm^2 of tissue are needed to be considered positive. The focus score is based on the number of mononuclear cell foci in at least four or five salivary gland lobules.

EPIDEMIOLOGY

Sjögren's syndrome occurs primarily in women during the fourth and fifth decades of life, with a female/male ratio of 9:1. The prevalence in the general population is not known. However, the disease affects approximately 30% of patients with rheumatoid arthritis.

DIAGNOSTIC CRITERIA

Table 40-2 lists the 1982 revised American College of Rheumatology criteria for diagnosing Sjögren's syndrome (Vitali et al, 1993). They are based on physical findings as well as laboratory

TABLE 40-2	Preliminary Criteria for the Classification of Sjögren's Syndrome*

1. Ocular symptoms
   Dry eyes for >3 months
   Use of artificial tears >3 times a day
   Recurrent sensation of sand in the eyes
2. Oral symptoms
   A daily feeling of dry mouth for >3 months
   Recurrent or persistently swollen salivary glands
   Frequent need for liquids to aid in swallowing dry foods
3. Ocular signs
   Objective evidence of ocular involvement, determined on the basis of a
     positive result on at least one of the following tests:
       Schirmer test (<5 mm of wetting in 5 minutes)
       Rose bengal score > 4
4. Salivary gland involvement
   Objective evidence of salivary involvement, determined on the basis of
     a positive result on at least one of the following tests:
       Salivary scintigraphy
       Parotid sialography
       Unstimulated salivary flow (<1.5 mL in 15 minutes)
5. Histopathology
   Focus score ≥2 on minor salivary gland biopsy. (Foci: at least 50
     mononuclear cells; focus score: number of foci/4 mm^2)
6. Autoantibodies
   Presence of at least one of the following serum autoantibodies:
     Antinuclear antibodies
     Antibodies to Ro/SSA, La/SSB
     Rheumatoid factor

* At least four of the six criteria must be met for diagnosis.
Vitali, C. Bombardieri, S. et al. (1993). Preliminary criteria for the classification of Sjögren's syndrome. *Arthritis and Rheumatism. 36* (3):340–347.)

findings, including histopathology. A definite diagnosis of Sjögren's syndrome can be made when four of the six criteria are met. Exclusion criteria include pre-existing lymphoma, AIDS, sarcoidosis, and graft-versus-host disease.

HISTORY AND PHYSICAL EXAM
History and Physical Exam

It is important to obtain a history of oral and ocular complaints. The patient should be asked about abnormalities of taste or smell, adherence of food to the buccal mucous membranes, difficulty chewing or swallowing, difficulty wearing dentures, and frequent ingestion of fluids. Ocular symptoms include a burning sensation, decreased tearing, a sensation of sand in the eyes, redness, and photosensitivity. The provider should also inquire about any parotid enlargement.

On physical examination, there is dryness of the buccal mucous membranes and lips and fissuring of the tongue. The normal pool of saliva under the tongue, visible when the tongue is elevated, is not present. Lesions such as oral candidiasis may be noted; it occurs with increased frequency in these patients.

Gross inspection of the eyes may be unrevealing. The results of a Schirmer's test, a crude measurement of tear formation, are abnormal. In this test, a strip of filter paper is placed in the lower palpebral fissure. After 5 minutes, the moistened portion normally measures 15 mm or more. Wetting less than 10 mm in 5 minutes indicates an abnormal test. Most patients with Sjögren's syndrome moisten less than 5 mm of the test paper. A more reliable diagnostic test is epithelial staining with rose bengal. Normally, no stain is visible a few minutes after dye instillation. Grossly visible or microscopic staining of the conjunctiva or cornea indicates the presence of small, superficial erosions.

The provider should differentiate between primary and secondary Sjögren's syndrome. Clinical features of rheumatoid arthritis, lupus, or systemic sclerosis in the context of sicca symptoms suggest a diagnosis of secondary Sjögren's syndrome. Sicca syndrome without evidence of another connective tissue disease indicates primary Sjögren's syndrome.

Primary Sjögren's syndrome presents with a rapid development of severe oral and ocular dryness, often accompanied by episodic recurrent parotid gland swelling and pain in an otherwise well patient. Secondary Sjögren's syndrome, on the other hand, develops insidiously. Approximately half of all Sjögren's syndrome patients have parotid gland enlargement, often recurrent and asymmetrical. Sometimes it is accompanied by fever, tenderness, or erythema. Rapid fluctuations in gland size are not unusual. However, salivary gland enlargement is not pathognomonic of Sjögren's syndrome (Table 40-3).

Salivary insufficiency can be very distressing to patients. Patients may require frequent ingestion of liquids, mainly at mealtime and at night. Many patients keep a water bottle by the bedside in case they are awakened by a dry mouth. Patients also experience difficulty chewing and swallowing dry foods such as crackers. Abnormalities of taste and smell may also occur.

Extraglandular involvement results in interstitial pneumonitis and fibrosis. When the lower respiratory tract is involved, there is hoarseness, chronic cough, and increased incidence of

TABLE 40-3	Diseases Associated With Parotid Enlargement

Viral infections (HIV, mumps, cytomegalovirus, Epstein-Barr, others)

Sarcoidosis

Chronic pancreatitis

Uremia

Amyloidosis

Endocrine disorders (acromegaly, diabetes mellitus, hypogonadism)

Alcoholism/hepatic cirrhosis

Tumors (lymphoma)

infection. Skin or vaginal dryness is common. Decreased vaginal secretions lead to vaginal and vulvar irritation and itching, decreased resistance to vaginal infections, and dyspareunia. Involvement of the gastrointestinal glands results in dysphagia and atrophic gastritis. Major renal complications include diabetes insipidus and renal tubular acidosis.

Disease Course

Although it is impossible to prevent the development of Sjögren's syndrome, patients need to be educated about the complications of Sjögren's and the increased risks of developing other diseases. (For more information on self-care resources, see the resource section at the end of this chapter.) Pregnant women who have Sjögren's syndrome should be tested for antibodies to SS-A. The presence of anti-SS-A antibodies is associated with congenital heart block and rash in newborns. In addition, the estimated risk that a patient with Sjögren's syndrome will develop malignant lymphoma is 43.8 times that of the general population (Kassan et al, 1978).

DIAGNOSTIC STUDIES

There are many laboratory aids for the diagnosis of Sjögren's syndrome. A complete blood count often shows anemia of chronic disease. Leukopenia has been reported in a third of patients with primary Sjögren's syndrome. Acute-phase reactants such as the erythrocyte sedimentation rate and C-reactive protein are elevated in most patients with primary Sjögren's syndrome.

Other laboratory studies may heighten suspicion of Sjögren's syndrome, although none are specific. Elevated serum immunoglobulin levels are present in half of the patients. Antinuclear antibodies are present in approximately 65% of patients: antinuclear antibodies to SS-A and SS-B are found in 25% to 45% of patients with Sjögren's syndrome. Positivity for rheumatoid factors is present in 90% of patients. Patients with Sjögren's syndrome exhibit high levels of antibodies to mitochondria, thyroid gland, and smooth muscle, as well as many other autoantibodies.

Sjögren's syndrome elicits a characteristic pattern on sialography, and radionucleotide scanning of the salivary gland demonstrates decreased function. A salivary gland biopsy demonstrates characteristic histology and confirms the diagnosis. Labial salivary gland biopsy is a safe, widely accepted method for ascertaining salivary gland inflammation. Major salivary gland biopsy is recommended only when there is a suspected malignancy or there are serious diagnostic doubts.

TREATMENT OPTIONS, EXPECTED OUTCOMES, AND COMPREHENSIVE MANAGEMENT

Teaching and Self-Care

The management of patients with Sjögren's syndrome should focus on improving sicca symptoms and treating associated disorders. It is important to avoid treating patients with Sjögren's syndrome with medications such as antihistamines, cyclic antidepressants, or other anticholinergic drugs that inhibit glandular secretion. Alcohol and smoking should also be avoided. However, the most important aspect of therapeutic management is regular outpatient care by the primary care provider, ophthalmologist, and dentist.

Frequent dental visits are advisable. Regular and frequent brushing with a soft-bristled toothbrush and fluoride toothpaste and the use of dental floss, oral fluoride gels, and mouthwash are strongly advocated for dental caries prophylaxis. Sugarless gum or candies should be used to stimulate saliva production.

Several over-the-counter and prescription tear substitutes are available for treating keratoconjunctivitis sicca. For patients with sensitivity to the preservatives, preservative-free solutions are available. Repeated instillation of drops may be necessary to control symptoms. A high-viscosity tear substitute may provide more comfort but can cause blurred vision. Lacriserts, a solid form of artificial tears that dissolve slowly when the eye is closed, may be useful at night.

If corneal ulceration is present, patching the eyes and applying a boric acid ointment may be necessary. Topical corticosteroids are generally avoided because corneal thinning and subsequent perforation may occur.

Xerostomia is difficult to treat. Several saliva substitutes are available, but they provide only temporary relief. Increasing fluid intake is an effective way of eliminating the symptoms. Sugarless gum or candy may promote salivary flow through masticatory stimulation. Pilocarpine in 2% solution may increase salivary flow too, but adverse side effects such as flushing, transient sweating, and urinary urgency may occur.

Nasal dryness is best treated with a humidifier in both the patient's house and office. Vaginal dryness may be treated by frequent applications of saline soaks, Replens, or even cooking oils. Lubricants are recommended for sexual activity. Skin dryness is managed with over-the-counter emollients and moisturizers. Postmenopausal estrogen replacement therapy may also be beneficial.

Medication Regimen

Treatment regimens are aimed at alleviating the symptoms of the disease, not at treating the disease itself. The management of rheumatoid arthritis or other associated disorders is not altered by the presence of Sjögren's syndrome. Nonsteroidal anti-inflammatory drug therapy may be useful for alleviating myalgias and arthralgia or arthritis. Hydroxychloroquine (Plaquenil), 400 mg/day, has been associated with improvement in energy level and joint and muscle pain but no change in sicca symptoms (St. Clair, 1992).

Oral candidiasis can be managed by oral miconazole, 100,000 to 400,000 units five times per day, or nystatin, 400,000 to 500,000 units swished and swallowed four times a day. Systemic therapy (with oral fluconazole) is indicated in severe recurrent oral candidiasis.

Surgical Intervention

Patients who have limited residual tear flow unresponsive to tear substitutes may benefit from nasolacrimal punctal occlusion by electrocautery or argon laser. Patients whose symptoms fail to improve with punctal occlusion may be candidates for soft contact lenses, creating a reservoir for the tears and the protective film over the corneal surface.

REFERRAL POINTS

Sjögren's syndrome is usually not a life-threatening illness but is extremely annoying and disabling. Symptoms are usually alleviated by the recommendations mentioned above. If, however, the patient is still symptomatic, advice from or referral to a rheumatologist or ophthalmologist is warranted. In addition, a referral to a rheumatologist may be needed to help control concomitant disease.

■ ■ ■ CLINICAL PEARLS

- Making the patient comfortable is the mainstay of treatment.
- Although symptoms are bothersome, patients are often reluctant to mention them to the provider, especially those related to vaginal dryness and sexual activity. The provider should inquire about symptoms in a nonjudgmental, compassionate fashion.
- Many of the treatments are self-initiated and do not require prescriptions, but patients need to know their options and what is and is not safe to use.
- Patients always seen sucking on hard candy or never parting from a water bottle should raise the suspicion of Sjögren's syndrome.
- Always look for associated connective tissue diseases such as rheumatoid arthritis and lupus.
- There is a small but real risk for B-cell lymphomas.
- Diuretics and anticholinergic medications should be avoided secondary to decreased tears and saliva.

Systemic Sclerosis

Systemic sclerosis is a connective tissue disease characterized by thickening and fibrosis of the skin (scleroderma), Raynaud's phenomenon, and widespread damage to the microvasculature. Musculoskeletal manifestations and distinctive internal organ involvement, notably of the gastrointestinal tract, lungs, heart, and kidneys, may be present.

ANATOMY, PHYSIOLOGY, AND PATHOLOGY

The pathologic features of scleroderma consist primarily of fibrosis, atrophy, inflammation, and a distinctive change in vasculature. These pathologic changes occur in all involved organs.

The excessive accumulation of collagen in the dermis is the pathologic hallmark of systemic sclerosis and leads to the clinical manifestations of taut skin. The fibrosis may be patchy or diffuse, and atrophy appears to represent an end-stage process. However, the vascular lesions appear to be the primary determinant of prognosis. It is theorized (Smith & Leroy, 1994) that some unknown inciting event triggers endothelial cell injury and immune system activation. The injury results in release of platelet constituents capable of causing fibroblast proliferation and matrix synthesis.

EPIDEMIOLOGY

The incidence of systemic sclerosis is 4.5 to 12 new cases per million per year. The female/male ratio is approximately 3:1. The usual age at onset is between the third and fifth decade, with 80% of cases occurring between ages 20 and 60 (Medsger & Masi, 1971, 1978). No significant racial differences have been observed (Medsger & Masi, 1971, 1978). Patients with systemic sclerosis are more often employed as laborers or other less-skilled jobs and have larger ethanol intakes than control patients (Medsger & Masi, 1978). Occupational exposures that may be related to development of systemic sclerosis include polyvinyl chloride, coal and gold mining, and silica dust exposure.

Although scleroderma occurs more often in females, males appear to have a poorer prognosis. African Americans without evidence of renal, cardiac, or pulmonary involvement have poorer survival rates than a comparable group of white patients (Medsger & Masi, 1971, 1978).

DIAGNOSTIC CRITERIA

The criteria used to make a definitive diagnosis of systemic sclerosis are listed in Table 40-5. The major criteria must be present, or two or more of the minor criteria. Once diagnosed, systemic sclerosis may be classified by clinical features, focusing primarily on skin thickness (Smith & Leroy, 1994). Table 40-4 describes the findings in each of the classes.

HISTORY AND PHYSICAL EXAM

The patient must be asked about systemic symptoms such as fever and weight loss; musculoskeletal complaints such as arthritis, arthralgia, and myalgias; cardiopulmonary complaints

TABLE 40-4	**Classification of Systemic Sclerosis**

1. Diffuse scleroderma—skin thickening present on the trunk in addition to the face and proximal and distal extremities
2. Limited scleroderma—skin thickening restricted to sites distal to the elbow and knee but also involving the face and neck.*
3. Sine scleroderma—no skin thickening but characteristic internal organ involvement
4. Overlap—systemic sclerosis occurring concomitantly with rheumatoid arthritis, lupus, or inflammatory muscle disease
5. Undifferentiated connective tissue disease—Raynaud's phenomenon with clinical or laboratory features of systemic sclerosis not meeting classification of definite systemic sclerosis.

(Leroy, EC, Black C. et al. (1998) Systemic sclerosis (scleroderma) classification, subsets and pathogenesis. *Journal of Rheumatology* 14:202-205.)
* Limited scleroderma is synonymous with CREST syndrome

(C, subcutaneous calcinosis; R, Raynaud's phenomenon; E, esophageal dysmotility; S, sclerodactyly; T, telangiectasis).

TABLE 40-5	Preliminary Criteria for Classification of Definite Systemic Sclerosis*

MAJOR CRITERION

Proximal scleroderma

MINOR CRITERIA

Sclerodactyly

Digital pitting scars or loss of substance on the digital finger pad

Bibasilar pulmonary fibrosis

---

* The major criterion or two of the minor criteria must be met for diagnosis.
(Leroy, E.C., Black C. et al. (1998) Systemic sclerosis (scleroderma) classification, subsets and pathogenesis. *Journal of Rheumatology* 14:202-205.)

such as chest pain and dyspnea; gastrointestinal complaints such as dysphagia, heartburn, or diarrhea; and cutaneous lesions such as hypopigmentation, thickening of the skin, or Raynaud's phenomenon.

The physical exam should focus on the organ systems that may be involved. The exam should begin with vital signs, including temperature, respirations, pulse, blood pressure, and weight. Weight loss is often noted through serial evaluations. The skin, hair, and scalp are usually examined first. Bilateral symmetrical swelling of the fingers or hands is seen early in the course of the disease. After several weeks to months, hard, thickened, indurated skin is seen in the digits, the dorsum of the hands, the face, and the trunk and is pathognomonic for systemic sclerosis. The provider should look for signs of Raynaud's phenomenon and nail capillaroscopy (see section on Raynaud's phenomenon). A thorough pulmonary and cardiac exam is required.

Systemic sclerosis incorporates two syndromes that are clinically different at early and late stages in the disease course. Limited scleroderma (previously called CREST syndrome) is typified by slowly progressing skin involvement. Internal organ involvement occurs with similar frequencies to that of diffuse scleroderma, but the onset of involvement is delayed for years. Clinical differences between limited and diffuse disease are listed in Table 40-6.

Early Disease

The earliest manifestations of scleroderma, including weakness, weight loss, easy fatigability, stiffness, and diffuse musculoskeletal aching, are often misinterpreted as being manifestations of

anxiety. The initial skin lesions are usually limited to the distal upper extremities. Also present is painless swelling of the fingers and hands, known as early "puffy" or edematous scleroderma. This stage usually lasts for several weeks to many months. Skin thickening virtually always begins on the fingers and hands. The skin may appear shiny or taut. Accompanying pruritus is common and may be intense.

Late Disease

The risk of developing new organ involvement late in the disease is reduced although still present. However, improvement in established internal organ dysfunction is uncommon.

CUTANEOUS INVOLVEMENT

Skin fibrosis occurs gradually as abnormal amounts of collagen are deposited in the dermis. The skin of the face and neck is usually affected after involvement of the hands and fingers. The loss of skin folds and wrinkles causes a characteristic mask-like, pinched face. The skin thickening limits the ability to open the mouth fully, impairing dental hygiene.

Skin thickening is usually accompanied by areas of hypo- and hyperpigmentation, particularly on the chest (called "salt-and-pepper" changes) and on the extremities. Fingertip ulcerations can result spontaneously from poor blood supply, trauma, or the development of subcutaneous calcifications that may intermittently extrude calcareous material. The ulcerations often become infected and are difficult to treat. Later in the disease course, the skin may become atrophic and more pliable, causing what seems to be an improvement of the skin.

MUSCULOSKELETAL

Although skin tightening is responsible for joint immobility, independent arthralgia occurs in most patients. Later in the course of the disease, absorption of tufts of the distal terminal phalanges is common. Tendon friction rubs from fibrin deposition are also seen in advanced disease. Subsequent swelling of tendons and tendon sheaths with resultant nerve compression (eg, carpal tunnel syndrome) is not uncommon. Myopathy occurs, affecting the proximal muscles with varying degrees of weakness and atrophy.

GASTROINTESTINAL

Involvement of the gastrointestinal tract frequently causes reflux of gastric acid and dysphagia of solid foods. Esophageal hypomotility or aperistalsis is common even when the patient

TABLE 40-6	Clinical Difference Between Limited and Diffuse Scleroderma	
	Limited Scleroderma	**Diffuse Scleroderma**
Common organs effected	Esophagus Small bowel Lungs	All systems involved. Renal crisis, heart and lung involvement are the most common causes of death
Tendon friction rubs	5%	70%
Arthralgias	90%	98%
Pulmonary hypertension	50%	Rare
Duration of Raynaud's phenomenon before development of disease	Long	Short
Anticentromere antibody	Up to 90%	<5%
Anti-Scl-70 antibody	10%	30%

is asymptomatic. Involvement of the small intestine may manifest as postprandial bloating, nausea and vomiting, and weight loss. Diarrhea may be present because the intestinal hypomotility associated with systemic sclerosis promotes bacterial overgrowth, resulting in malabsorption. On the other hand, colonic dysmotility may cause constipation.

PULMONARY

Pulmonary fibrosis is commonly seen on x-rays, even when the patient is asymptomatic. The diffusion capacity is typically reduced. Sclerosis of the pulmonary arteries results in severe pulmonary arterial hypertension, occurring most frequently in patients with limited disease.

CARDIAC

Cardiac involvement is now more frequently recognized (Follansbee, 1984). Cardiac involvement results in myocardial fibrosis, ventricular hypertrophy, cardiac arrhythmias, ischemia from small vessel disease, pericarditis, and pericardial effusions.

RENAL

Renal disease is a major cause of death in patients with systemic sclerosis. It is associated with rapidly progressive malignant hypertension and irreversible renal failure. Until a decade ago this complication was fatal. Survival today is much improved with early control of malignant hypertension and the use of angiotensin-converting enzyme inhibitors. Most renal episodes occur within the first 4 years of the disease and are rarely seen in limited scleroderma.

DIAGNOSTIC STUDIES

The typical patient with systemic sclerosis has unremarkable results on routine laboratory tests. There are no reliable laboratory tests of disease activity and progression. The erythrocyte sedimentation rate is generally normal or mildly elevated. Anemia may result from malabsorption or renal disease but is otherwise unusual. Ninety percent of patients with systemic sclerosis have serum antinuclear antibodies. The specificities of some of these antibodies have been identified. Antitopoisomerase I (anti-Scl-70) antibodies are found in 20% to 50% of patients with systemic sclerosis. Anticentromere antibodies are specific for limited scleroderma. They occur in more than 50% of patients with limited scleroderma, as opposed to less than 5% of patients with systemic sclerosis.

All patients deserve baseline testing to assess the extent and severity of internal organ involvement. Objective measures of organ involvement are essential to qualify disease changes and response to treatment. These would include measures of pulmonary, esophageal, myocardial, skin, and renal status, in addition to evaluating thyroid function.

Which test to chose is governed by the information sought and the expertise of the local laboratory. For example, there are diverse assessments available for esophageal function. Endoscopy measures lower esophageal function and assesses the degree of erosive esophagitis, esophageal ulcerations, and strictures. Cost and discomfort are considerable, making this exam impractical for serial assessment. Manometry is sensitive and quantitative but produces little information for managing the patient (Seibold, 1994). Pulmonary function tests, MUGA scans and echocardiograms, electrocardiograms, and urine creatinine clearance measurement are some reasonable baseline tests to evaluate the lungs, heart, and kidney.

TREATMENT OPTIONS, EXPECTED OUTCOMES, AND COMPREHENSIVE MANAGEMENT

Self-Care and Complementary Therapies

As with all diseases, treatment starts by teaching patients about the disease and what they can do to prevent flare-ups, progression, and complications. Rest and stress avoidance are suggested. Other self-care regimens are noted below, based on the organ system involved.

Systemic Therapy

No single agent has been proven to be effective in the treatment of systemic sclerosis. Evaluation of therapy is difficult because of the relative rarity of the disease and its slow, progressive course: some patients have spontaneous (incomplete) remissions, but others have a rapid downhill course. Therefore, therapy is tailored toward specific therapy for the underlying disease process and the organ systems affected.

Immunosuppressive agents are used to treat the underlying disease process. The use of corticosteroids has been disappointing. They may be of benefit for musculoskeletal symptoms and dermal involvement, but visceral involvement is not altered. D-penicillamine, an immunomodulating drug that interferes with collagen cross-links, has shown significant improvement in skin thickening after 2 years of therapy and improved 5-year survival rates (Steen et al, 1984). However, approximately 25% of the patients experience side effects and discontinue the medication.

Therapy According to Organ System

SKIN

Care to intact skin is essential. Patients must be taught that immediate and appropriate care of bruises and small wounds can prevent the development of more severe skin ulcerations. Antibiotic ointments such as neosporin or bacitracin may be of benefit. If self-care is not sufficient and the wound is persistent or worsening, the patient should contact the provider. In patients with Raynaud's phenomenon (see the section on Raynaud's), preventive measures such as avoiding cold, quitting smoking, and dressing warmly should be stressed. Dryness of the skin may be eased by frequent application of moisturizing agents such as lanolin-containing products. Most investigators report that D-penicillamine is beneficial for skin involvement in systemic sclerosis.

RENAL

Pharmacologic therapy with angiotensin-converting enzyme inhibitors is the preferred treatment for sclerodermal renal crisis. Unlike therapy with other antihypertensive medications such as propranolol or hydralazine, these agents appear to help prevent the progression of renal disease. However, renal failure may develop despite adequate blood-pressure control, and dialysis may become necessary.

PULMONARY

Pulmonary function tests, diffusion capacity, and ventilation perfusion scans should be obtained in all systemic sclerosis patients. Bronchial lavage and open lung biopsies suggestive of inflammation should be treated promptly with D-penicillamine or cyclophosphamide. Once interstitial fibrosis has occurred, there is usually little or no response to treatment. The general management of patients with pulmonary disease includes use of bronchodilators and smoking cessation.

MUSCULOSKELETAL

Stretching exercises, local heat applications, and the use of nonsteroidal anti-inflammatories may decrease arthralgia in patients with systemic sclerosis. Patients may try these therapies before they reach the provider's office. The patient should be encouraged to use these modalities at the onset of symptoms, before they are considered moderate to severe. Treatment for tenosynovitis includes nonsteroidal anti-inflammatories and local injections of corticosteroids. Treatment with systemic corticosteroids (prednisone 40 to 60 mg/day) is indicated in patients with a myopathy (manifested by mild weakness and myalgia).

Physical therapy is an important adjunct in the management of the patient with scleroderma. Active and passive range-of-motion exercises and the use of heat as stimulants improve circulatory flow and impede the contractures caused by fibrotic skin and joints.

GASTROINTESTINAL

Measures to reduce reflux should be tried, such as elevating the head of the bed, eating small, frequent meals, and avoiding food before going to bed. Patients may even self-medicate with antacids or over-the-counter histamine blockers to suppress acid secretion. Pharmacologic therapy to increase lower esophageal sphincter tone (eg, metoclopramide, cisapride) may be effective. Prescription medications such as proton pump inhibitors and histamine antagonists may also be of benefit (see Chap. 23). Therapy with tetracycline may reduce bacterial overgrowth and prevent subsequent malabsorption.

Surgical Intervention

Patients whose disease fails to respond to angiotensin-converting enzyme inhibitors and dialysis should be considered for total nephrectomy and transplantation. Nephrectomy, with or without renal transplantation, has been followed by rapid control of blood pressure and in some cases by apparent improvement in the skin and internal organ involvement. Surgery may be required in patients with esophageal stricture formation or reflux that does not respond to medical therapy.

REFERRALS AND CLINICAL WARNINGS

Therapy is tailored toward treatment of individual organ systems. Referrals should be made to the gastroenterologist for refractory cases and for endoscopies to rule out Barrett's esophagus, to the pulmonologist for follow-up of lung disease, and to the rheumatologist for overall guidance about management.

Renal crisis must be considered when the patient develops malignant hypertension with acute oliguric renal failure. Renal crisis is rare in limited disease and occurs typically in early (less than 4 years after onset) diffuse disease. A blood smear shows microangiopathic hemolytic anemia, and urinalysis shows proteinuria and microscopic hematuria. The key to treatment is early detection and normalization of blood pressure.

When a patient with scleroderma appears wasted, the provider must consider malabsorption. Malabsorption is caused by small bowel bacterial overgrowth and may be treatable with antibiotics.

■ ■ ■ CLINICAL PEARLS

- Skin tightening improves over time. Improvement in established organ dysfunction is very uncommon.
- Although Raynaud's phenomenon is very common (up to 90% of cases), scleroderma should not be excluded if it is absent.
- Routine laboratory tests are normal in most patients with scleroderma, including the erythrocyte sedimentation rate.
- Cardiac, pulmonary, or renal involvement indicates a poor prognosis.
- Limited scleroderma, although generally milder, still can produce severe complications from esophageal disease and pulmonary hypertension.

Rheumatoid Arthritis

Rheumatoid arthritis (RA) is a systemic disease that occurs in 1% of the adult population. It is characterized by inflammation of the diarthrodial joints (movable joints lined with synovial membrane). Arthritis represents the major expression of the disease, although it is often accompanied by a variety of extra-articular manifestations, such as Sjögren's syndrome and nodules.

ANATOMY, PHYSIOLOGY, AND PATHOLOGY

The synovium in RA has the propensity to become markedly hyperplastic and locally invasive at the synovial interface between cartilage and bone. This destructive tissue is called pannus and is unique to RA. The pannus is responsible for the marginal erosions seen on radiographic evaluation of the rheumatoid joints.

Like the other connective tissue disorders, RA is an autoimmune disorder. There are some suggestions, however, that it may be triggered by an infectious agent, which has not yet been identified.

EPIDEMIOLOGY

The overall prevalence of RA in the United States is approximately 1%. The prevalence, however, appears to increase with age in both men and women. The highest known prevalence rates are in Native Americans, the Chippewa (5.3%) and the Pima (5.3%) (Spector, 1990). Low prevalence rates of RA are reported in Asian populations. Prevalence rates for RA are similar in African American and white populations (Engel et al, 1966).

RA is two to three times more frequent in women than in men. It may begin at any age, but the peak onset is in the fourth and fifth decades of life. Patients over 50 years old at the onset of disease have a poorer prognosis than younger patients

(Sherrer et al, 1986). Prognosis is better in men than women (Sherrer et al, 1986).

DIAGNOSTIC CRITERIA

RA is a chronic (6 weeks or greater), symmetric polyarthritis (three or more joints). The American College of Rheumatology revised criteria for the classification of RA (Arnett, 1989), listed in Table 40-7, describe certain characteristics of the arthritis. If at least four of these criteria are satisfied, the patient has RA. Typically, RA affects the joints of the hands and wrists and is often associated with subcutaneous nodules and bony changes on x-rays. However, the manifestations of RA may be extra-articular as well.

Because the onset of RA may be insidious, the criteria for classification of RA may not always be present in the early stages of the disease. This often makes a definitive diagnosis difficult. In fact, over time, features of a different connective tissue disease may appear, and the presumptive diagnosis of RA may be proven incorrect.

HISTORY AND PHYSICAL EXAM

The history of a patient with RA includes pain and symmetrical swelling involving multiple joints. Any joint may be affected, but the joints most commonly involved are the metacarpophalangeal (MCP) joints of the hand, the proximal interphalangeal joints (PIP) of the hand, the foot metatarsophalangeal (MTP) joints, the wrists, the knees, and the elbows. A characteristic history also includes morning stiffness, which may last for several hours after arising.

Although RA is manifested primarily by joint involvement, it is a systemic inflammatory disease. Most patients note constitutional symptoms such as fatigue. Extra-articular involvement may be seen, including subcutaneous nodules, Sjögren's syndrome (dry eyes and dry mouth), and more rarely Felty's syndrome, with splenomegaly and leukopenia.

Swelling and tenderness are noted in at least three joints. The American College of Rheumatology identified five types of joint abnormalities for recording on the physical exam: swelling, tenderness, pain on motion, limited motion, and deformity. The primary changes associated with inflammation are tenderness and swelling for all joints except the shoulder and hip joints, in which pain on motion is a primary indicator of inflammation.

MCP involvement with the development of ulnar deviation is a characteristic deformity of RA. PIP deformities in RA in-

clude the boutonnière deformity (PIP flexion and dorsal interphalangeal [DIP] hyperextension) and the swan-neck deformity (MCP flexion, PIP hyperextension, and DIP flexion). Synovitis at the PIPs can produce any of these deformities. In the wrist, ulnar styloid swelling and loss of wrist extension indicate early involvement. Synovitis usually affects the ulnar side and results in carpal supination–subluxation, leading to prominence of the distal ulna and extensor tendon rupture. In the foot, the subtalar and talonavicular joints are frequently affected. Involvement of the MTP joints leads to reactivity of the extensor digitorum longus and clawing of the toes, with eventual dorsal dislocation of the MTP joints.

A general physical exam is indicated in all patients with RA. The physical exam should include a search for rheumatoid nodules on the extensor surfaces of the arms and legs, dry eyes and mouth associated with Sjögren's syndrome, splenomegaly associated with Felty's syndrome, and signs of vasculitis such as palpable purpura. Assessment of neurologic abnormalities and muscle weakness is also indicated.

Nerve compression is a common cause of neurologic impairment in RA. Peripheral entrapment neuropathies tend to correlate with the degree and severity of the local synovitis. The median, ulnar, and posterior tibial nerves and the posterior interosseous branch of the radial nerve are the most commonly affected nerves. Cervical atlantoaxial subluxation can cause a cervical myelopathy. This may manifest as neck and arm pains and paresthesias or as a sharp, shooting pain down the back when the neck is flexed (Lhermitte's sign). The presence of cord compression is indicated by a positive Babinski sign, hyperreflexia, and weakness.

Initially, there may be no clinical evidence of joint damage or radiographic signs of cartilage loss or bone erosions. However, several factors suggest an unfavorable prognosis and should be sought in the patient with early disease: uncontrolled polyarthritis, the presence of extra-articular features such as nodules, and a high level of rheumatoid factor (RF). When these factors are present, earlier and more aggressive therapy should be used.

In most cases the disease is chronic, lasting many years. Its damaging effects reflect the disease's severity and can be crippling. Patients with RA have an increase in work disability; 50% are disabled within 10 years of disease onset.

DIAGNOSTIC STUDIES

Laboratory Tests

Routine serum studies may suggest the diagnosis of RA. The complete blood count often shows anemia of chronic disease and thrombocytosis indicative of inflammation. Acute-phase reactants such as the erythrocyte sedimentation rate and C-reactive protein are elevated in most patients with active RA. Active RA may be associated with an elevation of liver enzymes (especially serum glutamic oxaloacetic transaminase and alkaline phosphatase). With control of the rheumatoid inflammation, the liver function abnormality returns to normal. As with many of the connective tissue disorders, an elevated globulin level with a polyclonal gammopathy may be present.

RF is an immunoglobulin (IgM) that binds the Fc portion of an immunoglobulin (IgG) as antiglobulin. It is found in 70% to 90% of patients with RA but can also be found in diseases such as infective endocarditis and hepatitis C. Therefore, the

TABLE 40-7	Revised Criteria for Classification of Rheumatoid Arthritis*

1. Morning stiffness of at least 1 hour
2. Arthritis of three or more joint areas
3. Arthritis of hand joints
4. Symmetric arthritis
5. Rheumatoid nodules
6. Serum rheumatoid factor
7. Radiographic changes typical of RA

* Four or more of the criteria must be met to make a diagnosis.
(Arnett, F.C. (1989). Revised criteria for the classification of rheumatoid arthritis. *Rheumatic Disease Clinics of North America 38*:1–6.)

presence of RF does not establish a diagnosis of RA, and the absence of RF does not exclude the diagnosis of RA.

HLA DR4 is present in 70% of patients with RA. People with a specific haplotype at the HLA-DR4 locus (*0401, *0101) have a fivefold increased risk of developing RA.

Radiographic Abnormalities

Early changes include juxta-articular osteopenia and soft-tissue swelling. As the disease progresses, there is cartilage destruction, manifested radiologically as erosions and joint space narrowing. Radiographic damage often occurs early in the course of RA (Fuchs et al, 1989); in fact, 70% of patients develop radiographic damage within 3 years of onset (Van der Heijde et al, 1992). However, a normal radiograph in the first 2 years of the disease does not exclude the diagnosis of RA. Quantifying radiologic changes is helpful in early diagnosis and in assessing disease progression.

The cervical spine is involved in 50% of RA patients (Brower, 1997). The most common abnormality is cervical subluxation, present in 30% of patients with severe erosive RA. The laxity becomes apparent in the flexed lateral view of the cervical spine; unless the radiograph is taken in this position, this abnormality may be missed. Because the presence of cervical subluxation presents a risk with the administration of general anesthesia, preoperative assessment by lateral flexion cervical radiographs is essential. Patients with RA complaining of occipital pain with or without neurologic symptoms should have evaluation of their cervical spine by computed tomographic scanning or magnetic resonance imaging.

TREATMENT OPTIONS, EXPECTED OUTCOMES, AND COMPREHENSIVE MANAGEMENT

Teaching and Self-Care

In addition to the pharmaceutical agents available for treating symptoms of RA and the disease itself, the comprehensive treatment of RA should include a variety of nonpharmacologic interventions. Application of heat or cold to the joints provides transient relief, as does the use of ultrasound techniques and electrical stimulation. Rest improves acute synovitis during a rheumatoid flare. Some patients find it helpful to integrate relaxation techniques into their daily routine.

Rehabilitation techniques are used when treating patients with RA. Patients should be advised about the availability of aids and durable medical equipment available to improve daily living. Exercise programs are also essential adjuncts. Joint protection methods must be taught. Patients are instructed to avoid positions that could lead to joint deformities and to use correct joint positioning during activity. They should avoid being in one position for a prolonged time. Patients should also learn to use the larger joints when possible and to avoid placing stress on the small joints.

Adaptive equipment is available, such as devices to open bottles and doors, tie shoelaces, and open buttons. Large-handled utensils and medicine bottles with easy-to-open tops help reduce stress on the small joints of the hands. Splints and braces are part of the rehabilitation treatment as well. They help properly position and protect joints and prevent deformities.

RA patients may be forced into muscular inactivity, resulting in weakness and wasting of muscles. Muscle wasting can de-

velop very rapidly, and it is important for RA patients to maintain physical activity. Each joint must be evaluated individually. Aquatic exercises and isometric strengthening are good exercises for RA patients. A joint that is normal or had undergone bony fusion does not need exercise.

Psychological intervention should be integrated into the management of RA. Psychological factors are implicated in pain perception and ability to cope with the disease. Counseling about work is also important, because a patient's self-esteem often depends on the ability to continue working. Patients may also be referred to the organizations listed in the resource section at the end of this chapter for self-help, support groups, and further information.

Many alternative and complementary approaches have been used to treat RA—collagen, cartilage, antioxidant, and magnesium supplements are but a few. In addition, prescription antibiotics have been suggested to be helpful because of the possibility that an infectious etiology is the cause of the disease. These studies have not been validated, and further investigation needs to be performed before conclusions can be reached.

Medication Regimen

Traditional therapy, usually referred to as the pyramid model, begins with nonsteroidal anti-inflammatory drugs (NSAIDs). For patients unable to tolerate NSAIDs, acetaminophen or even narcotics such as tramadol may be used. If these are ineffective, they are replaced or supplemented with second-line antirheumatic medications.

Over the past several years, a new approach to the treatment of RA has evolved. Because the rate of radiographic progression is highest in the first year of disease activity, the opportunity to intervene and modify the course of the disease before structural damage appears occurs earlier rather than later. Rheumatologists, therefore, advocate earlier use of disease-modifying antirheumatic drugs (DMARDs), also called second-line therapies or slow-acting antirheumatic drugs. These drugs include methotrexate, sulfasalazine, azathioprine, cyclophosphamide, cyclosporine, gold salts, D-penicillamine, and hydroxychloroquine. Each has a significant side effect profile with which the primary care provider must be familiar.

Toxicity indices for NSAIDs and most DMARDs have recently been shown to be similar. Thus, exposure of patients to possible adverse reactions is probably not in itself a reason to withhold treatment with DMARDs (Egsmose et al, 1995). Patients treated by a rheumatologist had a lower rate of functional disability than patients managed exclusively by a nonspecialist (Ward et al, 1993). This difference in the disability rate was associated with more intensive use of the second-line therapies and joint surgery among patients treated by a rheumatologist.

The use of corticosteroids in the management of RA is controversial. Initial enthusiasm for moderate doses was dampened by long-term toxicity. Although their use in the treatment of severe extra-articular features of RA is generally accepted, the role of systemic corticosteroids in the treatment of RA is not well defined. Low doses have been advocated. Great variation was found in the use of corticosteroids in RA among rheumatologists in the United States (Schlesinger et al, 1997). The most common oral dose of prednisone used was 5 to 9 mg/day, with higher doses (10 to 20 mg/day) given during acute flares. Selective intra-articular instillation of corticosteroids has also been shown to be effective in monoarticular synovitis, as have short courses of high-dose intravenous pulse therapy (ie, methylprednisolone 100 to 250 mg over 1 hour for up to 3 consecutive days).

The decision about which second-line therapy to use is still arbitrary. There is no widely acceptable drug algorithm for the treatment of RA. Decisions are made on a case-by-case basis, and comanagement with a specialist may be beneficial.

Surgical Intervention

Surgical treatment is indicated in the following scenarios:

- Progressive severe synovitis that does not respond to medical therapy. A synovectomy can be considered.
- Constant severe pain in a joint
- Loss of function and radiographic evidence of bony destruction, or loss of joint motion from bony ankylosis (bony fusion)
- Severe deformities and destruction of the joints (for rehabilitation)
- Prevention of attrition and rupture of a tendon in a patient with severe tenosynovitis
- Correction of contractures and faulty alignment
- Decompression of nerve compression by rheumatoid swelling. The most common entrapment is in the wrist (carpal tunnel).

REFERRAL POINTS AND CLINICAL WARNINGS

Patients with uncontrolled or advancing RA should be comanaged with a rheumatologist, as should patients with extra-articular manifestations such as Sjögren's syndrome, nodules, and leukocytoclastic vasculitis. Patients with occipital symptoms, with or without neurologic signs, should have an evaluation of their cervical spine and should be evaluated by a neurosurgeon if indicated. Physical therapy referrals should be made to avoid muscle wasting.

■ ■ ■ ■ CLINICAL PEARLS

- The diagnosis of RA is made at the bedside. The patient must demonstrate synovitis.
- The presence of RF is not pathognomonic for RA, and the absence of RF does not exclude a diagnosis of RA. Patients with liver disease, sarcoidosis, chronic infections, and other diseases can demonstrate RF positivity. Up to 30% of patients with RA do not demonstrate RF.
- The most common extra-articular manifestations of RA include nodules, dry eyes and mouth, carpal tunnel syndrome, leukocytoclastic vasculitis, eye involvement, pulmonary involvement, and Felty's syndrome (splenomegaly and neutropenia).
- An aggressive course of RA is suggested by a high titer of RF, a positive test for antinuclear antibodies, and the presence of rheumatoid nodules.
- When surgery is planned, patients with RA should be evaluated for atlantoaxial subluxation before receiving general anesthesia.

Vasculitis

The vasculitides are a heterogeneous group of diseases with the common denominator of an inflammatory and sometimes necrotic process of the blood vessel walls. They are distinguished from one another by the size of the vessel involved, the organ systems affected, and the pathologic presence or absence of a granulomatous disease. A useful classification of the vasculitides is based on the size of arterial involvement (Table 40-8) (Fauci et al, 1978).

DIAGNOSTIC CRITERIA

Diagnosis of the vasculitides is based on a combination of parameters. A diagnosis usually cannot be made conclusively without correlation to the clinical history, physical exam, and laboratory tests, including autoantibodies. If the history, physical exam, and laboratory tests do not provide a clear diagnosis, a biopsy or an angiogram must be considered.

TABLE 40-8	Classification of the Vasculitides by Artery Size
Artery Size	**Disease**
Large vessels	Takayasu arteritis
	Giant cell arteritis
Small and medium-sized arteries	Systemic necrotizing vasculitis (SNV)
	Polyarteritis nodosa
	Wegener's granulomatosis
	Churg-Strauss syndrome
	SNV associated with Crohn's disease
	SNV associated with infection
	SNV associated with neoplasm
	SNV associated with connective tissue disorders
Arterioles	Infection
(Hypersensitivity/Leukocytoclastic vasculitis)	Serum sickness
	Neoplasms
	Connective tissue diseases (rheumatoid arthritis, lupus)
	Essential mixed cryoglobulinemia
	Henoch-Schönlein purpura

(Fauci, A.S., Hynes, B.F. et al. (1978). The spectrum of vesiculitis: clinical pathologic, immunologic and therapeutic considerations. *Annals of Internal Medicine.* 89:660–676.)

ANATOMY, PHYSIOLOGY, AND PATHOLOGY

Each of the vasculitic syndromes has its own histopathologic features, but overlap is common. A diagnosis cannot be made by biopsy alone; clinical correlation is essential.

Large vessel involvement, in both giant cell arteritis and Takayasu arteritis, is characterized by granulomatous tissue with a variable number of giant cells (more pronounced in giant cell arteritis) in the acute phase. Fibrosis with scanty infiltrate occurs in the chronic phase. In Takayasu arteritis aneurysms of the large vessels are seen in 20% of patients. They may result in rupture and dissection of the large vessels.

Involvement of small to medium-sized arteries is characteristically seen in the systemic necrotizing vasculitides (SNV). The histopathology of SNV evolves over time. Early lesions are characterized by panarteritis with infiltrating polymorphonuclear leukocytes, fibrinoid necrosis, endothelial cell injury, and thrombosis. Necrotizing granulomas with mixed cells are seen in Wegener's granulomatosis and Churg-Strauss syndrome. Eosinophils are prominent in Churg-Strauss syndrome. In the chronic stages, mainly mononuclear cells are seen. In polyarteritis nodosa (PAN), vascular injury tends to occur with a focal distribution, often at sites of arterial bifurcations, producing microaneurysmal dilatation (Zeek et al, 1948).

Small vessel involvement seen in hypersensitivity vasculitis involves predominantly the skin. In Henoch-Schönlein purpura, the gastrointestinal tract, kidney, and synovium are also involved. The inflammatory cell infiltrate characteristically consists of polymorphonuclear leukocyte debris (leukocytoclastic) and therefore is termed leukocytoclastic vasculitis.

HISTORY AND PHYSICAL EXAM

The patient must be asked about systemic symptoms such as fever and weight loss; musculoskeletal complaints such as arthritis, arthralgia, and myalgias; cardiopulmonary complaints such as chest pain and shortness of breath; cutaneous lesions such as alopecia (hair loss), rash, or skin nodules; and nervous system complaints such as headaches and seizures. Exposure to infectious agents such as hepatitis B should also be raised (PAN).

The exam should be a thorough general internal medicine exam, with special attention to specific organ systems that may be involved. The presence of a rash or other skin lesions should be noted. A thorough pulmonary and cardiac exam is required. A careful neurologic exam is also necessary, as is a thorough musculoskeletal exam.

The prevalence of specific target organ involvement varies with each vasculitic syndrome. Typical presentations of the different vasculitides are noted in Table 40-9.

Large Vessel Diseases

Temporal arteritis is a disease of the elderly. It is more common in women than men. Although characteristically it involves branches of the carotid artery (temporal artery) and of the proximal aorta, it is a systemic vasculitis and may involve any medium-sized or large artery. It usually presents with fever, localized headaches, temporal artery tenderness and decreased pulse, jaw claudication (pain when chewing), and tongue claudication. It may be complicated by sudden blindness. Muscle aches accompanied by morning stiffness (polymyalgia rheumatica) may accompany the headache. Very often a markedly elevated erythrocyte sedimentation rate is present.

Takayasu arteritis is more common in young women. Large and medium-sized vessels may be involved, with a predilection for the aortic arch and its branches. It is manifested by generalized systemic symptoms and local signs related to the occluded artery. Complications are related to the distribution of involved vessels. Death usually occurs from congestive heart failure and cerebrovascular accident.

Small and Medium-Sized Vessel Diseases

SNV can be divided into a number of syndromes, all of which overlap clinically. These include PAN, Wegener's granulomatosis, Churg-Strauss syndrome, and systemic necrotizing vasculitis associated with Crohn's disease, neoplasms, infections, and

TABLE 40-9	Typical Vasculitis Presentations
Vasculitis	**Presentation**
Takayasu arteritis	Arm claudication
Giant cell arteritis	Polymyalgia rheumatica Jaw claudication Fever of unknown origin
Polyarteritis nodosa	Hypertension, renal involvement Peripheral neurologic impairment
Wegener's granulomatosis	Ear, nose, and throat abnormalities Pulmonary disease (nodules) Renal failure
Churg-Strauss syndrome	Pulmonary, cardiac, and peripheral nerve involvement History of asthma, atopy Eosinophilia
Serum sickness	Fever Arthralgia/arthritis Rash
Henoch-Schönlein	Arthritis Rash Renal failure Abdominal pain

connective tissue diseases (ie, rheumatoid arthritis, lupus, Behçet's disease).

Renal disease is the most common feature of polyarteritis (occurs in 70% or more of cases) and is the result of vasculitis, glomerulonephritis, or hypertension. Aneurysms of the renal circulation may rupture, leading to spontaneous perirenal hemorrhage and hypotension (Smith & Wernick, 1989).

Neurologic involvement is common to all forms of SNV (Moore & Fauci, 1981). Peripheral neuropathy occurs in up to two thirds of patients, usually in the form of a diffuse sensory-motor polyneuropathy. Mononeuritis and isolated cutaneous neuropathies may also develop. The most common sites are the peroneal, sural, radial median, and ulnar nerves. The most common cranial neuropathies are of cranial nerves II, VII, and VIII. Central nervous system involvement is present in approximately 40% of the patients with SNV. It is either diffuse (encephalopathy, seizures) or focal (cerebrovascular accident).

Gastrointestinal manifestations include ischemia and infarction of the bowel, hepatobiliary tree, and pancreas (Camilleri et al, 1983). Clinically, patients usually present with fever, abdominal pain, gastrointestinal bleeding, peritonitis, and intrahepatic hemorrhage.

Pulmonary infiltrates characteristic of Churg-Strauss or Wegener's granulomatosis are typically not seen in classic polyarteritis but may be a manifestation of overlap SNV. Pleural effusions should suggest infection until proven otherwise. Cardiac disease is characterized by congestive heart failure, fibrosis and pericarditis, myocardial infarction, and arrhythmias.

The cutaneous lesions of SNV are pleomorphic and not distinct for any individual syndrome. These lesions include palpable purpura, urticaria, ulcers, livedo reticularis, and subcutaneous nodules.

Testicular vasculitis, common at autopsy (up to 86%), is symptomatic in up to 20% of patients with SNV (Shrbaji & Epstein, 1988).

Leukocytoclastic vasculitis involves predominantly the skin, manifested by palpable purpura, although any organ may be involved. It is usually traced to a precipitating antigen such as a drug or a microorganism and occurs a week to 10 days after antigen exposure. Usually it is self-limited, but it can recur or become chronic.

DIAGNOSTIC STUDIES

Certain studies may be helpful in evaluating vasculitic involvement (eg, muscle enzymes) or in quantifying the severity of known disease (eg, creatinine determination for renal dysfunction). A complete blood cell count may identify anemia. The white blood cell count is usually not affected by vasculitis, except in Churg-Strauss syndrome, where eosinophilia is present. An elevated white cell count may suggest a superimposed infection. Thrombocytosis is seen with Wegener's granulomatosis. An elevated erythrocyte sedimentation rate is typical in all forms of vasculitis. A normal erythrocyte sedimentation rate in an untreated patient should raise a question as to whether the patient has vasculitis. A proper examination of urinary sediment is required to detect glomerulonephritis. Hepatitis B plays a role in the development of PAN, and hepatitis C is associated with cryoglobulinemia; therefore, they should be screened for hepatitis B and C when the diagnosis of vasculitis is in question.

Immunologic studies, including antinuclear antibodies and rheumatoid factor, may be positive. A high titer of rheumatoid factor is suggestive of cryoglobulinemia. Serum complement components may be consumed and thus lowered in cases of vasculitis. Assessment of CH50, an indicator of total complement consumption, may be useful in these circumstances.

The antineutrophil cytoplasmic antibodies (ANCA) are present in the sera of most patients with systemic necrotizing vasculitis. The ANCA represent a class of autoantibodies directed against leukocyte lysosomal enzymes. Antibodies with a perinuclear pattern are directed against myeloperoxidase and elastase and are found with greatest frequency in patients with disease confined to the kidney (crescentic glomerulonephritis). In contrast, antibodies with a central pattern are found more often in patients with granulomatous lung disease (eg, Wegener's granulomatosis). The sensitivity of the ANCA is greatest in Wegener's granulomatosis, where they have been noted in a prevalence of 50% to 100%. The sensitivity rises during active disease and is decreased by approximately 30% in disease limited to the respiratory tract.

Electromyography, especially of the lower limbs, may be helpful in establishing a diagnosis of vasculitis by identifying peripheral neurologic disease. An abnormal electromyograph should be pursued with a sural nerve and adjacent gastrocnemius muscle biopsy. Combining muscle with nerve tissue increases the yield of positive diagnoses. The choice of a blind biopsy or visceral angiography depends on the clinical presentation and the risk/benefit analysis for a particular patient. The following is a proposed diagnostic approach to biopsy and angiography in systemic vasculitis (Kaufman & Kaplan, 1993):

- Biopsy site (in decreasing preference): Skin, sural nerve, muscle, rectum, kidney
- Angiography (in decreasing preference): Renal arteries, celiac axis, superior mesenteric artery.

Angiography may identify the aneurysms seen in PAN. It is helpful in identifying intra-abdominal vascular lesions when vasculitis is suspected in a patient with an acute abdomen and no easily obtainable tissue. Unfortunately, the finding of microaneurysms is nonspecific, and they may be present in disorders that mimic SNV, such as atrial myxoma and endocarditis.

Ultimately, the conclusive diagnosis depends on the histopathologic lesion. The selection of proper tissue for biopsy is crucial. Biopsy sites should be determined by clinical manifestations, and tissue should be obtained from the most accessible and involved organs. The easiest sites to reach are the skin and peripheral muscles and nerves. If these areas are not clinically involved, other areas should be considered for biopsy.

Echocardiograms are useful in identifying aneurysms, especially with large vessel disease. Ultrasonography has also been suggested as a tool to guide temporal biopsies, which may otherwise be blind, and possibly to diagnose large cell arteritis as well (Schmidt et al, 1997).

TREATMENT OPTIONS, EXPECTED OUTCOMES, AND COMPREHENSIVE MANAGEMENT

Self-Care

Therapy depends on the nature of the vasculitis. Some cases are simple to treat, with only minimal intervention; others require aggressive treatment. With mild hypersensitivity vasculitis from a drug reaction, discontinuing the offending drug may be adequate. Simple observation may be adequate for transitory vasculitis confined to the skin, as in mild Henoch-Schönlein purpura. Patients should be educated about vasculitis by the provider, but additional information can be obtained from the organizations listed in the resource section at the end of this chapter.

Often patients may try to self-medicate before they see the provider. Over-the-counter medications, such as nonsteroidal anti-inflammatories (NSAIDs), are appropriate in less severe cases. If NSAIDs need to be avoided (eg, in patients with ulcer disease), a trial of acetaminophen may be useful for treating pain.

Medication Regimen

Some cases of cutaneous vasculitis are chronic and prolonged and are not associated with any recognizable cause. In these patients, drugs such as colchicine, dapsone, and NSAIDs should be tried before using potent medications such as corticosteroids and cyclophosphamide.

For systemic vasculitides, the mainstay of therapy is corticosteroids. A daily dose in the range of 1 mg/kg of prednisone is often used. Once controlled, a slowly tapering dose (over months) is administered. For severe, acute attacks of temporal arteritis, high-dose steroids must be started immediately to prevent blindness.

In patients with severe, rapidly progressive disease, such as Wegener's granulomatosis or PAN, additional treatment with cyclophosphamide (Cytoxan) is recommended. If renal or abdominal vessels are involved, a cytotoxic drug should be started immediately. Cyclophosphamide's onset of action is delayed by several weeks; therefore, the provider must predict the future course and severity of the patient's vasculitis before starting the medication. Cyclophosphamide may be administered orally (1 to 2 mg/kg/day). Some advocate the monthly intravenous bolus route (500 to 750 mg/m²), which is associated with fewer side effects, including pancytopenia, immune suppression, hemorrhagic cystitis, and alopecia.

Azathioprine may be used in less severe forms of vasculitis. Methotrexate has been used in patients with Wegener's granulomatosis and Takayasu arteritis, but in most case of vasculitis it is less helpful than corticosteroids or cyclophosphamide therapy. Immunotherapy with intravenous immunoglobulins seems to be beneficial in Kawasaki disease (Kawasaki, 1993) and is still investigational in others.

REFERRAL POINTS AND CLINICAL WARNINGS

The vasculitides are serious and sometimes fatal diseases. Patients with suspected vasculitis should be referred to a rheumatologist and to a specialist as indicated (eg, a pulmonologist, nephrologist, or vascular surgeon).

■ ■ ■ CLINICAL PEARLS

Think of necrotizing vasculitis in the following clinical situations:
    Unexplained persistent fever and elevated erythrocyte sedimentation rate
    Multisystem disease
    Unexplained glomerulonephritis
    Major ischemic findings (especially central nervous system, cardiovascular system, bowel, or skin)
    Palpable purpura or other potentially vasculitic skin lesions

    Peripheral nerve lesions (polyneuropathy, mononeuritis multiplex)
    Sudden severe hypertension in young patients.
Look for involved tissue to biopsy, because vasculitis is a clinicopathologic disease. If no good biopsy site is noted, consider a visceral angiogram.

Raynaud's Phenomenon

Raynaud's phenomenon is a syndrome characterized by episodic vasospasm of the digital vessels in response to cold or emotional stress. Classically, a triphasic response occurs. In the first phase, the major vessels of the digits close, causing local blood flow to the tissues to cease. The skin of the digit appears pale as a consequence of absent cutaneous blood flow. The second phase involves cutaneous cyanosis; digits may appear blue, purple, or even black. The third phase is the recovery phase. This phase lasts 15 to 20 minutes, resulting in intense hyperemia.

ANATOMY, PHYSIOLOGY, AND PATHOLOGY

The regulation of blood flow to the dermal blood vessels is one mechanism by which normal body temperature can be maintained, particularly during exercise or during exposure to an unusually warm or cold environment. Changes in cutaneous blood flow are accomplished by a unique system of thermoregulatory blood vessels coupled to arteriovenous shunts that can quickly shift blood flow from superficial dermal vessels to a deep venous plexus. Control of these thermoregulatory vessels is complex and involves mediators from the endothelium, platelets, central nervous system, and peripheral nervous system. Digital arteries and cutaneous arteriolar vessels are abnormally sensitive to cold in patients with Raynaud's phenomenon (Amieson et al, 1971).

The pathophysiologic abnormalities in Raynaud's phenomenon are complex and have not yet been elucidated. Although increased activity of the sympathetic system may enhance the response to cold, a local defect or fault in the vessel or its local regulation is thought to be the main cause of Raynaud's phenomenon. Several mechanisms have been suggested as the pathophysiologic response causing Raynaud's phenomenon. Table 40-10 (Seibold, 1994) illustrates a number of abnormalities that have been identified and are being currently studied.

EPIDEMIOLOGY

Establishing the true prevalence of Raynaud's phenomenon in the general population is complex because there is no gold standard diagnostic test. The strictest criteria for a clinical diag-

TABLE 40-10	**Possible Causes of Raynaud's Phenomenon**

Abnormal prostaglandin metabolism

Increased number and sensitivity of serotonin receptors

Increased blood viscosity

Increased rigidity of red blood cells

Increase in number and sensitivity of alpha-adrenergic receptors and decrease in number and sensitivity of beta-adrenergic receptors

Decreased fibrinolysis

Increased platelet adhesiveness

TABLE 40-11	Criteria for the Diagnosis of Primary Raynaud's Phenomenon

1. Recurrent episodic attacks of digital pallor or cyanosis
2. Normal vascular examination with symmetrical peripheral pulses
3. No evidence of digital pitting, ulceration, or gangrene
4. No clinical evidence of connective tissue disease, such as sclerodactyly
5. Absence of a significant titer of antinuclear antibodies
6. Normal erythrocyte sedimentation rate

(Leroy, E.C., Medsger, T.A. Jr., (1992). Raynaud's phenomenon: A proposal for *classification. Clinical and Experimental Rheumatology* 10:10485.)

nosis of Raynaud's phenomenon would include a history of cold hands, at least one color change (pallor or cyanosis), and agreement with a standard color chart. Studies using these criteria have found that 5% to 20% of women and 3% to 14% of men have Raynaud's phenomenon (Wigley, 1993). The primary form, which is more common, is generally first noted in young women. The female/male ratio is 4:1, and the teenage years are the average age of onset.

DIAGNOSTIC CRITERIA

The diagnosis of Raynaud's phenomenon is made clinically, based on the manifestations noted in Table 40-11 (Leroy & Medsger, 1992). Patients should be classified as having either primary (also called Raynaud's disease) or secondary Raynaud's phenomenon (associated with a connective tissue disease). Patients who meet the criteria for primary Raynaud's disease are unlikely to develop a secondary cause for Raynaud's phenomenon (Kalleenberg, 1990). Symptoms generally present in the teenage years, are mild, and do not become clinically problematic until the third or fourth decade of life. It is rare for patients with this condition to experience tissue loss or necrosis.

Secondary Raynaud's phenomenon is associated with a variety of causes. It is seen in more than 90% of patients with scleroderma and in 30% to 50% of patients with systemic lupus erythematosus, Sjögren's syndrome, polymyositis, and dermatomyositis. A long-term follow-up study of patients with secondary Raynaud's phenomenon reported that 19% developed the diagnosis of a connective tissue disorder approximately 12 years after the onset of Raynaud's phenomenon (Priolett et al, 1987).

HISTORY AND PHYSICAL EXAM

The key to diagnosis of Raynaud's phenomenon is the patient's history. The classic description of Raynaud's phenomenon is that of a triphasic color change (white, then blue, then red)—the initial pallor replaced by cyanosis and followed by reactive hyperemia. Usually the early phases are painless, but the hyperemic period can be uncomfortable, with the symptoms ranging from numbness, paresthesias, and coldness to varying degrees of pain. Raynaud's phenomenon usually affects the hands, but 30% to 40% of patients have symptoms in both the hands and feet. Rarely the chin, ears, and nose are also involved.

After the diagnosis of Raynaud's phenomenon has been made, the provider must determine whether the symptoms are primary or secondary. Several characteristic differences between the two types are noted in Table 40-12.

In the primary form, episodes are usually symmetrical in fingers and toes and restricted to the distal aspects of the digits. Patients who have this disorder are otherwise healthy and find the cold sensitivity bothersome, but it does not cause ischemic ulcerations. Milder attacks, in the absence of complications, are typical of primary Raynaud's phenomenon. Dryness of the hand, fissures, and paronychia are not uncommon when the disorder is the primary type.

Secondary Raynaud's phenomenon is associated with more than five episodes a day. The attacks are intense and painful and may be associated with pain or ischemic digital lesions. Males with Raynaud's phenomenon are more likely than females to have a secondary form. The age is another important clue. Children with Raynaud's phenomenon almost always have a secondary form, and the diagnosis of Raynaud's phenomenon begs further investigation for an underlying, associated disorder. Conversely, in a 15- to 35-year-old female who is otherwise healthy and whose physical examination is unremarkable, further diagnostic evaluation is not indicated. If the onset of Raynaud's phenomenon is after the age of 35, an evaluation to rule out a secondary cause is indicated. Secondary Raynaud's phenomenon also can be bilateral when associated with a systemic disease or unilateral in conjunction with an occupational trauma and localized anatomic defects (Table 40-13).

When searching for a secondary cause for Raynaud's phenomenon, it is important to question the patient about symptoms consistent with a connective tissue disease such as arthralgia, morning stiffness, dry mouth, photosensitivity, muscle weakness, and skin changes. Occupational causes such as vibratory trauma from frequent use of tools (eg, jackhammers, pneu-

TABLE 40-12	Comparison of Primary and Secondary Raynaud's Phenomenon	
Characteristic	**Primary Raynaud's**	**Secondary Raynaud's**
Age of onset	Puberty	Third to fourth decade
Female/male ratio	20:1	4:1
Severity	Mild	Severe
Frequency of attacks	>10/day	<5/day
Distribution	Hands and feet, symmetric	Asymmetric
Nail-fold capillaries	Normal	Dilated, enlarged loops, areas of ischemia
Tissue necrosis	Rare	Common
Positive antinuclear antibodies	25%	>95%

TABLE 40-13	Conditions Associated With Secondary Raynaud's Phenomenon

CONNECTIVE TISSUE DISEASE

Systemic sclerosis and limited scleroderma (CREST)

Mixed connective tissue disease

Systemic lupus erythematosus

Sjögren's syndrome

Rheumatoid arthritis

Polymyositis and dermatomyositis

VASCULAR

Thromboangiitis obliterans

Accelerated arteriosclerosis

Thrombosis or embolism

NEUROVASCULAR

Thoracic outlet syndrome

HYPERVISCOSITY/HEMATOLOGIC

Cryoglobulinemia

Polycythemia

Multiple myeloma/Waldenstrom's macroglobulinemia

ENDOCRINE

Hypothyroidism

OCCUPATIONAL

Use of vibratory tools

DRUGS OR TOXIC SUBSTANCES

Beta blockers

Ergot

Oral contraceptives

Bleomycin

Polyvinyl chloride

(Kalleenberg, C.G. (1990). Early detection of connective tissue disease in patients with Raynaud's phenomenon. *Rheumatic Disease Clinics of North America 16*:11)

matic drills) and exposure to chemicals such as polyvinyl chloride need to be explored. A history of other vascular disorders such as angina and migraine headaches also needs to be obtained. Certain medications such as decongestants, antihistamines, and oral contraceptives have also been implicated in causing secondary Raynaud's phenomenon.

On the physical exam, routine vital signs should be obtained. A careful exam of peripheral pulses should be conducted. Sequelae of chronic peripheral vascular disease, such as skin stasis changes and ulcerations, should be sought. Patients should have a comprehensive exam to rule out a systemic disease.

Nail-fold capillary microscopy is a simple vehicle for viewing the microcirculation. A drop of microscope immersion oil is placed on the skin at the base of the fingernail, followed by visualization of the nail-fold capillaries with a microscope or at the bedside with an ophthalmoscope. Approximately 80% of scleroderma patients have abnormalities of capillary loops (distortion of normal thin vessel structure and reduction in the number of vessels). Patients with primary Raynaud's phenomenon have normal capillary microscopy.

DIAGNOSTIC STUDIES

There is no practical and reliable laboratory test that establishes a diagnosis of Raynaud's phenomenon. A cold pressor test, in which a hand is placed into ice water, is painful and potentially dangerous. A negative test does not exclude Raynaud's phenomenon because of the variability of patient responses to this maneuver.

Baseline complete blood count, erythrocyte sedimentation rate, chemistry profile, and urinalysis should all be normal in primary Raynaud's phenomenon, and this information could help in the initial evaluation of a secondary cause. Further blood serology should be obtained (eg, antinuclear antibodies) only if there is a suspicion of a connective tissue disease. Chest and hand radiographs can be useful to ascertain whether trauma had occurred or whether a cervical rib is present, causing arterial compression.

TREATMENT OPTIONS, EXPECTED OUTCOMES, AND COMPREHENSIVE MANAGEMENT

Teaching and Self-Care

Patient education regarding the nature of Raynaud's phenomenon is an essential first step, because patients are the ones who initiate and evaluate treatment. Several measures can be used to prevent an attack of Raynaud's phenomenon (Table 40-14). A few changes in lifestyle are the only interventions required when the disease is mild. The most important lifestyle changes

TABLE 40-14	Self-Care Measures in Raynaud's Phenomenon

Type of Measure	Description
Cold protection	Avoid exposure to cold temperatures and to abrupt temperature changes. Have someone warm up the car before a trip. Avoid touching cold objects, such as frozen foods. Keep entire body warm (not just hands): wear multilayered clothing, hat, scarf, mittens. Use special materials: down, Gore-Tex, Thinsulate, electric mittens and socks. Use warm-water soaks, hand shaking, arm whirling.
Behavior modification	Avoid emotionally stressful situations. Stress management training, biofeedback
Drug avoidance	Avoid caffeine and vasoconstrictive medications. Do not smoke: nicotine is a vasoconstrictor.
Occupational modification	Avoid vibratory machine use. Change job if needed.

TABLE 40-15	Treatment of Raynaud's Phenomenon
Severity	**Type of Treatment**
Mild	Preventive measures alone
Moderate	Calcium channel blockers Nitrates
Digital ulcers	Calcium channel blockers Nitrates Occlusive dressing: soak in antiseptic solution, air dry, and then apply antibiotic ointment and bandage.
Acute ischemia	Sympathectomy Prostaglandins and prostacyclines Microvascular surgery
Infected or gangrenous digits	Antibiotics Pain control Surgical debridement Amputation (last resort)

are to avoid smoking, stresses, cold exposure, and vasoconstrictive drugs. Only when these measures fail should drug therapy be considered.

Medication Regimens

Because vasoconstriction is the most obvious problem in Raynaud's phenomenon, drugs that cause peripheral vasodilatation are usually the first ones tried. The most commonly used are calcium channel blockers. These agents have a direct effect on smooth muscle relaxation of the peripheral arterioles. Nifedipine has a stronger vasodilating effect than the other calcium channel blockers and has a lesser effect on cardiac conduction. Nifedipine has been shown to reduce the frequency and severity of attacks (Sarkozi et al, 1986). Consequently, nifedipine is the drug of choice for treatment of Raynaud's phenomenon. Many agents other than calcium channel blockers have been used in the treatment of Raynaud's phenomenon but have been disappointing in their clinical usefulness or are not available in the United States.

When the disease is severe, surgical interventions are sometimes necessary. Table 40-15 lists several treatment options, corresponding to disease severity and manifestations.

REFERRAL POINTS AND CLINICAL WARNINGS

Although usually managed well by the primary care provider, if extra assistance is needed with patients with Raynaud's phenomenon, consultation with a dermatologist or a rheumatologist may be warranted. Immediate and appropriate care of bruises and small wounds can avoid development of more severe skin ulcerations.

■ ■ ■ CLINICAL PEARLS

- The key to diagnosis of Raynaud's phenomenon is the triphasic color changes noted by the patient.

- Primary Raynaud's is more common than secondary Raynaud's.

- Patients with Raynaud's have an increased risk of developing a connective tissue disease.

- Raynaud's phenomenon occurs in different conditions, such as lupus, scleroderma, and polymyositis.

- Nail-fold capillary microscopy helps visualize the microvasculature. It is normal in primary Raynaud's phenomenon and abnormal in scleroderma, polymyositis, and lupus.

COMMUNITY RESOURCES

Education is an essential part of caring for the patient with a connective tissue disorder. There are a multitude of organizations that focus on educating both patients and providers, in addition to providing support groups.

Lupus

- Arthritis Foundation, P.O. Box 19000, Atlanta, GA 30326, 800-283-7800: Publishes booklets and pamphlets about lupus, coping with stress, Raynaud's phenomenon, and medications. Local chapters supply these pamphlets or booklets free to anyone who requests them. Local chapters can also provide lists of arthritis specialists and offer 7-week classes on self-care. http://www.arthritis.org

- American Lupus Society, 260 Maple Ct., Suite 123, Ventura, CA 93003, 800-331-1802 and 805-339-0443: This is a national charitable foundation. Several states have local chapters of lupus societies.

- L.E. Support Club, 8039 Nova Ct., North Charleston, SC 29420, 803-764-1769: Publishes a newsletter, supplies information about medications, and distributes a list of recommended rheumatologists.

- Lupus Foundation of America, 4 Research Place, Suite 180, Rockville, MD 20850-3226, 800-558-0121 and 301-670-9292; http://internet-plaza.net/lupus/: This group, which has approximately 100 chapters, provides patient education and public awareness and funds lupus research. It also publishes *Lupus News*, a newsletter. The Web site includes current information about living with lupus, disease treatments, chat rooms, a calendar of events, an explanation of lupus, and a list of local chapters by region.

- National Arthritis and Musculoskeletal and Skin Diseases Information Clearing House, Box AMS, 9000 Rockville Pike, Bethesda, MD 20892, 301-495-4484: Collects and disseminates audiovisual and printed materials about arthritis and musculoskeletal diseases. Used by physicians, nurses, allied health professionals, patients, and others.

- Hamline University's Lupus Home Page: http://www.hamline.edu/lupus/index.html: Includes current information about living with lupus, disease treatments, research information, and a listing of conferences and abstracts.

Sjögren's Syndrome

- Arthritis Foundation (see above for address): Publishes booklets about coping with pain, coping with stress, and Sjögren's syndrome.
- National Sjögren's Syndrome Association, 5815 N. Black Canyon Highway, Suite 103, Phoenix, AZ 85015, 800-395-6772 and 602-433-9844: A volunteer organization dedicated to providing educational information to patients and health professionals worldwide. Publishes a national newsletter, a patient education series, and a patient guide.
- The Sjögren's Syndrome Foundation Inc., 333 N. Broadway, Jericho, NY, 11753, 516-933-6365; E-mail: NSSA@AOL.com.: Provides materials, educational programs, and support groups throughout the United States and abroad. Publishes a monthly newsletter.

Systemic Sclerosis

- Arthritis Foundation (see above for address): Publishes booklets about scleroderma, Raynaud's phenomenon, medications, diet and arthritis, and others.
- Scleroderma Federation, Peabody Office Building, 1 Newbury St., Peabody, MA 01960, 800-422-1113 and 508-535-6600; www.scleroderma.org.: An international, nonprofit federation of scleroderma support groups.
- United Scleroderma Foundation, Inc., P.O. Box 399, Watsonville, CA 95077-0399, 800-722-HOPE and 408-728-2202: Another support group.
- Scleroderma Research Foundation, Box 200, Columbus, NJ 08022, 609-261-2200 and 800-637-4005.

Rheumatoid Arthritis

- Arthritis Foundation (see above for address): Publishes booklets about rheumatoid arthritis, medications, and diet and a newsletter. The foundation has adopted three exercise programs: the Arthritis Foundation YMCA aquatic program (any adult with arthritis may participate; it is not necessary to swim), "Joint Efforts" (nondemanding exercise for people with very limited movement or those who are older and less active), and PACE (People with Arthritis Can Exercise; designed to increase joint flexibility and range of motion and maintain muscle strength). The foundation also sponsors support groups.
- PALS (Partners in Arthritis Lay Support): Telephone support line that patients with arthritis can call when the daily struggle of arthritis becomes frustrating.
- Patient Partners in Teaching Arthritis: Educates patients with typical histories and physical exam findings about their disease. The patients, in turn, become "professional patients," helping health care providers learn how to take a better history and perform a more accurate physical.

Vasculitis

- The Arthritis Foundation (see above for address): Publishes booklets about vasculitis, Wegener's granulomatosis, polyarteritis nodosa, coping with stress, Raynaud's phenomenon, medications, and others.
- National Arthritis and Musculoskeletal and Skin Diseases Information Clearinghouse (see above for address): Provides useful information (printed and audiovisual) about the vasculitides.
- National Stroke Association, 1420 Ogden St., Denver, CO 80218, 303-771-1700: Can be useful because vasculitis increases the risk of stroke.

Raynaud's Phenomenon

- The Arthritis Foundation (see above for address): Publishes booklets about Raynaud's phenomenon and coping with stress.

EDITOR'S NOTE:
COMPLEMENTARY APPROACHES

A general discussion of complementary approaches can be found in Chapter 3. The following, while not an exhaustive list, are some complementary approaches being used for this condition. Additional information on these approaches, including precautions, can be found in Appendices A and B. Providers need to assess for the use of complementary approaches as part of the patient's history, as they may impact conventional therapies, and patients may not volunteer this information unless specifically asked. Efficacy of many complementary approaches is not as well documented as that of conventional therapies. Providers need to read the literature before suggesting these complementary approaches.

- Vitamins, minerals, herbs, supplements
  - Echinacea
  - Fish oils
  - Ginger
  - Vitamin C
- Complementary Modalities
  - Massage therapy

References

Amieson, G.G., Ludbrook, J., & Wilson, A. (1971). Cold hypersensitivity in Raynaud's phenomenon. *Circulation, 44,* 254.

Arnett, F.C. (1989). Revised criteria for the classification of rheumatoid arthritis. *Bulletin of Rheumatic Diseases, 38,* 1.

Baker, S.B., Rovira, J.R., Campion, E.W., & Mills, J.A. (1979). Late-onset systemic lupus erythematosus. *American Journal of Medicine, 66,* 727.

Barron, K.S., Silverman, E.D., Gonzales, J., & Reveille, J.D. (1993). Clinical, serologic, and immunogenetic studies in childhood-onset systemic lupus erythematosus. *Arthritis & Rheumatism, 36,* 348.

Bennett, W.M., Bardana, E.J., Houghton, D.C., Pirofsky, B., & Striker, G.D. (1977). Silent renal involvement in systemic lupus erythematosus. *International Archives of Allergy & Applied Immunology, 55*(4), 420.

Brandt, K.D., & Lessel, S. (1978). Migrainous phenomenon in systemic lupus erythematosus. *Arthritis & Rheumatism, 21*(1), 7.

Brower, A.C. (1997). In *Arthritis in black and white,* 2d ed. Philadelphia: W.B. Saunders.

Callahan, L.F., & Pincus, T. (1990). Associations between clinical status questionnaire scores and formal education level in persons with systemic lupus erythematosus. *Arthritis & Rheumatism, 33,* 407.

Callan, J.P. (1988). Mucocutaneous changes in patients with lupus erythematosus: The relationship of these lesions to systemic disease. *Rheumatic Diseases Clinic of North America, 14*, 79.

Camilleri, M., Pusey, C.D., Chadwick, V.S., & Rees, A.J. (1983). Gastrointestinal manifestations of systemic vasculitis. *Quarterly Journal of Medicine, 52*, 141.

Cronin, M.E. (1988). Musculoskeletal manifestations of systemic lupus erythematosus. *Rheumatic Diseases Clinic of North America, 14*, 99.

Egsmose, C., Lund, B., Borg, G., et al. (1995). Patients with rheumatoid arthritis benefit from early 2nd-line therapy: 5-year follow-up of a prospective double-blind placebo controlled study. *Journal of Rheumatology, 22*, 2208.

Engel, A., Roberts, J., & Burch, T. (1960). Rheumatoid arthritis in adults: United States, 1960. Vital and Health Statistics, National Center for Health statistics, DHEW, Series 11, No. 17.

Fauci, A.S., Hynes, B.F., & Katz, P. (1978). The spectrum of vasculitis: Clinical, pathologic, immunologic, and therapeutic considerations. *Annals of Internal Medicine, 89*, 660.

Follansbee, W.P., Curtiss, E.I., Medsger, T.A. Jr., et al. (1984). Physiologic abnormalities of cardiac function in progressive systemic sclerosis with diffuse scleroderma. *N Engl J Med, 310*, 142.

Fuchs, H.A., Kaye, J.J., Callahan, L.F., Nance, E.P., & Pincus, T. (1989). Evidence of significant radiographic damage in rheumatoid arthritis within the first 2 years of disease. *Journal of Rheumatology, 16*, 867.

Furie, R.A., & Chartash, E.K. (1988). Tendon rupture in systemic lupus erythematosus. *Seminars in Arthritis & Rheumatism, 18*, 127.

Godman, G.C., & Deitch, A.D. (1957). A cytochemical study of the LE bodies of systemic lupus erythematosus. I. Nucleic acids. *Journal of Experimental Medicine, 106*, 1575.

Harley, J.B., & Reichlin, M. (1993). In D.J. Wallace & B.H. Hahn (Eds.). *Dubois' lupus erythematosus*, 4th ed. Philadelphia: Lea & Febiger.

Hochberg, M.C. (1990). Systemic lupus erythematosus. *Rheumatic Diseases Clinic of North America, 16*, 617.

Hull, B. (Ed.). (1975). Summary from questionnaires: History of diseases in members' families. *Lupus Lifeline.*

Kalleenberg, C.G. (1990). Early detection of connective tissue disease in patients with Raynaud's phenomenon. *Rheumatic Diseases Clinics of North America, 16*, 11.

Kassan, S.S., Thomas, T.L., Moutsopoulos, H.M., et al. (1978). Increased risk of lymphoma in sicca syndrome. *Annals of Internal Medicine, 89*, 888.

Kaufman, L.D., & Kaplan, A.P. (1993). Current concepts of systemic necrotizing vasculitis. *Mount Sinai Journal of Medicine, 60*(2), 104.

Kawasaki, T. (1993). Kawasaki disease. In *Primer on the rheumatic diseases*, 10th ed. Arthritis Foundation.

Klippel, J.H. (1997). Treatment of SLE. In: *Primer on the rheumatic diseases*, 11th ed. Arthritis Foundation.

Leroy, E.C., Black, C., Fleischmajer, R., et al. (1988). Systemic sclerosis (scleroderma) classification, subsets and pathogenesis. *Journal of Rheumatology, 15*, 202.

Leroy, E.C., & Medsger, T.A. Jr. (1992). Raynaud's phenomenon. A proposal for classification. *Clinical & Experimental Rheumatology, 10*, 1.

Medsger, T.A. Jr., & Masi, A.T. (1971). Epidemiology of systemic sclerosis (scleroderma). *Annals of Internal Medicine, 74*, 714.

Medsger, T.A. Jr., & Masi, A.T. (1978). Epidemiology of systemic sclerosis (scleroderma) among male U.S. veterans. *Journal of Chronic Diseases, 31*, 73.

Medsger, T.A. Jr., Masi, A.T., Rodnan, G.P., Renedek, T.G., & Robinson, H. (1971). Survival with systemic sclerosis (scleroderma): A life table analysis of clinical and demographic factors in 309 patients. *Annals of Internal Medicine, 75*, 369.

Miller, M.H., Urowitz, M.D., Gladman, D.D., & Killinger, D.W. (1983). Systemic lupus erythematosus in males. *Medicine (Baltimore), 62*, 327.

Moore, P., & Fauci, A. (1981). Neurologic manifestations of systemic vasculitis: A retrospective and prospective study of the clinicopathologic features and responses to therapy in 25 patients. *American Journal of Medicine, 71*, 517.

Pistiner, M., Wallace, D.J., Nessim, S., Metzger, A.L., & Klinenberg, J.R. (1990). Lupus erythematosus in the 1980s: A survey of 570 patients. *Seminars in Arthritis & Rheumatism, 21*(1), 55.

Priolett, P., Vayssairat, M., & Housset, E. (1987). How to classify Raynaud's phenomenon: Long-term follow-up study of 73 cases. *American Journal of Medicine, 83*, 494.

Prystowsky, S.D., Herndon, J.H. Jr., & Gilliam, J.N. (1976). Chronic cutaneous lupus erythematosus: A clinical and laboratory investigation of 80 patients. *Medicine (Baltimore), 55*, 183.

Reveille, J.D., Bartolucci, A., & Alarcon-Seegovia, D. (1990). Prognosis in systemic lupus erythematosus. Negative impact of increasing age of onset, black race, and thrombocytopenia, as well as causes of death. *Arthritis & Rheumatism, 33*, 37.

Sarkozi, J., Bookman, A.A., Mahon, W., Ramsay, C., Petsky, A.S., & Keystone, E.C. (1986). Nifedipine in the treatment of idiopathic Raynaud's syndrome. *Journal of Rheumatology, 13*, 331.

Schlesinger, N., Farrukh, K., Barrett, K., Hoffman, B.I., & Schumacher, H.R., Jr. (1997). A survey of corticosteroid use in rheumatoid arthritis. *Arthritis & Rheumatism, 40*:S981.

Schmidt, W.A., Kraft, H.E., Vorpahl, K., Volker, L., & Gromnica-Ihle, E.J. (1997). Color duplex ultrasonography in the diagnosis of temporal arteritis. *N Engl J Med, 337*, 1336.

Schur, P.H. (1993). Complement and systemic lupus erythematosus. In *Dubois' lupus erythematosus*, 4th ed. Philadelphia: Lea & Febiger.

Seibold, J.R. (1994). Systemic sclerosis: Clinical features. In J.H. Klippel & P.A. Dieppe (Eds.). *Rheumatology*. St. Louis: Mosby.

Sherrer, Y.S., Bloch, D.A., Mitchell, D.M., Young, D.Y., Fries, J.F. (1986). The development of disability in rheumatoid arthritis. *Arthritis & Rheumatism, 26*, 494.

Shrbaji, M.S., & Epstein, J.I. (1988). Testicular vasculitis: Implications for systemic disease. *Human Pathology, 19*, 186.

Smith, D.L., & Wernick, R. (1989). Spontaneous rupture of a renal artery aneurysm in polyarteritis nodosa: Critical review of the literature and report of a case. *American Journal of Medicine, 87*, 464.

Smith, E.A., & Leroy, E.C. (1994). Systemic sclerosis: Etiology and pathogenesis. In J.H. Klippel & P.A. Dieppe (Eds.). *Rheumatology*. St. Louis: Mosby.

Spector, T.D. (1990). Rheumatoid arthritis. *Rheumatic Diseases Clinic of North America, 16*, 513.

St. Clair, E.W. (1992). Sjögren's syndrome and autoimmunity. *Concepts in Immunopathology, 8*, 161.

Steen, V.D., Medsger, T.A. Jr., & Rodnan, G.P. (1984). D-penicillamine therapy in progressive systemic sclerosis (scleroderma). *Annals of Internal Medicine, 97*, 652.

Tan, E.M., Cohen, A.S., Fries, J.F., et al. (1982). The 1982 revised criteria for the classification of systemic lupus erythematosus. *Arthritis & Rheumatism, 25*, 1271.

Ter Borg, E.J., Horst, G., Hummel, E.J., Limburg, P.C., & Kalleenberg, C.G. (1990). Measurement of increases in anti-double-stranded DNA antibody levels as a predictor of disease exacerbation in systemic lupus erythematosus. *Arthritis & Rheumatism, 33*, 634.

Van der Heijde, D.M., Van Leeuwen, M.A., Van Riel, P.L., et al. (1992). Biannual radiographic assessments of hands and feet in a three-year prospective follow-up of patients with early rheumatoid arthritis. *Arthritis & Rheumatism, 35*, 26.

Vitali, C., Bombardieri, S., Moutsopoulos, H.M., et al. (1993). Preliminary criteria for the classification of Sjögren's syndrome. *Arthritis & Rheumatism, 36*, 340.

Ward, M.M., Leigh, J.P., & Fries, J.F. (1993). Progression of functional disability in patients with rheumatoid arthritis. Associations with rheumatology subspecialty care. *Archives of Internal Medicine, 153*, 2229.

Ward, M.M., & Studenski, S. (1990). Clinical manifestations of systemic lupus erythematosus. Identification of racial and socioeconomic influence. *Archives of Internal Medicine, 150*, 849.

Wigley, F.M. (1993). Raynaud's phenomenon. *Current Opinion in Rheumatology, 5*, 773.

Zeek, P.M., Smith, C.C., & Weeter, J.C. (1948). Studies on periarteritis nodosa. III. The differentiation between the vascular lesions of periarteritis nodosa and of hypersensitivity. *American Journal of Pathology, 24*, 889.

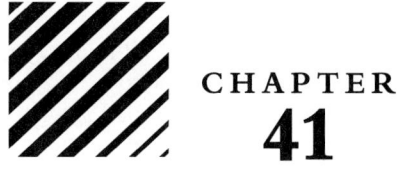

CHAPTER

41

HIV/AIDS

Debra A. Kosko, MN, FNP-C, Carla Alexander, MD, Karen Benker, MD, and Valery Hughes, BSN, RN

Human immunodeficiency virus type 1 (HIV-1) is an evolving disease. Its course and response to treatment are changing more quickly than the literature can describe these changes. The term "HIV positive" refers to a person who has been infected with the virus causing HIV. Acquired immunodeficiency syndrome (AIDS) refers to a person who has developed opportunistic diseases as a result of HIV or whose immune system, based on laboratory values, is shown to be significantly suppressed.

The estimated number of persons with AIDS and of persons infected with the HIV virus continues to increase. HIV, once considered a disease that quickly produced complications and death, is now a chronic disease. People with HIV and AIDS are living longer with more productive lives. Therefore, it is impossible for the subspecialist clinician alone to manage the care of this expanding population of patients.

This chapter provides an overview of HIV and AIDS from a primary care perspective. With a thorough knowledge of antiretroviral therapy and chemoprophylaxis, as well as key subspecialty consultation points along the disease process, the primary care provider can continue to provide needed, high-quality HIV care.

ANATOMY, PHYSIOLOGY, AND PATHOLOGY

The pathophysiology of HIV disease is quite complex, but an understanding of the basic progression of disease is necessary for optimal clinical management. Multiple sites in the reproductive cycle of the virus must be targeted simultaneously, and the immune system also needs to be bolstered. Understanding these concepts helps in the selection and sequencing of therapies (Fig. 41-1). Nucleoside reverse transcriptase inhibitors (NRTIs) block the production of viral DNA by inhibiting reverse transcriptase activity, thus preventing infection of new cells. Nonnucleoside reverse transcriptase inhibitors (NNRTIs) act at the same site as NRTIs, bind directly to reverse transcriptase, and also prevent infection of new cells. Protease inhibitors act at a later point in the HIV life cycle. These compounds inhibit protease from binding with the immature virions after they have budded from an HIV-infected cell, rendering them dysfunctional and noninfectious.

The pathogenesis of HIV-1 depends on the critical balance between viral factors and the host response. With current therapies, the time between primary infection and death can be extended for more than 10 years, depending on the patient's genetic makeup, the intrinsic health of the immune system, and the timing and choice of antiretroviral therapy. In persons with advanced disease, even after these defense mechanisms have apparently failed, prophylaxis against opportunistic infections alone may still prolong survival.

Course of Infection

After primary exposure to the virus, there is a burst of viral replication during which the virus is disseminated into lymphoid tissue. The immune system responds and in most patients can contain viral replication initially. A prolonged elevation of the amount of virus circulating in the bloodstream (the viral load or viral burden) is highly correlated with the rate of disease progression. This interval before the development of symptoms, termed "disease-free survival time," is quite variable from one person to the next. It is likely that both viral replication and host defenses are involved in the rate of progression of the disease (Fauci, 1996). With the current use of multidrug therapy, viral replication may remain unmeasurable for more than 10 years. However, what actually triggers the eventual decline of the immune system and resultant increase in viremia is still unclear.

Viral Factors

The virus enters the body as a direct injection (eg, blood transfusion or intravenous drug use) or through sexual contact via a mucosal surface. Concurrent infections, such as a sexually transmitted disease or tuberculosis (TB), increase the rate of transmission. Virus is produced at the rate of 10 billion virions per day, with infected cells having a life span of 2.2 days. The life cycle of the virus is 1.2 days, and it is this rapid growth, resulting in a high level of CD4 cell destruction, that has changed the way the disease is managed clinically (Perelson et al, 1996).

Immune System Response

Lymphoid tissue is the general reservoir for the virus. All immune cell types are affected, although the CD4 cells and monocytes are the main targets. Although the use of protease inhibitors usually decreases the amount of circulating virus, a simultaneous increase in CD4 cells does not always result. This may be because HIV not only causes direct cell destruction but also may have a role in producing programmed cell death (apoptosis).

The immune system is regulated by cytokines, soluble proteins that make up a complex messenger network to control gene activation and the expression of cell surface receptors. There are cytokines that stimulate the production of HIV and

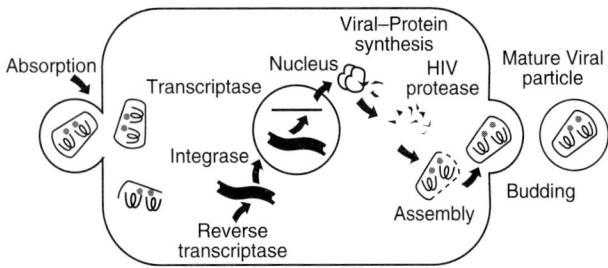

FIGURE 41-1 Life cycle of HIV. Reprinted with permission from Agouron Pharmaceuticals.

those that suppress replication. The same cytokine may produce opposite results at different times in the life cycle of cells. The complexity of the immune system and of HIV itself makes the development of useful clinical therapies a very difficult task.

EPIDEMIOLOGY

If current trends continue, 60 to 70 million adults will have been infected by the year 2000 (Centers for Disease Control & Prevention [CDC], 1997b). Sub-Saharan Africa has the most HIV-infected persons (18.5 million); Asia has the second highest number (4.7 million). The Americas have represented the third largest number of HIV infections (2 million in Latin America and the Caribbean and 1 million in North America). The United States has the highest number of reported AIDS cases in the world: 581,429 cases and 362,004 fatalities (CDC, 1996).

The pattern of HIV epidemiology in the United States is evolving. There has been a shift in the epidemic to minority populations, women, heterosexuals, and adolescents (CDC, 1997b). HIV infection is the second leading cause of death in persons ages 25 to 44. Approximately 1 in 300 persons in the United States is infected with HIV.

Some positive trends have also emerged. AIDS incidence among children has declined by 30%, probably the result of the use of zidovudine to prevent perinatal transmission (Quinn, 1996). For the first time, there has been a decline in the AIDS death rate (by 13% in 1996). However, the death rate declined by 15% for men while increasing by 3% for women. Death rates declined by 6% for injection drug users and by 18% for homosexual men while increasing 3% for persons infected through heterosexual contact (CDC, 1997b).

Cultural Factors

Within the context of the HIV/AIDS epidemic is the provider's obligation to understand how culture and subsequent belief systems affect health promotion. Often referred to as "special populations" issues, HIV has invaded every population and culture. Understanding diversity has a critical impact on a provider's ability to function effectively and treat appropriately. The effective outcome may be to prevent transmission, provide treatment or access to clinical trials, or to identify sources of support in special population communities. Table 41-1 is a brief summary of special populations, listing definitions, issues, and options for intervention. Specific referral sources may be found in the resources list toward the end of this chapter.

Socioeconomic Factors

HIV infection has crossed socioeconomic lines in ways that are uncharacteristic of other infectious diseases. Initially considered a disease of gay white males, HIV has infected and affected the wealthy and famous, the middle class, and the extremely disadvantaged. Epidemiologically in the United States, financial and social issues have had an impact on disease transmission, treatment, and survival.

HIV infection is now found along all racial, ethnic, gender, age, and economic lines. Particularly in urban areas, HIV infection is concentrated in people of minority groups in inverse proportion to their numbers in the population (CDC, 1994a; Byerly & Deardorff, 1994). Within racial and ethnic groups, women and adolescents are becoming infected at a faster rate than ever before.

Although injection drug use is practiced across socioeconomic lines, it is concentrated in areas where racial and ethnic minorities and economic disadvantage exist. These are the same neighborhoods where a lack of money and infrastructure makes it extremely difficult to increase HIV awareness and prevent transmission. Prevention strategies such as free needle exchanges or distribution of condoms have been opposed in some communities.

TABLE 41-1	HIV Care of Special Populations	
Special Population/Defining Characteristics	**Specific Issues**	**Possible Interventions**
Adolescents (Casey et al, 1996[1]) Ages 12–21	■ Time of growth, experimentation, and risk taking ■ Feeling of invulnerability ■ Concrete thinking without view to the future ■ Peer pressure ■ Lack of knowledge ■ Alcohol/substance use, sex for drugs, sex for survival	■ Peer educators ■ Maintenance of trusting relationship between provider and patient ■ Increase general knowledge base about transmission and treatment options ■ Involve peers in planning teaching and intervention programs. ■ *Early* education, targeted before teen years ■ Include safer sexual practices in teaching. ■ Include substance use education. ■ Identify adolescents at high risk—runaways, homeless, gay and lesbian, racial and ethnic minorities, young women.

(continued)

TABLE 41-1 HIV Care of Special Populations *(Continued)*

Special Population/Defining Characteristics	Specific Issues	Possible Interventions
African Americans (Casey et al, 1996) Majority are of West African descent; represent ~12% of US population but >33% of all AIDS cases (CDC, 1994)[1]	■ Distrust of health care providers ■ Lack of money to support prevention initiatives ■ Lack of culturally appropriate teaching tools ■ Myths and beliefs about origins and transmission of HIV ■ Lack of insurance ■ Poverty, especially in single-parent families with women head of household	■ Providers must understand their own values. ■ Assess patient's beliefs, traditions, and relationships with family, community, and church. ■ Providers must understand that the importance they place on certain aspects of treatment may not be the patient's main priority. ■ Support the patient's need to judge his or her own priorities. ■ Work with peer educators.
Hispanic communities (Casey et al, 1996) Multiple ethnicities (Puerto Rican, South American, Mexican, Cuban descent); represent ~8.4% of US population but >20% of US AIDS cases (CDC, 1994)[1]	■ Diversity of subgroups makes approaches harder to generalize. ■ Lower socioeconomic status ■ Lack of health insurance ■ Perceived lack of vulnerability by stigmatizing HIV as a "gay white" disease ■ Perception of health care as threatening to undocumented residents ■ Language barrier ■ Inferior role of women in many subgroups ■ Lack of family support in undocumented residents whose families are back in their country of origin	■ Target teaching material specifically for Hispanic subgroups to ensure validity. ■ Work with Hispanic community-based organizations to develop culturally sensitive approaches to care management. ■ Recognize that the threat of deportation often overrides health concerns. ■ Use peers for education. ■ Maintain a referral list of places that provide services regardless of residency status or ability to pay. Advocate for such access to care. ■ Teach women steps for risk reduction.
Gay men and lesbians (Casey et al, 1996)	■ Gay men and lesbians are not a uniform group of people. There are all levels of income, education, occupation, race/ethnicity, age; they may or may not use drugs; they may self-identify as gay or not; they may never have had a same-sex encounter but still identify as gay ■ The gay/lesbian community has suffered huge losses as a result of death from AIDS; lesbians without HIV infection have often had the role of caregiver to an infected friend or partner. ■ The caregiver/partner is often not accepted with the same status as a heterosexual spouse. ■ Often encounter stigma associated with sexual identity, to the point of harassment or even violence ■ May need to hide sexual identity to keep jobs, preserve harmony in the family, be accepted in religious observances, etc. ■ Once diagnosed HIV+, they may be fearful of increased prejudice; may handle diagnosis with denial and wait to seek medical intervention ■ Health care workers are often insensitive to gay/lesbian issues and needs. As the epidemic has progressed, there has been greater acceptance of gay men, but lesbians are often still the target of derision and insensitivity. ■ Self-identified lesbians may have sex with men for money or survival. ■ Providers' misinformation or insensitivity can result in inadequate safer sex education.	■ Recognize the diversity within the group and approach patient as the complex individual he or she is. ■ Acknowledge the person's losses. ■ Accept the partner as an important part of the patient's life; if the patient views the partner as a spouse, so should the provider. ■ Refer to community groups for issues that cannot be handled in primary care—such as support groups for coming out, handling antigay violence. ■ If uncomfortable with teaching safe sex, the provider should refer to someone who is able to provide the teaching in an effective and sensitive manner. ■ Maintain confidentiality; for instance, do not fax information until it is clear the receiving person has sole access to the material. ■ Explore issues of denial when they arise. ■ Recognize that women who self-identify as lesbians still require the same gynecologic care as straight women. ■ Recognize homophobic behavior in self or staff; obtain education and training to sensitize staff and self to perceive and change such behavior.
Deaf/Hearing impaired (Casey et al, 1996)	■ Lack of HIV/AIDS services for deaf people ■ Isolation secondary to communication barriers ■ Health care worker myths about the deaf/hearing impaired: writing information down will solve all communication problems; hearing problems imply lack of intelligence; any sign language is better than no sign language ■ Distrust of the health care system ■ Lack of self-esteem	■ Deaf people learn better by peer education and better in groups taught by a peer than in 1:1 session using an interpreter, so use deaf counselors. ■ Provide help in negotiating the system. ■ Recognize the diversity of subgroups among the hearing impaired—deaf gays, African Americans, injection drug users. ■ Refer to appropriate sources for information.

(continued)

TABLE 41-1   HIV Care of Special Populations *(Continued)*

Special Population/Defining Characteristics	Specific Issues	Possible Interventions
Homeless people (Casey et al, 1996)	■ Commonly have multiple health problems associated with or contributing to their homelessness: drug use, alcohol use, mental illness, victims or performers of abuse; respiratory, foot, skin, periodontal disease, TB, infestations ■ Limited access to hygiene facilities, inadequate clothing, poor diet ■ Discriminatory treatment by providers related to poor hygiene, infested clothing, uncontrolled or noncommunicative behavior, substance use ■ Decreased attendance for care related to fear of discrimination ■ Risk for HIV exposure via unsafe sex or needle sharing increases the longer a person is homeless. ■ At higher risk for violence, including rape ■ No insurance ■ Multiple barriers to care—as listed above, and inability to wait in a clinic setting secondary to substance use, mental illness, fear of losing place in shelter lines or food kitchens ■ Chaotic lives make active participation in medication taking virtually impossible. ■ Delays in treatment for HIV/opportunistic infections worsen prognosis.	■ Accept that developing a trusting relationship may take months. ■ Establish goals with the patient, taking into account the patient's real life. ■ Accept that basic needs will take priority before patient's acceptance into organized plan of care. ■ Use multidisciplinary team approach—the patient has many needs and the primary provider must refer out most of the social service coordination. ■ If patient has TB, the use of directly observed therapy after hospitalization is mandatory to prevention recurrence and development of resistance.
People who are incarcerated (Casey et al, 1996) All people in local, state, and federal detention	■ Transmission: few correctional facilities allow condoms or dental dams to be distributed; no provision for needle exchange even when injection of drugs is known to occur; HIV testing is inconsistent state to state, and testing is risky for inmates who may become the target for physical abuse secondary to racism and homophobia. ■ Disclosure may be mandatory to facility administrators. ■ Some states are not supportive of providing health care to inmates known to have HIV; inmates are not eligible for Medicaid or Medicare and therefore are without options for treatment. ■ Access to mental health or substance abuse rehabilitation often limited	■ Counseling re: risk reduction is more effective individually than in groups. ■ Inmates scheduled for release will need specific referrals for health care, mental health care, and substance abuse (where indicated). It is extremely useful to provide copies of medical records containing PPD results, immunizations, list of laboratory tests, and past and current medications. ■ Provide education re: prevention of exposure to organisms associated with opportunistic infections and in general about sexually transmitted diseases within the context of protecting the HIV-infected inmate from complications.
Substance users (Casey et al, 1996; Springer, 1992)	■ Transmission risk behavior is more likely when high or craving for drug. ■ Chaotic lifestyle secondary to altered mentation makes keeping appointments and medication schedules extremely difficult. ■ Medication gets lost, stolen. ■ Conflicts over pain medication create conflict with provider. ■ Rules about being clean and sober at clinic deters active users from seeking care. ■ Active users may have dual diagnosis of mental illness. ■ Nutrition ignored in favor of getting high ■ Self-medication with street drugs (including antiretrovirals) makes choosing regimens complicated. ■ Existence of drug interactions between street and prescribed medication also complicates care.	■ To treat active substance users, the provider has to be committed to dealing with the chaos and uncertainty that is the patient's real life. ■ Teach risk reduction. ■ Establish trust—it will take time. ■ Understand the patient's difficulty obtaining care, and work to overcome barriers; this may mean referral to a drop-in clinic, referral for detoxification or drug treatment. ■ If patient does not see the substance use as an issue, assess and if possible treat the presenting problem. ■ Manipulation is a survival tool for the active user—don't take it personally. ■ Decrease manipulation by establishing trust and setting limits where necessary. ■ Team approach with clear discussion among members decreases risk of "splitting."

(continued)

TABLE 41-1	HIV Care of Special Populations *(Continued)*

Special Population/Defining Characteristics	Specific Issues	Possible Interventions
Sex workers (Casey et al, 1996) People who exchange sex for money or drugs	■ Often considered disposable by the rest of society and lack power and self-esteem ■ May have mental illness or substance use issues ■ May be involved in a relationship that mandates continued sex work ■ Risk for workers higher than for customers because often the worker is in the receptive role ■ More money is offered for unprotected sex ■ High rate of STDs ■ Avoidance of care for fear of stigma attached to work ■ Poor nutrition and overall health maintenance	■ Establish trust by being nonjudgmental and respectful; make the clinical setting nonthreatening. ■ Teach risk reduction and negotiation of safer sex; screen often for STDs. ■ Refer to support groups that decrease feelings of hopelessness and isolation. ■ Address issues of substance use and mental illness. ■ Use team approach to address all needs—primary care, nursing, social work, and nutrition. ■ Work on health maintenance issues gradually.

[1] The CDC references from 1994 are used here to compare to census statistics, which were last gathered in 1990.

TABLE 41-2	Gynecologic Primary Care Considerations in the HIV-Positive Woman

CONTRACEPTION
(Carpenter, 1991)

Spermicides	■ In vitro activity against HIV ■ Ulcerative reactions with frequent use
Oral contraceptives	■ Possible drug interactions with rifampin, rifabutin, ampicillin, tetracycline
Intrauterine devices	■ Increased risk for HIV transmission ■ Increased risk for pelvic inflammatory disease ■ Should not be used in HIV+ women or women at risk for HIV

SEXUALLY TRANSMITTED DISEASES
(Augenbraun et al, 1995; Barbosa et al, 1997)

Herpes simplex virus	■ May demonstrate more severe, frequent, and atypical recurrences ■ Increased viral shedding while asymptomatic
Syphilis	■ Primary lesions probably more persistent ■ Abnormally high titers ■ Seroreconversion in advancing HIV disease ■ Increased risk of treatment failure
Pelvic inflammatory disease	■ HIV+ women are at increased risk ■ More severe presentation ■ Consider hospitalization for management, even if clinically mild case.

Human papilloma virus/Lower genital tract neoplasia
(Fruchter et al, 1996; Petry et al, 1996)
	■ Prevalence increases as CD4 count decreases.
	■ Repeat Pap smear twice within first year; if normal, repeat at least yearly.
	■ Repeat Paps more frequently when:
	  1. previous abnormal Pap smear
	  2. history of human papillomavirus infection
	  3. after treatment of abnormality
	  4. symptomatic HIV/CD4 < 500
	■ Refer for colposcopy when:
	  1. atypia/SIL on pap
	  2. history of untreated abnormal Pap
	  3. evidence of human papillomavirus

VULVOVAGINAL CANDIDIASIS
(Spinillo et al, 1994)

	■ Most common initial clinical manifestation of HIV ■ Tends to occur earlier than thrush or esophageal candida ■ At increased risk for species other than *Candida albicans*

Women and HIV

From 1990 to 1996, the incidence of AIDS rose three times faster in women than in men. Women now account for more than 92,200 (15%) of the cumulative AIDS cases in the United States (CDC, 1997b). For the first time, heterosexual sex rather than injection drug use is the leading cause of HIV transmission in women. African American and Hispanic women have consistently accounted for nearly 75% of AIDS cases, and in 1996 African American women represented more than half the new cases of AIDS (CDC, 1997b). As is the case for men, AIDS is the second leading cause of death for women ages 25 to 44. The prevalence of HIV infection among childbearing women nationwide is 1.6 per 1000, accounting for approximately 6500 births (Gwinn et al, 1991; Gwinn & Wortley, 1996).

Because the rate of HIV infection is disproportionately high among impoverished minority women, the social context of their lives is central to their experience and concerns about HIV. The primary care provider cannot separate the issues of poverty, minority status, substance use, gender, domestic violence, and isolation from medical care. Health care use is often sporadic and crisis-oriented as the competing concerns of housing, food, and health care for family members mesh (Anastasio et al, 1995; Hellinger, 1993; Casey et al, 1996; Ragsdale et al, 1995; Fox, 1995).

Although the natural history of HIV disease appears to be the same for both women and men, there tend to be some differences in clinical manifestations. Women appear to have a greater incidence of candidal esophagitis, a greater incidence of mucocutaneous herpes simplex ulcerations, and a low incidence of Kaposi sarcoma.

HIV may affect contraception as well as gynecologic problems (their frequency, presentation, natural history, and response to treatment). The primary care provider must be aware of the impact of HIV on these issues, for it can enable the identification of women at risk for HIV and can improve care to HIV-positive women (Table 41-2).

Studies in the United States show that HIV has not been demonstrated to affect the course or outcome of pregnancy; likewise, pregnancy does not affect HIV progression in woman (U.S. Public Health Service, 1997). Infection from the mother during pregnancy accounts for approximately 90% of cases of pediatric AIDS in the United States (CDC, 1994b). The use of zidovudine during pregnancy and labor and at delivery reduces the risk of HIV transmission by two thirds (CDC, 1994b). Before discussing a chemoprophylaxis regimen with the patient, the primary care provider should contact the CDC for the most current recommendation, as well as an obstetrician who specializes in HIV or an HIV subspecialist. Then the provider should discuss with and offer the patient the most current antepartum, intrapartum, and postpartum regimen (Casey et al., 1996; Landers, 1997).

In 1995, the U.S. Public Health Service (USPHS) issued recommendations for HIV counseling and voluntary testing of all pregnant women (CDC, 1995b). In addition, some states require testing of all newborns.

Occupational Hazards

As the AIDS epidemic expands, an increasing number of health care workers will encounter patients infected with HIV. The threat of occupational exposure to HIV is real but small. The average risk for HIV infection from all types of percutaneous exposures to HIV-infected blood is 0.3%, although it may be greater when the exposure involves a larger blood volume or a higher HIV titer in blood (*MMWR*, 1996).

Currently, there are 52 documented cases of HIV infection in health care workers as a result of occupational exposure (CDC, 1996). The Occupational Health and Safety Administration (OSHA), in an effort to minimize such exposures, developed the Bloodborne Pathogen Standard (*Rules and Regulations*, 1991). These government regulations require employers to protect employees by using universal precautions, having written exposure control plans, and adhering to the postexposure prophylaxis recommendations of the USPHS.

Postexposure prophylaxis with zidovudine (AZT) has been associated with a decrease of approximately 79% in the risk for HIV seroconversion after percutaneous exposure to HIV-infected blood (*MMWR*, 1996). Subsequently, the USPHS revised its recommendations to include lamivudine (3TC) and protease inhibitors, indinavir and/or nelfinavir (Table 41-3). In addition to chemoprophylaxis, the recommendations include the following:

- Postexposure prophylaxis should be implemented in consultation with persons having expertise in antiretroviral therapy and HIV transmission.
- Postexposure prophylaxis should be recommended in cases with the highest risk of HIV transmission and offered to those with lower-risk exposures.
- Postexposure prophylaxis should be administered within 1 to 2 hours after exposure for 4 weeks.

TABLE 41-3	Basic and Expanded Postexposure Prophylaxis Regimens	
Regimen Category	**Application**	**Drug Regimen**
Basic	Occupational HIV exposures for which there is a recognized transmission risk	4 weeks (28 days) of both zidovudine 600 mg every day in divided doses (ie, 300 mg twice a day, 200 mg 3 times a day, or 100 mg every 4 hours) **and** lamivudine 150 mg twice a day
Expanded	Occupational HIV exposures that pose an increased risk for transmission (eg, larger volume of blood and/or higher virus titer in blood)	Basic regimen plus **either** indinavir 800 mg every 8 hours **or** nelfinavir 750 mg 3 times a day*

* Indinavir should be taken on an empty stomach (ie, without food or with a light meal) and with increased fluid consumption (ie, drinking six 8-oz glasses of water throughout the day); nelfinavir should be taken with meals. (MMWR [1996]. Anergy skin testing and preventative therapy for HIV-infected persons: Revised recommendations. *MMWR 46* 1–10)

- If the patient's HIV status is unknown, postexposure prophylaxis should be administered on a case-by-case basis.
- Health care workers should receive counseling and medical evaluation at baseline and periodically for 6 months.
- If postexposure prophylaxis is used, drug toxicity monitoring (complete blood count, renal and hepatic function tests) should be done at baseline and at 2 weeks.
- Health care workers who receive postexposure prophylaxis should be enrolled in an anonymous registry developed by the CDC.

Prevention of exposure remains the key. Adherence to universal precautions and the use of needleless and protected needle intravenous systems can reduce the number of exposures in the workplace (Kelen et al, 1991; Ippolito et al, 1997).

HISTORY AND PHYSICAL EXAM

The finding of opportunistic infections makes it easier to diagnose HIV infection and AIDS. Patients, especially if asymptomatic, often do not know they are infected and may not even know they are at risk. A sexual history and a drug history should be part of every patient's evaluation. In addition, a history of blood transfusions before 1986 should be noted.

Screening for HIV

Early diagnosis of HIV with appropriate treatment can offer a patient many years of productive life. Making the diagnosis requires primary care providers to consider HIV screening for most patients and to suspect HIV infection in many situations (Table 41-4). With the spread of the epidemic into lower-risk

TABLE 41-4	Screening for HIV
Offer HIV testing to all patients	Sexually active/With history of chemical dependency
Strongly urge testing if patient	Is pregnant
	Is a male who has had sex with another man since 1976
	Has history of incarceration
	Has history of injecting drug use
	Received blood products in the US before 1986
	Received blood products while in developing country
	Has past or present sexually transmitted infection, including hepatitis B and C
	Has an abnormal Pap smear
	Has unexplained symptoms:
	fever
	persistent rash
	persistent diarrhea
	other symptoms of primary HIV infection
	Has unexplained laboratory findings:
	thrombocytopenia
	renal disease
	lymphopenia
	elevated serum protein
	Has any opportunistic condition, including:
	shingles
	thrush
	tuberculosis
	lymphoma

populations, it is prudent to offer HIV screening to all sexually active patients. In addition, it is good practice to offer testing to any patient with a history of chemical dependency because of the possibility of unprotected sex while intoxicated. The offer of testing provides an excellent opportunity to raise awareness of HIV among patients and to discuss the need for protection.

Risky behaviors can also be assessed during the history. Ownby, Ferri, and Vlahov (in Casey et al, 1996) stratified risky behavior as follows:

- The rate of HIV transmission is higher in injection drug use than in unsafe sex.
- The more sexual partners, the greater the risk for HIV exposure.
- Sexual activity has a high, medium, and circumstance-dependent HIV risk.

The most appropriate teaching strategy is one chosen by a provider who is aware of the patient's life, including cultural and socioeconomic factors. In addition, providers need to explore their own comfort with teaching risk-reduction behaviors. This is achieved by confronting their fears and prejudices as well as practicing such teaching.

Physical Exam

The standard physical exam includes serial assessments of weight and nutrition. A meticulous exam of the scalp and skin is essential (Table 41-5). The provider may first suspect HIV infection on finding specific conditions in the mouth. Oral hairy leukoplakia is a benign thickening of the mucosa in a corrugated pattern, often on the lateral surfaces of the tongue. Thrush (candidiasis) may present as erythema or more commonly as white, nonadherent plaques on the tongue, palate, buccal surfaces, or pharynx. The infection responds well to local or mild systemic antifungals. With more advanced immunosuppression, the infection involves the esophagus and may cause difficulty in swallowing solids. Severe, recurrent, or persistent herpes labialis is also common and responds to acyclovir and related drugs. Advanced gingivitis and periodontitis are also common and may interfere greatly with nutrition. Extensive treatment by a dentist is usually necessary. Kaposi sarcoma and bacillary angiomatosis can also present as oral lesions.

A funduscopic exam, a survey of lymph nodes, a neurologic exam (focusing on possible cognitive deficits and peripheral neuropathies), a routine cardiopulmonary exam, and a careful genital/rectal examination for coexisting diseases must also be done during the initial assessment, and any time there is a suspicion that one of these organ systems may have become involved.

Disease Course

ACUTE HIV INFECTION

Although a patient may present at any point during the disease, the first exposure to HIV infection typically manifests as a flu-like syndrome. From 50% to 90% of patients acutely infected will have some or all of the typical symptoms and signs, such as headache, fever, rash, and myalgias (Table 41-6). Symptomatic patients will have a marked transient drop in the CD4 count, and a few may even develop frank AIDS-defining conditions

TABLE 41-5		Common Skin Manifestations of HIV Disease	
Diagnosis	**CD4 Level**	**Appearance**	**Management**
Acute retroviral syndrome	Usually >200	Variable. Usually generalized nonpruritic, erythematous, maculopapular lesions, often with oral and genital ulcerative lesions	See text; consider aggressive, long-lasting combination antiretroviral medications
Seborrheic dermatitis	Any	Scaling lesions of scalp, face, chest, upper back, and groin	Topical steroids mixed with ketoconazole ointment. Refer for biopsy if no improvement.
Eosinophilic (pruritic) folliculitis	<200	Pruritic edematous or urticarial papules on face and upper torso with tiny central pustule	Refer for confirmatory biopsy. Bacterial culture of lesions for possible *S. aureus*. Continuous topical steroids and oral antifungal medication.
Shingles (herpes zoster)	Usually <500	Classic large and small grouped umbilicated vesicles on an erythematous base in dermatome distribution. If ophthalmic branch of trigeminal nerve involved, vision is threatened	Acyclovir, valacyclovir, or famcyclovir as soon as possible after onset of rash to minimize postherpetic neuralgia. If severe, refer for admission. May recur; may require suppressive therapy.
Herpes simplex	Any	Classic small grouped vesicles on erythematous base, usually on lips, in mouth, on genitals or perineum but may be on skin surface	Acyclovir, famcyclovir, or valacyclovir. May need suppressive therapy. If medication resistance develops or severe involvement, admit for intravenous medication.
Molluscum contagiosum	Usually <200	Pearly papules with central umbilication on face and groin	Benign. Dermatologist may curette for cosmetic purposes.
Scabies	Usually <200	Highly pruritic with very variable appearance, usually with scaling of palms and soles. Severe cases associated with bacterial sepsis.	Microscopic examination of scraping. Topical medication and environmental controls as in non-HIV patients.
Psoriasis	Any	Classic appearance but may be very severe in HIV patient	Treatment-resistant cases may respond to etretinate or zidovudine.
Hidradenitis suppurativa	Any	Classic appearance in axillae and groin but may be very severe in HIV patient	Aggressive management with bacterial cultures, I and D of abscesses, antibiotics. Smear and culture to rule out TB.
Photosensitivity reactions	Any	Classic, but more severe in HIV	Same as non-HIV patient
Drug reactions	Any	Classic, but more common and more severe in HIV	Same as in non-HIV patient
Kaposi sarcoma	Usually <350	Purple macules, papules, or nodules on any skin or mucosal surface. Very rare in women.	Refer suspect lesions for biopsy. Refer to oncologist for treatment.
Bacillary angiomatosis	Usually <200	Highly variable vascular proliferative lesion. May be indistinguishable from Kaposi sarcoma. May have associated necrotizing lymph node.	Refer suspect lesion for biopsy. Treat with oral macrolides.
Warts	Any	Same as in non-HIV but may show exuberant growth	Same as non-HIV patient

TABLE 41-6	Acute Retroviral Syndrome: Symptoms and Signs
Symptoms	Sore throat
	Myalgias or arthralgias
	Headache
	Nausea and vomiting
	Diarrhea
	Weight loss
Signs	Fever
	Lymphadenopathy
	Rash
	■ erythematous maculopapular lesions on face and trunk, sometimes on extremities including palms and soles
	■ mucocutaneous ulceration involving mouth, esophagus, or genitals
	Hepatosplenomegaly
	Thrush
	Neurologic symptoms
	■ aseptic meningitis or meningoencephalitis
	■ peripheral neuropathy or radiculopathy
	■ facial palsy
	■ Guillain-Barré syndrome
	■ Brachial neuritis
	■ Cognitive impairment or psychosis

Source: Panel, 1997.

that resolve with a rebound in the CD4 count and a drop in viral load. Patients with severe acute retroviral syndromes are more likely to have a rapidly progressive downhill course. This viral syndrome lasts several days and then resolves spontaneously.

EARLY DISEASE: ASYMPTOMATIC STAGE

With the resolution of any acute retroviral syndrome, the patient enters a phase of asymptomatic disease that usually lasts 5 or more years. Some patients, so-called nonprogressors, remain asymptomatic for 20 or more years, probably because a nonlethal, defective strain of virus has infected them. Other patients have a rapid downhill course and die within 2 or 3 years (the "crash and burn" syndrome), usually because mutations in the virus have produced a highly lethal strain.

HIV infection begins with acute transmission and primary infection, followed by seroconversion about 6 to 12 weeks later. Although there appears to be a period of clinical latency, we now know that viral replication is constant (see the section on pathophysiology below). The current staging of HIV disease is not clinically distinct. Although the CDC revised the AIDS-defining criteria in 1993 (CDC, 1993), this system does not take into account the amount of HIV present (the viral load or viral burden). As measures of circulating HIV RNA become more accessible, this staging system will need significant revision.

A prospective evaluation of gay men called the Multicenter AIDS Cohort Study has shown that persons with persistently high levels of viremia more rapidly progress to AIDS and death (Mellors et al, 1996). The advent of combination antiretroviral therapy has significantly affected the course of disease; thus,

prediction of survival is not as clear as it may have seemed before 1995. Even when the disease has failed to respond to these therapies, life can be prolonged simply by using recommended prophylaxis for known opportunistic infections.

MONITORING THE RATE OF PROGRESSION

The progression of HIV disease is quite variable. Newer therapies change the prognosis, and as providers become more adept at managing intercurrent illness, the course is prolonged (Kitahata et al, 1996). Both the durability and the magnitude of the virologic response affect progression to AIDS. Recent studies have shown that the viral load at baseline is a strong predictor of the rapidity of progression to AIDS, regardless of the CD4 count (Mellors et al, 1997; DHHS, 1997).

Persons infected with HIV-1 represent a normal distribution of response to the virus. A few are rapid progressors who develop full-blown AIDS in 2 to 3 years. Five percent to 12% are long-term nonprogressors who have lived for 10 or more years without symptoms or therapy (Cao et al, 1995; Pantaleo, 1995). The majority fall somewhere in between and need to be characterized by their immune response and their burden of viral activity.

STAGING THE DISEASE

Laboratory evaluation of the blood is especially important in staging the disease. Baseline screening for HIV-associated diseases such as syphilis, cervical cancer, and hepatitis B help stage HIV disease, as well as identifying anemia and neutropenia (see the section on diagnostic studies below). However, the most important blood tests for determining the patient's stage of HIV disease are the CD4 T-cell count and quantitative HIV RNA (viral loads). The CD4 count is known to be influenced by many factors such as diurnal variation, intercurrent infection, and substance use. Since the viral load has come into use, most surrogate markers are no longer as useful as they once were for staging. Viral quantitation should not be obtained when the person is ill or within 4 weeks of an immunization, because the viral burden is increased in those situations.

Originally, the definition of AIDS was made clinically, including multiple conditions of immunosuppression. In 1993, the definition was expanded to include invasive cervical carcinoma, recurrent bacterial infections, and *Mycobacterium tuberculosis* (Table 41-7). Persons with a CD4 count of less than 200 cells/mm³ were also classified as having AIDS, regardless of their clinical picture.

The current staging system for HIV disease uses the absence or presence of symptoms and is related to the CD4 count. However, staging and consequently management are more appropriately based on viral load. Exact correlations of these two measures have not been clearly established, but a change in the plasma viral load of 2.5-fold or more probably indicates a true biologic change (Casey et al, 1996).

LATE DISEASE

Later during the disease course, the patient may develop opportunistic infection, wasting syndrome, chronic diarrhea, or any of the other AIDS indicator diseases listed in Table 41-7. The primary care provider must be able to assess HIV-positive patients in a rapid and systematic manner, regardless of their CD4 count, and identify serious opportunistic complications. Table

TABLE 41-7	AIDS Indicator Diseases

Candidiasis—esophagus, trachea, bronchi, or lungs

Cervical cancer, invasive

Coccidioidomycosis, extrapulmonary

Cryptococcoses, extrapulmonary

Cryptosporidiosis with diarrhea >1 month

Cytomegalovirus outside of liver, spleen, or lymph nodes

Herpes simplex with mucocutaneous ulcer >1 month or in lungs or esophagus

Histoplasmosis, extrapulmonary

HIV-associated dementia

HIV-associated wasting: involuntary weight loss >10% of baseline plus chronic diarrhea; or chronic weakness and documented fever without cause >30 days

Isosporosis with diarrhea >1 month

Kaposi sarcoma if patient is <60 years

Lymphoma, non-Hodgkin's B cell or immunoblastic

Mycobacterium avium, disseminated

Mycobacterium tuberculosis, disseminated or pulmonary

Nocardiosis

Pneumocystis carinii pneumonia

Pneumonia, recurrent bacterial (>2 episodes/12 months)

Progressive multifocal leukoencephalopathy

Salmonella septicemia (nontyphoid), recurrent

Strongyloidosis, extraintestinal

Toxoplasmosis of an internal organ

Adapted from Bartlett, 1997.

41-8 presents one such approach. The primary care provider should be familiar with the manifestations of these diseases.

Opportunistic Infections

Although it is beyond the scope of this chapter to discuss all opportunistic infections in detail, the primary care provider should be familiar with the identification and significance of certain infections. The prevention of opportunistic infections is well defined. The guiding principle is simple: primary prophylaxis, when possible, is best (See Table 41-9). Currently, the USPHS and the Infectious Disease Society of America (CDC, 1997c) strongly recommend primary prophylaxis as a standard of care for *Pneumocystis carinii* pneumonia (PCP), *Mycobacterium avium* complex, *Toxoplasma gondii* infection, and TB. In addition, prophylaxis for *Streptococcus pneumoniae* and varicella is warranted.

TUBERCULOSIS

TB is common early and is often the initial manifestation of immunodeficiency. In some cities, as many as half of all cases of TB occur in HIV-infected persons. Its clinical course is more rapid, more virulent, and more varied in the presence of HIV, with the potential to kill patients within weeks of the onset of symptoms. Active TB in the HIV-positive patient often has an atypical presentation. Pulmonary TB may occur in the lower lobes with an x-ray picture that is negative or identical to other forms of pneumonia. Extrapulmonary TB commonly presents as meningitis, pericarditis, adenitis, or dermatitis. Any patient with a history of fever and cough should have at least three induced sputa cultured for TB. The workup of a lesion anywhere in the body likewise should usually include TB cultures and microscopic examination of biopsy samples or aspirates for acid-fast bacilli.

Once diagnosed, the treatment and prognosis of tuberculosis in the HIV-positive patient is the same as in other populations (see Chap. 75 for more information on TB).

Because active TB is particularly dangerous for the HIV-infected patient, each must be screened for the possibility of latent infection. Every patient with a positive PPD test on entry and without a history of previous full prophylaxis should receive a 6- to 12-month course of isoniazid (INH). In some areas, programs of directly observed preventive therapy are available for patients who are unlikely to adhere reliably to the regimen. Likewise, every patient with a history of a positive PPD test who has not received prophylaxis should receive a full course of INH. Patients with current or past positive skin tests should receive INH even if they give a history of BCG immunization. Reactivity to the tuberculin test protein wanes quickly with progression of immunodeficiency, so anergy testing is part of each PPD test (*MMWR*, 1997). If the patient is anergic, the provider must maintain a high level of vigilance for reactivation of latent infection and for the occurrence of new infection.

To prevent new infection with the tubercle bacillus, patients need to learn to avoid high-risk situations (prisons and homeless shelters) and persons (anyone with a chronic cough). Public health authorities have traced many outbreaks of TB in HIV-positive patients to exposure in clinic waiting rooms and on hospital wards. Patient care areas must maintain current standards for environmental controls and for isolation of potentially infectious persons to prevent transmission of TB among patients and staff (*MMWR*, 1994).

PNEUMOCYSTIS CARINII PNEUMONIA

PCP has changed from a major killer in AIDS to a usually preventable and treatable condition (see Table 41-9). Because the infection results in lasting damage to the lungs, diagnosis and treatment should be prompt. The provider should suspect the diagnosis in any patient with a fever and cough who is not receiving prophylaxis and has either a CD4 count of less than 200 or previous symptoms of immunodeficiency, such as thrush. The typical history is one of gradually worsening dyspnea, nonproductive cough, and constitutional symptoms, but rapid development of symptoms and productive cough from secondary bacterial infections can occur. Examination of the lungs may be normal or may reveal basilar rales. The chest x-ray may be normal or may show bilateral reticular infiltrates with thin-walled pneumatoceles, pneumothorax, or other patterns. Serum lactate dehydrogenase levels are often high. The clinical presentation can be indistinguishable from TB and many other opportunistic infections. Diagnosis depends on identification of the organism, either in bronchoalveolar lavage specimens obtained at bronchoscopy or occasionally in induced sputa, if the laboratory technician is specially trained. Patients suspected of having PCP should be admitted to the hospital for evaluation and treatment.

TABLE 41-8 Partial Guidelines for a Symptom-Based Approach to the HIV-Positive Patient

Symptom	Differential Diagnosis	Workup	Management
COUGH			
CD4 > 300	TB, sinusitis, bronchitis, bacterial pneumonia, other conditions same as non-HIV	CBC, sputum cultures: routine* and AFB, blood cultures,* chest x-ray, possible chest and sinus CT scan**	Treat aggressively; refer if working diagnosis not confirmed or if cough does not abate with treatment. For infiltrate on chest x-ray refer for bronchoscopy; if sinusitis persists or recurs, refer to ENT.
CD4 < 300	All of above; if thrush present include PCP in differential	Same as above, plus induced sputum for PCP***	Same as above; admit if febrile; refer rapidly for bronchoscopy if diagnosis not confirmed or symptoms persist
CD4 < 200	All of above plus fungal pneumonias and Kaposi sarcoma	Same as above	Same as above; refer rapidly—rapid decompensation possible
CD4 < 100	All of above plus atypical mycobacteria and other uncommon organisms	Same as above	Same as above
WEIGHT LOSS			
CD4 > 500	Acute retroviral syndrome, depression, social problems, TB	Full dietary and social history, induced sputa for AFB, chest x-ray, CBC, SMA20	Referrals to social worker and dietitian, possible psychiatric referral, monitor weight carefully
CD4 200–500	Depression, social problems, TB, dental problems, anorexia or nausea as medication side effects, oroesophageal candidiasis, any other opportunistic infection or malignancy	Same as above; medication review, chest x-ray, possible barium swallow, blood and induced sputa for AFB cultures, symptom-related workup (eg, for diarrhea)	Same as above; dental referral as warranted, aggressive nutritional support, refer rapidly if no etiology for weight loss identified
CD4 < 200	Same as above plus oral ulcers, hepatobiliary disease, and malabsorption	Same as above; culture oral ulcers for herpes	Same as above; refer as needed for biopsy of oral lesions or endoscopy, consult for possible pharmacologic intervention for anorexia or wasting
CD4 < 100	Same as above, plus disseminated atypical mycobacterial infection	Serial blood cultures for mycobacteria	Same as above; possible referral for bone marrow biopsy and culture for mycobacteria
VISUAL CHANGES			
CD4 > 200	Aseptic cerebromeningitis from acute retroviral syndrome, neurosyphilis, zoster ophthalmicus, intracranial mass	Serum VDRL/RPR/STS, serum toxoplasmosis titer, full ophthalmoscopic and neurologic exam and cognitive screening, head CT	Refer immediately to ophthalmologist or neurologist, admission likely for lumbar puncture
CD4 < 200	Neurosyphilis, intracranial mass, especially toxoplasmosis or lymphoma, HIV cerebrovasculitis or stroke	Same as above	Refer immediately as above
CD4 < 100	Same as above plus cytomegalovirus retinitis and PML	Same as above	Refer immediately as above
HEADACHE			
CD4 > 200	Same as non-HIV patient especially sinusitis plus aseptic cerebromeningitis from acute retroviral syndrome, neurosyphilis, TB meningitis, intracranial mass, and side effect of medication	Medication review, full neurologic exam with cognitive screening, CT of head and sinuses, serum VDRL/RPR/STS, serum toxoplasmosis titer	Refer quickly for lumbar puncture if diagnosis not established or not responding to treatment
CD4 < 200	Neurosyphilis, sinusitis, intracranial mass, side effect of medication, TB meningitis, viral encephalitis (herpes simplex, cytomegalovirus), fungal meningitis (cryptococcus, histoplasmosis, coccidioidomycosis, other)	Same as above plus serum cryptococcal antigen	Refer quickly for admission/lumbar puncture, rapid decompensation possible
Fever	Acute retroviral syndrome, TB, any infection or neoplasm	CBC, SMA20, induced sputa for AFB, routine and AFB blood and urine cultures, chest x-ray	Pursue diagnosis aggressively; if no specific diagnosis confirmed, refer or consult with infectious disease specialist

(continued)

TABLE 41-8	Partial Guidelines for a Symptom-Based Approach to the HIV-Positive Patient *(Continued)*		
Symptom	**Differential Diagnosis**	**Workup**	**Management**
DIARRHEA			
CD4 > 200	Lactose intolerance, medication side effect, food poisoning, bacterial infection****, common viral infections (eg, rotavirus, adenovirus), giardiasis, amebiasis, *Blastocystis hominis*, gonococcal and chlamydial colitis	Full dietary and household history, medication review, CBC, stool cultures, stool for *Calostridium difficile*, stools for ova and parasites, routine blood cultures if febrile	Consider adjusting offending medications, nutritional support, weight monitoring, specific treatment for pathogen and symptom relief, refer to gastroenterologist if diarrhea persists
CD4 < 200	All of above plus unusual parasitoses, atypical mycobacteria, cytomegalovirus colitis	Same as above; blood cultures for mycobacteria	Same as above; aggressive management indicated

* Consult with lab on specimen submission for *Streptococcus pneumoniae, Staphylococcus aureus, Haemophilus influenzae, Moraxella catarrhalis, Mycoplasma pneumoniae, Bordatella* species, *Rhodococcus equi*, and *Legionella pneumophilia.*

** Sinus films not sensitive enough for diagnosis of sinusitis

*** Consult with lab on specimen submission; requires specially trained technician.

**** *Salmonella* species, *Shigella* species, *C. difficile, Campylobacter jejeuni*, enteropathic *E. coli*

SKIN AND ORAL LESIONS

Rashes and oral lesions are particularly bothersome. Oral lesions, such as candidal lesions, especially when they cause esophagitis, may cause severe dysphagia. Even when hungry, the patient may not be able to eat. In addition, lesions of hairy oral leukoplakia may be uncomfortable. Skin lesions, such as herpes, Kaposi sarcoma, or even seborrheic dermatitis, may be noticeable by friends and colleagues. This may make patients extremely uncomfortable, especially when their HIV status is not disclosed (see Table 41-5).

CYTOMEGALOVIRUS INFECTION

Cytomegalovirus is a systemic viral infection in late-stage disease that can present as esophagitis, colitis, encephalitis, or chorioretinitis. For the primary care provider, infection of the eye is of primary concern because it can lead to rapid, irreversible destruction of vision. Retinal lesions have a characteristic appearance on funduscopy and are an indication for immediate hospital admission for prolonged intravenous treatment. Patients with a CD4 count below 100 need evaluation by an ophthalmologist every 3 to 6 months.

DISSEMINATED ATYPICAL MYCOBACTERIAL INFECTIONS

When the CD4 count drops to less than 100, the patient is at risk for the development of disseminated atypical mycobacterial infections. A group of bacteria related to TB bacteria, but less virulent, can colonize the intestinal tract and later penetrate the gut wall for hematogenous spread to all organs, especially the liver, spleen, and marrow, with resultant severe anemia. It is a common cause of death in late-stage patients. Symptoms are diarrhea, intermittent night sweats, fevers, weight loss, and fatigue. Diagnosis is by repeated blood cultures with special media. Suppressive therapy is suboptimal, so prevention is the goal (see Table 41-9).

TOXOPLASMOSIS

Toxoplasmosis is caused by the intracellular parasite *T. gondii.* It is usually transmitted orally. When the immune system is intact, infection is usually undetected. However, in a patient with AIDS, it may be rapidly fatal if left untreated. Clinical manifestations of *T gondii* infection are often that of central nervous system infection, including seizures, headaches, encephalitis, altered mental status, and focal neurologic deficits, mimicking a stroke. In addition, ocular infections occur, with chorioretinitis and blindness.

Testing for titers can be done. Elevated IgM titers are significant for acute infection, as are circulating IgA antibodies. The IgG titers will always be elevated once the patient is infected, but an acute rise in titers may represent recrudescent infection. Most cases of encephalitis occur when the CD4 count falls to less than 100.

DIAGNOSTIC STUDIES

Methods for Making the Diagnosis

The standard method for diagnosing HIV disease is to detect antibodies to HIV-1 using a plasma ELISA screening assay. The Western blot is used by the laboratory as a confirmatory test. Both tests can produce false-negative results in the 6 to 12 weeks after an acute exposure and should be repeated in 3 months. Infrequently, there are subtypes of HIV not detected by standard assays. Persons who are suspected of being positive or who are symptomatic with persistently negative tests should be referred to an HIV-experienced provider or to the CDC.

There are alternative testing methods available. Home test kits are commercially available for $33 to $50 from Direct Access Diagnostics (1-800-HIV-TEST). The sensitivity and specificity approach 100%. Results are given over the phone, and those with positive tests speak with a counselor. Currently, three FDA-licensed rapid HIV testing methods are available (Irwin et al, 1996). In addition, a salivary test (1-800-ORASURE, ext. 302) is available to providers (Gall et al, 1997). All of these tests are accurate and can serve as reasonable alternatives to the ELISA/Western blot method.

It is important to consider the amount of counseling available before and after the test. Although laws concerning consent for testing differ among states, most states require that a multitude of topics regarding risk factors, safer sex techniques, and discrimination possibilities (eg, employment, insurance, and relationship or living situations) be discussed before and after testing is done. Essential parts of informing a patient of a positive test result are shown in Table 41-10.

TABLE 41-9	Prophylaxis for First Episode of Opportunistic Disease in HIV-Infected Adults and Adolescents

		Preventive Regimens	
Pathogen	Indication	First Choice	Alternatives
STRONGLY RECOMMENDED AS STANDARD OF CARE			
Pneumocystis carinii	CD4+ count <200μL or oropharyngeal candidiasis or unexplained fever $\geq$2 weeks	Trimethoprim-sulfamethoxazole (TMP-SMZ), 1 DS po q.d. (AI); TMP-SMZ, 1 SS po q.d. (AI)	TMP-SMZ, 1 DS po t.i.w. (BIII); dapsone, 50 mg po b.i.d. or 100 mg po q.d. (BI); dapsone, 50 mg po q.d. plus pyrimethamine, 50 mg po q.w. plus leucovorin, 25 mg po q.w. (BI); dapsone, 200 mg po plus pyrimethamine, 75 mg po plus leucovorin, 25 mg po q.w. (BI); aerosolized pentamidine, 300 mg q.m. via Respirgard II™ nebulizer (BI)
Mycobacterium tuberculosis isoniazid-sensitive	TST reaction $\geq$5 mm or prior positive TST result without treatment or contact with case of active tuberculosis	Isoniazid, 300 mg po plus pyridoxine, 50 mg po q.d.x 12 mo (A1) or isoniazid, 900 mg po plus pyridoxine, 50 mg po b.i.w. × 12 mo (BIII)	Rifampin, 600 mg po q.d. × 12 mo (BII)
Isoniazid-resistant	Same; high probability of exposure to isoniazid-resistant tuberculosis	Rifampin, 600 mg po q.d. × 12 mo (BII)	Rifabutin, 300 mg po q.d. × 12 mo (CIII)
Multidrug- (isoniazid and rifampin) resistant	Same; high probability of exposure to multidrug-resistant tuberculosis	Choice of drugs requires consultation with public health authorities	None
Toxoplasma gondi	IgG antibody to Toxoplasma and CD4+ count <100/μL	TMP-SMZ, 1 DS po q.d. (AII)	TMP-SMZ, 1 SS po q.d. (BIII): dapsone, 50 mg po q.d. plus pyrimethamine, 50 mg po q.w. plus leucovorin, 25 mg po q.w. (BI)
Mycobacterium avium complex	CD4+ count <50/μL	Clarithromycin, 500 mg po b.i.d. (AI) or azithromycin, 1,200 mg po q.w. (AI)	Rifabutin, 300 mg po q.d. (BI); azithromycin, 1,200 mg po q.w. plus rifabutin, 300 mg po q.d. (CI)
Streptococcus pneumoniae	All patients	Pneumococcal vaccine, 0.5 mL im × 1 (CD4+ $\geq$200/μL [AII]; CD4+ <200/μL [CIII])	None
Varicella zoster virus (VZV)	Significant exposure to chickenpox or shingles for patients who have no history of either condition or, if available, negative antibody to VZV	Varicella zoster immune globulin (VZIG), 5 vials (1.25 mL each) im, administered $\leq$96 h after exposure, ideally within 48 h (AIII)	Acyclovir, 800 mg po 5 times/d for 3 weeks (CIII)
GENERALLY RECOMMENDED			
Hepatitis B virus	All susceptible (anti-HBc-negative) patients	Engerix B®, 20 μg im × 3 (BII); or Recombivax HB®, 10 μg im × 3 (BII)	None
Influenza virus	All patients (annually, before influenza season)	Whole or split virus, 0.5 mL im/yr (BIII)	Rimantadine, 100 mg po b.i.d. (CIII) or amantadine, 100 mg po b.i.d. (CIII)

Source: CDC. (1997). US Public Health Service/Infectious Disease Society of America guidelines for the prevention of opportunistic infections in persons infected with HIV. MMWR, 46 28–29.

Recently, two assays for measuring the plasma HIV RNA have become commercially available. The polymerase chain reaction and bDNA (branched DNA) essentially measure the number of replications of the virus in 1 mL of plasma. The viral concentration can usually be measured to the level of 400 copies/mL (Ho, 1996). The newer, more sensitive assays measure to less than 20 copies/mL, but the added expense is not warranted unless there is reason to suspect that the patient actually has progressive disease. Although the values from each test are similar, they cannot be directly compared. The levels appear to reflect true disease activity and are not always well correlated with the traditional CD4 cell count. Quantitative HIV RNA has become the standard for staging disease and monitoring response to retroviral therapy.

Once the patient begins an antiviral regimen, the viral load should be measured every 3 to 6 months using the same method and preferably the same laboratory. Response to therapy should be based on comparisons of samples evaluated in the same laboratory using the same method before and after changes in therapy.

The CD4 cell count remains a pivotal test for determining the stage of disease, providing guidelines for differential diagnosis of symptoms, and making therapeutic decisions regarding prophylaxis for opportunistic infections. Generally, the provider should perform a CD4 cell count and HIV RNA at the same time. Together, these tests more accurately interpret the patient's response to antiviral therapy. The normal CD4 value for most laboratories is a mean of 800 to 1050.

TABLE 41-10	Components of Informing a Patient With a Positive HIV Test Result

- Schedule a face-to-face meeting with the patient at the time the test is done to discuss the results.

- Encourage the patient to bring a supportive friend to the follow-up appointment in case the result is positive.

- Do not give positive results over the phone, but do reach out to patients who do not appear for their results.

- Be prepared to deal with the natural reactions of denial, anger, guilt, and sadness in the patient. Provide as much emotional support as possible and have available referral resources for ongoing supportive counseling.

- Determine with the patient what his or her immediate plan is:
  What will he or she do immediately on leaving your office?
  Is suicide a risk?
  Is relapse into self-destructive patterns, such as drinking or drugging, a risk?
  Who in the personal support system will be available to the patient that day? in the coming week?
  How will sexual or needle-sharing partners be informed of their risk?

- Offer to assist personally or through referral to public health programs with the notification and counseling of partners.

- Provide as much factual information as the patient is able to absorb. Emphasize the new advances in treatments, the value of regular medical follow-up, and your ongoing availability to the patient. Give literature for the patient to read later.

- Begin or schedule in the immediate future the needed baseline medical evaluation.

Routine Laboratory Studies for HIV-Positive Patients

Routine screening tests (complete blood count, urinalysis, liver function tests, and electrolytes; Table 41-11) are used to establish a baseline. Other special tests may be essential. In areas with a high TB prevalence, PPD testing every 6 months is appropriate; in other areas, yearly testing suffices. Screening for G-6-PD deficiency on the initial visit protects against inadvertent prescribing of hemolytic medications such as dapsone and trimethoprim–sulfamethoxazole for the prophylaxis of PCP and toxoplasmosis. A negative titer for toxoplasmosis indicates the need for education on preventing toxoplasmosis infection. Screening for syphilis (VDRL, RPR, STS) is vital because the course of infection may differ in patients with HIV from that in immunocompetent patients. In particular, all HIV patients with latent syphilis require a lumbar puncture to rule out neurosyphilis. The primary care provider should contact the CDC to ascertain the most recent treatment recommendations. Some providers also screen for cytomegalovirus IgG; others prefer active surveillance for infection in those with CD4 counts of less than 100.

Cervical disease is common in women with HIV, and progression to invasive cancer has occurred in less than 1 year after an abnormal Pap smear. The initial evaluation should include a full pelvic examination with a wet mount, as well as cultures for gonococcal and chlamydial infections.

Baseline ophthalmologic and dental examinations are recommended. The frequency of ophthalmologic evaluations should increase when the CD4 count is less than 100 (Sanda, 1997).

TABLE 41-11	Baseline Screening Tests
Test	**Comment**
HIV serology	1) Repeat test for patients with positive test results 2) Repeat if no confirmation is available 3) Repeat if denial of HIV risk factors
CBC with differential	
VDRL or RPR	
CD4 cell count and % Viral load	Perform tests concurrently at a time of clinical stability and >4 weeks from immunizations or infectious illness
Serum chemistries	To include liver function studies and BUN/creatinine
Hepatitis B serology	HbsAB, HbsAg, to determine if patient will need hepatitis B vaccination
PPD skin test	In previously negative patients
Pap smear, gonorrhea/ chlamydia cultures	
CMV IgG	Assists in differential diagnosis of possible CMV disease in latestage HIV infection
Toxoplasmosis serology	Assists in differential diagnosis of central nervous system complications; if seronegative, a candidate for counseling to prevent infection
Urinalysis	
Glucose-6-phosphate dehydrogenase level (G-6-PD)	Deficiency indicates a genetic disease (most prevalent in African Americans and men from Mediterranean areas, India, and Southeast Asia) that predisposes to hemolytic anemia after exposure to oxidant drugs; can be life-threatening.
Varicella zoster serology	Performed on patients with no history of chickenpox
OPTIONAL STUDIES	
Hepatitis C serology	With abnormal liver function tests
Chest x-ray	Indicated with a positive PPD or pulmonary symptoms

Adapted from Bartlett, 1997.

TREATMENT, EXPECTED OUTCOMES, AND COMPREHENSIVE MANAGEMENT

Establishing Care

The primary care provider should prepare for a long-term relationship marked by growing mutual trust and understanding. Table 41-12 lists some of the factors proven to correlate with the ability of a provider to engage a patient successfully in care. It is not unusual for patients to present for care for the first time many months or even years after they have learned of their HIV infection. The compassionate provider accepts the difficulty the patient has had in dealing with this diagnosis and praises the patient for coming for care. It is also not unusual for a patient to present for care after having been in treatment in one or more other locations. The reasons for transferring should be tactfully explored and the history of previous antiretroviral medications recorded. Any patient who requests care for HIV infection should supply documentation of a positive

TABLE 41-12	**Factors Promoting Patient Adherence to Medical Regimens**
Provider factors	Effective communication • Verbal, video, and written instructions including rationale for treatment • Clear, direct messages • Active listening skills Inclusion of patient in decision making • Tailor regimen to patient's schedule and needs • Contract with patient on what provider and patient will do • Negotiate goals and plan for reaching goals • Nonjudgmental follow-up and renegotiation as needed Use of cognitive–behavioral techniques • Schedule medications around daily cues (eg, brushing teeth, daily soap opera, etc.) • Give organizer boxes for weekly medications
System factors	Short waiting time in clinic Preappointment reminders Telephone follow-up Family, group, and individual counseling

Adapted from Miller et al, 1997; Haynes et al, 1996; Cramer, 1995.

test result or submit to retesting, because as many as 5% of people reporting the diagnosis are in fact uninfected (Haynes et al, 1996).

Maintaining Care

Patients present for care at all stages of infection. The well-prepared primary care provider who devotes the time to remaining current in HIV care can routinely manage the early stage of disease. Management of late-stage disease is much more complex: rapid changes in clinical knowledge and the use of specialized diagnostic techniques are the norm, and referrals to HIV specialists are often required. Both the primary provider and the health care setting need adaptation to provide this care. Maintaining a routine data base and summary sheet helps organize key elements of the patient's care for ready reference. Figure 41-2 is a sample summary sheet.

The relationship with the patient is one that will grow over years during contacts that vary from routine periodic screening to acute care visits to emergency care visits. The patient should be encouraged to bring significant family members and friends. The limits of what the patient wants disclosed to others should be clarified ahead of time. At every visit, the provider should continue to educate the patient about aspects of the disease, review measures to prevent transmission to others, and check self-care activities (see the section on teaching and self-care below). An integrated, multidisciplinary approach, using nurses, social workers, dietitians, dentists, psychiatrists, and HIV specialists, must be used (see the section on referrals below). At every visit, the provider monitors the progression of the disease, the response to treatment, and the possible emergence of new complications.

Adherence

Patients must understand that starting treatment means making a commitment to take full doses of all medications every time, every day, indefinitely. The primary care provider should initi-

ate treatment only when the patient is ready. Readiness implies not only a psychological willingness but also a practical ability to maintain a daily regimen of multiple doses of several medications. Some patients are eager to start medications but must wait until their prescription benefits are in place. Other patients prefer to delay starting medications until they leave homeless shelters for stable housing because they have no safe place to store medications. Others prefer to discuss the decision with family members and friends before making the commitment. Pressuring patients to start treatment before they are ready, or with medications that they distrust, leads to poor adherence to the regimen and a poor therapeutic effect. The medication regimens are very difficult to follow: some medications must be taken on an empty stomach and others with food. Because of the difficult timing and quantity of pills, there should be more than one source of teaching in the office or clinic. Patients must be counseled about the possible failure rates of the protease inhibitors when doses are missed or not taken as directed. Office contacts should be scheduled frequently enough that the patient receives support and encouragement for maintaining the regimen. These visits may be conducted by nurses or other knowledgeable staff members (Williams & Frieland, 1997).

Early Disease

If patients are diagnosed soon after exposure, they should be treated aggressively with a triple-drug regimen. Exactly which drugs to use is debated. This would be a time to contact the CDC or the National Institute of Allergy and Infectious Diseases to determine whether the patient should be entered in a treatment protocol.

Early treatment may be difficult because the patient often feels well. Despite recommendations for early aggressive therapy, the patient must be able to understand and accept the regimen. It is worth one or two preliminary office visits to discuss this at length before prescribing any regimen. Including supportive friends or family may also be helpful.

Current clinical trials will resolve the question of whether antiretroviral treatment should be started at this phase. The current treatment guidelines (Miller et al, 1997) note the theoretical rationale for early intervention with triple therapy:

- To suppress the initial burst of viral replication and check the degree of dissemination in the body
- To lessen the severity of the acute syndrome
- To alter potentially the theoretical viral "set point" that may determine the rate of progression
- To reduce possibly the rate of viral mutation by lowering the number of virus.

If the provider and patient agree to begin medications, the recommended combination is two NRTIs and one protease inhibitor. Some may also use an NNRTI. The goal is to drive the viral load below the detectable level. Once treatment begins, it should continue for at least 1 year and probably indefinitely, because viremia rapidly re-emerges.

Recommendations for treatment are rated on an alphabetic and numeric system. Both the strength of the recommendation and the basis for the recommendation are included (Table 41-13).

Name _____ Record # _____

Primary provider _____ Case manager _____

HIV positive test date __/__/__ Documented? [ ] yes [ ] no

Previous antiretroviral rx? [ ] no [ ] yes Meds/dates __

Intake CD4 _____ (%) Intake viral load (1ˢᵗ) _____, (2ⁿᵈ) _____

G6PD test: date __/__/__ Result [ ] normal [ ] low

Immunizations

Initial hepatitis B status: [ ] immune [ ] infected [ ] needs vaccine

HepB vaccine: Initial __/__/__ 1 month __/__/__ 6 months __/__/__

Varicella status: [ ] hx of chickenpox [ ] positive titer [ ] susceptible

Varicella vaccine: __/__/__ Pneumovax (once) __/__/__

Diphtheria/tetanus (q 10 yrs) __/__/__

TB history

Ever had active TB? [ ] no [ ] yes __/__/__ Tx: _____

Ever had +PPD? [ ] no [ ] yes Where?_____ When?_____

INH? [ ] no [ ] yes __ months

Ever incarcerated? [ ] no [ ] yes When? _____

Ever in homeless shelter? [ ] no [ ] yes When? _____

Ever in contact with known case of TB? [ ] no [ ] yes; Comments _____

Baseline CXR (if appropriate) __/__/__ Results _____

Substance abuse history

Hx injection drug use [ ] no [ ] yes Tx [ ] no [ ] yes _____

Hx alcohol use? [ ] no [ ] yes Tx [ ] no [ ] yes _____

Hx tobacco use? [ ] no [ ] yes Tx [ ] no [ ] yes _____

Hx other drug abuse? [ ] no [ ] yes Tx [ ] no [ ] yes _____

Psychiatric history

Hx psych hospitalization? [ ] no [ ] yes Tx [ ] no [ ] yes _____

Hx suicide attempt? [ ] no [ ] yes Tx [ ] no [ ] yes _____

Hx psych meds? [ ] no [ ] yes Tx [ ] no [ ] yes _____

FIGURE 41-2 Initial data base for HIV care.

Health Maintenance Flow Sheet

Date								
Physical q 1 yr								
Rectal q 1 yr								
Mammo* q 1 yr								
Dental q 1 yr								
Ophtho q 1 yr**								
RPR q 1 yr								
Toxo titer***								
PPD q 1 y+								
CXR (anergy) q 1 y								
Pap q 1 y++								
Flu vaccine q 1 y								
Contraception/ Safe sex education given (q 1 y minimum)								

* Women $\geq$ 50 yrs and/or family history breast cancer and/or history other breast disease
** CD4 <100
*** Repeat yearly if unable to take TMP/SMX
+ Q6 mos in areas with high rates of TB and/or patient with history of homelessness/incarceration
++ Q6 mos with CD4 $\leq$ 500 and/or history of abnormal PAP smear

Health care proxy: Discussed ___/___/___ Copy in chart ___/___/___

Updates ___/___/___, ___/___/___, ___/___/___, ___/___/___

Other advanced directives: Discussed ___/___/___ Copy in chart ___/___/___

Child custody arrangements: Discussed ___/___/___ Papers signed ___/___/___

Problem List

Date	OIs/HIV-Related Problems	Date	Other Medical Problems

FIGURE 41-2 *(continued)*

TABLE 41-13	Rating Scheme for Clinical Practice Recommendations

Strength of recommendation

A   Strong, should always be offered
B   Moderate, should usually be offered
C   Optional
D   Should generally not be offered
E   Should never be offered

Quality of evidence for recommendation

I   At least one randomized trial with clinical end points
II   Clinical trials with laboratory end points
III Expert opinion

Source: Feinberg, M.D., Carpenter, C., Favi, A. et al. (1998). Guidelines of the use of antiretroviral agents in HIV-infected adults and adolescents. *Annals of Internal Medicine.* 128(12 part 2)108.

Opinions vary as to when to initiate antiretroviral therapy in the asymptomatic patient with a CD4 count of more than 500 and a low viral load. All agree, however, that when the CD4 count drops to less than 500 or the viral load is elevated, medications should be offered. Table 41-14 lists the risks and benefits of initiating therapy in the asymptomatic patient (CDC, 1998).

Late Disease

When the patient develops symptoms of immunosuppression, then the consensus is strong that antiretroviral treatment must begin as soon as the patient is willing and able to do so. Again, the goal of treatment is to reduce the viral load to an undetectable level, or as low as possible, for as long as possible.

The problems that a patient develops reflect the degree of immunosuppression. It is convenient to consider problems most likely to occur at CD4 counts of less than 500, less than 200, and less than 100. The lowest historical CD4 count should be used in assessing patients, because an increase in the count after treatment does not necessarily restore immunologic memory—in other words, the new CD4 cells may not be of the same quality as those lost.

Late-stage AIDS becomes more difficult to treat, and appropriate provider education and referral sources and practice settings are necessary. Table 41-15 lists some provider and system requirements for treating patients with late-stage disease. Primary care providers who see few patients with HIV are wise to refer those with late-stage disease to special treatment centers for ongoing management (see referral points below) Stephenson, 1996).

Prophylactic treatment of opportunistic infections was discussed earlier in this chapter.

End-Stage Disease

Since the onset of multidrug therapy, both hospitalization and death rates have decreased by 15% to 19% throughout the United States. Even day-care programs and long-term care facilities have seen fewer patients. It is still too early to know whether these figures can be sustained (Standards & Accreditations Committee, 1996). For those whose disease has not responded to current therapies, the best care involves the use of prophylaxis and aggressive palliative treatment of symptoms that might interfere with quality of life (Gottlieb, 1997). For these patients, access to clinical trials of new therapies and com-

binations is extremely important; as many as possible should have access to such treatments.

Because HIV is now a chronic condition, and predicting the prognosis is becoming more difficult, the primary care provider will need to know how to manage the full continuum of disease. For people who have advanced disease and a poor response to highly active antiretroviral therapy (Williams & Frieland, 1997), day care, home care, and long-term care are useful options. The patient's and the family's concept of quality of life should serve as the guiding principle. This requires adjusting the treatment goals to value comfort and level of daily activity, much as one pursued the achievement of normal laboratory values earlier in the disease.

Providing aggressive palliative care, or symptom management, may improve the quality of life without increasing survival. Patients at this stage may become depressed as others around them are responding to recent therapeutic changes. It may be prudent to see them every 4 to 6 weeks to add moral support and preclude bothersome symptoms. They may also need a mental health referral or a trial of antidepressant therapy.

Medication Regimens

Decisions about when to initiate or change antiretroviral therapy should be based on the viral load and the CD4 count measured at a time when the person is generally symptom-free. The goal of therapy is to achieve a 1.5 to 2 log reduction in plasma HIV concentration or at best to maintain an undetectable viral load. A change in viral load can be detected 3 weeks after initiation of or a change in antiretroviral therapy, but it may take 12 to 24 weeks to see the full response. Once the level is undetectable, the viral load and CD4 count should be measured every 3 months. During this time, the CD4 count may increase, decrease, or remain the same. Although this measure may be useful as a guide to the function of the immune system, it does not necessarily correlate with clinical disease (O'Brien et al, 1997). In fact, patients may exhibit a discordance in their viral load and the CD4 count in either direction. A declining CD4

TABLE 41-14	Risks and Benefits of Early Initiation of Antiretroviral Therapy in the Asymptomatic HIV-Infected Patient

POTENTIAL BENEFITS

Control of viral replication and mutation, reduction of viral burden
Prevention of progressive immunodeficiency; potential maintenance or reconstition of a normal immune system
Delayed progression to AIDS and prolongation of life
Decreased risk of selection of resistant virus
Decreased risk of drug toxicity

POTENTIAL RISKS

Reduction in quality of life from adverse drug effects and inconvenience of current maximally suppressive regimens
Earlier development of drug resistance
Limitation in future choices of antiretroviral agents due to development of resistance
Unknown long-term toxicity of antiretroviral drugs
Unknown duration of effectiveness of current antiretroviral therapies

Panel on Clinical Practices for the Treatment of HIV Infection. (1997). Department of Health and Human Services draft guidelines on use of antiretroviral agents in HIV-infected adults. *The Hopkins HIV Report (Suppl. 9*(4), 2–7.

TABLE 41-15	Recommendations for Managing Late-Stage HIV

MAINTENANCE OF PROVIDER COMPETENCE

- Several hours a week of professional education (either independent reading or formal activities) on HIV and related topics
- Participation in one or more professional conferences a year on HIV

REQUIREMENTS OF THE PRACTICE SETTING

- Patient access to system by telephone 24 hours a day
- Ready access to hospital admission
- Ready access to laboratory able to do specialized stains and cultures for unusual bacteria, fungi, and viruses
- Referral network of specialists knowledgable about and interested in HIV
    Infectious disease specialist to consult on diagnosis of difficult cases and treatment decisions
    Dermatologist to consult on difficult cases and to biopsy and culture lesions (if primary provider not able)
    Visiting Nurses' Association to provide in-home evaluations, ongoing assessments, and home care
    Psychiatrist to assess and manage depression, anxiety, psychosis, and chronic mental illness
    Dentist or oral surgeon to treat gum disease and dental abscesses as well as perform biopsies of suspicious lesions
    Otolaryngologist to perform indirect laryngoscopy, needle aspiration of some sinus infections, and biopsy of masses
    Surgeon for general biopsies and placement of feeding tubes and indwelling venous catheters
    Neurologist to evaluate changes in mental status, new seizures, and unusual developments such as Guillain-Barré syndrome
    Gastroenterologist to perform endoscopies and biopsies
    Pulmonologist to perform bronchoscopies
    Nephrologist for evaluation for possible HIV nephropathy and renal failure
    Colposcopist to biopsy and follow cervical lesions
    Heme-oncologist to perform marrow aspirations and biopsies, to evaluate and comanage HIV-related neoplasms
    Radiologist with interventional capability to suggest and perform special studies

count may reflect the demise of cells that had already been infected before therapy, but the true explanation is not clear. Thus, relying on the rise and fall of the CD4 count alone can be misleading.

CHOICE OF MEDICATIONS

Combination therapy is recommended. This refers to using more than one antiviral drug at one time; the drugs come from two or more different classes. The number and type of antiretroviral drugs must be adapted for the patient. There are currently three classes of antiretroviral therapies; NRTIs, protease inhibitors, and NNRTIs. Current recommendations are to select two NRTIs plus one or more protease inhibitors, with or without an NNRTI (Table 41-16). In the future, there will be new classes of medications that will target other sites of viral replication. The idea is to use multiple methods of attacking the virus to prevent rapid mutation and early resistance. At this time, the three classifications of antiretroviral drugs found in Tables 41-17, 41-18, and 41-19 are the mainstays of therapy. Because each medication has its own set of side effects and best ways to be administered (eg, with or without food, needs refrigeration), the provider should be familiar with each medication and apply this information when choosing a medication.

CHANGING THERAPY

When the disease is no longer responding to therapy, it is wise to repeat the viral load studies because an intercurrent virus or missed medication doses may result in a burst of viral activity that could be controlled in the short term (International Workshop, 1997). If the patient has an adverse reaction to a specific drug, it may be best to halt all therapy until the effects resolve or until new therapy can be instituted. At no time should the patient be receiving a protease inhibitor alone, because the rate of viral resistance is quite rapid (Condra, 1997). Taking two drugs alone is like taking monotherapy if the patient is already resistant to one of the medications.

Choosing new therapy must be done methodically. Ideally, at least two drugs should be changed at any time; otherwise, the patient may be completely resistant to one of the two drugs. Viral burden should be measured about 4 weeks after any change in therapy.

Alternative Treatments

In addition to the FDA-approved medications, a collage of therapeutic approaches exists for HIV disease. These include Western, traditional, alternative and complementary therapies, clinical trials, and an underground of experimental medicines. Some alternative approaches are used to enhance immune restoration and to limit wasting (Abrams, 1997). Others are aimed at stress management.

Primary care providers should discuss the patient's concept of health promotion and holistic care therapies. The primary care provider should explain that complementary or alternative therapies combined with traditional treatment are a highly effective approach in the care of HIV disease, compared with complementary strategies alone. The primary care provider, however, needs to remember that the choice of treatment strategies lies with the patient. Table 41-20 is an abbreviated list of complementary therapies. See also the resources section below.

Care of the Care Giver

Many young and creative people have died of AIDS. Their care providers have been friends, parents, and relatives. Particularly in this disease, it is important to make sure that these people, as well as the staff, have emotional support when dealing with difficult issues surrounding death and dying. Ensuring that there is time for appropriate acknowledgment of feelings and grief helps prevent burnout among care providers. Rituals such as making quilt panels have become part of the culture of HIV. Some programs hold a monthly memorial service to remember those who have died, both that month and in previous years during that same month.

TEACHING AND SELF-CARE

In an ideal world, teaching and self-care would be the beginning from which all health care emanates. HIV disease has been a particularly clear demonstration of this, from issues of safer sex

TABLE 41-16 Recommended Antiretroviral Agents for the Treatment of Established HIV Infection

Preferred: Strong evidence of clinical benefit and/or sustained suppression of plasma viral load

One choice each from column A and column B. Drugs are listed in random, not priority, order:

Column A	Column B
Indinavir (AI)	ZDV + ddI (AI)
Nelfinavir (AII)	d4T + ddI (AII)
Ritonavir (AI)	ZDV + ddC (AI)
Saquinavir-SGC* (AII)	ZDV + 3TC§ (AI)
Ritonavir + Saquinavir-SGC or HGC† (BII)	d4T + 3TC§ (AII)

Alternative: Less likely to provide sustained virus suppression

1 NNRTI (Nevirapine)¶ + 2 NRTIs (Column B, above) (BII)

Saquinavir-HGC + 2 NRTIs (Column B, above) (BI)

Not generally recommended: Strong evidence of clinical benefit, but initial virus suppression is not sustained in most patients

2 NRTIs (Column B, above) (CI)

Not recommended:** Evidence against use, virologically undesirable, or overlapping toxicities

All monotherapies (DI)

d4T + ZDV (DI)

ddC + ddI†† (DII)

ddC + d4T†† (DII)

ddC + 3TC (DII)

Virologic data and clinical experience with saquinavir-sgc are limited in comparison with other protease inhibitors.

Use of ritonavir 400 mg bid with saquinavir soft-gel formulation (Fortovase™) 400 mg bid results in similar areas under the curve (AUC) of drug and antiretroviral activity as when using 400 mg bid of Invirase™ in combination with ritonavir. However, this combination with Fortovase has not been extensively studied and gastrointestinal toxicity may be greater when using Fortovase.

§ High-level resistance to 3TC develops within 2–4 wks. in partially suppressive regimens; optimal use is in three-drug antiretroviral combinations that reduce viral load to <500 copies/mL.

¶ The only combination of 2 NRTIs + 1 NNRTI that has been shown to suppress viremia to undetectable levels in the majority of patients is ZDV + ddI + Nevirapine. This combination was studied in antiretroviral-naive persons (36).

** ZDV monotherapy may be considered for prophylactic use in pregnant women who have low viral load and high CD4+ T cell counts to prevent perinatal transmission.

†† This combination of NRTIs is not recommended based on lack of clinical data using the combination and/or overlapping toxicities.

Source: Carpenter: Antiretroviral therapy for HIV infection in 1997: Updated recommendations of the International AIDS Society. *JAMA 227*(24), 1962–1969.

TABLE 41-17 Nucleoside Reverse Transcriptase Inhibitors (NRTIs)

Generic Name/Trade Name	Zidovudine (AZT/ZDV)/ Retrovir	Didanosine (ddI)/Videx	Zalcitabine (ddC)/Hivid	Stavudine (d4T)/Zerit	Lamivudine (3TC)/Epivir
Dosing Recommendations	300 mg BID or 200 mg TID	>60 kg, 200 mg BID or 400 mg qhs <60 kg, 125 mg BID	0.75 mg TID	>60 kg, 40 mg BID <60 kg, 30 mg BID	150 mg BID
Oral Bioavailability	60%	40%	85%	86%	86%
Intracellular Half-life	3 hours	12 hours	3 hours	3.5 hours	12 hours
Elimination	Renal	Renal 50%	Renal 70%	Renal 50%	Renal (unchanged)
Common Side Effects	Anemia or neutropenia, nausea, headache, insomnia, asthenia	Pancreatitis, peripheral neuropathy, nausea, diarrhea	Peripheral neuropathy, stomatitis, oral ulcers	Peripheral neuropathy	Minimal toxicity
Administration/ Storage	Store in dark container	Take 1 hour before or 2 hours after a meal	Take 1 hour before or 2 hours after a meal	N/A	N/A

Source: Panel on Clinical Practices for the Treatment of HIV Infection. (1997). Department of Health and Human Services draft guidelines on use of antiretroviral agents in HIV-infected adults. *The Hopkins HIV Report (Suppl. 9*(4), 2–7.

TABLE 41-18	Nonnucleoside Reverse Transcriptase Inhibitors (NNRTIs)	
Generic Name/Trade Name	Nevirapine/Viramune	Delaverdine/Rescriptor
Dosing Recommendation	200 mg QD × 14 then 200 mg BID	400 mg TID
Elimination	p450; 80% renal excretion	p450; 51% renal excretion
Drug Interactions	Requires dose increase for nelfinavir	Many drug interactions; cannot administer with ddI
Common Side Effects	Rash	Rash

Source: Panel on Clinical Practices for the Treatment of HIV Infection. (1997). Department of Health and Human Services draft guidelines on use of antiretroviral agents in HIV-infected adults. *The Hopkins HIV Report (Suppl. 9*(4), 2–7.

and risk reduction to patient–provider collaboration regarding combination therapy. There are some specific topics, however, that should be addressed relatively early in the patient–provider relationship.

COMMITMENT TO ACTIVE PARTICIPATION IN CARE

Often patients are not accustomed to being asked to participate actively in their health care. Therefore, it is important to spend time during the initial and subsequent visits establishing this concept. The primary care provider should request input as to the feasibility of the plan of care being discussed at every opportunity. Some patients may not accept this philosophy. Statements such as, "You make the decision; I don't know what to think," might be the response to the request for input. By establishing this concept early and building on it over time, the primary care provider may gradually stimulate the active participation of the patient. This will become critical as the self-care decisions become more complex over time.

TABLE 41-19	Protease Inhibitors (PIs)			
Generic Name/Trade Name	Saquinavir/Invirase Saquinavir/Fortovase	Ritonavir/ Norvir	Indinavir/Crixivan	Nelfinavir/ Viracept
Dosing Recommendations	3 × 200 mg q 8 hrs (Invirase) 6 × 200 mg q 8 hrs (Fortovase)	3 × 100 mg Day 1–2 4 × 100 mg Day 3–5 5 × 100 mg Day 6–13 6 × 100 mg Day 14+ BID dosing	2 × 400 mg q 8 hrs	3 × 250 mg q 8 hrs
Dose Adjustments	With ritonavir, decrease to 400 mg BID	With saquinavir, decrease to 400 mg BID	With nevirapine	With nevirapine
Oral Bioavailability	4% (improved w/ fat or ritonavir) (Invirase) Not determined (Fortovase)	Not determined	30%	20%–80%
Route of Metabolism	p450 cytochrome 3A4	p450 cytochrome 3A4, 2D6, 2C9/10	p450 cytochrome 3A	p450 cytochrome 3A4
Common Side Effects	Nausea, diarrhea, headache; increased liver function tests ok if asymptomatic or <5× elevated	GI intolerance, circumoral paresthesias if dose escalated too quickly, asthenia, increased triglycerides & liver function tests	Renal stones, GI intolerance, headache, metallic taste	Diarrhea
Administration Storage	Room temp; taken with high-fat meal, (Invirase) Refrigerate or store at room temperature (up to 3 mo) (Fortovase)	Gelcaps need refrigeration unless taken within 12 hrs, liquid form does not; taken with food	Packaged with silicon, deteriorates with moisture; taken on an empty stomach but ok w/skim milk or low-fat food; increase fluid intake; cannot be taken within 2 hours of ddI	Room temp; taken with food
Drug Interactions (All in this class have multiple drug interactions that must be checked carefully before prescribing)	Ritonavir, ketoconazole, & grapefruit juice increase levels of saquinavir; many drug interactions—need to check individually	Increases levels of multiple drugs metabolized by p450; check with Abbott if not listed; side effects are decreased when dose decreased in combo with other PI	Avoid rifampin, rifabutin, some benzodiazepines, cisopride, terfenadine.	Rifampin & rifabutin decrease nelfinavir levels; check interaction with contraceptive agents.

Source: Panel on Clinical Practices for the Treatment of HIV Infection. (1997). Department of Health and Human Services draft guidelines on use of antiretroviral agents in HIV-infected adults. *The Hopkins HIV Report (Suppl. 9*(4), 2–7.

TABLE 41-20	Complementary Therapies	
Wellness and holistic nursing	Qi chong (breathing exercises)	Psychotherapy
Therapeutic Touch and healing touch	Reflexology (based on the theory that there are reflex areas in the hands and feet that correspond to all parts of the body)	Exercise
Traditional Chinese medicine		Support groups
		Experimental or not yet FDA-approved medications such as mega-vitamin C, DNCB, SPV-30
Acupuncture	Yoga	
Chinese herbal medicine	Massage	

Source: Casey et al, 1996

Patients who are newly diagnosed may be in shock or denial and incapable of making decisions. The weeks between the initial diagnosis and the follow-up appointment can serve as a period of adjustment. The provider should arrange for the patient to be seen by other members of the HIV team, such as the registered nurse, dietitian, and social worker.

HOME INFECTION CONTROL

- HIV is not spread by living with someone who is HIV-positive unless the activities include intimate sexual encounters or sharing injection equipment.
- Preventive cleaning procedures performed with any household items (dishwashing, laundry, bathtub, toilet) are sufficient to prevent HIV transmission.
- The HIV-positive household member should never share toothbrushes or razors; they can provoke bleeding and, therefore, are potential vectors.
- All body fluids of the HIV-positive household member should be handled using the universal precautions guidelines. The home should be equipped with latex gloves.

DENTAL HYGIENE

- Daily oral care should include brushing at least twice a day and flossing daily.
- Gum pain or excessive bleeding should be reported (Hughes, 1996).
- An evaluation by a dentist should be performed every 6 months.

PETS

- People with HIV disease can keep or acquire pets.
- Gloves should be used for handling the waste of any pet. Place the waste in a plastic bag and dispose of it immediately.
- When changing a cat litter box (risk of toxoplasmosis), cleaning cages (risk of salmonellosis for lizards, snakes, turtles; risk for psittacosis with birds), or cleaning aquariums (risk for *Mycobacterium avium* complex), gloves should be worn and hands washed immediately after completing the task.
- Pets should be examined annually and vaccinated by the veterinarian. New pets or those who become ill should be evaluated as soon as possible.

- Pets with diarrhea should be tested for *Salmonella*, *Campylobacter*, and cryptosporidiosis.

NUTRITION

It is important to educate patients about eating a balanced diet. All patients with HIV infection should be evaluated by a registered dietitian (Position statement of the American Dietetic Association and the Canadian Dietetic Association, 1994). Patients who are considering radical dietary changes (from fruitarianism to strict macrobiotics) should be warned appropriately. Dietitians who have expertise in HIV/AIDS are often aware of these diets and can educate patients about false claims and potential dangers. Nutritional supplements and anabolic steroids, although controversial, have been used to prevent wasting syndrome (Kotler, 1994).

FOOD PREPARATION

People with HIV infection are more susceptible to foodborne illnesses (eg, *Salmonella*, *Shigella*). The following information should be shared by the dietitian or another member of the HIV team with the patient, household members, and care attendants:

- Careful handwashing must be performed before and after food preparation and before eating.
- All raw meat, fish, or poultry should be cut on boards and with knives that are thoroughly washed in hot soapy water and completely dried.
- After food shopping, refrigerate or freeze food immediately.
- To reduce the risk of *Salmonella* and other enteric pathogens, avoid foods that contain undercooked or raw eggs (eg, Hollandaise sauce, Caesar salad dressing, fresh mayonnaise).
- Do not eat rare or raw meat, fish, or poultry; all should be prepared well done.

DRINKING WATER

Cryptosporidium is a waterborne pathogen that can cause life-threatening diarrhea in the immunocompromised HIV-positive patient. Although this pathogen is usually a concern only at the time of rare outbreaks, the following information about drinking water should be discussed:

- Water that has been filtered to 4 microns or boiled for at least 1 minute is recommended.
- Distilled water is also acceptable.
- Bottled waters are not the same; it is important to know which brands in your area are filtered and which are not.
- Some people who drink boiled water put it through a home filtering system to remove the flat taste. However, some home filtering systems cannot to filter *Cryptosporidium*.

EXERCISE

The HIV-positive patient should be encouraged to participate in some form of exercise. Anecdotally, increasing lean muscle mass in HIV disease improves overall wellness. Currently, there are several studies underway to establish a link between immune function and lean muscle mass, and between survival and body mass.

VACCINATIONS

A general principle for the primary care clinician is that HIV-infected persons and their household contacts should not receive live virus or live bacteria vaccines. However, killed or inactive vaccines are of no danger to the immunosuppressed person. The following is a list of vaccines recommended for persons with HIV by the USPHS/Infectious Disease Society of America (CDC, 1997c):

- Pneumococcal vaccine (revaccination should be considered at 6-year intervals)
- Influenza vaccine (yearly mid-October to mid-November; probably of little value to anyone with a CD4 count of less than 200)
- Hepatitis B vaccine (if the patient is seronegative for hepatitis B and at risk for hepatitis B)
- Tetanus–diphtheria (Td) vaccine (for those who completed the primary series, a booster every 10 years).

COMMUNITY RESOURCES

Community-based resources are available outside the formal health care delivery system. They are intended to assist the HIV-positive patient, family members, and care partners, as well as the primary care provider, by providing information, psychosocial services, and complementary therapies. The following is a list of HIV-focused, community-based resources throughout the United States:

- National AIDS Hotline, 800-342-AIDS (2437): Data base of all HIV/AIDS community-based resources in the United States
- San Francisco AIDS Foundation, 10 United Nations Plaza, Suite 220, San Francisco, CA 94102, 415-487-3000, 415-487-8009 (fax): Education, referrals, outreach
- Shanti Project, 1546 Market St., San Francisco, CA 94102, 415-864-2273, 415-864-6584 (fax): Volunteer programs, transportation, emotional support, activities
- Project Open Hand, 730 Polk St., San Francisco, CA 94109, 415-447-2300: Food bank, home meal delivery
- American Red Cross, 8111 Gatehouse Rd., Falls Church, VA 22042, 703-206-7180: Education
- African American AIDS Network, 307 South Wabash Ave., Chicago, IL 60605, 312-786-2226: Educational seminars, referrals, technical assistance
- Chicago Women's AIDS Project, 5249 North Kenmore, Chicago, IL 60640, 773-271-2070, 773-863-8711: Case management, support group, home-based services
- Minority AIDS Information Network, 84 Walton St. NW, Atlanta, GA 30303, 404-651-8187: Education and technical assistance for African American youth and young adults
- SisterLove, 713 Cascade Ave. SW, Atlanta, GA 30310, 404-753-7733: Support groups for women and children, counseling, transitional housing
- AIDS Action Council, 1875 Connecticut Ave. SW, Suite 700, Washington DC 20009, 202-986-1300, 202-986-1345 (fax): Community outreach, government affairs

- AIDS National Interfaith Network, 1400 "I" St. NW, #1220, Washington DC 20005, 202-842-0010, 202-842-3323 (fax), aninken@aol.com: Data base of AIDS ministries in the United States, AIDS ministry handbook, referrals to local ministries around the country
- American Civil Liberties Union, National Legislative Office, 122 Maryland Ave. NE, Washington DC 20002, 202-544-1681: HIV discrimination in employment, housing, treatment by government
- Blacks Educating Blacks About Sexual Health Issues (BEBASHI), 1233 Locust St., Philadelphia, PA 19107, 215-546-4140: HIV testing, outreach education
- National AIDS Minority Information and Education Program, 2139 Georgia Ave. NW, Washington DC 20001, 202-865-3720: Education about HIV/AIDS, with a focus on African Americans
- National Minority AIDS Council, 1931 13th St. NW, Washington DC 20009, 202-483-6622: National and international technical assistance to AIDS community-based organizations within communities of people of color
- National Urban League, 500 E. 62d St., 10th Floor, New York, NY 10021, 212-310-9238: Advocacy, education; outreach in New York City only
- Gay Men's Health Crisis, 119 W. 24th St., New York, NY 10011, 212-807-7035: serves gay and nongay people with HIV/AIDS; education, advocacy, legal services, residency and immigration services, support groups, day treatment referrals, hot lunches, hotline services, nutritional counseling, information and referral to agencies in other cities
- UCSF AIDS Health Project, 1930 Market St., San Francisco, CA 94102, 415-476-6430, 415-476-7996 (fax): HIV testing and counseling, mental health services, case management, referrals
- Asian and Pacific Islander Coalition on HIV/AIDS, Inc., 275 Seventh Ave., 12th Floor, New York, NY 10001-6708, 212-620-7287 (voice), 212-627-5598 (TTY): Immigration issues, financial assistance, emergency needs, support groups, Asian ethnic food pantry, recreational activities, advocacy
- Harlem United, 306 Lenox Ave., 3d Floor, New York, NY 10027, 212-803-2850: Advocacy, housing, social services, crisis intervention, home visits, information, education and referral to other health-related services, referral/advocacy for job training and placement, advocacy with landlords, referral/advocacy for substance abuse services, referral for individual, family, or group therapy, referral for GED preparation and testing. Bilingual English/Spanish; sensitive to gay, lesbian, transgender issues. Eligibility: residence in Central Harlem, East Harlem, Inwood, Washington Heights, Bronx; Medicaid eligible
- American Indian Community House (AICH) HIV/AIDS Project, 708 Broadway, 8th Floor, New York, NY 10003, 212-598-0100, 212-598-4909 (fax), http:\\www.abest.com/aichnyc: Native community prevention education and information, outreach, referrals, case management

   AICH—Walk in Self Harmony (WISH), 306 S.

Salina St., Suite 201, Syracuse, NY 13202, 315-478-8532, 315-478-3850 (fax)

AICH—Akwesasne Care Together/Natives Oppose Wipeout (ACT NOW), Box 747, Hogansburg, NY 13655, 518-358-2001, 518-358-2540 (fax)

AICH—Sewanaka Place, 573 Roanoke Ave., Riverhead, NY 11901, 516-369-3426, 516-369-8082 (fax)

AICH—Vision Quest, 2495 Main St., Suite 524, Buffalo, NY, 14214, 716-832-2302, 716-832-2735 (fax)

- Treatment Action Group, 200 E. 10th St., Suite 601, New York, NY 10003, http:\\www.thebody.com, 212-260-0300: Mail request to receive monthly paper on research and policy, newsletter designed to keep patients aware of research and options for treatment; highly involved in political action; bilingual English/Spanish
- New York State Dept. of Health, Harm Reduction Unit, 5 Penn Plaza, New York, NY 10001, 212-613-2431: Information about current needle exchange program sites and hours
- American Holistic Nurses Association, P.O. Box 2130, Flagstaff, AZ 86003-2130, 800-278-2462: Wellness and holism
- Council of Colleges of Acupuncture and Oriental Medicine, 8403 Colesville Rd., Suite 370, Silver Spring, MD 20910, 301-608-9175, 301-608-9576 (fax): Acupuncture, academic and clinical guidelines
- International Academy for Reflexology Studies, 4759 Cornell Rd., Suite D, Cincinnati, OH 45241, 513-489-9328, 513-489-9354 (fax): School of reflexology, clinical services
- American Psychiatric Association, 1400 K St. NW, Washington DC 20005, 202-682-6800, 202-682-6850 (fax), http:\\www.psych.org: Referrals to district branches who can refer to local psychotherapists and support groups
- AIDS Treatment Data Network, 611 Broadway, Suite 613, New York, NY 10012, 800-734-7104, 212/260-8869 (fax), http://www.aidsnyc.org/network: Information about alternative, experimental, and not-FDA-approved medications and drugs in development
- National AIDS Treatment Advocacy Project, 580 Broadway, Suite 403, New York, NY 10012, 888-26-NATAP, 212-219-8473 (fax), http://www.aidsnyc.org/natap: Patient education about HIV treatments; brochures, newsletters, educational conferences

RESOURCES FOR THE PRIMARY CARE PROVIDER

The challenge for the primary clinician providing care to HIV-positive patients is staying abreast of new information being discovered daily that directly affects clinical decision making. Communication via the Internet, World Wide Web, and even the telephone is imperative for reaching this information in a timely and efficient manner. The following resources have been developed to support health care providers in their quest for the most current HIV clinical information:

- AIDS Clinical Trials Information Service, 800-TRIALS-A (800-874-2572), http://www.actis.org: Information about clinical trials, study protocols and locations, patient enrollment and eligibility
- National Clinician's Post-Exposure Prophylaxis Hotline (PEPLine), 888-448-4911: Free 24-hour hotline offered by the San Francisco General Hospital to clinicians in need of advice on how to treat health care workers accidentally exposed to bloodborne diseases such as HIV and hepatitis
- CDC National AIDS Clearinghouse, 800-458-5231, 301-738-6616 (fax), http://www.cdcnac.org; Gopher: gopher://gopher.cdcnac.org:72; AIDSNEWS Listserv: listserv@cdcnac.org; File Transfer Protocol: ftp://ftp.cdcnac.org/pub/cdcnac; Email: aidsinfo@cdcnac.org: Organizational reference and referral service, publication distribution (*MMWR, HIV/AIDS Surveillance Report*), 24-hour access to CDC NAC online, NAC FAX, Internet services, training and technical assistance
- HIV/AIDS Treatment Information Services, 800-HIV-0440 (Monday through Friday, 9 a.m. to 7 p.m. EST), http://www.hivatis.org: USPHS information about federally approved HIV/AIDS treatment options
- National AIDS Education and Training Centers, HIV/AIDS Telephone Consultation Service, 800-933-3413 (Monday through Friday, 8:30 a.m. to 6 p.m. MST, voice mail at other times): Telephone consultation service for health professionals with questions concerning clinical care. Staffed by a physician, nurse practitioner, and pharmacist operating out of San Francisco General Hospital.
- Johns Hopkins University AIDS Service, http://www.hopkins-aids.edu: *The Hopkins HIV Report*: Mail subscription request to JHU Division of Infectious Diseases, Ross Bldg., Room 1159, 720 Rutland Ave., Baltimore, MD 21205. Attn: Newsletter Subscription. This bimonthly publication compiles current HIV information for the clinician. It is free to Maryland residents and $20 to non-Maryland residents.
- Clinical Care Options for HIV, http://www.healthcg.com: An interactive online HIV medical resource developed by an independent national scientific advisory board of health care professionals. The three major resource sections are interactive treatment modules using case studies that provide free CME/CEU/ACPE hours; a full-text, online HIV journal, *Clinical Care Options for HIV*; and next-morning HIV conference briefings.
- CDC, Division of HIV/AIDS Prevention, http://www.cdc.gov/nchstp/hiv aids/dhap.htm: General AIDS information, publications, resources, statistics
- American Red Cross, http://www.redcross.org/hss: Community-level HIV/AIDS education programs and materials
- Harvard AIDS Institute, http://www.hsph.harvard.edu/organizations/hai/hai.html: Information on basic and clinical sciences, clinical care, epidemiology, public health, and prevention
- *JAMA* HIV/AIDS Information Center, http://www.ama-assn.org/ special/hiv: Journal scan, practice

guidelines, training resources, treatment resources, patient support group information. *JAMA*'s "Best of the Net" lists top selected resources on HIV/AIDS.

- International Association of Physicians in AIDS Care, http://www.iapac.org: News about antiviral therapies, opportunistic diseases, conferences, and AIDScan (summary reports from major international AIDS conferences). Index of articles from the *Journal of the International Association of Physicians in AIDS Care.*
- JRI Health Information Systems, http://www.jri.org/infoweb: Links to the online community with information about HIV/AIDS treatment, infoweb library with articles focusing on the treatment of HIV
- The National Clinician's Post Exposure Prophylaxis Hotline (PEPline). 1-888-448-4911. Free 24-hr hotline offered by San Francisco General Hospital advising clinicians how best to treat health care workers exposed to bloodborne diseases.
- National Institutes of Health, National Institutes of Allergy and Infectious Diseases, http://www.niaid.nih.gov, gopher://odie.niaid.nih.gov: Press releases, newsletter fact sheets
- National Pediatric & Family HIV Resource Center, http://www.wdcnet.com/PedsAIDS: Information about the care of children and families living with HIV, catalog of books and videos
- Rural Center for AIDS/STD Prevention, http://www.indiana.edu/aids: HIV/AIDS issues in rural areas, fact sheets, articles, references

BULLETIN BOARDS

- AIDS Education and Global Information System (AEGIS), 714-248-2836, AEGIS World HQ: AIDS education and prevention, treatment, and legal information
- Boston AIDS Consortium, Service Provider Information Network (SPIN), 617-432-0885, Dataline: 617-432-2511, username SPIN: AIDS treatment news, statistics from CDC
- CDC WONDER/PC, 888-496-8347: A link to epidemiologic data, public health reports and guidelines, and Email communication with CDC staff and other public health officials. Statistics can be downloaded and converted into graphs, charts, and maps.
- Norman Brown's Consolidated List of AIDS/HIV Bulletin Boards, ftp://tde.com/abbs.dir, listserv: abbs-request@ tde.com: Comprehensive listing of publicly accessible HIV/AIDS bulletin board services.

REFERRAL POINTS AND CLINICAL WARNINGS

Information about antiretroviral medications expands daily. This precludes the possibility of using a "cookbook" approach to the treatment for HIV disease. Therefore, the primary care provider may wish to consult an HIV specialist for decisions regarding the initiation of antiretroviral therapy. If a regimen fails, a complete review with a specialist of all laboratory data and the medication history is warranted as well. The primary care provider should consider consulting an HIV specialist,

either verbally or by having the patient make an appointment with the specialist, at the following clinical points:

1. After the initial history, physical, and laboratory results have been obtained, to determine the plan of care, including use of antiretroviral therapy
2. After the first 3 months of antiviral therapy (unless the viral load is undetectable, the CD4 count is stable or rising, and the patient is tolerating the treatment) and every 6 to 12 months thereafter, to review the case
3. If the CD4 count decreases or the viral load increases (Carpenter et al, 1997).
4. If the patient develops toxicity to antiretroviral therapy.
5. When an opportunistic infection is diagnosed, to determine treatment strategies
6. When recommending postexposure prophylaxis to a health care worker.

HIV/AIDS case management using a multidisciplinary team approach provides the best care for the patient living with this disease. Nursing provides a solid base for education, support, and symptom management of this complex disease. Nursing also contributes by integrating the patient's life situation with the plan of care. A referral to a social worker for a comprehensive psychosocial evaluation should be performed at the start of treatment and at regular intervals. Referral to a registered dietitian, experienced with HIV/AIDS, is also essential.

EDITOR'S NOTE:
COMPLEMENTARY APPROACHES

A general discussion of complementary approaches can be found in Chapter 3. The following, while not an exhaustive list, are some complementary approaches being used for this condition. Additional information on these approaches, including precautions, can be found in Appendices A and B. Providers need to assess for the use of complementary approaches as part of the patient's history, as they may impact conventional therapies, and patients may not volunteer this information unless specifically asked. Efficacy of many complementary approaches is not as well documented as that of conventional therapies. Providers need to read the literature before suggesting these complementary approaches. See Table 41-20.

- Vitamins, minerals, herbs, supplements
  Echinacea
- Complementary Modalities
  Aromatherapy

References

Abrams, D. (1997). Alternative therapies for HIV. In M. Sande, P. Volberding (Eds.). *Medical management of AIDS*, 5th ed. Philadelphia: W.B. Saunders.

Anastasio, C., McMahan, T., Daniels, A., Nicholas, P. K., & Paul-Simon, A. (1995). Self-care burden in women with human immunodeficiency virus. *Journal of the Association of Nurses in AIDS Care*, *6*(3), 31–42.

Augenbraun, M., Feldman, J., Chirgwin, K., et al. (1995). Increased genital shedding of herpes simplex virus type 2 in HIV-seropositive women. *Annals of Internal Medicine*, *123*(11), 845–847.

Barbosa C., Macaset, M., Brockmann, S., Sierra, M. F., & Duerr, A. (1997). Pelvic inflammatory disease and human immunodeficiency virus infection. *Obstetrics & Gynecology*, *89*(1), 65–70.

Bartlett, J.G. (1997). *Medical management of HIV infection*. Baltimore:.

Byerly, E.R., & Deardorff, K. (1995). *National and state populations estimates: 1990–1994*, U.S. Bureau of the Census, Current Population Reports. Washington DC: U.S. Government Printing Office.

Cao, Y., Quin, L, Zhang, L., et al. (1995). Virologic and immunologic characterization of long-term survivors of human immunodeficiency virus type 1 infection. *N Engl J Med, 332*(4), 201–208.

Carpenter, C.C.J., Fischl, M.A., Hammer, S.M., et al. (1997). Antiretroviral therapy for HIV infection in 1997: Updated recommendations of the International AIDS Society–USA Panel. *JAMA, 277*(24), 1962–1969.

Carpenter, C.C., Mayer, K.H., Stein, M.D., Leibman, B.D., Fisher, A., & Fiore, T.C. (1991). Human immunodeficiency virus infection in North American women: Experience with 200 cases and a review of the literature. *Medicine, 70*(5), 307–325.

Casey, K., Cohan, F., & Hughes, A. (Eds.). (1996). ANAC's *Care Curriculum for HIV/AIDS Nursing*. Philadelphia: Nursecom.

CDC (1998). Public Health Service guidelines for the management of health-care worker exposure to HIV and recommendations for post exposure prophylaxis, *Morbidity and Mortality Weekly Report, 47*(RR-7).

CDC. (1997a). Department of Health and Human Services draft guidelines on use of antiretroviral agents in HIV-infected adults.

CDC. (1997b). Update: Trends in AIDS incidence, deaths, and prevalence—United States, 1996. *MMWR, 46*, 165–192.

CDC. (1997c). U.S. Public Health Service/Infectious Disease Society of America guidelines for the prevention of opportunistic infections in persons infected with HIV. *MMWR, 46*, 28–29.

CDC. (1996). *HIV/AIDS Surveillance Report* (Year-end edition), *8*(2).

CDC. (1995a). Case-control study of HIV seroconversion in healthcare workers after percutaneous exposure to HIV-infected blood—France, United Kingdom, and United States, January 1988–August 1994. *MMWR, 44*, 929–933.

CDC. (1995b). U.S. Public Health Service recommendations for human immunodeficiency virus counseling and voluntary testing for pregnant women. *MMWR, 44*, 1–15.

CDC. (1994a). *HIV/AIDS Surveillance Report, 6*(1), 9–10.

CDC. (1994b). Zidovudine for the prevention of HIV transmission from mother to infant. *MMWR, 43*, 285–287.

CDC. (1993). Revised classification system for HIV infection and expanded surveillance case definition for AIDS among adolescents and adults. *MMWR, 41*, 1–18.

Condra, J.J., & Emini, E.A. (1997). Preventing HIV-1 drug resistance. *Science & Medicine, 4*(1), 14–23.

Cramer, J.A. (1995). Optimizing long-term patient compliance. *Neurology, 45*(2 Suppl 1):S25–28.

Fauci, A.S. (1996). Host factors and the pathogenesis of HIV-induced disease. *Nature, 384*, 529–534.

Fox, L.J., Williamson, N.E., Cates, W., Jr., & Dallabetta, G. (1995). Improving reproductive health: Integrating STD and contraceptive services. *Journal of the American Medical Women's Association, 50*(3-4), 129–136.

Fruchter, R.G., Maiman, M., Sedlis, A., Bartley, L., Camilien, L., & Arrastia, C.D. (1996). Multiple recurrences of cervical intraepithelial neoplasia in women with the human immunodeficiency virus. *Obstetrics & Gynecology, 87*(3), 338–344.

Gallo, D., George, D., Fitchen, J.H. et al. (1997). Evaluation of a system using oral mucosa transudate for HIV-1 antibody screening and confirmation testing. *JAMA, 277*(3), 254–261.

Gottlieb, M.S., & Schofferman, J.A. (1997). Hospice care and pain management. In S. Broder, T.C. Merigan, & D. Bolognes (Eds.). *Textbook of AIDS medicine*. Baltimore: Williams & Wilkins.

Gwinn, M., & Wortley, P.M. (1996). Epidemiology of HIV infection in women and newborns. *Clinical Obstetrics and Gynecology, 39*(2), 292–304.

Gwinn, M., Pappaioanou, M., George, J.R., et al. (1991). Prevalence of HIV infection in childbearing women in the United States: Surveillance using newborn blood samples. *JAMA, 265*(13), 1704–1708.

Haynes, R.B., McKibbon, K.A., & Kanani, R. (1996). Systematic review of randomized trials of intervention to assist patients to follow prescriptions for medications. *Lancet, 348*(9024), 383–6.

Hellinger, F. (1993). The use of health services by women with HIV infection. *Health Services Research, 28*, 543–561.

Ho, D.D. (1996). Viral counts count in HIV infection. *Science 272*, 1124–1125.

Hughes, M.D., Johnson, V.A., Hirsch, M.S. et al. (1997). Monitoring plasma HIV-1 RNA levels in addition to CD4 + lymphocyte count improves assessment of antiretroviral therapeutic response. *Annals of Internal Medicine, 126*, 929–938.

International Workshop on HIV Drug Resistance. *Treatment strategies and eradication*, St. Petersburg, Florida, June 25–28, 1997.

Ippolito, G., Puro, V., Petrosillo, N., et al. (1997). *Prevention, management & chemoprophylaxis of occupational exposure to HIV*. Charlottesville, VA: International Health Care Worker Safety Center.

Irwin, K., Olivo, N., Schable, C.A., et al. (1996). Performance characteristics of an HIV antibody assay in a hospital with a high prevalence of HIV infection. *Annals of Internal Medicine, 125*, 471–475.

Kelen, G.D., Green, G.B., Hexter, D.A., et al. (1991). Substantial improvement in compliance with universal precautions in an emergency department following institution of policy. *Archives of Internal Medicine, 151*, 2051–2056.

Kitahata, M.M., Koepsell, T.D., Deyo, R.A., Maxwell, C.L., Dodge, W.T., & Wagner, E.H. (1996). Physicians' experience with the acquired immunodeficiency syndrome as a factor in patients' survival. *N Engl J Med, 334*(11), 701–706.

Kotler, D.P. (1994). Wasting syndrome: Nutritional support in HIV infection. *AIDS Research and Human Retroviruses, 10*(8): 931–934.

Landers, D.V., & Shannon, M.T. (1997). Management of pregnant women with HIV infection. In M. Sande & P. Volberding (Eds.). *The medical management of AIDS*, 5th ed. Philadelphia: W.B. Saunders.

Mellors, J.W., Rinaldo, C.R. Jr., Gupta, P., et al. (1996). Prognosis in HIV-1 infection predicted by the quantity of virus in plasma. *Science, 272*(5265), 1167–1170.

Mellors, J.W., Kingsley, L.A., Rinaldo, C.R., Jr., et al. (1995). Quantitation of HIV-1 RNA in plasma predicts outcome after seroconversion. *Annuals of Internal Medicine, 122*(8), 573–579.

Miller, N.H., Hill, M., Kottke, & Ockene, I.S. (1997). The multilevel compliance challenge: Recommendations for a call to action. A statement for healthcare professionals. *Circulation, 95*(4), 1085–1090.

MMWR. (Sept. 5, 1997). Anergy skin testing and preventive therapy for HIV-infected persons: Revised recommendations. *MMWR, 46*, 1–10.

MMWR. (June 7, 1996). Update: Provisional public health service recommendations for chemoprophylaxis after occupational exposure to HIV. *MMWR, 45*(22), 469–472.

MMWR. (Oct. 28, 1994). Guidelines for preventing the transmission of *Mycobacterium tuberculosis* in health-care facilities. *MMWR, 43*.

O'Brien, W.A., Hartigan, P.M., Daar, E.S., et al. (1997). Changes in plasma HIV RNA levels and CD4 + lymphocyte counts predict both response to antiretroviral therapy and therapeutic failure. *Annals of Internal Medicine, 126*, 939–945.

Panel on Clinical Practices for Treatment of HIV Infection. (1997). Department of Health and Human Services draft guidelines on use of antiretroviral agents in HIV-infected adults. *The Hopkins HIV Report (Supp), 9*(4), 2–7.

Pantaleo, G., Stefano, M., Menzo, S., et al. (1995). Studies in subjects with long-term nonprogressive human immunodeficiency virus infection. *N Engl J Med, 332,* 209–216.

Perelson, A.S., Avidon, U.N., Neuman, A.U., et al. (1996). HIV-1 dynamics in vivo: Virion clearance rate, infected cell life-span, and viral generation time. *Science, 271,* 1582–1586.

Position Statement of the American Dietetic Association and the Canadian Dietetic Association. (1994). Nutritional intervention in the care of persons with human immunodeficiency virus infection. *Journal of the American Dietetic Association, 94*(9), 1042–1045.

Quinn, T. (1996). Global burden of the HIV pandemic. *Lancet, 348,* 99–106.

Ragsdale, D., Kotarba, J.A., Morrow, J.R., Jr., & Yarbrough, S. (1995). Health locus of control among HIV-positive indigent women. *Journal of the Association of Nurses in AIDS Care, 6*(5), 29–36.

Rules and regulations for bloodborne pathogens, FP 1910.1030, December 6, 1991.

Sande, M.A., & Volberding, P.A. (1997). *The medical management of AIDS.* Philadelphia: W.B. Saunders.

Spinillo, A., Michelone, G., Cavanna, C., Colonna, L., Capuzzo, E., & Nicola, S. (1994). Clinical and microbiological characteristics of symptomatic vulvovaginal candidiasis in HIV-seropositive women. *Genitourinary Medicine, 70*(4), 268–272.

Springer, E. (1992). Effective AIDS prevention with active drug users: The harm reduction model. In M. Shernoff (Ed.). *Counseling chemically dependent people with HIV illness.* New York: Hawthorne Press.

Standards & Accreditation Committee/Medical Guidelines Task Force. (1996). *Medical guidelines for determining prognosis in selected non-cancer diseases,* 2d ed. Arlington, VA: National Hospice Organization.

Stephenson, J. (1996). Survival of patients with AIDS depends on physicians' experience treating the disease. *JAMA, 275*(10), 745–746.

U.S. Public Health Service recommendations for use of antiretroviral drugs during pregnancy for maternal health and reduction of perinatal transmission of human immunodeficiency virus type 1 in the United States, Vol. 62, FR 36809, July 9, 1997.

Williams, A., & Frieland, G. (1997). Adherence, compliance, and HAART. *AIDS Clinical Care, 9*(7), 51–55.

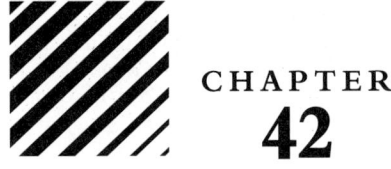

CHAPTER
42

Anterior Knee Pain

Sanjiv Bansal, MD, and William Urban, MD

Anterior knee pain is a common musculoskeletal complaint seen by primary care providers. It describes a large spectrum of clinical entities whose predominant symptoms include pain from the patellofemoral joint and surrounding structures. The term "anterior knee pain" can be used to describe primary painful syndromes as well as pain secondary to instability of the patellofemoral articulation. Classically, pain derived from the patellofemoral joint has been described under the broad category of "patellofemoral syndrome."

In the past, "chondromalacia patellae" has mistakenly been used as a "wastebasket" term for patellofemoral syndrome. This term should be used only as a specific pathologic description of abnormal patellar articular cartilage after arthroscopic, gross, or microscopic visualization. Chondromalacia patellae can also be used to describe changes in the articular cartilage visualized on magnetic resonance imaging. By age 30, one third to one half of patients have chondromalacia patellae; nearly 100% do by age 60. Pathologic changes of the articular surface, however, are not always clinically significant.

To describe the origin of the pain, patellofemoral syndrome is divided into specific clinical entities: malalignment, lateral hypercompression syndrome, and excessive lateral pressure syndrome.

This chapter will focus on painful syndromes of the patellofemoral joint. The term "patellofemoral syndrome" is used to encompass all the painful entities of this joint except those secondary to instability. It is imperative to determine the exact etiology of anterior knee pain to develop a precise and effective treatment protocol.

ANATOMY, PHYSIOLOGY, AND PATHOLOGY

Patellofemoral Joint Anatomy

The patellofemoral joint consists of the femoral trochlear and the patellar articular surface. The trochlear surface or sulcus is divided into medial and lateral condyles, by which the patella articulates with the femur (Figs. 42-1 and 42-2). The lateral condyle is higher than the medial and helps prevent lateral subluxation of the patella. The femoral sulcus is flatter proximally than distally. As it deepens distally, the femoral sulcus provides greater conformity for the patella. There is a greater propensity for the patella to sublux or dislocate in extension than in flexion, where it is captured in the femoral sulcus.

The patella is the largest sesamoid bone in the body and has the thickest articular surface. As a sesamoid bone, the patella

should not be considered as a separate osseous structure, but should be viewed in the context of the entire extensor mechanism. It is divided into lateral and medial facets by the middle ridge or crest. The extensor mechanism begins proximally at the pelvis at the insertion of the rectus femoris. The mechanism is responsible for dynamic control of the patellofemoral joint in the superior–inferior plane. The vastus medialis oblique muscle (VMO) inserts into the superomedial aspect of the patella. It is the primary dynamic force responsible for medial movement of the patella and is important in stabilizing the patella both in extension and internal rotation of the femur on the tibia. The vastus lateralis and part of the iliotibial band (ITB) provide the lateral dynamic force. Static constraints include the conformity of the facets within the sulcus of the femur and the patellofemoral ligaments. These ligaments represent thickening in the capsule medially and laterally. They are located both inferiorly and superiorly on the medial and lateral patella. They extend from the anterior surface of the patella to the posterior aspect of the femoral condyles.

Vascular and Nervous Supply of the Patellofemoral Joint

Six major arteries form a plexus of blood vessels that supply the patella. The blood supply to the patella is predominantly from the distal to the proximal aspect.

The anterolateral cutaneous aspect of the knee is innervated by the genitofemoral, femoral, obturator, and saphenous nerves. No nerve root endings have been identified within the body of the patella or the femoral sulcus. There is significant controversy over the exact mechanism responsible for patellofemoral pain. Nerve endings in the subchondral bone, increased interosseous pressure, venous congestion, synovitis, and shear stresses have all been implicated. Pain may be retinacular in nature or secondary to synovitis from progressive articular breakdown and release of enzymatic factors. To date, no single entity has been proven.

Biomechanics of the Patellofemoral Joint

The patella's most important function is to facilitate extension of the knee by biomechanically increasing the movement arm. The patella increases the quadriceps strength by as much as 50%. The patella protects the patellar and the quadriceps tendons against large shear and compressive forces. In full exten-

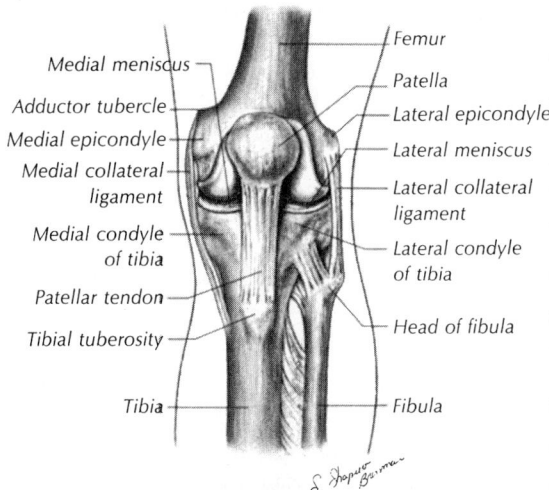

FIGURE 42-1 The anterior aspect of the knee joint. (Bates B. (1995). *A guide to physical examination and history taking*, 6/e. Philadelphia: J.B. Lippincott).

sion, the patella sits at the proximal aspect of the trochlear against the suprapatellar fat pad. As the knee flexes, the patella first articulates with the trochlear groove at about 10° in patients with normal patellar tendon length. On increasing knee flexion, the lateral facet contacts the lateral trochlear and the medial facet contacts the medial trochlear at 20° of flexion. With increased knee flexion, the patellar contact area increases and shifts proximally. At 90° of flexion, the patella enters the condylar fossa, where the contact areas are on both the lateral and medial trochlears of the femur. At 135° of knee flexion, the odd facet of the patella contacts the trochlear.

EPIDEMIOLOGY

Of 16,748 patients who presented to primary care providers with musculoskeletal complaints secondary to sports-related activities, approximately 10% had anterior knee pain (Ruffin &

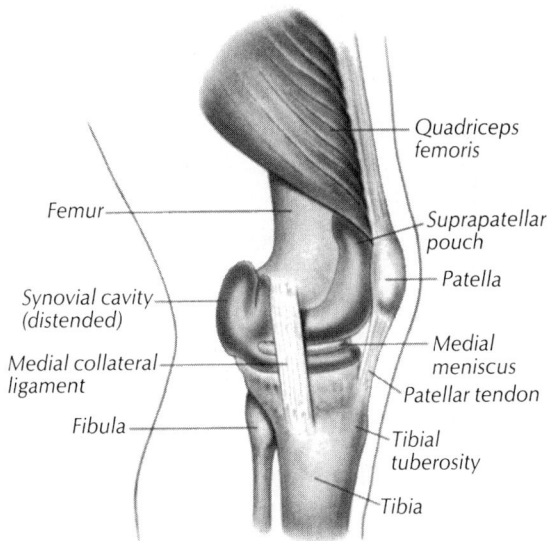

FIGURE 42-2 The medial aspect of the knee joint. (Bates B. (1995). *A guide to physical examination and history taking*, 6/e. Philadelphia: J.B. Lippincott).

Kinningham, 1993). Anterior knee pain is most common in young adults, runners, and women. In 32% of patients with anterior knee pain, running was thought to be the major cause (Davidson, 1993). Women appear to be more often affected than men because of the gynecoid pelvis, which increases their Q angle (the Q angle is formed by a line drawn from the anterior superior iliac spine of the pelvis to the center of the patella and from the center of the patella to the tibial tubercle).

HISTORY AND PHYSICAL EXAM

Patients with anterior knee pain complain of pain, crepitus, "giving way," locking, and swelling of the knee. The quality of pain must be assessed. Pain may be described as sharp, dull, burning, or aching. Patients can usually locate the pain to the kneecap, but complaints of pain referred to the back of the knee are not uncommon. The pain is worse on increased knee flexion, especially when sitting for a prolonged period. The pain is exacerbated on ascending and descending stairs. The level of pain should be assessed by discerning whether the pain prevents patients from performing activities they enjoy.

TABLE 42-1	Physical Examination

Observation
Gait: limping—weak abductors, painful joint or leg length discrepancy
Muscular atrophy
Joint effusion

Standing exam
Alignment
Q angle
Hip: femoral version
Knee: genu varum, valgum, recurvatum or flexion
Ankle/feet: valgus hindfoot or pronated foot
    Ankle equinus

Sitting exam
Observe for muscular atrophy
Measure quadriceps girth
Patella position: upward—patella alta; camelback sign
    Upward and externally rotated—"grasshopper eyes" sign
    Downward—patella baja

Supine exam
Examine for pain, swelling, masses, instability, or defect
Palpate knee joint; be systematic
    Anterior superior aspect—quadriceps tendinitis or defect
    Distal aspect—over patella, patellar tendon, and tibial tubercle
    Lateral aspect—lateral epicondyle, lateral collateral ligament, fibula head, lateral joint line, lateral retinaculum, and undersurface of the lateral facet
    Medial aspect—medial epicondyle, medial collateral ligament, medial retinaculum, medial facet, vastus medialis, or pesanserinus tendons
    Posterior aspects—hamstring tightness, Baker cyst or other masses, popliteal pulse
Q angle
Tubercle—sulcus angle
Patellofemoral grind test: chondromalacia patellae
Passive patellar tilt and glide
Ober test—ITB tendinitis
Lachman, anterior drawer, and pivot shift tests—anterior cruciate laxity
Posterior drawer and reverse pivot shift—posterior cruciate laxity
Varus and valgus stress test in 0° and 30° of knee flexion 0—LCL and MCL laxity
McMurray and Apley test—meniscus pathology

Prone exam
Quadriceps muscle tightness
Hip rotation—femoral version

Crepitus is a common finding even in normal knees. It should be considered significant only if it is associated with pain. Crepitus in patients with anterior knee pain could be secondary to synovitis, quadriceps tendon, or chondrosis.

After a careful history, a thorough exam should be done, not only of the knee joint but of the hip and ankle as well. Referred pain from the hip and ankle can present as patellofemoral pain. The patient must be examined walking, standing, sitting, and in supine, prone, and functional positions. Examine the hip and ankle first before proceeding to the more painful knee joint. The physical exam should begin with inspection of the patient (Table 42-1).

Inspection

When examining the patient, shoes, socks, and clothing should be removed to allow clear visualization of the entire pelvis and lower extremity. Observe the gait carefully as the patient enters the examining room. Limping could signify weak abductors, leg length inequality, or a painful joint in the lower extremity.

STANDING EXAM

During this phase, examine both legs. Standing alignment should be assessed for any pelvic, femoral, tibial, or pedal abnormalities that could alter the biomechanics of the knee and cause patellofemoral pain. Examine the pelvis first. The Q angle must be assessed (Fig. 42-3). The normal Q angle is 8° to 10° for a man and 10° to 20° for a woman. Women have a broader pelvis, which increases the Q angle. An increased Q angle indicates an increase in a laterally directed force on firing of the extensor mechanism. These patients frequently have malrotation of the patella with subluxation.

Next, examine the femur. The femur is normally slightly anteverted. With the feet in neutral position, the patella should point straight ahead. With increased anteversion, there is increased internal rotation of the hip, which increases the Q angle. This results in an inward-pointing patella, described as the "squinting" patella (Scuderi, 1995) (Fig. 42-4). Femoral anteversion should be evaluated by examining the hip for increased internal rotation when in supine and prone positions.

Examine the knee for genu varum (bowed legs), genu valgum (knock knees), or genu recurvatum (back knees). Genu valgum increases the Q angle and may cause patellar subluxation and lateral patellar compression syndrome. Patients may have unilateral or bilateral genu recurvatum. Those with bilateral genu recurvatum should be examined for generalized ligamentous laxity. Patients with unilateral genu recurvatum should be evaluated for possible anterior or posterior cruciate ligament insufficiency. Patients with a flexion contracture of the knee may have an untreated displaced meniscus tear, fat pad syndrome (Hoffa's disease), hamstring tightness, or contusion (Scuderi, 1995). Flexion increases the patellofemoral contact pressures and leads to patellofemoral syndrome.

Next, assess the tibia for rotation. Tibial rotation is evaluated with the patella pointing straight and the examiner looking at the direction the feet are pointing. The feet should be in neutral position. If they are pointing outward, then the patient has external tibial torsion; if the feet are pointing inward, then the patient has internal tibial torsion. In patients with external tibial torsion, the tibial tubercle moves laterally and the Q angle increases. This increases the risk of patellar subluxation and lateral patellar compression syndrome. Internal tibial torsion is generally not associated with patellofemoral disorders (Scuderi, 1995).

Finally, examine the ankles and feet. Valgus hindfoot, as in pronated foot, may be associated with genu valgus (Scuderi, 1995). This increases the Q angle and leads to patellofemoral pain. In addition, pronated feet may lead to internal tibial torsion, which causes increased femoral anteversion and increased patellofemoral pressure. Equinus deformity of the ankle, as in a tight Achilles tendon, may cause anterior knee pain by placing the knee in hyperextension during the stance phase of walking (Scuderi, 1995).

SITTING EXAM

Examine both legs as they hang loosely over the table. Look for asymmetrical muscular atrophy, and measure the girth of the quadriceps muscles on both legs at consistent locations.

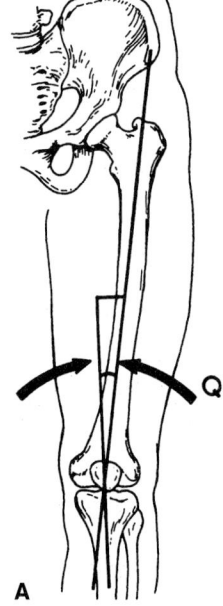

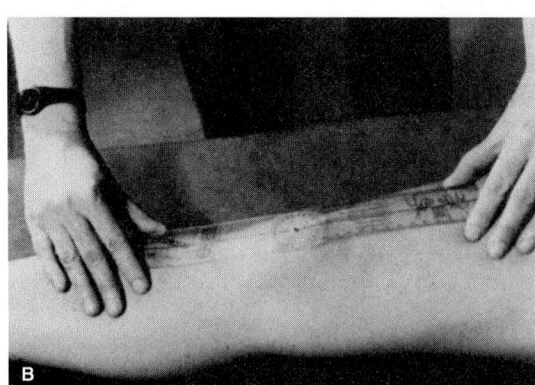

FIGURE 42-3A **(A)** The quadriceps angle (Q angle) is formed by a line drawn from the superior iliac spine of the pelvis to the center of the patella and from the center of the patella to the tibial tubercle. **(B)** Measurement of the Q angle. Source: Palmer, M.L. & Epler, M.E. (1998). *Fundamentals of musculoskeletal assessment techniques, 2/e.* Philadelphia: Lippincott-Raven Publishers.

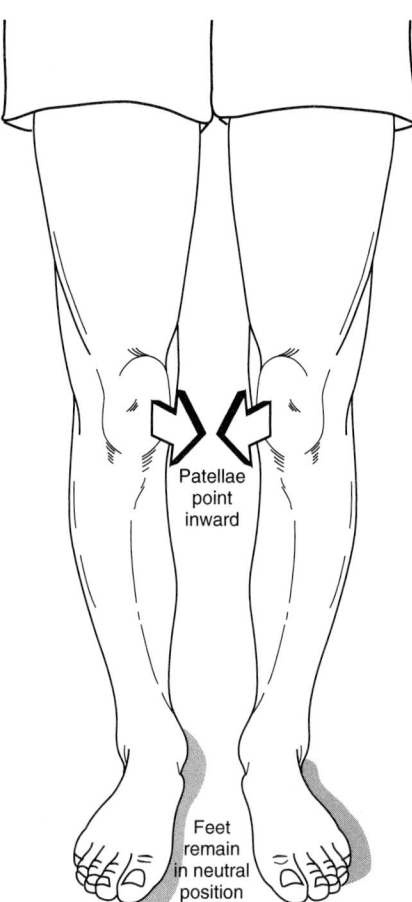

FIGURE 42-4 Squinting patallae. Rotational malalignment of the limb leads to an increased Q-angle. (Adapted from Scuderi, G. (1995). *The Patella*. New York: Springer.)

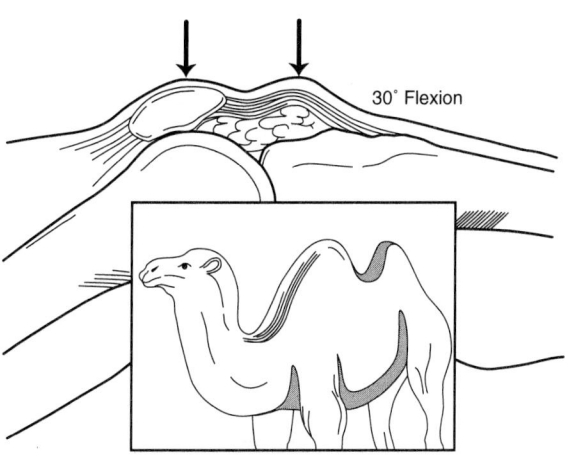

FIGURE 42-5 Camelback sign. Prominence of the infrapatellar fat pad is often associated with patella alta. (Adapted from Scuderi, G. (1995). *The Patella*. New York: Springer.)

Examine the vastus medialis muscle and its insertion area for any atrophy that may help in making a diagnosis of patellofemoral disorder.

Normally, the patella points straight forward, but in patients with a high-riding patella (patella alta), the patella points upward. In these patients, there is a prominence of the infrapatellar fat pad in extension that gives the knee a double prominence when viewed from the side; this is known as the camelback sign (Scuderi, 1995) (Fig. 42-5). These patients tend to have more patellofemoral symptoms because of the increased laxity at the patellofemoral joint. In addition, some patients with proximally riding patellae also have externally rotated patellae consistent with patella alta and lateral tilt. This is known as the "grasshopper eyes" sign (Scuderi, 1995) (Fig. 42-6).

The normal medial and lateral depression at the level of the inferior and superior poles of the patella may not be appreciated if an effusion is present. To confirm the presence of an effusion, the knee should be milked and palpated. A large effusion may allow the patella to be balloted. If swelling is present over the patellar tendon, then the patient may have patellar tendinitis or prepatellar bursitis. The tibial tubercle should be evaluated for any prominence or tenderness that would suggest chronic patellar tendinitis in the adult.

Range of motion is assessed both passively and actively. A normal range of motion of the knee is −5° to 0° of extension

to 120° to 135° of flexion. Active and passive range of motion is documented and compared to the nonpainful knee. While testing range of motion, document any abnormal tracking of the patella or any patellofemoral crepitus. Normally, the patella engages the femoral sulcus at 30° to 40° of flexion. At terminal extension, the patella may sublux or jump laterally, which is referred to as the J sign (Fig. 42-7). This usually indicates excessive pull by the vastus lateralis because of a weak vastus medialis.

SUPINE EXAM

In the supine exam, the patellofemoral area is systematically examined for pain, swelling, mass, instability, and defect. The entire joint is palpated (see Table 42-1). The Q angle is measured and documented. An increased Q angle alone is not a reliable indicator of patellar malalignment. The Q angle is greatest in full extension; a Q angle with the knee flexed is more significant.

The patellofemoral grind test is performed as the provider gently compresses the patella against the femoral sulcus and then has the patient contract the quadriceps. Any pain elicited on compression may signify articular injury, such as chondromalacia patellae. To increase specificity, the test should be performed again in 30° of flexion, because the grind test may be positive in an asymptomatic knee.

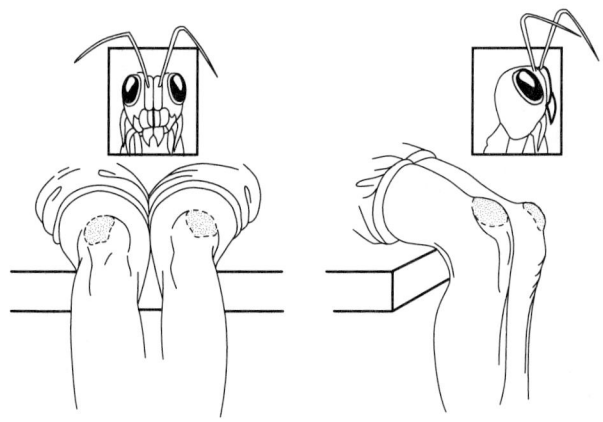

FIGURE 42-6 Grasshopper eyes. Proximal- and lateral-facing position of the patella associated with patella alta and lateral tilt. (Adapted from Scuderi, G. (1995). *The Patella*. New York: Springer.)

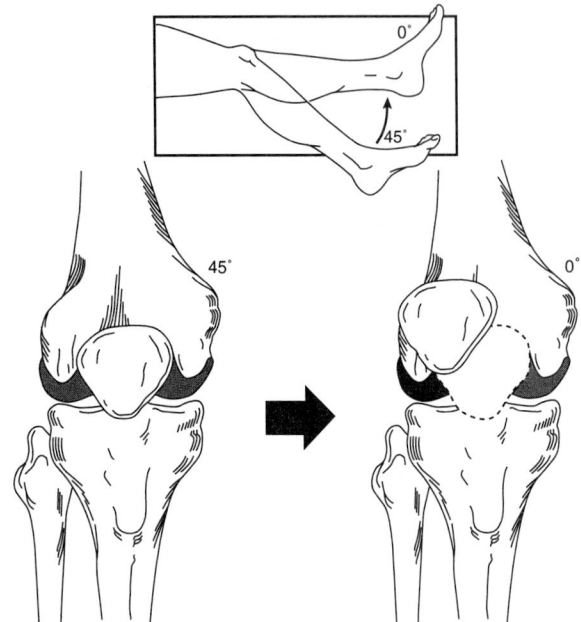

FIGURE 42-7 The J sign. Lateral deviation of the patella, with terminal extension rather than normal straight proximal line of pull. (Adapted from Scuderi, G. (1995). *The Patella*. New York: Springer.)

Assessments of passive patellar tilt and glide are important to determine the mobility of the patella. The passive patella tilt test evaluates the tightness of the lateral retinaculum (Fulkerson, 1997) (Fig. 42-8). With the patient supine and the quadriceps fully relaxed, the patella is grasped between the examiner's index finger and thumb at the midportion of the patella. The amount of upward tilt of the patella laterally is assessed. The normal tilt is 0°. A neutral tilt angle is one in which the lateral patellar edge is parallel to the floor. A negative tilt of less than 0° is consistent with an excessively tight lateral retinaculum and elevated lateral pressure syndrome (ELPS; Aglietti & Insall, 1993; Fulkerson, 1997; Parker, 1995). This should be compared to the asymptomatic knee. A passive patella glide test indicates medial or lateral retinacular laxity or tightness (Fig. 42-9). With the quadriceps relaxed and with the knee supported in 30° of flexion, the patella is displaced medially or laterally. Considering the patella in four longitudinal quadrants, a lateral glide of three or more quadrants indicates an incompe-

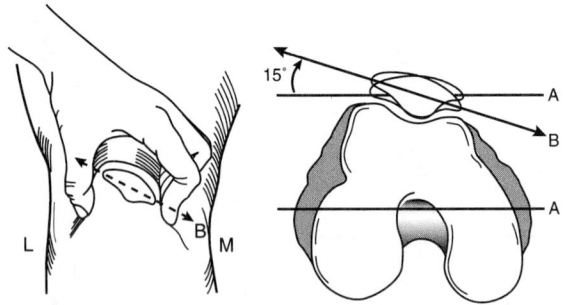

FIGURE 42-8 The passive patella tilt test. The inability to tilt the patella beyond a line parallel to the transepicondylar axis is consistent with a contracted lateral retinaculum. (**A′** transepicondylar axis; **A**, patella horizontal to transepicondylar axis; **B**, patella tilted beyond horizontal.) (Adapted from Scuderi, G. (1995). *The Patella*. New York: Springer.)

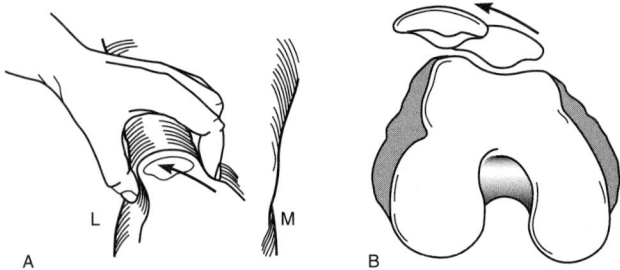

FIGURE 42-9 The passive patella glide test. With the knee flexed to 30° and the quadricep relaxed, the patella is pushed medially (**A**) then laterally (**B**). Medial deviation of one quadrant or less is consistent with a contracted lateral retinaculum. Lateral deviation of greater than two quadrants is consistent with a lax or ruptured medial retinaculum. (Adapted from Scuderi, G. (1995). *The Patella*. New York: Springer.)

tent medial retinaculum (Parker, 1995). A medial glide of one quadrant or less is consistent with a tight lateral retinaculum or ELPS (Parker, 1995). When the patella displaces medially three or more quadrants, a hypermobile patella is diagnosed, the result of congenital disorders or lateral retinacular release (Parker, 1995).

The patella can also be in a laterally tilted position if there is a tight ITB. Normally, the ITB falls posteriorly when the knee is flexed. With a tight ITB, the fibers attaching to the lateral retinaculum increase the pull between the patella and the ITB when the knee is flexed; this causes a laterally tilted patella and will cause ELPS. The Ober test is used to evaluate ITB tightness (described in the section on ITB syndrome below).

Each knee is tested for laxity of the anterior cruciate, posterior cruciate, medial collateral (MCL), and lateral collateral ligaments (LCL) and meniscal pathology by performing the appropriate tests. Patients with ligament insufficiency often complain of patellofemoral pain and of the knee "giving way." It is vital to differentiate giving way from quadriceps inhibition and instability. Reflex inhibition of the quadriceps may be caused by an effusion or patellofemoral pain. The anterior cruciate ligament is tested by performing the Lachman test, anterior drawer test, and pivot shift test. The posterior cruciate ligament can be tested by performing the posterior drawer test and reverse pivot shift and looking for posterior sag when the knee is flexed 90°. The collateral ligaments are tested by applying either varus or valgus force to the knee in 0° and 30° of knee flexion. Both patellofemoral syndrome and meniscal pathology can cause joint line tenderness in the anterior third of the medial and lateral joint line. To evaluate the meniscus, provocative tests such as those described by McMurray (Fig. 42-10) and Apley (Fig. 42-11) should be performed. A palpable or audible click produced in the joint by the McMurray test suggests a posterior medial meniscus tear. Pain produced by the Apley test suggests a tear related to the location of pain (Hoppenfeld, 1976).

PRONE EXAM

The patient should be examined in the prone position to determine quadriceps muscle tightness. To determine quadriceps flexibility, stabilize the pelvis to prevent compensatory hip flexion and allow the patient to touch the heel to the buttock. Comparison should be made to the contralateral normal leg. Hip rotation to assess femoral anteversion is easier in the prone

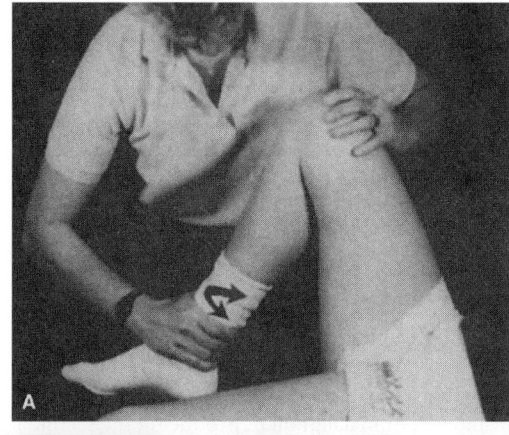
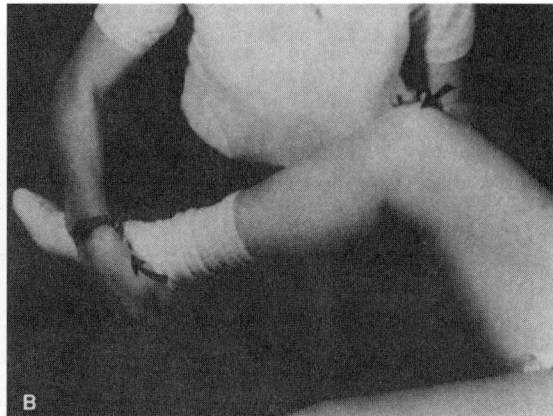
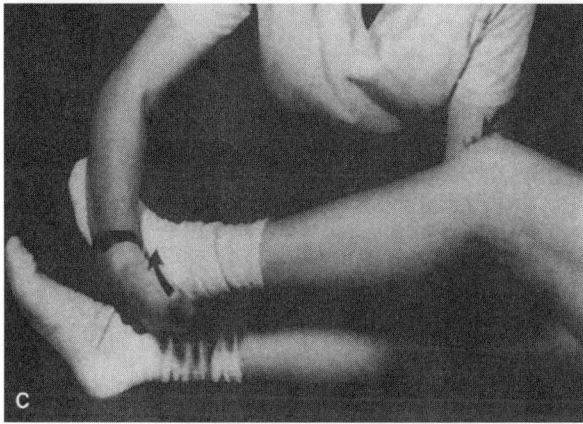

FIGURE 42-10 The McMurray test for meniscal tears. (**A**) Flex the knee. With the knee flexed, internally and externally rotate the tibia on the femur. (**B**) With the leg externally rotated, place a valgus stress on the knee. (**C**) With the leg externally rotated and in valgus, slowly extend the knee. If click is palpable or audible, the test is considered positive for a torn medial meniscus, usually in the posterior position. (Palmer, M.L. Epler, M.E. (1998). *Fundamentals of musculoskeletal assessment techniques. 2/e.* Philadelphia: Lippincott-Raven Publishers.)

position than in the supine position. With the knee flexed to 90°, rotate the leg internally until the greater trochanter is maximally prominent laterally. At this degree, the femoral neck is parallel to the table and the angle between the vertical and the tibia is the angle of hip anteversion. Both legs should be examined for femoral rotation.

Radiographic Imaging

The initial evaluation of the patellofemoral joint requires three radiographic views: an extension weight-bearing view, a lateral view with the knee in 30° of flexion, and a Mercer-Merchant view (Table 42-2). These views normally suffice for the provider to initiate treatment. Additional studies include computed tomographic (CT) scans with the knee in 15° and 30° of flexion, magnetic resonance imaging (MRI), radionuclide scans, and even venography.

The standing anteroposterior (AP) view of the knee is important in assessing the medial and lateral joint space for narrowing or widening. In patients with arthrosis, there may be bilateral joint space narrowing or single compartment narrowing. Mild degrees of cartilage loss may be detected in weight-bearing x-rays versus supine AP views. The AP view provides limited information on the patellofemoral joint. The patellar

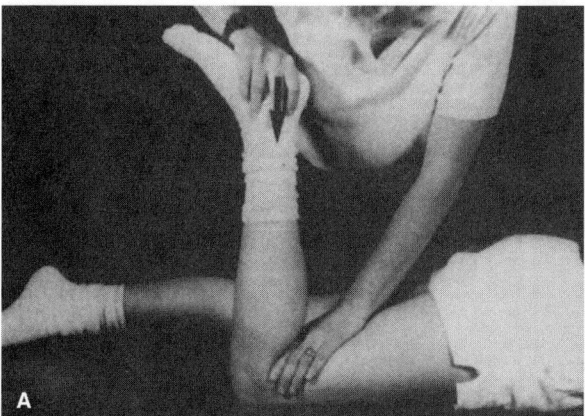
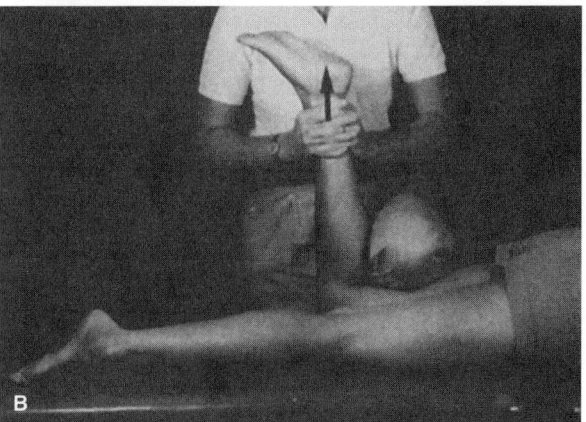

FIGURE 42-11 (**A**) Apley's compression test for meniscal tear. Compression force through the leg combined with medial tibial rotation. (**B**) Apley's distraction test for ligamentous damage. (Palmer, M.L. Epler, M.E. (1998). *Fundamentals of musculoskeletal assessment techniques. 2/e.* Philadelphia: Lippincott-Raven Publishers.)

TABLE 42-2	Radiographic Imaging

AP view
  Medial and lateral spaces
  Patellar length and width
  Femoral condyle symmetry
Lateral view (30°)
  Patellar height and thickness
  Subchondral patella sclerosis
  Patellofemoral arthrosis
  Soft-tissue calcifications in quadriceps or patellar tendon, infrapatellar fat pad, bursae, and muscles
  Patella position—Blumensaat's line and Insall-Salvati method
Mercer-Merchant axial view:
  Sulcus and congruence angle

length and width can be measured. Anatomic variations such as bipartite patella, patellar fracture, and the size and symmetry of the femoral condyle can be determined.

The 30° lateral view is critical in evaluating the patellofemoral joint. Patellar height and thickness can be measured. The presence of subchondral patellar sclerosis, evidence of patellofemoral arthrosis, can be determined. Abnormal soft-tissue calcification or ossification can be visualized in the quadriceps or patellar tendon, the infrapatellar fat pad, the bursae, and the muscles. Calcifications in the quadriceps muscle or tendon may represent myositis ossificans or an old tear. Calcifications or ossifications in the proximal or distal patellar tendon insertion may represent Sinding-Larson-Johansson disease or Osgood-Schlatter disease in the adolescent (Sinding-Larson, 1921; Osgood, 1903). Swelling or calcification in the prepatellar area may represent "housemaid's knee," and swelling in the suprapatellar area represents a joint effusion.

The lateral view in 30° of flexion places the patellar tendon under tension and demonstrates the functional relations of the patella to the tibia and to the femoral trochlear groove. The vertical patellar height is important in the integrity and stability of the extensor mechanism and the patellofemoral joint.

Axial tangential views, such as Mercer-Merchant, Laurin, or Jaroschy views, are important for assessing the contour of the patellar facets and their relation to the femoral trochlear sulcus (Laurin et al, 1979; Merchant et al, 1974). Although many axial views are described, Merchant's view is the most widely used. Two angles are measured on this view, the sulcus and the congruence angles. The average sulcus angle is 138°, with a standard deviation of 6°. The greater the sulcus angle, the less lateral buttressing the lateral condyle imparts to the patella and more likely for the patient to sublux the patella. The congruence angle is measured by bisecting the sulcus angle; then a line is drawn to the median crest of the patella (Merchant et al, 1974). The angle between the bisected angle of the sulcus and the median crest line indicates the congruence angle. A lateral congruence angle is considered positive, a medial angle negative. A congruence angle greater than +16° is considered abnormal, indicating lateral patellar subluxation.

TREATMENT OPTIONS, EXPECTED OUTCOMES, AND COMPREHENSIVE MANAGEMENT

After a thorough history and physical exam, a diagnosis can be made. Combining knowledge of the anatomy, biomechanics, and natural history of patellofemoral problems with the history

and physical exam, a logical treatment protocol can begin. Radiographic studies are used to corroborate the clinical diagnosis and must not be relied on in the absence of confirmatory clinical data (Table 42-3).

Chondromalacia Patellae

Chondromalacia patellae is defined as soft cartilage of the patella. The patient usually complains of anterior knee pain, but the origin of pain is difficult to define and localization of pain on the clinical exam does not coincide. The provider should look for the etiology of the chondromalacia patellae and should not assume that the anterior knee pain is secondary to cartilage softening. A primary condition such as trauma, patellofemoral instability, or malalignment producing the secondary chondromalacia patellae should be sought. In many cases, x-rays must include Merchant's axial view of both knees, and sometimes CT or MRI is helpful. The ultimate diagnosis requires arthroscopy. To begin treatment, the primary cause of chondromalacia patellae must be diagnosed. If a course of nonoperative treatment of at least 3 months' duration fails to produce a result, then arthroscopic evaluation is warranted.

Excessive Lateral Pressure Syndrome

ELPS or lateral patellar compression syndrome is diagnosed when the physical exam and radiographic studies indicate that the patient's complaints are associated with patellar malalignment without any gross patellofemoral instability consistent with dislocation (Fulkerson, 1990a, 1990b). The patella is laterally tilted secondary to a tight lateral retinaculum without evidence of patellar subluxation. On the physical exam, the patellar facets are usually tender, as is the lateral retinaculum. The passive patella tilt is less than 0°. Patients may have a J sign, and when they contract the quadriceps the patella moves laterally. Radiographic evaluation includes Merchant's axial view to determine if patellar tilt or subluxation is present. X-rays will show lateral tilting of the patella without subluxation, although minor subluxation secondary to malalignment may result in patellofemoral pain and should be included under the diagnosis of patellofemoral syndrome.

The treatment for ELPS consists of activity modification, nonsteroidal anti-inflammatories (NSAIDs), and a systematic rehabilitation protocol. The rehabilitation includes quadriceps strengthening and in particular vastus medialis oblique muscle strengthening. If a course of nonoperative treatment of at least 3 months' duration does not produce results, the patient may be a surgical candidate, although the vast majority of patients can be treated without surgery. Before surgery, the lateral retinaculum can be injected with lidocaine as a diagnostic test. If the pain is relieved, then lateral retinacular release may be of benefit.

Plica

Entities other than patellofemoral syndrome may be responsible for anterior knee pain. Patients with symptomatic plicae present with anterior knee pain in the medial infrapatellar or lateral suprapatellar region (Broom, 1986). This is common in runners and jumpers, whose activities lead to thickening and inflammation of the plicae normally found in the knee joint.

TABLE 42-3	Differential Diagnosis of Knee Pain				
Disorder	**Presentation**	**Physical Findings**	**Radiography**	**Pathophysiology**	**Treatment**
Chondromalacia patellae	Chronic anterior knee pain Pain worse climbing and descending stairs Older patients	Patellar tenderness on axial compression	AP/lat and axial view MRI is often helpful in making a diagnosis. Ultimate diagnosis requires arthroscopy.	Trauma Patellofemoral instability Patellofemoral malalignment	Phase I-IV rehab. Emphasis on quad. strengthening
Excessive lateral pressure syndrome	Pain over the lateral parapatellar region J sign	Lateral tilted patella Negative passive patella tilt	AP/lat and axial*	Patellofemoral malalignment No patellofemoral instability	Activity modifications NSAIDs VMO strengthening Surgery if rehab. fails
Plica	Pain in the medial infrapatellar or lateral suprapatellar region Painful medial click on range of motion	Palpable tender band along the superolateral aspect of the medial retinaculum	AP/lat and axial to exclude other causes of anterior knee pain MRI most useful	Repetitive lateral patella subluxation	Activity modification Training error correct. NSAIDs Rehabilitation Cortisone injection if rehab. fails Plica excision if conservative tx. fails
Patella tendinitis	Pain at the inferior aspect of the patella	Inferior pole of the patella tenderness Limited knee flexion	AP/lat and axial* Look for calcifications in the patella tendon insertion area	Overuse syndrome Training error	Activity modification Rest Training error correct. NSAIDs Cryotherapy Rehab. for quadriceps strengthening and stretching exercises Iontophoresis with hydrocortisone CHOPAT strap Surgery if conserv. tx. fails
Quadriceps tendinitis	Pain at the quadriceps insertion Limited knee flexion	Tenderness at the quadricep insertion	AP/lat and axial	Overuse syndrome Training error Forceful quad. contraction	Same as patella tendinitis
Bursitis	Anterior knee pain with swelling Pain localized to affected bursa	Acute bursitis: swollen, boggy and tender knee Chronic bursitis: skin thickening and swelling	AP/lat and axial	Prolonged kneeling Overuse Sports related: football and wrestling	NSAIDs Activity modification Rest Stretching and strengthening ex. Cortisone injection In acute cases with overlying abrasion start antibiotics
Fat pad syndrome	Pain peripatellar tendon region	Tenderness deep to the peripatellar tendon area	AP/lat and axial to exclude other causes	Direct trauma Fat pad compressed between femoral condyles and tibial plateaus in extension	Activity modification Anterior knee padding Cryotherapy Surgery if conserv. tx. fails
Iliotibial band friction syndrome		Pain on the lateral aspect with flexion and extension of the knee		Improper shoe wear Training error	Stretching ITB Local hot packs NSAIDs Orthotics Cortisone injection over lat. epicondyle Surgery if conserv. tx. fails
Patellar osteochondritis dissecans	Diffuse pain Swelling Locking Giving way	Crepitus and pain with patellar compression Quadriceps wasting Effusion Knee motion not limited	AP/lat* and axial MRI may be useful to determine viability and staging of fragment	Unknown, but possibly microtrauma, genetic, ischemia, endocrine, etc.	Stage I: Extension casting or arthroscopic drilling Stage II or III: small fragment-excise large fragment-drill and fix Stage IV: remove and abrade defect

On exam, the patient's pain is associated with a palpable tender band along the medial retinaculum superolaterally. This may also be associated with a painful click as the knee is flexed and extended. Isokinetic testing may reveal quadriceps muscle inhibition in the flexion zone where the pain is elicited.

Many conditions can mimic this condition. Conditions such as chondrosis, subluxation, and dislocation of the patella and ELPS need to be excluded. Theoretically, repetitive lateral subluxation of the patella may cause friction of a medial plica, which then becomes fibrotic and inflamed.

Treatment begins with modification of activities, rehabilitation, and correction of training errors. NSAIDs and icing should be used to decrease inflammation and swelling. A local steroid injection into the surrounding capsule may be warranted if other conservative measures fail. Arthroscopic surgical excision of the symptomatic plica is indicated if conservative measures fail.

Patellar Tendinitis (Jumper's Knee)

Patellar tendinitis is a common cause of anterior knee pain in athletes involved in jumping sports such as basketball, volleyball, and tennis. On exam, there is tenderness of the patellar tendon on palpation. The pain is usually located at the origin of the tendon from the inferior pole of the patella or at its insertion into the tibial tubercle. The deep portion of the patellar tendon should also be examined by fully extending the knee and allowing the quadriceps muscle to relax, thus allowing the examiner to palpate the deep portion of the patellar tendon (Roels et al, 1978). Examining the patellar tendon with the knee flexed may produce a false-negative result.

Initial management is the same as for any overuse syndrome: correcting training errors, relative rest, icing, progressive strengthening exercises, stretching (especially of the quadriceps tendon), and the use of NSAIDs. Modalities directed to the patellar tendon area such as iontophoresis with hydrocortisone cream, ice massage, ultrasonography, and even a patellar tendon strap may be helpful.

In most instances, tendinitis of the patellar tendon resolves with nonoperative treatment. In chronic cases, the inflammation may lead to a necrotic focus within the tendon. If the patient cannot perform normal activities after a prolonged trial of conservative treatment, then surgical exploration of the tendon is indicated. There is no place for cortisone injection in the patellar tendon.

Quadriceps Tendinitis

Quadriceps tendinitis is not as common as patellar tendinitis but is treated in a similar fashion. Typically it is seen in overuse situations, or after a forceful contraction of the quadriceps muscle causes a localized injury in the tendon. On exam, the patient has tenderness at the quadriceps tendon insertion. The patient can do the straight leg raise (SLR) but may have a mild extension lag. A partial or complete quadriceps rupture needs to be ruled out by palpating for any defect. Surgery is rarely indicated.

Bursitis

Bursae are synovium-lined cavities that help reduce friction between tendons and other soft tissues or bones. Bursae can become inflamed and symptomatic from acute trauma or chronic irritation. The bursae found around the knee include the suprapatellar, superficial prepatellar, superficial, deep infrapatellar, and pes anserinus bursae. Two of the most common types of bursitis, superficial prepatellar and pes anserinus, will be discussed.

Prepatellar bursitis is the most common bursitis of the knee, especially in patients who have a history of prolonged kneeling (eg, carpet cleaners or wrestlers). There is skin thickening and swelling of the anterior patella. In acute cases, prepatellar bursitis presents as a swollen, boggy, and tender knee. In subacute cases, there is pronounced thickening and tenderness of the skin.

In patients with acute cases, such as football players or wrestlers, it is important to examine for and treat abrasions because infection can occur. If abrasions are found at the anterior aspect of the knee with bursitis, then broad-spectrum antibiotics should be prescribed (Parker, 1995). If this area is aspirated, a sterile compressive dressing should be used to prevent reaccumulation of blood or fluid. Rarely, cortisone should be injected in the prepatellar bursa. Cortisone should not be used if infection is possible (Parker, 1995). If recurrent swelling prevents the patient from performing activities, then surgical excision of the prepatellar bursa is indicated.

The pes anserinus bursa is located underneath the insertion of the sartorius, gracilis, and semitendinosus tendon at the proximal medial tibial metaphysis. This pain is often present at the medial compartment area but can radiate to the anterior knee. Palpation of the pes anserinus region will often elicit pain. This form of bursitis responds to NSAIDs, ice, stretching, and physical therapy. A local injection of cortisone may be necessary if other conservative measures fail.

Hoffa's Disease (Fat Pad Syndrome)

Anterior knee pain caused by induration of the infrapatellar fat pad as a result of hemorrhage and fibrosis was first described by Hoffa in 1904. The infrapatellar fat pad can be traumatized by a direct blow or by chronic compression between the femoral condyles and the tibial plateaus on extension (Parker, 1995). Treatment includes activity modification, cryotherapy, and padding of the anterior knee to reduce trauma. In chronic cases where these methods are not beneficial, then surgical excision of the infrapatellar fat pad is warranted.

ITB Friction Syndrome

The ITB is both a flexor and an extensor of the knee, depending on the starting position of the knee. The ITB inserts at Gerdy's tubercle and moves posteriorly to the axis of rotation as the knee is flexed. In doing so, the ITB rubs over the lateral epicondyle and if unduly tight may cause the ITB friction syndrome.

The ITB should be palpated for tenderness as it slides over the lateral femoral epicondyle. The Ober test is performed to confirm the diagnosis (Ober, 1936) (Fig. 42-12). With the patient lying on the contralateral side, the hip is flexed and allowed to fall into an adducted position. If the ITB is tight, the leg will fail to fall into adduction and pain can be elicited over the femoral condyle by extending and flexing the knee. Improper shoes and genu varum may increase ITB tightness, causing the ITB syndrome.

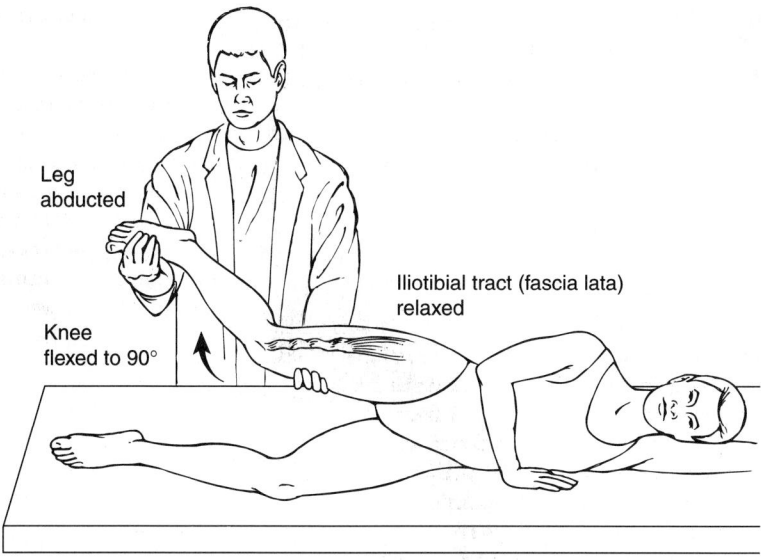

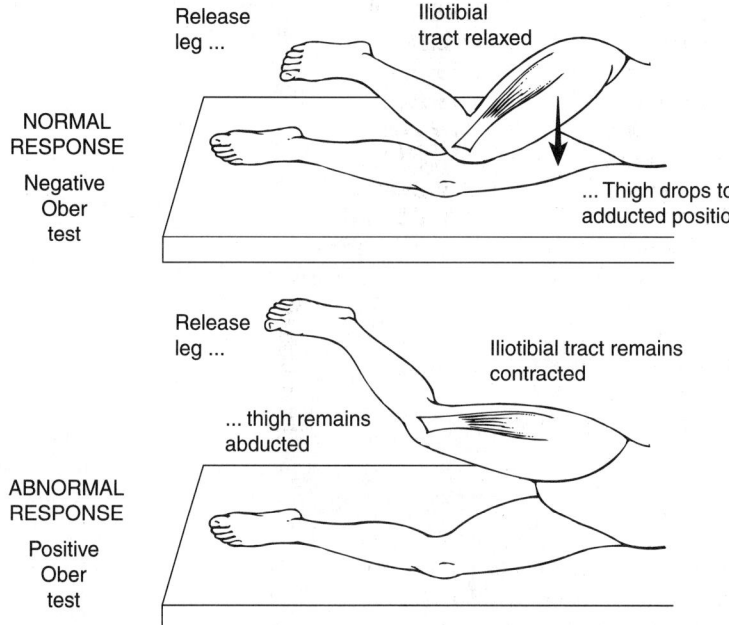

FIGURE 42-12 Ober's test. Tests for contraction of the iliotibial band (ITB). (Scuderi, G. (1995). *The Patella*. New York: Springer.)

Treatment begins with stretching of the ITB, local hot packs, NSAIDs, orthoses, and finally a cortisone injection over the lateral epicondyle. If conservative treatment fails, then surgical exploration and resection of a portion of the ITB is warranted.

Patellar Osteochondritis Dissecans

The middle and lower thirds of the medial facet are commonly affected in this rare disorder. The exact etiology is unknown. Common complaints are anterior knee pain, swelling, locking, and giving way; 30% of patients recall a history of trauma (Scuderi, 1995). On exam, the most notable sign is crepitus, as well as pain with compression of the patella, quadriceps wasting, and effusion. Knee motion is not usually restricted. The diagnosis is confirmed by AP, lateral, and Merchant's axial views of the patella. The lesion is most easily seen on the lateral x-ray. MRI is warranted in some cases to determine the viability and stage of the affected fragment. Treatment consists of immobilization in an extension cast or arthroscopic drilling to increase the vascularity and healing.

REHABILITATION

Rehabilitation is the initial treatment for anterior knee pain. A rehabilitation plan is initiated after an accurate diagnosis is established. Rehabilitation is recommended for at least 3 months before opting for surgical intervention. A phased system allows a comprehensive and individualized approach to treatment (Andrews, 1991; Brunet, 1989; Parker, 1995; Scuderi, 1995; Sheldon & Thigpen, 1991). This phased system allows the patient's specific goals to be met and results in func-

TABLE 42-4	Rehabilitation

Phase I: Acute or immediate postoperative phase
 Goals
  Reduce pain and swelling
  Retard muscular atrophy
  Maintain and improve range of motion
 Modalities
  NSAIDs
  Cryotherapy
  Acitivity modifications
  TENS
  Patella immobilization and mobilization
  Gentle range of motion
  Bracing and taping, including McConnell taping
  Stretching
 Exercises
  Isometric—supine and standing
  SLR (straight leg raise)
 Progress to phase II once symptoms diminished

Phase II: Intermediate or strengthening phase
 Goals
  Regain full pain-free range of motion
  Restore normal gait
  Increase muscular strength
 Exercises
  Continue isometric and SLR with weights
  Isotonic—concentric and eccentric
  Isokinetic
 70% to 80% of quadriceps muscle strength obtained after phase II
 Proceed to phase III once range of motion, pain, and swelling are within
  normal range

Phase III: Functional activity stage
 Goals
  Maximum strength
  Muscular endurance
  Muscular power
  Functional activities
 Modalities
  Aquatic exercises
  Sport-specific drills
 Progress to phase IV after returning to previous level of activities

Phase IV: Maintainance stage
 Goals
  Maintain range of motion, strength, and function
 Exercises
  Flexibility (stretching) emphasized
  Functional exercises continued two or three times/week

If patient cannot progress through phases, re-examine and change rehabilitation
  accordingly or refer to specialist for alternative treatment, such as surgery.

---

tional progress. There are four phases: acute or postoperative, intermediate or strengthening, functional activities, and maintenance (Table 42-4).

Phase I

In phase I, the acute injury or immediate postoperative phase, multiple modalities are used. Cryotherapy has been the most successful modality to reduce inflammation, swelling, and pain.

Rest, avoidance of aggravating activities, and the judicious use of NSAIDs are imperative to decrease pain, swelling, and inflammation. The next goal in this phase is to restore normal passive and active range of motion. Once the range of motion of all the joints is restored, then selective muscle-stretching exercises can begin. The patient is educated in appropriate soft-tissue stretching, with incorporation of strapping and taping for soft-tissue balancing.

Stretching of the hip, knee, and ankle musculature is very important in the initial phase. Improved flexibility is achieved through stretching to the point of mild muscle tension; it should not produce muscular pain. Each muscle group, such as the hamstrings, quadriceps, gastrosoleus, and ITB, should be stretched statically for 30 to 60 seconds, and the stretch should be repeated four times. Many runners have anterior knee pain secondary to poor stretching before running. Patients with ITB friction syndrome and ELPS should perform extensive stretching of the ITB.

Isometric exercises are also an important aspect of phase I. An isometric exercise involves a muscle contraction in which the length of the muscle remains constant while tension develops toward maximal force against an immovable resistance. Exercises such as isometric quadriceps muscle contractions at multiple angles and joint positions, with incorporation of biofeedback, are very useful for muscle contraction and strength. Both supine and standing isometric exercises can be performed to mimic functional activities. Another common exercise for rehabilitation of the patellofemoral joint is the SLR. The SLR is a effective way of increasing the quadriceps strength early, when range of motion of the knee is limited. SLR is initiated while the patient is still in the knee immobilizer.

Phase II

When the patient's symptoms have diminished, phase II can be started. The main goals of this phase are to regain full pain-free range of motion, to restore normal gait, and to increase muscular strength. The isometric quadriceps sets and SLR exercises are continued with weights. Isotonic (concentric and eccentric) and isokinetic exercises are started. Concentric contraction is when the muscle shortens when generating force; eccentric contraction is when the muscle lengthens on generating force. An isokinetic exercise is one in which the speed of motion is set and resistance accommodates to move the force applied. Strengthening exercises incorporating both concentric and eccentric contractions with endurance training of the total lower extremity are emphasized. Dynamic strengthening exercises should be performed in both a closed- and an open-chain manner. A closed kinetic chain is a series of connecting joints, creating an intricate motor system in which the distal segment is fixed; in the open kinetic chain, the distal segment is free. Closed-chain exercises involve weight bearing, or a planted foot; open-chain exercises do not involve weight bearing. Because closed-chain exercises mimic functional activities and activities of daily living, they are more important. Exercises include leg presses, unilateral and bilateral squats, step-downs, walk stance positions, wall slides in various positions, and step-ups. Isokinetic exercises can be started once isotonic exercises are performed without pain. By the end of this phase, quadriceps muscle strength should be 70% to 80% that of the contralateral normal leg.

Phase III

Phase III, or the functional activities stage, is initiated once range of motion, pain, and swelling are within the normal range. The goal of this phase is to reach maximal strength while developing muscular endurance, power, and functional activities. Aquatic exercises and sport-specific drills are imperative. Functional exercises are broken down into running, jumping, cutting, and agility drills, which then can be combined to re-create sport-specific movements. Continuation of these exercises returns the patient to the preinjury level.

Phase IV

Phase IV, or the maintenance stage, is continued once the patient has returned to the previous level of activity. Flexibility exercises used before and after sports activities are stressed. Functional exercises for specific muscle groups and resistance exercises are performed two or three times per week.

A patient who cannot progress through the phases should be re-examined and re-evaluated for any appropriate rehabilitation changes or for alternative treatments, such as surgery.

COMMUNITY RESOURCES

- Chondromalacia Links: http://www.fcg.net/darla/chondro/index.html: General information on chondromalacia, Swedish cartilage regeneration program, MRI of knee disorders, braces and supports, Aircast infrapatellar band
- YSMC Sports Injuries Page: http://info.med.yale.edu/ortho/ysmc/injuries/knee.htm: Anterior knee pain and patellofemoral syndrome
- Enid Family Medicine (Outpatient Orthopedics): http://www.fammed.uokhsc.edu/Enid/chondro.htm
- American Academy of Orthopaedic Surgeons: http://www.aaos.org/wordhtml/home2.htm
- American Academy of Orthopaedic Surgeons, 6300 N. River Rd., Rosemont, IL, 60018-4262, 847-823-7186, 800-346-AAOS, Fax: 847-823-8125

REFERRAL POINTS AND CLINICAL WARNINGS

The use of braces for the treatment of patellofemoral problems remains a controversial issue: there are just as many studies proving beneficial effects of bracing as there are showing a minimal effect. The various functions of these braces include dissipation of force, improved patellar tracking, maintenance of patellofemoral alignment, and prevention of patellar subluxation and dislocation (Cherf, 1990). Several braces should be tried to find one that provides symptomatic relief. When braces are used, they should be considered only an adjunct to other therapeutic techniques, such as physical therapy; they should never be the sole means of treating the patellofemoral problem.

Foot orthoses can be used in patients who have foot abnormalities. Orthoses have helped reduce anterior knee pain in patients with abnormal ankle and subtalar motion. Like braces, orthoses are an adjunct to the physical therapy program and should not be the sole means of treating patellofemoral disorders.

■ ■ ■ ■ **CLINICAL PEARLS**

- Referred pain from the hip and ankle can present as patellofemoral pain. The exam must include the hip, ankle, and knee.
- Internal tibial torsion is generally not associated with patellofemoral disorders.
- If the patient has a history of recent trauma, inability to extend the knee fully, and a palpable defect in the quadriceps tendon, a quadriceps tendon rupture should be suspected.

TEACHING AND SELF-CARE

The emphasis of teaching and self-care for the patient with anterior knee pain focuses on rehabilitation, as discussed above.

EDITOR'S NOTE:
COMPLEMENTARY APPROACHES

A general discussion of complementary approaches can be found in Chapter 3. The following, while not an exhaustive list, are some complementary approaches being used for this condition. Additional information on these approaches, including precautions, can be found in Appendices A and B. Providers need to assess for the use of complementary approaches as part of the patient's history, as they may impact conventional therapies, and patients may not volunteer this information unless specifically asked. Efficacy of many complementary approaches is not as well documented as that of conventional therapies. Providers need to read the literature before suggesting these complementary approaches.

- Vitamins, minerals, herbs, supplements
    Glucosamine sulfate
- Complementary Modalities
    Acupuncture
    Aromatherapy
    Biofeedback

References

Aglietti, P., & Insall, J.N. (1993). Disorders of the patellofemoral joint. In Insall JN (Eds.). *Surgery of the Knee.* NY: Churchill Livingstone, 246–251.

Broom, J.M. (1986). The plica syndrome: A new perspective. *Orthopedic Clinics of North America, 17*(2), 279–281.

Cherf, J. & Paulus, L. (1990). Bracing for patella instability. *Clinical Sports Medicine, 9,* 813–821.

Davidson, K. (1993). Patellofemoral pain syndrome. *American Family Physician, 48*(7), 1254–1262.

Fulkerson, J.P. (1990a). Biomechanics of the patellofemoral joint. *Disorders of the patellofemoral joint.* Baltimore: Williams and Wilkins, 25–41.

Fulkerson, J.P. (1990b). Disorders of patellofemoral alignment. *Journal of Bone & Joint Surgery, 72A,* Baltimore: Williams and Wilkins, 1424–1429.

Fulkerson, J.P. (1997). *Disorders of the patellofemoral joint.*

Laurin, C.A., Dussault, R., & Levesque, H.P. (1979). The tangential x-ray investigation of the patellofemoral joint: X-ray technique, diagnostic criteria and their interpretation. *Clinical Orthopaedics, 144,* 16–26.

Merchant, A.C., Mercer, R.L., Jacobsen, R.J., & Cool, C.R. (1974). Roentgenographic analysis of patello-femoral congruence. *Journal of Bone & Joint Surgery, 56A,* 1391–1396.

Ober, F.R. (1936). The role of the iliotibial band and fascia lata as a factor in the causation of low-back disabilities and sciatica. *Journal of Bone & Joint Surgery, 18A,* 106.

Osgood, R.B. (1903). Lesions of the tibial tubercle occurring during adolescence. *Boston Medical & Surgical Journal, 148,* 114–117.

Parker, G.C. (1995). Anterior knee pain. *Knee Surgery.* Baltimore: Williams and Wilkins, 929–951.

Roels, J., Martens, M., & Mulier, J.C. (1978). Patellar tendinitis (jumper's knee). *American Journal of Sports Medicine, 6,* 362–368.

Ruffin, M.T. IV, & Kinningham, R.B. (1993). Anterior knee pain: The challenge of patellofemoral syndrome. *American Family Physician, 47*(1), 185–194.

Scuderi, G. (1995). *The patella.* New York: Springer-Verlag.

Sheldon, G., & Thigpen, L.K. (1991). Rehabilitation of patellofemoral dysfunction: A review of the literature. *Journal of Orthopedics in Sports & Physical Therapy, 14,* 243–249.

Sinding-Larson, C. (1921). A hitherto unknown affection of the patella in children. *Acta Radiologica, 1,* 171–179.

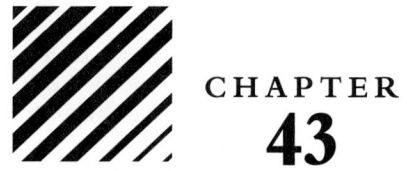

CHAPTER
43

Articulation Injuries of the Ankle and Hip

Robert Keith, PA-C, and Karen Anderson Keith, PhD, RN,CS, FNP

Articulation injuries, also known as joint injuries, occur where two bones join. The injury may result from acute or chronic trauma or from the destruction of articular cartilage. This chapter focuses on the examination of an injured joint in general, and specifically on the evaluation of the ankle and hip joints. Conditions that result in or may be associated with articulation injuries of the upper extremities, lower back, and knee, or those that result from underlying degenerative or destructive processes, are discussed in separate chapters in this unit.

Primary care providers frequently encounter patients with articulation injuries, making basic competency in their evaluation and management a necessity. Through the relationships they have established with their patients, primary care providers are often in the best position to assess the immediate impact of acute articular injuries on the patient's activities of daily living and social life. Also, awareness of predisposing or complicating underlying medical problems can allow nuanced management of the problem. This chapter provides an overview of how to examine an injured joint, followed by specific information on evaluating the ankle and hip. Definitions of articulation injuries are presented in Table 43-1.

GENERAL APPROACH TO THE JOINT EXAM

Some exam criteria are unique to each joint, but the following items are important in the evaluation of injury to any joint. The physical exam of the presenting joint should be undertaken as soon as feasible. As time progresses, edema, muscle spasm, pain, and joint effusion make the accurate elicitation of physical findings more difficult. The joint may also become less tractable over time, especially for injuries where closed reduction is the treatment of choice.

Inspection may reveal deformity, erythema, ecchymosis, and edema. Palpate for point tenderness, crepitus, deformity, increased warmth, and pulses. Ask the patient to move the joint through the full range of motion (active range of motion). Whether the patient is successful or unsuccessful in moving the joint, attempt passive range of motion. Motion against resistance can be used to assess neuromuscular function. Document the vascular status of the area by recording pulses and capillary refill time at a site distal to the injury.

To evaluate the functional status of a joint on physical exam, it is necessary to stress the involved joint and evaluate it for stability. In almost all cases, the differential diagnosis includes osteoarthritis and rheumatoid arthritis. When monoarticular pain is present in the absence of a clear-cut instance of trauma or gout, an infected joint is a clear possibility. Should an infected joint become prominent in the differential diagnosis, joint aspiration must be done to rule out an infectious or crystal-induced etiology.

ANKLE INJURIES

Anatomy, Physiology, and Pathology

The ankle is a complex joint that carries the full weight of the body. The ankle joint is formed by the articulation of the distal ends of the tibia and fibula with the calcaneus in the foot. The ankle is composed of four major ligaments, which are of concern during acute injury. Because the overwhelming majority of ankle sprains are the result of inversion of the foot during plantar flexion, the three ligaments on the lateral aspect of the foot are most in need of evaluation. The anterior talofibular ligament (ATFL) (Fig. 43-1) extends from the anterior aspect of the distal fibula to its insertion on the lateral talus. This ligament is the one most often injured when the ankle is suddenly inverted, typically while in plantar flexion. Posteriorly is the calcaneal fibular ligament (CFL), which links the posterior–inferior area of the fibula with the middle of the calcaneus. The posterior talofibular ligament (PTFL) is a short, strong, intracapsular ligament that runs posteriorly from the posterior lateral malleolus and attaches to the posterolateral surface of the talus. During inversion injuries, the ligaments are usually injured sequentially (ATFL then CFL, and finally PTFL) as increasing force is applied to invert the ankle.

On the medial side of the ankle, the deltoid ligament is a strong, five-component band that joins the distal medial malleolus of the tibia to the talus. This ligament is so strong that it often yields an avulsion fracture of the medial malleolus rather than rupture when force is applied to it in an eversion type of injury.

Epidemiology

Foot problems increase with age (Greenberg & Davis, 1993). In one study, people 65 years or older were found to have three times more problems than those between 18 and 44 (Greenberg & Davis, 1993). In this same study, during a 12-month period, 5.6 million patients over age 65 suffered from foot or ankle injuries (fracture, dislocation, sprain, or strain), a rate of 23 per 1000. No significant differences in the rates of foot and ankle injuries between women and men were found (22 and 23 per 1000, respectively); however, an unexplained higher rate of foot and ankle injuries was found in whites versus African Americans (15/1000 vs. 24/1000 in whites) (Greenberg & Davis, 1993).

Diagnostic Criteria

Fractures are ruled out with x-rays of the ankle, foot, and lower leg, as indicated by the history and physical exam. Stress testing provides the diagnosis for strains and sprains in the absence of radiographic abnormalities.

TABLE 43-1	**Definitions of Conditions Related to Articulation Injuries**
Term	Definition
Sprain	Complete or partial tear in a ligament or joint capsule
	Grade I: mild stretching of fibers
	Grade II: partial tear
	Grade III: complete tear
Strain	A torn muscle–tendon unit
Tendinitis	Inflammation of tendon
Tenosynovitis	Inflammation of the tendon sheath
Bursitis	Inflammation of a bursa
Fracture	Any break in the continuity of a bone
Dislocation	Complete loss of continuity between two opposing articular surfaces
Delayed union	A fracture that takes greater than 6 months to heal
Nonunion	Failure of a fracture to heal after 1 year
Subluxation	Partial dislocation
Epicondylosis	Arthritic changes in a joint

History and Physical Exam

The history should begin with questions directed at determining the mechanism of injury. How the injury occurred gives important insights about the magnitude of the forces involved and the likelihood of significant injury. Other key points include:

- Did the patient hear or feel any snap or pop?
- Was weight bearing or continued activity possible just after the injury?
- Is there numbness or tingling in the involved extremity?
- Was the onset sudden? If chronic, was it associated with a specific overuse activity?
- How does the injury affect the patient's activities of daily living?
- Is the injury to the dominant limb?

General questions about overall physical activity and fitness help to situate the injury in the context of the patient's life and anticipate the response to rehabilitation efforts. Ask about any chronic or recurrent joint pain, fever, or rash; review any medications the patient takes; check for allergies. Explore previous surgery or rehabilitation for orthopedic problems.

Patients present most commonly with a history of having had their foot inverted as a result of weight bearing on an uneven surface. The patient often describes a popping sensation when significant injury occurs. This does not necessarily mean the ligament has ruptured or a fracture is present, but it does increase the likelihood of significant injury. Injuries that are isolated to the ATFL are three times more common than injuries that include the CFL or the PTFL (Li & Meals, 1992). As a result, most ankle injuries are stable and can be treated conservatively.

Inspect the foot and ankle for edema and ecchymosis: the rapidity and extent of these conditions are helpful clues in judging the extent of injury. Careful palpation of the lateral margin of the foot over the site of the ATFL insertion will elicit pain if significant injury is present. The ability to bear weight for at least four steps has been highly correlated with grade I or II sprains. Stress testing by inverting and everting the foot has also been shown to be predictive of abnormalities on x-ray. If the foot can be inverted and has a talar tilt of less than 15°, then most likely only the ATFL is involved. If the tilt is 15° to 30°, then the ATFL and the CFL are affected. With more than 30° of tilt, all three lateral ligaments of the ankle are torn, and the risk of associated fracture is high (Seligson & Voos, 1997).

Diagnostic Studies

In the past, evaluation of a sprained ankle almost always included x-rays; however, only 15% of ankle x-rays were found to be positive for a fracture (Stiell et al, 1992). Ongoing efforts to reduce the number of unnecessary x-rays have resulted in several promising decision rules to guide x-ray usage. The Ottawa clinical decision guidelines, possibly the most widely

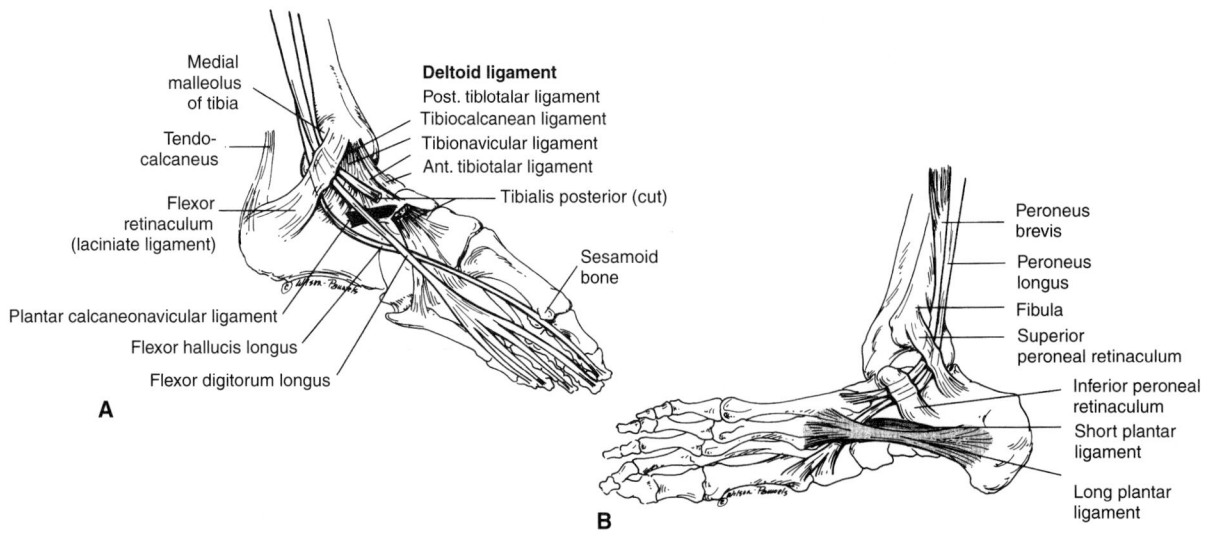

FIGURE 43-1 **(A)** Medial longitudinal arch of the left foot showing plantar calcaneonavicular (spring) ligament. **(B)** Lateral longitudinal arch showing long and short plantar ligaments, (Akesson, E.J., Loeb, J.A. & Wilson-Pauwels, L. (1990). *Thompson's Core Textbook of Anatomy, 2/e.* Philadelphia: J.B. Lippincott)

known, include the following:

- Inability to bear weight immediately after the injury
- Inability to take at least four unsupported steps during the office evaluation
- Point tenderness on palpation of the posterior aspect of either malleolus (Stiell et al, 1994).

By using these guidelines, all patients with ankle fractures were identified (sensitivity 100%), but specificity for ankle fracture was low (49%) (Stiell et al, 1994). In the absence of the above findings, however, there is virtually no chance that a fracture is present (negative predictive value of 100%). Implementation of these rules in follow-up studies with more than 2300 patients led to a 28% decrease in ankle x-rays, decreased time for evaluation, and no untoward outcomes (Stiell et al, 1994).

When indicated, x-rays should include anteroposterior, lateral, and mortise views. The mortise view is performed with the foot internally rotated 15°; this allows the ankle joint to be visualized without overlapping of the distal tibia and fibula on the calcaneus. When a mortise view is done, it is easy to check for even spacing throughout the joint. Stress films are advisable if the initial films are negative but the physical exam suggests a significant injury. After local anesthesia is administered, the ankle is inverted and everted to evaluate the extent of talar tilt. Magnetic resonance imaging plays no role in the evaluation of acute ankle injuries in the primary care setting. If concern remains after evaluation, prompt orthopedic referral while initiating conservative management is indicated.

Treatment Options, Expected Outcomes, and Comprehensive Management

Injuries to major joints are frequent, and common underlying principles of evaluation and management allow the provider to manage safely and effectively the early phases of the overwhelming majority of these cases. The acronym PRICE (protection, rest, ice, compression, elevation) is useful in guiding the initial care of articular injuries.

- Protection is most often accomplished by the application of some type of external support, such as a splint. Preventing further injury is a paramount concern when evaluating injuries at the scene of an accident. A patient who arrives at the office with an unsplinted joint injury should have a splint applied immediately.
- Rest is a natural continuation of protection. Rest is not always complete inactivity, but usually involves significant reduction in the intensity or frequency of use of the involved joint.
- Ice is the most common form of cryotherapy. Cold applied during the first 24 to 48 hours after injury has several beneficial effects. Pain reduction and decreased edema set the stage for rapid mobilization of the joint. Rapid mobilization has significant advantages over prolonged immobilization. Ideally, cold should be applied for 15 to 30 minutes every 3 hours.
- Compression and elevation serve to decrease edema and pain. When using compression in the form of an elastic bandage, care should be exercised to avoid circulatory compromise. Only moderate tension should be applied

to the bandage; if discomfort ensues, the bandage should be released.

Pain management with nonsteroidal anti-inflammatories (NSAIDs) or opioid derivatives should be guided by the patient's perception of the pain. Undertreatment of pain is a common mistake that can lead to prolongation of recovery, because the patient who is fearful of pain resists early mobilization of the joint.

PRICE and NSAIDs are appropriate for grade I and II sprains (see Table 43-1). General measures such as physical therapy and early mobilization improve the outcome. Anytime after 24 to 48 hours, the patient should begin ambulation and should slowly increase the ambulation time as tolerated. Many types of splinting devices are available—taping, air casts, and ankle braces, to name a few. The goal of splinting is to restrict the motion of the ankle in the direction that caused the injury while otherwise allowing full range of motion.

Rehabilitation after joint injury can be conveniently divided into four phases:

- Phase 1 focuses on the acute injury and involves PRICE and pain control.
- Phase 2 has as its central theme the early initiation of active range of motion, with the goal of preserving and restoring muscle strength. Specific graded exercises are used for each injury (Housner & Schwenk, 1997).
- Phase 3 is for injuries that have a prolonged recovery period. Exercises are devised to maintain cardiovascular fitness, increase flexibility, and limit stress on the recovering joint. Swimming, or bicycling when the upper extremities are involved, can be a useful way to accomplish this goal.
- Phase 4 has the prevention of future injuries as its primary goal. Often this involves evaluation of the patient's biomechanics while engaging in the activity that led to the injury. Patient education can help when poor body positioning (eg, while lifting heavy loads) contributes to the problem.

TEACHING AND SELF-CARE

Specific exercises to help recovery from an ankle injury and prevent future injuries are illustrated in Figure 43-2. This information should be carefully reviewed with patients when they are first seen for the injury and at subsequent visits.

Referral Points and Clinical Warnings

Sometimes the initial evaluation of a joint injury should not be done in an outpatient or office setting. Table 43-2 provides information regarding emergency care of potentially serious complications of articulation injuries. The problems listed can result in permanent disorders if they are not recognized and treated as quickly as possible. Any patient with these signs should be referred to an emergency room for immediate orthopedic consultation.

HIP

Anatomy, Physiology, and Pathology

The hip is a complex weight-bearing joint to which pain is often unduly ascribed. When a patient complains about hip pain, the etiology can be anything from a hernia to a fractured

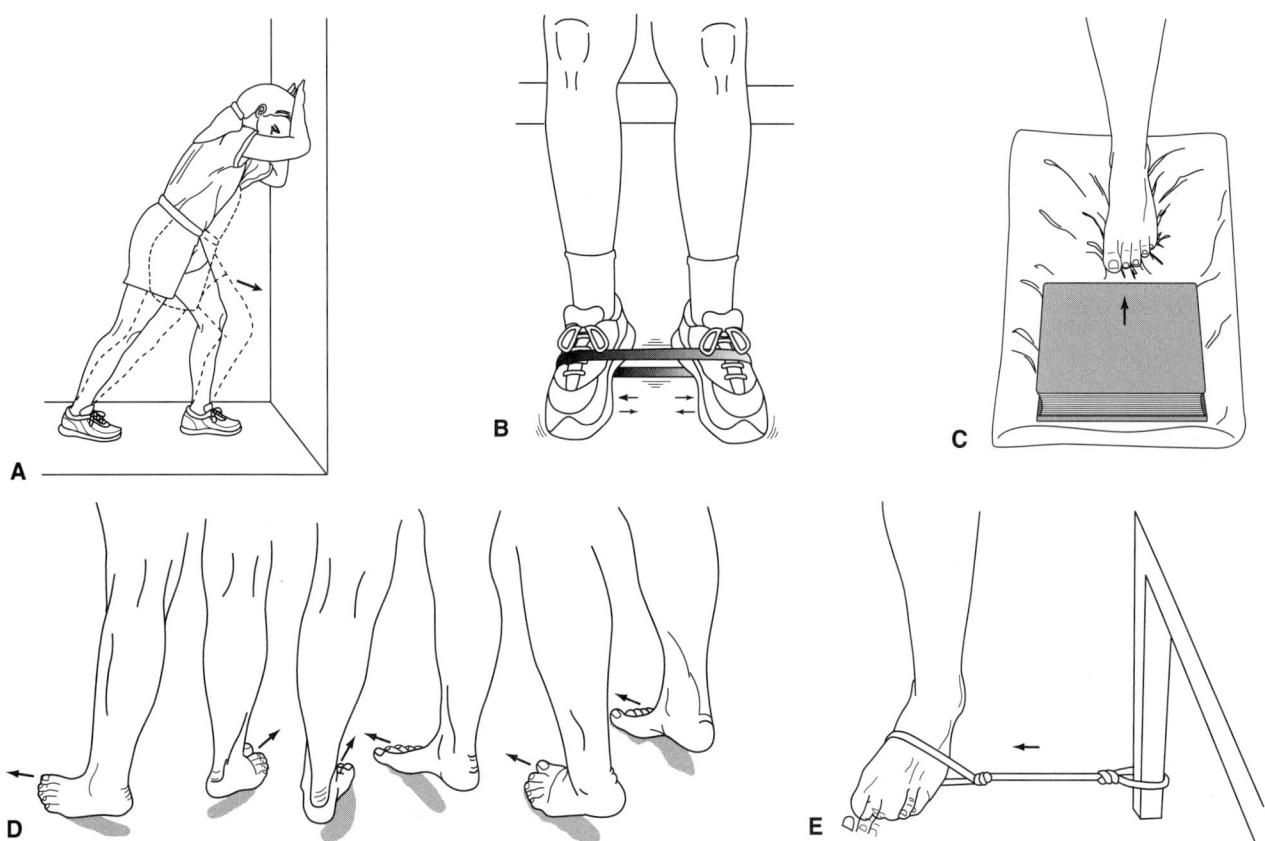

FIGURE 43-2 (A) To stretch the heel cord, stand at arm's length from a wall with your hands against the wall at about shoulder height. The foot to be stretched is extended behind you. Keep the foot flat on the floor, point your toes straight ahead and extend your knee. Bending the arms at the elbow, flex forward by bending the knee of the opposite leg and stretch the tight calf muscles and heel cord. Hold this stretch for about 30 seconds for each leg, 3 or 4 times a day. (B) Sit so that feet clear the floor, and place a slightly stretched cord around feet at about the midfoot. Move both legs apart at the same time so that you can feel the resistance against the cord. Repeat this 20 to 30 times, 3 or 4 times a day. (C) Sit in a chair, and put a towel on the floor in front of you. Keep your heel flat on the floor while you pull the towel toward you with the toes of your injured foot. Straighten out the towel, and repeat the exercise 10 to 15 times twice a day. You can make your ankle work harder if you put a book on the towel and pull it toward you. You can also try to pull the towel to the right and to the left. (D) Stand flat on the floor, then slowly rise up on tiptoes. Do this with your toes pointed straight ahead, then inward and, finally, outward. Try these heel raises about 30 times in each position, 3 times a day. (E) Tie one end of some rubber tubing to a heavy piece of furniture (a table, for example). Loop the other end of the tubing around your injured foot. Then, while you are sitting, stretch the tubing toward you as far as it will go; repeat this 20 times, 3 times a day. (Consultant, August 1996:36, 1644–1646. © 1996 by Ciggott Publishing Co.)

TABLE 43-2	Emergency Situations That May Be Encountered in a Patient With Joint Trauma		
Disorder	**Potential Problem**	**Diagnostic Studies**	**Usual Treatment**
Pulseless extremity	Severed artery	Angiography	Surgical repair
	Compartment syndrome	Measure compartment pressure	Fasciotomy
Change in level of consciousness or decreased neurologic function	Compression	CT scan; possibly electromyography	Surgical decompression
Dislocation of a major joint		Radiography	Closed (preferred) or open reduction of the joint

Always follow the ABCs (airway, breathing, circulation) and manage them first.

femur. Because of this, it is important to localize the origin of the pain and, based on the history, restrict the workup. Because of the many structures that constitute and surround the hip, the anatomy is best reviewed by reference to Figure 43-3.

Epidemiology

The causes of hip pain vary over the life cycle. In the young adult, etiologies such as lupus, rheumatic fever, avascular necrosis, reactive arthritis, gout, Lyme disease, hernias, bursitis, and radiculopathies are common. In the over-50 age group, osteoarthritis, dislocations and fractures of the femur, osteitis deformans, and cancers are most common. Entities such as rheumatoid arthritis and referred pain (eg, from pelvic infections, renal stones) tend to cut across the age spectrum. Athletic patients are at increased risk for overuse problems, which often manifest as bursitis or tendinitis. Women (especially African Americans) have an increased risk of hip problems caused by lupus and rheumatoid arthritis. Common causes of hip pain are outlined in Table 43-3.

Diagnostic Criteria

Diagnostic criteria vary based on the specific etiology of the pain; most important for a correct diagnosis is a good history and physical exam, with judicious use of adjunctive tests. The complexity of the hip prevents the identification of a routine workup for hip pain.

History and Physical Exam

Patients with hip pain are often unclear in their description of the pain: back pain, flank pain, and upper thigh problems are often described as hip pain. The key to the history is to determine the location and patterns of radiation of pain. Narrowing the differential by attributing the pain's origin to one of three areas (the lateral hip, the anterior hip, or the posterior hip) is

TABLE 43-3	Conditions That May Cause Hip Pain
	Avascular necrosis
	Gout/pseudogout
	Iliopectineal bursitis
	Ischial bursitis
	Osteoarthritis
	Septic arthritis
	Fracture of the femoral head or neck
	Hernia
	Iliopsoas tendinitis
	Lumbar radiculopathies
	Trochanteric bursitis
	Autoimmune disorders (lupus)

helpful. Each area is listed below with probable causes of pain in the area.

- Anterior hip pain is most likely the result of hernias, iliopectineal bursitis, fractures of the femoral neck, septic arthritis, crystal-induced arthritis, and avascular necrosis. These should be considered based on the demographic characteristics of the patient. Other considerations for anterior pain include iliopsoas bursitis, inguinal adenopathy, lupus, osteomyelitis, and adductor muscle strains.
- Posterior hip pain is frequently caused by sacral or ischial fractures, gluteal muscle strains, ischial bursitis, osteoarthritis, radiculopathies, and tumors. Posterior pain can often radiate from such structures as the rectum, pelvis, and lower back.
- Lateral hip pain is usually the result of iliotibial tendinitis, trochanteric bursitis, radiculopathies, and femoral fractures just superior and inferior to the greater trochanter.

Once the location of the pain is clear, the next task is to determine the character of the pain. Pain made worse by activity and better with rest is often seen with muscle strains, tendinitis, bursitis, and osteoarthritis. Paresthesias suggest a radiculopathy. Sharp pains with sudden onset associated with even minor trauma may be a fracture, especially in the older patient. In the patient who reports a fever and associated hip pain, septic arthritis must be ruled out. Other components in the history relevant to the evaluation of hip pain are history of past trauma, previous joint pains, medication use, sexual history, intravenous drug use, and significant medical or surgical problems.

With the history completed, the physical exam is conducted to determine the extent of disability and to reproduce gently the patient's pain. Inspection for erythema, edema, limb length discrepancies, the ability to arise from a chair, and observation of gait for a limp must be completed. This is followed by palpation of the painful area for increased warmth, point tenderness over a particular bursa or muscle insertion point, bony deformity, muscle spasm, or inguinal adenopathy. Helpful maneuvers include assessing range of motion, checking deep tendon reflexes and muscle strength, and the straight leg raise test to check for referred pain. By careful reference to the underlying anatomic structures, the etiology of the pain can be determined.

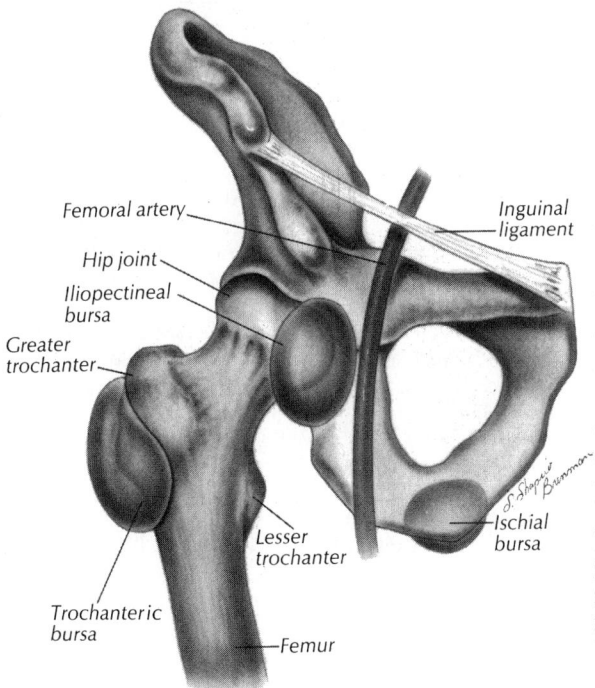

FIGURE 43-3 Anatomy of the hip, (Bates, B. (1995). *A guide to physical examination and history taking, 6/e.* Philadelphia: J.B. Lippincott)

Labels in figure: Femoral artery · Hip joint · Iliopectineal bursa · Greater trochanter · Trochanteric bursa · Femur · Lesser trochanter · Ischial bursa · Inguinal ligament

Diagnostic Studies

Test selection is based solely on the active differential diagnosis after the history and physical exam. The most common tests ordered are x-rays. Although not needed for mild or self-limiting conditions, x-rays can be helpful in fractures, infections, changes associated with arthritis, and cancers. If the diagnosis of septic or crystal-induced arthritis is entertained, it is mandatory to aspirate the joint. Bone scans for occult fractures may be ordered if needed. Blood work may include rheumatoid factor, HLA typing, ASLO titers, Lyme titers, RPR, complete blood count, ANA, and blood cultures. Computed tomography or magnetic resonance imaging may also be needed if more routine studies are uninformative or to define a soft-tissue or bony abnormality detected on plain x-ray.

Treatment Options, Expected Outcomes, and Comprehensive Management

For minor problems such as muscle strain, bursitis, tendinitis, gout, pseudogout, and acute exacerbations of arthritis, rest, warm soaks, protective devices (eg, pads, splints), and NSAIDs are often sufficient.

TEACHING AND SELF-CARE

Patients with problems such as tendinitis and bursitis can often be taught to modify athletic activities in a way that reduces the risk of recurrence. Treatment of alcoholism may prevent the occurrence of falls; alcoholism is also a risk factor for avascular necrosis (Meals, 1992). The incidence of hip fractures can be reduced in the elderly by exercise programs that increase muscle strength and coordination. Elimination of potentially hazardous obstacles (eg, floor rugs, toys, and stairs without banisters) can also help eliminate fractures. Formal fall-prevention measures should be instituted with the cooperation of the patient's family or roommates.

Clinical Warnings and Referral Points

In serious conditions such as fractures, septic joints, avascular necrosis, or neoplasms, hospitalization and specialty consultation and comanagement may be indicated.

COMMUNITY RESOURCES

- American Academy of Orthopaedic Surgeons, 6300 N. River Rd., Rosemont, IL 60018, 847-823-7186, 800-346-AAOS, http://www.aaos.org/wordhtml/home2.htm: Medical education, educational resources catalog, library, research

■ ■ ■ CLINICAL PEARLS

- How the injury occurred gives important insights into the magnitude of the forces involved and the likelihood of significant injury.
- The presenting joint should be examined as soon as feasible: as time progresses, edema, muscle spasm, pain, and joint effusion make the accurate elicitation of physical findings more difficult.
- Foot problems increase with age.
- The ATFL is the one most often injured when the ankle is suddenly inverted, typically while in plantar flexion.
- The provider should inspect the foot and ankle for edema and ecchymosis: the rapidity and extent of these conditions are helpful clues in judging the extent of injury.

EDITOR'S NOTE:
COMPLEMENTARY APPROACHES

A general discussion of complementary approaches can be found in Chapter 3. The following, while not an exhaustive list, are some complementary approaches being used for this condition. Additional information on these approaches, including precautions, can be found in Appendices A and B. Providers need to assess for the use of complementary approaches as part of the patient's history, as they may impact conventional therapies, and patients may not volunteer this information unless specifically asked. Efficacy of many complementary approaches is not as well documented as that of conventional therapies. Providers need to read the literature before suggesting these complementary approaches.

- Complementary Modalities
  Acupuncture
  Craniosacral therapy

References

Greenberg, L., & Davis, H. (1993). Foot problems in the U.S.: The National Health Interview Survey. *Journal of the American Podiatric Medical Association, 83*, 475–483.

Housner, J.A., & Schwenk, T.L. (1997). Musculoskeletal injuries: 10 principles of rehabilitation. *Consultant, 37*(7), 1777–1800.

Li, J., & Meals, R. (1992). Hoop fever. In R.A. Meals. *One hundred orthopaedic conditions every doctor should understand.* St. Louis: Quality Medical Publishing.

Meals, R.A. (1992). *One hundred orthopaedic conditions every doctor should understand.* St. Louis: Quality Medical Publishing.

Seligson, D. & Voos, K. (1997). *The primary management of musculoskeletal trauma.* Philadelphia: Lippincott-Raven.

Stiell, I.G., Greenberg, G.H., & McKnight, R.D. (1992). A study to develop clinical decision rules for the use of radiography in acute ankle injuries. *Annals of Emergency Medicine, 21*, 384–390.

Stiell, I.G., McKnight, R.D., & Greenberg, G.H. (1994). Implementation of the Ottawa ankle rules. *JAMA, 271*(16), 827–832.

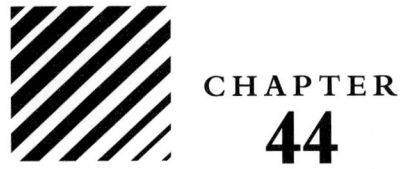

CHAPTER

44

Cumulative Trauma Disorder

Nancy S. Morris, PhD, RN, CS, ANP

Cumulative trauma disorder (CTD) is a collective term for a range of soft-tissue injuries and conditions that primarily involve tendons, tendon sheaths, muscles, or nerves and are characterized by discomfort, paresthesia, numbness, weakness, impairment, or persistent pain in the joints, muscles, tendons, and other soft tissues, with or without physical manifestations. Although they have been described in the literature since the 1700s, CTDs have received increased attention over the last 10 to 15 years because of changes in occupational and recreational activities, as well as advances in the field of ergonomics. The legal profession and issues of workers compensation have also been driving factors in this resurgence. This chapter focuses on the common CTDs of the upper extremity that a primary care provider is likely to encounter.

Many common daily activities at home, at work, and in the community require functional upper extremities. The upper extremities are used to perform basic activities such as dressing and eating, to communicate with others through gesturing and writing, to operate machinery and recreational equipment, and to meet the many demands inherent in a tactile world. When the upper extremity cannot function as desired because of pain, weakness, numbness, or paresthesias, problems can occur. Concerns may arise regarding ability to meet demands at home, at work, and in social or recreational situations. Given the impact that upper extremity dysfunction can have, thorough evaluation, proper diagnosis, and adequate treatment are essential.

ANATOMY, PHYSIOLOGY, AND PATHOLOGY

Anatomy and Physiology

The provider needs a working knowledge of the bones, muscles, tendons, nerves, and vessels of the upper extremity, neck, and back (Figures 44-1 through 44-4). The hand is innervated by the median, ulnar, and radial nerves. Each nerve passes through a muscle in the forearm, and each passes through potential points of entrapment. These nerves are involved in the control of the wrist, fingers, and thumbs. The sensory branches of the nerves are depicted in Figure 44-5.

Pathology

Although the etiology of CTDs remains controversial, there are two distinct views emerging. One perspective is that CTDs are the result of a musculotendinous injury caused by force, repetition, abnormal postures, and vibrations over time. The second perspective is that psychosocial and political factors account for conditions identified as CTDs. A single explanation for the diversity of disorders and the multiplicity of symptoms

is lacking, but there is consensus that these disorders develop gradually and are not the result of a single episode of trauma (Armstrong et al, 1987a; Higgs et al, 1993; Mackinnon & Novak, 1994; Putz-Anderson, 1988).

PHYSIOLOGIC PERSPECTIVE

Three hypothesis support the perspective that CTDs are a result of a musculotendinous injury (Mackinnon & Novak, 1994). The first hypothesis purports that muscle and tendon overuse is the primary etiology of CTDs. The second hypothesis maintains that there is a neurogenic origin to CTDs. The third hypothesis is based on an integration of neuropathic compression, myofascial pain, and muscle imbalance. A summary of each is provided below.

Muscle and Tendon Overuse

The premise behind the first hypothesis is that pain results directly from an overused muscle or as a result of pathologic changes that occur in the muscle fibers of overused muscles. With repetitive motion, there is reduced relaxation and increased tension in these tissues, reducing essential blood supply. This can lead to a rapid rate of wear and tear, with a greatly reduced ability to repair. Over time, a cumulative overload results in inflammation, edema, compression, ischemia, tearing, and fibrosis of affected tissues.

When muscles hold their contraction at more than about 15% to 20% of their maximal capability, they pull on their tendons and compress their joints, which decreases the blood supply to the tissues (Hebert, 1993). This can result in tissue ischemia and delayed dissipation of metabolites, causing irritation and inflammation. Additionally, overstrain of the muscles can cause microtears at the tendinous insertions; this leads to less diffusion, which causes a relative ischemia and subsequent inflammation at the tendon insertion. This results in mechanical attrition, a thickening of the tendon with irregular surfaces, and further abrasions and tearing (Childre & Winzeler, 1995). When there is insufficient time between episodes of heavy usage for a tissue to recover or repair itself, CTD can occur (Frederick, 1992; Hebert, 1993).

When a muscle or tendon unit is repeatedly tensed, the end result can be tendinitis. Tendons have both a biomechanical and a physiologic response to stressors. Tendons function as mechanical links that transmit forces, stabilize movements, and move the kinematic chains of the extremities. Consequently, tendons are subjected to tensile stresses by the muscle and to compressive and shearing stresses from adjacent bones and ligaments. Tendons respond mechanically to these stresses; if the stresses exceed a certain point, the tendons can become deformed.

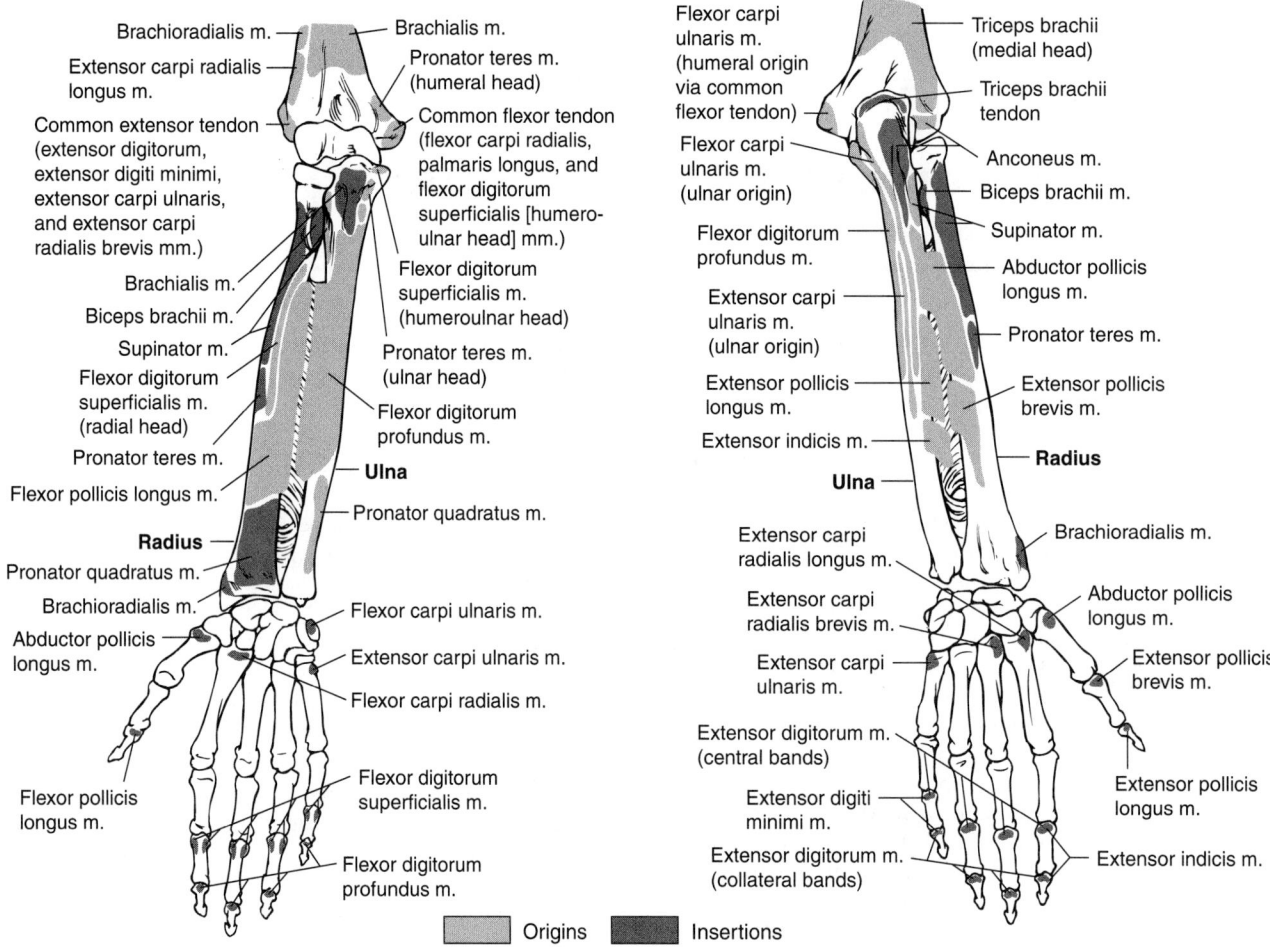

FIGURE 44-1 Muscles of forearm. (Adapted from the Ciba Collection of Medical Illustrations by Frank Netter, MD)

Normal tendon structure can be disrupted in response to three stressors: tension, compression, and abrasion secondary to friction (Gross, 1992). Mechanisms of injury may involve stressors that are too high in magnitude, too frequent in repetition, or both. Local mechanical stresses can also irritate tendons via excessive force or high frequency of physical contact between soft tissues and an object or tool in the work environment.

Tendons also respond physiologically to stressors. Physiologic responses include metabolic, circulatory, and adaptive changes in the accessory tissues, synovial and mesenteric membranes, and adjacent ligaments. The changes are likely to be related to the occlusion of blood flow and the subsequent deprivation of nutrients that can occur with compression of a tendon against adjacent surfaces, thickening of tendon sheaths, or increased diffusion distances because of thickened sheaths (Manske et al, 1985). The amount of deprivation is a result of the intensity, duration, and frequency of exertion, or the forcefulness and repetitiveness of the activity (Armstrong et al, 1987a).

Many of the tendons in the upper extremity are surrounded by a sheath that contains synovial fluid. This allows easy gliding of the tendon within its sheath. If there is insufficient fluid in the sheath, overuse may lead to friction between the tendon and sheath, initiating the protective response of inflammation. The tendon area will swell and feel warm, tender, and painful. Movement is limited as a result of increased muscle tension and muscle spasm. If this occurs repeatedly, the frequent episodes of acute inflammation may prompt the formation of extraneous fibrous tissue, which is largely responsible for establishing a permanent or chronic condition. Chronic overuse often results in a thickened tendon sheath that impedes tendon movement, particularly in tight areas such as the wrist and fingers.

Compression Neuropathy

A second hypothesis points to a neurogenic origin for cumulative trauma disorders, targeting multilevel compression neuropathy as the primary etiology. The mechanism by which acute compression affects the peripheral nerve is not completely understood but is thought to involve both ischemic and mechanical factors. Nerve entrapment syndromes result from repeated or sustained compression of a peripheral nerve between ligaments or constricted anatomic structures. In addition to external compression, nerve entrapment may also be caused, aggravated, or precipitated by posture (Mackinnon & Novak, 1994).

It is proposed that the hypoxia from compression of the blood supply by muscles and tendons leads to problems with the nerves (Mackinnon & Novak, 1994; Ranney, 1993). With compression of a nerve, there is obstruction of venous return.

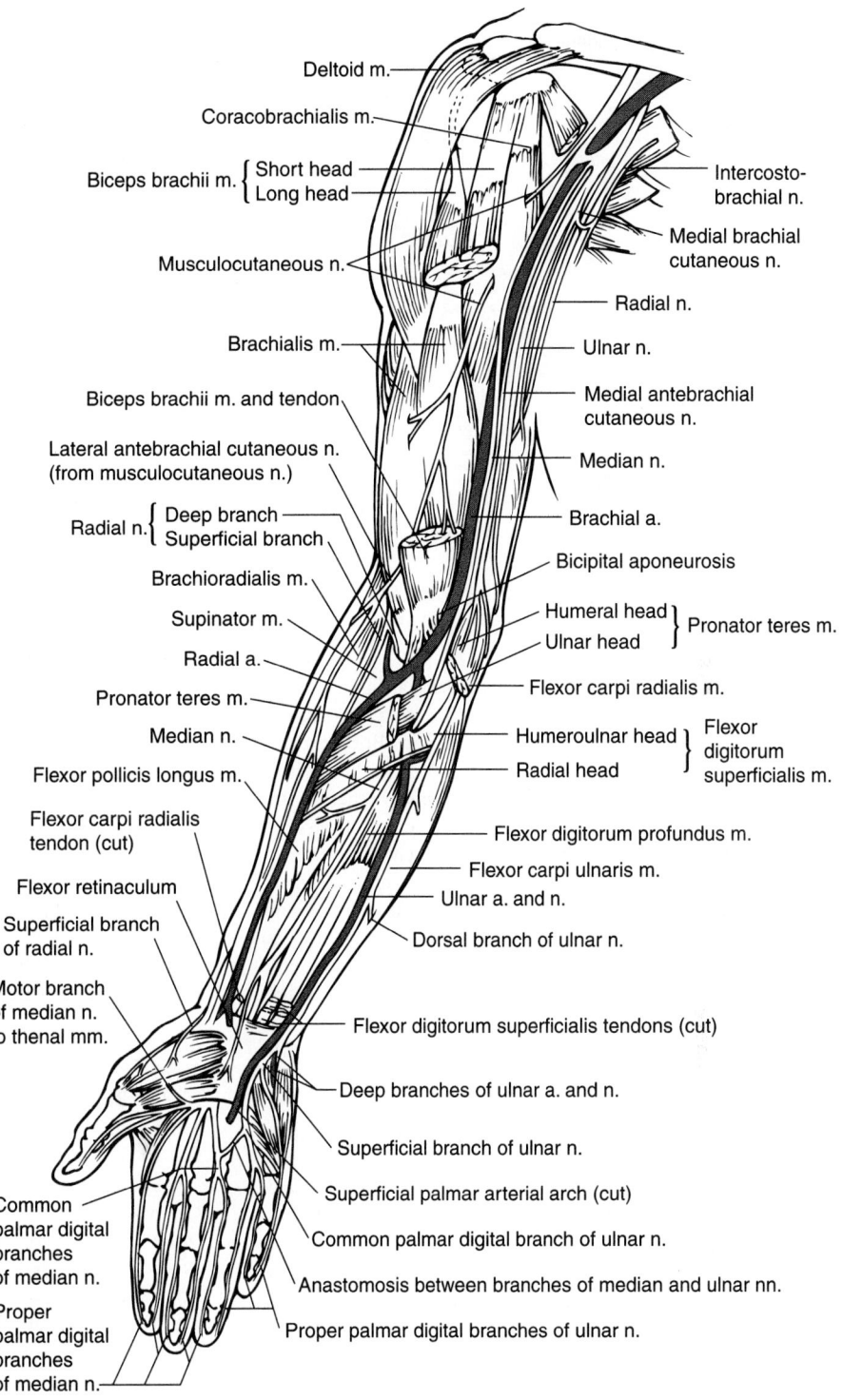

FIGURE 44-2 Arteries and nerves of upper limb (anterior view). (Adapted from the Ciba Collection of Medical Illustrations by Frank Netter, MD)

The increased venous pressure results in slowed circulation in the nerve complex and dilatation of the small vessels and capillaries within the nerve segment. There is edema, proliferation of fibroblasts, and scarring in the nerve segment, which compresses the nerve (Childre & Winzeler, 1995).

Critics of this hypothesis raise concerns regarding lack of an explanation for the etiology of the muscular component seen with CTDs.

Neuropathic Compression, Myofascial Pain, and Muscle Imbalance

The third hypothesis is an integration of the existing hypotheses relating to neuropathic compression and myofascial pain, with the addition of muscle imbalance (Higgs & Mackinnon, 1995; Mackinnon & Novak, 1994). The basic tenet of this hypothesis is that prolonged and frequent assumption of abnormal postures, positions, or movements of the head, neck, and upper extremity has two major influences on the body. First, specific

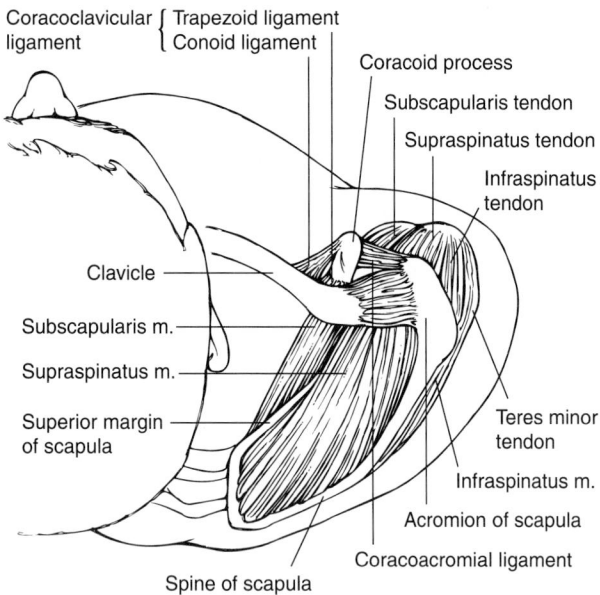

FIGURE 44-3 Shoulder and acromioclavicular joints. (Adapted from the Ciba Collection of Medical Illustrations by Frank Netter, MD)

extremity positions cause increased pressure around certain nerves and, if encountered frequently and for long periods, will eventually result in chronic nerve compression. Both chronic tension and direct mechanical compression decrease blood flow to the nerve, producing fibrosis in and around the nerve; this in turn inhibits full excursion during normal extremity movement. In addition, placing the nerve on stretch will cause increased tension within the nerve, provoking symptoms from both sensory and motor fibers. Nerve compression at one point along the nerve may cause both distal and proximal sites to be less tolerant to the effects of compression. Chronic nerve compression is thought to be progressive unless specific interventions are initiated.

Second, abnormal postures can result in a set of muscles being maintained and used in shortened positions, which can lead to muscle imbalance. Underuse of some muscles subsequently leads to a weak set of muscles; this ultimately results in a compensatory overuse of a second set of muscles, and a cycle of muscle imbalance will be established. The muscles maintained and used in shortened positions become tight and painful, especially when stretched. Some muscles secondarily compress neurovascular structures when in a tightened position. It is this self-perpetuating cycle of tight muscles becoming tighter and weak muscles becoming weaker that explains why rest alone will not relieve all the symptoms of CTDs (Mackinnon & Novak, 1994).

NONPHYSIOLOGIC PERSPECTIVE

The second perspective on CTDs is denial of their very existence. Proponents of this explanation (Ferguson, 1987; Hadler, 1990; Ireland, 1995; Lam, 1995; Ranney, 1993; Weiland, 1996) believe that CTDs are not primarily physiologic in nature but rather are based on psychosocial and sociopolitical factors. As such, they suggest that CTDs are a reflection of modern society without clearly identifiable pathology. The difficulty in the objective determination of the work-relatedness of CTDs and the frequently associated financial compensation

factor add to the difficulty of accepting CTD as a diagnosis. For the most part, supporters of this perspective recommend that syndromic titles such as CTD be abandoned in favor of clearly definable and diagnosable entities with a known histologic appearance and etiology.

Although there are different perspectives on the causative factors of CTDs, all but the psychosocial theory accept that both biomechanical and physiologic factors are involved. Most would agree that repeated or sustained exertion, in combination with certain postures, causes, precipitates, or aggravates chronic upper extremity tendon and nerve disorders. Additional contributing factors may include the force used in performing movements, increased muscle tension associated with mental stress, and factors external to the person (eg, faulty work station, equipment, task design, and maintenance of equipment).

EPIDEMIOLOGY

The overall incidence and prevalence of CTDs, as well as the distribution and determinants, are difficult to ascertain. No definition of CTD has been agreed on. Use of such a broad term does not specify the exact anatomic or pathologic involvement. This creates difficulty when the provider is pressed to determine an etiology and recommend a treatment plan. To complicate matters, there are several terms used synonymously with CTD, including repetitive strain injuries, overuse syndromes, and repetitive motion injuries. For clarity, the term CTD is used throughout this chapter.

In addition to variations in diagnostic terminology and criteria, differences in attitudes of health care providers about reporting CTDs contribute to the inadequacies of the epidemiologic data. Many of the published data involve occupation-related CTDs, but occurrence can also be related to intrinsic factors of the person and recreational activities. The epidemiologic literature also separates clinically well-defined disorders such as tendinitis and carpal tunnel syndrome from the more nonspecific diagnoses referred to as CTDs (Hales & Bernard, 1996).

The Bureau of Labor Statistics (U.S. Department of Labor, 1995) reports that the incidence rates for CTDs increased from 5.1 to 39 cases per 10,000 full-time workers from 1984 to 1994. This change is attributed to increased awareness among employees, employers, and health care providers that these disorders may be work-related, thereby resulting in more complete recording and an actual increase in the number of cases (Hales & Bernard, 1996). Given the inconsistencies in reporting and the occurrence of CTDs that are not work-related, these data are most useful for interpreting trends and identifying high-risk industries.

The prevalence of upper extremity CTDs depends on the occupation studied, the risk factors present, and the specific body part studied. The recent increase in prevalence may be related to ergonomic factors. Nearly two thirds of all occupational illnesses reported to the Bureau of Labor Statistics in 1994 were caused by exposure to repeated trauma to the upper body (wrist, elbow, or shoulder) (U.S. Department of Labor, 1996). The following five industries have had the highest rank of CTDs during the last 10 years: meat packing, knit underwear manufacturing, automobile manufacturing, poultry processing, and house slipper manufacturing (U.S. Department of Labor,

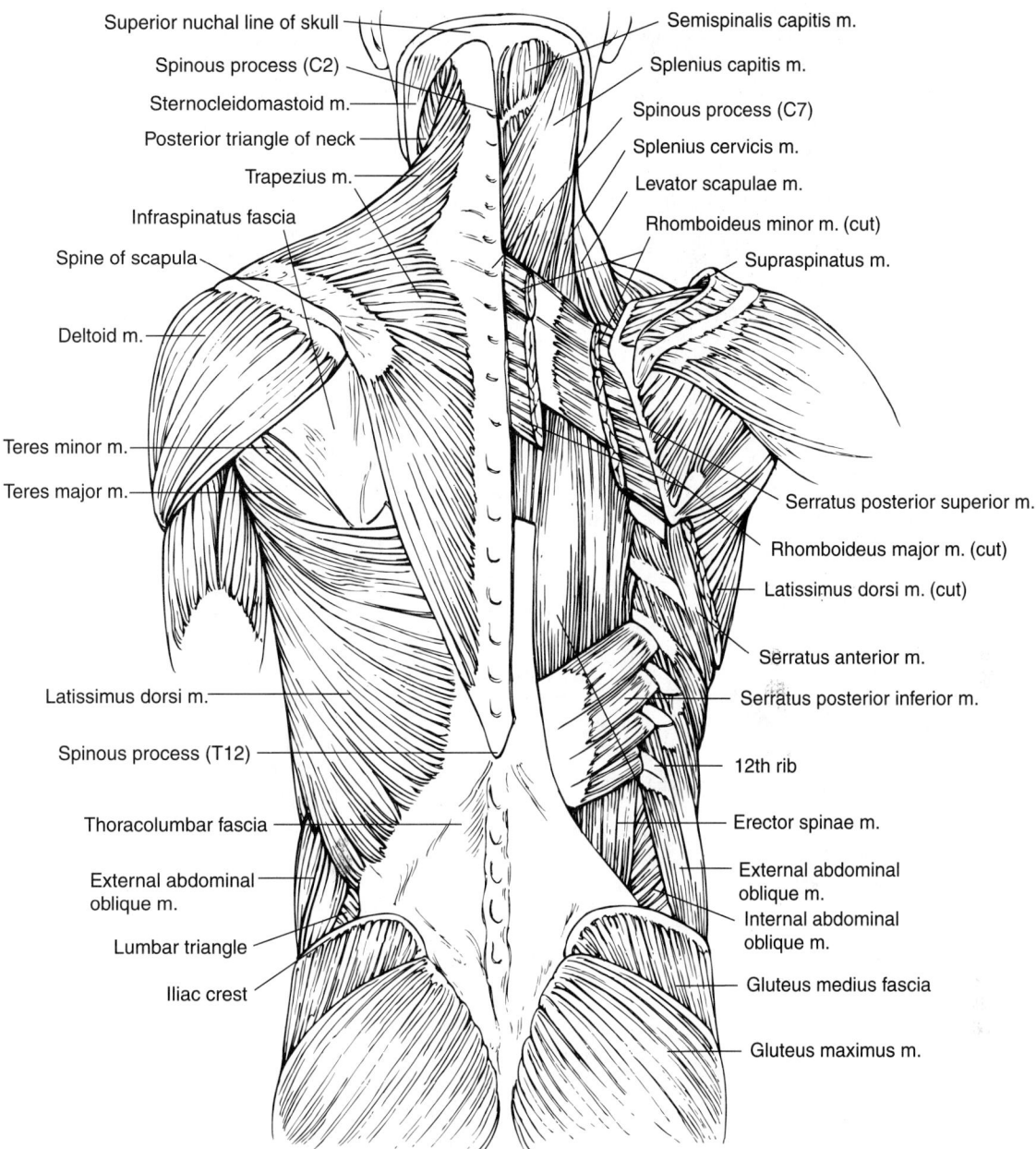

FIGURE 44-4 Musculature of back. (Adapted from the Ciba Collection of Medical Illustrations by Frank Netter, MD)

1995). However, the reporting of CTDs is inconsistent, and there may be other industries with a high occurrence.

Many factors, both occupational and nonoccupational, have been reported to cause, precipitate, or aggravate conditions categorized as CTDs. The specific contribution of occupational and nonoccupational factors has not been determined. Occupational factors include repetitive motion, forceful exertions, mechanical insult, sustained and awkward postures, and frequent exposure to low-frequency vibrations and cold temperatures, as well as lack of training and experience, poor work station design, and inappropriate tools. The association of job demand and workplace psychosocial factors should also be considered. Factors that have the most consistent association include high workloads, perceived time pressure, work pressure, high workload variability, poor work content, and monotonous work

(Hales & Bernard, 1996). Examples of nonoccupational factors thought to contribute to CTDs include congenital defects, use of birth-control pills, pregnancy, chronic disease, and recreational factors (Armstrong et al, 1987a; Hebert, 1993; Kroemer, 1992; Putz-Anderson, 1988). There are few epidemiologic data available to determine how age relates to CTDs; the influence of age and gender on the susceptibility to CTDs is controversial.

DIAGNOSTIC CRITERIA

CTDs include a variety of familiar clinical entities, such as tenosynovitis, tendinitis, epicondylitis, trigger finger, and carpal tunnel syndrome, as well as vague complaints of pain. Assessment and management of these familiar conditions are better

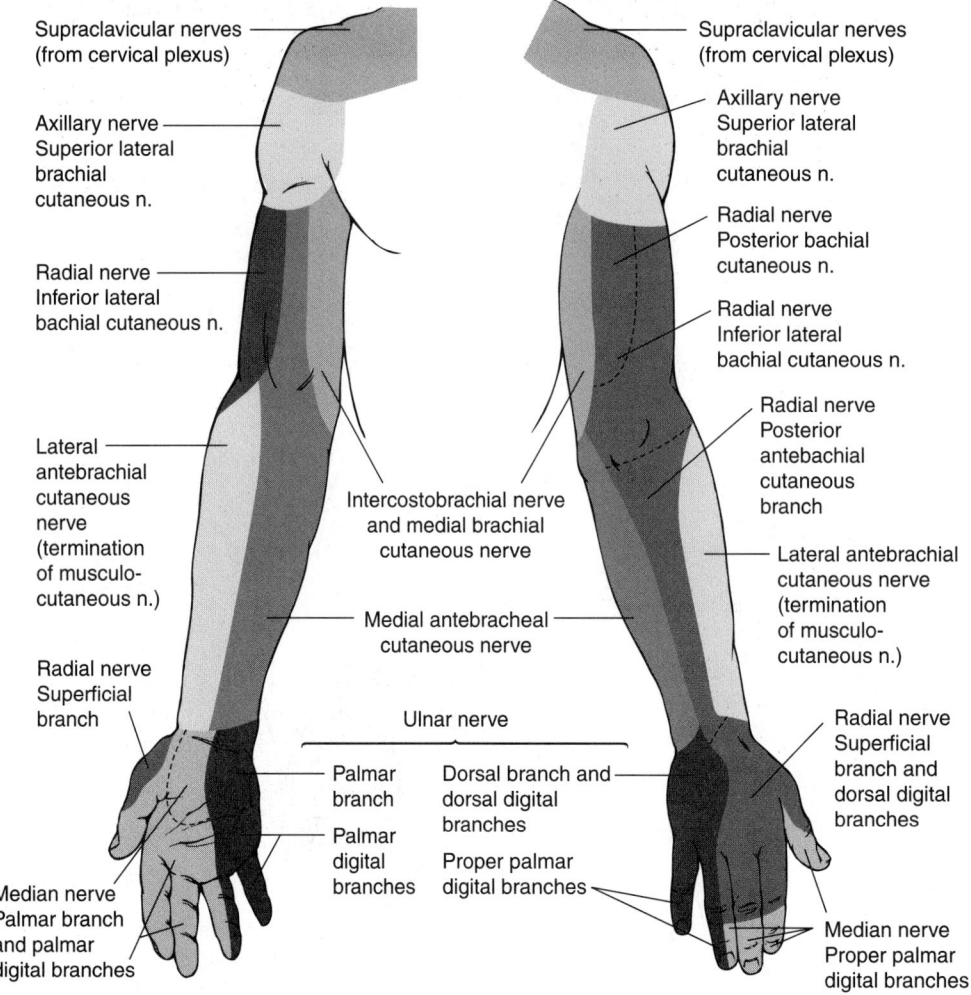

FIGURE 44-5 Cutaneous innervation of upper limb. (Adapted from the Ciba Collection of Medical Illustrations by Frank Netter, MD)

understood in contrast to the more challenging and often per-plexing disorders associated with compressive neuropathies and nonspecific complaints of pain. The major problem in assessing and managing CTDs occurs when paresthesias are accompanied by ambiguous complaints, such as pain in the entire upper extremity, neck, back, subscapular area, and shoulder (Higgs & Mackinnon, 1995).

Diagnosis is based on a careful history, physical exam, and the exclusion of other well-described entities. There are no specific pathologic or radiologic features to support a diagnosis of CTD, and definitive diagnostic criteria have not been established. There is, however, a distinct history that is suggestive of CTD:

- Symptoms come on gradually.
- Symptoms worsen over weeks, months, or even years.
- Initially the symptoms may subside with rest, but as time goes on, symptoms worsen and are no longer relieved with rest (Armstrong et al, 1987a; Higgs et al, 1993; Mackinnon & Novak, 1994; Putz-Anderson, 1988).

Subjective and objective signs and symptoms consistent with the diagnosis of CTD include:

- Soft-tissue swelling and muscle atrophy
- Pain and tenderness
- Decreased range of motion

- Loss of grip strength
- Reproduction of paresthesia and numbness by provocative maneuvers
- Decline in work performance
- Functional impairment
- Fatigue
- Sensory changes (Browne et al, 1984; Isernhagen, 1992; Millender et al, 1996; Putz-Anderson, 1988).

One of the difficulties in evaluating these disorders is trying to establish a diagnosis in the absence of objective physical findings or confirmatory diagnostic imaging or laboratory data. For the most part, authorities advocate using the diagnostic label that is most specific to the presenting condition (eg, de Quervain's tenosynovitis), reserving CTD for situations that do not meet the criteria of other known clinical entities (Millender et al, 1996) but contain the signs and symptoms described here.

HISTORY AND PHYSICAL EXAM

Early diagnosis and prompt treatment require adequate assessment. Key aspects of the history and physical exam are delineated in Table 44-1.

TABLE 44-1	Physical Examination of the Upper Extremity
Exam	**Findings**
INSPECTION Note skin turgor, color, swelling, wrinkles, scars, atrophy, contractures, masses, obvious deformity, symmetry, arm length discrepancies, and posture.	–Swelling and erythema are indicative of inflammation, often seen with tendinitis. –Atrophy is suggestive of nerve denervation or muscle imbalance. –Asymmetry and arm length discrepancy are suggestive of muscle imbalance and guarding. –Specific abnormalities associated with upper extremity compressive neuropathies include a poked-forward position of the chin, flexed position of the neck, sloping of the shoulders indicating internal rotation and a forward-flexed position. –If the palms face posteriorly when the arms are held by the side, suspect pronator teres tightness in the forearm and internal rotation of the shoulders.
PALPATION Assess skin temperature, moisture, and areas of tenderness.	–Warmth and tenderness are indicative of inflammation. –Localized tenderness over a tendon, while the adjacent bone and ligaments are nontender, is suggestive of tendinitis.
RANGE OF MOTION (passive, active, resisted) Assess flexion, extension, hyperextension, opposition, abduction, adduction, supination, pronation, ulnar deviation, radial deviation, and internal and external rotation. Compare right and left extremities. Determine joint stability and presence of crepitation. Assess for muscle tenderness by assessing pain with resisted activity.	–Localized pain with resisted muscle contraction is suggestive of a significant muscle strain. –Pain with active or passive tendon movement through the sheath indicates tenosynovitis. –Pain with passive stretching of the affected tendon is suggestive of tendinitis. –Pain over a tendon with contraction of the associated muscle against resistance indicates tendinitis. –Crepitus is indicative of inflammation. –Decreased range of motion from pain is suggestive of inflammation or injury to the muscle, tendon, or ligament. –The following altered range of motion and movement patterns are seen with some CTDs: scapulae are in an abducted position, and scapular movement is discoordinated; passive stretching of tight scalene, sternocleidomastoid, and pectoralis minor muscles elicits tenderness; chin retraction, which stretches the scalene, sternocleidomastoid, and suboccipital muscles, causes discomfort.
MOTOR STRENGTH Conduct gross muscle strength testing with right to left comparison. Measurement of grip and pinch strength to establish a baseline and subsequently as an indicator of improving or worsening condition. Use a grip dynamometer and a pinch dynamometer to make three successive determinations and calculate percentage relative to pretreatment value, if available, as well as to value from contralateral hand.	–Decreased strength is consistent with CTD. –Motor complaints vary from aching to weakness to atrophy.
SENSIBILITY Assess radial, median, and ulnar nerve distribution. Standard sensory testing includes two-point discrimination and threshold testing of vibration and pressure (Table 44-2).	–Sensory nerve changes may appear earlier than motor impairment. –Sensory complaints progress from occasional paresthesia to persistent paresthesia to numbness. –Decreased sensibility is suggestive of nerve compression or entrapment.
VASCULAR STATUS Assess ulnar, radial, and brachial pulse as appropriate See Figure 44-9 for Allen test to determine patency of the arteries supplying the hand.	–Decreased or absent pulse indicates a vascular condition.

Source: American Society for Surgery of the Hand, 1990; Higgs & Mackinnon, 1995; Messer & Bankers, 1995; Ranney, 1993; Rempel et al, 1992.

Focused History

- Elicit general information: age; hand dominance; past medical, surgical, and injury history; and current medications.
- Identify usual activity level and note any current impairment (occupational, recreational, exercise routine, and activities of daily living).
- Elicit the location, duration, frequency, intensity, and onset of discomfort (pain, swelling, aching, tingling, numbness, burning, or stiffness).
- Determine relieving and exacerbating factors.
- Assess the impact the condition is having on the person's life (activities of daily living, family relationships, economic, work, and social situations).
- Identify existing stressors and current coping techniques.
- Elicit sleep patterns and sleep positions.

TABLE 44-2	Standard Sensory Testing

Two-point discrimination: A subjective measure of cutaneous sensibility. With a blunt instrument, gently apply pressure, beginning at 6 mm between the two points. Increase or decrease to determine the distance at which the person can distinguish two points from one. Applied pressure should not blanch the skin. Responses are recorded with specific measurements or as normal, < 6 mm; fair, 6–10 mm; poor, 11–15 mm; protective, one point perceived; and anesthetic, no point perceived (American Society for Surgery of the Hand, 1990).

Tuning fork: A subjective measure of vibration. It can be used on each digit to determine a baseline and change in perception of vibration.

Semmes–Weinstein monofilament test: An objective measure of cutaneous sensibility involving light touch–deep pressure testing with monofilaments of increasing force. Standardized nylon filaments of specific length and diameter are applied three times to the same spot to ascertain perception. The filament design controls the force and velocity of application. The standardized testing instrument has 20 filaments, each a different size. This test can be used serially to determine changes in neural status or as an initial evaluation of touch threshold in areas of normal sensibility and areas of diminution. Responses are recorded as normal, diminished light touch, diminished protective sensation, loss of protective sensation, and untestable based on responses to application of the monofilaments (Bell-Krotoski, 1995). This test is often conducted by an occupational therapist.

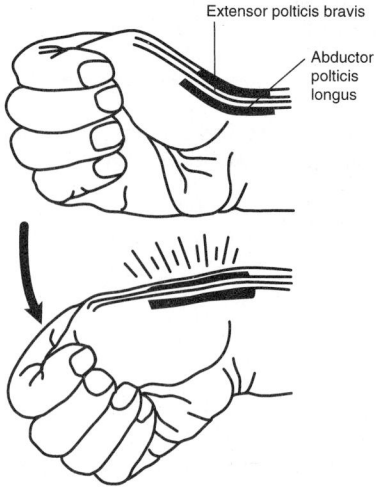

FIGURE 44-7 Finkelstein's test. Finkelstein's test is ulnar deviation of the hand with the thumb flexed against the palm and the fingers flexed over the thumb. A positive response is pain at the radial styloid due to stretching of the abductor pollicis longus and extensor pollicis brevis. A positive response is indicative of de Quervain's tenosynovitis.

If the condition appears to be related to occupational activities, include the following:

- Exposure to occupational risk factors (high force, repetitive motions, awkward or sustained positioning, local mechanical contact stress, exposure to low-frequency vibration and cold temperatures)
- Length of time in current occupation

- Previous occupations with similar risk factors
- Relation of symptoms to work; duration of work at a particular task before the onset of symptoms.

Physical Exam

Examination of the upper extremity includes inspection, palpation, and evaluation of range of motion, motor strength, sensibility, neurologic function, and vascular status. Tables 44-1 and 44-2 outlines key aspects of the exam and interpretation of common findings. Provocative tests to elicit specific findings are illustrated in Figures 44-6 through 44-10.

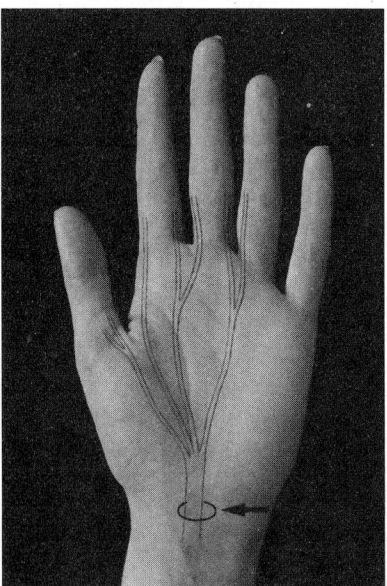

FIGURE 44-6 Tinel's test consists of a gentle tapping over the nerve. A positive response is pain or paresthesia in the distribution of the nerve. A positive response is indicative of compression or entrapment of the nerve. (Bates B. (1995). *A guide to physical examination and history taking, 6/e.* Philadelphia: J.B. Lippincott.) (Adapted from the Ciba Collection of Medical Illustrations by Frank Netter, MD)

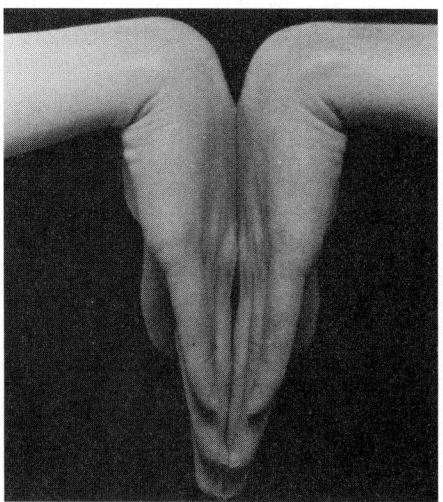

FIGURE 44-8 Phalen's sign involves flexion of both wrists 90° with the dorsal aspect of the hands held in apposition for 60 seconds. A positive response is pain or anesthesia in at least one finger innervated by the median nerve. A positive response is suggestive of entrapment of the median nerve.

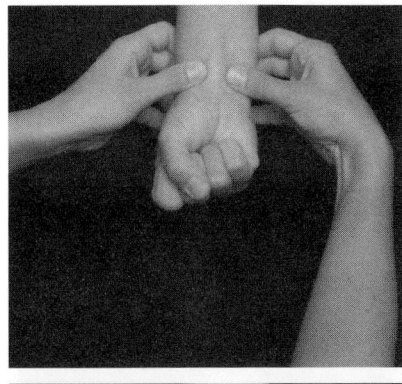
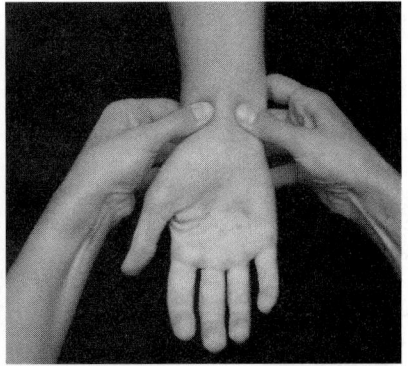
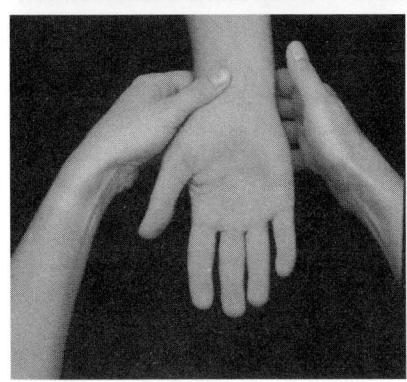
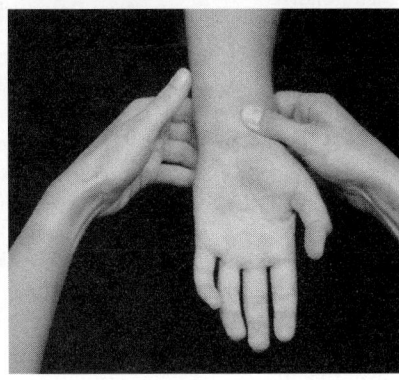

FIGURE 44-9 The Allen test is used to determine patency of the arteries supplying the hand. It is done as follows: (**1**) Compress the radial and ulnar arteries at the wrist; (**2**) Have the person make a fist, open and close it several times to exsanguinate the hand, and then open the hand again into a relaxed position, avoiding hyperextension; (**3**) Release the radial artery only. If the entire hand pinks up in color, the radial artery is patent with good collateral flow into the ulnar artery system. (**4**) Repeat the first two steps. (**5**) Release the ulnar artery only. If the entire hand pinks up in color, the ulnar artery is patent with good collateral flow into the radial artery system.

DIAGNOSTIC STUDIES

Electrodiagnostic studies can be performed to confirm the clinical diagnosis, to assess the severity of nerve compression, and to rule out more proximal compression sites. Traditionally this involved electromyelography and nerve conduction velocity studies. With the advent of portable electrical and vibrometric tests, more options are now available. An electroneurometer is a portable nerve conduction testing instrument that can measure distal motor and sensory latencies of nerves by direct stimulation of the nerve. The sensitivity and specificity of the electroneurometer are equal to those of conventional nerve conduction studies (Atroshi & Johnsson, 1996). A digital vibrometer

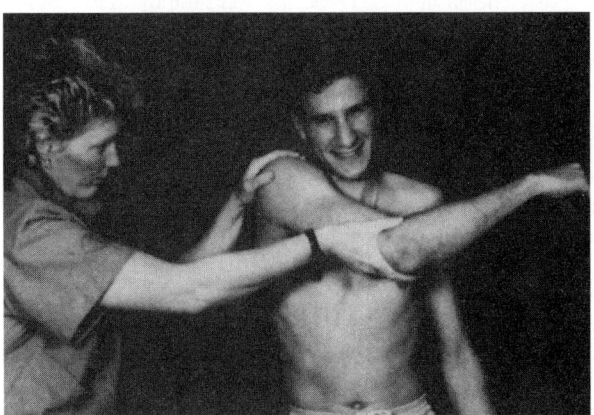

FIGURE 44-10 A positive impingement sign is pain at 90° with resisted abduction and normal strength or forcibility forward elevating the affected arm while stabilizing the scapula; pinching of the supraspinatus tendon between the humeral head and the anterior–inferior aspect of the acromion. (Neer, 1983).

provides an assessment of perception thresholds for a vibratory stimulus applied at a designated frequency. Results of a comparison study of traditional electrodiagnostic studies, electroneurometry, and vibrometry in the diagnosis of carpal tunnel syndrome, however, indicate the need for further evaluation before considering electroneurometry or vibrometry for screening of common entrapment disorders (Cherniack et al, 1996).

The clinical history and physical exam are the primary methods of identifying nerve entrapment or compression such as carpal tunnel syndrome. The correlation of electrodiagnostic test results and outcome after carpal tunnel release shows no advantage to obtaining electrodiagnostic testing before surgical release (Glowacki et al, 1996). Electrodiagnostic testing is recommended for patients with confounding symptoms or those in whom the diagnosis is suspected but who do not present with strict diagnostic criteria.

Radiographs in general are not necessary unless accurate location of the pain is uncertain or if there is a history of trauma. Use of magnetic resonance imaging, computed tomography, and vascular testing in assessment of nerve compression and other CTDs should be restricted to special diagnostic problems (Seyfert et al, 1994).

TREATMENT OPTIONS, EXPECTED OUTCOMES, AND COMPREHENSIVE MANAGEMENT

Primary Prevention

Primary prevention of CTDs requires both health promotion and health protection interventions. Health promotion interventions have as a goal the achievement and maintenance of strong upper extremity muscles. Health protection interventions focus on the avoidance of known causative factors. The acquisition of a CTD occurs over time, and thus prevention is an ongoing process.

HEALTH PROMOTION AND SPECIFIC PROTECTION

General recommendations for health promotion—a healthy diet, regular aerobic and strengthening exercise, and achievement and maintenance of ideal body weight—are all considered beneficial for the prevention of CTDs (Nathan et al, 1995). An awareness of risk and nonrisk positions for nerve compression and muscle imbalance (Mackinnon & Novak, 1995) would also be helpful. The prevention and the resolution of CTDs require an all-encompassing approach: CTDs and cumulative life experiences cannot be viewed in isolation from each other.

Most of the CTD prevention literature is related to the occupational environment. The same principles, however, apply regardless of the setting. Recognition of the potential for injury is the first step, followed by specific strategies (outlined below) to minimize the risk associated with both occupational and recreational activities.

Systematic analysis of work sites to identify ergonomic hazards is an aspect of primary prevention for occupational risk factors. A checklist can be used to determine the presence of ergonomic risk factors associated with the development of upper extremity CTDs (Keyserling et al, 1993). The checklist should address the presence of and duration of exposure to the following stressors: repetitiveness, local mechanical contact stress, forceful manual exertions, awkward upper extremity posture, vibration, cold temperature, and hand tool use. It should be regarded as an initial screening tool used to increase awareness of potential risk factors.

Hebert (1993) suggested the five "E's" of injury elimination: engineering, education, exposure reduction, exercise, and enforcement. Engineering refers to the correction of faulty design in work processes, tools, materials, and procedures to avoid stressful motions or postures. Exposure reduction refers to job rotation frequent enough to provide effective interruption of stressful job demands and to provide a variety of movements and posture loads. Education refers to the training of managers, supervisors, and workers so that they might be motivated to adopt CTD avoidance behaviors. Exercise refers to stretching musculoskeletal tissues frequently to reduce fatigue and restore circulation. Enforcement implies a structure of expectations and responsibility for all involved to carry out their CTD prevention roles. As isolated initiatives, each action has limited effect. However, when all are applied in a coordinated and controlled manner, successful outcomes can be achieved.

The role of the primary care provider is to identify persons at risk and encourage an adequate conditioning program, with a focus on the upper extremity. Also, provision of information specific to certain postures and motions that are thought to be causative factors may be beneficial. Tables 44-3, 44-4, and 44-5 give specific examples. Persons whose job activities include:

- Repetitive motion
- Prolonged or repeated forceful exertion
- Sustained or awkward positioning
- Exposure to low-frequency vibration
- Exposure to cold temperatures
- Maintenance of the same posture for long periods of time

should be advised to discuss ergonomic issues with their supervisor and the occupational health provider at their place of work (Kroemer, 1992). Preventing a problem is much easier than resolving one.

Secondary Prevention

Two factors are critical in developing treatment plans for persons with CTDs: first, identifying the specific musculoskeletal problem, and second, determining the degree to which the disorder is work-related. It is best to describe the clinical entity with a straightforward diagnostic label whenever possible. An accurate diagnosis allows treatment specific to the problem and facilitates evaluation of the outcome.

CTDs with a work-related component as part of the causality become compounded by the workers compensation system or legal system as well as by psychosocial issues. The causes of prolonged disabilities are multifactorial and include musculoskeletal, ergonomic, and psychosocial factors. Early recognition and proper management of work-related disorders result in more rapid alleviation of symptoms (Millender et al, 1996).

A comprehensive approach to the management of CTDs requires a thorough assessment of risk factors associated with work and recreational activities, in addition to person-specific conditions such as pregnancy. Appropriate diagnostic labeling is important for the patient, the employer, and the provider. A treatment plan that incorporates measures to reduce inflammation, manage pain, restore strength and flexibility, alleviate symptoms, and prevent recurrence is a prudent approach. For work-related CTDs, communication with all parties involved is important, as is appreciation of ergonomic factors. In all situations, psychosocial aspects and the effect on function should be addressed.

Treatment options for CTDs are generally conservative and lengthy. The onset of CTDs occurs over time and the rehabilitation, likewise, can take several months. Many times the treatment approach requires lifestyle changes and incorporation of a regular exercise routine. If conservative measures are unsuccessful and a definitive etiology can be pinpointed that is amenable to surgical intervention, it should be considered. Otherwise, a multidisciplinary approach focusing on physical, ergonomic, and psychological factors is warranted, especially in chronic or repeated circumstances.

Acceptable treatment of inflammatory disorders, a component of many CTDs, is well established. A general approach is to rest the injured part while maintaining activity in other areas to minimize overall deconditioning. Rest may require immobilization of the extremity or simply restricted activity. Control inflammation with ice, supplemented with anti-inflammatory medication where possible. Avoid causative factors to prevent recurrence. Corticosteroid injections and involvement of an occupational or physical therapist may be indicated if progress toward healing is not occurring. A graded part-time resumption of former activities is important to permit conditioning, as is done frequently after sports injuries. For patients with a work-

TABLE 44-3	Maintain Nonrisk Positions
▪ Keep wrists neutral	▪ Do not elevate or roll shoulders forward
▪ Supinate forearms	▪ Hold neck erect
▪ Extend elbows	▪ Maintain lordosis of the back

Source: Higgs & Mackinnon, 1995.

TABLE 44-4	Eliminate Awkward Postures	
Goals	**Actions**	**Rationale**
Alleviate shoulder and arm fatigue	Minimize reaching above shoulder height. Avoid reaching above the head. Keep the elbow close to the body and bent 90° to 110°. Use adjustable chairs and work stations. Avoid sustained applications of force. Minimize force exerted. Move parts and tools within easy reach.	Muscle fatigue accelerates as the arm extends away from the body.
Minimize problems with the hand and wrist	Use properly designed tools and equipment that will allow the wrist to be kept in a neutral posture while working. Ensure correct work height. For precision work, the work piece should be 2″ to 4″ above elbow height; for light assembly work, the work piece should be 2″ to 4″ below elbow height; for heavy work, the work piece should be 4″ to 5″ below elbow height.	Awkward positioning can lead to tendinitis, compression of nerves.
Alleviate neck pain	Avoid neck extension & flexion. Tilt or raise the work piece if fine vision is required. Enlarge print of text. Adjust height of chair or workbench. Schedule frequent, short rest breaks.	Head inclination angles greater than 20° to 30° lead to fatigue and pain.

Source: Carson, 1994.

related CTD, treatment should stress ergonomic training, focusing on the early symptoms of CTDs, the necessity of using proper work methods from an ergonomics perspective, and the value of reporting early signs and symptoms of CTDs so that interventions can be initiated in a timely manner (Carson, 1993).

Medications

The role of medications in the treatment of CTDs is limited. If there is an inflammatory component, anti-inflammatory medications may be considered. If nonsteroidal anti-inflammatory medications are selected for this purpose, the dosage must be sufficient to provide an anti-inflammatory and not just an analgesic effect. For example, 2400 mg/day in three or four divided doses would be an appropriate oral anti-inflammatory dose of ibuprofen for an adult. Consideration should be given to frequency of dosing, concurrent medications, comorbidity, and cost when determining which drug to recommend. Analgesics may also be necessary to manage pain during acute periods.

TABLE 44-5	Safe Positioning for Keyboard Users

1. Keep head erect, with the line of vision horizontal with the first line of the draft document or screen characters.

2. Keep shoulders relaxed, upper arms by the side of the trunk, and forearms level with the ASDF row of the keyboard.

3. Keep the wrist straight when the fingers are resting on the ASDF row of the keyboard.

4. Keep the angle of the elbows 90° or greater, with the upper arm parallel to the body.

5. Support the feet, either on the floor or on a footstool with the knees at 90°.

6. Ensure leg room to allow unrestricted movement.

7. Support the lower back curve with the backrest of the chair.

Source: Harris & Gianacakes, 1994; Isernhagen, 1992.

Corticosteroid injections have value in specific situations. They are used predominantly for their potent anti-inflammatory effects. However, the potential benefit of reduced inflammation can have negative effects on healing, because inflammation is an important component of the normal healing process; thus, judicious use of corticosteroids is recommended. Some CTDs, such as tenosynovitis of the thumb and fingers, de Quervain's tenosynovitis, and lateral epicondylitis, respond well to corticosteroid injection. However, the injection must be part of a treatment plan that includes rest, a structured exercise program, and close follow-up.

There are no firm guidelines with regard to the choice of a corticosteroid or the dosage. Some general guidelines are to select a more water-soluble preparation or a mixture of short- and long-acting compounds for acute inflammatory conditions and to select a more water-insoluble preparation for chronic inflammatory conditions (Fadale & Wiggins, 1994). Commonly accepted practice is to select the dose on the basis of the size of the area that will receive the injection. Sterile gloves and sterile technique should be used for all injections. Cutaneous anesthesia can be obtained with lidocaine, bupivacaine, or ethyl chloride spray. After the injection, the extremity should be rested or immobilized for a few days to minimize pain and to reduce systemic absorption (Fadale & Wiggins, 1994). The treatment plan should include a program to improve flexibility, range of motion, and strength of the involved extremity.

The primary complications of steroid injection are tendon rupture, subcutaneous atrophy, loss of skin pigmentation, cartilage damage, and infection (Swain & Kaplan, 1995). Infection and acute local tissue trauma are two absolute contraindications to corticosteroid injection. Care should be taken not to inject directly into a blood vessel, ligament, or tendon. Injections into small joints, such as the fingers, can be difficult and may best be referred to a hand specialist.

Teaching and Self-Care

Education can help patients assume the responsibility for participating fully in their care. Information about both prevention and treatment of CTDs is valuable. Ergonomics training and knowledge of risk factors would be valuable prevention strategies. Once a CTD has been diagnosed, treatment should start with patient education, including a description of the disorder, an explanation of the muscle and nerve abnormalities, and the mechanism by which proximal problems may produce peripheral symptoms. Safe positions and the positions of the extremity that increase pressure around the nerves or potentiate positions of muscle imbalance should be explained. Nonrisk positions include wrists in neutral, forearms supinated, elbows extended, shoulders not elevated or rolled forward, neck not flexed, and back with an appropriate lordosis (Mackinnon & Novak, 1994). The patient must be aware of these postures during both work and nonwork activities, as well as their relation to sleep patterns.

Education should also include the specific exercises necessary to restore muscle balance. A physical therapist can provide the guidance and structure necessary to carry out the exercise program on a regular basis. Initially, stretches are the mainstay of the program; only after achieving a full and pain-free range of motion should strengthening exercises be initiated (Mackinnon & Novak, 1994).

Specific Entities

CTDs encompass conditions involving tendons, tendon sheaths, muscles, blood vessels, and nerves. The treatment approach depends on the actual tissue or nerve involved. Tendinitis, stenosing tenosynovitis, lateral epicondylitis, medial epicondylitis, and subacromial impingement syndrome are some of the common tendon-related disorders categorized as CTDs that are likely to be seen in a primary care setting. Common upper extremity nerve entrapments categorized as CTDs include carpal tunnel syndrome and cubital tunnel syndrome. A common presentation of a CTD includes nonspecific complaints of pain, paresthesia, numbness, and weakness in the upper extremities. Assessment and care of each of these entities is summarized below. It is worthwhile to determine the effect on function both at work and with recreational and daily activities. Attention should also be given to pain control, modification of functional impairments, emotional support, and stress management, because these injuries are often frustrating and may pose a financial difficulty, especially if the patient cannot work.

TENDONS

Tendinitis is a global term used to indicate the inflammation of tendon tissue. It is based more on a clinical finding than on a pathoanatomic observation. No matter which tendon is involved, the signs and symptoms of tendinitis include pain at rest and with particular activities, localized tenderness and swelling in the area of the tendon, erythema, and restricted movement of the affected joint. Pain is increased by passively stretching the affected tendon or contracting the associated muscle against resistance. With tendinitis, the provider can expect to see a dystrophic, an atrophic, or an overtly inflammatory state. Treatment goals are to reduce inflammation and pain, regain range of motion, strengthen, and return to function. Cold application is useful for pain relief and swelling reduction. All treatments should involve the avoidance of activities that would result in repetitive loading of the involved tendon until

---

TABLE 44-6	Lateral Epicondylitis

Lateral epicondylitis is inflammation of the common extensor origin of the extensor muscles of the forearm.

PRESENTATION
- Aching and deep tenderness on the extensor aspect of the forearm

EVALUATION
- Point tenderness over the lateral epicondyle
- Increased pain with resisted wrist extension
- Increased pain with resisted supination with the wrist in extension
- Increased pain with radial deviation

TREATMENT CONSIDERATIONS
- Eliminate all activities that reproduce symptoms, and avoid wrist extension and forearm pronation.
- Recommend local ice treatment with an ice cup massage over the lateral epicondyle for 3 minutes several times daily. An alternative would be application of a cold pack for 30 minutes three times daily.
- Initiate anti-inflammatory medication as appropriate.
- If pain is severe, start range of motion exercises with pendulum exercises until comfortable.
- Begin elbow extension and flexion, forearm pronation and supination, and wrist flexion and extension. These should all be done as slow active range of motion, with a passive terminal stretch held for at least 5 seconds each repetition. Work towards two sets of up to 20 repetitions in each plane three times daily.
- Once range of motion is pain-free, begin resisted exercises. A physical therapist can help patients learn to do these independently, which is important so that they can work toward two sets of 15 repetitions once or twice daily.
- Begin work on grip strength with a soft ball and work up to Thera-putty and racquetball squeezes three to five times daily, working up to 50 repetitions. Exercises should be done at a subfatigue level until they have been done asymptomatically for 4–8 weeks, after which point the patients can work up to fatigue of their muscles.
- If little progress is being made, consideration should be given to a corticosteroid injection.
- Use of a counterforce brace or a forearm band may be beneficial.
- If symptoms continue (1–2 years) and pain is incapacitating, surgical intervention may be necessary.
- Consider recreational or job site analysis with ergonomic adjustments as appropriate

Source: Gellman, 1992; Kraay, 1994; Thomas et al, 1995.

---

symptoms have resolved. Tables 44-6 through 44-9 provide specific examples.

TENDON SHEATHS

Two common presentations of stenosing tenosynovitis are trigger finger and de Quervain's tenosynovitis. Early symptoms are tenderness, warmth, and pain, all suggestive of inflammation. Pain occurs when the tendon moves through the sheath. Specific examples are given in Tables 44-10 and 44-11.

NERVES

Nerve entrapment syndromes result from compression of a peripheral nerve between ligaments or constricted anatomic structures. Symptoms vary depending on the nerve involved but in general include pain, numbness, tingling, cramping, and swelling. Tables 44-12, 44-13, and 44-14 provide specific examples.

Work-Relatedness

Musculoskeletal disorders are considered to be work-related when the work environment and the performance of work contribute significantly to their development (World Health Organization, 1995). Occupations that involve forceful exertion, repetitive motions, sustained and awkward postures, and possibly exposure to low-frequency vibration and cold temperatures have been identified as risk factors for CTDs of the upper extremity. The role of these occupational factors in the onset of CTDs, however, remains controversial; the relative contribution of occupational and nonoccupational factors is not clear. Many believe scientific data are insufficient to establish a definitive causal relation between the patient's occupation and CTDs (Lister, 1995; Millender et al, 1996; Vender et al, 1995). When

---

TABLE 44-7   Medial Epicondylitis

Medial epicondylitis is inflammation of the common flexor origin of the flexor muscles of the forearm.

PRESENTATION

- Burning and tenderness on the flexor aspect of the forearm

EVALUATION

- Point tenderness over the medial epicondyle (may be worse 1–2 cm distal and slightly anterior to the medial epicondyle)
- Increased pain with resisted pronation
- Increased pain with resisted wrist flexion
- Increased pain when lifting objects with the wrists supinated

TREATMENT CONSIDERATIONS

- Eliminate all activities that reproduce symptoms, and avoid wrist flexion and forearm supination.
- Recommend local ice treatment with an ice cup massage over the lateral epicondyle for 3 minutes several times daily. An alternative would be application of a cold pack for 30 minutes three times daily.
- Initiate anti-inflammatory medication as appropriate.
- If pain is severe, start range of motion exercises with pendulum exercises until comfortable.
- Begin elbow extension and flexion, forearm pronation and supination, and wrist flexion and extension. These should all be done as slow active range of motion, with a passive terminal stretch held for at least 5 seconds each repetition. Work toward two sets of up to 20 repetitions in each plane three times daily.
- Once range of motion is pain-free, begin resisted exercises. A physical therapist can help patients learn to do these independently, which is important so that they can work toward two sets of 15 repetitions once or twice daily.
- Begin work on grip strength with a soft ball and work up to Thera-putty and racquetball squeezes three to five times daily, working up to 50 repetitions. Exercises should be done at a subfatigue level until they have been done asymptomatically for 4–8 weeks, after which point patients can work up to fatigue of their muscles.
- If little progress is being made, consideration should be given to a corticosteroid injection.
- Use of a counterforce brace or a forearm band may be beneficial.
- If symptoms continue (1–2 years) and pain is incapacitating, surgical intervention may be necessary.
- Consider recreational or job site analysis with ergonomic adjustments as appropriate.

Source: Gellman, 1992; Kraay, 1994; Thomas et al, 1995.

TABLE 44-8   Supraspinatus Tendinitis

Supraspinatus tendinitis is inflammation of the supraspinatus tendon and is often the result of repetitive arm elevation at the glenohumeral joint and static abduction of the arm. Subdeltoid bursitis is a common concomitant inflammation because the inner synovial wall of the subdeltoid bursa is the outer wall of the supraspinatus tendon.

PRESENTATION

- Achiness to pain in the shoulder and upper arm with activity, especially with overhead use
- Decreased motion in the shoulder

EVALUATION

- Point tenderness over the greater tuberosity and anterior acromion
- Painful arc of motion between 60° and 120° of abduction and decreased internal rotation
- Shoulder pain increased against resistance
- Decreased strength of shoulder external rotators and scapular stabilizers
- Pain with shoulder adduction suggests involvement of the acromioclavicular joint.
- Weakness in the absence of shoulder pain suggests a rotator cuff tear.

TREATMENT CONSIDERATIONS

- Avoid overhead activities and all activities that aggravate symptoms.
- Use a cold pack or ice massage for symptom reduction.
- Initiate anti-inflammatory medication as appropriate.
- Begin Codman pendulum exercises with passive and active range of motion. Consider referral to physical therapy for initial guidance and support with the exercise program.
- Consider subacromial corticosteroid injection if pain interferes with stretching exercises or if pain is significant.
- Initiate strengthening exercises to correct any muscle imbalances within the shoulder.
- Failure to progress over 6–12 weeks may necessitate referral for further evaluation and more definitive treatment.

Source: Childre & Winzeler, 1995; Curtis & Wilson, 1996; Dalton, 1994; Frieman, et al, 1994.

---

a provider is asked to comment on the causal relation, it is best to state that the condition is causally related to the job or is aggravated by the job, or that no definite determination can be made (Millender et al, 1996).

When a patient has upper extremity symptoms that seem related to work activities, it is worthwhile to ask about working conditions to identify any potential ergonomic stressors. It would be of value to consider modification and adaptation of job tasks, tools, and techniques to diminish the effects of repetition, resistance, and sustained postures, which appear to play a role in precipitating complaints of upper extremity disorders (Higgs et al, 1993). Industrial occupational health departments and ergonomic specialists may be able to minimize or prevent many of the upper extremity complaints of their workers by evaluating job tasks, modifying the environment to meet ergonomic standards, and providing education regarding ergonomic positioning.

Rehabilitation

Although there are no large-scale epidemiologic studies on chronic work-related upper extremity disorders, clinical observation suggests a pattern of persistent pain, high perceived disa-

TABLE 44-9 Subacromial Impingement Syndrome

Subacromial Impingement Syndrome represents a narrowing of the subacromial space with impingement of the subacromial bursa, long head of the biceps, and rotator cuff on the undersurface of the acromion.

PRESENTATION

- Constant pain in the anterolateral aspect of the deltoid with radiation toward the elbow
- Aggravation of pain with overhead activities and at night
- Decreased shoulder motion, especially reaching behind the back
- Decreased strength in the affected extremity

EVALUATION

- Tenderness over the greater tuberosity and anterior aspect of the acromion
- Crepitation may be felt or heard with shoulder motion.
- Positive impingement sign and painful arc of motion between 60° and 120° of abduction
- May have weakness of the supraspinatus or external rotator muscles with loss of internal rotation
- Consider radiograph evaluation (anteroposterior, axillary, supraspinatus outlet views) when symptoms persist beyond 4–6 weeks of treatment.
- Injection of a local anesthetic agent into the subacromial bursa with reduction of pain can provide confirmation of diagnosis.
- Weakness in the absence of shoulder pain suggests a rotator cuff tear.
- Pain caused by shoulder adduction suggests involvement of the acromioclavicular joint.

TREATMENT CONSIDERATIONS

- Avoid overhead activities and all activities that aggravate symptoms.
- Use a cold pack or superficial or deep heat for symptom reduction.
- Initiate anti-inflammatory medication as appropriate.
- Stretching and range of motion (active and passive) of arm and shoulder. Consider referral to physical therapy for initial guidance and support with the exercise program.
- Consider subacromial corticosteroid injection if pain interferes with stretching exercises or if pain is significant.
- Strengthening of internal and external rotators (subscapularis, infraspinatus, and teres minor muscles) performed with the extremity at the side once normal range of motion has been achieved.
- Consider referral to physical therapy for ultrasound.
- Consider recreational or job site analysis with ergonomic adjustments as appropriate.
- Failure to progress over 6–12 weeks, and the extent of the functional demands required or desired, may necessitate referral for further evaluation and possible surgical intervention.

Source: Blair, et al, 1996; Klaiman & Gerber, 1996; Morrison et al, 1997; Neer, 1983.

bility, loss of function, distress, and dysphoria similar to that observed in the person with work-related disabling low back pain (Feuerstein et al, 1993). The psychosocial and economic impact can create a burden for injured workers and their families. An accurate diagnosis must be established. If the CTD becomes a chronic problem, the disorder is best examined from an overall functional impairment perspective rather than from the standpoint of recognized syndromes or clinical disorders (Higgs et al, 1992).

Persistent pain, loss of function, and associated work disability in patients with work-related upper extremity disorders ap-

TABLE 44-10 Trigger Finger or Thumb

Trigger finger or thumb is incompatibility between the tendon and its sheath that interferes with the normal gliding excursion of the tendon within its sheath.

PRESENTATION

- Painful triggering or snapping when the involved digit is flexed and then extended

EVALUATION

- Triggering of the digit when flexed and then extended
- Palpable nodule on the tendon surface

TREATMENT CONSIDERATIONS

- Intrasynovial injection with a steroid compound; repeat once if necessary.
- Possible short-term splinting of the digit
- Surgical intervention—open and percutaneous release of the A-1 pulley. Indications for surgery include failure of conservative management and possibly locking of a digit.

Source: Freiberg et al, 1989; Kirkpatrick & Lisser, 1995; Marks & Gunther, 1989; Ross, 1994.

pear to be affected by multiple factors, including physical capabilities in relation to work demands, ergonomic risk factors on the job, psychological factors related to worker traits, psychological readiness to return to work, and ability to manage symptoms (Feuerstein et al, 1993). A multidisciplinary approach that focuses on the physical, ergonomic, and psychological factors that may contribute to prolonged work disability has been associated with return-to-work rates greater than those found

TABLE 44-11 de Quervain's Tenosynovitis

de Quervain's tenosynovitis is inflammation and effusion of the abductor pollicis longus and the extensor pollicis brevis tendons in the first dorsal compartment of the wrist.

PRESENTATION

- Pain with thumb and wrist movement
- Pain may radiate into the forearm and over the thumb surface.
- Subjective paresthesia over the dorsum of the hand

EVALUATION

- Tenderness, thickening, and crepitus of the common tendon sheath
- Erythema and localized swelling over the radial styloid
- Decreased pinch and grip strength
- Positive Finkelstein's test

TREATMENT CONSIDERATIONS

- Immobilize the thumb.
- Initiate anti-inflammatory medications as appropriate to reduce pain and inflammation.
- Ice massage
- Cortiocosteroid injection into the synovial sheath of the first dorsal compartment
- If resistant, surgical release may be required.
- Consider recreational or job site analysis with ergonomic adjustments as appropriate.

Source: American Society for Surgery of the Hand, 1990; Guidotti, 1992; Kirkpatrick & Lisser, 1995; Messer & Bankers, 1995; Ranney, 1993.

with usual care for the person with a chronic work-related musculoskeletal disorder (Feuerstein et al, 1993).

When the cause of the CTD is work-related, the role of the provider expands beyond the diagnosis and treatment of the injured worker (Millender et al, 1996). An understanding of the factors that affect an injured worker's response to treatment, and communication with employers, insurers, and case managers to identify the job functions and requirements of the injured worker, will ultimately yield a positive outcome for all parties involved. Persons from the work site health services department who know the specifics of the work site requirements can be a great resource for the primary care provider.

COMMUNITY RESOURCES

- A Patient's Guide to Carpal Tunnel Syndrome, http:// www.sechrest.com/mmg/cts/ctsinfo.html: Overview of CTD, anatomy, diagnosis, treatment
- A Patient's Guide to Cumulative Trauma Disorders, http://www.sechrest.com/mmg/ctd/index.html: Overview of CTD, additional information on CTDs of neck, shoulder, elbow, wrist, and hand
- American Association of Orthopaedic Surgeons, 6300 N. River Rd., Rosemont, IL 60018, 847-823-7186, 800-346-AAOS, http://www.assos.org/wordhtml/ homew.htm

TABLE 44-12	Carpal Tunnel Syndrome

Carpal tunnel syndrome is compression of the median nerve at the wrist as it passes through the carpal bones.

PRESENTATION
- Numbness and tingling in distribution of median nerve (especially at night)
- Aggravation of symptoms with high force, high repetitions, and wrist flexion
- Weakness or clumsiness in holding small objects

EVALUATION
- Self-administered hand pain diagram indicating location and quality of symptoms
- Positive Phalen's test
- Positive Tinel's sign
- Thenar atrophy if severe
- Increase in two-point discrimination with worsening of symptoms
- Abnormal nerve conduction studies showing slowed nerve impulses

TREATMENT CONSIDERATIONS
- Splint the wrist in neutral position at night.
- Decrease repetitive wrist flexion and extension; avoid ulnar deviation loading, as with carrying a plastic grocery bag; avoid forceful gripping and loading of wrist, avoid finger extension with forearm supination.
- Initiate anti-inflammatory medication as appropriate.
- Consider corticosteroid injection.
- Surgical release of the transverse carpal ligament if poor response to 6–8 weeks of conservative measures.
- Consider recreational or job site analysis with ergonomic adjustments as appropriate.

Source: Childre & Winzeler, 1995; Gelberman, et al, 1980; Guidotti, 1993; Katz et al, 1990; Mackinnon & Novak, 1994; Messer & Banders, 1995; Siebenaler & McGovern, 1992; Szabo & Madison, 1992; Weiss et al, 1994.

TABLE 44-13	Cubital Tunnel Syndrome

Cubital tunnel syndrome is compression of the ulnar nerve just distal to the medial epicondyle as it passes through the two heads of the flexor carpi ulnaris. Resting the arm or hand on hard surfaces for prolonged periods or working with the arms in a constant flexed position can compress and damage the ulnar nerve.

PRESENTATION
- Initially, intermittent paresthesias in the ulnar nerve distribution with repetitive elbow flexion
- Numbness more constant as condition worsens
- Elbow and medial forearm pain
- Decreased endurance and awkwardness

EVALUATION
- Diminished grip and pinch strength
- Intrinsic wasting
- Anterior subluxation of the ulnar nerve over the medial epicondyle
- Positive Tinel's sign
- Increased pain and paresthesia with elbow flexion and pressure on the ulnar nerve in the region of the cubital tunnel
- Electrodiagnostic nerve conduction studies show evidence of significant slowing of conduction in the ulnar nerve across the elbow, confirming the clinical diagnosis if necessary.

TREATMENT CONSIDERATIONS
- Initiate anti-inflammatory medication as appropriate.
- Minimize frequent and forceful elbow flexion.
- Avoid direct pressure on flexed elbow.
- Recommend use of an elbow pad.
- Persistence of symptoms despite conservative therapy may lead to operative care, which includes decompression, anterior transposition, and medial epicondylectomy.
- Consider recreational or job site analysis with ergonomic adjustments as appropriate.

Source: Childre & Winzeler, 1995; Higgs & Mackinnon, 1995; Novak et al, 1994; Spinner, 1995.

REFERRAL POINTS AND CLINICAL WARNINGS

Because CTDs are a progressive entity, they do not generally present as emergency situations. However, significant sensory deficits, motor deficits, and muscle atrophy warrant further and timely evaluation by an orthopedist or hand specialist. Situations resistant to the usual interventions should also prompt referral to a specialist.

■ ■ ■ CLINICAL PEARLS

- A comprehensive approach to the management of CTDs requires a thorough assessment of the risks associated with work and recreational activities, in addition to person-specific conditions such as pregnancy.
- Workers whose job activities include exposure to cold temperatures or low-frequency vibration, sustained or awkward positioning, repetitive motion, or prolonged or repetitive exertion should discuss ergonomic issues with their supervisor and the occupational health provider at their place of work.

- Treatment options for CTDs are generally conservative and lengthy.
- Education can help patients assume the responsibility for participating fully in the plan of care for their CTD.
- A multidisciplinary approach that takes into account physical, ergonomic, and psychological factors results in greater return-to-work rates than other approaches.

TABLE 44-14	**Compressive Neuropathies and Nonspecific Pain Complaints**

Compressive neuropathies are vague complaints of discomfort in the neck, across the shoulders and upper back, and in both upper extremities.

PRESENTATION

- Vague complaints of pain, weakness, and numbness and tingling in the upper extremity, neck, back, subscapular area, and shoulder
- History of a job or regular activity that requires highly stereotypic activity or static postures for a substantial portion of the day
- Complaints of headaches and difficulty sleeping through the night
- Complaints of tingling in the hand and forearm

EVALUATION

- Painful limitation of shoulder and neck movement
- Paresthesias do not follow a pattern of a single nerve.
- Muscle weakness
- Nerve conduction studies are normal or show only borderline abnormalities.

TREATMENT CONSIDERATIONS

- Education regarding description of the disorder, causative factors, and positions of the extremity that increase pressure around the nerves or potentiate positions of muscle imbalance
- Teach nonrisk positions (wrists neutral, forearms supinated, elbow extended, avoid elbow flexion, minimize elevation and use of arms above head, do not elevate or roll shoulders forward, avoid neck flexion, and support the back with an appropriate lordosis).
- Ergonomic changes at the work station
- Postural changes
- Restore muscle balance with specific stretching and strengthening exercises to correct the imbalance between the strong and overused muscles and the weak and underused muscles.
- Once a pain-free range of motion is achieved, initiate strengthening exercises of the middle and lower trapezius and serratus anterior muscles.
- Splints may be provided to maintain a neutral wrist position while sleeping.
- Soft splints may be used to support the wrist during working hours.
- Elbow pads may be used to protect the ulnar nerve and as a reminder of the need to avoid elbow flexion.
- Soft neck ruffs may be worn at night to support the head and decrease tightness and spasm in neck muscles.
- Advocate a general exercise program.
- Recommend weight reduction if overweight.
- Continue to perform stretching and strengthening exercises as long as involved in activities that provoke abnormal positions.
- Consider recreational or job site analysis with ergonomic adjustments as appropriate.

Source: Higgs & Mackinnon, 1995; Mackinnon & Novak, 1994.

EDITOR'S NOTE:
COMPLEMENTARY APPROACHES

A general discussion of complementary approaches can be found in Chapter 3. The following, while not an exhaustive list, are some complementary approaches being used for this condition. Additional information on these approaches, including precautions, can be found in Appendices A and B. Providers need to assess for the use of complementary approaches as part of the patient's history, as they may impact conventional therapies, and patients may not volunteer this information unless specifically asked. Efficacy of many complementary approaches is not as well documented as that of conventional therapies. Providers need to read the literature before suggesting these complementary approaches.

- Complementary Modalities
  Acupuncture
  Massage therapy

References

American Society for Surgery of the Hand. (1990). *The hand: Examination and diagnosis*, 3d ed. New York: Churchill-Livingstone.

Armstrong, T.J., Fine, L.J., Goldstein, S.A., Lifshitz, Y.R., & Silverstein, B.A. (1987a). Ergonomics considerations in hand and wrist tendinitis. *The Journal of Hand Surgery, 12A*, 830–837.

Armstrong, T.J., Fine, L.J., Radwin, R.G., & Silverstein, B.A. (1987b). Ergonomics and the effects of vibration in hand-intensive work. *Scandinavian Journal of Work Environment and Health, 13*, 286–289.

Atroshi, I., & Johnsson, R. (1996). Evaluation of portable nerve conduction testing in the diagnosis of carpal tunnel syndrome. *Journal of Hand Surgery, 21A*, 651–654.

Bell-Krotoski, J.A. (1995). Sensibility testing: Current concepts. In J.M. Hunter, E.J. Mackin, & A.D. Callahan (Eds.). *Rehabilitation of the hand: Surgery and therapy*, 4th ed. Boston: Mosby-Year Book, pp. 109–128.

Blair, B., Rokito, A.S., Cuomo, F., Jarolem, K., & Zuckerman, J. D. (1996). Efficacy of injections of corticosteroids for subacromial impingement syndrome. *The Journal of Bone and Joint Surgery, 78A*, 1685–1689.

Browne, C.D., Nolan, B.M., & Faithfull, D.K. (1984). Occupational repetition strain injuries. Guidelines for diagnosis and management. *Medical Journal of Australia, 140*, 329–332.

Carson, R. (1993). Proper medical management can reduce cumulative trauma disorder incidence. *Occupational Health & Safety, 62*(12), 41–44.

Carson, R. (1994). Reducing cumulative trauma disorders, use of a proper workplace design. *AAOHN Journal, 42*(6), 270–276.

Cherniack, M.G., Moalli, D., & Viscolli, C. (1996). A comparison of traditional electrodiagnostic studies, electroneurometry, and vibrometry in the diagnosis of carpal tunnel syndrome. *Journal of Hand Surgery, 21A*, 122–131.

Childre, F., & Winzeler, A. (1995). Cumulative trauma disorder: A primary care provider's guide to upper extremity diagnosis and treatment. *Nurse Practitioner Forum, 6*(2), 106–119.

Dalton, S.E. (1994). The conservative management of rotator cuff disorders. *British Journal of Rheumatology, 33*, 663–667.

Fadale, P.D., & Wiggins, M.E. (1994). Corticosteroid injections: Their use and abuse. *Journal of the American Academy of Orthopaedic Surgeons, 2*(3), 133–140.

Ferguson, D.A. (1987). RSI: Putting the epidemic to rest. *Medical Journal of Australia, 147*, 213–214.

Feuerstein, M., Callan-Harris, S., Hickey, P., Dyer, D., Armbruster, W., & Carosella, A.M. (1993). Multidisciplinary rehabilitation of chronic work-related upper extremity disorders, long-term effects. *Journal of Occupational Medicine, 35*, 396–403.

Frederick, L.J. (1992). Cumulative trauma disorders, an overview. *AAOHN Journal, 40*(3), 113–116.

Freiberg,, A., Mulholland, R.S., & Levine, R. (1989). Nonoperative treatment of trigger fingers and thumbs. *Journal of Hand Surgery, 14A*, 533–558.

Frieman, B.G., Albert, T.J., & Fenlin, J.M. (1994). Rotator cuff disease: A review of diagnosis, pathophysiology and current trends in treatment. *Archives in Physical Medicine and Rehabilitation, 75*, 604–609.

Gelberman, R.H., Aronson, D., & Weisman, M.H. (1980). Carpal tunnel syndrome: Results of a prospective trial of steroid injection and splinting. *Journal of Bone and Joint Surgery, 62A*, 1181–1184.

Gellman, H. (1992). Tennis elbow (lateral epicondylitis). *Orthopedic Clinics of North America, 23*, 75–81.

Glowacki, K.A., Breen, C.J., Sachar, K., & Weiss, A.P. (1996). Electrodiagnostic testing and carpal tunnel release outcome. *Journal of Hand Surgery, 21A*, 117–121.

Gross, M.T. (1992). Chronic tendinitis: Pathomechanics of injury, factors affecting the healing response, and treatment. *Journal of Orthopaedic Sports Physical Therapy, 16*, 248–261.

Guidotti, R.L. (1992). Occupational repetitive strain injury. *American Family Physician, 45*(2), 585–592.

Hadler, N.M. (1990). Cumulative trauma disorders: An iatrogenic concept. *Journal of Occupational Medicine, 32*(1), 38–41.

Hales, T.R., & Bernard, B.P. (1996). Epidemiology of work-related musculoskeletal disorders. *Orthopedic Clinics of North America, 17*, 679–709.

Harris, N.R., & Gianacakes, N. (1994). Repetitive motion disorders of the upper extremity: Strategies for computer keyboard operators. *Journal of Florida Medical Association, 81*, 831–832.

Hebert, L. (1993). Analytical focus reduces anxiety over CTD claims. *Occupational Health and Safety, April*, 56–62.

Higgs, P.E., Edwards, D.F., Seaton, M.K., Feely, C.A., & Young, V.L. (1993). Age-related differences in measures of upper extremity impairment. *Journal of Gerontology, 48*(4), M175–M180.

Higgs, P.E., & Mackinnon, S.E. (1995). Repetitive motion injuries. *Annual Review of Medicine, 46*, 1–16.

Higgs, P., Young, V.L., Seaton, M. D., Edwards, D., & Feely, C. (1992). Upper extremity impairment in workers performing repetitive tasks. *Plastic and Reconstructive Surgery, 90*, 614–620.

Ireland, D.C. (1995). Repetition strain injury: The Australian experience—1992 update. *Journal of Hand Surgery, 20A*, S53–56.

Isernhagen, S.J. (1992). Principles of prevention for cumulative trauma. *Occupational Medicine, 7* (1), 147–153.

Katz, J.N., Larson, M.G., Sabra, A., et al. (1990). The carpal tunnel syndrome: Diagnostic utility of the history and physical examination. *Annals of Internal Medicine, 112*, 321–327.

Keyserling, W.M., Stetson, D.S., Silverstein, B.A., & Brouwer, M.L. (1993). A checklist for evaluating ergonomic risk factors associated with upper extremity cumulative trauma disorders. *Ergonomics, 36*(7), 807–831.

Kirkpatrick, W.H., & Lisser, S. (1995). Soft-tissue conditions: Trigger fingers and de Quervain's disease. In J.M. Hunter, E.J. Mackin, & A.D. Callahan (Eds.). *Rehabilitation of the hand: Surgery and therapy*, 4th ed. Boston: Mosby-Year Book, pp. 1007–1016.

Klaiman, M.D., & Gerber, L.H. (1996). General considerations for managing tendon injuries. *Bulletin on the Rheumatic Diseases, 45*(1), 1–6.

Kraay, M.A. (1994). The painful elbow: Causes to consider. *Hospital Medicine, 30*, 25–34.

Kroemer, K.H.E. (1992). Avoiding cumulative trauma disorders in shops and offices. *American Industrial Hygiene Association Journal, 53*(9), 596–604.

Lam, S.J.S. (1995). Repetitive strain injury or cumulative trauma disorder as legal and clinical entities. *Medicine, Science & the Law, 35*(4), 279–286.

Lister, G. (1995). Ergonomic disorders. *Journal of Hand Surgery, 20A*, 353.

Mackinnon, S.E., & Novak, C.B. (1994). Clinical commentary: Pathogenesis of cumulative trauma disorder. *Journal of Hand Surgery, 19A*(5): 873–883.

Mackinnon, S.E., & Novak, C.B. (1995). Comment to letter in Nathan, P.A., Keniston, R.C., Meadows, K.D., & Lockwood, R.S. (1995). Therapeutic value of repetitive motion: Work fitness hypothesis, a response to Mackinnon and Novak (Letter; comment). *Journal of Hand Surgery, 20A*, 513–514.

Manske, P.R., Ogata, K., & Lesker, P.A. (1985). Nutrient pathways to extensor tendons of primates. *Journal of Hand Surgery, 10B*, 8–10.

Marks, M.R., & Gunther, S.F. (1989). Efficacy of cortisone injection in treatment of trigger fingers and thumbs. *Journal of Hand Surgery, 41A*, 722–727.

Messer, R.S., & Bankers, R.M. (1995). Evaluating and treating common upper extremity nerve compression and tendonitis syndromes without becoming cumulatively traumatized. *Nurse Practitioner Forum, 6*(3), 152–166.

Millender, L.H. (1992). Occupational disorders: The disease of the 1990's: A challenge or a bane for hand surgeons? *Journal of Hand Surgery, 17A*, 193–194.

Millender, L.H., Tromanhauser, S.G., & Gaynor, S. (1996). A team approach to reduce disability in work-related disorders. *Orthopedic Clinics of North America, 17*, 669–677.

Morrison, D.S., Frogameni, A.D., & Woodworth, P. (1997). Nonoperative treatment of subacromial impingement syndrome. *The Journal of Bone and Joint Surgery, 79A*, 732–737.

Nathan, P.A., Keniston, R.C., Meadows, K.D., & Lockwood, R.S. (1995). Therapeutic value of repetitive motion: Work fitness hypothesis, a response to Mackinnon and Novak (letter; comment). *Journal of Hand Surgery, 20A*, 513–514.

Neer, C.S. II (1983). Impingement lesions. *Clinical Orthopaedics, 173*, 70–77.

Putz-Anderson, V (Ed.). (1988). *Cumulative trauma disorders: A manual for musculoskeletal diseases of the upper limbs*. London: Taylor & Francis Ltd.

Ranney, D. (1993). Work-related chronic injuries of the forearm and hand: Their specific diagnosis and management. *Ergonomics, 36*(8), 871–880.

Rempel, D.M., Harrison, R.J., & Barnhard, S. (1992). Work-related cumulative trauma disorders of the upper extremity. *JAMA, 267*(6), 838–842.

Ross, P. (1994). Ergonomic hazards in the workplace, assessment and prevention. *AAOHN Journal, 42*(4), 171–176.

Seyfert, S., Boegner, F., Hamm, B., Kleindienst, A., & Klatt, C. (1994). The value of magnetic resonance imaging in carpal tunnel syndrome. *Journal of Neurology, 242*, 41–46.

Siebenaler, M.J., & McGovern, P. (1992). Carpal tunnel syndrome: Priorities for prevention. *AAOHN Journal, 40*(2) 62–71.

Spinner, M. (1995). Nerve lesions in continuity. In J.M. Hunter, E.J. Mackin, & A.D. Callahan (Eds.). *Rehabilitation of the hand: Surgery and therapy*, 4th ed. Boston: Mosby-Year Book, pp. 627–634.

Swain, R.A., & Kaplan, B. (1995). Practices and pitfalls of corticosteroid injection. *The Physician and Sportsmedicine, 23*(3), 27–39.

Szabo, R.M., & Madison, M. (1992). Carpal tunnel syndrome. *Orthopedic Clinics of North America, 23*, 103–109.

Thomas, D.R., Plancher, K.D., & Hawkins, R.J. (1995). Prevention and rehabilitation of overuse injuries of the elbow. *Clinics in Sports Medicine, 14*, 459–477.

U.S. Department of Labor. (Sept. 11, 1996). Occupational Safety & Health Administration. News Release USDL: 96-377.

U.S. Department of Labor, Bureau of Labor Statistics. (1995). Occupational injuries and illnesses in the United States by injury. Washington DC: U.S. Government Printing Office.

Vender, M.I., Kasdan, M.L., & Truppa, K.L. (1995). Upper extremity disorders: A literature review to determine work-relatedness. *The Journal of Hand Surgery, 20A,* 534–541.

Weiland, A.J. (1996). Repetitive strain injuries and cumulative trauma disorders (editorial). *Journal of Hand Surgery, 21A,* 337.

Weiss, A.P., Sachar, K., & Gendreau, M. (1994). Conservative management of carpal tunnel syndrome: A reexamination of steroid injection and splinting. *Journal of Hand Surgery, 19A,* 410–415.

World Health Organization. (1995). *Identification and control of work-related diseases* (Technical report series no. 714). Geneva: World Health Organization.

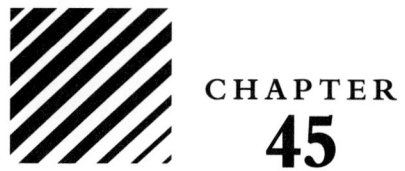

CHAPTER

45

Fibromyalgia and Diffuse Illnesses

Karen Anderson Keith, PhD, RN,CS, FNP, and Robert Keith, PA-C

One of the most puzzling and frustrating problems confronting primary care providers is the evaluation of vague symptoms such as weakness, fatigue, or widespread pain. Often these complaints are self-limiting, and because a complete evaluation would require an in-depth workup, patients may be given a preliminary evaluation and asked to come back if the problems persist. If the problem does persist, patients are frequently referred to specialists for evaluation, with variable results. This chapter provides a framework for the initial assessment and evaluation of fibromyalgia, polymyositis, and myasthenia gravis, three conditions in which the chief complaints are weakness, fatigue, and widespread pain. Table 45-1 lists these and other diseases that can present with weakness. Primary care providers, through a relationship-centered approach to care, play an important role in the initial workup, ongoing management, and when indicated comanagement of patients with diffuse illnesses.

FIBROMYALGIA

Anatomy, Physiology, and Pathology

Although there is no clearly identified pathophysiologic process related to the development of fibromyalgia (FM) (Bennett, 1995), some believe that the syndrome is partially the result of aberrant central pain mechanisms (Bendtsen et al, 1997). FM has been identified as a systemic disease process associated with a dysfunctional limbic system or neuroendocrine axis (Schneider, 1995). Focal blood flow decreases, and low cerebral blood flow has been found in patients with FM (Johansson et al, 1995; Mountz et al, 1995). This has led to the conclusion that abnormal pain perception (a low pain threshold) in women with FM may be the result of central nervous system dysfunction. Patients with FM exhibit disturbances in three areas: their stress response systems (low basal cortisol levels), their hypothalamic–pituitary–adrenal axis (increased release of corticotropin [adrenocorticotropic hormone, or ACTH] to endogenous or exogenous corticotropin-releasing hormone with blunted cortisol response to ACTH and exercise), and their sympathetic nervous systems (lowered activity, particularly related to norepinephrine and serotonin), reflecting a possible stress-related pathophysiologic response (Crofford et al, 1996). FM can be a sequela to trauma (Waylonis & Perkins, 1994), resulting in typical facet joint inflammation (Bassan et al, 1995). The prevalence of carpal tunnel syndrome is higher in women diagnosed with FM than in the general population, along with a higher level of undiagnosed carpal tunnel syndrome in those with FM. Although traditional wisdom suggests that there is no weakness associated with FM, reduced quadriceps muscle strength in patients with FM has been reported (Norregaard et al, 1995a).

FM can be a complication of hypothyroidism, rheumatoid arthritis, or (in men) sleep apnea (Hellmann, 1997); phenobarbital use has been noted as a reversible cause of FM (Goldman & Krings, 1995). A sport-induced FM with facet joint irritation has also been identified as a cause (Bassan et al, 1995). In the final analysis, the etiology of FM is unknown; hypotheses include hypothyroidism, sleep disorders, depression, viral infection, or an abnormal perception of stimuli.

Epidemiology

FM is seen mostly in women (66% to 90% of those diagnosed with FM are women), aged 20 to 50. The disease affects 3% to 10% of the population (Hellmann, 1997). Of the 6 million Americans diagnosed with FM, 4 million are women (Bennett, 1995). FM is seen in the elderly but may present without specific complaints beyond physical decline or confusion (Michet et al, 1995); this seriously complicates the diagnostic challenge.

Diagnostic Criteria

The American College of Rheumatology (Wolfe et al, 1990) has developed classification criteria for FM based on a history of widespread pain for at least 3 months and pain in 11 of 18 identified points. Both criteria must be satisfied for the patient to be diagnosed with FM.

The history of diffuse pain must include:

- Pain in the left side of the body
- Pain in the right side of the body
- Pain above the waist
- Pain below the waist
- Axial skeletal pain (cervical spine or anterior chest, or thoracic spine, or low back).

Pain in 11 of the 18 tender points must be bilateral and must be described as painful, not simply tender. Tender points (Fig. 45-1) are identified as:

- Occiput at the suboccipital muscle insertion
- Low cervical at the anterior aspect of the intertransverse spaces of C5 to C7
- Trapezius at the midpoint of the upper border
- Supraspinatus above the spine of the scapula near the medial border
- Second rib at the second costochondral junctions, just lateral to the junctions on the upper surface
- Lateral epicondyle 2 cm distal to the epicondyle
- Gluteus in the upper outer quadrants of the buttocks in the anterior fold of the muscle

TABLE 45-1	Disorders Presenting With Muscle Weakness
Disorder	**Presentation: Muscle Weakness and . . .**
Fibromyositis	Fatigue Numbness Chronic, widespread, aching pain Headaches Symptoms of irritable bowel syndrome
Polymyositis	Weakness begins in legs, goes to upper extremities and possibly neck May have cutaneous manifestations
Myasthenia gravis	Double vision Asymmetric ptosis Difficulty chewing or swallowing Weakness varies diurnally; improves with rest Waxing and waning course Weak voice Choking Sensation and reflexes normal
Rhabdomyolysis	Muscle pain History of a crushing injury, alcohol abuse, muscle necrosis, or seizures Dark-brown urine
Guillain-Barré syndrome (acute idiopathic polyneuropathy)	Weakness begins in legs, spreads to arms, then face Difficulty breathing, swallowing, chewing Distal paresthesias Palpitations/tachycardia Facial flushing Sweating Loss of sphincter control Hyper- or hypotension (Aminoff, 1997)
Lyme disease	Exposure to deer tick Neurologic deficits Rash Polyarthritis (Gorroll, 1994)
Postpoliomyelitis syndrome	New weakness Fatigue Pain Occurs decades after paralytic poliomyelitis (Trojan & Cashman, 1995)
Myofascial pain syndrome	Discrete muscular trigger points that, when stimulated, produce referred regional pain patterns Taut bands of skeletal muscle with a nodular texture when palpated (Schneider, 1995)
Hypernatremic myopathy	Dry skin Axillary and pubic hair loss Decreased libido Not thirsty Elevated serum sodium level Elevated CPK level Myogenic changes on electromyelogram (Hiromatsu et al, 1994)
Rheumatoid arthritis	Morning stiffness Fatigue Focal tenderness Abnormal laboratory studies (Goroll, 1994)
Hypothyroidism	Muscle weakness Cold intolerance Goiter Dry skin and hair Weight gain Elevated level of thyroid-stimulating hormone

(continued)

TABLE 45-1	Disorders Presenting With Muscle Weakness *(continued)*
Disorder	**Presentation: Muscle Weakness and . . .**
Depression or somatization syndrome	Fatigue No tender points Psychopathology of the condition present
Chronic fatigue syndrome	Presents very similarly to fibromyalgia Viral titers may be elevated Tender points sometimes present
Viral infection	Usually acute onset Myalgias Usually resolves within 4 weeks

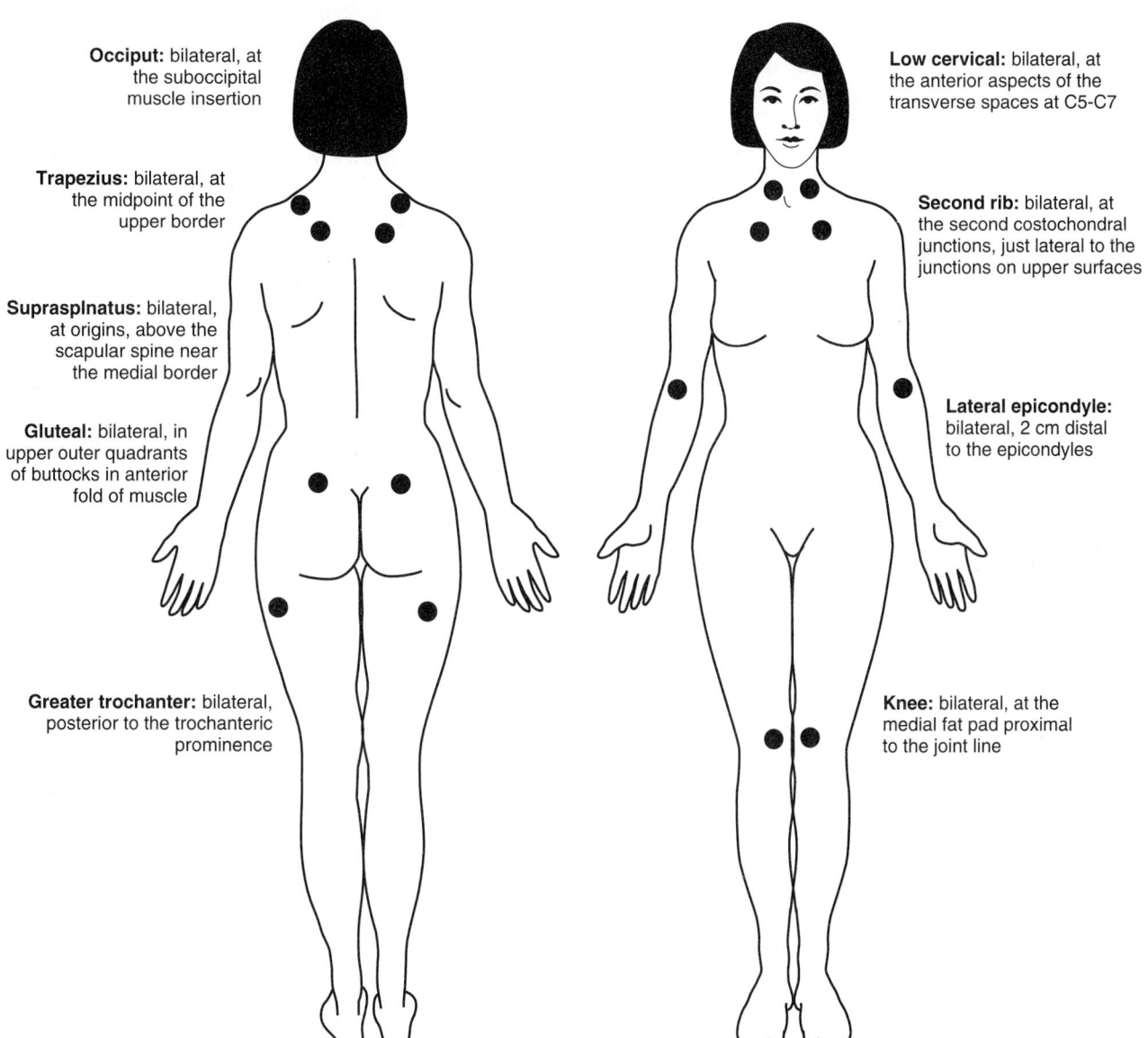

Occiput: bilateral, at the suboccipital muscle insertion

Trapezius: bilateral, at the midpoint of the upper border

Supraspinatus: bilateral, at origins, above the scapular spine near the medial border

Gluteal: bilateral, in upper outer quadrants of buttocks in anterior fold of muscle

Greater trochanter: bilateral, posterior to the trochanteric prominence

Low cervical: bilateral, at the anterior aspects of the transverse spaces at C5-C7

Second rib: bilateral, at the second costochondral junctions, just lateral to the junctions on upper surfaces

Lateral epicondyle: bilateral, 2 cm distal to the epicondyles

Knee: bilateral, at the medial fat pad proximal to the joint line

FIGURE 45-1 Eighteen tender point sites on digital palpation as identified by the American College of Rheumatology. (© 1996, by the Arthritis Foundation. Used by permission of the Arthritis Foundation. For more information, please call the Arthritis Foundation information line at 800-283-7800.)

- Greater trochanter posterior to the trochanteric prominence
- Knee at the medial fat pad proximal to the joint line.

These are consensus criteria until more definitive findings are set out (Wolfe et al, 1990).

History and Physical Exam

A comprehensive approach to the history is essential in the evaluation of FM because of the diffuse nature of the symptoms. A detailed review of systems should be conducted. Complaints of fatigue, numbness, stiffness, chronic widespread aching pain (usually without perceived weakness), headaches, and symptoms of irritable bowel syndrome predominate. A sleep history, with particular attention to the quality, not just the amount, of sleep, should be elicited (Schaefer, 1995). Many patients with FM complain of waking from sleep unrefreshed. Symptoms of depression (feelings of sadness, change in sleeping or eating patterns, difficulty falling asleep, early morning awakening, difficulty completing normal daily activities, decreased libido, suicidal ideation, as well as weakness and fatigue) should be explored, as should those of hypothyroidism (cold intolerance, constipation, weight change, hoarseness, dry skin, menorrhagia, as well as weakness, fatigue, and depression). The impact of the symptoms on the patient's relationships, employment, and social life and current stressors and coping methods should be assessed. Any history of fever, muscle injury, rash, or symptoms of arthritis must be elicited.

Ascertaining the location of the pain is very important; the pain of FM is located by applying pressure to the tender points (see Fig. 45-1) until the provider's fingers blanch slightly. The pain or tenderness elicited is diffuse as opposed to the localized, regional pain of myofascitis. Symptoms of FM wax and wane and may be exacerbated by weather changes as well as poor sleep and other stressors.

The patient is usually afebrile and exhibits no weight loss. A complete physical exam should include in-depth musculoskeletal and neurologic exams. On the general exam, the skin, nails, mucous membranes, and fundi should be carefully evaluated for rheumatoid disease, myopathy, osteoarthropathy, thyroid disease, and focal pathology (Goroll, 1994). The findings on the physical exam are typically normal, except for the usually symmetrical tenderness elicited by pressure on the tender points.

Diagnostic Studies

The results of laboratory studies are usually normal, but these studies are important to eliminate other conditions as the cause of symptoms. Customary laboratory studies include a complete blood count (CBC) and erythrocyte sedimentation rate (ESR) (may show an elevated ESR in arthritis or lupus), thyroid function tests (because FM may be a result of hypothyroidism) (Hellmann, 1997), and creatine phosphokinase level (usually elevated in polymyositis). Further testing becomes costly and is usually noncontributory. Lyme titers can be useful if the patient has symptoms of Lyme disease (rash, fever, neurologic symptoms, arthritis symptoms, exposure to deer ticks). If fatigue is the outstanding complaint and the history and physical exam do not point to a diagnosis, a more extensive workup is necessary.

The diagnosis of FM is one of exclusion. The differential includes rheumatoid arthritis (early morning stiffness that may improve during the day and worsens after exercise; symmetrically erythematous, edematous joints, particularly of the fingers and toes; elevated ESR, rheumatoid factor), systemic lupus erythematosus (rash over exposed areas; decreased hemoglobin, platelets, and white cells; positive antinuclear antibody preparation), polymyositis (weakness, not pain), and polymyalgia rheumatica (patient usually older than 50; shoulder and hip girdle pain; elevated ESR; frequently associated with temporal arteritis) (Hellmann, 1997).

Treatment Options, Expected Outcomes, and Comprehensive Management

Because patients frequently seek many opinions before they are diagnosed with FM, feelings of shame and embarrassment may predominate. These feelings can be increased when health care providers have expressed frustration, impatience, or suspicions of malingering in reaction to the patient's symptoms. An atmosphere of support must be provided for patients diagnosed with FM. Often just the knowledge that they have a recognizable syndrome shared with others produces comfort (Hellmann, 1997). Patients with FM are often depressed and frustrated because of the difference between their symptoms and their perception of illness and the objective findings (Henriksson, 1995a). This can prevent a patient from taking an active part in the treatment of FM. Patients must be assured that the duration of symptoms does not predict the long-term outcome (Wigers, 1996) and that FM is not a progressive disease. Patients must be made aware that there is not one, single treatment option that works in all cases (Hellmann, 1997). Any approach to treatment must be holistic and empathetic (Bennett, 1995); the goal of any therapeutic regimen is the resumption of normal or near-normal activity levels.

Pharmacologic treatment of FM is generally unsatisfactory. Nonsteroidal anti-inflammatories and other pain relievers are generally not effective, but individual patients may report feeling better when taking them. The possible benefits of over-the-counter or prescription pain relievers should be discussed with the patient in the context of the therapeutic benefits versus the effects of prolonged use and the risk of side effects. Amitriptyline has been used with some success; the dose is titrated beginning at 10 mg at bedtime and gradually building to 40 or 50 mg at bedtime (Hellmann, 1997). Tricyclic antidepressants can cause heart conduction problems, and an electrocardiogram should be obtained before the tricyclic is begun (Retfalvi et al, 1997). Tricyclics and nonsteroidal anti-inflammatories have been shown to work synergistically in relieving pain (Goldenberg, 1989). Although some advocate the use of selective serotonin reuptake inhibitors, their efficacy is still in question (Norregaard et al, 1995b). Lidocaine injection, although recommended by some (Bassan et al, 1995), is not always effective (Scudds et al, 1995). For patients with severe, debilitating pain, a pain management consultation may be required.

Patients frequently request antibiotics, with the notion that there must be something "going on" that causes their symptoms. Providers should work with patients to explain the use and efficacy of antibiotic treatment and the toxicities that can result from antibiotic treatment. Some patients may also question the role of magnesium and selenium in their condition, but at this time there is no conclusive information on their effectiveness (Eisinger et al, 1994).

Most useful to patients with FM is a gradually progressive exercise regimen. The exact mechanism by which this helps is not clear, but many patients report feeling better when engaged in a regular exercise program. Contradictory results, however, have been noted, and general feelings of fatigue, exercise-induced extremity pain, and exertion were found to be significantly higher for women with FM than for normal controls, although there was no difference in their pre-existing cardiovascular fitness (Mengshoel et al, 1995b). Stress reduction is an important aspect of the treatment of FM. Some useful methods include a regular exercise regimen (as noted previously), yoga (although stretching has not been shown to benefit FM, the relaxation of yoga can be useful), biofeedback, acupuncture, acupressure, transcutaneous electrical nerve stimulation, scheduled recreational activities, and other individualized activities. To identify these activities, patients must be questioned about their favorite recreational activities, which may include active participation in social events or quiet activities such as crossword puzzles, sewing, or reading.

Teaching and Self-Care

Patients must be informed of the possibility that symptoms of FM may never completely resolve, but that increasing age and physical activity have been associated with decreased symptoms (although a negative outcome is associated with many negative life events and the receipt of a disability pension) (Wigers, 1996). Patients are often relieved when a primary care provider takes their complaints seriously and provides the time and attention necessary to develop a plan with them. Guidance regarding necessary habit, role, and lifestyle changes must be addressed. Both the health care environment and the outside environment must be structured to provide as much support as possible (Henriksson, 1995b). Patients and providers should plan together how patients can "take charge of their lives" and actively seek friends and social situations that may be stress-reducing. Psychological support and counseling are also possible ways for patients to feel more secure in their ability to affect their health. The benefits of relaxation techniques and adequate nutrition should be underscored when working with patients battling FM. In one study, patients who were able to make adjustments to their daily lives (exercise, relaxation, nutrition) had reductions in pain intensity (Mengshoel et al, 1995a).

Self-efficacy on the part of patients in the areas of pain control and physical activities has been associated with less pain and less impairment of activities (Buckelew et al, 1995). Any teaching that will promote pain control and increased physical activity should help patients diagnosed with FM. An association between FM and depression, anxiety, and personality disturbances suggests that psychotherapy is indicated (Martinez et al, 1995).

Community Resources

- Arthritis Foundation, http://www.arthritis.org/: Facts about FM; support and self-help groups by state; state and local chapters

- Fibromyalgia syndrome: A source of information and support: http://www.clark,net/pub/tbear/fms: Articles, NIH handout, tender point map, support groups, links to other FM sites
- Fibromyalgia Network, 5700 Stockdale Hwy, Ste. 100, Bakersfield, CA 93309, 805-631-1950 (10 a.m. to 2 p.m. Pacific time)
- Arthritis Foundation, National Office, 1330 W. Peachtree St., Atlanta, GA 30309, 404-872-7100
- Arthritis Answers: 800-283-7800

Referral Points and Clinical Warnings

Some patients have serious problems sustaining employment and can be completely disabled with FM. There are great difficulties in adequately documenting the existence of FM because many health care providers do not believe it is a true diagnosis (Bohr, 1995; Capen, 1995; Liu & Canoso, 1996; White et al, 1995). This can prove very difficult for the primary care provider and absolutely devastating to the patient. Patients and providers may have to work together to educate other health care providers, the employment environment, friends, and family members who are not supportive.

POLYMYOSITIS

Anatomy, Physiology, and Pathology

Polymyositis (PM) is an acquired inflammatory disorder of the skeletal muscle that causes bilateral muscle weakness and sometimes pain. Muscles are necrotic and invaded by phagocytes and show evidence of degenerative and regenerative changes (Ytterberg, 1996). The etiology is unknown, although PM has been linked to infection with a number of viruses, including HIV, HTLV-I (Hellmann, 1997), coxsackieviruses, picornaviruses, and adenoviruses, among others (Ytterberg, 1996). PM is one of the idiopathic inflammatory myopathies; another is dermatomyositis, which resembles PM but also exhibits dermatologic manifestations (Ytterberg, 1996).

The initial presentation of PM is typically a complaint of muscle weakness, usually without pain. The progression of the weakness is insidious and typically begins in the lower extremities, moves to the upper extremities, and may ultimately involve the neck muscles (about 66% of the time). Pain or tenderness in the weak muscles develops in about 25% of cases (Hellmann, 1997). Pericardial disorders occur in about 11% of cases (Langley & Treadwell, 1994), and severe respiratory failure is an infrequent occurrence (Sano et al, 1994).

Epidemiology

PM occurs in twice as many women as men. It may occur at any age, but incidence peaks in the 40s and 50s. The exact incidence is unknown, although it is considered the most frequent primary myopathy in adults (Hellmann, 1997). Two million to 3 million people in the United States are diagnosed with PM; about four times as many African American than whites have PM. There may be a seasonal variation in the onset of PM. There is an association (not a causal relation) between idiopathic inflammatory myopathies and malignancy (incidence of about 15% overall), although no one kind or category of malignancy is found. The malignancy may occur before or after the onset of the myositis and is more likely in those with the onset of myositis after age 45 (Ytterberg, 1996). Malignancy is more likely in dermatomyositis than PM and is associated with a poorer prognosis (Hellmann, 1997).

Diagnostic Criteria

The diagnosis depends on the characteristic presentation of bilateral proximal muscle weakness (usually in the upper and lower extremities and the muscles of the neck) (Ytterberg, 1996) and the laboratory findings of elevated CPK and aldolase levels. Further workup would reveal inflammation and necrosis of the muscle fibers evident on muscle biopsy and electromyelographic changes (Hellmann, 1997).

History and Physical Exam

The initial complaint of weakness must be thoroughly explored. In PM, weakness usually first develops in the legs, so patients should be asked if they are having difficulty climbing stairs or rising from a chair. Specific questions must follow regarding symptoms of weakness in the arms and the neck muscles. Because cutaneous manifestations may indicate dermatomyositis, specific questions regarding rashes, erythema, and edema must be asked.

A complete physical should include in-depth examination of the musculoskeletal and neurologic systems. Raynaud's phenomenon (as a secondary effect of the connective tissue disease of PM) is possible, and atrophy or contractures are late results of PM. Signs suggestive of dermatomyositis include a malar maculopapular rash of the face; a maculopapular rash on the arms, neck, shoulders, and back; periorbital edema with a purplish discoloration ("heliotrope"); subungual erythema, cuticles with telangiectases; and scaling of the dorsum of the fingers (interphalangeal and metacarpal joints) (Hellmann, 1997).

Diagnostic Studies

Typical laboratory tests include a CBC and ESR (50% of patients have an elevated ESR), CPK and aldolase (used for diagnosis and to follow the disease progression), rheumatoid factor (may be positive), antinuclear antibody preparation (many patients have antinuclear antibodies), chest x-ray (often normal; some patients have interstitial fibrosis), electromyelography (abnormalities of conduction occur in PM), and muscle biopsy of affected muscle (may show nonspecific changes or may reveal inflammatory cells and muscle necrosis). Occult malignancy is a concern and must be investigated, although many times malignancies do not show up until months after symptom onset (Hellmann, 1997). To this end, a stool guaiac and urine dipstick are necessary, and the complete blood count must be assessed for signs of malignancy-induced anemia. Depending on the history and physical exam, a bone scan may be ordered. The provider should ensure that the patient has had all age- and gender-appropriate health maintenance screening tests (eg, mammogram, cervical Pap smear, sigmoidoscopy).

The differential diagnosis of PM includes hypothyroidism (elevated levels of thyroid-stimulating hormone [TSH]), hyperthyroidism (elevated T_3, T_4, thyroid resin uptake, and free thyroxin levels), polymyalgia rheumatica (pain, not weakness;

usually over age 50), central or peripheral nervous system disorders (myasthenia gravis, multiple sclerosis, amyotrophic lateral sclerosis), and substance ingestion (alcohol, corticosteroids, clofibrate, penicillamine, tryptophan, hydroxychloroquine, colchicine in elderly with renal impairment, rarely lovastatin) (Hellmann, 1997). As noted above, the possibility of malignancy should be investigated.

Treatment Options, Expected Outcomes, and Comprehensive Management

Steroids are the mainstay of treatment. Typically treatment is begun with 40 to 60 mg/day of prednisone, and the dose is titrated downward while being correlated with muscle enzyme (CPK and aldolase) levels. Because symptoms may recur, long-term steroid treatment is often needed, and adverse effects of prednisone must be vigilantly pursued. If steroids do not help, or if the patient cannot tolerate steroids, methotrexate, azathioprine, or intravenous immune globulin may be used (Hellmann, 1997). Physical or occupational therapy may be helpful in assisting a patient to regain function and participate fully in activities of daily living. Primary care providers should follow treatment not only with muscle enzyme levels but also with subjective and objective measures of muscle strength.

TEACHING AND SELF-CARE

Patients need to know that symptoms of PM may begin abruptly or have a gradual onset; the disease may have a progressive course. Those diagnosed with PM have an increased chance of malignancy, particularly if dermatomyositis is present or if the patient is over 50 at the time of diagnosis. Patients must be vigorously encouraged to follow recommended screening procedures for age and gender; the provider should work with the patient to develop a reasonable approach to scheduling screenings within the limitations of disability (Hellmann, 1997). Regular exercise may improve a patient's functioning because it prevents muscle atrophy. PM is a frustrating and debilitating disease; the support of family, friends, and coworkers is vital, and professional counseling or psychotherapy may be needed.

Community Resources

- The Myositis Association of America, 1420 Huron Ct., Harrisonburg, VA 22801, 540-433-7686, http://www.myositis.org/: Classification and diagnosis information, support for those diagnosed with PM and dermatomyositis

Referral Points and Clinical Warnings

Patients with rapidly progressive disease or disease unresponsive to steroid treatment within 2 months should be referred, as should patients who develop cardiac or respiratory problems.

MYASTHENIA GRAVIS
Anatomy, Physiology, and Pathology

The symptoms of myasthenia gravis (MG)—weakness and easy fatigability—are the result of the blockage of neuromuscular transmission. Between 90% and 95% of cases of MG are caused by autoimmune dysfunction, in which acetylcholine receptors are blocked by antibodies that selectively bind to them. The result is that fewer receptors are available for normal functioning. Affected muscles are usually those influencing extraocular movements, cranial muscles, and facial, pharyngeal, and masticatory muscles. The respiratory, arm, and leg muscles are also affected (Aminoff, 1997; Hart, 1996).

Epidemiology

MG occurs most often in young women, although it occurs in all ages. Young women may have their first manifestation after an infection, just after menses, or after pregnancy (Aminoff, 1997). Most patients with MG have a hyperplastic thymus, and 10% to 15% have thymomas that require removal (Messing, 1997). The number of cases has increased from 41 per 1 million in 1950 to 77 per 1 million in 1988, with a predicted rate of 83 per 1 million in the year 2000. These numbers reflect the improved prognosis for those with MG (Somnier, 1996).

Diagnostic Criteria

A single test is not considered adequate for diagnosis; rather, an acetylcholine antibody assay, an edrophonium test, and an electromyelogram must be used together (Hart, 1996). In a patient with generalized MG, the acetylcholine antibody level is elevated in about 95% of cases (fewer in those with ocular MG). In the edrophonium test, the anticholinesterase is administered intravenously and the patient is observed for improvement in symptoms. If the patient's muscle strength increases, then the test result is positive. The edrophonium test is most useful for those with generalized MG; it does not work well with ocular MG. The third test, the electromyelogram, shows a decreased response to nerve stimulation in patients with MG (Aminoff, 1997; Hart, 1996; Kernich & Kaminski, 1995). The diagnostic sensitivity of the acetylcholine antibody test is 88%, with the positivity correlated with the clinical severity of MG. The specificity of the antibody test for MG exceeds 99.9%. Confirmation of the diagnosis of MG should be made in collaboration with a neurologist (Skarf, 1996).

History and Physical Exam

A comprehensive approach to the history is essential in the evaluation of MG. Patients with MG usually have a history of localized or generalized weakness and fatigue. There is fluctuating weakness in the voluntary muscles, including ptosis, diplopia, and difficulty swallowing. The weakness is episodic and progressive and increases with activity (Aminoff, 1997; Kernich & Kaminski, 1995; Petit & Barkhaus, 1997). There are often diurnal variations in the weakness, and the symptoms may disappear for a period and then reappear (Aminoff, 1997). Patients often have weak voices and complain of choking (Kernich & Kaminski, 1995). A careful and detailed review of systems should be obtained, and each symptom uncovered should be thoroughly investigated.

The physical exam should include an exhaustive evaluation of the musculoskeletal and neurologic systems, which may be very tiring for the patient. The provider assesses for asymmetric ptosis (which can be induced by having the patient look up to the ceiling for several minutes) with normal pupillary reactions,

intact sensation, and normal reflexes. Keen observation of the patient's level of difficulty and fatigability when performing musculoskeletal maneuvers, as well as any improvement in function with rest, is obligatory (Aminoff, 1997).

Diagnostic Studies

The three key diagnostic studies were listed above. A chest x-ray with anteroposterior and lateral views should be ordered to look for a coexisting thymoma (although a normal chest x-ray does not exclude the diagnosis) (Aminoff, 1997).

Treatment Options, Expected Outcomes, and Comprehensive Management

Primary care providers should work with specialists in neurology to manage the patient with MG. Anticholinesterase drugs may diminish the symptoms of MG but do not change the course of the disease. Anticholinesterases used in individually determined doses are neostigmine (7.5 to 30 mg four times a day; average 15 mg) and pyridostigmine (30 to 180 mg four times a day; average 60 mg). A thymectomy is recommended for any patient under age 60 with MG (unless the symptoms are confined to the extraocular muscles); a thymectomy usually provides symptomatic benefit or remission of the MG. In new-onset, slowly progressive disease, the thymectomy can be delayed in the hope of a spontaneous remission (Aminoff, 1997).

Corticosteroids can be used in patients who do not respond to the anticholinesterases and who have had a thymectomy. Corticosteroid treatment is initiated in the hospital because the weakness of MG may be aggravated. The dose of prednisone is begun at 60 to 100 mg/day. This is tapered as the patient improves, but it is very difficult to wean a patient with MG from corticosteroids entirely. Azathioprine 2 to 3 mg/kg/day can be helpful (beginning with a low dose and slowly increasing). Plasmapheresis or intravenous immune globulin therapy may also be used in acute exacerbations or for patients, before thymectomy, who did not respond to the above therapy (Aminoff, 1997).

TEACHING AND SELF-CARE

Patients must be aware of the variety of drugs they take and their possible adverse effects. Pyridostigmine may cause diarrhea, bradycardia, sweating, and salivation, and prednisone can predispose the patient to subclinical infections. Overexertion or heat exposure can exacerbate MG, so patients must be warned to develop defensive strategies to stay cool. Stress, physiologic or psychological, can exacerbate MG, as can many common medicines (aminoglycosides, polymyxins, tetracyclines, verapamil, beta blockers, phenytoin, and chlorpromazine).

Because the symptoms of MG are so devastating, patients may be desperate to maintain whatever gains they have achieved through the use of anticholinesterase medications. They must be warned that overmedication with anticholinesterases may temporarily increase muscle weakness (which cannot be reversed with intravenous edrophonium) (Aminoff, 1997; Hart, 1996).

Patients must be supported in their adjustment to MG and must know that although medication can reduce the symptoms, it does not alter the course of the disease. Family, friends, and other associates must be told of the patient's physical limitations and learn to be supportive of the activities the patient can enjoy. Major lifestyle changes may be necessary.

Community Resources

- Myasthenia Gravis Links, http://pages.prodigy.com/ myasthenia/#INDEX: MG organizations around the world, including the MG Foundation of America
- Neuromuscular Disease Center—Myasthenia Gravis: Treatment information on pyridostigmine, prednisone, azathioprine, cyclosporine A, plasma exchange, human immune globulin, thymectomy
- Myasthenia Gravis Foundation of America, 222 S. Riverside Plaza, Suite 1540, Chicago, IL 60606, 312-248-0522, 800-541-5454, http://www.med.unc.edu/ mgfa/welcome.htm: Summary of illness, diagnosis, common treatments, chapter and support group listings, research and educational services

Referral Points and Clinical Warnings

MG is relatively rare and may present with very subtle manifestations. Health care providers must be alert for the signs of MG to refer patients to a neurologist (Kernich & Kaminski, 1995). Providers must also be aware that aminoglycosides can exacerbate MG; these drugs must be prescribed with caution in patients exhibiting questionable symptoms of MG (Aminoff, 1997).

■ ■ ■   **CLINICAL PEARLS**

- Diffuse illnesses are chronic conditions that currently lack cures, and they must be approached as such. Management requires both short- and long-term interventions developed with the patient in the context of family and community.
- Multiple approaches are necessary in the treatment and management of patients with diffuse illnesses.
- Patients with FM must participate in the treatment plan to achieve pain relief, maintain function, and manage fluctuating symptoms.
- There may be a seasonal variation in the onset of PM.
- A weak voice and history of choking may be suggestive of MG.

EDITOR'S NOTE:
COMPLEMENTARY APPROACHES

A general discussion of complementary approaches can be found in Chapter 3. The following, while not an exhaustive list, are some complementary approaches being used for this condition. Additional information on these approaches, including precautions, can be found in Appendices A and B. Providers need to assess for the use of complementary approaches as part of the patient's history, as they may impact conventional therapies, and patients may not volunteer this information unless specifically asked. Efficacy of many complementary approaches is not as well documented as that of conventional therapies. Providers need to read the literature before suggesting these complementary approaches.

- Complementary Modalities
  Acupuncture
  Aromatherapy
  Chiropractic
  Massage therapy

References

Aminoff, M.J. (1997). Nervous system. In L.M. Tierney, S.J. McPhee, & M.A. Papadakis (Eds.). *Current medical diagnosis and treatment*, 36th ed., pp. 892–948. Stamford, CT: Appleton & Lange.

Bassan, H. Niv, D., Jourgenson, U., Wientroub, S., & Spirer, Z. (1995). Localized fibromyalgia in a child. *Paediatrica Anaesthesia, 5*(4), 263–265.

Bendtsen, L., Norregaard, J., Jensen, R., & Olesen, J. (1997). Evidence of qualitatively altered nociception in patients with fibromyalgia. *Arthritis and Rheumatology, 40*(1), 98–102.

Bennett, R.M. (1995). Fibromyalgia: The commonest cause of widespread pain. *Comprehensive Therapy, 21*(6), 269–275.

Bohr, T.W. (1995). Fibromyalgia syndrome and myofascial pain syndrome: Do they exist? *Neurology Clinics, 13*(2), 365–384.

Buskila, D., Neumann, L., Hershman, E., Gedalia, A., Press, J., & Sukenik, S. (1995). Fibromyalgia syndrome in children: An outcome study. *Journal of Rheumatology, 22*(3), 525–528.

Capen, K. (1995). The courts, expert witnesses and fibromyalgia. *Canadian Medical Association Journal, 153*(2), 206–208.

Crofford, L.J., Engleberg, N.C., & Demitrack, M.A. (1996) Neurohormonal perturbations in fibromyalgia. *Baillieres Clinical Rheumatology 10*(2), 365–378.

Eisinger, J., Plantamura, A., Marie, P.A., & Ayavou, T. (1994). Selenium and magnesium status in fibromyalgia. *Magnesium Research 7*(3-4), 285–288.

Goldenberg, D.L. (1989). Treatment of fibromyalgia syndrome. *Rheumatic Disease Clinics of North America, 15*, 61–71.

Goldman, S.I., & Krings, M.S. (1995). Phenobarbital-induced fibromyalgia as the cause of bilateral shoulder pain. *Journal of the American Osteopathic Association, 95*(8), 487–490.

Goroll, A.H. (1994). Approach to the patient with fibromyalgia. In A.H. Goroll L.A. May & A.G. Mulley (Eds.), (1995). Primary Care Medicine, 3rd. ed, 799–801, Philadelphia: J.B. Lippincott.

Hart, J.J. (1996). Myasthenia gravis. In R.E. Rakel (Ed.). *Saunders manual of medical practice*, pp. 1056–1057. Philadelphia: W.B. Saunders.

Hellmann, D.B. (1997). Arthritis and musculoskeletal disorders. In L.M. Tierney, S.J. McPhee, & M.A. Papadakis (Eds.). *Current medical diagnosis and treatment*, 36th ed., pp. 750–799. Stamford, CT: Appleton & Lange.

Henriksson, C.M. (1995a). Living with continuous muscular pain—patient perspectives. Part I: Encounters and consequences. *Scandinavian Journal of Caring Science, 9*(2), 67–76.

Henriksson, C. M. (1995b). Living with continuous muscular pain—patient perspectives. Part II: Strategies for daily life. *Scandinavian Journal of Caring Science, 9*(2), 77–86.

Hiromatsu, K., Kobayashi, T., Fujii, N., Itoyama, Y., Goto, I., & Murakami, J. (1994). Hypernatremic myopathy. *Journal of Neurologic Science, 122*(2), 144–147.

Johansson, G., Risberg, J., Rosenhall, U., Orndahl, G. Svennerholm, L., & Nystrom, S. (1995). Cerebral dysfunction in fibromyalgia: Evidence from regional cerebral blood flow measurements, otoneurological tests and cerebrospinal fluid analysis. *Acta Psychiatrica Scandinavica, 91*(2), 86–94.

Kernich, C.A., & Kaminski, H.J. (1995). Myasthenia gravis: Pathophysiology, diagnosis and collaborative care. *Journal of Neuroscience Nursing, 27*(4), 207–215.

Langley, R.L., & Treadwell, E.L. (1994). Cardiac tamponade and pericardial disorders in connective tissue diseases: Case report and literature review. *Journal of the National Medical Association, 86*(2), 149–153.

Liu, N.Y.N., & Canoso, J.J. (1996). Periarticular rheumatic disorders. In J.Noble (Ed.). *Textbook of primary care medicine*, 2d ed., pp. 1112–1129. St. Louis: Mosby.

Martinez, J.E., Ferraz, M.B., Fontana, A.M., & Atra, E. (1995). Psychological aspects of Brazilian women with fibromyalgia. *Journal of Psychosomatic Research, 39*(2), 167–174.

Mengshoel, A.M., Forseth, K.O., Haugen, M., Walle-Hansen, R., & Forre, O. (1995a). Multidisciplinary approach to fibromyalgia. A pilot study. *Clinics of Rheumatology, 14*(2), 165–170.

Mengshoel, A.M., Vollestad, N.K., & Forre, O. (1995b). Pain and fatigue induced by exercise in fibromyalgia patients and sedentary health subjects. *Clinical Experiments in Rheumatology, 13*(4), 477–482.

Messing, R.O. (1997). Nervous system disorders. In S.J. McPhee, V.R. Lingappa, W.F. Ganong, & J.D. Lange (Eds.). *Pathophysiology of disease: An introduction to clinical medicine*, 2d ed., pp. 124–164. Stamford, CT: Appleton & Lange.

Michet, C.J. Jr., Evans, J.M., Fleming, K.C., O'Duffy, J.D., Jurisson, M.L., & Hunder, G.G. (1995). Common rheumatologic diseases in elderly patients. *Mayo Clinic Proceedings, 70*(12), 1205–1214.

Mountz, J.M., Bradley, L.A., Modell, J.G., et al. (1995). Fibromyalgia in women. Abnormalities of regional cerebral blood flow in the thalamus and the caudate nucleus are associated with low pain threshold levels. *Arthritis Rheumatism, 38*(7), 926–938.

Norregaard, J., Blow, P.M., Vestergaard-Poulsen, P., Thomsen, C., & Danneskiold-Same, B. (1995a). Muscle strength, voluntary activation and cross-sectional muscle area in patients with fibromyalgia. *British Journal of Rheumatology, 34*(10), 925–931.

Norregaard, J., Volkmann, H., & Danneskiold-Same, B. (1995b). A randomized controlled trial of citalopram in the treatment of fibromyalgia. *Pain, 61*(3), 445–449.

Petit, J., & Barkhaus, P.E. (1997). Evaluation and management of polyneuropathy: A practical approach. *Nurse Practitioner 22*(5), 131–148.

Retfalvi, P.M., Rosse, R.B., & Deutsch, S.I. (1997). Fibromyalgia: A neuropsychiatric perspective. *The Journal of Musculoskeletal Medicine, 14*(10), 52–61.

Sano, M., Suzuki, M., Sato, M., Sakamoto, T., & Uchigata, M. (1994). Fatal respiratory failure due to polymyositis. *Internal Medicine, 33*(3), 185–187.

Schaefer, K.M. (1995). Sleep disturbances and fatigue in women with fibromyalgia and chronic fatigue syndrome. *Journal of Obstetric, Gynecologic, and Neonatal Nursing, 24*(3), 229–233.

Schneider, M.J. (1995). Tender points/fibromyalgia vs. trigger points/myofascial pain syndrome: A need for clarity in terminology and differential diagnosis. *Journal of Manipulative Physiological Therapy, 18*(6), 398–406.

Scudds, R.A., Janzen, V., Delaney, G. et al. (1995). The use of topical 4% lidocaine in spheno-palatine ganglion blocks for the treatment of chronic muscle pain syndromes: A randomized controlled trial. *Pain, 62*(1), 69–77.

Skarf, B. (1996). Neuro-ophthalmology. In J.Noble (Ed.). *Textbook of primary care medicine*, 2d ed., pp. 1502–1516. St. Louis: Mosby.

Somnier, F.E. (1996). Myasthenia gravis. *Danish Medical Bulletin, 43*(1), 1–10.

Trojan, D.A., & Cashman, N.R. (1995). Fibromyalgia is common in a postpoliomyelitis clinic. *Archives of Neurology, 52*(6), 620–624.

Waylonis, G.W., & Perkins, R.H. (1994). Post-traumatic fibromyalgia: A long-term follow-up. *American Journal of Physical Medicine and Rehabilitation, 73*(6), 403–412.

White, K.P., Harth, M., & Teasell, R.W. (1995). Work disability evaluation and the fibromyalgia syndrome. *Seminars in Arthritis and Rheumatology, 24*(6), 371–381.

Wigers, S.H. (1996). Fibromyalgia outcome: The predictive values of symptom duration, physical activity, disability pension, and critical life events—a 4.5-year prospective study. *Journal of Psychosomatic Research, 41*(3), 235–243.

Wolfe, F., Smythe, H.A., Yunus, M. B. (1990) The American College of Rheumatology 1990 criteria for the classification of fibromyalgia: The multicenter criteria committee. *Arthritis and Rheumatology, 33*, 160.

Ytterberg, S.R. (1996). Idiopathic inflammatory myopathies. In J.Noble (Ed.). *Textbook of primary care medicine*, 2d ed., pp. 1084–1093. St. Louis: Mosby.

CHAPTER

46

Low Back Pain

Steve Weintraub, DO

Low back pain (LBP) remains one of the leading reasons for primary care visits. It usually resolves with nonspecific treatment within 6 weeks in 75% to 90% of cases, but there is a high likelihood of recurrence. LBP continues to be a costly condition in terms of both actual health care dollars spent and time lost from work.

Pain is subjective, and there may be few if any objective findings. In fact, a precise pathognomonic diagnosis can be given in only 10% to 20% of patients with LBP (Margo, 1994; Brady, 1996). Because back pain may spontaneously resolve on its own, the back pain sufferers who seek health care attention are those for whom the pain is severe or disabling or lasts beyond a reasonable time, or for those seeking secondary gain. In most cases, LBP is labeled as lumbar strain because the physical exam reveals no gross abnormalities and recovery is often quick.

This chapter discusses the etiologies of LBP and the evaluation and treatment of patients. Primary care providers must have a good understanding of the anatomic, biomechanical, and physiologic factors of back pain, for this will aid in the evaluation and treatment of patients with LBP.

ANATOMY, PHYSIOLOGY, AND PATHOLOGY

Anatomy of the Spine

The spine is divided into four sections: there are 7 cervical, 12 thoracic, and 5 lumbar vertebral sections and the fused sacrum (Hainline, 1995) (Fig. 46-1). The bony vertebral bodies and intervertebral discs provide weight bearing and shock absorption. The posterior elements—vertebral arches, transverse and spinous processes, and facet joints—protect the spinal cord and nerve roots. The facets, ligaments, and paraspinal muscles provide stability and balance (Wipf & Deyo, 1995; Brady, 1996). Pain may arise from any of these structures. The combined anterior and posterior elements are referred to as a functional unit.

The lumbar vertebra is a static structure that is made up of the anterior vertebral body and posterior elements (spinous process, articular facets, and transverse process). There is a strong potential for pain at the vertebral body and facet articular cartilage secondary to increased pain sensitivity. The most common etiologies are degenerative joint disease and fracture of any part of the vertebra (body, compression fraction secondary to osteoporosis, pars interarticularis stress fractures).

The intervertebral disc plays a major role in LBP. It is composed of the outer annulus fibrosis, made up of multiple layers of collagen fibers, and the inner nucleus pulposus, made up of a colloidal gel of proteoglycans and collagen. It is 80% fluid (Hainline, 1995; Cyriax, 1991; Al-Magdassy, 1996). Its functions are absorbing shock, providing resistance to compression, and allowing flexibility of the vertebral column (Hainline, 1995). A compromised disc lends itself to abnormal motion

and disc herniation, with potential radiculopathy and pain. The neurologic components of spinal anatomy are discussed below.

Degenerative disc disease is usually secondary to an annular tear, with subsequent leakage of nuclear material and dehydration of the disc (Hainline, 1995). Large annular tears may lead to prolapse or herniation of the nuclear material and subsequent nerve root compression. With aging, the percentage of water decreases and the disc becomes less able to function normally, decreasing the risk of disc herniation in the older population.

The superior and inferior posterior lumbar facets are synovial articulations situated between each vertebral body (Margo, 1994; Wipf & Deyo, 1995; Hainline, 1995; Cyriax, 1991). They play a potential role, along with the intervertebral discs, which play a major role, in lower back dysfunction and pain.

Ligaments play a major role in stability and restriction of motion in the lumbar spine. The key ligamentous structures include the anterior and posterior longitudinal ligaments, which help reinforce the annulus. As the ligament descends toward the sacrum, it narrows, increasing the risk of a herniated nucleus pulposus. The ligamentum flavum and the interspinous and supraspinous ligaments all provide further support to spinal movement (Hainline, 1995; Al-Magdassy, 1996).

Muscles can be divided into anterior and posterior muscle groups. Most posterior is the erector spinae, which is made up of the lateral iliocostals, the intermediate longissimus, and the medial spinalis. The middle layer is the thick multifidus, and the deep posterior muscles include the rotators, interspinalis, and intertransversarii (Fig. 46-2). The anterior muscle group includes the abdominal muscles, which play a major role in lumbar stabilization. They include the psoas (which is a primary hip flexor), the outer external obliques, the intermediate internal obliques, and the inner transversus abdominis. The remaining anterior muscles include the midline rectus abdominis and the lateral quadratus lumborum, which functions as a lateral trunk flexor (see Fig. 46-2). All these muscles play a role in trunk motion and stabilization.

The anatomy of LBP is a combination of fact and theory. Studies have shown that pain can be reproduced by injecting hypertonic saline into the ligamentum flavum in facet joint capsules. Supra- and infraspinous ligaments are innervated by afferent branches of the posterior primary rami, and muscle spasms are thought to be a motor reflex to pain. The role of muscle injury as it relates to back pain has not been fully elucidated. Strains and sprains, however, remain the leading diagnosis.

Sciatic pain requires both mechanical and inflammatory stimuli. The sciatic nerve arises from L4–S3 nerve roots (common peroneal and fibial nerves), passes over the lower edge of the sciatic notch, and lies just beneath the piriformis muscle and just above the obturator internus muscle (see Fig. 46-2). The nerve innervates the gluteus medius and minimus as well

526

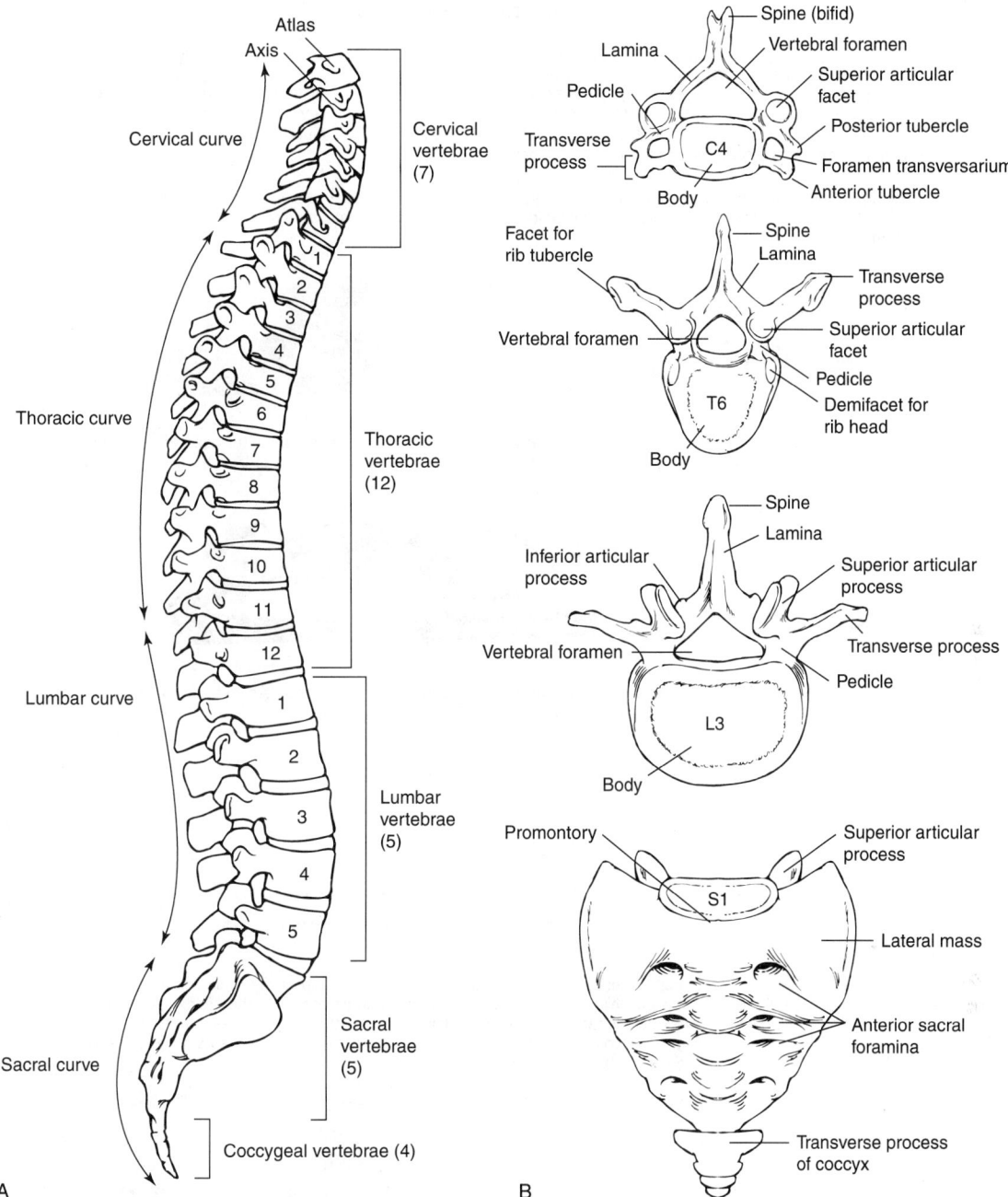

FIGURE 46-1 (**A**) Lateral view of vertebral column. (**B**) General features of different kinds of vertebrae. (Snell, R. (1992). *Clinical anatomy for medical students, 4/e.* Boston: Little, Brown.)

as the tensor fasciae latae before passing beneath the piriformis muscle. After passing through the main branch of the sciatic nerve, it innervates the hamstring and the muscles of the lower leg, and provides sensory innervation of the leg and foot (Borenstein et al, 1995).

EPIDEMIOLOGY

Approximately 75% to 85% of the U.S. population will experience LBP at some point in their lives (Wheeler, 1995; Margo, 1994; Wipf & Deyo, 1995; Hainline, 1995). The prevalence

of back pain ranges from 60% to 90%, with an annual incidence of 5% (Beattie, 1996; Daltroy & Iverson, 1997). The prevalence of LBP in both men and women 25 to 74 years of age is 16%, with an increase in prevalence in persons ages 45 to 64. There is a greater incidence in whites (16.5%) than African Americans (13.2%) or other racial groups (11.3%). Men and women are equally affected (Daltroy & Iverson, 1997), but women complain of back pain more often after the age of 60.

The prevalence of back pain alone and back pain with sciatica (defined as pain radiating along the course of the sciatic nerve to below the knee in one or both legs) is summarized in Table 46-1. Back pain, especially back pain with features of sciatica,

Back Extension Exercises

The following exercises are to be performed in accordance with the comfort of the patient. Perform only one exercise on any one particular day. Progress to the next exercise only when the pain from the previous one decreases. For patients with sciatic-type conditions, IF SYMPTOMS INTENSIFY IN EITHER OR BOTH LEGS (increased pain, numbness, or tingling) DISCONTINUE THAT EXERCISE UNTIL YOU SPEAK WITH YOUR PHYSICAL THERAPIST OR YOUR PRIMARY CARE PROVIDER. If symptoms diminish in the legs, continue as instructed, even if this is accompanied by a temporary increase in lower back pain.

1. **Lying on the stomach:** Lie on your stomach with your arms close to your body and your head turned to one side or supported by a towel roll or small pillow under your forehead. Take a deep breath, then relax for 5 minutes. Perform 1–2 times per day.

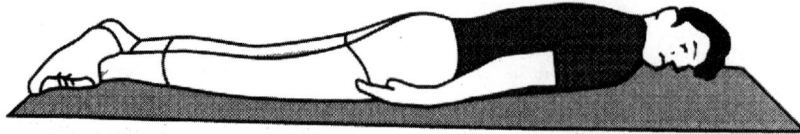

2. **Pillow under the chest:** Lie on your stomach with your arms close to your body and your head turned to one side. While in this position a pillow should be placed directly under the chest. Take a deep breath, then relax for 5 minutes. Perform 1–2 times per day.

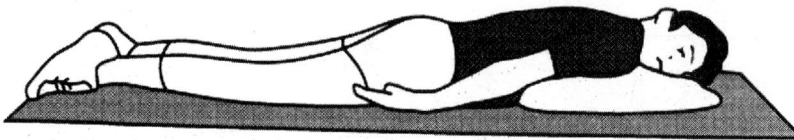

3. **Prone on elbows:** While lying on your stomach, place your elbows under your shoulders so that you are resting on your forearms. Take a deep breath, then relax for 30 seconds. Perform 10 repetitions, 1–2 times per day.

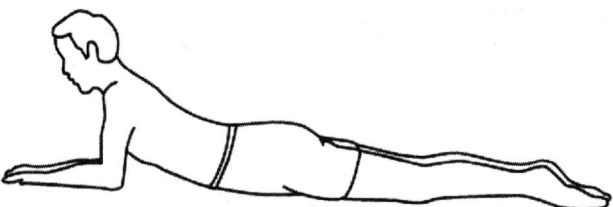

4. **Press-ups:** While lying on your stomach, place your hand under the shoulders and slowly straighten your elbows. Keep the lower part of the body relaxed while raising the back upwards as far as possible. Then relax and return to the starting position. Only raise the back as far as the pain will allow. Perform 10 repetitions, 1–2 times per day.
5. **Back bending:** While standing, place your hands on your low back. Slowly bend backwards as far as possible, then relax and return to the starting position. Perform 10 repetitions, 1–2 times per day.

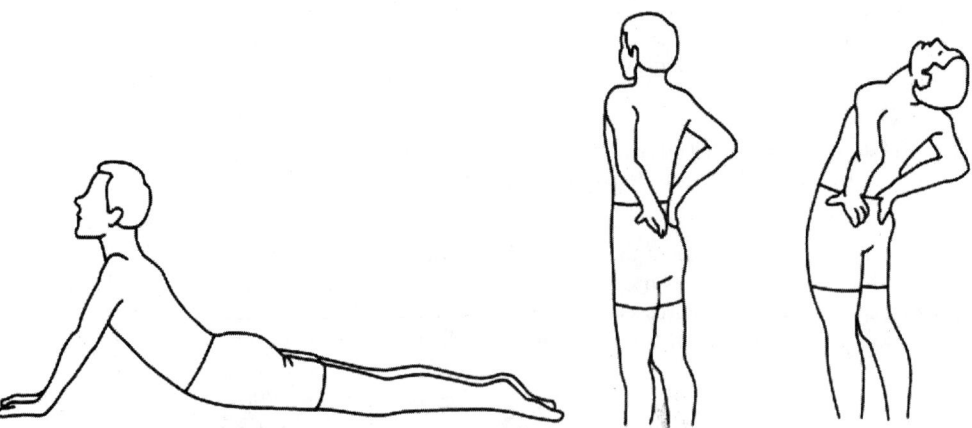

6. **Back strengthening exercises:**

(A) Lying on your stomach, with your forehead supported by a rolled towel or a pillow, raise one arm off the floor, keepig it straight. Do not lift your head. Hold for 10 seconds. Relax. Repeat 5–10 times, then do the other arm.

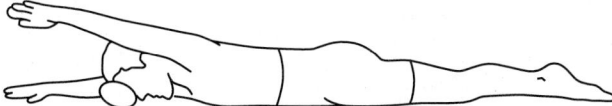

(B) Lying on your stomach, raise one leg off the floor, keeping it straight. Hold for 10 seconds. Relax. Repeat 5–10 times, then do the other leg.

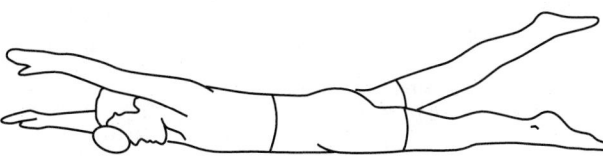

(C) Lying on your stomach, with your forehead supported by a rolled towel or a pillow, raise both arms off the floor, keeping them straight. Do not lift your head. Hold for 10 seconds. Relax. Repeat 5–10 times.

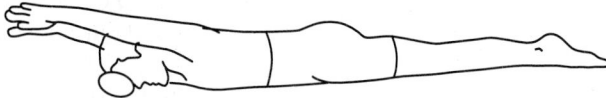

(D) Lying on your stomach, with your forehead supported by a rolled towel or a pillow, raise one arm and the opposite leg off the floor at the same time, keeping them straight. Do not lift your head. Hold for 10 seconds. Relax. Repeat 5–10 times, then do the other arm and leg.

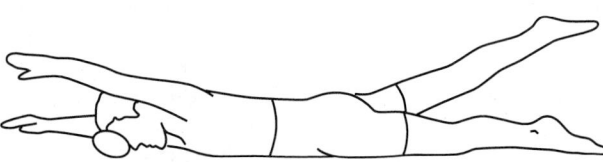

(E) Support yourself on both hands and knees. From this position, raise one arm and the opposite leg at the same time, as shown below, keeping them straight. Hold for 10 seconds. Relax. Repeat 5–10 times, then do the other arm and leg.

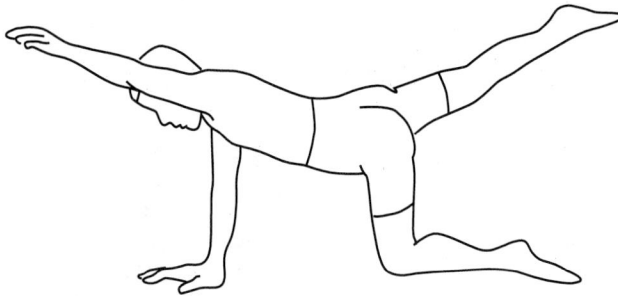

7. **Hip flexor stretching:** Lie down on your back near the right edge of the table. Pull the left knee to your chest and let the right leg hand off the side of the table. You may use a weight on the right ankle. Be sure to hold your left knee as close to the chest as you can throughout the exercise. Hold for 10 seconds, then relax. Repeat 5–10 times, then move to the other edge of the table and stretch the other side.

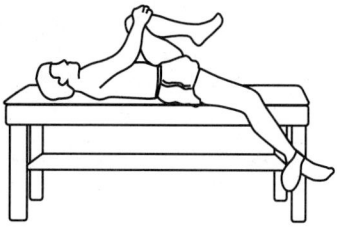

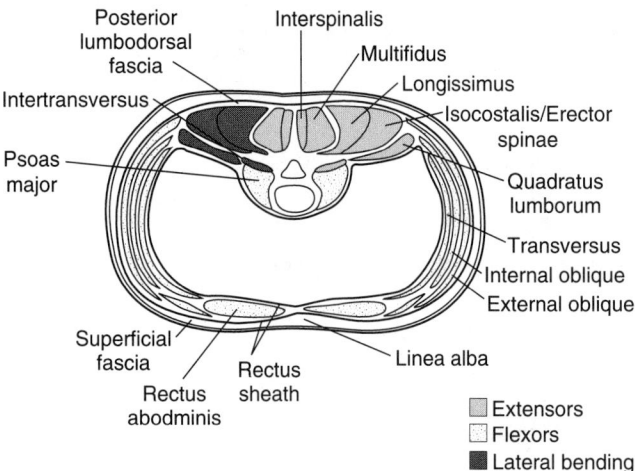

FIGURE 46-2 Cross-section of body musculature and fascia through the third lumbar vertebra. The primary motions of the lumbar spine are flexion, extension, and lateral bending (only a small portion of rotation occurs in the lumbar spine). Flexors are anterior to the spine and extensors are posterior. The muscles that cause lateral bending are contiguous to the vertebral bodies in a lateral position.

usually does not last longer than 2 weeks. As a result of back pain, there are 7 million people missing work at any one time in the United States alone.

LBP has numerous etiologies. Fewer than 3% of cases are secondary to a serious medical disease. Most cases of LBP are mechanical in origin. Mechanical conditions of the spine, including disc disease, spondylosis, spinal stenosis, and fractures, account for up to 98% of cases of LBP, with the remaining cases the result of systemic and visceral disease (Wheeler, 1995; Margo, 1994). There are many opinions as

to the actual neurogenic etiology of LBP, and only 10% to 20% of cases can actually be attributed to an anatomically defined lesion.

Epidemiologic studies also reveal distinct characteristics in the occupational and psychological profiles of people disabled by LBP. Many of these patients view their jobs as boring and dissatisfying (Daltroy & Iverson, 1997). They present with depression, anxiety, hypochondriasis, and hysteria. There also appear to be increased rates of alcoholism, divorce, headaches, and ulcers in this population (Turner & Denny, 1993). When working with patients with LBP, providers must keep in mind the possibility of secondary gain—either financial gain (through a lawsuit for a motor vehicle accident or other liability) or the desire to remain off work and collect disability. These issues must be carefully and sensitively discussed if the provider has evidence that this is the nature of the patient's LBP disability.

There are equal numbers of reports of LBP in heavy laborers compared to those in sedentary occupations. The loss of productivity, however, and time lost from work are greater in heavy laborers. The risk factors in both settings may be biomechanical (twisting and other repetitive motions that occur on the job). In sedentary occupations, there is an increased risk secondary to muscular deconditioning or the chronic mechanical stress from sitting positions (Beattie, 1996). Other risk factors include obesity, cigarette smoking, lower socioeconomic status, and lower educational attainment.

Osteoporosis increases the risk of spinal compression fractures. Genetics may play a role in osteoporosis as well as congenital isthmic spondylolisthesis, spinal osteochondrosis (Scheurmann's disease), and spinal stenosis associated with achondroplasia. Also, certain athletic activities, such as gymnastics and football, may increase the risk of spondylolysis and isthmic spondylolisthesis because they involve repetitive hyperextension.

TABLE 46-1	Classification of Low Back Pain Syndromes
Mechanical or Activity-Related Causes	**Referred Pain**
Segmental and discal degeneration	Gastrointestinal disorders
Myofascial or soft tissue injury disorder	Genitourinary disorders, including nephrolithiasis,
Disc herniation, with possible radiculopathy	prostatitis, and pyelonephritis
Spinal instability, with possible spondylolisthesis or	Gynecologic disorders, including ectopic pregnancy and
fracture	pelvic inflammatory disease
Vertebral body fracture	Abdominal aortic aneurysm
Spinal canal or lateral recess stenosis	Hip pathology
Arachnoiditis, including postoperative scarring	Psychosocial causes
	Compensable injury
Systemic Disorders	Somatoform pain disorder
Primary or metastatic neoplasm, including myeloma	Psychiatric syndromes, including delusional pain
Osseous, discal, or epidural infection	Drug seeking
Inflammatory spondyloarthropathy	Abusive relationships
Metabolic bone disease, including osteoporosis	Seeking disability or out-of-work status
Vascular disorders such as atherosclerosis or vasculitis	
Neurologic Syndromes	
Myelopathy from intrinsic or extrinsic processes	
Lumbosacral plexopathy, especially from diabetes	
Neuropathy, including inflammatory demyelinating type (ie, Guillain-Barré)	
Mononeuropathy, including causalgia	
Myopathy, including myositis and metabolic causes	

Wheeler, A. (1995). Diagnosis and management of low back pain and sciatica. *American Family Physician* 52(5), 1333–1343.

DIAGNOSTIC CRITERIA

Differential Diagnosis

Although there are no true diagnostic criteria for LBP, Table 46-1 shows the multitude of LBP syndromes. This section focuses on the more common etiologies, or specific diagnoses of secondary back pain. The provider must be able to differentiate between benign causes, such as lumbar strain and disc disease, and the more ominous and life-threatening disorders that need quick referral, such as cauda equina syndrome, malignancy, and vertebral fracture with neurologic compromise. A thorough history and a detailed physical exam, including a neurologic exam, are warranted.

LBP can be divided into three clinical courses: acute, subacute, and chronic. It is useful to differentiate these three categories when approaching treatment protocols. The definitions are as follows:

- Acute: 0 to 6 weeks
- Subacute: 6 to 12 weeks
- Chronic: More than 12 weeks.

It is also important to categorize back pain along with its etiology for correct treatment and accurate referral.

Mechanical or Activity-Related Causes

DEGENERATIVE DISC DISEASE

There appears to be a correlation between annular tears of the disc and degenerative disc disease. As previously stated, there is also a correlation with herniated nucleus pulposus. A slow leak over time of the nuclear material will lead to desiccation of the disc. How does this lead to back pain? One explanation is an inflammatory pathway involving chemical factors. This pathway may explain why pain is relieved when a corticosteroid or nonsteroidal anti-inflammatory agent is administered (Saal, 1995). The other theory is an immunologic phenomenon, described by in vitro studies. It is theorized that the nuclear material, previously sheltered from the immune system, generates an autoimmune response once it is exposed.

Degenerative disc disease may present with isolated LBP or with radicular symptoms. The diagnosis can be made with plain radiographs, noting diminished disc space between the vertebral bodies, or by magnetic resonance imaging (MRI), which notes changes on T_2-weighted images.

LUMBAR SOFT-TISSUE INJURY/STRAIN, SPRAIN

Most cases of LBP fall into this category, known as nonspecific back pain. This pain usually resolves spontaneously in 2 to 6 weeks. If the pain persists longer than this, a secondary cause must be considered (ie, disc versus facet). In this type of pain, the most common etiologic factors are poor conditioning, excess weight, and sudden overuse or overload activities.

HERNIATED LUMBAR INTERVERTEBRAL DISC

Herniated disc is diagnosed in a small percentage of patients with LBP. Lumbar disc herniation is most common in persons ages 30 to 40; it is less common in adolescents and young adults and rare in the older population (Lazara & Quinet, 1994;

Rothman & Simeone, 1992; Beattie, 1996). Acute herniation of the nucleus pulposus may result from sudden overload of the intervertebral disc or from repetitive microtraumatic loading (Hainline, 1995). For most patients with a herniated disc, back pain precedes the onset of sciatica. The back pain may or may not linger as the pain and paresthesias begin to radiate down the leg (Beattie, 1996).

The onset of sciatic pain may be gradual or sudden. Pain and radicular symptoms may be worsened by sitting for a long period, rising from a sitting or supine position, or coughing or sneezing.

Herniated discs occur at the L4-5 or L5–S1 level in 95% of cases (Wipf & Deyo, 1995; Beattie, 1996). The neurologic examination should focus on the L5 and S1 nerve roots. A herniated disc at the L5 nerve root may cause pain and numbness radiating from the back to the anterior thigh, anterolateral leg, medial foot, and great toe. There are no reflex changes, and the motor exam reveals weakness in the great toe extensor as well as the dorsiflexors of the foot (Table 46-2).

Patients with an L5–S1 disc herniation (sacroiliac root) have pain and numbness of the posterior thigh and leg, posterior-lateral foot, and lateral toes; a diminished ankle reflex; and weakness of the plantar flexors of the foot, which can be seen with difficulty on toe walking (see Table 46-2). It is rare to see clinical herniations above the level of L4.

A positive straight leg raise (SLR) test helps confirm nerve root irritation. This test has a sensitivity of 95% with proven disc herniation, and its absence can actually rule out disc herniation. A crossover test or crossed SLR is less sensitive but more specific for disc herniation (Fig. 46-3). Electromyography may aid in the diagnosis of a particular radiculopathy, but it is better used to discriminate radicular pain from peripheral neuropathy.

Plain x-rays are not helpful in diagnosing a herniated disc, but they should be used to rule out tumor, infection, fracture, and spondylolisthesis. A herniated disc is usually confirmed when an imaging study such as myelography, computed tomography (CT), or MRI shows an abnormality corresponding to the clinical exam. However, these sophisticated and expensive studies should not be ordered too early in the course of a workup for LBP, especially if the patient is not considered a surgical candidate. These tests should be ordered in patients who have a long protracted course, or early in the case of cauda equina syndrome, a progressive neurologic deficit, or the suspicion of tumor or infection (Beattie, 1996).

SPINAL STENOSIS

Spinal stenosis (narrowing of the spinal canal) may be secondary to hypertrophy of the facet joints (osteoarthritis), hypertrophy of the ligamentum flavum, or spondylosis of the intervertebral disc, which is often superimposed on a congenitally narrow canal (Wipf & Deyo, 1995; Lazara & Quinet, 1994).

Spinal stenosis is most likely in the older population. Patients present with an insidious onset of pain and numbness that worsens with walking. The pain of spinal stenosis is referred to as pseudoclaudication because of its similarity to vascular claudication (Wipf & Deyo, 1995). Patients may have a dermatomal distribution of pain and sensory deficit as well as an abnormal SLR test. To differentiate this from a herniated disc, the factors that exacerbate and relieve the pain should be noted. Spinal stenosis is relieved by sitting and aggravated by standing; a

TABLE 46-2   Presentations of Disc Herniation with Nerve Root Involvement

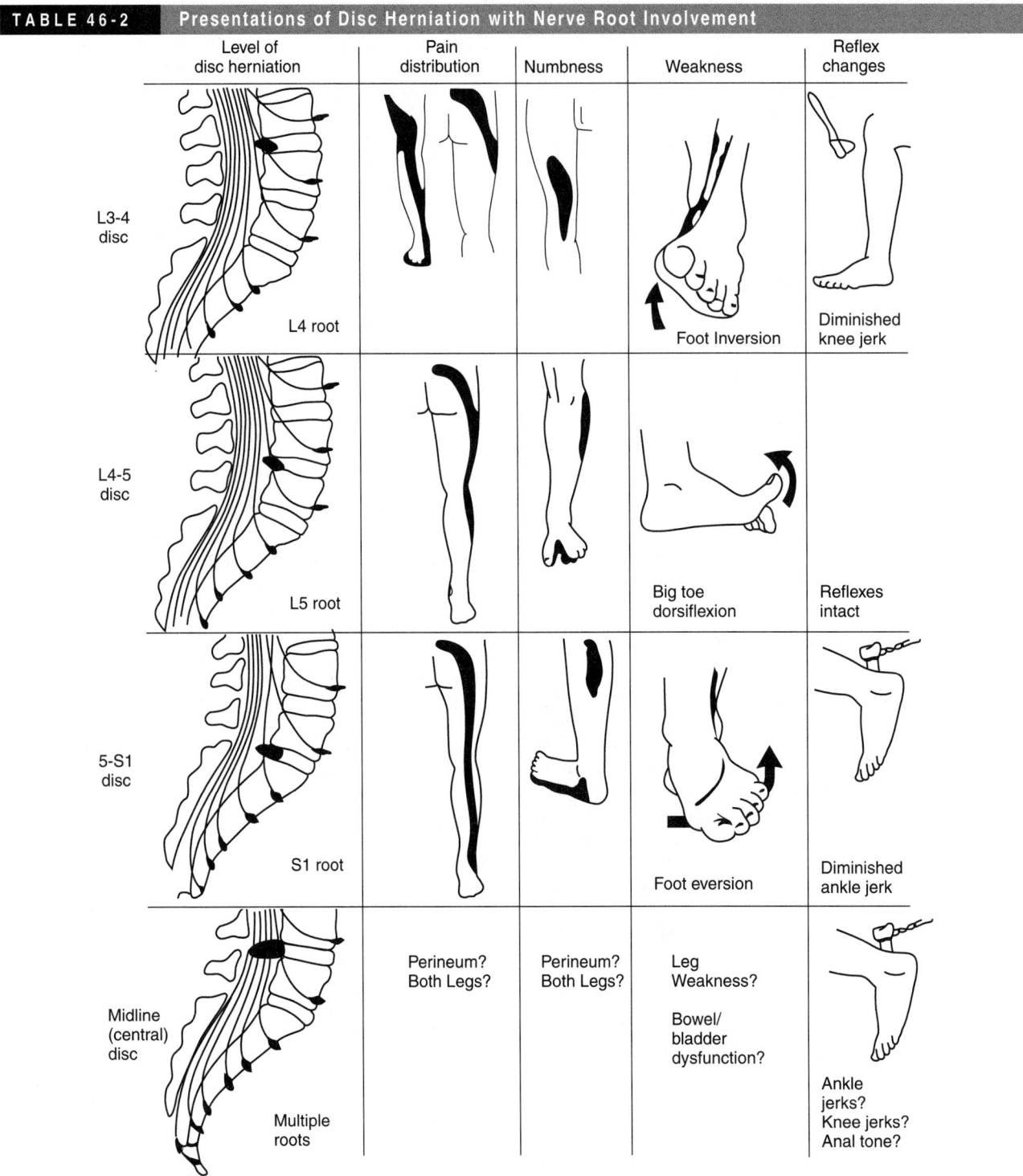

Level of disc herniation	Pain distribution	Numbness	Weakness	Reflex changes
L3-4 disc	L4 root		Foot Inversion	Diminished knee jerk
L4-5 disc	L5 root		Big toe dorsiflexion	Reflexes intact
5-S1 disc	S1 root		Foot eversion	Diminished ankle jerk
Midline (central) disc / Multiple roots	Perineum? Both Legs?	Perineum? Both Legs?	Leg Weakness? Bowel/ bladder dysfunction?	Ankle jerks? Knee jerks? Anal tone?

Reilly, B.M. (1991). *Practical strategies in outpatient medicine*. Philadelphia: WB Saunders.

herniated disc is exacerbated by sitting and relieved by standing (Wipf & Deyo, 1995).

In spinal stenosis, deep tendon reflexes may be decreased, with weakness in one or both lower extremities. The diagnosis is confirmed by MRI imaging revealing a narrow spinal canal. Plain films would point out only the degenerative changes that lead to spinal stenosis.

SPONDYLOLYSIS/SPONDYLOLISTHESIS

These disorders are most common in young adolescents and young adults who are involved in sports, such as gymnastics, tennis, weight lifting, and football (linemen). These sports put the lumbar spine into hyperextension. Spondylolisthesis is the slipping of one vertebral body forward on the one below. The extent of slippage is graded from grade I to grade IV (total

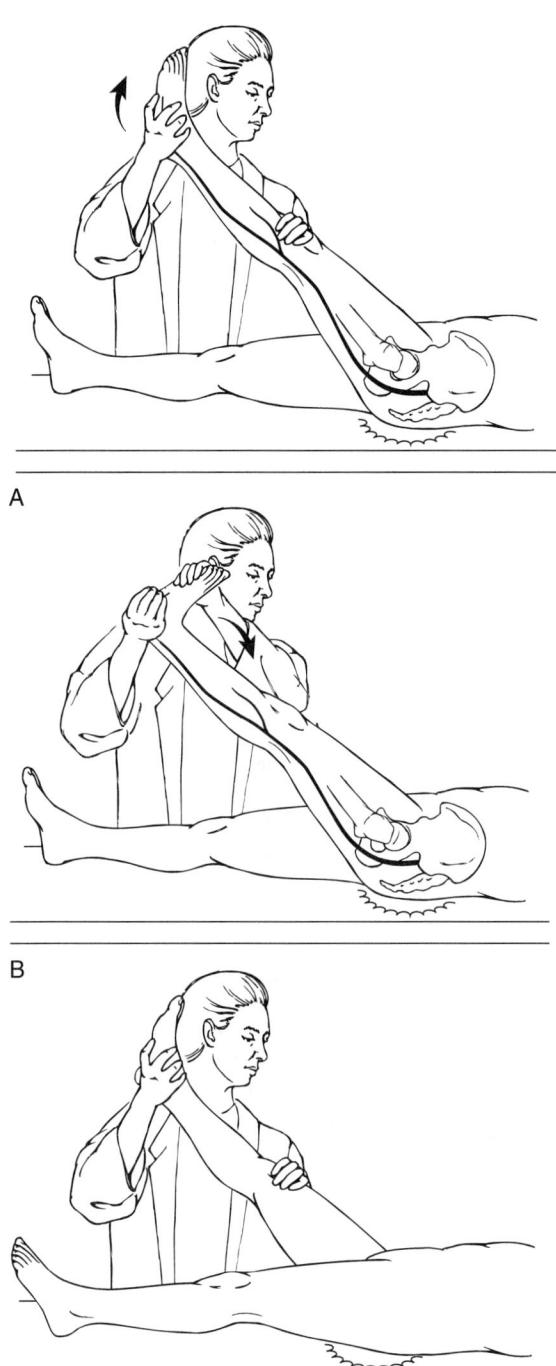

FIGURE 46-3 (A) Straight-leg raising. **(B)** In this position, dorsiflexion of the foot reproduces sciatic pain. **(C)** A positive crossed SLR test: Back pain on the involved side induced by straight-leg raising the noninvolved leg. (Adapted from Hoppenfeld, S. [1976]). Physical exam of the spine and extremities. Stamford, CT: Appleton & Lange.

forward displacement). Often spondylolisthesis is secondary to bilateral spondylolysis. Spondylolisthesis is best seen on plain lateral radiographs.

Spondylolysis is a stress fracture or fatigue fracture of the pars interarticularis. This stress fracture is usually caused by repetitive overload of the pars with repeated hyperextension.

The symptoms may include LBP with or without radiation, a tight hamstring, and relief of symptoms with rest. The severity and extent of the defect may change the clinical findings. For example, a unilateral defect may be found in an asymptomatic person. This lesion would be considered inactive, whereas a patient with an active lesion or significant spondylolisthesis may have severe hamstring tightness, gait disturbance, and neurologic symptoms. X-rays may reveal a defect through the pars interarticularis. This may be seen on standard anteroposterior and lateral views but is usually seen better on oblique radiographs, which truly outline La Chapele's "Scotty dog" (Rothman & Simeone, 1992).

VERTEBRAL COMPRESSION FRACTURE

Vertebral compression fractures are most consistent with osteoporosis in women over age 65 and men over age 75 with decreased bone mass. Osteoporosis in itself has no signs and symptoms and may progress silently for years until an ominous compression fracture leads to pain and disability. The patient may have pain and a tender point at the level of fracture and may splint the back to avoid mobility at the fracture site. Plain films may reveal the fracture or a decrease in vertebral height. Bone mineral densitometry can be used to diagnose osteoporosis by calculating the patient's bone mineral density and comparing it to the normal bone density for age (see Chap. 48).

FACET SYNDROME (ARTHROPATHY)

Arthropathy of the facet joints may be difficult to diagnose. Patients may have LBP with or without radiation to the buttocks. Hyperextension may precipitate facet impingement and exacerbate symptoms (Hainline, 1995). The physical exam may be unremarkable except for pain on extension of the trunk. SLR and the neurologic exam are usually unremarkable. A plain radiograph may or may not demonstrate changes at the facet joints. MRI demonstrates degenerative changes at the intervertebral discs and at the facet joints.

PIRIFORMIS SYNDROME

Piriformis syndrome has become a common diagnosis, especially when it relates to buttock pain without LBP symptoms. The piriformis muscle is an external rotator of the hip. It traverses over the sciatic notch and inserts on the greater trochanter of the femur. Piriformis syndrome is common in athletes, persons who excessively abduct the hip or overuse the muscles of the buttock, and persons who have excessive compression over the sciatic notch (eg, sitting on an overstuffed wallet). The physical exam may reveal tenderness over the sciatic notch, pain with forced internal rotation of the hip, and pain and weakness with simultaneous abduction and external rotation of the hip. The neurologic exam is normal (Hainline, 1995), as are plain radiographs.

SACROILIAC SPRAIN

The sacroiliac (SI) joints are often overlooked as an etiology for LBP. There is controversy as to whether the sacroiliac joints can be sprained, because they are among the strongest joints in the body. True subtle motion at this joint may predispose a person to injury of this joint. Clinically, the patient may present with pain at the sacroiliac joint. This SI pain should be differentiated from that of piriformis syndrome or other pathology, which may be referred to the groin and posterior thigh. Pain may increase when the patient lies on the affected side

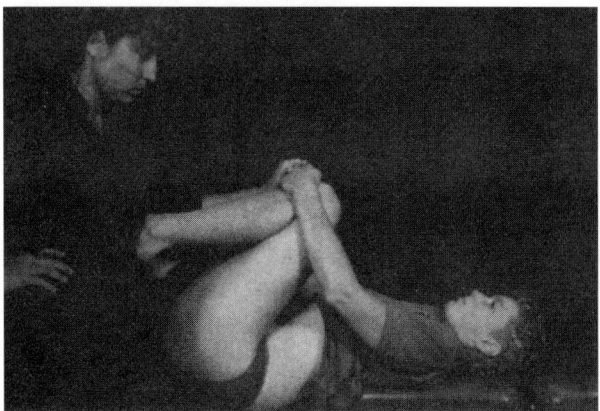

FIGURE 46-4 Gaenslin's test. (Palmer, M.L. and Epler, M.E. [1998]. *Fundamentals of musculoskeletal assessment techniques, 2/e.* Philadelphia: Lippincott-Raven Publishers.)

(LeBlanc, 1992). There are several provocative tests, including Gaenslen's extension test (Fig. 46-4), the Patrick/Fabere test (Fig. 46-5), and the sacroiliac compression test. Unlike patients with sciatica and piriformis syndrome, there is no tenderness at the sciatic notch. Plain radiographs may or may not show changes at the sacroiliac joint; nevertheless, they are valuable in ruling out other potential diagnoses (eg, fracture, malignancy, infection, ankylosing spondylitis).

Degenerative Disorders: Osteoarthritis

Osteoarthritis is the most common degenerative disorder. Degeneration of the articular cartilage involving both the facet joints (as previously described) and vertebral columns occurs. It is easily diagnosed by correlation of symptoms and plain x-ray findings. Other possibilities that cause back pain must still be considered before making a diagnosis.

Systemic Disorders

INFLAMMATORY DISEASES

The seronegative arthropathies, rheumatoid arthritis, ankylosing spondylitis, psoriatic arthritis, Reiter's syndrome, and arthritis associated with inflammatory bowel disease are a few

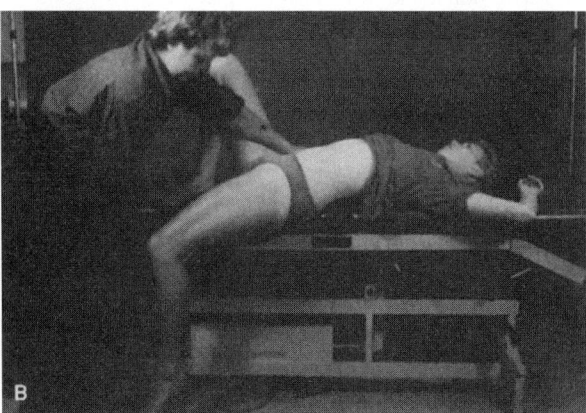

FIGURE 46-5 Patrick/Fabere test—lower limb of the unsupported side is lowered over the side of the table. Pain upon execution of this maneuver indicates pathology in the area of the sacroiliac joint. (Palmer, M.L. and Epler, M.E. [1998]. *Fundamentals of musculoskeletal assessment techniques, 2/e.* Philadelphia: Lippincott-Raven Publishers.)

of the inflammatory arthropathies that may lead to LBP. The diagnosis is made usually after the failure of other diagnoses. The workup includes laboratory tests specific for each disorder (see the diagnostic studies section below).

MALIGNANCY

Malignancies are most often the result of metastatic carcinoma from the breast, lung, or prostate. They may include, however, multiple myeloma, lymphoma, leukemia, and primary spinal cord or extradural tumors (Wheeler, 1995; Wipf & Deyo, 1995).

INFECTION

Sepsis leading to discitis, sacroiliitis, vertebral osteomyelitis, and epidural abscess must be suspected in patients with fever and LBP. Tuberculosis (Pott's disease) also may infect the spine.

Other LBP Etiologies

Other etiologies of LBP include:

- Gastrointestinal disorders
- Hip pathology
- Psychosocial causes
- Seeking disability
- Drug seeking
- Abdominal aortic aneurysm
- Genitourinary Disorders (eg, renal stones)
- Gynecologic disorders (eg, pelvic inflammatory disease)
- Neurologic syndrome: myelopathy
- Neuropathy
- Myopathy.

HISTORY AND PHYSICAL EXAM

The history plays a major role in the evaluation of the back pain sufferer. In most cases, the diagnosis can be made by a thorough history. The history is of utmost importance to rule out organic, nonmechanical causes. The following questions may be helpful in ruling out organic causes (Margo, 1994):

- Is the pain worse at rest?
- Are there significant associated symptoms, such as weight loss or fever?
- Is the pain associated with urinary incontinence or retention and caudal anesthesia?
- Is the pain so severe that it causes writhing?
- In the elderly patient, is the onset of pain new?

If causes such as infection, tumor, or the cauda equina syndrome are ruled out, attention should be focused on mechanical causes.

The rest of the history should focus on the pain:

- What is the quality of pain?
- What is the location of pain?
- Is the pain referred?
- Are there radicular components to the pain?
- What (if anything) relieves the pain? (eg, sitting in the flexed position worsens discogenic pain but may relieve the pain of spinal stenosis.)
- Does the pain radiate? If so, does it follow a dermatomal pattern?

- How did the pain start? Was there trauma or a specific injury, or a cumulative effect (eg, frequent lifting of small loads or twisting in an awkward position)? Knowing the cause of the pain also helps with the prognosis.
- Was the cause occupational or recreational? This may aid in determining the degree of disability and the prognosis.

Risk factors for LBP are listed in Table 46-3.

A history of worsening pain or radiating pain with coughing, sneezing, or the Valsalva maneuver may point toward a discogenic origin. These maneuvers increase intra-abdominal pressure and lead to increased disc pressure.

It is important to assess the severity of pain and the impact on daily function. This will guide the treatment plan and assessment for improvement of functional status.

In the older adult, osteoporotic stress fractures are usually associated with constant pain that is localized and severe. Pain increases with certain movements and activities and is never completely relieved. A radicular component may be secondary to posterior displacement of a bone fragment with impingement on a nerve root or cord (Lazara & Quinet, 1994).

The pain of spinal stenosis is usually associated with worsening pain with walking and standing. The opposite is noted with disc herniations and nerve entrapment. If pain is not relieved at rest (eg, the fetal position), the provider must consider infection, a metastatic process, or a compression fracture.

Leg pain may be true radiculopathy versus referred pain. Radiculopathy is associated with pain that follows a dermatomal pattern, consistent with a specific nerve root, whereas referred pain is nonspecific and achy, is confined to the buttock or posterior thigh, and does not radiate past the knee.

The rest of the history may focus on the medical etiologies. For example, renal stones may be associated with back pain and blood in the urine. Abdominal pathology, such as an abdominal aortic aneurysm or pancreatitis, may present as back pain.

The physical exam is initiated as the patient walks into the office. Observe the gait for the presence of limp or a particular stance. For example, a patient with severe spinal stenosis may assume a "simian stance," with the hips, knees, and back flexed. The patient should be undressed for the physical exam. The provider must be able to observe the back with the patient standing. Inspect to see if the patient is leaning to either side, if the iliac crest heights are equal, if there is paraspinal spasm or muscle atrophy, and if there are abnormal markings or discolorations on the back.

The next part of the physical exam is palpation. Palpate along the paraspinal muscles, spinous processes, lumbo–sacral

TABLE 46-3	**Risk Factors for Low Back Pain**

Increasing age up to age 55
White race
Living in Western states
Smoking
Prolonged driving of a motor vehicle
Hard physical labor (ie, exposure to vibrations or repetitive lifting of >40 lb)
Psychological stress
Job dissatisfaction
Previous episode of low back pain
Osteoporosis (causing vertebral fractures)

Margo, K. (1994). Diagnosis, treatment, and prognosis in patients with low back pain. *American Family Physician 49*(1), 171–184.

transition, sacrum, coccyx, sacroiliac joints, and bilateral buttocks (sciatic notch). Point tenderness on palpation and percussion at the level of involvement may be consistent with a vertebral compression fracture, whereas tenderness or spasm along the paraspinals is nonspecific.

Assessment of range of motion in all planes of motion (eg, flex-extend, lateral side bend) is important in the functional evaluation and in follow-up assessment of improvement. It is also helpful in differentiating the etiology of back pain. For instance, increased pain on flexion is often associated with discogenic back pain, whereas pain in extension is associated with posterior element back pain (eg, facet joints, pars interarticularis stress fractures).

Next, check for the ability to toe walk, as an assessment of gastrocnemius muscle strength (nerve root level, S1, S2), and the ability to heel walk, assessing the tibialis anterior muscle strength (nerve root level L4-5).

The neurologic exam should further consist of sensation to light touch and pin prick of the lower extremities, which must be compared to the contralateral extremity. Abnormal sensation that does not follow a specific dermatome is highly nonspecific. If it follows a specific dermatome pattern, it may be secondary to nerve root entrapment of the corresponding nerve.

The motor exam should be performed with the patient in either a seated or supine position. Any specific weakness or atrophy should be recorded.

The next test is the SLR test (see Fig. 46-3). This test helps in differentiating disc pain from other causes. This test is performed preferably in both the seated and supine positions, which may help rule out a malingering patient. In both cases, the knee is kept in full extension while the hip is passively flexed. This tests specifically for L5, S1 nerve root entrapment and sciatica. The SLR test is positive if the patient's radicular symptoms (numbness, tingling down the affected leg) are reproduced. It is negative if only LBP or pain consistent with hamstring tightness is reproduced. The crossed or contralateral SLR test is highly specific for disc pathology. A LeSeague maneuver (see Fig. 46-3B) is specific for sciatic nerve involvement. Sensitivity to palpation over the sciatic notch may also lead to a diagnosis of sciatica; however, the piriformis syndrome or sacroiliac pathology must also be considered.

A thorough hip exam must also be performed to rule out hip pathology. The hip exam should include inspection and palpation and range of motion in all planes (flexion, extension, abduction, adduction, and internal and external rotation). Look for pain as well as restrictions in motion. Always compare to the contralateral side.

The Patrick/Fabere test is another provocative test to differentiate sacroiliac pathology from hip pathology. Evaluate the hip with the patient lying supine on the examining table. Have the patient place the foot on the involved side on the opposite knee. The hip joint is now flexed, abducted, and externally rotated. In this position, inguinal pain is a general indication that there is pathology in the hip or the surrounding muscles. To stress the sacroiliac joint, extend the range of motion by placing one hand on the flexed knee joint and the other hand on the anterior superior iliac spine of the opposite side. Pressing down on each of these points places stress on the sacroiliac joint, and pain may be an indicator of sacroiliac pathology. Gaenslen's test is another provocative test to evaluate for sacroiliac pathology; it involves stressing the sacroiliac joint with extension of the ipsilateral hip in the supine position (Fig. 46-4) (Hoppenfeld, 1976) (Fig. 46-5).

DIAGNOSTIC STUDIES

Laboratory Testing

Laboratory testing usually produces a low yield and should be used only if clinically indicated. If infection is suspected, a complete blood count should be ordered. A chemistry panel may be useful to rule out underlying renal or hepatic disorders or crystalline arthropathy. The erythrocyte sedimentation rate and levels of C-reactive protein may initially be abnormal with tumor, infection, or other inflammatory processes, but they would be normal in most other causes of back pain. An elevated alkaline phosphatase level may indicate abnormal bone turnover, as in Paget's disease or osteoporosis. If an occult compression fracture is diagnosed, ruling out bone malignancy such as multiple myeloma with a serum protein electrophoresis is warranted. Other studies, such as a protein specific antigen level to rule out prostate cancer, should be ordered if clinically warranted.

Radiographic Evaluation

Plain x-rays of the lumbar spine generally have a low yield, especially early in the course of LBP. However, in older patients with LBP, or in patients with chronic LBP, x-rays are often required (Al-Magdassy, 1996), especially if trauma, infection, malignancy, or a metabolic disorder is suspected. X-rays may reveal lytic or blastic lesions, fractures, degenerative joint disease, facet arthropathy, degenerative disc disease, or dislocation/subluxation (spondylolisthesis). In younger patients, the yield is extremely low, but x-rays may be necessary if the pain is chronic and fracture is suspected.

Bone scans may be useful, especially if malignancy is suspected. They may also be abnormal in metabolic bone disease, ankylosing spondylitis, or severe degenerative joint disease of the spine.

An initial episode of back pain present for less than 7 weeks, with either no treatment or improvement with treatment, does not require x-rays (Glimer et al, 1993). The following are exceptions to this rule:

- Age over 65
- History of high risk for osteoporosis
- Symptoms of urinary tract dysfunction
- Pain that worsens despite adequate treatment
- Intense pain at rest
- Pain worse at night
- Fever or chills
- Unexplained weight loss
- History of injury of sufficient violence or force
- History of repetitive stress or increased risk of stress fracture
- Recurrent back pain with no x-rays in 2 years or more
- Prior lumbar surgery or fracture
- History of radiographic abnormality
- Anticipation of need for another study or treatment that would be facilitated by preliminary x-rays (eg, epidural injection)

- Patient who cannot give a reliable history
- Atypical physical findings (eg, significant motor deficit or unexplained deformity).

These are only guidelines; good clinical judgment must be used in each case.

When x-rays are deemed necessary, five views of the lumbar spine should be obtained:

- Anteroposterior and lateral
- Spot view
- Lumbosacral level
- Right oblique
- Left oblique.

Other Imaging Techniques

CT scan, MRI, and myelography should be performed only after conservative management has failed and if the results will change the course of treatment (eg, surgery).

MRI is becoming the optimal imaging modality because it provides the maximum amount of information when evaluating patients with suspected spinal disorders. MRI produces superb delineation of soft-tissue structures and excellent characterization of medullary bone, it allows direct multiplanar imaging, and it does not involve radiation exposure (Nachemson, 1993). MRI is readily available in most of the United States. It is noninvasive, is risk- and pain-free for most people, and requires no special preparation. In degenerative disease, MRI provides an abundance of information about the intervertebral discs, facet joints, and end plates. When nuclear material is displaced, MRI can differentiate among a contained, noncontained, or sequestrated disc herniation (Nachemson, 1993). In spinal stenosis, MRI permits the evaluation of true sagittal dimensions and cross-sectional areas. MRI is also the optimal exam to detect primary and metastatic neoplasms in the spinal column, cord, or paravertebral soft tissues. It is also an excellent tool in diagnosing spinal infection. The use of MRI with gadolinium contrast is preferable after surgery.

Criticisms of MRI include its cost and its false-positive yields, which lead to unnecessary surgery and treatments. However, MRI lends considerable importance to information gained from other tests and complements the provider's clinical judgment. It is hoped that ongoing research and technology development will reduce the cost of MRI.

Bone scans (radionuclide scintigraphy) are useful in identifying bone tumors and infections (Lazara & Quinet, 1994). Bone scans are more useful than MRI in poorly defined tumors or infections. If the location is not well defined, the MRI is limited to one region and may miss abnormalities that may be picked up by a radionuclide scan.

CT scan is the test of choice for showing bony abnormalities, such as bone destruction from malignancy or infection. It can also reveal lesions of discs and other soft tissues but is not as sensitive or specific for this as MRI.

CT myelography in general has been replaced by MRI. It is still used, however, for presurgical evaluation and for definition of the level of nerve root compression and extent of herniation. It may also be used to evaluate for a tumor or spinal abscess that may be mistaken for a disc.

Discography is a specialized testing method that may help in evaluating disc disease and identifying patients who may benefit from spinal fusion (Jenner & Barry, 1995). It is a time-tested procedure used for pain provocation. Typically, a small needle is placed within the three lower lumbar discs, and each is separately injected with contrast. The test has two parts. The first is a subjective evaluation of familiar pain provocation. If pain is initiated, it can also be alleviated by lidocaine administration into the disc. The second part is an objective evaluation for degeneration of the annulus or a complete annular tear (radial tear). Both plain films and CT scan are obtained. The indications for discography are three: to assess a single degenerative lumbar disc on MRI or CT, to determine the number of levels to include in a posterior lumbar fusion, and to evaluate failed back syndrome after surgery.

Electromyelography (nerve conduction test) should be performed if there is concern about nerve involvement or when the neurologic exam is equivocal for radiculopathy. It may confirm the presence and level of nerve root involvement and may differentiate the condition from a neuropathy (eg, diabetic neuropathy). Electromyelograms are generally performed by a neurologist or physical medicine and rehabilitation specialist (Wipf & Deyo, 1995).

TREATMENT OPTIONS EXPECTED OUTCOMES, AND COMPREHENSIVE MANAGEMENT

Most patients with LBP can be treated conservatively, and pain will resolve spontaneously in 6 to 8 weeks. Surgery is undertaken only when conservative management has failed, when progressive pain cannot be relieved with conservative treatment, and when neurologic deficits progress in quality and severity.

The treatment of LBP can be outlined in algorithmic form. Figure 46-6 provides a general overview of diagnostic and treatment considerations when caring for the patient with LBP. It is also important to recognize extraneous factors, such as patient motivation, psychological factors, litigation, and hope for secondary gain, that may affect treatment outcomes of what is essentially a benign condition. (Sihorsh, 1996).

The goals of treating back pain should be the same for every patient:

- Relief of pain
- Increased strength
- Increased motion
- Increased endurance
- Return to preinjury functional status.

The initial treatment of bed rest remains controversial. Multiple studies have shown that bed rest for 2 to 3 days has the same or greater benefit than longer periods of rest and that shorter bed rest leads to an earlier return to functional activity, whether work or other physical activities (Wipf & Deyo, 1995; Chilton & Nisenfeld, 1993; Jenner & Barry, 1995). Further disadvantages of prolonged bed rest include rapid muscle atrophy, deconditioning, and an increased risk of thrombophlebitis. Also, musculoskeletal problems may benefit from motion and early mobilization, further supporting limited bed rest (Margo, 1994).

Medications

Medications continue to be a mainstay in the treatment of LBP, along with physical therapy, exercise, and mobilization. Low doses of narcotics such as propoxyphene may be used for short periods in the initial phases of acute LBP. Nonsteroidal anti-inflammatory agents are useful in the acute relief of pain as well as pain management for chronic sufferers. There are many of these agents. Their efficacy may be based on trial and error, and the provider must always consider the risk of side effects. Dosage and choice of agent are based on these factors. Aspirin and acetaminophen are effective agents for acute LBP as well.

Muscle relaxants have no proven efficacy in the treatment of LBP. Sporadically, however, they may be used for their sedative side effects, especially at night. A bedtime dose is often sufficient. As with narcotics, there is a risk of dependency over a long period, so only a short course, such as 1 week, should be prescribed (Margo, 1994).

For chronic LBP, low doses of tricyclic antidepressants such as imipramine have proven effective in some cases. There have been no definitive studies to support the use of these drugs in the treatment of LBP, however. As with muscle relaxants, they have a sedative side effect that may allow a patient to sleep, especially at night (Turner & Denny, 1993).

Injection Therapy

Injections may include trigger point injection, facet joint injection, and epidurals. Any provider can be trained in injection therapy, but most injections are done by physiatrists (providers trained in physical and musculoskeletal medicine) or anesthesiologists trained in pain management. Pain management centers staffed by these specialists have been established recently, and often patients are referred to these centers after conservative treatment has failed.

Trigger point injections with a local anesthetic such as lidocaine, with or without steroids, have no real proven benefit, but anecdotally they are effective in many patients. These injections remain controversial (Margo, 1994). This also holds true for facet joint injections: although widely used, they are costly (because of the equipment and time needed) and are of little value when compared with saline injections (Wipf & Deyo, 1995).

Epidural injections have shown moderate effects in some studies. They have been shown to be effective in LBP that is associated with sciatica and lower limb symptoms. Anecdotally, they appear to be effective in random patients, with no specificity toward a certain personality or psychological type (Wipf & Deyo, 1995).

Physical Therapy and Exercise

Physical therapy combines therapeutic exercises, mobilization, and other physical modalities. It may also include education in proper body mechanics, lifting techniques, and preventive measures. This mode of treatment requires the patient to become an active participant in self-care rather than a passive recipient of treatment (Wheelor & Hanley, 1995).

The modalities used in physical therapy include:

- Heat and cold therapy for symptomatic relief of pain by reducing spasm
- Ultrasound
- Phonophoresis
- Iontophoresis
- Electric stimulation
- Therapeutic exercise.

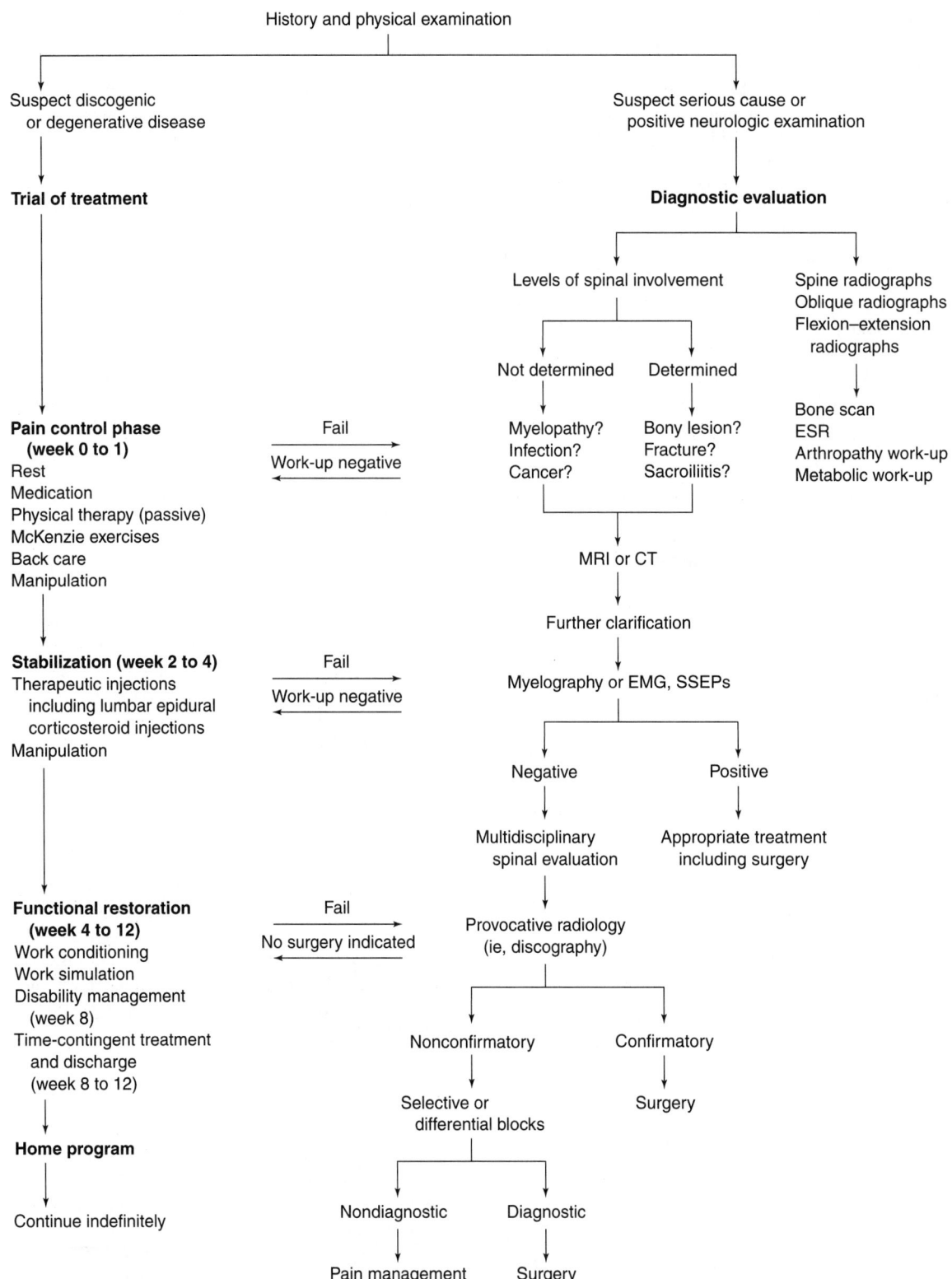

FIGURE 46-6 Algorithm for management of low-back pain and sciatica. ESR - erythocyte sedimentation rate; MRI - magnetic resonance imaging; CT - Computed tomography; EMG - electromyography; SSEPs - somatosensory evoked potentials.

Although extensive scientific data on all these modalities are not available, anecdotally and in theory they appear to be effective (Margo, 1994; Drez, 1990).

Patients can be instructed to perform therapeutic exercises on their own, or they may be guided and monitored by a physical therapist. Factors that determine the approach used include the extent of the injury and the patient's disability. A realistic plan should be developed with the patient, because if the exercises are not going to be performed, or if they are performed incorrectly, they will have limited or no benefit.

The exercises most frequently used in the treatment of LBP include William's flexion, McKenzie's extension, and isometric exercises (eg, pelvic tilts). Flexion exercise needs to be avoided in early injury, especially if disc pathology is the cause of LBP, because these exercises may increase intradiscal pressures. They are of great benefit, however, in posterior element disorders,

as well as in acute or chronic muscle spasm. McKenzie extension exercises are usually contraindicated in posterior element disorders (eg, facet arthropathy or spondylolysis) but are an excellent method of strengthening muscles and stabilizing the back element when pain arises from anterior element structures, such as a herniated intervertebral disc. A McKenzie program will lead into a lumbar stabilization program (McKenzie, 1981).

The exercise program is initially used as a treatment modality. After the patient has recovered from the acute episode, a routine maintenance program should be established. The goal is a lifetime of health, not just for the back, but for the whole patient.

Education in appropriate sitting and standing postures is an integral part of the entire treatment plan for the patient with LBP. There are long-term benefits from educating workers about ways to prevent low back injury. "Back schools" initially

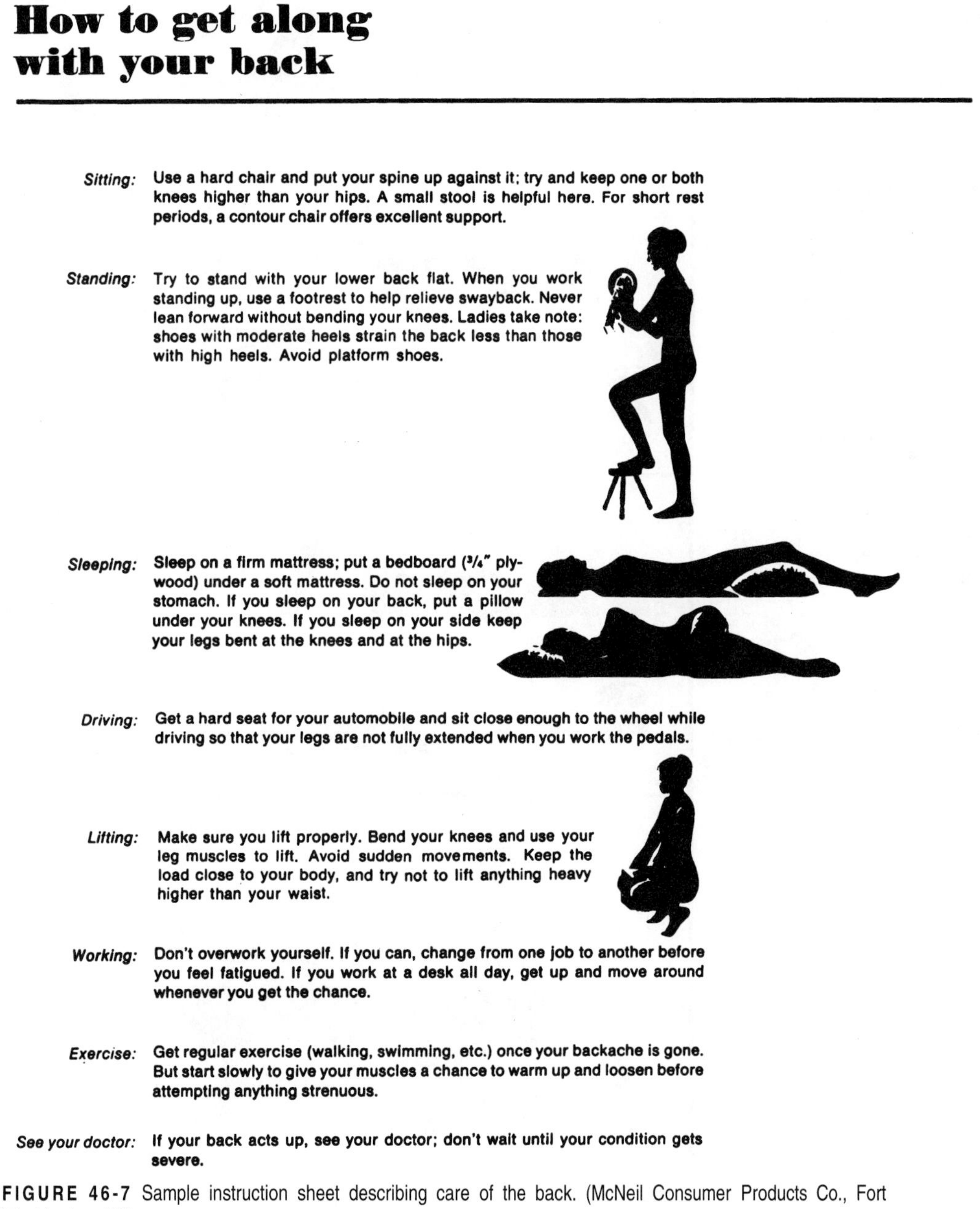

How to get along with your back

Sitting: Use a hard chair and put your spine up against it; try and keep one or both knees higher than your hips. A small stool is helpful here. For short rest periods, a contour chair offers excellent support.

Standing: Try to stand with your lower back flat. When you work standing up, use a footrest to help relieve swayback. Never lean forward without bending your knees. Ladies take note: shoes with moderate heels strain the back less than those with high heels. Avoid platform shoes.

Sleeping: Sleep on a firm mattress; put a bedboard (¾" plywood) under a soft mattress. Do not sleep on your stomach. If you sleep on your back, put a pillow under your knees. If you sleep on your side keep your legs bent at the knees and at the hips.

Driving: Get a hard seat for your automobile and sit close enough to the wheel while driving so that your legs are not fully extended when you work the pedals.

Lifting: Make sure you lift properly. Bend your knees and use your leg muscles to lift. Avoid sudden movements. Keep the load close to your body, and try not to lift anything heavy higher than your waist.

Working: Don't overwork yourself. If you can, change from one job to another before you feel fatigued. If you work at a desk all day, get up and move around whenever you get the chance.

Exercise: Get regular exercise (walking, swimming, etc.) once your backache is gone. But start slowly to give your muscles a chance to warm up and loosen before attempting anything strenuous.

See your doctor: If your back acts up, see your doctor; don't wait until your condition gets severe.

FIGURE 46-7 Sample instruction sheet describing care of the back. (McNeil Consumer Products Co., Fort Washington, PA)

developed in Sweden are effective in quickly returning the injured industrial worker to normal activities (Jenner & Barry, 1995). This model involves intensive physical, psychological, and behavioral reconditioning (Wheelor & Hanley, 1995). Part of the education process includes teaching patients proper terminology. For example, terms such as "backache," "mild strain," or "sprain" may reduce the patient's fear and the psychological factors that may increase disability and their recovery time, whereas the term "bulging disc" or "degenerative disc" may frighten the patient and have the reverse effect. The last important factor in education is lifestyle changes: people who are sedentary or obese and smokers are at increased risk for back pain.

Teaching and Self-Care

In general, LBP resolves within the first 6 to 8 weeks, regardless of treatment. For the vast majority of patients, LBP can be treated with conservative management. An exercise program

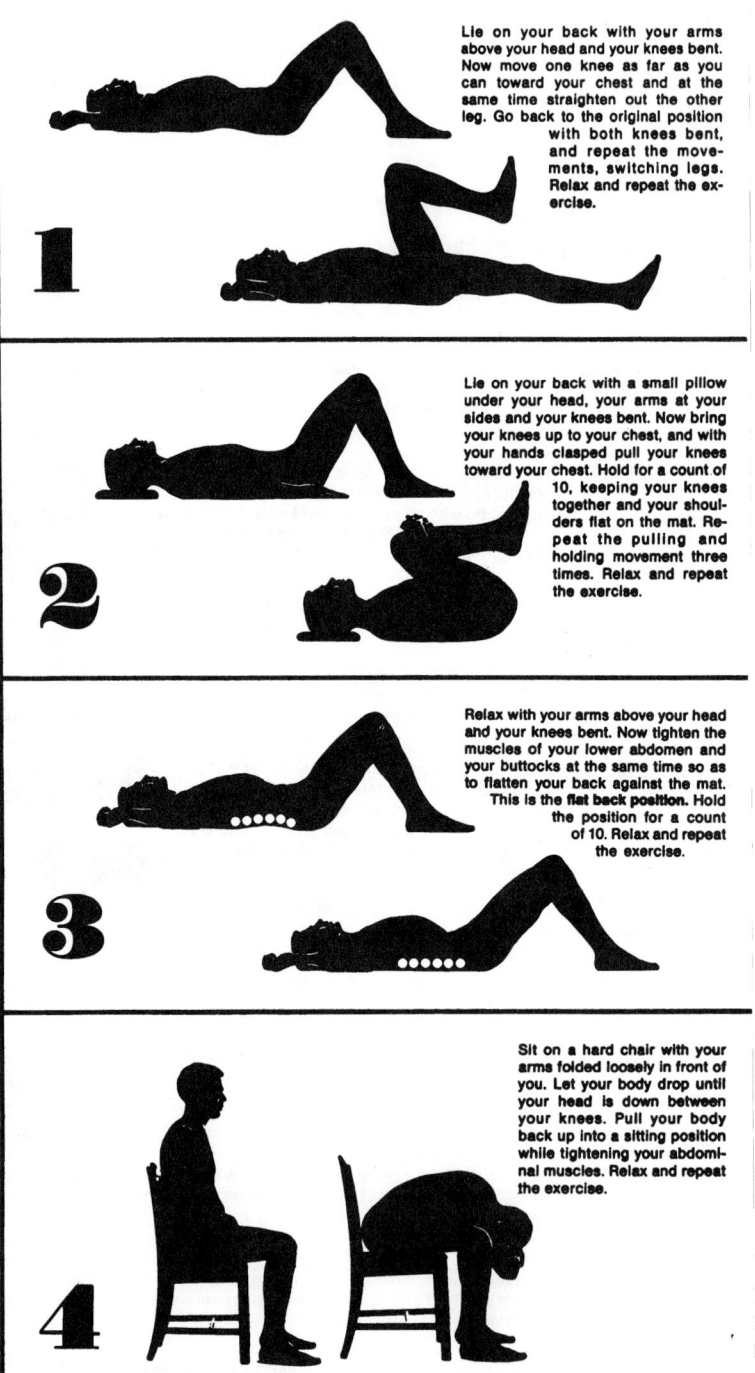

Exercises for low back pain

General Information:

Don't overdo exercising, especially in the beginning. Start by trying the movements slowly and carefully. Don't be alarmed if the exercises cause some mild discomfort which lasts a few minutes. But if pain is more than mild and lasts more than 15 or 20 minutes, *stop* and do no further exercises until you see your doctor.

Do the exercises on a hard surface covered with a thin mat or heavy blanket. Put a pillow under your neck if it makes you more comfortable. Always start your exercises slowly—and in the order marked—to allow muscles to loosen up gradually. Heat treatments just before you start can help relax tight muscles. Follow the instructions carefully; it will be well worth the effort.

Do exercises marked (X)

in numerical order

for _____ minutes

_____ times a day.

Take the medication

prescribed for you

_____ times daily

for_____.

1 Lie on your back with your arms above your head and your knees bent. Now move one knee as far as you can toward your chest and at the same time straighten out the other leg. Go back to the original position with both knees bent, and repeat the movements, switching legs. Relax and repeat the exercise.

2 Lie on your back with a small pillow under your head, your arms at your sides and your knees bent. Now bring your knees up to your chest, and with your hands clasped pull your knees toward your chest. Hold for a count of 10, keeping your knees together and your shoulders flat on the mat. Repeat the pulling and holding movement three times. Relax and repeat the exercise.

3 Relax with your arms above your head and your knees bent. Now tighten the muscles of your lower abdomen and your buttocks at the same time so as to flatten your back against the mat. This is the flat back position. Hold the position for a count of 10. Relax and repeat the exercise.

4 Sit on a hard chair with your arms folded loosely in front of you. Let your body drop until your head is down between your knees. Pull your body back up into a sitting position while tightening your abdominal muscles. Relax and repeat the exercise.

FIGURE 46-8 Sample instruction sheet describing exercises for low back pain. (McNeil Consumer Products Co., Fort Washington, PA)

and education in body mechanics, lifting, and preventive measures are self-care essentials for patients with LBP. Anatomic, biomechanical, and psychological factors must all be considered in working with patients to develop a comprehensive and realistic treatment and management plan aimed at returning them to and maintaining them at their optimal level of functioning. Figures 46-7 and 46-8 provide sample instructions for providers to use with their patients.

Exercise for LBP sufferers usually involves a combination of William's flexion exercises and an extension exercise program. The idea is to strengthen anterior supporting structures such as the abdominal muscles and posterior supporting structures such as the erector spinae muscles. Flexibility and range of motion exercises are incorporated into the program to increase range of motion.

Complementary Approaches

Spinal manipulation, associated by most lay people with chiropractic medicine, has evolved into a standard of treatment for selected cases of LBP. Manipulation was actually first proposed by osteopathic physicians as early as 1874. In addition, some allopathic providers as well as physical therapists use manipulative techniques (Margo, 1994). The communication between these disciplines has improved over the last two decades, and in general manipulation is becoming more accepted as a treatment.

Controversy as to the frequency and duration of spinal manipulation remains. The only agreement found in the literature relates to what constitutes an appropriate trial of manipulative therapy: the conclusion is that 12 manipulations lasting up to 1 month is appropriate. There are studies underway to define conditions for which spinal manipulation is appropriate, the optimal duration of treatment, and the relative effectiveness and cost-effectiveness of manipulation compared to other treatments (Shekelle, 1994).

Other alternative therapies that have proven to be effective for selected patients include the VAX-D therapeutic table, which lowers the pressure in the nucleus pulposus of herniated discs (Ramos & Martin, 1994). However, studies are limited, and this modality needs to be compared to others, such as pelvic traction. Less well-studied treatments for LBP are massage therapy, Rolfing, Feldenkreitz, acupuncture, and neural therapy. These are not fully understood but have benefited selected groups of patients.

COMMUNITY RESOURCES

- LBP (Eyckle's Physiotherapy), http://home.hkstar.com/eyckle/lbp.html: Common causes, signs and symptoms, diagnosis, treatment
- The Virtual Hospital, http://www.vh.org/Beyond/PeerReviews/30BackPain.html: Links to sites containing information on LBP
- LBP Problems, http://www.pe.net/sawshy/lbp.htm: Pain causation, arthritis, disc surgery, spine surgery
- National Chronic Pain Outreach Association, Inc., 7979 Old Georgetown Rd., Ste. 100, Bethesda, MD 20814-2429, 301-652-4948

- American Chronic Pain Association, P.O. Box 850, Rocklin, CA 95677, 916-632-0922, 916-632-3280
- International Association for the Study of Pain, 909 NE 43d St., Ste. 306, Seattle, WA 98105-6020, 206-547-6409, 206-547-1703
- American Pain Society, P.O. Box 468, Des Plaines, IL 60016-0468, 708-966-5595
- The American Back Pain Association, P.O. Box 135, Pasadena, MD 21122-0135, 410-255-3633

CLINICAL WARNINGS AND REFERRAL POINTS

Patients with persistent, progressive, or severe neurologic deficits should be referred for neurologic and surgical evaluation. Bowel or bladder dysfunction, saddle anesthesia, and bilateral leg weakness and numbness are clinical warnings suggestive of the compression that may occur secondary to central disc herniation, known as cauda equina syndrome. This syndrome is considered a surgical emergency and requires immediate referral.

■ ■ ■ ▫ **CLINICAL PEARLS**

In patients with lower extremity pain, think "back."

- Sitting and flexing the back worsen disc pain but may relieve pain in spinal stenosis. In spinal stenosis, pain may worsen with walking and standing.
- Increased pain on flexion is associated with discogenic back pain, whereas pain on extension is associated with posterior element pain.
- If pain is not relieved at rest, infection, a metastatic process, or a compression fracture must be considered.
- Flexion exercise needs to be avoided in early injury, especially if disc pathology is the cause of LBP, because these exercises may increase intradiscal pressure.

EDITOR'S NOTE:
COMPLEMENTARY APPROACHES

A general discussion of complementary approaches can be found in Chapter 3. The following, while not an exhaustive list, are some complementary approaches being used for this condition. Additional information on these approaches, including precautions, can be found in Appendices A and B. Providers need to assess for the use of complementary approaches as part of the patient's history, as they may impact conventional therapies, and patients may not volunteer this information unless specifically asked. Efficacy of many complementary approaches is not as well documented as that of conventional therapies. Providers need to read the literature before suggesting these complementary approaches.

- Complementary Modalities
  Acupuncture
  Aromatherapy
  Biofeedback
  Craniosacral therapy
  Chiropractic
  Massage therapy

References

Al-Magdassy, E.G. (1996). The role of plain radiography in the diagnosis of low back pain. *Journal of Neurologic & Orthopedic Medicine & Surgery, 16,* 222–226.

Beattie, P. (1996). The relationship between symptoms and abnormal magnetic resonance images of lumbar intervertebral discs. *Physical Therapy, 76*(6), 601–608.

Borenstein, D., Wiesel, S., & Boden, S. (1995). *Low back pain: Medical diagnosis and comprehensive management,* 2d ed. Philadelphia: W.B. Saunders.

Brady, M. (1996). Low back pain. *Annals of Emergency Medicine, 27*(4), 454–456.

Chilton, M., & Nisenfeld, M. (1993). Nonoperative treatment of low back injury in athletes. *Clinics in Sports Medicine, 12*(3), 547–555.

Cyriax, J. (1991). *Textbook of orthopaedic medicine,* 8th ed. London: Balliere Tindall.

Daltroy, L., & Iverson, M. (1997). A controlled trial of an educational program to prevent low back injuries. *N Engl J Med, 337*(5), 322–328.

Drez, D. (1990). *Therapeutic modalities in sports injuries.* Chicago: Year Book Medical.

Frymoyer, J., Nelson R., Strangford, E., & Waddell, G. (1991). Clinical tests applicable to the study of chronic lower back disability. *Spine, 16*(6), 681–682.

Glimer, H., Papdopolos, S., & Tuite, G. (1993). Lumbar disk disease: Pathophysiology, management, and prevention. *American Family Physician, 47*(5), 1141–1152.

Hainline, B. (1995). Low back injury. *Clinics in Sports Medicine, 14*(1), 241–265.

Hoppenfeld, S. (1976). *Physical examination of the spine and extremities.* New York: Appleton-Century-Crofts.

Jenner, J., & Barry, M. (1995). Low back pain. *British Medical Journal, 310*(6984), 929–932.

Lazara, L., & Quinet, R. (1994). Low back pain: How to make the diagnosis in the older patient. *Geriatrics, 49*(9), 48–53.

LeBlanc, K. (1992). Sacroiliac sprain: An overlooked cause of back pain. *American Family Physician, 46*(5), 1459–1463.

Margo, K. (1994). Diagnosis, treatment and prognosis in patients with low back pain. *American Family Physician, 49*(1), 171–184.

McKenzie, R. (1981). *The lumbar spine: Mechanical diagnosis and therapy.* Waikanae, N.Z.: Spinal Publications.

Nachemson, A. (1993). Lumbar disc herniation: Conclusions. *Acta Orthopaedica Scandinavica, 251*(Suppl), 49–50.

Ramos, G., & Martin, W. (1994). Effects of vertebral axial decompression on intradiscal pressure. *Journal of Neurosurgery, 81*(3), 350–353.

Rothman, R., & Simeone, F. (1992). *The Spine,* 3d ed. Philadelphia: W.B. Saunders.

Saal, J. (1995). The role of inflammation in lumbar pain. *Spine, 20*(16), 1821–1827.

Shekelle, P. (1994). Spinal manipulation. *Spine, 19*(7), 858–861.

Shorsh, J.M. (1996). Psychological aspects of chronic low back pain. *Australia J Surg, 66*: 294–297.

Turner, J., & Denny, M. (1993). Do antidepressant medications relieve chronic low back pain? *Journal of Family Practice, 37*(6), 545–553.

Wheeler, A. (1995). Diagnosis and management of low back pain and sciatica. *American Family Physician, 52*(5), 1333–1343.

Wheelor, A., & Hanley, E. (1995). Nonoperative treatment for low back pain: Rest to restoration. *Spine, 20*(3), 375–378.

Wipf, J., & Deyo, R. (1995). Low back pain. *Medical Clinics of North America, 79*(2), 231–243.

Suggested Reading List

Cailliet, R. (1995). *Low back syndrome,* 5th ed. Philadelphia: F.A. Davis.

Cavanaugh, J. (1995). Neural mechanism of lumbar pain. *Spine, 20*(16), 1804–1809.

Deyo, R. (1993).Back pain revisited: Newer thinking on diagnosis and therapy. *Consultant, 33*(2), 88–100.

Escalante, A. (1993). Ankylosing spondylitis: A common cause of low back pain. *Postgraduate Medicine, 94*(1), 153–161.

Frank, A. (1993). Low back pain. *British Medical Journal, 306*(6882), 901–909.

Herzog, R., Guyer, R., & Graham-Smith, A. (1995). Magnetic resonance imaging: Use in patients with low back pain or radicular pain. *Spine, 20*(16), 1834–1838.

Jensen, M., Brant-Zawadski, M., Obuchowski, N., Modic, M., Malkasion, D., & Ross, J. (1994). Magnetic resonance imaging of the lumbar spine in people without back pain. *N Engl J Med, 331*(2), 69–73.

Keim, H,, & Kirkaldy-Willis, W.H. (1987). *Low back pain.* Clinical Symposium, CIBA Gergy.

Kopec, J., & Esdaile, J. (1995). Spine update: Functional disability scales for back pain. *Spine, 20*(17), 1943–1949.

Kummel, B. (1996). Nonorganic signs of significance in low back pain. *Spine, 21*(9), 1077–1081.

Payne, W., & Ogilvie, J. (1996). Back pain in children and adolescents. *Pediatric Clinics of North America, 43*(4), 899–917.

Porter, R. (1996). Spinal stenosis and neurogenic claudication. *Spine, 21*(17), 2046–2052.

Sikorski, J., Stampfer, H., Cole, R., & Wheatley, A. (1996). Psychological aspects of chronic low back pain. *Australian & New Zealand Journal of Surgery, 66*(5), 294–297.

Simmons, E., Guyer, R., Graham-Smith, A., & Herzog, R. (1995). Radiographic assessment for patients with low back pain. *Spine, 20*(16), 1839–1841.

Twomey, L., & Taylor, J. (1994). Spine update: Exercise and spinal manipulation in the treatment of low back pain. *Spine, 20*(5), 615–619.

Waddell, G. (1991). Occupational low back pain, illness, behavior and disability. *Spine, 16*(6), 683–685.

CHAPTER
47

Osteoarthritis

Dennis A. Cardone, DO, and Alfred F. Tallia, MD, MPH

Osteoarthritis (OA) is a clinical condition of diarthroidal joints characterized by pain, stiffness, and structural alteration. Underlying this condition are destruction and abnormal repair of articular cartilage, followed by deposition of new bone and cartilage at the margins of the joint. The process may lead to joint deformity, decreased range of motion, and in later stages severe functional impairment. Although all diarthroidal joints may be affected, OA is most commonly seen in hand, hip, and knee joints.

Primary care providers are at the front line of diagnosing and treating OA. The national ambulatory medical care survey reveals that problems of the musculoskeletal system are one of the most frequent reasons for office visits. With proper attention to details of diagnosis, treatment, and outcomes, the primary care provider is best suited to care for patients with OA and to coordinate the use of other specialists.

The pain of OA is characteristically worsened with activity and relieved by rest. Conversely, the stiffness associated with OA is worse after rest of the affected joint and better with motion. The bony structural alteration of joints associated with OA and seen in radiographic studies may or may not be associated with pain or stiffness. Hence, the diagnosis of OA is clinically based on more than just the radiologic features of a joint.

OA is classified as either primary/idiopathic (without a discernible explanatory event such as joint trauma) or secondary (to a specific insult to the joint). OA may affect one or more joints simultaneously. Although OA is not characterized as a systemic inflammatory illness, recent studies have suggested a local inflammatory component to this protean condition (Smith et al, 1997).

ANATOMY, PHYSIOLOGY, AND PATHOLOGY

Three types of joints exist within the body: diarthroidal or synovium-lined joints, which are involved in the movement of limbs; synarthrosis or pseudojoints; and amphiarthroses or cartilaginous joints. OA is a disease strictly of diarthrodial joints. Examples of diarthrodial joints are the knee, hip, and joints of the hands. The bony articular prominences of diarthrodial joints are lined by articular cartilage, which facilitates motion at the joint. The biochemical composition of adult cartilage is roughly 70% water and 30% solids. Current understanding of the pathophysiology of OA suggests that articular cartilage trauma, possibly complicated by normal aging, results in alteration of the water/solid ratio. An inflammatory process involving a variety of biochemically initiated cellular events leads to cartilage breakdown. Further joint response leads to changes in bone, resulting in osteophyte formation and bone reconstruction. The exact role that aging plays in OA is uncertain.

Joint remodeling occurs initially at the edge of the affected joint. Osteophyte formation (new bone at the edge of joints) is thought to be the result of endochondral ossification of existing and new cartilage. The relation between osteophyte formation and the development of clinical symptoms is not known. Osteophytes are often present in radiologic studies of asymptomatic persons and may represent a normal response to a variety of joint stressors. Osteophyte formation and other bone remodeling, however, are generally present in advanced OA.

EPIDEMIOLOGY

OA is thought to result from a complex interplay between a variety of host-specific characteristics, such as immunologic, biomechanical, or bioinflammatory variables, and functional characteristics, such as joint use, environmental trauma, or stresses. OA is the most prevalent joint disease.

Within the past 15 years, the American College of Rheumatology has developed and published criteria for the classification of OA of the knee, hip, and hand (Table 47-1). These criteria have proven helpful in establishing a uniform definition for the diagnosis and the extent to which the condition is present within populations. Efforts to discern the prevalence and incidence of OA in this country and worldwide have been hampered by the lack of such a definition.

Exact data are lacking, but the overall incidence of OA appears to increase with age. Because of the chronicity of the condition, prevalence also increases with age. OA is the most prevalent chronic condition in middle and older adulthood (Verbrugge, 1995). In general, age and gender are the most important risk factors for OA, with the rate for women exceeding that of men at all ages (Hughes & Dunlop, 1995; Verbrugge, 1995).

Death associated with OA is most often a direct result of functional impairment of the joint and resulting injury or immobility. The complications associated with OA, at least in terms of its economic affect, and the overall financial impact of musculoskeletal conditions are both high. Given the aging of the population in the United States, and the resultant increase in the prevalence of OA, the financial impact of this illness can be expected to rise in the next 20 to 30 years. There is a significant earning loss from work disruption in patients with OA less than 65 years old. Specific risk factors associated with OA include:

- Age: Prevalence is directly related to advancing age.
- Obesity: Although the exact mechanism has yet to be described, overweight people have higher rates of OA of

TABLE 47-1	The American College of Rheumatology Criteria for the Classification and Reporting of Osteoarthritis of the Hand, Hip, and Knee

CLASSIFICATION CRITERIA FOR OSTEOARTHRITIS OF THE HAND, TRADITIONAL FORMAT*

Hand pain, aching, or stifness
    and
3 or 4 of the following features:
    Hard tissue enlargement of 2 or more of 10 selected joints
    Hard tissue enlargement of 2 or more DIP joints
    Fewer than 3 swollen MCP joints
    Deformity of at least 1 of 10 selected joints

* The 10 selected joints are the second and third DIP, the second and third proximal interphalangeal, and the first carpometacarpal joints of both hands. This classification method yields a sensitivity of 92% and a specificity of 98%.

CRITERIA FOR CLASSIFICATION OF IDIOPATHIC OSTEOARTHRITIS OF THE KNEE*

Clinical and Laboratory	Clinical and Radiographic	Clinical†

Knee pain + at least 5 of 9:
  Age >50 years
  Stiffness <30 minutes
  Crepitus
  Bony tenderness
  Bony enlargement
  No palpable warmth
  ESR <40 mm/hour
  RF <1:40
  SF OA
	Knee pain + at least 1 of 3:
	  Age >50 years
	  Stiffness <30 minutes
	  Crepitus
	    +
	  Osteophytes
		Knee pain + at least 3 of 6:
		  Age >50 years
		  Stiffness <30 minutes
		  Crepitus
		  Bony tenderness
		  Bony enlargement
		  No palpable warmth

92% sensitive	91% sensitive	75% sensitive
75% specific	86% specific	69% specific

* ESR = erythrocyte sedimentation rate (Westergren); RF = rheumatoid factor; SF OA = synovial fluid signs of OA (clear, viscous, or white blood cell count <2,000/mm³).
† Alternative for the clinical category would be 4 of 6, which is 84% sensitive and 89% specific.
Altman R, Alarcón G, Appelrouth D, et al: The American College of Rheumatology criteria for the classification and reporting of osteoarthritis of the hand. Arthritis Rheum. 33:1601–1610, 1990; Altman R, Alarcón G, Appelrouth D, et al: The American College of Rheumatology criteria for the classification and reporting of osteoarthritis of the hip. Arthritis Rheum 34:505–514, 1991; Altman R, Asch E, Bloch G, et al: Development of criteria for the classification and reporting of osteoarthritis: classification of osteoarthritis of the knee. Arthritis Rheum 29:1039–1049, 1986.

COMBINED CLINICAL (HISTORY, PHYSICAL EXAM, LABORATORY) AND RADIOGRAPHIC CLASSIFICATION CRITERIA FOR OSTEOARTHRITIS OF THE HIP, TRADITIONAL FORMAT*

Hip pain
    and
At least 2 of the following 3 features
    ESR <20 mm/hour
    Radiographic femoral or acetabular osteophytes
    Radiographic joint space narrowing (superior, axial, and/or medial)

* This classification method yields a sensitivity of 89% and a specificity of 91%. ESR = erythrocyte sedimentation rate (Westergren).
Altman, R. et al. (1991). American College of Rheumatology Criteria for the Classification and Reporting of Osteoarthritis in the Hand, Hip and Knee. *Arthritis and Rheumatism 34(5).*

the hips and knees (Felson, 1996). Although this may make biomechanical sense in terms of the increased stress that being overweight may place on these joints, what is less well understood is the increased association between obesity and hand OA. It is suspected but not clinically proven that weight loss may be an opportunity for clinical prevention of OA in later ages.

■ Exercise: Several studies have suggested a link between specific forms of exercise and sports and OA (Lane & Buckwalter, 1993), but none have been conclusive. More recent research has suggested that exercise may have a beneficial effect in the treatment of established OA. Given the multiple beneficial effects of exercise on other aspects of health, recommendations for the curtailment of specific types of exercise to reduce the risks of OA seem unwarranted. More recent studies suggest just the opposite—that exercise in moderate forms may be beneficial in primary prevention.

■ Genetics and family history: The genetic risk for the development of OA is likely to involve multiple genes (Cicuttini & Spector, 1996; Jimenez & Dharmavaram, 1994). Familial tendencies in the development of joint deformities such as Heberden's nodes were first described earlier this decade. Although genetic factors are most likely polygenic, specific gene mutations resulting in changes of joint components that may lead to the development of OA also have been described. For example, a variety of collagen disorders linked to gene defects are thought to be involved in the development of certain forms of OA. As the molecular genetic revolution progresses, more genes will be elucidated as playing a role in this disease. In the interim, more research on the complex interaction between genetics and family history and environment needs to be performed.

- Occupation: Occupation is a risk factor for OA (Creamer & Hochberg, 1997) Work-related activity has been linked to the development of OA of the knee and other joints. This is thought to be the result of repeated minor trauma, exacerbating an already increased risk at a joint predisposed from underlining mechanical factors such as joint deformity or malalignment.
- Trauma: A history of major trauma to the knees is strongly associated with the development of OA. The same is true for injuries to other joints. In general, any injured joint is at risk for the later development of OA.

DIAGNOSTIC CRITERIA

The American Arthritis Association's diagnostic criteria appear in Table 47-1.

HISTORY AND PHYSICAL EXAM

Pain is the most common presenting complaint in OA. The pain is usually localized to the involved joint, but it may be referred. An example of referred pain is cervical OA presenting as pain in the shoulder, or lumbar facet joint OA causing pain in the buttock or hip regions. Early in the course of OA, pain may have a nagging or aching quality that varies in intensity according to the level of activity. Pain usually occurs with activity or motion and is relieved by rest. In early disease, the pain is not severe, but as the disease progresses pain may be present with minimal motion or even at rest.

Stiffness is very common. Early in the disease, it is felt when the patient resumes activity after a period of rest, and later it may become a permanent complaint. Bony swelling and joint deformity, especially of affected knees and interphalangeal joints, are common later in the disease. Muscle wasting, bowing of the legs, and knock knees are also late manifestations. Bony swelling of the interphalangeal joints may make it difficult to perform activities requiring fine motor skills, such as writing, as well as gross motor skills, such as opening jars or grasping objects. Patients complain of loss of function according to the site involved.

The cause of pain in OA may include muscle spasm and fatigue, joint contracture, capsular fibrosis, and in some cases mild to moderate synovitis. Acute inflammatory flares can be related to trauma or crystal-induced synovitis.

On the physical exam, there may be multiple joints involved. The patient's gait should be evaluated for disturbances related to OA of the hip and knees. A limp or stiff-kneed gait may be present. Bony swelling and deformity are usually easily recognized, especially at the interphalangeal joints of the hand and the knees. In the later stages of the disease, muscle wasting may become obvious. During acute flares, there may be signs of inflam-

mation, including erythema, warmth, and swelling. Passive joint motion is restricted and painful, and there may be crepitus or a feeling of crackling as the joint is moved through its range of motion. On palpation, joint tenderness, intra-articular effusions, synovial thickening, and marginal osteophytes may be present. In most cases, there is no joint instability.

Hand

The most commonly affected joints of the hand are the first carpometacarpal joint and the distal and proximal interphalangeal joints. Heberden's nodes are spurs formed at the distal interphalangeal joints. Bouchard's nodes are present at the proximal interphalangeal joints. Deformity or loss of motion tends to be gradual (Fig. 47-1). There is a lateral deviation of the joints involved. Hand OA may progress or remain stable over time. The progression is usually fastest in the distal interphalangeal joints. When the first carpal metacarpal joint is involved, there is tenderness at the site and later a squared appearance of the hand. The trapezioscaphoid joint is also commonly involved. Metacarpophalangeal involvement is rare. Despite the development of bony deformities, function of the hands remains relatively good.

Knee

OA of the knee tends to be gradual in onset. There may be a stiff-kneed gait. Visual inspection may reveal bony swelling or genu varus or genu valgus deformity. Any of the three compartments (medial, lateral, tibiofemoral) or the patellofemoral joints may be involved; most commonly, the medial compartment is affected. Medial compartment OA involves joint line tenderness and a loss of articulator cartilage, leading to joint space narrowing and a varus deformity of the knee. With pro-

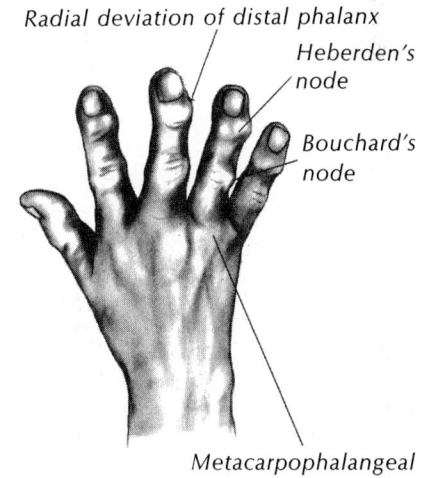

Radial deviation of distal phalanx
Heberden's node
Bouchard's node
Metacarpophalangeal joints uninvolved

FIGURE 47-1 Nodules on the dorsolateral aspects of the distal interphalangeal joints (*Heberden's nodes*) are due to the bony overgrowth of osteoarthritis. Usually hard and painless, they affect the middle-aged or elderly and often, although not always, are associated with arthritic changes in other joints. Flexion and deviation deformities may develop. Similar nodules on the proximal interphalangeal joints (*Bouchard's nodes*) are less common. The metacarpophalangeal joints are spared. (Bates, B (1995). *A guide to physical examination and history taking, 6/e.* Philadelphia: JB Lippincott.)

gression of disease, there is a loss of active and passive motion in both flexion and extension. Crepitus may be present, especially at the patellofemoral joint. In more advanced cases, a flexion contracture, quadriceps atrophy, and joint effusion may be present. Knee OA does not progress in all persons, and in some joint symptoms may improve with time.

Hip

OA of the hip usually begins with a gradual onset of pain, often followed by a limp. The pain typically occurs in the groin or anterior thigh, but occasionally it is in the buttock or even in the knees because of pain referred along contiguous nerves. Range of motion in the hip, especially internal rotation, becomes limited. In chronic OA, weak abductor muscles may result in a positive Trendelenburg sign and an ataxic gait. Some patients with OA of the hip experience radiologic and symptomatic improvement.

Spine

The intervertebral disc, intervertebral osseous bodies, and posterior apophyseal articulations are involved in OA of the spine. Physical findings include restricted range of motion, localized paraspinal muscle tenderness and spasm, and radicular pain from nerve root compression. Nerve root compression can also lead to other signs presenting at the extremities, including muscle weakness and atrophy, reflex changes, and positive tension signs such as positive straight leg raising tests. There is restricted motion because of pain, stiffness, and bony changes.

Foot

The first metatarsophalangeal joint is the most commonly involved joint of the foot. Joint tenderness, bony swelling, irregular joint contours, and restricted motion, especially in dorsiflexion, usually occur.

Disease Course

The course of OA is variable. Although it is a slowly progressive disease, some patients can improve, especially over the short term. Those with multiple affected joints appear to have a more rapid progression. This increased risk of progression is especially seen in the knee. Crystal deposition (calcium pyrophosphate, hydroxide apatite, or a mixture) in the joints of patients with OA is associated with an increased risk of progressive disease. Age is also a risk factor for progression of OA. Elderly persons are more likely to have rapid deterioration of their joints than younger persons with the same degree of OA. Other factors associated with progression include obesity, muscle weakness, joint instability, and peripheral neuropathy.

DIAGNOSTIC STUDIES

The diagnosis of OA is usually made clinically. To differentiate OA from other arthritides definitively, synovial fluid analyses and joint imaging may be used.

OA generally does not cause any abnormal laboratory results. The erythrocyte sedimentation rate may be mildly elevated in patients with inflammatory OA. Tests for rheumatoid factor or antinuclear antibodies are sometimes positive in normal elderly persons (Sack, 1995). In a few patients, the C-reactive protein level is moderately elevated (Spector et al, 1997).

Joint aspiration may be performed when the diagnosis is unclear. If infection is suspected, aspiration must be performed. Synovial fluid obtained by aspiration from joints affected by OA is characteristically noninflammatory, with normal viscosity and few leukocytes and a normal differential count.

Plain radiographs are the most useful form of imaging in OA. They may be helpful in establishing the diagnosis (see Table 47-1) but are not alone sufficient to make the diagnosis. This is because there is a poor correlation between radiologic changes and clinical symptoms. Many people with radiographic evidence of OA have no symptoms or disability. Despite this, radiographic changes are still helpful for classifying OA. The changes associated with OA on plain radiographs are pathognomonic. The most common features of OA on plain radiographs include asymmetrical joint space narrowing, subchondral bone sclerosis, subchondral cysts, osteophyte formation, and bone remodeling (Solomon, 1997).

Further imaging studies are rarely needed but may include radionucleotide scintigraphy, computed tomography, and magnetic resonance imaging; they are not recommended for routine use. Technetium-99m scintigraphy is a sensitive indicator of OA and may be useful in diagnosing early OA or identifying involved joints before symptoms and radiographic changes of OA occur. Magnetic resonance imaging reveals the entire spectrum of osteoarthritic changes much more accurately and earlier than conventional radiography. However, conventional radiography remains a sensitive and cost-effective modality and is the initial imaging study of choice in the routine evaluation of OA. Biochemical markers of OA will probably play an increasing role in the diagnosis and monitoring of disease activity.

TREATMENT OPTIONS, EXPECTED OUTCOMES, AND COMPREHENSIVE MANAGEMENT

The management of OA continues to evolve. Although no cure exists for OA, many interventions exist to relieve pain, maintain or improve functional status, and minimize disability. Today there is greater emphasis on individualized treatment and on exercise rather than the use of nonsteroidal anti-inflammatory drugs (NSAIDs). Because of the protean biomedical and psychosocial manifestations of this disease, the condition is best managed in the primary care provider's office. However, when the diagnosis is in doubt or treatment is unsuccessful, appropriate consultation with other specialists is indicated.

Applications of heat or cold are widely used by patients with OA. Moist heat is generally preferable to dry heat for relief of joint pain. Most modalities of superficial heat do not penetrate to the deeper tissues. Deep heat, such as ultrasound, can be beneficial in relieving pain. Cold is usually recommended after strenuous activity and can be effective in decreasing pain and muscle spasms.

Exercise has taken on an increasingly important role in the treatment of OA. The goals of an exercise program for the patient with OA include a reduction of joint pain, an increase in range of motion and strength, improved performance of daily activities, and prevention of disability and poor health from inactivity (Brandt, 1995). Muscle surrounding the involved joint should be strengthened. For example, knee exercises are directed at strengthening the quadriceps muscles. Isometric exercises are preferable to isotonic exercises because of decreased joint stresses. Patients should be encouraged to exercise on a daily basis. Aerobic exercises that can be recommended for patients with OA include cycling, swimming, and aerobic pool exercises. Resistance training, cross-country exercisers, and walking can be instituted as tolerated by the patient. Patients with moderately severe knee OA who perform isometric strengthening exercises for the lower extremities usually have a decrease in their joint pain and a decreased need for analgesics or NSAIDs.

Braces can provide stability, increase proprioception, and decrease joint stress. They are especially useful for patients with moderate to severe knee OA. Custom-fitted knee braces, which are intended to unload the medial compartment of the knee, are available.

The most commonly prescribed oral agents include NSAIDs, acetaminophen, and corticosteroids. NSAIDs have shown no advantage over acetaminophen in controlling pain in OA. Acetaminophen should be taken in doses up to 4000 mg/day to control pain. Until recently, NSAIDs were the first choice for oral agents in the treatment of OA. However, they should be used less commonly because they have a high incidence of gastrointestinal and renal side effects, they may produce deleterious effects on articular cartilage, and there is only a mild degree of synovial inflammation in OA (Kraus, 1997). Topical NSAIDs are commonly used in Europe, but they have not been approved for use in the United States.

Pain management, a fundamental aspect of treatment in OA, requires careful attention to nonpharmacologic interventions, which are often more important than medications. However, if first-line oral agents given for analgesia fail, second-line agents should be considered as useful adjuncts to nonpharmacologic modalities. Second-line therapy for pain has been enhanced with the arrival of nonnarcotic, nonsedating agents such as tramadol. In severely advanced cases, narcotics can be used as adjuncts for pain management, particularly in anticipation of joint replacement or other surgical procedures. Systemic corticosteroid treatment is not indicated for OA.

Intra-articular corticosteroid injections are sometimes used in the treatment of OA, but improvement after an intra-articular injection is likely to be only temporary. There have not been any studies showing lasting benefit from corticosteroid injections. High doses or repeated doses of corticosteroids may, in fact, impede the cartilage repair process, including the biosynthesis of glycosaminoglycans and hyaluronic acid. Intra-articular corticosteroids are generally not given at intervals shorter than 3 months.

Newer concepts in the treatment of OA include chondroprotective agents, which conserve cartilage or stimulate cartilage repair within the OA joint. These agents include tetracyclines, glycosaminoglycans, hyaluronic acid, and gene therapy. In animal studies, tetracyclines and tetracycline derivatives have been shown to have chondroprotective effects. Chemically modified tetracyclines have been developed that eliminate the antimicrobial effect while retaining the chondroprotective ef-

fects (Kraus, 1997). Oral supplements of glycosaminoglycans (glucosamine and chondroitin sulfate) have been compared in short-term trials with NSAIDs and have been found to be as effective, with fewer side effects, in reducing the clinical symptoms of OA (Noack et al, 1994). Daily dosages used in the studies were 1500 mg of glucosamine and 1200 mg of chondroitin sulfate.

Another new therapeutic approach to OA is viscosupplementation therapy. Hyaluronan preparations are injected into the knee in an attempt to return to normal the elasticity and viscosity of the synovial fluid (Adams, 1993). Several studies have reported beneficial effects and minimal side effects with this intra-articular therapy.

For patients with more severe OA who have persistent pain and significantly impaired function, other therapeutic interventions may be indicated. Tidal irrigation (saline flushes) of the knee using normal saline has been shown to be effective in patients with milder OA refractory to other measures. Tidal irrigation, which may be performed in the office, is much less expensive than arthroscopy of the knee and may provide similar pain relief and improved functional results. Patients with radiographically advanced OA, however, do not appear to benefit from this procedure (Brandt, 1995).

Surgery is reserved for cases in which advanced symptomatic OA has proved refractory to optimal medical management and other less invasive therapies. Arthroscopic débridement of osteoarthritic joints sometimes offers temporary relief of symptoms. This relief may be in large part the result of the lavage inherent in the procedure. Arthroplasty is the most common and effective surgery for OA of the weight-bearing joints. Other approaches under investigation include harvesting of mesenchymal stem cells to induce cartilage regeneration, allogenic cartilage transplantation, and the stimulation of in vitro cartilage matrix elaboration by harvested cadaver chondrocytes.

Teaching and Self-Care

Educating patients with OA about the disease leads to a better understanding of the physical limitations, a more positive attitude, and increased participation in exercise. The provider's support can also directly affect the level of disability. Interventions such as regular phone calls or office visits have been shown to lead to a reduction in joint pain (Brandt, 1995). Patients should be instructed in the principles of joint protection. For example, those with OA of the knees or hips should be advised against squatting, kneeling, and activities that repetitively stress the joints (eg, stairs, running). For patients with more advanced OA, the use of a cane, crutches, or a walker may help reduce joint pain. Orthotic supports such as wedge insoles can also help relieve pain and distribute joint forces.

Obese patients with OA should be encouraged to lose weight. Weight loss may reduce the severity of joint pain and slow the progression of the disease.

Complementary Approaches

Antioxidants may protect against the progression of OA. Vitamin C, an antioxidant essential for type II collagen synthesis, has been shown to protect against the progression of knee OA. In one study, a threefold reduction in risk of OA progression was observed in persons consuming more than 150 mg of vitamin C compared to those not taking vitamin C. However, there was no effect on the overall incidence of OA (Mc Alindon, 1996).

Over-the-counter topical preparations are commonly used by patients with OA. Evidence of efficacy, however, is limited. Capsaicin cream (capsaicin is the active ingredient in Tabasco sauce) stimulates local depletion of substance P, the main chemical responsible for stimulating pain nerve fibers. Clinical trials have shown relief of joint pain in patients with OA of the hand or knee using capsaicin cream (Deal et al, 1991). The cream needs to be applied as often as three or four times daily. A maximal benefit may not be achieved until 3 to 4 weeks of use.

Other substances and modalities that have been used in the treatment of OA include ginger, shark cartilage, acupuncture, and biofeedback. Clinical trials on each of these are limited. Some health insurance plans provide coverage for one or more of these approaches. Primary care providers must maintain a flexible disposition toward these and other investigational, complementary therapies.

COMMUNITY RESOURCES

- The Arthritis Foundation, 1330 W. Peachtree St., Atlanta, GA 30309, 404-872-7100, http://www.arthritis.org: State and federal legislation updates, links to legislators, frequently asked questions about arthritis, local support and self-help group information Arthritis Answers: 800-283-7800
- Health Promotion on the Internet (OA and Exercise), http://www.monash.edu.au/health/pamphlets/osteo arthritis2/: General exercise information and illustrations
- Consumer Health and Patient Information Resources, http://buddy.library.mun.ca/elaine/arthriti.htm: Links to sites containing information about arthritis

CLINICAL WARNINGS AND REFERRAL POINTS

Patients who use NSAIDs, especially the elderly, must be carefully monitored for signs of bleeding. Referrals are indicated when a therapeutic response is not achieved, or when surgical intervention for OA is contemplated. There are a multitude of new therapies for OA, and it is important for the primary care provider to keep an open mind and work with the patient. Additional referrals may result when the provider identifies positive results from a new therapy.

▪ ▪ ▪ CLINICAL PEARLS

- OA can affect anyone.
- The clinical picture in OA is more important than the radiologic picture.
- Good functional performance and maximal capacity are important treatment outcomes for patients with OA.
- The degree of dysfunction is not always directly related to the clinical findings.
- The use of acetaminophen for patients with OA has been undervalued and should be considered before prescribing NSAIDs.

EDITOR'S NOTE:

COMPLEMENTARY APPROACHES

A general discussion of complementary approaches can be found in Chapter 3. The following, while not an exhaustive list, are some complementary approaches being used for this condition. Additional information on these approaches, including precautions, can be found in Appendices A and B. Providers need to assess for the use of complementary approaches as part of the patient's history, as they may impact conventional therapies, and patients may not volunteer this information unless specifically asked. Efficacy of many complementary approaches is not as well documented as that of conventional therapies. Providers need to read the literature before suggesting these complementary approaches.

- Vitamins, minerals, herbs, supplements
  - Ginger
  - Glucosamine sulfate
  - Vitamin C
- Complementary Modalities
  - Aromatherapy
  - Massage therapy

References

Adams, M.E. (1993). An analysis of clinical studies of the use of cross-linked hyaluronan, hylan, in the treatment of osteoarthritis. *Journal of Rheumatology, 39*(suppl), 16–18.

Brandt, K.D. (1995). Nonsurgical management of osteoarthritis with an emphasis on nonpharmacologic measures. *Archives of Family Medicine, 4*, 1057–1064.

Cicuttini, F.M., & Spector, T.D. (1996). Genetics of osteoarthritis. *Annals of the Rheumatic Diseases, 55*(9), 665.

Creamer, P., & Hochberg, M.C. (1997). Osteoarthritis. *The Lancet, 350*(9076), 503.

Deal, C.L., Schnitzer, T.J., Lipstein, E. et al. (1991). Treatment of arthritis with topical capsaicin: A double-blind trial. *Clinical Therapeutics, 13*, 383.

Hughes, S.L., & Dunlop, D. (1995). The prevalence and impact of arthritis in older persons. *Arthritis Care and Research, 8*(4), 257–264.

Jimenez, S.A., & Dharmavaram, R.M. (1994). Genetic aspects of familial osteoarthritis. *Annals of the Rheumatic Diseases, 53*(12), 789.

Kraus, V.B. (1997). Pathogenesis and treatment of osteoarthritis. *Medical Clinics of North America, 81*, 85–112.

Lane, N.E., & Buckwalter, J.A. (1993). Exercise: A cause of osteoarthritis? *Rheumatic Diseases Clinics of North America, 19*(3), 617–633.

McAlindon, T.E. (1996). Do antioxidant micronutrients protect against the development and progression of knee osteoarthritis? *Arthritis & Rheumatism, 39*(4), 648–656.

Nelson, D.T. (1996). Weight and osteoarthritis. *American Journal of Clinical Nutrition, 63*(suppl), 430–436S.

Noack, W., Fischer, M., Forster, K.K. et al. (1994). Glucosamine sulfate in osteoarthritis of the knee. *Osteoarthritis Care, 2*(1), 51–59.

Sack, K.E. (1995). Osteoarthritis: A continuing challenge. *Western Journal of Medicine, 163*(6), 579–586.

Smith, M.D., Triantafillou, S., Parker, A., Youssef, P.P., & Coleman, M. (1997). Synovial membrane inflammation and cytokine production in patients with early osteoarthritis. *Journal of Rheumatology, 24*(2), 365–371.

Spector, T.D., Hart, D.J., Nandra, D. et al. (1997). Low-level increases in serum C-reactive protein are present in early osteoarthritis of the knee and predict progressive disease. *Arthritis and Rheumatism, 40*(4), 723–727.

Solomon, L. (1997). Clinical features of osteoarthritis. In W.N. Kelley, E.D. Harris, S. Ruddy, & C.B. Sledge (Eds.). *Textbook of rheumatology*, 5th ed. Philadelphia: W.B. Saunders.

Verbrugge, L.M. (1995). Women, men, and osteoarthritis. *Arthritis Care and Research, 8*(4), 212–220.

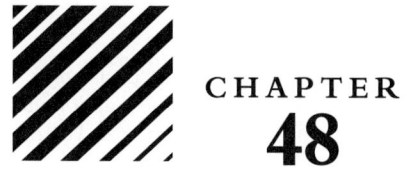

CHAPTER
48

Osteoporosis

Ellen R. Rich, PhD RN, CS, FNP

Osteoporosis is a generalized metabolic disease characterized by both diminished bone mineral density (BMD) and deterioration of the microarchitecture of remaining bone. Because bone strength is proportional to its density, the consequences of these changes are bone fragility and an increased rate of fractures.

Osteoporosis is a silent disease, usually asymptomatic until a fracture occurs. Because lifelong habits can influence susceptibility to osteoporosis, it has been considered to be a pediatric disease with geriatric manifestations (New York State Department of Health, 1996). There are no early warning symptoms; when fractures occur, bone density has already been lost. Osteoporosis is preventable through a lifelong commitment to proper nutrition, adequate and appropriate exercise, and early intervention for those at risk.

ANATOMY, PHYSIOLOGY, AND PATHOLOGY

The matrix of bone comprises organic and inorganic components. Collagen, proteins, and lipids constitute the organic portion of the bone matrix. The inorganic matrix, which represents 65% of bone's total weight, is largely composed of calcium and phosphate, with smaller amounts of magnesium, sodium, and potassium. Hydroxyapatite is the principal mineral component of bone and is 40% calcium by weight. Histologically, bone can be subdivided into two types: cancellous (spongy) and cortical (compact). Cancellous bone has a large surface area, and its metabolic activity is much more rapid than that of cortical bone. Viewed microscopically, bone of normal strength and density has a honeycomb appearance, whereas osteoporotic bone appears less dense, with a weaker, more spindly structure.

Bone mass is the total quantity of bone tissue in the skeleton. Greater bone mass equals more bone, which indicates a stronger skeleton. Most diagnostic studies for osteoporosis measure bone density of a part of the skeleton, another indicator for osteoporosis because high density also is representative of bone strength. Although bone mass and density differ slightly in meaning, these terms are used interchangeably in this chapter.

Bone mass undergoes predictable changes throughout the life cycle. During the first several decades of life, active growth occurs, building toward peak bone mass, the maximal bone density a person achieves. Peak bone mass is usually achieved by age 30. In women after this age, there is a plateau or very slow decline from peak bone mass until menopause. Declining ovarian function accelerates the loss of bone mass at a rate of approximately 2% to 4% per year; this loss is most rapid in the first 2 years after menopause and gradually subsides within 5 to 10 years. This decline in bone loss then slows, but bone mass continues to decrease over the years. Total loss of bone can approach 50%. For men, bone mass decreases gradually,

particularly after age 50, as testosterone levels diminish, without the sharper dip associated with menopause. However, men with hypogonadism also experience an accelerated rate of bone loss. All adults after age 30 are on a lifelong course of decreasing bone mass leading to senile osteoporosis, but women have the additional burden of postmenopausal osteoporosis from estrogen deficiency.

Osteoporosis may be etiologically divided into primary and secondary types. Primary osteoporosis is further subdivided into three types: postmenopausal (type I), principally affecting cancellous bone; age-associated disease (type II), a slower loss of cancellous and cortical bone seen in both sexes, especially past the age of 70; and idiopathic osteoporosis, in which bone loss occurs in young and middle-aged men and premenopausal women. Secondary osteoporosis is the result of underlying conditions (Table 48-1).

Bone is continually replaced by a process called bone remodeling. Humans remodel their skeletons to a greater degree than most other mammals at a rate that increases with age. Each year, approximately 20% of the skeleton is remodeled. Bone remodeling can be divided into two processes: resorption and formation. During resorption, osteoclasts excavate the bone surface by dissolving the mineral component of the bone and hydrolyzing the organic matrix. Saucer-shaped cavities are produced on the surface of cancellous bone; tunnels are formed in cortical bone. Cancellous bone is subject to more remodeling activity and quicker turnover than cortical bone because its large surface area provides a greater number of remodeling sites and its metabolic rate is more rapid. Menopause actually causes increased activation of these remodeling sites, intensifying resorption and producing deeper cavities in cancellous bone.

Formation is carried out by osteoblasts, which migrate to the pits and tunnels and begin to fill them in by secreting collagen fibrils to form the bone matrix. After this protein matrix is formed, it becomes mineralized through the deposition of calcium hydroxyapatite crystals. Adequate intake of vitamin D and calcium is required for mineralization. During both the resorption and formation phases of remodeling, biochemical markers reflective of these processes are released into the bloodstream.

In the pathogenesis of osteoporosis, the most important aspect of remodeling is the rate of formation relative to resorption. During childhood and early adulthood, as bone mass builds, the rate of formation exceeds that of resorption; it then plateaus until about the age of 40. Thereafter, resorption outpaces formation, and bone density continues to decrease.

Also significant is each person's peak bone mass, which becomes the starting point for later loss. Slow decreases in mass in someone who achieved a relatively low peak may ultimately yield the same net bone mass as a more rapid decline in someone whose peak mass was high. This highlights the importance of

TABLE 48-1	Causes of Secondary Osteoporosis
Malignancy (especially multiple myeloma)	Pharmacologic agents
Chronic liver or renal disease	Glucocorticoids
Malabsorption	Thyroid hormone
Cushing's syndrome	Anticonvulsants
Hyperthyroidism	Heparin
Hyperparathyroidism	Lithium
Hypogonadism (in men)	Chemotherapy drugs
Athletic amenorrhea	Some diuretics
Eating disorders	GnRH agonists
Systemic mastocytosis	Aluminum-containing antacids
Rheumatoid arthritis	Parenteral nutrition
Osteogenesis imperfecta	Early oophorectomy
Hyperprolactinemia	Subtotal gastrectomy
	Major organ transplantation

proper nutrition and exercise during the years of active bone growth to attain maximal peak mass.

Osteoporotic changes are more significant at certain body sites. Because cancellous bone has greater remodeling activity than cortical bone, it is subject to a more rapid loss of density. The vertebral body, femoral neck, and distal radius are composed of cancellous bone, and they are therefore the most common sites of osteoporotic fractures. Other fracture sites are the pelvis, tibial plateau, proximal humerus, and ribs.

The fragility of porous bone predisposes not only to fractures from trauma but also to nonviolent fractures. Nonviolent fractures, caused by minimal trauma that would not result in fracture in a young adult, are responsible for 90% of hip and wrist fractures in the elderly. Overall, the spine is the most common site for osteoporotic fractures. Secondary to vertebral compression, spinal fractures may occur in the absence of recognizable trauma, triggered perhaps by a cough or sneeze. In fact, 50% of people with vertebral fractures from osteoporosis have no recollection of back pain, and only one third of persons with vertebral fractures are clinically diagnosed. Fractured vertebrae assume a wedge shape, narrowing anteriorly, causing kyphosis, height and waistline loss, and abdominal protrusion.

EPIDEMIOLOGY

Osteoporosis affects an estimated 25 million Americans, 80% of whom are women. Approximately 1.5 million osteoporotic fractures occur each year (Galsworthy & Wilson, 1996; Kessenich, 1996b). Fifty percent of women and 20% of men over age 65 will experience an osteoporotic fracture during their lifetime. Only one woman in nine between the ages of 60 and 70 has normal BMD, nearly one third have osteoporosis, and the remainder have osteopenia, which is subnormal BMD not severe enough to be classified as frank osteoporosis (Ross, 1996). Men over age 50 have a higher risk of suffering an osteoporotic fracture than of developing prostate cancer ("Men are at risk," 1996). In America, the cost of acute and long-term care for patients with osteoporotic fractures is estimated to be $10 to $18 billion per year (Kessenich, 1996a).

The most common osteoporotic fracture is the vertebral crush fracture; approximately 500,000 of these occur per year

in the United States. Mostly affecting women over age 55, vertebral fractures may result in chronic back, rib, or abdominal pain, kyphosis, and poor body image (Galsworthy & Wilson, 1996). For 60% to 87% of those with symptomatic vertebral fractures, activities such as carrying, lifting, walking, shopping, and house cleaning are difficult (Ross, 1996). Although less debilitating in the long term, Colles' fractures of the distal radius, occurring at a rate of 200,000 per year, may hinder the patient's ability to function in the workplace, because those affected are often young enough still to be employed (Lindsay, 1992).

Most significant in terms of complications, death, and cost is osteoporotic hip fracture. Each year in the United States, more than 7 million days of restricted activity, 3.4 million hospital bed days, and 60,000 nursing home admissions are attributable to hip fractures. Nineteen percent of patients with hip fractures require long-term nursing home care (Ross, 1996). Hip fractures, which occur at a rate of approximately 250,000 per year, claim the lives of 25% of those affected within the first year after the fracture. This death rate is attributable to peri- and postoperative complications, including pneumonia, deep vein thrombosis, and pulmonary embolism. Of those who survive, only 20% have a complete return of function (Lindsay, 1992). The vast majority suffer permanent disability, with compromised ability to perform activities of daily living.

A few studies have demonstrated an association between osteoporosis and an increased death rate from stroke in elderly women, although it is not clear why this is so. Every decrease of one standard deviation of BMD was associated with a 70% increase of risk of death from stroke (Browner et al, 1993).

Cultural Factors

Much of the variation in BMD and bone geometry is attributable to heredity. Small frame size (weight less than 125 lb) is an example of a type of bone geometry that presents a high risk for osteoporosis. Hip geometry, which varies among races, may influence the risk for hip fracture. BMD tends to be higher in African American and Hispanic women and lower in whites and Asians. Whites have twice the incidence of hip fractures as African Americans. The BMD of an African American woman is typically equivalent to that of a white male (Arnaud, 1996; Kessenich, 1996a; New York State Department of Health, 1996; Ross, 1996).

Other factors may moderate the effects of heredity. Although being Asian is a risk factor for osteoporosis when compared to whites, the Japanese have a lower incidence of hip and other nonspinal fractures. This finding was attributed to different hip geometry and a decreased rate of falls. BMD differences have been observed between persons of the same race living in different locations, suggesting that environmental or lifestyle influences may override hereditary factors (Ross, 1996).

Type of diet is another cultural factor that could enhance the risk of osteoporosis. A group that does not consume dairy products or other calcium sources would be unlikely to achieve maximal peak bone density.

Socioeconomic Factors

Those who lack the resources for adequate nutritional intake could be at higher risk for osteoporosis.

DIAGNOSTIC CRITERIA

Definitive diagnostic criteria are:

- Dual energy x-ray absorptiometry (DEXA) bone density reading more than 2.5 standard deviations below the young adult mean (Hurst, 1996; Ross, 1996)
- Radiographic evidence of decreased bone density (x-ray changes usually not detectable until at least 30% of bone mass is lost) (Galsworthy & Wilson, 1996; Kessenich, 1996a; Riggs & Melton, 1995).

Suggestive diagnostic criteria are:

- Fractures that occur with minor trauma (usually a fall from standing height or lower) or no known trauma (Hurst, 1996; Ross, 1996)
- Loss of height and kyphotic spinal curvature (Kessenich, 1996a).

HISTORY AND PHYSICAL EXAM

Historical findings related to osteoporosis differ based on whether the patient is presenting before or after an osteoporotic fracture. Those evaluated before the fracture stage are likely to be asymptomatic; the history, therefore, is directed at risk factor evaluation. Those who have had osteoporotic fractures are more likely to have related complaints, although they, too, may be asymptomatic. Table 48-2 lists pertinent historical data for the assessment of osteoporosis.

The physical exam should include measurement of height and careful inspection of the posture and spinal curves. Kyphosis and loss of space between the inferior portion of the anterior rib cage and the iliac crests are indicators of collapse of the vertebral bodies. A protuberant abdomen may also be noted. Mild to moderate scoliosis may appear, particularly if there have

TABLE 48-2	Historical Data for Assessment of Osteoporosis

- Age
- Gender (female at greater risk)
- Family history of osteoporosis or nonviolent fractures
- Exercise habits (sedentary or lacking weight-bearing exercise)
- Nutritional history (calcium and vitamin D intake)
- Caffeine intake (consumption of 2 or more caffeinated beverages/day increases risk for hip fracture)
- Alcohol abuse (greater than moderate intake increases fracture risk)
- Smoking habits (some association with bone loss and fracture)
- Personal history of fractures (traumatic and nonviolent)
- Recent or past falls or injuries and related symptomatology
- Perceived loss of height (past medical records may be referenced), waistline, or difficulty fitting into clothes
- Early satiety, abdominal or anterior rib discomfort (skeletal cause increased pressure on the abdomen, iliac crests may hit the lower ribs, causing pain)
- Acute pain at or radiating from a fracture site
- Chronic back pain (often lumbar) from skeletal changes
- Coexistent visual or neurologic disorders (these may predispose the patient to falls; correction could reduce fracture risk)
- History of any of the conditions listed in Table 48-1

been fractures of vertebrae between T2 and T11. A complete musculoskeletal exam should be performed, including palpation of the spine, paravertebral muscles, and other involved areas for tenderness or deformity, range of motion, and assessment of gait. Assessments of muscle mass, strength, and balance help identify deficits that may be correctable. The examiner should also look for physical manifestations of diseases that could cause secondary osteoporosis (see Table 48-1).

DIAGNOSTIC STUDIES

The most reliable diagnostic tool for osteoporosis is DEXA, a measure of BMD. BMD is the strongest indicator of future fracture risk; in fact, low BMD is more strongly predictive of future fracture than elevated cholesterol levels and high blood pressure are for myocardial infarction and stroke, respectively. DEXA provides a high-resolution, very reproducible image of the lumbar spine, intertrochanteric regions of the hip, and the wrist. Radiation exposure from DEXA is less than 3 mrem, one-tenth that of a routine chest x-ray. DEXA is less costly than quantitative computed tomography, which exposes the patient to 100 to more than 1000 mrem. Other positive attributes of BMD measurement are ease and noninvasiveness, reproducibility for reliable follow-up measurements, a strong correlation between bone density and bone strength, and evidence of treatment response through BMD readings. Changes in bone density significant enough to show on DEXA (variations of at least 2% to 4%), however, may not be evident for at least a year. This limits the utility of DEXA in terms of assessing immediate or short-term response to treatment.

Interpretation of BMD readings is based on comparison to expected values for young healthy adults between ages 30 and 40. Table 48-3 depicts the bone density states depending on the number of standard deviations from the mean of the healthy comparison group. A 1.5-fold to twofold increase in fracture risk is associated with each drop of one standard deviation of bone density.

There are no universal guidelines for the use of DEXA in the assessment of osteoporosis. Expense is a limiting factor. The National Osteoporosis Foundation recommends BMD measurements in estrogen-deficient women, when a vertebral abnormality is detected on x-ray, on initiation of glucocorticosteroid therapy, and in primary hyperparathyroidism (Lindsay, 1992). Others suggest BMD studies for those with several risk factors for osteoporosis, for establishment of a pretreatment baseline, and for those who have had prior osteoporotic fractures. DEXA measurements may help when treatment decisions, such as whether to begin estrogen replacement therapy (ERT), need to be made. Follow-up measurements at appropriate intervals (no more frequently than every 14 to 18 months) can gauge response to treatment.

TABLE 48-3	Classification of Bone Density Results

Diagnostic Category	Standard Deviations Below Young Adult Mean
Osteopenia	1 to 2.5
Osteoporosis	Greater than 2.5
Severe osteoporosis	Greater than 2.5 *and* a history of nonviolent fracture

Osteoporosis may also be detected through simple x-ray readings; however, osteoporotic changes become evident only after 30% to 40% of bone density has been lost. X-rays are valuable in the diagnosis of osteoporotic fractures. Osteoporotic fractures of the spine cause compression; fractured vertebrae become wedge-shaped and narrow anteriorly. Decrease in vertebral height of 15% to 20%, seen on x-ray, is one indicator of vertebral fracture.

Under investigation is the diagnostic use of biochemical markers found in blood and urine. Indicators of the process of bone formation are serum alkaline phosphatase, serum osteocalcin, and serum carboxy terminal propeptide of type I procollagen. Markers reflective of bone resorption are urinary hydroxyproline, urinary hydroxylysine glycosides, and urinary pyridinium cross-links (Kessenich, 1996a). At the present level of development, these markers are useful only in highly specialized practice and for pharmacologic research. With improved specificity, these tests may be more immediate indicators than DEXA of both rapid changes in bone density and response to treatment. Quantitative ultrasound measurement of bone density, currently lacking FDA approval, may also become a useful modality in the future.

In addition to these studies, some fairly routine laboratory tests should be performed when osteoporosis is diagnosed to rule out conditions associated with secondary osteoporosis. A complete blood count may reveal malignant disease when the erythrocyte sedimentation rate is high and red blood cell indices are consistent with anemia. Urinalysis, serum creatinine, protein, and thyroid and liver function tests may indicate renal, hepatic, or thyroid disease. Serum calcium levels may be elevated in hyperparathyroidism and malignant disease and diminished in osteomalacia, malnutrition, hypoparathyroidism, and renal disease. Increased serum alkaline phosphatase levels may be associated with hyperparathyroidism, Paget's disease, thyrotoxicosis, neoplasm, malabsorption, vitamin D deficiency, alcohol abuse, anticonvulsant therapy, and chronic renal or hepatic disease. Hyperparathyroidism, malabsorption, malnutrition, and osteomalacia can result in hypophosphatemia. Ruling out other causes of secondary osteoporosis may require more specialized testing. Serum 25-hydroxy vitamin D assessment may be indicated in cases where gastrointestinal disease or osteomalacia is suspected, and adrenal function studies will help detect Cushing's disease.

TREATMENT OPTIONS, EXPECTED OUTCOMES, AND COMPREHENSIVE MANAGEMENT

Primary Prevention

Because osteoporosis is a silent disease for which risk may begin to manifest as early as childhood, primary prevention is critical for reducing its incidence. So many people are affected by osteoporosis later in life that it would be ideal for all to follow preventive guidelines. Primary prevention is of significantly greater importance for those at risk.

Health promotion and protection measures for osteoporosis are principally focused on proper nutrition, physical exercise, and avoidance of habits that contribute to risk. Because healthy bone is largely composed of calcium, this is the nutritional element of principal concern. Vitamin D is necessary for calcium absorption, so adequate intake is also important.

TABLE 48-4	Dietary Sources of Calcium
Source	**Calcium (mg)**
Milk, whole, 1 cup	288
Milk, skim or buttermilk, 1 cup	296
Cottage cheese, 12 oz.	320
Yogurt (whole milk), 1 cup	272
Yogurt (part skim), 1 cup	294
Cheese, Swiss, natural, 1 cubic inch	139
Cheese, cheddar, 1 cubic inch	129
Sardines, canned in oil, drained, 3 oz.	372
Oysters, raw, 1 cup	226
Salmon, pink, canned, 3 oz.	167
Broccoli, cooked, 1 cup	158
Collards, cooked, 1 cup	289
Mustard greens, cooked, 1 cup	193
Peanuts, roasted, 1 cup	107
Spinach, 1 cup	200
Turnip greens, cooked, 1 cup	252
Rhubarb, cooked, 1 cup	212
Apricots, dried, 1 cup	100
Dates, pitted, 1 cup	105
Farina, cooked, 1 cup	147
Pizza, cheese, 5.5-inch section	107
Molasses, blackstrap, 1 tbsp.	137
Almonds, 1/2 cup	160
Tofu, 3.5 oz.	128

Peak bone mass is usually attained by age 30, but a few studies have suggested it may be reached in some by age 16, illustrating the importance of sufficient calcium and vitamin D intake beginning in childhood. Vitamin D supply is usually adequate in childhood because of outdoor activities with exposure to sunlight and fortification of dairy products. If there is limited exposure to sunlight and inadequate intake of dairy products, some supplementation with vitamin D may be indicated. Ample calcium intake through dietary consumption is optimal. Table 48-4 lists foods that are rich sources of calcium. Recommended calcium intake for various age groups is listed in Table 48-5. If the requisite amount of calcium cannot be obtained through dietary intake, supplementation is recommended.

TABLE 48-5	Recommendations for Calcium Intake
Age	**Milligrams per day**
18–24 years	1200–1500
Men 25–65 years	900
Men over 65 years	1500
Women 25–50 years	1000
Women treated with estrogen	1000
Postmenopausal women (not on ERT)	1500
Pregnant or lactating women	1600

A sedentary lifestyle is considered a risk factor for osteoporosis. The skeleton must be "loaded" by weight bearing or other resistance to maintain its density. Most studies have shown that the magnitude of this loading is more important than its frequency. Immobility from prolonged bed rest after a fracture may result in up to a 40% loss of bone density, and this may persist. Physical exercise throughout childhood is a significant determinant of the degree of peak bone density attained. Continued physical activity during adulthood helps increase or maintain bone density at skeletal sites that are loaded. With the exception of swimming, most types of aerobic exercise load the lower extremities and the spine (through weight-bearing exercise). Resistance training can load the upper extremities. A lifetime program of physical exercise is critical for primary prevention of osteoporosis.

Attending to risk factors is a prime component of osteoporosis prevention and detection of those with particular susceptibility to osteoporotic fractures. For those at high risk, interventions can halt and possibly reverse bone loss and decrease the risk of future fractures. Because these fractures have multifactorial origins, elimination of even one risk factor may be influential. Alterable risk factors include sedentary lifestyle or lack of weight-bearing exercise, inadequate intake of calcium and vitamin D, consumption of two or more caffeinated beverages per day, alcohol abuse (greater than moderate intake), and smoking.

Obviously, other risk factors, such as female gender, small frame size, race, advancing age, and family history of osteoporosis cannot be altered. Persons with these unalterable risk factors should be even more attentive to the alterable risk factors that are responsive to lifestyle modifications.

Secondary Prevention

Those at high risk for osteoporosis should be screened for the disease. Because interventions at almost any stage can to some degree improve bone density or reduce the risk of fractures, case finding is beneficial. It has been estimated that only 4% of persons with osteoporosis are receiving treatment specific for their disease. Greater awareness of the risk factors, signs, symptoms, and diagnostic testing for osteoporosis should increase the number of persons receiving appropriate care. See the sections on history and physical exam and diagnostic studies for information regarding disease detection.

Tertiary Prevention

TREATMENT OPTIONS AND EXPECTED OUTCOMES

Goals of the various treatment modalities for osteoporosis are to enhance the bone mass still of normal quality, to avoid additional bone loss, and to prevent fractures. The therapeutic regimen should include lifestyle modifications as well as medical interventions. Although most of the studies regarding therapeutic agents for osteoporosis have included patients up to age 80, researchers generally agree that the very elderly are also likely to benefit from therapy. Very small changes in bone mass (halting further loss or increasing mass) decrease the fracture risk. It is never too late to initiate treatment. Before initiating treatment, the provider must evaluate the patient for correctable causes of secondary osteoporosis.

COMPREHENSIVE MANAGEMENT RECOMMENDATIONS

An algorithm for the comprehensive management of osteoporosis is shown in Figure 48-1. These guidelines combine BMD and bone resorption testing. If bone resorption testing is unavailable, management may be based solely on the BMD assessment.

Calcium

Adequate intake of calcium (see Tables 48-4 and 48-5) must be ensured. In well-nourished populations in developed nations, where protein and phosphorous intake is adequate, calcium is the limiting nutrient for the process of bone growth. Our calcium intake is less than that of our primitive predecessors, and our intestinal absorption and renal excretion are less efficient. Because the principal mineral component of bone is calcium, ample calcium intake must undergird any therapeutic recommendations for osteoporosis (Riggs & Melton, 1995).

Throughout the life span, whenever intake through diet is inadequate (see Tables 48-4 and 48-5), calcium supplementation is indicated. When dietary sources are insufficient, calcium is pulled from the bones to maintain normal serum levels. There are various forms of calcium supplements. Calcium carbonate is the least expensive and contains the most elemental calcium by weight (40%). Other forms include dicalcium phosphate (30% elemental), calcium citrate (24% elemental), calcium lactate (9% elemental), and calcium gluconate (10% elemental). Supplementation using bone meal or dolomite should be avoided because these sources have been associated with contamination by arsenic and lead. Calcium carbonate may cause gastrointestinal symptoms such as bloating, gas, and constipation, especially in those with low levels of gastric hydrochloric acid. Calcium citrate is better tolerated in persons with these symptoms.

Calcium should be taken in divided doses with meals because the release of hydrochloric acid associated with food consumption assists in absorption. Some commercial brands of calcium are less soluble than others. The solubility of a calcium supplement can be tested by placing it in vinegar and observing for dissolution. Calcium supplements that fail to dissolve in 30 minutes are unlikely to dissolve in the stomach (Maher et al, 1994).

Some foods affect the absorption of calcium. Lactose and vitamin D enhance absorption, whereas fats, fiber, and oxalates decrease absorption. Therefore, low-fat (1% milk fat or less) dairy products contain higher levels of calcium than high-fat sources and are better absorbed. Fats from other sources also interfere with calcium absorption. High protein or caffeine intake enhances excretion of calcium. Phytates, sodium, and phosphorous probably do not significantly affect calcium absorption (New York State Department of Health, 1996).

Osteoporosis patients with calcium oxalate renal calculi have been successfully supplemented with calcium citrate (at least 700 mg/day of elemental calcium). They experienced favorable changes in bone density with no change in renal parameters. In fact, decreased calcium intake was associated with more stone formation because of excess oxalate (New York State Department of Health, 1996).

Vitamin D

Calcium is poorly absorbed from the gastrointestinal tract and requires vitamin D for successful absorption and use. A vitamin D precursor is present on the skin and is converted first by

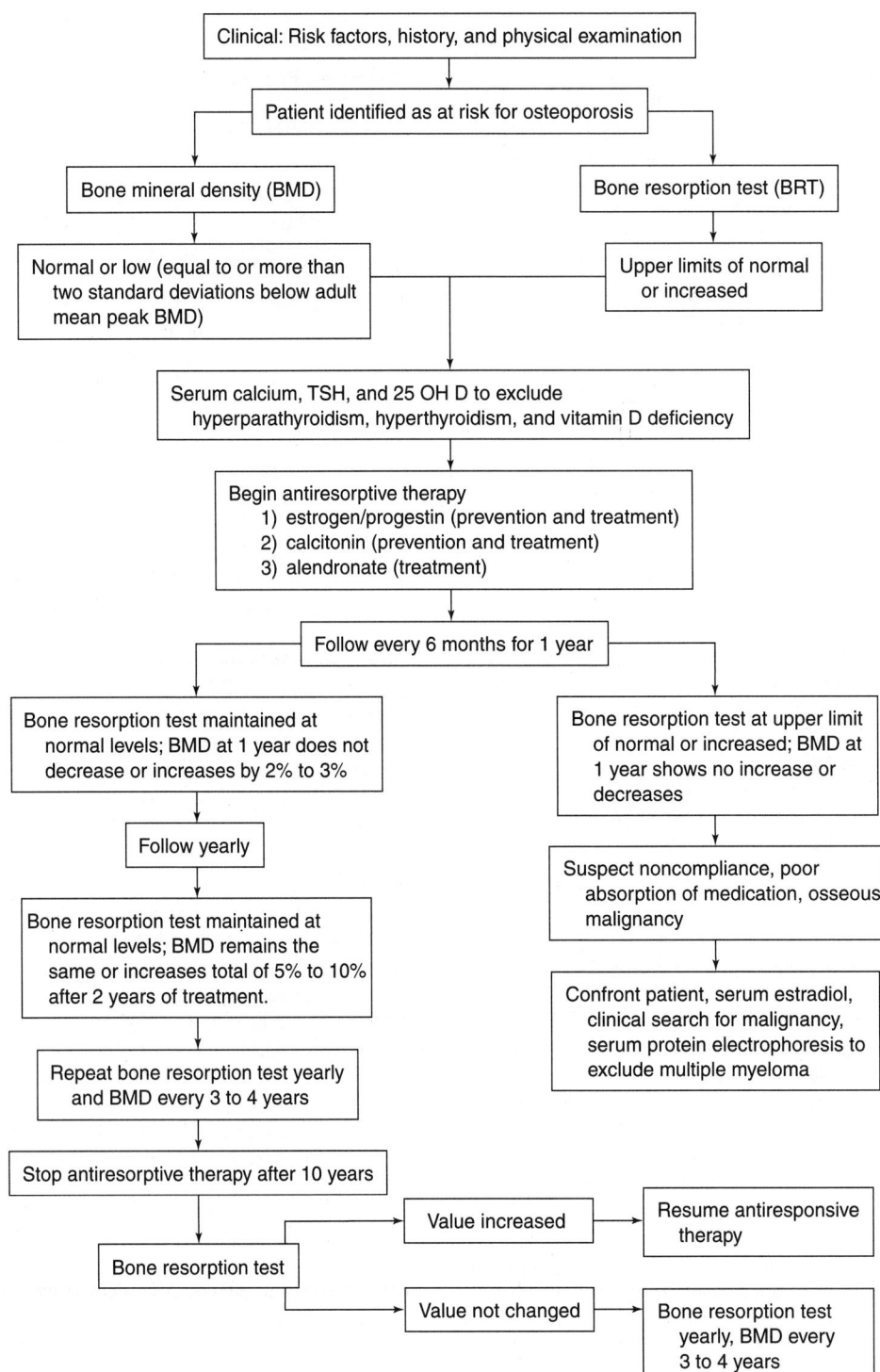

FIGURE 48-1 Osteoporosis: Guidelines for the use of bone mineral density and bone resorption testing. (Reproduced with permission from Geriatrics, Vol. 51, No. 4, April 1996, p 27. © Advanstar Communications Inc., Advanstar Communications Inc. retains all rights to this article.

sunlight and later by the liver and kidneys to its active form, 1,25 dihydroxyvitamin D, which functions in the intestine to enhance calcium absorption. Persons with inadequate exposure to sunlight or the elderly require supplemental vitamin D. Many foods are enriched with vitamin D, and calcium supplements often contain vitamin D. The recommended dosage is typically 200 to 400 IU/day, but higher doses may be required for patients with special needs.

Estrogen Replacement Therapy

Estrogen is an antiresorptive agent that reverses the metabolic changes of menopause by slowing the bone remodeling process and thus preventing bone loss. Some studies have actually indicated modest increases in bone mass secondary to estrogen use. ERT has also been associated with increased efficiency of calcium absorption.

ERT is most effective when implemented early, as close as possible to the onset of estrogen deficiency, before the bulk of the menopausal bone loss occurs; with early use, bone mass is maintained at a higher level. However, ERT has been shown to prevent bone loss even when therapy is initiated 10 to 15 years after menopause. The benefits of ERT persist only for the duration of treatment, so it should be taken indefinitely. When ERT is withdrawn, hormonal effects mirror those secondary to oophorectomy. Long-term therapy has been associated with the most favorable outcomes in terms of osteoporosis. Women receiving ERT for at least 6 years showed bone mass values 10% higher than those of untreated women and had a 50% reduction in hip and other fractures (Ross, 1996).

ERT is the most commonly prescribed treatment for women with osteoporosis. It has been estimated that widespread use of ERT could prevent 80% of vertebral fractures and lead to a 50% reduction in hip and distal radius fractures.

The effective dose for treatment of osteoporosis is 0.625 mg/day of conjugated equine estrogen. Some women may temporarily require doses of up to 1.25 mg/day to suppress menopausal symptoms. The minimal equivalent dose for synthetic estrogen is 20 μg/day. Transdermal delivery has been shown to be as effective as oral dosing. To prevent endometrial hyperplasia or cancer in women with intact uteri, exogenous estrogen must be opposed with a progestin (see Unit 11).

Many women are fearful of or reluctant to try ERT. Nonhormonal agents that are active at estrogen receptors are under investigation. When ERT is being considered, careful education will help the patient make an informed decision. The provider should present risk/benefit data and various dosing options (including continuous estrogen therapy, which is generally not associated with monthly bleeding). Obtaining a DEXA result may be an important influence on the decision to begin ERT.

Selective Estrogen Receptor Modulators

The selective estrogen receptor modulators (SERMs) have estrogenic activity in some tissues but not others. Raloxifene (Evista) is the first drug in this class to receive marketing approval. Large-scale studies have shown that raloxiphene prevented bone loss and increased bone mineral density in the total body, lower spine, and hip when compared to calcium-supplemented placebo. These skeletal benefits were achieved without estrogenic stimulation of uterine or breast tissue, and therefore there was no increased risk of endometrial or breast cancer. Increased rates of venous thrombotic events were similar to those associated with estrogen replacement therapy. The recommended dosage for raloxifene is 60 mg once daily ("FDA Committee Recommends Evista for Osteoporosis Prevention" (Nov. 21, 1997). Doctor's Guide to Medical and Other News; http://pslgroup.com/dg/47996.htm.)

Alendronate

Alendronate (Fosamax) is a third-generation biphosphanate, a synthetic analogue of endogenous pyrophosphate. It is an antiresorptive that is approved for the treatment of osteoporosis in postmenopausal women. Alendronate has been shown to increase bone density at all skeletal sites progressively and to reduce the incidence of vertebral fractures. Indications include DEXA results at least two standard deviations below young normal and a history of osteoporotic fracture. Future use for prophylaxis of osteoporosis is a possibility. Alendronate is a viable alternative for those who have contraindications to or are unwilling to use ERT. The effects of ERT given concurrently with alendronate have not been evaluated, although these drugs have, in practice, been used in combination.

The effective dosage for alendronate is 10 mg/day, taken a half-hour before breakfast with a full glass of water to maximize bioavailability. To protect the esophagus, the patient should refrain from eating or drinking and should remain in an upright position for 30 minutes after it is taken. The relatively few adverse effects include mild gastrointestinal symptoms, musculoskeletal pain, and headache. Persons with esophageal obstruction or a creatinine clearance of less than 30 should not take alendronate. Adequate intake of calcium and vitamin D is important to support the process of increasing bone density.

Calcitonin

Calcitonin, a naturally occurring polypeptide, inhibits osteoclast activity and thus diminishes bone resorption. Miacalcin is an intranasal form of calcitonin that has virtually replaced the less convenient injectable type. In addition to its antiresorptive qualities, calcitonin has an analgesic effect for osteoporotic fracture pain in many patients and is therefore useful in established osteoporosis. Studies evaluating intranasal calcitonin's effect on fracture risk are underway.

Because Miacalcin's effect on BMD principally involves the vertebrae and is more modest than that of ERT or alendronate, it is usually used when those alternatives are contraindicated or when its analgesic effect is sought. One puff (0.09 mL) contains the daily dose of 200 IU. Nostrils should be alternated daily. In contrast to the injectable form, which is associated with several side effects, Miacalcin is well tolerated. Adverse effects include nasal irritation, fatigue, and flulike symptoms.

Sodium Fluoride

Sodium fluoride has preceded many of the medications currently used in the treatment of osteoporosis: it has been used in Europe for more than 30 years. It has the effect of actually increasing bone formation. Some earlier studies, however, showed that this newly formed bone was inelastic and brittle and was possibly associated with an increased risk of hip fracture. As a result, sodium fluoride fell into disfavor in the United States. Newer research, using a slow-release form of sodium fluoride combined with calcium supplementation, has shown promising results in terms of increased spine and hip density and reduction in vertebral fracture risk (Pak et al, 1995).

Testosterone

Testosterone therapy may be a treatment option for osteoporosis in elderly men or those with hypogonadism who have low testosterone levels. Administration of this hormone has been associated with an increase in bone mass; however, long-term effects have not been fully investigated. Modes of administration include intramuscular injection every 2 to 3 weeks or a transdermal scrotal patch every 24 hours.

Complementary Approaches

The effect of soy protein on bone density is under investigation. Soy protein is a rich source of isoflavones, vegetable substances also present in other plants, that are called phytoestrogens because they have weak estrogenic activity. A vegetarian diet high in phytoestrogens may afford protection against cancer and heart disease (Knight & Eden, 1995). Animal studies suggest that phytoestrogens inhibit bone resorption and stimulate bone mineralization (Tsutsumi, 1995). A daily intake of 25 to 40 g of soy has been recommended for women wishing to use this approach to osteoporosis prevention or amelioration (Jaret, 1995). Complementary modalities that improve strength, flexibility, or balance should be considered for the osteoporosis patient. Yoga, t'ai chi, and other movement therapies may be helpful.

REHABILITATION

The psychological effects of osteoporosis often lead to adaptations that may actually speed the progression of the disease. Aside from issues related to negative body image from vertebral fractures, those with any type of prior osteoporotic fracture may be very fearful of reinjury and its resultant disability. Another fracture could signify permanent loss of independence or nursing home admission. To avoid reinjury, people with osteoporosis often tend to limit activity by remaining at home and keeping exercise to a minimum, moving carefully and as little as possible. These measures hinder the maintenance of bone density and lead to loss of protective factors such as strength, balance, and flexibility. Staying indoors deprives the person of sunlight exposure, a source of vitamin D. Inactivity and social isolation often eventually lead to depression.

Rehabilitative measures should address both physical and psychological needs. Because treatment at virtually any point during the disease process can help prevent further bone loss, and even small increases in bone mass decrease future fracture risk, appropriate therapy should be promptly initiated. If pain is an issue, analgesia, ranging from acetaminophen and anti-inflammatory agents to a comprehensive, multimodal approach, should be prescribed. A lumbar support cushion or other type of back orthotic device may help improve lumbar extensor strength and relieve the symptoms of back pain related to osteoporosis (Huffman, 1996).

Exercise is a key component of both rehabilitative and preventive approaches. A physical therapy referral for evaluation of exercise capacity and creation of an individualized exercise program may be helpful. Strength training (weight-bearing activity), the principal element of an exercise program for women of any age, imparts the following benefits:

- Maintenance of bone density
- Flexibility, balance, and agility, leading to reduced risk of falls and enhanced vigor and coordination

- Increased muscle mass, which cushions the skeleton and lowers fracture risk in the event of a fall.

High-impact exercise, such as jogging or jumping rope, may need to be avoided by those with significant disease or a history of fractures, because such exercise may overstress the vertebrae. Likewise, exercises involving flexion or rotation of the spine (eg, golf, bowling) may be contraindicated. Milder weight-bearing exercises, such as walking or cycling, are preferable. Exercises that strengthen the musculature supporting the spine are beneficial. These include back extension and isometric, non-flexion abdominal strengthening maneuvers. Sit-ups are contraindicated for those with osteoporotic vertebral fractures.

Patients should be encouraged to engage in activities outside the home that include exposure to sunlight, exercise, and maintenance of social contacts. Persons with social attachments have displayed better prognoses after hip fractures than those who are socially isolated.

Prevention of falls is important in reducing the incidence of fractures. Specific suggestions are noted in the section on self-care below. Analgesic medications that cause drowsiness or affect coordination may need to be avoided because they could lead to a greater potential for injury from falls.

Special Diagnostic and Treatment Considerations

AGE

Because osteoporosis is a disease associated with aging, this theme is woven throughout the sections of this chapter. One outstanding consideration, however, is vitamin D. Plasma levels of several forms of vitamin D have been found to decline with age. This has been attributed to decreased exposure to sunlight and diminished intestinal absorption of vitamin D. Other conjectures include decreased ability of the skin to produce vitamin D in response to light and increased use of sunscreen to prevent skin cancer (Riggs & Melton, 1995). Whatever the cause, the provider must ensure that elderly patients being treated for osteoporosis receive adequate amounts of vitamin D.

CULTURE

Culture may influence the treatment of osteoporosis. The principal consideration is nutrition. Culturally specific dietary intake should be carefully evaluated for calcium content, because dairy products may be excluded. Supplementation is indicated for persons with inadequate calcium intake.

Teaching and Self-Care

Once the diagnosis has been established, patients with osteoporosis must first be instructed regarding the nature of the illness and its complications. It is important to inform them of the potential effectiveness of interventions initiated at virtually any time during the course of the disease. The clinician should strive to enhance patients' feelings of hopefulness, motivation, and personal efficacy related to care of the disease.

Patients should be well informed regarding their treatment options, which are now diverse and offer alternatives for the patient unwilling to take ERT. If medical therapy is prescribed, careful instructions regarding the mechanism of action, administration, and adverse effects should be provided. Patients should understand the importance of calcium therapy as an adjunct to the prescribed modalities. Knowing the calcium content in common foods (see Table 48-4) will help the provider and the patient evaluate dietary calcium intake to determine supplemental needs (see Table 48-5). Adequate intake of vitamin D must also be ensured.

Lifestyle modifications were noted above. Smokers or those with high alcohol or caffeine intake may require further education and behavioral support to deal with their habits. Those new to exercise should have appropriate health clearance and a clearly outlined, gradually progressive program. Patients should be informed to report any pain or extreme breathlessness associated with exercise. Instruction on proper body mechanics, with particular emphasis on avoidance of spinal flexion, should be provided. Patients should be advised to report new musculoskeletal pain because it may indicate a fracture.

Fall-prevention strategies are important for those with osteoporosis, especially those with a history of osteoporotic fractures. Alcohol intoxication and hypothermia both contribute to altered mental status and increased risk of falling. Patients should avoid lightheadedness by getting up slowly from a lying or sitting position. Adequate illumination, including night lights, should be available to prevent falls when ambulating at night. Footwear should be well fitted, with low, broad heels. Walking in socks or stockings on stairs, wood, or waxed floors should be avoided. Hip pads may be used for cushioning and preventing hip fractures. Clutter, wires, small pieces of furniture, and loose throw rugs should be removed from halls and walkways. Area rugs should be well anchored, and nonskid mats or strips should be used on surfaces that may get wet. Nonskid wax should be used on floors. Older or more debilitated persons may benefit from grab bars and a padded shower seat.

COMMUNITY RESOURCES

- National Osteoporosis Foundation, 1150 17th St. NW, Washington DC 20036, 202-223-2226, 800-223-9994: Information for patients and health care providers
- Calcium Information Center, Clinical Nutrition and Research Unit, Division of Nephrology, Hypertension, and Clinical Pharmacology, Oregon Health Sciences University, 3314 SW U.S. Veterans Hospital Rd., Portland, OR 97201, 800-321-2681: Patient information, "Hot Topics" educational messages, consultation for clinicians, opportunity for patients to talk with a health care provider
- Older Women's League, 666 Eleventh St. NW, Suite 700, Washington DC 20001, 202-783-6686, 800-TAKE-OWL: Patient booklet and fact sheet
- Endocrine Nurses Society, 2258 SE Darling Ave., Gresham, OR 97080, 503-215-1082: Speakers' bureau for osteoporosis educational programs presented by nurses

REFERRAL POINTS AND CLINICAL WARNINGS

Because osteoporosis is a chronic, degenerative disease, emergency referral is generally not an issue. The only indication for an immediate referral would be in the case of an acute fracture that requires evaluation and intervention. Signs and symptoms of fractures are discussed in Chapter 43. Minimal trauma can cause a fracture in an osteoporotic person.

■ ■ ■ CLINICAL PEARLS

- Fifty percent of people with vertebral fractures from osteoporosis have no recollection of back pain.
- BMD tends to be higher in African American and Hispanic women and lower in whites and Asians.
- Changes in bone density that are significant enough to show on DEXA may not be evident for at least 1 year.
- Osteoporosis may be detected on simple x-rays, but the changes become evident only after 30% to 40% of bone density has been lost.
- Attending to alterable risk factors is a prime component of osteoporosis prevention and detection of those with particular susceptibility to osteoporotic fractures.
- Throughout the life span, whenever calcium intake through diet is inadequate, supplementation is indicated.
- Lactose and vitamin D enhance the absorption of calcium, whereas fats, fiber, and oxalates decrease absorption.
- Plasma levels of vitamin D decrease with aging. Elderly persons being treated for osteoporosis must receive adequate amounts of vitamin D.
- Persons at high risk for osteoporosis should be screened for the disease because interventions at almost any stage can improve bone density or reduce the risk of fractures. Case finding is beneficial.

References

Arnaud, C. (1996). Osteoporosis: Using "bone markers" for diagnosis and monitoring. *Geriatrics, 51*(4), 24–30.

Browner, W.S., Pressman, A.R., Nevitt, M.C., Cauley, J.A., & Cummings, S.R. (1993). Association between low bone density and stroke in elderly women: The study of osteoporotic fractures. *Stroke, 24*(7), 940–946.

Galsworthy, T.D., & Wilson, P.L. (1996). Osteoporosis: It steals more than bone. *American Journal of Nursing, 96*(6), 27–33.

Huffman, G.B. (1996). Use of back orthotics in patients with osteoporosis. *American Family Physician, 54*(8), 2536.

Hurst, J.W. (Ed.). (1996). *Medicine for the practicing physician*, 4th ed. Stamford, CT: Appleton & Lange.

Jaret, P. (1995, October). The miracle bean. *Health*, pp. 30–32.

Kessenich, C.R. (1996a). Breaking the osteoporosis cycle. *Advance for Nurse Practitioners, 4*(8), 16–20.

Kessenich, C.R. (1996b). Update on pharmacologic therapies for osteoporosis. *Nurse Practitioner, 21*(8), 19–24.

Knight, D.C., & Eden, J.A. (1995). A review of the clinical effects of phytoestrogens. *Obstetrics and Gynecology, 87*(5), 897–904.

Lindsay, R. (1992). *Osteoporosis: A guide to diagnosis, prevention, and treatment.* New York: Raven Press.

Maher, A.B., Salmond, S.W., & Pellino, T.A. (Eds.). (1994). *Orthopaedic nursing.* Philadelphia: W.B. Saunders.

Men are at risk for osteoporosis too. (1996). *Medical World News, 64*(10), 8.

New York State Department of Health (producer). (March 22, 1996). *Osteoporosis teleconference.* Albany: New York State Department of Health.

Pak, Y.C., Kakhaee, K., Adams-Hunt, B., Piziak, V., Petersen, R.D., & Poindexter, J.R. (1995). Treatment of postmenopausal osteoporosis with slow-release sodium fluoride. *Annals of Internal Medicine, 123*(6), 401–408.

Riggs, B.L., & Melton III, L.J. (Eds.) (1995). *Osteoporosis: Etiology, diagnosis, and management.* Philadelphia: Lippincott-Raven.

Ross, P.D. (1996). Osteoporosis: Frequency, consequences, risk factors. *Archives of Internal Medicine, 156,* 1399–1411.

Tsutsumi, N. (1995). Effect of coumestrol on bone metabolism in organ culture. *Biological and Pharmacological Bulletin, 18*(7), 1012–1015.

Suggested Reading List

Browner, W.S., Seeley, D.G., Vogt, T.M., & Cummings, S.R. (1991). Non-trauma mortality in elderly women with low bone density. *Lancet, 338,* 355–358.

Goroll, A.H., May, L.A., & Mulley, A.G. (1995). *Primary care medicine: Office evaluation and management of the adult patient.* Philadelphia: J.B. Lippincott.

Kessenich, C.R. (1997). Preventing and managing osteoporosis. *American Journal of Nursing, 97*(1), 16B–16D.

Kirk, J.K., & Spangler, J.G. (1996). Alendronate: A biphosphanate for treatment of osteoporosis. *American Family Physician, 54*(6), 2053–2060.

Lieberman, U.A., Weiss, S.R., Broll, J., et al. (1995). The effect of oral alendronate on bone mineral density and the incidence of fractures in postmenopausal osteoporosis. *N Engl J Med, 333*(22), 1437–1443.

Nelson, M.E., & Wernick, S. (1997). *Strong women stay young.* New York: Bantam.

Optimal calcium intake. (1994). *National Institute of Health Consensus Statement, 12*(4).

Sambrook, P.N. (1995). The treatment of postmenopausal osteoporosis. *N Engl J Med, 333*(22), 1495–1496.

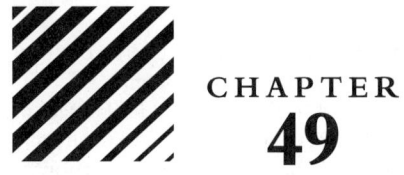

CHAPTER
49

Plantar Fasciitis

Maria Procopio Dugan, DO

Plantar heel pain is one of the most common orthopedic pain syndromes seen in a primary care practice. The true prevalence is not known. It affects both male and female patients of all ages but usually occurs in middle-aged to elderly patients or athletes. There are a multitude of potential causes of the painful heel syndrome (also known as heel spur syndrome and subcalcaneal pain), which can lead to some diagnostic uncertainty.

ANATOMY, PHYSIOLOGY, AND PATHOLOGY

The plantar fascia, or aponeurosis, is a fibrous band of connective tissue in the sole that extends proximally from the medial calcaneal tuberosity to the metatarsal heads. The central portion, which originates from the medial calcaneus, is the thickest and narrowest, with fibers arranged longitudinally. The thinner and smaller lateral and medial portions cover the abductor digiti minimi and abductor hallucis muscles. Distally, the fascia widens and thins, dividing into five rays that attach to each toe (Fig. 49-1).

The plantar fascia provides stability to the arch of the foot and functions through a windlass-type mechanism to depress the metatarsal heads and raise the longitudinal arch (Hicks, 1954). This occurs when the toes are dorsiflexed, passively pulling the fascia under the metatarsal heads, which causes the fascia to tighten, thereby shortening the distance between the heel and the forefoot and increasing the height of the arch. The work of raising the arch is done by body weight; no muscle is directly involved in the mechanism. Through the windlass effect, the plantar fascia and the bony and ligamentous support of the foot maintain the arch during weight bearing. During normal gait, the foot pronates at heel strike to become flexible enough to conform to the ground and partially absorb the initial contact force (Karr, 1994). At toe-off, the plantar fascia becomes taut, which aids in the resupination of the foot.

Inflammation and microtears of the plantar fascia near its origin from the medial calcaneal tubercle appear to be the pathologic process responsible for pain. If left untreated, or if trauma is permitted to continue, the inflammatory response will progress and thickening, fibrosis, chronic granulomatous tissue, or mucinoid degeneration of the plantar fascia will ensue (Furey, 1975; Davis et al, 1994; Schepsis et al, 1991).

Entrapment of the medial calcaneal nerves, the lateral plantar nerve, or the nerve to the abductor digiti minimi has also been implicated in the etiology of plantar heel pain. Chronic inflammation and subsequent changes in the plantar fascia may predispose a person to nerve entrapment. A heel spur also may play a role in the development of an entrapment neuropathy of the nerve to the abductor digiti minimi because this nerve passes close to the bony ridge of the medial calcaneal tubercle,

the site of the spur, if present. Chronic inflammation, fibrosis, and thickening of the plantar fascia at its origin, with formation or growth of a heel spur, may cause compression of the nerve (Fig. 49-2).

EPIDEMIOLOGY

The most common etiology of plantar heel pain is plantar fasciitis, an inflammation of the plantar fascia at its insertion on the calcaneus. Additional etiologies include stress fractures and entrapment of the lateral plantar nerve. More remote causes are fracture, calcaneal periostitis, plantar fascia rupture, fat pad syndrome (heel pad atrophy), seronegative spondyloarthropathies, gout, and rheumatoid arthritis. The painful heel syndrome remains a difficult problem to manage because of its protracted clinical course. Fortunately, 90% of the patients respond to conservative measures, leaving just 10% who require further evaluation and consideration for surgical intervention (Davis et al, 1994).

DIAGNOSTIC CRITERIA

The diagnosis of plantar fasciitis can generally be made on clinical grounds with a careful history and physical exam:

- Unilateral medial plantar pain in patients (70% to 80%)
- Gradual onset
- Aching or burning
- Maximal pain during the first few steps from bed or from rising after prolonged sitting
- Pain initially improves after 5 to 10 minutes of walking
- Pain recurs as the day progresses
- Training errors or sudden increase in activity
- Occupation that requires a lot of standing or walking
- Sudden weight gain
- Localized tenderness at the insertion of the plantar fascia onto the medial tubercle of the calcaneus
- Thickened, tight, or nodular plantar fascia
- Biomechanical abnormalities—pes planus (flat foot), pes cavus (high arch), excessive pronation
- Worsening of pain with passive dorsiflexion of toes
- Restricted dorsiflexion of the ankle from tight Achilles tendon or soleus and gastrocnemius muscles.

HISTORY AND PHYSICAL EXAM

The typical patient with plantar heel pain describes pain that is of gradual onset, not associated with a specific traumatic event. In the nonathletic patient, the pain may occur sponta-

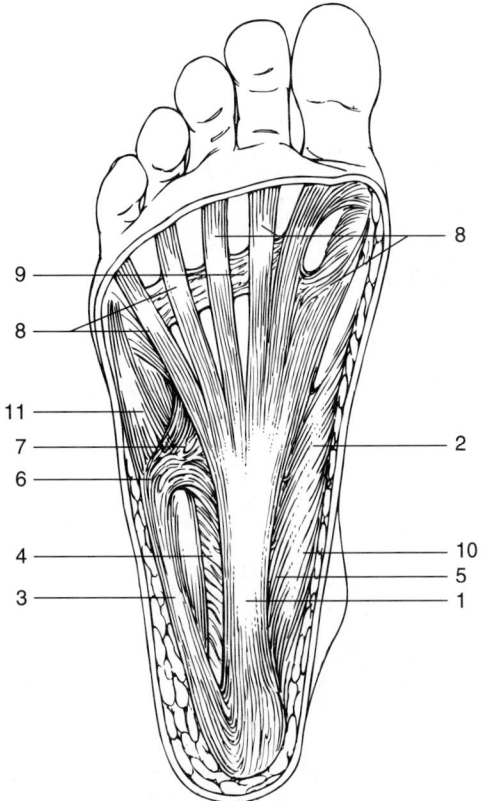

FIGURE 49-1 Plantar aponeurosis. (*1*) Central component, ie, plantar fascia, (*2*) Medial component, (*3*) Lateral component, (*4*) Lateral plantar sulcus, (*5*) Medial plantar sulcus, (*6*) Lateral crux, (*7*) Medialcrux, (*8*) Superficial longitudinal tracts, (*9*) Transverse superficial tract, (*10*) Abductor hallucis muscle, and (*11*) Abductor digiti quinti muscle. (Sarrafian, S.K. (1983). *Anatomy of the foot and ankle.* Philadelphia: JB Lippincott.)

neously, or it may follow a sudden weight gain, the start of an exercise program, or a sudden increase in activity. It is a common condition late in pregnancy. In athletes, the condition is usually related to training errors such as rapidly increasing the mileage, intensity, or duration of workouts, running on steep hills, changing shoes or training surfaces, and biomechanical factors (Davis

et al, 1994). The continued use of shoes with a badly worn heel also contributes to the development of plantar fasciitis.

The pain is usually localized to the plantar medial aspect of the heel at the site of the plantar fascial attachment to the medial tubercle of the calcaneus (DeMaio et al, 1993). Radiation of the pain into the arch and the medial side of the foot occasionally occurs. The pain is described as burning or aching and will gradually worsen if left untreated.

Patients characteristically complain of pain that is maximal during the first few steps from bed or from rising after prolonged sitting. This pain eases after 5 to 10 minutes of walking but recurs later in the day with normal activities, especially with walking on concrete or hard surfaces. The condition is usually not disabling, but it may limit weight-bearing activities, especially running and jumping. The pain is usually unilateral; therefore, if bilateral heel pain occurs, a systemic disorder must be ruled out (Table 49-1).

The physical exam should include the entire lower extremity, with attention to the anatomic and biomechanical factors that predispose to plantar fasciitis. The patient should be examined standing and walking to evaluate the arch during weight bearing. This may reveal the existence of static biomechanical abnormalities such as pes planus and pes cavus, or an abnormality of gait such as excessive pronation of the foot. Range of motion testing, motor and sensory testing, vascular evaluation, and palpation for the location of tenderness should be included in the exam.

Localized tenderness at the insertion of the plantar fascia onto the medial tubercle of the calcaneus is pathognomonic for plantar fasciitis. Tenderness less commonly occurs in the medial longitudinal arch of the foot and the central heel. Passive dorsiflexion of the toes and ankle, or having the patient stand on the toes, may reproduce or worsen symptoms by tightening the plantar fascia (Davis et al, 1994; Karr, 1994). Passive abduction and eversion of the foot is another provocative test that indicates involvement of the lateral plantar nerve (Davis et al, 1994). Patients often have restricted dorsiflexion of the ankle because of a tight Achilles tendon or gastrocnemius and soleus muscle tightness. Localized swelling is usually absent, but the plantar fascia may be thickened, tight, or nodular (Seto & Brewster, 1994).

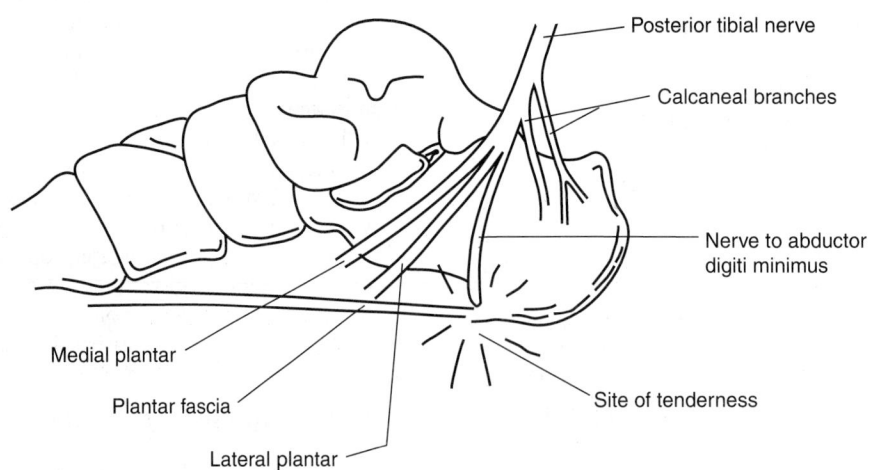

FIGURE 49-2 Plantar fasciitis. Note site of tenderness on plantar aspect of heel at origin of plantar fascia off calcaneus. Also note course of nerve abductor digiti minimus. (Adapted from Baster, D.E. Thigpen, C.M. (1984). Heel pain: operative results. *Foot and Ankle 5*(1), p 16–25. Fig. 9-18.)

TABLE 49-1	Differential Diagnosis of the Painful Heel Syndrome
LOCAL FACTORS	**SYSTEMIC FACTORS**
Plantar fasciitis	Rheumatoid arthritis
Stress fracture	Juvenile rheumatoid arthritis
Nerve entrapment	Gout/pseudogout
Adductor digiti minimi	Sarcoidosis
Medial calcaneal nerve	Ankylosing spondylitis
Lateral plantar nerve	Idiopathic skeletal hyperostosis
Heel pad atrophy	Reiter's syndrome
Tarsal tunnel syndrome	Psoriatic arthritis
Calcaneal apophysitis (Sever's disease)	Behçet's syndrome
Calcaneal fracture	Infections
Plantar fascia rupture	Tuberculosis
Osteomyelitis	Gonorrhea
Tumors	
Osteoid osteoma	
Osteoblastoma	
Simple and aneurysmal cysts	

Other etiologies for plantar heel pain (see Table 49-1) must be excluded. If the pain has an acute onset and there is localized swelling or ecchymosis of the plantar fascia or heel, the provider must suspect a calcaneal fracture or plantar fascia rupture. The latter is also associated with prior corticosteroid injection into the planter fascia (Sellman, 1994). A patient with tarsal tunnel syndrome will have a burning pain radiating into the toes that is worse at night and is often associated with paresthesias and motor deficits. It is more common in women, and there should be a Tinel's sign over the tarsal tunnel. Systemic inflammatory disorders are not uncommon in patients with plantar heel pain. Patients with seronegative spondyloarthropathies are especially prone to develop plantar heel pain, and the foot is second only to the knee as the site of initial presentation in rheumatoid arthritis. Gout can also cause plantar fascia inflammation. These should be ruled out if the provider is clinically suspicious or if a course of treatment 6 to 12 months long produces no results.

DIAGNOSTIC STUDIES

Most cases of plantar heel pain or plantar fasciitis can be diagnosed by the history and physical exam alone. X-rays, bone scans, and blood tests are used when patients have atypical presentations.

X-rays of the heel and foot should be obtained in the oblique and standing anteroposterior and lateral projections. The radiograph is usually normal, but it can rule out unusual causes of heel pain such as fracture, tumor, or calcaneal cysts. It may reveal a traction heel spur in up to 50% of patients with plantar fasciitis. It is important to note, however, that 15% to 25% of asymptomatic adults also have heel spurs (Wolgin et al, 1994; Tanz, 1963). A heel spur is a common finding in rheumatoid arthritis, idiopathic skeletal hyperostosis, ankylosing spondylitis, psoriatic arthritis, and Reiter's syndrome. Although once thought to be an etiology of heel pain, the heel spur is now believed to be more likely the result of inflammation or trauma (Davis et al, 1994; DeMaio et al, 1993; Seto & Brewster, 1994). Heel spur is not considered the cause of the pain. A bone scan is useful when a calcaneal stress fracture is suspected or when the pain fails to respond to treatment within 6 months. Use of magnetic resonance imaging in the evaluation of recalcitrant heel pain is investigational.

TREATMENT OPTIONS, EXPECTED OUTCOMES, AND COMPREHENSIVE MANAGEMENT

Plantar fasciitis is best treated conservatively. Effective management requires the use of multiple treatment modalities, patient education, and patience (Table 49-2). Improvement is slow and gradual and may take up to a year. Initial treatment should address the local inflammatory process, underlying mechanical problems, and training errors.

Because plantar fasciitis is viewed as an overuse syndrome that causes inflammation of the plantar fascia, rest should be the first-line treatment in both athletes and nonathletes. Running and jumping should be avoided in the acute stages and cross-training (eg, swimming, bicycling) encouraged. Patients whose jobs require a lot of walking or standing may need a period of time off work, or job modification. When symptoms have improved, patients should be instructed to increase their activity or exercise levels slowly, using exacerbation of symptoms as their guide. Patients who did not exercise regularly should begin a walking program.

Nonsteroidal anti-inflammatory drugs (NSAIDs) and ice massage applied for 20 minutes three or four times a day, espe-

TABLE 49-2	Treatment of Plantar Fasciitis	
STEP 1: 1st VISIT		**STEP 3: 7–24 WEEKS**
Rest—limitation of activity		*Improved/resolved*
NSAID		Continued stretching
Ice		Strengthening
1/4″–1/2″ heel cup/arch support (over the counter)		Prevent recurrence—avoid overuse or training errors
Stretching—plantar fascia and Achilles tendon stretch, gastrocnemius and soleus stretch		*No improvement*
		Night splint or casting
Massage to the heel and arch of the foot		Continue stretching, orthotics, and NSAID
Proper footwear		**STEP 4: 6–12 MONTHS**
Weight loss if indicated		*Continued pain*
STEP 2: 4–6 WEEKS		Confirm diagnosis
Improvement		Rule out systemic disease
Continue stretching		Bone scan—Rule out stress fracture/DJD
Taper NSAID		EMG—Rule out entrapment neuropathy
Increase activity		Consider surgery (12 months)
No improvement		
X-ray		
Steroid injection (methylprednisolone acetate; may repeat in 2–3 weeks)		
Address abnormal biomechanics		
Custom orthoses if indicated		
Stretching		
NSAID		
Arch taping		

Source: DeMaio et al, 1993.

cially after activity, will help to decrease the inflammation. No one NSAID is more effective than another. Although NSAIDs appear to be more useful early in the course of disease and are less beneficial in chronic, recalcitrant cases, they remain helpful throughout as part of a comprehensive treatment plan.

Stretching and strengthening exercises of the foot and lower leg are vital to successful treatment and have been cited by patients as the most effective treatment, with an 83% response rate (Steinberg et al, 1992). Stretching exercises should emphasize the plantar fascia, Achilles tendon, gastrocnemius, and soleus (Table 49-3). Invariably, patients with plantar fasciitis have tight calf muscles, Achilles tendons, and heel cords. Stretching will reduce tension on the plantar fascia, improve flexibility, and thus help to prevent recurrence. Proper stretching should create a gentle pulling sensation in the stretched muscle and tendon. There should be no increase in pain and no bouncing. Because the most intense pain occurs with the first morning step, stretching should be done on arising, and the patient should step into shoes with a heel lift or cushion or arch support (eg, Birkenstocks or running shoes). The exercise prescription should be as follows:

- Gentle sustained stretch for 10 to 30 seconds
- At least 10 repetitions of each exercise five or six times daily, including before getting out of bed and before standing after prolonged sitting (Davis et al, 1994; Quaschnick, 1996).

The rehabilitation program to strengthen the intrinsic and extrinsic muscles of the foot should not begin until symptoms improve (DeMaio et al, 1993; Chandler & Kibler, 1993). These simple but important exercises are toe and towel curls, picking up objects off the floor with just the toes, resisted ankle dorsiflexion, and heel raises. The exercises should be done three or four times a day for at least 6 to 8 weeks (DeMaio et al, 1993; Quaschnick, 1996; Chandler & Kibler, 1993). The role of other physical therapy modalities appears limited.

The importance of proper footwear should not be overlooked. Athletic shoes should have a firm heel, good heel cushioning, and arch support to help eliminate stress on the plantar fascia. Flat, flimsy, nonsupportive shoes and high heels must be avoided. Old shoes with worn heels should be discarded. An in-shoe heel cup or pad of $\frac{1}{4}''$ to $\frac{1}{2}''$ decreases tension on the plantar fascia and should be used in step 1 of treatment. In general, the pad should be placed in both shoes to avoid creating a leg length discrepancy. Arch taping or strapping may also be used, and if helpful a more permanent device can be prescribed. Patients in need of arch support should initially be instructed to try the over-the-counter variety. The orthosis is designed to restore normal biomechanics by maintaining the subtalar joint in the neutral position and supporting the longitudinal arch. If pain continues in patients with pes planus or hyperpronation, then custom orthoses may be indicated. The treatment of pes cavus with orthotic devices has not been very successful (Quaschnick, 1996).

If there has been no improvement in symptoms after 4 to 6 weeks of treatment, a corticosteroid injection into the calcaneal attachment of the plantar fascia may be beneficial. A local anesthetic, preferably a long-acting one, should be administered with the corticosteroid (eg, methylprednisolone acetate 20 to 40 mg/1 cc bupivacaine). Pain should be localized and the needle inserted into the medial aspect of the heel and directed to the tender point. The injection is extremely painful and must never be given directly through the sole or into the heel pad. No more than two injections should be given because of the associated risk of plantar fascia rupture and heel pad atrophy (Karr, 1994; Sellman, 1996).

The use of night splints or casting is of benefit to those with recalcitrant pain and should be used before contemplating surgery (Gill & Kiebzak, 1996; Tisdel & Harper, 1996; Wapner & Sharkey, 1991). Patients studied had heel pain for an average of 12 months. The night splint is designed to hold the ankle in 5° of dorsiflexion, thus preventing the contraction of the Achilles tendon and plantar fascia when the foot naturally assumes a plantar-flexed position during sleep. The night splint is worn for 3 months only while asleep and has a response rate of approximately 80% (Wapner & Sharkey, 1991). A short-leg walking cast with the foot slightly dorsiflexed and a toe plate extension distally provides constant stretch to the plantar fascia. Its use for 4 to 6 weeks has been shown to be 85% effective (Tisdel & Harper, 1996).

Most cases of plantar heel pain resolve with nonsurgical management. A minimum of 6 months of conservative care should be given before considering a surgical option. If even limited improvement is seen, nonoperative modalities should continue for another 6 months (Davis et al, 1994; Karr, 1994). Patients for whom surgery is considered usually have significant pain and disability in activities of daily living or in activities considered to be important to them.

TABLE 49-3   Stretching Exercises

STRETCHING EXERCISES FOR PLANTAR FASCIITIS

Plantar Fascia	Dorsiflexion of toes—knee bent and straight Friction massage to heel and arch of foot Cylinder roll—with cylinder (can, bottle, weight) on floor, roll it back and forth across the arch
Achilles tendon	Slant box—stand on board with block under front edge Flex knee while keeping heel on floor Sitting—dorsiflexion of ankle using rubber tubing across ball of foot
Gastrocnemius	Dorsiflexion of ankle while keeping knee extended; may be done standing leaning against a wall, on a stair, or sitting using a rubber tubing or towel
Soleus	Dorsiflexion of ankle while the knee is flexed; may be done standing leaning against a wall, on a stair, or sitting using a rubber tubing or towel

STRENGTHENING EXERCISES FOR MUSCLES OF THE FOOT

Toe curls	Curl toes, squeeze and hold, then extend
Towel curls or gathers	Patient sits with feet on a towel and curls the toes to gather the towel under the arch
Pick-ups	Pick up marbles, pens, pencils off the floor using only the toes
Resisted dorsiflexion of the ankle	Second person uses a towel or rubber tubing wrapped around the dorsal aspect of the foot to gently resist the patient's dorsiflexion
Heel raises	Standing on step or stair, raise heel to stand on toes and drop heel past horizontal

The type of surgical procedure used varies with the patient. The goal is to decompress the site of the origin of the plantar fascia. Commonly used procedures include limited plantar fascia release and decompression of the lateral plantar nerve, the medial calcaneal nerve, or the nerve to the adductor digiti minimi. Procedures are done with and without excision of the heel spur. Regardless of technique, risks of surgery include continued pain and decreased strength and function of the plantar fascia and arch by disruption of the windlass mechanism (De-Maio et al, 1993).

TEACHING AND SELF-CARE

Prevention of plantar heel pain, whether primary or secondary, relies on patient education and the principles discussed above. Stretching and strengthening of the ankle and foot must continue. Normal range of motion of the ankle is helpful in avoiding functional biomechanical deficits that contribute to heel pain development. Running on hard surfaces (concrete) or sand and climbing or running hills also are strongly associated with heel pain. Weight loss may be appropriate. The key features of prevention are:

- Maintain strength and flexibility of the ankle, calf musculature, and foot.
- Correct biomechanical abnormalities with permanent orthoses.
- Participate in a proper training regimen.
- Use proper footwear with an extended heel counter; discard worn shoes. Avoid flat, nonsupportive shoes and high heels.
- Maintain proper body weight.

COMMUNITY RESOURCES

- *Runner's World* Online/Runner's Guide to Home Remedies—Plantar Fasciitis, www.runnersworld.com: Definitions, symptoms, causes, self-treatment, alternative exercises, preventive measures
- *Wheeler's Textbook of Orthopaedics*—Plantar Fasciitis, http://medmedia.com/o12/104.htm: General information, pathophysiology, symptoms, laboratory studies, x-rays, nonoperative and surgical treatment
- Virtual Podiatry Hospital—Heel Pain/Plantar Fasciitis, http://www.podiatryinfo.com/vphtml/heel.html: General information, self-help tips
- American Podiatric Medical Association, 9312 Old Georgetown Rd., Bethesda, MD 20814-1698, 301-571-9200, askapma@apma.org

REFERRAL POINTS AND CLINICAL WARNINGS

A referral to an orthopedic surgeon or a podiatrist is needed in only a few instances: patients with biomechanical abnormalities who require custom orthoses, and those who have had no response to treatment after 6 to 12 months. Depending on the primary care provider's resources and expertise, a patient may also need referral for treatment with a night splint or cast. Referral is also needed for patients with clear symptoms of nerve entrapment (a positive Tinel's sign or paresthesias) that have not responded to the initial treatment plan. Referral should be made to an orthopedic surgeon with expertise in foot and ankle surgery or to a skilled podiatric surgeon.

■ ■ ■ □ **CLINICAL PEARLS**

- Examine the heels of the patient's shoes: badly worn heels can contribute to the development of plantar fasciitis.
- Pain associated with plantar fasciitis is usually unilateral. If bilateral pain occurs, a systemic disorder must be ruled out.
- Localized tenderness at the insertion of the plantar fascia onto the medial tubercle is pathognomonic for plantar fasciitis.
- Heel spurs are no longer thought to be an etiology of heel pain.

EDITOR'S NOTE:
COMPLEMENTARY APPROACHES

A general discussion of complementary approaches can be found in Chapter 3. The following, while not an exhaustive list, are some complementary approaches being used for this condition. Additional information on these approaches, including precautions, can be found in Appendices A and B. Providers need to assess for the use of complementary approaches as part of the patient's history, as they may impact conventional therapies, and patients may not volunteer this information unless specifically asked. Efficacy of many complementary approaches is not as well documented as that of conventional therapies. Providers need to read the literature before suggesting these complementary approaches.

- Complementary Modalities
  Acupuncture
  Massage therapy

References

Chandler, T., & Kibler, W. (1993). A biomechanical approach to the prevention, treatment, and rehabilitation of plantar fasciitis. *Foot and Ankle International, 17*(9), 527–532.

Davis, P., Severus, E., & Baxter, D. (1984). Painful heel syndrome: Results of nonoperative treatment. *Foot and Ankle International, 15*(10), 531–534.

DeMaio, M., Paine, R., Mangine, R., & Drez, D. (1993). Plantar fasciitis. *Orthopedics, 16*(10), 1153–1163.

Furey, J. (1975). Plantar fasciitis: The painful heel syndrome. *Journal of Bone Joint Surgery, 57A,* 672–673.

Gill, L., & Kiebzak, G. (1996). Outcome of nonsurgical treatment for plantar fasciitis. *Foot and Ankle International, 17*(9), 527–532.

Hicks, J. (1954). Mechanics of the foot II: The plantar aponeurosis and the arch. *Journal of Anatomy, 88,* 25–31.

Karr, S. (1994). Subcalcaneal heel pain. *Orthopedic Clinics of North America, 25*(1), 161–174.

Quaschnick, M. (1996). The diagnosis and management of plantar fasciitis. *Nurse Practitioner, 21*(4), 50–63.

Schepsis, A., Leach, R., & Gorsyca, J. (1991). Plantar fasciitis: Etiology, treatment, surgical results, and review of literature. *Clinical Orthopedics, 266,* 185–196.

Sellman, J. (1994). Plantar fascia rupture associated with corticosteroid injection. *Foot and Ankle International, 15*(7), 376–381.

Seto, J., & Brewster, E. (1994). Treatment approaches following foot and ankle injury. *Sports Medicine, 13*(4), 713–714.

Steinberg, G., Akins, C., & Baron, D. (1992). *Ramamurti's ortho-*

paedics in primary care, 2d ed. Baltimore, MD: Williams & Wilkins.

Tanz, S. (1963). Heel pain. *Clinical Orthopedics, 28,* 169–177.

Tisdel, C., & Harper, M. (1996). Chronic plantar heel pain: Treatment with a short leg walking cast. *Foot and Ankle International, 17*(1), 41–42.

Wapner, K., & Sharkey, P. (1991). The use of night splints for treatment of recalcitrant plantar fasciitis. *Foot and Ankle, 12*(3), 135–137.

Wolgin, M., Cook, C., Graham, C., & Mauldin, D. (1994). Conservative treatment of plantar heel pain: Long-term follow-up. *Foot and Ankle, 15*(3), 97–102.

CHAPTER

50

Temporomandibular Disorders

Edgar Fayans, DDS

Vague pain relating to the temporomandibular joint (TMJ) that resembled otalgia was first described by Costen in 1934. Since that time, temporomandibular disorders (TMDs) have been identified as Costen's syndrome, TMJ disease, TMJ syndrome, and trigeminal syndrome. Although TMD is mainly treated by dentists, this entity is complex and often requires a multidisciplinary approach. The primary care provider may elect to initiate immediate care and refer cases that recur to specialists. Frequently, patients seek different providers for diagnosis and relief.

TMJ articulation disorders and masticatory muscle disorders appear in the differential diagnosis of headache disorders, cranial neuralgias, and facial pain. Pain in and around the jaw can also be infective, metabolic, neoplastic, systemic, or referred. Diagnosis of jaw pain must progress by first ruling out the most significant or life-threatening findings. Pain from myocardial perfusion insufficiency can radiate to the mandible and be a sole finding (Balchelder et al, 1987). Intracranial and cervical spine lesions can cause pain around the jaw and can have significant consequences if undiagnosed (Polette, 1992). However, most TMDs are not related to these problems.

Pain from TMD of nonneurogenic origin is most often muscular, which may be a contributory factor in tension headaches. Another common origin of pain is the TMJ structure. Lack of concrete, agreed-on diagnostic criteria, however, has led to confusion in diagnosis and management. Patients may be referred from provider to provider in a continuous loop. Primary care providers, dentists, orthopedists, otolaryngologists, neurologists, rheumatologists, chiropractors, anesthesiologists, and acupuncturists all treat patients with chronic facial pain, but most management options are performed by dentists.

Recent literature about and recognition of this condition have brought significant changes in the management of TMDs. Recognition of related disorders has produced advances in management, although in certain patients the diagnosis and treatment are elusive. Common TMDs (especially those aggravated by stress) seem to be cyclic and diminish with age (NIH, 1996). Successful therapy may be simple palliation until symptoms abate and remission occurs.

ANATOMY, PHYSIOLOGY, AND PATHOLOGY

Facial pain relating to TMD may arise from neurogenic sources, muscles, the salivary glands, bone, the TMJ, the vascular system, the pharynx, the tongue, the mucosa, the eustachian tubes and ears, the skin, the teeth, the gingiva, or the ligaments. The following discussion focuses on the bones, the joint, the muscles, and other important structures (Fig. 50-1).

Anatomy

Both jaws—the maxilla and the mandible—have alveolar processes that connect to the roots of teeth with ligaments. The mandible has attachments from all the major muscles of mastication. It articulates with the maxillary teeth (occlusion) and the cranium at the temporal bone's glenoid fossa, just anterior to the ear.

The TMJ is a unique joint in the body. Unlike others, it has cartilaginous end plates and a hyaline cartilage disc between the bones. The TMJ is composed of a capsule surrounding the cartilaginous head of the mandible, the articular disc, and the articulating temporal bone surface. It has a muscle-assisted interarticular disc that has almost no healing capacity. The disc is mainly fibrous and is attached posteriorly to a superior elastic vascular bed (which produces synovial fluid) and to a ligament-like fibrous band inferiorly (which limits movement forward). The disc is bathed in synovial fluid, which lubricates, hydrates, and protects it from compression, deformation, and shear forces.

Physiology and Pathology

The TMJ slides completely out of its socket over the articular eminence as it translates forward almost two times the anterior-posterior width of the condylar head. The joint is under load even during sleeping hours. Jaw tone, in addition to being constantly adjusted with changes in head position and posture, is highly prone to increased tonus during stress. Microtrauma and repetitive abuse can also lead to significant joint derangement and joint crepitus and noises. If excessive pressure occurs, permanent deformation may cause surface contour irregularities, leading to pain, crepitus, clicking, or other noises. Acute trauma, when not absorbed by injuring the dentition or fracturing the jaw, may cause significant trauma in the joint. This may lead to hemarthrosis, perforations, disc separations, and inflammatory states, which may be temporary or permanent. Inflammation can lead to intersynovial volume increase (synovitis, capsulitis) without reabsorption. Fluid in one joint may increase the distance from the temporal bone and cause a lack of occlusion (space between posterior teeth) on this side and pain.

The ligaments that attach to the mandible and joints do not control movement until the extremes of motion (Posselt, 1989). When the jaw protrudes, the posterior fibrous zone that holds the disc, the temporomandibular ligament, the sphenomaxillary ligament, and the stylomandibular ligament prevent joint laxity. These ligaments, together with muscular tone, prevent dislocation of the jaw. Muscle and ligament laxity may lead to dislocation. The muscles and ligaments act bilaterally

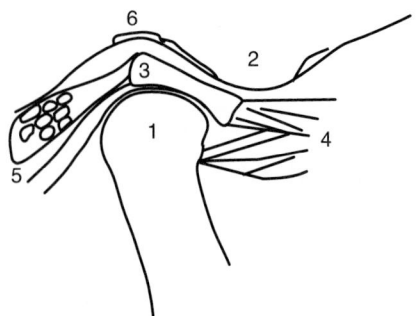

FIGURE 50-1 Anatomy of the jaw: (*1*) Condylar head, (*2*) Articular eminence, (*3*) Disc, (*4*) Lateral ptyerigoid muscle, (*5*) Retrodiscal tissues, (*6*) Glenoid fossa.

in straight protrusive movements and unilaterally during lateral excursions of the mandible. When going into a lateral movement, the joint on the same side as the jaw is moving rotates as the other joint translates. End points of closure and initial movement of the jaw are guided by planes established by the intermeshing of the dentition. If jaw movement is not synchronized with disc movement, the joint can malalign, causing pain.

The musculature is the cause of most TMDs (Sciffman et al, 1989). Joint movement irregularities or joint problems often create resultant myospasm or myositis. Myospasm and myositis often exist with relatively asymptomatic joints. The large elevator muscles (medial pterygoid, masseter, and temporalis) are responsible for the powerful crushing actions of the jaw.

Reflexes, which cause the jaw to snap open when the biting surfaces close into a hard object, synapse from the trigeminal spinal tract nucleus to the motor nucleus without any cortical input and cause sudden changes in muscle tone. A current explanation of the TMD condition is that it may be caused by brain stem inflammation along these tracts. Muscles also suddenly relax during the yawn reflex. Overstretching of muscles has been demonstrated to be an etiology in myospasm. The identifiable painful area in a muscle is often not the area that is in spasm; this is called a trigger point. Myospasm can occur because of protective muscle splinting. This muscle guarding is often a response to avoidance of a painful input.

Patients with persistent overuse of the masticatory muscles may demonstrate muscular hypertrophy. This is evident mainly in the masseter and temporalis muscle. Dental etiology should always be ruled out. Occlusion may cause disruption of normal biting. Premature contacts of teeth (teeth that do not allow the joint to settle completely in the fossa) can cause disharmony of the joint and musculature. The patient should be questioned as to the date of the last dental visit to rule out prosthetic dental interference. Continuous muscle splinting and other parafunctional habits can cause pressure spots in the joint apparatus and pain. Bruxism, the continuous intermeshing of teeth under force, usually at night, can overload the normal physiologic homeostasis of the joint.

Spasms in the stylohyoid and digastric muscles occur with some frequency and can mimic the symptoms of submandibular lymphadenopathy. Muscles in the soft palate or ligaments near the joint can cause abnormal pressures on the eustachian tube, causing altered hearing or "clogging" of the ears. Perhaps the most common muscles to go into spasm and demonstrate pain

are the masseter and the lateral pterygoid. The lateral pterygoid probably is responsible for disc and capsule movement, along with the initiation of movement of the mandible in opening. Because this muscle is short, powerful, and deep, pain here is not easily localized to its origin. When the masseter or temporalis goes into spasm, the patient can more easily identify the site of pain. Traction of the lateral pterygoid on the joint (from spasm) can cause otalgia. Incoordination of this muscle has been implicated in joint noises as well as deviation in the uniformity of jaw opening. If the lateral pterygoid suddenly contracts strongly when the jaw is initiating its closure stroke, a sudden anterior disc displacement can occur, causing acute pain, a popping noise, and malocclusion.

Drugs such as butyrophenones, phenothiazines, levodopa, anticholinergics, antihistamines, amphetamines, and cocaine have also been implicated in acute-onset jaw pain, deviations, and malocclusions. Serotonin reuptake inhibitors have been implicated in clenching, which may be resolved by dose adjustments or the addition of buspirone to the regimen (Ellison & Stanziani, 1993).

Other etiologies for TMDs can be from many sources. Neurogenic pain such as trigeminal neuralgia, glossopharyngeal neuralgia, and postherpetic pain are well documented but have unique presentations. Burning, throbbing pain of the mouth and surrounding structures can have several etiologies. This pain, if not fungal or the result of vitamin deficiencies or an allergic response, may be related to the sympathetic nervous system's effect on vascular beds.

Salivary gland dysfunction may relate to arthritis (Sjögren's syndrome); as a whole, TMDs have a much higher prevalence in patients with arthritis. Lyme disease with an arthritic presentation should be ruled out in a TMD workup. Viral infections such as wryneck and mumps may produce symptoms similar to those of TMDs. The patient with severe pain of sinus origin usually has a previous history, point tenderness, positional pain, and congestion. Pain over the temporal artery (overlying the TMJ) should alert the provider to obtain a sedimentation rate to rule out temporal or cranial arteritis, which can swiftly lead to ipsilateral blindness, or central nervous system involvement.

EPIDEMIOLOGY

Patients with TMDs number more than 10 million (NIH, 1996). TMDs are difficult to discuss from an epidemiologic viewpoint because of their multiple diagnoses and presentations. Diverse pain conditions such as arthritis, growth disorders, connective tissue diseases, Lyme disease, injuries, muscular disorders, Eagle syndrome, and vascular, neurogenic, dental, salivary, and bone problems complicate any study of frequency and distribution.

Epidemiologic studies suggest a greater incidence in women; however, women are more frequent users of health care in general (Levitt & McKinney, 1994). Peak prevalence of TMDs is in persons ages 20 to 40. TMDs may be self-limiting: the incidence, signs, and symptoms diminish in older age. Clicking or other joint noises or jaw deviation occurs in up to 50% of normal persons (Wabeke & Spruijt, 1994) and may be disregarded if no other symptoms are present. In addition, up to 15% of asymptomatic joints that were silent (no clicking) were found to have joint displacements (Westesson et al, 1989).

Osteoarthritis and rheumatoid arthritis can occur in patients susceptible to these diseases, but arthritis rarely occurs only in the TMJ. Patients with progressive TMD do not follow epidemiologic norms. There is little information as to the ethnic and racial prevalence of TMDs. Societal barriers and prejudice may also exist, as in all chronic pain states. Even though signs and symptoms may occur in up to 50% of the population, only a few seek treatment.

DIAGNOSTIC CRITERIA

Definitive diagnostic criteria have not been established for TMDs. TMD is often a diagnosis of exclusion.

HISTORY AND PHYSICAL EXAM

Information from the history and physical exam is paramount in the assessment of TMD. Because of the plethora of TMD etiologies, a thorough history of past and present illnesses, including current use of prescription and nonprescription medications, is very important. These findings, identified in a nonprejudicial manner, provide information by which the diagnosis may be established. Temporal sequencing, location of pain areas, factors that increase or decrease severity, limitation of normal activities, limitation of socialization, and psychological factors affecting the disease should be analyzed and recorded.

If the patient has seen multiple providers, a detailed course of treatment, specific medications, and diagnostic tests previously performed must be examined within the context of the patient's overall improvement. Patient defenses (eg, "Nothing helped!") should be fully explored and qualified to assess what, if anything, has led to improvement during treatment. Anesthesia, dysesthesia, hyperesthesia, photophobia, nausea, intracranial pain, fainting, and significant postural findings should prompt suspicions of neurologic involvement. Eagle syndrome may be uncovered if the patient has dizziness or becomes lightheaded with rapid positional changes of the head. This may be caused by a calcified stylomandibular ligament that is putting pressure on the internal carotid. Burning, throbbing pain not associated with dental pain should raise suspicions of vascular sympathetic or inflammatory involvement. When treating chronic pain, it is important to inform patients that although a complete cure is usually not possible, pain can be managed and improved.

Inspection of the internal and external ear, nose, and throat should be performed, even when involvement is not indicated by the symptoms. The provider should palpate the areas of lymphatic drainage (submandibular, submental, triangles of the neck, auricular and mastoid areas) to rule out infective phenomena. Palpation producing pain in the salivary glands or along vascular tracts may lead to clinical suspicions warranting blood studies (sedimentation rate, amylase, antinuclear antibodies). Joint line tenderness is often a problem associated with TMD. This finding does not eliminate the influence of musculature on the disorder.

The physical exam may uncover knotting or trigger points in the muscle. These findings should be recorded for overall analysis. Trigger points may not be the site of spasm, but they are usually close and almost always on the same side. Referral of pain may be to distant sites on the same side. Muscle splinting, usually done unconsciously to prevent painful stimuli, may be evident on exam. Chronic muscle splinting, often for long periods, may lead to myositis and decreased range of motion. Chronic myositis with muscular hypertrophy usually produces little significant pain. If the muscles have calcific degeneration, the state is referred to as myositis ossificans.

Joint tenderness, pain on palpation, pain on biting, and joint noises may help in the diagnosis of joint problems. Joint noises may be insignificant to the treatment unless significant internal derangement has occurred.

The masseter and fan-shaped temporalis are broad surface muscles that may be easily palpated. The medial pterygoid makes a sling to the inferior body of the mandible and may be palpated from the submandibular area under the angle of the jaw, or in the pharynx. The gag reflex often reveals information about the anterior aspect of the medial pterygoid. The lateral pterygoid is often a site of significant discomfort on palpation. Lateral pterygoid spasms are quite painful when palpated, and the patient may have pain radiating to the joint. The lateral pterygoid is palpated by having the patient laterally deviate the jaw to the side of the exam to swing the coronoid complex of the mandible out of the way. Then the provider's pinky finger is moistened, placed lateral to the maxilla, and pressed upward and inward toward the pterygoid plates behind the last tooth. Comparison to the contralateral side should be evaluated. Although many patients state that they become swollen when they have pain (when no significant inflammation or infection is noted), in most cases no obvious swelling is evident.

The posterior belly of the digastric muscle and the stylohyoid muscle also frequently go into spasm. These are palpated under the angle of the mandible. The suprahyoid, the mylohyoid, and the anterior belly of the diagastric may be bimanually palpated along the floor of the mouth and externally from the hyoid to the anterior mandible. Spasm in these muscles may produce symptoms of difficulty in tongue movement, pain in the anterior teeth, or possibly pain under the tongue when swallowing.

Movement of the jaw should next be evaluated, along with neck range of motion. The sternocleidomastoid and occipital muscles may alert the provider to neck posture problems. Opening of the jaw should be in a relatively straight line when viewed from the anterior aspect. The patient should be able to fit three or four fingers sideways into the mouth when it is wide open. Limitation of opening can indicate joint problems, especially if the joint rotates but does not translocate out of the glenoid fossa.

Deviation (movement toward one side only, with no return to midline) on wide opening is usually a joint problem on the side of the deviation. This may be a unilateral joint problem such as disc trapping, especially if anteriorly displaced, only on the side of the deviation. Deflection (movement lateral, then returning to midline) on opening may connote irregularities in disc morphology or muscular incoordination. If there is limitation of opening, no deviation or deflection on pushing the jaw open, and no significant joint pain, myositis is usually the cause.

Diagnosis of closed locks of the TMJ may be established by tight end-point feel. The provider mobilizes the jaw in an attempt to slide the joints out of their sockets. When cross-fingered pressure (thumb on the top teeth, index finger on the bottom) is applied to the side, no movement should occur. Muscle problems causing inability to open usually have a softer end-point feel.

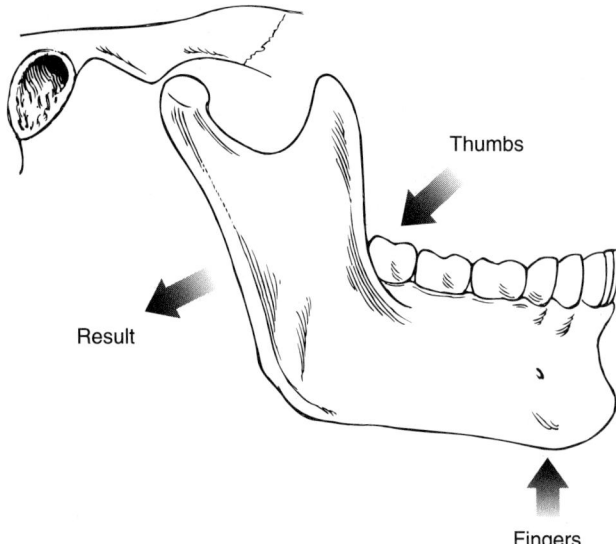

Thumbs

Result

Fingers

FIGURE 50-2 Forces applied to reduce dislocation of jaw.

Open locks or dislocations are easy diagnoses: the patient cannot self-reduce without some external force applied. The condyles, when palpated, usually are not in their fossa but are in an anterior position. The provider may rock the condyles over the prominence of the articular eminences of the temporal bone by applying downward force with the thumbs intraorally in the areas of the mandibular third molar and lifting the point of the chin while pushing back (Fig. 50-2). If the joints reduce, this confirms that a dislocation had occurred. Dislocation is a problem of muscle and ligament laxity. Laxity of ligaments may be a finding on the physical exam. Hypermobile joints generally do not cause significant pain unless internal derangement occurs and bone-to-bone contact ensues.

Abnormal tenderness in the teeth may also indicate regional inflammation from excessive chronic occlusion trauma. Simultaneous joint problems often appear with excessive muscular pressure, leading to joint overloading. Sinusitis may also give rise to inflammation in the maxillary teeth, where occlusion of the teeth may create pain. Carotid artery auscultation should be performed when a typical rhythmic noise is reported by the patient.

DIAGNOSTIC STUDIES

Once the physical exam is completed, studies may be ordered to validate or eliminate diseases in the differential diagnosis. TMD usually is a clinical diagnosis of muscle and joint problems. Open- and closed-jaw TMJ radiographic views may show osseous changes or failure to translocate on the open-jaw view. Diagnostic anesthetic blockade (auriculotemporal block) often helps in the diagnosis of true joint pain. Transcranial, TMJ, and panoramic dental radiographs are often of diagnostic value. Computed tomography scans can demonstrate the best view of osseous morphology and can also help to rule out intracranial, cervical, TMJ, sinus, and otologic pathology where indicated. In controlled studies, magnetic resonance imaging (MRI) resulted in positive findings of internal derangement in a third of asymptomatic persons. MRI cannot demonstrate disc perforations predictably (Moses et al, 1993). Blood tests are usually nonconclusive, although sedimentation rate, complete blood count, methionine level, mean corpuscular volume, amylase, eosinophil count, antinuclear antibodies, and Lyme disease testing may help rule out uncommon etiologies. Electromyelography has not been used with predictable results (Lund et al, 1995). Thermometry has shown some application, especially in arthritis (Kawano et al, 1993).

TREATMENT OPTIONS, EXPECTED OUTCOMES, AND COMPREHENSIVE MANAGEMENT

Treatment in most cases should be reversible, should provide symptomatic relief, and if possible should ameliorate the etiologic factors (Table 50-1). Aggressive surgical or prosthetic care should be reserved for recalcitrant cases. Presenting signs and symptoms usually improve with nonaggressive therapy. For some patients, symptoms worsen and signs increase over time; these patients may need more aggressive therapy. Disruption of normal life activities by the condition or by the perception of pain may be the precipitating factor that leads to aggressive therapy. Patients with chronic pain appear to suffer with their condition, and depression often occurs with suffering.

Muscle Spasms

Providers with knowledge of muscle pain states can usually treat muscle spasms effectively. Muscle spasms of an acute nature may be halted by various means. This is gratifying to both patient and provider, because relief can be instantaneous. Massaging of the muscle in spasm with intermittent spraying often breaks the spasm, although it may recur. Observe the skin to watch for icing, because this may cause frostbite. Ethyl chloride spray should be used with great caution in the office because it is packaged in glass and must be carefully stored; breakage demands evacuation of the area. Never allow direct inhalation, because it can act as a general anesthetic with myocardial irritation. Fluor-Methane spray is canned and is less dangerous. It can be used for therapy in the office and with proper guidance by the patient at home. Vapor coolant spraying is used with a "spray and stretch" technique, with care not to get agents in the eyes, ears, nose, or mouth. As follow-up for several days, a soft diet should be eaten and drugs with muscle-relaxing ability taken; diazepam remains one of the best. Injections of long-acting local anesthetics into the muscle bed or trigger points are also effective. Deep spasms, such as those in the pterygoids, may be better treated by this approach. Transcutaneous electrical nerve stimulation (TENS), at a low rate and broad pulse to capture muscle, is effective and may be used for therapy in the office or at home with proper guidance.

Physical therapy modalities such as infrasound and thermal pulsing should be considered but are often unnecessary. For pain management, nonsteroidal anti-inflammatories or narcotics may be used, along with relaxants. Patients with repetitive spasms may need referral to a dentist for the construction of an intraoral device to "deprogram" the muscles from repetitive overuse (clenching, bruxism, parafunctional activities and habits). Muscle training may be advisable when the incidence of spasm has stopped. This may be done by advising the patient to place a 4″ piece of tape vertically on a mirror at home. A pen is then used to ink one edge of the tape to create a line

TABLE 50-1	Simplified TMD Management				
Pain Causes	**Presentation**	**Mechanisms and Etiologies**	**Positive Diagnostic Findings**	**Treatment and Referral***	**Expected Outcome**
Acute myospasm	Limited mobility Pain Deviation	Muscular overcontraction Tension Drug side effect Protection of painful area	Jaw deviation Pain in muscle beds Soft end point painful Pain on opening	Rule out other pain sites. Vapocoolant spray and stretch TENS, trigger point injections, NSAIDs, diazepam, analgesics Occlusal splints	Immediate relief or relief in several days to 1 week
Chronic myospasm myositis	Limited mobility Muscle tightness deviation Dull diffuse pain Pain may present in joint.	Protective splinting Tension Protection of painful area Clenching Bruxism	Limitation of opening Masseteric hypertrophy Tight non-rigid end point—usually not very painful	Rule out pain site. Rule out drug side effect. Avoid stimulants. TENS, occlusal splints	General improvement; not a great increase in opening
Joint problem	Deviation Joint line pain may radiate.	Myospasm Old injury Clenching Bruxism Repetitive overuse	Often a click, pop, or creptic Past history of same Uneven opening Disruption of occlusion	Refer to dentist for workup. Warm moist compresses NSAIDs, analgesics, possibly diazepam TENS, soft diet, exercises but limit pain-producing motions; consider like closed mouth lock treatment	Cyclic pain should reduce its intensity slowly.
Dislocation or open mouth lock	Unable to close and open greater than 10 mm Agitation	Arthritis Joint in deep fossa Chronic overuse Internal derangement	Radiographic finding Palpation demonstrates joints ant. to fossa Often past history	Reduce and stabilize Refer to dentist for follow-up. Soft diet, NSAIDs Modifications of opening	Reduction = relief, but recurrence possible
Closed mouth lock	Patient unable to open Joint pain	Arthritis Severe myospasm Internal derangement	Often tight end point Radiograph and CT scan may confirm MRI confirmation	Soft diet Refer to dentist. NSAIDs, analgesics, diazepam, trigger point injections Intrasynovial steroids Arthrocentesis Arthroscopic or open surgery Occlusal splints Progressive opening Exercise Hourly glucose ingestion Avoid nicotine, caffeine, alcohol.	Gradual relief and increase in opening Recurrence likely
Acute joint trauma	Unable to open Malocclusion Hemorrhage Hematoma Laceration	Hemarthrosis Bone fracture Capsulitis Internal derangement	Injury Radiographic finding Pain on joint palpation Possible edema or hematoma	Refer to oral surgeon. Reduction of fracture Possible reduction for hemarthrosis Liquid diet Rest	Recovery after healing

* If diazepam is too sedating, other muscle relaxants may be used.

for the lower jaw to follow. The patient should then open and close very slowly along a direct line for 2 minutes five times per day. Exercises aiming to increase range of motion should not be painful. As exercises increase blood flow, improvement and healing should occur.

Joint problems combined with excessive muscular activity will overload the disc. Treatment consists of a soft diet, anti-inflammatories, pain-reducing drugs, compresses, rest, thermal packs (ice in acute, warm moist in chronic), and avoidance of pain-stimulating activities. When these fail, appliances worn intraocclusally (occlusal splints or night guards) have a good record of success in managing overloaded joints and abating

muscular spasms. These devices are usually adapted to the maxillary teeth and have also been called antibruxism devices. Several "boil and adapt" products are available over the counter, but the patient should be referred to a dentist. Irreversible alterations of occlusion (prosthetically) should be seldom done. In some cases, splint therapy can worsen the situation; if so, use of the device should be promptly halted and the diagnosis reevaluated.

For the patient who has no relief of joint pain with routine measures, interarticular steroid injections (on a limited basis) have shown beneficial effects. Subdermal injections of steroid compare favorably in some reports and may have a better profile because of decreased side effects. Closed (disc displacement without reduction) and open mouth block (dislocation of condyle) may respond to the injection of local anesthetics into the joint that dilate joint volume and allow reduction with less pain. Manipulation, under sedation or general anesthesia, has also been used to mobilize joints that are locked. Some closed mouth blocks need surgical intervention. Arthrocentesis is a procedure that has recently been shown to have promising effects. Arthrocentesis may remove metabolic joint toxins or gelated joint fluids, break adhesions, and stimulate repair in this nonvascular space.

Patients with chronic dislocation may benefit from reduction and stabilization. The primary care provider may wish to apply extra oral wraps (Barton bandage) to prevent recurrence. Patients with acute joint injury with hemarthrosis should be referred and may be stabilized with extra oral wraps or wiring the jaws for short periods. As a last resort, open joint surgery, repositioning of the disc, or plication to correct disc location may be used for painful chronic cases of joint derangement that do not respond to conventional treatment.

Arthroscopic diagnosis and surgery should usually precede open procedures. Arthroscopes have been successfully used in most procedures done in open fashion. Some allograft implants in the past have resulted in disastrous fragmentation of the implant in the joint. Newer implant designs and materials are being used, but in a few patients the implant deteriorates despite all surgical efforts.

Psychosocial management should start at the initial consultation. Patients are usually upset when told there is a psychological component of their disease. Life stress, recurrent pain, lack of a concrete explanation, hopelessness, and negative self-image require supportive treatment and psychosocial interventions.

Biofeedback, hypnosis, stress reduction, and progressive relaxation should be emphasized. If complicating factors are part of the etiology, they should be addressed and treated. Lifestyle changes may be necessary in chronic cases. Keeping the respiratory rate below 20 at rest; avoiding alcohol, nicotine, and caffeine; and ingesting glucose on an hourly basis have been shown to be effective. These approaches may quell brain stem inflammation and lessen the severity of pain. Posture (eg, protrusion of the jaw, clenching, holding a phone laterally against the head and shoulder, cheek chewing, lip biting, tongue rubbing, nail biting, pipe smoking) may aggravate the symptoms or even be the etiology. Such habits should be discussed and repetitive abuse syndromes identified and abolished.

Drug therapy consisting of anti-inflammatories, opiates, and muscle relaxants is often accepted by patients. Antidepressants can be quite useful to elevate the pain threshold in much lower dosages than those used for depression. Tricyclics, anticonvulsants, and central membrane stabilizers are often effective in management, although use of these drugs is usually supervised by a neurologist.

It remains unclear why bite splints (night guards) ameliorate facial tension and pain, but referral to a dentist for this therapy is advised.

As long as patients understand that the goal of TMD treatment is to decrease pain, increase range of motion, increase social interaction and self-dependence, and decrease reliance on medications, this syndrome is quite amenable to therapy. In one study, approximately 90% of patients whose pain stabilized 6 to 12 months after conservative treatment commenced had lasting relief (Garafis et al, 1994). For many patients with diagnosed joint derangement, jaw functions are possible with no significant pain (Vichaichalermvong & Nilner, 1993).

TEACHING AND SELF-CARE

Self-care and teaching for patients with TMDs begins with a discussion of treatment and management focused on palliation of symptoms and nonaggressive therapy. Patients can be instructed in jaw massage, use of warm moist compresses, hourly glucose ingestion, and muscle training, as previously described. Biofeedback, hypnosis, stress reduction, and progressive relaxation are supportive techniques that can be used for symptom management.

COMMUNITY RESOURCES

- TMJ and Facial Pain Center, http://www.netset.com/docws/
- American Academy of Head, Neck and Facial Pain, 520 W. Pipeline Rd., Hurst, TX 76053-4924, 817-282-1501, http://www.aahnfp.org/
- ENT Information Center, http://www.netdor.com/entinfo/tmjaao.html
- Healthtouch—TMJ and Jaw Joint Disorder, http://www.healthtouch.com/level1/leaflets/106358/106358.htm

CLINICAL WARNINGS AND REFERRAL POINTS

Referrals or consultations are indicated when there is suspicion that the jaw pain is the result of myocardial perfusion insufficiency, intracranial or cervical spinal lesions, or temporal arteritis. Referral or consultation may also be indicated in recurrent cases.

■■■□□ CLINICAL PEARLS

- Common TMDs (especially those aggravated by stress) seem to be cyclic and diminish with age.
- Successful therapy may consist of simple palliation until the symptoms abate and remission occurs.
- The musculature is the most common cause of most TMDs.
- Drug use may be implicated in acute-onset jaw pain, deviations, malocclusions, and clenching of teeth; therefore, a thorough history, including prescription and nonprescription medications, is essential in the evaluation of patients presenting with these signs and symptoms.
- In the absence of other symptoms, clicking or other joint noises or jaw deviation, which occurs in 50% of the population, does not lead to the diagnosis of TMD.
- Trigger points identified on the physical exam may not be the actual site of the spasm; however, they are usually close to the site and almost always on the same side.
- Disruption of normal life activities by the condition or by the perception of pain may be the precipitating factor that leads to aggressive therapy.

References

Balchelder, B., Krutchkoff, D., & Amara, J. (1987). Mandibular pain as the internal and sole clinical manifestation of coronary insufficiency: Report of case. *Journal of the American Dental Association, 115,* 710.

Costen, J. (1934). Syndrome of sinus and ear symptoms dependent upon disturbed function of the temporomandibular joint. *Annals of Otology Rhinology and Laryngology, 43,* 1.

Ellison, J., & Stanziani, P. (1993). SSRI-associated nocturnal bruxism in four patients. *Journal of Clinical Psychiatry, 54,* 11.

Garafis, P., Gregoriadon, E., Zarafi, A., et al. (1994). Effectiveness of conservative treatment for craniomandibular disorders: A two-year longitudinal study. *Journal of Orofacial Pain, 8,* 309–314.

Kawano, W., Kawazoe, T., Tanaka, M., et al. (1993). Deep thermometry of the temporomandibular joint and masticatory muscle regions. *Journal of Prosthetic Dentistry, 51,* 1–8.

Levitt, S., & McKinney, M. (1994). Validating the TMJ scale in a national sample of 10,000 patients: Demographic and epidemiologic characteristic. *Journal of Orofacial Pain, 8,* 23–35.

Lund, J., Widmer, C., & Feine, J. (1995). Validity of diagnostic and monitoring tests used in temporomandibular disorders. *Journal of Dental Research, 74,* 1133–1143.

Moses, J., Salinaa, E., Georgen T., et al. (1993). Magnetic resonance imaging or arthrographic diagnosis of internal derangement of the temporomandibular joint: Correlation comparison study with arthroscopic surgical conformation. *Oral Surgery, Oral Medicine, and Oral Pathology, 75,* 268–272.

NIH. (1996). Management of temporomandibular disorder. *NIH Technology Access Statement.*

Polette, C.E. (1992). C2 and C3 radiculopathies. Anatomy, patterns of cephalic pain and pathology. *APS Journal, 1,* 272.

Schiffman, E., Friction, J.R., Haley, D, et al. (1989). The prevalence and treatment needs of subjects with temporomandibular disorders. *JADA 120:* 295–304.

Vichaichalermvong, S., & Nilner, M. (1993). Clinical follow-up of patients with different disc positions. *Journal of Orofacial Pain, 7,* 61–67.

Wabeke, K., & Spruijt, R. (1994). On temporomandibular joint sounds. Dental and psychological studies. Thesis, University of Amsterdam, pp. 91–103.

Westesson, P., Eriksson, L., & Kurita, K. (1989). Reliability of a negative clinical temporomandibular joint examination: Prevalence of disk displacement in asymptomatic temporomandibular joints. *Oral Surgery, 68,* 551.

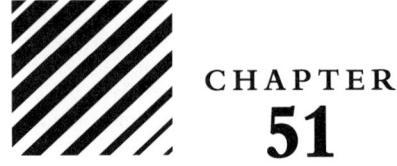

CHAPTER
51

Dementia and Delirium

Joseph Scarpa, MD, CMD, and Peter Sanna, PA-C, MPH

Dementia, a syndrome of deterioration of cognition in alert persons that results in their impaired performance of activities of daily living (Fleming et al, 1995), is difficult to recognize, especially in the early stages, as evidenced by the failure of clinicians to detect this disease in 21% to 72% of patients who have it (Pinholt et al, 1987; Fleming et al, 1995). The importance of early recognition cannot be emphasized strongly enough because with early recognition and aggressive management, the outcome for reversible disease may be improved, and incurable dementias may be better managed (Fleming et al, 1995).

The cost of caring for persons with dementia is high: according to Ernst and Hay (1994), direct costs of Alzheimer's disease (separate from other dementing illnesses) in the United States in 1991 were an estimated $20.6 billion, and unpaid caregiver costs were an estimated $33.3 billion.

Dementia and delirium were previously thought to be related, but now it is well established that these are, indeed, two separate disease entities. Delirium, also known as acute confusional state, is a transient disorder involving cognitive impairment with attentional deficit resulting in behavioral phenomena; like dementia, it is frequently misdiagnosed (Caine et al, 1995). Delirium is discussed in the second part of this chapter.

Dementia is distinguished from delirium because dementia is an acquired loss of or impairment in intellectual function whose nature is persistent and stable, whereas delirium is associated with altered consciousness, fluctuating deficits, and usually rapid onset (Caine et al, 1995).

Because of the vast body of literature in this field, the references used for this article were mainly recent, comprehensive review articles addressing the various subtopics presented below. The interested reader may wish to gather further, more detailed information from the references cited.

DEMENTIA

Dementia is an acquired loss of multiple cognitive functions and is usually, but not always, progressive, resulting in the deterioration of social, occupational, and functional abilities. At least two domains of intellectual function are affected: one is memory, and the other may be language, perception, visuospatial function, calculation, judgment, abstraction, and problem-solving skills. Patients may present with the full array of psychiatric symptoms (Caine et al, 1995; Fleming et al, 1995).

Anatomy, Physiology, and Pathology

One useful scheme of classifying the dementias is by the structures involved, because each dementia is associated with a typical pattern of neuropsychological deficits correlated with specific brain sites (Tien et al, 1993). The three major categories of dementias are cortical, subcortical, and mixed (Table 51-1).

CORTICAL DEMENTIA

Cortical dementia affects predominantly the cerebral cortex and includes dementia of the Alzheimer's type (DAT) and Pick's disease. The clinical correlates include agnosia, apraxia, aphasia, amnesia, abnormal cognition, and abnormal affect (classically, disinhibition); the motor system is unaffected (Tien et al, 1993).

Pathologic studies of brains of patients with DAT reveal diffuse atrophy of the brain, with widespread loss of neurons, especially in the temporal, parietal, and anterior frontal lobe cortices. The degree of atrophy tends to correspond to the clinical stage of DAT. Microscopic studies show neurofibrillary tangles, senile plaques, and granulovacuolar degeneration, usually in the pyramidal neurons of the hippocampus. A definitive diagnosis can be made only at autopsy or on cerebral biopsy (Tien et al, 1993).

In Pick's disease, which is 10 to 15 times less common than DAT, cortical lobar atrophy is highly focal, usually affecting the frontal and temporal lobes (both in approximately 50% of cases, and approximately evenly divided between the two in the rest of the cases). Histopathologic studies reveal intracytoplasmic Pick bodies (composed of neural filaments and tubules) and neuronal loss accompanied by cortical and subcortical gliosis (Tien et al, 1993).

SUBCORTICAL DEMENTIA

Subcortical dementia is caused by diseases that produce dysfunction in the basal ganglia, thalamus, and brain stem. It includes extrapyramidal syndromes, hydrocephalus, and white matter disease. Clinical manifestations include not only forgetfulness, slowing of cognition, and abnormal affect (classically, depression), but also motor symptoms such as disorders of posture, increased tone with tremors or dystonia, and gait disturbance (Tien et al, 1993).

Parkinson's Disease

Dementia is identified in 20% to 90% of patients with Parkinson's disease, a disease that affects approximately 1% of the population over age 50. Subcortical dementia of this type is

TABLE 51-1	Dementia Processes by Site of Involvement

Cortical dementia
    Dementia of the Alzheimer's type
    Pick's disease
Subcortical dementia
    Parkinson's disease
    Parkinsonian syndromes
        Progressive supranuclear palsy
        Olivopontocerebellar degeneration
        Striatonigral degeneration
        Multiple system atrophy
    Huntington's disease
    Wilson's disease
    Hydrocephalus
    Multiple sclerosis
    HIV encephalopathy
Combined cortical and subcortical dementia
    Vascular dementia (eg, multi-infarct dementia, Binswanger's disease, cerebral lacunae)
    Infectious dementias (eg, Creutzfeldt-Jakob disease)
    Hypoxic encephalopathy
    Miscellaneous (eg, toxic and metabolic encephalopathy, post-traumatic events, neoplastic conditions)

Tien, RD, Felsberg, G. et al. (1993). The dementias: correlation of clinical features, pathophysiology and neuroradiology. Amer J. Radiology 161:245–255.

associated with a reduction of pigmented cells of the substantia nigra, which results in malfunction of the efferent nigrostriatal tract; this loss of nigral input to the striatal dopamine receptors further results in disruption of normal coordination of basal ganglionic activity. The interruption of dopaminergic pathways from the ventral tegmentum to the frontal lobe may cause the clinically identifiable cognitive abnormalities. The remaining neuronal cells may contain eosinophilic cytoplasmic inclusions called Lewy bodies (Tien et al, 1993).

Parkinsonian Syndromes

Patients with parkinsonian syndromes (including progressive supranuclear palsy, striatonigral degeneration, multiple system atrophy, Shy-Drager syndrome, and olivopontocerebellar atrophy) may show typical subcortical dementia, including forgetfulness, slowness of thought, and personality changes, usually with depression, but they may also have varied clinical presentations, depending on the specific disease. Patients with parkinsonian syndromes respond poorly to antiparkinsonian therapy, a feature that may be used diagnostically (Tien et al, 1993).

One of the main pathologic differences between patients with Parkinson's disease and patients with parkinsonian syndromes is the presence of striatal nerve cell degeneration in the latter. The dopamine content of the striatum and substantia nigra is decreased, and there is degeneration of cells in the putamen and pars compacta of the substantia nigra—this is associated with rigid bradykinesia. Degeneration of cells in the intermediolateral columns of the spinal cord is associated with progressive autonomic failure, and degeneration of cells in the inferior olivary and pontine nuclei and of cerebellar Purkinje cells is associated with olivopontocerebellar atrophy. The cerebral cortex seems to be histologically and anatomically unaffected (Tien et al, 1993).

Other Subcortical Dementias

Huntington's disease, Wilson's disease, hydrocephalus, multiple sclerosis, and HIV encephalopathy are also considered underlying causes of subcortical dementias.

The pathologic changes associated with Huntington's disease are gross atrophy of the head of the caudate nucleus, with less severe changes in the putamen and globus pallidus. Histologically, neuronal loss and gliosis in the caudate nucleus, putamen, and globus pallidus can be observed (Tien et al, 1993).

Wilson's disease (hepatolenticular degeneration), resulting from a genetic inability to synthesize ceruloplasmin, is associated with pathologic evidence of atrophy, gliosis, edema, and occasionally necrosis in the lentiform nuclei (globus pallidus and putamen) (Tien et al, 1993).

Hydrocephalus is an uncommon cause of dementia, and can be corrected with resultant reversal of intellectual deficits. Dilation of the ventricular system is the main pathologic feature (Tien et al, 1993).

Multiple sclerosis is associated with multiple scattered lesions (plaques) involving the white matter—especially subependymal veins in the periventricular white matter, although the distribution of the plaques in the white matter could be random—but not the subcortical U fibers, cortex, and deep gray matter.

HIV encephalopathy is the most common infection-related dementia and the most common cause of dementia in young adults (excluding trauma). It is associated with multinucleated giant cells in the white matter and, to a lesser extent, the gray matter. Demyelination can be seen on neuroimaging (Tien et al, 1993).

MIXED DEMENTIA

Mixed dementia includes conditions involving both cortical and subcortical structures; vascular dementia and infectious dementia are included in this category (Tien et al, 1993).

Vascular Dementia

Vascular dementia includes syndromes of mental insufficiency related to multiple infarcts, small single strategically placed infarcts, posthemorrhagic states, and ischemic states not necessarily resulting in infarction. The vessels involved determine the signs and symptoms. Multi-infarct dementia, subcortical arteriosclerotic encephalopathy or Binswanger's disease, and cerebral lacunae are the main vascular dementia syndromes. Of patients with vascular dementia, approximately 20% have cortical infarcts, approximately 70% have lacunar infarcts, approximately 60% to 100% have small-vessel ischemia, and approximately 30% have a mixture (Tien et al, 1993).

In the brains of patients with Binswanger's disease, demyelination, axonal loss, and hyalinoid thickening of small artery walls in the deep white matter can be observed (Tien et al, 1993).

Cerebral lacunae result from lesions of the lenticulostriate and thalamoperforating arteries (which show arterial disorganization and fibrinoid destruction), and refer to the presence of multiple, small, deep, focal infarcts in the deep gray matter and internal capsule (Tien et al, 1993).

Creutzfeldt-Jakob Disease

In Creutzfeldt-Jakob disease, there is diffuse cerebral atrophy with no evidence of inflammation. Neuronal loss and gliosis are widespread, accompanied by spongiform change (Tien et al, 1993).

Hypoxic Encephalopathy

Neuronal loss can be observed after both acute and chronic cerebral hypoxia; if acute, neuronal injury tends to be focal and of a characteristic pattern visible on neuroimaging.

DEMENTIA WITH LEWY BODIES

Recently, another category of dementia has been recognized: dementia with Lewy bodies. Neuropathologic autopsy studies found that 15% to 25% of elderly demented patients have Lewy bodies in their brain stem and cortex, possibly making this the second most common pathologic subgroup among the dementias (after Alzheimer's disease) (McKeith et al, 1996). Patients with dementia with Lewy bodies tend to have rapidly progressing clinical symptoms, especially attentional impairments, problem-solving difficulties, and visuospatial impairments. Persistent visual hallucinations and spontaneous motor features of parkinsonism are hallmarks of the early development of this disease.

The identification of the specific cause of dementia is important in improving both the treatment and the prognosis of the patient.

Epidemiology

Dementia affects 3% to 11% of community-dwelling older adults over 65 years of age (severe in 5%, mild in 10% [Andreasen & Black, 1995]), but the prevalence in persons over 80 is 20% to 50%, with lower rates among community dwellers and higher rates among hospitalized and institutionalized patients. Almost 60% of people over 100 years of age are reported to have dementia (Fleming et al, 1995; Andreasen & Black, 1995).

Although more than 60 causes of dementia have been identified, DAT accounts for approximately 50% to 60% of cases (Tien et al, 1993) and affects approximately 2.5 million Americans (Andreasen & Black, 1995). It is the most common dementing disorder in North America, Scandinavia, and Europe (Caine et al, 1995). In Japan and Russia, however, vascular dementia is the more common type (Caine et al, 1995). Among persons over 75, the risk for DAT is six times greater than for vascular dementia (Caine et al, 1995).

Diagnostic Criteria

Diagnostic criteria according to *DSM-IV* are listed in Tables 51-2, 51-3, 51-4, and 51-5.

Risk factors for Alzheimer's disease include those that are definite, such as old age, Down syndrome, family history, ApoE genotype 4; those that are less definite, such as female, history of head injury, Down syndrome in the family, and vascular risk factors; and those that are least definite, such as aluminum and herpes simplex virus I (Writing Committee, 1996; Eastwood, 1997). "Protective factors" include ApoE 2 genotype, high IQ or educational achievement, postmenopausal estrogen use, and use of nonsteroidal anti-inflammatory drugs (Eastwood, 1997).

History and Physical Exam

HISTORY

Advanced age and a family history of DAT are the most important risk factors for Alzheimer's disease; however, a family history of Down syndrome and hematologic malignancies (eg,

TABLE 51-2	Diagnostic Criteria for Dementia Due to Other General Medical Conditions

A. The development of multiple cognitive deficits manifested by both
  (1) memory impairment (impaired ability to learn new information or to recall previously learned information)
  (2) one (or more) of the following cognitive disturbances:
    (a) aphasia (language disturbance)
    (b) apraxia (impaired ability to carry out motor activities despite intact motor function)
    (c) agnosia (failure to recognize or identify objects despite intact sensory function)
    (d) disturbance in executive functioning (i.e., planning, organizing, sequencing, abstracting)

B. The cognitive deficits in criteria A1 and A2 each cause significant impairment in social or occupational functioning and represent a significant decline from a previous level of functioning.

C. There is evidence from the history, physical examination, or laboratory findings that the disturbance is the direct physiological consequence of one of the general medical conditions listed below.

D. The deficits do not occur exclusively during the course of a delirium.

DEMENTIA DUE TO HIV DISEASE
Coding note: Also code HIV infection affecting central nervous system on Axis III.

DEMENTIA DUE TO HEAD TRAUMA
Coding note: Also code injury on Axis III.

DEMENTIA DUE TO PARKINSON'S DISEASE
Coding note: Also code Parkinson's disease on Axis III.

DEMENTIA DUE TO HUNTINGTON'S DISEASE
Coding note: Also code Huntington's disease on Axis III.

DEMENTIA DUE TO PICK'S DISEASE
Coding note: Also code Pick's disease on Axis III.

DEMENTIA DUE TO CREUTZFELDT-JAKOB DISEASE
Coding note: Also code Creutzfeldt-Jakob disease on Axis III.

DEMENTIA DUE TO . . . *[INDICATE THE GENERAL MEDICAL CONDITION NOT LISTED ABOVE]*
For example, normal-pressure hydrocephalus, hypothyroidism, brain tumor, vitamin B_{12} deficiency, intracranial radiation. **Coding note:** Also code the general medical condition on Axis III.

American Psychiatric Association: Diagnostic and Statistical Manual of Mental Disorders, 4/e. Washington, DC: American Psychiatric Association, 1994.

leukemia, myelolymphoma, Hodgkin's disease) is also important. Although familial predisposition appears to be a risk factor for vascular dementia, the association is not as strong with DAT. As would be expected, family history is extremely important in hereditary dementias such as Huntington's disease, Wilson's disease, and metachromatic leukodystrophy.

Suspicion of dementia related to head trauma should be raised in patients with a history of severe head trauma or multiple traumas acquired over a period of time. Suspicion of neurosyphilis should be raised if the patient has had an untreated or partially treated sexually transmitted disease; similarly, AIDS dementia complex should be suspected if the patient has risk factors for HIV (eg, homosexuality, multiple sex partners, intravenous drug use).

TABLE 51-3	Diagnostic Criteria for Substance-Induced Persisting Dementia

A. The development of multiple cognitive deficits manifested by both
   (1) memory impairment (impaired ability to learn new information or to recall previously learned information)
   (2) one (or more) of the following cognitive disturbances:
      (a) aphasia (language disturbance)
      (b) apraxia (impaired ability to carry out motor activities despite intact motor function)
      (c) agnosia (failure to recognize or identify objects despite intact sensory function)
      (d) disturbance in executive functioning (ie, planning, organizing, sequencing, abstracting)

B. The cognitive deficits in criteria A1 and A2 each cause significant impairment in social or occupational functioning and represent a significant decline from a previous level of functioning.

C. The deficits do not occur exclusively during the course of a delirium and persist beyond the usual duration of substance intoxication or withdrawal.

D. There is evidence from the history, physical examination, or laboratory findings that the deficits are etiologically related to the persisting effects of substance use (eg, a drug of abuse, a medication).

Code (Specific substance)-induced persisting dementia: (alcohol; inhalant; sedative, hypnotic, or anxiolytic; other [or unknown] substance)

American Psychiatric Association: Diagnostic and Statistical Manual of Mental Disorders, 4/e. Washington, DC: American Psychiatric Association, 1994.

TABLE 51-4	Diagnostic Criteria for Dementia Due to Multiple Etiologies

A. The development of multiple cognitive deficits manifested by both
   (1) memory impairment (impaired ability to learn new information or to recall previously learned information)
   (2) one (or more) of the following cognitive disturbances:
      (a) aphasia (language disturbance)
      (b) apraxia (impaired ability to carry out motor activities despite intact motor function)
      (c) agnosia (failure to recognize or identify objects despite intact sensory function)
      (d) disturbance in executive functioning (ie, planning, organizing, sequencing, abstracting)

B. The cognitive deficits in criteria A1 and A2 each cause significant impairment in social or occupational functioning and represent a significant decline from a previous level of functioning.

C. There is evidence from the history, physical examination, or laboratory findings that the disturbance has more than one etiology (eg, head trauma plus chronic alcohol use, dementia of the Alzheimer's type with the subsequent development of vascular dementia).

D. The deficits do not occur exclusively during the course of delirium.

Coding note: Use multiple codes based on specific dementias and specific etiologies (eg, dementia of the Alzheimer's type, with late onset, uncomplicated; vascular dementia, uncomplicated).

American Psychiatric Association: Diagnostic and Statistical Manual of Mental Disorders, 4/e. Washington, DC: American Psychiatric Association, 1994.

TABLE 51-5	Diagnostic Criteria for Dementia Not Otherwise Specified

This category should be used to diagnose a dementia that does not meet criteria for any of the specific types described in this section. An example is a clinical presentation of dementia for which there is insufficient evidence to establish a specific etiology.

American Psychiatric Association: Diagnostic and Statistical Manual of Mental Disorders, 4/e. Washington, DC: American Psychiatric Association, 1994.

A history of chronic medical illnesses such as epilepsy, renal failure, or hepatic cirrhosis, especially if poorly controlled, as well as a history of occupational exposure to heavy metals or other toxins, should also raise the index of suspicion for dementia (Caine et al, 1995).

As mentioned earlier, a history of the clinical pattern of the disease may provide clues as to whether the dementia is of a degenerative or vascular type. The former tends to progress insidiously and slowly, whereas the latter tends to occur in a stepwise fashion (probably coinciding with cerebrovascular events). Interviews of family members often yield additional information regarding the patient's deteriorating memory, changes in language skills, and functional impairment, if any, providing more clues that could aid in pinpointing the diagnosis (Fleming et al, 1995).

Early signs of dementias include problems with the performance of personal care tasks, changes in personality (eg, indifference, regression, impulsiveness, withdrawal), and behavioral changes (eg, agitation, aggression, restlessness, wandering, delusions, paranoia, hallucinations, and sleep cycle disturbances) (Fleming et al, 1995).

PHYSICAL AND LABORATORY STUDIES

A thorough physical exam may disclose evidence of a systemic disease to which dementia or the risk thereof may be associated. Examples include enlarged liver and hepatic encephalopathy, Kaposi sarcoma, and focal neurologic findings (eg, asymmetrical hyperreflexia or weakness, seen more often in vascular dementia than in degenerative diseases) (Caine et al, 1995; Fleming et al, 1995).

Neurologic and psychiatric histories should also be taken and tests performed, but a diagnosis should be reserved until results from several tests or questionnaires have been obtained and correlations can be made with results of the physical exam (Fleming et al, 1995). Neurologic exams should include mental status testing, brief screening tests, and formal cognitive testing (eg, 30-point Mini-Mental State Examination—a score of 25 or less suggests impairment; a score of 20 or less usually indicates definite impairment [Andreasen & Black, 1995], or the 38-point Short Test of Mental Status).

Table 51-6 reviews some of the abnormalities that may be present on an elementary neurologic exam and their possible causes (Sandson & Price, 1996). Psychiatric evaluation should take into consideration that depression and dementia, both of which are common in elderly patients, may coexist, especially in the early stages of degenerative dementias; pseudodementia (reversible dementia resulting from depression) should be ruled

TABLE 51-6	Neurologic Findings and Associated Dementias in Adults
Finding	**Associated Dementing Illness**
Ataxia	AzD, cerebellar degenerations, GM2 gangliosidosis, Med, MS, prion disease, PML, WK, WD
Dysarthria	AzD, dementia pugilistica, dialysis dementia, HS, MND, MS, PML, PSP, WD
Dystonic or choreoathetotic movements	AzD, HS, HD, ICBG, PD, WD
Extrapyramidal signs	Alzheimer's disease, ALS–parkinsonism–dementia complex, ALSPDG, AzD, dementia pugilistica, diffuse Lewy body disease, GM1 gangliosidosis type III, HS, HD, ICGB, Med, MID, multiple systems atrophy, neuroacanthocytosis, NPH, PD, postencephalitic parkinsonism, PSP, striatonigral degeneration, SSPE, WD
Extraocular movements	Gaucher's disease type 1, Kearns-Sayre syndrome, MID, MS, Niemann-Pick disease type IIc, PSP, WK
Gait disorder	AMN, ADC, AzD, dementia pugilistica, MID, MS, NPH, PD, PSP, syphilis, WK
Neuropathy	AMN, ADC, B_{12} deficiency, MLD, porphyria, Med, thyroid disease, uremia
Myoclonus	Dialysis dementia, HS, Kufs's disease, Lafora's disease, MERRF, prion disease, SSPE
Pyramidal tract signs	AMN, ADC, B_{12} deficiency, GM2 gangliosidosis, HS, Kufs's disease, MLD, MND, MID, MS, PML, syphilis, spinocerebellar degenerations

ADC, AIDS dementia complex; AMN, adrenomyeloneuropathy; AzD = Azorean disease; HS, Hallerverden-Spatz; HD, Huntington's disease; ICBG, idiopathic calcification of the basal ganglia; Med, medications and toxins; MERRF, myopathy and encephalopathy with ragged red fibers; MLD, metachromatic leukodystrophy; MID, multi-infarct dementia; MND, motor neuron disease; MS, multiple sclerosis; PD, Parkinson's disease; PML, progressive multifocal leukoencephalopathy; PSP, progressive supranuclear palsy; SSPE, subacute sclerosing panencephalitis; WK, Wernicke-Korsakoff syndrome; WD, Wilson's disease. (Sandson, TA, Price, BH. (1996). Diagnostic testing in dementia. *Neurologic Clinics* 14:45–56.)

out (Table 51-7). In these cases, neuropsychological evaluation may be helpful to distinguish depression from dementia. DAT is associated with withdrawal, paranoia, and anxiety; depression, delusions, and "emotional incontinence" are common in patients with vascular dementias; and personality changes, disinhibited behaviors, social withdrawal, and lack of insight are associated with Pick's disease (Fleming et al, 1995).

Selected laboratory studies (eg, blood chemistry studies, complete blood cell counts, erythrocyte sedimentation rate, thyroid function tests, HIV screening [in the presence of risk factors], drug screening, urinalysis for heavy metals, and collagen vascular profile) may help in identifying the etiology, but these should follow clinical suspicion as raised by the results of the history, physical, and mental exams (Caine et al, 1995; Fleming et al, 1995; Andreasen & Black, 1995). Table 51-

TABLE 51-7	Clinical Features Differentiating Dementia From Delirium	
Dementia	**Delirium**	
Chronic or insidious onset	Acute or rapid onset	
Level of consciousness unimpaired early on	Level of consciousness clouded	
Normal level of arousal	Agitation or stupor	
Usually progressive and deteriorating	Often reversible	
Common in nursing homes and psychiatric hospitals	Common on medical, surgical, and neurologic wards	

Andreasen, NC, Black, DW. (1995). Introductory Textbook of Psychiatry, 2/e. Washington, DC: American Psychiatric Association.

8 lists the recommended laboratory evaluations for dementia (Fleming et al, 1995).

Neuroimaging studies are performed to exclude reversible causes of dementia (eg, tumors or other types of mass lesions, ischemic disease, and normal-pressure hydrocephalus). Most of the reversible dementias caused by structural lesions can be detected by computed tomography (CT) without contrast media, but CT findings are not suitable for determining the presence or absence of Alzheimer's disease, for distinguishing Alzheimer's disease from normal aging, or for clearly diagnosing normal-pressure hydrocephalus.

Although it is easier to evaluate atrophy and various lesions with magnetic resonance imaging (MRI), the clinical usefulness of MRI is questionable because white matter hyperintensities are evident in 30% of patients with Alzheimer's disease and in 10% to 90% of nondemented healthy elderly subjects (Drayer, 1988; Fleming et al, 1995).

Some investigators believe that routine neuroimaging studies are unwarranted, especially if management of the patient's disease will not be affected by the findings. Exceptions include CT scanning in patients with recent (less than 1 year) onset of dementia or acute deterioration, patients with unexplained or atypical neurologic findings, and patients with a reasonable probability of intracranial disease (Fleming et al, 1995).

In cases of acute or subacute onset of dementing illnesses, dementia in a patient less than 55 years old, atypical or progressive manifestations, suspected infection or lesion of the central nervous system, suspected syphilis, hydrocephalus, demyelinating disease, immunosuppression, or vasculitis, cerebrospinal fluid analysis is recommended after neuroimaging of the brain to determine the safety of the procedure (Fleming et al, 1995).

TABLE 51-8	Recommendations for Laboratory Evaluation of Dementia

American Academy of Neurology (1995). Corey-Bloom J., Thal, L.J., Galasko, D., et al. (1995). Diagnosis and evaluation of dementia. *Neurology, 45*, 211–218.

   Routine: CBC, ESR, electrolytes, BUN, creatinine, liver function tests, serum vitamin B_{12}, syphilis serology, urinalysis, HIV testing

National Institute on Aging Task Force (1980). Senility reconsidered: treatment possibilities for mental impairment in the elderly. *JAMA, 244*, 259–263.

   Routine: CBC, ESR, syphilis serology, serum vitamin B_{12} and folate, SMA-12, serum phosphate, thyroid screen, urinalysis, chest roentgenography, ECG

Larson E.B., Reifler, B.V., et al. (1986). Diagnostic tests in the evaluation of dementia: A prospective study of 200 elderly outpatients. *Archives of Internal Medicine, 146*, 1917–1922.

   Routine strategy 1: CBC, chemistry panel (glucose, calcium, creatinine, sodium, potassium, chloride, bicarbonate), thyrotropin

Routine strategy 2: Same as strategy 1 plus syphilis serology, ESR, serum folate

In selected patients: Serum folate and vitamin B_{12} (if CBC abnormal), TSH,* syphilis serology

Siu, A.L. (1991). Screening for dementia and investigating its causes. *Annals of Internal Medicine, 115*, 122–132.

   Routine: Initial chemistry panels, CBC, and thyroid function tests have a reasonable yield in identifying clinically significant problems that complicate dementia.

   Chest roentgenography, ECG, and urinalysis: Selective ordering for exclusion of coexisting nondementing medical problems (frequently indicated because of high prevalence of cardiopulmonary and urologic disorders)

   ESR: If evidence of decline in health status

   Serum vitamin B_{12}: If evidence of anemia, macrocystosis, or abnormal findings on exam (impaired vibration or position sense, abnormal gait, clouded consciousness) suggest deficiency

   Serum folate: Probably indicated only in patients with dementia who also have anemia

   Syphilis serology: Only if the history or signs suggest a moderate pretest probability of neurosyphilis; even if serum nonreactive, additional tests are necessary if suspicion for neurosyphilis is high.

BUN, blood urea nitrogen; CBC, complete blood cell count; ECG, electrocardiography; ESR, erythrocyte sedimentation rate; HIV, human immunodeficiency virus; SMA-12, 12-factor automated chemical analysis; TSH, thyroid-stimulating hormone (thyrotropin).

* Updated by the authors.

Fleming, KC, Adams, AC et al. (1995). Dementia: Diagnosis and evaluation; *Mayo Clinic Proceedings* 70:1093–1107.

Electroencephalography (EEG) tends to be of limited value in the initial evaluation of dementia but may be helpful in cases of suspected Creutzfeldt-Jakob disease and in cases of delirium, complex partial seizures, and certain encephalitides (Fleming et al, 1995).

Diagnostic Studies

First, it is necessary to establish that a patient with a stable level of consciousness does, indeed, have multiple cognitive deficits (Caine et al, 1995). This implies that a diagnosis of delirium, whose chief feature is disturbance of consciousness, is excluded at the outset. Next, dementia must be distinguished from focal cognitive impairments (eg, in amnestic or aphasic patients) and

from mood disorders (possibly major depressive disorder) (Caine et al, 1995). The various diagnostic tests that can be used in this evaluation were discussed in the previous section.

Treatment Options, Expected Outcomes, and Comprehensive Management

The progress and prognosis of dementia vary with its etiology. In general, treatment options are limited because, even though dementia itself does not necessarily mean that deterioration will be progressive, the processes underlying many of the dementias are degenerative, and to date there are no known means of halting or altering their progress. However, in cases of vascular dementias and drug-related or toxin-related (but not radiation-related) dementias, if their associated risk factors can be controlled or eliminated, the progress of these dementias may be abated, halted, or in some cases even reversed.

Infection-related dementias are usually acute, although this may not be the case with infections such as syphilis and cryptococcal meningitis. Degenerative dementias tend to have a slow, stealthy onset and are usually gradually progressive, but some patients with DAT exhibit one or more plateaus in functional impairment during the course of the disease. Vascular dementias are characterized by abrupt, progressive episodes associated with new vascular events, even though, like most degenerative dementias, the overall progress of the disease tends to be steadily progressive (Caine et al, 1995).

Confirmation that the diagnosis is correct is the first step in treating dementias. In vascular dementias, preventive measures such as dietary changes and exercise regimens may be instituted, along with measures to control blood pressure and blood glucose levels. Beta-blockers, but not diuretics and angiotensin-converting enzyme inhibitors, have been associated with an exaggeration of cognitive impairment, as has low blood pressure. Unfortunately, with respect to the degenerative dementias, no conclusive evidence regarding preventive measures or even direct therapies to retard or halt the disease processes has been found.

In DAT, which has been the most studied, as well as in dementias resulting from chronic alcohol-related disorders, vascular dementia, Parkinson's disease, and Huntington's disease, decreases in the levels of various neurotransmitters (eg, acetylcholine, dopamine, norepinephrine, gamma-aminobutyric acid [GABA], serotonin) and neuropeptides (eg, somatostatin, substance P) have been observed. These decreases are far greater than those observed during the course of normal aging. Neurotransmitter replacement therapy with, for example, acetylcholine precursors, cholinergic agents, and cholinesterase inhibitors has been the most common strategy used to attempt to improve memory in patients with Alzheimer's disease. Some therapies have shown limited, although statistically significant, improvement.

With an eye toward preserving neuronal integrity and function, antioxidant therapy, in the form of monoamine oxidase B inhibitors, has been used to slow the progression of Parkinson's disease. Experimental antioxidant therapies are being studied in patients with dementias associated with Huntington's disease and vascular dementia (Caine et al, 1995).

Consistent daily schedules and environments appear to be helpful in managing the behavior of patients with symptoms of dementia. At times these patients display mood disorders or behavioral symptoms; the same pharmacologic agents used for idiopathic psychiatric disorders can also be used in patients with dementias (Kaplan & Saddock, 1995). Individual psychotherapy begun during the early stages of dementia has been found beneficial in helping patients not only in the short term when they cope with losses, but also in the long term when their cognitive deficits become more severe (Caine et al, 1995). Cognitive training early in the disease is helpful to both the patient and the caregiver, as assessed by quality of life measurements (Fig. 51-1) (Writing Committee, 1996).

Teaching and Self-Care

Caring for the caregivers is an essential part of caring for people with dementia and includes counseling, educational courses, self-help groups, respite care, day care for the patients, and inpatient admission as ways to complement without undermining the coping mechanisms (emphasis on positive aspects and moral obligation) of the caregivers (Writing Committee, 1996).

The importance of family education, support, and involvement cannot be overemphasized as part of the treatment plan, because everyone benefits from the knowledge of the patient's prognosis and progress. If the family members need help with their adjustment to new roles as they care for and interact with the patient, the appropriate network will already be in place (Caine et al, 1995).

Referral Points and Clinical Warnings

Early in the course of Alzheimer's disease, extrapyramidal symptoms and delusions may be present, although the former are associated with greater severity and a more rapid progression of the disease. Delusions tend to foreshadow a more rapid decline in cognitive function, as do aggressive behavior, sleep disturbances (especially nocturnal awakening), and language impairment. Predictors of a more rapid functional decline include paranoia, delusions, hallucinations, wandering, inappropriate or purposeless activities, extrapyramidal symptoms, and lower scores on nonverbal cognitive tests. Functional losses in dementia have been suggested to follow a sequence that seems

TABLE 51-9	Factors That Predict Institutionalization in Patients With Dementia

Patients with cognitive or behavioral problems (especially aggressive behavior, delusions, incontinence)

Unmarried patients

Son or daughter as caregiver (especially if employed)

Greater number of family and friends involved as caregivers*

High caregiver stress or burden

Poor caregiver health

Increased use of health care and home help services

Increased functional impairments (by ADL scales)

Lower cognitive status at baseline

Death of a spouse

Hospitalization

Prior institutionalization

ADL, activities of daily living

* The greater the number, the higher the risk of institutionalization.

Fleming, KC, Adams, AC et al. (1995). Dementia: Diagnosis and evaluation. *Mayo Clinic Proceedings* 70:1093–1107.

to be the reverse of normal early development—in other words, the deterioration appears as a sequential loss of speech, ambulation, continence, sitting, smiling, posture, and feeding. Late manifestations of the disease, including incontinence and impaired hygiene, suggest a more advanced stage of dementia (Fleming et al, 1995).

It seems that patients with a shorter duration of disease before evaluation have a faster progression of the disease over time, whereas those with a longer duration of disease before evaluation have a slower progression of the disease process, possibly because the disease went unnoticed until its manifestations became apparent. When abrupt changes in behavior, cognitive status, or loss of function occur, prompt and thorough reevaluation is recommended to rule out an underlying medical illness (Fleming et al, 1995).

Factors that predict institutionalization in patients with dementia are listed in Table 51-9. One community-based prospective study (Severson et al, 1994) showed that half of the

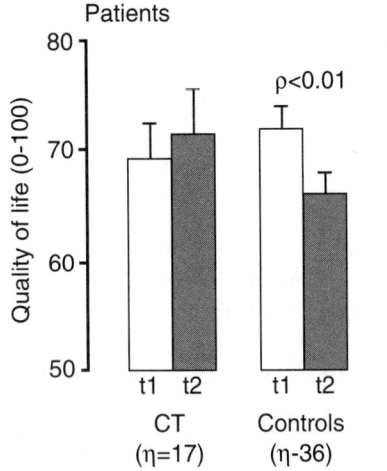
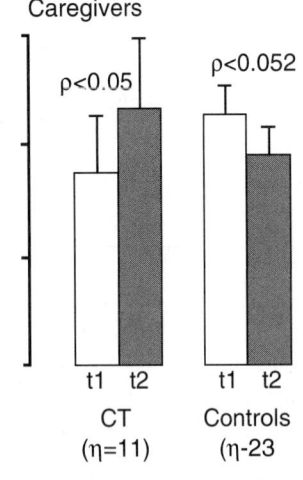

FIGURE 51-1 Effect of cognitive training on quality of life in people with dementia and their caregivers. (t1 = baseline, t2 = 12 months later, CT = cognitive training) Writing committee, Lancet Conference 1996. The challenge of the dementias. Lancet 347: 1303–1307.

patients with dementia were institutionalized within 2.5 years after diagnosis, and that the median time from estimated onset of dementia to placement in a nursing home was 5.6 years.

Several trends regarding survival rates of patients with dementia have become apparent (Fleming et al, 1995). Community-based patients had higher 1-year and 5-year survival rates than did residents of long-term care facilities, who in turn had higher survival rates than did mental hospital patients. The mortality rate associated with dementia increased with advancing age. Women with dementia have longer survival than do men with dementia, possibly because of an overall higher life expectancy and possibly because dementia is recognized earlier in women because of loss of home-management skills.

DELIRIUM

Delirium, also known as acute confusional state, is a primary disorder of attention characterized by fluctuating features of abrupt onset of inattention, variable psychomotor activity (from lethargy to hypervigilance), disorganized sleep–wake cycles, and global cognitive impairment. It is usually associated with a serious underlying medical disorder or illness (eg, infection, drug toxicity, myocardial infarction) and has an increased mortality rate (40% to 50% of patients with delirium die within 1 year).

An underlying dementia may be an important risk factor for the development of delirium, but when a patient presents with an acute state of confusion, the diagnosis of dementia must be deferred (Fleming et al, 1995; Caine et al, 1995; Andreasen & Black, 1995). Usually, dementia is a transient syndrome (although not by DSM-IV criteria) that resolves within a few days to a few weeks (Caine et al, 1995), but its course is largely affected by the course of the underlying cause (Casey et al, 1996).

Anatomy, Physiology, and Pathology

The pathophysiology of delirium is not well understood. Dysfunction of the reticular activating system has been suggested because of its role in arousal. Hypofunction of cholinergic systems has been demonstrated in the basal forebrain and pons, and there is some evidence for dysfunction of several other neurochemical systems, including noradrenergic, GABA-ergic, and serotonergic. Much research remains to be conducted to elucidate the pathways and mechanisms by which delirium is manifested (Caine et al, 1995).

Epidemiology

Few studies have been performed to determine the incidence and prevalence of delirium, especially in a community or nonpatient setting. Because delirium is often unrecognized or misdiagnosed (as depression, schizophrenia, or other psychiatric disorders), rates of delirium are at best approximations. It is estimated that at any given time, 10% to 15% of general medical inpatients are delirious. Thirty percent to 50% of acutely ill geriatric patients are estimated to become delirious at some point during their hospitalization (Caine et al, 1995). Risk factors for delirium include increased severity of physical illness, advanced age, and baseline cognitive impairment (eg, because of dementia) (Caine et al, 1995).

Diagnostic Criteria

The core features of delirium include altered consciousness (eg, decreased level of consciousness), altered attention (may include inability to focus, sustain, or shift attention), impairment in other areas of cognitive function (may present as disorientation, especially to time and space, and decreased memory), relatively rapid onset (usually hours to days), brief duration (usually days to weeks), and marked and unpredictable fluctuations in severity during the day (ranging from periods of lucidity to severe cognitive impairment). Sometimes the confusion, agitation, and psychotic episodes are worse at night (''sundowning'') (Caine et al, 1995; Andreasen & Black, 1995; Casey et al, 1996; Inouye & Charpentier, 1996).

Disorganization of thought processes (ranging from mild tangentiality to outright incoherence), perceptual disturbances (illusions, hallucinations), psychomotor hyperactivity and hypoactivity, disruption of the sleep–wake cycle, mood alterations (ranging from subtle irritability to obvious dysphoria, anxiety, or even euphoria), and other evidence of altered neurologic function (eg, autonomic hyperactivity or instability, myoclonic jerking, and dysarthria) are associated clinical features of delirium (Caine et al, 1995; Casey et al, 1996).

Although the core syndrome for delirium remains the same regardless of etiology, diagnostic criteria are organized into groups by etiologies in *DSM-IV*: delirium due to a general medical condition (Table 51-10), substance intoxication (Table 51-11), substance withdrawal (Table 51-12), multiple etiologies (Table 51-13), and "not otherwise specified" (Table 51-14). Whenever a patient displays a new onset of or a rapid change in a psychiatric sign or symptom, delirium should be suspected (Caine et al, 1995).

Differentiating delirium from other psychiatric disorders that share signs and symptoms is often challenging. Table 51-15 presents a few characteristics that might help distinguish delirium from dementia, depression, and psychosis (Casey et al, 1996).

TABLE 51-10	Diagnostic Criteria for Delirium Due to a General Medical Condition

A. Disturbance of consciousness (ie, reduced clarity of awareness of the environment) with reduced ability to focus, sustain, or shift attention.

B. A change in cognition (such as memory deficit, disorientation, language disturbance) or the development of a perceptual disturbance that is not better accounted for by a preexisting, established, or evolving dementia.

C. The disturbance develops over a short period of time (usually hours to days) and tends to fluctuate during the course of the day.

D. There is evidence from the history, physical examination, or laboratory findings that the disturbance is caused by the direct physiological consequences of a general medical condition.

Coding note: If delirium is superimposed on a preexisting dementia of the Alzheimer's type or vascular dementia, indicate the delirium by coding the appropriate subtype of the dementia (eg, dementia of the Alzheimer's type, with late onset, with delirium).

Coding note: Include the name of the general medical condition on Axis I (eg, delirium due to hepatic encephalopathy); also code the general medical condition on Axis III.

American Psychiatric Association: Diagnostic and Statistical Manual of Mental Disorders. 4/e. Washington, DC: American Psychiatric Association, 1994.

TABLE 51-11	Diagnostic Criteria for Substance Intoxication Delirium

A. Disturbance of consciousness (ie, reduced clarity of awareness of the environment) with reduced ability to focus, sustain, or shift attention.

B. A change in cognition (such as memory deficit, disorientation, language disturbance) or the development of a perceptual disturbance that is not better accounted for by a preexisting, established, or evolving dementia.

C. The disturbance develops over a short period of time (usually hours to days) and tends to fluctuate during the course of the day.

D. There is evidence from the history, physical examination, or laboratory findings of either (1) or (2):
(1) The symptoms in criteria A and B developed during substance intoxication
(2) Medication use is etiologically related to the disturbance.

Note: This diagnosis should be made instead of a diagnosis of substance intoxication only when the cognitive symptoms are in excess of those usually associated with the intoxication syndrome and when the symptoms are sufficiently severe to warrant independent clinical attention.

Note: The diagnosis should be recorded as substance-induced delirium if related to medication use.

Code (Specific substance) intoxication delirium: (Alcohol; amphetamine [or amphetamine-like substance]; cannabis; cocaine; hallucinogen; inhalant; opioid; phencyclidine [or phencyclidine-like substance]; sedative, hypnotic, or anxiolytic; other [or unknown] substance [eg, cimetidine, digitalis, benztropine])

American Psychiatric Association: Diagnostic and Statistical Manual of Mental Disorders, 4/e. Washington, DC: American Psychiatric Association, 1994.

History and Physical Exam

Delirium is the result of brain dysfunction that is almost always caused by an identifiable systemic or cerebral disease or by drug intoxication or withdrawal. The most frequently encountered etiologies are listed in Table 51-16. Several of these may be present simultaneously, and although one might be sufficient

TABLE 51-12	Diagnostic Criteria for Substance Withdrawal Delirium

A. Disturbance of consciousness (ie, reduced clarity of awareness of the environment) with reduced ability to focus, sustain, or shift attention.

B. A change in cognition (such as memory deficit, disorientation, language disturbance) or the development of a perceptual disturbance that is not better accounted for by a preexisting, established, or evolving dementia.

C. The disturbance develops over a short period of time (usually hours to days) and tends to fluctuate during the course of the day.

D. There is evidence from the history, physical examination, or laboratory findings that the symptoms in criteria A and B developed during, or shortly after, a withdrawal syndrome.

Note: This diagnosis should be made instead of a diagnosis of substance withdrawal only when the cognitive symptoms are in excess of those usually associated with the withdrawal syndrome and when the symptoms are sufficiently severe to warrant independent clinical attention.

Code (Specific substance) withdrawal delirium: (alcohol; sedative, hypnotic, or anxiolytic; other [or unknown] substance)

American Psychiatric Association: Diagnostic and Statistical Manual of Mental Disorders, 4/e. Washington, DC: American Psychiatric Association, 1994.

TABLE 51-13	Diagnostic Criteria for Delirium Due to Multiple Etiologies

A. Disturbance of consciousness (ie, reduced clarity of awareness of the environment) with reduced ability to focus, sustain, or shift attention.

B. A change in cognition (such as memory deficit, disorientation, language disturbance) or the development of a perceptual disturbance that is not better accounted for by a preexisting, established, or evolving dementia.

C. The disturbance develops over a short period of time (usually hours to days) and tends to fluctuate during the course of the day.

D. There is evidence from the history, physical examination, or laboratory findings that the delirium has more than one etiology (eg, more than one etiological general medical condition, a general medical condition plus substance intoxication, or medication side effect).

Coding note: Use multiple codes reflecting specific delirium and specific etiologies (eg, delirium due to viral encephalitis, alcohol withdrawal delirium).

American Psychiatric Association: Diagnostic and Statistical Manual of Mental Disorders, 4/e. Washington, DC: American Psychiatric Association, 1994.

to result in delirium, often it is the combination of etiologies, any of which alone might not have resulted in delirium, that may cause the syndrome (Caine et al, 1995). Because delirium is a syndrome and not a disease, it may be viewed as a final common pathway of many possible causes (Andreasen & Black, 1995).

Diagnostic Studies

Once delirium is suspected, a history gleaned from the family, nursing staff, and prior medical and nonmedical caregivers, together with a mental status exam, may disclose cognitive disturbances and associated clinical events that may suggest an etiology and influence the patient's management. A careful medical history, including medications and drug history, a physical exam, and a neurologic exam should be performed. In some cases, additional procedures such as laboratory tests (including routine blood and urine studies), neuroimaging procedures (CT, MRI), lumbar puncture, blood gas analysis, electrocardiogram, and EEG are useful. For example, an EEG may demonstrate diffuse brain function, even though it provides no clues as to etiology. Several minor abnormalities (eg, slight hypercalcemia plus slight hyponatremia plus mild anemia) may contribute to produce delirium, even when any single abnormality would not have done so (Andreasen & Black, 1995; Caine et al, 1995).

TABLE 51-14	Diagnostic Criteria for Delirium Not Otherwise Specified

This category should be used to diagnose a delirium that does not meet criteria for any of the specific types of delirium described in this section.

Examples include:

1. A clinical presentation of delirium that is suspected to be due to a general medical condition or substance use but for which there is insufficient evidence to establish a specific etiology

2. Delirium due to causes not listed in this section (eg, sensory deprivation)

American Psychiatric Association: Diagnostic and Statistical Manual of Mental Disorders, 4/e. Washington, DC: American Psychiatric Association, 1994.

TABLE 51-15	Differential Diagnosis of Delirium			
Observation	Delirium	Dementia	Depression	Psychosis
Onset	Acute	Insidious	Variable	Variable
Orientation	Impaired	Impaired	Intact	Intact
Short-term memory	Impaired	Impaired	Intact	Intact
Sensorium	Fluctuating	Variable	Intact	Intact
Attentiveness	Impaired	Variable	Usually intact	Variable
Delusions (eg, paranoia)	Common	Sometimes	Rare	Common
Hallucinations	Visual, tactile, or olfactory	Uncommon	Rare	Auditory
Duration	Short	Chronic	Variable	Variable

Casey, DA, Defazio, JV et al. (1996). Delirium: Quick recognition, careful evaluation and appropriate treatment. *Postgraduate Medicine* 100:121–134.

Treatment Options, Expected Outcomes, and Comprehensive Management

It is first necessary to identify and treat any medical conditions that could be underlying or contributing to the delirium. To that end, dosages of all sedatives and medications active in the central nervous system should be reduced as much as possible. The exception is delirium resulting from alcohol withdrawal or sedative/hypnotic withdrawal, in which case a cross-tolerant agent such as a benzodiazepine should be administered.

TABLE 51-16	Etiologies of Delirium

Drug Intoxication
Anticholinergics
Lithium
Antiarrhythmics (eg, lidocaine)
H_2-receptor blockers
Sedative–hypnotics
Alcohol

Drug Withdrawal
Alcohol
Sedative–hypnotics

Tumor
Primary cerebral

Trauma
Cerebral contusion (as an example)
Subdural hematoma

Infection
Cerebral (eg, meningitis, encephalitis, HIV, syphilis)
Systemic (eg, sepsis, urinary tract infection, pneumonia)

Cardiovascular
Cerebrovascular (eg, infarcts, hemorrhage, vasculitis)
Cardiovascular (eg, low output states, congestive heart failure, shock)

Physiologic or Metabolic
Hypoxemia, electrolyte disturbances, renal or hepatic failure, hypo- or hyperglycemia, postictal states (as examples)

Endocrine
Thyroid or glucocorticoid disturbances (as examples)

Nutritional
Thiamine or vitamin B_{12} deficiency, pellagra (as examples)

Caine, Ed, Grossman, H, Lyness, JM, (1995). Delerium, Dementia and amnesia and other cognitive disorders. In Kaplan, HI, Saddocl, BJ. (1995). Comprehensive Textbook of Psychiatry, 6/e, Vol 1. Baltimore, MD: Williams & Wilkins.

Special attention should be paid to ensure that the patient's nutritive needs (both fluid and food) are met. The environment should be kept as quiet and undistracting as possible to reduce agitation. A brightly lit room has been found helpful (Carter et al, 1996).

Delirious patients often require much reassurance by family, friends, and staff members that their behavioral state is the result of a physical illness and that they are not going crazy. Orientation cues are also very helpful. Attention should be paid to the patient's legal capacity to make informed clinical choices (Kaplan & Sadock, 1995).

In cases of intermittent or persistent psychomotor agitation, physical restraints may be used temporarily if necessary to prevent the patient from inflicting self-harm. If sedation is required, low doses of high-potency antipsychotics (eg, haloperidol [Haldol] 0.5 to 1 mg orally or parenterally) may be administered. Low-potency agents, benzodiazepines, and other sedatives such as antihistamines and barbiturates should be avoided because they tend to worsen the delirium, but in cases of life-threatening agitation in which patients pull out arterial lines, for example, various combinations that achieve sedation safely have been used (Caine et al, 1995).

Teaching and Self-Care

Caring for the caregiver with a patient experiencing delirium is similar to the concerns identified with dementia. Involvement of the family in all aspects of care is essential for success in the plan of care.

Referral Points and Clinical Warnings

Precipitating factors for delirium in older patients may include:

- Use of physical restraints
- Malnutrition
- Medications.

These concerns need to be reviewed with family members.

Accidents are a primary area of concern as patients become uncertain about what activities they can participate in safely.

Family members and other caregivers will need respite during long-term care of the patient with dementia.

COMMUNITY RESOURCES

- Internet Mental Health—Delirium, http://www.mentalhealth.com/dis/p20-or01.html: Research (1991 to May 1995), booklets, magazine articles, Internet links to cognitive disorders sites
- Internet Mental Health—Dementia, http://www.mentalhealth.com/dis/p20-or05.html: Research (1991 to May 1995), booklets, magazine articles, Internet links to cognitive disorders sites
- The Institute for Brain Aging and Dementia, http://www.apa.uci.edu/dement.html: What is dementia, what causes dementia, how is dementia diagnosed
- National Mental Health Association, 1021 Prince St., Alexandria, VA 22314-2971, 1-800-969-NMHA (6942)
- National Institute of Mental Health, Public Inquiries, 5600 Fishers Lane, Room 7C-02, MSC 8030, Bethesda, MD 20892-8030

EDITOR'S NOTE:

COMPLEMENTARY APPROACHES

A general discussion of complementary approaches can be found in Chapter 3. The following, while not an exhaustive list, are some complementary approaches being used for this condition. Additional information on these approaches, including precautions, can be found in Appendices A and B. Providers need to assess for the use of complementary approaches as part of the patient's history, as they may impact conventional therapies, and patients may not volunteer this information unless specifically asked. Efficacy of many complementary approaches is not as well documented as that of conventional therapies. Providers need to read the literature before suggesting these complementary approaches.

- Vitamins, minerals, herbs, supplements
  Ginkgo
  Vitamin B_{12}
- Complementary Modalities
  Aromatherapy

References

Andreasen, N.C., & Black, D.W. (1995). *Introductory textbook of psychiatry*, 2d ed. Washington, D.C.: American Psychiatric Press, Inc.

Caine, E.D., Grossman, H., & Lyness, J.M. (1995). Delirium, dementia, and amnestic and other cognitive disorders and mental disorders due to a general medical condition. In H.I. Kaplan, B.J. Dock (Eds.). *Comprehensive textbook of psychiatry*, Vol. 1, 6th ed. Baltimore: Williams & Wilkins.

Casey, D.A., DeFazio, J.V., Varsickle, K., et al. (1996). Delirium: Quick recognition, careful evaluation, and appropriate treatment. *Postgraduate Medicine, 100*, 121–134.

Drayer, B.P. (1988). Imaging of the aging brain. Part I. Normal findings. *Radiology, 166*, 785–796.

Eastwood, R. (1997). Dementia: Current developments. *Biomedicine & Pharmacotherapy, 51*, 112–117.

Ernst, R., & Hay, J. (1994). The U.S. economic and social costs of Alzheimer's disease revisited. *American Journal of Public Health, 8*, 1261–1264.

Fleming, K.C., Adams, A.C., Peterson, R.C., et al. (1995). Dementia: Diagnosis and evaluation. *Mayo Clin Proceedings, 70*, 1093–1107.

Inouye, S.K., & Charpentier, P.A. (1996). Precipitating factors for delirium in hospitalized elderly persons. Predictive model and interrelationship with baseline vulnerability. *JAMA, 275*. 852–857.

Kaplan, H.I., & Sadock, B.J. (1995). *Comprehensive textbook of psychiatry/VI*, vol. 1 (6th ed). Baltimore: Williams & Wilkins.

McKeith, L.G., Galasko, D., Kosaka, K., et al. (1996). Consensus guidelines for the clinical and pathologic diagnosis of dementia with Lewy bodies (DLB): Report of the consortium on DLB international workshop. *Neurology, 47*, 1113–1124.

Pinholt, E.M., Kroenke, K., Hanley, J.F., et al. (1987). Functional assessment of the elderly: A comparison of standard instruments with clinical judgment. *Archives of Internal Medicine, 147*, 484–488.

Sandson, T.A., & Price, B.H. (1996). Diagnostic testing in dementia. *Diagnostic Testing in Neurology, 14*, 45–56.

Severson, M.A., Smith, G.E., Tangalos, G.E., et al. (1994). Patterns and predictors of institutionalization in community-based dementia patients. *Journal of the American Geriatric Society, 42*, 181–185.

Tien, R.D., Felsberg, G.J., Ferris, N.J., et al. (1993). The dementias: Correlation of clinical features, pathophysiology, and neuroradiology. *American Journal of Radiology, 161*, 245–255.

Writing Committee, *Lancet* conference. (1996). The challenge of the dementias. *Lancet, 347*, 1303–1307.

Demyelinating Disease/Multiple Sclerosis

Ann Higgins, MS, RN, ANP

Multiple sclerosis (MS) is a chronic disease of the central nervous system (CNS) that typically appears in late adolescence or early adulthood. Although the etiology is unknown, it is believed to be autoimmune in nature, after a viral infection, with genetic and environmental factors involved. During what could be their most productive and active years, affected persons become partially or completely disabled; this has a profound social, emotional, and financial impact on their lives.

The neurologic abnormalities that constitute MS may be acute or subacute in onset and may wax and wane over time. Early symptoms include numbness, double vision, paresis, bladder control problems, ataxia, and tremor. The clinical course of the disease may be benign, relapsing and remitting, or progressive. Treatment is based on the progression of the disease and symptoms, including fatigue, spasticity, urinary dysfunction, emotional problems, cognitive dysfunction, and pain. Management of chronic symptoms helps the patient remain functional even when the problems are severe. Medication designed to reduce a specific immune response and medications that assist in the stimulation of remyelination are being developed.

Other neurologic conditions, not emphasized in this chapter, may be similar in some ways to MS. Table 52-1 compares Guillain-Barré syndrome, Huntington's disease, and amyotrophic lateral sclerosis. These diseases also have an impact on the sensory and motor functioning of patients and may be diagnosed in primary care settings.

ANATOMY, PHYSIOLOGY, AND PATHOLOGY

Oligodendroglia cells of the CNS and Schwann cells of the peripheral nervous system are responsible for forming lipoprotein layers of nerve fibers in early life known as myelin sheaths. There are chemical and immunologic differences between central and peripheral myelin sheaths, but they serve the same function: to promote nerve transmission along the axon. Demyelination, a feature of many neurologic disorders, can result from neuronal damage, as well as damage to the myelin itself, whether it is the result of local injury, ischemia, toxic agents, or metabolic disorders (Berkow, 1992).

Extensive myelin loss is usually followed by axonal degeneration and cell body degeneration and may be irreversible. However, there are instances in which remyelination occurs, and repair, regeneration, and complete recovery of neural function are possible. This is often seen after the segmental demyelination that characterizes many peripheral neuropathies and may explain the exacerbations and remissions of MS. Central demyelination is the predominant finding in several disorders of uncertain etiology that are known as primary demyelinating diseases (Berkow, 1992). The most prominent of these demyelinating diseases is MS, the focus of this chapter.

The pathologic hallmarks of MS are plaques, areas of demyelination restricted to the white matter of the CNS. These sites lack myelin and contain perivascular inflammation. Plaques are frequently found in the white matter of the optic nerves, the brain stem, the cerebellum, and the spinal cord. They are also found in the cerebrum, usually in a perivascular distribution. Occasionally plaques are seen in the gray matter. The location of the plaques correlates with the patient's symptoms (Lynch & Rose, 1996). The reasons for the patterns of lesion location are not known. However, proximity to the flow of cerebrospinal fluid or vascular perfusion might result in a high concentration of circulating inflammatory proteins in these areas (Sobel, 1995).

Currently, pathologists believe that demyelination is secondary to inflammation. The inflammatory response is perivenular, with a lesser response at the edges of or within plaques. Features of the cellular immune response that may be seen in MS are cells such as mononuclear cells, lymphocytes, and monocytes. These cells are engaged in reactions in the perivascular cuffs, in the leptomeninges, and diffusely in the CNS parenchyma (Sobel, 1995).

Lymphocytes probably contribute to the inflammatory process through antibody and cell-mediated immunity. Secretion of lymphokines and cytokines may be an indirect mechanism (Lynch & Rose, 1996). Cytokines may influence macrophage activation, stimulating the phagocytosis of myelin. Products of the immune response, including immunoglobins, interleukins, interferon, and tumor necrosis factor, accompany the acute MS lesion. After the initial events, immature oligodendrocytes appear and presumably participate in remyelination.

MS lesions may vary in size, the extent of CNS involvement, and the stage of evolution. These lesions may evolve through multiple remyelinating and demyelinating episodes, with the result being a chronic burned-out plaque. An autopsy of a patient with MS may show old inactive plaques, along with actively inflamed lesions and ongoing demyelination (Sobel, 1995).

EPIDEMIOLOGY

There are more than 300,000 people with the diagnosis of MS in the United States. Most cases appear during the third and fourth decades of life, with the risk of the first episode peaking at about age 30 (Vollmer & Waxman, 1991). The incidence of the disease before the age of 10 and after the age of 50 is less than 5%. The risk for development of MS for women is two to three times greater than that for men. The onset of the disease occurs in women at a younger age. The higher incidence

TABLE 52-1	Comparisons of Guillain-Barré Syndrome, Huntington's Disease, and Amyotrophic Lateral Sclerosis		
Disease	**Genetics/Onset Prognosis**	**Symptoms**	**Major Care Considerations & Treatment Approaches**
Guillain-Barré syndrome (acute polyneuritis with facial diplegia, acute infectious polyneuritis, and Landry-Guillain-Barré syndrome)	Acute autoimmune response to a febrile (viral) infection	1 to 3 weeks after a febrile episode, symmetrical pain and muscle weakness involving one or many muscle groups. Loss of deep tendon reflexes	Respiratory support may be necessary during the recovery phase (weeks to months). Swallowing difficulties may precede respiratory and fluid/electrolyte problems. Plasmapheresis (2–4 plasma exchanges) and intravenous immunoglobulin (IVIg) may decrease recovery time and improve recovery.
Huntington's disease	Inherited CNS (corticospinal) neuro-degenerative disease, often occurring between 30–50 years	Progressive dementia and involuntary muscular movements of limbs and facial muscles (choreiform movements)	No specific therapy; motor control may be aided by occupational and physical therapy. End-stage disease includes loss of activities of daily living, including bowel and bladder control. Associated emotional/psychiatric conditions can be treated. Emotional concerns of presymptomatic testing need to be fully considered but not exaggerated.
Amyotrophic lateral sclerosis (Lou Gehrig's disease, motor neuron disease)	Possible association with a genetic defect	Muscular spasticity and weakness, hyperreflexia secondary to degeneration of motor neurons of cortex, medulla, and spinal cord	No specific therapy; motor control may be aided by occupational and physical therapy. Discussion of end-of-life issues may be necessary.

Source: Asbury & McKhann, 1997; Bundey, 1997; Goroll et al, 1995; French Cooperative, 1997; Thomas, 1993.

of MS in women may reflect a hormonal factor that increases susceptibility (Matthews, 1991).

There appears to be a distinct geographic difference in the incidence and prevalence of MS. In general, these rates escalate with increasing distance from the equator, the highest prevalence being between 40° north and 40° south from the equator. People of higher socioeconomic status are at higher risk, and the relation to urbanization remains unknown (Vollmer & Waxman, 1991).

MS occurs among whites and other ethnic groups, but a higher frequency has been reported in whites than in non-whites. African Americans are at a lower risk than whites (Sibley et al, 1989). Asians manifest low rates of disease (2 per 100,000 people). There have been no reported cases of MS in the native-born people of Alaska and Greenland (Matthews, 1991).

There has been support for the idea that environment may be related to the development of the disease. In studies on immigrants, it was found that those who moved after age 15 from a high-risk area retained much of the high-risk status of their place of origin. Those moving at a younger age acquired the low-risk status of their new home (Hopkins, 1993). A latent period of approximately 20 years follows before the development of the chronic illness (Vollmer & Waxman, 1991).

Genetic factors have long been recognized to play a role in the development of MS. An increased prevalence of MS in fam-ily members of MS patients has been observed. Fifteen percent of patients are known to have an affected relative. Siblings of an affected person are at a higher risk than parents or children (Matthews, 1991).

However, the tendency to consider all diseases with increased familial incidence as hereditary may be erroneous. Virus infection as a possible cause for MS has been studied. Elevated antibody levels to measles are found in MS patients compared with controls. The measles antibody level is also raised in siblings of MS patients. Raised titers of antibodies to other viruses have been reported in cases of MS, including rubella, herpes zoster, herpes simplex, and Epstein-Barr virus (Matthews, 1991).

ETIOLOGY

MS is an immune-mediated disease, acquired by a genetically predisposed persons near the time of puberty. Epidemiologic and pathologic aspects, as well as a host of immunologic and experimental observations, must be taken into account when considering the mechanism of demyelination (Hopkins, 1993). An immune-mediated inflammatory demyelination, probably genetically determined, may be the basis for the disease. Markers for immunopathologic processes, such as perivascular infiltration by lymphocytes, class II major histocompatibility com-

TABLE 52-2	Indicators of a Possible Autoimmune Response

- Immune abnormalities in blood and CSF—high frequency of activated lymphocytes, reduced number of suppressor cells, antimyelin antibody responses
- Similarities between MS and experimental allergic encephalitis—an animal model in which inflammatory demyelination can be induced by inoculating animals with basic myelin protein
- Association between MS and certain MHC class II allotypes
- Clinical response of patients to immunosuppressive drugs

Source: Lynch & Rose, 1996.

plex antigen expression by cells in the lesions, lymphokines and cytokines secreted by activated cells, and absence of evidence of infection, are all noted on pathology exams. Other indicators of a possible autoimmune response and theories of autoimmune pathogenesis are listed in Tables 52-2 and 52-3.

DIAGNOSTIC CRITERIA

No specific test for MS exists. The evidence supporting diagnosis rests on multiple signs and symptoms and characteristic remissions and exacerbations. MS is characterized by dissemination in time and space—in other words, there are multiple episodes of dysfunction and multiple areas of involvement within the CNS. The diagnosis cannot be made with assurance at the first attack. Table 52-4 lists the criteria for diagnosis.

Course of Disease

Although the course of MS is unpredictable in any given patient, for most patients it is more benign than generally thought. Twenty-five years after diagnosis, an estimated 75% of patients are alive, 66% are ambulatory, and 33% are productively employed (Vollmer & Waxman, 1991). The various courses MS can take are presented in Tables 52-5 and 52-6.

TABLE 52-3	Theories of Autoimmune Pathogenesis

The following theories, alone or in combination, are under consideration by researchers searching for the basis for the disease:

- **Molecular mimicry.** The term arises from the demonstration of shared homology between human myelin proteins and viral polypeplides. In MS, homology between myelin antigens and viral peptides has been established; thus, this mechanism could result in CNS demyelination after viral infection.
- **Altered immunity.** Patients tend to have higher antibody titers in serum and CSF for measles virus. Patients and siblings also have higher serum titers of antibodies to many other viruses, such as rubella and varicella.
- **T lymphocytes.** Infection activates T lymphocytes, resulting in the production of gamma interferon, a substance that enhances antigenic recognition.
- **Genetic predisposition.** 5% of patients have a sibling with MS. Overall, about 15% have some close relative with the illness. When one of a pair of monozygote twins develops MS, the other member develops clinical MS in 40% of the cases, with evidence of 70% on MRI. The precise interplay among genetic, environmental, and immunologic factors remains to be determined.

Source: Rudnick, 1996.

Clinical Symptoms

The initial symptoms may occur alone or in combination. The distribution of pathologic lesions accounts for the wide variety of symptoms. The clinical picture objectifies the loss, permanent or temporary, of normal impulse-conduction properties in myelinated nerve fibers. The fibers can be in the long ascending and descending tracts of the spinal cord, the shorter white matter tracts within the brain stem, or the subcortical white matter of the cerebrum and cerebellum (Vollmer & Waxman, 1991).

The incidence of initial symptoms is as follows: weakness in one or more limbs, 40%; optic neuritis, 22%; paresthesia, 21%; diplopia, 12%; vertigo, 5%; and disturbance of micturition, 5%. There is usually asymmetric distribution of the clinical defects, but as the disease progresses and lesions become more widely distributed, the symptoms become bilateral (Matthews, 1991).

MOTOR SYMPTOMS

Motor symptoms often occur early in the disease. Patients may complain of weakness or heaviness of the involved limb. They may initially complain of weakness on exertion, gradually increasing until it is constantly present. They may describe a tendency to trip or fall or may drag the affected limb (Hickey, 1992). The symptoms may last for minutes to hours and therefore cannot always be observed during an ordinary clinical exam (Matthews, 1991). There may be no abnormal signs on the clinical exam at rest except for the absence of abdominal reflexes, an indication of cortical tract dysfunction. On exercise, weakness, spasticity, and extensor plantar reflexes rapidly appear, only to become reversible at rest (Matthews, 1991). Uhthoff's phenomenon is a worsening of motor function after a hot shower or a hot bath. This can be of diagnostic significance.

Pyramidal tract involvement produces characteristics of upper neuron disease: spasticity, hyperreflexia, clonus, and extensor plantar responses. Deep tendon reflexes are exaggerated, sustained clonus may be elicited (usually at the ankles), and extensor plantar responses may be observed. Commonly, these signs are asymmetric. Deep tendon reflexes can be decreased if the reflex arc has been interrupted by a lesion at a certain segmental level of the spinal cord. The Achilles reflex may be absent, and sphincter and sexual dysfunction may be present if lesions are found in sacral segments (Gordon et al, 1991).

Triceps jerks are lost more frequently in the upper extremities; ankle jerks are lost more frequently than knee jerks. In established disease in the upper limbs, biceps and supinator jerks may be associated with finger flexion and Hoffman's sign. Flicking or nipping the nail of the second, third, or fourth finger, if the reflex is present, causes flexion of these fingers and possibly the thumb. Its presence indicates that the tendon reflexes are hyperactive. An increased jaw jerk suggests involvement above the level of the foramen magnum (Matthews, 1991).

Increased muscle tone is an important factor in this disease. In less severe cases, there is spasticity of the extensor muscles of the legs. This occurs in bed at night or when trying to rise in the morning. The legs are held rigidly extended, usually for several minutes. These spasms are seldom painful but are inconvenient. As the disease progresses, the flexor muscles become spastic. The patient may fall without warning while walking. Flexor spasms are frequently painful (Matthews, 1991).

TABLE 52-4	Revised Criteria for the Diagnosis of MS
Clinically Definite MS	Two attacks of neurologic symptoms, each lasting 24 hours, separated by 1 month involving different parts of the nervous system. There must be clinical evidence of two separate lesions on physical exam or clinical evidence of one and paraclinical evidence (ie, neuroimaging, electrophysiologic, and neuropsychiatric techniques) of another.
Laboratory Definite MS	Two attacks, clinical or paraclinical evidence of one lesion, and the presence of oligoclonal bands. One attack, clinical evidence of one lesion, and paraclinical evidence of another separate lesion and oligoclonal bands. Progressive course for 6 months, sequential discrete involvement clinically or paraclinically and the presence of oligoclonal bands.
Clinically Probable MS	Two attacks and clinical evidence of one lesion. One attack and clinical evidence of two lesions. One attack, clinical evidence of one lesion, and paraclinical evidence of another.
Laboratory-Supported Probable MS	Two attacks and presence of oligoclonal bands.

Source: Hopkins, 1993; Vollmer & Waxman, 1991.

Bilateral involvement of the corticobulbar tracts occurs in some patients; this leads to dysarthria, dysphagia, hyperactive jaw jerks, bifacial paralysis, and apparent emotional lability. Spastic weakness of the muscles of speech is common. In the early stages, speech is often slurred. As the disease progresses, speech becomes explosive or staccato and unintelligible. Scanning speech—slow and measured speech with pauses between syllables—is seen in later stages of the disease (Hickey, 1992).

SENSORY SYMPTOMS

Sensory symptoms are the most common initial features of MS and occur throughout the course of the disease. These symptoms are varied and the onset may be symmetrical. The sensations are described as tingling, numbness, a pins-and-needles sensation, tightness, coldness, or swelling of the limbs or trunk. Complaints of tight bands or straps around the trunk or limbs are characteristic symptoms (Gordon et al, 1991). A common pattern is for unusual sensations to begin in one foot and spread to both lower limbs, the buttock, the perineum, and the trunk within a few days.

The normal sensation of micturition and defecation may be affected, but control remains normal. Vaginal sensation is also diminished. The exam may reveal no loss of light touch or pinprick, but the pinprick may feel distant, as if something is between the pin and the skin. An intensely itching pain, especially in the cervical dermatomes, usually unilateral and occurring in young women, is suggestive of MS (Gordon et al, 1991).

The most frequent sensory signs are varying degrees of impairment of vibration and joint position sense, decrease of pain and light touch in a stocking-and-glove distribution in the four extremities, and patchy areas of reduced pain and light touch perception in the limbs and trunk (Gordon et al, 1991).

Lhermitte's sign consists of an electric feeling passing down the back to the legs on flexing the neck. This is common in MS but can occur in other conditions (compressive myopathies). The usual course of a sensory episode is toward complete remission within 6 to 8 weeks; for patients who have frequent attacks, these episodes may clear in 10 days. Observant patients may recognize sensory symptoms of a more localized nature that last for only 1 to 2 days, unrelated to exercise, infection, or environmental temperatures (Matthews, 1991). Sensory symptoms tend to remit more frequently than do symptoms involving other systems.

CEREBELLAR INVOLVEMENT

Cerebellar dysfunction is characterized by gait imbalances, difficulty in performing coordinated actions with the arms, and slurred speech. Cerebellar signs are usually uncommon at the

TABLE 52-5	Courses of MS

Benign MS is manifested with a single bout, followed by no new episodes. It is not clear how many patients fall into this category because many do not seek medical attention, thereby eluding diagnosis.

Relapsing and remitting course is the classic form of the disease, in which relapses are clearly distinguished from remissions. During remissions, symptoms resolve or partially resolve. After each relapse, there may be an increasing degree of fixed clinical defect.

Chronic progressive MS is manifested by relentless progression without distinct relapses. Ten percent of patients may exhibit this form of disease from onset.

TABLE 52-6	Some Patients With Relapsing Remitting Course May Deteriorate to the Chronic Progressive Form of MS

- Relapsing–remitting patients may convert to progressive disease, and approximately the same percentage of progressive patients will change to relapsing–remitting disease.

- Prognostically, shorter intervals between the initial relapses are associated with progressive disease. Risk of relapse is high for the first year, as well as for the 5 years following. There is no consistent relation between rate of relapse and outcome of disease.

- Fifty percent of patients with MS have a clinically manifested bout of optic neuritis at some time during their illness. Ninety percent of MS patients exhibit electrophysiologic evidence of optic nerve involvement.

- Patients of older age at onset tend to have a chronically progressive course more frequently than younger patients.

- Cerebellar or multiple system involvement at onset is common in patients with severe disease. Severe ataxia as an initial symptom indicates severe disease. Tremor, incoordination, or disturbance of mobility as initial symptoms have a poor prognosis.

Source: Matthews, 1991; Vollmer & Waxman, 1991.

onset of the disease (Matthews, 1991). The early appearance of cerebellar ataxia is an indication of a poor prognosis, and cerebellar signs often persist. There may be difficulty in distinguishing cerebellar signs from those of weakness, spasticity, sensory loss, and vertigo. Cerebellar ataxia naturally affects the gait, but spasticity and weakness are more important causes of disability.

Conventional heel–knee shin tests are poorly performed by weak and spastic legs. Truncal ataxia and gait are not obvious when sitting but contribute to poor balance. These abnormalities may be observed by having the patient stand or walk normally. Cerebellar incoordination in the upper limbs may be terribly disabling, especially when combined with any significant degree of intentional tremor. Severe degrees of intentional tremor may render the hands useless; voluntary movement can be disturbed by violent deviations of the arms that may render the patient unapproachable (Matthews, 1991).

VISUAL INVOLVEMENT/OPTIC NEURITIS
Many patients with MS display abnormalities of vision. These defects are the result of lesions of the optic nerve or chiasm. Even patients who do not demonstrate a clinically detectable visual defect often do so electrophysiologically through the measurement of visual evoked potentials. Evoked potentials are considered extensions of the clinical exam and allow objective measurement of lesions in specific pathways (Rudnick, 1996).

Uthhoff, in a classic paper on the ophthalmic findings in MS, found a high incidence of optic atrophy in patients with chronic disease; central scotoma and loss of visual acuity were observed (Matthews, 1991). Optic neuritis may be acute or subacute, with the acute form being more common, and may represent a presenting episode of MS. Visual blurring or haziness may resolve rapidly, stabilize, or progress to complete visual loss (Vollmer & Waxman, 1991).

Pain most commonly precedes the onset of visual symptoms but can occur simultaneously with the onset or develop subsequently. The pain is felt in the eye or is supraorbital and is often accompanied by unilateral or generalized headaches. Tenderness may be elicited by putting pressure on the globe. The pain varies in intensity. It can be aggravated by movement of the eye or may be present only on movement. Absence of pain does not exclude the diagnosis, nor does the severity of pain represent a poor prognosis. Treatment with steroids or ACTH often relieves the pain. The period from the onset of visual symptoms to peak loss of acuity is usually 3 to 7 days (Matthews, 1991).

In mild cases, where the lesion is retrobulbar, the optic disc may appear normal. In more severe cases, the disc shows indistinct margins and may be pinker during the acute stages. There may be edema or slight swelling of the disc. If there have been previous attacks of optic neuritis, pallor of the disc can progress to the chalk white of optic atrophy (Vollmer & Waxman, 1991).

In two thirds of cases, there is some degree of pupillary dilation. The Marcus Gunn pupillary response, also known as afferent pupillary defect, is noted in these patients. When light is shined in the normal eye, bilateral pupillary constriction results. Shining the light into the diseased eye, however, produces delayed or incomplete direct pupillary constriction. If the light is moved from the unaffected eye to the abnormal eye, the pupil appears to dilate on illumination (Williams & Schneiderman,

1996). The visual field defect in most patients is either a central scotoma or generalized impairment of the whole field (Matthews, 1991).

Recovery of visual acuity is the rule after an initial attack of optic neuritis, although there are exceptions. Optimal acuity is achieved after a mean of 2 months from onset. Improvement can continue, but at a decelerating rate. Recovery of normal vision does not mean full recovery of function of the optic nerve or complete freedom from symptoms. There may be a slight dulling of visual images and lack of appreciation of brightness of colors (Matthews, 1991).

BRAIN STEM FUNCTIONS
Demyelination of the third, fourth, and sixth cranial nerves before they leave the brain stem is the cause for diplopia. Diplopia may also occur as a result of demyelination of the medial longitudinal bundle, which links the third, fourth, and sixth nuclei (Hopkins, 1993). Characteristic of such a lesion is internuclear ophthalmoplegia (weakness of adduction with nystagmus of the abducting eye on lateral gaze) (Vollmer & Waxman, 1991).

Nystagmus occurs in 50% of MS patients. Different forms of nystagmus occur. Horizontal nystagmus on lateral gaze is most common. Jelly nystagmus can be detected only when inspecting the fundus with an ophthalmoscope; the optic disc can be seen to jerk rapidly from side to side over a small range (Matthews, 1991).

Facial numbness may accompany symptoms of sensory relapse. Facial weakness occurs in up to 5% of patients (Vollmer & Waxman, 1991). The lack of pain and preservation of taste distinguish it from Bell's palsy. Facial myokymia occurs in MS and also in other conditions (eg, Guillain-Barré, posterior fossa tumors, pontine glioma). The onset is sudden: the patient complains of stiffness of the face that makes certain movements difficult, even though there is no weakness or pain. Patients may observe their own reflections and see that their face is drawn up on the affected side; the palpebral fissure is slightly narrowed and the nasolabial fold deepened. Slight contraction of all the muscles on one side of the face is accompanied by an extraordinary rapid flickering that passes over the face in undulating waves. Remission occurs within 1 week to 6 months (Matthews, 1991).

Vertigo occurs as an initial symptom in 5% of cases. It is usually of acute onset and is prostrating. When the patient lies perfectly still, it subsides, but it is immediately aggravated by any movement of the head. Nystagmus is seen and increased with head movement. The duration of the attack is variable, from a few days to several weeks. During the course of the disease, vertigo occurs in up to 40% to 50% of patients. In many patients, vomiting accompanies vertigo (Vollmer & Waxman, 1991). Demyelination may occur in the olfactory and auditory nerves, the only other cranial nerves in which oligodendroglial cells are present.

AUTONOMIC NERVOUS SYSTEM
Bladder
Loss of bladder control is the most important autonomic disturbance to MS patients. The initial presentation includes bladder problems in at least 5% of patients, and in some patients it is the only initial symptom (Vollmer & Waxman, 1991). Isolated instances of retention or incontinence may be realized in retro-

spect as the first evidence of the disease. When evaluating bladder incontinence or urgency, the provider must rule out other causes of these problems. Usually there is urgency of micturition in mild relapses involving the spinal cord. If there is a remission, bladder function is restored, but if a mild motor disability persists, urgency continues (Matthews, 1991).

Small quantities of urine are passed with urgency accompanied by hesitancy. Frequency also is a problem with increasing disability. The nature of the urgency changes and large quantities of urine are passed without warning, without sensation, leading to a state of constant dribbling. Acute retention can occur at any stage of the disease but usually resolves. Recurrence is common. The degree of bladder disorder is usually related to the severity of motor and sensory impairment, but there are exceptions (Mastwin, 1990). Urinary infections are common in MS patients, especially in women. They do not usually cause fever and back pain but present as an increase in bladder or neurologic dysfunction (Gordon et al, 1991).

Bowel
Fecal incontinence is uncommon. As the disease advances, constipation becomes a major manifestation, reflecting upper and lower motor neuron impairment in addition to decreased general mobility (Gordon, 1991). Patients with paraplegia usually need a bowel regimen to maintain regular bowel movements.

SEXUAL FUNCTION
Sexual dysfunction can affect the quality of life in MS patients, who are usually of childbearing age (Mattson, 1995). Disorders of sexual function are common. Mattson found sexual dysfunction in 57% of MS patients; 78% of these patients were men and 45% women. Thirty-five percent of patients expressed less interest in sex since their diagnosis. Among the commonly reported problems in men were erectile dysfunction, trouble achieving orgasm, and inability to ejaculate. Women reported decreased vaginal lubrication, trouble achieving orgasm, and decreased vaginal sensation. Patients who began receiving steroids for nonsexual exacerbation had a lower incidence of sexual dysfunction. There was no relation between the presence of sexual dysfunction and age, duration of disease, type of disease, or degree of disability.

Issues of sexual function should be an important consideration in the care of these patients. Although impotence is usually associated with prolonged disease, it can occur in the first episode. There is a clear relation between impotence and sphincter disturbance and also the duration of the disease. In men totally impotent, sweating was absent below the waist; in partial impotence, sweating was absent below the groin (Matthews, 1991).

CORTICAL FUNCTION
Rao and Leo (1991) found that 43% of MS patients tested had an overall cognitive decline, with impairment in recent memory, sustained attention, verbal fluency, cognitive reasoning, and visuospatial perception. However, even before dementia is demonstrated by testing, patients often complain of not being able to perform certain tasks that they had been able to do before illness (Vollmer & Waxman, 1991).

Depression in MS patients is probably not caused by the disease process; instead, it is a reaction to the prospect of chronic progressive disability and isolation (Matthews, 1991). Pathologic laughing and weeping are extreme examples of lability of affective display. The patient cannot modulate affective expression, so even mild emotional stimuli bring on an emotional display that is exaggerated in its intensity. These displays are socially disabling and are likely to disrupt personal relationships. Emotional communication can be disrupted because facial expression may not be reflecting what the patient is saying. While patients are laughing, it is hard to recognize depression or to appreciate that they are feeling bad (Johnson et al, 1987).

SEIZURES
Seizures appear on every list of symptoms at the onset or during the course of the disease. Tonic-clonic or partial motor seizures occur in about 5% of MS patients. Demyelinating disease is the cause in some patients; however, MS patients can also be affected by other disorders of the CNS, so it is important to determine the etiology of seizures (Matthews, 1991).

DIAGNOSTIC STUDIES

No laboratory test is universally diagnostic for MS, but some studies are helpful in confirming the presence of lesions over time. These are listed in Table 52-7.

DIFFERENTIAL DIAGNOSIS

The vast assortment of signs, symptoms, and clinical entities of MS tax even the most experienced providers, affording ample opportunity for misdiagnosis. However, with careful investigation, a correct conclusion can be established. Table 52-8 lists key diseases that should be ruled out in the diagnosis of MS.

TREATMENT OPTIONS AND COMPREHENSIVE MANAGEMENT

The diagnosis of MS should be given to the patient as soon as it has been established. Basic information should be given on the disease process. With subsequent visits, more information can be disseminated and any questions regarding the condition can be answered. Questions concerning long-term prognosis and degree of handicap can be answered when patients ask them, suggesting they are ready to hear the answers (Lynch & Rose, 1996). General health measures for MS patients are listed in Table 52-9. Table 52-10 provides guidelines for the treatment of symptoms.

Neurobehavioral Disorders

Depression, emotional lability, dementia, and cognitive impairment are some of the neurobehavioral problems seen in MS patients. Depression occurs in 27% to 54% of MS patients. The etiology of the depression is probably multifactorial (biologic, psychological, and social) (Mitchell, 1993). The suicide rate in MS patients is 7.5 times that of the normal population. Providers should be alert for signs of depression (Lynch & Rose, 1996). If the depression is a reaction to illness, counseling and appropriate pharmacotherapy should be considered.

Euphoria in MS is a persistent change in mood consisting of cheerfulness and optimism. It is seen in up to 63% of patients. No treatment is required. On the other hand, pathologic laughing and crying can be very distressing. Psychosis in MS is rare

TABLE 52-7	Laboratory Studies
CSF	A common finding in MS is an elevation of the CSF immunoglobin level relative to the other protein components. There is good evidence of synthesis of immunoglobin G (IgG) within the blood–brain barrier of patients with MS. The ratio between CSF IgG and albumin is increased (IgG fraction) in about two thirds of patients with MS. An increased CSF IgG fraction is not specific for MS; however, an increased percentage of CSF gamma globulin, together with normal or slightly elevated CSF protein, greatly increases the likelihood of MS. Electrophoresis of CSF shows several fractions that are not found in the blood. The presence of these fractions, which form bands on electrophoresis, is known as oligoclonal banding. These are stable and persistent throughout the disease course and do not correlate with the clinical progression of the disease. Oligoclonal bands are found in 85% to 95% of cases of clinically definite MS. The presence in CSF of myelin components (myelin basic protein) and antibodies directed against MBP have been reported.
Evoked Potentials	Clinical electrophysiologic methods are useful noninvasive tools. These tests reveal a CNS abnormality that may be clinically undetectable. A good example is a finding of abnormal visual evoked potentials in a patient with progressive paraparesis and no symptoms of disease beyond the cord, suggesting disease in both the spinal cord and the optic nerve.
Neuroimaging	MRI is a potent diagnostic tool in the detection of MS. Early studies of MRI indicated a higher rate (80% to 100%) of lesion detection compared to CT (50%). The number of patients with lesions increased; the number of detectable lesions in individual patients also increased. The MRI is positive in 85% to 95% of cases of clinically definite MS. Other diseases such as lupus erythematosus, diabetes, hypertension, Behçet's disease, Sjögren's syndrome, Lyme disease, progressive multifocal leukoencephalopathy, and multi-infarct dementia may be indistinguishable from MS on MRI. Patchy areas of abnormal white matter are most commonly found in the periventricular areas of the cerebral hemispheres. Gadolinium enhancement can be seen around some lesions, especially if the patient is having an exacerbation or a fairly rapid chronic progression. Decreased cognitive function is correlated with an increase of lesions in the cerebral hemispheres. Use of MRI for follow-up is extremely important in the management of MS patients to measure treatment effectiveness and disease progression.

Source: Gordon et al, 1991; Hopkins, 1993; Lynch & Rose, 1996; Vollmer & Waxman 1991.

but may be associated with agitated depression or complications of steroid therapy (Mitchell, 1993).

Patients with cognitive problems show a larger number and size of lesions in the white matter of the cerebral hemispheres (Lynch & Rose, 1996). Determining the area and degree of cognitive difficulty may help in the care of the patient. Ways of working around the problem can be sought. If the patient is having a problem on the job, altering the job to suit the patient's abilities may be a solution. In discovering the areas of cognitive deficit, the family may be better able to understand and help the patient deal with these problems.

Effects on Relationships

How a person adjusts to MS may be determined by income and social networks. Spouse, children, relatives, friends, and organizations such as a house of worship or a community group can help keep the patient anchored. The divorce rate for MS patients is double that of the population at large. Sexual difficulties and altered life plans may result in anger and frustration for patient and partner alike. Couples should be encouraged to seek counseling and join groups that foster a positive approach to physical and emotional health (Murray, 1995). Referral or consultations with other health care professionals should be made to help patient and spouse or significant other cope with these issues. Most children adjust to and accept dealing with a disabled person (Murray, 1995).

The caregiver is an important persons in the long-term health and functioning of the patient with MS. However, the caregiver must take on complex roles. Burnout can occur if the caregiver feels helpless, misunderstood, or undervalued, and the caregiver may become resentful toward the patient. Women traditionally assume the caregiver role, and some men are reluctant to take this role. It is important that the caregiver be involved in discussions with the health care providers, because MS is a disorder that affects not only the patient but also the caregiver.

Immunosuppressive Therapy

These treatments, aimed at reducing inflammation in the CNS, have been used for both relapsing and remitting and chronic progressive types of MS.

TREATMENT OF RELAPSE

A relapse is an onset of new neurologic symptoms or marked worsening of old symptoms lasting longer than 24 hours. The following conditions may mimic an exacerbation and should be ruled out or treated before any therapy is given: fever, infection (usually urinary tract or viral), overheating, fatigue, and severe emotional stress. When these disorders are treated, the patient's condition will improve (Lynch & Rose, 1996). Mild relapses are treated with steroids. Any new abnormality that does not interfere with a patient's ability to perform daily activities may not require steroid therapy. Rest may be helpful. Patients with severe worsening of symptoms require steroids.

STANDARD THERAPY

ACTH and steroids have been the medications used in treating acute exacerbations. The primary effect is to shorten the attack, but no overall benefit has been noted on the outcome. Predni-

(text continued on page 592)

TABLE 52-8	Key Diseases That Should Be Ruled Out in the Diagnosis of MS
Collagen Vascular Disease	Systemic lupus erythematosus and polyarteritis nodosa may present with signs of involvement of CNS and peripheral nerves. Fever, leptocytosis, increased ESR, and visceral (renal, pulmonary, cardiac) involvement may provide important data for diagnosis.
Behçet's Disease	Behçet's disease is a connective tissue disorder that has neurologic components (seizures, corticospinal abnormalities, ataxia, bulbar palsy). The characteristic mucocutaneous ulceration of the mouth and perineum usually precedes neurologic symptoms but may occur later in the disease. The clinical features to direct diagnosis are headache, fever, elevated ESR, and less commonly meningeal irritation.
HIV/AIDS	Spastic paralysis and sensory ataxia are part of AIDS-related myelopathy. Cerebral white matter lesions on MRI can be indistinguishable from those of MS. CSF findings of total protein concentration and cell count are increased within range of parameters for MS, but oligoclonal bands are uncommon.
Intracranial Tumor	Neoplasms of the cerebellum may present with nystagmus, diploplia, facial numbness, dysarthria, and signs of corticospinal tract dysfunction. In some cases of MS, temporary improvement suggests a remission. Increased CSF proteins without abnormalities of gamma globulin or oligoclonal bands suggest a tumor.
Acute Disseminated Encephalomyelitis (ADEM) or Postinfectious Encephalomyelitis (PIEM)	ADEM may occur after either an infectious process or an immunization after an interval of 3–21 days. Fever, stiff neck, headache, radicular pain, stupor, or convulsions suggest ADEM. CSF proteins and cell counts may be higher in this entity than in MS.
Neurosyphilis	The diagnosis of MS can be confused when the patient suffers from impaired sensation in the lower extremities, ataxia, and sphincter dysfunction. Optic atrophy can also be present. Areflexia, hypotonia, normal superficial abdominal and plantar reflexes, and trophic changes of neurosyphilis contrast with the spastic, hyperflriric paresis seen together with absent abdominal reflexes and extensor plantar responses in MS. Argyll Robertson pupils are seen in syphilis and not in MS.
Lyme Disease	Progressive neurologic syndrome can be seen in Lyme disease. MRI reveals white matter lesions. The infection can cause a vasculitis that affects the CNS, causing meningitis polyradiculitis and peripheral neuropathy. Lyme disease does not usually present with a remitting–relapsing course. Anti-*Borrelia* antibodies may be detected in CSF, which may aid diagnosis. However, *Borrelia burgdorferi* has been associated with optic neuritis and oligoclonal immunoglobin found in CSF.
Vitamin B$_{12}$ Deficiency	The patient usually complains of paresthesias in distal parts of lower and upper limbs. Deep tendon reflexes may be reduced or absent but later in the disease may become increased. Optic neuritis and mental symptoms occur in B$_{12}$ deficiency. Diagnosis can be made by obtaining vitamin B$_{12}$ serum level; if doubtful, a Schilling test would help distinguish it from MS.

Source: Matthews, 1991; Motomura et al, 1980; Vollmer & Waxman, 1991

TABLE 52-9	General Health Measures
Alcohol	Alcohol should be avoided because it aggravates cerebellar deficits.
Heat	Exposure to heat, hot baths, or the sun can have destabilizing effects on the CNS.
Exercise	Proper exercise leads to fitness and decreased fatigue. Exercising to the point of pain increases fatigue and weakness; increasing core body temperature worsens fatigue and increases symptoms. It is important for the patient to have a carefully developed individualized exercise program. Exercises that increase mobility through stretching and range of motion will ultimately relieve stiffness and fatigue. Balancing exercises help maintain upright stance. Swimming and water aerobics are best because the patient is cooled while exercising.
Physical and Occupational Therapy	Devices that provide assistance with walking reduce the risk of falls, allowing greater independence and increased activity. Bracing disabled portions of limbs helps provide stability and improve function. Exercise programs and mobility can improve strength. A consultation with rehabilitative medicine can help the patient with everyday activities.
Nutrition	One of the most common concerns of most people, including patients with MS, is weight control. Patients with motor sensory or coordination deficits have an added risk of falls or serious injury if overweight. In many patients, the capacity to exercise is limited. It is commonly suggested that patients with MS restrict cholesterol and fat in the diet. This, with as much activity as possible, will help lessen the problem of obesity.
Pregnancy	Most studies have reported a decrease in disease activity, as reflected by remissions during pregnancy, especially the second and third trimesters. The effect of pregnancy on MS is similar to the effect of pregnancy on other autoimmune diseases. There is an increase in the relapse rate during the postpartum period, which may be caused by a return to normal immune function.

Source: Abramsky, 1994; Lynch & Rose, 1996; Shapiro, 1994.

TABLE 52-10	Symptom-Directed Therapy

Spasticity: Although patients with earlier or mild disease may not have spasticity, it may accumulate over time or with severe disease. Spasticity can appear in different forms. It may be seen as a "catch" in the muscles with passive rapid movement of the limbs, or it may cause stiffness or tightening of the affected limb. Most commonly, the lower limbs are affected as well as the trunk. Spasticity results in pain, increased fatigue, and difficulty in ambulation. Asymptomatic bladder infections can cause spasticity to flare. Treatment for spasticity includes physical therapy, stretching exercise, and medication.

- Baclofen is the most common antispasticity drug used in MS. The medication should be started at a low dose (10 mg) at bedtime or 10 mg twice daily and slowly increased weekly or biweekly by 10 mg per day as tolerated. Common side effects consist of drowsiness, confusion, and nausea. Baclofen cannot be discontinued abruptly, but should be tapered over weeks. The baclofen pump is an intrathecal pump with a subcutaneous reserve of baclofen that administers continuous doses directly into the spinal canal. The pump is reserved for patients with severe spasticity or those who have complications from oral therapy.
- Benzodiazepines can be used initially as therapy to prevent spasticity and clonus induced by movements during sleep, although they can cause somnolence during the day. They are very effective and can be combined with baclofen for severe spasticity or when a patient cannot tolerate high doses of baclofen.
- Dantrolene (Dantrium) is of limited value because of hepatotoxicity and increased weakness associated with its use.
- Surgical intervention may be considered when the above medications do not control spasticity or when they are contraindicated. These include percutaneous radiofrequency, foraminal rhizotomy, sciatic neurectomy, intramuscular neurolysis, tenotomy, neurotomy and myelotomy.

Fatigue is the most common and annoying symptom for patients with MS. The classic disruption is of increasing weakness that progresses as the day goes on. Other disruptions include sudden attacks of sleepiness or excessive chronic sleepiness even after adequate night's sleep. Spasticity and weakness may contribute to fatigue. Insomnia may be responsible for daytime fatigue. Depression may cause fatigue. Hot environments may increase fatigue. Planning work schedules and performing tasks in an energy-efficient manner can conserve energy.

Fatigue can be managed with medications:
- Amantadine offers modest reduction of fatigue in most patients; side effects may include headache, dizziness, nervousness, and edema.
- Pemoline is a CNS stimulant with abuse potential, which precludes its long-term use; anxiety and anorexia also occur with this drug.

Tremor and Incoordination

Tremor is one of the most difficult symptoms to treat. Treatment with medications has frequently proved unsuccessful.
- Medications that may prove useful include clonazepam, propranolol, pirmidone, and diazepam.
- Isoniazid (INH) in high dosages has shown some value but is associated with a high risk of hepatic toxicity.
- Surgical intervention (stereotaxic thalatomy) is controversial and has been used in the past for severe cases. However, this procedure tends to superimpose a new disability on already impaired persons.
- No drug therapy exists for ataxia.
- Gait training and use of aids for ambulation are approaches to dealing with ataxia.

Bladder Dysfunction: Most patients experience symptoms of bladder dysfunction at some time during illness:
- Difficulty in storing urine result in symptoms of urgency, frequency, nocturia, and incontinence and is treated with anticholinergic drugs.
- Difficulty in emptying the bladder results in symptoms such as hesitancy and retention of urine and is treated by intermittent catheterization or use of cholinergic drugs such as bethamechol.
- Bladder infections, due to residual urine and bacteruria, are common in patients with MS; prophylaxis may be required with recurrent infections.

- Acidification of urine can be accomplished with vitamin C (4 g/day) or cranberry juice.
- Orange juice and other citrus juices should be avoided because they raise urinary pH.
- Patients with severe bladder problems may require an indwelling catheter and rarely surgical diversion such as an ileal conduit.

Bowel Problems: Constipation is a frequent problem.

- Bulk formers such as Metamucil can be used; increase or decrease liquid intake depending on the presence of constipation or diarrhea.
- If bulk formers do not work, a glycerin suppository can be used; enemas may have to be given to patients restricted to bed.

Sexual Problems: It is important that patients maintain their sexual activity.

Women may suffer decreased sensation, lack of vaginal lubrication, difficulty achieving orgasm, or painful muscle spasms in legs or pelvis during intercourse.

Men should be interviewed to rule out other causes of erectile dysfunction.

Women
- Vaginal lubricants can be used.
- Vibrators may enhance sensation.
- Clitoral stimulation will help women achieve orgasm.

Men
- Medications that affect erectile function should be eliminated if possible.
- Treatment for impotence may be considered.

(continued)

TABLE 52-10	*(Continued)*
Swollen Ankles: Another common complaint of MS patients is swollen ankles. The reason for the edema is that the kneading action of the muscles to the blood vessels does not occur in MS patients, and thus fluid accumulates by gravity. Giving diuretics does not solve the problem and may even create intravascular dehydration.	■ Elevating the legs will help increase absorption of fluid into the systemic vascular system. ■ The Jobst pump is contained within a zippered stocking measured to fit over swollen legs. The pump action of this device alternates contraction with relaxation, giving a natural kneading process to the muscles.
Pain: Pain may be a primary concern for patients with MS.	■ Musculoskeletal pain may be related to abnormal use of muscles and joints. Anti-inflammatory medications and physical therapy will help. ■ Pain of dysesthetic nature—burning sensation or even electric shock pain—can occur anywhere but mostly occurs in the lower extremities. This pain may be controlled with cyclic antidepressants, a tight wrap over the painful area (ie, glove or stocking), and acupuncture. ■ Trigeminal neuralgia occurs in 1% to 2% of MS patients. These paroxysmal episodes may be triggered or nontriggered. It occurs at a higher incidence and at a younger age and is often bilateral in MS patients. Carbamazepine alone or in combination with phenytoin or baclofen reduces the pain in most patients and gives complete relief in others.

Source: Francis, 1991; Lynch & Rose, 1996; Mitchell, 1993; Schapiro, 1994; Werner, 1995.

sone is commonly used for mild to moderate exacerbations. There is no standard regimen; however, some recommend prednisone in a daily dosage of at least 1 mg/kg, continued for 7 to 10 days (Lynch & Rose, 1996).

Methylprednisolone is beneficial in severe relapses or when the patient's condition worsens after high doses of prednisone. High doses of methylprednisolone (500 to 1000 mg/day for 3 to 5 days) are given intravenously, followed by high oral doses of prednisone, which are then tapered over weeks. The dosage and regimen may vary with the provider. This treatment appears to decrease relapses and slow progression in most patients (Lynch & Rose, 1996).

The results of the Optic Neuritis Treatment trial suggested that high-dose methylprednisolone produced more favorable results than oral prednisone. Visual function recovered faster, but there was no overall difference in final outcome. The trial suggested that methylprednisolone can prolong the time between attacks (Beck et al, 1992). It was also discovered that patients receiving oral steroids were at a higher risk for further episodes of optic neuritis in the next 18 months; the reason is unknown (Hopkins, 1993). Precautions that are helpful when administering steroids are listed in Table 52-11.

PREVENTING ACUTE ATTACKS

The only treatment that has been proven to reduce the frequency and severity of acute attacks is interferon-bIb (Betaseron). This drug is a genetically engineered version of human interferon-beta. It has been shown to decrease the number of acute attacks of MS by about one third and to decrease their severity. Reduction in the appearance of new lesions on magnetic resonance imaging was another result of the drug. However, it has been shown to have no significant effect on progression (Herndon, 1990). The drug has been studied only in the relapsing and remitting form of disease (Lynch & Rose, 1996).

Betaseron is administered by subcutaneous injection every other day in a dose of 8.3 million IU. Flulike symptoms and injection site reactions were the most troublesome adverse effects (Keating & Ostby, 1996). Side effects generally decrease over time (Herndon, 1990) but can last as long as a year (Lynch & Rose, 1996). Although infrequent, depression is a potentially serious side effect and requires prompt treatment. There have also been liver function abnormalities and leukopenia. Blood should be monitored periodically for these abnormalities (Lynch & Rose, 1996).

Copolymer 1

Copolymer 1 (COP-1) is a synthetic random polymer designed to resemble myelin basic protein. Studies indicate that it reduces the number of acute attacks and slows progression of the disease. Its effectiveness is similar to that of interferon-beta. It is given twice a day by subcutaneous injection. Its side effects are mainly local redness and irritation at the injection site. Formal approval from the FDA is pending; therefore, the cost of this expensive drug is not covered by medical insurance (Herndon, 1990).

Treatment of Chronic Progression

Most treatment regimens for chronic progression remain experimental. Immunosuppressant drugs used in MS include cyclophosphamide (Cytoxan), azathioprine (Imuran), methotrexate, and cyclosporine A (Sandimmune).

Azathioprine is an immunosuppressive antimetabolite that has been used to treat aggressive MS. It appears to reduce the frequency and severity of attacks and overall progression of the disease (Herndon, 1990). However, it is debatable whether the slight clinical benefits of azathioprine outweigh its side ef-

TABLE 52-11	**Precautions When Administering Steroids**

■ Administration of calcium and vitamin D

■ Restriction of foods high in sugar or sodium

■ Increase of intake of potassium-rich foods, such as bananas, orange juice, and tomatoes

■ Because of mood swings, anxiety, or sleeplessness, patients may need sedation.

■ Monitor for hypertension, electrolyte imbalance, and hyperglycemia.

Source: Lynch & Rose, 1996.

fects. The actual drug benefit probably takes months to develop, with increased value after 2 years of treatment. Patients who take the drug should be monitored for leukopenia and hepatotoxicity (Lynch & Rose, 1996). About 15% of patients cannot take the drug because of fever, rash, and nausea. One of the greater concerns is decreased tumor surveillance with an increase in malignancies, especially non-Hodgkin's lymphoma (Mitchell, 1993).

Cyclophosphamide is an alkylating agent with cytotoxic and immunosuppressive activities, affecting both cellular and humoral immunity. Cyclophosphamide may be reserved for very aggressive disease that has not responded to other measures. Its use is highly controversial. In some drug trials, the disease was found to stabilize in many patients for approximately 2 to 4 years. Most of the patients who did better were younger, with a shorter total disease duration. Side effects include alopecia, hemorrhagic cystitis, nausea, vomiting, leukopenia with complicating infections, and pulmonary fibrosis. The tumor surveillance may be affected and the number of malignancies increased because of decreased immune function (Mitchell, 1993).

Cyclosporine is a fungal antimetabolite that appears to enhance T-cell suppressor cell function while reducing the number of T-helper cells. Slight benefits have been reported from the use of the drug, including decreased progression of disease, relapse rate, and relapse severity. The efficacy of the drug is equal to that of azathioprine, but the side effects are doubled. Plasma exchange may provide some benefit in terms of disease stabilization and decreased severity of flares, but only when used with other immunosuppressive drugs. Coupled with the expense and time involved, this treatment modality appears less feasible.

In conclusion, there is no therapy that shows long-term clinical benefit. The use of immunosuppressive agents, except for steroids and ACTH, is limited to clinical trials (Mitchell, 1993). More specific immune mechanisms of the disease need to be identified, and therapies need to be developed that are more focused on the immune modulation and that have fewer side effects.

Rehabilitation

In the past decade, the survival time of persons with MS has risen to a mean of 40 years, resulting in an almost normal life expectancy. This has been largely the result of modern symptom-management methods. For the MS patient, rehabilitation should become a way of life, not an on/off modality. Rehabilitation should be initiated early, and the patient needs to become an active member of the rehabilitation team, not simply relying on the advice or activities of the health care team (Mertin, 1994).

Working with the patient to cope with the disease's physical, psychological, and social consequences is an integral role of the provider. Helping the patient adapt to and accept the disease will go a long way to improving the quality of life. Early modifications, ranging from changes in physical activities to altered dietary attitudes, may help influence the course of disease. Rehabilitation is not the last resort, but rather a preventive aspect of treatment. It should be viewed as fundamental to the care of the MS patient. MS patients must be, within their own limits, as active as possible in all ways of life to counteract complications (Mertin, 1994).

Spasticity is a prominent impairment in MS. The mainstay of treatment of this impairment is active exercise under the guidance of a therapist. Exerting control on the muscle activity of the spastic patient can provoke reflex-inhibiting motor patterns, facilitating normal movement. Regular repetition of such exercises initiates the process of motor learning, which leads to reducing spasticity and regaining selective motor function. Standing in an upright position in and of itself can reduce spasticity.

Special programs, as part of the treatment regimen, should be carried out regularly. Noncompetitive sports (eg, gymnastics, ball games, or swimming) with groups of disabled patients help counteract inactivity and dispel social isolation (Mertin, 1994). Efforts to counteract disease-related inactivity are an important part of successful, comprehensive rehabilitation therapy. Daily therapy regimens, in conjunction with behavioral changes, initiated early in the disease course may help delay disability and maintain independence.

Prevention and Future Prospects

Discoveries about the cause of MS do not seem to be on the horizon. The genes that determine susceptibility to MS may soon be defined. However, these will not be mutant genes, amenable to gene therapy, but rather essential elements for the maintenance of vital systems. The evidence points to the probability that more than one gene contributes to MS susceptibility; probably several genes are involved and need to be identified. There also seems to be little prospect of identifying a trigger in susceptible persons that could be a target for vaccination or antimicrobial treatment (Compston, 1994).

If heredity and environment do not provide us with the means to avoid the devastation of this disease in the foreseeable future, then other avenues must be scrutinized. Promoting repair of demyelinated axons or interfering with the pathogenesis on a cellular level may prove efficacious in stabilizing and reversing clinical defects.

Interventions that may thwart the development of this disease may be to block or deplete functional populations of T cells that initiate the inflammatory lesion in MS. Tissue necrosis factor has been identified as being directly cytotoxic to oligodendrocytes and in tissue cultures. It is responsible for the toxic effects of macrophages and microglia (Compston, 1994) on oligodendrocytes. The answer to preventing the pathogenesis of MS may be in interfering in this cascade of events.

Another topic for research in MS would be limiting the damage to the axon through remyelination. Glial cells that act as progenitors for oligodendrocytes retain the ability to proliferate, migrate, survive, and differentiate. Growth factors for these cells may hold the answer. Using glial cells for repair of myelin may hold the best hope for the MS patient in the near future (Compston, 1994).

TEACHING AND SELF-CARE

Every patient and family responds differently to the plan of care generated from living with a demyelinating disease. Taking time to plan routine activities like bathing, dressing, and ambulating should decrease frustration and avoid accidents. A family/caregiver support group in the local area where the patient lives may provide the most practical help with teaching and self care.

COMMUNITY RESOURCES

Treatments for demyelinating diseases, similarly with cancer therapy, may include a wide variety of experimental and nutritional approaches to care. Patients should be encouraged to discuss alternative treatment options.

- National Multiple Sclerosis Society
  733 Third Avenue
  New York, NY 10017

  http://www.nmss.org

EDITOR'S NOTE:
COMPLEMENTARY APPROACHES

A general discussion of complementary approaches can be found in Chapter 3. The following, while not an exhaustive list, are some complementary approaches being used for this condition. Additional information on these approaches, including precautions, can be found in Appendices A and B. Providers need to assess for the use of complementary approaches as part of the patient's history, as they may impact conventional therapies, and patients may not volunteer this information unless specifically asked. Efficacy of many complementary approaches is not as well documented as that of conventional therapies. Providers need to read the literature before suggesting these complementary approaches.

- Complementary Modalities
  Aromatherapy
  Massage therapy

References

Abramsky, O. (1994). Pregnancy and multiple sclerosis. *Annals of Neurology*, S36, 538–541.

Asbury, A.K., & McKhann, G.M. (1997). Changing views of Guillain-Barré syndrome. *Annals of Neurology, 41*(3), 287–288.

Beck, R. & Cleary, P. (1992). A randomized controlled trial of corticosteroids in the treatment of acute optic neuritis. *N Engl J Med, 326,* 581–588.

Berkow, R. (Ed.). (1992). Demyelinating diseases. *The Merck manual of diagnosis and therapy*, pp. 1487–1490. New Jersey: Merck Research Laboratories.

Bundey, S. (1997). Few psychological consequences of presymptomatic testing for Huntington disease. *Lancet, 349*(9044), 4.

Compston, A. (1994). Future prospects for the management of multiple sclerosis. *Annals of Neurology*, S36, 5146–5149.

Gordon, F., Antel, J., & Daquette, P. (1991). Inflammatory demyelinating diseases of the central nervous system. In W. Bradley (Ed.). *Neurology in clinical practice: Principles of diagnosis and management*, pp. 1134–1157. Boston: Butterworth-Heinemann.

Goroll, A.H., May, L.A., & Mulley, A.G. (1995). *Primary care medicine: Office evaluation and management of the adult patient,* 3d ed. Philadelphia: J.B. Lippincott.

Hauser, S. (1994). Prevention strategies for multiple sclerosis. *Annals of Neurology,* S36, 5157–5161.

Herndon, R. (1990). Multiple sclerosis. In R. Johnson (Ed.). *Current therapy In neurologic disease*, pp. 159–164. Philadelphia: B.D. Decker.

Hickey, J.V. (1992). Degenerative diseases of the nervous system. In *The clinical practice of neurological and neurosurgical nursing*, pp. 627–633. Philadelphia: J.B. Lippincott.

Hopkins, A. (1993). Multiple sclerosis. In *Clinical neurology*, pp. 240–245. New York: Oxford University Press.

Keating, M., & Ostby P. (1996). Education and self-management of interferon beta-1b therapy for multiple sclerosis. *Journal of Neuroscience Nursing, 28*(6), 350–385.

Kelley, C. (1996). The role of interferons in the treatment of multiple sclerosis. *Journal of Neuroscience Nursing, 28*(2), 114–120.

Lynch, S., & Rose, J. (1996). Multiple sclerosis. *Disease-a-Month, 42*(1), 1–54.

Mallson, D., et al. (1995). Multiple sclerosis: Sexual dysfunction and its response to medications. *Archives of Neurology, 52,* 862–867.

Mastwin, J. (1990). Urinary problems in multiple sclerosis and other spinal diseases. In R. Johnson (Ed.). *Current therapy in neurologic disease*, pp. 159–164. Philadelphia: Decker.

Matthews, W.B. (Ed.). (1991). *McAlpine's multiple sclerosis*. Edinburgh: Churchill-Livingstone.

Mertin, J. (1994). Rehabilitation in multiple sclerosis. *Annals of Neurology*, S36, 5130–1533.

Mitchell, G. (1993). Update on multiple sclerosis therapy. *Medical Clinics of North America, 77*(1), 231–245.

Motomura, S., et al. (1980). A clinical comparative study of multiple sclerosis and neuro-Behçet's syndrome. *Journal of Neurology, Neurosurgery and Psychiatry, 43,* 210–213.

Murray, T.J. (1995). The psychosocial aspect of multiple sclerosis. *Neurologic Clinics, 13*(1), 197–218.

Rao, S., Leo, G.J., Bernardin, L. et al. (1991). Cognitive dysfunction in multiple sclerosis: Frequency, patterns and prediction. *Neurology, 41*(5), 685–690.

Rudnick, R. (1996). Multiple sclerosis and related conditions. In J. Bennett (Ed.). *Cecil textbook of medicine*, pp. 2106–2113. Philadelphia: W.B. Saunders.

Schapiro, R. (1994). Symptom management in multiple sclerosis. *Annals of Neurology*, S36, 5123–5129.

Sibley, W., Posner, C., & Alter, M. (1989). Multiple sclerosis. In L. Rowland (Ed.). *Merrit's textbook of neurology*, pp. 741–760. Philadelphia: Lea & Febiger.

Sobel, R. (1995). The pathology of multiple sclerosis. *Neurologic Clinics, 13*(1), 1–16.

Thomas, C.L. (Ed.). (1993). *Taber's cyclopedic medical dictionary,* 17th ed. Philadelphia: F.A. Davis.

Vollmer, T., & Waxman, S. (1991). Multiple sclerosis and other demyelinating disorders. In R. Rosenberg (Ed.). *Comprehensive neurology*, pp. 489–511. New York: Raven.

Weiner, H., Hohol, M., Khoury, S. et al. (1995). Therapy for multiple sclerosis. *Neurologic Clinics, 13*(1), 173–192.

Williams, J., & Schneiderman, H. (1996). *Pocket guide to physical diagnosis*. Baltimore: Williams & Wilkins.

Bibliography

Anderson, M., et al. (1994). Cerebrospinal fluid in the diagnosis of multiple sclerosis: a case report. *Journal of Neurology, Neurosurgery and Psychiatry, 57,* 897–902.

Bornstein, M. (1992). Hopeful prospects in multiple sclerosis. *Hospital Practice,* 83–106.

Brod, S.A., et al. (1996). Multiple sclerosis: Clinical presentation, diagnosis and treatment. *American Family Physician, 54*(4), 1301–1311.

Chelmicka-Schorr, E., (1994). Nervous system–immune system interactions and their role in multiple sclerosis. *Annals of Neurology,* S36, 529–532.

Chipps, E., & Skinner, C. (1994). Intravenous immunoglobin: Implications for use in neurologic patient. *Journal of Neuroscience Nursing, 26*(1), 8–17.

French Cooperative Group on Plasma Exchange in Guillain-Barré Syndrome. (1997). Appropriate number of plasma exchanges in Guillain-Barré syndrome. *Annals of Neurology, 41*(3), 298–306.

Gould, J. (1982). Multiple sclerosis. *Lancet, 2*, 1208–1210.

Janisen, R., et al. (1989). Neurological and neuropsychological manifestations of HIV infection: Association with AIDS-related complex but not asymptomatic HIV infection. *Annals of Neurology, 26*(5), 592–599.

Johnson, R. et al. (1987). Myopathies and retroviral infections. *Annals of Neurology, 21*(2), 113–115.

Johnson, R., (1994). The virology of demyelinating diseases. *Annals of Neurology, S36*, 554–558.

Kesselring, J., et al. (1990). Acute disseminated encephalomyelitis: MRI findings and the distinction from multiple sclerosis. *Brain, 113*, 291–302.

Khoury, S.J. (1994). Longitudinal MRI in multiple sclerosis. *Neurology, 44*(11), 2120–2124.

Koldewyn, E., Hommes, O., et al. (1995). Relationships between lower urinary tract abnormalities and disease related parameters in multiple sclerosis. *Journal of Neurology, 154*, 169–173.

Kurtzke, J. (1985). Optic neuritis or multiple sclerosis? *Archives of Neurology, 42*, 704–709.

Ludwin, S. (1994). Central nervous system remyelination: Studies in chronically damaged tissue. *Annals of Neurology, S36*, 143–145.

McDonald, W.I. (1989). Diagnosis of multiple sclerosis. *British Medical Journal, 299*, 635–637.

Miller, D. et al. (1989). The early risk of multiple sclerosis following isolated acute syndromes of the brain stem and spinal cord. *Annals of Neurology, 26*(5), 635–639.

Poser, C., et al. (1983). New diagnostic criteria for multiple sclerosis: Guidelines for research protocols. *Annals of Neurology, 13*(3), 227–231.

Schapiro, R. (1994). *Symptom management in multiple sclerosis*, 2d ed. New York: Demos.

Scheinberg, L. (1994). Therapeutic strategies. *Annals of Neurology, S36*, 5122.

Sibley, W. (1985) Clinical viral infections and multiple sclerosis. *Lancet*, 1313–1315.

Thompson, A., et al. (1990). Patterns of disease activity in multiple sclerosis: Clinical and resonance imaging study. *British Medical Journal, 300*, 631–634.

Dizziness, Vertigo, and Ataxia

Henry Cohen, MS, PharmD, and Salah M. Mesad, MD

DIZZINESS AND VERTIGO

Vertigo is a precise term, defined as a sensation of spinning or whirling motion; it implies a definite sensation of rotation of subject or of objects about the subject in any plane (Spraycar, 1991; Basmajian et al, 1992). Dizziness is an imprecise term, appropriately and commonly used by patients in an attempt to describe various subjective symptoms such as faintness (analogous to the feelings that precede syncope), giddiness, lightheadedness, and unsteadiness; it may include vertigo (Spraycar, 1991; Basmajian et al, 1992). Dizziness is not mental confusion, blurred vision, headache, or tingling. Dizziness is one of the most common complaints causing patients to seek medical attention (Woodwell, 1989). In a United States national survey, dizziness was the 13th most common individual reason to visit a primary care provider (Herr et al, 1989). In a study from a general internal medicine outpatient clinic, dizziness was the third most frequent complaint (Kroenke & Mangelsdorff, 1989).

Anatomy, Physiology, and Pathology

Vertigo and dizziness can represent several different overlapping sensations; the pathophysiologic mechanisms are multifactorial. The vestibular nuclei, which are in the medulla and lower pons, receive input from the vestibular labyrinth via the vestibular branch of cranial nerve VIII and from the cerebellum (Herr et al, 1989). Vertigo is an illusion of motion without external stimuli, and it always indicates an imbalance within the vestibular system, although the symptom itself does not indicate where the imbalance originates. The maintenance of the sense of balance depends primarily on input from the vestibular labyrinth, visual system, and proprioceptive nerves arising from tendons, muscles, and joints (Frederick, 1973; Kelly, 1985). Therefore, vertigo and the sensation of dizziness can result from lesions in the inner ear, the deep paravertebral stretch receptors of the neck, the visual–vestibular interaction centers in the brain stem and cerebellum, the thalamus, or the cortex (Frederick, 1973; Baloh & Honrubia, 1990).

Nausea as a result of motion sickness is initiated by stimulation of the labyrinthine mechanism of the inner ear, which sends impulses to the chemoreceptor trigger zone (CTZ), in turn stimulating the vomiting center (VC). The CTZ, located in the area postrema of the fourth ventricle of the brain, is a major chemosensory organ for emesis. The VC is made up of a nucleus of cells located within the medulla. Vomiting is triggered by afferent impulses to the VC. Impulses are received from the sensory centers (eg, CTZ, gastrointestinal tract) and integrated by the VC, resulting in efferent impulses to the salivation center, respiratory center, and the pharyngeal, gastrointestinal, and abdominal muscles, ensuing in vomiting. The VC

may also be directly stimulated by gastrointestinal irritation and vestibular neuritis. Enhanced activity of the central neurotransmitters, including dopamine in the CTZ, and acetylcholine in the VC, are major mediators for the emesis (Frederick, 1973; Baloh & Honrubia, 1990).

History and Physical Exam

Information from the history and physical exam can play a major role in determining the etiology of dizziness. Unfortunately, patients often have difficulty describing precise symptoms of dizziness. Therefore, the provider must take a careful history and perform a meticulous physical and neurologic exam to determine the type of dizziness; this will serve as a guide for confirmatory diagnostic studies (Herr et al, 1989; Adams & Victor, 1985; Lehrer & Poole, 1987). A cardiovascular exam should be done, including supine and standing blood pressure measurements in both arms, peripheral pulses, carotid bruits, heart murmur, and heart rate and rhythm. An ear exam is necessary to detect impacted cerumen or infection. Cerebellar function should be tested by performing the finger-to-nose test and having the patient tandem-walk while performing rapid alternating movements. Cranial nerves should be examined carefully by observing for any extraocular movement abnormality or nystagmus.

Dizziness when standing may be the result of vertigo, cerebral hypoperfusion, or disequilibrium (Kroenke et al, 1992). Dizziness when turning, and especially when rolling over in bed, is usually the result of vertigo. If the patient reports having symptoms of dizziness primarily while standing, both supine and standing blood pressure measurements and pulse rates should be determined. The patient should be allowed to be in both the supine and standing positions for at least 5 minutes before checking blood pressure and pulse rate. If there is an orthostatic decrease in blood pressure, the symptom is probably the result of impaired central nervous system (CNS) blood perfusion. Unsteadiness while walking, particularly in elderly patients, is often the result of disequilibrium, and its etiology is generally multifactorial. The presence of decreased visual acuity and signs of peripheral neuropathy or abnormal vestibular function supports a diagnosis of disequilibrium.

Psychogenic dizziness is a diagnosis of exclusion that should be especially considered in patients with psychiatric disorders, such as major depression, mania, anxiety disorder, and somatization disorders. The diagnosis of a hyperventilation syndrome can be established if symptoms of dizziness are reproduced by having the patient hyperventilate for 2 to 3 minutes.

Once the provider can establish that the patient is describing vertigo, further questioning will aid in determining the specific etiology. The provider must determine if vertigo is a recurrent or monophasic symptom and must assess the duration of the episodes, the circumstances in which vertigo occurs, and the presence of other otologic or neurologic symptoms (Herr et al, 1989; Lehrer & Poole, 1987).

Acute spontaneous vertigo can result from sudden loss of peripheral input caused by damage to the labyrinth or vestibular nerve, or it can be caused by a sudden unilateral impairment of vestibular nuclear or vestibulocerebellar activity (Kelly, 1985; Baloh & Honrubia, 1990). The patient experiences an intense sense of rotation aggravated by head motion and often by lying down, whereas sitting upright and keeping the head motionless relieves the vertigo. The patient usually notices that the visual world is moving slowly in one direction and quickly back in the other direction; this is the result of spontaneous nystagmus. Standing and walking are difficult, and the patient may fall toward the affected side. Acute spontaneous vertigo is almost always accompanied by autonomic symptoms, including malaise, pallor, diaphoresis, nausea, vomiting, and occasionally diarrhea.

The history often provides critical information that will aid in determining whether vertigo is peripheral (labyrinth) or central (brain stem or cerebellum) in origin (Table 53-1) (Herr et al, 1989; Frederick, 1973; Lehrer & Poole, 1987). Generally, peripheral vertigo is more severe than central vertigo and is more likely to be associated with autonomic symptoms, ear fullness or pressure, tinnitus, and hearing loss. Central vertigo is typically associated with neurologic symptoms such as diplopia, dysarthria, incoordination, numbness, and weakness. Lesions within the internal auditory canal produce a combination of vertigo, hearing loss, and facial weakness because of the involvement of cranial nerves VII and VIII. A prior history of cardiovascular disease (ie, hypertension) or stroke may suggest cerebral or brain stem vascular insult—hence, a central etiology. However, a prior history of ear trauma or ear infection accompanied by unilateral hearing loss suggests a peripheral etiology. Patients with central vestibular lesions often cannot stand or even walk a single step without falling.

Patients with peripheral vestibular lesions have impaired balance, but they are able to ambulate, even during the acute phase. Spontaneous nystagmus of peripheral origin does not change direction with gaze in either side, although it increases in amplitude with gaze away from the fast phase. In contrast, spontaneous nystagmus of central origin typically changes direction when the patient looks away from the direction of the fast phase. Further, spontaneous nystagmus of peripheral vertigo is inhibited with fixation and therefore is usually prominent for only the first 12 to 24 hours. Spontaneous nystagmus of central vertigo often persists for weeks to months.

Magnetic resonance imaging (MRI) of the brain is indicated in patients with vertigo and focal neurologic findings, new-onset severe headaches, or vertical spontaneous or positional nystagmus. In the patient with acute vertigo and profound imbalance, cerebellar infarct or hemorrhage must be ruled out. Any central lesions or hemorrhaging must be identified immediately, because they can culminate in a mass effect with compression of the brain stem. If the indications for an MRI after a physical and neurologic exam are nebulous, the patient should be observed for 24 to 48 hours; on repeat neurologic examination without improvement, an MRI is indicated.

Recurrent attacks of vertigo may occur when there is a sudden temporary and largely reversible impairment of the labyrinth or its central connections (Herr et al, 1989; Frederick, 1973; Lehrer & Poole, 1987). Such attacks typically last minutes to hours rather than days and terminate through restoration of normal neural activity. The duration of vertigo episodes provides additional relevant diagnostic information. Vertigo of vascular origin, such as a transient ischemic attack, typically last minutes, whereas those of peripheral inner ear etiology generally persist for hours. On the neurologic exam, if focal neurologic findings are present, imaging studies of the head are warranted. However, patients with vertebrobasilar transient ischemic attacks often have a completely normal neurologic exam between attacks, and MRI of the brain is usually normal.

A screening audiogram and an electronystagmogram are indicated in all patients with recurrent vertigo that is likely to be of peripheral origin (eg, hearing loss) (Herr et al, 1989; Frederick, 1973; Lehrer & Poole, 1987). Vertigo accompanied by hearing loss is common in patients with otosclerosis. Episodes of vertigo with hearing loss, tinnitus, and the sensation of ear fullness occur in patients with Meniere's disease. Patients

TABLE 53-1	Features of Peripheral and Central Vertigo	
Sign or Symptom	Peripheral (Labyrinth)	Central (Brain Stem or Cerebellum)
Direction of associated nystagmus	Unidirectional; fast phase opposite lesion	Bidirectional or unidirectional
Purely horizontal nystagmus without torsional component	Uncommon	Common
Vertical or purely torsional nystagmus	Never present	May be present
Visual fixation	Inhibits nystagmus and vertigo	No inhibition
Severity of vertigo	Marked	Often mild
Direction of spin	Toward fast phase	Variable
Direction of fall	Toward slow phase	Variable
Duration of symptoms	Finite (minutes, days, weeks) but recurrent	May be chronic
Tinnitus or deafness	Often present	Usually absent
Associated central abnormalities	None	Extremely common
Common causes	Infection (labyrinthitis), Meniere's, neuronitis, ischemia, trauma, toxin	Vascular, demyelinating neoplasm

with acoustic neuromas usually have hearing loss rather than vertigo. Neurologic symptoms, which are generally referable to the posterior fossa, include diplopia, facial paresthesia or weakness, and dysarthria, as well as symptoms resulting from dysfunction of the motor and sensory tracts. Patients with vestibular neuronitis, benign paroxysmal positional vertigo, and recurrent vestibulopathy have normal hearing. Patients with benign positional vertigo (BPV) have intermittent episodes of vertigo with head turning. Vestibular neuronitis is characterized by a relatively sudden onset of severe constant vertigo that resolves after days or weeks. Patients with recurrent vestibulopathy have intermittent episodes of constant vertigo lasting for minutes or hours. Vertigo with or without hearing loss in a patient who has recently received aminoglycoside antimicrobials may be the result of an inherent toxic effect on the vestibular labyrinth (Jackson & Arcieri, 1971).

Benign Positional Vertigo

BPV is the most common cause of acute episodes of vertigo. It is characterized by brief (minutes or less) attacks of vertigo and nystagmus with certain head positions, such as lying down or turning over in bed, or tilting the head backward (Baloh et al, 1987). The patient can often identify a head position that can trigger symptoms. Symptoms may recur periodically for several days or months. Hearing is not affected. Diagnosis is confirmed by performing the Nylen-Barany maneuver, during which the patient is moved from the sitting position to a lying position with the head extended 45° backward. This maneuver is repeated with the head extended and turned to the right and to the left. The Nylen-Barany maneuver usually produces a brief attack of vertigo and nystagmus.

Positional vertigo nearly always is a benign condition. However, in rare cases, it is a symptom of a central lesion (in particular, the brain stem), including multiple sclerosis, tumors, stroke, or drug intoxications (alcohol and antiepileptic drugs). The Nylen-Barany maneuver helps distinguish benign positional nystagmus from more ominous central conditions. In BPV, there is a latency period for several seconds before the appearance of a transient vertigo and nystagmus, which dissipates on repetition of the Nylen-Barany maneuver. In BPV, nystagmus lasts less than 30 seconds and is unidirectional (Baloh et al, 1987). Any deviation from this characteristic nystagmus profile should raise suspicion that a central lesion may exist. Central positional nystagmus typically is nonfatiguing and purely vertical (either up- or downbeating). Most cases of central positional nystagmus have different neurologic findings.

Acute Vestibular Neuronitis

Acute vestibular neuronitis is characterized by a sudden and severe attack of vertigo, often accompanied by nausea, vomiting, and apprehension (Lehrer & Poole, 1987). The symptoms are exacerbated and pronounced on head movements or changes in position. Spontaneous nystagmus occurs with the slow phase toward the abnormal ear. Tinnitus or a sensation of fullness in the ear occurs in about 40% of cases, but hearing remains unimpaired. With the exception of unsteadiness, there are no neurologic signs. Vertigo usually resolves spontaneously over several hours, but it, may recur within days or weeks. Acute vestibular neuronitis affects adults of all ages. The cause of acute

vestibular neuronitis has not been elucidated, but a viral etiology has been postulated.

Meniere's Disease

The onset of Meniere's disease usually occurs in the third or fourth decade of life. It generally presents with a history of antecedent head trauma or otic infection, followed by a constellation of episodes of vertigo, nausea, and ataxia that persist for hours (Paparella, 1991). Fullness or pressure in the ear, tinnitus, and fluctuating hearing loss usually precede (but may follow) the episodes of vertigo. There are no associated neurologic symptoms. Examining the patient during an episode of vertigo reveals a typical horizontal–torsional nystagmus of the peripheral type. It is of paramount importance to perform an audiogram in patients with symptoms suggestive of Meniere's disease because a characteristic, subclinical, low-frequency sensorineural loss may be present (Horner, 1991).

Disequilibrium Without Vertigo

Patients with diminished perception in the lower extremities can experience severe unsteadiness and imbalance when attempting to walk. They often use the term dizziness to describe their disequilibrium; vertigo is not present. These patients are particularly unsteady when walking in the dark because there are few visual cues to compensate for their loss of perception. Disequilibrium without vertigo is often termed multisensory dizziness and occurs when there is partial loss of multiple sensory inputs (eg, diabetic peripheral neuropathy and retinopathy) (Lehrer & Poole, 1987). Loss of proprioception commonly occurs in patients with peripheral neuropathy, vitamin B_{12} deficiency, tabes dorsalis, and myelopathies.

Drug-induced peripheral neuropathies have been associated with many agents, including phenytoin, phenobarbital, primidone, nitrofurantoin, dapsone, metronidazole, oral contraceptives, colchicine, podophyllin, hydralazine, didanosine, stavudine, zalcitabine, paclitaxel, carboplatin, altretamine, vincristine, vinblastine, and isoniazid (Gallagher, 1994). Toxin-induced peripheral neuropathies have been associated with arsenic, gold, lead, and mercury (Gallagher, 1994). The normal deterioration in gait and balance that occurs with aging can mimic potentially treatable disorders such as occult hydrocephalus, Parkinson's disease, and the multi-infarct syndrome. An MRI of the brain helps distinguish among these entities.

ATAXIA

Disturbances of coordination are typically caused by dysfunction of the cerebellum or its major input systems—the frontal lobes or the posterior columns of the spinal cord. Ataxia is an abnormality of movement characterized by errors in rate, range, direction, timing, duration, and force of motor activity. The ataxic gait is characterized by unsteadiness and staggering and wide-based movements in all directions. When primarily the truncal muscles are involved, ataxia is not as obvious. Ataxias may be classified by their localization, etiology, or mode of

TABLE 53-2	Features of Ataxic Disorders	
Localization	Etiology	Presentation
Cerebral	Degenerative	Acute
Cerebellum	Infectious	Subacute
Spinal cord	Vascular	Chronic
Peripheral nerve	Neoplastic/paraneoplastic	Intermittent
	Traumatic	
	Demyelinating	
	Idiopathic	

onset (Table 53-2). Ataxia of short duration suggests a toxic (eg, drug-induced) or infectious etiology.

Slowly progressive ataxia may occur in patients with posterior fossa tumors, but they may also be present in a plethora of hereditary degenerative disorders. These disorders are characterized by a chronic, slowly progressive ataxia that usually begins in the legs (Harding, 1984). Also, signs and symptoms of lesions of the posterior columns, pyramidal tracts, basal ganglia, and other regions of the brain are common (Harding, 1993).

Friedreich's Ataxia

Friedreich's ataxia is a familial and hereditary disease characterized by ataxia, areflexia, impaired proprioception, and the involvement of cardiac and skeletal abnormalities (Harding, 1993). Friedreich's ataxia presents with degenerative changes of the dorsal half of the spinal cord and the cerebellum. This condition usually begins in the first or second decade of life. It is usually inherited as an autosomal recessive disorder; however, sporadic cases have been reported.

Ataxia of gait, the most common symptom, is usually the first to appear. Involvement of the posterior funiculi is present in almost all patients. Loss of the appreciation of vibration is an early sign. Some impairment of position sense in the legs and later in the arms is almost always present. Muscle weakness is common and may lead to an almost complete or complete paralysis of the legs. Deep tendon reflexes in the legs are almost always absent, but they may be present in the arms, particularly during the early stages of the disease. The plantar responses are extensor in practically all patients. The abdominal and cremasteric reflexes are preserved in most patients.

Optic atrophy, cranial nerve palsies, mental deficiency, and dementia are less commonly noted (Harding, 1993). Pes cavus (clubfoot) and kyphoscoliosis are common skeletal deformities. Pes cavus is not an absolute feature of Friedreich's ataxia, but the foot deformity is present in 75% of patients; it is occasionally found in other family members as the only sign of the disease. Dysrhythmia, muscle atrophy, and degeneration of the optic nerve may occur in the late stages of the disease. Cardiomyopathy is often present, and diabetes mellitus is reported in over 10% of cases (Thilenius & Grossman, 1961). The laboratory findings in Friedreich's ataxia are generally normal (Harding, 1993; Thilenius & Gorssman, 1961). In the cerebrospinal fluid (CSF), there is an occasional slight increase in the protein content and rarely a mild pleocytosis.

In most cases, disease onset occurs in the early years of life, and the disease progresses to complete incapacity by the age of 20. Death usually occurs as a result of intercurrent infections, and to a lesser extent as a result of cardiomyopathy. Unfortunately, no specific treatment influences the course of Friedreich's ataxia. Tenotomies or other orthopedic operations are indicated for relief of the foot deformity. Physical therapy focusing on muscle training is of value in the abortive forms and in the rare cases with spontaneous remissions.

Olivopontocerebellar Atrophy

Olivopontocerebellar atrophy is differentiated from Friedreich's ataxia by its relatively late onset (late middle life) and the absence of signs and symptoms of spinal cord disease. The clinical syndrome of olivopontocerebellar atrophy is characterized by the development of progressive ataxia of the trunk and limbs, impairment of equilibrium and gait, slowness of voluntary movements, scanning speech, nystagmoid jerks, and oscillatory tremor of the head and trunk. Dysarthria, dysphagia, and oculomotor and facial palsies may also occur. Extrapyramidal symptoms include rigidity, immobile facies, and a parkinsonian-like tremor. The reflexes are usually normal, but knee and ankle jerks may be lost and extensor responses may occur. Dementia is not rare, but it is usually mild. Impairment of sphincter function commonly occurs, producing urinary incontinence and less commonly fecal incontinence. MRI of the brain typically reveals significant atrophy of the cerebellum and the pons (Klockgether et al, 1993).

Infection-Induced Ataxia

The most common cerebellar syndrome that has been attributed to viral infections is acute cerebellar ataxia of childhood (Harding, 1984; Harding, 1993). It usually occurs in children between the ages of 1 and 8 years, but older children and adults with similar illness have been reported. The neurologic illness may be preceded by a trivial respiratory or gastrointestinal tract infection. Over hours or a few days, the patient develops severe truncal ataxia, with less prominent limb involvement. There is often static and kinetic tremor of the head, trunk, and limbs. Myoclonus and opsoclonus or ocular flutter occur in some cases, causing the clinical syndrome to resemble that of a neuroblastoma. Recovery is usually complete but may take up to 6 months. A mild mononuclear pleocytosis in the CSF may be present. Implicated viruses include coxsackie groups A and B, poliovirus, Epstein-Barr, and herpes simplex.

Subacute or chronic cerebellar ataxia has been described in adults with a variety of infections. Infections caused by *Mycoplasma pneumoniae* or *Legionella pneumoniae*, CNS infections with AIDS such as *Toxoplasma gondii*, and meningitis, typhoid fever, and tick paralysis have all been implicated. Cerebellar ataxia, combined with bilateral facial palsy and a lymphocytic CSF pleocytosis, has also been described in Lyme disease. In adults, cerebellar dysfunction may dominate the clinical picture of Creutzfeldt-Jakob disease for several months. Other features of Creutzfeldt-Jakob disease include dementia and myoclonus. Also, involvement of the cerebellum is particularly prominent in postinfectious disseminated encephalomyelitis after certain viral infections, such as varicella, rubella, and mumps.

Neoplastic and Paraneoplastic Cerebellar Lesions

Tumors of the cerebellum such as astrocytomas, blastomas, and ependymomas often cause cerebellar ataxia in addition to signs of increased intracranial pressure (Posner & Furneaux, 1990). Metastatic cerebellar tumors originate from lung, breast, and gastrointestinal tract cancers, and present similarly. Paraneoplastic cerebellar degeneration is a rare nonmetastatic complication of malignancy. The most common type of tumor accompanying this syndrome is lung cancer (particularly small cell), followed by carcinoma of the ovary, breast, uterus, stomach, and colon, and Hodgkin's lymphoma (Posner & Furneaux, 1990). Symptoms develop 3 months to 2 years after the tumor develops; however, neurologic symptomatology may precede the discovery of the malignancy by 2 months to 3 years.

The typical neurologic presentation includes subacute ataxia, progressing to severe disability over several months or even weeks, and then often remitting. Onset may be acute and is sometimes accompanied by vertigo, mimicking a vascular event. There is severe truncal, gait, and limb ataxia, and dysarthria. Abnormal eye movements are common, with nystagmus and occasionally opsoclonus. Mental status changes are common, including euphoria, confusion, and dementia. MRI of the brain often shows cerebellar atrophy and excludes metastases, which exhibits a greater prevalence for cerebellar dysfunction in patients with cancer. The CSF shows an elevated protein concentration in about 50% of patients and a moderately increased lymphocyte count in about a third of patients.

Vascular Causes of Cerebellar Ataxia

Cases of ataxia induced by cerebellar infarction or hemorrhage are relatively rare. They are difficult to distinguish from each other on clinical presentation and are often misdiagnosed unless a computed tomography or MRI scan of the head is performed early. The presentation of cerebellar infarction can mimic that of hemorrhage, with an abrupt onset of headaches, vomiting, vertigo, and ataxia (Harding, 1984; Harding, 1993). However, many patients have vertigo or dizziness and have few cerebellar-like signs despite radiologic evidence of cerebellar hemisphere infarction. Facial weakness, gaze palsies, and a deteriorating level of consciousness may occur in hemorrhage and infarction, the latter the result of hydrocephalus secondary to hematoma or cerebellar edema. Late diagnosis of cerebellar hemorrhage is associated with a poor prognosis, and approximately 20% of patients die before reaching medical assistance. Both infarction and hemorrhage may be amenable to surgical therapy.

Metabolic Ataxic Disorders

Various metabolic disorders with an early onset (infancy or early childhood), such as disorders of the urea cycle, some aminoacidurias, and disorders of pyruvate and lactate metabolism, give rise to a constellation of symptoms including intermittent ataxia (Harding, 1984). Hyperammonemia is the most common metabolic abnormality associated with intermittent ataxia. Valproic acid may cause hyperammonemia, Fanconi syndrome with aminoaciduria, and disturbances of the urea cycle. These effects are more commonly seen in children than adults (Davis et al, 1994).

The metabolic ataxic disorders have a similar clinical picture, comprising intermittent ataxia, dysarthria, vomiting, headache, ptosis, involuntary movements, confusion, and seizures. These episodes may be precipitated by high protein loads and intercurrent illness. There is a variable degree of associated mental retardation. Ataxia may be a minor feature of storage and other metabolic neurodegenerative disorders developing in early childhood. Some disorders have been identified in patients with predominantly ataxic features developing in late childhood or early adult life. These include adrenoleukodystrophy, the sphingomyelin lipidoses, metachromatic leukodystrophy, and the hexosaminidase deficiencies.

Acquired metabolic disorders include hepatic encephalopathy, pontine and extrapontine myelinolysis related to hyponatremia, hypothyroidism, vitamin E deficiency, and thiamine deficiency (Harding, 1984). Hypothyroidism may be associated with a cerebellar syndrome in both children and adults. Symptoms of hypothyroidism precede loss of balance and clumsiness. Neurologic signs and symptoms usually resolve completely after thyroid replacement therapy.

Severe and prolonged vitamin E deficiency produces spinocerebellar degeneration in a number of inherited and acquired disorders. The most severe vitamin E deficiency state is abetalipoproteinemia. Abetalipoproteinemia causes severe malabsorption of fat-soluble vitamins A, D, E, and K. Symptoms of fat malabsorption may be mild and overlooked. Patients may then present in the second decade of life with a progressive neurologic syndrome resembling Friedreich's ataxia, consisting of ataxia, areflexia, and proprioceptive loss (Harding, 1984). In abetalipoproteinemia, serum vitamin E concentrations are low or undetectable from birth. Treatment with high doses of vitamin E prevents the development of neurologic signs or symptoms and leads to improvement if present.

Alcoholics with thiamine deficiency are almost invariably malnourished, often giving a history of profound weight loss before developing neurologic symptoms. Ataxia may develop during periods of abstinence, and identical cerebellar degeneration has been observed in nonalcoholic patients with severe malnutrition. Cerebellar ataxia is a common finding in the Wernicke-Korsakoff syndrome. Typically patients present with encephalopathy, confabulation, and ophthalmoplegia. The cerebellar syndrome predominantly affects stance and gait, sometimes with truncal ataxia and titubation. Peripheral neuropathy may be present. Wernicke's encephalopathy often presents contemporaneously with Korsakoff's psychosis, a disorder of learning and processing new information (anterograde amnesia is common). The administration of parenteral thiamine 100 mg daily offers improvement in the early stages of alcoholic cerebellar degeneration; some authorities suggest up to 1 g may be administered in the first 24 hours. In the late stages of Wernicke's encephalopathy, Korsakoff's psychosis is generally irreversible.

Drug- and Toxin-Induced Ataxias

Cerebellar dysfunction can occur as a consequence of exposure to a wide range of toxins, including drugs, solvents, and heavy metals (Harding, 1984; Harding, 1993). The most common cause of toxicity is that associated with antiepileptic drugs, particularly phenytoin. Transient ataxia, dysarthria, and nystagmus usually develop when serum concentrations of phenytoin, carbamazepine, or barbiturates are above the therapeutic range.

Chronic phenytoin toxicity may cause persistent cerebellar dysfunction and is pathologically associated with loss of Purkinje cells. High doses of 5-fluorouracil or cytosine arabinoside also cause reversible cerebellar ataxia. Recreational or accidental exposure to a number of solvents, including carbon tetrachloride and toluene, may cause cerebellar ataxia and other neurologic problems, including psychosis, cognitive impairment, and pyramidal signs.

Hysterical Gait

Patients with hysterical gait may be unable to stand or walk despite the absence of paralysis (Harding, 1984; Harding, 1993). Tests for power, tone, and coordination may be normal if carried out while the patient is lying down. The gait is often bizarre, irregular, and changeable, and does not conform to a specific organic disease pattern. Patients may appear to be falling, but can usually regain and maintain their balance.

TREATMENT OPTIONS, EXPECTED OUTCOMES, AND COMPREHENSIVE MANAGEMENT

Pharmacotherapy

The management of dizziness, vertigo, and ataxia requires treatment of the underlying etiology. For example, neoplastic and infectious causes must be treated pharmacologically or surgically; vascular and traumatic causes must be treated supportively; drug- and toxin-induced causes must be managed by successful withdrawal of the offending agent; and metabolic disorders must be corrected with appropriate supplementation. If these interventions are contraindicated, unsuccessful, or only partially successful, persistent residual dizziness or vertigo may be managed with the use of several pharmacologic agents. Only meclizine, dimenhydrinate, and diphenidol are available and approved by the FDA for the management of vertigo (Kastrup, 1997; McEvoy, 1997) (Table 53-3).

Antivertiginous agents are chosen based on their pharmacologic effects and on the severity and time course of the patient's symptoms. Dimenhydrinate is used principally for the prevention and treatment of nausea, vomiting, and vertigo of motion sickness; however, meclizine, scopolamine, and promethazine may be more effective and less sedating (McEvoy, 1997). Scopolamine is considered the most effective agent for motion sickness. However, because of its potent anticholinergic effects, meclizine is preferred (McEvoy, 1997).

Patients with severe acute vertigo are often in severe distress and require immediate sedation. Diazepam, a rapid-acting benzodiazepine, may be used as an adjunct in this setting.

For the management of vestibular disturbances, diphenidol may be the most effective agent; however, because of its high propensity for neurotoxicity, it is considered a refractory agent, and meclizine is preferred (McEvoy, 1997).

Antivertiginous agents not approved by the FDA include promethazine and prochlorperazine. Because these agents are less effective than the FDA-approved antivertiginous agents and they have a high propensity to cause extrapyramidal adverse effects (eg, dystonia, akinesia, akathesia), they are not recommended for the initial treatment of vertigo. However, when nausea and vomiting are prominent, they may be administered solely or adjunctively for their potent antiemetic effects.

Although the antivertiginous agents are used to treat dizziness and vertigo, they may initiate or exacerbate same. These agents have been associated with paradoxical restlessness, irritability, insomnia, euphoria, auditory and visual hallucinations, and diplopia. Paradoxical effects are most common in children and older patients. Antivertiginous agents are CNS depressants and may cause drowsiness, lethargy, and hypersomnia. If possible, use of these agents should be avoided when operating heavy machinery or a motor vehicle. Concomitant administration of other CNS depressant agents such as alcohol, barbiturates, benzodiazepines, sedative–hypnotics, and tricyclic antidepressants is relatively contraindicated.

The antivertiginous agents possess anticholinergic activity and are relatively contraindicated in patients with narrow closure glaucoma, prostatic hypertrophy, and gastric or genitourinary obstruction. Patients should be counseled regarding the signs of anticholinergic toxicity: xerostomia, blurred vision, constipation, urinary retention, and mental status changes. Concomitant administration of anticholinergic agents such as atropine, hyoscyamine, neuroleptics, and tricyclic antidepressants is relatively contraindicated.

TABLE 53-3	FDA-Approved Antivertiginous Agents		
Drug	**Onset of Action**	**Dosage**	**Comments**
Dimenhydrinate	Oral: 15–30 min IV: immediate	Prophylaxis: 50 mg before exposure, then 50–100 mg q4–6h; max 400 mg daily. Treatment: 25–50 mg TID/QID	Oral and IV are equipotent Oral available over-the-counter Metabolic fate unknown.
Diphenidol	Oral: within 90 min	25–50 mg q4h; max 300 mg daily	Completely eliminated renally; contraindicated in renal failure patients
Meclizine	Oral: 20–60 min	Prophylaxis: 25–50 mg before exposure and once daily thereafter. Treatment: 25–100 mg BID/TID	Available over-the-counter Metabolic fate not well elucidated Metabolized to renally eliminated; norchlorcyclizine; norchlorcyclizine has unknown activity.

MECLIZINE

Meclizine is a piperazine-derivative CNS depressant with antihistaminic, antiemetic, anticholinergic, and antispasmodic effects (Kastrup, 1997; McEvoy, 1997). Meclizine is indicated for the prevention and treatment of nausea, vomiting, and dizziness of motion sickness. The FDA considers meclizine "possibly effective" for the management of vertigo associated with diseases affecting the vestibular system (eg, labyrinthitis, Meniere's disease). The antiemetic and antimotion sickness effects of meclizine result, in part, from its central antimuscarinic and CNS depressant properties. The antivertigo action of meclizine occurs as a result of depressed labyrinth excitability and conduction in the vestibular–cerebellar pathways.

DIMENHYDRINATE

Dimenhydrinate is an ethanolamine-derivative antihistamine that contains approximately equimolar concentrations of diphenhydramine and chlorotheophylline. Dimenhydrinate's pharmacologic effects are primarily caused by the diphenhydramine moiety. Dimenhydrinate is a CNS depressant with antihistaminic, antiemetic, and anticholinergic properties. Dimenhydrinate is indicated for the prevention and treatment of nausea, vomiting, and vertigo from motion sickness. Dimenhydrinate may be used for the management of vertigo associated with diseases affecting the vestibular system (eg, Meniere's disease).

Dimenhydrinate has been associated with photosensitivity reactions. Patients should be counseled to wear protective clothing, use sunblock with a sun protection factor (SPF) of 15, and avoid artificial sunlamps while using this agent. Dramamine chewable tablets, a brand of dimenhydrinate, contain the dye tartrazine (FD&C yellow No. 5), which may cause anaphylactic reactions. Patients with a history of asthma or aspirin sensitivity are most likely to be at risk for a tartrazine reaction. Moreover, the chewable tablets contain aspartame (NutraSweet), which is metabolized in the gastrointestinal tract to phenylalanine. Phenylketonurics who must restrict their phenylalanine intake should avoid this product.

DIPHENIDOL

Diphenidol is a refractory antiemetic that is structurally unrelated to the antihistamines or phenothiazines. Diphenidol exerts its antivertigo effects via conduction inhibition of the vestibular pathways. It exerts its antiemetic effect via inhibition of the CTZ. Diphenidol is indicated for the control of nausea and vomiting associated with surgery, malignant neoplasms, antineoplastic chemotherapy, radiation sickness, infectious diseases, and labyrinthine disturbances. Diphenidol is also used in the management of labyrinthine vertigo-associated nausea and vomiting in conditions such as Meniere's disease and labyrinthitis (Kastrup, 1997; McEvoy, 1997).

Diphenidol is considered a refractory agent because of its high propensity for mental status changes, particularly hallucinations, disorientation, and confusion. The risk of auditory and visual hallucinations is at least 1 in 350. The reaction onset usually occurs 3 days after starting the drug, and symptoms dissipate within 3 days after discontinuation. Because of diphenidol's neurotoxicity profile, its use is generally limited to hospitalized patients or those with comparable continuous professional supervision. Diphenidol has weak anticholinergic properties; nevertheless, relative contraindications are similar to those for meclizine and dimenhydrinate. Diphenidol contains tartrazine and should be avoided in tartrazine-sensitive patients.

Vestibular Rehabilitation

Permanent vestibular damage results in an initial state of imbalance, presenting as acute vertigo. The patient will gradually adapt to the imbalance through a process called compensation. Compensation requires intact vision, depth perception, sensation in the lower extremities, and normal proprioception. Generally, vestibular compensation requires 3 to 6 months. Vestibular compensation can be maximized by initiating exercises as soon as possible after the vestibular lesion. Vestibular exercises should commence as soon as the acute stage of nausea and vomiting is complete and the disease process has begun to subside. Vestibular exercises may be initiated twice daily for several minutes and increased gradually and as often as tolerated. Vestibular exercises often cause dizziness, but because it is a necessary sensation for effective compensation, the use of antivertiginous agents should be avoided. Also, compensation is accelerated by CNS stimulant drugs and slowed by sedative drugs, reaffirming the need to avoid antivertiginous agents.

TEACHING AND SELF-CARE

Special care to make the home environment as accident-proof as possible for the patient with dizziness, vertigo, or ataxia is a priority. Throw rugs, furniture with sharp edges, and stairs without a reinforced handrail are potential sources of danger. The environment is also important to assess when the patient is traveling, as well as when hospitalized.

Patients with dizziness, vertigo, or ataxia should keep with them at all times a list of the medications they take. If they see a provider with another concern, this can eliminate possible drug interaction problems.

COMMUNITY RESOURCES

Patients and their families can obtain information from local medical centers concerning their problems with dizziness, vertigo, and ataxia. The following are regional or national resources:

- The Vestibular Disorders Association (VEDA), http://www.teleport.com/veda/index.shtml
- Johns Hopkins University, Research and Training Center for Hearing and Balance, http://www.bme.jhu.edu/labs/chb/faq/faq.html
- House Ear Institute, http://www.hei.org/hei/balance.htm
- Healthtouch: Headaches and Dizziness, http://www.healthtouch.com/level/leaflets/104947/104948.htm
- The EAR Foundation, 1817 Patterson St., Nashville, TN 37203-2110, 615-329-7807
- Vestibular Disorders Association, P.O. Box 4467, Portland, OR 97208-4467, 503-229-7705, Fax 503-229-8064
- National Institute of Neurological Disorders and Stroke, 31 Center Drive, MSC 2540, Building #31,

Room 8A-06, Bethesda, MD 20892-2540, 301-496-5751, 800-352-9424, Fax 301-402-2186

EDITOR'S NOTE:

COMPLEMENTARY APPROACHES

A general discussion of complementary approaches can be found in Chapter 3. The following, while not an exhaustive list, are some complementary approaches being used for this condition. Additional information on these approaches, including precautions, can be found in Appendices A and B. Providers need to assess for the use of complementary approaches as part of the patient's history, as they may impact conventional therapies, and patients may not volunteer this information unless specifically asked. Efficacy of many complementary approaches is not as well documented as that of conventional therapies. Providers need to read the literature before suggesting these complementary approaches.

- Complementary Modalities
  Aromatherapy

REFERENCES

Adams, R.D., & Victor, M. (1985). Deafness, dizziness, and disorders of equilibrium. In *Principles of neurology*, 3d ed., pp. 216–218. New York: McGraw-Hill.

Baloh, R.W., & Honrubia, V. (1990). Clinical neurophysiology of the vestibular systems, 2d ed. Philadelphia: F.A. Davis.

Baloh, R.W., Honrubia, V., & Jacobson, K. (1987). Benign positional vertigo: Clinical and oculographic features in 240 cases. *Neurology, 37,* 371.

Basmajian, J.V., Burke, M.D., Burnett, G.W. et al. (1992). *Stedman's Medical Dictionary*, 25th ed. Baltimore: Williams & Wilkins.

Davis, R., Peters, D.H., & McTavish, D. (1994). Valproic acid: A reappraisal of its pharmacological properties and clinical efficacy in epilepsy. *Drugs, 47,* 332–372.

Frederick, M.W. (1973). Central vertigo. *Otolaryngology Clinics of North America, 6,* 267–285.

Gallagher, E.J. (1994). Neurologic principles. In L.R. Goldfrank, N.E. Flomenbaum, N.A. Lewin, et al. (Eds.). *Goldfrank's toxicologic emergencies*, pp. 205–227. Norwalk, CT, Appleton & Lange,

Harding, A.E. (1984). *The hereditary ataxias and related disorders.* Edinburgh: Churchill-Livingstone.

Harding, A.E. (1993). Clinical features and classification of inherited ataxias. *Advances in Neurology, 61,* 1–14.

Herr, R.D., Zun, L., & Matthews, J.J. (1989). A directed approach to the dizzy patient. *Annals of Emergency Medicine, 18,* 664–672.

Horner, K.C. (1991). Old theme and new reflections: Hearing impairment associated with endolymphatic hydrops. *Hearing Research, 52,* 147–156.

Jackson, G.G., & Arcieri, G. (1971). Ototoxicity of gentamicin in man: A survey and controlled analysis of clinical experience in the United States. *Journal of Infectious Diseases, 124* (suppl), S130–S137.

Kastrup, E.K. (Ed.). (1997). *Facts and Comparisons drug information.* St. Louis: Facts and Comparisons.

Kelly, J.P. (1985). Vestibular system. In E.R. Kandel, J.H. Schwartz (Eds.). *Principles of Neural Science*, 2d ed., pp. 591–595. New York: Elsevier.

Klockgether, T., Wuellner, U., Dichgans, W., et al. (1993). Clinical and imaging correlations in inherited ataxias. *Advances in Neurology, 61,* 77–96.

Kroenke, K., Lucas, C.A., Rosenberg, M.L., et al. (1992). Causes of persistent dizziness: A prospective study of 100 patients in ambulatory care. *Annals of Internal Medicine, 117,* 898–904.

Kroenke, K., & Mangelsdorff, A.D. (1989). Common symptoms in ambulatory care: Incidence, evaluation, therapy, and outcome. *American Journal of Medicine, 86,* 262–266.

Lehrer, J.F., & Poole, D.C. (1987). Diagnosis and management of vertigo. *Comprehensive Therapy, 13,* 31–40.

McEvoy, G.K. (Ed.). (1997). *American Hospital Formulary Service Drug Information.* Bethesda, MD: American Society of Health-System Pharmacists, Inc.

Paparella, M.M. (1991). Pathogenesis and pathophysiology of Meniere's disease. *Acta Otolaryngology, 485,* 26–35.

Posner, J.B., & Furneaux, H.M. (1990). Paraneoplastic syndromes. In B.H. Waxman. *Immunological mechanisms in neurologic and psychiatric disease*, pp. 187–219. New York: Raven Press.

Spraycar, M. (1991). *PDR Medical Dictionary.* Montvale, N.J.: Medical Economics.

Thilenius, O.G., & Grossman, B.J. (1961). Friedreich's ataxia with heart disease in children. *Pediatrics, 27,* 246–254.

Woodwell, D.A. (1992). Office visits to internists, 1989. *Advance Data, 209,* 1–10.

CHAPTER

54

Headache

Virginia E. Robertson, MD, and Mary E. McCormack, RNCS, FNP-C, MPH

Headache is a challenging symptom for both patient and provider. Etiologies are varied and include idiopathic and specific conditions, with prognoses ranging from benign to life-threatening. Further, depending on the nature of the headache syndrome, the impact on the patient and on society may be minimal or major. Nearly 15 million people in the United States in 1994 had headaches (National Center for Health Statistics, 1995), and headache is among the top 10 causes for primary care visits (Kumar & Cooney, 1995). Thus, it is important to recognize serious secondary causes of headache and manage the benign yet potentially disabling primary headaches.

The primary headache syndromes are those headaches that are considered idiopathic, including migraine, tension-type headache, and cluster headache. Secondary headache syndromes usually can be found to have a treatable cause, which will result in "cure" of the headache. These headaches may be caused by a wide variety of conditions, from the relatively rare brain tumor and subarachnoid hemorrhage to the more common and benign systemic viral syndromes. Diagnostic classifications of headaches are discussed below, using the International Headache Society (IHS) criteria (International Headache Society, 1988).

ANATOMY, PHYSIOLOGY, AND PATHOLOGY

The symptom of headache arises when pain is referred to the surface of the head from either intra- or extracranial sources. Although the anatomy and pathophysiology of all headache syndromes have not been fully elucidated, certain structures and contributing physiology are understood and aid the provider in both diagnosis and treatment.

Anatomic Sources for Headache

Intracranial structures that are implicated in some headaches include the periosteum, the dura at the base of the skull, the venous sinuses, the anterior and middle meningeal arteries, and the upper cervical nerves and cranial nerves V, VII, IX, and X. Pain from intracranial sources above the tentorium is usually referred via cranial nerve V to the frontal, orbital, and temporal regions. Pain originating below the tentorium and in the posterior fossa is typically transmitted via the facial, glossopharyngeal, and vagus nerves and the upper cervical nerves to the ear, nose, throat, and occiput. The brain parenchyma and bony skull themselves are almost completely insensitive to pain, as are certain cranial nerves (I, II, and VIII).

Extracranial structures that can give rise to headache include the skin, fascia, muscles, extracranial vasculature, ears, nasal mucosa, eyes, teeth, and cervical spine (Goroll et al, 1995;

Stevens, 1993). Pain referred from these structures usually directly overlies the structure.

Pathophysiologic Mechanisms for Headache

Several types of stimuli affect these structures and become detected as pain. Dilatation of intra- and extracranial vasculature occurs in migraine, giant cell arteritis, malignant hypertension, eclampsia, transient ischemic attacks, arteriovenous malformation, and alcohol or drug withdrawal. Contraction or tension of cranial and cervical muscles is implicated in tension-type headache, temporomandibular joint dysfunction, and head or neck trauma.

Distention, stretching, or displacement of the dura or cranial nerves may be associated with an increase or decrease in intracranial pressure, mass lesions, or mass effect from bleeding. Inflammation of the meninges, as in meningitis or meningoencephalitis, or of cranial or spinal nerves, as in trigeminal neuralgia, mass lesions, and cervical radiculopathy, also can cause headache. Iritis and angle-closure glaucoma may yield headache along the trigeminal nerve (cranial nerve V, first division), in addition to eye pain (Wyngaarden, 1992).

The known pathophysiology of the primary headache syndromes reveals complex neurohormonal and neurochemical contributors. Migraine, for example, involves both vascular and neurologic factors. Vascular changes include constriction of branches of the carotid artery, causing the prodromal symptoms, followed by arterial dilation, causing the pain, and ending with arterial wall edema, which accounts for the sometimes protracted pain. However, regional blood flow does not explain all aspects of migraine. A neurologic component may be mediated by a phenomenon called cortical spreading depression, which decreases the excitability of central neurons to neurochemical transmitters.

One transmitter currently under focus is serotonin, which has been found to be released abnormally from platelets during migraine. A rich supply of serotonergic nerve endings are found in the meningeal vasculature, as well as in the peripheral trigeminal nerve (Zagami, 1994). Such findings have helped to create new treatments, including sumatriptan, a serotonin-1d receptor agonist.

Hormonal and neurohormonal changes are also thought to be involved in some headaches. For example, hypothalamic and neurohormonal alterations, as well as vasomotor disturbances, have been implicated in the pathophysiology of cluster headaches (Kudrow, 1994). Also, the preponderance of women migraine sufferers after menarche, as well as the variation in migraine occurrence for some women taking birth-control pills, have long implicated estrogens as contributory to migraine.

TABLE 54-1	Prevalence of Primary Headache Syndromes	
Type of Headache	One-Year Prevalence (%)	Lifetime Prevalence (%)
Migraine	10–16	
With aura	0–4.6	
Tension-type	20–30	66
Chronic		3
Cluster		0.1

Adapted from Rasmussen & Olesen, 1994; Rasmussen, 1995.

EPIDEMIOLOGY

Epidemiologic surveillance of headache has improved since the advent of the IHS classification system because it provides specific diagnostic criteria for different headache syndromes. However, other methodologic differences between studies remain problematic. Studies using general versus referral populations, differing age ranges, self-administered headache questionnaires versus structured interviews, and self-reported versus provider-reported diagnoses have yielded varying interpretations of prevalence and sociodemographic data. The use of IHS diagnostic criteria to study general populations, however, has shown some consistent headache patterns between studies and has challenged certain prior concepts.

Prevalence

Estimates of headache prevalence for the U.S. population have been derived by the National Health Interview Survey, most recently conducted in 1994 (National Center for Health Statistics, 1995). In household interviews, nearly 4 million people reported that they experienced acute nonmigraine headaches in the prior 3 months that were severe enough to limit their activities or prompt medical attention. Of these, 30% were among people ages 5 to 17 and 34% were between ages 25 and 44. For migraine, 11 million people reported that they have migraine as a chronic condition. Of these migraine sufferers ("migraineurs"), 10% were younger than 18 years old, and 60.5% were 17 to 44 years old. The predominance of headache among working-age adults creates great financial impact in the United States as a result of work lost from absences and disability (Stang & Osterhaus, 1993). Table 54-1 shows typical prevalences for the primary headache syndromes.

Among secondary headache syndromes, many of the relatively benign types are highly prevalent. The more serious secondary headache syndromes are, fortunately, relatively rare.

TABLE 54-2	Lifetime Prevalence of Selected Secondary Headaches
Alcohol withdrawal (hangover)	70%
Associated with fever	63
Intracranial mass	0.5
Vascular disorders (eg, aneurysm, cerebrovascular accident)	1
Head trauma	4

Ramusen, BK. (1995). Epidemiology of headache. *Cephalalgia. 15* 45–68.

Table 54-2 provides prevalence rates of some secondary headaches.

Age

Primary headache syndromes can have their onset at any age, but typical patterns are seen. Migraines tend to present in the second and third decades, whereas tension-type headaches usually have an onset in the second decade. The peak prevalence of migraines tends to be around age 40 years in women and 35 in men (Stewart et al, 1992), whereas tension-type headaches peak in the middle to late 40s for both men and women. Peak age of presentation for episodic tension headaches occurs a few years before the peak for chronic tension headache (Rasmussen, 1995). This trend has contributed to the controversial idea that episodic headaches may transform into chronic headaches (Ziegler, 1995).

Both types of headache show decreasing prevalence with aging, especially after the 50s, although it is unclear whether this trend is related to the natural history of these headaches, to increased treatment, or to other factors (Rasmussen & Olesen, 1994). The proportion of migraineurs reporting disability with headaches appears to remain constant regardless of age (Stewart et al, 1992).

In contrast, vascular and other secondary headaches are more prevalent in the elderly, necessitating close attention to the presentation, or change in pattern, of headache in the elderly.

Gender

Among the primary headache syndromes, migraines and tension-type headaches disproportionately affect women. The 1-year prevalence for migraines is 3% to 9% in men and 13% to 20% in women. The gender differences are further accentuated by age and subtype of headache, as shown in Table 54-3.

Cultural Factors

Headache, with its major symptom being pain, is subject to cultural differences in patient experience, meaning, and outcomes. Until recently, migraines and tension-type headaches were thought to be more common in industrialized countries or in certain ethnic groups, but this conclusion has not, in fact, been supported in population-based studies (Rasmussen, 1995). In contrast, for migraine, the similarity of prevalence between different populations has been cited as partial evidence for the underlying biologic, rather than cultural, basis of migraine (Goadsby, 1994).

TABLE 54-3	Gender Differences Among Headache Types
Type of Headache	Female : Male Distribution
Migraine (all)	3:1 (1:1 until puberty, 2:1 after menopause)
With aura	2:1
Without aura	7:1
Tension-type	5:4 (1:1 until puberty)
Cluster	1:7

Adapted from Rasmussen, 1995; Stewart et al, 1992.

Socioeconomic Factors

Early studies on headache prevalence concluded that migraines were more common in higher socioeconomic classes, but more recent studies have challenged this finding (Rasmussen, 1995; Stang & Osterhaus, 1993; Stewart et al, 1992). However, several studies have shown that migraine patients with higher income do have more physician visits (Lipton et al, 1992; Rasmussen & Olesen, 1994) and have been given an IHS-consistent diagnosis from a physician (Lipton et al, 1992).

In terms of socioeconomic impact, migraine headaches contributed to 1.5 million person-days of work lost as a result of patients being bedridden and 2.8 million person-days of restricted activity in 1989 (Stang & Osterhaus, 1993). For non-migraine headaches, the 1994 National Health Interview Survey data attributed 3.5 million bed-days and more than 8 million restricted activity days (similar data were not cited for migraines).

DIAGNOSTIC CRITERIA

In 1988, the IHS published "Classification and Diagnostic Criteria for Headache Disorders, Cranial Neuralgias, and Facial Pain" in an effort to facilitate headache research and to improve clinical care. Although diagnostic criteria for headache had been established before, the IHS classifications and criteria are the current standards because of their comprehensive and organized approach, permitting more precise diagnoses of the symptom of headache.

The IHS classifies headaches according to their unique definition or pathologic basis (Table 54-4). The IHS system then provides a list of diagnostic criteria that characterize each headache syndrome by its specific features—its history, pattern of recurrence, and known contributing factors.

Clinical use of the IHS system, therefore, relies on the ability of the provider to elicit a sound and complete history. Indeed, because primary headaches have no physical markers, the history is the provider's prime tool for diagnosis. The physical exam and laboratory workup are used selectively to detect other illnesses or specific treatable entities when indicated.

TABLE 54-4	Classification of Headaches
1. Migraines	
2. Tension-type headache (HA)	
3. Cluster HA and chronic paroxysmal hemicrania	
4. Miscellaneous HA unassociated with structural lesion	
5. HA associated with head trauma	
6. HA associated with vascular disorders	
7. HA associated with nonvascular intracranial disorder	
8. HA associated with substances or their withdrawal	
9. HA associated with noncephalic infection	
10. HA associated with metabolic disorder	
11. HA or facial pain associated with disorder of facial or cranial structures	
12. Cranial neuralgias, nerve trunk pain, and deafferentation pain	
13. HA not classifiable	

Adapted from IHS, 1988.

HISTORY AND PHYSICAL EXAM

As many as 50% to 85% of headache sufferers, depending on the type of headache, do not seek care or obtain a formal diagnosis (Lipton et al, 1992; Rasmussen & Olesen, 1994). Those who do seek care may have already had headaches for some time; others come in very early, at the first sign of headache. In general, the secondary headache syndromes present more acutely or can have more serious consequences, whereas the primary headache syndromes often have a benign prognosis but can be quite limiting if not well diagnosed or treated.

The headache history (Table 54-5) should be used to characterize the headache and discern any acute or serious features. Unusual symptoms should be assessed: headache that flares during coughing, sneezing, or physical exertion (including sex); headache described as the "worst ever"; ongoing neurologic symptoms and signs during or after the headache; seizures or syncope; red eye; and others (see "Referral Points and Clinical Warnings" below). Headache that awakens the patient from sleep is a another feature that should alert the provider to possible intracranial mass.

Additional essential elements of the history include:

- Medications, including all prescribed medications and over-the-counter drugs. Some cause headache as a direct side effect, such as nitrates and calcium channel blockers; others contribute to rebound headache, such as analgesics containing caffeine or ergotamine.
- Substance use, including any recent use of alcohol or other substances that cause acute or withdrawal headache
- Trauma, acute or distant
- Concurrent fever and change in mental status
- Family history, especially of migraines
- Nutritional and occupational histories
- Recent stressors or symptoms of anxiety and depression
- Personal medical history of hypertension, chronic lung diseases, diabetes, and other chronic diseases that put the patient at risk for metabolic or medication-induced headaches.

TABLE 54-5	Key Elements of the Headache History
Laterality	Unilateral, bilateral, "side-locked" (recurrence on same side always)
Location	Site of pain on cranium, generalized vs. focal
Quality	Throbbing/pulsating, achy, burning, bandlike, stabbing, pressurelike
Severity	Graded from 0 (no pain) to 10 (extreme pain, worst ever)
Frequency	Number of headaches in specified time frame
Triggers	Foods, food additives, medications, sleep patterns, stress, specific activities, sex, chemical exposures
Timing	Patterns related to work, activities, or menstrual cycle
Prodromal changes	Change in sleep or appetite, moodiness, yawning, hyperactivity, hypoactivity
Aura symptoms	Blurred vision, scotomata or fortifications, hemianopsia or quadrantanopsia, auditory or olfactory hallucinations, weakness
Worsening factors	Light or noise exposure, physical activity, Valsalva maneuver
Relieving factors	Medications, massage, exercise, sleep or rest

The physical exam is used to find any secondary causes of headache and to screen for warning signs of serious etiologies. A general exam including a complete neurologic exam is essential. Fever, abnormal mental status, restricted range of motion on neck exam, hypoxia, purulent nasal discharge, and clicks on jaw movements may all point to secondary causes of headache. Warning signs of neurologic compromise include persistent visual field defects, focal weakness or sensory loss, seizures, orbital bruits, change in mental status (confusion, drowsiness), asymmetrical pupillary response, and papilledema. Any unusual finding on the history or physical exam should prompt the provider to consider a more sophisticated workup, which may include immediate consultation with a neurologist or infectious disease specialist or referral to the emergency department.

Primary Headache Syndromes

MIGRAINE HEADACHES

Both migraine without aura (common migraine, Table 54-6) and migraine with aura (classic migraine, Table 54-7) are typically recurrent, unilateral, throbbing or pulsating headaches accompanied by nausea or vomiting, or by photophobia and phonophobia. They tend to last 4 to 72 hours if untreated. The site, intensity, and features can vary from headache to headache.

Patients can often identify certain precipitating factors that seem to trigger the headaches. Common triggers include excess or lack of sleep, irregular eating habits, and certain foods or food additives. The most common trigger is stress and "mental strain" (Rasmussen, 1995). Women may find that headaches occur with menstrual periods. The so-called menstrual migraine commonly arises during the few days before the onset of menses and resolves at menstruation.

Some patients also notice premonitory symptoms 1 to 2 days before the headache, which can include hyper- or hypoactivity, depression, cravings, and repetitive yawning. Such symptoms are distinct from a true aura. Migraines with aura are further characterized by typical neurologic symptoms shortly preceding the headache: visual scotomata (flashing lights), visual field defects (hemianopsia, quadrantopsia), fortification scintillations (zigzag lines or waves), vertigo, and (rarely) aural or olfactory hallucinations. Typically, the symptoms of an aura cease soon after the headache begins and leave no permanent sequelae.

TABLE 54-6	Migraine Without Aura, Diagnostic Criteria

Headache attack lasts 4–72 hrs (untreated or unsuccessfully treated).

At least 2 of the following characteristics:

1. Unilateral location
2. Pulsating quality
3. Moderate or severe intensity (inhibits or prohibits activities of daily living)
4. Aggravation by walking stairs or similar routine physical activity

During headache, at least one of the following:

1. Nausea or vomiting
2. Photophobia and phonophobia

At least 5 attacks fulfilling above

No evidence of organic disease OR, if comorbid, no temporal relation

Adapted from IHS, 1988.

TABLE 54-7	Migraine With Aura, Diagnostic Criteria

See Table 54-6. Additionally . . .

At least 3 of the following characteristics:

1. One or more fully reversible aura symptoms indicating focal cerebral, cortical, or brain stem dysfunction
2. At least one aura symptom develops gradually over >4 min OR 2 or more symptoms occur in succession
3. No aura symptoms last more than 60 min. If >1 aura symptom is present, accepted duration is proportionally increased
4. Headache begins before, concurrent with, or follows aura in <60 min

No evidence of organic disease OR, if comorbid, no temporal relation

Adapted from IHS, 1988.

Migraine variants exist. Occasionally, a patient notes a typical aura that is *not* followed by a headache, considered a migraine equivalent. In complicated migraines, the neurologic symptoms or focal deficits of the aura persist through the headache and may leave neurologic impairments. Other causes for lasting deficits (stroke, intracranial bleeds, vascular malformations, or brain tumors) must be excluded before this migraine variant is diagnosed. Ophthalmoplegic, hemiplegic, and basilar artery migraines are rarer forms with more unusual focal neurologic symptoms and signs such as ocular palsies, persistent weakness or sensory losses, or symptoms suggestive of basilar artery involvement (vertigo, ataxia, tinnitus, diplopia, disturbed consciousness).

TENSION HEADACHES

Tension-type headaches can be episodic (Table 54-8) or chronic (Table 54-9). The typical tension-type headache is a bilateral, dull, bandlike or pressing pain of mild to moderate intensity that lasts from minutes to days. The pain gradually builds with time. Routine physical activity should not make it worse, but noise or light exposure may exacerbate the pain. Frank nausea is typically absent, although the patient may be anorexic. Actual muscular tension (eg, cervical muscle spasm) may or may not be present.

TABLE 54-8	Episodic Tension-Type Headache, Diagnostic Criteria

Headache lasting from 30 min–7 days

At least 2 of the following characteristics:

1. Pressing/tightening (nonpulsating) quality
2. Mild or moderate intensity (may inhibit but does not prohibit activities of daily living)
3. Bilateral location
4. No aggravation by walking stairs or similar routine physical activity

Both of the following:

1. No nausea or vomiting. Anorexia may occur.
2. Phonophobia OR photophobia OR neither but not both

At least 10 prior headache episodes as above, no more than 15/month or 180/year

No evidence of organic disease OR, if comorbid, no temporal relation

Adapted from IHS, 1988.

TABLE 54-9	Chronic Tension-Type Headache, Diagnostic Criteria

At least 2 of the following characteristics:
1. Pressing/tightening quality
2. Mild or moderate severity (may inhibit but does not prohibit activities)
3. Bilateral location
4. No aggravation by walking stairs or similar routine physical activity

Both of the following:
1. No vomiting
2. Nausea **OR** photophobia **OR** phonophobia (no more than one)

Average headache frequency 15 days/month (180 days/year) for 6 months

No evidence of organic disease **OR,** if comorbid, no temporal relation

Adapted from IHS, 1988.

Many studies have looked at the relation of mood disorders and both tension-type and migraine headaches. Stressful events or emotional upset have been found to be common triggers for both tension-type and migraine headaches (Rasmussen, 1995; Stevens, 1993), but depression as a true comorbidity for tension-type headache is controversial. The independent association of depression with headaches at all seems to be stronger for migraines than tension-type headaches (Merikangas, 1995).

Recognizing and carefully treating both migraine and episodic tension-type headache is critical to interceding in the development of chronic tension-type headache. The patient with chronic tension-type headache may have originally had periodic headaches but a chronic, daily pattern has evolved; analgesic overuse may contribute to as many as 20% of cases (Rapoport et al, 1996). Analgesic overuse, especially of analgesics containing caffeine, ergot, and barbiturates, can lead to withdrawal and cyclic headaches. Careful diagnosis and prescription of medications will help to prevent analgesic rebound headaches; treatment may be complicated and will require consultation with a headache specialist.

Careful evaluation for mood disorders (most commonly depression) is also indicated for patients with chronic, daily headaches; in these cases the headache is a somatic component of the depression. The symptom of headache may precede or even mask the psychiatric diagnosis. Such patients often awake with headache and have other indicators for psychiatric illness on history, such as anhedonia, sleep disturbance, eating disorder, difficulty with concentration, and so forth.

OTHER HEADACHE SYNDROMES

Other primary headache syndromes are quite rare; however, cluster headache should be recognized by the primary care provider because the syndrome is often easily diagnosed and is highly treatable. The headache is strictly unilateral, intense, ocular or temporal, and relatively short (15 to 180 minutes) but recurrent, usually several times each day. The headache may come at a highly predictable time of the day, every day. Ocular symptoms may include lacrimation, miosis, ptosis, conjunctival injection, or eyelid edema. Nasal congestion or frank rhinorrhea on the affected side may occur, as can forehead and facial sweating. The headaches are clustered in series over weeks or months, often occurring in the spring or fall, but with remission periods between clusters. Alcohol ingestion may trigger the headaches once a cluster has begun.

Secondary Headache Syndromes

SUBDURAL HEMATOMA

The section "Referral Points and Clinical Warnings" below discusses classic findings related to many urgent and serious, although mostly rare, causes of secondary headache syndromes. Of the mass lesions, subdural hematoma may have a particularly subtle presentation, especially in the elderly or alcoholic patient. Antecedent trauma may have been relatively mild in the elderly person or forgotten by the alcohol-abusing patient. The headache may overlie the site of the hematoma as it forms or be more generalized and bandlike. Neurologic symptoms and signs will present gradually.

TUMORS

Other mass lesions include primary brain tumors and metastatic tumors from other primary cancers. The headache is "side-locked" (without variation in its location) in about 30% of patients, or it may present more variably with characteristics similar to tension-type headache or migraine (Kumar & Cooney, 1995). Activities that involve a Valsalva maneuver worsen the headache, as do sudden position changes. The patient reports being awakened at night by the headache. Mental status changes and neurologic symptoms and signs present gradually. Infections that cause mass lesions (eg, toxoplasmosis) or abscesses (eg, tuberculosis) are typically accompanied by fever. Pseudotumor cerebri can present like a mass lesion.

SUBARACHNOID HEMORRHAGE

The "sentinel headache" is the sudden, unusual headache that may precede or herald serious conditions such as stroke or subarachnoid hemorrhage from a ruptured arteriovenous malformation or aneurysm. In subarachnoid hemorrhage, patients may report the "worst headache" of their lives or a "thunderclap" headache. Nuchal rigidity is an unreliable sign on physical exam (Edmeads, 1995). A computed tomography (CT) scan followed by lumbar puncture (if the scan is negative) is indicated when there is strong clinical suspicion based on the history.

OTHER SECONDARY HEADACHES

The most common secondary headache—indeed, the most common headache of all in most populations—is alcohol withdrawal (the hangover). Patients usually diagnose themselves accurately and are unlikely to present to the primary care provider. Headache associated with noncranial infections, such as influenza and other systemic viral syndromes, should also be identifiable based on the history of the illness and supportive findings on the physical exam. Meningitis and encephalitis have varied infectious etiologies; outcomes depend on the rapidity of diagnosis and treatment. Headache related to concussion can be either acute, immediately after trauma, or more persistent, as in postconcussive syndrome.

Acute sinusitis may be accompanied by a dull frontal or maxillary headache that typically worsens with bending over and is accompanied by purulent nasal discharge. In contrast, chronic sinusitis is not classified by the IHS as a source of headache (Coutin & Glass, 1996). Headaches may also be a symptom in some collagen vascular diseases, such as systemic lupus erythematosus.

Age and Gender Considerations

The onset of headaches or a change in headache pattern in those over age 50 deserves special consideration. Most of the primary headaches present at a younger age and show established, recognizable patterns. Serious intracranial conditions and some of their contributing comorbidities (such as hypertension) increase with aging; thus, headache in a patient over age 50 generally warrants a particularly careful history and physical exam. Diagnostic testing is generally more frequently indicated in the older patient.

One subtype of headache clearly is more common in the older patient: giant cell, or temporal, arteritis. The headache can be quite variable but classically is unilateral, throbbing (but evolving into a dull ache), and temporal. Intermittent jaw claudication occurs in about half of patients. Temporary visual disturbances may occur, such as blurring, diplopia, or amaurosis fugax (transient unilateral blindness, classically described as "a shade being pulled down" in the patient's field of vision). Scalp tenderness may be noted by the patient when combing the hair. On exam, some patients have a palpable temporal artery, which may be nodular or tender. Fever occurs in about 25% of patients. There may be evidence of more diffuse arteritis on the general exam. Polymyalgia rheumatica is a common comorbidity.

A major complication of temporal arteritis, inflammation of the ophthalmic or retinal artery, can lead to blindness. Prompt diagnosis of this type of headache, via detection of an elevated erythrocyte sedimentation rate and characteristic pathology on temporal artery biopsy, is critical. Prednisone, starting at 40 to 60 mg/day and tapering to the lowest possible maintenance dose, reduces and controls inflammation.

Gender-based prevalence of the various headache types was noted in the section on epidemiology. Migraine may be a risk factor or risk marker for cerebral ischemia for people less than 45 years old, especially women less than 35 (Carolei et al, 1996); transient ischemic attacks and stroke in young adults are extremely rare, however. Migraine is considered a relative contraindication for the prescription of oral contraceptives.

Nutritional Considerations

Regular meals and adequate fluid intake are an important part of preventing certain headache syndromes. Fasting, with resultant hypoglycemia, has been found to precipitate migraines (Guyton, 1991). Dehydration, either from poor fluid intake or from febrile illness, may be the source of headache in some patients. Excessive intake of alcohol and caffeine or withdrawal

TABLE 54-10	Substances in Foods That May Contribute to Headache
Substance	**Found in**
Tyramine	Aged cheese, red wine, chocolate
Phenylalanine	Artificial sweetener
Nitrites	Food preservatives, hot dogs, luncheon meats
Sulfites	Food preservatives, red wine
Monosodium glutamate (MSG)	Chinese food, commercial flavor enhancers
Caffeine	Coffee, tea, chocolate, certain sodas

TABLE 54-11	Occupational Risk Factors for Headache
Exposure	**Type of Job or Job Setting**
CHEMICAL EXPOSURE	
Carbon monoxide	Truck/cab driver, mechanics, construction crews
Heavy metals	Battery factories, firing ranges
Irritant gases (eg, ammonia, methylene chloride)	Painters, chemical plant workers, housekeepers
PHYSICAL AGENTS	
Temperature extremes	Firefighters, bakers, foundry workers
Noise	Construction crews, firing range workers/users
Vibration	Construction crews, firing range workers/users
Muscle strain	Secretaries, data entry clerks, construction crews

from these substances is an important source of headaches that should not be overlooked.

There are also many substances in food that are known to produce headache in those sensitive to them when ingested even in small amounts (Table 54-10). Other foodstuffs that have been reported to trigger headaches include Champagne, vinegar, nuts and peanut butter, yogurt, buttermilk, sour cream and other fermented foods, shellfish, citric acid, beans, garlic and onions, sugar, and freshly baked yeast products (Balch & Balch, 1990). A thorough nutritional assessment is essential to the evaluation of headache in primary care.

Occupational Considerations

Many occupations pose an increased risk for headache. In the nonindustrial office setting, headaches are often associated with poor indoor air quality in buildings with insufficient ventilation. Other factors include tobacco secondhand smoke exposure, poor lighting, and eye strain or musculoskeletal strain associated with work at computer stations (Zenz, 1988). Industrial and other high-risk settings for occupational headaches include, but are not limited to, construction, fire fighting, and chemical production (Table 54-11).

DIAGNOSTIC STUDIES

The primary headache syndromes have no unique biologic markers, although serotonin abnormalities, cervical muscle contractions, and other pathophysiologic findings have been implicated (Ziegler, 1995). The secondary syndromes do have associated abnormalities on laboratory, radiologic, or biopsy testing that can be helpful in clarifying the source of the headache. The provider's main task is to distinguish when such studies are warranted and to use them in an efficacious manner. No particular diagnostic study is considered routine for headache workup. One particular test used for the workup of some headaches, the lumbar puncture, is in itself associated with headache. The "post-LP headache," which occurs after dural puncture because of a slow leak of cerebrospinal fluid, may be prevented by the use of small cannulae needles aimed along the long axis of the spine during insertion (Leibold et al, 1993). Lying down immediately after the procedure also may help.

Laboratory Testing

Most patients with headache have normal or unrelated basic hematology and chemistry laboratory findings. The white cell count and differential are helpful if meningitis (high white count, left shift if bacterial) or viral syndrome (moderately elevated white count, lymphocytosis) is suspected. For patients with HIV, the white count and CD4 count will help to indicate risk for opportunistic infections that might cause meningitis (eg, *Cryptococcus*).

The provider will need more focussed laboratory testing in certain circumstances. If meningitis is suspected, lumbar puncture with opening pressure, chemistries, cell count, and cultures are needed. Cultures may need to include bacteria, viruses, mycobacteria, and more unusual organisms (eg, fungi), depending on the patient's risk factors. Latex agglutination, India ink, and titers for syphilis or other organisms should be considered. If a subarachnoid bleed is suspected, the lumbar puncture will be confirmatory, although it should be done after a CT scan (to rule out mass lesion). When temporal arteritis is suspected, an elevated erythrocyte sedimentation rate (above 80 in all but 1% to 2% of patients) will support the diagnosis; temporal artery biopsy can confirm the diagnosis. To detect significant headache-causing metabolic abnormalities, a glucose tolerance test (to rule out hypoglycemia) or arterial blood gas analysis (to rule out hypoxia or hypercapnia) is indicated on rare occasions.

Radiologic Studies

The need for radiologic studies should be carefully reviewed for each patient. The vast majority of patients will not need x-rays, CT scans, or magnetic resonance imaging (MRI); the latter two tests, because of their cost and potential discomfort to the patient, should be ordered only if an intracranial mass, vascular lesion, or bleed is strongly suspected based on the history and physical exam. A CT scan should be considered in the following circumstances (Kumar & Cooney, 1995; Frishberg, 1994):

- When there is a change in the characteristics, frequency, or severity of headaches in a person with known migraines
- When headaches are refractory to proper treatment
- If headaches are accompanied by focal neurologic symptoms or signs, especially seizure or papilledema
- If the headache is worsened by the Valsalva maneuver (sneeze, cough, bowel movement, physical exertion, sex)
- When headaches begin after age 50, especially if there are atypical features
- If headaches persistently localize to one location (side-locked headaches)
- If there is an orbital bruit.

Most intracranial lesions will be revealed on CT scan, but MRI may be more useful when posterior fossa lesions or craniospinal lesions (eg, Arnold-Chiari malformations) are suspected (Kumar & Cooney, 1995).

Simple cervical x-rays may be indicated for some patients, depending on the trauma or injury history and any focal cervical impingement findings on the physical exam. When sinusitis is suspected and is not responding to antibiotics, consider a CT scan of the sinuses, particularly in high-risk patients such as those with HIV.

Other Studies

The need for biopsy of brain masses discovered on CT scan or MRI will depend on whether there is a known primary cancer and the likelihood of that primary to metastasize to the brain. An electroencephalogram may be indicated for headaches presenting with seizure, especially if the CT scan fails to reveal a source. Electromyelography, blood levels of substance P and serotonin, personality inventories, and other studies have been used in research protocols but are not used routinely.

TREATMENT OPTIONS, EXPECTED OUTCOMES, AND COMPREHENSIVE MANAGEMENT

Prevention

Primary prevention of headaches such as migraine is elusive. Even though family histories usually reveal that up to 50% of migraineurs have first-degree relatives with migraines (Rasmussen, 1995), there is no actual prophylactic task or early diagnostic test for unaffected relatives. Similarly, structural or metabolic causes of headache may not have any specific prophylaxis. However, although few types of headaches may be considered fully preventable, most have risk factors that may be modified or recognized early. For example, migraineurs, once their triggers are recognized, can strive to avoid them and thus prevent some headaches. Headaches related to certain injuries and occupational hazards should be avoidable to a large extent.

HEAD INJURY PREVENTION

Bicycle and motorcycle safety helmets are critical to prevent head injury and, hence, headache associated with concussion. Review Chapter 3 for discussion of this hazard.

OCCUPATIONAL HAZARDS

Prevention of occupational headaches includes the use of glare screens on computer terminals to reduce eye strain, proper ergonomics at work stations to decrease muscle strain, good ventilation systems in work sites with significant exposure to chemical fumes, and protective gear for noise and inhalants.

Therapeutic Interventions

A comprehensive approach to the patient with recurrent or chronic headache includes both preventive and abortive measures, which must be individually tailored. General strategies for care of most of the primary headaches include encouraging adequate nutrition and rest, avoidance of known triggers, regular exercise, proper posture, and relaxation. A physical therapy regimen incorporating exercise, stretching, and ergonomic adjustments for usual activities is particularly useful for reducing the frequency and intensity of tension-type headaches (Hammill et al, 1996). For patients with cluster headaches, avoidance of alcohol during a cluster period is helpful.

Further nonmedication treatment for headaches such as topical cold or heat applications, rest or sleep in a dark quiet room, and relaxation techniques should be attempted with all drug regimens. Alternative and complementary therapies are discussed below.

Before initiating a medication, the provider should find out what the patient may have already tried. The medication history

TABLE 54-12 Abortive Medications

MIGRAINE

Analgesics/NSAIDs

Aspirin (ASA) or acetaminophen 325 mg: 2 tabs q4–6h

Naproxen 250–500 mg BID

Ibuprofen 300–800 mg TID

Analgesic Combinations

ASA/butalbital/caffeine (Fiorinol): 1 or 2 tab/cap q4h
(max 6/24 h)

Acetaminophen/isometheptene/dichlorolphenazone
(Midrin): 2 caps then 1 cap q1h (max 5/12 h)

Narcotics/Opioids

Acetaminophen/codeine (various fixed dosages): 1 or 2
tabs q4h

Butorphanol nasal spray: 1 spray unilateral to HA, can
repeat once in 3–5 h

Ergot Alkaloids

Ergotamine/caffeine tablets: 2 tabs then q30min
(max 6)

Ergotamine/caffeine rectal suppositories: 1 at onset,
may repeat once in 1 h

Dihydroergotamine mesylate: 1 mL IV/IM at onset, then
q1h (max 2 mL IV or 3 mL IM)

Serotonin Receptor Agonist

Sumatriptan 6 mg/0.5 cc: 6 mg SC, may repeat once
(max 2 injections/24 hs)

Sumatriptan tablets: 25 mg PO, may give up to 100 mg
2 h later (max 300 mg/day, 200 mg if SC injection
used initially)

Anticonvulsants

Phenytoin 300–600 mg QD

Carbamazapine 200 mg QD

TENSION-TYPE

Analgesics/NSAIDs

See Migraine

Analgesic Combinations

ASA/butalbital/caffeine: See Migraine

Acetaminophen/isometheptene/dichlorolphenazone: 1 or
2 tabs q4h (max 8/24 h)

Antidepressants

Amitriptyline 50–100 mg HS

Buspirone 15–80 mg QD

Sertraline 50–200 mg QD

Muscle Relaxant

Cyclobenzaprine 10–40 mg QD

CLUSTER

Oxygen Therapy

100% O_2 at 7 L/min $\times$ 15 min

Lidocaine

Viscous lidocaine 2–4%: 1 inhalation q4h

Ergot Alkaloids

Ergotamine/caffeine: 2 tabs then q30min (max 6
tabs/attack)

Dihydroergotamine mesylate: 1 mL IV/IM at onset, then
q1h (max 2 mL IV or 3 mL IM)

Serotonin Receptor Agonist

Sumatriptan: See Migraine

---

should include prescribed as well as over-the-counter agents, the sequence of agents attempted, and the relative success of each agent. The provider must also evaluate whether abortive or prophylactic medications or both are warranted, usually based on the frequency of the headaches and the degree of functional limitations the patient is having. Any new medication choice must, of course, be reviewed for contraindications, precautions, and drug interactions with other headache medications or medications for other conditions. A headache diary with a severity scale can be useful for initial diagnosis and for tracking therapeutic response. It is wise to prepare the patient for a certain amount of "trial-and-error" in identification of the most successful regimen.

ABORTIVE THERAPY

For abortive agents (Table 54-12), the earlier the treatment is initiated at the onset of headache, the more likely it will be effective. Many migraineurs can recognize actual early warning signs of impending headache, based on premonitory symptoms or true prodromal symptoms in those with aura. For other headaches, beginning medication appropriately during the first phase of pain will limit the extent of the headache.

Choice of therapy will be guided by the type of headache, prior use of typical medications, the patient's preference and needs as to route of delivery, and concurrent symptoms or problems that may restrict the use of certain agents or routes.

Patients with significant nausea or frank vomiting during headache will need an injected, inhaled, or rectal medication or the addition of antiemetics to their oral regimen.

Many different classes of drugs have been used for abortive therapies. As theories of headache pathophysiology have changed, so too have the medications. Some agents have the potential for addiction (eg, the opioids and some of the analgesic combinations containing barbiturates), others for contributing to rebound headaches (those with caffeine or ergots). However, all the agents in Table 54-12 can be useful for individualized therapy.

For migraines, sumatriptan is considered to be particularly effective for headache control. It has been shown to improve the quality of life for migraineurs and to decrease clinic visits and health care costs for migraine (Litaker et al, 1996). However, the effects of sumatriptan therapy are limited by frequent recurrent headaches (as much as 40%), as well as by side effects and patient inconvenience when administered in the more rapid-acting subcutaneous form (Goadsby, 1994). Both the side effect profile and patient acceptance have improved with the release of the oral form.

Other agents that work on the serotonergic system, perhaps on more selective receptors, are expected. Additionally, an inhaled route of dihydroergotamine with a good response rate and a low recurrence rate of headache will be available soon (Gallagher, 1996).

TABLE 54-13	Prophylactic Medications	
Migraine	**Tension-Type**	**Cluster**
BETA-ADRENERGIC BLOCKERS Propranolol; 40–160 mg QD Timolol: 10–30 mg BID	**ANTIDEPRESSANTS** Amitriptyline: 25–200 mg QD Nortriptyline: 25–200 mg QD	**CALCIUM CHANNEL BLOCKER** Verapamil: 120 mg TID
CALCIUM CHANNEL BLOCKERS Verapamil: 40–120 mg TID Nifedipine: 10–30 mg TID	**MUSCLE RELAXANT** Cyclobenzaprine: 10–40 mg QD	**ANTIDEPRESSANT** Lithium carbonate: 300 mg TID
ANTIDEPRESSANTS Amitriptyline: 50–200 mg QD Sertraline HCl: 50–200 mg QD Buspirone: 15–80 mg QD	**NSAIDs** Naproxen: 250 mg BID Ibuprofen: 200 mg BID	**CORTICOSTEROIDS** Prednisone: 40–60 mg QD Triamcinolone: 12–16 mg QD
SEROTONIN INHIBITORS/ERGOT ALKALOIDS Methysergide: 2–4 mg BID (max 8 mg/day) Cyproheptadine: 4–20 mg QD		**ERGOT ALKALOIDS** Methysergide: 4–8 mg QD

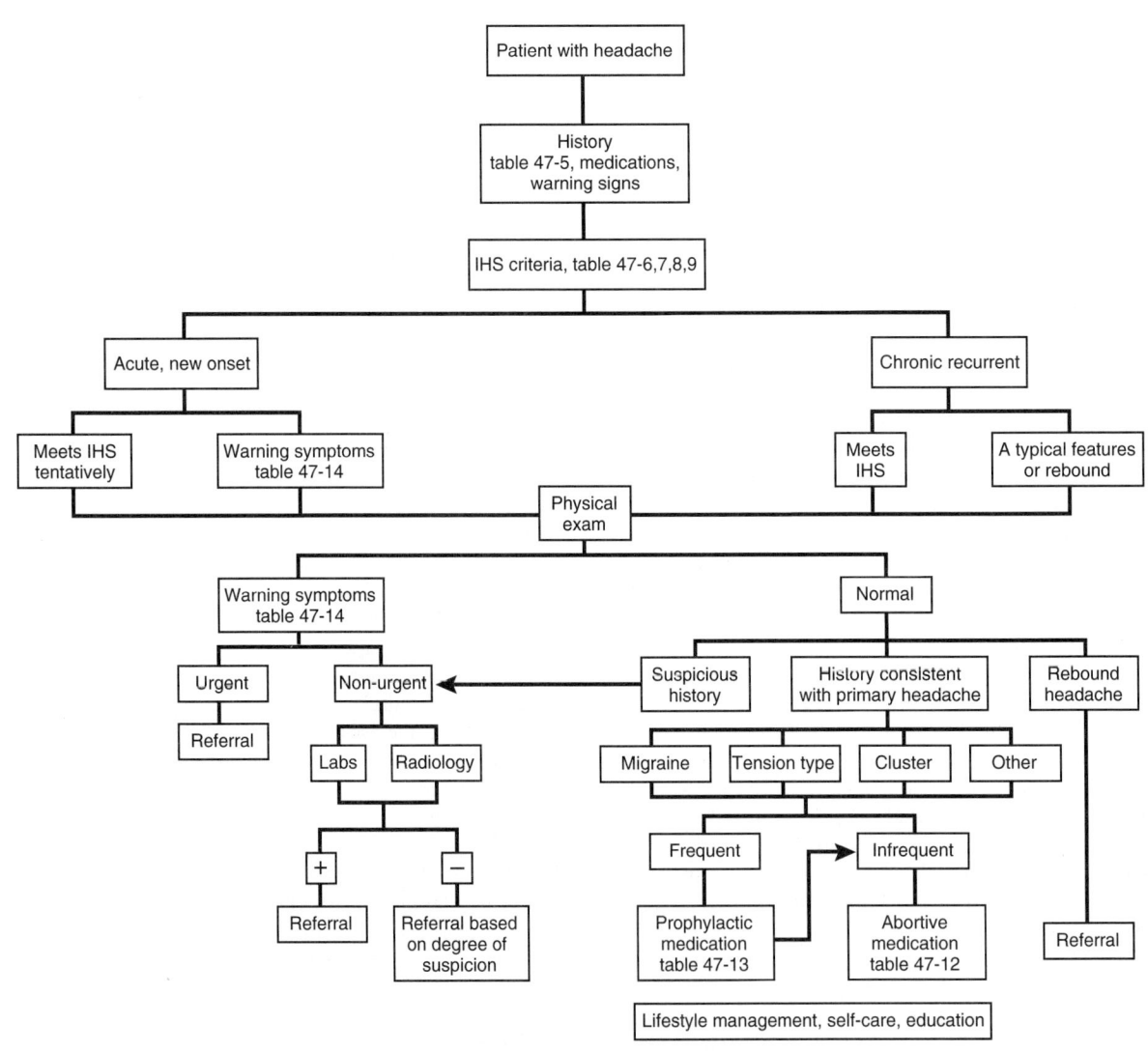

FIGURE 54-1 Comprehensive management recommendations for the patient with a headache.

TABLE 54-14	Referral Points and Clinical Warnings	
Associated Symptoms/Signs	**Possible Urgent or Serious Causes**	**Possible Workup or Referral**
Exacerbated by exertion (Valsalva maneuver, strain, cough, sneeze)	CNS mass lesion, leaking aneurysm, increased intracranial pressure	Lumbar puncture, CT scan, neurology consult
Altered mental status, confusion, drowsiness	Toxic exposure, CNS mass lesion, cerebrovascular accident, encephalitis, metabolic disorders	Bloodwork, lumbar puncture, CT scan, neurology consult
Abnormal neurologic signs (pupil/reflex/extraocular movement inequality, papilledema, facial asymmetry)	Cerebrovascular accident, mass lesion	CT scan or MRI depending on features, neurology consult
Stiff neck/nuchal rigidity and fever	Meningitis	Lumbar puncture, infectious disease consult
Onset after age 50 (in patient with no prior Hx)	Mass lesion, leaking aneurysm, temporal arteritis	Consider neurology consult
Described as the "worst ever" with a sudden onset	Subarachnoid hemorrhage	CT scan without contrast, possible lumbar puncture, neurology consult
Red eye, eye pain, and dilated pupils	Acute angle-closure glaucoma	Ophthalmology consult
Headache on rising or orthostatic	Decreased cerebrospinal fluid	Lumbar puncture (likely a diagnosis of exclusion)
Seizures	Mass lesion, toxic exposure	Electroencephalogram, CT scan, neuro consult
Pulsatile temporal artery, jaw claudication, scalp tenderness, elevated erythrocyte sedimentation rate	Giant cell (or temporal) arteritis	Temporal artery biopsy; vascular surgery and neuro-ophthalmology consult

PROPHYLACTIC THERAPY

The use of prophylactic medications (Table 54-13) should be considered for patients who have at least one headache per week that interferes with their daily living. Prophylaxis is essential for the patient who has already evolved a chronic headache pattern, defined by the IHS as headache that is present for at least 15 days per month for at least 6 months.

The provider first should assess whether the chronic headache sufferer is having rebound headaches associated with too-frequent dosing with analgesics, especially preparations containing caffeine or ergotamine. These patients need to be weaned entirely off these medications before proper evaluation and management can be completed, which rarely requires hospitalization for management of withdrawal. Consultation with a neurologist is particularly helpful for all patients who are suspected of having significant rebound headaches.

In general, a prophylactic agent should be tried for 2 to 3 months before switching to an alternative. As with the abortive therapies, there are many classes of drugs to try. The tricyclic antidepressants and serotonin reuptake inhibitors are often reasonable first agents to try for prophylaxis, but it may take several trials to identify the best agent. Medications such as the beta-blockers, although often effective, must be carefully prescribed in patients with concurrent asthma, diabetes, or other conditions that may be adversely affected by the addition of a beta-blocker. Once a successful drug regimen has been found, it is recommended that the patient remain on it for 6 months before a trial without it.

Comprehensive management recommendations are shown in Figure 54-1.

TEACHING AND SELF-CARE

Any recurrent type of primary headache offers ample opportunity for patient education about the illness and self-care. The patient should be encouraged to recognize triggers and early warning signs of the headaches, to use medications and other therapeutic modalities carefully and discriminately, and to seek provider input early when therapies do not seem to work. The provider should educate the patient about the benefits, proper use, and side effects of the medications and other treatments chosen. Using headache diaries, distributing educational literature, and referring patients to community resources are integral to helping patients toward self-care.

COMMUNITY RESOURCES

The following organizations provide information about treatment options, dispense educational materials, supply a list of their physician members, and direct headache sufferers to support groups in their area.

- The National Headache Foundation, 428 W. St. James Place, 2d floor, Chicago, IL 60614-2750, 800-843-2256, www.headaches.org
- American Council for Headache Education, 875 Kings Highway, Suite 200, Woodbury, NJ 08096-3172, 800-255-ACHE, 609-845-0322

REFERRAL POINTS AND CLINICAL WARNINGS

Headache is usually a benign symptom: research has shown that only 0.5% to 4% of headaches have a serious organic origin (Rasmussen, 1995). The majority of headaches are the result of migraine, tension, or other benign causes. The most important step in the primary care setting is to identify emergent situations requiring immediate care. Table 54-14 presents key points and approaches for semiurgent or urgent headache syndromes requiring consultation.

EDITOR'S NOTE:
COMPLEMENTARY APPROACHES

A general discussion of complementary approaches can be found in Chapter 3. The following, while not an exhaustive list, are some complementary approaches being used for this condition. Additional information on these approaches, including precautions, can be found in Appendices A and B. Providers need to assess for the use of complementary approaches as part of the patient's history, as they may impact conventional therapies, and patients may not volunteer this information unless specifically asked. Efficacy of many complementary approaches is not as well documented as that of conventional therapies. Providers need to read the literature before suggesting these complementary approaches.

- Vitamins, minerals, herbs, supplements
  - Magnesium
  - Peppermint
- Complementary Modalities
  - Acupuncture
  - Aromatherapy
  - Biofeedback
  - Chiropractic
  - Massage therapy

References

Balch, J.F., & Balch, P.A. (1990). *Prescription for nutritional healing.* Garden City, NY: Avery Publishing Group.

Carolei, A., Marini, C., DeMatteis, G. et al. (1996). History of migraine and risk of cerebral ischaemia in young adults. *Lancet, 347,* 1503–1506.

Coutin, I.B., & Glass, S.F. (1996). Recognizing uncommon headache syndromes. *American Family Physician, 54*(7), 2247–2252.

Edmeads, J.G. (1995). Headache as a symptom of organic disease. *Current Opinion in Neurology, 8,* 233–236.

Frishberg, B.M. (1994). The utility of neuroimaging in the evaluation of headache in patients with normal neurologic examinations. *Neurology, 44,* 1191–1197.

Gallagher, R.M., for the Dihydroergotamine Working Group. (1996). Acute treatment of migraine with dihydroergotamine nasal spray. *Archives of Neurology, 53*(Dec), 1285–1291.

Goadsby, P.J. (1994). The challenges of headache for the 1990s. *Current Opinion in Neurology, 7,* 255 257.

Goroll, A.H., May, L.A., & Mulley, A.G., Jr. (1995). *Primary care medicine: Office evaluation and management of the adult patient,* 2d Ed. Philadelphia: J.B. Lippincott.

Guyton, A.C. (1991). *Textbook of medical physiology,* 8th ed. Philadelphia: W.B. Saunders.

Hammill, J.M., Cook, T.M., & Rosecrance, J.C. (1996). Effectiveness of a physical therapy regimen in the treatment of tension-type headache. *Headache, 36,* 149–153.

International Headache Society, Headache Classification Committee. (1988). Classification and diagnostic criteria for headache disorders, cranial neuralgias and facial pain. *Cephalalgia, 8,* supplement 7.

Kudrow, L. (1994). The pathogenesis of cluster headaches. *Current Opinion in Neurology, 7,* 278–282.

Kumar, K.L., & Cooney, T.G. (1995). Headaches. *Medical Clinics of North America, 79*(2), 261–286.

Leibold, R.A., Yealy, D.M., Coppola, M., & Cantees, K.K. (1993). Post-dural puncture headache: Characteristics, management, and prevention. *Annals of Emergency Medicine, 22*(12), 1863–1870.

Lipton, R.B., Stewart, W.F., Celentano, D. et al. (1992). Undiagnosed migraine headaches: A comparison of symptom-based and reported physician diagnosis. *Archives of Internal Medicine, 152,* 1273–1278.

Litaker, D.G., Solomon, G.D., & Genzen, J.R. (1996). Impact of sumatriptan on clinic utilization and costs of care in migraineurs. *Headache, 36,* 538–541.

Merikangas, K.R. (1995). Association between psychopathology and headache syndromes. *Current Opinion in Neurology, 8,* 248–251.

National Center for Health Statistics. (1995). *Current estimates from the National Health Interview Survey, 1994.* Hyattsville, MD: US Department of Health and Human Services, Publication No. (PHS) 96-1521.

Rapoport, A., Stang, P., Gutterman, D. et al. (1996). Analgesic rebound headache in clinical practice: Data from a physician survey. *Headache, 36,* 14–19.

Rasmussen, B.K., & Olesen, J. (1994). Epidemiology of migraine and tension-type headache. *Current Opinion in Neurology, 7,* 264–271.

Rasmussen, B.K. (1995). Epidemiology of headache. *Cephalalgia, 15,* 45–68.

Stang, P.E., & Osterhaus, J.T. (1993). Impact of migraine in the United States: Data from the National Health Interview Survey. *Headache, 33,* 29–35.

Stevens, M.B. (1993). Tension-type headaches. *American Family Physician, 47*(4), 799–806.

Stewart, W.F., Lipton, R.B., Celentano, D. et al. (1992). Prevalence of migraine in the United States: Relation to age, income, race, and other sociodemographic factors. *JAMA, 267*(1), 64–69.

Wyngaarden, J.B., Smith, L.H., & Bennett, J.C. (Eds.). (1992). *Cecil textbook of medicine,* 19th ed. Philadelphia: W.B. Saunders.

Zagami, A.S. (1994). Pathophysiology of migraine and tension-type headache. *Current Opinion in Neurology, 7,* 272–277.

Zenz, C. (1988). *Occupational medicine: Principles and practical applications,* 2d ed. Chicago: Yearbook.

Ziegler, D.K. (1995). Some unsolved problems in the epidemiology of headache. *Current Opinion in Neurology, 8,* 231–232.

BIBLIOGRAPHY AND FURTHER READING

Adams, R.D., & Victor, M. (1993). *Principles of neurology,* 5th ed. New York: McGraw-Hill.

Barrett, E. (1996). Primary care for women: Assessment and management of headache. *Journal of Nurse-Midwifery, 41*(2), 117–124.

French, M.A. (1996). The mind-body-spirit connection: An introduction to alternative therapies. *Advance for Nurse Practitioners, 4*(11), 38–46.

Isselbacher, K.J., Braunwald, E., Wilson, J. et al. (1994). *Harrison's principles of internal medicine,* 13th ed. New York: McGraw-Hill.

Heinerman, J. (1988). *Heinerman's encyclopedia of fruits, vegetables and herbs.* West Nyack, NY: Parker Publishing Co.

McCance, K.L., & Heuther, S.E. (1990). *Pathophysiology: The biologic basis for disease in adults and children.* St. Louis: C.V. Mosby.

Moltyaner, Y., & Tenenbaum, J. (1996). Temporal arteritis: A review and case history. *Journal of Family Practice, 43*(3), 294–300.

Newman, L.S. (1995). Occupational illness. *N Engl J Med, 333*(17), 1128–1134.

Sellers, R.H. (1996). *Differential diagnosis of common complaints,* 3d ed. Philadelphia: W.B. Saunders.

Solomon, G.D., Skobieranda, F.G., & Gragg, L.A. (1994). Does quality of life differ among headache diagnoses? Analysis using the medical outcomes study instrument. *Headache, 34,* 143–147.

Stang, P.E., & Von Korff, M. (1994). The diagnosis of headache in primary care: Factors in the agreement of clinical and standardized diagnoses. *Headache, 34,* 138–142.

CHAPTER

55

Parkinson's Disease

Daisy Arce, MD, Steven Kaner, MD, Felix Enabosi, OT, PhD, and Bayo Sedenu, PT, PhD

Nearly one million people in the United States have Parkinson's disease. This is a disease with no known cause or cure. It is essential to recognize that "Parkinsonism" refers nonspecifically to syndromes of akinetic rigidity. Several different kinds of parkinsonism can be mentioned: postencephalic, arteriosclerotic, post-traumatic, secondary to medications, atrophic encephalopathies, and as part of a wider involvement of the nervous system in olivopontocerebellar atrophy and other neurodegenerative diseases. Idiopathic PD is the most common form of parkinsonism and accounts for more than 75% of patient visits to most large movement disorder centers. It is the focus of this chapter.

James Parkinson's "An Essay on the Shaking Palsy" in 1817 formally described features of PD. His account of six patients was a remarkably accurate assessment of the clinical features of the disease that bears his name. Actually, PD is referred to as a distinct clinicopathologic disorder usually defined by cardinal clinical features: resting tremor, rigidity, bradykinesia, and postural instability associated with neuropathologic evidence of cell loss in the substantia nigra and the presence of Lewy bodies (Langston, 1987).

ANATOMY, PHYSIOLOGY, AND PATHOLOGY

The primary neurochemical lesion of PD results from the deficiency of striatal dopamine. There is a loss of nerve cells in the pigmented substantia nigra pars compacta, in the locus ceruleus in the midbrain, and in the globus pallidus and putamen. Other monoaminergic systems besides the dopaminergic system can be affected in PD. Histochemical studies confirm degeneration of both the noradrenergic locus ceruleus system and the serotonergic raphe nuclear groups. The cholinergic system is affected as well, most notably with the nucleus basalis of Meynert (Langston, 1992). It is estimated that the loss of 70% or greater of substantia nigra neurons and a loss of 80% or more of striatal dopamine are necessary to have the clinical symptoms of PD. This suggests a longer presymptomatic phase during which selective neuronal cell death progresses.

The cause of PD is unknown. The role of genetics in the disease has been debated for many years, and that controversy continues. Studies of monozygotic and dizygotic twins with an index case of PD have been variably interpreted and suggest that genetics may not bear a strong influence on the cause of PD (Ward et al, 1983).

Positron emission tomography (PET) studies have shown that asymptomatic twins of parkinsonian patients commonly have abnormalities of striatal dopamine uptake. If these findings are valid, a genetic predisposition for PD would be supported. Attempts to identify the gene or genes that may be involved in the development of PD are in progress. One large family with parkinsonism, the Contursi kindred, has been well studied

for several years (Golbe et al, 1990). In 1996, researchers announced that the region of the chromosome responsible for the genetic transmission of parkinsonism in the Contursi family was found, probably with an autosomal dominant type of genetic inheritance. However, this chromosome area cannot be linked to all cases of familial PD (Polymeropoulos, 1996).

Recently, a team of researchers at Washington University School of Medicine in St. Louis has characterized a rare disease, aceruloplasminemia, that causes a rare form of Parkinsons. Aceruloplasminemia is caused by a mutation in the ceruloplasmin gene located in chromosome 3, which is involved in iron transport. Patients with this disease do not make ceruloplasmin, a protein that removes iron from the cells. Then the iron accumulates in cells in the brain's basal ganglia region and causes neurological problems. These include the tremors and gait abnormalities associated with PD. This genetic form of PD was discovered during a study of a Japanese family with Parkinson's symptoms and low levels of ceruloplasmin. This finding gives researchers important new information that could lead to innovation in the diagnosis and treatment of PD. (Harris et al, 1998)

There is also a mitochondrial genetic hypothesis that reported the activity of Complex I of mitochondria from both substantia nigra and platelets of patients with PD to be less than that of controls. This decrease is also noted in Huntington's disease and Leber's disease. Thus, while the fall in Complex I is not specific, it may still be a useful marker of idiopathic parkinsonism. The mitochondrial genetic hypothesis suggests that there could be a biochemical test to identify PD in an early stage. (Langston, 1992)

Many researchers have focused their interest on the possibility that PD may be caused, at least in part, to environmental factors. This fact was supported by the development of Parkinsonian symptoms in several young people after they used an illegal drug (1-methyl-4-phenyl-1,2,3,6-tetrahydropyridine, abbreviated MPTP) related to the narcotic meperidine. A single dose of this compound can cause selective destruction of the nigrostriatal dopaminergic neurons. (Langston et al, 1983). It is thought that the sequence of events involves MPTP successive oxidation by monoamine oxidase B to the dihidropyridinium and pyridinium ion derivatives. The latter compound (1-methyl-4-phenylpyridium; MPP+) is actively and specifically accumulated in the dopaminergic terminals by the dopamine uptake system. It is also accumulated nonspecifically by mitochondria and acts as a reversible inhibitor of mitochondrial oxidative phosphorylation at the level of NADH dehydrogenase (complex I). It appears that the resultant loss of ATP-generating capacity, with consequent changes in the ability to maintain membrane potentials, calcium ion homeostasis, and consequent free radical generation, may be sufficient to cause neuronal degeneration (Taipton et al, 1993).

There is no investigation that supports a viral etiology for PD. After the pandemic of encephalitis lethargica (1919–1926), many cases of parkinsonism were observed but no definite causal relation was established to a specific virus. Transient parkinsonian features may occur during the acute or convalescent phases of a variety of viral encephalitides, including measles, Japanese B, and western equine. Rarely, parkinsonism may remain as a permanent sequela (Langston et al, 1992).

Unrecognized environmental toxins structurally similar to MPTP may play a role in the etiology of PD. The major culprits are suspected to be industrial chemicals, herbicides, and pesticides in well water. Exposure to manganese dust or carbon disulfide causes parkinsonian symptoms, and the diagnosis is suggested by an accurate occupational history. Parkinsonism sometimes occurs as a result of severe carbon monoxide poisoning.

Endogenous toxins may also be responsible. In particular, the normal neurotransmitter dopamine readily oxidizes to produce free radicals that destroy the dopaminergic nerves. Although the precise role of dopamine itself remains unclear, the evidence relating PD to damage by free radicals remains compelling. This evidence includes increased iron levels, increased lipid peroxidation, decreased peroxidase and catalase levels, increased superoxide dismutase levels, and decreased glutathione levels.

NEUROANATOMY

Movement disorders result from disease of the basal ganglia. This consists of the caudate and the putamen (together called the striatum), the internal and external segments of the globus pallidus, the subthalamic nucleus, and the substantia nigra. Cortically initiated movements are facilitated and competing movements are inhibited through the influence of the basal ganglia.

The activity of the output structures of the basal ganglia (the internal segment of the globus pallidus and the pars reticulata of the substantia nigra) is controlled by two opposing striatal pathways, the so-called direct and indirect routes. The direct pathway consists of the striatal projections to the substantia nigra pars reticulata and the globus pallidus interna. This pathway is (gamma-aminobutyric acid) GABA-ergic and inhibitory, expressed mainly on the dopamine D_1 receptor. This direct route then functions to facilitate thalamocortical projections that reinforce cortically initiated movement. An alternative polysynaptic (indirect) pathway involves striatal GABA-ergic, inhibitory neurons that express the dopamine D_2 receptors and project to the globus pallidus externa, which has an inhibitory effect on the subthalamic nucleus (Hutchinson et al, 1997). This nucleus has excitatory glutamatergic feedback on the globus pallidus externa and excitatory glutamatergic input on the substantia nigra pars reticulata and the globus pallidus interna. The final effect of the indirect pathway is that striatal activity would lead to disinhibition of the subthalamic nucleus, which in turn, through its excitatory projections, leads to a higher activity of the neurons in the basal ganglia output nuclei and a stronger inhibition of their targets.

A balance between direct and indirect pathways is crucial to the normal functioning of the basal ganglia–thalamocortical circuits. It is also important to the balance among dopamine receptors in each pathway because, interestingly, dopamine has opposing effects on the two striatal output pathways—a stimulatory effect on the D_1 receptor-containing direct pathway and a suppressing effect on the D_2 receptor-containing indirect pathway) (Groenewegen, 1997).

In PD, loss of dopaminergic cells in the substantia nigra leads to striatal dopamine depletion. This depletion results in decreased activity of the direct pathway and increased activity of the indirect pathway. This results in reduced thalamic excitation of the motor cortex and loss of facilitation of cortically initiated movement. (The two striatal output pathways are out of balance and act in the same direction.) This may be explained, at least in part, the hypokinesia characteristic of PD. The resting tremor of PD is less readily explained by the model but may result from effects on cholinergic interneurons in the striatum (Olney & Aminoff, 1998).

EPIDEMIOLOGY

PD usually commences in middle or late life and leads to progressive disability with time. One study reported that compared with nondemented elderly people in the same community, patients with PD have a two- to fivefold increased risk of death. The risk is strongly related to the presence of severe extrapyramidal symptoms, especially bradykinesia (Louis et al, 1997); the mean time of survival is 13 to 14 years after the onset of clinical signs (Eichhorn & Oertel, 1994).

There is some discrepancy in the ethnic and sex distribution of PD. Some authors consider that the disease occurs more commonly in men than women; others insist it has an equal sex distribution. Although the disease occurs in all ethnic groups, most reports show that PD is more common among whites than nonwhites (Lanska et al, 1997). The prevalence is 1 to 2 per 1000 for the general population and 1 per 100 among people older than 65 years. A recent study indicated that 15% of persons ages 65 to 74, and more than half of all persons over 85, have some extrapyramidal disorders (Aminoff, 1998). The disease occurs with less frequency among the young, although about 5% of PD patients develop the illness before the age of 40.

HISTORY AND PHYSICAL EXAM

So gradual and insidious is the onset of PD that patients can rarely pinpoint the precise date it began. Initial manifestations are often noted by someone other than the patient. Usually it is someone close to the patient who notices some subtle changes, perhaps in posture or manner of walking or moving. Eventually the patient becomes aware that something is indeed wrong. There may be persistent tiredness, minor aches and pains, or a vague sense of malaise. Perhaps the patient feels a lack of energy or a sense of nervousness and irritability. Performance on the job may be declining for no apparent reason. The patient may notice that things that were formerly performed easily, without a thought, now require conscious effort.

Diagnostic mistakes may occur early in the course of the disease because there are almost as many initial symptoms as there are patients. The diagnosis can be made with certainty only when three characteristic signs are present: tremor, rigidity, and bradykinesia.

Tremor is usually the first to appear, is relatively slow (4 to 6 Hz), is present when the limb is supported or suspended (arm resting in lap or hanging by the side), and is abolished by complete relaxation (such as during sleep), or by voluntary movement of the limb (Nutt, 1997). The tremor generally begins in one hand, to-and-fro flexion movement of the wrist, hand, thumb, and fingers that is most apparent when patient sits comfortably. The cupped hand's appearance of shaking pills gave rise to the name "pill-rolling" tremor (Friedman, 1994). Then from one hand, the tremor spreads to the ipsilateral foot, subsequently to the contralateral limbs, and perhaps to the tongue and jaw. In addition to the resting tremor, many patients have a faster 6 to 9 Hz postural tremor (Nutt, 1997). It is important to distinguish the Parkinson's resting tremor, which is frequently asymmetrical, from the essential tremor, which is symmetrical, and commonly affects upper extremities, head and voice, but only rarely the legs. The handwriting is large and irregular (tremorous), rather than small (micrographia) as in parkinsonism.

Rigidity, defined as an increase in resistance to passive movement, is a common clinical feature that accounts for the flexed posture of many patients. The most disabling feature is bradykinesia, a slowness of voluntary movement associated with a reduction in coordinated automatic movements, such as the swinging of both arms when walking. Other findings can include a masklike facies with widened palpebral fissures and infrequent blinking. There may be blepharoclonus (fluttering of the closed eyelids), blepharospasm (involuntary closure of the eyelids), and drooling of saliva from the mouth. Patients have difficulty rising from bed or an easy chair and tend to assume a flexed posture when erect.

Many patients with PD have difficulty turning over in bed. This difficulty in turning when lying flat is the result of inability to execute the sequence of axial movements required to achieve the task. This disability becomes more prominent with longer disease duration (Steiger et al, 1996). Walking is often difficult to initiate, and patients may have to lean forward increasingly until they can advance. The tension reflexes are unaltered, and the plantar responses are flexor. Repetitive tapping over the glabella produces a sustained blink response (Myerson's sign), in contrast to the response of normal subjects. Other findings include psychomotor retardation, fatigue, sleep disorder, and unilateral findings. This presentation may lead to the misdiagnosis of depression or stroke.

Fifty percent of tremor patients do not have PD, and a broader differential diagnosis needs to be considered. The history should focus on the development of neurologic symptoms, depression, other concurrent medical illnesses (eg, hypothyroidism), medications, injuries (eg, falls), and occupational hazards. Drug-induced disease should be ruled out by the elimination of offending drugs such as neuroleptics, antiemetics (eg, metoclopramide), and antihypertensives (eg, reserpine, methyldopa). The physical exam should include a thorough mental status and neurologic exam. Typical physical signs: the tremor usually at rest, accompanied by "pill rolling" movement of the thumb and finger. Passive movement of the wrist or elbow may reveal cogwheel rigidity.

The gait features *marche a petit pas* (characterized by short steps with a tendency to accelerate), shuffling, lack of arm swing, and the turning of the body *en bloc*. Speech is often soft and monotonal, and it may be inaudible. Autonomic insufficiency may result in constipation, impotence, and orthostatic hypotension.

Mental changes such as dementia occur in about 15% to 20% of people with PD, and in 40% of patients older than 70 years (Kaufman, 1995; Aarsland et al, 1996). The so-called subcortical dementia of PD is distinguished from the cortical dementia of Alzheimer's disease. In cortical dementias, cognitive deficits are characterized by impairments in language and memory, agnosia and apraxia. In subcortical dementias, cognitive deficits are characterized by a general slowness of the thought process and impaired manipulation of acquired knowledge (deficits in abstracting abilities, retrieval, and neurospatial functions) (Starkstein et al, 1996; Kuzis et al, 1997).

Depression affects almost 50% of PD patients, and psychosis is present in at least 10%. Visual hallucinations, delusions, and chronic confusion are the most common psychotic features. This psychosis is most often attributable to a combination of dementia, antiparkinsonian medications, and the toxic–metabolic encephalopathy from other illnesses (eg, pneumonia).

DIAGNOSTIC STUDIES

Early detection of PD is useful from the viewpoint of addressing patients about their future. The recent claims that a medication (deprenyl) may slow the progression of the underlying pathology provides a new justification for attempting to make a diagnosis as soon as possible, perhaps even while the patient is still clinically normal. The majority of the tests and possible early markers for idiopathic PD are still under research. The clinical diagnosis rests on the history and physical exam, finding the cardinal features of tremor at rest, postural and balance dysfunction, akinesia, bradykinesia, rigidity, and gait abnormalities.

Brain Imaging

In single photon emission computed tomographic imaging (SPECT), radioactive iodine (^{123}I Beta-CIT) is used to label dopamine transporters and is therefore a marker of the neurons that degenerate in PD. SPECT with ^{123}I Beta-CIT showed that the radioactivity in striatal regions in healthy subjects increased during a 2-day imaging study, whereas that in parkinsonian patients peaked earlier at lower levels than in healthy subjects. Kinetic analysis of the radioactivity in plasma and the brain suggested that this decrease was the result of an approximately 65% loss of target sites in patients versus healthy subjects; greater losses occurred in the putamen than in the caudate. These preliminary results suggests that ^{123}I Beta-CIT is a marker for the loss of striatal dopamine terminals in patients with PD and may be useful for early diagnosis of the disorder, monitoring the progression of the disease, and distinguishing the idiopathic disorder from other parkinsonian syndromes with more widespread pathology (Innis et al, 1993).

PET scanning (PET with fluorodopa) reveals a reduction in striatal uptake in idiopathic parkinsonism and in both humans and cynomolgus monkeys with the clinical features of parkinsonism induced by MPTP. More relevant to the current issue, PET with fluorodopa also displays a decrease in uptake, although less severe in cynomolgus monkeys and humans exposed to MPTP in doses insufficient to result in any parkinsonism deficits, and may detect subclinical impairment of nigrostriatal integrity before the expression of clinical features (Calne & Snow, 1992).

Magnetic Resonance Imaging

Magnetic resonance imaging with high field strength allows localization of certain regions of the brain that have a high concentration of iron. Initial reports indicate that in idiopathic parkinsonism, the image of the substantia nigra is blurred, reflecting an increased accumulation of iron (Calne & Snow, 1992).

Blood Analysis

Parker et al reported a reduction of mitochondrial complex I (NADH ubiquerone oxidoreductase) in the platelets of patients with idiopathic parkinsonism. Others have reported reduced S-oxidation capacity in patients with idiopathic parkinsonism. There is also an increase in the ratio of cysteine to sulfate, and this may impair the body's ability to metabolize environmental toxins.

MAO-B in platelets deaminates endogenous dopamine. It may also activate environmental protoxins. The oxidation of dopamine may produce increased free radicals, which in turn may damage dopaminergic neurons. Researchers have found a highly significant increase in the generation of oxygen free radicals (in leukocytes) in idiopathic parkinsonism. Malondialdehyde is a product of tissue injury by lipid peroxidation of membrane phospholipids, and levels are elevated in the serum of patients with idiopathic PD (Calne & Snow, 1992).

Physiologic Testing

Long latency stretch reflexes, increased latency of the visual evoked potential, and a deficit in olfactory discrimination have been found in patients with PD. Lewy bodies are not limited to the substantia nigra in PD; they can be found in sympathetic ganglia and in the mesenteric plexi of the whole gastrointestinal tract, particularly the lower esophagus. This may lead to a possible diagnostic evaluation for idiopathic parkinsonism through biopsy of a more accessible location and may be the subject of further exploration (Calne & Snow, 1992).

DIFFERENTIAL DIAGNOSIS

Multiple neurologic and psychiatric disorders, some associated with exposure to medications or toxins as well as other clinical conditions, can mimic and share similar features with idiopathic PD. Table 55-1 lists the most commonly prescribed medications that can cause secondary parkinsonism. Table 55-2 summarizes

TABLE 55-1	Drug-Induced Parkinsonism

All anti-psychotics (neuroleptics) except clozapine
    Phenothiazines (Compazine, Mellaril, Phenergan, Prolixin, Stelazine, Thorazine)
    Butyrophenones (Haldol, fentanyl)
    Thioxanthines (Navane)

Antiemetics
    Metoclopramide (Reglan)
    Droperidol

Lithium
Antihypertensives
    Reserpine
    Methyldopa (Aldomet)
    Some calcium channel blockers (available in Europe and Latin America: flunarizine and annarize)

Antidepressant
    Amoxapine

other causes of secondary parkinsonism and lists the neurologic system degenerations that may have parkinsonism as a major component of the clinical picture. It is important to differentiate between the various parkinsonian syndromes because there is prognostic significance. For instance, idiopathic PD responds to levodopa, but in other forms of parkinsonism levodopa is less beneficial and may produce major side effects (Nutt, 1997).

TREATMENT, EXPECTED OUTCOMES, AND COMPREHENSIVE MANAGEMENT

Nutrition

Although in general there is no diet or food that is known unequivocally to have a beneficial effect on the symptoms of PD, patients should eat as normally as possible, including a well-balanced diet with fruits, vegetables, cereal, high amounts of fiber, and adequate protein. Because patients with PD tend to develop constipation, liberal water intake (six to eight glasses per day) and a diet rich in high-fiber foods are well-known practices that can be more palatable and effective than regular laxative use (Duvoisin, 1991).

For many years, providers had prescribed restrictions on protein for patients with PD. Because large neutral amino acids and levodopa share the same transport mechanism across the blood–brain barrier, there can be a decreased supply of levodopa crossing from the blood if the carrier system is saturated by a large protein load. However, a low-protein diet must be used with caution, especially in the elderly, because it may lead to a negative nitrogen balance (Vilming, 1995). The development of sustained-release versions of the levodopa/carbidopa combination medication has also had an impact on the need for dietary protein modification.

There is no reason to prohibit the use of alcoholic beverages in normal amounts. Alcoholism seems to be rare in patients with PD. The reason is not known.

With regard to vitamins and minerals, the body requires these in minute amounts and there is nothing specific about the PD patient to indicate an increased susceptibility to vitamin deficiencies (Duvoisin, 1991). It is always a good idea, however, to encourage patients, especially elderly ones, to take a multiple vitamin each day. A growing body of literature suggests an association between vitamin E use (at doses above those found in the typical multivitamin tablet) and the retarding of aging as well as PD and Alzheimer's disease. A high intake of dietary vitamin E (maybe 2000 IU) may protect against the occurrence of PD, but these data are still under critical review (Derijk et al, 1997).

In summary, for PD patients the provider should:

- Lower protein intake to the minimum daily requirement (0.5 to 0.8 g/kg) to improve the response to levodopa
- Restrict vitamin B_6, alcohol, and caffeine intake
- Encourage the intake of high-biologic-value proteins at dinner to promote the absorption of levodopa during the day
- Encourage intake of foods rich in vitamins B_{12} and C
- Improve the patient's ability to eat by providing small meals of chopped or puréed foods as necessary; the rigidity of pharyngeal muscles may result in chewing or swallowing problems.
- Provide adequate calories to prevent weight loss and avoid constipation.

TABLE 55-2	Differential Diagnosis of Parkinson's Disease
Cause or Neurologic Disorder	**Features Differentiating from PD**
Encephalitis	History, pupillary and extraocular abnormalities, oculogyric crises, other neurologic signs
Head trauma	History of boxing, other neurologic signs, cerebellar and corticospinal signs
Toxins	History of carbon monoxide, carbon disulfide, cyanide, manganese, mercury, methanol, or MPTP exposure (neurotoxic meperidine analogue used by drug addicts)
Normal-pressure hydrocephalus	Urinary urgency, gait disorder, but with relatively intact arm swing. CT or MRI.
Essential senile tremor	Positive family history; present during maintenance of posture (postural tremor) and aggravated by stressful situations flexion/extension type; decreases tremor with ethanol; treatment: propranolol, primidone
Atherosclerotic parkinsonism	Akinetic rigid state without tremor; corticospinal signs. Dx: CT, MRI. PD "from waist down"
Striatonigral degeneration; Shy Drager syndrome and olivopontocerebellar atrophy	Autonomic dysfunction (particularly orthostatic hypotension), cerebellar ataxia, corticospinal tract signs
Progressive supranuclear palsy	Paresis of voluntary vertical gaze (particularly downward gaze). Pseudobulbar palsy; marked postural instability with relatively preserved locomotion.
Corticobasal ganglionic degeneration	Asymmetric in onset; aphasia and apraxia without memory dysfunction. Resting tremor does not occur; corticospinal tract signs and limb dystonia are common; gaze palsies.
Alzheimer's disease	Early and prominent dementia preceding motor abnormalities; aphasia, apraxia, agnosia; less depression associated
Creutzfelt-Jakob disease	Rapidly progressive dementia; myoclonus, ataxia, pyramidal signs, visual disturbance. Electroencephalogram is characteristic.
Rigid Huntington's disease	Family history of Huntington's disease
Depression	Abnormal effect without rigidity or resting tremors. Good response to antidepressant therapy.
Diffuse Lewy body disease	Cortical dementia, aphasia, apraxia; labile effect

Pharmacologic Treatment

The initial treatment of PD should be addressed at improving symptoms, slowing the progression of the illness, and avoiding long- and short-term complications. Without treatment, PD progresses over 5 to 10 years to a rigid, akinetic state in which patients are incapable of caring for themselves. The availability of effective pharmacologic treatment has altered the natural course of the disease, and the life expectancy is substantially increased.

The drugs currently available for symptomatic patients are levodopa, dopaminergic agonists, and anticholinergics (amantadine). The newer dopamine agonists and inhibitors of catechol-O-methyltransferase are under development. Selegiline, a MAO-B inhibitor with a possible neuroprotective effect, should also be considered as an initial option (Kulisevsky & Lopez-Villegas, 1997).

LEVODOPA

Levodopa is also known as L-Dopa; its trade names are Larodopa and Dopar and its chemical makeup is L-3,4-dihydroxy-phenylalanine. Although itself largely inert, its therapeutic as well as adverse effects result from its decarboxylation to dopamine. When administered orally, it is rapidly absorbed from the small bowel by an active transport for aromatic amino acid. The concentration of the drug in plasma usually peaks 0.5 to 2 hours after the oral dose. Administration with meals delays absorption and reduces peak plasma concentrations.

Entry of the drug into the central nervous system across the blood–brain barrier also is an active process mediated by a carrier aromatic amino acid. Once in the brain, levodopa is converted to dopamine by decarboxylation, primarily within the presynaptic terminals of dopaminergic neurons in the striatum. The dopamine produced is responsible for the therapeutic effectiveness of the medication in PD. If levodopa is administered alone, it is largely decarboxylated peripherally by enzymes in the intestinal mucosa that are rich in MAO; probably less than 1% of the unchanged drug could reach the central nervous system. The most commonly prescribed form of carbidopa/levodopa is available in 25/100-, 10/100-, and 25/250-mg strengths.

■ ■ ■ **CLINICAL PEARL**

Usually the starting dosage for carbidopa/levodopa is 25/100 mg three or four times per day, 1 hour before or 2 hours after meals to maximize absorption and transport across the blood–brain barrier. It is best given during the waking hours when the patient is expected to be physically active.

Levodopa therapy early in the course of the disease can have a dramatic effect, with improvement of tremor, rigidity, and bradykinesia. With long-term use of levodopa, this efficacy may be lost, and the patient's motor state can fluctuate dramatically with each dose of levodopa. Providing a continuous supply of dopamine by intravenous or intestinal infusion of levodopa, or by subcutaneous infusion of a dopamine agonist, can overcome this type of fluctuation by maintaining constant plasma levels (Fahn, 1992).

The "on–off" phenomenon is an important late complication of levodopa therapy. Abrupt but transient fluctuations in the clinical state occur commonly during the day, without warning or an obvious relation with the dosing schedule, resulting in alternating periods of marked akinesia (off period) and disabling dyskinesias (on period). The on–off phenomenon can be controlled in part by reducing dosing intervals, administering levodopa 1 hour before meals, and restricting dietary protein intake, or by treatment with dopamine agonists. The addition of selegiline (5 mg at breakfast and lunch) reduces the metabolic breakdown of dopamine and may be helpful (Aminoff, 1998).

When to start levodopa remains controversial, especially because of the concern that early introduction of levodopa might accelerate the death of nigrostriatal neurons because of the hypothetical increase in dopamine-mediated neurotoxicity secondary to the production of free radicals during dopamine metabolism. Some providers argue that levodopa therapy should be started as soon as is warranted by the patient's clinical state rather than postponed out of concern for this theoretical possibility (Aminoff, 1998).

In addition to motor fluctuations and nausea, several other adverse effects may be observed with levodopa therapy—for example, hallucinations and confusion, especially in the elderly and in those with pre-existing cognitive dysfunction. Antipsychotic medications such as phenothiazines are effective for this levodopa-induced psychosis but cause marked worsening of parkinsonism symptoms. Lately, clozapine has been used with good response.

Orthostatic hypotension is another adverse effect associated with the use of levodopa. This is thought to be the result of the peripheral decarboxylation of the drug and the release of dopamine into the peripheral circulation and the subsequent stimulation of the vascular dopamine receptors. The action of dopamine at alpha- and beta-adrenergic receptors may produce cardiac arrhythmias. The use of MAO inhibitors such as pargyline is contraindicated in combination with levodopa therapy because of the incidence of hypertensive crisis and hyperpyrexia. Nonspecific MAO inhibitors must be discontinued 14 days before starting treatment with levodopa (this contraindication does not include the MAO-B subtype-specific inhibitor selegiline, which can be administered safely with levodopa). Acute withdrawal of levodopa or other dopaminergic medications may precipitate neuroleptic malignant syndrome, which is commonly observed after treatment with dopamine antagonists.

DOPAMINE AGONISTS

Two dopamine agonists, ergot derivatives, are available in the United States. Bromocriptine (Parlodel) is a strong agonist of the D_2 class of dopamine receptors and a partial antagonist of D_1 receptors. Pergolide (Permax) is an agonist at both D_1 and D_2 receptors. Both are well absorbed orally and have a plasma half-life in the range of 3 to 7 hours. Unlike carbidopa/levodopa, which needs to be converted to dopamine, the agonists work directly on the dopamine receptors, do not need conversion, and subsequently do not generate potentially toxic byproducts. Agonists may, however, cause orthostatic hypotension, confusion, or hallucinations. Bromocriptine and pergolide share some properties with ergot compounds, including the ability to induce pleuropulmonary and retroperitoneal fibrosis, erythromyalgias, and digital vasospasm (Standaert & Young, 1996).

In current practice, the most common use of dopamine agonists is their early introduction in conjunction with low-dose carbidopa/levodopa therapy (25/100 mg three times daily). This combination yields sustained benefit and a lower incidence of late complications.

Pramipexole (Mirapex) and ropinirole (Requip) are newer dopamine agonists. They differ from bromocriptine and pergolide in that they are not ergot derivatives, and in addition to binding to D_2-like receptors they also bind to D_3 receptors (*Medical Letter*, 1997).

Recently, a study reported the efficacy of short-term monotherapy with a new dopamine agonist, pramipexole, that could be useful in patients with early PD who are not receiving levodopa (Kieburtz et al, 1997). This drug has good gastrointestinal absorption, with peak serum concentrations occurring in 2 hours in a fasting patient and about 3 hours when taken with food. Excretion is via a renal route. The drug is excreted in the urine unchanged, with a half-life of 8 to 12 hours. The initial dosage is 0.125 mg three times daily; this dose can be doubled at weekly intervals to 0.75 mg three times daily in the fourth week. Subsequently, it can be increased by 0.75 mg/day each week to a maximum of 4.5 mg/day. Side effects are similar to those found in other medications of this class; hallucinations may be more common, ranging from 10% in patients with early disease to 21% in those with advanced disease (*Medical Letter*, 1997).

Ropinirole also has rapid oral absorption, with peak concentrations in 1 to 2 hours. However, it is metabolized in the liver to inactive metabolites, which are excreted in the urine; the half-life is approximately 6 hours. The initial dosage is 0.25 mg three times a day, which may be increased by 0.25 mg per dose each week for the first 4 weeks, then by 0.5 mg per dose per week up to 3 mg three times a day, and then by 1 mg per dose each week to a maximum of 8 mg three times a day. Syncope, occasionally associated with bradycardia, has been observed in approximately 12% of patients with early disease; this was associated with an increase in dosage more than 4 weeks after the start of treatment (*Medical Letter*, 1997).

Drug interactions include dopamine antagonists such as antipsychotics or metoclopramide. Cimetidine, by interfering with renal tubular secretion, may affect serum concentrations of pramipexole. Ciprofloxacin, by interfering with hepatic metabolism, may increase the serum concentrations of ropinirole (*Medical Letter*, 1997).

MUSCARINIC RECEPTOR ANTAGONISTS

Anticholinergics are usually helpful with tremor, but the biologic basis for their therapeutic actions is not completely understood. Used in early PD, they sometimes postpone the need for carbodopa/levodopa by 1 or 2 years. The adverse effects of these drugs include sedation and mental confusion (frequently seen in the elderly); they may also produce constipation, urinary retention, and blurred vision and must be used with caution in patients with narrow-angle glaucoma. Examples are trihexyphenidyl (Artane), benztropine (Cogentin), and amantadine. The latter, an antiviral agent used for the prophylaxis and treatment for influenza A, also has antiparkinsonian actions. It acts by potentiating the release of endogenous dopamine. Although the effects of amantadine in PD are modest, it is used as initial therapy for mild PD. It may be helpful as an adjunct in patients taking levodopa who are having dose-related performance fluctuations. Usually the dosage is 100 mg twice daily; it is generally well tolerated. Dizziness, lethargy, and sleep disturbance, as well as nausea and vomiting, have been reported as side effects, but these adverse reactions are mild and reversible (Standaert & Young, 1996).

Neuroprotective Treatment

The isoenzyme MAO-B is the predominant form in the striatum and is responsible for most oxidative metabolism of dopamine in that area. Selective inhibitors of MAO-B such as selegiline (Eldepryl, Deprenyl) may reduce oxidative damage and thus slow disease progression, but the evidence for this is incomplete. Selegiline has a mild effect on symptoms and can be given in a standard dosage of 5 mg with breakfast and lunch. Acute toxic interactions may occur with meperidine, tricyclic drugs, or serotonin reuptake inhibitors, so selegiline is contraindicated in combination with those medications. Selegiline is

metabolized to amphetamine or methamphetamine, so some patients may experience anxiety and insomnia.

Tocopherol (vitamin E) is an important scavenger of free radicals. It may have some role in neuroprotective therapy but at higher doses than the ones usually found in supplemental vitamin preparations.

Table 55-3 lists some of the commonly used antiparkinsonian medications, as well as the estimated cost for these drugs. As can be seen, medications for the treatment of PD are quite costly, and in more advanced stages of the disease, when multiple drugs from different classes are combined, the monthly medication cost can exceed several hundred dollars.

Surgical Treatment

There has been a recent worldwide renaissance in neurosurgical treatment for PD based on substantial progress in the basic sciences. Pallidotomy and thalamotomy have evolved with the use of better neuroradiologic and electrophysiologic targeting. Posteroventral pallidotomy is considered a useful treatment for levodopa-induced dyskinesias and bradykinesia and has been demonstrated to improve rigidity, tremor, postural instability, and gait disturbance (Krauss et al, 1997).

Thalamotomy is an operation that has proven to be efficient for tremor. A lesion (destruction) placed in a nucleus of the thalamus has been found to reduce tremor significantly, but not the slowness of parkinsonism. The procedure may be associated with a 25% risk of several speech problems and mental side effects.

A new surgical approach to the treatment of essential and parkinsonian tremor is called deep brain stimulation of the VIM nucleus of the thalamus. A thin wire (the lead) is placed in the brain during a neurosurgical operation, and a frame is placed on the patient's head. An implantable pulse generator (pacemaker) is placed underneath the skin under the collarbone and connected to the lead. It was found that high-frequency stimulation (more than 100 pulses per second) can block neuronal activity and have the same effect as a destructive lesion, resulting

TABLE 55-3	Drugs Used in PD			
Generic Name	Strength	Form	Price/Tab/Cap	Note Brand Price/Tab
Trihexyphenidyl HCl	2 mg/5 mg	Tablets	$00.33 (HCFA 5 mg)	0.18 (2 mg)/0.29 (5 mg)
Procyclidine HCl	5 mg	Tablets	0.46	0.46
Biperiden HCl	2 mg	Tablets	0.18 (PTC)	0.28
Benztropine mesylate	0.5 mg/2 mg	Tablets	0.02 (0.5)/0.03 (2 mg)	0.18 (0.5 mg)/26 (2 mg)
Amantadine HCl	100 mg	Capsules	0.17 (HCFA)	0.87
Bromocriptine	2.5 mg/5 mg	Tab/Cap	$1.68 (2.5-mg tab)	
Pergolide	0.05–.25–1 mg	Tablets	0.51 (0.05 mg)/$1.06 (.25 mg)	
Levodopa	0.1g–0.25g–0.5g	Tab/Cap	0.23(1g)/0.36(0.25g)/0.63(0.5g) 0.28(0.1g)/0.49(0.25g)/0.75(0.5g)	
Carbidopa/ levodopa	10/100 mg or 25/50 mg	Tablets	0.63(10/100 mg) 0.91(25/250 mg)	
Carbidopa/ levodopa (CR)	25/100 mg or 50/200 mg	Tablets	0.73(25/100 mg) $1.53(50/200 mg)	
Selegiline	5 mg	Cap	$2.24	

in a dramatic reduction of tremor. Follow-up studies indicate that the effectiveness persists for many years (Koller, 1996).

There has been recent interest in dopaminergic reinnervation and increased dopaminergic output of the striatum. This has been seen only after transplantation of fetal cells that have the capacity to send out new processes and form such dopaminergic synaptic contacts. This method, however, carries immunologic and ethical problems (Diederich & Alesh, 1997). Transplantation of autologous adrenal medullary tissue has also been attempted for Parkinson's disease with mixed results; benefits seem most likely to occur in individuals younger than 50 years of age.

There are also other surgical options that continue to be studied such as injection into the fluid-filled space in the brain of pharmacologic agents that enhance the survival and growth of nerve cells (nerve growth factors). Researchers at the Karolinska Institute in Stockholm conducted a series of experiments in mice using a cloned version of a natural protein associated with nerve cell growth called glial cell line-derived neurotrophic factor (GDNF). They concluded that intracerebral GDNF administration exerts both protective and reparative effects on the nigrostriatal dopamine system, which may have implications for the development of new treatment strategies for Parkinson's disease (Beck et al, 1995).

Therapeutic Approach

Before drug therapy is initiated, it is important to educate the patient and the family or caregivers. The provider should reassure patients that they are not alone with this disease, that there is ongoing research to identify not only the cause but also better treatments, and finally that although the disorder is progressive, usually this progression is slow. There is an extreme variability of the disease, and drug response or lack thereof will also play a major role in the progression (Friedman, 1996). Because of these factors, changes in lifestyle have to be considered: dietary issues, rehabilitation, and exercise at home. Speech therapy and alterations in the home environment to make it safer are also important. The goal is always toward making patients active participants in their treatment, as well as providing good quality of life.

Nationwide, drug therapy alone costs nearly $6 billion dollars per year, and the cost of hospital care and other consequences associated with PD is estimated at $25 to $50 billion per year (Isaacson, 1996). Symptomatic treatment should be tailored to each patient. If there is only a slight disability, treatment may be started with amantadine alone or with a dopaminergic agonist. If the patient is less than 60 years old and there is a conspicuous tremor, consider anticholinergic agents. If there is greater disability, consider levodopa or the simultaneous use of levodopa and a dopaminergic agonist. In advancing disease, when after adjustment of medications there is no improvement, consider the neurosurgical approach.

Rehabilitation

PD patients tend to withdraw from their usual activities. They are somewhat disabled in nearly every aspect of their lives. Increased immobility leads to a sedentary and isolated lifestyle unless there is a conscious effort to intervene. Symptoms do not respond equally with medical treatment, and it is important

to introduce adjuvant therapies such as physiotherapy, occupational therapy, and speech therapy.

Preventive rehabilitation should start early in the course of the illness and requires a team effort, involving the patient, the family or caregivers, therapists, and primary care providers. Patient and family support groups (eg, the Parkinson's Disease Society) are important resources for helping to meet all the needs of neurologic rehabilitation (Auff et al, 1995). Physical therapy should be directed at helping patients deal with specific PD symptoms, such as stooped posture, the tendency to shuffle when walking, trouble getting out of a deep chair, or various other difficulties in carrying out ordinary tasks of daily life.

Gait and balance training emphasizes a safe gait and improved balance (Fig. 55-1). The patient should be taught to keep the head up, to counter the flexed posture consciously, and to lift the toes during the swing phase of the gait. It also may help to take longer steps and widen the base. The therapist often prescribes a home program of regular exercises to maintain or improve strength, range of motion, and flexibility (Basmajian & DeLuca, 1985).

Physical Therapy

When treating patients with PD, the physical therapist develops strategies to break the vicious cycle of physiologic changes, which if allowed to continue gradually decreases the patient's quality of life (Tappan, 1988; Jacobson, 1929; Kisner & Colby, Schultz & Little, 1959; Brummel-Smith, 1997). Greater benefit is derived if the treatment is begun as soon as a diagnosis is established.

REDUCING RIGIDITY (RELIEVING MUSCLE TENSION)
Massage
A combination of kneading, wringing (Mennel's petrissage), and deep stroking techniques stimulates sensory receptors, improves muscle nutrition, stretches the muscles, and prevents contractures and stagnation of body fluid.

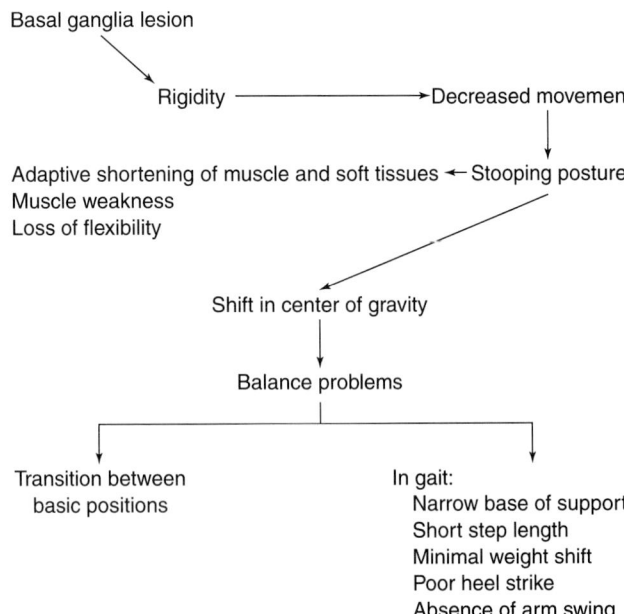

FIGURE 55-1 Physiological charges in Parkinson's disease.

Relaxation Techniques

- Active range of motion: The caregiver encourages the patient to move body parts in a direction counter to the posture that part tends to adopt and to perform exercises that promote activity of antigravity muscles. Resistance may be used in these exercises to strengthen these muscles, which keep the body in erect posture.
- Flexibility exercises for muscles that tend to shorten: A patient who is alert and aware may be taught to perform these exercises independently. In some cases, the caregiver may assist with or perform these stretches on the patient.
- Local and general conscious relaxation techniques: When patients can move the body part through full range of motion, they should be encouraged to move it several times, paying particular attention to the feel of the contracting and relaxing muscles. In a quiet surrounding, with comfortable clothing and position, patients can be taught to perform deep-breathing exercises in a relaxed manner. They are also taught to experience local or general voluntary muscle contraction and relaxation, as well as awareness of the state (rigidity or relaxation) of the body or body part. Biofeedback and the development of kinesthetic awareness (postural training) are helpful.

Patient Education

- Teach the patient what the correct posture should be.
- Reinforce education as you interact with the patient daily.
- Let patients know what they should be feeling in relaxed or contracted muscle.
- Use mirrors to let patients see how they look when properly aligned.
- Touch the muscle that needs to contract to elicit contraction of the muscle.

GAIT TRAINING

- Body alignment: use of mirrors
- Base of support: stepping on designated floor tiles
- Walking on parallel bars with abduction partition
- Heel strike: Emphasize picking up the swing foot and landing on the heel, pointing the toes upward.

WALKING AIDS/ADAPTIVE DEVICES

Patients may become dependent on assistive devices if the condition progresses. These devices, which are recommended to improve mobility, balance, and safety, may include:

- Gliding walker
- Raised chairs
- Raised toilet seat
- Handrails.

◼ ◼ ◼ ◻ CLINICAL PEARL

Canes should be avoided because of the posture of PD; protraction and internal rotation of the shoulder may place the tip of the cane between the legs, causing a fall. If a walker is necessary, it should have front wheels to avoid backward falls. The wheels should be retractable to avoid forward falls.

Attention to the disposition of furniture around the house helps prevent falls. There should be an adequate rail on stairways. Hand bars on the wall near the bathtub and toilet should be installed. The toilet seat can be raised with blocks an inch or two high, and a rubber bath mat in the tub should help reduce falls. A specially designed bath chair can be placed in the shower to ensure easier and safer bathing. Shag or throw rugs should be removed to prevent slips and falls. Modifications of clothing, such as zippers or adhesive cloth instead of buttons, should be considered for patients who have difficulty dressing.

A few more severely affected patients with PD may need more intensive physical therapy. In these patients, the use of rehabilitation services in an institution or daily home visits from a physical therapist may be necessary. The goal is to keep the patient as independent as possible for as long as possible.

Speech Therapy

Patients whose speech is difficult for others to understand may benefit from practicing singing and reading out loud. Short courses of speech therapy have shown great improvements in dysarthria scores, volume, and other measurements of speech efficiency. Intensive voice and respiration treatment, focusing on increased vocal fold adduction and respiration, is more effective than respiration treatment alone for improving vocal intensity and decreasing the impact of PD (Ramigs et al, 1995).

TEACHING AND SELF-CARE

Patients and families experiencing Parkinson's disease may have some additional time to prepare for some social and physical limitations. Patients should be encouraged to participate in care to the maximum of their ability. Professional counseling may be helpful for the patient facing increasing limitations.

Summary

The treatment of patients with PD requires an interdisciplinary approach. The primary care provider must work closely with neurology consultants to provide the patient with up-to-date interventions. Because of the systemic involvement of this disease and the medications used to treat it, the manifestations of the disease as well as the side effects of the drugs used must be monitored. Rehabilitative services are crucial in terms of providing additional interventions to maintain the patient's level of function. As the disease progresses, caregiver burnout becomes a serious problem, and the availability of adequate social and community supports becomes as important for the care of the patient as any medical intervention.

Because many patients with PD take multiple medications, both for PD and other comorbid conditions, the risk of potentially adverse drug interactions exists. The patient, family, primary care provider, and other ancillary members of the team must function in an organized and goal-directed way to keep the patient at the highest level of function possible.

COMMUNITY RESOURCES

- The American Parkinson's Disease Association, 1250 Hyalan Boulevard, Suite 4B, Staten Island, NY 10305-1946, 800-223-2732, 800-908-2732 (West Coast office), 718-981-8001, Fax: 718-981-4399, E-mail AP DA@ADMIN.CON2.COM

- The National Parkinson Foundation, Inc., 1501 N.W. 9th Ave./Bob Hope Road, Miami, FL 33136-1494; Parkinson Information Lines: 800-327-4545 (in the United States and Canada, except Florida and California), 800-433-7022 (in Florida), 305-547-6666 (in Miami), 818-981-2233 (in Los Angeles), http://www.parkinson.org/
- Parkinson's Disease Foundation, 650 West 168th Street, NY, NY 10032-9982, 800-457-6676, 212-923-4700.
- United Parkinson Foundation, 833 West Washington Boulevard, Chicago, IL 60607, 312-733-1893

Local divisions of these major organizations provide patient information, counseling, group discounts on medication purchases, and support groups for patients and families. Newsletters published by national and regional groups provide updates regarding therapy, conferences, and experimental treatment programs.

EDITOR'S NOTE:

COMPLEMENTARY APPROACHES

A general discussion of complementary approaches can be found in Chapter 3. The following, while not an exhaustive list, are some complementary approaches being used for this condition. Additional information on these approaches, including precautions, can be found in Appendices A and B. Providers need to assess for the use of complementary approaches as part of the patient's history, as they may impact conventional therapies, and patients may not volunteer this information unless specifically asked. Efficacy of many complementary approaches is not as well documented as that of conventional therapies. Providers need to read the literature before suggesting these complementary approaches.

- Complementary Modalities
  Massage therapy

REFERENCES

Aarsland D., Tandberg E., Larsen, J.P., Cummings, J.L. (1996). Frequency of dementia in Parkinson disease. *Archives of Neurology, 53*(6):538–542.

Aminoff, M.J. (1998). Parkinson's disease and other extrapyramidal disorders. In *Harrison's principles of internal medicine*, 14th ed., Vol. 2, pp. 2356–2359.

Auff, E., Ferth, E., & Schnieder, P. (1995). Parkinson's disease and neurological rehabilitation. *Wiener Mediunische Wochenscheift, 145*(R), 302–305.

Basmajian, J.V., & DeLuca, C.J. (1985). *Muscles alive: Their function revealed by electromyography*, 5th ed. Baltimore: Williams & Wilkins.

Beck, K.D., Valverde, J., Alexi, T. et al. (1995). Mesencephalic dopaminergic neurons protected by GDNF from axotomy-induced degeneration in the adult brain. *Nature 373* (6512):339–341.

Block, G., et al. (1997). Comparison of immediate-release and controlled-release carbidopa/levodopa in Parkinson's disease: A multicenter 5 year study. *European Neurology, 37*(1), 23–27.

Brummel-Smith, K. (1997). Rehabilitation. Geriatric medicine. Cassel, C. (ed.) 3d ed. New York: Springer-Verlag, pp. 223–224.

Calne, D.B., & Snow, B.J. (1992). Early markers of idiopathic parkinsonism. In C.W. Olanow & A.N. Lieberman (Eds.). *The scientific bases for the treatment of Parkinson's disease*, pp. 3–11. N.J.: Parthenon.

Cassel, C. (Ed.). (1997). *Geriatric medicine*, 3d ed. New York: Springer-Verlag.

Derijk, Mc., Breteler, MMB., Denbreeijen, J.H. et al. (1997). Dietary antioxidants and Parkinson's disease. The Rotterdam Study. *Archives of Neurology 54* (6):762–765.

Diederich, N.J., & Alesh, F. (1997). Neuro-surgical methods in treatment of Parkinson's disease. *Nervenarzt, 68*(6), 466–476.

Dirijk-McBreteler, M.M.B., Der Breeijer, J.H., Laerier, L.J., Grobbe, D.E., Vandermecke, F.G.A., & Hofman, A. (1997) Dietary antioxidants and Parkinson's disease. The Rotterdam Study. *Archives of Neurology, 54*(6), 762–765.

Duvoisin, R.C. (1991). Parkinson's disease: A guide for patient and family. 3rd ed. New York: Raven Press.

Eichhorn, T., & Oertel, W.H. (1994). Incidence, differential diagnosis, work capacity, mortality and cause of death in Parkinson's disease. *Verse Cherungs Reedeger, 46*(4), 122–128.

Fahn, S. (1992). Adverse effects of levodopa. In C.W. Olanow & A.N. Lieberman (Eds.). *The scientific basis for the treatment of Parkinson's disease*. N.J.: Parthenon.

Friedman, J.H. (1994). Parkinson's disease and other akinetic rigid syndromes. Current diagnosis in neurology. St. Louis: Mosby, pp. 185–188.

Friedman, J.H. (1996). Parkinson's disease in the elderly. In J.I. Sage & M.H. Mann (Eds.). *Practical neurology of the elderly*, pp. 625–663.

Golbe, L.I., DiIorio, G., Bonavita, V., et al. (1990). A large kindred with autosomal dominant Parkinson's disease. *Annals of Neurology 27*(3):276–282.

Groenewegen, H.J. (1997). Cortical-subcortical relationships and the limbic forebrain. In M.R. Tremble & J.L. Cummings (Eds.). *Contemporary behavioral neurology*, pp. 35–37. Newton, Mass.: Butterworth-Heinemann.

Harris, Z.L., Klomp, L.W., Gintlin, J.D. (1998). Aceruloplasminemia: An inherited neurodegenerative disease with impairment of iron homeostasis. *American Journal of Clinical Nutrition 67*(5 Suppl): 972S–977S.

Hutchinson, W.D., Levy, R., Dostrovsky, J.O., et al. Effects of apomorphine on globus pallidus neurons in parkinsonian patients. *Annals of Neurology 42*:767–775.

Innis, R.B., Suzyl, J.P., Scanley, B.E., et al. (1993) Single photon emission computed tomographic imaging demonstrates loss of striatal dopamine transporters in Parkinson's disease. *Proceedings of the National Academy of Sciences USA, 90*(24), 11965–11969.

Isaacson, O. (1996). On the causes and treatment of Parkinson's Disease. *Parkinson Report, 17,* 8–12.

Jacobson, E. (1929). *Progressive relaxation*. Chicago: University of Chicago Press.

Kaufman, D.M. (1995). *Clinical neurology for the psychiatrist*, pp. 419–429. Philadelphia: W.B. Saunders.

Kieburtz, K., Shoulson, I., Mcdermott. (1997). Safety and Efficacy of Pramipexole in early Parkinson's disease: A randomized dose ranging study. *Journal of the American Medical Association 278*(2), 125–130.

Kisner, C. & Colby, L. (1985). *Therapeutic Exercise: Foundations and techniques*, Philadelphia: F.A. Davis.

Koller, W.C. (1996). Deep brain stimulation of the thalamus for the treatment of tremor disorder. *Parkinson Report, 17*(1), 1–4.

Krauss, J.K., Jankovic, J., Lai, E.C., Retting, G.M., & Grossman, R.G. (1997). Postoventral medial pallidotomy in levodopa-unresponsive parkinsonism. *Archives of Neurology, 54,* 1026–1029.

Kulisevsky, J., & Lopez-Villegas, D. (1997). Initial treatment of Parkinson's disease. *Reresta de Neurologia, 25*(Suppl. 2), S163–169.

Kuzis, G., Sabe, L., Tiberti, C., Leiguarda, R. (1997). Cognitive functions in major depression and Parkinson Disease. *Archives of Neurology 54*(8) 982–986.

Langston, J.W. (1987). Etiology. In W.C. Koller (Ed.). *Handbook of Parkinson's disease,* pp. 297–308. New York: Marcel-Dekker.

Langston, J.W. (1992). Etiology of Parkinson's disease. In C.W. Olanow & A.N. Lieberman (Eds.). *The scientific basis for the treatment of Parkinson's disease*, pp. 33–58. N.J.: Parthenon.

Langston, J.W., Ballard, P., Te Trud, J.W., & Irwin, I. (1983). Chronic parkinsonism in humans is due to a product of meperidine-analog synthesis. *Science, 219*, 979–980.

Lanska, D.J. (1997) The geographic distibution of Parkinson's disease mortality in the United States. *Journal of the Neurological Sciences 150*(1):63–70.

Louis, E.D., Marder, N., Cote, L., Tang, M., & Majeux, R. (1997). Mortality from Parkinson's disease. *Archives of Neurology, 54*(3), 260–264.

The Medical Letter (November 21, 1997). Pramipexole and ropinirole for Parkinson's disease. Vol. 39(1014), pp. 109–110.

Nutt, J.G. (1997). Abnormalities of posture and movement. Geriatric medicine. Cassell, C. (Ed.) 3d Ed., pp. 939–947. New York: Springer-Verlag.

Olney, R.K., & Aminoff, M.J. (1998). Weakness, abnormal movements, and imbalance. In *Harrison's principles of internal medicine*, 14th ed., Vol. 1, pp. 112–113. New York: McGraw-Hill.

Parker Jr, W.D., Boyson, J.J., & Parks, J.K. (1989). Abnormalities of the electron transport chain in idiopathic Parkinson's disease. *Annals of Neurology 26*, pp. 719–723.

Polymeropoulos, M.H., Higgins, J.J., Gulbe, L.I., et al. (1996). Mapping of a gene for PD to chromosome 4q21-q23. *Science 274* (5290), pp. 1197–1199.

Ramig, L.O., Countryman, S., Thompson, L.L., & Horii, Y. (1995). Comparison of two forms of intensive speech treatment for Parkinson's disease. *Journal of Speech and Hearing Research, 39*(6), 1232–1251.

Sanchez-Ramos, J.R., Ortoll, R., Paulson, G.W. (1996) Visual hallucinations associated with Parkinson disease. *Archives of Neurology 53*(12):1265–1268.

Schultz, J.H., & Little, W. (1959). *Autogenic training: A psychophysiological approach in psychotherapy.* New York: Grune & Stratton.

Standaert, D.G., & Young, A.B. (1996). Treatment of central nervous system, degenerative disorders. Goodman & Gilman's The pharmacological basis of therapeutics, 9th ed. New York: McGraw-Hill. pp. 509–512.

Starkstein, S., et al. (1996). Neuropsychological and psychiatric differences between Alzheimer's disease and Parkinson's disease with dementia. *Journal of Neurology & Neurosurgical Psychiatry, 61*, 381–387.

Steiger, M.J., Thompson, P.D., & Marsden, C.D. (1996). Disordered axial movement in Parkinson's disease. *Journal of Neurology & Neurosurgical Psychiatry, 61*, 645–648.

Taipton, K.F., McCrodden, J.M., & Sullivan, J.P. (1993). Metabolic aspects of the behavior of MPTP and some analogues. In H. Narabayashi, T. Nagatsu, N. Yanagisawa, & Y. Mezuro (Eds.). *Advances in neurology*, Vol. 60, pp. 186–193. New York: Raven Press.

Tappan, F.M. (1988). *Healing massage techniques: Holistic, classic, and emerging methods*, 2d ed. Norwalk, Conn.: Appleton & Lange.

Vilming, S.T. (1995). Diet therapy in Parkinson's disease. *Tiedssurft for Der Noiske Laleporenirg (Norway), 115*(10), 1244–1247.

Ward, C.D., Duvoisin, R.C., Ince, S.E, Nutt, J.D., Eldridge, R., & Calne, D. (1983). Parkinson's disease in 65 pairs of twins and in a set of quadruplets. *Neurology, 33*, 815–824.

Peripheral Neuropathy

Henry Cohen, MS, PharmD, Dalia Abdelmacksoud, PharmD, and Joanne V. Hickey, PhD, RN, CS,
ACNP, CNRN, FAAN

Peripheral neuropathy (PN) is a serious complication that occurs in a myriad of clinical conditions treated by the primary care provider. PN is defined as deranged function and structure of peripheral motor, sensory, and autonomic neurons, involving either the entire neuron or selected levels. The disorders of the peripheral nervous system are clinically diverse and depend on the severity of the pathologic process, the rate of progression, the population of neurons or Schwann cells affected, the level within the neurons affected, and the subcellular pathologic events involved (Ziegler, 1996; Brew, 1994).

PN may manifest a wide variety of signs and symptoms, including burning sensations, paresthesias and dysesthesias, and a "pins and needles" sensation. Underlying disease states that may cause PN include diabetes mellitus (DM; Llewelyn, 1995; Ziegler, 1996), HIV infection, uremia, neoplasms, and chronic alcohol abuse. Nutritional deficits in thiamine, pyridoxine, or cyanocobalamin may cause PN (Kelly, 1994). Drugs have also been implicated in causing PN and are listed in Table 56-1. Environmental toxins, including heavy metals such as lead and mercury, have also been implicated.

ANATOMY, PHYSIOLOGY AND PATHOLOGY

Each peripheral nerve has a well-defined anatomic course, supplies a dermatome (although there is some overlap), and innervates specific muscles. The proximity of some nerves to bony structures makes them particularly vulnerable to compression or entrapment injury. Although there are several etiologies for PN, the pathologic processes can generally be divided into four categories: wallerian degeneration, axonal degeneration, neuropathy, and segmental demyelination (Bosch & Mitsumoto, 1991).

An injury that causes interruption of the axon and myelin, as in a transection of a nerve, results in *wallerian degeneration* distal to the injury site. In this distal segment, the myelin and axon degenerate, resulting in a loss of electrical conduction. Proximal to the transection, regrowth may occur, but it is slow and often incomplete, and the recovery of the nerve is limited. *Axonal degeneration* refers to distal axonal breakdown resembling wallerian degeneration, but it is the result of metabolic derangement within neurons (eg, DM, toxins). This results in denervation of the muscle and muscle atrophy.

Neuropathy refers to primary loss or destruction of nerve cell bodies, along with degeneration of their entire peripheral and central processes. Inherited conditions such as spinal muscular atrophies (lower motor neurons) and hereditary sensory neuropathies (primary sensory neurons) may be affected. Tox-

ins and organic compounds such as mercury and pyridoxine overdose can result in primary neuronal degeneration (Bosch & Mitsumoto, 1991). *Segmental demyelination* (eg, Guillaine Barré syndrome) is an injury of the myelin sheath or the myelin-producing Schwann cells, resulting in breakdown of myelin with relative sparing of axons so that no atrophy occurs unless nerve fibers are affected, as can occur in severe cases.

There are two broad classes of peripheral nerve injury. Mononeuropathies are focal lesions of peripheral nerves (eg, traumatic or ischemic). Polyneuropathies are bilateral symmetric disturbances of function (eg, toxic, hereditary, inflammatory, or metabolic). Multifocal isolated lesions are termed "mononeuropathy multiplex" and most commonly affect peroneal, median, and ulnar nerves.

Most PNs are associated with a loss of function, either sensory, motor, or both, and are typically not painful. Pain is characteristic of diabetic, alcoholic, and nutritional deficiency neuropathies.

Diabetic PN

The exact etiology and pathogenesis of diabetic PN has not been well elucidated and may be multifactorial. Chronic hyperglycemia has been associated with diminished nerve conduction velocity and the clinical presentation of PN. Glucose is usually metabolized by hexokinase to glucose-6-phosphate. In the presence of constant hyperglycemia, saturation of the hexokinase enzymatic pathway occurs, and excess glucose is converted to sorbitol by the polyol pathway.

A likely mechanism for the pathogenesis of human diabetic neuropathy is increased polyol pathway activity secondary to diabetic hyperglycemia. During hyperglycemia, however, the cellular level of glucose increases in tissues such as the peripheral nerve, where glucose entry is independent of insulin.

In peripheral nerve tissues, the excess glucose is metabolized predominantly by aldose reductase. Increased flux of glucose through the polyol pathway may be associated with myoinositol depletion, decreased sodium-potassium ATPase activity, decreased nitric oxide synthetase, tissue hypoxia, and subsequent structural lesions.

Aldose reductase inhibitors block the flux of glucose through the pathway and prevent these abnormalities. Aldose reductase inhibitors are under clinical investigation for the treatment and prophylaxis of diabetic PN.

HIV PN

PNs are a common complication of HIV disease, occurring at all stages of infection. Acute PN in HIV disease may be an early feature of the infection, especially around the time of serocon-

TABLE 56-1	Categories and Etiologies of Peripheral Neuropathies
Metabolic/Nutritional	Diabetes mellitus, hypothyroidism, acromegaly, uremia, liver disease, vitamin B_{12} deficiency
Drug-Induced	*Antineoplastics:* cisplatin, vincristine *Antimicrobials:* chloroquine, dapsone, isoniazid, metronidazole, nitrofurantoin *Cardiovascular:* amiodarone, hydralazine *Central nervous system:* alcohol, lithium, phenytoin *Other:* cimetidine, colchicine, disulfiram, gold, pyridoxine
Industrial/Environmental Toxins	*Organic and industrial compounds:* acrylamide, carbon disulfide, dimethylamino-proprionitrile, ethylene oxide, hexacarbons, organophosphates, thallium, trichlorethylene, vacor *Heavy metals:* arsenic, lead, mercury, gold, platinum
Connective Tissue Processes/Vasculitis	Polyarteritis nodosa, rheumatoid arthritis, systemic lupus erythematosus, scleroderma, ischemic neuropathies, systemic necrotizing vasculitis, giant cell arteritis, Wegener's granulomatosis
Infections/Infectious Processes	Leprosy, HIV; diphtheria, Epstein-Barr virus, rabies, sarcoidosis
Inflammatory Processes	Acute idiopathic polyneuropathy (Guillain-Barré syndrome), chronic inflammatory demyelinating polyneuropathy
Neoplasms	Compression and infiltration by tumor, multiple myeloma, nonhereditary amyloidosis
Trauma/Compression	Severance contusion, stretching, compression, crushing, ischemia, electrical, thermal, and radiation injuries and drug injection, stretch injuries from orthopedic traction, compression from prolonged pressure, herniated discs, osteophytes, or fractures
Entrapment Syndromes	*Lower extremities:* sciatic and peroneal entrapment syndromes *Upper extremities:* carpal tunnel syndrome, ulnar entrapment syndrome, radial nerve entrapment, thoracic outlet syndrome
Hereditary	Hereditary motor and sensory neuropathies, hereditary sensory and autonomic neuropathies types I–IV, Friedreich's ataxia, porphyria, hereditary amyloidosis

version (Brew, 1993). HIV-related PN may manifest in a variety of forms: a predominantly sensory neuropathy, an autonomic neuropathy, a mononeuritis multiplex, or an inflammatory demyelinating polyneuropathy. One of the distinguishing features of the neuropathies that occur in HIV patients is the relative specificity of the individual neuropathic syndromes with the stages of infection.

Neuropathies may be the result of immunopathogenic events, such as the inflammatory demyelinating polyneuropathies. During the early stages of infection, the immune system is relatively competent but is stimulated and has altered responsiveness. A vasculitic syndrome occurs mainly during the early symptomatic phase of infection and has been postulated to be the result of circulating immune complexes of HIV-1 antibody and antigen that are deposited in vessel walls.

Distal symmetric polyneuropathy occurs mainly in the late phase of HIV infection (AIDS), when there is severe immunosuppression. At this stage the mechanisms that have been proposed include productive infection of neural tissue with HIV-1 or cytomegalovirus or toxic or metabolic abnormalities as a result of advanced systemic disease.

Another possible mechanism for HIV PN is a dysregulation of macrophages within the peripheral nerve, resulting in excessive production of tumor necrosis factor and other interleukins. Additional factors that may damage the peripheral nerves in

HIV patients include gp-120 (the coat protein of HIV virus) or a nutritional deficiency (eg, vitamin B_{12}).

The most common neuropathy is a predominantly sensory neuropathy presenting distally and symmetrically with little functional weakness. Predominantly sensory neuropathies are a common feature of advanced HIV disease, with an estimated prevalence of 45% in AIDS patients.

Toxin-Induced PN

Exposure to environmental, biologic, and experimental toxins, metals, and drugs can produce neurologic manifestations resulting from impaired function of the central and peripheral nervous systems. Metals that are associated with PN include mercury, lithium, gold, and platinum. Sources of human exposure to neurotoxins include occupational exposure, environmental contamination, drug therapy, and food poisoning. *Botulinum* toxin, a potent neurotoxin, causes paralysis when ingested in contaminated foods.

Neoplasm PN

Neoplasm PN is most common in carcinoma of the lung, but it is also associated with carcinoma of the stomach, colon, rectum, and other organs. It is difficult to ascertain the prevalence of PN in malignancy, because it depends on the pathologic type and site of the tumor, the stage and duration of the illness, the techniques for diagnosis used, and the criteria for diagnosis. Pathogenic mechanisms for neoplasm-associated PN include direct infiltration of roots and nerves by tumor cells, toxic factors released by the tumor, alterations in protein and fat metabolism as a result of the tumor, nutritional deficiencies, vascular causes, viral infections, and immunologic disturbances.

Alcoholic PN

Despite the observation that chronic excessive alcohol ingestion is associated with peripheral nerve disease, there is still controversy about whether the neuropathy is the result of a direct toxic effect of alcohol, malnutrition, or both. Human studies have not been able to differentiate a direct toxic action of alcohol on the peripheral nervous system from the effects of poor nutrition. The neuropathy observed may be the result of a deficiency in vitamin B_1, niacin, vitamin B_6, vitamin B_{12}, or vitamin E.

Neuropathy Associated With Renal Failure

PN became clearly established as a complication of chronic renal failure in the early 1960s. In progressive chronic renal failure, slowing of nerve conduction tends to occur when creatinine clearance is approximately 10% of normal. Nerve conduction continues to worsen as renal function deteriorates. The diminished nerve conduction occurs proximally and distally to the same degree. Uniform generalized slowing of conduction tends to occur subclinically and does not predict the appearance of clinical signs and symptoms of neuropathy.

The subclinical diminished nerve conduction in chronic renal failure is functional and is not accompanied by evident renal morphologic change; thus, it is readily reversible by restoration of normal renal function. Chronic dialysis may prevent, stabilize, or improve uremic neuropathy, but dialysis has relatively little effect on nerve conduction velocity. Other observations suggest widespread axonal dysfunction in chronic renal failure (Aminoff et al, 1996).

EPIDEMIOLOGY

An accurate accounting of the epidemiology of PN is unknown because, in most instances, the neuropathy is part of a clinical presentation or a complication associated with a long-term, chronic condition (eg, DM, alcoholism, or exposure to toxins). DM is the most common human metabolic disease (5 million cases in the United States), and diabetic neuropathy is the most common complication of DM.

Forty percent of patients with insulin-dependent DM for greater than 20 years and 5% to 10% of patients with noninsulin-dependent DM develop neuropathies. The incidence is declining, perhaps as a result of improved glycemic control (Greene, 1994).

Neuropathies associated with toxic substances used in industries such as farming or the oil industry are seen in such workers

TABLE 56-2	Sensory, Motor, Reflex, or Autonomic/Trophic Disturbances

- *Sensory:* Decreased or loss of light touch and pin prick sensation along the involved dermatome; tingling, numbness, and dyesthesias are common. Loss of appreciating vibration and position are also seen. Pain is a feature of some neuropathies, especially if small fibers within the nerves are affected. Polyneuropathies with pain include those related to diabetes, alcoholism, porphyria, rheumatoid arthritis, and AIDS. Pain is also common with many entrapment syndromes.

- *Motor:* Involvement of the motor fibers of a purely motor nerve or a mixed nerve results in lower motor neuron weakness, paresis, or paralysis of the muscles innervated by the involved peripheral nerve. Atrophy of the specific muscle groups and related deformities may follow. Fasciculations may also be noted.

- *Reflexes:* Deep tendon reflexes of the involved muscle or muscle groups are decreased or absent.

- *Autonomic/Trophic:* Skin in the affected area may become dry, thin, scaly, inelastic, and cold and may cease to sweat. The nails may become curved and brittle; nail and hair growth becomes stunted. Orthostatic hypotension is a less common symptom.

(Table 56-2). The incidence of toxin-related neuropathies is not known, partly because of the long delay (often more than 20 years) between exposure and development of symptoms.

Thirty percent of all cases of PN are attributed to alcoholic neuropathy. A close association between alcoholic neuropathy and nutritional deficiency has also been noted (Bosch & Mitsumoto, 1991).

Entrapment syndromes are more common in persons who use their hands in repetitive motions, such as musicians, hairdressers, and computer users. The risk of developing carpal tunnel syndrome is more than doubled in persons with DM.

Although a few conditions produce mononeuropathy and mononeuropathy multiplex, there are many etiologies of polyneuropathy. Diagnosis often depends on obtaining a thorough history (eg, alcohol abuse or occupational exposures and risk factors), identifying systemic conditions associated with neuropathies (eg, DM, systemic lupus erythematosus), and conducting a careful physical and neurological exam.

DIAGNOSTIC CRITERIA

Disorders of one or more peripheral nerves cause various signs and symptoms that correspond to the anatomic distribution and normal function of the peripheral nerve. Some peripheral nerves are purely motor, some are purely sensory, and others are mixed. Diagnostic accuracy depends on a thorough knowledge of specific sensory dermatomes, muscle innervations, reflexes, and autonomic function related to a particular nerve. The signs and symptoms of a peripheral nerve disorder may include sensory, motor, reflex, or autonomic/trophic disturbances (Table 56-3) (Brazis et al, 1990; Aminoff et al, 1996):

Classification of Neuropathies

PNs are classified based on the number of peripheral nerves involved and the pattern of involvement (eg, symptoms may be confined to one side or both). The classification includes:

TABLE 56-3 Commonly Used Therapeutic Agents in the Treatment of Peripheral Neuropathy

Drug	Dosage	Established Efficacy	Adverse Drug Reactions	Generic Availability	Cost per Month to Pharmacist
ANTIDEPRESSANTS					
Amitriptyline	10–25 mg/day PO initially, then titrate to a max of 150 mg/day	+ + +	Cardiac dysrhythmias, orthostatic hypotension, dry mouth, constipation, blurred vision, urinary retention, sedation, seizures	Yes	50 mg daily Elavil: $21.50 Generic (CMC-Cons): $0.97
Clomipramine	10–25 mg/day PO initially, then titrate to a max of 250 mg/day	+ + +	Same as amitriptyline	Yes	50 mg daily Anafranil: $35.78 Generic (Taro): $27.86
Desipramine	10–25 mg/day PO initially, then titrate to a max of 300 mg	+ +	Same as amitriptyline except less antimuscarinic side effects and less sedation	Yes	50 mg daily Norpramin: $36.61 Generic (Major): $14.25
Imipramine	10–25 mg/day PO initially, then titrate to a max of 200 mg/day	+ + +	Same as amitriptyline	Yes	75 mg daily Tofranil PM: $34.24
Paroxetine	40 mg/day	+	Visual disturbances, headache, fatigue, nausea, diarrhea, vomiting, sexual dysfunction	No	40 mg daily Paxil: $67.35
CAPSAICIN CREAM	0.075% applied 3 or 4 times daily	+ + +	Transient burning, sneezing, coughing, irritation, rash, erythema, dry skin, increased pain	No	Zostrix 60 g: $17.68
1B ANTIARRHYTHMICS					
Lidocaine	5 mg/kg IV infusion over 30 min	+	Lightheadedness, confusion, dizziness, drowsiness, tinnitus, hallucinations, seizures, hypotension, bradycardia, cardiovascular collapse	Yes	70 Kg patient dose = 350 mg 0.8% (8 mg/mL) 250 mL: $10.83
Mexiletine	450–600 mg PO daily	+ +	Nausea, headache, diarrhea, vomiting, itching, pain, palpitations, cardiovascular abnormalities, CNS side effects similar to lidocaine	Yes	450 mg daily Mexetil: $62.00 Generic (Geneva): $53.74
ANTIEPILEPTICS					
Carbamazepine	600–900 mg PO daily	+/−	Dizziness, drowsiness, unsteadiness, nausea, vomiting, leukopenia, thrombocytopenia, SIADH, dysrhythmias, rash, Stevens-Johnson syndrome, hepatic dysfunction, anticonvulsant hypersensitivity syndrome	Yes	600 mg daily Tegretol: $34.06 Generic (Allscrips): $23.33
Phenytoin	200–400 mg PO daily	+/−	Ataxia, nystagmus, slurred speech, drowsiness, fatigue, nausea, vomiting, diarrhea, constipation, gingival hyperplasia, hepatic dysfunction, rash, thrombocytopenia, leukopenia, granulocytopenia, pancytopenia, anticonvulsant hypersensitivity syndrome, lymphadenopathy, hypertrichosis, hyperglycemia	No	300 mg daily Dilantin: $21.50
Gabapentin	300–900 mg PO daily	+	Somnolence, dizziness, ataxia, nystagmus, fatigue	No	300 mg daily Neurontin: $29.62
FLUPHENAZINE	1 mg twice daily max 2 mg twice daily	+ +	Extrapyramidal symptoms, sedation, antimuscarinic effects, quinidine-like cardiovascular effects	Yes	1 mg twice daily Prolixin: $48.78 Generic (Parmed): $14.38

+/−, conflicting data; +, one study available; + +, several studies available with limitations; + + +, established efficacy; several studies available.

- Mononeuropathy simplex involves a single peripheral nerve (eg, the median nerve in carpal tunnel syndrome)
- Mononeuropathy multiplex involves several isolated, unilateral nerves, often widely separated in location. Mononeuropathy multiplex is usually the result of disseminated vasculitis, as in DM or polyarteritis.
- Polyneuropathy describes impairment of multiple peripheral nerves simultaneously, resulting in a symmetric, bilateral pattern of functional loss, usually distal. Polyneuropathy is seem with many systemic processes. The presentation may be mainly sensory (eg, amyloidosis, leprosy), mainly motor (GBS, porphyria), or both.

Distribution of Involvement

DISTAL SYMMETRIC POLYNEUROPATHY

A distal distribution of motor and sensory deficit is the most common pattern observed in generalized symmetric polyneuropathies. Distal symmetric polyneuropathy can be mixed (sensory-motor autonomic) or predominantly sensory. With motor involvement, weakness and wasting begin distally in the limbs and spread proximally. The lower limbs are affected before the upper limbs. Distal symmetric polyneuropathy that is predominantly motor is less common than mixed or sensory polyneuropathy. For sensory involvement, the distal distribution produces glove-and-stocking sensory loss in the limbs.

With advanced neuropathy, sensory loss appears in the midline of the anterior abdominal wall and spreads laterally. Later, the vertex of the head and central face are affected. In severe sensory neuropathy, there may be virtually universal sensory loss, with the exception of the midline area over the posterior trunk and neck and peripheral aspects of the face.

Sensory polyneuropathies are usually symmetric, involving both sides of the body, and involve distal rather than proximal sensory nerves. Sensory neuropathy may involve large (myelinated) or small (nonmyelinated) fibers, or both. When sensory polyneuropathy involves small fibers, pain and paresthesias in the legs and feet most commonly occur. The pain is described as dull, burning, lancinating, crushing, aching, or cramplike. Paresthesia is also observed. In addition, temperature and pain perception may be decreased or lost, especially in the legs and feet.

Large-fiber neuropathies produce deficits in proprioception. Abnormalities in gait and Charcot joints occasionally occur with the involvement of proprioceptive fibers. Sensory polyneuropathies are often more intense in the evening. Extremely painful periods are often limited to a few months or years.

Distal polyneuropathy may present with a predominantly autonomic involvement, affecting gastrointestinal motility, bladder and anal sphincter control, sexual function, perspiration, and pupillary accommodation reactions. Cardiovascular autonomic dysfunction can lead to tachycardia at rest, orthostatic hypotension, and painless myocardial infarction.

PROXIMAL SYMMETRIC POLYNEUROPATHY

In symmetric polyneuropathies, a proximal distribution of motor involvement is occasionally observed. This is encountered in GBS and in rare cases of chronic progressive inflammatory demyelinating polyneuropathy. Proximal symmetric motor neuropathy may result in bilateral or unilateral weakness and wasting of pelvifemoral muscles. A proximal distribution of sensory loss is less frequent.

Proximal motor neuropathies may possess asymmetric or symmetric patterns, and are subdivided clinically into acute, subacute, and chronically evolving. Sudden onset of asymmetric weakness of the hip and thigh muscles with or without pain characterizes acute and subacute presentations. The reason for selective proximal involvement is unknown. A possible cause may be that the proximal portions of the limbs are supplied by nerve fibers of larger diameter than those in the more distal regions and the trunk. These fibers may have differing susceptibility to metabolic aberrations or immunologic insult.

CRANIAL MOTOR NEUROPATHY

Focal and multifocal cranial nerve lesions can occur alone or in combination with a generalized polyneuropathy. In progressive polyneuropathies, the cranial nerves tend to be involved late in the evolution of the disease, being preceded by symptoms distally in the legs and arms. Cranial motor neuropathy results from occlusion of the vascular supply. This neuropathy is usu-ally asymmetric and involves mononeuropathy of cranial nerves III (oculomotor), IV (trochlear), and VI (abducens), which are responsible for ocular movement and pupillary accommodation and constriction, resulting in extraocular muscle palsies. Cranial neuropathies involving cranial nerves III and VI are common.

ENTRAPMENT SYNDROMES

Entrapment syndromes occur in the limbs and are mononeuropathies involving the median, ulnar, common peroneal, and femoral nerves. Entrapment syndromes are characterized by sudden wrist or foot drop. The carpal tunnel syndrome (median nerve) is prevalent and commonly affects the hands. Carpal tunnel syndrome characteristically presents with pain and paresthesia that worsens at night. Etiologies include occupational trauma, DM, amyloidosis, rheumatoid arthritis, and hypothyroidism.

DIABETIC PN

The classification of PN in the diabetic patient has been categorized based on the characteristics of the pain. These categories include muscular pain, superficial pain, and deep pain. Muscular pain, described as muscle cramping and spasm, is believed to be caused by damage to the reflex loop or to the motor neurons. Superficial pain is described as burning or allodynia (ordinarily nonpainful stimuli evoke pain) and is believed to be caused by an increased firing of damaged or abnormally excitable nociceptive fibers. Deep pain, described as pins and needles, is believed to be caused by spontaneous activity or increased sensitivity of damaged afferent fibers in the dorsal root ganglion and loss of inhibition of large myelinated and small nonmyelinated fibers.

HISTORY AND PHYSICAL EXAM

The health care provider must take a careful medical history to determine risk factors. A careful, detailed neurologic exam should include sensory (pin prick, temperature, position, light touch), motor (strength; look for weakness, atrophy, or fasciculations), reflexes (hypo- or hyperactive), and autonomic function (anhidrosis) of both the proximal and distal extremities, as well as the cranial nerves and abdominal/truncal areas.

A functional assessment by observing the patient and asking questions such as, "Do you drag your toe or trip easily?" can suggest distal leg weakness. If a median nerve entrapment at the wrist is suspected (carpal tunnel syndrome), a Tinel sign and Phalen maneuver are done. The diagnostic goals are to isolate the peripheral nerve or nerves involved, determine the overall pattern of neuropathy (eg, stocking-and-glove weakness), and identify the underlying cause.

DIAGNOSTIC STUDIES

Electrophysiologic nerve conduction velocity studies are usually diagnostic of PN. However, the more important concern is to identify the underlying etiology so that the primary problem can be addressed. Referral to a neurologist may also be considered.

The laboratory exam should include an evaluation of hematologic status, including vitamin B_{12} and folate levels. Once these diagnostic steps are taken and evaluated, an etiology for the PN can be established in most cases. The classification of the types of PN on the basis of pathologic process or etiology is of limited clinical value because the management algorithm is patient-specific and based on the type of pain, not on the etiology or pathologic process.

TREATMENT OPTIONS, EXPECTED OUTCOMES, AND COMPREHENSIVE MANAGEMENT

Generally, treatment is directed at addressing the underlying problem and providing patient education. Drug therapy with nonsteroidal anti-inflammatory drugs (NSAIDs) and analgesics, including topical creams, may be helpful. If an entrapment syndrome is present, removal of pressure on the nerve is the goal. In carpal tunnel syndrome, use of splints at night, use of NSAIDs, and a possible ergonomics consultation in the home and workplace may be helpful. If symptoms persist, a neurosurgical referral may be indicated for evaluation for surgical decompression.

Pharmacotherapy

The following principles should be considered in the management of neuropathic pain:

- Remove the cause where possible.
- Promote healing or fiber regeneration.
- Correct metabolic parameters and normalize the nerve microenvironment.
- Normalize sensory input and nerve transmission.
- Modulate centrally acting inhibitory pathways.
- Reduce sympathetic overactivity or its effects.
- Modify emotional or behavioral components of pain interpretation (changing the pain threshold).

Damaged peripheral nerves become spontaneously active. The damaged nerve is excessively mechanosensitive and responds to mild mechanical deformation and sympathetic activation with an increased rate of firing. This increase can be inhibited by alpha-adrenergic blockade, resulting in vasodilation and increased vascular permeability, which may benefit the traumatized nerve. The mechanism of action of neuroleptics, prazosin, and antidepressants may include an alpha-adrenergic blockade that reduces neuronal firing.

Symptomatic treatment does not alter the underlying cause of PN. The underlying cause of PN should be addressed and remedied in all patients. Patients may have spontaneous resolution of PN and thus should be re-evaluated periodically.

The patient with chronic lancinating, epicritic, and well-localized pain should be treated with carbamazepine. If the response is inadequate, a combination of phenytoin and carbamazepine may be tried. Pain described as a diffuse burning that is nonlancinating, protopathic, and poorly localized should be treated with amitriptyline or imipramine. For the patient with severe, intractable neuropathic pain that is unresponsive to amitriptyline, fluphenazine may be added. Over-the-counter analgesic agents may be used for breakthrough pain.

Antidepressants are first-line drug therapy for the treatment of symptomatic diabetic PN. Amitriptyline, clomipramine, and imipramine are ideal agents whose efficacy has been established in controlled clinical trials. They may be given once daily and are inexpensive because they are available in generic form. If symptoms improve but the side effects are unacceptable, an alternative cyclic antidepressant agent with milder side effects (fewer antimuscarinic and sedative effects) is desipramine. The role of paroxetine in the management of PN is less well established. Paroxetine appears to exert a weaker therapeutic effect than other antidepressant agents because it lacks pharmacologic action on norepinephrine reuptake. Paroxetine is relatively devoid of any antimuscarinic and sedative side effects, but its role remains to be elucidated. Patients must be instructed to take tricyclic antidepressants (TCAs) or paroxetine on a daily basis, because sporadic use is not effective.

Patients with focal or small localized areas of neuropathy may be candidates for topical capsaicin treatment. Topical therapy may be advantageous because it avoids the systemic adverse effects and potential drug and disease interactions seen with TCAs or other oral agents. Capsaicin is not recommended for patients with extensive areas of PN because of its high cost, inconvenient application method, and irritating side effects. Patients with larger PN involvement may benefit from therapy with TCAs.

The sodium channel antagonists carbamazepine and phenytoin are recommended in patients who cannot tolerate antidepressants or whose symptoms do not improve with cyclic antidepressant treatment. These agents are more expensive than antidepressants and are administered several times a day (in certain settings, phenytoin may be given once a day). The efficacy of mexiletine, carbamazepine, and phenytoin for the treatment of PN is not well established. Therapy with lidocaine should be reserved for refractory PN pain in the hospital setting.

If an adequate response is not achieved with sodium channel antagonists for the treatment of lancinating pain, a trial of antidepressants, gabapentin, or prazosin may be initiated.

Therapy for PN is patient-specific and should be based on the nature of the pain in addition to individual patient factors, such as tolerance of adverse effects, likelihood of adherence to the therapeutic plan, and financial status. The dose, adverse reactions, established efficacy data, and cost of the commonly used therapeutic agents in the treatment of PN may be found in Table 56-3.

ANALGESICS

NSAIDs, acetaminophen, and salicylate analgesics may also be used in the treatment of PN. Patients may self-medicate with these agents because they are easily accessible and fairly inexpensive, although they are not recommended because of a lack of established efficacy in the treatment of PN. The NSAIDs exert their analgesic effects by inhibiting prostaglandins produced by the arachidonic acid cascade in response to noxious stimuli in the periphery and may also affect serotonin, substance P, bradykinin, and histamine. Adverse reactions with NSAIDs include nausea, vomiting, and dyspepsia. NSAIDs can also cause a rash, a burning sensation in the esophagus and stomach, edema, hypertension, constipation, and vertigo. NSAIDs should be avoided in patients with a history of peptic ulcer disease, asthma, or renal dysfunction.

Aspirin or aspirin-like compounds are the most widely used peripherally acting analgesics worldwide. Aspirin also exhibits analgesic and anti-inflammatory activity that is mediated through the inhibition of prostaglandin synthesis. Acetaminophen appears to have no role in the treatment of PN, apparently because it lacks anti-inflammatory activity. Complications associated with the use of aspirin include gastric ulcers, gastrointestinal bleeding, tinnitus, and hypersensitivity reactions in patients with asthma. Salicylates have similar precautions as with NSAIDs.

Patients with signs and symptoms suggestive of PN should be extensively evaluated before beginning drug therapy, particularly with over-the-counter analgesics, whose efficacy in this setting is not established.

ANTIDEPRESSANTS

Cyclic antidepressants are the most extensively studied agents in the treatment of PN (Wright, 1994). They serve as analgesics in the setting of PN and result in improved symptomatology. The analgesic effect of TCAs is mediated by blocking the central neuronal reuptake of serotonin or norepinephrine, therefore potentiating the inhibitory effect of these neurotransmitters on nociceptive pathways. The catecholamine reuptake inhibition of the TCAs may be the mechanism of analgesia because of the existence of an endogenous pain-suppressing system (dependent on opiates, serotonin, and norepinephrine). TCAs also have a peripheral alpha-adrenergic receptor blocking action at high doses. The TCA-induced analgesia appears to be independent of the antidepressant effect of these agents.

Adverse effects associated with TCAs include cardiac dysrhythmias, orthostatic hypotension, and peripheral and central antimuscarinic side effects (eg, dry mouth, constipation, blurred vision, urinary retention, and sedation). Use of TCAs should be avoided in patients with heart block, left bundle branch block, heart failure, or recent myocardial infarction. Other contraindications include symptomatic prostatic hypertrophy, neurogenic bladder dysfunction, and narrow angle glaucoma.

■ **CLINICAL WARNING:** A possibly fatal reaction that may potentially occur with the use of antidepressants is the serotonin syndrome (Table 56-4).

The serotonin syndrome is a constellation of mental status changes and nervous system and neuromuscular effects that result from an increase in serotonin concentrations. The excess serotonin most often occurs as a result of the concurrent ingestion of two serotonergic agents, which often have different mechanisms of action. An increase in dose of either agent may

also result in the serotonin syndrome. The diagnosis of the serotonin syndrome should be considered when three of the following occur: agitation, diaphoresis, diarrhea, fever, hyperreflexia, incoordination, mental status changes, myoclonus, shivering or tremor, in the setting of an increase in dose of a known serotonergic agent. Other manifestations include seizures and muscle rigidity.

Because the presentations of neuroleptic malignant syndrome and serotonin syndrome are similar, distinguishing between these syndromes can be perplexing. The onset of symptoms in serotonin syndrome is more rapid than in neuroleptic malignant syndrome (within minutes to hours). Neuroleptic malignant syndrome generally presents with extrapyramidal symptoms. Resolution of the serotonin syndrome is also rapid compared to the neuroleptic malignant syndrome. Death is possible but rare.

CAPSAICIN

An alternative to oral cyclic antidepressants for the treatment of PN is topical capsaicin. Capsaicin is a natural substance derived from plants of the Solaraceae family and is found in capsicum peppers. Capsaicin yields the characteristic flavor found in peppers. When applied to the skin, capsaicin first produces a sensation of warmth, and with increasing concentrations a burning sensation. Repeated application results in desensitization. Capsaicin appears to alleviate pain and burning by stimulating the release and subsequent depletion of substance P from sensory fibers. Capsaicin may also block substance P axonal transport. Capsaicin treatment does not alter vibration, temperature, and touch perception (Wright, 1994).

Adverse effects may include transient burning, sneezing, coughing, irritation, rash/erythema, dry skin, and increased pain. No systemic adverse effects have been reported. Although capsaicin appears to be a promising agent for the treatment of PN, patients may have problems following the guidelines for use, and this may hinder its efficacy. Capsaicin must be applied three or four times daily; it is expensive; its side effects are often intolerable; and cosmetic acceptance may be a problem. Patients should be advised not to expect relief for up to 6 weeks after initiating capsaicin treatment. Symptoms may worsen transiently for 2 to 3 days during the initiation of therapy. Appropriate application of capsaicin includes wearing gloves, applying only a thin layer of cream, avoiding rubbing or agitating the area, and avoiding exposing the eye and mouth area to the cream.

SODIUM CHANNEL ANTAGONISTS

Vaughn-Williams class 1B antiarrhythmic agents and antiepileptic drugs are sodium channel antagonists that produce their membrane-stabilizing and subsequent analgesic effects by altering neuronal membrane sodium currents and suppressing neuronal firing and generation of the pain impulse. Of the Vaughn-Williams class 1B antiarrhythmic agents, both mexiletine and lidocaine have been studied for the treatment of PN.

Depression of synaptic transmission and subsequent elevation of the threshold for repetitive firing of nociceptive neurons is considered the mechanism for analgesia produced by antiepileptic agents. Central effects on pain modulatory systems have also been observed experimentally and may be related to their general effect on the reduction of neuronal excitability.

TABLE 56-4	**Selected Serotonergic Agents**
Increased synthesis	**Serotonin agonists**
L-tryptophan	Buspirone
Serotonin reuptake inhibitors	LSD
Amphetamines	Lithium
Cocaine	Mescaline
Dextromethorphan	Sumatriptan
Meperidine	**Increased serotonin release**
SSRIs	Amphetamines
TCAs	Cocaine
Venlafaxine	Fenfluramine
Inhibits serotonin metabolism	Mirtazapine
MAOIs	
Selegiline	

Mexiletine

The efficacy of mexiletine in the treatment of PN has not been well elucidated. Mexiletine may be used in patients without evidence of heart disease who have sensations of burning, heat, formication, or stabbing pain and in whom standard therapy has been ineffective. The frequency of mexiletine side effects appears to be dose-dependent. Common adverse effects reported include nausea, headache, diarrhea, vomiting, itching, pain, and palpitations. Until prospective trials are conducted, mexiletine should be considered second-line therapy for patients who are unresponsive to first-line therapy and in whom the benefit from therapy must outweigh the potential adverse effects. Mexiletine should not be used in patients who have cardiac dysfunction.

Lidocaine

Lidocaine, by stabilizing nerve membranes, may reduce or impair the spontaneous activity in the damaged small myelinated fibers and therefore may be efficacious in the management of PN. Intravenous lidocaine may have a beneficial effect on the symptoms but not on the objective measures of neuropathy. This may be the result of a central effect of the drug, as opposed to a peripheral effect. Although intravenous lidocaine may be a promising agent, its use is not practical because it is not available as an oral agent.

Antiepileptics

Phenytoin and carbamazepine appear to be effective in the treatment of pain and paresthesia associated with PN. Common side effects include nystagmus, ataxia, slurred speech, mental confusion, transient nervousness, dizziness, fatigue, irritability, tremor, headache, and depression. Gastrointestinal manifestations are also common, including nausea, vomiting, and abdominal pain and discomfort.

CLINICAL WARNING: A possibly fatal adverse effect that may occur with both agents is the anticonvulsant hypersensitivity syndrome. Hallmark clinical features of this syndrome are fever, rash, hepatitis, and lymphadenopathy. Diagnostic criteria for the syndrome include fever, rash, lymphadenopathy, periorbital or facial edema, hepatitis, hematologic abnormalities, multiorgan system involvement, myalgias, and arthralgias.

The incidence of the anticonvulsant hypersensitivity syndrome is unknown because of its variable presentation and diverse clinical features. The onset usually occurs within 3 months of initiating treatment, most often within 2 to 4 weeks. The onset for each feature of this syndrome may be variable, which may lead to a delay in diagnosis. The onset of fever, rash, and lymphadenopathy is presumptive evidence for the syndrome, warranting discontinuation of therapy.

Patients should take phenytoin and carbamazepine with food to reduce gastrointestinal upset. Patients should be cautious while driving or performing other tasks that require mental alertness. Patients should notify the physician if they experience a rash, unexplained fever, severe nausea or vomiting, swollen glands, bleeding, swollen or tender gums, joint pain, yellowish discoloration of the eyes, and any indication of infection or malaise.

Gabapentin is an oral antiepileptic agent introduced in 1994 as adjunctive therapy for partial seizures with or without secondary generalization. The rationale for its use is based on the effect of other anticonvulsants (carbamazepine and phenytoin) in the treatment of certain types of pain. Gabapentin is an anticonvulsant agent structurally related to the inhibitory central nervous system neurotransmitter gamma-aminobutyric acid (GABA). Although gabapentin was developed as a structural analogue of GABA that would penetrate the blood–brain barrier (unlike GABA) and mimic the action of GABA at inhibitory neuronal synapses, the drug has no direct GABA-mimetic action; its precise mechanism of action has not been elucidated. Gabapentin does not exhibit hematologic or hepatic toxicity and does not interact with other medications. It should be considered an agent used in the treatment of refractory PN.

ANTIPSYCHOTICS AS ADJUNCT THERAPY TO ANTIDEPRESSANTS

Antipsychotic agents have been used successfully in conjunction with antidepressant agents in the treatment of PN. The mechanism of action is not known, although a possible mechanism is alpha-adrenergic blockade. Fluphenazine is often used in combination with amitriptyline. Fluphenazine is categorized as a high-potency antipsychotic and exhibits a low incidence of sedation, antimuscarinic adverse effects, and quinidine-like cardiovascular effects. Fluphenazine is likely to produce extrapyramidal side effects, such as tardive dyskinesia, neuroleptic malignant syndrome, and dystonias. Antipsychotics such as fluphenazine should be reserved as adjunctive therapy with TCAs in patients who do not respond to TCAs alone.

CLONIDINE AND PENTOXIFYLLINE

Clonidine has analgesic effects in postherpetic neuralgia and therefore may be an effective analgesic in the management of diabetic PN. Clonidine is an alpha-2-adrenoreceptor agonist. There is a high concentration of alpha-2-adrenergic receptor binding sites in rat and human dorsal horn. Clonidine inhibits the firing of dorsal horn nociceptors. Pentoxifylline may improve blood flow through the microvasculature by decreasing erythrocyte stiffness and increasing erythrocyte flexibility, thus causing a secondary reduction in the viscosity of whole blood. It is therefore a potential treatment for diabetic neuropathy.

Clonidine and pentoxifylline should be reserved for refractory cases of PN. Further randomized prospective trials are warranted to establish the role of these agents in the treatment of PN.

PYRIDOXINE

It is postulated that pyridoxine deficiency may be responsible for abnormal glucose metabolism. A deficiency in pyridoxine may result in increased gluconeogenesis as a result of abnormal tryptophan metabolism. Alternatively, several metabolites of tryptophan, which is produced in excess because of pyridoxine deficiency, have been observed to bind insulin and decrease its biologic effect.

PRAZOSIN

Prazosin is a selective alpha-1-adrenoreceptor antagonist. Its use in the treatment of painful neuropathy is based on the suggested upregulation of alpha-adrenoreceptors in injured nerves. Alpha-1-adrenoreceptor antagonists may also act on postsynaptic receptors at the medulla oblongata.

CLINICAL WARNING: A high first dose may result in syncope from postural hypotension. The first dose should not exceed 1 mg. The dose is increased in increments of 1 mg/week. Benefit usually occurs at a dose of 4 to 8 mg. Prazosin should be used only when all other treatment modalities fail.

TEACHING AND SELF-CARE

Patients and their families need to be encouraged to participate fully in their care. As with other sensory and motor problems, special care is needed to assess the environment for potential problems with safety. Patients with PN should make every effort to identify activities in which they will need to ask for help.

The various symptoms and variations in response to treatment make PN frustrating for many patients. The primary care provider needs to encourage the patient to engage in the usual activities of daily living. Patients must be monitored for depression and activity limitations secondary to pain. Validating the patient's pain may help the patient participate fully in the plan of care.

COMMUNITY RESOURCES

- The Neuropathy Association, 60 E. 42d St., Suite 942, New York, NY 10165, 212-692-0662, http://www.neuropathy.org/explaining/index.html
- Seattle Treatment Education Project, http://www.thebody.com/step/neuro.html
- Project Inform Sensory Neuropathy Hotline Handout, http://www.projinf.org/hh/sneuro.html
- National Institute of Neurological Disorders and Stroke, 31 Center Dr. MSC 2540, Building 31, Rm. 8A16, Bethesda, MD 20892, 301-496-5751, Fax 301-402-2186, 800-352-9424

SUMMARY

Care of the patient with PN is a challenge because signs and symptoms of this condition vary widely. Poor glycemic control, alcoholism, nutritional deficiencies, including folate, pyridoxine, and cyanocobalamin, drug-induced PN, and HIV-related PN are common scenarios in which underlying issues should be addressed. Pharmacologic management has been directed toward improving nerve function or providing symptomatic relief of neuropathic pain. Depletion, stimulation, antagonism, or other alterations of neuropeptides such as substance P, norepinephrine, serotonin, and endorphins may alter the transmission or perception of neural impulses. Agents that have been used include analgesics, antidepressants with or without pheno-

thiazines, topical capsaicin, pentoxifylline, phenytoin, carbamazepine, mexiletine, gabapentin, prazosin, and clonidine. Experimental agents include aldose reductase inhibitors and alpha-lipoic acid.

EDITOR'S NOTE:

COMPLEMENTARY APPROACHES

A general discussion of complementary approaches can be found in Chapter 3. The following, while not an exhaustive list, are some complementary approaches being used for this condition. Additional information on these approaches, including precautions, can be found in Appendices A and B. Providers need to assess for the use of complementary approaches as part of the patient's history, as they may impact conventional therapies, and patients may not volunteer this information unless specifically asked. Efficacy of many complementary approaches is not as well documented as that of conventional therapies. Providers need to read the literature before suggesting these complementary approaches.

- Complementary Modalities
  Acupuncture

References

Aminoff, M.J., Greenberg, D.A., & Simon, R.P. (1996). *Clinical neurology*, 3d ed., pp. 192–204. Stamford, CT: Appleton & Lange.

Bosch, P.E., & Mitsumoto, H. (1991). Disorders of peripheral nerves, plexuses, and nerve roots. In W.G. Bradley, R.B. Daroff, G.M. Fenichel, & C.D. Marsden (Eds.). *Neurology in clinical practice*, pp. 1719–1818. New York: Butterworth-Heinemann.

Brazis, P.W., Masdeu, J.C., & Biller, J. (1990). *Localization in clinical neurology*, 2d ed. Boston: Little, Brown.

Brew B. (1993). HIV-1 related neurological disease. *Journal of Acquired Immune Deficiency Syndromes, 6*, S10–S15.

Brew J. (1994). The clinical spectrum and pathogenesis of HIV encephalopathy, myelopathy, and peripheral neuropathy. *Current Opinion in Neurology, 7*, 209–216.

Green, F.A. (1994). Mono-/amyoradiculopathy. In H.E. Lebovitz (Ed.). *Therapy for diabetes mellitus and related disorders*, 2d ed., pp. 283–287. Alexandria, VA: American Diabetic Association.

Wright J. (1994). Review of symptomatic treatment of diabetic neuropathy. *Pharmacotherapy, 14*, 689–697.

Ziegler D. (1996). Diagnosis and management of diabetic peripheral neuropathy. *Diabetic Medicine, 13*, S34–S38.

Bibliography

Hickey, J.V. (1997). Peripheral nerve injuries. In J.V. Hickey. *The clinical practice of neurological and neurosurgical nursing*, 4th ed., pp. 487–497. Philadelphia: J.B. Lippincott.

Kelley, W. (1994). *Essentials of internal medicine*. Philadelphia: J.B. Lippincott.

Llewelyn, J. (1995). Diabetic neuropathy. *Current Opinion in Neurology, 8*, 364–366.

Miller, R.S., Iverson, D.C., Fried, R.A., Green, L.A., & Nutting, P.A. (1994). Carpal tunnel syndrome in primary care: A report from ASPN. *Journal of Family Practice, 38*(4), 337–344.

Trellis, J.K. (1990). *The peripheral nerves: Structures, function, and reconstruction*. New York: Raven Press.

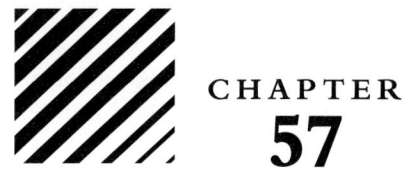

CHAPTER

57

Seizure Disorders

Henry Cohen, MS, PharmD, and Salah M. Mesad, MD

Seizures are the clinical manifestations of excessive and hypersynchronous, usually self-limiting, abnormal activity of neurons in the cerebral cortex. The behavioral features of a seizure reflect the cerebral cortical areas where the abnormal neuronal activity originates and spreads (Engel, 1989). A convulsion implies a violent, involuntary contraction or series of contractions of voluntary muscles. Epilepsy is a chronic condition characterized by two or more unprovoked recurrent seizures. Epilepsy implies a periodic recurrence of seizures with or without convulsions (Engel, 1989).

ANATOMY, PHYSIOLOGY, AND PATHOLOGY

The excitability of the neuronal cell membrane depends on the maintenance of an electrical charge, or potential difference, between the intracellular and extracellular environments, analogous to the cardiac cell. This is achieved through the maintenance of different concentrations of negatively charged ions on either side of the membrane in the resting state, with the outside having a net positive charge relative to the inside.

The membrane is thus polarized in its resting state, usually with a membrane potential of -60 to at least -80 millivolts. During depolarization, the permeability of the membrane changes to allow positive ions to flow in, eliminating the potential difference. The membrane is subsequently repolarized when the ions that flowed in are pumped back out. The movement of ions during these phases is extremely complex and involves many different channels that are governed by various influences and are operative at different phases of the process (Engel, 1989).

Excitatory postsynaptic potentials generally are caused by excitatory neurotransmitters, which include the excitatory amino acids glutamate and aspartate, acetylcholine, and the less potent histamine and corticotropin-releasing factor (Engel, 1989; Meldrum, 1992). These substances modify Na^+, K^+, or Ca^{++} channels to reduce the potential difference across the membrane and facilitate rapid depolarization (Fig. 57-1). Inhibitory postsynaptic potentials are caused by inhibitory neurotransmitters, primarily gamma-aminobutyric acid (GABA) and glycine, and the less potent dopamine, norepinephrine, and serotonin. These substances move K^+ out of the cell or Cl^- into the cell, increasing the relative intracellular negativity and hyperpolarizing the membrane, making rapid depolarization less likely.

Any imbalance in excitatory or inhibitory influence may lead to hypersynchronous neuronal firing. The action potential spreads to neighboring cells, causing them to fire at the same time and to have concurrent refractory periods. All the neurons emerge from refractoriness simultaneously and are susceptible to firing simultaneously again; the process is thus repeated and perpetuated (Engel, 1989). This coordinated firing spreads until a critical mass is reached and a seizure ensues. The term "seizure threshold" corresponds to the limit beyond which the patient can be made to seize, when subjected to a sufficient number of epileptogenic factors.

During a generalized tonic-clonic seizure, there is a 300% increase in cerebral oxygen consumption and a 900% increase in cerebral blood flow. The increased brain blood flow is necessary to supply neurons with oxygen, glucose, and other necessary nutrients while removing the enormous amounts of carbon dioxide and metabolic waste products. Unfortunately, the brain has a limited capacity to increase brain blood flow, and a state of sequential neuronal hypoxia, anoxia, ischemia, and impending necrosis develops. Hypoxia-induced lactate synthesis causes the production of free radicals (eg, superoxides, peroxides), damaging and destroying the neuronal cells. In patients with status epilepticus (a convulsive seizure or series of seizures lasting longer than 10 to 15 minutes), cardiac collapse and rhabdomyolysis may occur with renal failure as a consequence of prolonged ictal activity (Dodson et al, 1993; DeLorenzo et al, 1992).

EPIDEMIOLOGY

Epilepsy and seizures are among the most common neurologic disturbances. The prevalence of epilepsy ranges from 4 to 8 per 1000. By age 20, about 1% of the population in the United States will have epilepsy, and this cumulative incidence increases to 3% to 4% by 80 years of age (DeLorenzo et al, 1992; Hauser & Annegers, 1992). The annual incidence of epilepsy in the U.S. population is about 50 per 100,000 people (DeLorenzo et al, 1992; Hauser & Annegers, 1992; Hauser et al, 1991). The prevalence of epilepsy increases to 65 per 100,000 people per year if single unprovoked seizures are included, and up to 85 per 100,000 people per year if nonfebrile reactive seizures are added. Of those afflicted, 75% experience their first seizure before the third decade of life (Department of Health, Education & Welfare, 1978).

HISTORY AND PHYSICAL EXAM

The diagnosis of epilepsy is clinical and is based on a detailed description of events experienced by the patient before, during, and after a seizure and, more importantly, on an eyewitness account. Three questions need to be answered when the provider is evaluating a patient with possible epileptic seizures:

- Is it epilepsy?
- What type of epilepsy?
- What is the etiology?

The Na⁺ Action Potential

A

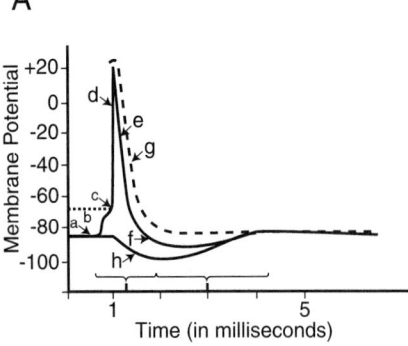

B

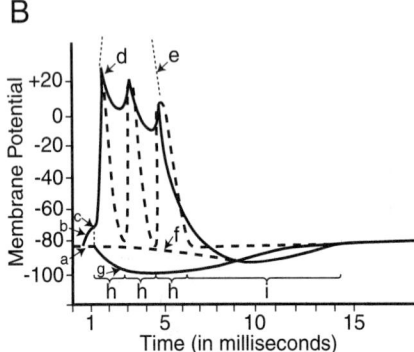

FIGURE 57-1 This graph shows the phases of the Na⁺ action potential as afterhyperpolarization as recorded at the neuronal cell body (soma). "a" shows the resting membrane potential of approximately −85 mV; "b" shows the phase of graded Na⁺-mediated depolarization, during which a slow moderate inward flow of Na⁺ ions begins to reduce the membrane potential; "c" indicates the level of the threshold (approximately −65 mV) at which "explosive" or rapid depolarization "d" occurs; this is also known as the rising phase of the all-or-none regenerative spike. "e" is the repolarization phase, during which the Na⁺ current "g" and voltage-dependent K⁺ current "h" reestablish the resting membrane potential; in fact, the potential transiently becomes greater than the resting potential, in the phase known as afterhyperpolarization "f". "i" indicates the absolute refractory period, and "j" indicates the relative refractory period, during which an appropriate change in the electrophysiologic environment can induce a depolarization to occur prematurely.

DIAGNOSTIC TESTS

The electroencephalogram (EEG) provides supportive evidence for the clinical diagnosis of epilepsy by demonstrating epilepiform discharges; however, normal studies do not exclude seizures. The EEG aids in the classification of seizures, the selection of appropriate antiepileptic drugs (AEDs), and the analysis of the patient's response to therapy.

Magnetic resonance imaging (MRI) and computed tomography (CT) of the brain can complement electrophysiologic studies by identifying structural brain lesions that may be causally related to the development of epilepsy. MRI is more sensitive than CT in detecting cerebral lesions related to epilepsy, such as cortical heterotopias or mesial temporal sclerosis, and hamartomas. Some abnormalities, such as calcified or bony abnormalities, may be easier to interpret on CT than MRI. Positron emission tomography and single photon emission computed tomography are less readily obtainable. These tech-

niques can identify areas of cerebral hypometabolism interictally in patients with partial epilepsy, even when MRI and CT have been normal (Engel, 1989).

DIFFERENTIAL DIAGNOSIS

Differentiating epileptic seizures from other paroxysmal nonepileptic events is a common problem. Not all paroxysmal behaviors that include shaking, stiffening, or staring are epileptic seizures. Paroxysmal behavioral changes can result from many different medical, neurologic, and psychiatric disorders. In some cases, these disorders coexist, further confounding the diagnosis and therapy.

Nonepileptic seizures are common and are reported to occur in approximately 5% to 20% of epileptic outpatients (Commission, 1989; Gates et al, 1991). Patients whose nonepileptic episodes are mistaken for epilepsy face a variety of potential iatrogenic hazards. Patients with undiagnosed nonepileptic seizures usually receive AEDs, whose behavioral toxicity may actually exacerbate nonepileptic seizures (Gates et al, 1991). Physiologic nonepileptic seizures such as syncope are commonly misdiagnosed as seizures (Table 57-1).

TABLE 57-1	**Nonepileptic Seizures Presenting as Syncope**

I. Syncope of cardiac origin
  A. Dysrhythmias
    1. Supraventricular dysrhythmias
    2. Atrial flutter/fibrillation
    3. Paroxysmal atrial tachycardia
    4. Sick sinus syndrome
    5. Ventricular dysrhythmias
    6. Paroxysmal bradycardia or tachycardia
    7. Heart block or asystole
  B. Congenital heart disease
  C. Cardiomyopathy
  D. Drug-induced cardiac abnormalities
II. Syncope of noncardiac origin, from diminished cerebral perfusion
  A. Vasovagal
    1. Micturition
    2. Cough
    3. Carotid sinus disturbance
  B. Valsalva maneuver
  C. Drug-induced (decreased systemic vascular resistance)
    1. Antipsychotics
    2. Tricyclic antidepressants
    3. Antihypertensives
  D. Orthostatic
    1. Antihypertensive agents
    2. Hypovolemia
    3. Parkinson's disease
    4. Shy-Drager syndrome
    5. Autonomic dysfunction
      a. Diabetes
      b. Amyloidosis
      c. Porphyria
  E. Benign paroxysmal vertigo
  F. Breath-holding
  G. Hyperventilation
  H. Migraine headaches
  I. Cerebrovascular disease
    1. Stroke
    2. Transient ischemic attack

Syncope is defined as a sudden transient loss of consciousness resulting from a reduction of cerebral blood flow. It is associated with a loss of postural tone and spontaneous recovery. The diagnosis of syncope is supported if episodes:

- Are precipitated by anxiety or pain (eg, venipuncture) or assumption of the upright position
- Exclusively occur while standing or sitting
- Are associated with pallor and diaphoresis
- Are not associated with sustained tonic or clonic movements, bladder incontinence, or tongue or cheek bites
- Are not followed by postepisode confusion, lethargy, muscle soreness, and headache.

Although incontinence strongly suggests an epileptic seizure, if the bladder is overdistended when syncope occurs, there also may be incontinence. Prodromal symptoms such as abdominal sensations (eg, "butterflies" or nausea), flushing and warmth, dizziness and lightheadedness, bilateral paresthesia, and a feeling of fear and unreality occur with both syncope and epileptic seizures. Symptoms such as formed visual or auditory hallucinations, olfactory hallucinations, déjà vu, or focal sensory or motor phenomena strongly suggest partial seizures.

A prodrome lasting several seconds, followed by loss of consciousness for 15 to 60 seconds, followed by a rapid return to a normal level of attentiveness, is typical of syncope. The greatest source of error in distinguishing seizures from syncope is failure to recognize that brief tonic or clonic movements often occur in syncope (convulsive syncope), especially when the patient is maintained in the upright or sitting position (Ziegler et al, 1978; Pacia et al, 1994).

The physical exam in patients with possible syncope includes a brief survey of general medical and neurologic systems, specifically palpation of the pulse and measurement of orthostatic heart rate and blood pressure. An electrocardiogram may help detect abnormalities such as arrhythmias, conduction blocks, and prolonged Q–T syndrome (Pacia et al, 1994).

Classification of Seizures

A seizure is not a diagnosis; it is a series of signs and symptoms. Similar seizures can result from multiple underlying cerebral processes. In some cases, seizures are the sole manifestation of the disorder; in others, they are only one of several signs and symptoms present. Certain seizures affect patients of a select age group and produce a characteristic clinical and EEG profile but are idiopathic. The International League Against Epilepsy classifies epileptic seizures based on clinical symptoms and EEG features (Tables 57-2 and 57-3) (Commission, 1989 & 1981). This classification subdivides epileptic seizures into two major categories: partial and generalized. Defining the seizure type and epilepsy syndrome helps determine whether medication is necessary, the likelihood of complete response to AED treatment, and the potential duration of treatment.

Partial seizures have clinical or EEG evidence of a focal onset from one or more areas of the cerebral cortex. Generalized seizures begin in both sides of the brain simultaneously and may arise in subcortical pacemaker regions (eg, thalamus). Partial seizures are subdivided into simple partial seizures (without impairment of consciousness) and complex partial seizures (with impairment of consciousness). A simple partial seizure

TABLE 57-2	**International Classification of Epileptic Seizures**

I. Partial seizures (focal or local onset)
  A. Simple partial seizures (consciousness is preserved)
    1. With motor signs
    2. With special sensory or somatosensory symptoms
    3. With autonomic symptoms or signs
    4. With psychic symptoms
  B. Complex partial seizures (consciousness is impaired)
    1. Simple partial onset followed by impairment of consciousness
    2. With impairment of consciousness at onset
  C. Partial seizures evolving to secondarily generalized seizures
    1. Simple partial seizures evolving to generalized seizures
    2. Complex partial seizures evolving to generalized seizures
    3. Simple partial seizures evolving to complex partial seizures evolving to generalized seizures
II. Generalized seizures (bilateral symmetric onset; convulsive or nonconvulsive)
  A. Absence seizures
    1. Typical absences (no motor involvement)
    2. Atypical absences (motor involvement)
    3. Myoclonic seizures
  B. Clonic seizures
  C. Tonic seizures
  D. Tonic-clonic seizures
  E. Atonic seizures (static seizures)
III. Unclassified epileptic seizures

Source: Commission, 1989.

may evolve into a complex partial seizure, and both types may evolve into a secondarily generalized tonic-clonic (grand mal) seizure. Auras are simple partial seizures.

Generalized seizures can be further categorized as convulsive or nonconvulsive (Commission, 1989 & 1981). The typical convulsive generalized seizure is the tonic-clonic seizure. Some convulsive seizures may be characterized by only clonic, only tonic, or myoclonic manifestations. The major group of nonconvulsive seizures is absence attacks, which consist of brief lapses of consciousness. Absence seizures that last less than 10 seconds, are associated with bilaterally synchronous 3-Hz spike-and-wave complexes on the EEG, and have no postictal EEG or behavioral disturbances are referred to as typical. Absence seizures that last longer, have slower or more irregular EEG correlates, or are followed by varying periods of postictal dysfunction are referred to as atypical. Absence seizures are generally a disease of childhood; they rarely commence before age 3 and exist after age 15.

Seizure Etiology

The etiology for epileptic seizures is multifactorial. In approximately 50% of cases, no specific cause is identified; these are termed idiopathic. Most other epileptic seizures have a single etiology, such as genetic or environmental (eg, head trauma) factors. Some patients have more than one underlying disturbance, a multifactorial etiology. Any injury to the brain can cause epilepsy, including infections, head trauma, stroke, and tumors. Brain injuries can occur at any age but have age-related predilections: infections such as meningitis are prevalent in children; head trauma is prevalent in young adults; stroke and degenerative disorders are prevalent in the elderly. Many patients with epilepsy secondary to these causes, particularly if the damage

TABLE 57-3	International Classification of Epilepsies, Epileptic Syndromes, and Related Seizure Disorders

1. Localization-related (focal, local, partial)
   1.1 Idiopathic (primary)
      A. Benign childhood epilepsy with centrotemporal spikes
      B. Childhood epilepsy with occipital spikes
      C. Primary reading epilepsy
   1.2 Symptomatic (secondary)
      A. Temporal lobe epilepsies
      B. Frontal lobe epilepsies
      C. Parietal lobe epilepsies
      D. Occipital lobe epilepsies
      E. Chronic progressive epilepsia partialis, continuation of childhood syndromes characterized by seizures with specific modes of precipitation
   1.3 Cryptogenic, defined by:
      A. Seizure type
      B. Clinical features
      C. Etiology
      D. Anatomic localization
2. Generalized
   2.1 Idiopathic (primary)
      A. Benign neonatal familial convulsions
      B. Benign neonatal convulsions
      C. Benign myoclonic epilepsy in infancy
      D. Childhood absence epilepsy (pyknolepsy)
      E. Juvenile absence epilepsy
      F. Juvenile myoclonic epilepsy (impulsive petit mal)
      G. Epilepsies with grand mal seizures on awakening
      H. Other generalized idiopathic epilepsies
      I. Epilepsies with seizures precipitated by specific modes of activation
   2.2 Cryptogenic or symptomatic
      A. West syndrome (infantile spasms, Blitz-Nick-Salaam Kraempfe)
      B. Lennox-Gastaut syndrome
      C. Epilepsy with myoclonic astatic seizures
      D. Epilepsy with myoclonic absences
   2.3 Symptomatic (secondary)
      Nonspecific etiology
      A. Early myoclonic encephalopathy
      B. Early infantile epileptic encephalopathy with suppression bursts
      C. Other symptomatic generalized epilepsies
      Specific syndromes
      A. Epileptic seizures may complicate many disease states.
3. Undetermined epilepsies
   3.1 With both generalized and focal seizures
      A. Neonatal seizures
      B. Severe myoclonic epilepsy in infancy
      C. Epilepsy with continuous spike-waves during slow-wave sleep
      D. Acquired epileptic aphasia (Landau-Kleffner syndrome)
      E. Other undetermined epilepsies
   3.2 Without unequivocal generalized or focal features
4. Special syndromes
   4.1 Situation-related seizures
      Febrile convulsions
      A. Isolated seizures or isolated status epilepticus
      B. Seizures occurring only when there is an acute or toxic event due to factors such as alcohol, drugs, eclampsia, nonketotic hyperglycemia

Source: Commission, 1981.

is extensive, have other mental or neurologic handicaps that limit their participation in active sports programs.

Seizures in the patient with extensive brain damage may be multiple in type and are difficult to control with medications. Nonspecific predisposing factors (eg, inconsistent medication regimen, sleep deprivation, intercurrent illnesses, especially with fever, stress, alcohol, illicit drug use, hormonal changes) determine differences in individual susceptibility to epileptic seizures, whereas specific predisposing factors (eg, flashing lights, reading) can provoke epileptic seizures in susceptible persons. Precipitating factors are endogenous or exogenous perturbations capable of acutely evoking epileptic seizures in persons with chronic epilepsy and, in some cases, reactive seizures in nonepileptic persons (Hauser et al, 1991).

Head trauma increases the risk for seizures and epilepsy in proportion to the severity of the injury. The occurrence of seizures is highest in the first few years after injury. Patients with penetrating head injuries or a loss of consciousness longer than 24 hours have a risk of seizures 5 to 15 times above the baseline population rates, even 15 years or more after the injury (Annegers et al, 1988). Early seizures, those occurring within the first week after injury, occur in approximately 5% of patients with brain trauma. Early seizures are associated with an increased risk of epilepsy later in life; this occurs in adults but not children.

Seizures occur in 10% to 15% of patients with acute stroke, especially patients with cortical infarcts. Epilepsy develops in 15% to 20% of stroke survivors. Seizures in the week after stroke are associated with an increased risk for epilepsy, when compared with stroke patients without early seizures (Hauser & Annegers, 1991).

Persons with encephalitis or bacterial meningitis have a four- to sixfold risk for epilepsy compared with the general population (Gates et al, 1991; Annegers et al, 1988). The risk of epilepsy for patients with meningitis is increased only in the setting of persistent neurologic deficits, suggesting structural brain damage. About 5% of patients have seizures contemporaneously with meningitis. Patients with aseptic meningitis have no subsequent discernible increase in risk for epilepsy.

Intracranial tumors can cause epilepsy, particularly in adult patients. Seizures frequently are the presenting manifestation of a central nervous system (CNS) tumor. Although seizures occur in approximately 30% of persons with brain tumors, they account for less than 5% of new cases of adult-onset epilepsy. Brain tumors are a cause of epilepsy at all ages, but their impact is proportionately greatest between ages 25 and 64 (Franceschetti et al, 1988).

Ten percent to 15% of patients with Alzheimer's disease have unprovoked seizures in the course of their illness, a rate at least 10 times more than expected in the general population over age 60 (Hauser et al, 1986). Patients with multiple sclerosis have a risk of epilepsy at least threefold greater than the general population. Up to 5% of patients with multiple sclerosis are reported to have seizures or epilepsy (Kinnunen & Wikstrom, 1986).

Alcohol withdrawal seizures, described as the occurrence of seizures during abstinence, when alcohol intake is reduced, is well recognized (Hauser & Annegers, 1991). The risk of seizures increases with increasing alcohol consumption; persons who drink less than 50 g of alcohol daily are not at increased risk, but the risk of epilepsy is 20 times greater than expected in persons who drink more than 300 g of alcohol daily. In a study of adult patients with newly diagnosed epilepsy, a history of chronic alcoholism was the only factor that could be identified in 20% of cases (Hauser & Annegers, 1991).

Other factors that can precipitate seizures include metabolic disturbances. Carbamazepine, a potent AED, commonly causes the syndrome of inappropriate antidiuretic hormone. This syndrome presents with serum hyponatremia, a known sei-

TABLE 57-4	**Selected Seizuregenic Agents**
Epinephrine	Beta-blockers (O.D.)
Amphetamines	Calcium channel blockers (O.D.)
Antipsychotics	Type 1B antiarrhythmics
Cyclic antidepressants	Cocaine
Carbamazepine (toxicity)	Phencyclidine
Phenytoin (chronic toxicity?)	Carbon monoxide
Lithium (toxicity)	DEET (eg, OFF!)
Folic acid (high dose)	Ipecac (toxicity)
Methylxanthines	Baclofen (O.D.)
Penicillins (high dose)	Cyclobenzaprine (O.D.)
Cephalosporins (high dose)	Metoclopramide
Imipenem/Cilastatin	Isoniazid (O.D.)
Quinolones	Terfenadine (O.D.)
Ondansetron (toxicity)	Astemizole (O.D.)
Granisetron (toxicity)	Lindane
Meperidine	Oral contraceptives
Na Bisulfite	

O.D., generally occurs only in the overdose setting.

TABLE 57-5	**First Aid for a Person With Convulsive Seizures**

1. Keep calm, and explain to other people around the area that a seizure is occurring.
2. Clear the area around the seizing patient, especially of hard, sharp, or other harmful objects.
3. Loosen the tie or any object that may make breathing difficult.
4. Place a soft object (eg, pillow, blanket, folded jacket) under the head.
5. Turn the person gently onto the side—this will aid in maintaining a clear airway and preventing aspiration. Do not attempt to force the mouth open with any hard objects or your fingers; this can lead to airway obstruction or significant trauma, hemorrhage, and aspiration. A person seizing cannot swallow the tongue.
6. Do not attempt to restrain the person and prevent movements. Allow the convulsion to take its course.
7. During a seizure, do not attempt artificial respiration.
8. Stay with the person until the seizure ends naturally, consciousness is regained and the patient is alert and can ambulate.
9. If the patient seems confused (postictal state), offer to call a taxi, friend, or relative to help the person get home.

zuregenic metabolic disturbance. Other agents that commonly cause this syndrome include chlorpropamide, tolbutamide, antidepressants, neuroleptics, and less commonly barbiturates (Hoffman, 1994).

A severe hypoglycemic episode may present with syncope and seizures; often the provider misdiagnoses the patient with epilepsy. Agents other than sulfonylureas that have potent hypoglycemic properties include pentamidine, disopyramide, high-dose sulfonamide antimicrobials, aspirin (more than 3 g daily), and the angiotensin converting enzyme inhibitors (Hoffman, 1994). Other metabolic disturbances that can precipitate seizures include hypernatremia, hyperglycemia, hypomagnesemia, hypocalcemia, and hypophosphatemia (Hoffman, 1994).

Sudden withdrawal of AEDs may precipitate seizures. All AEDs must be withdrawn slowly; the longer a patient has been taking an AED, the longer the weaning schedule should be. Abrupt withdrawal of benzodiazepines, meprobamate, cyclic antidepressants (excluding serotonin selective reuptake inhibitors), and neuroleptics all may precipitate seizures (Hauser & Annegers, 1991). Also, many drugs have inherent seizuregenic potential. Drug-induced seizures can occur at normal or toxic doses with some agents (eg, amphetamines) and only at toxic concentrations with others (eg, chronic phenytoin, carbamazepine). Table 57-4 lists drugs that can induce seizures.

TREATMENT OPTIONS, EXPECTED OUTCOMES, AND COMPREHENSIVE MANAGEMENT

Pharmacologic Treatment

Once the diagnosis of epilepsy has been confirmed, long-term treatment with an AED is recommended. However, of tantamount importance is the need to instruct the patient's family in first-aid techniques for a convulsive seizure (Table 57-5). The goal of pharmacotherapy is to achieve complete seizure control with a minimum of adverse drug effects, thereby maximizing the patient's quality of life. AEDs are approximately 70% effective as monotherapy (Holmes, 1993).

Most first-line AEDs indicated for a specific seizure type are equally effective. Table 57-6 lists first-line and alternative agents for specific seizure disorders. Selecting the best agent for the epileptic patient is often based on pharmacokinetic and adverse reaction profiles. To maximize adherence with the therapeutic plan, AEDs that may be administered once or twice daily are preferred. For most AEDs, an adequate trial consists of achieving serum concentrations at the upper therapeutic range or until intolerable adverse effects develop.

Because the AEDs readily penetrate the blood–brain barrier, neurologic adverse effects are common. All AEDs, with the exception of phenytoin at concentrations less than 20 mcg/mL, are known CNS depressants. Common CNS adverse effects include sedation, drowsiness, dizziness, headaches, confusion, and diplopia (Cascino, 1993).

The traditional, most effective, and best studied AEDs include phenytoin, phenobarbital, carbamazepine, and valproic acid. All of these agents are associated with cognitive impairment and behavioral disturbances (Cascino, 1993; French, 1994). The greatest offender is phenobarbital, and to a lesser extent and in descending order, phenytoin, carbamazepine, and

TABLE 57-6	**Drugs of Choice for Specific Seizure Disorders**	
Epilepsy Type	First-Line Agents	Second-Line Agents
Simple partial	Carbamazepine Phenytoin	Gabapentin Lamotrigine Topiramate Valproic acid
Complex partial	Carbamazepine Phenytoin	Gabapentin Lamotrigine Topiramate
Tonic–clonic	Phenytoin Valproic acid Carbamazepine	Phenobarbital
Absence	Ethosuximide Valproic acid	Clonazepam Acetazolamide

valproic acid. Cognitive impairment is subtle and difficult to recognize, and is most pronounced in children. Altered cognition manifests with memory deficits, causing learning disabilities and affecting intelligence. Behavioral disturbances include lethargy, irritability, peevishness, disobedience, obstinacy, depression, and cantankerousness. A paradoxical hyperactive, excitable, and insomniac state often occurs in children and the elderly.

With the exception of valproic acid, all three traditional agents have been associated with the AED hypersensitivity syndrome (Cascino, 1993; French, 1994). The hypersensitivity syndrome presents with a generalized rash, lymphadenopathy, low-grade fever, malaise, fatigue, eosinophilia, thrombocytopenia, and symptoms of hepatotoxicity. These symptoms wax and wane progressively, engendering a life-threatening hepatotoxicity. Before beginning an hepatotoxic AED, baseline liver enzyme tests must be obtained, with periodic monitoring. If a patient develops an increase in liver enzymes (ALT, AST) greater than three times the upper limit of normal, the AED should be discontinued. Patients must be counseled regarding the signs and symptoms of hepatic disease (eg, protracted nausea, vomiting, and anorexia, abdominal pain, dark urine and stool, fatigue).

All four traditional AEDs have been associated with a generalized urticaria, which can progress to the life-threatening Stevens-Johnson syndrome or toxic epidermal necrolysis (Cascino,

1993; French, 1994). If a rash develops secondary to AED therapy, the agent should be immediately discontinued and an alternative agent initiated. Specific drug information pertaining to dosing, pharmacokinetics, and adverse effects may be found in Table 57-7.

In approximately one third of patients, no single drug or combination of drugs can control seizures (Mattson et al, 1992). Switching or adding AEDs with different mechanisms of action is recommended. Until recently, the major AEDs were barbiturates, benzodiazepines, carbamazepine, ethosuximide, phenytoin, and valproate. Most of the established AEDs were developed before 1980 and generally act on sodium or calcium channels or the gamma-aminobutyric acid type A (GABA-A) receptors (Holmes, 1993; Cascino, 1993). Although their mechanisms of action have not been completely established, all appear to decrease membrane excitability. By decreasing membrane excitability, the tendency of neurons to produce abnormal, high-frequency, repetitive action potentials is reduced. Such patterns of firing have been associated with the presence of epilepsy and may serve as a trigger for further abnormal electrical activity in the nervous system.

The benzodiazepines and barbiturates act at the GABA-A receptor, enhancing the inhibitory action of the neurotransmitter (Holmes, 1993; Cascino, 1993). Phenytoin, carbamazepine, and possibly valproate enhance the influx of sodium via sodium channels, thereby decreasing the high-frequency, re-

TABLE 57-7 Pharmacologic Data

Drug	Usual Maximum Daily Dose	Therapeutic Range	Route of Elimination	Time to Steady State	Side Effects (Dose-Related)	Side Effects (Not Dose-Related)
Carbamazepine	400–2400 mg/d (tid or qid)	4–12 mg/L	>95% metabolized to active epoxide	Initiation: 4–6 weeks after induction: 2–4 days	Diplopia, dizziness, lethargy, ataxia, cardiac dysrhythmias, seizures, rash, GI	Leukopenia, SIADH
Felbamate	3600 mg (tid or qid)	22–140 mg/L	50% metabolized; 50% renally unchanged	5–7 days	GI, insomnia, headaches	Aplastic anemia, hepatic failure
Gabapentin	4800 mg/d (tid or qid)	Not established	Completely renal	1–2 days	Fatigue, dizziness, ataxia, drowsiness	None known
Lamotrigine	100–150 mg/d if on VPA; 300–500 mg/d if not on VPA (bid)	Not established	85% metabolized to inactive metabolites; 10% unchanged in urine	3–15 days	Diplopia, dizziness, drowsiness, ataxia	Rash, Stevens-Johnson syndrome
Phenobarbital	180–300 mg/d (qd–tid)	10–40 mg/L	75% metabolized; 25% unchanged in urine	7–28 days	Sedation, dizziness, cognitive impairment, behavioral impairment	Rash, paradoxical excitement
Phenytoin	200–400 mg/d (qd–qid)	5–20 mg/L	>90% metabolized to inactive metabolites	22 days	Diplopia, dizziness, drowsiness, ataxia, gingival hyperplasia	Rash, blood dyscrasias, osteomalacia, hypertrichosis
Valproic acid	3000–5000 mg/d (bid–qid)	50–100 mg/L	>95% metabolized	5–10 days	Nausea, vomiting, tremor, weight gain	Hepatic dysfunction, alopecia, pancreatitis
Topiramate	200–400 mg/d	Not established	70% unchanged in urine	4–5 days	Psychomotor slowing, cognitive impairment, drowsiness, fatigue, nephrolithiasis, dysgeusia, paresthesia	None known

petitive firing of action potentials. Ethosuximide and possibly valproate act by reducing the low threshold (T-type) calcium channel current, thereby affecting the neuron's excitability (Holmes, 1993; Cascino, 1993).

Over the past several years, a number of AEDs have obtained FDA approval for marketing or are in the late stages of clinical development. The four newly marketed agents are felbamate, gabapentin, lamotrigine, and topiramate. All four agents are approved for adjunctive therapy in the treatment of adults with partial-onset seizures with or without secondary generalization (Bazil & Bazil, 1997). These agents may also be considered as monotherapy when two or more first-line agents have failed as monotherapy or combination therapy, or when first-line agents are contraindicated. Drug interactions associated with these agents are listed in Table 57-8.

FELBAMATE

Felbamate was introduced in the United States in August 1993; however, by August 1994, several serious cases, with fatalities, of aplastic anemia and hepatotoxicity occurred (Faught et al, 1993). Subsequently, felbamate has been relegated as an agent used for refractory partial epilepsy and as an adjunct in the Lennox-Gastaut syndrome in children—and only when the risk/benefit ratio warrants its use (Faught et al, 1993; Felbamate, 1993). Written informed consent should be obtained from all patients before using this agent. Felbamate may cause gastrointestinal disturbances, including dysgeusia, and should be taken with food. Felbamate is phototoxic. It is associated with many hepatic cytochrome P450 inducer and inhibitor interactions (Bazil & Bazil, 1997).

GABAPENTIN

Gabapentin is structurally similar to the inhibitory neurotransmitter GABA but does not appear to interact with the GABA system. Gabapentin's binding site in the CNS and complete mechanism of action are unknown (French, 1994; Mattson et al, 1992). Gabapentin may have a relatively low potential for neurologic and gastrointestinal adverse effects. It is primarily eliminated renally and is not known to be hepatotoxic. Gabapentin is not associated with any hematologic or biochemical adverse effects. It does not affect the hepatic cytochrome P450 system and is less than 3% plasma protein-bound. Because gaba-pentin is relatively devoid of drug interactions, it is an easy "add-on" drug. Because of its short half-life, it must be given three or four times a day (Felbamate, 1993; U.S. Gabapentin, 1993).

LAMOTRIGINE

Lamotrigine appears to decrease the sustained high-frequency, repetitive firing of voltage-dependent sodium action potentials, an action that may preferentially decrease the release of presynaptic glutamate and aspartate (Bazil & Bazil, 1997; Risner, 1994). Although approved only for use in partial epilepsy, it has been studied and proven effective in generalized epilepsy, including absence seizures. Lamotrigine appears to be well tolerated, although neurologic and gastrointestinal effects are common. Approximately 10% of patients develop a rash, but it is usually transient despite continued therapy. In 1% to 2% of patients, the rash represents a more serious hypersensitivity reaction and may progress to Stevens-Johnson syndrome or toxic epidermal necrolysis. Concomitant use of lamotrigine with valproic acid or carbamazepine may increase the likelihood of a serious rash (Hoffman, 1994; Cascino, 1993). Because of the risk of a life-threatening dermal reaction, if a rash develops with the use of lamotrigine, the agent should be discontinued. Lamotrigine is phototoxic and has been associated with the AED hypersensitivity syndrome. Lamotrigine is an autoinducer and is associated with a plethora of hepatic cytochrome P450 inducer and inhibitor interactions (Bazil & Bazil, 1997). Lamotrigine is generally administered once or twice daily (Risner, 1994).

TOPIRAMATE

Topiramate is a carbonic anhydrase inhibitor that may work primarily by enhancing GABA activity at the GABA-A receptors (Holmes, 1994; Bazil & Bazil, 1997). Topiramate, like the barbiturates, is associated with significant cognitive impairment. Topiramate has been associated with dysgeusia, paresthesias, and nephrolithiasis. To minimize the risk of nephrolithiasis, patients must maintain an adequate fluid intake. To date, topiramate has not been associated with any hematologic or biochemical toxicities. Topiramate is associated with hepatic cytochrome P450 inducer and inhibitor interactions (Bazil & Bazil, 1997). Topiramate is a potent CNS depressant; to mini-

TABLE 57-8	Interactions of New Antiepileptic Drugs			
	Effect on the Plasma Levels of Other Drugs			
Drug	*PHT*	*CBZ*	*VPA*	*PB*
FBM	FBM↓ PHT↑	FBM↓ CBZ↓*	FBM↑ VPA↑	FBM↓ PB↑
GPT	GPT NC PHT NC	GPT NC CBZ NC	GPT NC VPA NC	GPT NC PB NC
LTG	LTG↓ PHT NC	LTG↓ CBZ NC	LTG↑ VPA NC	LTG↓ PB NC
TPM	TPM↓ PHT NC or ↑	TPM↓ CBZ NC	TPM↓ VPA↓	Effect on TPM unknown; PB NC

PHT, phenytoin; CBZ, carbamazepine; VPA, valproate; PB, phenobarbital; FBM, felbamate; GPT, gabapentin; LTG, lamotrigine; TPM, topiramate; NC, no change.

* The 10,11-epoxide metabolite increases, so CBZ dose may require reduction.

Bazil, M.K. and Bazi, C. (1997). Recent advances in the pharmacotherapy of epilepsy. *Clinical Therapeutics*, 19(3), 372.

mize neurotoxic effects, it must be initiated at low doses and titrated upward slowly for 8 weeks. Topiramate's half-life is approximately 21 hours, but to minimize neurotoxicity, twice-daily dosing is recommended.

TEACHING AND SELF-CARE

Patients and their family and friends must plan ahead to maintain safety at work and at home. Many patients are hesitant to discuss their medical condition, in part because of the stigma associated with seizure disorders. Patients need to be encouraged to discuss their condition with the health-related staff at work or school so that proper care can be provided in the event of a seizure.

Having sufficient supplies of medications is critical. Patients should be encouraged to carry medications in at least two separate pieces of luggage in case one is misplaced. Having a sufficient amount of medication mailed to a destination is another way to avoid missing doses.

Patients need to know that any change in medication needs to be made gradually. A calendar or days-in-the-week pill box may help the patient avoid missing doses of medication.

Some patients who experience an aura may find it helpful to practice getting to the ground to avoid injury from a fall. Practicing moving to a safe area, away from sharp objects, may decrease the chance of an accident.

COMMUNITY RESOURCES

Local resources may be available related to support groups as well as more controversial subjects like seizure-alert dogs.

Epilepsy Foundation, 4351 Garden City Drive, Landover, MD 20785-2267, 301-459-3700, 800-EFA-1000.

References

Annegers, J.F., Hauser, W.A., Beghi, E., Nicolosi, A., & Kurland, L.T. (1988). The risk of unprovoked seizures after encephalitis and meningitis. *Neurology, 38,* 1407–1410.

Bazil, M.K., & Bazil, C.W. (1997). Recent advances in the pharmacotherapy of epilepsy. *Clinical Therapeutics, 19,* 369–382.

Cascino, G.D. (1993). Antiepileptic drug management in patients with seizure disorders. *Hospital Formulary, 28,* 154–172.

Commission on Classification and Terminology of the International League Against Epilepsy. (1981). Proposal for revised clinical and electroencephalographic classification of epileptic syndromes. *Epilepsia, 22,* 489–501.

Commission on Classification and Terminology of the International League Against Epilepsy. (1989). Proposal for revised classification of epilepsies and epileptic syndromes. *Epilepsia, 30,* 389–399.

DeLorenzo, R.J., Towne, A.R., Pellock, J.M., et al. (1992). Status epilepticus in children, adults, and the elderly. *Epilepsia, 33*(suppl. 4), S15–S25.

Department of Health, Education and Welfare. (1978). *Plan for nationwide action on epilepsy* (DHEW publication NIH 78-726).

Dodson, W.E., DeLorenzo, R.J., Pedley, T.A. et al. (1993). Treatment of convulsive status epilepticus. *JAMA, 270,* 854–859.

Engel, J., Jr. (1989). *Seizures and epilepsy.* Philadelphia: F.A. Davis.

Faught, E., Sachdeo, R.C., Remler, M.P., et al. (1993). Felbamate monotherapy for partial-onset seizures: An active-control trial. *Neurology, 43,* 688–692.

Felbamate Study Group in Lennox-Gastaut Syndrome. (1993). Efficacy of felbamate in childhood epileptic encephalopathy (Lennox-Gastaut syndrome). *N Engl J Med, 328,* 29–33.

Franceschetti, S., Battagha, G., Lodrini, S., et al. (1988). Relationship between tumors and epilepsy. In G. Groggi (Ed.). *The rational basis of surgical treatment of epilepsies.* London: John Libbey.

French, J. (1994). The long-term therapeutic management of epilepsy. *Annals of Internal Medicine, 120,* 411–422.

Gates, J.R., Luciano, D., & Devinsky, O. (1991). The classification and treatment of nonepileptic events. In O. Devinsky & W.H. Theodore (Eds.). *Epilepsy and behavior,* pp. 251–263. New York: Wiley-Liss.

Hauser, W.A., & Annegers, J. (1991). Risk factors for epilepsy. *Epilepsy Research,* Suppl 4, 45–52.

Hauser, W.A., & Annegers, J.F. (1992). Epidemiology of epilepsy. In J.P. Laidaw, A. Reichens, & D. Chadwick (Eds.). *Textbook of epilepsy,* 4th ed. New York: Churchill-Livingstone.

Hauser, W.A., Annegers, J.F., & Kurland, L.T. (1991). Prevalence of epilepsy in Rochester, Minnesota: 1940–1980. *Epilepsia, 32,* 429–445.

Hauser, W.A., Morris, M.L., Heston, L.L., et al. (1986). Seizures and myoclonus in patients with Alzheimer's disease. *Neurology, 36,* 1226.

Hoffman, R.S. (1994). Fluid, electrolyte, and acid–base principles. In L.R. Goldfrank, N.E. Flomenbaum, N.A. Lewin, et al (Eds.). *Goldfrank's toxicologic emergencies,* pp. 283–295. Norwalk, CT: Appleton & Lange.

Holmes, G.L. (1993). Critical issues in the treatment of epilepsy. *American Journal of Hospital Pharmacy, 50* (suppl 5), S5–16.

Kinnunen, E., & Wikstrom, J. (1986). Prevalence and prognosis of epilepsy in patients with multiple sclerosis. *Epilepsia, 27,* 729.

Mattson, R.H., Cramer, J.A., Collins, J.F., and the Department of Veterans Affairs Epilepsy Cooperative Study No. 264 Group. (1992). A comparison of valproate with carbamazepine for the treatment of complex partial seizures and secondarily generalized tonic-clonic seizures in adults. *N Engl J Med, 327,* 765–771.

Meldrum, B.S. (1992). Excitatory amino acids in epilepsy and potential novel therapies. *Epilepsy Research, 12,* 189–196.

Pacia, S.V., Devinsky, O., Luciano, D.J., & Vazquez, B. (1994). The prolonged QT syndrome presenting as epilepsy: A report of two cases and literature review. *Neurology, 44,* 1408–1410.

Risner, M., and the Lamictal Study Group. (1994). Multicenter, double-blind, placebo-controlled, add-on, crossover study of lamotrigine (Lamictal) in epileptic outpatients with partial seizures. *Epilepsia, 31,* 619–620.

U.S. Gabapentin Study Group No. 5. (1993). Gabapentin as add-on therapy in refractory partial epilepsy: A double-blind, placebo-controlled, parallel-group study. *Neurology, 43,* 2292–2298.

Ziegler, D.K., Lin, J., & Bayer, W.L. (1978). Convulsive syncope: Relationship to cerebral ischemia. *Transactions of the American Neurologic Association, 103,* 150–154.

CHAPTER
58

Stroke, Transient Ischemic Attacks, and Carotid Stenosis

Willem Wisselink, MD, and Thomas F. Panetta, MD

Stroke is the third leading cause of death in the United States. Approximately 2 million people are affected annually, with the highest incidence in elderly men—1440 cases annually per 100,000 men over 75 years old. The estimated yearly cost of stroke disability is $16.8 billion in the United States. Stroke, also referred to as cerebrovascular accident (CVA) or brain attack, is associated with an initial death rate of 15% to 35%. Of those who survive, approximately one third will recover to near-normal function; another third will have residual deficits but can return to work. Twenty-five percent of stroke victims are permanently disabled to a degree that they cannot perform their professional duties; the remaining 6% to 8% require custodial care. Only 50% of patients who suffer a CVA are alive 5 years later, and 25% will have a second stroke, for which the death rate is 62%.

Because of these devastating sequelae, prevention of stroke is a primary concern. Early recognition and treatment of persons at risk may lead to a decreased incidence. Risk factors for cerebrovascular arterial disease include hypertension, smoking, obesity, aging, male gender, and hyperlipidemia. With regard to etiology, a stroke can be ischemic or hemorrhagic. Ischemic strokes, in turn, can be caused by embolization or hypoperfusion. Embolic strokes frequently result from migration of a thrombus from the heart or from an ulcerated lesion in the carotid artery to the brain. Hypoperfusion may result from a tight stenosis in the carotid artery, causing brain ischemia in the corresponding hemisphere. Hemorrhagic stroke, accounting for some 25% of cases, is caused by hypertensive intracerebral hemorrhage, ruptured saccular intracranial aneurysm, hemorrhage associated with bleeding disorders, or arteriovenous malformations.

DEFINITIONS

Patients with ischemic cerebrovascular disease are usually classified by clinical presentation:

- Asymptomatic carotid stenosis
- Transient ischemic attacks (TIA)
- Reversible ischemic neurologic deficits
- Chronic cerebral ischemia
- Vertebrobasilar symptoms
- Stroke in evolution
- Completed stroke.

Patients with hemorrhagic strokes are categorized by the location of the bleeding: intracerebral, subarachnoid, subdural, or epidural.

An *asymptomatic carotid stenosis* is any preocclusive atherosclerotic plaque in the common carotid artery, the carotid bifur-

cation, or the internal carotid artery in a patient with no ipsilateral monocular or cerebral hemispheric symptoms. A number of asymptomatic carotid stenoses are detected by the presence of a bruit during simple auscultation of the neck. Alternatively, a patient may undergo a carotid imaging test as part of routine screening or a preoperative workup (eg, a patient who is prepared for coronary artery bypass grafting), or because of contralateral hemispheric symptoms.

TIAs are focal neurologic deficits that resolve within 24 hours. TIAs are quite variable and may cover the entire spectrum of neurologic dysfunction, ranging from complete hemiparesis to just a small loss of sensation in an extremity. *Amaurosis fugax* (transient blindness) is a type of transient attack in which the patient experiences an episode of monocular blindness, usually described as "a shade coming down over the eye." During the funduscopic exam, small, bright-yellowish material may be seen in the retinal arteries. Hollenhorst, an ophthalmologist at the Mayo Clinic, first identified these plaques as small emboli consisting of cholesterol crystals, which were most likely to originate from a diseased carotid bifurcation.

Amaurosis fugax in the absence of Hollenhorst plaques can be caused by platelet fibrin complex emboli that have subsequently dissipated, emboli in the choroidal circulation that cannot be visualized on funduscopic examination, or symptomatic low flow states. White, nonscintillating calcific emboli and diffuse pallor of the disc have also been described. Plaques in the retina have been associated with all forms of cerebrovascular disease and are a marker for both systemic atherosclerosis and atherosclerotic coronary artery disease.

Crescendo TIAs are monocular or hemispheric symptoms that resolve within minutes after each episode but increase in frequency, eventually occurring multiple times on a daily basis.

Reversible ischemic neurologic deficits is an obsolete term for symptoms that persist longer than 24 hours but resolve within 72 hours. These patients are now referred to as having sustained a stroke with full recovery.

Chronic cerebral ischemia is a term reserved for patients with less specific symptoms such as lightheadedness, (pre)syncope, ataxia, or even a subjective impression of compromised cerebral function. It is associated with the presence of multiple extracranial cerebrovascular occlusions.

Disease of the *vertebrobasilar system* can result in any combination of motor dysfunction, sensory loss, homonymous visual field deficits, or, more specifically related to the posterior circulation, loss of balance, vertigo, dysequilibrium, diplopia, dysarthria, and dysphagia.

A *stroke in evolution* is a neurologic deficit that progresses or fluctuates while the patient is under observation.

A frank *stroke* is defined as a sudden, nonconvulsive, focal neurologic deficit that is no longer changing and has persisted for more than 72 hours. Hemorrhagic stroke is subdivided into *primary intracerebral hemorrhage*, believed to originate from arteries weakened by chronic hypertension, and *spontaneous subarachnoid hemorrhage*, resulting from a ruptured saccular aneurysm.

ANATOMY, PHYSIOLOGY, AND PATHOLOGY

Blood supply to the brain occurs through paired carotid and vertebral arteries, all of which contribute to the circle of Willis. From the circle of Willis, which lies in the subarachnoid space at the base of the skull and is a complete circle in only 30% of people, the anterior, middle, and posterior cerebral arteries arise (Fig. 58-1). The carotid bifurcation, by far the most common site of atherosclerotic disease of the extracranial cerebral vessels, is located at the midcervical level (usually between C3 and C4). Occasionally, it may be as high as C1 or as low as T2. The internal carotid artery normally lies posterolateral to the external carotid and can be distinguished by its complete lack of branches in the neck. The vertebral arteries fuse at the base of the skull to form the basilar artery, which in turn gives rise to the posterior communicating arteries.

Anatomic variations include the so-called bovine arch, where the common carotid artery arises directly from the innominate artery (10%), an aberrant right subclavian artery originating distal to the left subclavian artery and passing behind the esophagus (0.5 to 1%), and, less commonly, a right or double aortic arch. Rarely, the internal carotid artery is congenitally absent or hypoplastic. The vertebral arteries may arise directly from the aorta, from various locations of the subclavian arteries, or directly from the carotids. Kinks and coils of the carotid arteries, seen in 10% to 15% of patients, are the result of disproportionate embryonic migration of these arteries in relation to the central nervous system. Unless associated with atherosclerotic disease, kinking and coiling are usually benign conditions and are not related to either age or hypertension.

More than any other organ, the brain depends from minute to minute on an adequate blood supply. If deprived of oxygenated blood for 4 to 5 minutes, irreversible damage occurs in the form of ischemic necrosis or infarction. This common end point, also referred to as softening of the brain or encephalomalacia, can be the result of many different pathologic alterations in the circulation, including atherosclerosis, thrombosis, atheroembolism, fibromuscular dysplasia, arteritis, hypertensive hemorrhage, hemorrhage from intracranial aneurysms or arteriovenous malformations, trauma, and hematologic disorders.

Although atherosclerosis is a generalized process, specific vessels, such as the abdominal aorta and the orifices of its major branches, are particularly susceptible. The superficial femoral artery and the coronary and carotid arteries also are frequently involved. Even within susceptible arteries, certain areas are particularly likely to be affected: carotid plaque is usually confined to the bifurcation of the common carotid artery and the bulbar, proximal area of the internal carotid artery. This is one of the reasons carotid endarterectomy can be relatively easily performed: only a short segment of carotid artery is usually involved, which enables the surgeon to reach "clean" end points proximal and distal to the endarterectomy site.

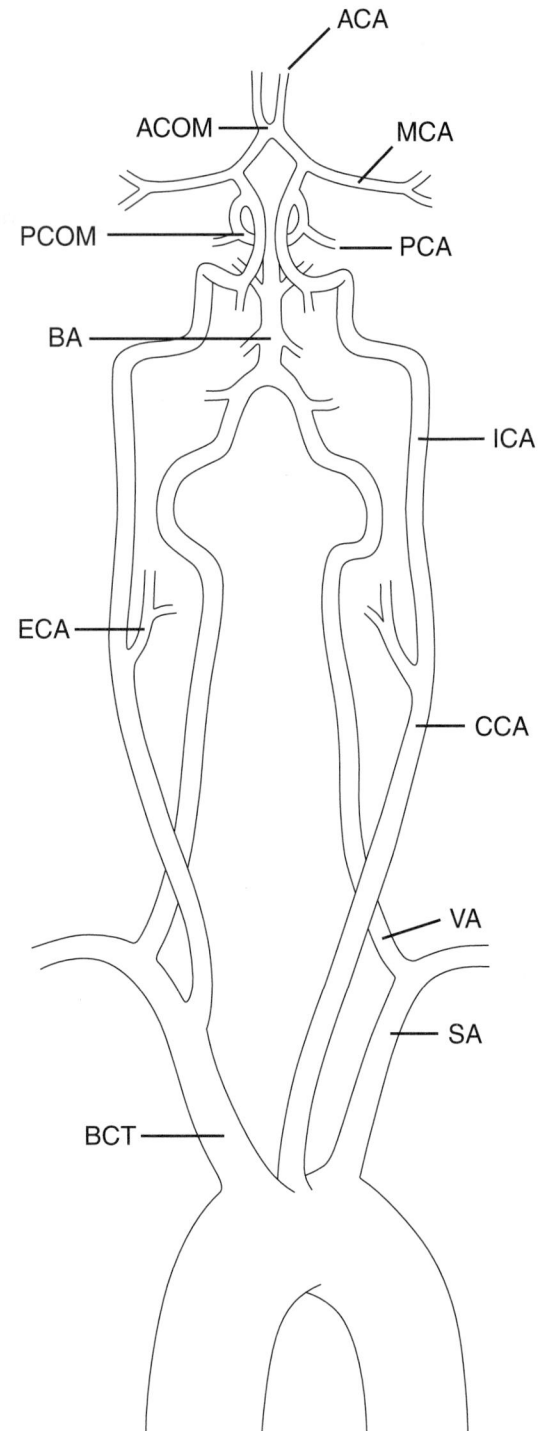

FIGURE 58-1 Schematic representation of the arterial circulation to the brain. ACA, anterior cerebral artery; MCA, middle cerebral artery; ACOM, anterior communicating artery; PCOM, posterior communicating artery; PCA, posterior cerebral artery; BA, basilar artery; ICA, internal carotid artery; ECA, external carotid artery; CCA, common carotid artery; VA, vertebral artery; SA, subclavian artery; BCT, brachiocephalic trunk (Wolf PA, Kannel WB, Verter J. [1983]. Current status of risk factors for stroke. *Neurol Clin*, 1: 317–343.)

Thrombosis occurs if flow in a diseased artery decreases to a critical threshold. Emboli may arise from the heart in the form of mural thrombi or valvular vegetations. Mural thrombus may be the result of atrial fibrillation or myocardial infarction. Alternative sources for emboli to the brain are atherosclerotic plaques and ulcers in the aortic arch or the carotid arteries. Fibromuscular dysplasia is a disease that affects mainly women in their third or fourth decade of life and leads to a classic "chain of beads" appearance of the internal carotid artery.

The term "arteritis" covers a mixed bag of disorders, including the connective tissue diseases, such as polyarteritis nodosa, lupus erythematosus, temporal arteritis, and Takayasu disease, and infectious processes, such as syphilis or tuberculosis.

Hemorrhagic stroke may occur as a result of a hypertensive crisis or from rupture of a saccular aneurysm or an arteriovenous malformation. The problem may also lie in the blood itself (bleeding disorders such as thrombocytopenia or the use of anticoagulants and fibrinolytic agents).

Primary (hypertensive) intracerebral hemorrhage occurs almost without exception within the brain tissue itself. Rupture of arteries in the subarachnoid space is unheard of unless aneurysms are present. The extravasated blood forms a roughly circular or oval mass that disrupts and compresses the surrounding tissue and increases in size as the bleeding continues. In the first hours after a bleed, edema accumulates around the clot, adding to its mass effect. If the mass effect is significant, shift of the midline structures and compression of the brain stem may occur, leading to coma and death. A satisfactory explanation as to why these intracerebral arteries rupture does not exist, but rupture is believed to occur in areas in the arteries that have been weakened by the effects of chronic hypertension.

Spontaneous subarachnoid hemorrhage from a saccular aneurysm of one of the arteries of the circle of Willis is the second most common cause of hemorrhagic stroke. Extravasated blood floods the subarachnoid space (in which these arteries reside) and increases intracranial pressure. Because the hemorrhage is confined to the subarachnoid space, there are few or no lateralizing symptoms, which may greatly delay the correct diagnosis.

EPIDEMIOLOGY

Stroke is generally considered a disease of middle-aged and elderly persons. In the Framingham study (Kiely et al, 1993; Wolf et al, 1983), stroke rates gradually increased with age in men and escalated dramatically after menopause in women. National surveys (Weinfield, 1981) have indicated that no more than 3% of cerebral infarctions occur in patients younger than 45 years. In contrast, however, a recent study evaluating a large number of hospital admission records found that 25% of patients admitted with the diagnosis of cerebral infarction were 50 or younger. A possible explanation is the improved recognition of stroke-related symptoms in young people.

In the United States, stroke incidence has been nearly equally distributed across racial lines; however, African American men have much higher age-adjusted stroke death rates than do men and women of other races. Recently, however, hospitalized stroke was found to be twice as frequent in African Americans compared to whites, both men and women, in a study in northern Manhattan (Sacco et al, 1991). In another study, ethnic differences appeared to reflect the impact of various stroke risk factors in patients with nonhemorrhagic infarcts. The study population was divided into white, African American, or Hispanic patients. Recurrent stroke, death from stroke, or both were most frequent in whites and least frequent in Hispanics, especially in the first year after stroke. Hypertension was more prevalent in African Americans and Hispanics. The incidence of cardiac disease was highest in whites and lowest in Hispanics. Thus, African Americans and Hispanics may have an increased burden of stroke risk factors to account for their increased incidence of stroke. Ongoing case-control and cohort studies are aimed at determining whether these differences persist after controlling for differences in socioeconomic status and access to medical care. Knowledge of the varying effects of risk factors in ethnic groups, however, may raise the level of suspicion and promote more aggressive treatment of such factors in persons of different ethnicity.

DIAGNOSTIC CRITERIA

The mode of presentation of cerebrovascular disease is so distinctive that the diagnosis is seldom in doubt. Stroke may vary in presentation from, most severely, hemiplegia or even coma to milder forms, such as numbness of a small part of the body. The key factor in the diagnosis of acute stroke, however, is the distinction between hemorrhage and ischemia. Treatment goals for each condition are linearly opposed: in hemorrhagic stroke, the aim is to limit further extravasation of blood by controlling blood pressure and promoting coagulation, whereas treatment of ischemic stroke is directed toward augmenting blood supply to the affected area. Needless to say, treatment modalities for one condition are likely to be harmful for the other.

HISTORY AND PHYSICAL EXAM

The denominative feature in the patient history is the temporal profile of neurologic events. The abruptness of onset of neurologic deficits is the hallmark of a vascular cause. Embolic strokes usually occur suddenly, without warning, and the deficit reaches its peak almost instantly. Thrombotic strokes usually develop slightly more gradually and sometimes in stepwise fashion. Hypertensive hemorrhage is almost always preceded by severe headaches and may cause a steadily progressive deficit over a period of minutes or hours.

Another important aspect of the temporal profile of stroke, as opposed to for example a brain tumor, is the arrest and then regression of the neurologic deficit. Embolic deficits, in particular, may improve dramatically over a period of hours to days, whereas reversal of thrombotic deficits is characteristically more gradual over weeks to months. A history of vomiting and seizures with the onset of the neurologic deficit points to a hemorrhagic cause, whereas severe headaches and altered consciousness without lateralizing symptoms may be the first symptoms of a subarachnoid bleed from a saccular arterial aneurysm.

On physical exam, hemiplegia stands out as the classic sign of all cerebrovascular disease. In addition, particular symptoms and physical findings are strongly related to the location of ischemic lesions in specific areas in the brain and their respective blood supply. Defects in areas supplied by the middle cerebral artery typically involve the cortex, basal ganglia, and internal capsule and result in contralateral hemiplegia, global aphasia when the dominant hemisphere is involved, head and eye deviation toward the side of the infarct, hemianesthesia, and hemianopsia (neglect of the opposite side).

Less typical signs include mental confusion, sensory deficits, aphasia, dysarthria, visual deficits, diplopia, and dizziness. Aphasia is a language impairment that commonly accompanies a CVA in the dominant hemisphere and may be receptive or expressive. Dysarthria is a speech impairment resulting from disturbances in muscular control. Neck rigidity is frequently found in the early stages of hemorrhagic stroke.

DIAGNOSTIC STUDIES

The combination of history and physical findings frequently allows for an accurate determination of the size and localization of the lesion, as well as a differentiation between hemorrhage and infarction. However, more definitive and highly accurate information is derived from imaging techniques such as computed tomography (CT), magnetic resonance imaging (MRI), magnetic resonance angiography (MRA), Doppler ultrasound (duplex scanning), transcranial Doppler, and arteriography.

With CT scanning, small hematomas, hemorrhagic infarcts, subarachnoid blood, clots surrounding aneurysms and arteriovenous malformations, shifts of the midline, and deformities of the ventricles can be diagnosed. Acute ischemic stroke is usually not visualized with CT until frank infarct necrosis occurs, usually 15 to 30 hours after the initial insult. MRI demonstrates all of the above lesions, with the additional ability to image areas of hypoperfusion (eg, fresh ischemic infarctions). With MRA, all cervical and intracranial arteries can be seen. If available, MRI is currently preferred over CT for the diagnosis and localization of ischemic stroke (Warach et al, 1995; Muto et al, 1996).

Duplex scanning (a combination of ultrasound and Doppler techniques) is used to image plaques and stenoses in the carotid and vertebral arteries, whereas transcranial Doppler allows visualization of the circle of Willis and its major branches. Both imaging modalities, depending on the skills of the person performing the study, provide not only an image but also real-time characteristics of blood flow in the arteries studied. Flow velocity—the actual speed of blood particles in a sample area of the blood vessel—is directly related to the degree of narrowing. For example, peak systolic velocities in the range of 150 to 200 cm/sec or above correspond to a hemodynamically significant lesion. Another indicator of vascular disease on duplex scanning is the presence of turbulent flow.

Although it is often replaced by duplex ultrasonography and MRA, contrast arteriography is still the gold standard in imaging both the cervical and intracranial circulation. Echocardiography is important in the workup of stroke patients because cardioembolism is the cause of roughly 25% to 30% of ischemic strokes.

Positron emission tomography and single photon emission computed tomography are newer imaging studies that measure the cerebral concentration of systemically administered radioactive isotopes. Cerebral blood flow, oxygen uptake, and glucose use can be measured. These tests have proved to be of value in grading brain tumors and localizing epileptic foci. As yet, this technology is found in relatively few medical centers and is not commonly used for routine diagnosis.

Laboratory tests are mostly nonspecific in patients with stroke. A mildly elevated white blood cell count may be seen in patients with ischemic stroke, whereas in hemorrhagic stroke counts may go up as high as 20,000 cells/mm^3. Blood coagulation studies may unmask a bleeding disorder or a hypercoagulable state.

TREATMENT OPTIONS, EXPECTED OUTCOMES, AND COMPREHENSIVE MANAGEMENT

Treatment options for patients at risk for stroke or those who have actually sustained a CVA can be divided into several categories: treatment of acute stroke, prevention, and rehabilitation. In the acute phase of stroke, the choice of therapy depends entirely on the underlying pathologic mechanism, as was stressed earlier. In ischemic stroke, the goal is to improve circulation, whereas in hemorrhagic stroke, therapy is geared toward eliminating bleeding. Therapy, in general, may be divided into two parts: management of the acute phase and arrest of the pathologic process, and stroke prevention (primary, secondary, and tertiary).

Management of Acute Ischemic Stroke

Even when an ischemic stroke has developed, some of the affected brain tissue at the edges of the infarct (the so-called ischemic penumbra) may not be irreversibly damaged and will survive if blood flow can be re-established. On the assumption that cerebral perfusion is optimal in the horizontal position, patients are urged to lie down in the acute phase. Hypertension, if present, is treated only if the blood pressure is high enough to pose a risk to other organs, such as the heart and the kidneys. Although intuitively the concept of immediate restoration of blood flow is attractive, it is also fraught with potential dangers.

First, before attempting to improve circulation, hemorrhage needs to be ruled out by CT. Technical means to improve or restore cerebral circulation include the use of anticoagulant and fibrinolytic drugs, angioplasty, and carotid endarterectomy. Warfarin and heparin administration, although widely used to prevent TIAs and impending stroke, seems to be of little value in the acute phase of a completed stroke (Sandercock et al, 1993). Fibrinolytic drugs such as urokinase and recombinant tissue plasminogen activator (t-PA), however, have recently appeared to have a role in the treatment of acute stroke. Although in earlier studies the risk of bleeding complications outweighed the benefits, more recently a 30% increase in the number of patients recovering without a deficit was found if the drug was administered within 3 hours of the onset of symptoms (Del Zoppo et al, 1992). Similarly, the effects of early carotid angioplasty and endarterectomy have been disappointing unless performed within 2 or 3 hours of the onset of symptoms. Practically, this has been the case only for patients who developed their initial symptoms while in the hospital for other reasons.

Management of Acute Hemorrhagic Stroke

There is currently no specific therapy for acute cerebral hemorrhage. Cerebral hemorrhage is a space-occupying lesion and thus induces intracranial hypertension. To maintain adequate perfusion pressure, hypertension is treated only if mean arterial blood pressure rises to more than 130 to 150 mmHg. An immediate neurosurgical consultation should be obtained to evaluate the need for surgical decompression (Blecic & Bogousslavsky, 1995).

Preventive Strategies

Core preventive strategies relate to modification of risk factors amenable to change, including tobacco use, hypertension, cerebrovascular disease, and cardiac disease. In addition, health teaching and support efforts for populations thought to be at particular risk for these conditions may offer a major opportunity in stroke prevention.

Hypertension is the most readily recognized factor in the pathogenesis of intracerebral hemorrhage. Recent studies (Collins et al, 1990) have clearly demonstrated that long-term control of hypertension decreases the incidence of both intracerebral hemorrhage and atherothrombotic infarction. Congestive heart failure and coronary atherosclerosis greatly increase the probability of stroke in general; arrhythmias such as atrial fibrillation promote the occurrence of embolic stroke, in particular. Warfarin is currently the agent of choice in patients with nonvalvular atrial fibrillation to prevent embolic stroke.

In one study (Weinberger et al, 1983), diabetic patients were found to be twice as susceptible to stroke as their nondiabetic age-matched controls. The relation between long-term cigarette smoking and carotid atherosclerosis has been well documented, and recent clinical trials have demonstrated the effectiveness of cholesterol-lowering drug regimens in the prevention of stroke.

Aspirin is commonly prescribed for patients with a history of TIAs on the basis of prospective, randomized clinical trials showing a reduction in stroke rate in these patients. Dosages as low as 80 mg/day have shown effectiveness in recent clinical trials (Gorelick, 1995). Ticlopidine, a newer platelet inhibitor, also has been demonstrated to reduce stroke rates in patients with TIAs and minor strokes (Hass et al, 1989).

In addition, recent large, multicenter, prospective, randomized trials have clearly demonstrated the benefits of carotid endarterectomy as a measure for stroke prevention in both symptomatic and asymptomatic patients. In the North American Asymptomatic Carotid Atherosclerosis Study, patients with an asymptomatic carotid stenosis of 60% or greater (found on routine physical exam or screening) were prospectively assigned to undergo carotid endarterectomy and to receive aspirin, or to receive aspirin only. The number of strokes was reduced from 11% to 5% over 5 years in patients who had undergone endarterectomy compared to those who received aspirin only.

In the North American Symptomatic Carotid Endarterectomy Trial (1991), patients with a carotid stenosis of 70% or greater and a history of ipsilateral TIAs were randomized to undergo endarterectomy or not. The trial was interrupted when patients who had undergone the operation were found to have a 66% reduction in stroke rate over 5 years.

An estimated 30% to 50% of patients presenting with ischemic stroke are found to have surgically correctable extracranial cerebrovascular disease. Carotid endarterectomy is commonly performed under general anesthesia (local or regional anesthesia is reserved for certain high-risk patients) with intraoperative electroencephalography and transcranial Doppler monitoring. Shunting during the endarterectomy is performed selectively in patients with inadequate collateral circulation. The operation may last 1.5 to 3 hours, depending on the local anatomy and the extent of the dissection. Patients are monitored overnight to control blood pressure and to watch the neurologic status. Most patients leave the hospital the next day. Combined death and complication rates of the procedure are less than 2% in most modern series (Executive Committee, 1995). Carotid angioplasty and stenting is currently considered an experimental procedure, and relatively high complication rates have raised concern about the feasibility of this procedure (Konstadinos et al, 1996).

Warfarin has been shown to be beneficial in the prevention of recurrent stroke in the presence of atrial fibrillation and possibly in myocardial infarction (Beebe et al, 1996).

TEACHING AND SELF-CARE

Rehabilitation of patients with stroke is aimed toward a return to the highest level possible. Often, people who have had a stroke have chronic or long-lasting residual deficits that make full recovery impossible. In these situations, patients are encouraged to lead a full life within the constraints of disability.

Physiotherapy traditionally is begun within 2 to 4 weeks after stabilization of the clinical course. Occupational, speech, and language therapy, reorientation to visuospatial relations, and re-establishment of the patient's role in family life are all addressed early if appropriate. It is commonly recognized that recovery of ambulation and other important motor skills does not usually extend beyond 8 to 12 months. Interestingly, there is very little scientific basis for the effectiveness of various rehabilitation programs, despite the billions of dollars spent annually by third-party health insurance carriers. Although not proven, most providers agree that physiotherapy should begin promptly after the onset of symptoms. Passive range-of-motion exercises to prevent contractures require little or no cooperation from the patient and should be started within the first 24 hours of the diagnosis. Progression to active range of motion and strengthening exercises and re-education in activities of daily living should occur as soon as the patient can cooperate.

COMMUNITY RESOURCES

Community-based resources include organizations that provide direct aid to persons with stroke and their caregivers, those that furnish mail-order catalogs, and those that provide technology-related assistance. In the United States, many organizations can be called on to provide help for those who have suffered a stroke or who are at risk for doing so. A list of such organizations is made available by the National Stroke Association (NSA), a national voluntary health care organization committed to the prevention and treatment of stroke and the rehabilitation of stroke survivors. Activities include sponsoring research, promoting national awareness of stroke warning signs and risks, providing education, heightening awareness of the effectiveness of rehabilitation, and providing general support to people who have had a stroke and their families. The address is 300 E. Hampden Ave., Suite 240, Englewood, CO 80110-2654, 800-STROKES.

REFERRAL POINTS AND CLINICAL WARNINGS

Any patient with signs of a focal neurologic deficit such as hemiplegia, but also more subtle findings such as localized numbness or unexplained alterations in mental status, aphasia, dysarthria, visual defects, or dizziness, should be considered to have a stroke until proven otherwise. Immediate referral to an emergency room for further evaluation and prompt treatment is indicated.

Approximately 75% of stroke victims experienced some episodes of transient focal neurologic dysfunction that were ignored because "it went away." Recognition of these prodromal episodes may prevent a catastrophe.

EDITOR'S NOTE:

COMPLEMENTARY APPROACHES

A general discussion of complementary approaches can be found in Chapter 3. The following, while not an exhaustive list, are some complementary approaches being used for this condition. Additional information on these approaches, including precautions, can be found in Appendices A and B. Providers need to assess for the use of complementary approaches as part of the patient's history, as they may impact conventional therapies, and patients may not volunteer this information unless specifically asked. Efficacy of many complementary approaches is not as well documented as that of conventional therapies. Providers need to read the literature before suggesting these complementary approaches.

- Complementary Modalities
  Aromatherapy
  Craniosacral therapy

References

Beebe, H.G., Archie, J.P., et al. (1996). Concern about safety of carotid angioplasty. *Stroke, 27,* 197–198.

Blecic, S., & Bogousslavsky, J. (1995). Current management of acute stroke. In M. Fisher (Ed.). *Stroke therapy.* London: Butterworth.

Collins, R., Peto, R., Macmahon, S., et al. (1990). Blood pressure, stroke and coronary artery disease. *Lancet, 335,* 827.

Del Zoppo, G.J., Poek, K., et al. (1992). Recombinant tissue plasminogen activator in acute thrombotic and embolic stroke. *Annals of Neurology, 32,* 78–86.

Executive Committee for the Asymptomatic Carotid Stenosis Study. (1995). Endarterectomy for asymptomatic carotid artery stenosis. *JAMA, 273,* 1421–1428.

Gorelick, P.B. (1995). Stroke prevention. *Archives of Neurology, 52,* 347–355.

Hass, W.K., Easton, J.D., Adams, H.P., et al. (1989). A randomized trial comparing ticlopidine with aspirin for the prevention of stroke in high-risk patients. *N Engl J Med, 321,* 501.

Kiely, D.K., Wolf, P.A., Cupples, L.A., et al. (1993). Familial aggregation of stroke: The Framingham Study. *Stroke, 24,* 1366–1371.

Konstadinos, A.P., Kantis, G., et al. (1996). Carotid endarterectomy with homologous vein patch angioplasty: A review of 1006 cases. *Journal of Vascular Surgery, 24,* 109–119.

Muto, P.M., Welch, H.J., Mackey, W.C., & O'Donnel, T.F. (1996). Evaluation of carotid artery stenosis: Is duplex ultrasonography sufficient? *Journal of Vascular Surgery, 24,* 17–24.

North American Symptomatic Carotid Endarterectomy Trial Collaborators. (1991). Beneficial effect of carotid endarterectomy in symptomatic patients with high-grade stenosis. *N Engl J Med, 325,* 445–453.

Sacco, R.L., Hauser, W.A., & Mohr, J.P. (1991). Hospitalized stroke incidence in blacks and Hispanics in Northern Manhattan. *Stroke, 22,* 1491–1496.

Sandercock, P.A.G., van den Belt, A.G.M., Lindley, R.I., & Slattery, J. (1993). Antithrombotic therapy in acute ischaemic stroke: An overview of the completed randomized trials. *Journal of Neurology, Neurosurgery & Psychiatry, 56,* 17–25.

Warach, S., Gaa, J., Siewert, B., et al. (1995). Acute human stroke studied by whole brain echo planar diffusion weighted MRI. *Annals of Neurology, 37,* 231–241.

Weinberger, J., Biscarra, V., & Weisberg, M.K. (1983). Factors contributing to stroke in patients with atherosclerotic disease of the great vessels: The role of diabetes. *Stroke, 14,* 709.

Weinfield, F.D. (1981). National Survey of Stroke. *Stroke, 12,* 1–55.

Suggested Reading

Stroke prevention in atrial fibrillation investigators. (1994). Warfarin vs. aspirin for prevention of thromboembolism in atrial fibrillation. *Lancet, 343,* 687–691.

Yatsu, F.M., Grotta, J.C., Pettigrew, L.C. (1995). *Stroke: 100 maxims in neurology,* p. 7. St. Louis: Mosby.

CHAPTER
59

Anxiety Disorders, With an Emphasis on Panic Disorder

David S. Resch, MD

Anxiety is a nonspecific symptom that is a frequent experience in life. In a large case study, 24.4% of patients described themselves as nervous people, whereas 9.3% of the population described having a panic attack during their lifetime (Robins & Reiger, 1991; Wolfe & Mase, 1994). Anxiety becomes a disorder when it impairs a person's interpersonal, occupational, or social functioning (American Psychiatric Association [APA], 1994).

The APA's *Diagnostic and Statistical Manual,* 4th edition (DSM-IV), defines 12 types of anxiety disorders: panic disorder (PD) with agoraphobia, PD without agoraphobia, agoraphobia without history of PD, generalized anxiety disorder (GAD), specific phobia, social phobia, obsessive-compulsive disorder (OCD), post-traumatic stress disorder (PTSD), acute stress disorder (ASD), anxiety disorder due to a general medical condition, substance-induced anxiety disorder, and anxiety disorder not otherwise specified (APA, 1994).

These disorders can lead to significant disability and create a disproportionate number of office visits and medical care use. PD, GAD, OCD, and simple phobias are seen in 38.5% of primary care visits (Katon et al, 1986) and equate to 31.5% of the total costs of psychiatric disorders in the United States (Katon et al, 1992). Patients with PD have the highest rates of use of general medical, emergency, and psychiatric services of all psychiatric disorders (Katon et al, 1992).

Eighty-five percent to 88% of the time, these patients present to their primary care provider with a constellation of somatic complaints: palpitations, dizziness, shortness of breath, diarrhea, epigastric pain, chest pain, headache, hot flashes, or numbness of an extremity (Barbee et al, 1997). This variability in presentation can present a major clinical challenge to primary care providers. For example, 33% of patients with chest pain and negative angiograms suffer from PD. The extra costs of testing these patients exceed $33 million per year (Katon et al, 1992). Unnecessary emergency room visits are another cost associated with undiagnosed PD. Patients with PD may see as many as 10 different health care professionals before receiving the correct diagnosis (Katon et al, 1992).

ANXIETY DISORDERS IN GENERAL

The primary care provider will care for a large number of patients with anxiety disorders. The prevalence of these will rival other illnesses traditionally expected in a primary care clinic.

Table 59-1 lists the rates of incidence and prevalence for some common illnesses found a primary care clinic.

The responsibility for accurately diagnosing and subsequently treating patients requires a firm understanding of the various medical conditions and medications that can create an anxiety syndrome. The DSM-IV defines these disorders as anxiety disorder due to a general medical condition and substance-induced anxiety disorder, respectively. Tables 59-2 and 59-3 list some of the more common conditions and medications that can create anxiety.

These symptoms, individually or together, can mimic a number of medical conditions. Attempting to ascertain whether the patient's complaints result from an underlying anxiety disorder or other medical illness is difficult. The necessary screening tests for PD include a complete blood count, urinalysis, renal and hepatic studies, measurement of serum calcium and phosphorus levels, and an electrocardiogram (Raj & Sheehan, 1987). A thorough history of symptoms and temporal profile, combined with a physical exam, can effectively rule out a majority of medications, illicit drugs, and medical conditions that can produce an anxiety syndrome. Features such as onset after age 45 years or the presence of atypical symptoms during a panic attack (eg, vertigo, loss of consciousness, loss of bladder or bowel control, headaches, slurred speech, or amnesia) suggest the possibility that a general medical condition or a substance may be causing the panic attack symptoms.

PANIC DISORDER

PD is a chronic, often debilitating condition that can have devastating effects on a person's life, family, work, and social interactions. Because its symptoms mimic a variety of medical conditions, this disorder frequently goes undiagnosed. Fortunately, with increased education and awareness, the frequency of identification of PD has increased from 5% in 1980 to 59% in 1990. However, delayed diagnosis and high medical care use are still common (Gerdes et al, 1995).

Anatomy, Physiology, and Pathology

Theories regarding the nature and etiology of PD range from the biologic to the psychological: false suffocation alarms, serotonin dysregulation, respiratory drive dysregulation, and locus

TABLE 59-1	Prevalence of Common Primary Care Disorders in the United States	
Disorder/Illness	Lifetime Prevalence (%)	Primary Care Group Prevalence Diagnosed[c] (%)
Any substance abuse disorder	26.6[a]	
Hypertension	25.3[d]	
Smoking	25[c]	
Any anxiety disorder	24.9[a]	
Obesity	20[e]	
Major depressive disorder	20[b]	7.3–14.1
Phobias	14.3[b]	
Alcohol abuse/dependence	13.8[b]	3.2–5.2
Social phobia	13.3[a]	
Specific (simple) phobia	11.3[a]	
Generalized anxiety disorder	8.5[b]	2.8–3.7
Mitral valve prolapse	5–10[g]	
Drug abuse/dependence	6.2[b]	2.4
Diabetes mellitus	2–6[e]	
Asthma	4[c]	
Panic disorder	3.5[a]	4.8–6.2
Coronary artery disease	3.1[f]	
Obsessive-compulsive disorder	2.6[a]	1.4–2.2
Hypothyroidism	0.8[b]	

[a] Kessler et al, 1994

[b] Robins & Reiger, 1991

[c] Leon et al, 1995; Olfson et al, 1996; Wyngaarden et al, 1992

[d] Kaplan, 1992

[e] Farmer & Gotto, 1992

[f] Rutherford et al, 1992

[g] Braunwald, 1992

ceruleus dysfunction (Barlow & Lehman, 1996; Grove et al, 1997; Klein, 1993; Klein, 1996). Among the anxiety disorders, PD has been studied more often from a biologic perspective because there is an easy means of provoking panic attacks in vulnerable people: lactate infusions or inhalation of 5% to 35% CO_2 (Gorman et al, 1994). However, these research efforts have failed to identify consistently the presence of a specific neuroendocrine or other neurobiologic correlate of anxiety or panic attacks.

The role of genetics in PD has also been studied. Multiple family studies have found a higher rate of PD in the relatives of probands with the disorder. This finding has been seen consistently in all studies and in different countries. The risk to first-degree relatives of PD patients ranged from 2.6- to 20-fold, with a median value of 7.8 times that of the general population (Maier et al, 1993; Mendlewicz et al, 1993). Most of the studies were done on samples ascertained from treatment settings, and so this relative risk may be of a more severe form of PD.

Epidemiology

PD has been found in cultures throughout the world with prevalence rates of 0.4% to 3.5% (Weissman et al, 1997). PD without agoraphobia is diagnosed twice as often and PD with agora-phobia three times as often in women as in men. Approximately one third to one half of persons diagnosed with PD in community samples also have agoraphobia, although a much higher rate of agoraphobia is encountered in clinical samples (APA, 1994).

Age at onset for PD varies considerably but is usually between late adolescence and the mid-30s (Weissman et al, 1997). The mean age at onset of the disorder is earlier for women, at 25 to 34 years (30 to 44 years for men). The prevalence of existing cases steadily declines in age groups greater than 60 (1-month prevalence rates ranging from 0% to 0.3% compared with a peak prevalence rate of 0.7% in the 25-to-44-year-old age group) (Myers et al., 1984). In addition, illness such as chronic obstructive pulmonary disease can raise the risk of PD (to a level about five times that of the general population) (Karajgi et al, 1990).

Diagnostic Criteria

PD has two subtypes: with and without agoraphobia.

DIAGNOSTIC CRITERIA FOR PANIC DISORDER

- Recurrent unexpected panic attacks
- At least one of the attacks has been followed by one or more of the following for at least 1 month:
- Persistent concern about having additional attacks
- Worry about the implications of the attack
- A significant change in behavior.

SYMPTOMATOLOGY OF PANIC ATTACKS

- Shortness of breath/smothering sensations
- Dizziness, unsteady feelings, or faintness
- Palpitations/tachycardia
- Trembling/shaking
- Sweating
- Choking
- Nausea/abdominal distress
- Depersonalization (being detached from oneself)
- Derealization (feelings of unreality)
- Paresthesias (numbness or tingling sensations)
- Flushes/chills
- Chest pain or discomfort
- Fear of dying
- Fear of going crazy or doing something uncontrolled.

DIAGNOSTIC CRITERIA FOR AGORAPHOBIA

- Anxiety about being in places or situations from which escape might be difficult or embarrassing
- Situations are avoided or else endured with significant distress.

Natural History of Illness/Comorbidity

Patients receiving ongoing, established treatments for PD show a higher rate of recovery; many of these patients continue to have mild to moderate symptoms (Barlow, 1990). Relapse rates

TABLE 59-2	Medical Causes of Anxiety or Anxiety Disorder Due to General Medical Conditions	
Cardiology	Angina pectoris	Hypovolemia
	Arrhythmias	Myocardial infarction
	Congestive heart failure	Valvular heart disease
	Hypertension	
Dietary	Caffeinism	Monosodium glutamate
Hematologic	Anemia	
Immunologic	Anaphylaxis	Systemic lupus erythematosus
Infectious	Brucellosis	Lyme borreliosis
	Cerebral syphilis	Poliomyelitis
	Encephalitis	
Metabolic	Acute intermittent porphyria	Hypocalcemia
	Addison's disease	Hypoglycemia
	Cushing's disease	Hyponatremia
	Hypercalcemia	Hypopituitarism
	Hyperparathyroidism	Hypothyroidism
	Hyperthermia	Virilization syndromes
	Hyperthyroidism	
Neurologic	Dementia	Myopathies
	Essential tremor	Polyneuritis
	Intracranial mass/tumors	Postconcussive syndrome
	Meniere's disease	Partial complex seizure disorders
	Multiple sclerosis	Vertigo
	Myasthenia gravis	Wilson's disease
Respiratory	Asthma	Pneumonia
	Chronic obstructive pulmonary disease	Pulmonary edema
	Chronic pulmonary hypertension	Pulmonary emboli
		Hypoxemia
Secreting Tumors	Carcinoid	Pheochromocytoma
	Insulinoma	

Adapted from Gorroll et al, 1995, with additional data from Fallon et al, 1993; Ballentine & Kettle, 1998.

are high after discontinuation of effective treatment (Noyes et al, 1992), which suggests that PD is a chronic condition with a very low rate of spontaneous recovery.

Although agoraphobia may develop at any point, its onset is usually within the first year of occurrence of recurrent panic attacks. The course of agoraphobia and its relation to the course of panic attacks are variable. In some cases, a decrease or remission of panic attacks may be followed closely by a corresponding decrease in agoraphobic avoidance and anxiety. In others, agoraphobia may become chronic regardless of the presence or absence of panic attacks (Noyes et al, 1990).

At the present state of our knowledge, there are few signs and symptoms that predict with certainty the onset of PD. The age of risk for onset extends well into middle age, with the 20th percentile at about 25 years and the median at about 35 years. The prodromal period is about 10 to 15 years long, with 20% of affected persons reporting their first panic attack at about age 14 years, and about 50% reporting a panic attack by about 20 years. The simple question, "Are you a nervous person?" would help identify more than 60% of persons with onset of PD in the next year. The occurrence of a panic attack accompanied by tachycardia would identify 45% of the cases of PD over the next year (Eaton et al, 1995).

Factors associated with increasing impairment were fewer years of education, increasing age, the presence of major depression, and a higher level of neuroticism and to a lesser extent male gender and being non-Hispanic (Hollifield et al, 1997; Karajgi et al, 1990). Patients with PD are at a higher risk than the general population for major depression, substance abuse, suicide attempts, marital problems, and financial dependency.

■ ■ ■ CLINICAL PEARL

In addition to morbidity, patients with PD also have a higher rate of death from suicide, cardiovascular disorders, and stroke.

Suicide accounts for approximately 20% of deaths of patients with PD. This rate is considerably higher than the rate for the general population (Noyes, 1991). The rate of suicide attempts in uncomplicated PD is considerably higher than in subjects with no psychiatric disorder. Even more alarming is the rate at which patients with comorbid major depression and PD kill themselves (19.5%) compared to the rate for patients with uncomplicated PD (7%) (Johnson et al, 1990).

Death from other causes is also increased in PD patients. Patients with PD had a risk of stroke twice that of persons with other psychiatric disorders or no psychiatric disorder (Weissman et al, 1990). PD has been shown to be associated with hypertension (Weissman et al, 1990), increased resting heart rate (Chignon et al, 1993; Freeman et al, 1995), increased cardiac ventricular size (Kahn et al, 1990), and decreased cerebral blood flow (Gibbs, 1992). All these physiologic changes have been theorized to play a role in the increased death rate for cerebrovascular and cardiovascular events, by arguing an abnormality in the sympathetic nervous system that leads to increased reactivity and poor tonal control.

Treatment Options, Expected Outcomes, and Comprehensive Management

Treatment options can be divided into pharmacologic and psychological interventions; often these two modalities can be used concomitantly. The most common psychological interventions

TABLE 59-3	Medications That Can Cause Anxiety or Substance-Induced Anxiety Disorders

Aminophylline	Estrogens
Amphetamines	Hallucinogens
Anesthetics	Insulin
Anorectics	Interferon alpha
Fenfluramine	Isoniazid
Dexfenfluramine	Levodopa
Phenteramine	Mefloquine
Anticholinergics	Metrizamide
Anticonvulsants	Metronidazole
Antidepressants	Muscle relaxants
Isocaboxazid	Cyclobenzaprine
Tricyclics	Narcotics
SSRIs	Neuroleptic agents
Buproprion	Prochlorperazine
Antihistamines	Metoclopramide
Antihypertensives	Nonsteroidal anti-inflammatory
ACE inhibitors	agents
Captopril	Norfloxacin
Enalapril	Pergolide
Alpha antagonists	Procaine derivatives
Calcium channel blockers	Quinacrine
Nifedipine	Salicylate overdose
Hydralazine	Sympathomimetics
Baclofen	Phenylephrine
Bromocriptine	Pseudoephedrine
Bronchodilators (methylxanthines)	Ephedrine
Buspirone	Phenylpropylamine
Caffeine	Theophylline
Chronic elemental mercury	Thiabendazole
exposure	Thyroid preparations
Cocaine	Withdrawal syndromes
Corticosteroids	Alcohol
Cycloserine	Benzodiazepines
Dapsone	Barbiturates
Digitalis toxicity	Ethchlorvynol
Disopyramide	
Dronabinol	

Adapted from Gorroll et al, 1995; *Medical Letter,* 1993.

are cognitive-behavioral therapy (CBT), exposure therapy, and psychodynamic therapy. Pharmacologic options can include benzodiazepines, selective serotonin reuptake inhibitors (SSRIs), tricyclic antidepressants (TCAs), or monoamine oxidase inhibitors (MAOIs).

The provider, in consultation with the patient, should select as the initial treatment one with demonstrated efficacy. Attitudes and concerns regarding various treatment options must be explored and decisions negotiated with the patient. Patients should be educated about the disorder and encouraged to re-enter phobic situations gradually when medication alone is chosen as the initial treatment. Current practice suggests that an absence of any noticeable improvement after about 6 to 8 weeks of any treatment should lead to a reassessment, consultation, or change of modality.

COGNITIVE-BEHAVIORAL THERAPY

CBT teaches patients to anticipate the situations and bodily sensations associated with their panic attacks. This awareness sets the stage for helping the patient to control the attacks. Specially trained therapists tailor CBT to the specific needs of each patient. The therapy usually includes the following components:

- Informational overview of the cycle of anxiety and the anticipation of further anxiety episodes, and rationale for the treatment
- Helping patients to identify and change patterns of thinking that cause them to misperceive common events or situations as dangerous and to think the worst. For example, the therapist can help the patient to replace alarmist thoughts such as, "I'm dying" with more appropriate ones, such as "I'm hyperventilating; I can handle this."
- Teaching the patient relaxation exercises to prevent or minimize the symptoms commonly felt during a panic attack
- Helping patients becomes less fearful by safely and gradually exposing them to situations they previously avoided or found frightening. This step provides an opportunity to have patients practice their coping and relaxation skills in the anxiety-provoking event.

CBT is a short-term treatment, typically lasting 12 to 15 sessions over several months. Patients who undergo CBT demonstrate a high maintenance of treatment gains over time. Follow-up studies of 1 to 3 years have found patients to be free of panic attacks at least 81% of the time (Barlow, 1997; Beck et al, 1992; Brown et al, 1997). Fifty percent to 70% of the patients maintain a high level of functioning (minimal if any disability) during this same time frame. These numbers compare to 45% with imipramine for the same time frame (Clark et al, 1994; Craske et al, 1995). Some authors have argued that such comparisons are not valid because they fail to compare the treatments in a truly double-blind fashion within a single protocol (McNally, 1996).

PHARMACOTHERAPY

Anxiety disorder patients tend to be sensitive to medication and often experience exacerbation of their symptoms with medication, especially if too large an initial dose is used. The initial treatment goal is to block the panic attacks with pharmacotherapy, then to encourage the patient to enter phobic situations to help extinguish the avoidance behavior. Pharmacotherapy should be continued for 1 year after remission of the panic attacks to prevent relapse. After 12 months, the medication can be tapered. Two thirds of the patients will not relapse immediately after cessation of pharmacotherapy (Noyes et al, 1990). CBT can improve a patient's ability to be tapered off the drug and maintain control of symptoms at 6 months after discontinuation (Bruce et al, 1995).

Boyer (1995) performed a meta-analysis contrasting the effectiveness of the SSRIs (paroxetine, zimelidine [not available in the United States], fluvoxamine, and clomipramine) to imipramine and alprazolam in the treatment of PD. All treatments were superior to placebo in alleviating panic, and the SSRIs were superior to imipramine and alprazolam in alleviating panic.

Initially, SSRIs can be panicogenic. As such, they need to be initiated at low doses and slowly tapered up. For example, the titration rate for fluoxetine should be 5 mg/day for week 1, 10 mg/day for weeks 2 through 4, and 15 to 20 mg/day for week 5 and thereafter.

The dosage of imipramine may be as low as 25 mg/day. A total imipramine plasma concentration (imipramine plus desipramine level) of 110 to 140 ng/mL or a target imipramine dose of 2.25 mg/kg/day are optimal in the acute treatment of patients with PD with agoraphobia (Mavissakalian & Perel, 1995). The drug can be initiated at 10 to 25 mg/day, which can be increased to 150 to 200 mg/day over a 2- to 4-week period. Doses of other TCAs in the management of PD are typically in the antidepressant range.

Treatment with MAOIs is usually initiated at 15 mg/day and increased by 15 mg/day every week until a positive response or a maximum of 90 mg/day. Tranylcypromine is begun at 10 mg/day in the morning. The dose is raised 10 mg/day every week until a response is seen or a maximum of 80 mg/day. Because of the dietary restrictions and significant drug–drug interactions, these medications are usually reserved for patients who do not respond to the SSRIs or TCAs.

Symptoms responding to benzodiazepines include anxiety, the frequency and severity of panic attacks, and phobic fear and avoidance. With alprazolam, the number of panic attacks per week decreased by an average of 81% and were sometimes eliminated completely. More patients experienced moderate to marked improvement than with any other class of drugs. A decrease in anticipatory anxiety and disability at work and in family life and social life was reported. Unfortunately, a common complaint regarding the benzodiazepines is the difficulty in tapering patients off them. Slow benzodiazepine tapering results in re-emergent symptoms in 20% to 38% of patients (Sheehan & Raj, 1990).

This effect has led researchers to look at alternate agents that work on gamma-aminobutyric acid (GABA) receptors without the associated risk of withdrawal difficulty. Valproic acid also enhances GABA transmission. Two studies (Keck et al, 1993; Woodman & Noyes, 1994) using valproate show a 31% to 59% reduction in anxiety scores. However, these studies were not placebo-controlled, and with placebo responses of up to 50% (Cross National Collaborative Panic Study, 1992) in some studies, routine use of these agents cannot currently be recommended.

COMBINED THERAPY

Use of brief dynamic psychotherapy (15 weekly sessions) in conjunction with clomipramine therapy significantly reduces the 9-month relapse rate for PD (Wiborg & Dahl, 1996). A recent meta-analysis of studies comparing seven different treatment options (high-potency benzodiazepines, antidepressants, psychological panic management, exposure in vivo, pill-placebo combined with exposure, antidepressants combined with exposure, and psychological panic management combined with exposure in vivo) demonstrated that exposure in vivo was not effective. The remaining six treatments had the same effect in decreasing panic. Antidepressant use plus exposure in vivo was superior to all other treatments (van Balkrom et al, 1997).

- To differentiate PD from other medically important conditions, the patient should have a thorough physical exam. PD symptoms can mimic those of other conditions, such as myocardial infarction, cardiac arrhythmias, hyperthyroidism, and certain types of epilepsy.
- Patients may focus on only one or two symptoms as they describe the attacks, concentrating only on their physical sensations and not on the fears they experience.
- Panic attacks can also be triggered by large doses of caffeine, some cold medicines, and cocaine and marijuana. If a patient has a substance abuse problem, it will have to be treated before PD can be addressed fully.
- Even though panic attacks do not represent an immediate danger to the life of the patient, patients with PD have a higher death rate from vascular events.
- Patients with psychiatric comorbidities should be referred for further evaluation and treatment to a psychiatrist familiar with PD.

GENERALIZED ANXIETY DISORDER

GAD is an illness characterized by at least 6 months of persistent and excessive anxiety and worry. Adults with GAD often worry about everyday, routine life circumstances such as possible job responsibilities, finances, the health of family members, misfortune of their children, or minor matters such as household chores, car repairs, or being late for appointments. Although persons with GAD may not always identify their worry as excessive, they report objective distress from constant worry, have difficulty controlling the worry, or have related impairment in social, occupational, or other important areas of functioning (APA, 1994).

Epidemiology

In clinical settings, GAD is diagnosed somewhat more frequently in women than in men (about 55% to 60% of those presenting with the disorder are female) (APA, 1994). In a community sample, the 1-year prevalence rate for GAD was approximately 3% and the lifetime prevalence rate was 5.1% to 6.6% (Robins & Reiger, 1991; Wittchen et al, 1994).

Diagnostic Criteria

- Excessive anxiety and worry, occurring more days than not for the last 6 months, about a number of events or activities
- Difficulty controlling the worry
- The anxiety and worry are associated with three of the following six symptoms:
    Restlessness or feeling keyed up or on edge
    Irritability
    Being easily fatigued
    Muscle tension
    Difficulty concentrating or mind going blank
    Sleep disturbance.

Natural History of Illness/Comorbidity

Most persons with GAD report feeling anxious and nervous all their lives. Although more than half those presenting for treatment report onset in childhood or adolescence, onset occurring after age 20 is not uncommon (Keller et al, 1992; Robins & Reiger, 1991). The course is chronic but fluctuating and often worsens during times of stress (Angst & Dobler-Mikola, 1991). The mean duration of the illness is reported to be about 6 to 10 years, with 40% of patients reporting durations of illness of greater than 5 years (Robins & Reiger, 1991). GAD may have a more chronic course than PD (Massion et al, 1993; Noyes et al, 1992). Thirty-one percent of patients who have a remission subsequently have another episode (Keller et al, 1992).

GAD patients report physical symptoms as often as PD patients (Barbee et al, 1997). The most common symptoms reported include palpitations, joint pain, chest pain, shortness of breath, headaches, dizziness, and excessive gas (Barbee et al, 1997; Logue et al, 1993). GAD interferes with the patient's life substantially in 49% of cases (Wittchen et al, 1994).

The comorbidity of GAD in community samples is fairly significant. In outpatient clinics, 36% to 51% of patients with GAD also met the criteria for PD, 29% to 46% for major depressive disorder, and 17% to 29% for social phobia (Brown & Barlow, 1992; Massion et al, 1993; Noyes et al, 1992). Personality disorders have been reported to occur in 30% to 60% of patients with GAD (Noyes et al, 1992; Sanderson et al, 1994). The comorbidity with substance abuse is lower than other anxiety disorders, about 10% to 20% in clinic samples and lower in community samples (Massion et al, 1993; Noyes et al, 1992; Robins & Reiger, 1991). Overall, 90.4% of persons with a lifetime diagnosis of GAD have at least one other lifetime psychiatric diagnosis, whereas 66.3% of those with a current diagnosis of GAD had another comorbid disorder (Wittchen et al, 1994). The strongest comorbidities were found for mood disorders, PD, and agoraphobia. Because of this significant comorbidity, management of GAD can be difficult.

Treatment Options, Expected Outcomes, and Comprehensive Management

With pure GAD, patients should be asked to avoid caffeine and alcohol and stop using all possible sympathomimetic medications. If symptoms do not significantly improve with these changes, alternative treatments may be considered. Benzodiazepines have been the mainstay of treatment of GAD, but little data are present to suggest any long-term benefit of these agents. Short-term use of diazepam appears to help with the physical symptoms of anxiety but not the psychic symptoms. However, discontinuation can create rebound anxiety—anxiety that is greater than the original symptoms and not related to withdrawal effects (Pourmotabbed et al, 1996).

The only FDA-approved medication for the treatment of GAD is buspirone (Table 59-4). There are several studies demonstrating its efficacy in the short and long term. The best placebo-controlled trial demonstrated that buspirone at 15 to 45 mg/day produced improvement in 54.9% of patients, compared with 34.6% of patients taking placebo (Schweizer & Rickels, 1997; Sramek et al, 1996). However, patients who have been treated with benzodiazepines and then changed to buspir-

TABLE 59-4	Medications for Generalized Anxiety Disorder	
Medication	Daily Dose (mg)	Response Rate (%)
Buspirone[a]	15–60	55
Diazepam[b]	5–40	66
Chlordiazepoxide[c]	5–60	55
Paroxetine[d]	10–60	66
Nefazodone[e]	300–600	80
Imipramine[b]	50–200	66–73
Trazodone[f]	200–450	69
Placebo[g]	Not applicable	35–47

[a] Sramek et al, 1996
[b] Rickels et al, 1993; Rocca et al, 1997
[c] Kahn et al, 1986
[d] Rocca et al, 1997
[e] Hedges et al, 1996
[f] Rickels et al, 1993
[g] Rickels et al, 1993; Sramek et al, 1996

one are five times less likely to respond to buspirone (Schweizer et al, 1986). This phenomenon has prompted some authors to argue for the use of buspirone in benzodiazepine-naïve patients only.

Open label trials conducted with paroxetine (Rocca et al, 1997) and nefazodone (Hedges et al, 1996) both suggested benefit in reducing the psychic anxiety associated with GAD. When anxiety symptoms present for the first time in later life, there is a high rate of comorbidity with depressive disorders. In this case, one of the antidepressants used to treat GAD should be used rather than benzodiazepines (Flint, 1997).

Cognitive and behavioral therapies and relaxation training have also demonstrated efficacy in treating GAD. Patients taught anxiety-reduction techniques showed stable or improved symptoms at 6 months of follow-up. The degree of symptom reduction exceeded the greatest reported amount for short-term benzodiazepine treatment. A comparative trial of CBT, anxiety-management training, benzodiazepines, and a wait list control demonstrated that psychological interventions produced sustained improvement and the benzodiazepine group had minimal improvement, but all were superior to the control group (Harvey & Rapee, 1995).

Referral Points and Clinical Warnings

- GAD is a highly prevalent condition. The course of illness is often chronic and fluctuates in severity.
- Buspirone is probably the treatment of choice when prolonged pharmacotherapy is indicated, because it does not produce physical dependence.
- CBT or anxiety-management techniques may offer longer-term gains than medications. Referral to an appropriate mental health specialist may be indicated.
- SSRIs and imipramine are effective in treating GAD.

SPECIFIC PHOBIA

The term "phobia" is used frequently in conversation to imply several different ideas. The clinical diagnosis of a phobia is appropriate only if the fear or anticipation of encountering the phobic stimulus interferes significantly with the person's daily routine, occupational functioning, or social life; this may vary with culture and ethnicity (APA, 1994). The phobia can be diagnosed only if it exceeds the usual cultural norms.

Epidemiology

Specific phobias are one of the most common psychiatric diagnoses. Approximately 5.1% to 13.3% of the population will meet the symptom criteria for a specific phobia, but rarely are they significant enough to impair a person's life (Magee et al, 1996; Robins & Reiger, 1991). The gender ratio varies with different types of phobias. Approximately 75% to 90% of persons with animal, natural environment, and situational subtypes are female, compared to 55% to 70% of blood injection injury or height subtypes (APA, 1994). Multiple phobias are reported in 5.4% of women and 1.5% of men (Fredrikson et al, 1996).

Diagnostic Criteria

- Marked, persistent fear, dread, or horror in a situation when the person is in a harmless situation
- Exposure to the phobic stimulus almost invariably provokes an immediate anxiety response.
- The person recognizes the fear as unreasonable.
- The person avoids exposure to the object or situation and has anxious anticipation or distress in the feared situation that interferes significantly with the person's normal routine.
- Many subtypes of specific phobias exist:
  Animals
  Natural environmental events (heights, storms, lightning, water)
  Blood injection injury
  Situational (public transportation, tunnels, bridges, elevators, flying, driving).

Natural History of Illness/Comorbidity

Age of onset tends to be bimodal in distribution, with a peak in childhood and a second peak in the mid-20s. Predisposing factors to onset tend to be traumatic events, unexpected panic attacks, observation of others undergoing trauma, fearfulness in others (eg, observing others becoming fearful around certain animals), and informational transmission (parental warnings) (Fredrikson et al, 1997). Feared objects tend to represent things that may have a potential threat or have represented a threat in the past. Phobias that persist into adulthood tend to remit less than 20% of the time (APA, 1994).

Treatment Options, Expected Outcomes, and Comprehensive Management

BEHAVIORAL THERAPY
Behavioral (exposure) therapy relies on exposing the person to the feared objects or situations. There are two common methods: systemic desensitization and flooding. In both, the patient meets with a trained therapist and confronts the feared object or situation. By confronting rather than fleeing the object of fear, patients become accustomed to it and can lose the terror, horror, panic, or dread they once felt.

Systemic desensitization is a more gradual form of exposure therapy. In a series of steps, patients first learn relaxation techniques to control the physical manifestations of fear. Then they imagine the feared object, work their way up to looking at pictures of the object or situation, and finally experience the situation or being in the presence of the feared object. With each incremental increase in exposure, patients are asked to implement the relaxation techniques they have learned. During flooding, patients are exposed directly and immediately to the most feared object or situation. They stay in that situation until their anxiety is markedly reduced.

PHARMACOTHERAPY
With the exception of agoraphobia (discussed above) and social phobia (discussed below), there are no data to support the routine use of medications for specific phobias. Benzodiazepines have been used in acute situations where patients must confront their phobic stimulus—for instance, a person must take a transatlantic flight for business reasons. Agents such as diazepam, lorazepam, and alprazolam are common choices. Dose equivalents are about 5 mg of diazepam (0.5 to 1 mg lorazepam, 0.25 to 0.5 mg of alprazolam).

Referral Points and Clinical Warnings

Long-term use of anxiolytic agents is not indicated.

SOCIAL PHOBIA

Social phobia is characterized by significant anxiety provoked by exposure to certain types of social or performance situations, often leading to behavior to avoid the situation. In the feared social or performance situation, patients have concerns about embarrassment and are afraid that others will judge them to be anxious, weak, crazy, or stupid. They may fear public speaking because of concern that others will notice their trembling hands or voice, or they may experience extreme anxiety when talking with others because of fear that they will appear inarticulate (APA, 1994; Judd, 1994).

Clinical presentation and resulting impairment may differ across cultures, depending on social demands. In certain cultures (Japan and Korea), persons with social phobia may develop persistent and excessive fears of giving offense to others in social situations, instead of being embarrassed. These fears may take the form of extreme anxiety that blushing, eye-to-eye contact, or body odor will be offensive to others (APA, 1994). Lifetime rates of social phobia vary from 2.6% in the United States to 0.5% in Korea (Weissman et al, 1996).

Social phobia is subdivided into two categories: generalized and nongeneralized. In the generalized type, the patient fears most social situations, whereas in the nongeneralized type the patient's fear is evoked only in certain events (eg, public speaking) (APA, 1994; Heimberg et al, 1993).

Epidemiology

Epidemiologic studies suggest that social phobia has a 12-month prevalence rate of 7.9% (6.6% for men and 9.1% for women) and a lifetime prevalence rate of 13.3% (11.1% for men and 15.5% for women) (Kessler et al, 1994; Magee et al, 1996). Generalized social phobia is about three times more likely to occur among relatives of patients with social phobia (16% to 36%) versus those with nongeneralized social phobia (6% to 13%) and controls without mental illness (6% to 19%) (Fyer et al, 1993; Mannuzza et al, 1995).

Diagnostic Criteria

- A marked and persistent fear of one or more social or performance situations in which the person is exposed to unfamiliar people and to the possible scrutiny of others.
- Exposure to the feared social situation almost invariably provokes anxiety, which may take the form of a situationally bound panic attack.
- The person recognizes that the fear is excessive or unreasonable.
- The feared social or performance situations are avoided or else are endured with intense anxiety or distress.
- Subtypes include:
  Generalized
  Nongeneralized
  Performance.

Natural History of Illness/Comorbidity

Generalized social phobia has an average age of onset at about age 11, compared to age 17 for nongeneralized social phobia. Half of those with generalized social phobia had an onset before age 10 (Mannuzza et al, 1995). Onset after age 25 is rare (Schneier et al, 1992). Onset may abruptly follow a stressful or humiliating experience, or it may be insidious. Social phobia appears to follow a chronic and unremitting course. In a naturalistic study, Reich et al (1994) followed 140 patients with social phobia for 65 weeks. Approximately 88% of the study participants received some form of psychotherapy or pharmacotherapy, but only 11% achieved full remission of social phobia symptoms by 65 weeks.

Persons with social phobia may manifest poor social skills (poor eye contact) or observable signs of anxiety (cold clammy hands, tremors, shaky voice). Students often underachieve in school because of test anxiety or avoidance of classroom participation. Affected persons may underachieve at work because of anxiety about or avoidance of speaking in groups, in public, or to authority figures and colleagues. Because those with social phobia tend to withdraw, because they fear scrutiny, they often have decreased social support and are less likely to get married (64% are unmarried). More than 50% are unable to complete high school, and 22.3% receive some financial assistance (Mannuzza et al, 1995). Social phobia has been associated with suicidal ideation and multiple other comorbidities (Table 59-5).

Treatment Options, Expected Outcomes, and Comprehensive Management

GENERALIZED SOCIAL PHOBIA

Cognitive-behavioral group therapy (CBGT) uses the same premises as cognitive therapy but is administered to small groups (usually six people). The patient, in a group situation, identifies feared situations and with the group's feedback develops a treatment plan. Response rates are 81% for CBGT versus 47% for educational support groups at 6 months and 89% versus

TABLE 59-5	Comorbidities of Social Phobia
Comorbidity	**Frequency (%)**
Simple phobia	59
Agoraphobia	45
Atypical depression[a]	36
Alcohol abuse	19
Major depressive disorder	17
Drug abuse	13
Dysthymia	12
Obsessive-compulsive disorder	11.1
Panic disorder	4.7

[a] Atypical depression is manifested by hypersomnia, anergia, weight gain, and rejection sensitivity.
Source: Aimes et al, 1983; Judd, 1994; Mannuzza et al, 1995; Schneier et al, 1992; Smail et al, 1984.

44% at 5 years (Heimberg & Juster, 1994). CBGT is effective for both generalized and nongeneralized social phobia at up to 5 years after treatment (Juster & Heimberg, 1995).

Multiple medications have been used in social phobia, but the most effective are the MAOIs. These agents are typically used only by experienced health care professionals because of dietary restrictions and frequent drug–drug interactions that must be monitored. Because of this, SSRIs, although slightly less effective, are frequently used by primary care providers.

NONGENERALIZED SOCIAL PHOBIA

For stage fright or nongeneralized social phobia, beta-blockers (propranolol, atenolol, nadolol, or timolol) are effective in most cases (Liebowitz, 1993). Beta-blockers taken 1 hour before the performance situation can decrease performance anxiety. Successful use requires a stressful situation that can be identified, is predictable in timing, and occurs so infrequently that intermittent dosing can be used (Gorman & Gorman, 1987). Nonselective beta-blockers may be more effective for symptoms of tachycardia and tremor. Propranolol at 20 to 40 mg/day is the usual dose. A test dose should be tried in a nonperformance setting to assess for side effects and untoward reaction.

Referral Points and Clinical Warnings

- MAOIs are effective but carry side effects of drug–drug interactions, low blood pressure, weight gain, edema, and change in sexual desire. Tyramine in the diet can cause potentially dangerous rises in blood pressure.
- SSRIs are a second-line choice for pharmacotherapy.

OBSESSIVE-COMPULSIVE DISORDER

OCD is characterized by obsessions (which cause marked anxiety or distress), compulsions (which serve to neutralize the anxiety), or both. Obsessions are persistent ideas, thoughts, impulses, and images that are experienced as intrusive and inappropriate and that cause marked anxiety or distress. The obsessions are out of the patient's control and are not the type of thoughts the patient would expect to have. Compulsions are repetitive behaviors (eg, hand washing, ordering, and checking) or mental acts (praying, counting, and repeating words silently) performed to prevent or reduce anxiety or distress, not to provide pleasure or gratification (APA, 1994).

Anatomy, Physiology, and Pathology

Neurobiologic evidence indicates that central serotonergic dysregulation is a feature of OCD. Several different brain lesions have been associated with OCD. A high prevalence of obsessive-compulsive symptoms is noted in patients with Sydenham's chorea compared to other poststreptococcal illnesses (Swedo et al, 1989). This finding led to the speculation that dysfunction in the striatum may occur in OCD patients. The close association of Tourette's syndrome with OCD also lends credence to the striatal dysfunction etiology. Some authors have speculated that Tourette's and OCD are both disorders of the striatum, with the precise area of damage within the striatum and the size of the lesion determining the clinical symptoms (Baxter, 1990; Goodman et al, 1990).

Further evidence that this portion of the brain is involved is the presence of autoantibodies against the caudate and putamen at levels two to three times those of clinical controls (Kiessling et al, 1994). Functional brain studies with single photon emission computed tomography are strongly suggestive of abnormalities in the basal ganglia (particularly the caudate), in orbitofrontal cortical function, or both; these abnormalities may normalize during treatment (Machlin et al, 1991; Rubin et al, 1992).

Epidemiology

The 1-year prevalence is 1.5% to 2.1% and the lifetime prevalence is 2.5% (Rasmussen & Eisen, 1992). Annual prevalence rates range from 1.1% in Korea to 1.8% in New Zealand (Weissman et al, 1994). The disorder is equally common in men and women (Rasmussen & Eisen, 1992). Family studies have suggested an increase in anxiety disorders in general, and OCD specifically, in first-degree relatives compared to matched comparisons. Anxiety disorders are found in 16% of first-degree relatives versus 3.5% of controls (Black et al, 1992). OCD is found in 10.3% of first-degree relatives compared to 1.6% of controls (Pauls et al, 1995).

Diagnostic Criteria

- Either obsessions or compulsions
- At some point during the disorder the person recognizes that the obsessions or compulsions are excessive or unreasonable.
- The obsessions or compulsions cause marked distress, are time-consuming (take more than 1 hour per day), or significantly interfere with the person's normal routine, occupational functioning, or usual social activities or relationships.

Of persons with OCD, 50% suffer from obsessions only, 34% have compulsions only, and 16% have both obsessions and compulsions. Twenty-seven percent to 63% of patients with OCD have major depressive disorder and 43% to 49% have another anxiety disorder (Hollander et al, 1997; Weissman et al, 1994).

Natural History of Illness/Comorbidity

The age at onset is earlier in males (19.5 ± 9.2 years) than in females (22 ± 9.8 years) (Rasmussen & Eisen, 1992). For the most part, onset is gradual, but acute onset has been noted in some cases. Patients wait up to 10 years on average before telling a health care professional about their obsessive-compulsive symptoms (Hollander et al, 1997). Embarrassment may cause patients to present with complaints other than their obsessions or compulsions (Rasmussen & Eisen, 1994), such as chapped hands, eczema, trichotillomania, hypochondriasis, Tourette's syndrome, episodes during pregnancy, difficulty in school, associated with Sydenham's chorea, body dysmorphobia, lesions from excessive cleaning of teeth, or reports from a family member of excessive cleaning. Primary care providers may misdiagnose the condition as depression or PD (Shahady, 1994).

Most patients have a chronic waxing and waning course; exacerbation of symptoms may be related to stress. About 15% show progressive deterioration in occupational and social functioning. Sixty-four percent of patients report a negative impact on their spouse, with 23.7% of patients reporting that their symptoms led to the breakup of their marriage or relationship (Hollander et al, 1997). About 5% of patients have an episodic course, with minimal or no symptoms between episodes (APA, 1994).

OCD may be associated with major depressive disorder, other anxiety disorders, eating disorder, substance dependence, and obsessive-compulsive personality disorder (Douglas et al, 1995). Thirteen percent of patients report a history of suicide attempts (Hollander et al, 1996). There is a high incidence of OCD in persons with Tourette's disorder, with estimates ranging from approximately 35% to 50%. The incidence of Tourette's disorder in patients with OCD is lower, with estimates ranging from 5% to 7%. Between 20% and 30% of OCD patients have reported current or past tics.

Predicting the development of OCD can be difficult. Retrospective reviews have identified several factors; however, a recent prospective study did not support any of those items. The only identifiable prospective risk factors were a history of depression or substance abuse (Douglas et al, 1995).

Treatment Options, Expected Outcomes, and Comprehensive Management

The National Consensus Group has created a recommended treatment algorithm for OCD (Table 59-6) (March et al, 1997):

- For milder OCD symptoms, start with CBT. For more severe symptoms, combine CBT and an SSRI, or use an SSRI alone.
- If there is an inadequate response in 8 weeks, add CBT to medication or add medication to CBT.
- If there is still an inadequate response, switch to an alternate SSRI or change the CBT approach. Use clomipramine after two or three failed trials of SSRIs and CBT.
- If there is still a poor response, consider intravenous clomipramine, electroconvulsive therapy, or neurosurgery.

Exposure therapy is effective in the short term when combined with fluvoxamine; after 18 months, there was 80% reduction in symptoms compared to 40% with fluvoxamine

TABLE 59-6	Medications for Obsessive-Compulsive Disorder	
Medication	Usual Daily Dose	Response Rate (%)
Clomipramine[a,b,f]	100–250 mg	38–95
Fluoxetine[a,b,c]	20–80 mg	40–56
Fluvoxamine[d]	100–300 mg	40
Paroxetine[c]	40–60 mg	40
Sertraline[g]	50–200 mg	27
Phenelzine[d]	60 mg	41
Amitriptyline[f]	100–250 mg	56
Doxepin[f]	100–250 mg	36
Exposure Therapy[d]	29 months	76
Placebo[d]	Not applicable	5–6

[a] Koran et al, 1996
[b] Malanfranchi et al, 1997
[c] Mundo et al, 1997
[d] Barlow & Lehman, 1996; Jenike et al, 1997
[e] Jenike et al, 1997
[f] Jenike, 1993
[g] Piccinelli et al, 1995

alone (Cottraux et al, 1993). At 1 year, 87% of the patients remaining on medication showed improvement (Orloff et al, 1994). CBT is used for OCD symptoms. The process is identical to that described for PD, although the cognitive constructs identified are different. The behavioral component of CBT involves exposure therapy or response prevention. Exposure is based on the fact that anxiety usually diminishes after sufficient contact with something feared (usually greater than 20 to 25 minutes). For example, people with obsessions about germs are told to stay in contact with germy objects until their anxiety is extinguished. The anxiety tends to decrease after repeated exposure until the patient no longer fears the contact.

For exposure to be most helpful, it needs to be combined with response or ritual prevention. In response prevention, the person's rituals or avoidance behaviors are blocked. For example, those with excessive worries about germs must not only stay in contact with germy things, but also must refrain from ritualized washing. Exposure is generally more helpful in decreasing anxiety and obsessions, whereas response prevention is more helpful in decreasing compulsions.

For patients whose disorder is refractory to all medications and psychotherapeutic interventions, cingulotomy has been used with significant success for reducing obsessive-compulsive symptoms. Symmetry obsessions, ordering compulsions, or hoarding rituals predicted which intractable patients responded better with cingulotomy (Baer et al, 1995; Jenike, 1993).

Referral Points and Clinical Warnings

- Patients are hesitant to disclose their symptoms for fear of being labeled crazy.
- Many patients are misdiagnosed initially with PD disorder or depression. The health care provider must maintain a high index of suspicion to be able to diagnose OCD.
- Effective treatment is typically a combination of CBT and medications.
- Untreated OCD carries a high morbidity rate.

POST-TRAUMATIC STRESS DISORDER AND ACUTE STRESS DISORDER

In 1994, the diagnostic categories for traumatic stress disorders were separated into two categories: PTSD and ASD. Both will be described together because there is significant overlap; one of the main differences is the duration of symptoms.

As a response to the traumatic event, a person may develop dissociative symptoms. Persons with ASD have a decrease in emotional responsiveness, often finding it impossible to experience pleasure in previously enjoyable activities; they frequently feel guilty about pursuing usual life tasks. They may have difficulty concentrating, feel detached from their bodies, experience the world as unreal or dreamlike, or have increasing difficulty recalling specific details of the traumatic event (dissociative amnesia) (APA, 1994).

Anatomy, Physiology, and Pathology

Trauma is thought to be a psychobiologic event that produces not only adverse psychological effects but also potentially long-term neurobiologic changes in the brain. PTSD seems to be associated with changes in the noradrenergic and serotonergic systems, the hypothalamic–pituitary–adrenocortical axis, and the endogenous dopaminergic/opioid system (Sutherland & Davidson, 1994). The current state of understanding has been thoroughly reviewed, but with no definitive answers (Friedman et al, 1995).

Epidemiology

The lifetime incidence of PTSD has been estimated at 1% to 14% (Solomon et al, 1992). This wide variation depends on the study performed and the diagnostic interview instrument used in the study. Another confounding factor associated with the prevalence of this disease is that some patients receive secondary gain from having a PTSD diagnosis because of potential disability compensation. The most reasonable estimate was achieved in the National Co-Morbidity Survey, which yielded a lifetime PTSD rate of 7.8% in the general population (Kessler et al, 1995).

PTSD rates of 59% to 66% were reported among crime victims exposed to a life threat combined with injury (Kilpatrick & Resnick, 1993). The National Co-Morbidity Study found lifetime PTSD rates among those exposed to severe trauma ranging from 39% for combat to 65% for rape (Kessler et al, 1995).

Studies in which exposure to trauma has been less severe, however, suggest that most subjects exposed to trauma do not develop PTSD (Breslau et al, 1991; Helzer et al, 1987; Southwick et al, 1993). Factors that contribute to PTSD include:

- Prior exposure to trauma (Bremner et al, 1993)
- Pretrauma personality (Schnurr et al, 1993)
- Heritability (True et al, 1993)
- Age at exposure to trauma (King et al, 1996; Speed et al, 1989)
- Amount of social support after the traumatic event
- Exposure to reactivating stressors (Solomon et al, 1992).

Diagnostic Criteria

DIAGNOSTIC CRITERIA FOR POST-TRAUMATIC STRESS DISORDER

- Person who has been exposed to a traumatic event in which both of the following were present:
- The person experienced, witnessed, or was confronted with an event or events that involved actual or threatened death or serious injury, or a threat to the personal integrity of self or others.
- The person's response involved intense fear, helplessness, or horror.
- The traumatic event is persistently re-experienced via:
    Intrusive recollections of the event
    Recurrent distressing dreams of the event
    Feeling as if the event is recurring
- Persistent avoidance of the stimuli associated with the trauma and numbing of general responsiveness
- Persistent feelings of increased arousal suggested by:
    Difficulty falling or staying asleep
    Irritability or outbursts of anger
    Difficulty concentrating
    Hypervigilance
    Exaggerated startle response
- Duration of the symptoms is greater than 1 month.

DIAGNOSTIC CRITERIA FOR ACUTE STRESS DISORDER

- Symptoms similar to those of PTSD that can occur immediately after an extremely traumatic event
- The person has been exposed to a traumatic event in which both of the following were present:
- The person experienced, witnessed, or was confronted with an event or events that involved actual or threatened death or serious injury, or a threat to the physical integrity of self or others.
- The person's response involved intense fear, helplessness, or horror.
- Either during or after the traumatic event, the person has three of the following dissociative symptoms:
    A subjective sense of numbing, detachment, or absence of emotional responsiveness
    A reduction in awareness of surroundings
    Derealization
    Depersonalization
    Dissociative amnesia
- The traumatic event is persistently re-experienced.
- There is marked avoidance of the stimuli that arouse recollections of the trauma.

Natural History of Illness/Comorbidity

PTSD can be divided into three stages. Stage 1 involves the response to trauma. Nonsusceptible persons may experience an adrenergic surge of symptoms immediately after the trauma but do not dwell on the incident. Predisposed persons have higher levels of anxiety at baseline, an exaggerated response to trauma, and an obsessive preoccupation with it afterward.

If the symptoms persist beyond 4 to 6 weeks, the patient enters stage 2, or acute PTSD. Feelings of helplessness and loss of control, symptoms of increased autonomic arousal, reliving of the trauma, and somatic symptoms may occur. The patient's life becomes centered around the trauma, with subsequent changes in lifestyle, personality, and social functioning. Phobic avoidance, startle response, and angry outbursts may occur.

In stage 3, chronic PTSD develops, with disability, demoralization, and despondency. The patient's emphasis changes from preoccupation with the actual trauma to preoccupation with the physical disability resulting from the trauma. Somatic symptoms, chronic anxiety, and depression are common complications at this time, as well as substance abuse, disturbed family relations, and unemployment. The patient may focus on compensation and lawsuits. By 6 months, the natural history is for avoidance and numbing to decline, but not the hyperarousal events (Blanchard et al, 1995).

Commonly, the person has recurrent and intrusive recollections of the event or recurrent distressing dreams during which the event is replayed. In rare instances, the person has dissociative states that last from a few seconds to several hours, or even days, during which the components of the event are relived and the person behaves as though the event is being experienced at that moment. The person commonly makes deliberate efforts to avoid feelings, thoughts, and conversations about the traumatic event and to avoid activities, situations, or people who arouse recollections of it (APA, 1994; Breslau et al, 1995).

There is some evidence that social supports, family history, childhood experiences, personality variables, and pre-existing mental conditions may influence the development of PTS. However, this disorder can develop in persons with no predisposing conditions, particularly if the stressor is extreme (Barton et al, 1996). The highest predictors of development of PTSD from ASD are emotional numbing and derealization (Eriksson & Lundin, 1996; Staab et al, 1996). Of patients with PTSD, 82.3% meet the criteria for at least one other disorder (OCD, PD with agoraphobia, major depression, social phobia, specific phobia, somatization disorder, substance-related disorder) (APA, 1994; Breslau et al, 1992).

Treatment Options, Expected Outcomes, and Comprehensive Management

It is not yet clear that gains can be made in preventing PTSD by early intervention; nonetheless, the face validity of such an argument is frequently accepted. By the use of endorsed rituals (religious or otherwise), psychotherapy, formal crisis intervention, or psychopharmacology, the acute symptoms can be reduced (Lundin, 1994). Treatment incorporates psychotherapy, behavioral therapy such as systemic desensitization, and medications.

The primary approach for the treatment of PTSD should be psychotherapy. The principles for managing acute stress reactions are best summed up by the mnemonic BICEPS (Wise, 1983). At first, the treatment should be *brief*, completed within a few days. Second, it should be *immediate*. By delaying treatment, there is a greater chance that complications, secondary gain, and avoidance will set in. Third, it is best to provide a *central* location for treatment. The fourth factor is *expectation* that the victim of acute trauma will be able to return to good functioning or to the situation that originally provoked the traumatic reaction. A fifth consideration is *proximity*: treatment should be given as close to the "combat zone" as possible. The sixth element is *simplicity*. Treatment should be focused on the current problems—the trauma and the patient's response to it.

An intervention termed eye movement desensitization and reprocessing has been purported to have significant benefits for patients with PTSD. The premise is that while patients are reliving the traumatic event, they have saccadic (rapid, intermittent) eye movements. In this intervention, the vividness of the distressing image is decreased, as well as the associated emotional intensity. The efficacy has been reported to be from 100% to negligible (Andrade et al, 1997; Oswall et al, 1993; Rothbaum, 1997; Shapiro, 1996; Shapiro et al, 1994; Vaughn et al, 1994; Wilson et al, 1995).

Referral Points and Clinical Warnings

- Acute intervention is helpful. Crisis intervention personnel, or those trained in these techniques, should care for persons with this diagnosis.
- There is a high risk of complications if intervention is delayed; long-term disability can occur without intervention.
- Treatment by a provider experienced with the disorder is essential.

TEACHING AND SELF-CARE

The patient experiencing anxiety disorders may present problems in learning how to change behavior or care for himself or herself. The provider should pay special attention to the environment to decrease stressors and thereby decrease anxiety. The patient and family should be encouraged to tell providers what activities assist with learning and providing self care.

COMMUNITY RESOURCES

- Anxiety Disorders Association of American, 6000 Executive Blvd., Suite 513, Rockville, MD 20852-4004, 301-231-8368
- National Anxiety Foundation, 3135 Custer Dr., Lexington, KY 40517-4001
- American Psychiatric Association, 1400 K St., NW, Washington, DC 20005, 202-682-6220
- American Psychological Association, 750 First St., NE, Washington, DC 20002, 202-336-5500
- National Panic/Anxiety Disorder Newsletter, 1718 Burgandy Place, Santa Rosa, CA 95403, 707-527-5738
- Obsessive-Compulsive Foundation, Box 70, Milford, CT 06460-0070, 203-878-5669
- OC Information Center, Allen Boulevard, Middleton, WI 53562, 608-836-8070

In addition, the bibliography lists books and other publications that may be useful for patients and their families.

SUMMARY

Anxiety disorders are prevalent in the United States and represent a disproportionate share of contacts with primary care providers. These disorders can carry a high rate of complications but are treatable. Interventions ranging from psychotherapeutic to pharmacologic are helpful, and the entire array of interventions should be used. Patient participation is essential when planning treatment. The potential risks and benefits of each activity should be explained to the patient. For most anxiety

disorders, any intervention will take a few weeks to work; making patients aware of this can improve their long-term adherence to the treatment plan.

The provider must bear in mind the large number of medical and pharmacologic interventions that can mimic anxiety disorders. A thorough history of symptoms and their temporal profile combined with a physical exam can effectively rule out most medications, illicit drugs, and medical conditions that can produce an anxiety syndrome. Features such as onset after age 45 years or the presence of atypical symptoms during a panic attack (eg, vertigo, loss of consciousness, loss of bladder or bowel control, headaches, slurred speech, or amnesia) suggest that a general medical condition or a substance may be causing the panic attack symptoms.

EDITOR'S NOTE:
COMPLEMENTARY APPROACHES

A general discussion of complementary approaches can be found in Chapter 3. The following, while not an exhaustive list, are some complementary approaches being used for this condition. Additional information on these approaches, including precautions, can be found in Appendices A and B. Providers need to assess for the use of complementary approaches as part of the patient's history, as they may impact conventional therapies, and patients may not volunteer this information unless specifically asked. Efficacy of many complementary approaches is not as well documented as that of conventional therapies. Providers need to read the literature before suggesting these complementary approaches.

- Complementary Modalities
  Acupuncture
  Aromatherapy
  Biofeedback
  Craniosacral therapy
  Massage therapy

References

Aimes, P., Gelder, M. et al. (1983). Social phobia: A comparative clinical study. *Br J Psychiatry 142*, 174–179.

American Psychiatric Association. (1994). *Diagnostic and statistical manual of mental disorders*, 4th ed. Washington, DC: American Psychiatric Press.

Andrade, J., Kavanagh, D., & Baddeley, A. (1997). Eye movements and visual imagery: A working memory approach to the treatment of post-traumatic stress disorder. *British Journal of Clinical Psychology*, *36*(Pt 2), 209–223.

Angst, J., & Dobler-Mikola, A. (1991). The natural history of anxiety disorders. *Acta Psychiatrica Scandinavica*, *84*, 446–452.

Baer, L., Rauch, S., Ballantine, H., et al. (1995). Cingulotomy for intractable obsessive-compulsive disorder: Prospective long-term follow-up of 18 patients. *Archives of General Psychiatry*, *52*, 384–392.

Ballentine, N. & Kettle, P. (1998). Medical illness in psychiatric patient. In Medical consultation: The internist on surgical, obstetrical, and psychiatric services. 3rd ed., Gross, R. & Caputo, G., eds. Baltimore: Williams & Wilkins.

Barbee, J., Todorov, A., Kuczmierczyk, A., et al. (1997). Explained and unexplained medical symptoms in generalized anxiety and panic disorder: Relationship to the somatoform disorders. *Annals of Clinical Psychiatry*, *9*(3), 149–155.

Barlow, D. (1990). Long-term outcome for patients with panic disorder treated with cognitive-behavioral therapy. *Journal of Clinical Psychiatry*, *51*, 17–23.

Barlow, D. (1997). Cognitive-behavioral therapy for panic disorder: Current status. *Journal of Clinical Psychiatry, 58*(Suppl), 32–36.

Barlow, D., & Lehman, C. (1996). Advances in the psychosocial treatment of anxiety disorders: Implications for national health care. *Archives of General Psychiatry, 53,* 727–735.

Barton, K., Blanchard, E., & Hickling, E. (1996). Antecedents and consequences of acute stress disorder among motor vehicle accident victims. *Behav Res Ther, 34*(10), 805–813.

Baxter, L. (1990). Brain imaging as a tool in establishing a theory of brain pathology in obsessive compulsive disorder. *Journal of Clinical Psychiatry, 51*(Suppl), 22–25.

Beck, A., Clark, D., Berchick, R., & Wright, F. (1992). A crossover study of focused cognitive therapy for panic disorder. *American Journal of Psychiatry, 149*(6), 778–783.

Black, D., Noyes, R., Goldstein, R., & Blum, N. (1992). A family study of obsessive compulsive disorder. *Archives of General Psychiatry, 49,* 362–368.

Boyer, W. (1995). Serotonin uptake inhibitors are superior to imipramine and alprazolam in alleviating panic attacks: A meta-analysis. *International Clinical Psychopharmacology, 10,* 45–49.

Braunwald, E. (1992) Valvular heart disease. In E. Braunwald (Ed.). *Heart disease: Textbook of cardiovascular medicine,* 4th ed. Philadelphia: W.B. Saunders.

Bremner, J., Southwick, S., Johnson, D., Yehuda, R., & Charney, D. (1993). Childhood physical abuse and combat-related posttraumatic stress in Vietnam veterans. *American Journal of Psychiatry, 150,* 235–239.

Breslau, N., Davis, G. et al. (1992). Traumatic events and post-traumatic stress disorders in an urban population of young adults. *Arch Gen Psych 48,* 216–220.

Breslau, N., Davis, G., & Andreski, P. (1995). Risk factors for PTSD-related traumatic events: A prospective analysis. *American Journal of Psychiatry, 152*(4), 529–535.

Brown, G., Beck, A., Newman, C., Beck, J., & Tran, C. (1997). A comparison of focused and standard cognitive therapy for panic disorder. *Journal of Anxiety Disorders, 11*(3), 329–345.

Brown, T., & Barlow, D. (1992). Comorbidity among anxiety disorders: Implications for treatment and DSM-IV. *Journal of Consulting & Clinical Psychology, 60,* 835–844.

Bruce, T., Spiegel, D., Gregg, S., & Nuzzarello, A. (1995). Predictors of alprazolam discontinuation with and without cognitive behavior therapy in panic disorder. *American Journal of Psychiatry, 152,* 1156.

Chignon, J., Lepine, J., & Ades, J. (1993). Panic disorder in cardiac outpatients. *American Journal of Psychiatry, 150,* 780–785.

Clark, D., Salkovskis, P., Hackmann, A., et al. (1994). A comparison of cognitive therapy, applied relaxation and imipramine in the treatment of panic disorder. *British Journal of Psychiatry, 164,* 759–769.

Cottraux, J., Mollard, E., Bouvard, M., & Marks, I. (1993). Exposure therapy, fluvoxamine, or combination treatment in obsessive-compulsive disorder: One-year follow-up. *Psychiatry Research, 49*(1), 63–75.

Craske, M., Maidenberg, E., & Bystritsky, A. (1995). Brief cognitive-behavioral versus nondirective therapy for panic disorder. *Journal of Behav Ther Exp Psychiatry, 26*(2), 113-120.

Cross National Collaborative Panic Study, & Second Phase Investigators. (1992). Drug treatment of panic disorder: Comparative efficacy of alprazolam, imipramine and placebo. *British Journal of Psychiatry, 160,* 191–202.

Douglas, H., Moffitt, T., Dar, R., McGee, R., & Silva, P. (1995). Obsessive-compulsive disorder in a birth cohort of 18-year-olds: Prevalence and prediction. *Journal of the American Academy of Child & Adolescent Psychiatry, 34*(11), 1424–1431.

Eaton, W., Badawi, M., & Melton, B. (1995). Prodromes and precursors: Epidemiologic data for primary prevention of disorders with slow onset. *American Journal of Psychiatry, 152,* 967–972.

Eriksson, N., & Lundin, T. (1996). Early traumatic stress reactions among Swedish survivors of the Estonia disaster. *British Journal of Psychiatry, 169*(6), 713–716.

Fallon, B., Nields, J., Parsons, B., Liebowitz, M., & Klein, D. (1993). Psychiatric manifestations of Lyme borreliosis. *Journal of Clinical Psychiatry, 54*(7), 263–268.

Farmer, J., & Gotto, A. (1992) Risk factors for coronary artery disease. In E. Braunwald (Ed.). *Heart disease: Textbook of cardiovascular medicine,* 4th ed. Philadelphia: W.B. Saunders.

Flint, A. (1997). Epidemiology and comorbidity of anxiety disorders in later life: Implications for treatment. *Clinical Neuroscience, 4*(1), 31–36.

Fredrikson, M., Annas, P., Fischer, H., & Wik, G. (1996). Gender and age differences in the prevalence of specific fears and phobias. *Behav Res Ther, 34*(1), 33–39.

Fredrikson, M., Annas, P., & Wik, G. (1997). Parental history, aversive exposure, and the development of snake and spider phobia in women. *Behav Res Ther, 35*(1), 23–28.

Freeman, R., Ianni, P. et al. (1985). Ambulatory monitoring of panic disorder. *Arch Gen Psych 42,* 244–248.

Friedman, M., Charney, D., & Deutch, A. (1995). *Neurobiological and clinical consequences of stress: From normal adaptation to PTSD.* Philadelphia: Lippincott-Raven.

Fyer, A., Mannuzza, S. et al. (1993). A direct interview family study of social phobia. *Arch Gen Psychiatry 50*(4), 286–293.

Fyer, A., Mannuzza, S., Chapman, T., Liebowitz, M., & Klein, D. (1993). A direct interview family study of social phobia. *Archives of General Psychiatry, 50.*

Gerdes, T., Yates, W., & Clancy, G. (1995). Increasing identification and referral of panic disorder over the past decade. *Psychosomatics, 36,* 480–486.

Gibbs, D. (1992). Hyperventilation-induced cerebral ischemia and panic disorder and effect of nimodipine. *American Journal of Psychiatry, 149,* 1589–1591.

Goodman, W., McDougle, C., Price, L., et al. (1990). Beyond the serotonin hypothesis: A role for dopamine in some forms of obsessive-compulsive disorder? *Journal of Clinical Psychiatry, 51*(Suppl), 36–43.

Gorman, J. & Gorman L. (1987). Drug treatment of social phobia. *J Affect Disord 13,* 183–192.

Gorman, J., Papp, L., Coplan, J., et al. (1994). Anxiogenic effects of CO_2 and hyperventilation in patients with panic disorder. *American Journal of Psychiatry, 151*(4), 547–553.

Gorroll, A., May, L., & Mulley, A. (Eds.). (1995). *Primary care medicine: Office evaluation and management of the adult patient,* 3d ed. Philadelphia: J.B. Lippincott.

Grove, G., Coplan, J., & Hollander, E. (1997). The neuroanatomy of 5-HT dysregulation and panic disorder. *Journal of Neuropsychiatry and Clinical Neurosciences, 9*(Spring), 198–207.

Harvey, A., & Rapee, R. (1995). Cognitive-behavior therapy for generalized anxiety disorder. *Psychiatric Clinics of North America, 18*(4), 859–870.

Hedges, D., Reimherr, F., Strong, R., Halls, C., & Rust, C. (1996). An open trial of nefazodone in adult patients with generalized anxiety disorder. *Psychopharmacology Bulletin, 32*(4), 671–676.

Heimberg, R., Holt, C., Schneier, F., Spitzer, R., & Liebowitz, M. (1993). The issue of subtypes in the diagnosis of social phobia. *Journal of Anxiety Disorders, 7,* 249–269.

Heimberg, R., & Juster, H. (1994). Treatment of social phobia in cognitive-behavioral groups. *Journal of Clinical Psychiatry, 55*(Suppl), 38–46.

Helzer, J., Robins, L. et al. (1987). Post-traumatic stress disorder in the general population. *N Engl J Med 317,* 1630–1634.

Hollander, E., Kwon, J., Stein, D., Broatch, J., Rowland, C., & Himelein, C. (1996). Obsessive-compulsive and spectrum disorders: Overview and quality of life issues. *Journal of Clinical Psychiatry, 57*(Suppl), 3–6.

Hollander, E., Stein, D., Kwon, J., et al. (1997). Psychosocial function and economic costs of obsessive-compulsive disorder. *CNS Spectrums, 2*(10), 16–25.

Hollifield, M., Katon, W., Skipper, B., et al. (1997). Panic disorder and quality of life: Variables predictive of functional impairment. *American Journal of Psychiatry, 154,* 766–772.

Jenike, M. (1993). Obsessive-compulsive disorder: Efficacy of specific treatments as assessed by controlled trials. *Psychopharmacology Bulletin, 29,* 487–499.

Jenike, M., Baer, L., Minichiello, W., Rauch, S., & Buttolph, M. (1997). Placebo-controlled trial of fluoxetine and phenelzine for obsessive-compulsive disorder. *American Journal of Psychiatry, 154*(9), 1261–1264.

Johnson, J., Weissman, M., & Klerman, G. (1990). Panic disorder, comorbidity, and suicide attempts. *Archives of General Psychiatry, 47,* 805–808.

Judd, L. (1994). Social phobia: A clinical overview. *Journal of Clinical Psychiatry, 55*(Suppl), 5–9.

Juster, H., & Heimberg, R. (1995). Social phobia: Longitudinal course and long-term outcome of cognitive-behavioral treatment. *Psychiatric Clinics of North America, 18*(4), 821–842.

Kahn, J., Groman, J. et al. (1990). Cardiac left ventricular hypertrophy and chamber dilitation in panic disorder patients: Implications for idiopathic dilated cardiomyopathy. *Psychiatr Res 32,* 657–666.

Kahn, R., McNair, D. et al. (1986). Imipramine and chlordiazepoxide in depressive and anxiety disorders. II. Efficacy in anxious outpatients. *Arch Gen Psychiatry 43,* 79.

Kaplan, N. (1992) Systemic hypertension: Mechanisms and diagnosis. In E. Braunwald (Ed.). *Heart disease: Textbook of cardiovascular medicine,* 4th ed. Philadelphia: W.B. Saunders.

Karajgi, J., Rifkin, A. et al. (1990). The prevalence of anxiety disorders in patients with chronic obstructive pulmonary disease. *Am J Psych 147,* 200–201.

Katon, W., Vitaliano, P. et al. (1986). Panic disorder: Epidemiology in primary care. *J Family Prac 23,* 233–239.

Katon, W., Von Korff, M., & Lin, E. (1992). Panic disorder: Relationship to high medical utilization. *American Journal of Medicine, 92*(Suppl 1A), 7S–11S.

Katzelnick, D., Kobak, D., Griest, J., Jefferson, J., Mantle, J., & Serlin, R. (1995). Sertraline in social phobia: A double-blind, placebo-controlled crossover study. *American Journal of Psychiatry, 152,* 1368–1371.

Keck, P., Taylor, V., & Tugrul, K. (1993). Valproate treatment of panic disorder and lactate-induced panic attacks. *Biological Psychiatry, 33,* 542–546.

Keller, M., Lavori, P., Wunder, J., et al. (1992). Chronic course of anxiety disorders in children and adolescents. *Journal of the American Academy of Child & Adolescent Psychiatry, 31,* 595–599.

Kessler, R., McGonagle, K., Zhao, S., et al. (1994). Lifetime and 12-month prevalence of DSM-III-R psychiatric disorders in the United States. *Archives of General Psychiatry, 51,* 8–19.

Kessler, R., Sonnega, A., Bromet, E., Hughes, M., & Nelson, C. (1995). Posttraumatic stress disorder in the National Comorbidity Survey. *Archives of General Psychiatry, 52,* 1048–1060.

Kiessling, L., Marcotte, A., & Culpepper, L. (1994). Antineuronal antibodies: Tics and obsessive-compulsive symptoms. *Journal of Dev Behav Pediatr, 15*(6), 421–425.

Kilpatrick, D., & Resnick, H. (1993). PTSD associated with exposure to criminal victimization in clinical and community populations. In J. Davidson & E. Foa (Eds.). *Posttraumatic stress disorder: DSM-IV and beyond,* pp. 113–146. Washington, DC: American Psychiatric Press.

King, D., King, L., Foy, D., & Gudanowski, D. (1996). Prewar factors in combat-related posttraumatic stress disorder: Structural equation modeling with a national sample of female and male Vietnam veterans. *Journal of Consulting & Clinical Psychology, 64,* 520–531.

Klein, D. (1993). False suffocation alarms and spontaneous panic attacks: Subsuming the CO_2 hypersensitivity theory. *Archives of General Psychiatry, 50,* 306–317.

Klein, D. (1996). Panic disorder and agoraphobia: Hypothesis hothouse. *Journal of Clinical Psychiatry, 57*(Suppl), 21–27.

Koran, L., McElroy, S., Davidson, J., Rasmussen, S., Hollander, E., & Jenike, M. (1996). Fluvoxamine versus clomipramine for obsessive-compulsive disorder: A double-blind comparison. *Journal of Clinical Psychopharmacology, 16*(2), 121–129.

Leon, A., Olfson, M., Broadhead, W., et al. (1995). Prevalence of mental disorders in primary care. Implications for screening. *Archives of Family Medicine, 4*(10), 857–861.

Liebowitz, M. (1993). Pharmacotherapy of social phobia. *Journal of Clinical Psychiatry, 54*(12[Suppl]), 31–35.

Logue, M., Thomas, A., Barbee, J., et al. (1993). Generalized anxiety disorder patients seek evaluation for cardiologic symptoms at the same frequency as patients with panic disorder. *Journal of Psychiatric Research, 27,* 55.

Lundin, T. (1994). The treatment of acute trauma. Post-traumatic stress disorder prevention. *Psychiatric Clinics of North America, 17*(2), 385–391.

Machlin, S., Harris, G., Pearlson, G., et al. (1991). Elevated medial-cortical blood flow in obsessive-compulsive patients: A SPECT study. *American Journal of Psychiatry, 148,* 1240–1242.

Magee, W., Eaton, W., Wittchen, H.-U., McGonagle, K., & Kessler, R. (1996). Agoraphobia, simple phobia, and social phobia in the National Comorbidity Survey. *Archives of General Psychiatry, 53*(2), 159–168.

Maier, W., Lichtermann, D., Meyer, A., et al. (1993). A controlled family study in panic disorder. *Journal of Psychiatric Research, 27*(Suppl 1), 79–87.

Malanfranchi, A., Ravaglis, S., Lensi, P., Marazziti, D., & Cassano, G. (1997). A double-blinded study of fluvoxamine and clomipramine in the treatment of obsessive-compulsive disorder. *International Clinical Psychopharmacology, 12*(3), 131–136.

Mannuzza, S., Schneier, F., Chapman, T., Liebowitz, M., Klein, D., & Fyer, A. (1995). Generalized social phobia: Reliability and validity. *Archives of General Psychiatry, 52,* 230–237.

March, J., Frances, A., Carpenter, D., & Kahn, D. (1997). Treatment of obsessive-compulsive disorder. *Journal of Clinical Psychiatry, 58*(Suppl), 11–28.

Massion, A., Warshaw, M., & Keller, M. (1993). Quality of life and psychiatric morbidity in panic disorder and generalized anxiety disorder. *American Journal of Psychiatry, 150,* 600–607.

Mavissakalian, M., & Perel, J. (1995). Imipramine treatment of panic disorder with agoraphobia: Dose ranging and plasma level-response relationships. *American Journal of Psychiatry, 152,* 673–682.

McNally, R. (1996). Methodological controversies in the treatment of panic disorder. *Journal of Consulting & Clinical Psychology, 64*(1), 88–91.

Medical Letter. (1993). Drugs that cause psychiatric symptoms. *Medical Letter, 35*(901), 65–70.

Mendlewicz, J., Papadimitriou, G., & Wilmotte, J. (1993). Family study of panic disorder: Comparison with generalized anxiety disorder, major depression, and normal subjects. *Psychiatric Genetics, 3,* 73–78.

Mundo, E., Blanchi, L., & Boelloti, L. (1997). Efficacy of fluvoxamine, paroxetine, and citalopram in the treatment of obsessive-compulsive disorder: A single-blind study. *Journal of Clinical Psychopharmacology, 17*(4), 267–271.

Noyes, R. (1991). Suicide and panic disorder: A review. *Journal of Affective Disorders, 22,* 1–11.

Noyes R., Reich, J. et al. (1990). Outcome of panic disorder: Relationship to diagnostic subtypes and comorbidity. *Arch Gen Psych 47,* 809–818.

Noyes, R., Woodman, C., Garvey, M., et al. (1992). Generalized anxiety disorder vs. panic disorder: Distinguishing characteristics and patterns of comorbidity. *Journal of Nervous & Mental Disease, 180*, 369–379.

Olfson, M., Broadhead, W., & Weissman, M. (1996). Subthreshold psychiatric symptoms in a primary care group practice. *Archives of General Psychiatry, 53*(10), 880–886.

Orloff, L., Battle, M., Baer, L., Ivanjack, L., Pettit, A., Buttolph, M., & Jenike, M. (1994). Long-term follow-up of 85 patients with obsessive-compulsive disorder. *American Journal of Psychiatry, 151*(3), 441–442.

Oswall, R., Anderson, M., Hagstrom, K., & Berkowitz, B. (1993). Evaluation of the one-session Eye-Movement Desensitization Reprocessing procedure for eliminating traumatic memories. *Psychology Report, 73*(1), 99–104.

Pauls, D., Alsobrook, J., Goodman, W., Rasmussen, S., & Leckman, F. (1995). A family study of obsessive-compulsive disorder. *American Journal of Psychiatry, 152*(1), 76–84.

Piccinelli, M., Pini, S., Bellantuono, C., & Wilkinson, G. (1995). Efficacy of drug treatment in obsessive-compulsive disorder. A meta-analytic review. *British Journal of Psychiatry, 166*(4), 424–443.

Pourmotabbed, T., Mclead, D., Hoehn-Saric, R., Hipsley, P., & Greenblatt, D. (1996). Treatment, discontinuation, and psychomotor effects of diazepam in women with generalized anxiety disorder. *Journal of Clinical Psychopharmacology, 16*(3), 202–207.

Raj, A. & Sheehan, D. (1987). Medical evaluation of panic attacks. *J Clin Psych 48*, 309–313.

Rasmussen, S., & Eisen, J. (1992). The epidemiology and clinical features of obsessive-compulsive disorder. *Psychiatric Clinics of North America, 15*, 743–758.

Rasmussen, S., & Eisen, J. (1994). The epidemiology and differential diagnosis of obsessive-compulsive disorder. *Journal of Clinical Psychiatry, 55*(Suppl 4), 5–10.

Reich, J., Goldenberg, I., Vasile, R., et al. (1994). A prospective follow-along study of the course of social phobia. *Psychiatry Research, 54*, 249–258.

Rickels, K., Downing, R., Schweizer, E., & Hassman, H. (1993). Antidepressants for the treatment of generalized anxiety disorder. A placebo-controlled comparison of imipramine, trazodone, and diazepam. *Archives of General Psychiatry, 50*(11), 884–895.

Robins, L., & Reiger, D. (1991). *Psychiatric disorders in America: The Epidemiologic Catchment Area Study.* New York: The Free Press.

Rocca, P., Fonzo, V., Scotta, M., Zanalda, E., & Ravizza, L. (1997). Paroxetine efficacy in the treatment of generalized anxiety disorder. *Acta Psychiatrica Scandinavica, 95*(5), 444–450.

Rothbaum, B. (1997). A controlled study of eye movement desensitization and reprocessing in the treatment of posttraumatic stress disordered sexual assault victims. *Bulletin of the Menninger Clinic, 61*(3), 317–334.

Rubin, R., Villanueva-Meyer, J., Ananth, J., et al. (1992). Regional Xenon-133 cerebral blood flow and cerebral technetium 99m HMPAO uptake in unmedicated patients with obsessive-compulsive disorder and matched normal control subjects. *Archives of General Psychiatry, 49*, 695–702.

Rutherford, R., Braunwald, E., & Sobel, B.. (1992) Chronic ischemic heart disease. In E. Braunwald (Ed.). *Heart disease: Textbook of cardiovascular medicine*, 4th ed. Philadelphia: W.B. Saunders.

Sanderson, W., Wetzler, S., Beck, A., & Betz, F. (1994). Prevalence of personality disorders among patients with anxiety disorders. *Psychiatry Research, 51*, 167–174.

Schneier, F., Jihad, B., Campeas, R., et al. (1993). Buspirone in social phobia. *Journal of Clinical Psychopharmacology, 13*, 251–256.

Schneier, F., Johnson, J. et al. (1992). Social phobia: Comorbidity and morbidity in an epidemiological sample. *Arch Gen Psychiatry 49*, 282–288.

Schnurr, P., Friedman, M., & Rosenberg, S. (1993). Premilitary MMPI scores as predictors of combat-related PTSD symptoms. *American Journal of Psychiatry, 150*, 479–483.

Schweizer, E., & Rickels, K. (1997). Strategies for treatment of generalized anxiety in the primary care setting. *Journal of Clinical Psychiatry, 58*(Suppl 3), 27–31.

Schwiezer, E., Rickels, K. et al. (1986). Resistance to the anti-anxiety effect of buspirone in patients with a history of benzodiazepine use. *N Engl J Med 313*, 719–720.

Shahady, E. (1994). Obsessive-compulsive disorder in primary care. *Journal of Clinical Psychiatry, 55*(Suppl), 79–82.

Shapiro, F. (1996). Eye movement desensitization and reprocessing (EMDR): Evaluation of controlled PTSD research. *J Behav Ther Exp Psychiatry, 27*(3), 209–218.

Shapiro, F., Vogelmann-Sine, S., & Sine, L. (1994). Eye movement desensitization and reprocessing: Treating trauma and substance abuse. *Journal of Psychoactive Drugs, 26*(4), 379–391.

Sheehan, D., & Raj, A. (1990). Benzodiazepine treatment of panic disorder. In R. Noyes, M. Roth, & G. Burrows (Eds.). *Handbook of anxiety*, Vol. 4, pp. 169–206. New York: Elsevier.

Solomon, S., Gerrity, E., & Muff, A. (1992). Efficacy of treatments for posttraumatic stress disorder: An empirical review. *JAMA, 268*, 633–638.

Southwick, S., Morgan A. et al. (1993). Trauma-related symptoms in veterans of Operation Desert Storm: A preliminary report. *Am J Psychiatry 150*, 1524–1538.

Southwick, S., Morgan, A., Nagy, L., et al. (1993). Trauma-related symptoms in veterans of Operation Desert Storm: A preliminary report. *American Journal of Psychiatry, 150*, 1524–1538.

Sramek, J., Tansman, M., Suri, A., et al. (1996). Efficacy of buspirone in generalized anxiety disorder with coexisting mild depressive symptoms. *Journal of Clinical Psychiatry, 57*(7), 287–291.

Staab, J., Grieger, T., Fullerton, C., & Ursano, R. (1996). Acute stress disorder, subsequent posttraumatic stress disorder and depression after a series of typhoons. *Anxiety, 2*(5), 219–225.

Sutherland, S., & Davidson, J. (1994). Pharmacotherapy for post-traumatic stress disorder. *Psychiatric Clinics of North America, 2*, 409–423.

True, W., Rice, J., Eisen, S., et al. (1993). A twin study of genetic and environmental contributions to liability for posttraumatic stress symptoms. *Archives of General Psychiatry, 50*, 257–264.

van Balkrom, A., Bakker, A., Spinhoven, P., Blaauw, B., Smeenk, S., & Ruesink, B. (1997). A meta-analysis of the treatment of panic disorder with or without agoraphobia: A comparison of psychopharmacological, cognitive-behavioral, and combination treatments. *Journal of Nervous & Mental Disease, 185*(8), 510–516.

Vaughn, K., Weise, M., Gold, R., & Tarrier, N. (1994). Eye-movement desensitization. Symptom change in post-traumatic stress disorder. *British Journal of Psychiatry, 164*(4), 533–541.

Weissman, M., Bland, R., Canino, G., et al. (1994). The cross national epidemiology of obsessive-compulsive disorder. The Cross National Collaborative Group. *Journal of Clinical Psychiatry, 55*(Suppl 3), 5–10.

Weissman, M., Bland, R., Canino, G., et al. (1997). The cross-national epidemiology of panic disorder. *Archives of General Psychiatry, 54*, 305–309.

Weissman, M., Bland, R., Canino, G., et al. (1996). The cross-national epidemiology of social phobia: A preliminary report. *International Clinical Psychopharmacology, 11*(3, Suppl), 9–14.

Weissman, M., Markowitz, J. et al. (1990). Panic disorder and cardiovascular/cerebrovascular problems: Results from a community survey. *Am J Psych 147*, 1504–1508.

Wiborg, I., & Dahl, A. (1996). Does brief dynamic psychotherapy reduce the relapse rate of panic disorder? *Archives of General Psychiatry, 53*(8), 689–694.

Wilson, S., Becker, L., & Tinker, R. (1995). Eye movement desensitization and reprocessing (EMDR) treatment for psychologically traumatized individuals. *Journal of Consulting & Clinical Psychology, 63*(6), 928–937.

Wittchen, H.-U., Zhao, S., Kessler, R., et al. (1994). DSM-III-R generalized anxiety disorder in the National Comorbidity Survey. *Archives of General Psychiatry, 51*, 8–19.

Wolfe, B., & Mase, J. (Eds.). (1994). *Treatment of panic disorder: A consensus development conference.* Washington, DC: American Psychiatric Press.

Woodcock, J. (1990). Psychiatry. *Medical consultation: The internist on surgical, obstetric, and psychiatric services.* W. Kammerer and R. Gross. Baltimore, MD: Williams & Wilkins.

Woodman, C., & Noyes, R. (1994). Panic disorder: Treatment with valproate. *Journal of Clinical Psychiatry, 55*, 134–136.

Wyngaarden, J., Smith, L., & Bennett, J. (Eds.). (1992). *Cecil's textbook of medicine,* 19th ed. Philadelphia: W.B. Saunders.

Bibliography

Anxiety disorders. (1994/1995). NIH Publication No. 95-3879.

Babior, S., & Goldman, C. (1990). *Overcoming panic attacks: Strategies to free yourself from the anxiety trap.* Duluth, MN: Pfeifer-Hamilton Publishers/Whole Person Associates.

Baer, L. (1991). *Getting control.* Boston: Little, Brown & Co.

Barlow, D.H., & Craske, M.G. (1994). *Mastery of your anxiety and panic II. (a workbook),* 2d ed. Albany, NY: Graywind Publishers.

Black, D., Uhde, T., & Tancer, M. (1992). Fluoxetine for treatment of social phobia. *Journal of Clinical Psychopharmacology, 12,* 293–295.

Black, D., Wesner, R., Bowers, W., & Gabel, J. (1993). A comparison of fluvoxamine, cognitive therapy and placebo in the treatment of panic disorder. *Archives of General Psychiatry, 50,* 44–50.

Blanchard, E., Hickling, E., Vollmer, A., Buckley, T., & Jaccard, J. (1995). Short-term follow-up of post-traumatic stress symptoms in motor vehicle accident victims. *Behav Res Ther, 33*(4), 369–377.

Bland, R., Newman, S., & Orn, H. (1988). Prevalence of psychiatric disorders in elderly persons in Edmonton. *Acta Psychiatrica Scandinavica, 77,* 57–63.

Bourne, E.J. (1991). *The anxiety and phobia workbook.* Oakland, CA: New Harbinger.

Buchanan, A., Meng, K., & Marks, I. (1996). What predicts improvement and compliance during behavioral treatment of obsessive compulsive disorder? *Anxiety, 2*(1), 22–27.

Ciarrocchi, J. (1995). *The doubting disease.* New Jersey: Paulist Press.

Clark, D., & Agras, W. (1991). The assessment and treatment of performance anxiety in musicians. *American Journal of Psychiatry, 148*(5), 598–605.

Davidson, J., Ford, S., Smith, R., & Potts, N. (1991). Long-term treatment of social phobia with clonazepam. *Journal of Clinical Psychiatry, 52*(Suppl), 16–20.

Davidson, J., Kudler, H., & Saunders, W. (1993). Predicting response to amitriptyline in posttraumatic stress disorder. *American Journal of Psychiatry, 150,* 1024–1029.

Davidson, J., Potts, N., Richichi, E., et al. (1993). Treatment of social phobia with clonazepam and placebo. *Journal of Clinical Psychopharmacology, 13*(6), 423–428.

Foa, E., & Wilson, R. (1991). *Stop obsessing!* New York: Bantam.

Getting treatment for panic disorder. (1994). NIH Publication No. 94-3641.

Griest, J.H., & Jefferson, J.W. (1992). *Panic disorder and agoraphobia: A guide.* Madison, WI: Anxiety Disorders Center and Information Centers, University of Wisconsin.

Herman, J.L. (1992). *Trauma and recovery.* New York: Basic Books.

Hoehn-Saric, R., McLeod, D., & Hipsley, P. (1993). Effect of fluvoxamine on panic disorder. *Journal of Clinical Psychopharmacology, 13*(5), 321–326.

Hoffart, A., Due-Madsen, J., Lande, B., Gude, T., Bille, H., & Torgerson, S. (1993). Clomipramine in the treatment of agoraphobic inpatients resistant to behavioral therapy. *Journal of Clinical Psychiatry, 54*(12), 481–487.

Kernodle, W.D. (1995). *Panic disorder: The medical point of view.* Richmond, VA: Cadmus Publishing.

Lecrubier, Y., & Judge, R. (1997). Long-term evaluation of paroxetine, clomipramine and placebo in panic disorder. Collaborative Paroxetine Panic Study Investigators. *Acta Psychiatrica Scandinavica, 95*(2), 153–160.

Liebowitz, M., Schneier, R., Campeas, R., et al. (1992). Phenelzine vs. atenolol in social phobia. A placebo-controlled comparison. *Archives of General Psychiatry, 49*(4), 290–300.

Louie, A., Lewis, T., & Lannon, R. (1993). Use of low-dose fluoxetine in major depression and panic disorder. *Journal of Clinical Psychiatry, 54,* 435–438.

Mallinger, A., & DeWyze, J. (1992). *Too perfect: When being in control gets out of control.* New York: Ballantine Books.

Marks, I.M. (1978). *Living in fear.* New York: McGraw-Hill.

Marshall, J.R. (1994). *Social phobia: From shyness to stage fright.* New York: Basic Books.

Modigh, K., Westberg, P., & Eriksson, E. (1992). Superiority of clomipramine over imipramine in the treatment of panic disorder with agoraphobia: A placebo-controlled trial. *Journal of Clinical Psychiatry, 12,* 251–259.

Neziroglu, F., & Yaryura-Tobias. (1990). *Over and over again: Understanding obsessive-compulsive disorder.* Lexington, MA: Lexington Books.

Pollack, M., Otto, M., Tesar, G., Cohen, L., Meltzer-Brody, S., & Rosenbaum, J. (1993). Long-term outcome after acute treatment with alprazolam or clonazepam for panic disorder. *Journal of Clinical Psychopharmacology, 13*(4), 257–263.

Rapoport, J. (1991). *The boy who couldn't stop washing.* New York: Penguin Books.

Ravaris, C., Friedman, M., Hauri, P., et al. (1991). A controlled study of alprazolam and propranolol in panic disordered and agoraphobic outpatients. *Journal of Clinical Psychopharmacology, 11,* 344–350.

Ross, J. (1994). *Triumph over fear: A book of help and hope for people with anxiety, panic attacks and phobias.* New York: Bantam.

Schneier, F., & Welkowitz, L. (1996). *The hidden face of shyness: Understanding & overcoming social anxiety.* New York: Avon Books.

Schwartz, J. (1996). *The brain lock.* New York: Regan Books/HarperCollins.

Sheehan, D., Raj, A., Harnett-Sheehan, K., et al. (1993). The relative efficacy of high-dose buspirone and alprazolam in the treatment of panic disorder: A double-blind-controlled study. *Acta Psychiatrica Scandinavica, 88,* 1–11.

Sheehan, D.V. (1986). *The anxiety disease.* New York: Bantam.

Steketee, G., & White, K. (1990). *When once is not enough.* Oakland, CA: New Harbinger Publications.

Shelton, R., Harvey, D., Stewart, P., & Loosen, P. (1993). Alprazolam in panic disorder: A retrospective analysis. *Progress in Neuropsychopharmacology & Biologic Psychiatry, 17*(3), 423–434.

Spiegel, D., Saeed, S., & Bruce, T. (1996). An open trial of fluvoxamine therapy for panic disorder complicated by depression. *Journal of Clinical Psychiatry, 57*(Suppl), 37–40.

Understanding panic disorder. (1993). NIH Publication No. 93-3509.

Van der Kolk, B., Dreyfuss, D., Michaels, M., et al. (1994). Fluoxetine in posttraumatic stress disorder. *Journal of Clinical Psychiatry, 55*(12), 517–522.

Van Vliet, I., den Boer, J., & Westenberg, H. (1994). Psychopharmacological treatment of social phobia: A double-blind, placebo-controlled study with fluvoxamine. *Psychopharmacology, 115,* 128–134.

Versiani, M., Nardi, A., Mundim, F., Alves, A., Liebowitz, M., & Amrien, R. (1992). Pharmacotherapy of social phobia. A controlled study with moclobemide and phenelzine. *British Journal of Psychiatry, 161,* 353–360.

Weissman, M., Wickramaratne, P., Adams, P., et al. (1993). The relationship between panic disorder and major depression: A new family study. *Archives of General Psychiatry, 50,* 767–780.

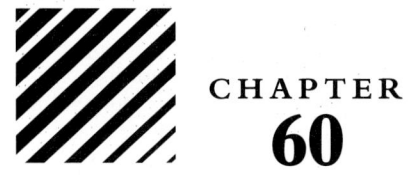

CHAPTER
60

Depression and Bipolar Disorder

Diane M. Snow, PhD, RN, CS, CARN, PMHNP

Depression and bipolar disorder (BPD; formerly called manic-depressive disorder) are mood disorders characterized by predominant affective or mood symptoms along with a variety of cognitive and behavioral symptoms. Occurring for specified periods of time, mood disorders cause variable but significant problems in social and occupational functioning. They are prevalent in all age groups and are more commonly diagnosed in women. The majority of suicides occur in persons with serious depression.

Patients with mood disorders are frequently seen in primary care, often presenting with somatic symptoms or coexisting acute or chronic medical illnesses that complicate the clinical picture. Substance abuse, medications, and serious stressors may be precipitating factors. Frequently a family history of depression is reported.

Primary care providers, in a managed care environment, are usually expected to treat depression rather than refer the patient to a psychiatrist. However, depressive illnesses often are underdiagnosed, untreated, and undertreated in primary care settings. Often patients hesitate to discuss symptoms because of embarrassment or fear, or thinking they are there for "physical problems only." The provider may avoid asking about suicidal ideation despite recognition of depressed mood. Patients with chronic physical illnesses are often not asked about mood and other behaviors indicative of masked depression. Men are rarely asked about depression, as if it is a disease of women only.

Elderly patients are assumed to have dementia when there are any memory or concentration difficulties. Moreover, unless the provider develops adequate rapport with the patient and views the patient "holistically," the disorder may go undetected. Finally, if the patient is irritable or hostile or shows poor judgment, the provider may dismiss the patient as uncooperative. Adequate treatment and prevention of further episodes are mandatory. Collaborative relationships must be maintained with psychiatric services, and prompt referrals and emergency care must be implemented when warranted. Strategies for prevention include building healthy coping skills, early detection, and relapse prevention, often with help from community resources.

ANATOMY, PHYSIOLOGY, AND PATHOLOGY

There are numerous biologic changes that occur in depression and BPD, and they have helped create a new understanding of these painful, often life-threatening disorders. Genetic factors, neuroendocrine, neurotransmission, structural, and functional brain changes are all important aspects of the pathology of depression. Physical illness, medication effects, electrolyte disturbances, and nutritional deficits play an important role as well. Life events such as recent stressors, when combined with

genetic factors, are also important (Kendler et al, 1992). More traditional psychological theories support the role of personalities and problem-solving skills in depression and BPD.

Genetics

Family studies have demonstrated that monozygotic twins have a higher rate of concordance (agreement) for depression and BPD than dizygotic twins (Andrews et al, 1990). Family aggregation studies point to the increased risk of depression and BPD in first-degree relatives. Major depressive disorder (MDD) is 1.5 to 3 times more common in first-degree relatives. Rates of BPD exceed those of depression, with a 25% to 27% chance that a child with one parent with BPD will have the disorder (versus 10% to 13% for depression) and a 50% to 75% chance if both parents have bipolar disorder (American Psychiatric Association [APA], 1994). Moreover, early-onset depression, when symptoms occur as early as childhood, is more familial; patients are likely to have more genetic vulnerability (Overaschel, 1990).

Linkage genetic studies demonstrate that certain chromosomes may show a single gene for certain disorders. Chromosome 11 was first thought to be the genetic marker for BPD, but this was not supported in later studies. More recently, a corticotrophin receptor and a subunit of a G protein on chromosome 18 have been implicated, but this is still under investigation. No single gene has been associated with MDD, probably because of genetic heterogeneity (Berrettini et al, 1994).

Neurobiologic Changes

Neurobiologic changes in mood disorders primarily involve dysfunction of the limbic system, the basal ganglia, and the hypothalamus. The limbic system, specifically the amygdala, modulates emotions, whereas the hippocampus is implicated in memory and concentration difficulties. Changes in the basal ganglia involve motor changes such as stooped posture, motor slowness, and cognitive impairment. Dysfunction of the hypothalamus involves three axes: the hypothalamic–pituitary–adrenal (HPA) axis, the hypothalamic–pituitary–thyroid axis, and the hypothalamic–pituitary–gonadal axis.

Dysregulation of several neurotransmitter systems has been found in depression and BPD. Neurotransmitters are molecules that carry messages between neurons. They are released into the synaptic cleft from the presynaptic neuron. From here, they either occupy a receptor site on the postsynaptic membrane of the target neuron or are stored or metabolized by the presynaptic neuron (Restak, 1988). The biogenic amines, particularly serotonin (5HT) and norepinephrine, interact and modulate a variety of functions, such as cognitive, sexual, motor, neuroendocrine, mood, and sleep, and have been found to be abnormally regulated in depression.

Serotonin, whose precursor is the dietary amino acid tryptophan, originates in the raphe nuclei of the pons and upper brain stem and travels widely throughout the brain and spinal cord. Serotonin depletion may precipitate depression; receptor sensitivity increases during a depressive episode, and modulation with other neurotransmitters may be out of balance. Serotonin's major metabolite, 5-hydroxyindoleacetic acid (5H1AA), was lower than normal in a study of depressed persons who committed suicide (Goodwin & Jamison, 1990). Serotonin dysregulation, then, may be related to suicide, impulsivity, and aggressive behavior.

Depletion of norepinephrine is shown in most, but not all, depressed persons. Norepinephrine, whose precursor is the dietary amino acid tyrosine, is produced in the locus ceruleus and projects through six noradrenergic tracts through various parts of the brain. Dopamine levels are believed to increase in mania and decrease in depression. Gamma-aminobutyric acid (GABA), an inhibitory amino acid neurotransmitter, and acetylcholine (ACTH) also are dysregulated in depression. In BPD, excessive baseline calcium may contribute to a mixture of symptoms as a compensatory response (Dubovsky et al, 1992).

Neuroendocrine changes in the HPA axis include consistent findings of elevated cortisol secretion from the adrenal glands associated with the stress response. Levels of corticotrophin-releasing factor (CRF), the hypothalamic peptide that regulates pituitary secretion of corticotrophin, and cortisol have been found to be elevated in the cerebrospinal fluid of depressed persons (Nemeroff et al, 1984). CRF release depends on neurotransmitters such as serotonin, norepinephrine, acetylcholine, and GABA (Beeber, 1996). Corticotrophin, by attaching to cells in the adrenal cortex, causes the release of cortisol. In a feedback loop, cortisol then inhibits the secretion of corticotrophin in the anterior pituitary and CRF in the hypothalamus. Increased CRF levels, therefore, may explain the hypercortisolism and HPA axis overactivity seen in MDD. Elevated CRF levels in depression normalize after electroconvulsive therapy and after treatment with selective serotonin reuptake inhibitor medications (SSRIs).

Levels of somastatin, a growth hormone release inhibitor hormone, decrease in both MDD and depressive episodes of BPD (Rubinow et al, 1983); in manic episodes, this change has not been documented. Along with hypercortisolemia, somastatin underactivity is a consistent finding in depression.

Hypothalamic–pituitary–thyroid axis changes frequently occur with depression and BPD. In 25% of people with depression, there is blunting of the thyroid-stimulating hormone (TSH) response to thyroid-releasing hormone in the thyroid-releasing hormone stimulation test (Nemeroff, 1990). Elevation of thyroxin, or T4, may be significant in severely depressed patients. Moreover, there are some indications that in postpartum women and women with rapid-cycling BPD (four or more episodes a year), there are thyroid changes that may precipitate bipolar episodes. Lastly, thyroid hormone replacement is used to augment antidepressant therapy in MDD and is sometimes used in rapid-cycling BPD.

Biologic Rhythm Changes

Sleep alterations frequently occur in both depressive and manic episodes; both insomnia and hypersomnia reflect circadian rhythm dysregulation. Sleep problems may include many if not all of the following: delayed sleep onset, shortened rapid eye movement (REM) latency (the time before falling asleep and the first REM period), increased length of first REM period, increased frequency of eye movements during REM sleep, increased spontaneous awakenings, and abnormal delta sleep. Sleep electroencephalographic recordings are abnormal in many depressed persons even before the onset of clinical depression (Giles et al, 1989). This finding may explain why depressed persons report feeling tired even after a night's sleep. Antidepressant medications are helpful in resetting sleep circadian rhythms.

Additional biologic rhythm disturbances are seen in depression that has seasonal variation, rapid-cycling BPD, and premenstrual mood changes. More common is seasonal depression that recurs in the fall and winter, although some persons have a reverse pattern of depression in the spring and summer. Thought to be related to the changes in light and temperature, seasonal depression is currently being treated or "reset" with phototherapy or light therapy. Rapid-cycling BPD involves rapidly switching to mania or depression in rhythmic cycles that may be days, weeks, or months long. Many women note increased mood variations based on the biologic rhythm and hormonal changes during their menstrual cycles.

Electrophysiologic Process of Kindling

A recent advance in understanding the nature of relapse in depression and BPD has been through the phenomenon of "kindling," or sensitization. Repeated subthreshold stimulation of neurons in seizure disorders eventually can precipitate a seizure, and the same electrophysiologic process is believed to occur with depression and BPD (Keltner et al, 1998). Kindling in the temporal lobes, possibly based on genetic predisposition, causes a return of symptoms, even more so if there has been inadequate treatment. Each subsequent episode tends to have worse symptoms, and episodes occur closer together.

Although earlier episodes often require triggering from external stimulation, later episodes kindle by repetition and become an autonomous process. Continued prophylactic pharmacotherapy after the reduction or elimination of symptoms will help prevent chronicity and worsening of symptoms. Particularly useful for prophylaxis of BPD are the anticonvulsant medications used as mood stabilizers (carbamazepine, valproax sodium, lamotrigine, and gabapentin).

Structural and Functional Brain Changes

Structural changes in the brain, interpreted in neuroimaging studies using magnetic resonance imaging and computed tomography, include decreased size of the caudate nuclei and putamen of the basal ganglia and decreased prefrontal cortex volume. There are abnormal hippocampal times in magnetic resonance imaging T_1 images, which are short-time sequences used to define the brain and spinal cord anatomy. The hippocampus is the major area of the limbic system for memory and learning. Temporal lobe volume is reduced and there are deep white matter lesions in BPD. Changes in the orbitofrontal cortex during a manic episode are probably responsible for the impulsivity, social inhibition, and lability of mood of these periods (Cummings, 1993).

Cerebral blood flow and metabolism are measures of brain function that are seen in photon emission tomography and single photon emission computed tomography. Decreased cerebral blood flow and hypometabolism in the frontal cortex, where logical thought and reasoning occur, have been consistent findings in depression (Keltner et al, 1998). Increased metabolic activity, as well as cerebral asymmetries indicating hypometabolism limited to the left frontal lobe, have been found in these scans in patients with BPD. Also, abnormal regulation of phospholipid metabolism has been found in BPD patients.

Physical Illness and Depression

Certain physical illnesses that involve the same brain structures that are altered in depression will cause symptoms of depression. For example, in Huntington's disease there is a high rate of depression, based on the reduction of volume in the putamen and caudate nuclei. In cerebrovascular accidents that involve the frontal and temporal lobes, manic symptoms are more common with right-sided lesions, whereas depressive symptoms are more common with left-sided lesions (Keltner et al, 1998).

Psychological Theories

Psychological theories of depression include the psychoanalytic explanation of depression as anger directed internally, based on the introjection of an ambivalently held lost object. Early attachment difficulties, based on the impact of separation and loss, may precipitate depression (Bowlby, 1980). Behavioral theory views vulnerability to depression as a lack of social support, causing loneliness and isolation (Skinner, 1953). Inadequate social skills that prevent positive reinforcement from others contribute to depression under this model (Lewinsohn, 1974). Cognitive theory proposes that depression is precipitated and maintained by negative thoughts and attitudes; a cognitive triad of negative views of self, others, and the future; and negative schemas or belief systems (Beck, 1976).

EPIDEMIOLOGY

Depression and BPD are serious mental health problems that must be addressed in primary care. MDD affects 15% of the population, with prevalence rates as high as 25% in women (APA, 1994). The National Institute of Health estimates that 15 million Americans become depressed in any given year (Hall & Wise, 1995). It is estimated that 1 in 5 women and 1 in 10 men seen in primary care have recently been depressed (Rowe et al, 1995). The rate may be even higher (12% to 36%) when the person has a general medical condition (Depression Guideline Panel, 1993a).

Women suffer depression at a rate twice that of men, and younger women are at greater risk than any other age group (Depression Guideline Panel, 1993a). Particular points of vulnerability for depression in women are rhythm-disrupting events such as the perinatal, menopausal, and menstrual periods and seasonal light changes (Beeber, 1996). Treatment may involve restoration of normal rhythms through endocrine treatment and phototherapy.

Depression and BPD are found in all cultures. Cultural expressions of symptoms vary and should be considered during all aspects of care. True psychosis must be distinguished from culturally specific experiences. Treatment choices must be sensitive to the cultural needs of patients.

Increased rates of alcoholism are seen in adult first-degree relatives of persons with MDD; the incidence of ADHD is also increased in children of adults with MDD (APA, 1994).

In older adults, the rate of depression seen in primary care is 5%; the rate seen in long-term care facilities is 15% to 25% (NIH, 1992). A study of long-term care patients found that the presence of MDD raised the risk of rapid death by 59% (Rover et al, 1991).

The lifetime rate of dysthymic disorder has been found to be 4.1% for women and 2.2% for men. The diagnosis of depression not otherwise specified has a point prevalence of 8.4% to 9.7% in primary care patients (Depression Guideline Panel, 1993a).

Suicide is the eighth leading cause of death among all age groups, and at least 50% of suicides can be attributed to MDD. For persons aged 15 to 24, suicide is the third leading cause of death. More than 70% of all suicides in the United States are committed by white men. Suicide rates are alarmingly high in very old men, with 75.1 suicides per 100,000 population versus an overall suicide rate of 11.8 per 100,000. The group at highest risk for suicide is elderly American men (Moscicki, 1995). (See Table 60-5.)

BPD type I disorder has a lifetime risk of close to 1%, with approximately equal gender distribution and no association with race or ethnic origin. Combining types I and II, there is a 1.2% lifetime prevalence rate (Regier et al, 1990). Interestingly, in men the first episode is more likely to be a manic episode, whereas in women the first episode is more likely to be a major depressive episode. Women with type I have an increased risk for further episodes postpartum. First-degree biologic relatives have 4% to 24% higher rates of type I (APA, 1994).

Cyclothymic disorder has a lifetime prevalence of 0.4% to 1% (Depression Guideline Panel, 1993a).

BPD in children and adolescents, although underdiagnosed, is considered to occur at least as frequently as in adults (Geller & Luby, 1997). Comorbidity includes ADHD, conduct disorder, substance abuse, and anxiety disorders.

DIAGNOSTIC CRITERIA

Screening, assessment, accurate diagnosis, adequate treatment, frequent follow-up, and referrals for psychotherapy and psychiatric evaluation (if needed) are critical for patients with symptoms of depression and BPD. Any patient with a history of depression or BPD needs to be assessed on a regular basis for treatment response, side effects, new symptoms, and recurrence of symptoms. Patients need encouragement to obtain and continue treatment. Providers need a thorough understanding of the diagnostic categories and the complexity and variability of depressive symptoms. Widely available self-report screening tools for depression that are useful for measuring treatment response include the Beck Depression Inventory, Zung Depression and Anxiety Scales, Center for Epidemiological Studies Depression Scale, and Geriatric Depression Scale. The Symptoms-Driven Diagnostic System for Primary Care (SIDDS-PC) is a computer-based tool; the Hamilton Depression Rating Scale and Montgomery-Asberg Depression Rating Scale are provider-rated tools that are completed during the interview.

Next, the history and clinical interview address target symptoms from the *Diagnostic and Statistical Manual of Mental*

Disorders, fourth edition (DSM-IV; APA, 1994), including age, gender, family system, and cultural considerations. The results of the screening tools, mental status exam, laboratory values, and physical exam will help determine the presence of depression or BPD. Medical illnesses and medications that may precipitate depression must also be evaluated (Tables 60-1 and 60-2).

Major Depressive Disorder

MDD, or unipolar depression, is the most frequently diagnosed mood-related disorder. It signifies there has been at least one major depressive episode and no manic or hypomanic episodes. Symptoms have occurred every day for 2 weeks or longer. Significant distress or impairment in psychosocial or work functioning must be present. For a diagnosis of MDD to be made, substance use, medication, and medical conditions must be ruled out. A mood disturbance must be present with a number of alterations from normal mood (eg, depressed mood with typical sadness, agitation and anger, irritability, dysphoria, numbing of feelings, or somatic preoccupation). Of equal importance is the loss of pleasure in activities that were previously enjoyed, such as hobbies, work, or sexual activity. One of these two symptoms—mood disturbance or loss of pleasure—must be present for a diagnosis of MDD.

Additional symptoms must also be present. Three neurovegetative symptoms are evaluated: sleep, appetite, and psychomotor activity. Sleep alteration may be present (insomnia or hypersomnia). Insomnia can take the form of difficulty falling asleep (initial insomnia), frequent waking without being able to fall back to sleep quickly (middle insomnia), or waking several hours earlier than usual (terminal insomnia). Hypersomnia means the person sleeps several more hours a day than is usual for that person. A key concern is whether the person feels rested after a night's sleep. Psychomotor activity may be observed as either very sluggish, slow movements or agitation or pacing, where the person cannot stop moving. An increase or decrease in appetite or weight gain or loss of 5% or more of body weight must be assessed.

TABLE 60-1	General Medical Conditions Associated With Depression

Neurologic
  Parkinson's disease
  Huntington's disease
  Stroke
  Multiple sclerosis
  Sleep apnea
  Cerebral tumors
  Alzheimer's disease

Infectious
  Influenza
  Viral hepatitis
  General paresis
    (tertiary syphilis)
  Tuberculosis
  Infectious mononucleosis
  Chronic fatigue syndrome

Collagen
  Systemic lupus erythematosus
  Scleroderma
  Rheumatoid arthritis

Nutritional
  Vitamin B_{12} deficiency
  Pernicious anemia

Cardiovascular
  Coronary artery disease

Endocrine
  Cushing's disease
  Addison's disease
  Diabetes mellitus
  Hypo- and hyperthyroidism

Neoplastic
  Carcinoma of head of pancreas
  Oat cell carcinoma

TABLE 60-2	Medications Associated With Depressed Mood and Manic Symptoms
Depressed Mood	**Manic Symptoms**
Reserpine	Levodopa
Propranolol	Amphetamines
Glucocorticoids	Bromide
Alcohol	Bromocriptine
Physostigmine	Captopril
Sedative–hypnotics	Cimetidine
Amphetamine or cocaine withdrawal	Cocaine
Benzodiazepines	Corticosteroids
Neuroleptics	Cyclosporine
Anti-inflammatories	Disulfiram
Anticonvulsants	Hallucinogens
Antihypertensives	Hydralazine
Antineoplastics	Isoniazid
Antiparkinsonian drugs	Methylphenidate
Stimulants	Metrizamide (following myelography)
Antihistamines	Monoamine oxidase inhibitors
Cimetidine	Opiates and opioids
Ranifidine	Procarbazine
Disulfiram	Procyclidine
Methysergide	Tricyclic antidepressants
Antibiotics	Thyroid hormones

Other evaluated symptoms include a feeling of fatigue or loss of energy, expressed as a loss of will. Also, feelings of worthlessness and guilt are common, sometimes manifested in psychotic delusions. Difficulty with concentration, thinking, or making decisions is distressing. A patient may forget to bathe or change clothes or complain of not being able to complete tasks. In the older person, memory loss may appear to be dementia when in fact it is pseudodementia or memory loss caused by depression.

Suicidality is an extremely serious symptom of MDD and must be assessed in anyone who has mood alteration. Hopelessness and thoughts of death without specific suicidal thoughts (eg, "Death would be such a relief; why go on?"). More serious are suicidal thoughts or ideation (eg, "I keep thinking that everyone would be better off without me"), while some persons have made actual suicide attempts. Asking the patient about suicidal thoughts will not cause the person to become suicidal. Frequency of thoughts, presence of a plan, methods, previous attempts, and history of suicide in the family are important assessment factors (Table 60-3).

There are subtypes of MDD that delineate the severity and type of depression. These include mild, moderate, and severe, referring to the severity of impairment in functioning; psychosis with hallucinations or delusions, catatonic features, melancholic features, and atypical features are other specifiers.

The onset of MDD in the postpartum period (within 4 weeks of delivery), with symptoms that last 2 to 12 months after delivery, is a specifier and is likely to recur with later deliveries. Guilt is a major component of this type of depression.

Seasonal pattern delineation is made when there is a 2-year pattern of recurrence during the winter (or, more rarely, during

TABLE 60-3	Criteria for Major Depressive Episode

A. Five (or more) of the following symptoms have been present during the same 2-week period and represent a change from previous functioning; at least one of the symptoms is either (1) depressed mood or (2) loss of interest or pleasure. **Note:** Do not include symptoms that are clearly due to a general medical condition, or mood-incongruent delusions or hallucinations.

   (1) Depressed mood most of the day, nearly every day, as indicated by either subjective report (eg, feels sad or empty) or observation made by others (eg, appears tearful). **Note:** In children and adolescents, can be irritable mood.
   (2) Markedly diminished interest or pleasure in all, or almost all, activities most of the day, nearly every day (as indicated by either subjective account or observation made by others)
   (3) Significant weight loss when not dieting or weight gain (eg, a change of more than 5% of body weight in a month), or decrease or increase in appetite nearly every day. **Note:** In children, consider failure to make expected weight gains.
   (4) Insomnia or hypersomnia nearly every day
   (5) Psychomotor agitation or retardation nearly every day (observable by others, not merely subjective feelings of restlessness or being slowed down)
   (6) Fatigue or loss of energy nearly every day
   (7) Feelings of worthlessness or excessive or inappropriate guilt (which may be delusional) nearly every day (not merely self-reproach or guilt about being sick)
   (8) Diminished ability to think or concentrate, or indecisiveness, nearly every day (either by subjective account or as observed by others)
   (9) Recurrent thoughts of death (not just fear of dying), recurrent suicidal ideation without a specific plan, or a suicide attempt or a specific plan for committing suicide.

B. The symptoms do not meet criteria for a Mixed Episode (see p. 335).

C. The symptoms cause clinically significant distress or impairment in social, occupational, or other important areas of functioning.

D. The symptoms are not due to the direct physiologic effects of a substance (eg, a drug of abuse, a medication) or a general medical condition (eg, hypothyroidism).

E. The symptoms are not better accounted for by Bereavement, ie, after the loss of a loved one, the symptoms persist for longer than 2 months, or are characterized by marked functional impairment, morbid preoccupation with worthlessness, suicidal ideation, psychotic symptoms, or psychomotor retardation.

American Psychiatric Association: Diagnostic and Statistical Manual of Mental Disorders, 4/e. Washington, DC: American Psychiatric Association, 1994.

the summer). Characteristics are weight gain, low energy, hypersomnia, and carbohydrate craving. Remission requires 2 months without symptoms.

Dysthymic disorder is a chronic milder form of depression that lasts 2 years in adults and 1 year in children and adolescents. Two or more of the following must be present: poor appetite or overeating; insomnia or hypersomnia; low energy or fatigue; low self-esteem; poor concentration or difficulty making decisions; and feelings of hopelessness.

Adjustment disorder with depressed mood is a direct result of a designated stressor occurring within 3 months; as such, the cause must be identified. The distress is more than would be expected and causes significant impairment in functioning.

Depressive disorder not otherwise specified (NOS) refers to depressed persons who do not meet the criteria for MDD, dysthymia, or adjustment disorder with depressed mood. Included are premenstrual dysphoric disorder, which occurs each month, 1 or 2 weeks before the onset of menses, and has the

same symptoms as MDD. Symptoms completely remit when menses begins.

Bipolar Disorders

BPDs are defined by the presence of depressive and manic, hypomanic, or mixed episodes.

BPD type I means the person has had a major depressive episode and a manic episode. Manic episodes refer to periods of abnormally elevated, expansive, "top of the world" or irritable, dysphoric mood, along with marked impairment in judgment, social function, and occupational function, that lasts at least 1 week. Three of the following symptoms must also be present: inflated self-esteem or unrealistic grandiosity; a decreased need for sleep; loud, rapid, pressured speech; flight of ideas or racing thoughts; distractibility; increased goal-directed activity, including sex, work, school, or social events; and excessive involvement in pleasurable experiences that have a high potential for painful consequences. Typically, these experiences include buying sprees, sexual indiscretions, and foolish business investments. Impaired judgment and an inability to anticipate consequences often warrant hospitalization to prevent harm to self or others. There may be psychotic symptoms of hallucinations and delusions. Frequently weight loss and dehydration occur, related to insomnia and hyperactivity.

BPD type II is characterized by a major depressive episode and hypomanic (milder manic) episodes. Hypomanic episodes include an elevated expansive mood that lasts at least 4 days, with three or more of the same symptoms as in BPD type I, although the episode is not severe enough to cause major impairment in social or occupational functioning, hospitalization, or psychosis.

Cyclothymic disorder is a chronic, milder type of BPD in which there are numerous periods of hypomanic symptoms and numerous periods of depressive symptoms that do not meet the criteria for MDD.

Depression Related to Medical Conditions and Medications

Mood disorder due to a medical condition is a disturbance in mood that is a direct result of a general medical condition. This diagnosis involves establishing a diagnosis of a medical condition as a direct physiologic cause of the depressed or manic mood (see Table 60-1). An example would be "Mood disorder due to hyperthyroidism, with manic features."

Mood disorders induced by substances such as medications, illicit drugs, or toxins are classified as substance-induced mood disorders. They must be directly caused by a substance—in other words, they must develop within a month of intoxication or withdrawal. The implicated drug is part of the diagnosis—for instance, "Alcohol-induced mood disorder with depressive features, with onset during intoxication" (or withdrawal).

HISTORY AND PHYSICAL EXAM

Using the DSM-IV criteria to guide the evaluation of signs and symptoms, to make a correct diagnosis, and to formulate a plan of care is a challenge to all primary care providers. Mnemonics may be helpful in identifying symptoms of depression (Fig. 60-

S = Is your sleep disturbed?

I = Have you noted a loss of libido or interest in your usual activities?

G = Are you feeling guilty or having self-deprecatory thoughts?

E = Have you noticed a decrease in your energy level?

C = Have you been having trouble concentrating?

A = Have you experienced changes in your appetite?

P = Have you been physically slowed down or sped up (i.e., psychomotor abnormalities)?

S = Have you had thoughts of suicide, feelings of hopelessness or preoccupation with issues related to death?

FIGURE 60-1. Mnemonics *SIG E CAPS* for Major Depressive Disorder. Rauch, S.L., Hyman, S.E. (1995) Approach to the patient with depression. In: Goroll A.H., May LA, Mully AG, Jr. Eds. *Primary Care Medicine: Office Evaluation and Management of the Adult Patient.* Philadelphia, PA: JB Lippincott, 1033–43.

1) and a manic episode of bipolar disorder (Fig. 60-2). If the patient has cognitive dysfunction (memory loss, agitation, or psychotic symptoms), getting a complete history from the patient may not be possible. Family members and care providers can offer premorbid subjective data.

When obtaining the history of the presenting illness, suicidal ideation must be carefully assessed. Even if a patient does not initiate the discussion or does not look seriously depressed, questions about suicide must be asked of anyone with signs of depression or mania. This questioning should continue at each visit throughout the treatment period. A specific question such as, "Do you have thoughts of killing yourself?" should be followed by focused questions to obtain a careful suicide history. Having a plan and the means to carry it out indicates serious lethality, as does a history of previous suicide attempts. Questions about suicide should not be asked in a negative way ("You are not thinking about suicide, are you?") because this might keep the patient from admitting the thoughts.

Inquiring about current and past life stressors, such as family issues, abuse issues, work-related stress, financial concerns, and health concerns, is critical and will help in determining the appropriate referrals. If there are no new stressors, this should not be considered unusual because of the largely biologic origins of the disorders, especially in later episodes. All current medications must be listed, including prescription and over-the-counter drugs, alcohol, illicit drugs, and herbal medications. Patients being treated for depression or BPD must be asked at each visit about all medications, because depression is a side effect of some medications (see Table 60-2).

A thorough psychiatric history should reveal previous episodes of depression or mania or comorbid conditions such as

G = Grandiosity

I = Increased activity

D = Decreased judgment

D = Distractibility

I = Irritability

N = Need for sleep decreased

E = Elevated mood

S = Speedy thoughts

S = Speedy talk

FIGURE 60-2. Mnemonic GIDDINESS for bipolar disorder, manic episode. Wise, M. (1995) in Basco, M.R., Biggs, M.M. and Davies, D. DSM-IV Life Charts and Pocket Guide. Dallas, TX: University of Texas Southwestern Medical Center at Dallas.

anxiety disorders or substance abuse. The response to previous treatment, including medications, therapy, electroconvulsive therapy, or hospitalization, should be evaluated. If treatment was not received, the symptoms should be described in terms of the level of impairment. Also, the family history of psychiatric illness will denote the type of problems, severity, type of treatment received, and response to treatment in family members.

Objective data are important in confirming the diagnosis and monitoring for response to treatment. Along with a physical exam, weight, height, laboratory work, and screening tools for depression and anxiety, a mental status exam is used to confirm the findings (Table 60-4). Scores on the Mini-Mental Status Exam provide a baseline for symptoms of cognitive loss, including memory, orientation, and constructional ability. A depressed patient may have "pseudodementia" or cognitive loss that improves with treatment of the depression. The depressed patient typically says, "I don't know" and is very distressed, whereas in dementia the patient becomes defensive or gives a wrong answer. Other objective data come from observations of appearance, mood, dress, behavior, thought process, thought content, perception, judgment, and insight.

DIAGNOSTIC STUDIES

Laboratory studies that may help substantiate the diagnosis of depression include a complete blood count with differential, electrolyte analysis, kidney and liver function screening, and thyroid function studies. Levels of vitamin B_{12} and folate are of value in ruling out vitamin deficiency, especially in the elderly. A urinalysis in an older adult helps rule out a urinary tract infection when agitation and confusion are present. A urine drug screen may be necessary to determine if symptoms are arising from or are complicated by drug intoxication or withdrawal.

An electrocardiogram is necessary to provide a baseline of cardiac function when tricyclic antidepressants (TCAs) are ordered. Conduction delays should be monitored; these could cause heart block when therapeutic levels are achieved. An annual electrocardiogram is advised for patients taking TCAs. Plasma concentrations are often tested with TCAs, especially if there is a poor response at normal dose ranges and when it is important to know if levels are therapeutic or toxic. Samples should be drawn 10 to 14 hours after the last dose.

Blood pressure must be followed in all patients on antidepressant therapy.

Before starting lithium, the following should be done: TSH assay, electrolyte levels, white blood cell count, renal function (specific gravity or urine osmolality, blood urea nitrogen, and serum creatinine), and an electrocardiogram. Regular serum lithium measurements are a continuing part of treatment; samples should be drawn 8 to 12 hours after the last dose. Levels are needed once or twice a week during stabilization and every 6 months on maintenance. The therapeutic range is 0.8 to 1.2 mEq/L. In the maintenance phase of treatment, a lower range is usually therapeutic.

When starting carbamazepine (Tegretol), a complete blood count with platelet count is done, along with a serum iron measurement and a reticulocyte count, and is repeated weekly during the first 3 months of therapy, then monthly. Liver function tests should be done every 3 to 6 months. There is a danger of aplastic anemia, agranulocytosis, thrombocytopenia,

TABLE 60-4	Mental Status Assessment	
	Depression	**Manic Episode**
APPEARANCE	Disheveled Lack of attention to clothing Poor hygiene No make-up	Bright, colorful Flamboyant Heavy make-up and jewelry Poor grooming Provocative
POSTURE	Stooped Rigid	Varies
MOTOR ACTIVITY	Minimum spontaneous movement Agitation, pacing	Fast-moving Intrusive Hyperactive Extreme goal-directed "Have to be doing something"
MOOD/AFFECT	Depressed Dysphoric Irritable Angry Sad Apathetic Lack of eye contact	Labile Elated, euphoric Angry, dysphoric Expansive Humorous Intolerant of criticism
ATTITUDE	Negative about self Blames others Negative view of future	Arrogance Inflated self-esteem
SPEECH	Slow Agitated Quiet, mute Alogia (few words)	Fast Pressured, loud
INSIGHT	Varies	Lack of shame or guilt No awareness of others' feelings
JUDGMENT	May drink excessively Indecisive	High-risk behavior Poor judgment Irresponsible Sexually inappropriate Spends money excessively Drinking, using drugs
MEMORY	Short-term loss	Varies
CONCENTRATION	Forgetful	Easily distracted
THOUGHT PROCESS	Slowed thinking Thought blocking	Loose associations Racing thoughts

THOUGHT CONTENT	Preoccupation
	Rumination
	Hopelessness, suicide
	Delusions
	   Mood congruent
	   Mood incongruent
	Guilt
	Worthlessness
	Hopelessness
	Suicide
		Grandiose delusions
		Flight of ideas
		Illusions
		Hypersexuality
		Persecutory delusions
		
		Suicide

PERCEPTION	Hallucinations (only when psychotic)	Hallucinations possible

and leukopenia. The target serum level of carbamazepine is 8 to 12 mg/mL.

TREATMENT OPTIONS, EXPECTED OUTCOMES, AND COMPREHENSIVE MANAGEMENT

There are three phases of treatment for depression and BPD. Goals of the acute phase traditionally are relief of mood alterations and associated symptoms and return to previous level of functioning. Treatment should alleviate any medical causes of depressive or manic symptoms, improve self-management skills, and improve quality of life. Continuation phase treatment focuses on psychoeducation, pharmacotherapy, and other modalities to prevent relapse and recurrence. If symptoms return within 6 months of remission, a relapse is declared (Depression Guideline Panel, 1993b). The maintenance phase is directed toward preventing future episodes of depression. Interventions should be sensitive to the patient's age, gender, and culture, and the plan of care should be individualized.

Having a model of care that addresses possible chronicity reinforces the need for ongoing, vigilant care. Because there is still a stigma attached to having a mental disorder, patients need support and guidance to build trust and rapport with their care provider and to feel safe, knowledgeable, and confident discussing their symptoms, side effects, and overall progress. They also benefit from positive therapeutic relationships (Keltner et al, 1998) that build hope and that engage support. They should have the benefit of a caring, compassionate team that includes professionals, support groups, family, friends, and co-workers

Figures 60-3 gives an algorithm for the treatment of BPD.

Antidepressant Therapy

Antidepressants are used to treat the depressive disorders, including MDD, dysthymia, adjustment disorder with depressed mood, and mood disorder due to general medical illness or substance abuse. The latter two are treated with antidepressants only after the medical illness or substance abuse is addressed. Antidepressants are also frequently given to BPD patients during depressive episodes and prophylactically between episodes. Decisions regarding the choice of antidepressant therapy are made based on several factors: age, general health status, previous response to antidepressants, side effect profile, and cost (Keltner et al, 1998) Other factors include symptom profile, family history of response to antidepressants, and personal preference.

There is no one optimal antidepressant for all patients, and all have the potential to be effective. Antidepressants should be started at low doses and increased based on response. A general rule is with partial response, increase the dose; with no response within 4 weeks, change the medication; with good response, stay at the same dose. If a medication produces a partial response and the side effect profile is minimal, then the dose should be raised gradually until the maximum recommended dose is given, providing it is tolerated, before switching to another antidepressant. Once-a-day dosing of the newer drugs can be timed to fit the symptoms or side effects. For instance, if a patient complains of drowsiness from the medication, it can be given in the evening. If it produces restless sleep and insomnia, it should be given in the morning to see if the symptoms are relieved.

Target symptoms such as the neurovegetative symptoms (sleep, appetite, and psychomotor symptoms) are usually the first to improve, usually within 1 to 2 weeks. Next, cognitive symptoms such as concentration improve over 1 to 2 weeks, and finally mood disturbance improves by the fourth to sixth week. In older patients, a longer trial is needed to evaluate response to treatment.

For partial response, the provider should add one or more of the following: an antidepressant from a different class, lithium carbonate, a thyroid preparation such as levothyroxine, a neuroleptic such as olanzapine, buspirone, a mood stabilizer such as valproic acid/valproate, and other choices. Decisions about augmentation are based on the symptom profile, comorbid mental and physical disorders, and personal choice. Patients must give informed consent to all medications, based on thorough knowledge of the actions and side effects of each medication. Primary care providers should use psychiatric consultation and referral for complicated diagnostic and management decisions and, most certainly, with refractory depression.

First-line choice of pharmacotherapy for depression includes the SSRIs as well as heterocyclic and other newer agents. These drugs are safer than older medications (TCAs and monoamine oxidase inhibitors [MAOIs]) in overdoses, have improved side effect profiles, and are well tolerated by most people. As with all antidepressants, activation of mania is always possible in patients with a history of mania. Patients with a high risk for suicide should be monitored for response, and only small quantities should be prescribed to prevent intentional overdoses. All patients receiving antidepressant therapy should have renal and liver profiles done regularly.

Serum drug levels can be measured for any antidepressant if there is danger of an overdose or toxic effects. Medications most commonly monitored in this way are the TCAs. Generally, dose changes are made no more often than every 1 to 2 weeks. No other antidepressants are safe to give with MAOIs, and MAOIs must be discontinued for 2 weeks before starting another antidepressant.

None of the antidepressants are considered totally safe during pregnancy; the risk/benefit ratio must be weighed for each patient. Breastfeeding is not advised for any woman taking antidepressants because they pass into the breast milk.

Initial dosages in the elderly should be reduced.

SSRIS

The SSRIs inhibit the reuptake of serotonin and have no significant interactions with the muscarinic, histaminic, adrenergic, and serotonergic receptors, which means that the side effects common with TCAs are avoided. SSRIs are usually given once a day in the morning to avoid insomnia. A trial of at least 2 weeks is required before their effectiveness can be determined. They are approved for the management of anxiety disorders as well, so depressed patients with anxiety symptoms should be started at a lower dose to minimize the stimulating side effects.

Common side effects of SSRIs are anxiety, insomnia, nausea, diarrhea, headache, decreased appetite, and sexual dysfunction (anorgasmia, delayed orgasm, erectile dysfunction, and decreased libido). The latter are frequent reasons for discontinuing the medications. Adding the sexual stimulant yohimbine (Yocon), cyproheptadine (Periactin, 4 to 8 mg 4 to 8 hours before sexual activity), low doses of bupropion (Wellbutrin),

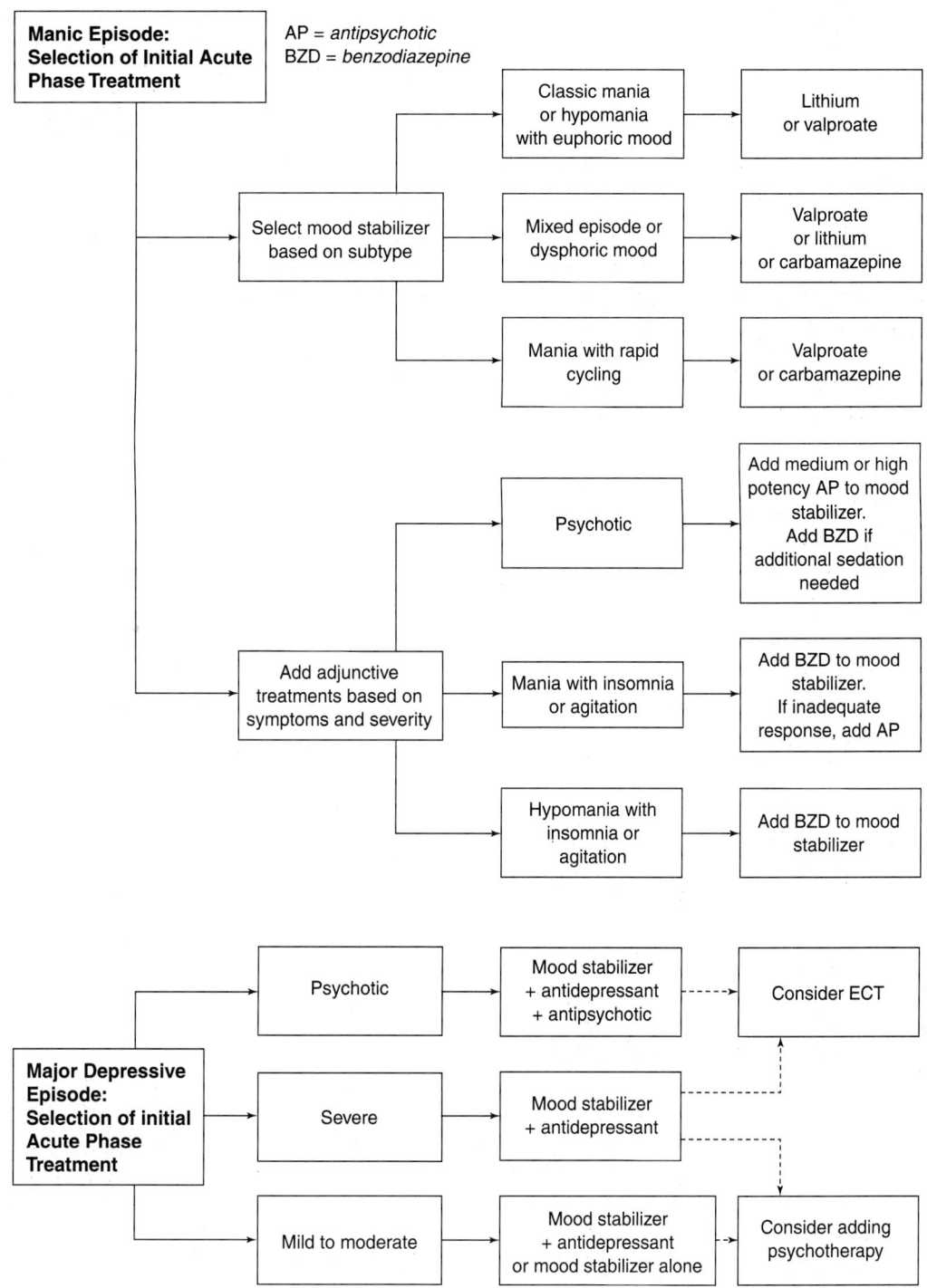

FIGURE 60-3 Bipolar Disorder Treatment Algorithm (Kahn et al. 1996. Expert consensus treatment guidelines for bipolar disorders: a guide for patients and families. *J Clin Psychiatry 57* (suppl 12A).

or buspirone (BuSpar) may be successful. Mechanical devices for producing erection or the use of alprostadil in a urethral suppository or an injectable form may be advised. Switching to nefazodone (Serzone) or bupropion are other options. Some providers recommend weekend "drug holidays," taking the last dose at noon on Thursday and starting the drug again on Sunday. For many patients, however, this causes a return of depressed mood and is not recommended.

Use of sildenofil (Viagra) may also be considered, providing the patient is not taking medications with nitrates or no other risk factors are present.

Because of the side effect profile, SSRIs may be helpful for premature ejaculation. They are also used in eating disorders and chronic pain. In women with premenstrual syndrome, the dosage may be increased from day 15 of cycle through onset of menses, or given intermittently instead of daily, taking the drug from day 15 of the cycle through the first day of menses, although data are limited on this type of treatment. SSRIs are also first-line choices for the depression phase of BPD, in conjunction with mood stabilizers such as lithium and valproate (Kahn et al, 1996).

Generally, SSRIs are safer than TCAs and MAOIs in patients with comorbid cardiovascular disorders, although caution should still be used. Generally, SSRIs are safer than TCAs and MAOIs in patients with comorbid cardiovascular disorders, stroke, or Parkinson's disease, although caution should be taken. Traditionally, chronic pain has been treated with TCAs; SSRIs have been used recently. Depressed patients with chronic constipation will not minimal anticholinergic problems with SSRIs. SSRIs, bupropion, or trazodone (Desyrel) may be prescribed for glaucoma patients.

Fluoxetine (Prozac) is highly protein-bound and is metabolized by the liver to an active metabolite, which is excreted by the kidneys. The half-life of fluoxetine is longer than most, at 2 to 3 days, whereas the metabolite norfluoxetine's half-life is 7 to 9 days. Because of its longer half-life, a period of 2 to 3 weeks is needed to attain steady-state plasma levels. Fluoxetine is not used as frequently in older adults because of its long half-life, although it is helpful in patients who miss doses. The daily dosage is 20 mg for adults and 10 mg for older adults (or lower doses using the liquid preparation). A trial of up to 6 weeks may be needed before effectiveness can be evaluated. Fluoxetine is more of a stimulating medication, so it is preferred for patients with lethargy or hypersomnia.

Paroxetine (Paxil) is a potent SSRI. It is 95% protein-bound and has a half-life of 24 hours. There are no active metabolites. Therapy is initiated at 20 mg/day; older adults, anxious patients, and those with renal and hepatic impairment are started at 10 mg. The dosage ranges from 10 to 60 mg. Because it may cause somnolence, it is particularly helpful in depressed patients with insomnia. Nausea, diarrhea, tremor, dry mouth, and headache are other side effects of paroxetine.

Sertraline (Zoloft) is stronger than fluoxetine in enhancing serotonergic neurotransmission. It has a half-life of 26 hours and has one weak metabolite. Dosage starts at 50 mg (25 mg in the elderly) and ranges from 50 to 200 mg. Side effects may include insomnia, diarrhea, and nausea. Weight loss may occur. It is tightly bound to plasma proteins and may cause a shift in the plasma concentration of other protein-bound drugs (Kaplan & Sadock, 1996).

Fluvoxamine (Luvox) is effective in depression as well as obsessive-compulsive disorder and other anxiety disorders. The half-life is 15.6 hours. Nine metabolites are present; however, it is only 80% protein-bound, so there is less risk of drug–drug interactions. The dosage range is 50 to 300 mg. The drug is usually given at night to minimize side effects, although twice-a-day dosing is advised for dosages of more than 100 mg. Side effects may include nausea, drowsiness, constipation, nervousness, abnormal ejaculation, asthenia, dry mouth, and dizziness. Fluvoxamine is not given with diazepam (Valium) because it causes reduced clearance of diazepam. It is a potent inhibitor of $P_{450}IIIA4$ enzyme. It interacts with alprazolam (Xanax), triazolam, and astemizole (Hismanal).

Venlafaxine (Effexor) has potent serotonin and norepinephrine reuptake inhibitor effects. It has one active metabolite and a short 5-hour half-life. It may be useful in ADHD and pain syndromes. The starting dosage is 25 mg two or three times a day, and the dosage is increased as necessary to maximum dose of 375 mg/day. A newer slow-release preparation allows once-a-day dosing. Possible side effects include nausea, somnolence, dry mouth, dizziness, and nervousness. Slow tapering to prevent withdrawal is recommended when discontinuing venlafaxine. Elevation of blood pressure may occur at higher doses, and blood pressure should be monitored regularly, especially with dosage increases. Venlafaxine is a weak inhibitor of $P_{450}IID6$; therefore, cimetidine (Tagamet) should be used with caution.

Trazodone is an atypical antidepressant. It has a half-life of 6 to 11 hours and is a serotonin reuptake inhibitor. It can be used for its antidepressant qualities and also improves sleep quality by increasing total sleep time, decreasing nighttime awakenings, and decreasing REM sleep (Kaplan & Sadock, 1996). In low doses (25 to 100 mg), it can be used as a hypnotic; this can be helpful when other antidepressants cause insomnia. The daily dosage range is 200 to 600 mg; the drug is given two or three times a day. Side effects may include sedation, orthostatic hypotension, dizziness, headache, nausea, and priapism.

Nefazodone is a heterocyclic agent that is an analogue of trazodone. It has three active metabolites. Its pharmacodynamic effects are antagonism of the 5-HT$_2$ receptor, sensitization of the 5-HT$_{1A}$ receptor, and weak inhibition of serotonin and norepinephrine reuptake. It does not suppress REM sleep in persons with MDD (Kaplan & Sadock, 1996), and it is effective in pain management and premenstrual syndrome as well as other depressive disorders. Dosage begins at 50 to 100 mg twice a day and can be increased up to 300 to 600 mg/day in two doses. Side effects may include dry mouth, nausea, drowsiness, dizziness, headache. Astemizole and cisapride (Propulsid) should not be used with nefazodone.

Mirtazapine (Remeron) is a tetracyclic compound that enhances both norepinephrine and serotonin. Mirtazapine produces its antidepressant effects by antagonizing the alpha$_2$-adrenergic inhibitory receptors and serotonin 5HT$_2$ and 5HT$_3$ receptors. Side effects may include drowsiness (from the histamine antagonist effect), increased appetite, weight gain, dizziness, and orthostatic hypotension. It has a half life of 20 to 40 hours, is 85% protein-bound, and is metabolized through the cytochrome 2D6 and 1A2 and 3A liver enzymes, which form three metabolites. It should be considered when target symptoms include weight loss and insomnia. The dosage is 15 mg/day to start, with a range of 15 to 45 mg, taken preferably in the evening before sleep.

Bupropion (Wellbutrim) is a unicyclic antidepressant that inhibits the reuptake of norepinephrine and dopamine. Along with depressive disorders, it has been found effective in treating ADHD. It is used as a first-line antidepressant for depression in BPD patients, especially when there is concern about a switch to mania (Kahn et al, 1996). It is contraindicated in patients with a history of seizures, head injuries, central nervous system tumors, electroencephalographic abnormalities, and medications that may contribute to seizures (eg, neuroleptics and lithium). Alcohol intake may increase the risk of seizures. Side effects may include weight loss, dry mouth, constipation, headache, nausea, restlessness, agitation, and menstrual irregularities. It does not cause the sexual side effects of the SSRIs. Dosage starts at 150 mg of the sustained-release formulation once a day and is increased to 150 mg of the sustained-release formulation twice a day, then to a maximum of 200 mg of the sustained-release formulation twice a day. The sustained-release tablet is believed to prevent side effects caused by the drop in blood levels throughout the day. Insomnia usually can be prevented by taking the second dose no later than 4 to 5 p.m. Caution should be used when this drug is administered with medications metabolized by the liver, such as carbamazepine, cimetidine, and phenytoin.

TCAS AND MAOIS

TCAs include tertiary amines (imipramine [Tofranil], amitriptyline [Elavil], doxepin [Sinequan, Adapin]) and secondary amines (desipramine [Norpramin], nortriptyline [Pamelor, Aventyl], protriptyline [Vivactil]). Protein-binding exceeds 75% with half-lives ranging from 10 to 70 hours. TCAs reduce reuptake of norepinephrine and serotonin and block muscarinic, acetylcholine and histamine receptors, with downregulation of receptors (reduction in number) occurring as symptoms improve.

All TCAs are equally effective, but they vary in responsiveness. They are particularly effective when there is severe depression with melancholia features. A therapeutic response to TCAs takes 3 to 4 weeks, and the trial should last 6 weeks. Plasma levels of TCAs help guide dosage and augmentation. A common mistake is not to raise the dosage to its maximum level. Most TCA doses can be given before bedtime because of their sedative effects and long half-life.

Overdose is a constant risk. Prescriptions should be written for no longer than 1 week, appointments should be weekly or more often, and availability by telephone must be part of the treatment for anyone at risk of overdose (U.S. Department of Health and Human Resources, 1993).

A physical exam, blood tests (complete blood count, white cell count, serum electrolyte measurements, liver function tests) should be done before starting a TCA. An electrocardiogram provides a baseline so that conduction changes can be monitored. Narrow angle glaucoma and cardiac illness are contraindications for TCA use. Birth-control pills may decrease the plasma concentration of TCAs through hepatic metabolism.

The tertiary amines produce more side effects, such as sedation, orthostatic hypotension, and anticholinergic effects. The secondary amine nortriptyline produces the least orthostatic hypotension, and desipramine has the least anticholinergic activity (Kaplan & Sadock, 1996). Anticholinergic syndrome caused by TCAs results in confusion and delirium. The elderly are particularly prone to falls and injuries from orthostatic hypotension. Cardiotoxic effects may include tachycardia, flattened T waves, prolonged Q–T intervals, and depressed ST segments. Desipramine and protriptyline are associated with psychomotor stimulation, presenting with myoclonic twitches and tremors of the tongue and upper extremities.

MAOIs are effective in patients with depression with atypical features. If phenelzine (Nardil) or tranylcypromine (Parnate) is prescribed, the provider must teach the patient about the dietary restrictions and potentially fatal reactions that may occur from interaction with sympathomimetic medications. This makes the MAOIs second- or third-line line treatments. Refractory depression that does not respond to other medications is an indication for MAOI use. A family history or personal history of MAOI responsiveness influences the decision. To prevent hypertensive crisis, the patient taking MAOIs must avoid foods that contain large amounts of tyramine, such as broad beans, aged cheese, beer, sherries, liquors, red wine, smoked or pickled fish, liver paté, sausage, sauerkraut, and yogurt. Foods that are prepared by smoking, pickling, fermenting, or aging must be avoided. Coffee, tea, and colas may have stimulant effects. Chocolate should be eaten in moderation only. Interactions with other medications must be avoided, including over-the-counter medications, other prescription medications, and illicit drugs; potentially fatal reactions can occur. Anesthesia cannot be administered for 2 weeks after MAOIs are discontinued.

MOOD STABILIZERS FOR BIPOLARITY

Lithium carbonate (Lithonate, Eskalith) is an alkali metal available as a carbonate (Li_2CO_3) and is used for the first-line treatment of BPD. It is not protein-bound, it has a half-life of 20 hours, it takes 5 to 7 days to reach equilibrium, and it is excreted by the kidneys. Lithium's action may be the result of blocking the enzyme inositol-1-phosphatase within neurons (Kaplan & Sadock, 1996), linked to second messenger systems. Lithium is used along with a neuroleptic such as haloperidol in acute manic episode, and is often used with an antidepressant in the depressive episodes, provided it does not induce a manic episode. Lithium is given prophylactically to help prevent further episodes. It is also used in MDD to augment the action of antidepressants (Keltner & Folks, 1997).

The dosage of lithium is usually 300 mg three times a day, with a maximum dosage of 900 to 2100 mg/day. Serum lithium levels should be .8 to 1.2 mEq/L in the acute phase, lower in the maintenance and continuation phases of treatment.

The patient must know to avoid dehydration. Excess sodium lowers lithium levels; conversely, too little sodium can cause lithium to reach a toxic level. Side effects include increased thirst, polyuria, nausea, vomiting, diarrhea, tremor, fatigue, weight gain, and cognitive impairment. Lithium toxicity may appear at blood levels of 2 mEq/L or lower. It causes severe vomiting, profuse diarrhea, muscle flaccidity, severe tremor, ataxia, coma, and seizures. This is a psychiatric emergency.

Levothyroxine (Synthroid, Levothroid, Levoxyl) may be added for patients with rapid-cycling BPD and if TSH levels are elevated. Polyuria, caused by decreased resorption of fluid from the distal tubules of the kidney, should be evaluated through a 24-hour creatinine clearance test. Electrocardiograms are needed at baseline and once a year because of possible T-wave changes, elevated as a result of lithium therapy. Skin eruptions are not uncommon with lithium treatment. Use during pregnancy may be dangerous and may cause Epstein's anomaly.

Valproate (Depakote) is also a first-line treatment for manic episodes of BPD. It is highly recommended by expert clinicians for euphoric "classic" mania and is the treatment of choice for mixed or dysphoric mania, rapid-cycling mania (Kahn et al, 1996), and mania from HIV/AIDS (Burack et al, 1997). A loading dose can be used in acute mania. Except in patients with liver disease (in which case lithium is recommended), valproate is recommended as first-line treatment for BPD patients with medical complications (Keltner & Folks, 1997).

Carbamazepine (Tegretol) is an anticonvulsant that is used as a mood-stabilizing agent in mixed episodes of mania or with dysphoric mood, mania with rapid cycling, and a major depressive episode of BPD (along with an antidepressant). It can be added to lithium if there is not a good response, and is effective as a prophylactic agent. Its half-life is 12 to 17 hours, and it is thought to prevent kindling or sensitization in the brain to the manic episode. The usual starting dose is 200 mg twice a day; the dose can be increased by 200 mg/day up to 600 to 1000 mg/day. Some patients need up to 2200 mg to obtain a therapeutic blood level. Serious symptoms of aplastic anemia and agranulocytosis can occur. Liver and renal function tests should be ordered at months 1, 3, 6, 9, and 12 during the first year of use.

Gabapentin (Neurontin) and lamotrigine (Lamictal) are two newer anticonvulsants that are producing good results in BPD. Gabapentin is similar to GABA in structure but is more lipophilic and is used in partial seizures. Lamotrigine blocks the sustained firing of neurons by prolonging the inactivation of sodium channels (Meldrum, 1994). Therapeutic levels of both medications is more than 2 mg/mL (Keltner & Folks, 1997).

Verapamil (Calan, Isopfin) and other calcium channel blockers have shown some effectiveness in patients with BPD when other medications are not tolerated or effective; they can also be used as an augmenting medication (Kaplan & Sadock, 1996).

Electroconvulsive Therapy

Electroconvulsive therapy is effective for the treatment of depression. It is a treatment of choice when there is an inadequate response to antidepressant therapy, when psychosis is present, and when there is a high risk of suicide from preoccupation and rumination. It is also recommended in cases of life-threatening mania, with failure of mood stabilizers, and in those who cannot tolerate mood stabilizers (Kahn et al, 1996). The major side effect is amnesia for the time of the treatment and several days before the treatment. Some patients complain of permanent memory loss, but studies have not supported this finding. Referral to a psychiatrist is necessary. Usually a series of 8 to 12 treatments is necessary, along with antidepressant medication to prevent recurrence of depression.

Phototherapy

Phototherapy, or light therapy, involves exposing patients with MDD with a seasonal component to 2500 lux of light for 1 to 2 hours after awakening. Within 4 to 7 days, there is some improvement in resetting the biologic clock and restoring circadian rhythm. Only experienced clinicians should administer this type of therapy. Symptoms of mania may result in patients vulnerable to type I bipolar disorder.

St. John's Wort

Hypericum, or St. John's Wort, is an herbal product sold in health food stores as "natural Prozac." Its forms include tablets or tea. Its effects are thought to be similar to those of MAOIs, and patients are cautioned to avoid foods high in tyramine. Patients with mild to moderate depression may begin to have some positive response after a month's time. The dosage needed is not clear. Patients should be cautioned that there is no regulation regarding the strength and processing of St. John's Wort. They should not take it with any other medications, especially cold products and other antidepressants, or there may be severe side effects.

Other Alternative Therapies

Because of the close connection of depression to the immune system and the endocrine system, several types of alternative therapies are thought to be beneficial. These include massage, therapeutic touch, Reiki, relaxation with imagery, acupressure, shiatsu, therapeutic movement, aromatherapy, water therapy, reflexology, acupuncture, and others. Many of the methods are thought to increase energy flow and restore health through healing of the chakras or energy fields of the body. Depression is viewed as an imbalance in the energy flow of the body.

Cognitive Therapy and Other Therapies

The acronym SPEAK is helpful in counseling depressed patients in primary care: **S**chedule, **P**leasurable activities, **E**xercise, **A**ssertiveness, and **K**ind thoughts about oneself (Christensen, 1997). Following a schedule "regardless of whether you feel like it" helps overcome the motivational deficits and anergia of depression. Pleasurable activities involve mobilizing the patient to do things once found enjoyable, to counteract anhedonia (lack of pleasure). Identifying 15 activities and writing them down may help in this process. Exercising several times a week will help with mood and overall health. Teaching assertiveness helps mobilize and discharge emotions externally as the patient becomes more direct at expressing thoughts and feelings and asking for what is needed. Thinking kind thoughts about oneself involves changing negative thought patterns to more positive ones.

Formal psychotherapy may be used alone or with medication in some cases of depression. In the acute phase of treatment, psychotherapy alone might be beneficial if: the depression is not severe, there has been a prior response to psychotherapy, there was an incomplete response previously to medication alone, there are chronic psychological problems, a competent therapist is available, and the patient prefers this type of treatment. Referring the patient for psychotherapy also has a beneficial effect if medication is used and will help with maintenance therapy for prevention of future episodes (Cole et al, 1997). Therapy may be individual, group, or family therapy.

Brief counseling of at least 3 minutes is associated with substantial improvement in functional outcomes and is a minimum recommendation in all settings (Meredith et al, 1996).

Rehabilitation

Depression and BPD are treatable illnesses with distinct episodes; reduction of symptoms, return to normal functioning, and improved quality of life are the goals of rehabilitation. Because of the chronic nature of mood disorders in most persons, these goals are evaluated on a regular basis when patients are taking medication as well as when and if they discontinue medication. With medication and other treatment, it is hoped that the person will feel "normal" again.

A holistic approach to rehabilitating the person with mood disorders takes into consideration healing of mind, body, and spirit. Depressed persons should be encouraged to exercise for the general sense of well-being it provides as well as for the positive effects on the immune system. During manic episodes, patients should be encouraged to rest and relax as much as possible because of the overactivity and exhaustion of the manic episode. They, too, benefit from regular exercise when not in a manic phase.

Proper nutrition becomes a way to restore the amino acids needed for neurotransmitter production. Having regular meals helps establish rituals that are healing in themselves. If weight changes are issues for the patient, then nutritional support is essential.

Self-esteem issues focus on building healthy relationships and a sense of connectedness or awareness of spirituality.

Concerns with Older Adults

Diagnosing and treating mood disorders in older adults can be particularly challenging. Despite the many life stresses of this developmental stage, depressive illnesses should never be considered a normal aspect of aging (Small, 1991). They are serious but treatable illnesses that increase the number of complications and speed death in this population, particularly through the high frequency of suicides (DeLeo & Diekstra, 1990) and the impact on coexisting illnesses. Recent studies show that 75% of elderly suicide victims saw their primary care provider in the month before death (Kelleher & Holmes, 1995).

Because of the variability of presenting symptoms and the frequency of medical illnesses in later life, masked depression, or focusing on physical rather than affective complaints, is common. Thorough assessment to uncover the depression is essential (Small, 1991). With multiple losses, tremendous changes in lifestyle, and loss of social support as contributing factors, many older adults have their first episode of depression, called late-onset depression, at this time. It is much less common, however, for BPD to have a late onset. In persons with a history of early-onset (before the age of 50 to 60 years) depression or BPD, there is an increased risk for episodes in later years (Georgotas et al, 1989), and an accurate history will help diagnose new or continuing episodes. Many older adults consider psychiatric treatment for "crazy people" and are reluctant to get the help they need.

Although there may be variations in the syndrome of depressive and manic episodes in the elderly, the same DSM-IV criteria are used as a guide to diagnosis (Small, 1991). Symptoms of depression in the older adult often resemble symptoms of other illnesses. Multiple somatic complaints are not uncommon in place of the severity of affective changes more typical of the mood disorders. Frequently, problems with memory, concentration, and confusion occur along with dementia, or they may in themselves be symptoms of depression that may go misunderstood and mislabeled.

As with all psychiatric presentations, a physical cause for the symptoms should be ruled out. However, if there is not a clear distinction of what is being presented, it may be wise, using caution, to try a low-dose antidepressant to help determine if the somatic complaints are signs of actual clinical depression.

The use of psychotropic medications in the older adult requires careful consideration of the aging process, the interactions among the multiple medications most older adults take for acute and chronic illnesses, increased side effects, and the patient's ability to participate in the plan. Because drugs are metabolized more slowly in the elderly, dosages should start low, usually about half the normal dose. The dosage should be raised at a slower rate until there is a therapeutic response or adverse side effects appear (Kaplan & Sadock, 1996). Many

older adults require usual dosages for a therapeutic response. Because most antidepressants are lipophilic, they may cause toxicity in the older adult who has decreased lean muscle and water and an increased proportion of fat.

Psychotherapy may be of particular benefit for the older adult to "process" their losses and their subsequent anger and frustration. Supportive therapy may be needed for reassurance that depression is not a "moral weakness." Persons in long-term care particularly benefit from reminiscence therapy as a means to restore lost self-esteem and connectedness with the past. Referrals should be made to a psychiatric specialist using the previously recommended guidelines, as well as whenever the patient requests a referral. Also, referrals should be made to psychotherapists who specialize in the geriatric population, geriatric partial-day programs for those who need short-term daily support, and inpatient psychiatric programs when there is a concern for safety or major functional loss.

Nutritional Considerations

Weight change is a major symptom of depression. A loss or gain of 5% of body weight in a month is considered significant and meets one of the DSM-IV criteria for MDD. The patient should be weighed at each visit, comparing the weight to that at previous visits, and a history of weight changes should be taken from the patient and family. Appetite changes are important, too: the patient may feel too fatigued to eat and not feel any pleasure from eating. When patients feel hopeless or angry, severe weight loss may be a type of passive suicide. This type of suicide attempt is seen quite often in long-term care settings.

A referral to a dietitian who can help the patient set small goals and determine ways to increase caloric intake can be beneficial for the symptoms of weight loss. Also, keeping a journal of food intake and feelings, rewarding oneself for weight gain, and eating several small meals a day are helpful strategies. Antidepressant medication will help restore normal mood, and in this setting weight gain becomes one of the outcomes of recovery. Nearly all the SSRIs can cause weight loss or weight gain as either a side effect or a therapeutic effect. Paroxetine may be an appropriate choice when there is weight loss, fluoxetine when there is weight gain. TCAs such as nortriptyline may be an appropriate choice because they tend to cause weight gain. In extreme cases, patients with severe weight loss may respond to cyproheptadine (Periactin) or megestrol (Megace).

Extreme weight gain may be a serious symptom of depression. Referrals can be made to support groups such as Overeaters Anonymous, Weight Watchers, and group therapy. Most of the SSRIs and bupropion are appropriate to use unless the patient has a side effect of increased hunger. Caution must be taken to assess for coexisting eating disorders, which have high rates of depression.

TEACHING AND SELF-CARE

Depression and BPD are treatable biologic illnesses, and patients should be taught the genetic factors, neurotransmitter actions, relation to stressors, types of symptoms, medication actions and side effects, and type of follow-up care. The more informed the patient and family are, the more likely they will seek help and make good choices. Patients should always be offered several options and helped to make choices that will move them along the mental health continuum. Keeping a mood chart is recommended, noting feelings, activities, sleep patterns, medication use and side effects, and important life events, or a visual scale of 1 to 10 can be used. Self-care can involve finding helpful resources, reaching out to support groups, and becoming a part of the movement toward an informed and caring attitude toward mental illness.

Teaching early signs and symptoms of behaviors that may indicate a recurrence of the illness and triggers that may contribute to the relapse is important for families, friends, coworkers, and the patient. For example, a patient with a history of BPD may stay on the telephone with friends all night, make large numbers of credit-card purchases, or begin promiscuous sexual behavior; these may be early symptoms of relapse. A depressed patient often withdraws and begins to have very sad, hopeless feelings. Patients and family members should be taught to call immediately if symptoms return. A support group can help the patient learn successful strategies for managing the illness.

A useful patient teaching handout is "Expert Consensus Treatment Guidelines for Bipolar Disorder: A Guide for Patients and Families" (Kahn et al., 1996).

COMMUNITY RESOURCES

The following organizations focus on depression and BPD. In addition, pharmaceutical companies offer tremendous resources for primary care providers in terms of teaching materials, videos, and so forth.

- National Alliance for Mentally Ill, 200 N. Glebe Rd., Suite 1015, Arlington, VA 22203-3754, 800-950-NAMI: Local and state chapters, consumer advocacy, patient and family education and support, grants for research on depression and other brain disorders
- National Foundations for Depressive Illness (NFDI), P.O. Box 2257, New York, NY 10116-2257, 800-248-4344
- National Mental Health Association (NMHA), 1021 Prince St., Alexandria, VA 22314-2971, 800-969-6642
- National Depression and Manic Depression Association, 730 N. Franklin St., #501, Chicago, IL 60601, 800-82-NDNMA, http://medhlp.netusa.net/agsg/agsg95 .htm: Educational resources, local chapters and support groups
- American Association of Child and Adolescent Psychiatry, 3615 Wisconsin Ave., NW, Washington, DC 20016: Practice guidelines
- Dean Foundation for Health Research and Education, 2711 Allen Blvd., Middleton, WI 53562-2215, 608-827-2390: Books on bipolar disorder
- D/ART (Depression Awareness, Recognition and Treatment), National Institute of Mental Health, 800-421-4211

REFERRAL POINTS AND CLINICAL WARNINGS

Providers should have a list of local psychiatrists and psychiatric nurse practitioners, including child and adolescent, adult, and geriatric specialists and noting those who will visit patients in their homes and in long-term care facilities. Providers should also have a list of therapists, including those who specialize in cognitive and behavioral therapy, marriage and family therapy, group therapy, play therapy, counseling for children and adolescents and older adults, those who deal with chronic physical illness, and other specialties; this will help the patient choose the best options. The list should include agencies that charge sliding-scale fees, providers approved by health insurance carriers, and those that accept private pay. Also, a list of local support groups that will help with emotional and spiritual issues for the patient and family should be readily available. The provider should also be familiar with community mental health centers, psychiatric home health agencies, private psychiatric facilities, detoxification and addictions treatment programs, and emergency facilities.

Primary care providers frequently refer patients to psychiatrists or psychiatric mental health nurse practitioners. Some referrals are made for emergencies that may necessitate hospitalization. In a situation deemed an emergency, the patient should not leave the office without an appropriate treatment plan. Threats of suicide and in rare cases homicide provide the greatest safety risks and should be treated as emergencies. Although there can be no guarantee a patient will not commit suicide, lower-risk patients can be managed using a "no harm" contract in which patients agree, for a designated period of time, that they will not hurt themselves in any way, and that they will notify the provider or other reliable person if they have suicidal thoughts. Asking the patient to write out the contract and date and sign it is beneficial (Table 60-5 lists suicide risk factors).

If psychotic features accompany the depression, an emergency referral for hospital evaluation is important, especially if the patient is paranoid, has command-type hallucinations threatening self-harm or harm to others, or has bizarre delusions. Psychosis in a manic episode requires hospitalization to protect the patient from poor judgment such as violence, and safety risks from not eating or sleeping.

Severe depression, with major impairment in functioning, and depression induced by illicit drugs, alcohol, or prescription drug dependency also are considered psychiatric emergencies. A medication overdose, whether taken accidentally or in a suicide attempt, requires emergency measures. High doses of TCAs are frequently used in intentional drug overdoses and can be fatal; MAOIs can be fatal as well. SSRIs are not lethal in themselves but can be dangerous when mixed with other medications. SSRIs and MAOIs together, as well as other combinations, may cause a serotonin syndrome, with symptoms of fever, rigidity, myoclonus, confusion, delirium, and coma (Kaplan & Sadock, 1996).

TABLE 60-5	Risk Factors for Suicide
Psychosocial	History:
Hopelessness	Prior suicide attempts
Male gender	Family history of suicide attempts
Advanced age	Family history of substance abuse
Living alone	History of childhood abuse and trauma
Adolescence	Diagnoses
	General medical illness
	Psychosis
	Substance abuse
	Mood disorder

Other causes of delirium complicating depression, whether medication-induced or from other causes, require hospital evaluation—for instance, lithium toxicity, with a serum level at 2 mEq/L or more, and anticholinergic delirium as a side effect of psychotropic medications.

In a psychiatric emergency, the patient may need to be transported to a psychiatric clinician or an emergency psychiatric setting for further evaluation. Hospitalization may be voluntary, or if the patient refuses help, commitment papers may be sought, in accordance with state and county mental health codes. Such papers allow the psychiatric hospital to hold patients against their will until an examination can be made to determine if the criterion of "danger to self or others" is met. Patients should be approached gently but firmly and told they are at significant risk and that the provider must make decisions for them at this time (Goldberg, 1995).

EDITOR'S NOTE:
COMPLEMENTARY APPROACHES

A general discussion of complementary approaches can be found in Chapter 3. The following, while not an exhaustive list, are some complementary approaches being used for this condition. Additional information on these approaches, including precautions, can be found in Appendices A and B. Providers need to assess for the use of complementary approaches as part of the patient's history, as they may impact conventional therapies, and patients may not volunteer this information unless specifically asked. Efficacy of many complementary approaches is not as well documented as that of conventional therapies. Providers need to read the literature before suggesting these complementary approaches.

- Vitamins, minerals, herbs, supplements
    Kava Kava
    St. John's Wart
- Complementary Modalities
    Acupuncture
    Aromatherapy
    Craniosacral therapy
    Massage therapy

References

American Psychiatric Association. (1994). *Diagnostic and statistical manual of mental disorders*, 4th ed. Washington, D.C.: American Psychiatric Association.

Andrews, G., Stewart, G., Morris-Yates, A., et al. (1990). Evidence for a general neurotic syndrome. *British Journal of Psychiatry, 157*, 6–12.

Beck, A.T. (1976). *Cognitive therapy and the emotional disorders.* New York: International Universities Press.

Beeber, L. (1996). Depression in women. In A.B. McBride & J.K. Austin (Eds.). *Psychiatric-mental health nursing: Integrating the biological and behavioral sciences.* Philadelphia: W.B. Saunders.

Berrettini, W.H., Ferraro, T.N., et al. (1994). Chromosome 18 DNA markers and manic-depressive illness. Evidence for a susceptibility gene. *Proceedings of the National Academy of Sciences of the U.S.A., 91*(13), 5918–5921.

Brent, D.A., Perper, J.A., Moritz, G., et al. (1993). Psychiatric risk factors for adolescent suicide: A case-control study. *Journal of American Academy of Child and Adolescent Psychiatry, 32*, 521–529.

Bowlby, J. (1980) *Attachment and loss*, Vol. 3: *Loss: Sadness and depression.* New York: Basic Books.

Burack, J.H., Feldman, M.D., & Coates, T.J. (1997). HIV/AIDS. In M.D. Feldman & J.F. Christensen (Eds.). *Behavioral medicine in primary care: A practical guide.* Stamford, CT: Appleton & Lange.

Cole, S.A., Christensen, J.F., Raju, M.A. & Feldman, M.D. (1997). In M.D. Feldman & J.F. Christensen. (Eds.). *Behavioral medicine in primary care: A practical guide.* Stamford: CT: Appleton & Lange.

Cummings, J.L. (1993). Frontal-subcortical circuits and human behavior [Summary]. *Archives of Neurology, 50*(8), 873–880.

DeLeo, D., & Diekstra, R.F.W. (1990). *Depression and suicide in late life.* Lewiston, N.Y.: Hogrefe & Huber.

Depression Guideline Panel (1993a). *Depression in primary care: Vol. 1: Detection and diagnosis.* Clinical Practice Guideline, Number 5. AHCPR Publication No. 93-0550. Rockville, MD: U.S. Department of Health and Human Services, Public Health Service, Agency for Health Care Policy and Research.

Depression Guideline Panel (1993b). *Depression in primary care: Vol. 2: Treatment of major depression.* Clinical Practice Guideline, Number 5. AHCPR Publication No. 93-0550. Rockville, MD: U.S. Department of Health and Human Services, Public Health Service, Agency for Health Care Policy and Research

Dubovsky, S.L., Murphy, J., Christian, J., & Lee, C. (1992). The calcium second messenger system in bipolar disorders: Data supporting new research directions. *Journal of Neuropsychiatry and Clinical Neurosciences, 4*(1), 3–14.

Expert Consensus Treatment guidelines for bipolar disorder: A guide for patients and families. (1996). *Journal of Clinical Psychiatry, 57*(suppl. 12A), 81–88.

Geller, B., & Luby, J. (1997). Child and adolescent bipolar disorder: A review of the past 10 years. *Journal of American Academy of Child and Adolescent Psychiatry, 36*(9), 1168–1176.

Georgotas, A., McCue, R.E., & Cooper, T.B. (1989). A placebo-controlled comparison of nortriptyline and phenelzine in maintenance therapy of elderly depressed patients. *Archives of General Psychiatry, 46*, 783–786.

Giles, D.E., Jarrett, R.B., Roff, H.P., et al. (1989). Clinical predictors of recurrence in depression. *American Journal of Psychiatry, 146*, 764–767.

Goldberg, R.J. (1995). *Practical guide to the care of the psychiatric patient.* St. Louis: Mosby.

Goodwin, G.K., & Jamison, K.R. (1990). *Manic-depressive illness.* New York: Oxford University Press.

Hall, R.C., & Wise, M.G. (1995). The clinical and financial burden of mood disorders. Cost and outcome. *Psychosomatics, 36*(2), 8–11.

Kahn, D.A., Carpenter, D., Docherty, J.P., & Frances, A. (1996). Treatment of bipolar disorder. *Journal of Clinical Psychiatry, 57*(Suppl 12 A), 1–88.

Kaplan, H.I., & Sadock, B.J. (1996). *Pocket handbook of psychiatric drug treatment*, 2d ed. Baltimore: Williams & Wilkins.

Kelleher, K., & Holmes, T.M. (1995). Major recent trends in mental health in primary care. In *U.S. HealthCare.* HHR Publications.

Keltner, N.L., & Folks, D.G. (1997). *Psychotrophic drugs*, 2d ed. St. Louis: Mosby.

Keltner, N.L., Folks, D.G., Palmer, C.A., & Powers, R.E. (1998). *Psychobiological foundations of psychiatric care.* St. Louis: Mosby.

Kendler, K.S., Neale, M.C. Kessler, R.C., et al. (1992). A population-based twin study of major depression in women. *Archives of General Psychiatry, 49*, 257–266.

Lewinsohn, P.M. (1974). A behavioral approach to depression. In R.J. Friedman & M.M. Katz (Eds.). *The psychology of depression: Contemporary theory and research.* New York: John Wiley & Sons.

Meldrum, B.S. (1994). Lamotrigine: A novel approach. *Seizure, 3*(suppl A), 41–45.

Meredith, L.S., Wells, K.B., Kaplan, S.H., & Mazel, R.M. (1996). Counseling typically provided for depression. *Archives of General Psychiatry, 53*, 905–912.

Moscicki, E. (1995). Epidemiology of suicide behavior. *Suicide and Life-Threatening Behavior, 25*(1), 22–35.

Nemeroff, C.B. (1990). The relevance of thyrotropin-releasing hormone to psychiatric disorders. In C.B. Nemeroff (Ed.). *Progress in psychiatry, neuropeptides, and psychiatric disease.* Washington, D.C.: American Psychiatric Press.

Nemeroff, C.B., Widerlov, E., Bisatte, G., et al. (1984). Elevated concentrations of CSF corticotrophin-releasing factor-like immunoreactivity in depressed patients. *Science, 226,* 1342–1344.

NIH Consensus Development Panel on Depression in Late Life (1992). Diagnosis and treatment of depression in late life. *JAMA, 268,* 1018–1024.

Overaschel, H. (1990). Early onset psychiatric disorder in high-risk children and increased familial morbidity. *Journal of the American Academy of Child and Adolescent Psychiatry, 29,* 184–188.

Regier, D., Farmer, M., Rae, D., et al. (1990). Comorbidity of mental disorders with alcohol and other drugs. Results from the Epidemiological Catchment Area (ECA) Study. *JAMA, 264,* 2511–2518.

Restak, R.M. (1988). *The mind.* New York: Bantam Books.

Rover, B.W., German, P.S., Brant, L.J., et al. (1991). Depression and mortality in nursing homes. *JAMA, 265,* 993–996.

Rowe, M.G., Fleming, M.F., Barry, K.L., et al. (1995). Correlates of depression in primary care. *Journal of Family Practice, 41,* 551–558.

Rubinow, D.R., Gold, P.W., & Post, R.M. (1983). CSF somastatin in affective illness. *Archives of General Psychiatry, 40,* 409.

Simpson, S.G., & Depaulo, J.R. Jr. (1993). Are you recognizing depression in your patients? *Postgraduate Medicine, 94,* 85–93.

Skinner, B.F. (1953). *Science and human behavior.* New York: Free Press.

Small, G.W. (1991). Recognition and treatment of depression in the elderly. *Journal of Clinical Psychiatry, 52*(6, suppl), 11–22.

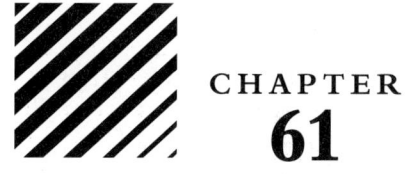

CHAPTER

61

Eating Disorders

Carmel Dato, MS, RN, CS, NPP

Eating disorders are common conditions that warrant the attention of primary care providers. Eating patterns are aspects of self-care, and as such should be part of every physical and emotional assessment. Alterations in eating patterns may be symptomatic of multiple conditions or may be a specific disorder of eating. Primary care providers have the opportunity to monitor changes in eating patterns and discuss them fully with patients. Care in recording nutritional concerns will allow for early intervention into problems with eating.

Anorexia nervosa and bulimia nervosa are potentially life-threatening eating disorders that are very common, particularly in young women. This chapter offers an overview of anorexia nervosa and bulimia nervosa, including diagnostic and treatment approaches.

ANATOMY, PHYSIOLOGY, AND PATHOLOGY

Anatomy and Physiology

The origins of eating disorders are not definitive; one line of research is in the area of neurobiology. The relations between eating disorders and mood disorders are being examined in terms of etiology based in the neuroendocrine or neurotransmitter systems. Neuroendocrine and metabolic abnormalities associated with anorexia nervosa may predate substantial weight loss, as evidenced by the development of amenorrhea before weight loss in one third of the women with anorexia nervosa. Serotonergic systems also remain altered after normal weight has been achieved (Irwin, 1993).

The complications of eating disorders are secondary to starvation or purging; these complications are not the underlying pathology. Complications become severe once adipose tissue reserves are depleted and there is more severe food refusal. At this point protein catabolism increases and water loss is accelerated, with metabolic and electrolyte disturbances. Other complications arise from vomiting or the use of laxatives or diuretics for purging.

Psychopathology

The etiology of both anorexia nervosa and bulimia nervosa is multifactorial and is associated with psychological determinants. Bruch's (1973) classic explanation of anorexia nervosa characterizes children of overinvolved mothers with poorly developed identities and a sense of ineffectiveness. Other models encompass additional individual, family, and cultural factors. Individual factors include emotional instability, anxiety (possibly social phobia or obsessive-compulsive symptoms), and personality disorders.

Depression is very common. It may predate the eating disorder symptoms or may be secondary to starvation, often improving with weight gain. Patients with anorexia nervosa typically have distortions in thinking and reasoning, with an extreme focus on their weight and eating behavior. Their sense of self-esteem is tied to their perception of being thin. Neuroendocrine and metabolic abnormalities associated with anorexia nervosa are related to starvation and have also been viewed as a potentially predisposing factor (Garner, 1993; Walsh & Devlin, 1992).

Some authors describe family factors, such as a dominant mother as well as a passive father (Bruch, 1973). Others downplay the relationship between parents and the patient. The young person with anorexia nervosa may be a stabilizing force in a family characterized by enmeshment, rigidity, and conflict avoidance (Garner, 1993).

Anorexia nervosa is frequently precipitated by dieting after either a perception of being plump or a comment by someone else. Depression and stressful experiences typically associated with greater autonomy (eg, puberty, parental divorce, graduating from high school, beginning college, leaving home) are all potential precipitating factors for anorexia nervosa. The patient has a sense of control of food in the face of feeling out of control in other areas. The effects of starvation provide perpetuating factors in anorexia nervosa (Beumont et al, 1993; Garner, 1993).

Bulimia has been recognized as a distinct disorder for only a relatively short period. A clear understanding of its history and determinants has yet to emerge. Patients do not demonstrate the rigidity and inflexibility of those with anorexia nervosa. Patients with bulimia frequently have impulse-control problems such as substance abuse, theft, and suicide. There is a high comorbidity with affective disorders, anxiety disorders, substance abuse, and personality disorders (Edwards, 1993).

Patients with bulimia nervosa typically come from families where there is parent–child conflict, sometimes with physical, verbal, or sexual abuse. Patients feel guilty and out-of-control after bingeing, and they purge to relieve this tension. They have marked fluctuations of weight but not the extremely low weights seen in anorexia nervosa.

EPIDEMIOLOGY

Most people with anorexia nervosa are women, with the illness developing most commonly in adolescence; however, 5% to 10% of patients seeking treatment for anorexia nervosa are men. Anorexia nervosa is the third most common chronic illness among teenage girls (Hoek, 1991; Lucas et al, 1991). It has a prevalence of 0.5% to 1% of women aged 15 to 30 in Western countries. Bulimia nervosa is also more common among young women, with a prevalence of 2% to 10% in women aged 15 to 30; men account for 10% of patients with the disorder (Mehler, 1996; Putukian, 1994).

Cultures that emphasize thinness can provide a predisposing factor for the development of eating disorders. The stigma attached to obesity and role conflicts of women are other cultural factors.

DIAGNOSTIC CRITERIA

The diagnostic criteria for anorexia nervosa include:

- Unwillingness to sustain body weight at or above the normal range for height and age (85% of the minimum)
- Extreme apprehension and dread of gaining weight or being fat, in an underweight person
- Distorted body image or denial of the danger of present low weight
- Amenorrhea (absence of three or more consecutive menstrual cycles).

There are two types of anorexia nervosa, the restricting type, in which the patient does not regularly binge or purge, and the binge-eating or purging type, where there is regular binge-eating or purging (American Psychiatric Association [APA], 1994).

The seriousness of the low weight is often denied. Restrictive behaviors common in dieting are used to a much greater extreme and with an inability to stop. Some patients also use more dangerous methods such as self-induced vomiting or large doses of laxatives, or they misuse diuretics and appetite suppressants. Other symptoms are those common to semistarvation, including depressed mood, irritability, social withdrawal, loss of libido, preoccupation with food, obsessional behavior, reduced alertness, and poor concentration (Beumont et al, 1993).

The diagnostic criteria for bulimia nervosa include:

- Current episodes of binge-eating, where the patient consumes very large quantities of food in a discrete period of time and feels a lack of control over ability to cease eating
- Repeated purging to prevent weight gain in the form of self-induced vomiting, fasting, extreme vigorous exercise, laxatives and diuretic abuse, or enemas
- Persistent overconcern with body image as self-evaluation.

The binge-eating and purging both occur at least twice a week for 3 or more months and do not occur exclusively during episodes of anorexia nervosa. There are two types of bulimia nervosa, the purging type and the nonpurging type. In the nonpurging type, the patient exercises or fasts but does not use purging to control weight (APA, 1994).

It is common for patients to progress from anorexia nervosa to bulimia nervosa, and some alternate between the two illnesses.

HISTORY AND PHYSICAL EXAM

A careful history and physical exam will provide information for the differential diagnosis and will raise suspicion of an eating disorder. A careful and detailed eating history is crucial (Powers, 1996). To differentiate the patient with an eating disorder from one who is perhaps dieting, it is important to elicit the extent of behavioral and psychological disturbances, such as distorted body image (Beumont et al, 1993).

Patients with anorexia nervosa may present with:

- Low weight
- Emaciation
- Cachexia
- Amenorrhea
- Bradycardia
- Orthostatic hypotension
- Lanugo
- Dry skin
- Hair loss
- Brittle hair and nails
- Cold intolerance.

These patients may appear younger than their age, have yellow-tinged skin due to carotenemia, and have cyanosis of the extremities (particularly when exposed to cold temperatures) (Carney & Andersen, 1996; Edwards, 1993; Herzog, 1992).

Other disorders must be ruled out in patients with weight loss. Medical illnesses with weight loss include brain tumors, malignancy, connective tissue disease, malabsorption syndromes, hyperthyroidism, and infection. Psychiatric diagnoses include affective disorders, obsessive-compulsive disorder, somatization disorder, and schizophrenia. In the absence of additional findings, the diagnosis of anorexia nervosa may be made by confirmation of the history and mental status exam rather than by ruling out all the possible diagnoses (Carney & Andersen, 1996).

The basic physical exam is important for both early detection and establishment of the severity of the illness. Many patients with anorexia nervosa disguise their appearance by wearing loose-fitting clothes. Patients who are resistant to gaining weight may add weighted objects when being weighed; the primary care provider must be careful to obtain accurate weights.

Patients with bulimia nervosa are more difficult to detect because they are not emaciated and appear more healthy. They often engage in bingeing and purging for years before seeking medical attention. They may complain of swelling of the hands and feet, abdominal fullness, fatigue, headaches, swelling of the cheeks, and fluid retention (Herzog, 1992).

Patients with eating disorders frequently have gastrointestinal complaints that are related to self-starvation, binge-eating, and purging and later to refeeding. These may include sore throat, abdominal pain, esophagitis, constipation, abdominal bloating, slowed intestinal mobility, and mild hematemesis (Carney & Andersen, 1996; Edwards, 1993; Herzog, 1992).

Evaluation for purging includes questions about:

- Sensitive teeth
- Periodontal disease
- Sore throat
- Gastroesophageal reflux
- Hematemesis
- Muscle weakness
- Orthostatic symptoms

- Abdominal pain
- Constipation
- Polyuria
- Cardiac palpitations.

Patients who have vomited extensively show perimolysis (dental enamel erosion), particularly on the lingual, palatal, and posterior occlusal surfaces of the teeth. In the early stages of the disease, before the patient learns to vomit reflexively, there may be skin changes, lesions, or calluses on the dorsal surface of the hand from induced vomiting (Russell's sign). Benign enlargement of the salivary glands, particularly the parotid gland, is also a common finding (Carney & Andersen, 1996; Herzog, 1992; Sharp & Freeman, 1993). Patients who purge through self-induced vomiting may have esophagitis and more rarely esophageal rupture, which is life-threatening. Ipecac abuse can be toxic, even fatal.

Abnormalities detected by electrocardiography are common in patients with anorexia nervosa and potentially life-threatening. These abnormalities include low voltage, bradycardia, T-wave inversions, and ST-segment depressions. Abnormalities that are more dangerous include dysarrhythmias (supraventricular premature beats, ventricular tachycardia, and prolonged Q–T intervals). These abnormalities normalize when the patient achieves a normal weight (Herzog, 1992).

With anorexia nervosa, there may be musculoskeletal complications, including cramps, tetany, muscle weakness, osteopenia, and stress fractures. Skeletal abnormalities may lead to advanced early osteoporosis, fracture, and disability (Carney & Andersen, 1996; Beumont et al, 1993). Bone density levels may not increase after weight restoration (Rigotti et al, 1991).

In both anorexia nervosa and bulimia nervosa, there may be weakness, confusion, nausea, palpitations, polyuria, abdominal pain, and constipation, secondary to hypokalemia (Carney & Andersen, 1996; Edwards, 1993; Herzog, 1992). Hyponatremia and hypochloremic alkalosis are also present from vomiting.

Many abnormal findings reverse with weight gain or cessation of vomiting. These include increased serum amylase, increased blood urea nitrogen, renal calculi, and amenorrhea. Emetic poisoning and metabolic acidosis secondary to laxative abuse are also reversible (Herzog, 1992).

In anorexia nervosa, there may be increased liver enzymes and hematologic abnormalities such as pancytopenia and decreased neutrophil levels. Decreased renal concentrating capacity and abnormal vasopressin secretion may result in partial diabetes insipidus with polyuria (that may lead to insomnia as well). Mild hypothyroidism and increased cholesterol levels (from disturbances in lipoprotein metabolism) are also present. All of these potential complications are reversible with weight gain, and there is usually no other treatment; iron supplements are sometimes indicated (Herzog, 1992).

DIAGNOSTIC STUDIES

The screening evaluation should include a complete blood count with red blood cell indices and white blood cell differential; screening electrolytes, including potassium, glucose, magnesium, calcium, and phosphorus; blood urea nitrogen level; creatinine level; and thyroid function tests. The endocrine evaluation is based on the presentation. Bone density measurements are indicated for patients with chronic anorexia nervosa.

Routine electrocardiography should be obtained; a thorough cardiac assessment is indicated when there is the possibility of ipecac misuse. Urine samples can be used to detect diuretic or laxative abuse. Toxicology screens and neurologic assessment may also be indicated. Liver function and renal function assessments and a chest radiograph are sometimes recommended (Beumont et al, 1993; Carney & Andersen, 1996; Edwards, 1993; Herzog, 1992).

Diagnostic studies of patients with anorexia nervosa may reveal anemia, iron deficiency anemia, elevated total cholesterol levels, elevated blood urea nitrogen level, thrombocytopenia, hypokalemia, malignant arrhythmias and other cardiac complications, endocrine disturbances, gastrointestinal effects such as hyperamylasemia, and elevated liver function tests (Beumont et al, 1993: Carney & Andersen, 1996; Edwards, 1993).

Patients with bulimia nervosa may have fluid and electrolyte imbalance related to vomiting or laxative abuse. Abnormal findings may include hypokalemia, hyponatremia, metabolic acidosis, elevated serum amylase levels, and hypochloremic alkalosis.

TREATMENT OPTIONS, EXPECTED OUTCOMES, AND COMPREHENSIVE MANAGEMENT

The primary care provider may be the first person to identify or suspect the disorder, and then to refer the patient. The primary care provider, along with psychiatric professionals, monitors the patient's physical and emotional status, particularly in the early and acute stages of the illness. Primary care providers are also actively involved in the refeeding treatment, which may take place in a hospital or outpatient setting.

The most efficient model of treatment for eating disorders is a multidisciplinary approach that involves an awareness of the complexity of the illness and the importance of teamwork. Patients frequently have contact with numerous health care providers who may not have information about prior treatment approaches. Opportunities to work together can be quite beneficial for the patient (Herzog, 1992).

Restoring normal weight, nutritional state, and eating patterns is a priority in the treatment of an emaciated patient with anorexia nervosa. The initial eating plan is a diet of approximately 1500 calories to prevent physical discomfort. Rapid weight gain may also cause the patient to become unable to participate in the plan of care. There is also a risk of congestive heart failure from rapid weight gain (Carney & Andersen, 1996). Caloric intake may be increased to 3500 calories to achieve weight goals. Patients should be warned about potential ankle edema and facial swelling, which responds to salt and water restriction (Herzog, 1992).

Patients who abused laxatives may have difficulties with laxative withdrawal as a result of reflexive constipation, fluid retention, and bloating. It may take weeks for normal bowel function to return, and they should avoid the use of laxatives during this time. A high-fiber diet and exercise should be prescribed, and glycerine suppositories can also be used.

Medications are not usually indicated for the emaciated patient with anorexia nervosa. Antidepressants may be used if depression does not improve with weight gain. Antidepressants are used more commonly in the short-term treatment of bulimia nervosa. They have been shown to be effective with both depression and bingeing (Walsh & Devlin, 1992).

The comprehensive management of eating disorders by the primary care provider includes referral for psychiatric treatment, management of medical complications, and patient education. The overall treatment may include support groups, individual psychotherapy, cognitive behavioral therapy, psychopharmacotherapy, inpatient hospitalization, family therapy, and nutritional counseling. Patients with bulimia nervosa rarely need inpatient hospitalization; their medical and psychiatric treatment can usually be managed on an outpatient basis.

Groups at Risk

Eating disorders are more prevalent among dancers and athletes, particularly in sports such as gymnastics, diving, and skating where there is an emphasis on thinness (Putukian, 1994). Primary care providers can provide health teaching and support for those particularly at risk. This may also be helpful when there is exaggerated concern about weight or shape or disturbed eating patterns.

Rehabilitation

Anorexia nervosa often has a chronic course, with relapses and hospitalizations. Family members and health care providers may become frustrated, particularly because patients usually are in denial about their illness and resist seeking or accepting treatment (Beumont et al, 1993; Herzog, 1992). The many potential medical and psychiatric complications can be quite serious. Starvation, cardiac abnormalities, sepsis, and suicide are responsible for deaths in 6% of patients with anorexia nervosa, with suicide accounting for the most deaths (Putukian, 1994). Mortality rates with anorexia nervosa increase the longer a patient has the illness; studies show mortality rates of 5% at 5 years, 16% at 20 years, and 18% at 33 years (Herzog et al, 1988 Ratnuriya et al, 1991; Theander, 1983).

Bulimia nervosa is also a chronic illness, with a high relapse rate and progressive symptoms (Edwards, 1993; Herzog, 1992). The prognosis is better than for anorexia nervosa, with the bulimic form of anorexia having the poorest outcomes (Sharp & Freeman, 1993). Patients with bulimia nervosa often feel a sense of shame and hide their illness from others.

TEACHING AND SELF-CARE

Many communities have educational, supportive, and treatment groups for people with eating disorders. They may be affiliated with clinics or other psychiatric treatment centers. Self-help groups, including anorexia and bulimia groups within Overeaters Anonymous, are very helpful for many patients.

The primary care provider can reinforce the progress patients are making with their recovery and can emphasize the role of proper eating in feeling better about themselves. Providers can help patients develop an exercise or activity program to reinforce a positive self-esteem. Spending some time every visit talking about progress in caring for the self is a positive interaction that can foster healthier behaviors.

COMMUNITY RESOURCES

Information for patients and their families and friends can be obtained from the following organizations:

- Eating Disorders Site Map, http://www.something-fishy, com/sitemap.htm: Information on anorexia nervosa, bulimia nervosa, compulsive overeating, other eating disorders, links, local treatments, national organizations, on-line support
- HealthGuide: Eating Disorders, http://www.health guide.com/eating/: General information, treatment options, symptoms, complications, resources
- Males and Eating Disorders, http://www.primenent .com/danslos/males.html: Information about men and eating disorders, links to the stories of men who have or have had eating disorders
- National Association of Anorexia Nervosa and Associated Disorders (ANAD), P.O. Box 7, Highland Park, IL 60035, 847-831-3438
- National Eating Disorders Organization, 6655 S. Yale Ave., Tulsa, OK 74136, 918-481-4044, fax 918-481-4076
- Anorexia Nervosa and Related Eating Disorders, Inc. (ANRED), P.O. Box 5102, Eugene, OR 97405, 541-344-1144: A clearinghouse for information about eating disorders
- National Association to Advance Fat Acceptance, Inc. (NAAFA), P.O. Box 188620, Sacramento, CA 95818, 800-442-1214, 916-558-6880
- Eating Disorders Awareness and Prevention, Inc. (EDAP), 603 Stewart St., Suite 803, Seattle, WA 98101, 206-382-3587, fax 206-292-9890
- Overeaters Anonymous, P.O. Box 44020, Rio Rancho, NM 87124-4020, 505-891-4320: Check the local phone listings in your area.
- Support And Assistance for Binge-Related Eating and Associated Disorders (SABRE), 726 Eglin Pkwy. N.E., #A6, Ft. Walton Beach, FL 32547
- American Anorexia/Bulimia Association, Inc. (AABA), 165 W. 46th St., Suite 1108, New York, NY 10036, 212-575-6200
- Compulsive Eaters Anonymous (H.O.W.), P.O. Box 4403, 10016 Pioneer Blvd., Suite 101, Santa Fe Springs, CA 90670, 562-942-8161, fax 562-948-3721
- Academy for Eating Disorders (AED), 111 E. 210th St., Bronx, NY 10467, 718-920-6782
- Mercy Center for Eating Disorders, 301 St. Paul Place, Baltimore, MD 21202, 410-332-9800, eatdis@mer cymed.com
- Food Addicts Anonymous, 4623 Forrest Hill Blvd., Suite 109-4, West Palm Beach, FL, 561-967-3871
- Mothers of Eating Disorder Children (of all ages), 39 Quail Ct., Walnut Creek, CA 94596, 510-210-0817

REFERRAL POINTS AND CLINICAL WARNINGS

- Patients suspected of having anorexia nervosa or bulimia nervosa should be referred for extensive psychiatric evaluation and treatment. The ideal referral would be to an eating disorders specialist.

- Close monitoring of eating patterns is essential.
- Special attention to weighing the patient in the same clothes at similar times of the day will provide more accurate weights.

EDITOR'S NOTE:
COMPLEMENTARY APPROACHES

A general discussion of complementary approaches can be found in Chapter 3. The following, while not an exhaustive list, are some complementary approaches being used for this condition. Additional information on these approaches, including precautions, can be found in Appendices A and B. Providers need to assess for the use of complementary approaches as part of the patient's history, as they may impact conventional therapies, and patients may not volunteer this information unless specifically asked. Efficacy of many complementary approaches is not as well documented as that of conventional therapies. Providers need to read the literature before suggesting these complementary approaches.

- Complementary Modalities
  Aromatherapy
  Acupuncture

References

American Psychiatric Association. (1994). *Diagnostic and statistical manual of mental disorders*, 4th ed. Washington, D.C.: APA.

Beumont, P.J.V., Russell, J.D., & Touyz, S.W. (1993). Treatment of anorexia nervosa. *Lancet, 341*, 1635–1640.

Bruch, H. (1973). *Eating disorders: Obesity, anorexia nervosa and the person within*. New York: Basic Books.

Carney, C.P., & Andersen, A.E. (1996). Eating disorders: Guide to medical evaluation and complications. *Psychiatric Clinics of North America, 19*(4), 657–679.

Edwards, K.I. (1993). Obesity, anorexia, and bulimia. *Medical Clinics of North America, 77*(4).

Garner, D.M. (1993). Pathogenesis of anorexia nervosa. *Lancet, 341*, 1631–1634.

Herzog, D.B. (1992). Eating disorders: New threats to health. *Psychosomatics, 33*(1), 10–15.

Herzog, D.B., Keller, M.B., & Lavori, P.W. (1988). Outcome in anorexia nervosa and bulimia nervosa: A review of the literature. *Journal of Nervous Mental Disorders, 176*, 131–143.

Hoek, H.W. (1991). The incidence and prevalence of anorexia nervosa and bulimia nervosa in primary care. *Psychological Medicine, 18*, 947–951.

Irwin, E.G. (1993). A focused overview of anorexia nervosa and bulimia. Part I: Etiological issues. *Archives of Psychiatric Nursing, 7*(6), 342–346.

Lucas, A.R., Beard, C.M., O'Fallon, W.M., & Kurland, W.M. (1991). 50-year trends in the incidence of anorexia nervosa in Rochester, Minnesota: A population-based study. *American Journal of Psychiatry, 148*, 917–922.

Mehler, P.S. (1996). Eating disorders: Bulimia nervosa. *Hospital Practice*, 107–126.

Powers, P.S. (1996). Initial assessment and early treatment options for anorexia nervosa and bulimia nervosa. *Psychiatric Clinics of North America, 19*(4), 639–655.

Putukian, M. (1994). The female triad: Eating disorders, amenorrhea, and osteoporosis. *Medical Clinics of North America, 78*(2), 345–356.

Ratnasuriya, R.H., Eisler, I., Szmukler, G.I., & Russell, G.F.M. (1991). Anorexia nervosa: Outcome and prognostic factors after 20 years. *British Journal of Psychiatry, 158*, 495–502.

Rigotti, N.A., Neer, R.M., Skates, S.J. et al.(1991). The clinical course of osteoporosis in anorexia nervosa: A longitudinal study of cortical bone mass. *JAMA, 265*, 1133–1138.

Sharp, C.E., & Freeman, C.P.L. (1993). The medical complications of anorexia nervosa. *British Journal of Psychiatry, 162*, 452–462.

Theander, S. (1983). Research on outcome and prognosis of anorexia nervosa and some results from a Swedish longterm study. *International Journal of Eating Disorders, 2*, 167–174..

Walsh, B.R. & Devlin, M.J. (1992). The pharmacologic treatment of eating disorders. *Psychiatric Clinics of North America, 15*(1), 149–159.

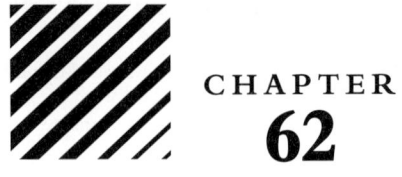

Sleeping Disorders

Carmel Dato, MS, RN, CS, NPP

Sleeping disorders are common conditions that warrant the attention of primary care providers. Sleep is an aspect of self-care that should be part of every assessment, because alterations may be symptomatic of many other conditions or actual specific disorders of sleeping. The importance of sleep and rest is well accepted, and complaints about the quality of sleep are very common.

There are 84 different sleep order entities (American Sleep Disorders Association, 1990). The crippling effects of disordered sleep can exacerbate a psychological state, can reduce the patient's quality of life, or can be dangerous as a result of daytime fatigue. This chapter offers an overview of insomnia, hypersomnia, and narcolepsy, including the most common causes and treatments.

ANATOMY, PHYSIOLOGY, AND PATHOLOGY

With normal physiologic sleep, a person feels adequately restored. The amount of sleep needed varies with the person but is generally about 7 hours a night, with a standard deviation of 1 hour. Many people are probably sleep-deprived (Barthlen & Stacey, 1994).

The stages of sleep follow a predictable pattern of rapid eye movement (REM) and nonrapid eye movement (NREM) sleep with corresponding physiologic functions. The neuroanatomy, neurophysiology, and biochemistry of sleep and wakefulness are not completely understood (Gillin et al, 1995).

Patients with primary insomnia may appear tired, exhausted, and weary; however, there may be no other characteristics on the physical exam. Polysomnography (PSG) may show alterations in sleep continuity and stages of sleep, increased muscle tension, and increased electroencephalographic (EEG) alpha activity.

Disorders that may cause insomnia include obstructive sleep apnea (OSA), periodic limb movement disorder (PLMD), and restless limb syndrome (RLS). PLMD and RLS are poorly understood disorders that interrupt sleep due to limb movements and sensations. They may be related to other medical conditions.

Obstructive sleep apnea (OSA) is caused by a collapse of the pharyngeal airway during sleep, despite continuous efforts to breathe. Airway muscles relax and the airway closes in a person with an anatomically small pharyngeal airway. Breathing resumes after a brief arousal or awakening. During apneic periods, there is a progressive blood oxygen desaturation and an increase in carbon dioxide. With each arousal, the person returns to a deeper stage of sleep, with subsequent periods of apnea and arousal. As the disease progresses, the duration of apneic periods and the degree of hypoxemia increase. Sequelae include:

- Bradycardia with rebound tachycardia on awakening
- Electrocardiogram abnormalities, such as premature ventricular contractions and sleep apnea-associated arrhythmias

- Cyclic changes in systemic and pulmonary arterial pressure
- Sustained pulmonary hypertension
- Right-sided heart failure
- Systemic hypertension
- Impaired cerebral functioning.

Symptoms increase when the person drinks alcohol, takes a depressant drug, or changes sleep patterns. There may also be a reduction in intellectual capacity, personality changes, sudden bursts of anger and hostility, and impairments in social and work life (Jaquis, 1987; Stradling, 1995; White, 1995; Williams et al, 1995).

The pathophysiology of narcolepsy results in a disturbance of control of both REM and NREM sleep onset and offset. There is resulting disruption of nighttime sleep and the impingement of sleep into daytime wakefulness (Mahowald, 1996). Narcolepsy is considered a disorder of REM sleep mechanisms. There has not been supporting evidence thus far for the hypothesis that narcolepsy is an autoimmune disorder, based on the extremely high rate (up to 100%) of occurrence with HLA DR2 (Barthlen & Stacey, 1994).

EPIDEMIOLOGY

Studies show a 1-year prevalence rate of insomnia complaints of 30% to 40% in adults (American Psychiatric Association [APA], 1994). The incidence of narcolepsy is estimated at 0.02% to 0.09% (Williams et al, 1995), with a prevalence of more than 50 per 100,000, and a genetic linkage. Narcolepsy occurs in 10% of first-degree relatives and excessive daytime sleepiness in up to 30% (Barthlen & Stacey, 1994).

OSA predominantly affects middle-aged, overweight men; however, it can occur at all ages and in both sexes (Williams et al, 1995). The prevalence is approximately 4% in men and 2% in women, with higher rates in African Americans, older people, obese people, and those with hypertension, hypothyroidism, and upper airway anatomic abnormalities (Young, 1993).

Restless leg syndrome (RLS) occurs in 5% to 10% of the population, with a strong family history. The rate of periodic limb movement disorder (PLMD) increases in patients older than age 60; it occurs rarely in patients younger than 30 and is found in nearly half of patients older than 65 (Barthlen & Stacey, 1994; Jamieson & Becker, 1992).

There is an increase in sleep disturbances in the elderly, with a greater number of awakenings, possibly as a result of the increased incidence of sleep-related breathing disorders (mild apnea) and PLMD. The elderly also sleep less efficiently and have more circadian rhythm changes (Moran & Stoudemire, 1992).

DIAGNOSTIC CRITERIA

Many patients with insomnia can be successfully managed by a primary care provider. An in-depth interview to obtain a full description of the problem is the most important diagnostic procedure. A sleep laboratory study (PSG) may also be indicated. Changes in sleep habits and patterns should alert the primary care provider to the possibility of a sleep disorder; however, not all disturbances in sleep are symptomatic of a primary sleep disorder. It is important to inquire about sleep as part of the routine assessments, because some patients will not describe problems otherwise. An accurate diagnosis can be difficult, because many different sleep disorders share signs and symptoms (Williams et al, 1995).

There is frequently a close connection and interaction between the quality of sleep and health problems (Moran & Stoudemire, 1992). The primary care provider should listen carefully for symptoms of depression, bipolar disease, anxiety disorder, panic disorder, substance abuse, or psychosis (Barthlen & Stacey, 1994). Disordered sleep is also found in dementia, parkinsonism, epilepsy, nocturnal cardiac ischemia, sleep-related gastroesophageal reflux, peptic ulcer disease, sleep-related asthma, and fibromyalgia (Barthlen & Stacey, 1994; Williams et al, 1995).

The APA's *Diagnostic and Statistical Manual of Mental Disorders*, 4th edition (1994), classifies sleep disorders into four main classes:

- Primary sleep disorders (dyssomnias and parasomnias)
- Sleep disorder related to another mental disorder (eg, a depressive or anxiety disorder)
- Sleep disorder due to a general medical condition
- Substance-induced sleep disorder.

Dyssomnias are basic disorders of initiating or maintaining sleep or of excessive sleepiness, characterized by a disturbance in the amount, quality, or timing of sleep. Parasomnias are disorders that include unusual behavior or physiologic events that occur in association with sleep.

Primary Insomnia

The diagnostic criteria for primary insomnia includes a complaint, lasting for at least 1 month, of difficulty initiating or maintaining sleep or of unrestful, nonrestorative sleep (APA, 1994). Many patients complain of a combination of symptoms. They may have increased physiologic or psychological arousal at nighttime, often associated with preoccupation, distress, and worry related to prior experiences with insomnia.

There are clinically significant consequences of the sleep disturbance in the form of distress or impairment in social, occupational, or other important areas of functioning. Patients may have irritability, difficulty concentrating, or problems with inattention. One diagnostic criterion is that the insomnia is not the result of another condition, such as another sleep disorder, a mental disorder, a medical condition, or the direct physiologic effects of a substance. Primary insomnia must also be distinguished from normal sleep variance—for instance, "short sleepers" who require less sleep but do not have other characteristics of primary insomnia.

Transient Insomnia

Transient insomnia is a form of insomnia that is not considered a sleep disorder but a symptom that lasts only a few consecutive nights or weeks. It is usually related to a temporary situational stressor or the effects of biologic clock disruptions. Internal or external stimuli may cause arousal and thus insomnia. The most common internal stimulus is a psychological stress that feels like imminent danger—for example, job pressures, relationship conflicts, or security fears (Barthlen & Stacey, 1994).

A chronic complaint of insomnia may be further evaluated in a sleep disorders center with PSG. This is indicated when there is suspicion of RLS, PLMD, or OSA. PSG may also be indicated when there is severe, excessive daytime sleepiness, when there is violent behavior during sleep, or when treatment has been unsuccessful. It may also be indicated when the clinical diagnosis is unclear, with suspicion of circadian rhythm disorder (Mahowald, 1996).

Other Sleep Disorders

Recent changes in sleep patterns as a result of time zone change, travel, or shift work may result in circadian rhythm sleep disorder, which manifests as difficulty falling asleep at socially normal times, with reduced alertness. Delayed or advanced sleep phase syndromes are patterns of sleeping several hours later or earlier than conventional times for sleep. Patients with this disorder have normal sleep but may be sleep-deprived because of insufficient hours of sleep.

Other specific types of insomnia include altitude insomnia, hypnotic-dependent sleep disorder, stimulant-dependent sleep disorder, alcohol-dependent sleep disorder, and medication-induced sleep disorders. It is important to evaluate the many potential contributing influences to insomnia (Barthlen & Stacey, 1994; Rosekind, 1992).

Narcolepsy

Excessive sleepiness is a common complaint in clinical practice and may be a sign of one of several treatable conditions. It differs from fatigue, an experience of tiredness and desire to sleep that does not usually lead to sleep. With insomnia, for example, there is fatigue, with difficulty initiating and maintaining sleep. The patient with true excessive daytime sleepiness, compared with fatigue, easily and involuntarily falls asleep quickly at troublesome times and places, such as when driving, working, or meeting with friends. This type of recurring pathologic sleepiness is serious and may be quite dangerous (Gillin et al, 1995). Insufficient sleep syndrome is caused by multiple problematic behavioral habits or environmental stimuli (Barthlen & Stacey, 1994).

Narcolepsy is characterized by excessive daytime sleepiness and is often associated with cataplexy. The cataplexic attacks may be either a barely perceptible, brief weakness of a muscle group, resulting in the jaw dropping or losing one's grip, or a total collapse after sudden paralysis. Narcolepsy usually develops in the second decade of life and progresses slowly but steadily. It is diagnosed by PSG (Williams et al, 1995). The sleep attacks are often irresistible and may last minutes to an hour, after which the person feels refreshed. The attacks may occur many times daily during periods of either activity or inactivity. The patient may collapse suddenly without warning. The patient may experience a sleep paralysis on falling asleep or awakening; in this situation, the patient is unable to move a muscle, or breathing feels paralyzed. The patient often experiences panic when this first begins to occur (Barthlen & Stacey, 1994).

Obstructive Sleep Apnea

OSA is a form of sleep-related breathing disorder characterized by repetitive intervals of upper airway obstruction. These episodes last longer than 10 seconds and occur more than 30 times during both REM and NREM sleep in a 7-hour sleep period. However, patients may more episodes than this, and the obstructive time periods may last up to 2 minutes (Jaquis, 1987; Williams et al, 1995). An OSA can be thought of as a continuum from normal sleep to severe, all-night OSA.

There are variations of the pattern on a night-to-night basis, with a long, gradual history (Stradling, 1995). An acute onset may be symptomatic of another disorder such as hypothyroidism (Stradling, 1995). OSA's principal manifestations are excessive daytime sleepiness with long and unrefreshing naps, disorientation, and periods of automatic behavior. It should be considered when the patient is obese and reports drowsiness, morning headaches, irritability, or erectile impotence, or a bed partner complains of loud snoring. The syndrome is usually associated with snoring; however, most snorers do not have sleep apnea. Bed partners report loud snoring with periods of apnea, when the patient continues to make breathing efforts. Patients with HIV disease are at particular risk in the early stages of the illness because of adenotonsillar hypertrophy (Epstein et al, 1995).

Periodic Limb Movement Disorder

PLMD, also known as nocturnal myoclonus, results in periodic, repetitive movements of the limbs during sleep. Patients complain of nonrefreshing sleep and are unaware of the movements, although they may have brief arousals or even full awakenings. Information from a bed partner can be very helpful in making this diagnosis. Both the quality and quantity of sleep are affected. PSG readings, including an electromyogram (EMG) and an EEG, are essential for diagnosis. An EMG shows either a series of bursts or single sustained contractions in the anterior tibialis muscles bilaterally, the biceps, or the triceps. The EEG shows a K complex followed by a brief alpha rhythm. The movements are stereotypical and rhythmic and include rapid flexion or jerking of the legs and feet (Barthlen & Stacey, 1994; Jamieson & Becker, 1992; Williams et al, 1995).

Restless Leg Syndrome

RLS is related to PLMD. Almost all patients with RLS also have PLMD, but the reverse is not true. The diagnosis of RLS can be made from the history and description of symptoms. Symptoms of RLS include pricking, tingling, creeping, and crawling sensations deep in the (usually lower) legs that escalate to an irresistible urge to move the legs. The symptoms occur at rest, usually when lying down, and worsen toward evening, thus interfering with both sleep onset and continuity of sleep. RLS is exacerbated by:

- Caffeine intake
- Pregnancy (third trimester)
- Use of tricyclic antidepressants, decongestants, or neuroleptics
- Benzodiazepine or barbiturate withdrawal
- Neuropathy

- Venous varicosities
- Iron deficiency
- Environmental temperature extremes
- Muscular fatigue.

Both RLS and PLMD are also related to other medical disorders, including uremia, emphysema, rheumatoid arthritis, fibromyalgia, amyotrophic lateral sclerosis, and myelopathies (Barthlen & Stacey, 1994; Jamieson & Becker, 1992; Williams et al, 1995).

HISTORY AND PHYSICAL EXAM

The interview can often elicit information that helps determine possible causes of sleep disturbances. The patient's sleep habits can be informative in making a diagnosis. Patients may be asked to keep a sleep diary or log that they fill out every morning for a week. The information in the diary is similar to the information sought during the interview. Table 62-1 lists items to be noted in a sleep history. The primary care provider should also review the use of sedatives, hypnotics, stimulants, and other medications in the history.

The primary care provider should ask the patient's partner whether the patient snores or makes other types of breathing noises or has abnormal or violent movements, such as very forceful thrashing and kicking. Information obtained from partners can be very useful for many diagnoses, because they may have information not known by the patient. When the patient complains of daytime sleepiness and dysphoria but not of insomnia, the partner's observations can prove useful. The patient may have interruptions in the continuity of sleep that are very brief and not remembered but still interfere with sleep.

TABLE 62-1	Sleep History

- Time patient went to bed
- Time patient turned off lights
- Time patient fell asleep
- Time patient awakened
- Total time spent in bed
- Total time asleep
- Any variations or changes in pattern of sleep
- Other activities in bed
- Number and duration of awakenings during night
- Estimate of sleep quality
- Comments on unusual events and any associated symptoms (eg, orthopnea, urinary frequency, pain, palpitations)
- Any sensations just before and during sleep (eg, sweating, feeling hot, pins and needles, restless legs and jerking)
- Type of mental activity patient participates in before going to sleep
- Evidence of excessive brooding, anxious or repetitive thoughts, or panic attacks while waiting to get to sleep
- Affective quality of dreams (eg, an increase in anxious dreams and nightmares)
- Alterations in diet, occupational and travel patterns, weight, lifestyle, alcohol intake, sexual habits, menstruation, and consumption of sleeping pills or other over-the-counter sleeping aids, other medications
- Daytime consequences of disturbed sleep

These may include patients who have problems with coughing, painful arthritis, OSA, or PLMD (Gillin et al, 1995).

Primary insomnia usually involves a sudden onset after a psychological, social, or medical stressor or crisis. It often continues after the original precipitating factors resolve because of heightened arousal and negative conditioning. The course is variable, often starting in young adulthood or middle age. The most typical course involves a period of incremental deterioration of the sleep pattern over weeks or months, replaced by a persistent period of steady sleep difficulty that may last for years.

Narcolepsy develops slowly and steadily, reaching a stable point where there is little variation. The symptoms may vary from mild to severe.

DIAGNOSTIC STUDIES

PSG is the only diagnostic test used in diagnosing sleep disorders (other than laboratory tests used to rule out other disorders). PSG is performed by a sleep disorders specialist in a sleep disorders center, where patients usually spend one or two nights sleeping. PSG involves synchronized, all-night, standard electrophysiologic recording. It includes an EEG, an EMG, and an electrocardiogram, and also measures electrical activity in the eyes, respiration, muscle tone, blood oxygen saturation, and respiratory air flow; occasionally other physiologic assessments are also done (eg, hormonal and biochemical estimations). For definitive diagnosis of OSA, other respiratory parameters are also monitored (Jaquis, 1987; Mahowald, 1996). Daytime sleepiness may be measured by the Multiple Sleep Latency Test, which uses the same parameters as PSG during daytime naps (Mahowald, 1996).

TREATMENT OPTIONS, EXPECTED OUTCOMES, AND COMPREHENSIVE MANAGEMENT

When treating a patient with more than one sleep disorder, the primary care provider uses a hierarchical approach, treating the disorder that presents the most immediate danger to the patient's health (Williams et al, 1995).

Sleep Hygiene

Good sleep hygiene habits are the mainstay of treatment in both chronic insomnia and transient insomnia (eg, after the resolution of an internal stressor). Transient, short-term insomnia can be effectively managed by the primary care provider. Patients can learn ways to improve their self-care with regard to sleep hygiene habits (Table 62-2). Patients may use remedies such as chamomile tea and warm milk to improve their sleep. The primary care provider may also recommend complementary modalities such as acupuncture, hypnosis, systematic desensitization, biofeedback, and progressive muscle relaxation to relieve muscle tension. Imagery training and meditation are used to control intrusive or racing thoughts and reduce cognitive arousal. Elimination of common performance anxiety is used by some insomniacs as a way to facilitate sleep (Barthlen & Stacey, 1994; Nino-Murcia, 1992).

Pharmacotherapy

Pharmacotherapy may be an appropriate intervention for transient insomnia. Sedative-hypnotic medications are judiciously used for transient insomnia when other diagnoses have been

TABLE 62-2	Good Sleep Hygiene

- Maintain a regular sleep schedule for going to sleep and getting up, regardless of the amount of sleep the previous night.
- If sleep doesn't occur within 20 to 30 minutes, get out of bed and do something relaxing (reading, music, television) and then return to bed when drowsy; repeat as necessary.
- Avoid napping.
- Maintain a sleep diary of sleep hours and factors that seem to influence sleep, such as exercise, caffeine and alcohol use, cigarette smoking, bedroom temperature, and noise.
- Avoid caffeine and stimulant xanthines found in coffee, tea, colas, and chocolate 6 hours before sleep.
- Avoid alcohol 6 hours before sleep.
- Minimize use of caffeine, alcohol, and nicotine.
- Participate in regular exercise (not later than 3 to 4 hours before bedtime).
- Create a comfortable sleep environment that is quiet, dark (avoid illuminated clocks), and moderate in temperature, with a comfortable bed and pillow.
- Avoid going to bed hungry or extremely full.
- Minimize fluid consumption in the evening, thus minimizing nocturia.
- Stop using over-the-counter sleeping aids.
- Avoid long periods of nonsleep time in bed; don't work, eat, read, or watch television in bed.
- Go to bed only when sleepy.

ruled out and modifications of sleep hygiene have not been effective. They are used in small doses and for the shortest possible time. Care is taken to avoid escalation of dosage and to prevent drug-dependency insomnia.

When a hypnotic is indicated, the smallest dose should be prescribed for a few nights up to a few weeks. Patients should be instructed to stop the medication after one or two nights of restful sleep. They should also be instructed not to exceed the recommended dose or length of treatment, even though hypnotics are a safe and effective treatment for insomnia.

Medications from various pharmaceutical classes may be useful (Table 62-3). Hypnotics can be useful in breaking a cycle of sleeplessness resulting from stress or altered sleep cycle by increasing total sleep time and improving the patient's perceptions of sleep. Benzodiazepines are the first choice; they have a high efficacy, a wide margin of safety, and a relatively low

TABLE 62-3	Drugs Used for Insomnia
Benzodiazepines	**Nonbenzodiazepine–Nonbarbiturates**
Estazolam	Choral hydrate
Flurazepam	Ethchlorvynol
Quazepam	Glutethimide
Temazepam	Methyprylon
Triazolam	Paraldehyde
Barbiturates	Zolpidem
Amobarbital	Tricyclic antidepressants
Aprobarbital	Antihistamine (diphenhydramine)
Butabarbital	Neurotin (gabapentin)
Pentobarbital	Clonazepam
Phenobarbital	
Secobarbital	
Talbutal	

abuse potential, cause minimal tolerance and physical dependence, present a minimal risk of suicide, and have few interactions with other drugs. Those with a longer half-life may produce next-day sedative effects or impaired daytime behavior. Shorter-acting benzodiazepines may cause hangover effects or rebound insomnia. The benzodiazepines decrease latency time in falling asleep, reduce awakenings, and increase total sleep time (Barthlen & Stacey, 1994).

Hypnotics should be used cautiously in patients with a history of alcohol or substance abuse, or with suicidal tendencies. They should be avoided in patients with OSA or other respiratory disorders, current depression, pregnancy, or current substance abuse. Low doses of antidepressants may also be used as hypnotic agents, especially for those with a history of depression or current depression, or abstinent alcoholics. Anxiolytic agents may be indicated for patients with both insomnia and anxiety; however, they should be avoided in the elderly (Rakel, 1993).

Obstructive Sleep Apnea

Treatment of OSA may include behavior modification, including weight loss (although this may not prevent OSA), avoidance of alcohol and sedatives, and avoidance of supine sleep positions. Continuous positive airway pressure and bilevel positive airway pressure are effective, inexpensive, and well-tolerated treatments; their use is initiated by a sleep disorders specialist. These therapies involve the continuous administration of air via a nasal mask, maintaining positive air pressure in the airway. This prevents it from collapsing during inhalation, when intrathoracic pressure become negative (Williams et al, 1995). Patients wear either a nasal mask (for mouth breathers), a triangle that fits over the nose, or a "nasal pillow" that rests below the nose (for patients who feel claustrophobic with the triangle) during the night. Patients are initially taught the use of the mask in a sleep laboratory for one or two nights. Some specialists also prescribe a sleeping medication for a few nights to ensure initial success by helping the patient relax and adjust to the equipment. After this instruction, patients use the equipment at home. Some patients need encouragement and support to use the equipment, because they may view it as unnatural and cumbersome. Most patients report having a refreshing night's sleep with the first use and continue the therapy. Patients may need to continue the therapy indefinitely. The primary care provider should continue to ask about sleep when seeing the patient for regular checkups because there may be a need to adjust the amount of pressure. In this case, the patient would be referred back to the specialist.

Oral appliances that modify the upper airway by repositioning the mandible and tongue are an alternative treatment. Oral appliances are useful for patients who cannot tolerate continuous positive airway pressure (Schmidt-Nowara et al, 1995). Surgical treatments may also be used (Williams et al, 1995).

Patients with OSA who need to undergo surgery should advise the anesthesiologist of the disorder; the anesthesiologist may want to review the results of the sleep study to make determinations about the choice of anesthesia and recovery (Ogan & Plevak, 1996).

Periodic Limb Movement Disorder and Restless Leg Syndrome

The treatment of PLMD and RLS should address the underlying conditions whenever possible. Small doses of benzodiaze-

pines taken at bedtime are successful with PLMD by suppressing arousals; although the movements continue, the sleep quality is unfragmented (Barthlen & Stacey, 1994; Jamieson & Becker, 1992; Williams et al, 1995).

Circadian Rhythm Sleep Disorders

Patients with circadian rhythm sleep disorders can be instructed to undergo a course of chronotherapy, following 27-hour-day cycles until conventional sleep hours are attained. Good sleep hygiene measures may then be effective long-term treatment.

TEACHING AND SELF-CARE

Patients with insomnia can be taught good sleep hygiene methods as a form of self-care (see Table 62-2). The primary care provider can review the history and sleep diary to make specific recommendations for behavioral changes.

Daytime sleepiness secondary to a sleep disorder can lead to potential hazards. Patients should be cautioned about driving and operating machinery; the provider should note any special hazards related to their occupation and interests.

Patients with OSA need education about the disorder, diagnostic tests, and treatments. Before treatment, they may have difficulty concentrating as a result of tiredness. They may need to discuss problems secondary to the disorder, such as relationship strain or negative self-concept. They may need reinforcement about the importance of treatment and the care of respiratory equipment (Jaquis, 1987). Instructions come with the equipment regarding washing the hose (weekly), changing the reservoir of distilled water (daily), and replacing the mask or nosepiece (every 6 months).

Patients taking medications for sleep should be taught about measures they should take for safety in getting to the bathroom at night, such as:

- Using a night light
- Wearing well-fitting slippers
- Moving scatter rugs out of the route to the bathroom.

Other safety measures include not driving or operating machinery while taking medications. Patients with fatigue or daytime sleepiness also need to be cautioned about driving and operating machinery.

COMMUNITY RESOURCES

- National Sleep Foundation, 729 Fifteenth St., NW, 4th Floor, Washington, D.C. 20005, Natsleep@erols.com, http://www.sleepfoundation.org: Sleep disorder information
- The Sleep Well, http://www-leland.stanford.edu/dement/: Sleep disorder information, list of accredited sleep disorder centers in the United States
- American Sleep Apnea Association, 2025 Pennsylvania Ave., NW, Suite 905, Washington, D.C. 20006: Sponsors local A.W.A.K.E. (Alert, Well, and Keeping Energetic) support groups and events such as informational meetings about insurance coverage. Members also receive bimonthly issues of *Wake-up Call: The Wellness Letter for Snoring and Apnea*, which gives medical information about snoring and sleep apnea.

- The Sleep Research Center, P.O. Box 111, Bancroft, MI 48414, 800-765-3360
- Tristate Sleep Disorders Center, 1275 E. Kemper Rd., Cincinnati, OH 45246, 513-671-3101, TDD: 311-111-6111, Sleepsat1@aol.com
- Big Apple Support and Education Group for Sleep Apnea, Robert Wood Johnson University Hospital, 1 Robert Wood Johnson Place, New Brunswick, NJ 08901; Community Education Department, 732-937-8820

REFERRAL POINTS AND CLINICAL WARNINGS

Referrals to a sleep disorders specialist may be indicated for complaints of excessive daytime sleepiness or chronic insomnia. Patients should be referred when traditional therapeutic measures, such as sleep hygiene techniques and medications, have not been effective or have resulted in unacceptable side effects. The referral may also be indicated for confirmation of a diagnosis such as OSA or PLMD (Moran & Stoudemire, 1992).

Referral to a psychotherapist is indicated for the evaluation of psychiatric disorders, many of which are accompanied by insomnia (Gillin & Byerley, 1990). Patients with transient insomnia may also be referred to a psychotherapist for further help in coping with the situations and emotions that triggered the insomnia. They may be able to learn additional coping methods and to increase their ability to manage stress. By uncovering internal conflicts, psychotherapy may be able to prevent future incidents of insomnia.

EDITOR'S NOTE:

COMPLEMENTARY APPROACHES

A general discussion of complementary approaches can be found in Chapter 3. The following, while not an exhaustive list, are some complementary approaches being used for this condition. Additional information on these approaches, including precautions, can be found in Appendices A and B. Providers need to assess for the use of complementary approaches as part of the patient's history, as they may impact conventional therapies, and patients may not volunteer this information unless specifically asked. Efficacy of many complementary approaches is not as well documented as that of conventional therapies. Providers need to read the literature before suggesting these complementary approaches.

- Vitamins, minerals, herbs, supplements
  Melatonin
- Complementary Modalities
  Acupuncture
  Aromatherapy
  Biofeedback

References

American Psychiatric Association. (1994). *Diagnostic and statistical manual of mental disorders*, 4th ed. Washington, D.C.: Author.

American Sleep Disorders Association. (1990). *International classification manual of sleep disorders: Diagnostic and coding manual*. Rochester, MN: Author.

Barthlen, G.M., & Stacey, C. (1994). Dyssomnia, parasomnias, and sleep disorders associated with medical and psychiatric diseases. *Mount Sinai Journal of Medicine, 61*(2), 139–159.

Epstein, L.F., Strollo, P.J., Donegan, R.B., Delmar, J., Hendrix, C., & Westbrook, P.R. (1995). Obstructive sleep apnea in patients with human immunodeficiency virus (HIV) disease. *Sleep, 18*(5), 368–376.

Gillin, J.C., & Byerley, W.F. (1990). The diagnosis and management of insomnia. *N Engl J Med, 322*(4), 239–248.

Gillin, J.C., Zoltoski, R.K., & Salin-Pascual, R. (1995). Basic science of sleep. In H.I. Kaplan & B.J. Sadock (Eds.). *Comprehensive textbook of psychiatry*, 6th ed., pp. 80–88. Baltimore: Williams & Wilkins.

Jaquis, J. (1987). Obstructive sleep apnea syndrome. *Nurse Practitioner, 12*(6), 50–56.

Jamieson, A.O. & Becker, P.M. (1992). Management of the 10 most common sleep disorders. *American Family Physician, 45*(3), 1262–1268.

Mahowald, M.W. (1996). Diagnostic testing. In R.W. Evans (Ed.). *Neurologic Clinics*, pp. 183–198. Philadelphia: W.B. Saunders.

Moran, M.G., & Stoudemire, A. (1992). Sleep disorders in the medically ill patient. *Journal of Clinical Psychiatry, 53*(Suppl. 6), 29–36.

Nino-Murcia, G. (1992). Diagnosis and treatment of insomnia and risks associated with lack of treatment. *Journal of Clinical Psychiatry, 53*(Suppl. 6), 43–47.

Ogan, O.U., & Plevak, D.J. (1996). Sleep apnea and anesthesia. *Wake-up call: The wellness letter for snoring and apnea*. Washington, D.C.: The American Sleep Apnea Association.

Rakel, R.E. (1993). Insomnia: Concerns of the family physician. *Journal of Family Practice, 35*(5), 551–557.

Rosekind, M.R. (1992). The epidemiology and occurrence of insomnia. *Journal of Clinical Psychiatry, 53*(Suppl. 6), 4–6.

Schmidt-Nowara, W., Lowe, A., Wiegand, L., Cartwright, R., Perez-Guerra, F. & Menn, S. (1995). Oral appliances for the treatment of snoring and obstructive sleep apnea: A review. *Sleep, 18*(6), 501–510.

Stradling, J.R. (1995). Obstructive sleep apnea: Definitions, epidemiology, and natural history. In P.M.A. Calverley (Series Ed.). *Thorasic, 50*, 683–689.

White, D.P. (1995). Pathophysiology of obstructive sleep apnea. In P.M.A. Calverley (Series Ed.). *Thorax, 50*, 797–804.

Williams, R.L., Karacan, I., Moore, C., & Hirshkowitz, M. (1995). In H.I. Kaplan & B.J. Sadock (Eds.). *Comprehensive textbook of psychiatry*, 6th ed., pp. 1373–1408. Baltimore, MD: Williams & Wilkins.

Young, T. (1993). The occurrence of sleep-disordered breathing among middle-aged adults. *N Engl J Med, 328*, 1230.

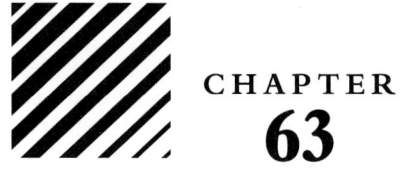

CHAPTER
63

Somatization Disorder

Timothy F. Landers, MA, MS, CRNP

Somatization disorder (SD) is a clinical syndrome characterized by the presence of multiple unexplained physical complaints without a known physical cause. SD is an important condition in primary care because it is responsible for unnecessary diagnostic testing and therapeutic interventions. It is well known in primary care that patients express emotional or psychological symptoms physically and respond to these symptoms differently.

Somatization can be seen as one end of a continuum in which physical complaints are perceived to be debilitating, either because of the patient's preoccupation with the symptoms or because the experience of the symptoms is intense. For these patients, somatic complaints tend to be more debilitating, involve a greater number of clusters of complaints, and occur over a longer period of time. At the other end of the continuum are patients who describe what has been called symptom sensitivity. These patients are acutely aware of the presence of physical symptoms to a greater degree than many other patients.

Patients with SD tend to have a greater-than-expected degree of disability from their complaints. In some cases, what appear to be minor complaints may cause such psychological distress that social or occupational functioning is compromised. This is one of the hallmarks of SD. Situation one provides an example of a patient with complaints that are seriously affecting his quality of life.

The diagnosis of SD must be made carefully to exclude underlying physical conditions that have not been diagnosed. Often years of medical records need to be reviewed to ensure that adequate testing has been undertaken to exclude physical complaints. Thorough attention must be paid to atypical presentations of common illnesses and to rarer illnesses. Treatment involves the development of a therapeutic relationship over an extended period of time, one in which patients feel that their complaints are taken seriously. Often, the development of a therapeutic relationship is troubled by doubt and frustration by both the patient and the provider. It is important that while this relationship is forming, the primary care provider maintains an open, nonjudgmental, and caring demeanor.

ANATOMY, PHYSIOLOGY, AND PATHOLOGY

As with many illnesses, there appears to be a strong familial link in SD. It is unknown whether this is the result of environmental or genetic influences. For example, some families may sanction the expression of physical complaints to a greater degree than other families. Researchers have postulated that there are biochemical influences on the expression of SD, but this has not been proven (Smith, 1995).

In SD, physical complaints are presented without adequate physical findings. This lack of presence of an organic pathology can be frustrating to even the most experienced primary care provider. There is little if any match between the symptoms and the actual physical findings (Barsky, 1995).

EPIDEMIOLOGY

Much has been written about the social, gender, and situation influences on somatization. SD has been found to be expressed differently in different cultural groups. It is thought to have a much higher prevalence among women than men. In general, the lifetime prevalence of SD is 0.2% to 2% (American Psychiatric Association [APA], 1994). However, rates of SD vary greatly depending on the population studied, the definition of the syndrome, and the practice setting. Rates as high as 8% have been reported in psychiatric settings, and higher rates tend to occur in patients with other conditions such as irritable bowel disease, polycystic ovary syndrome, and chronic pain, where the rate may be as high as 28% (Smith, 1995).

Recent research has suggested that environmental factors may play a role in the expression of SD (Gothe et al, 1995). Certain environmental factors, such as exposure to certain chemicals, are thought to cause or aggravate physical complaints. In cases of this environmental somatization syndrome, no cause can be found for these physical complaints based on the suspicious agent. An example of this syndrome is the association of disease or illness with office buildings. Although there are no environmental or physical causes for these beliefs, groups of people may come to see the building itself as the cause of this syndrome. In addition, patients tend to downplay the importance of other explanations for the cause of their symptoms. Patients become convinced that the facility is to blame for their illness and often refuse suggestions that other factors, such as stress or tobacco use, may be involved. Because of the link of this syndrome and geography, environmental somatization syndrome tends to appear in clusters (Gothe et al, 1995).

It is thought that because different social groups may sanction the expression of physical complaints through different symptoms, there is likely to be a large cultural component to the expression of SD. For example, in one study of African patients, common somatic complaints included heat radiating from the head, generalized aches and pains, crawling sensations, and muscle fasciculations (Ohaeri & Odejide, 1994). Among Hispanic patients, common complaints included headache, excessive gas, chest pain, and gynecologic complaints (Hulme, 1996). The differences in SD between men and women is being studied (Wool & Barsky, 1994).

DIAGNOSTIC CRITERIA

Widely recognized criteria for the diagnosis of SD are presented in Table 63-1. The diagnosis requires the presence of symptoms without a corresponding medical condition. Although the cri-

TABLE 63-1	Diagnostic Criteria for Somatization Disorder

A. A history of complaints beginning before age 30 years that occur over a period of several years and result in treatment being sought or significant impairment in social, occupational, or other important areas of functioning.

B. Each of the following criteria must have been met, with individual symptoms occurring at any time during the course of the disturbance:
1. Four pain symptoms: a history of pain related to at least four different sites or functions (eg, head, abdomen, joints, extremities, chest, rectum, during menstruation, during sexual intercourse, or during urination)
2. Two gastrointestinal symptoms: a history of at least two gastrointestinal symptoms other than pain (eg, nausea, bloating, vomiting other than during pregnancy, diarrhea, or intolerance of several different foods)
3. One sexual symptom: a history of at least one sexual or reproductive symptom other than pain (eg, sexual indifference, erectile or ejaculatory dysfunction, irregular menses, excessive menstrual bleeding, vomiting throughout pregnancy)
4. One pseudoneurologic symptom: a history of at least one symptom or deficit suggesting a neurologic condition not limited to pain (conversion symptoms such as impaired coordination or balance, paralysis or localized weakness, difficulty swallowing or lump in throat, aphasia, urinary retention, hallucinations, loss of touch or pain sensation, double vision, blindness, deafness, seizures, dissociative symptoms).

C. Either (1) or (2):
1. After appropriate investigation, each of the symptoms in Criterion B cannot be fully explained by a known medical condition or the direct effects of a substance (eg, a drug of abuse, a medication).
2. When there is a related general medical condition, the physical complaints or resulting social or occupational impairments are in excess of what would be expected from the history, physical exam, or laboratory findings.

D. The symptoms are not intentionally produced or feigned (as in factitious disorder or malingering).

Source: American Psychiatric Association: Diagnostic and Statistical Manual of Mental Disorders, 4/e, Washington, DC: American Psychiatric Association, 1994.

teria for diagnosis are widely accepted and were formed by consensus (APA, 1994), other researchers often use lower symptom thresholds to determine the number of patients within a population with somatization tendencies.

It is important to distinguish SD from complaints that occur in patients with coexisting anxiety disorders. Complaints associated with panic attacks are likely to be identified with the panic or anxiety; in contrast, in patients with SD, physical complaints tend to be the primary complaint. These physical complaints can cause a significant degree of anxiety. This distinction often must be made over a period of months to years, allowing the provider to make subtle distinctions.

Patients who present with multiple complaints often have been through multiple diagnostic procedures. It is important that before a referral is made for specialty care, the purpose of these visit be made clear with both the patient and the consultant. It is often helpful to present these consultations as a way to garner additional information for the patient and the provider; the patient should know that nothing definitive may be found.

HISTORY AND PHYSICAL EXAM

The history and physical exam are vital tools in the primary care management of SD. They can often exclude the most dangerous causes of the complaints and are likely to yield complaints across multiple systems that have been present for years. In addition, patients are likely to have had extensive workups for other conditions without any specific findings. Patient histories often fail to show any cluster of symptoms specific for any illness categories. The history can be a valuable tool when complaints involve multiple systems, occur over a long period of time, and are not associated with any identifiable illness. Above all, the physical exam should be conducted in a way that does not reinforce symptoms.

TREATMENT OPTIONS, EXPECTED OUTCOMES, AND COMPREHENSIVE MANAGEMENT

The treatment of SD must include a strong therapeutic alliance between the primary care provider and the patient. The development of a trusting relationship is crucial to the management of patients with SD because it reassures patients that their symptoms are being taken seriously. This may have the effect of reducing unnecessary referrals and testing.

Group therapy has been shown to be effective in reducing the morbidity associated with SD. In one study (Kashner et al, 1995), group therapy was shown to result in a 52% net savings in dollars spent on health care utilization for patients with SD. This treatment approach involved eight sessions that focused on group definition, strategies for dealing with physical complaints, assertiveness with health care providers, taking control of one's life, structured problem solving, and personal risk-taking instruction.

There are no specific pharmacotherapies for SD, although patients with other conditions that can present in a similar manner (eg, depression with anxious features) may benefit from pharmacotherapy. Occasionally, patients may benefit from selective symptomatic treatment of their complaints. The provider must keep in mind, however, that these patients are likely to be sensitive to the side effects of most medications, so the use of symptomatic treatment should be judicious.

All members of the team must have the same set of expectations for the care of the patient. It is the responsibility of the primary care provider to see that worrisome symptoms are evaluated while at the same time minimizing intrusive diagnostic testing. One common mistake made in the primary care setting is failing to take these patients' complaints seriously. Patients with SD want to know that their symptoms are taken seriously and that there is a strong therapeutic alliance. A balance must be sought between intrusive diagnostic testing and the benefit to be gained by the patient.

Perhaps one of the most challenging aspects of the care of patients with SD is the fact that health professionals are trained to identify health problems and work with the patient toward resolution or control of the problem. SD, however, is a chronic condition without a known cure, and it presents with many chief complaints. Complete symptom abatement may be an unrealistic goal; rather, the treatment process involves minimizing the effect of the disorder on the patient's social and occupational functioning.

Patients are often unable to accept the diagnosis of SD and may continue to search for a "cure" for their illness. Providing support and guidance is important during this process. In other patients, the insight gained from the presentation of their diagnosis may be helpful.

TEACHING AND SELF-CARE

Careful presentation of the diagnosis to the patient is recommended (McCahill, 1995). Care must be taken to present the diagnosis in an empathetic and nonjudgmental manner; avoid making the patient feel that the symptoms are "all in my head." A therapeutic relationship must be established before the diagnosis is presented.

Families and significant others may find counseling helpful to understand how to support the patient. The primary care provider may explore the meaning of illness in the family and encourage counseling if the family reinforces somatization behaviors.

COMMUNITY RESOURCES

Special counseling services may be availalbe locally for general psychosocial support. Special services for gender and age specific populations (eg, women's health, adolescent care, sports medicine) may have support groups for various psychosocial concerns.

REFERRAL POINTS

Somatic complaints can be found in conjunction with other psychiatric illnesses, including depression. A thorough interview for tendencies toward self-harm is important; any findings of suicidal ideation or plan warrant referral to a psychiatrist or psychologist.

Patient with somatizing tendencies often present symptoms profiles that are baffling to even the most experienced clinician. Often a telephone consultation with a specialist in the field of the patient's primary complaints can be helpful in defining a conservative treatment plan.

CLINICAL WARNINGS:

- Because patients rarely acknowledge the psychological component of their symptoms, psychiatric treatment is often rejected.
- Irregularly scheduled appointments with different providers may reinforce the symptomatic complaints. The interdisciplinary team needs to work together to foster a strong relationship between the patient and one provider, who can consult with other providers as necessary.

CLINICAL PEARLS

- Explain that coming to see a primary care provider does not require a physical complaint.
- Empathize with the patient and explain that adaptation to chronic symptoms may be the realistic goal of treatment (Barsky, 1995).

EDITOR'S NOTE:

COMPLEMENTARY APPROACHES

A general discussion of complementary approaches can be found in Chapter 3. The following, while not an exhaustive list, are some complementary approaches being used for this condition. Additional information on these approaches, including precautions, can be found in Appendices A and B. Providers need to assess for the use of complementary approaches as part of the patient's history, as they may impact conventional therapies, and patients may not volunteer this information unless specifically asked. Efficacy of many complementary approaches is not as well documented as that of conventional therapies. Providers need to read the literature before suggesting these complementary approaches.

- Complementary Modalities
  Craniosacral therapy
  Massage therapy

References

American Psychiatric Association. (1994). *Diagnostic and statistical manual of mental disorders*, 4th ed. Washington, D.C.: Author.

Barsky, A.J. (1995). Approach to the somatizing patient. In A.H. Goroll, L.A. May, & A.G. Mulley (Eds.). *Primary care medicine: Office evaluation and management of the adult patient*, pp. 1057–1060. Philadelphia: J.B. Lippincott.

Gothe, C.J., Odont, C.M., & Nilsson, C.G. (1995). The environmental somatization syndrome. *Psychosomatics, 36*(1), 1–11.

Hulme, P. (1996). Somatization in Hispanics. *Journal of Psychosocial Nursing and Mental Health, 34*(3), 33–37.

Kashner, T.M., Rost, K., Cohen, B., Anderson, M., & Smith, R. (1995). Enhancing the health of somatization disorder patients. *Psychosomatics, 36*(2), 462–479.

McCahill, M.E. (1995). Somatoform and related disorders: Delivery of diagnosis as first step. *American Family Physician, 52*(1), 193–204.

Ohaeri, J., & Odejide, O. (1994). Somatization symptoms among patients using primary health care facilities in a rural community in Nigeria. *American Journal of Psychiatry, 151*(5), 728–731.

Smith, G.R. (1995). Somatization disorder and undifferentiated somatization disorder. In G.O. Gabbard (Ed.). *Treatment of psychiatric disorders,* Vol. 2. Washington, D.C.: American Psychiatric Press.

Wool, C.A., & Barsky, A.J. (1994). Do women somatize more than men? *Psychosomatics, 35*(5), 445–452.

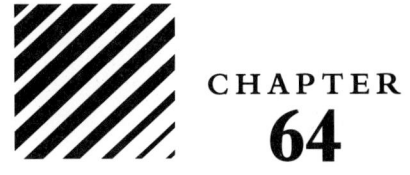

CHAPTER

64

Substance Abuse

Stephen Paul Holzemer, PhD, RN, and Joanne Singleton, PhD, RN, FNP-C

The use of alcohol and other legal as well as illegal chemical substances is a growing problem in many societies. Approximately 10% to 20% of a primary care provider's caseload involves patients with substance use disorders (Israel et al, 1996). Substance abuse has a profound effect on the mortality and morbidity of many patients, their families, and their communities. The social cost related to accidental death, violence, loss of productivity in the workforce, and unemployment can only be estimated. A definition of substance abuse must include the behavior of the patient and the effect of the abuse on all these variables.

This chapter is a general overview of substance abuse problems and challenges for the provider. A review of these issues should be made on a patient-by-patient basis because of the many complexities of substance abuse. Providers must construct an interdisciplinary approach based on the demographics of their practice locations.

The term *substance abuse* is used in this chapter to include concepts of use and misuse. Relationship-centered care would rely on assessing and intervening into patterns of substance use well before abuse patterns develop.

GENERAL PRINCIPLES FOR PLANNING CARE

Substance abuse is complicated because the drugs involved may be prescribed, purchased over the counter, or sold in illegal transactions. The addictive nature of these substances makes changing the using behavior difficult. Some patients may become physically or emotionally abusive if the pattern of their drug use changes, including withdrawal. Identifying, engaging, and managing the active substance user includes cooperation between generalist providers and an emerging cadre of specialists in substance abuse.

Primary care providers must first examine their own attitudes about substance abuse. Providers must define what is acceptable and unacceptable use and how to motivate or encourage patients to change their behavior. Exploring these issues with the patient allows care to be provided from a supportive but well-planned perspective. The plan of care involves family members and other support persons willing or able to participate in recovery.

Caring for the substance abuser is very expensive (Lewis, 1997). The challenges of cost containment in health care make providing comprehensive care to the substance abuser a concern for many providers. Fleming (1995) identified nine competencies needed by primary care providers in caring for the substance abuser, and these nine have been restructured into six (Table 64-1). These competencies should allow providers a framework to identify their strengths and limitations in caring for substance abusers.

ANATOMY, PHYSIOLOGY, AND PATHOLOGY

The effect of substance abuse on body systems ranges from temporary impairment to multisystem failure. Long-term drug use can cause diseases of the lungs (cancer), liver (cirrhosis), heart (cardiac myopathy, ischemia, hypertension), and gastrointestinal tract (gastritis, hemorrhage, malnutrition). Alcohol use has been associated with breast cancer in women (Smith-Warner et al, 1998), as well as demineralization of the bone (Chang et al, 1997). Cocaine has induced wide complex dysrhythmia in some patients (Kerns et al, 1997) and myocardial infarction. Patients may present only after serious health problems surface.

Changes in pleasure pathways occur in the brain and the number and receptivity of dopamine and serotonin receptors increase with substance use. These changes add to the physiologic challenge in substance use, which is sometimes overshadowed by the psychosocial aspects. Finding a chromosomal link to a biologic cause or predisposition to addiction would help predict who would be at risk for these health-related problems.

EPIDEMIOLOGY

Substance abuse accounts for 50% of the more than 1 million deaths attributed to unsafe or unhealthy lifestyle behaviors (Lewis, 1997). The morbidity often extends to include relatives and friends of the substance user. For example, children may have asthma attacks triggered by tobacco use (second-hand smoke). Family members may experience physical, emotional, and economic harm because of the behavior of the substance abuser. Family members and others may be the victims of crime when substance abusers seek money for drugs or are under the influence of drugs.

The differing effects of substance abuse on Hispanics, African Americans, and whites is still under study (Caetano, 1997; Herd, 1997). One predictor of substance abuse in women is childhood sexual abuse (Wilsnack et al, 1997) or victimization (Liebschutz et al, 1997). There is increasing research interest in how abuse affects the entire family (Ryan et al, 1997).

The wide variation in the physical, occupational, and economic attributes of drug users suggests that all patients should be screened for substance use and potential abuse. No clear profile of a typical substance user has emerged.

Alcohol Use

Approximately 70% of men and 60% of women drink (or have drunk) alcohol. Men are three times more likely to binge (five or more drinks on one occasion) than women and six to seven times more likely to be chronic drinkers. The disease occurs

TABLE 64-1	Competencies for Treating Substance Use Disorders
Relationship-centered care of the patient with a substance use disorder includes intervention into the effects of the disorder on family and significant others.	
Screen for alcohol and other drug use, including tobacco.	Screening needs to include the quantity and frequency of use.
Assess for problems related to drug use.	
Tobacco	Types of tobacco and level of dependence/addiction
Alcohol	Women >7 drinks/week or 3 drinks/occasion, men >14 drinks/week or 4 drinks/occasion, and level of dependence/addiction
Addictive prescription drugs	Current use and level of dependence/addiction
Illicit drugs	Used five times or more; current use and level of dependence/addiction
Initiate office-based treatment.	Treatment options should include brief intervention strategies, counseling, and pharmacotherapy
Pharmacotherapy	Drug treatment includes management of drug withdrawal, postwithdrawal abstinence syndromes, drug maintenance, and comorbid conditions.
Detoxification and community support programs	A wide range of services exist, from specialized in-house drug detoxification programs to community support programs such as Alcoholics Anonymous.
Counseling	Long-term, nonconfrontational, motivational strategies are effective for many patients.
Provide appropriate pain management.	Management of acute and chronic pain in substance abusers is a clinical challenge.
Use drug testing when appropriate.	Including drug testing as part of the patient's workup and ongoing treatment is a joint decision between the provider and patient.
Monitoring drug misuse by primary care providers	Assist colleagues in seeking help, and monitor one's own drug use.

Adapted from Fleming, 1995.

earlier in men but may be fatal earlier in women (Centers for Disease Control and Prevention [CDC], 1996, 1997a; Chang et al, 1997).

Smoking

About 25% of men and slightly fewer women smoke. Almost 33% of college students smoke. There is some evidence that the incidence of smoking (defined as being a current smoker and having had smoked at least 100 cigarettes) is decreasing in teenagers, both boys and girls (CDC, 1996, 1997a, 1997b). Tobacco industry promotions are considered a major contributor to adolescent smoking (Pierce et al, 1998).

Illegal Drug Use

Almost 40% of adults have used an illicit drug during their lives. Of these, 33% have used marijuana and 11% have used cocaine (Schorling & Buchsbaum, 1997). Among college students, 48% had smoked marijuana, 14.4% had used some form of cocaine, 9.1% had used inhalants (eg, glue, spray can contents), and 1.7% had injected illegal drugs in their lifetime (CDC, 1997b). These percentages may be low because of underreporting, making the problem much more serious.

DIAGNOSTIC CRITERIA

The criteria for substance abuse and dependence (including alcohol) are listed in Table 64-2 (American Psychiatric Association, 1994). This information can help the provider screen for substance use.

Toxicology screens do not differentiate between occasional use and dependence (Schorling & Buchsbaum, 1997). The presence of a drug in the body suggests the need for the provider to explore the impact of alcohol and drug use on the patient and family. For many patients, the impact of alcohol and other drugs on behavior and relationships defines the level of abuse. Events such as being arrested for driving while intoxicated are indicative of an alcohol-related problem that the provider must continue to explore.

Two illegal drugs that account for much drug abuse are heroin and cocaine (including crack cocaine). The characteristics and effects of their use are listed in Table 64-3. These drugs are highlighted because of the complex nature of their addictive potential. They are also closely tied to the spread of HIV infection (Academy for Educational Development, 1997). Individuals under the influence of these drugs may have unprotected sex more often.

HISTORY AND PHYSICAL EXAM

Screening for alcohol and other drug abuse is a sensitive part of the history and physical exam. An interpersonal relationship between the patient and the provider needs to be established before the provider can expect such questions to be answered in a thorough and honest manner. Some providers ask patients if they have experienced recent trauma (physical or emotional) as a way to elicit problem drinking behavior (Israel et al, 1996). Many accidents are alcohol-related, and the provider needs to

TABLE 64-2	DSM-IV Criteria for Substance Abuse and Dependence

Criteria for Substance Abuse: A maladaptive pattern of substance use leading to clinically significant impairments or distress, as manifested by 1 (or more) of the following, occurring within a 12-mo period:

- Recurrent substance use resulting in a failure to fulfill major role obligations at work, school, or home (eg, repeated absences or poor work performance related to substance use; substance-related absences, suspensions, or expulsions from school; neglect of children or household)
- Recurrent substance use in situations in which it is physically hazardous (eg, driving an automobile or operating a machine when impaired by substance use)
- Recurrent substance-related legal problems (eg, arrests for substance-related disorderly conduct)
- Continued substance use despite having persistent or recurrent social or interpersonal problems caused or exacerbated by the effects of the substance (eg, arguments with spouse about consequences of intoxication, physical fights)
- The symptoms have never met the criteria for Substance Dependence for this class of substance.

Criteria for Substance Dependence: A maladaptive pattern of substance use, leading to clinically significant impairment or distress, as manifested by 3 (or more) of the following, occurring at any time in the same 12-mo period:

- Tolerance, as defined by either of the following:
  A need for markedly increased amounts of the substance to achieve intoxification or desired effect
  Markedly diminished effect with continued use of the same amount of the substance
- Withdrawal, as manifested by either of the following:
  The characteristic withdrawal syndrome for the substance
  The same (or a closely related) substance is taken to relieve or avoid withdrawal symptoms
- The substance is often taken in larger amounts or over a longer period than was intended.
- There is a persistent desire of unsuccessful efforts to cut down or control substance use.
- A great deal of time is spent in activities necessary to obtain the substance (eg, visiting multiple physicians or driving long distances), use the substance (eg, chain-smoking), or recover from its effects.
- Important social, occupational, or recreational activities are given up or reduced because of substance use.
- The substance use is continued despite knowledge of having a persistent or recurrent physical or psychological problem that is likely to have been caused or exacerbated by the substance (eg, current cocaine use despite recognition of cocaine-induced depression or continued drinking despite recognition that an ulcer was made worse by alcohol consumption).

Source: American Psychiatric Association: Diagnostic and Statistical Manual of Mental Disorders, 4/e, Washington, DC: American Psychiatric Association, 1994.

screen for alcohol or other drug use when accidental or suspicious trauma occurs.

Questionnaire Assessments

Numerous questionnaires have been designed to identify substance abuse disorders. However, in the absence of a trusting patient–provider relationship, patients may harbor the truth when answering these highly personal questions; a "no" response may be meaningless. Providers must assess the impact of using these questions on their relationship with patients.

Ewing (1984) developed the CAGE questionnaire to detect alcoholism, and these questions have been adapted to screen for other drug dependencies. The CAGE questionnaire is thought to be a gold standard for drug abuse screening. The CAGE questions are:

- **C**: Have you ever felt that you should **C**ut down on your drinking?
- **A**: Have people **A**nnoyed you by criticizing your drinking?
- **G**: Have you ever felt bad or **G**uilty about drinking?
- **E**: Have you ever taken a drink first thing in the morning (**E**ye Opener) to steady your nerves or get rid of a hangover?

The TACE questions (Sokol et al, 1989) can be used to assess problem drinking:

- **T**: How many drinks does it take to make you feel high (**T**olerance)?
- **A**: Have people ever **A**nnoyed you by criticizing your drinking?
- **C**: Have you ever felt you ought to **C**ut down on your drinking?
- **E**: Have you ever had a drink first thing in the morning to steady your nerves or get rid of a hangover (**E**ye Opener)?

The two-question approach (Brown et al, 1997) suggests that an affirmative answer to both questions will identify the vast majority of alcohol and other drug abusers. The questions are:

- In the last year, have you ever drunk alcohol or used drugs more than you meant to?
- Have you felt you wanted or needed to cut down on your drinking or drug use in the last year?

■ ■ ■   **CLINICAL PEARL**

The most important concept to apply to the use of questionnaires is that a "yes" answer to any question requires further assessment of actual or potential problems related to drug use.

DIAGNOSTIC STUDIES

Gamma-Glutamyl Transferase

Gamma-glutamyl transferase (GGT, GGTP) measurement is used to identify and monitor the progression of liver disease, to screen for alcoholism, and to identify if drinking has resumed (Chernecky et al, 1993).

■   **CLINICAL WARNING:** For an accurate result, the patient should fast for 8 hours (except for water) and abstain from alcohol for 24 hours.

TABLE 64-3	Heroin, Cocaine, and Crack: Characteristics and Effects	
Heroin	**Cocaine**	**Crack**
■ Made from morphine, which is obtained from the opium poppy ■ High risk of developing physical and psychological dependence ■ Can be administered by injection, sniffing (snorting), or smoking ■ Commonly injected about three times a day (every 8 hours) ■ Effects last 3 to 6 hours ■ Typical behaviors under the influence include sleepiness ("nodding") after injection, sedate behavior, docile appearance, and shuffling gait. ■ Acute withdrawal symptoms begin 8 to 12 hours after last dose. ■ Withdrawal is severe, although generally not life-threatening. ■ Withdrawal symptoms include severe gastrointestinal distress, muscle cramping, and other flulike symptoms. Heroin users call this withdrawal being "drug sick." When these withdrawal symptoms are severe enough, addicts want to obtain and inject the drug as rapidly as possible, sometimes without concerns for possible HIV risks.	■ The most potent of the stimulants ■ High risk of developing physical and psychological dependence ■ Can be administered by smoking, or "freebasing" (onset of effect: less than 10 seconds), injection (onset of effect: 15–20 seconds), or snorting (onset of effect: 2–4 minutes) ■ Effects last 10 to 40 minutes, depending on purity and route of administration. ■ Typical behaviors under the influence include hyperactivity, elation, increased energy and alertness, and increased sexual activity. The user may feel invincible and is often difficult to deal with and quarrelsome. ■ Withdrawal symptoms occur several hours after last use and result in agitation and depression. ■ High risk of HIV transmission (contaminated needles and syringes; unprotected, prolonged sexual intercourse) ■ Sold in ready-to-use crystals that, when heated and smoked, cause a crackling sound	■ Prepared by heating cocaine, water, and bicarbonate (baking soda). This treatment chemically changes cocaine into a smokeable form. Costs less than freebase cocaine (also smoked), making it more accessible. ■ Use is now widespread in some urban and rural areas among both women and men. ■ Results in an intense rush in a matter of seconds. ■ Effects are short-lived (a few minutes), resulting in repeated use to achieve the initial rush again and to avoid severe postcocaine depression. ■ Typical behaviors under the influence include intense agitation and erratic activity, mood swings, confusion and disorientation, facial and body twitching ("tweaking"), and preoccupation with obtaining the next dose of crack. ■ Dependence on crack is thought to develop more rapidly than dependence on heroin and other forms of cocaine. ■ Crack sale and use can spread rapidly with devastating effects, including an increase in related violence, crime, and the exploitation of users, especially women. ■ Crack use is associated with increased sexual activity, often performed with little regard for HIV risks. As with cocaine use, male sexual performance is often affected due to delayed ejaculation and results in prolonged intercourse, with increase of genital injury and bleeding.

Academy for Educational Development. (1997). *HIV prevention among drug users: a resource book for community planners and program managers,* Washington, DC.: Centers for Disease Control and Prevention.

Toxicology Screening

Toxicology screening of the blood or urine for legal or illegal drugs is routine in patients who are stuporous or unconscious. Providers should follow protocols for obtaining consent from the patient for samples to be drawn.

> ■ **CLINICAL WARNING:** Specimens for legal evidence or criminal charges should be collected with a witness present. Every institution should have a procedure stating how specimens that may be used in such situations are collected, stored, and transferred to the police or proper authority.

Blood specimens to screen for alcohol ingestion should be collected using a povidone–iodine swab or wipe rather than an alcohol one.

Unannounced and periodic toxicology screenings may also be required for certain workers or athletes. The person takes a job or participates in sports knowing that urine samples will be required for drug screening. Some workers, such as government employees, may be required to provide on-the-spot routine specimens for analysis.

Electrocardiograms and X-Rays

Electrocardiograms can reveal cardiac ischemic changes and x-rays and echocardiograms can reveal cardiomyopathy in patients abusing alcohol or cocaine. However, old x-rays and electrocardiograms may be difficult to obtain if the patient uses multiple health care facilities.

TREATMENT OPTIONS, EXPECTED OUTCOMES, AND COMPREHENSIVE MANAGEMENT

Substance abuse is a chronic, context-dependent disorder that requires long-term treatment and support (Humphreys et al, 1997). Patients, primary care providers, substance abuse counselors, and recovery sponsors all should participate in the recovery plan. Plans for recovery may include 12-step programs, pharmacotherapy, addiction treatment, or psychiatric hospitalization. A combination of strategies may be most helpful at various stages of recovery.

Much attention is focused on the inadequacies of treatment facilities for substance abuse; less attention is given to the need for earlier intervention. The emphasis on treating advanced physical and psychiatric conditions seems misplaced because many of these conditions could have been prevented (Lewis, 1997).

TABLE 64-4	Four-Step Process to Monitor Alcohol Use

STEP 1.

ASK ABOUT ALCOHOL USE.

If consumption is 14 drinks per week or more than 4 drinks per occasion for men, or 7 drinks per week or more than 3 drinks per occasion for women	Go to Step 2.
OR	
A score of 1 or more on the CAGE questionnaire	

STEP 2.

ASSESS FOR ALCOHOL-RELATED PROBLEMS.

Medical	Go to Step 3.
Behavioral	
Alcohol dependence	

STEP 3.

ADVISE APPROPRIATE ACTION

| With alcohol dependence, advise patient to abstain and refer to a specialist. With identification of real or potential alcohol problems, advise patient to cut down and set a drinking goal. | Go to Step 4. |

STEP 4.

MONITOR PATIENT PROGRESS.

Source: National Institute on Alcohol Abuse and Alcoholism, 1995.

It is important to assess the patient's motivation to stop or change patterns of substance abuse. Factors that influence motivation may include the patient, the support network of family and friends, and the patient's living conditions.

Four-Step Monitoring Process

The National Institute on Alcohol Abuse and Alcoholism (1995) has suggested a four-step monitoring process (Table 64-4). Primary care providers should review these guidelines and how they can be applied to the substance-abusing population in their practice. The efficacy of the process varies with the mix of patients and providers.

Pharmacotherapy

Pharmaceutical treatment for alcohol, heroin, and cocaine abuse is summarized in Tables 64-5 and 64-6. Pharmacotherapy must be viewed as a dynamic process that requires continuous monitoring and re-evaluation.

Major Issues in Providing Primary Care to Substance Abusers

Several issues confront the primary care provider caring for substance abusers. The primary care provider needs to confront these issues and others as they arise.

TABLE 64-5	Pharmacotherapy for Alcohol Abuse	
Drug/Classification	**Choice for Therapy**	**Complications/Concerns**
Benzodiazepines	Drugs of choice to decrease symptoms of withdrawal, seizures, and delirium tremens	Sedation may occur with elderly or patients with liver disease. Decrease dosages slowly.
Barbiturates	Anticonvulsant properties well documented. May be used during pregnancy	Long-acting barbiturates may result in respiratory depression.
Sympatholytics	β-blockers may help with angina or anxiety.	β-blockers may correct hypertension and tachycardia, masking the advent of delirium tremens or seizures.
Carbamazepine	Anticonvulsant effect	Nausea and ataxia may result with high doses.
Neuroleptics	Used in adjunctive therapy for agitation, delirium, and hallucinations	Not appropriate for monotherapy
Thiamine and magnesium	Acute Wernicke's encephalopathy can be prevented by administering thiamine. Korsakoff's syndrome	Magnesium levels may be normal even with depletion in body reserves.
Alcohol-sensitizing drugs (disulfiram)	Disulfiram–ethanol reactions motivate abstinence.	Severe reactions can put patients at risk. Liver function studies need to be monitored. Reactions can occur with mouthwashes and other alcohol-containing substances.
Opiate antagonists (naltrexone)	Decreases craving and feeling of intoxication	Liver function studies need to be monitored. Patients scheduled for surgery with opioid-containing analgesics should discontinue opioid antagonist 72 hours before the procedure.

Adapted from Allen, 1996; Saitz & O'Malley, 1997.

TABLE 64-6	Pharmacotherapy for Heroin and Cocaine Abuse	
Drug/Classification	**Choice for Therapy**	**Complications/Concerns**
HEROIN AND DERIVATIVES		
Opioid agonists (methadone)	Detoxification is monitored in hospitals with tapering doses; maintenance occurs in ambulatory care settings. Urine testing validates taking of methadone and abstinence from other drugs.	Change of drug use without psychological and social supports has limited effect.
Long-acting methadone derivative (*l*-acetyl-α-methadol or LAAM)	Daily dosing is not necessary because of long half-life.	Drugs metabolized by the cytochrome p450 enzymes need to be monitored closely.
Opioid antagonists (naloxone, nalmefene, naltrexone)	Naloxone and nalmefene are used in acute opioid overdose. Naltrexone is withheld many days after methadone or heroin is stopped.	Significant withdrawal symptoms can occur.
COCAINE AND DERIVATIVES		
Dopamine agonists	Treatment of withdrawal and craving may increase success of staying drug-free.	Side effects may be a problem.
Antidepressants	Antidepressants with dopamine agonist properties may relieve symptoms of cocaine withdrawal.	Delay in onset of action may make relapse more likely.
Antihypertensives (clonidine)	Effects are immediate, without opiate euphoria; not a scheduled medication.	Not effective for muscle discomfort, drug craving, or problems with sleep.

Adapted from Allen, 1996; Saitz & O'Malley, 1997.

ABSTINENCE VERSUS RISK REDUCTION

Many primary care providers see the ultimate goal of intervention as abstinence from all drugs, but for some patients this approach is neither practical nor possible. Because of the nature of addiction and relapse, total abstinence is unrealistic for many users. Users should have their "nonuse" and "commitment to change" behaviors rewarded, as well as receiving support and concrete relapse-management strategies.

Risk reduction includes having patients place themselves in a position not to harm themselves or others. For instance, injection drug users should use condoms and clean needles to decrease the spread of HIV. Controlling drug use is also necessary for the proper care of children and other dependents. Criminal activity to acquire drugs needs to be addressed.

VICTIMIZATION AND VIOLENCE

Liebschutz et al argued that women who feel victimized are more likely to abuse substances, as seen in somatic complaints and more frequent medical problems (1997). It appears that many substance abusers have feelings of anger or psychological unrest. A sense of victimization and violence may have introduced the patient to substance use, and the resulting addiction may keep the patient exposed to these variables. Some abusers, men and women alike, report being physically abused as children by parents or other adults. Alcohol or drug use provides some escape from the violence in their lives, or the memory of it (Wyshak & Modest, 1996).

LIFE EXPERIENCES

For some patients, there is a connection among loss, troubled family relationships, and substance abuse. Patients may abuse drugs to avoid confrontations or problems in their families, or at times of personal loss (eg, a recent death or a death anniversary, holidays, loss of friends, income, or opportunity). The treatment of family problems and feelings of loss often requires a family therapy or support group approach; all people involved in the family problem or loss may need to be involved in the process. One challenge with this approach is that drug abusers often have alienated their family members and friends by their behavior. A therapeutic community or recovery support group may be effective once detoxification has begun.

PARENTAL ROLE MODELING AND PEER PRESSURE

Children whose parents were alcohol or drug abusers may be influenced to use as well. The social behavior of some substance users may promote their segregation from the social mainstream, which often reinforces their isolation and drug-using behavior. Culturally, many people are exposed to alcohol during family celebrations and religious ceremonies. The provider should ascertain how the patient and family members distinguish use from abuse. Children of parents who abuse drugs or alcohol are not likely to listen if the parents urge them to abstain.

As young adults take on more social responsibility, they are less likely to use substances (Chilcoat & Breslau, 1996). Many people in responsible positions may have to avoid or limit their use of substances to maintain their job. The provider must avoid thinking in stereotypes, because drug use is found in all socioeconomic and cultural groups.

DUAL DIAGNOSES

Many abusers have concurrent severe psychiatric problems. Increased depression and suicide risk may be a result of long-term drug use or may be exacerbated by the social situations in which users find themselves (eg, homeless, unemployed). Although the number who get medical or psychiatric treatment is unknown, many dual diagnoses are made. Addiction is often paired with depression, anxiety, personality disorders, somatoform disorders, eating disorders, attention deficit hyperactivity disorder, and psychotic disorders (Ziedonis & Brady, 1997). In one northeastern state, about half the Medicaid-eligible substance abusers also had schizophrenia; about 60% had bipolar disease. The cost to treat these abusers was 60% higher than that for nonusers (Dickey & Azeni, 1996). Careful coordination of primary care and mental health services is needed for prudent cost management (Institute of Medicine, 1996).

Mental health services are critical in substance abuse treatment. The key to success is to develop services with clear linkages among providers (Brach et al, 1995). Many referrals are generated between primary care providers and specialists for detecting new problems as well as working with chronic ones.

ELDERLY PATIENTS

As the population ages, more attention is paid to substance abuse among the elderly (Mirand & Welte, 1996). Some older people see multiple primary care providers and thereby have access to more prescription drugs. Chronic pain and other complaints can be controlled by various drug regimens. One of the best ways to decrease the misuse of prescription drugs in the elderly is to have providers communicate their plans of care to one another whenever possible. Patients should bring all medication bottles to each visit so that overuse or underuse can be assessed. Using one pharmacy may help because of the tracking mechanisms for drug refills. This system can also help monitor for the potential side effects of multiple drug regimens. This system also allows patients to develop a relationship with a pharmacist, adding this resource to their network of support.

Late-onset alcohol abuse may be triggered by loneliness, social isolation, pain, or change in routine (Reid & Anderson, 1997). An assessment of the patient's social setting and activities may warn of alcohol abuse problems and can help identify related issues such as neglect by the family. Taking time to assess older persons carefully is necessary, because many are losing their peer support network because of death, and they may live far from their children.

Peers and adult children of the older patient may not be able to assist with monitoring for substance abuse. Some children are preoccupied with raising their own children or managing their careers. Early signs of alcohol abuse may mimic some of the natural signs of aging, such as changes in memory and gait, and may be missed by family members or friends who see the older person less frequently.

LIFE SKILLS

Some people who misuse substances have poor life skills related to lack of employment and poor education. Job counseling may be necessary for former substance users seeking re-entry to the job market. A stable job can improve interpersonal relationships and housing possibilities and may spur the worker to seek additional education. Literacy is needed for successful education and employment: low literacy levels increase frustration and stress and decrease self-esteem and coping skills. The combination of these may encourage the patient to return to drug use as an escape from a no-win situation.

Improving life skills is difficult with this population because many abusers are homeless or are mistrusted by society if they are engaged in illegal actions to obtain drugs. Often these patients have no "safety net" or resources for support. Re-establishing life skills is the goal of therapeutic communities and is used to support recovery and avoid relapse.

COMMUNICABLE AND INFECTIOUS DISEASES

Substance abusers may be less concerned about illness and its prevention because of their drug use. The focus on the substance preoccupies the user; therefore, contact with the health care system may occur only with an overdose, a serious medical problem, or an injury.

The exact prevalence of tuberculosis and HIV infection, especially among homeless substance users, is difficult to quantify but is of critical concern. Prostitution for drug money is not uncommon during periods of use and relapse. Condoms and supplies to clean drug paraphernalia may be unavailable. Screening for other sexually transmitted diseases may not be done.

Poor diet is a concern in abusers. Eating may become an afterthought, especially if there is not enough money to buy both drugs and food. Drug use may also affect the appetite, making eating less pleasant. The long-term alcohol abuser may have deficiencies of thiamine, folate, and vitamin B_{12} because of the empty calories of alcohol.

Lack of immunizations poses additional problems. Substance abusers may not have had yearly flu vaccines, pneumococcal vaccine, or hepatitis vaccinations. They may not seek reimmunization when it is needed. Although the resurgence of childhood communicable diseases has not been studied in this population, it poses a serious public health concern, second only to HIV, tuberculosis, and hepatitis.

CARE OF CHILDREN

Many substance abusers retain custody of their children, even when they are unable to care for them. Substance abuse is a family issue. A history of child protection and court intervention may be difficult to construct. Minors may be cared for by various relatives for any length of time, making it difficult to prove parental neglect. Follow-up of the health care needs of children is important for their safety.

Children may also be used to support drug use patterns. They may be placed in harm's way if they are used as decoys to buy or deliver drugs. If they are placed in foster care, they may act out their frustration or anger with the parent by continuing to be involved in drug use or trafficking.

SELF-CARE FOR THE PROVIDER

Caring for patients with substance abuse problems is stressful for providers. These patients may have many more needs than the provider can meet, and the provider may feel resentful or overwhelmed. Relationship-centered care suggests that the provider may need support to provide effective care for specific patients as well as the general category of substance abusers.

TEACHING AND SELF-CARE

At each level of treatment, the provider should counsel the patient about healthy behaviors. The motivation of patients and their support systems is a key factor in working toward such behaviors, which may involve abstinence from some or all substances or the moderate use of legal substances.

COMMUNITY RESOURCES

- Academy for Educational Development, 1255 23rd St., NW, Suite 400, Washington, D.C. 20037, 202-884-8862, E-mail/Web site http://www.aed.org: Contracts with the CDC to develop community-based health information materials, primarily for community planners and program managers.
- Center for Alcohol and Addiction Studies, Brown University, Box G-BH, Providence, RI 02912, 401-444-1817, fax 401-444-1850
- The Century Council, 550 S. Hope St., Suite 1950, Los Angeles, CA 90071, 213-624-9898, fax 213-624-9012: Publishes a sourcebook, *Promising Practices: Campus Alcohol Strategies*, to promote responsible decisions about drinking or abstaining from alcohol, as well as fighting all forms of irresponsible drinking.
- Hazelden Publishing and Education, 15251 Pleasant Valley Rd., P.O. Box 176, Center City, MN 55012-0176, 800-328-9000, 612-257-4010, fax 612-257-1331, E-mail/Web site www.hazelden.org, webmaster@hazel den.org.: Provides a wide selection of video and print materials related to chemical dependency.
- Pride Institute at Solutions, 800-547-7433, 800-342-5429: Provides dual diagnosis treatment services to lesbian, gay, and bisexual adults.
- Substance Abuse and Mental Health Services Administration (SAMHSA), 301-443-8956, fax 301-443-9050, E-mail/Web site http://www.samhsa.gov: This group's mission is to improve the quality and availability of prevention, treatment, and rehabilitation services for persons with substance abuse and mental illness. Also administers grant programs.
- National Clearinghouse on Alcohol and Drug Information, 800-729-6686, fax 301-468-6433, E-mail/Web site http://www.health.org: A one-stop resource for federal alcohol and drug information.
- Web of Addictions, http://www.well.com/user/woa/
- Al-Anon/Alateen Family Group Headquarters, Inc., P.O. Box 862, Midtown Station, New York, NY 10018-0862, 800-344-2666, http:// solar.rtd.utk.edu/al-anon/
- Alcoholics Anonymous (AA) World Services, Inc., 475 Riverside Dr., New York, NY 100115, 212-870-3400
- Children of Alcoholics Foundation, Inc., Box 4185, Grand Central Station, New York, NY 10115, 800-359-2623

- Gamblers Anonymous, International Service Office, P. O. Box 17173, Los Angeles, CA 90017, 213-386-8789, E-mail isomain@gamblersanonymous.org
- Narcotics Anonymous (NA), P.O. Box 9999, Van Nuys, CA 91409, 818-780-3951
- Center for Substance Abuse, National Treatment Line, 800-662-HELP
- Center for Substance Abuse Prevention, Workplace Helpline, 800-WORKPLACE

REFERRAL POINTS AND CLINICAL WARNINGS

- Security procedures for drugs and supplies should be enforced in the same way for all patients. A pre-established security plan should be in place for the patient who exhibits signs of drug intoxication or violence.
- A motivational, not a confrontational, communication style is critical in many situations.
- Primary care providers may need some form of counseling themselves to help them care for substance users. The multiproblem presentation of these patients can be very stressful for the provider.
- Polydrug addiction requires immediate consultation with a substance abuse specialist.
- Patients withdrawing from alcohol and other drugs may be overhydrated or dehydrated. Special care is needed in monitoring parenteral and oral fluid intake. Fluids (intravenous or oral) should contain carbohydrates to prevent hypoglycemia and electrolytes to maintain electrolyte balance during detoxification.
- Providers must monitor their own substance use and that of their colleagues.
- Brief therapeutic interventions should follow mild to moderate at-risk use, with specialized treatment reserved for evidence of substance dependence (Kresper et al, 1997).

EDITOR'S NOTE:

COMPLEMENTARY APPROACHES

A general discussion of complementary approaches can be found in Chapter 3. The following, while not an exhaustive list, are some complementary approaches being used for this condition. Additional information on these approaches, including precautions, can be found in Appendices A and B. Providers need to assess for the use of complementary approaches as part of the patient's history, as they may impact conventional therapies, and patients may not volunteer this information unless specifically asked. Efficacy of many complementary approaches is not as well documented as that of conventional therapies. Providers need to read the literature before suggesting these complementary approaches.

- Complementary Modalities
  Acupuncture
  Aromatherapy
  Massage therapy

SUMMARY

Substance abuse is a complicated problem for the primary care provider. A strong interpersonal relationship is helpful in obtaining a complete picture of the patient and the possible solutions to their physical, emotional, familial, and financial problems. Specialists in substance abuse should be contacted. Referral to a specialist for comanagement ensures that the patient will receive comprehensive care and minimizes the chance of poor patient outcomes.

References

Academy for Educational Development. (1997). *HIV prevention among drug users: A resource book for community planners & program managers.* Washington, D.C.: Author.

Allen, K.M. (1996). *Nursing care of the addicted client.* Philadelphia: J.B. Lippincott.

American Psychiatric Association. (1994). *Diagnostic and statistical manual of mental disorders,* 4th ed. Washington, D.C.: Author.

Brach, C., Falik, M., Law, C., et al. (1995). Mental health services: Critical component of integrated primary care and substance abuse treatment. *Journal of Health Care for the Poor & Underserved, 6*(3), 322–341.

Brown, R.L., Leonard, T., Saunders, L.A., & Papasouliotis, O. (1997). A two-item screening test for alcohol and other drug problems. *Journal of Family Practice, 44*(2), 151–160.

Caetano, R. (1997). Prevalence, incidence and stability of drinking problems among whites, blacks and Hispanics: 1984–1992. *Journal of Studies on Alcohol, 58*(6), 565–572.

Centers for Disease Control and Prevention. (1996). State- and sex-specific prevalence of selected characteristics—behavioral risk factor surveillance system, 1992 and 1993. *MMWR, 45,* 4–7.

Centers for Disease Control and Prevention. (1997a). State- and sex-specific prevalence of selected characteristics—behavioral risk factor surveillance system, 1994 and 1995. *MMWR, 46,* 4.

Centers for Disease Control and Prevention. (1997b). Youth risk behavior surveillance: National college health risk behavior survey—United States, 1995. *MMWR, 46,* 10–15.

Chang, G., Behr, H., Goetz, M.A., Hiley, A., & Bigby, J. (1997). Women and alcohol abuse in primary care: Identification and intervention. *American Journal on Addictions, 6*(3), 183–192.

Chernecky, C.C., Krech, R.L., & Berger, B.J. (1993). *Laboratory tests and diagnostic procedures.* Philadelphia: W.B. Saunders.

Chilcoat, H.D., & Breslau, N. (1996). Alcohol disorders in young adulthood: Effects of transitions into adult roles. *Journal of Health and Social Behavior, 37*(4), 339–349.

Dickey, B., & Azeni, H. (1996). Persons with dual diagnoses of substance abuse and major mental illness: Their excess cost of psychiatric care. *American Journal of Public Health, 86*(7), 973–977.

Ewing, J.A. (1984). Detecting alcoholism: The CAGE questionnaire. *JAMA, 252,* 1905–1907.

Fleming, M. (1995). Competencies for substance abuse training. In C. Sirica (Ed.). *Training about alcohol and substance abuse for all primary care physicians.* New York: Josiah Macy, Jr. Foundation.

Herd, D. (1997). Sex ratios of drinking patterns and problems among blacks and whites: Results from a national survey. *Journal of Studies on Alcohol, 58*(1), 75–82.

Humphreys, K., Moos, R.H., & Cohen, C. (1997). Social and community resources and long-term recovery from treated and untreated alcoholism. *Journal of Studies on Alcohol, 58*(3), 231–238.

Institute of Medicine. (1996). *Primary care: America's health in a new era.* Washington, D.C.: National Academy Press.

Israel, Y., Hollander, O., Sanchez-Craig, M., et al. (1996). Screening for problem drinking and counseling by the primary care physician–nurse team. *Alcoholism, Clinical & Experimental Research, 20*(8), 1443–1450.

Kerns, W., Garvey, L., & Owens, J. (1997). Cocaine-induced wide complex dysrhythmia. *Journal of Emergency Medicine, 15,* 321–329.

Kresper, D.J., Riba, M.B., & Schweak, T.L. (1997). *Primary care psychiatry.* Philadelphia: W.B. Saunders.

Lewis, D.C. (1997). The role of the generalist in the care of the substance-abusing patient. *Medical Clinics of North America, 81*(4), 831–843.

Liebschutz, J.M., Mulvey, K.P., & Samet, J.H. (1997). Victimization among substance-abusing women: Worse health outcomes. *Archives of Internal Medicine, 157*(10), 1093–1097.

Mirand, A.L., & Welte, J.W. (1996). Alcohol consumption among the elderly in a general population, Erie County, New York. *American Journal of Public Health, 86*(7), 978–984.

National Institute on Alcohol Abuse and Alcoholism. (1995). *The physician's guide to helping patients with alcohol problems.* Washington, D.C.: U.S. Department of Health and Human Services.

Pierce, J.P., Choi, W.S., Gilpin, E.A., Farkas, A.J., & Berry, C.C. (1998). Tobacco industry promotion of cigarette and adolescent smoking. *JAMA, 279,* 511–515.

Reid, M.C., & Anderson, P.A. (1997). Geriatric substance use disorders. *Medical Clinics of North America, 81*(4), 999–1016.

Ryan, J.G., Verardo, L.T., Kidd, J.M., et al. (1997). Health outcomes of women exposed to household alcohol abuse: A family practice training site research network (FPTSRN) study. *Journal of Family Practice, 45*(5), 410–417.

Saitz, R. & O'Malley, S.S. (1997). Pharmacotherapies for alcohol abuse. *Medical Clinics of North America, 81*(4), 881–907.

Schorling, J.B., & Buchsbaum, D.G. (1997). Screening for alcohol and drug abuse. *Medical Clinics of North America, 81*(4), 845–865.

Smith-Warner, S.A., Spiegelman, D., Yaun, S.S., et al. (1998). Alcohol and breast cancer in women. *JAMA, 279,* 535–540.

Sokol, R.J., Martier, S.S., & Ager, J.W. (1989). The T-ACE questions: Practical prenatal detection of risk drinking. *American Journal of Obstetrics and Gynecology, 160,* 863–870.

Wilsnack, S.C., Vogeltanz, N.D., Klassen, A.D., & Harris, T.R. (1997). Childhood sexual abuse and women's substance abuse: National survey findings. *Journal of Studies on Alcohol, 58*(3), 264–271.

Wyshak, G., & Modest, G.A. (1996). Violence, mental health, and substance abuse in patients who are seen in primary care settings. *Archives of Family Medicine, 5*(4), 441–447.

Ziedonis, D., & Brady, K. (1997). Dual diagnosis in primary care: Detecting and treating both the addiction and mental illness. *Medical Clinics of North America, 81*(4), 1017–1036.

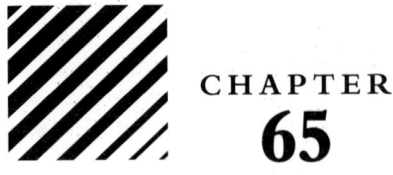

CHAPTER

65

Breast Mass

Seth P. Harlow, MD, and Hyman B. Muss, MD

Diseases of the breast are common clinical problems that are frequently seen in primary care practice. The most important aspect of managing breast problems is the early recognition of breast cancer. With the exception of skin malignancies, breast cancer is the most common malignancy affecting women in the United States today. Recently, a great deal of public attention has been focused on improving methods of early detection and developing new treatments for patients with breast cancer. Together with the patient, the primary care provider is the crucial first link in the effort toward prevention and early detection of breast cancer. Primary care providers must become adept at risk assessment and early diagnosis of these lesions. Breast cancer survival is clearly related to detection at an earlier stage of disease, which can best be insured by providing patient education and following screening guidelines. All women should be considered to be at risk for breast cancer and should undergo recommended screening. Use of screening guidelines has led in large part to a recent decrease in the annual mortality rate from breast cancer. Developing a systematic approach to the screening and evaluation of new breast problems is essential to provide the best possible patient care in this age of cost containment.

ANATOMY, PHYSIOLOGY, AND PATHOLOGY

Until puberty, the female breast is a rudimentary structure consisting of only a few ducts without acini. Under the influence of estrogens, progesterone, and the pituitary hormones, ductal tissue begins to grow, bud, and form acini at puberty. Glandular tissue separates into 12 to 20 lobes, or segments, extending from the nipple in a radial fashion. The ducts from each segment empty into a single lactiferous sinus that terminates at the nipple. The glandular tissues of the breast undergo cyclical changes in response to the hormone fluctuations during the menstrual cycle. At the start of the cycle, the ductal cells proliferate, there is an increase in interstitial fluid, and a lymphocytic infiltration is seen. This reaches a maximum just before the menses, at which time the ducts shrink and the ductal epithelium is shed. The cycle then repeats itself. These changes may lead to subsequent dilatation or hyperplasia of the ducts, hypertrophy of the surrounding connective tissue, and many benign pathologic conditions loosely referred to as fibrocystic changes.

During pregnancy, the breast lobules undergo maximal proliferation, and alveoli form. This proliferation is stimulated by the placental hormones. After delivery, the withdrawal of the placental hormones, along with prolactin secretion by the pituitary gland, stimulates lactation. Milk is produced by shedding of the alveolar cells. After the completion of lactation, the breast glandular tissue partially involutes. At menopause, there is further involution of the glandular tissue of the breast, with loss of the lobular outlines. Fibroglandular tissue is replaced by fatty tissue.

Common abnormalities of breast development include accessory nipples and ectopic glandular tissue. These abnormalities may occur anywhere along the "milk line," which extends from the axillae, through the nipple and down to the inguinal ligament. Accessory breast tissue (polymastia) is most often seen in the axilla; accessory nipples (polythelia) are most often seen in the midclavicular line below the normal breast.

The lymphatic drainage of the breast is predominantly toward the ipsilateral axillary lymph nodes. Lymphatic drainage in the medial aspect of the breast may also proceed toward the internal mammary nodes or the interpectoral nodes. Lymphatic spread of breast carcinoma cells may lead to enlargement of the axillary lymph nodes, which may be apparent on physical examination.

Breast lesions may be classified into five broad histopathologic categories:

1. Benign, nonproliferative lesions carry no increased risk of subsequent development of malignancy. Benign lesions include:
   Cystic hyperplasia (fibrocystic disease)
   Duct ectasia
   Galactoceles
   Lipomas
   Fat necrosis
   Fibroadenoma
   Hamartoma
   Papilloma
   Inflammatory lesions
2. Benign proliferative lesions include:
   Ductal hyperplasia without atypia, which carries no significant increased risk for subsequent malignancy (Dupont & Page, 1985)
   Atypical ductal hyperplasia, which carries an increased risk of subsequent malignancy (Dupont & Page, 1985)
   Atypical lobular hyperplasia, which also carries an increased risk of subsequent malignancy (Dupont & Page, 1985)
   Sclerosing adenosis, which has no significant link to subsequent malignancy (Jensen et al, 1989)

3. In situ carcinomas are malignant-appearing cells that lack evidence of invasion through the basement membrane. These include:

   Lobular carcinoma in situ (LCIS), considered a marker for increased risk of subsequent cancer development in either breast (Carson et al, 1994)

   Ductal carcinoma in situ (DCIS), considered a direct precursor to invasive ductal carcinomas

4. Invasive carcinomas are malignant cells that demonstrate invasion of the basement membrane. These lesions have the potential for metastatic spread.

   Invasive ductal carcinoma (80% of invasive carcinomas)

   Invasive lobular carcinoma (15%)

   Medullary carcinoma, tubular carcinoma, mucinous carcinoma, and papillary carcinoma (5%)

5. Other malignancies include:

   Phylloides tumors (20% to 30% have malignant features)

   Soft-tissue sarcomas

   Lymphomas

   Metastatic Tumors.

EPIDEMIOLOGY

The incidence of breast cancer steadily increases with age. Breast cancer is rare in patients under 20 years of age, but its incidence begins to rise rapidly during the childbearing years. The rate of breast cancer continues to increase after menopause but at a slower rate. Women in the United States currently have a lifetime risk of developing breast cancer of approximately 12% and a lifetime risk of dying of breast cancer of approximately 3.6% (Hankey et al, 1993).

The incidence of breast cancer in men is approximately 0.5% to 1% the rate of breast cancer in women. There are about 1000 new cases of these cancers per year in the United States. Male breast cancers typically present as palpable masses, with a pattern of spread and prognosis similar to those in women (Boring et al, 1994).

The incidence of breast cancer is higher in the United States and western Europe than in other parts of the world. In the United States, the rates are highest in whites and persons of Hawaiian descent. These rates decrease in women of African American, Asian American, and Hispanic American heritage. Native Americans have a particularly low rate of breast cancer (Muir et al, 1987).

■ **CLINICAL WARNING:** Women of African American background have a mortality rate about 10% higher than white women, even when matched for stage.

The incidence of breast cancer shows a steady increase from lower to middle to upper socioeconomic groups. The reason for this increase is not entirely clear, but it may be related to reproductive, dietary, or environmental factors (Krieger, 1990).

DIAGNOSTIC CRITERIA

Diagnostic criteria are defined by the pathologic findings.

HISTORY AND PHYSICAL EXAM

The primary care provider must document the following:

- Age (ie, postmenopausal)
- Age of menarche and, if applicable, menopause
- Age of first full-term pregnancy
- Use of hormones
- Family history of breast and other cancers
- Prior breast biopsies.

The provider should screen for the following symptoms:

- Palpable lesion
- Skin or nipple changes
- Nipple discharge
- Breast pain.

The clinical breast exam should focus on:

- Inspection
  Skin dimpling
  Skin redness
  Nipple retraction
  Nipple excoriation
  Visible masses
- Palpation
  Palpable masses
  Asymmetric thickening
  Nipple discharge
  Axillary lymph nodes.

DIAGNOSTIC STUDIES

Screening mammography is a routine component of health maintenance. Current recommendations for screening are discussed later in this chapter. Screening mammograms should include:

- Standard two views of each breast
- Additional views if abnormalities are seen.

Mammographic Abnormalities

Correct identification of any abnormalities will support effective, timely management.

Macrocalcifications are calcifications that measure more than 1 mm. They are usually benign. Microcalcifications measure less than 1 mm. It is suspicious for malignancy if there are more than five microcalcifications per cubic centimeter, if they are pleomorphic in appearance, or if they are increased in number from prior mammograms.

Lesions are classified as benign if:

- Calcifications show as meniscus on lateral views, are spherical or eggshell in appearance, or are large and rod-shaped.
- Mass lesions which are smooth-walled and well defined are usually benign but need further evaluation by ultrasound.

A border that is irregular or speculated is suspicious for malignancy. An asymmetric density may represent malignancy.

Figures 65-1 and 65-2 illustrate views of two breast malignancies visible on mammography.

Ultrasound

Ultrasound is a valuable adjunct to the physical exam and mammography. Its benefits include the following:

- It provides better resolution of mass lesions in dense breast tissue, or breasts that have been previously irradiated.
- It can distinguish solid from cystic lesions.
- It is portable and easily accessible.
- It does not expose the patient to radiation.
- It allows image-guided biopsies.

However, ultrasound will not identify calcifications or small masses in breasts with fat replacement. Figures 65-3, 65-4, and 65-5 illustrate views of three breast lesions visible with ultrasound.

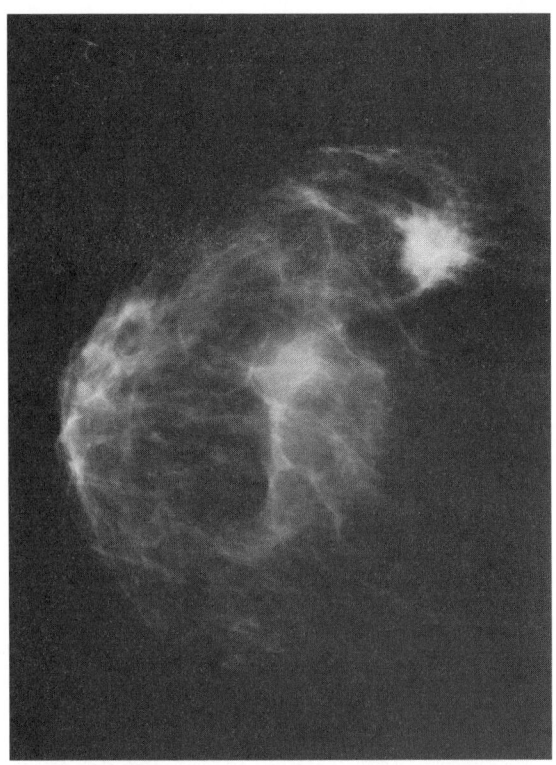

FIGURE 65-2 Mammographic appearance of an irregular spiculated mass lesion associated with an underlying breast malignancy (infiltrating ductal carcinoma). (Source: Vermont Cancer Center [authors' files])

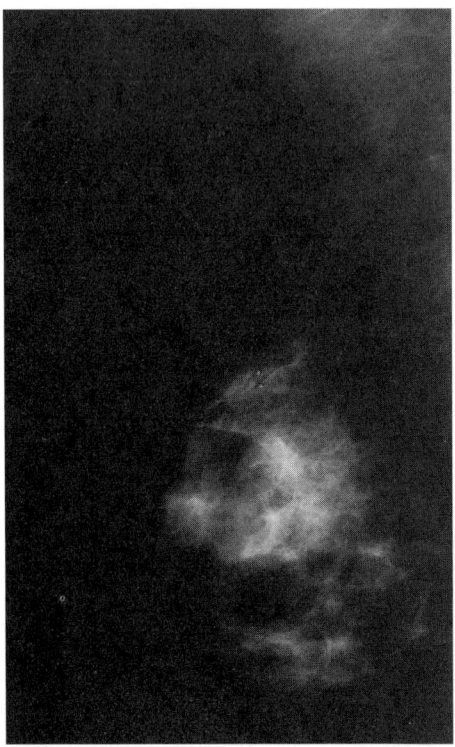

FIGURE 65-1 Mammographic appearance of clustered pleomorphic microcalcifications associated with an underlying breast malignancy (ductal carcinoma in situ). (Source: Vermont Cancer Center [authors' files])

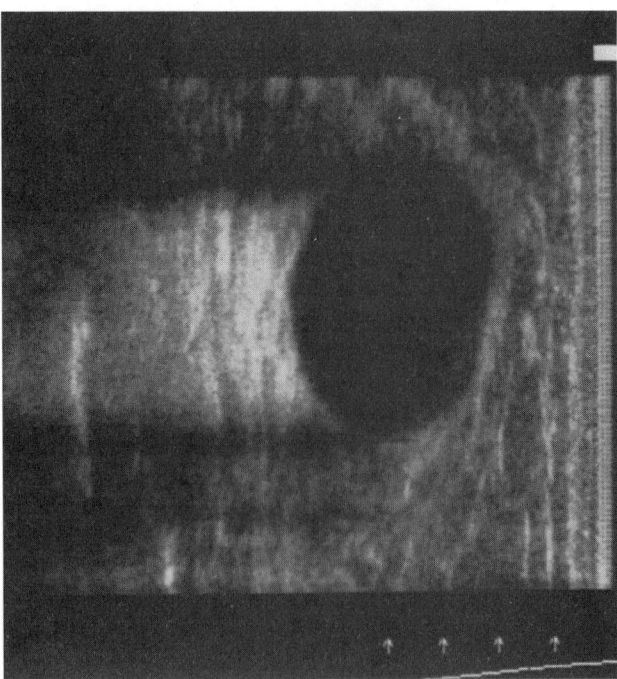

FIGURE 65-3 Ultrasound appearance of a simple cyst. Characteristic features include thin, sharply defined wall without nodularity, no internal echoes (anechoic), and strong posterior enhancement. (Source: Vermont Cancer Center [authors' files])

Magnetic Resonance Imaging

Several drawbacks make the use of magnetic resonance imaging (MRI) less than practical in most clinical screening situations. Significant among these drawbacks is its expense. MRI also has a relatively low specificity for breast cancer (30% to 40%) (Heywang-Kobrunner, 1994). Finally, MRI is not widely available outside of more metropolitan areas.

■ ■ ■ CLINICAL PEARL

MRI is useful in two situations: its high sensitivity for breast lesions (88% to 100%) and its value in detecting leaks from breast implants.

Biopsy Techniques

Fine-needle aspiration (FNA) is carried out using a 25- to 27-gauge needle. Little specialized equipment is needed. FNA is less traumatic than other biopsy techniques. Aspirated material must be interpreted by a cytopathologist skilled in this area.

Core needle biopsy is carried out using a 14- to 18-gauge needle; a specialized core biopsy needle is needed. A larger

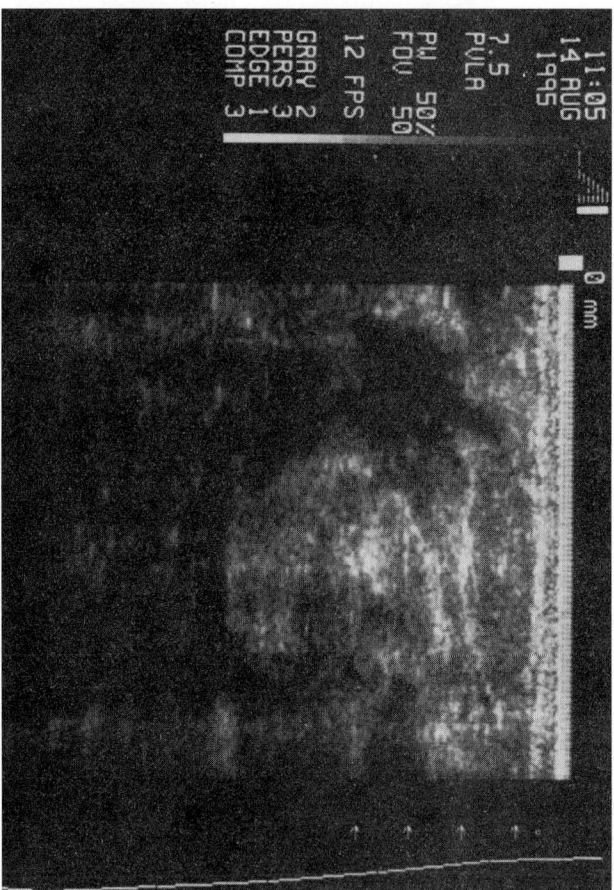

FIGURE 65-5 Ultrasound appearance of a malignant solid breast mass (infiltrating ductal carcinoma). Features include irregular jagged margins, height greater than width, heterogeneous internal echoes and posterior shadowing. (Source: Vermont Cancer Center [authors' files])

sample is required for standard histopathologic evaluation. This technique is more invasive than FNA.

Open surgical biopsy is the most invasive of the biopsy methods and is also the most costly. Potentially therapeutic, open surgical biopsy also produces fewer false-negative results.

TREATMENT OPTIONS, EXPECTED OUTCOMES, AND COMPREHENSIVE MANAGEMENT

The causes of breast cancer are not understood and are likely to be multifactorial. Several factors are known to increase a woman's risk for breast cancer:

- A family history of breast cancer, particularly if one or more first-degree relatives are affected. Specific genetic abnormalities, including mutations of the BRCA1 and BRCA2, genes have recently been described (discussed below). If present, such genetic abnormalities have been found to confer a high risk (50% to 90%) that the patient will develop breast cancer. Other genetic syndromes predisposing patients to breast cancer include Li-Fraumeni (p53 gene mutation), Cowden's, and ataxia–telangiectasia.
- Early onset of menarche: Higher breast cancer risks are seen in patients with onset of menses before age 12 than in those with menarche after age 15 (Brinton et al, 1988).

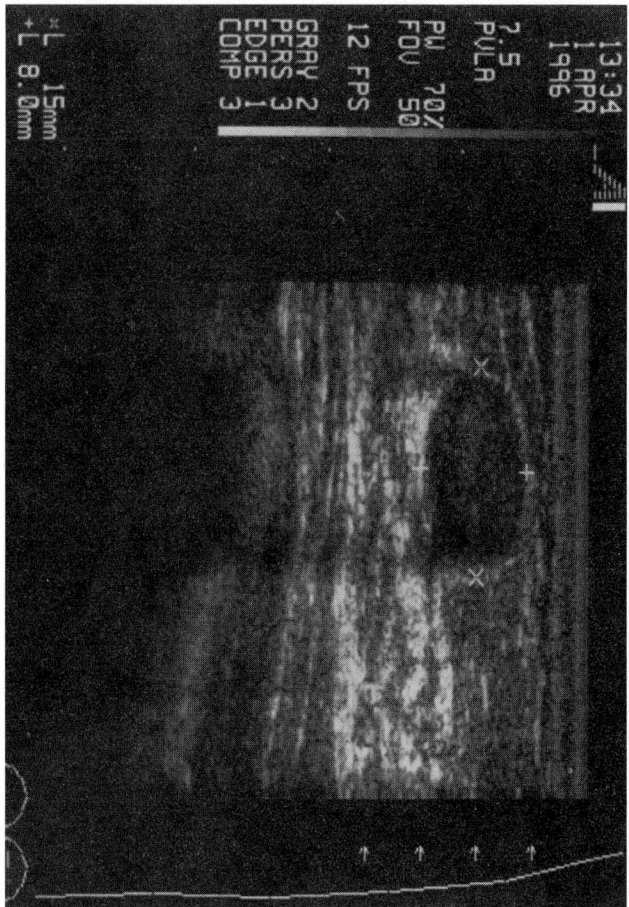

FIGURE 65-4 Ultrasound appearance of a benign solid breast mass (fibroadenoma). Features include well-defined smooth margins, oval shape, homogeneous interior, and weak posterior enhancement. (Source: Vermont Cancer Center [authors' files])

- Late onset of menopause: Higher breast cancer risks are seen in patients with natural menopause after age 55 than in those with menopause before age 45 (Trichopoulos et al, 1972).
- Late age at first pregnancy: Women who have their first pregnancy after age 30 have been seen to have a small but significantly increased risk of developing breast cancer (MacMahon et al, 1970).
- Postmenopausal obesity
- Previous history of radiation to the chest
- Higher socioeconomic status
- Previous history of ovarian or endometrial cancer.

Many of the known risk factors for breast cancer can be altered, including diet and lifestyle habits. Altering these may lead to a slight reduction in breast cancer risk. For example, eating a diet that includes foods such as soybeans, which have large quantities of the phytoestrogens genistein and daidzein, may block the proliferative effects of endogenous estrogens. This in turn decreases the risk of breast cancer development (Barnes et al, 1994; Ingram et al, 1997).

Factors that may increase the risk for breast cancer include increased alcohol consumption (Longnecker et al, 1988) and a sedentary lifestyle (Bernstein et al, 1994). Several studies have suggested that women who follow a moderate exercise program may have a decreased risk for breast cancer, probably as a result of a decrease in their overall total body fat content (Bernstein et al, 1994; McTiernan et al, 1997). However, to date there is no convincing relation between dietary fat intake and breast cancer risk.

Chemopreventive Agents

Because of the hormonal influences associated with the development of breast cancer, much effort has been expended in designing chemopreventive agents that result in hormonal manipulation. The drug that has shown the greatest promise is the antiestrogen tamoxifen, which is used in the treatment of breast cancer. There are several large multicenter trials underway, including the National Surgical Adjuvant Breast and Bowel Project prevention trial, to determine the efficacy of tamoxifen in reducing the incidence of breast cancer. (A recent preliminary report by the NSABP has shown a 45% reduction in breast cancer incidence in short-term followup of high-risk patients treated with tamoxifen vs. placebo [Wickerham et al, 1998]).

Other agents are also being investigated as potential chemopreventive agents, including retinoids and newly discovered phytochemicals. Again, it is likely to be several years before significant information is available as to the efficacy of these compounds.

Screening

Breast cancer screening has been the subject of much recent controversy. Like all other screening efforts, screening for breast cancer is used to identify disease at an earlier stage, before it becomes symptomatic. Early staging is important because it improves the patient's chances for survival.

The first large study to suggest any improvement is breast cancer survival with screening was the Health Insurance Plan (HIP) of New York study (Shapiro et al, 1988). The HIP study showed an improvement in survival in women undergoing two-

view mammography and physical exam every 12 months during a 4-year period compared with women not screened. Additional studies from Sweden have confirmed this improvement in breast cancer survival associated with the systematic use of screening mammography (Nystrom et al, 1993).

■ ■ ■ **CLINICAL PEARL**

The most significant improvement in survival in all studies to date has been in women older than 50. Annual mammography may decrease the risk of dying of breast cancer by as much as 30% in this age group.

The value of routine mammography in patients age 40 to 50 has not been completely resolved. Several randomized studies have produced conflicting results, leading to different recommendations for screening in this population. Current recommendations from the American College of Radiology, the American Cancer Society (Mettlin & Smart, 1994), and the American College of Obstetricians and Gynecologists suggest performing mammography every 1 to 2 years in women ages 40 to 49 and yearly after age 50, along with yearly clinical breast exams beginning at age 40. The recommendations from the National Cancer Institute and the American Board of Family Practice for women aged 40 to 49 with average risk is that the benefit of screening mammography is uncertain and should be discussed with each patient before proceeding (Fletcher et al, 1993).

■ **CLINICAL WARNING:** Mammography alone will detect only 85% to 90% of breast cancers. The remainder will be detected only with a careful clinical breast exam.

■ ■ ■ **CLINICAL PEARL**

Effective breast cancer screening requires a combination of high-quality mammography and well-performed clinical breast exams.

Breast Self-Exam

Breast self-exam has been recommended as a method of early breast cancer detection. Numerous trials have evaluated the influence of breast self-exam on breast cancer mortality rates, but there are no convincing data to support this screening strategy (O'Malley & Fletcher, 1987).

■ ■ ■ **CLINICAL PEARLS**

- Because breast self-exam has minimal risk and low cost, it is likely to be worthwhile and should be encouraged, provided the technique can be taught carefully.
- The primary care provider should encourage all women to undergo recommended screening. It has been shown that such women have a higher rate of participation in accepted screening practices (Kerlikowske et al, 1993; Rimer et al, 1989).

■ **CLINICAL WARNING:** Women thought to be at excessive risk should be screened by mammography on an annual basis and not more often. More frequent mammograms have not been shown to lower mortality rates (Kerlikowske et al, 1993). Patients at higher risk may benefit from more frequent clinical breast exams.

Genetic Testing

Up to 20% of breast cancer patients have a positive family history for breast cancer. About 5% of patients demonstrate a clear pattern of autosomal dominant inheritance. These latter 5% are likely to have either the BRCA1 or BRCA2 gene and are likely to develop breast cancer at a younger age (Shattuck-Eidens et al, 1995). The BRCA1 gene has been cloned and resides on chromosome 17.

■ **CLINICAL WARNINGS:**

- Women who have a strong family history of breast or ovarian cancer and who inherit a mutation in this gene have a greater than 50% chance of developing breast cancer by age 50 and an 80% chance by age 70. Moreover, they have a 30% chance of developing ovarian cancer by age 50 and an almost 50% chance by age 70.
- Women who inherit this gene but who lack a family history of breast or ovarian cancer have a lower risk of breast cancer, probably about 50%.

The BRCA2 gene has also been recently cloned and resides on chromosome 13. Patients with mutations in this gene have a similar risk for breast cancer as those with the BRCA1 gene but a lower risk of ovarian cancer (probably less than 20%).

■ **CLINICAL WARNING:** There is an increased frequency of male breast cancer in BRCA2 carriers (Couch et al, 1996). The BRCA1 and BRCA2 genes can be carried and passed to offspring by men as well as women.

Numerous mutations in both the BRCA1 and BRCA2 genes have been identified. Some mutations have been found to be more prevalent in certain groups. These include the 185delAG mutation and the 5382inc2 mutation of the BRCA1 gene and the 6174delT mutation of the BRCA2 gene. These genes account for the vast majority of hereditary breast cancers in women of Ashkanazi Jewish heritage. A mutation in the gene that results in the recessive disorder ataxia–telangiectasia may also make patients more susceptible to radiation-induced breast cancer.

■ ■ ■ **CLINICAL PEARL**

Commercial vendors now offer genetic testing for BRCA1 and BRCA2 mutations to all providers.

■ **CLINICAL WARNING:** Genetic testing should generally be offered only to women whose family history is suggestive of a familial pattern of breast or ovarian cancer. Such patients should generally be referred to centers experienced in genetic testing so that they might receive appropriate counseling before making a decision concerning testing. In addition to psychosocial issues related to testing, there are unresolved issues concerning insurance coverage. Many women who are offered testing refuse for a variety of reasons (Lerman et al, 1996). Consideration of genetic testing is appropriate for women who develop breast cancer at a young age, women with a family history of breast or ovarian cancer in first-degree relatives, or women who have a blood relative with a known BRCA1 or BRCA2 mutation. Guidelines are available to help in the selection of patients for testing (American Society of Clinical Oncology, 1996). Information is also readily available to providers for calculating risk based on the patient's family history of breast and ovarian cancer (Claus et al, 1996).

Evaluation of Breast Problems

The algorithms in Figures 65-6 through 65-10 are guidelines for the primary care evaluation and management of specific breast problems. It is up to providers to decide to what extent they will evaluate breast problems before referring the patient to a breast care specialist. These guidelines are not meant to supplant sound clinical judgment. Deviations from these recommendations may be appropriate for an individual patient.

Treatment of Invasive Breast Cancer and Carcinoma In Situ

It is now clear that breast-conserving therapy (lumpectomy and breast radiation) is as effective as mastectomy in providing the opportunity for cure in most women with early-stage breast cancer (Early Breast Cancer Trialists' Collaborative Group, 1995; Fisher et al, 1996). Women with newly diagnosed breast cancer should be given information and guidance concerning their options for primary therapy. Collaboration and coordination before surgery by the primary care provider, surgeon, pathologist, and radiation oncologist are necessary. Women who wish to proceed with mastectomy should be given information concerning breast reconstruction, which can be done in many patients concurrent with mastectomy. This is called immediate reconstruction.

Women with invasive breast cancers less than 4 to 5 cm in largest diameter are excellent candidates for lumpectomy (also called partial mastectomy, or tylectomy). Lumpectomy consists of removing the tumor mass with clear surgical margins. Patients who choose lumpectomy should have postoperative radiation therapy to the involved breast to minimize the likelihood of ipsilateral tumor recurrence (Morrow et al, 1995). Postoperative breast irradiation minimizes subsequent recurrence in the involved breast and has no major adverse impact on cosmesis. The risk of ipsilateral recurrence after lumpectomy and breast irradiation is less than 10% and probably less than 5% in women who also receive adjuvant systemic therapy. Without

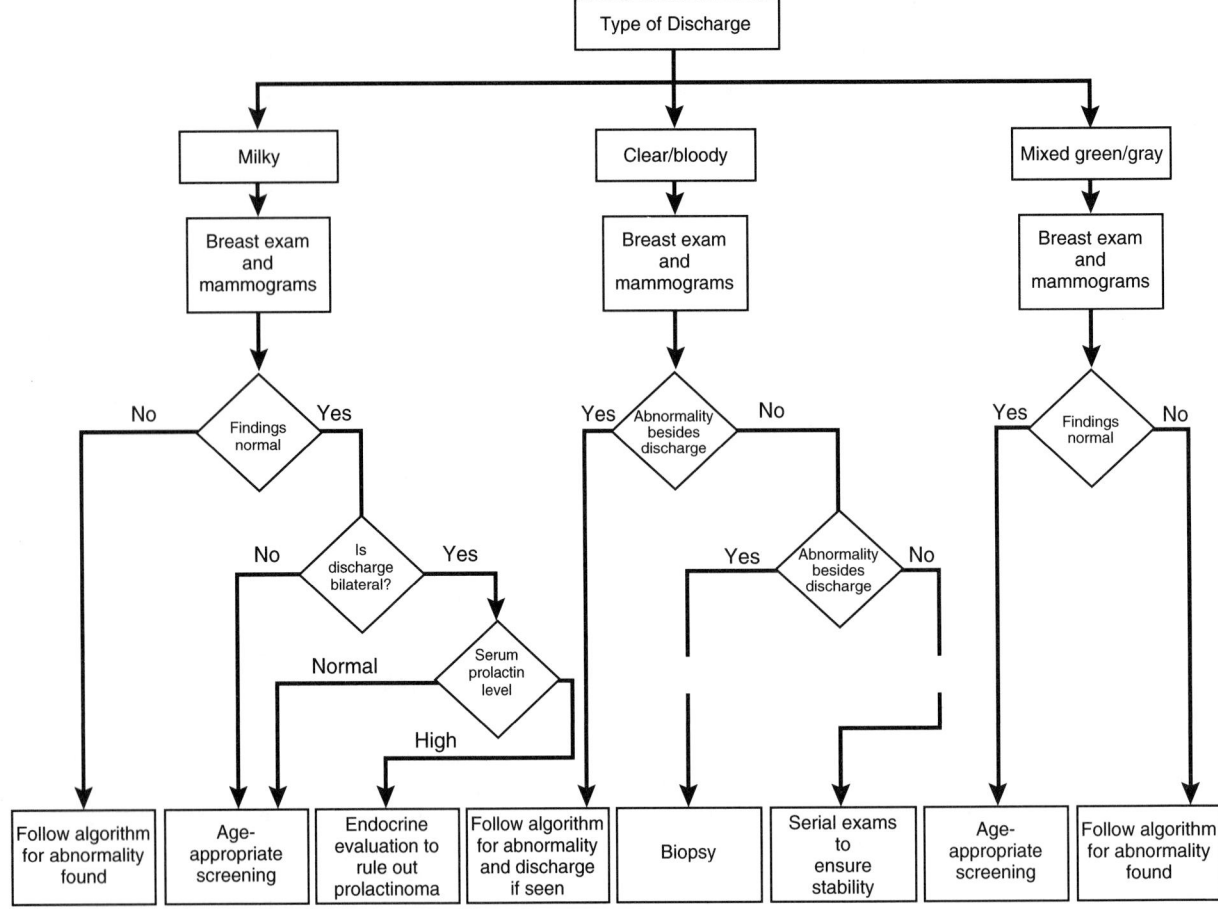

FIGURE 65-6 Algorithm 1: Evaluation of nipple discharge. (Source: Author's work.)

breast irradiation, recurrence at the lumpectomy site occurs in up to 40% of patients (Fisher et al, 1995).

Patients with larger breast cancers who desire breast preservation may be treated with preoperative chemotherapy to make this more feasible. Preoperative chemotherapy results in shrinkage of the primary lesion of more than 50% in more than 75% of patients. Thus, the majority of patients may be suitable candidates for lumpectomy (Bonadonna & Valagussa, 1996).

Women with invasive breast cancer commonly have carcinoma in situ adjacent to or commingled with their invasive lesion. Such women should be treated similar to women who pathologically have only invasive breast cancer. Carcinoma in situ without any invasive component now accounts for about 20% of all breast cancers; there are two main types, LCIS and DCIS (see above). Historically, patients with both LCIS and DCIS underwent mastectomy, but more recently patients with DCIS have been managed with lumpectomy and radiation, selected patients with lumpectomy alone (Solin et al, 1991; Page & Jensen, 1996). Metastatic disease occurs in only 1% to 3% of such patients. Despite the better prognosis of this lesion compared to invasive breast cancer, primary treatment remains controversial. Such patients should be managed by surgeons and radiation oncologists who are expert in the care of breast cancer.

For women with invasive breast cancer, pathologic determination of the extent of axillary node involvement is the most effective predictor of metastatic risk. Axillary dissection is gen-

erally well tolerated, but a few patients develop arm edema and other complications. No other single or combination of prognostic factors can reliably predict the likelihood of axillary node involvement (Ravdin et al, 1994). Even for patients with small invasive lesions (less than 5 mm in largest diameter) and without evidence of adenopathy on the clinical exam, positive axillary nodes are found in 5% to 15% of patients.

The recent identification of a sentinel node using radioactive colloid or a blue dye before dissection may minimize the extent of axillary surgery. Less than 5% of patients with sentinel nodes that are negative are likely to have higher axillary nodes involved after more extensive axillary dissection. The sentinel node technique is currently being evaluated in many centers and has great promise. At present, axillary node dissection should be performed on all women who are suitable candidates for systemic adjuvant therapy, and in whom the oncologist will use these data to make major decisions in treatment.

Axillary node dissection is also therapeutic. The risk of recurrence in the axilla is extremely low (less than 5%) in patients who have had such a procedure. At least six lymph nodes need to be removed for accurate staging (Dixon, 1994).

For women who are treated with mastectomy, postoperative radiation to the chest wall has been shown to decrease the rate of local skin recurrence but has little if any impact on overall survival (Early Breast Cancer Trialists' Collaborative Group, 1995). In general, such treatment is now reserved for women with large primary lesions (5 cm or greater) or four or more

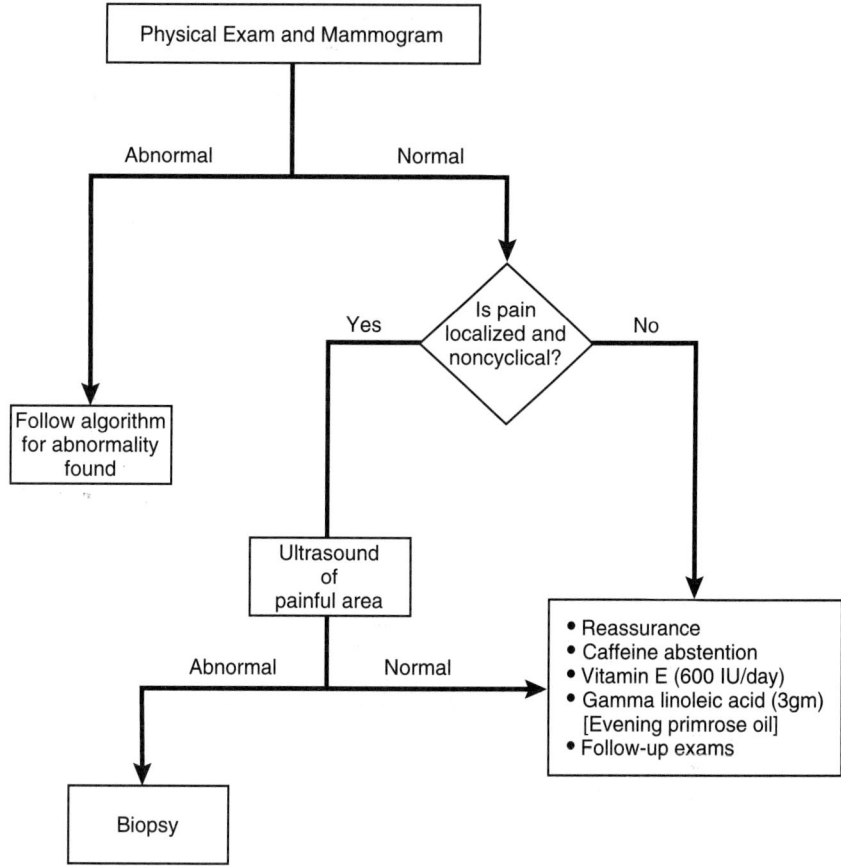

FIGURE 65-7 Algorithm 2: Evaluation of breast pain. (Source: Author's work.)

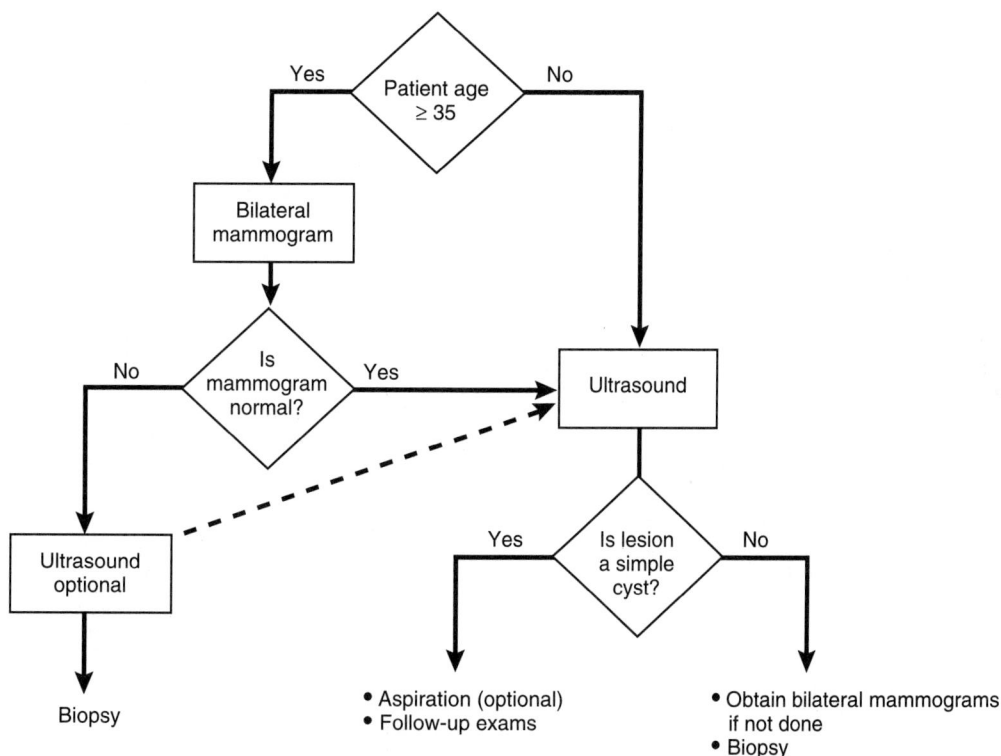

FIGURE 65-8 Algorithm 3: Palpable abnormality. (Source: Author's work.)

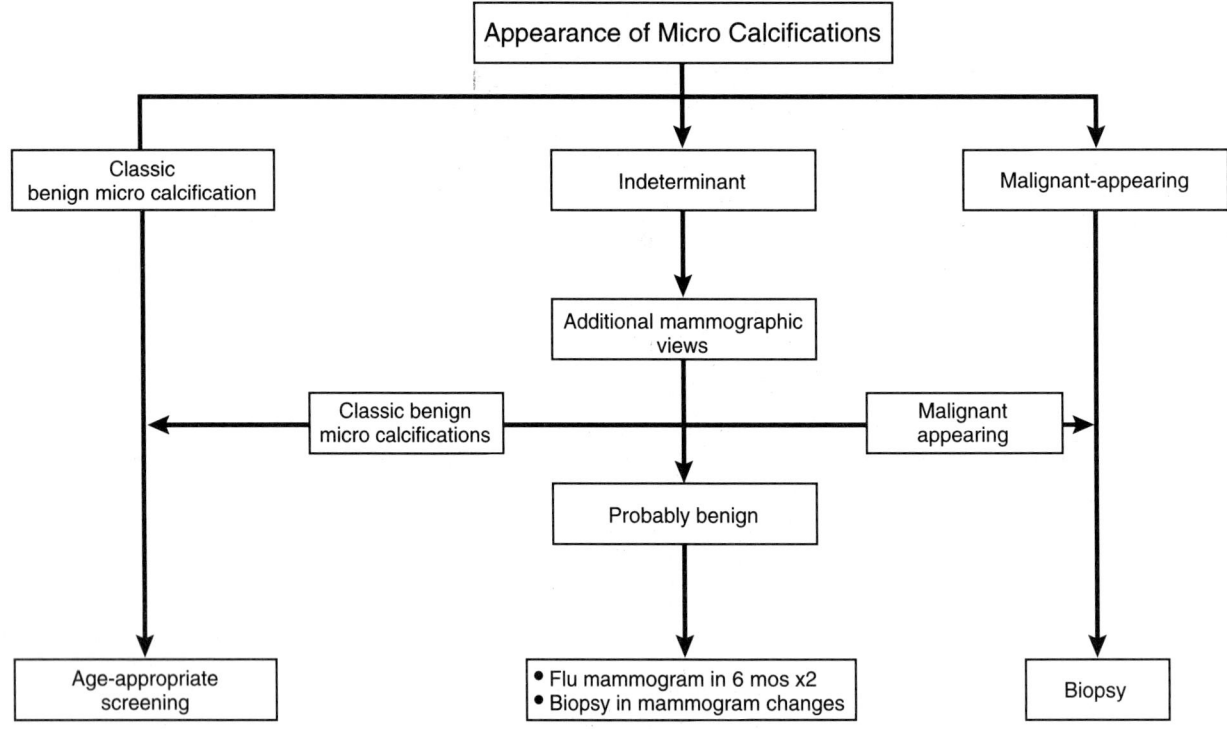

FIGURE 65-9 Algorithm 4: Mammographic abnormality microcalcifications. (Source: Author's work.)

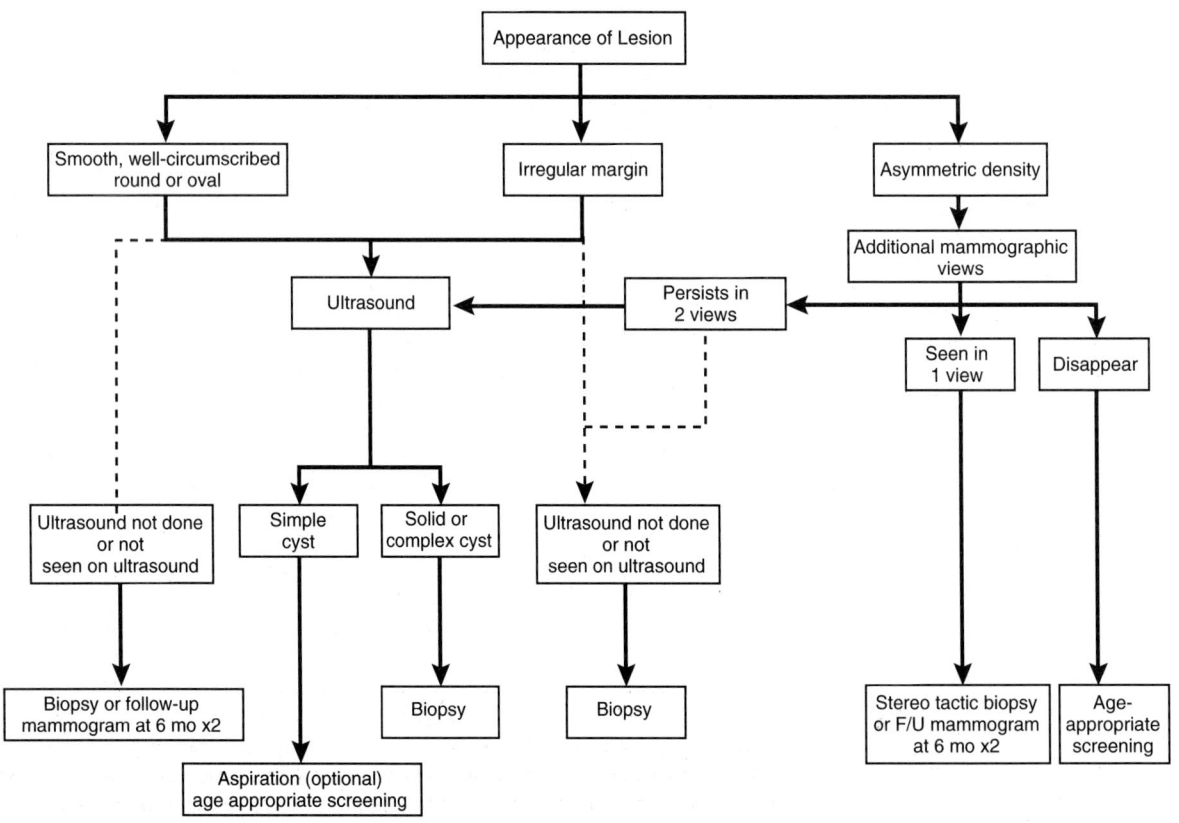

FIGURE 65-10 Algorithm 5: Mammographic abnormality (nonpalpable nodule/density). (Source: Author's work.)

involved axillary nodes, or in cases where tumor involves the margins of the mastectomy specimen.

Staging

Staging of breast cancer is based on tumor size, extent of breast involvement, axillary lymph node involvement, and the presence or absence of distant metastases. These criteria describe the TNM system (American Joint Committee on Cancer [AJCC], 1992). Tumor size can be estimated by physical examination or mammogram. The most accurate determination of primary tumor size, and the one that should be used for staging, is made by the pathologist on review of the biopsy, lumpectomy, or mastectomy specimen. The largest diameter of the invasive component is used to determine tumor size. The staging system suggested by the AJCC in 1992 is the most current.

At diagnosis, more than 50% of patients have disease confined to the breast alone, about 30% to 40% have ipsilateral regional lymph node involvement, and less than 10% present with distant disease. About 60% of those with lymph node involvement have fewer than four nodes involved by tumor.

Preoperative Management

A careful history and physical exam, complete blood count and chemistry profile, and chest x-ray constitute an appropriate preoperative workup for asymptomatic women with breast cancer. Women with symptoms such as bone pain or abdominal pain should have imaging studies of symptomatic sites. Bilateral mammograms should be obtained in all women with biopsy-proven breast cancer. This is necessary to look for disease in the opposite breast.

Adjuvant Systemic Therapy for Early-Stage Breast Cancer

Adjuvant therapy is defined as the use of chemotherapy, hormonal therapy, or immunotherapy in conjunction with definitive treatment of the primary lesion. Adjuvant therapy is used to lower the risk of distant metastases. The goal of adjuvant therapy is to eliminate small, clinically occult micrometastases arising from the hematogenous spread of malignant cells from the primary lesion before diagnosis. An excellent review of these concepts is available (Bonadonna, 1992).

Most adjuvant therapy is currently given after lumpectomy or mastectomy. The effectiveness of adjuvant therapy is judged by measuring recurrence-free (ie, relapse-free) survival as well as overall survival. Current therapy decreases the annual odds of breast cancer recurrence by about 25% to 30% and the odds of dying of breast cancer by about 20%. Adjuvant therapy also delays recurrence and in some trials has lowered the risk of ipsilateral recurrence in women who have had lumpectomy and breast radiation as their primary therapy.

Current adjuvant therapy regimens can cure only about 20% of women at risk of developing metastases. Many potential prognostic factors have been evaluated in an attempt to identify the women most likely to benefit from treatment. However, no prognostic factors yet have been found that can clearly identify women who have only a minimal risk for recurrence.

CLINICAL WARNING: Careful estimation of the risks versus the benefits of therapy is mandatory before placing patients on adjuvant treatment regimens.

The percentage of patients likely to benefit from adjuvant therapy is similar regardless of the risk of recurrence. For instance, assume a 30% reduction in relapse rate for a group of patients at a very low (10%) risk of systemic recurrence. For every 100 patients treated, only 3% ($0.3 \times 0.1 \times 100$) would be helped. For a group at a very high (80%) risk of developing metastases, 24% ($0.3 \times 0.8 \times 100$) would be helped.

CLINICAL PEARL

Recommendations for adjuvant therapy are based on menopausal status, the number of positive lymph nodes, and the estrogen and progesterone receptor status of the tumor. The selection of adjuvant therapy is complex and frequently controversial; consensus guidelines are now available (Goldhirsch et al, 1995).

The most commonly used endocrine agent in the adjuvant setting is tamoxifen (Jaiyesimi et al, 1995). Tamoxifen is an antiestrogen with weak estrogen agonist properties. It is generally recommended for both pre- and postmenopausal women with estrogen receptor-positive primary lesions. Current data suggest that tamoxifen should be used for 5 years to achieve maximum benefit (Fisher et al, 1996).

CLINICAL WARNING: The major toxicities of tamoxifen include hot flashes, thromboembolic phenomena (occurring in about 1% of patients), and endometrial cancer (occurring in an estimated 1% of patients for every 5 years of use) (Fisher et al, 1994; Muss, 1992). Weight gain is not a side effect of tamoxifen but is a common observation in many women after breast cancer. Asymptomatic patients taking tamoxifen who have an intact uterus should have pelvic exams yearly. Further evaluation, including possible endometrial biopsy, should be considered for patients with symptoms. Other toxicities include vaginal dryness or discharge and mood changes; these problems are usually mild. Retinopathy is rare. Although of concern from animal data, no increased risk of hepatocellular carcinoma has been noted.

In addition to its adjuvant effects, tamoxifen's weak estrogen agonist activity results in a significant reduction in serum cholesterol levels (about 15%) and decreases the concentration of low-density lipoproteins in postmenopausal women (Spicer et al, 1990). In at least two clinical trials, the incidence of cardiac disease was significantly reduced in postmenopausal women taking tamoxifen (McDonald & Stewart, 1991; Rutqvist & Mattsson, 1993). In women who have had breast cancer, tamoxifen also significantly decreases the risk of developing contralateral breast cancer by approximately 40%. Bone density may be maintained in postmenopausal women taking tamoxifen (Love et al, 1992).

Adjuvant chemotherapy is usually reserved for higher-risk patients. These include women whose nodes were negative, but have large or estrogen receptor-negative tumors, and those whose nodes were positive. In patients with estrogen receptor-positive tumors, the combination of tamoxifen and chemotherapy results in superior survival compared to the use of tamoxifen or chemotherapy alone. Combination regimens using several chemotherapeutic agents are commonly used for a period of 3 to 6 months. The use of adjuvant chemotherapy in women 70 years or older has not been defined; it should be considered for older women in good health who are at high risk for recurrence. There is now major interest in defining the role of high-dose chemotherapy and autologous stem cell support in high-risk patients in the adjuvant setting.

Recent data show that ovarian ablation is similar to chemotherapy in improving breast cancer survival in premenopausal women who have receptor-positive tumors. Many providers and patients find ovarian ablation by surgical or radiotherapeutic means objectionable, and ablation has not been widely used in the United States. The introduction of gonadotropin-releasing hormone agonists has provided a more acceptable and potentially reversible means of providing ablative therapy.

■ ■ ■ **CLINICAL PEARL**

All patients with early-stage breast cancer should be referred to an oncologist for discussion and decisions regarding adjuvant therapy.

Follow-Up After Primary Breast Cancer

Early detection of distant metastases improves survival. The most common sites of metastatic disease include the chest wall (in patients with mastectomy, local recurrence), bone, local lymph nodes, lung and pleura, and liver. Isolated recurrence in the central nervous system and meningeal involvement are uncommon.

Almost all investigators have demonstrated that a brief follow-up visit, which includes an interim history and physical exam, will detect recurrence in more than 75% of patients. In asymptomatic patients, chemistry profiles, complete blood counts, routine chest x-rays, radionuclide bone scans, and other expensive imaging studies add great cost but only a small additional yield in detecting early recurrence (Muss et al, 1988).

Two large randomized trials have compared intensive (history and physical exam, chest x-ray, and bone scan) and clinical (history and physical exam only) follow-up strategies (Rosselli et al, 1994; GIVIO Investigators, 1994). Neither showed a survival advantage for intensive follow-up, although in one trial imaging studies detected bone and intrathoracic relapse earlier. This earlier detection of relapse did not translate into improved survival (Rosselli et al, 1994). In the second trial, quality of life, emotional well-being, social functioning, symptoms, and satisfaction with care were similar among the intensively followed and clinically followed groups (GIVIO Investigators, 1994). More recently, tumor marker studies have become available for monitoring early-stage patients for relapse. Again, there is no convincing evidence that early detection of relapse using marker studies improves survival. In short, limiting the use of high-cost imaging and laboratory studies for routine follow-up will lower the costs of medical care for women with early-stage breast cancer without compromising their quality of life.

TABLE 65-1	Guidelines for Follow-Up in Asymptomatic Patients
Procedure or Test	**Frequency**
History and physical exam*	Every 3–6 months for 3 years, then every 6–12 months for 2 years, then yearly
Mammography	
Mastectomy patients	Yearly
Lumpectomy patients	Involved breast: every 6 months for 2 years and then yearly
Uninvolved breast	Yearly
Pelvic exam	Yearly

* Limited evaluation: Assess for pain, dyspnea, weight loss, other major changes in function. Limited examination to include nodal assessment, breast axillary, and lumpectomy or mastectomy site, chest, abdomen. Patients should be instructed regarding symptoms of recurrence.

The literature does not support the use of complete blood counts and chemistry studies. Bone scans, liver imaging, and marker studies are not recommended for routine follow-up in asymptomatic patients.

Source: American Society of Clinical Oncology, 1997.

Guidelines for follow-up evaluation in asymptomatic patients have been recently developed by the American Society of Clinical Oncology and are presented in Table 65-1.

TEACHING AND SELF-CARE

All patients should be instructed in breast self-exam and the need for appropriate screening studies to minimize the risk of breast cancer mortality. It has been clearly shown that patients who are well informed are more likely to follow screening recommendations. Patients should be encouraged to notify the primary care provider if any new breast abnormality is identified that persists beyond 1 month. Such a waiting time will probably reduce the number of benign lesions requiring evaluation without jeopardizing the patient if the lesion is malignant. Table 65-2 presents several self-care strategies providers can discuss with their patients.

Breast cancer support groups are available in most regions of the country and may be of great benefit to the patient trying to cope with the psychological and physical aspects of breast cancer treatment (Maunsell et al, 1995; Speigel et al, 1997).

TABLE 65-2	Self-Care Strategies for Women with Breast Cancer

Take time out to explore your feelings and gather information. Share this with family and friends. Get feedback. Reduce stress as much as possible (Speigel, 1997). Express yourself; feel angry, cry, laugh. Meditate. Use affirmations. Engage in emotionally satisfying activities. Join a breast cancer support group (Maunsell, et al., 1995). Participate in an enjoyable exercise (McTiernan, 1997). Eat right. Get plenty of sleep.

Initiate a calorie-balanced diet (intake matches energy requirements). Add a weight-reduction component according to BMI/waist-to-hip ratio. Supplements (research is inconsistent; prudence is advised) (Kimmick, et al, 1997). Include soy products freely (Ingram, et al, 1997). Drink at least 8 glasses of water daily. Limit alcohol and caffeine. Avoid tobacco and recreational drugs.

See also Table 67-9, Self-Care Strategies for the Menopausal Woman, for additional ideas.

COMMUNITY RESOURCES

- American Cancer Society: A strong proponent for breast cancer screening and multidisciplinary breast cancer care. They offer several support services and are an excellent source of information for finding cancer-related treatment services.

- Reach to Recovery, 800-ACS-2345: An organization staffed by volunteers who have been treated for breast cancer. Their members visit newly diagnosed or postsurgical patients and give moral support, answer questions, and demonstrate rehabilitative exercises.

- National Cancer Institute, 800-4-CANCER, TTY 800-332-8615, Web site http://rex.nci.nih.gov: Provides excellent, up-to-date information for providers and patients concerning breast and other cancers through the Physician's Data Query system. The Cancer Information Service, the NCI's national information and education network, is the source for the latest, most accurate cancer information. Specially trained staff provide scientific information in understandable language and are bilingual (English and Spanish).

- Cancer Care Inc., 800-813-HOPE: A hotline staffed by professionally trained social workers who can provide immediate help during times of crisis and can refer patients to a nationwide network of local community resources.

- YWCA's Encore Plus, 800-95E-PLUS, 202-682-3636: Offers exercise programs and support groups.

- The Wellness Community, 310-314-2555: Has 14 centers in the United States, offering support groups, exercise programs, classes in stress reduction and nutrition, social get-togethers, and workshops.

- Office of Technology Assessment, www.wws.princ ton.edu/ota: Information on unconventional cancer treatments.

- National Library of Medicine, www.nlm.nih.gov: Provides free Internet access to MEDLINE via PubMed or Grateful Med.

REFERRAL POINTS AND CLINICAL WARNINGS

This information is integrated throughout the chapter.

References

American Joint Committee on Cancer. (1992). *Manual for staging of cancer*, 4th ed. Philadelphia: J.B. Lippincott.

American Society of Clinical Oncology. (1996). Genetic testing for cancer susceptibility. *Journal of Clinical Oncology, 14,* 1730–1736.

American Society of Clinical Oncology. (1997). Recommended breast cancer surveillance guidelines. *Journal of Clinical Oncology, 15,* 2149–2156.

Barnes, S., Peterson, G., Grubbs, C., et al. (1994). Potential role of dietary iso-flavones in the prevention of cancer. In M.M. Jacobs (Ed.). *Diet and cancer: Markers, prevention and treatment*, p. 135. New York: Plenum.

Bernstein, L., Henderson, B.E., Hanisch, R., et al. (1994). Physical exercise and reduced risk of breast cancer in young women. *Journal of the National Cancer Institute, 86,* 1402.

Bonadonna, G. (1992). Evolving concepts in the systemic adjuvant treatment of breast cancer. *Cancer Research, 52,* 2127–2137.

Bonadonna, G., & Valagussa, P. (1996). Primary chemotherapy in operable breast cancer [Review]. *Seminars in Oncology, 23,* 464–474.

Boring, C., Squires, T., Tong, T., et al. (1994). Cancer statistics 1994. *CA: A Cancer Journal for Clinicians, 44,* 18.

Brinton, L.A., Schairer, C.S., Hoover, R.D., et al. (1988). Menstrual factors and risk of breast cancer. *Cancer Investigation, 6,* 245.

Carson, W., Sanches-Forgach, E., Stomper, P., Penetrante, R., Tsang-aris, T.N., & Edge, S.B. (1994). Lobular carcinoma *in situ* without surgery as an appropriate therapy. *Annals of Surgical Oncology, 1,* 141–146.

Claus, E.B., Schildkraut, J.M., Thompson, W.D., & Risch, N.J. (1996). The genetic attributable risk of breast and ovarian cancer. *Cancer, 77,* 2318–2324.

Couch, F.J., Farid, L.M., DeShano, M.L., et al. (1996). BRCA2 germ-line mutations in male breast cancer cases and breast cancer families. *Nature Genetics, 13,* 123–125.

Dixon, J.M. (1994). Role of axillary dissection in women with early breast cancer. Current medical literature: Breast cancer. *Royal Society of Medicine, 6,* 99–104.

Dupont, W.D., & Page, D.L. (1985). Risk factors for breast cancer in women with proliferative breast disease. *N Engl J Med, 312,* 146.

Early Breast Cancer Trialists' Collaborative Group. (1995). Effects of radiotherapy and surgery in early breast cancer. An overview of the randomized trials. *N Engl J Med, 333,* 1444–1455.

Fisher, B., Anderson, S., Redmond, C.K., Wolmark, N., Wickerham, D.L., & Cronin, W.M. (1995). Reanalysis and results after 12 years of follow-up in a randomized clinical trial comparing total mastectomy with lumpectomy with or without irradiation in the treatment of breast cancer. *N Engl J Med, 333,* 1456–1461.

Fisher, B., Costantino, J.P., Redmond, C.K., Fisher, E.R., Wickerham, D.L., & Cronin, W.M. (1994). Endometrial cancer in tamoxifen-treated breast cancer patients: Findings from the National Surgical Adjuvant Breast and Bowel Project (NSABP) B-14. *Journal of the National Cancer Institute, 86,* 527–537.

Fisher, B., Dignam, J., Bryant, J., et al. (1996). Five versus more than five years of tamoxifen therapy for breast cancer patients with negative lymph nodes and estrogen receptor-positive tumors. *Journal of the National Cancer Institute, 88,* 1529–1542.

Fletcher, S., Black, W., Harris, R., et al. (1993). Special article: Report of the international workshop on screening for breast cancer. *Journal of the National Cancer Institute, 85,* 1644.

GIVIO Investigators. (1994). Impact of follow-up testing on survival and health-related quality of life in breast cancer patients. A multicenter randomized controlled trial. *JAMA, 271,* 1587–1592.

Goldhirsch, A., Wood, W.C., Senn, H., Glick, J.H., & Gelber, R.D. (1995). Meeting highlights: International consensus panel on the treatment of primary breast cancer. *Journal of the National Cancer Institute, 87,* 1441–1445.

Hankey, B.F., Brinton, L.A., Kessler, L.F., et al. (1993). Breast cancer statistics review, 1973–1990. In B.A. Miller, L.A.G. Ries, B.F. Hankey, et al. (Eds.). NIH publication No. 93-2789, p. 1. Bethesda, MD: U.S. Department of Health and Human Services, National Cancer Institute.

Heywang-Kobrunner, S.H. (1994). Contrast-enhanced magnetic resonance imaging of the breast. *Investigative Radiology, 29,* 94.

Ingram, D., Sanders, K., Kolybaba, M., & Lopez, D. (1997). Case-controlled study of phyto-oestrogens and breast cancer. *Lancet, 350,* 990–994.

Jaiyesimi, I.A., Buzdar, A.U., Decker, D.A., & Hortobagyi, G.N. (1995). Use of tamoxifen for breast cancer: 28 years later [Review]. *Journal of Clinical Oncology, 13,* 513–529.

Jensen, R.A., Page, D.L., Dupont, W.D., et al. (1989). Invasive breast cancer risk in women with sclerosing adenosis. *Cancer, 64,* 1977.

Kerlikowske, K., Grady, D., Barclay, J., et al. (1993). Positive predictive value of screening mammography by age and family history of breast cancer. *JAMA, 270,* 1.

Krieger, N. (1990). Social class and the black/white crossover in the age-specific incidence of breast cancer: A study linking census-derived data to population-based registry records. *American Journal of Epidemiology, 131,* 804.

Lerman, C., Narod, S., Schulman, K., et al. (1996). BRCA1 testing in families with hereditary breast-ovarian cancer. A prospective study of patient decision making and outcomes. *JAMA, 275,* 1885–1892.

Longnecker, M., Berlin, J.A., Orza, M.D., et al. (1988). A meta-analysis of alcohol consumption in relation to breast cancer risk. *JAMA, 260,* 642.

Love, R.R., Mazess, R.B., Barden, H.S., et al. (1992). Effects of tamoxifen on bone mineral density in postmenopausal women with breast cancer. *N Engl J Med, 326,* 852–856.

MacMahon B., Cole, P., Lin, T.M., et al. (1970). Age at first birth and breast cancer risk. *Bulletin of the World Health Organization, 43,* 209.

Maunsell, E., Brisson, J., & Deschenes, L. (1995). Social support and survival among women with breast cancer. *Cancer, 76,* 631–637.

McDonald, C.C., & Stewart, H.J. (1991). Fatal myocardial infarction in the Scottish adjuvant tamoxifen trial. The Scottish Breast Cancer Committee. *British Medical Journal, 303,* 435–437.

McTiernan, A. (1997). Exercise and breast cancer—time to get moving? [Editorial]. *N Engl J Med, 336,* 1311–1312.

Mettlin, C., & Smart, C.R. (1994). Breast cancer detection guidelines for women aged 40–49 years: Rationale for the American Cancer Society reaffirmation of recommendations. *CA: A Cancer Journal for Clinicians, 44,* 248.

Morrow, M., Harris, J.R., & Schnitt, S.J. (1995). Local control following breast-conserving surgery for invasive cancer: Results of clinical trials [Review]. *Journal of the National Cancer Institute, 87,* 1669–1673.

Muir, C., Waterhouse, J., Mack, T., et al. (Eds.). (1987). *Cancer incidence in five continents,* Vol. 5. IARC Scientific (No. 88). Lyon: IARC.

Muss, H.B. (1992). Endocrine therapy for advanced breast cancer: A review. *Breast Cancer Research & Treatment, 21,* 15–26.

Muss, H.B., McNamara, M.J., & Connelly, R.A. (1988). Follow-up after stage II breast cancer: A comparative study of relapsed versus nonrelapsed patients. *American Journal of Clinical Oncology, 11,* 451–455.

Nystrom, L., Rutqvist, L.E., Wall, S., et al. (1993). Breast cancer screening with mammography; overview of Swedish randomized trials. *Lancet, 341,* 973.

O'Malley, M.S., & Fletcher, S.W. (1987). Screening for breast cancer with breast self-examination: A critical review. *JAMA, 257,* 2197.

Page, D.L., & Jensen, R.A. (1996). Ductal carcinoma *in situ* of the breast: Understanding the misunderstood stepchild. *JAMA, 275,* 948–949.

Ravdin, P.M., De Laurentiis, M., Vendely, T., & Clark, G.M. (1994). Prediction of axillary lymph node status in breast cancer patients by use of prognostic indicators. *Journal of the National Cancer Institute, 86,* 1771–1775.

Rimer, B.K., Keintz, M.K., Keller, H.B., et al. (1989). Why women resist screening mammography: Patient-related barriers. *Radiology, 172,* 243.

Rosselli-Del Turco, M., Palli, D., Cariddi, A., Ciatto, S., Pacini, P., & Distante, V. (1994). Intensive diagnostic follow-up after treatment of primary breast cancer. A randomized trial. National Research Council Project on Breast Cancer Follow-Up. *JAMA, 271,* 1593–1597.

Rutqvist, L.E., & Mattsson, A. (1993). Cardiac and thromboembolic morbidity among postmenopausal women with early-stage breast cancer in a randomized trial of adjuvant tamoxifen. The Stockholm Breast Cancer Study Group. *Journal of the National Cancer Institute, 85,* 1398–1406.

Shapiro, S., Venet, W., Strax, P., et al. (1988). Current results of the breast cancer screening randomized trial: The health insurance plan (HIP) of greater New York study. In *Screening for breast cancer.* Toronto: Sam Huber Publishing.

Shattuck-Eidens D., McClure M., Simard J., et al. (1995). A collaborative survey of 80 mutations in the BRCA1 breast and ovarian cancer susceptibility gene. Implications for presymptomatic testing and screening. *JAMA, 273,* 535–541.

Solin, L.J., Recht, A., Fourquet, A., et al. (1991). Ten-year results of breast-conserving surgery and definitive irradiation for intraductal carcinoma (ductal carcinoma *in situ*) of the breast. *Cancer, 68,* 2337–2344.

Speigel, D. (1997). Psychosocial aspects of breast cancer treatment. *Seminars in Oncology, 24*(Suppl. 1), S36–47.

Spicer, D., Pike, M.D., Henderson, B.E. (1990). The question of estrogen replacement therapy in patients with a prior diagnosis of breast cancer. *Oncology, 4,* 49–59.

Trichopoulos, D., MacMahon, B., & Cole, P. (1972). Menopause and breast cancer risk. *Journal of the National Cancer Institute, 48,* 605.

Wickerham, D.L., Costantino, J.C, Fisher, B. et al. (1998). The initial results from NSABP protocol P-1: A clinical trial to determine the worth of tamoxifen for preventing breast cancer in women at increased risk. [Abstract] *Proceedings American Society of Clinical Oncology, 3A.*

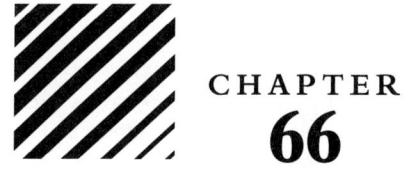

CHAPTER

66

Gynecologic Cancers

Miriam Shustik, MD

Gynecologic malignancies represent 13% of all cancers affecting women. They are the fourth most common cancers in American women. Cervical, endometrial, and ovarian cancers make up the majority of these tumors and contribute significantly to the morbidity and mortality of the female population. Whereas cervical and endometrial cancers can be detected early in their development, many patients with ovarian cancer present with already advanced disease. If detected early, cancer is more easily treated and the possibility of long-term cure is greatest. All cancer survivors face the issue of uncertainty.

This chapter reviews gynecologic cancers, including cervical, vaginal, vulvar, endometrial, ovarian, and trophoblastic disease, and also addresses how the primary care provider can work effectively with patients having any of these conditions. Family and community resources will also be discussed.

CARCINOMA OF THE CERVIX

Anatomy, Physiology, and Pathology

The cervix is a fusiform cavity that communicates below with the vagina and above with the uterine body. The epithelium of the upper two thirds is cylindrical, whereas the lower third gradually changes to squamous close to the external os. The junction between the primarily columnar epithelium of the endocervix and the squamous epithelium of the ectocervix is a site of continuous metaplastic change. This change is most active in utero, at puberty, and during the first pregnancy, and then declines after menopause. The greatest risk of neoplastic transformation coincides with periods of vast metaplastic activity, and most carcinomas arise from this zone of metaplastic transformation in the squamocolumnar junction.

EARLY DISEASE

Preinvasive disease is usually detected during routine screening from cervical cytology. Patients with early invasive disease may also be asymptomatic.

> **CLINICAL WARNING:** The first symptom of invasive cervical cancer is usually abnormal bleeding, often after coitus. This may be associated with clear or foul-smelling vaginal discharge. Pelvic pain may result from invasion of the disease or from coexistent pelvic inflammatory disease.

LATE DISEASE

The triad of sciatic pain, leg edema, and hydronephrosis is almost always associated with extensive pelvic involvement by the tumor. Hydronephrosis may cause flank pain and may be associated with pyelonephritis.

> **CLINICAL WARNING:** Patients with very advanced tumors may present with hematuria or incontinence from a vesicovaginal fistula caused by extension of the tumor to the bladder. Constipation could be a consequence of external compression of the rectum by the tumor.

Epidemiology

The American Cancer Society estimates that there are 15,800 new cases of invasive cervical cancer and 65,000 cases of carcinoma in situ diagnosed in the United States per year. Forty-eight hundred patients are expected to die of cervical cancer; this represents approximately 2% of all cancer deaths in women and 18% of all gynecologic cancers. Cervical cancer is the third most common gynecologic cancer in the United States.

Squamous cell carcinoma of the cervix follows a pattern of sexually transmitted disease. The risk of cervical cancer is increased in female prostitutes. The risk also is high for women whose first episode of sexual intercourse occurred at less than age 17, those with a history of multiple sex partners or sexually transmitted diseases, or those who bear children at less than age 17. Molecular studies have demonstrated a strong relation between human papillomavirus (HPV), cervical intraepithelial neoplasia, and invasive carcinomas of the cervix. HPV has been identified in more than 60% of cervical cancers (Duggan et al, 1995; Zur Hausen, 1997). Other important risks include having a male partner whose sexual behavior is promiscuous or who is uncircumcised and has poor hygiene. Several significant personal risk factors are also associated with an increased incidence of cervical cancer. These include cigarette smoking, immunodeficiency, vitamin A and C deficiency and, possibly, oral contraceptive use. In the United States, the incidence of cervical cancer is higher among women of Native American, African, and Hispanic heritage.

Cervical cancer continues to be the leading cause of cancer deaths for women in underdeveloped countries. Incidence and death rates are particularly high in South and Central America, Africa, India, and Eastern Europe (Kurman & Solomon, 1994). Twenty-five percent of all cancer-related deaths in Mexican women are caused by cervical cancer. Screening and prevention programs are not yet completely effective in developing countries.

Diagnostic Criteria

Several systems have been developed to classify cervical cytology. The Bethesda system is now used commonly in the United States for classifying cervical changes (Berek & Hacker, 1994).

History and Physical Exam

All patients with cervical cancer should be evaluated with a careful history and physical exam, with particular attention to inspection and palpation of pelvic organs with bimanual and rectovaginal exams. Attention to the psychosocial aspect of the patient is very important. The provider must consider the difficulties of this moment and should be comfortable and knowledgeable enough to encourage patients to express and discuss their concerns.

Diagnostic Studies

PAP SMEAR

The false-negative rate of the Pap smear is about 10% to 15% in women with invasive cancer. The sensitivity of the test may be improved by proper sampling of the squamocolumnar junction and the endocervical canal. Smears without endocervical cells or metaplastic cells are inadequate and must be repeated. Because adenocarcinoma in situ originates near or above the transformation zone, it may not be sampled by a conventional smear. Detection of high endocervical lesions might be improved with the use of a cytobrush. Also, because hemorrhage, tissue necrosis, and inflammation may obscure the cytology report, the Pap is not a good test to diagnose gross lesions; they should always be biopsied (Miller et al, 1993).

COLPOSCOPIC EXAM

Patients with abnormal cytology and no gross lesion must be evaluated by colposcopy and directed biopsy. The skilled colposcopist can often differentiate between LSIL and HSIL, but microinvasive disease and intraepithelial lesions cannot be consistently distinguished (Burger & Hollema, 1993).

ENDOCERVICAL CURETTAGE

If the entire squamocolumnar junction cannot be visualized on colposcopy in a patient with an atypical Pap smear, endocervical curettage is indicated.

CONE BIOPSY

Cervical cone biopsy is used to diagnose occult endocervical lesions and is an important step in the diagnosis of microinvasive carcinoma of the cervix. It is indicated in the following cases.

- When the squamocolumnar junction is poorly visualized on colposcopy and a high-grade lesion is suspected
- When a high-grade dysplastic epithelium extends into the endocervical canal
- When cytology results suggest carcinoma in situ
- When endocervical curettage shows HSIL
- When there is suspicion of adenocarcinoma in situ (Morris et al, 1993).

LABORATORY STUDIES

Standard laboratory studies should include a complete blood count and renal and liver function tests in all patients with invasive cervical cancer.

RADIOLOGIC STUDIES

All patients with invasive cervical cancer should have a chest radiograph to rule out metastatic disease to the lungs, and an intravenous pyelogram to determine the kidney's location and to rule out ureteral obstruction by the tumor. The value of computed tomography (CT) or magnetic resonance imaging (MRI) is uncertain because the accuracy of these studies is compromised by their failure to detect small metastases and because patients with bulky tumors often have enlarged, reactive lymph nodes (Lien et al, 1993).

Treatment Options, Expected Outcomes, and Comprehensive Management

Several factors may influence treatment options, including tumor size, stage, and histology; evidence of lymph node involvement; risk factors for surgery or radiation; and patient preference. The International Federation of Gynecology and Obstetrics (FIGO) has defined the most widely accepted staging system for carcinomas of the cervix; it was last updated in 1994 (FIGO, 1995). As a rule, intraepithelial lesions are treated with superficial ablative techniques such as cryosurgery, laser therapy, or loop excision. These are all outpatient procedures that maintain fertility and carry a low recurrence rate; progression to invasion is rare. Lifelong surveillance of these patients is necessary, however, to detect early signs of recurrence.

Microinvasive cancers invading less than 3 mm (stage IA1) are managed with conservative surgery, such as excisional conization or extrafascial hysterectomy. Total or vaginal hysterectomy is the standard treatment for this stage of disease. For those who wish to maintain fertility, conization is the choice. Conization is performed with a cold knife or carbon dioxide laser under general or spinal anesthesia. Complications occur in 2% to 12% of patients and include sepsis, hemorrhage, infertility, stenosis, and cervical incompetence.

Early invasive cancers (stages IA2 and IB1 and some small stage IIA tumors) are managed with either radical surgery or irradiation. Locally advanced cancers (stages IB2 through IVA) are managed with radiation therapy (Landoni et al, 1995; Matthews et al, 1993). The prognosis is influenced by tumor characteristics such as bulk and diameter, lymph node metastasis, histology, and hemoglobin level (Eifel et al, 1994; FIGO, 1994; Matthews et al, 1993).

SCREENING

The long preinvasive stage of cervical cancer, the relatively high prevalence of the disease in unscreened populations, and the sensitivity of cytologic screening all have made cervical carcinoma an ideal target for cancer screening. In the United States, screening with cervical cytology, as well as performing frequent pelvic exams, has led to a decrease in the mortality rate from cervical cancer of more than 70% since 1940 (Boring et al, 1996; Koss, 1993). Only countries that have invested in screening programs have experienced this kind of result.

Authorities disagree about the optimal frequency of screening for cervical cancer. Since the time of a 1988 consensus statement, the American Cancer Society has recommended annual Pap smears beginning at age 18 years or with the onset of sexual activity. After three consecutive normal exams, the evaluation could be performed less frequently at the discretion of the provider. The U.S. Preventive Task Force (1994) has recommended that screening be discontinued at age 65 if results have been consistently normal. Because of a lack of objective measurement of low- and high-risk patients, physicians continue to recommend that patients be screened more often than recommended by national guidelines.

Patients who were diagnosed and treated for cervical cancer should be followed by the provider over their lifetime to maintain health. Periodic exams will prevent or at least delay the recurrence of the disease and further complications.

Referral Points and Clinical Warnings

Patients with abnormal Pap smears should be followed closely by the primary care provider with periodic Pap smears, colposcopy, and biopsy in case of LSIL. When needed, referral should be made to a gynecologic oncology practice that performs cone biopsies and loop and laser procedures; surgical procedures such as hysterectomy in case of HSIL or invasive carcinoma come under the venue of such a practice.

CLINICAL WARNING: Any abnormal bleeding is suspicious and must be investigated.

CARCINOMA OF THE VAGINA

Anatomy, Physiology, and Pathology

The vagina extends from the vulva to the uterus. It is situated in the pelvic cavity behind the bladder and in front of the rectum. It is about 2″ along its anterior wall and 3″ inches along its posterior wall. The vaginal epithelium is of the squamous type.

Squamous cell carcinomas account for 80% to 90% of primary vaginal malignancies, adenocarcinomas for 5% to 10%, vaginal melanomas for 3%, and vaginal sarcomas for another 3% (Kurman & Solomon, 1994).

Epidemiology

Vaginal intraepithelial neoplasms often accompany cervical intraepithelial neoplasia and are thought to have similar etiology. Carcinomas of the vagina are rare and represent 2% to 3% of gynecologic malignancies. Approximately 50% of vaginal cancers arise in the upper third of the vagina (Kirkbride et al, 1995; Stock et al, 1995). The vagina is a common site of metastasis or direct extension from tumors originating in other genital sites, such as the cervix and endometrium, or extragenital sites, such as rectum and bladder. Primary invasive carcinoma of the vagina is predominantly a disease of elderly women, with 70% to 80% of cases presenting in women older than age 60 (except for clear cell carcinomas, which are associated with maternal exposure to diethylstilbestrol [DES]) (Kirkbride et al, 1995). Predisposing factors for carcinoma of the vagina are chronic vaginitis, HPV, herpes simplex virus, and prior pelvic irradiation.

Diagnostic Criteria

Most patients with vaginal intraepithelial neoplasms are asymptomatic at diagnosis. The carcinoma is usually diagnosed during an investigation of an abnormal Pap smear. The FIGO categories are used for staging vaginal cancers (FIGO, 1995).

 CLINICAL WARNING: About 50% to 60% of patients with invasive cancer present with abnormal vaginal bleeding, frequently after coitus. Vaginal discharge, a palpable mass, dyspareunia, and perineal or pelvic pain are other complaints that may be expressed at presentation (Kirkbride et al, 1995).

History and Physical Exam

The workup should include a careful exam of the cervix and vagina, including a bimanual exam. A careful history and assessment of the woman's psychosocial status and needs should be included.

Diagnostic Studies

All patients should have a chest radiograph, complete blood count, and biochemical profile. Cystoscopy and ureteroscopy are strongly recommended for patients with large tumors and tumors involving the anterior wall of the vagina. Proctoscopy is recommended for lesions involving the posterior wall of the vagina.

Treatment Options, Expected Outcomes, and Comprehensive Management

- Stage 0: Management ranges from no treatment for type 1, to laser ablation for type 2, to surgery for type 3.
- Stage I: Radiotherapy is the treatment of choice. Survival rates are 75% to 95%.
- Stage II: Radiotherapy or radical surgery is indicated. Survival rates are 50% to 80%.
- Stages III and IV: Radiotherapy is indicated. Survival rates are 30% to 50% for stage III and 15% to 30% for stage IV (Chyle et al [in press]; Kirkbride et al, 1995; Lee et al, 1994).

CANCER OF THE VULVA

Anatomy, Physiology, and Pathology

The female external genitalia include the mons pubis, labia majora, labia minora, clitoris, vestibular bulb, vestibular glands, and vestibule of the vagina. Together these structures form the vulva.

Vulvar intraepithelial neoplasia is characterized by disruption of the normal epithelial architecture, with giant cells and abnormal nuclei. Squamous cell carcinomas account for more than 90% of vulvar malignancies; atypical keratinization is its hallmark. Anaplastic carcinomas account for 5% of all vulvar cancers, and vulvar melanoma is found in 2% to 4% of vulvar malignancies. Vulvar sarcomas are seen in 1% to 2% of vulvar malignancies (Loret de Mola et al, 1993; Weinstock, 1994).

Epidemiology

Invasive carcinoma of the vulva is a rare disease that accounts for 5% of gynecologic cancers. The median age at diagnosis is 65 to 70 years, and the incidence peaks in women older than 75. In contrast, vulvar carcinoma in situ tends to occur in younger women (ages 45 to 50). Recent studies suggest that HPV could play a role in the etiology of vulvar cancer because it is present in 30% to 50% of diagnosed cases. About 70% of vulvar squamous carcinomas involve the labia majora or minora, most frequently the labia majora. About 15% to 20% involve the clitoris, and a similar proportion arises in the perineum (Ansink et al, 1994; Monk et al, 1995).

Diagnostic Criteria

Patients with vulvar intraepithelial neoplasia may complain of vulvar pruritus, irritation, or a mass, but up to 50% of cases are asymptomatic at the time of diagnosis. Patients with invasive vulvar cancer usually complain of a vulvar mass and chronic vulvar pruritus. Advanced lesions may bleed. In 1983, FIGO adopted a clinical TNM staging system for vulvar cancer (FIGO, 1995).

Diagnostic Studies

- Wedge biopsy: Diagnosis of invasive vulvar cancer requires a wedge biopsy with surrounding skin and underlying dermis and connective tissue so the pathologist can evaluate the depth of stromal invasion. This procedure can be done in the office under local anesthesia.
- Excisional biopsy: This is the preferred method for lesions smaller than 1 cm in diameter. It is done to avoid the possibility of total eradication of the lesion.
- Chest radiograph: All patients with invasive disease require a chest radiograph to rule out metastatic disease.
- Biochemical profile: Standard laboratory work should be obtained in all patients.
- Cystoscopy and proctoscopy: These procedures should be performed in patients with advanced lesions or tumors that are near the urethra or anus, respectively.
- CT or MRI: Because of poor correlation between radiologic and pathologic lymph node findings, the FIGO staging system was modified in 1988 to incorporate more accurate information gained from surgical assessment (FIGO, 1995).

Treatment Options, Expected Outcomes, and Comprehensive Management

The traditional surgical approach to invasive carcinoma of the vulva was radical resection of the vulva and inguinal-femoral nodes. This was the standard of care until the early 1980s. However, because of significant psychological and physical complications, less radical procedures are now used that achieve comparable cure rates. Radiation therapy is gaining popularity as a treatment option (FIGO, 1995).

Referral Points and Clinical Warnings

Vulvar intraepithelial neoplasia is a multifocal disease with a propensity for recurrence. Frequent follow-up by the primary care provider will be necessary for the rest of the woman's life.

ENDOMETRIAL CARCINOMA

Tumors of the uterine fundus represent the most common group of gynecologic malignancies. The incidence is 35,000 cases a year. Four to five thousand women die each year from this disease. Most of the survivors are those who receive treatment early on, when symptoms first occur, using well-established diagnostic guidelines.

Anatomy, Physiology, and Pathology

The uterus is a pear-shaped intrapelvic organ, situated between the bladder and the rectum. It is retained in its position by the round and broad ligaments on each side. Its lumen is covered by a columnar ciliated epithelium intimately connected with the innermost layer, the muscularis mucosae. Uterine fundal cancers are divided into epithelial tumors (90% of all endometrial cancers, typically adenocarcinomas), mesenchymal tumors (5%), mixed tumors (3%), and secondary tumors (2%) (Parker et al, 1996).

Epidemiology

Endometrial carcinoma is a disease of postmenopausal women. The average age at diagnosis is 60 years. Abnormal proliferation and neoplastic transformation of the endometrium have been associated with unopposed estrogen stimulation. It is believed that estrogen-associated cancers progress through a premalignant phase called adenomatous hyperplasia. It is estimated that at least one third of those progress to carcinoma. The best-recognized risk factors for endometrial cancer are chronic estrogen exposure, including oral intake of exogenous estrogen (without progestins); estrogen-secreting tumors; low parity; extended periods of anovulation; early menarche; and late menopause. Morbidly obese women also have a great risk of developing endometrial cancer because their adipocytes can convert androstenedione from the adrenals into estrone, a weak estrogen. Also, women with diabetes and hypertensive disease have been found to have an increased risk of endometrial cancers. The reason for this increased risk is not yet known (Kupelian et al, 1993; Miller et al, 1994).

Diagnostic Criteria

A diagnosis of endometrial carcinoma should be considered in postmenopausal women with any vaginal bleeding, perimenopausal women with heavy or prolonged bleeding, and premenopausal women with abnormal bleeding patterns who are obese or oligo-ovulatory. Before 1988, uterine cancers were staged clinically, but this system was abandoned and replaced by the FIGO surgical staging system (FIGO, 1995).

Diagnostic Studies

- Dilatation and curettage (D&C): This has been the standard technique for tissue collection but is being replaced by endometrial biopsy. D&C is done in the operating room, under anesthesia.
- Endometrial biopsy: When done correctly, with enough tissue obtained, biopsy has a diagnostic accuracy equiva-

lent to that of D&C. It can be performed in the office with no anesthesia.

CLINICAL WARNING: Endometrial biopsy cannot be performed in patients with cervical stenosis or in those unable to tolerate the outpatient procedure.

Treatment Options, Expected Outcomes, and Comprehensive Management

Resection of the primary tumor by total abdominal hysterectomy and bilateral salpingo-oophorectomy is the treatment of choice. Salpingo-oophorectomy is recommended because the ovaries are common sites of occult metastasis and because most women are already postmenopausal and no longer have hormonal function from the organ. Removal of the uterus is curative in most stage I cases (Kupelian et al, 1993).

The survival rate for patients with endometrial carcinoma is clearly related to the surgical stage. Representative 5-year survival rates by stage are 90% for stage I, 60% for stage II, 40% for stage III, and 5% for stage IV (Miller et al, 1994).

Referral Points and Clinical Warnings

Any postmenopausal woman with vaginal bleeding must undergo an endometrial biopsy. If this is not possible, she should be referred for a D&C to obtain a tissue sample for prompt diagnosis.

OVARIAN CARCINOMA

Approximately 15,000 women die of ovarian cancer each year, making this tumor the leading cause of gynecologic deaths. It is estimated that 27,000 new cases of ovarian cancer will be diagnosed annually in the United States (Parker et al, 1996).

Anatomy, Physiology, and Pathology

The ovaries are oval bodies of an elongated form, situated on either side of the uterus. The ovarian fimbria attaches the tubes to the ovaries. Each ovary is attached to the uterus by the ovarian ligament. The surface of the ovary is not covered by peritoneum—hence, the oocyte is expelled into the peritoneal cavity. The ovary consists of a number of graafian follicles that develop and mature uninterruptedly from puberty to the end of the fertile period of a woman's life. Epithelial tumors account for 90% of all ovarian malignancies; the remaining 10% arise from germ or stromal cells (Parker et al, 1996).

Epidemiology

The vast majority of ovarian carcinomas are epithelial in origin and are diagnosed in postmenopausal women (median age 63 years). In the past two decades, there has been an increase in the incidence of ovarian cancers of 0.1% (National Cancer Institute [NCI] Surveillance, 1995). African American women have a lower incidence than white women in the United States (John et al, 1993), with an overall survival rate of 38% for the former and 44% for the latter (NCI Surveillance, 1995). Hormonal, genetic, and environmental factors have all been identified as playing a role in the development of ovarian cancer. Pregnancy decreases the risk and multiple pregnancies have an increasingly protective effect.

Infertility increases the risk for ovarian cancer, as do drugs that stimulate ovulation (Rossing et al, 1994; Whittemore, 1994). A history of breast cancer increases the risk of ovarian cancer. There is a two- to threefold increased risk for breast cancer in women with ovarian cancer. Women who use oral contraceptives have a decreased incidence of ovarian cancer.

With the exception of Japan, industrialized countries have the highest incidences of ovarian cancer. This led to epidemiologic studies examining the association between diet and industrial exposure to carcinogens. Some studies have shown a relation between a diet high in meat and animal fat and a risk of ovarian cancer. No studies have shown an association between exposure to industrial carcinogens and an increased risk of ovarian cancer.

FAMILY HISTORY

The vast majority of ovarian cancers are sporadic; less than 5% of cases can be defined as hereditary ovarian cancers. In contrast to the hereditary ovarian cancer syndromes, in which lifetime probability approaches 50%, a woman with a single family member affected by ovarian cancer has a lifetime risk of 4% to 5% (Carlson et al, 1994; National Institutes of Health [NIH], 1994). This is an increased risk compared with the general population.

CLINICAL WARNING: Family history is the single most important risk factor for the development of ovarian cancer.

Diagnostic Criteria

Epithelial cancers of the ovaries have been described as a silent killer. In the majority of patients, the disease has spread outside the ovary and pelvis at the time of initial presentation. Approximately 70% of patients with epithelial cell tumors will present with stage III or IV disease. Sixty percent of all patients diagnosed with ovarian cancer will be dead in 3 years. Abdominal discomfort and bloating are the most common symptoms, followed by vaginal bleeding, gastrointestinal symptoms, and urinary tract symptoms (Carlson et al, 1994; John et al, 1993; NIH, 1994).

Diagnostic Studies

- Ultrasound: Ultrasound is indicated on discovery of any palpable adnexal mass.
- CT: CT is useful in the preoperative evaluation of the extent of the disease when a pelvic mass is present.
- Serum CA-125: Level is elevated in 80% of patients with an ovarian malignancy. This measurement is also used postoperatively to confirm the effectiveness of treatment.
- Diagnostic laparoscopy: Laparoscopy is used to evaluate unexplained pelvic pain and small masses.
- Peritoneal cytology: Ascitic fluid is aspirated for cytologic exam (Carlson et al, 1994).

Treatment Options, Expected Outcomes, and Comprehensive Management

EARLY-STAGE DISEASE

Patients with early-stage ovarian cancer require no additional therapy after surgical removal of the tumor. For patients with residual disease after surgery, chemotherapy with cisplatin or paclitaxel has become the initial treatment. However, a number of studies have demonstrated that whole-abdominal radiotherapy is also a highly effective treatment. Patients with stage IA and IB disease have a 90% 5-year survival rate with no adjuvant therapy (NIH, 1994).

ADVANCED-STAGE DISEASE

The generally accepted treatment for patients with stage III or IV ovarian cancer has been cytoreductive surgery (aggressive surgery to reduce the bulk of the tumor) followed by chemotherapy. Since 1990, combination chemotherapy with paclitaxel and a platinum compound has been the standard of care in the United States (NIH, 1994).

Referral Points and Clinical Warnings

Patients diagnosed with ovarian cancer should be referred to a gynecologic oncologist for treatment to increase survival rates. Patients should be followed for life with CA-125 measurements at regular intervals to detect recurrence.

GERM CELL TUMORS

Germ cell tumors are much less common than epithelial tumors, but because they affect primarily young women and are highly curable, they should be managed by a gynecologic oncologist promptly. They account for 2% to 3% of all ovarian cancers. Serum tumor markers for alpha-fetoprotein and human chorionic gonadotropin (hCG) are useful in the diagnosis and management of these tumors. Abdominal pain, pelvic fullness, and urinary symptoms are common. In contrast to epithelial tumors, about 60% to 70% of germ cell tumors are stage I at diagnosis. The treatment is surgery, and its importance cannot be overemphasized (Williams, 1996). Most patients can have their fertility conserved by preserving the contralateral ovary and the uterus.

FALLOPIAN TUBE CANCER

Primary malignant neoplasms of the fallopian tubes are exceedingly rare, making this the least common site of a malignant neoplasm in the female tract.

GESTATIONAL TROPHOBLASTIC DISEASE

Gestational trophoblastic disease is a group of conditions resulting from an abnormal fertilization, leading to highly malignant lesions such as choriocarcinoma. Four different entities have been described: molar pregnancy, invasive mole, placental site trophoblastic tumors, and choriocarcinoma.

Metastatic disease occurs in 4% of patients. Rapid growth and a high propensity for hemorrhage make this tumor a medical emergency. Metastases are found in the lungs (80%), vagina (30%), pelvis (20%), brain (10%), and liver (10%) (Williams, 1996).

Epidemiology

Although they constitute less than 1% of gynecologic malignancies, it is important to recognize these lesions: they are potentially life-threatening, but they are highly curable if treated early. The incidence varies widely among populations, with figures as high as 1:120 in Asia and South America, compared with 1:1200 in the United States. The risk is fivefold greater in women 40 years and older and is also increased in those younger than 20 years. Women with prior molar pregnancies, women of lower socioeconomic status, and women with blood group A who are married to group O men are at a higher risk (Carlson et al, 1994; NCI Surveillance, 1995).

Diagnostic Criteria

A molar pregnancy is suspected with first-trimester bleeding, a uterus larger than expected for gestational age, and an absence of fetal heart sounds in association with a markedly elevated hCG level. After evacuation of a molar pregnancy, titers of hCG should disappear in 8 to 10 weeks (Roberts & Mutter, 1994). Persisting hCG may indicate metastatic disease.

Diagnostic Studies

- Diagnostic ultrasound: Ultrasound reveals a "snowstorm" pattern. Vesicular spaces are demonstrated within the uterine cavity, with no evidence of a fetal pole.
- hCG titers: These are useful for diagnosis and follow-up.
- D&C: A diagnostic and therapeutic D&C will furnish tissue for the final diagnosis (Roberts & Mutter, 1994).

Treatment Options, Expected Outcomes, and Comprehensive Management

Chemotherapy is highly effective for all forms of trophoblastic disease. Molar pregnancies should be treated with D&C and close follow-up with hCG titers for a year. In cases of invasion of the myometrium, if hysterectomy was performed, or if fertility is to be preserved, methotrexate alone or in combination with dactinomycin is achieving curative rates. Standard practice includes follow-up with monthly hCG titers until negative for 1 year. Conception can be planned after 1 year free of disease (Berkowitz et al, 1994).

TEACHING AND SELF-CARE

Women should be taught periodically about cervical cancer and its risk factors. This should be part of regular office visits, focusing on a healthy lifestyle. Every women who is sexually active is a potential target for cervical cancer: as noted above, it is directly related to the number of sexual partners a woman has. Other risk factors include cigarette smoking. These habits can be modified if identified early. Women should be taught about protected intercourse to decrease the risk of contracting sexually transmitted diseases. Young women and teenagers should be taught about the risks of early intercourse and pregnancy. They should be given information about the benefits of delaying sexual activity until a later age, when they will be more mature and their bodies as well as their minds will be ready. Also, smoking cessation programs should be readily available and the cause-and-effect correlation of smoking and cervical cancer should be emphasized.

As for all cancers, the patient who is recovering from gynecologic cancer needs to have immediate and ongoing access to support services. Community resources (listed below) should be supplemented by personal support mechanisms. The provider should try to identify whether the patient lacks reliable social support. Patient-centered primary care is never more important than when the patient has a potentially life-threatening disease. The compassionate provider is a good listener, from the time of the initial history-taking, through the time of diagnosis and treatment, and beyond.

The primary care provider should work with the patient in planning a self-care program that is both salient and manageable. Dietary intake will wax and wane with treatment. Referral to a registered dietitian may be needed to support the woman's nutritional requirements throughout this period and beyond. Maintaining a reasonable exercise program—even if minimal at times—can help maintain function as well as promote a sense of well-being.

The provider must be familiar with local counseling resources and support groups. The local office of the American Cancer Society can provide this information. Both counseling and support groups may be important to the patient's emotional and psychological health, and she should consider these services. Outward Bound can be a resource for the recovering woman who desires a personally and physically challenging way of confronting her cancer head-on. Groups are available for women who have survived breast and gynecologic cancers.

For the terminally ill, local hospice services can be recommended.

EDITOR'S NOTE:
COMPLEMENTARY APPROACHES

A general discussion of complementary approaches can be found in Chapter 3. The following, while not an exhaustive list, are some complementary approaches being used for this condition. Additional information on these approaches, including precautions, can be found in Appendices A and B. Providers need to assess for the use of complementary approaches as part of the patient's history, as they may impact conventional therapies, and patients may not volunteer this information unless specifically asked. Efficacy of many complementary approaches is not as well documented as that of conventional therapies. Providers need to read the literature before suggesting these complementary approaches.

- Vitamins, minerals, herbs, supplements
  Betacarotene
- Complementary Modalities
  Aromatherapy

COMMUNITY RESOURCES

- American Cancer Society, 800-ACS-2345, http:/www.cancer.org
- Gilda Radner Familial Ovarian Cancer Registry, 800-682-7426: Information on risk factors, warning signs, and diagnostic tests
- Information and Treatment on Ovarian Cancer, 800-422-6237

- Survivors of Ovarian Cancer, 888-682-7426
- National Cancer Institute, 800-4CANCER
- CanCom—Women's Cancer Information Project, http://www.eurohealth.iecancom/contents.htm: Information on gynecologic cancers, complementary approaches, support groups
- Gynecologic Cancer Inquirer, http://members.sol.com/GynCancer/index.htm: Information on gynecologic cancers
- Introduction to Gynecologic Oncology, http://www.GynCancer.com/: General cancer information and statistics
- OncoLink, University of Pennsylvania Cancer Center, http://www.oncolink.upenn.edu/disease/gynecologic1/: Information on gynecologic cancers
- Gynecologic Cancer Foundation Information Hotline, 800-444-4441
- Society of Gynecologic Oncologists, 1 N. Michigan Ave., Chicago, IL 60611, 312-644-6610, http://www.sgo.org/
- Women's Cancer Center, http://www.wccenter.com/wcctoc.html

REFERRAL POINTS AND CLINICAL WARNINGS

This information is integrated throughout the text.

References

Ansink, A.C., Krul, M.R., De Weger, R.A., et al. (1994). Human papillomavirus, lichen sclerous and squamous cell carcinoma of the vulva: Detection and prognostic significance. *Gynecologic Oncology, 52,* 180.

Berek, J.S., & Hacker, N.F. (1994). *Practical gynecologic oncology.* Baltimore: Williams & Wilkins.

Berkowitz, R.S., Bernstein, M.R., Laborde, O., et al. (1994). Subsequent pregnancy experience with gestational trophoblastic disease. New England Trophoblastic Disease Center, 1965–1992. *Journal of Reproductive Medicine, 39,* 228.

Boring, C.C., Squires, T.S., & Tong, T. (1996). Cancer statistics. *CA: A Journal for Clinicians, 44,* 7.

Burger, M.P.M., & Hollema, H. (1993). The reliability of the histologic diagnosis in colposcopically directed biopsy: A plea for LETZ. *International Journal of Gynecological Cancer, 3,* 385.

Carlson, K.J., Skates, S.J., & Singer, D.E. (1994). Screening for ovarian cancer. *Annals of Internal Medicine, 121,* 124.

Chyle, V., Zagars, G.K., Wheeler, J.A., Wharton, J.T., & Delclos, L. (1998). Definitive radiotherapy for carcinoma of the vagina: Outcome and prognostic factors. *International Journal of Radiation, Oncology, Biology, Physics.*

Duggan, M.A., McGregor, S.E., Benoit, J.L., Inoue, M., Nation, J.G., & Stuart, G.C. (1995). The human papillomavirus status of invasive cervical adenocarcinoma: A clinicopathological and outcome analysis. *Human Pathology, 26,* 319.

Eifel, P.J., Morris, M., Wharton, J.T., & Oswald, M.J. (1994). The influence of tumor size and morphology on the outcome of patients with FIGO stage IB squamous cell carcinoma of the uterine cervix. *International Journal of Radiation, Oncology, Biology, Physics, 29,* 9.

International Federation of Gynecology and Obstetrics. (1994). *Annual report on the results of treatment in gynecologic cancer.* Stockholm: Radium Hemmet.

International Federation of Gynecology and Obstetrics. (1995). Staging announcement: FIGO staging of gynecologic cancers: Cervical and vulva. *International Journal of Gynecological Cancer, 5,* 319.

John, E.M., Whittemore, A.S., Harris, R., et al. (1993). Characteristics relating to ovarian cancer risk: Collaborative analysis of seven U.S. case-control studies: Epithelial ovarian cancer in black women. *Journal of the National Cancer Institute, 85,* 142.

Kirkbride, P., Fyles, A., Rawlings, G.A., et al. (1995). Carcinoma of the vagina: Experience at the Princess Margaret Hospital (1974–1989). *Gynecologic Oncology, 56,* 435.

Koss, L.G. (1993). Cervical (Pap) smear: New directions. *Cancer, 71,* 406.

Kupelian, P.A., Eifel, P.J., Tornos, C., Burke, T.W., Delclos, L., & Oswald, M.J. (1993). Treatment of endometrial carcinoma with radiation therapy alone. *International Journal of Radiation, Oncology, Biology, Physics, 27,* 817.

Kurman, R.J., & Solomon, D. (1994). *The Bethesda system for reporting cervical/vaginal cytologic diagnosis: Definitions, criteria, and explanatory notes for terminology and specimen adequacy.* New York: Springer-Verlag.

Landoni, F., Maneo, A., Colombo, A., et al. (1995). Radical surgery or radiotherapy for cervical carcinoma stage IB-IIA. *International Journal of Gynecological Cancer, 5*(Suppl.), 14.

Lee, W.R., Marcus, R.B., Sombeck, M.D., et al. (1994). Radiotherapy alone for carcinoma of the vagina: The importance of overall treatment time. *International Journal of Radiation, Oncology, Biology, Physics, 29,* 983.

Lien, H.H., Blomlie, V., Iversen, T., Trope, C., Sundfor, K., & Abeler, V.M. (1993). Clinical stage I carcinoma of the cervix: Value of MRI in determining invasion into the parametrium. *Acta Radiologica, 34,* 130.

Loret de Mola, J.R., Hudock, P.A., Steinetz, C., Jacobs, G., McFee, M., & Abdul-Karim, F.W. (1993). Merckel cell carcinoma of the vulva. *Gynecologic Oncology, 51,* 272.

Matthews, C.M., Burke, T.W., Tornos, C., et al. (1993). Stage I adenocarcinoma: Prognostic evaluation of surgically treated patients. *Gynecologic Oncology, 49,* 19.

Miller, B., Morris, M., & Silva, E. (1994). Nucleolar organizer regions: A potential prognostic factor in adenocarcinoma of the endometrium. *Gynecologic Oncology, 54,* 137.

Miller, B.E., Flax, S.D., Arheart, K., & Photopulos, G. (1993). The presentation of adenocarcinoma of the uterine cervix. *Cancer, 72,* 1281.

Monk, B.J., Burger, R.A., Lin, F., Parham, G., Vasilev, S.A., & Wilczynski, S.P. (1995). Prognostic significance of human papillomavirus (HPV) DNA in primary invasive vulvar cancer. *Obstetric Oncology, 85,* 709.

Morris, M., Mitchell, M.F., Silva, E.G, Copeland, L.J., & Gershenson, D.M. (1993). Cervical conization as definitive therapy for early invasive squamous carcinoma of the cervix. *Gynecologic Oncology, 51,* 193.

National Institutes of Health Consensus Development Conference Statement. (1994). Ovarian cancer: Screening, treatment and follow-up. April 5–7, 1994. *Gynecologic Oncology, 55,* S4.

National Cancer Institute Surveillance. (1995). *Epidemiology and end results programs.*

Parker, S.L., Tong, T., Bolden, S., & Wingo, P.A. (1996). Cancer statistics. *CA: A Journal for Clinicians, 46,* 5.

Roberts, D.J., & Mutter, G.L. (1994). Advances in the molecular biology of gestational trophoblastic disease. *Journal of Reproductive Medicine, 39,* 201.

Rossing, M.A., Daling, J.R., Weiss, N.S., et al. (1994). Ovarian tumors in a cohort of infertile women. *N Engl J Med, 331,* 771.

Stock, R.G., Chen, A.S.J., & Seski, J. (1995). A 30-year experience in management of primary carcinoma of the vagina: Analysis of prognostic factors and treatment modalities. *Gynecologic Oncology, 56,* 45.

Weinstock, M.A. (1994). Malignant melanoma of the vulva and vagina in the United States: Patterns of incidence and population-based estimates of survival. *American Journal of Obstetric Oncology, 171,* 1225.

Whittemore, A.S. (1994). The risk of ovarian cancer after treatment of infertility. *N Engl J Med, 331,* 805.

Williams, S.D. (1996). Current management of ovarian germ cell tumors. *Oncology, 8,* 53.

Zur Hausen, H. (1997). Human papillomaviruses and their possible role in squamous cell carcinomas. *Current Topics in Microbiology and Immunology, 78,* 1.

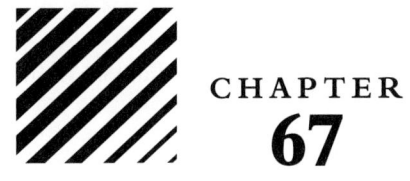

CHAPTER
67

Menopause

Elena M. Umland, PharmD

Menopause is the cessation of ovarian function and the consequent ending of menstruation. Estrogen previously produced by the ovaries is absent. This may occur naturally as part of the female life process or by surgical removal of the ovaries. The number and severity of symptoms experienced vary from woman to woman. Therapy is determined only after close examination of menopausal symptoms, risk factors for the long-term effects of menopause, side effects of the therapeutic agents, and patient preferences. Therapeutic management specific to menopause can be augmented and sometimes replaced by other preventive and health management strategies.

Because women are living longer, the long-term consequences of estrogen depletion in menopause have been identified, along with the short-term menopausal symptoms. Shorter-term symptoms include vasomotor hot flashes and urogenital atrophy. These symptoms occur in up to 85% of menopausal women in the United States (Bonk, 1996; Greendale & Judd, 1993). Long-term complications, which may not occur until years after menopause, include osteoporosis and coronary heart disease (CHD). Understanding which patients are at risk for developing these complications is important in undertaking the management of menopause in primary care.

ANATOMY, PHYSIOLOGY, AND PATHOLOGY

Besides cessation of menstruation and ovarian function, menopause also includes cessation of production of the potent estrogen estradiol. The total production of estrogen, however, does not cease entirely: estrogen production continues in the form of estrone, a weaker form of estrogen. Estrone is produced from the conversion of androstenedione in extraglandular tissue, particularly fat tissue (Wilson & Foster, 1992).

Before menopause, the ovary is very responsive to the two pituitary gonadotropins, follicle-stimulating hormone (FSH) and luteinizing hormone (LH). In high enough concentrations, estrogen produced by the ovary signals the pituitary not to release FSH and LH through negative feedback. As the ovaries age and the follicles produced diminish, estrogen concentrations decline, and the release of FSH and LH is no longer blocked. The concentrations of these hormones rise in an attempt to stimulate the ovary. This period of reduced estrogen production and increased concentrations of FSH and LH may occur 10 years or more before the woman's final menses (Greendale & Judd, 1993). This period is referred to as the perimenopause (Wilson & Foster, 1992).

In understanding the consequences of menopausal estrogen depletion, it is important to know the location of estrogen receptors. Estrogen receptors can be found in the urogenital system, cardiovascular system, and bone. Therefore, the lack of stimulation of these receptors results in certain sequelae.

Table 67-1 presents the manifestations of menopause and its relative estrogen deficit.

SIGNS AND SYMPTOMS

Early manifestations of menopause may begin in the perimenopausal period. Among the most common are vasomotor symptoms. These symptoms may extend for years; urogenital atrophy, another sequela of estrogen depletion, may last an indefinite period of time.

Vasomotor Symptoms

Vasomotor symptoms result from vasomotor instability caused by estrogen depletion and occur in the majority of menopausal women. Eighty percent experience these symptoms for more than 1 year, whereas 25% to 50% continue to experience them for 5 years or more (American College of Obstetrics and Gynecology [ACOG], 1992; Bonk, 1996). Symptoms range in frequency and severity from mild annoyances to true disruptions of everyday life. Some women experience occasional symptoms; others are affected more than three times daily. Difficulty sleeping and concentrating are not uncommon (Leppert & Howard, 1997). This may occur through mood changes and perceived changes in energy level. As may be expected, all of this has the potential to affect a woman's personal life, affecting her relationships with family and close friends.

Urogenital Atrophy

Although not all women experience vasomotor symptoms, urogenital atrophy is a sequela of menopause that is difficult to avoid. Such atrophy normally occurs within 2 or 3 years after menopause (Lemcke et al, 1995). Estrogen receptors are located throughout the urogenital system in the vagina, urethra, and bladder. Urogenital atrophy occurs in the absence of estrogen stimulation. However, not all women will report to the provider the related symptoms, which include thinning and drying of the vaginal epithelium and loss of its elasticity, resulting in pruritus and dyspareunia (Leppert & Howard, 1997). Urinary incontinence is a symptom that is more likely to be reported. Each of these symptoms may hinder the woman's sexual functioning.

Hypoestrogenism also contributes to a decrease in cellular glycogen, with a resultant increase in vaginal pH. This predisposes women to bacterial vaginoses after menopause (Greendale & Judd, 1993).

TABLE 67-1	Manifestations of Menopause	
Early	**Late**
Vasomotor symptoms: hot flashes, night sweats, changes in skin temperature, changes in core body temperature, fluctuations in pulse rate	CHD: angina, stroke, myocardial infarction
Urogenital atrophy: pruritus, dyspareunia, bacterial vaginoses, stress or urge incontinence, dysuria, urgency, or frequency of urination	Osteoporosis: reduced height, fractures, increased mortality risk with fracture (especially hip), reduced quality of life and increased morbidity

Sources: ACOG, 1992; Greendale & Judd, 1993; Leppert & Howard, 1997.

■ ■ ■   **CLINICAL PEARL**

Some of the indications of bacterial vaginosis are the absence of lactobacilli on vaginal microscopy, or the presence of a very low number, and an elevated pH ($>$4.5). The provider should encourage hygiene that helps to keep the vaginal pH in the normal range ($<$4.5 [3.8 to 4.2]). Refer to Chapter 69 for more information.

The late sequelae of menopause are identified in Table 67-1. They include CHD and osteoporosis.

Coronary Heart Disease

CHD is the leading cause of death among women in the United States (ACOG, 1992; Carson, 1994; Lemcke et al, 1995). Forty-six percent of deaths in women were secondary to cardiovascular disease, defined as heart disease, stroke, and atherosclerosis (Greendale & Judd, 1993); this figure is 40% in men. Studies have reported a clear association between the loss of ovarian function and CHD. Because menopause is a gradual process, this increased CHD risk is generally not abrupt. It commonly takes several years for the ovary to cease functioning completely. Women who have undergone bilateral oophorectomy are at risk of developing CHD earlier (Greendale & Judd, 1993).

Several mechanisms of cardioprotection afforded by estrogen include improved lipid metabolism, vasodilation, and positive effects on platelet function, endothelial-derived relaxing factor, prostacyclin, and others (Carson, 1994). Some of these functions are related to estrogen receptor stimulation. Estrogen receptors are located throughout the cardiovascular system. Estrogen receptor stimulation may contribute to vasodilation. In the absence of estrogen and estrogen receptor stimulation, vasodilation may not occur to the greatest extent possible.

Osteoporosis

Osteoporosis is a late manifestation of menopause. Its incidence clearly rises after menopause, when bone loss accelerates to 2% to 3% per year. This loss rate continues for 6 to 10 years, exceeding the premenopausal loss rate of 0.3% to 1.2% (Leppert & Howard, 1997). Increased bone loss and the subsequent development of symptomatic osteoporosis are directly related to reduced estrogen production. The effect of estrogen on bone is

direct. Estrogen receptors are located throughout bone tissue. When stimulated, they inhibit osteoclastic activity (ie, bone resorption) (Carson, 1994). In the absence of estrogen, osteoclastic activity increases, contributing to enhanced bone breakdown and increased fracture risk.

EPIDEMIOLOGY

The average age of menopause in the United States is 52 years. Because the average female life expectancy is 78 years or more, a woman can expect to spend one third of her life in the postmenopausal stage (Greendale & Judd, 1993). The baby-boomers are now entering their fifth decade of life, with 1.2 million women becoming menopausal annually (Ojeda, 1995). Among the factors found to contribute to early menopause (before the average age of 50 to 52 years) are undernourishment and living at high altitudes. Cigarette smoking and the duration of smoking have also been found to correlate with early menopause (Leppert & Howard, 1997; Wilson & Foster, 1992). Some evidence suggests that the age of maternal menopause may correlate with the age of menopause in the daughter (Torgerson et al, 1987). An exhaustive review of the literature indicated that there is little evidence to suggest that race or socioeconomic status affects the age of menopause.

DIAGNOSTIC CRITERIA

The diagnosis of menopause is based on multiple components. The occurrence of irregular cycles, followed by amenorrhea for 1 year, is a hallmark symptom. Within an age-related context, the presence of perimenopausal or menopausal symptoms of estrogen deficiency is classic. Age, however, is not always indicative of menopause: menopause may occur before 40 or as late as 60 (Speroff, 1994). In addition to symptoms and age, laboratory evaluations may also be performed to help confirm the diagnosis.

HISTORY AND PHYSICAL EXAM

The history is important in the diagnosis of menopause. Questions to be asked are listed in Table 67-2. The physical exam includes a Pap smear and pelvic exam. These can assist in the

TABLE 67-2	Questions for Patient History

- Age
- Last menstrual period
- Family history regarding menopause (ie, experience of mother and sister)
- Symptoms and their severity (eg, hot flashes, moodiness, difficulty sleeping, irregular menstrual periods, vaginal dryness)
- Length of time for changes in or absence of menstrual cycle
- Use of tobacco, caffeine, alcohol, recreational drugs
- Typical diet (include salt use and beverage types, including carbonated beverages)
- Complementary therapies, including herbs and dietary or herbal sources for phytoestrogens and progesterones
- Exercise, noting activities, frequency, and typical duration
- Emotional stressors and their management
- Typical sleep pattern, noting any changes

Source: Author

evaluation of the physiologic changes that occur secondary to menopause.

DIAGNOSTIC STUDIES

Ovarian failure is detected by rises in FSH and LH levels (Lemcke et al, 1995; Leppert & Howard, 1997; Northrup, 1994). The concentrations of these hormones rise in response to the failing ovary. They increase in an attempt to stimulate the ovary to produce a dominant follicle. The rise in FSH is 10- to 20-fold; the increase in LH is approximately three times the concentration found before menopause (Leppert & Howard, 1997).

■ ■ ■ CLINICAL PEARL

FSH concentrations greater than 30 mIU/mL are indicative of menopause (Lemcke et al, 1995). LH is not routinely measured for the diagnosis of menopause.

TREATMENT OPTIONS, EXPECTED OUTCOMES, AND COMPREHENSIVE MANAGEMENT

Although menopause itself cannot be prevented, interventions exist to ease this transitional period. It is possible to prevent or alleviate early and late manifestations. Many preventive interventions are related to diet, exercise, and general health promotion.

Vasomotor Symptoms

The vasomotor symptoms of menopause may be prevented or reduced by simple dietary adjustments. These include avoiding foods that may trigger hot flashes (eg, hot, spicy foods, hot drinks, and caffeine). This intervention may be most helpful in reducing the severity of hot flashes (Ojeda, 1995).

Breathing exercises have also been studied in preventing the vasomotor symptoms of menopause (Bonk, 1996; Ojeda, 1995). One exercise consists of taking six to eight deep breaths per minute, inhaling down to the chest or abdomen. This should be done for 15 minutes twice a day. The theory behind this preventive technique is that breathing lowers the arousal of the central nervous system that occurs at the beginning of a hot flash (Bonk, 1996).

Urogenital Symptoms

Urogenital atrophy has numerous consequences, including dyspareunia, increased risk of bacterial vaginoses and urinary tract infection, and incontinence.

■ ■ ■ CLINICAL PEARLS

Dyspareunia can be prevented through continued regular, frequent intercourse. This contributes to lubrication and the improvement of muscle tone (Ojeda, 1995). Techniques to prevent urinary tract infections and bacterial vaginoses

TABLE 67-3	Lifestyle Interventions to Help Prevent UTIs and Bacterial Vaginoses

- Void the bladder completely and without delay.
- Empty the bladder after sexual intercourse.
- Avoid tight clothes such as jeans and pantyhose worn without cotton panties.
- Wear cotton-crotch underpants and pantyhose.
- Increase fluid intake.
- If prone to or currently experiencing bacterial vaginosis, use a condom during intercourse to minimize exposure to the alkaline spermatic fluid.
- Avoid douching.

Source: Ojeda, 1995.

include various lifestyle interventions (Table 67-3). These topics are also covered extensively in Chapters 34 and 69.

The prevention of urinary incontinence centers around strengthening and developing the urogenital muscles by means of techniques such as Kegel exercises (see Chap. 34). These exercises may also help to improve sexual satisfaction (Ojeda, 1995).

Coronary Heart Disease and Osteoporosis

CHD and osteoporosis can be prevented. Preventive measures should start before menopause and continue through and after menopause. Regular visits to the primary care provider throughout this time can ensure early diagnosis of menopause, leading to the initiation of preventive measures and prompt treatment for its manifestations. Prevention begins by reducing or eliminating risk factors for CHD and osteoporosis (Table 67-4).

General preventive guidelines include eating a diet low in saturated fats and cholesterol that includes adequate amounts

TABLE 67-4	Risk Factors for the Long-Term Consequences of Menopause

CHD	Osteoporosis
Age >55 years or postmenopausal and not taking estrogen	Age >65 years
Tobacco use	Reduced weight for height
Hypertension	Premature or surgical menopause
Diabetes mellitus	Race: Asian or White
High-density lipoprotein <35 mg/dL	Sedentary lifestyle
Family history (mother or first-degree female relative diagnosed with CHD before 65 years; father or first-degree male relative diagnosed with CHD before 55 years)	Low calcium intake
	High alcohol consumption
	Tobacco use
	Consumption of carbonated beverages daily
Obesity	

Source: Lemcke et al, 1995, Eckel et al, 1998.

of calcium and vitamin D. Smoking cessation and regular aerobic, weight-bearing exercise are also of extreme importance in the prevention and treatment of osteoporosis and CHD.

Treatment Options, Expected Outcomes, and Comprehensive Management

In conjunction with the dietary and lifestyle changes, pharmacologic interventions are common. Estrogen hormonal replacement therapy (HRT) can prove useful for some women. Table 67-5 lists the contraindications to HRT.

Estrogen products are manufactured in various formulations, such as oral tablets, transdermal patches, vaginal creams, and vaginal ring inserts. Choosing the most appropriate formulation depends on the indication. HRT may be used for menopausal symptom management, reduction of CHD and osteoporosis risk, and treatment of osteoporosis.

Table 67-6 lists common estrogen and progesterone formulations currently available and their place in therapy.

Estrogen alone has been shown to reduce the risk of developing CHD by 56% (Leppert & Howard, 1997). When combined with a progestin, this reduction in risk declines to 20% to 25% (Gibaldi, 1996). There is insufficient evidence to indicate the age after which primary prevention with estrogen would no longer be effective. Certain investigators support the use of estrogen, regardless of age, if one or more risk factors for CHD are present (Gibaldi, 1996).

Secondary prevention of CHD has also been described. Estrogen afforded a 96% survival rate at 10 years in women with mild to moderate CHD, compared with 85% in women not receiving estrogen. In women with severe CHD, estrogen users had a 97% 10-year survival, compared with 60% in women not receiving estrogen (Gibaldi, 1996).

Osteoporosis also has been prevented and treated with HRT. Although data initially indicated a need to take estrogen for 7 to 10 years after menopause, the longer a woman is treated with estrogen, the greater her reduction in osteoporosis risk (Belchetz, 1994; Gibaldi, 1996; Felson et al, 1993). Very recent data have supported the position that estrogen started after age 60 and continued indefinitely offers bone-conserving effects similar to those in women who started estrogen at menopause and continued (Arky, 1997; Schneider et al, 1997). Regardless of when it is initiated, HRT confers conserving effects on bone density (Gibaldi, 1996).

Despite the observed CHD and osteoporosis risk reduction, much discussion exists regarding the prescription of HRT in women with a personal or family history of breast cancer. Both issues are controversial. The role of estrogen use in increasing breast cancer risk has not been clearly illustrated. Studies vary,

TABLE 67-5 Contraindications to HRT

- Active thrombophlebitis or thromboembolic disorder
- Known or suspected breast cancer or estrogen-dependent neoplasia
- Pregnancy
- Liver disease
- Undiagnosed or abnormal vaginal bleeding
- Migraine headaches
- Cholelithiasis

Source: Carson, 1994.

showing no increase in risk to up to a 30% risk increase (Isaacs & Swain, 1994).

CLINICAL PEARL

The approach often taken to HRT includes risk assessment. A woman's risk factors for breast cancer are compared to the potential benefits regarding CHD and osteoporosis. A 50-year-old woman has a 46% lifetime risk of developing CHD, a 15% hip fracture risk, and an 8% risk for breast cancer. HRT with estrogen and progestin appears to reduce the risk of CHD to 20% to 25% and the hip fracture risk to 5% to 10% (Gibaldi, 1996). The maximum potential increase in breast cancer risk is 30% above baseline (Isaacs & Swain, 1994). Risks and benefits must be assessed. Patient and provider alike need to ask whether the woman's risk of breast cancer outweighs the potential benefits to be gained in terms of prevention or mitigation of CHD and osteoporosis.

CLINICAL WARNING: It is currently recommended that a woman with an intact uterus receiving oral or transdermal estrogen also receive progesterone to reduce her risk of developing endometrial hyperplasia, a risk factor for the development of endometrial cancer. The landmark trial of postmenopausal estrogen and progestin interventions (PEPI) assessed the risk of estrogen-related endometrial hyperplasia. The researchers concluded that a woman's risk of developing endometrial hyperplasia secondary to receiving progesterone and estrogen is comparable to that observed when given placebo (Writing Group for the PEPI Trial, 1996). These results occurred whether the progesterone (medroxyprogesterone acetate) was cycled at 10 mg/day for 12 days of the month or given continuously at 2.5 mg/day. None to 1% of those receiving placebo developed endometrial hyperplasia. The risk of hyperplasia in those receiving estrogen alone was as high as 27.7%.

The side effects that may result from these therapeutic interventions vary widely and are affected by the choice of HRT regimen and the duration of use (Table 67-7). The side effects of HRT use are listed in Table 67-8.

CLINICAL PEARL

One of the effects of HRT is menstrual bleeding. This is to be expected when a woman with an intact uterus begins HRT. The pattern of bleeding, however, varies depending on the regimen chosen. Generally, spotting is noted throughout the 28-day cycle of a woman receiving the continuous combined or cyclic combined regimen. This effect can be expected to occur for several months, even up to a year, before the woman becomes amenorrheic. Alternatively, a regular cyclic menstrual period can be anticipated in women who receive the continuous sequential or cyclic sequential regimen.

Teaching and Self-Care

The menopausal woman should be made aware of the following vitamin and mineral requirements in an effort to reduce her risk of osteoporosis:

TABLE 67-6 — Common Estrogen Formulations and FDA-Approved Uses

Agent	FDA-Approved Uses[1,2]	Dosage Forms[3]	Common Starting Doses
ESTROGEN			
Estradiol	s,o	tab, td, vcr	tab = 1–2 mg/day td = 0.05 mg/day patch applied weekly vcr = 2–4 g/day
Ethinyl estradiol	s	tab	tab = 0.02–0.05 mg/day
Estrone sulfate/conjugated equine estrogen	s,o	tab, vcr, iv, im	tab = 0.625 mg/day vcr = 1–2 gm/day
Estropipate	s,o	tab, vcr	tab = 0.75–3 mg/day vcr = 2–4 g/day
Estrone sulfate/conjugated equine estrogen combined with medroxyprogesterone acetate	s,o	tab	tab = 0.625 mg/day estrogen plus 2.5 mg/day progesterone component
PROGESTERONE			
Medroxyprogesterone acetate	*	tab	tab = 2.5–10 mg/day**

Sources: Northrup, 1994, and Arky, 1997.

[1] The FDA-approved indications may not apply to all the brand-name drugs. For specific brand-name indications, see the package insert of that specific agent.

[2] s, symptoms including vasomotor and urogenital; o, osteoporosis prevention. CHD is not included here because it is not an approved indication for HRT use.

[3] tab, oral tablet; td, transdermal patch; vcr, vaginal cream; iv, intravenous; im, intramuscular.

* Indicated for use in conjunction with estrogen for the prevention of endometrial hyperplasia in postmenopausal women who have an intact uterus and are receiving estrogen therapy.

** Dose depends on the HRT regimen chosen (ie, sequential versus combined).

TABLE 67-7 — HRT Regimens

Regimen	How Administered	Compliance	Notes
Continuous combined	e = every day p = every day	Best	Vaginal bleeding pattern irregular; majority of women amenorrheic after 8–12 months
Continuous sequential	e = every day p = first 9–14 days of the month	Favorable	Vaginal bleeding regular and predictable in 50% to 80% of women
Cyclic combined	e = 25 of 30 days p = 25 of 30 days No therapy on days 26–30	Not ideal	Vaginal bleeding extremely unpredictable; estrogen deficiency symptoms possible days 26–30
Cyclic sequential	e = 25 of 30 days p = last 10–14 days of the 25 days No therapy on days 26–30	Not ideal	Vaginal bleeding predictable around the end of the progesterone therapy; estrogen deficiency symptoms possible days 26–30

e, estrogen; p, progesterone
Sources: Northrup, 1994; Young & Koda-Kimble, 1995.

TABLE 67-8	Side Effects of HRT

- Nausea, vomiting
- Dizziness
- Weight gain
- Breast tenderness, and enlargement
- Endometrial hyperplasia (when estrogen is used alone in a woman with an intact uterus)
- Increased risk of breast cancer (not conclusively established)

Sources: Northrup, 1994; Young & Koda-Kimble, 1995.

- 400 to 800 IU/day of vitamin D and at least 1000 mg/day of calcium (1500 mg/day of calcium in a woman not receiving HRT) (Ojeda, 1995). These requirements can be met through either supplementation or diet.
- Boron (a trace element) may be beneficial in preventing osteoporosis. In a dose of 2 to 12 mg/day, it may reduce urinary calcium loss and increase serum levels of estradiol (Torgerson et al, 1987). One study showed a 44% reduction in urinary calcium excretion with a dose of 3 mg daily (Ojeda, 1995). It can be found naturally in foods, including fruits, nuts, and vegetables.

Other self-care strategies for managing the symptoms associated with menopause are listed in Table 67-9. More information is given in the "Editor's Note: Complementary Ap-

TABLE 67-9	Self-Care Strategies for the Menopausal Woman

LIFESTYLE CHANGES

Following approval of the provider, exercise for 25–30 minutes 3 to 6 days/week.

Weight-bearing exercise such as walking, jogging, or bike-riding is preferable.

Cross-train with site-specific exercises to upper and lower extremities.

Balance and strength-building exercises such as tai chi or yoga are often helpful.

Try to revise lifestyle, being aware of sources for stress.

Develop stress-relieving interventions.

DIET AND NUTRITION

Eat a well-balanced diet that includes adequate dairy intake, fresh fruits and vegetables, and grains and pastas.

Use the food pyramid as a guide to serving sizes.

Limit fats and sweets, avoid fried foods, and limit serving sizes of meats.

Limit daily caffeine and alcohol intake, and avoid tobacco products and recreational drugs.

HOT FLASHES

In addition to lifestyle interventions, dress in layers.

Avoid stimuli that trigger hot flashes, including caffeine and alcohol.

Eat smaller, more frequent meals.

Avoid spicy foods if these seem to trigger flashes.

Some women report that drinking a cold beverage at the beginning of a flash is cooling.

Keep a log to determine triggers if needed.

VAGINAL ATROPHY/DRYNESS

Continue sexual activity/vaginal stimulation.

Maintain adequate fluid intake—at least 8 to 10 8-oz glasses of water/day.

Water-soluble lubricants such as Astroglide, K-Y jelly, and Replens (a bioadhesive vaginal moisturizer) are very effective. Dietary oils (eg, vegetable oils) are inexpensive alternatives to commercial lubricants, but they will stain fabrics.

■ **CLINICAL WARNING:**
Clinical Warning: Vaseline and other brands of petroleum-based products are insoluble in water. Their intravaginal use could pose a theoretical risk for embolus.

INSOMNIA

Decrease emotional stress, exercise regularly, and avoid eating before bedtime.

Limit caffeine and alcohol, and avoid altogether before bedtime if these interfere with rest.

Develop a bedtime routine.

Use the bedroom for sleep or sexual activity only—watch television, listen to music, or read in a different space.

Sleep disturbances can become opportunities. If sleep is delayed for 30 minutes, get up and undertake some sort of quiet activity until sleepiness returns. Sometimes warm milk or herbal tea may be soothing.

MOOD SWINGS AND FUZZY THINKING

Decrease emotional stress, exercise regularly, and eat as outlined earlier.

Limit caffeine and alcohol.

Avoid tobacco and recreational drugs.

Make lists for organizing. Some women find that keeping lists in a consistent place (such as the right-hand pocket of a coat worn that day) can help prevent forgetting where one has put the list.

Join a menopause support group.

Become involved in community volunteer efforts.

■ **CLINICAL WARNING:**
Clinical Warning: Advise the patient to seek out help from the primary care provider if depression develops.

DECREASED LIBIDO

Treat vaginal atrophy/dryness as previously discussed.

Use a water-soluble lubricant with intercourse.

Increase foreplay before intercourse.

Plan to have intercourse when rested rather than when tense or tired.

Refer to Chapter 34 for management strategies for urinary incontinence issue.

Sources: Butler et al., 1994; Doughty, 1996; Lichtman, 1996; Nachtigall, 1994; Ravnikar, 1994; Wolfson et al., 1996.

proaches" box, which appears at the end of the chapter. As Table 67-9 demonstrates, the range of therapeutic options for menopause management is extensive and can include changes in diet, exercise, and sleep patterns. These options help the provider to individualize therapy.

CLINICAL WARNING: Decisions about the choice of interventions must take into account various factors, including age and concomitant disease states.

COMMUNITY RESOURCES

Clinics specializing in women's health are becoming more popular, and providers should determine whether their local area has such a clinic. Two such clinics are:

- Center for Climacteric Studies, University of Florida, 901 N.W. 8th Ave., Suite B1, Gainesville, FL 32601
- North American Menopause Society, University Hospitals Dept. of OB/GYN, 2074 Abington Rd., Cleveland, OH 44106

Information on the compounding of natural estrogen products and estrogen and progesterone products that are not commercially available can be obtained from:

- Bajamar Women's Health Care, 800-255-8025
- Women's International Pharmacy, 800-279-5708

Menopause-related newsletters include:

- *Berkeley Wellness Newsletter*, University of California, Berkeley, P.O. Box 10922, Des Moines, IA 50340
- *Midlife Wellness*, Center for Climacteric Studies, University of Florida, 901 N.W. 8th Ave., Suite B1, Gainesville, FL 32061
- *Hot Flash: Newsletter for Midlife and Older Women*, School of Allied Health Professionals, State University of New York, Stony Brook, NY 11794

Internet resources include:

- Endocrine Metabolic Consultants, http://www.endocrineconsultants.com/page1[htm]
- North American Menopause Society, P.O. Box 94527, Cleveland, OH 44101, 216-844-8748, http://www.menopause.org/home.htm
- Doctor's Guide to Menopause Information and Resources, Http://www.pslgroup.com/menopause.htm
- Menopause Matters, http://world.std.com/susan207/
- Women's Health Hot Line Home Page, Http://www.soft-design.com/softinfo/womens-health.html: An on-line newsletter on women's health issues
- Healthtouch Menopause Information Page, Http://www.healthtouch.com/level1/leaflets/101323/110367.htm

REFERRAL POINTS AND CLINICAL WARNINGS

The primary care provider is an important resource for education and care during menopause and its sequelae. Sometimes referral to a specialist may be necessary, for instance for a woman who has a history of breast, uterine, or ovarian cancer (Leppert & Howard, 1997). If HRT is being considered, a consulting specialist may be invaluable in assessing the appropriateness of therapy and the patient's risks and benefits. The advice of a registered dietitian can be helpful because nutritional considerations directly affect the woman's risk for CHD and osteoporosis. The dietitian can offer tips about food choice and preparation.

EDITOR'S NOTE:
COMPLEMENTARY APPROACHES

A general discussion of complementary approaches can be found in Chapter 3. The following, while not an exhaustive list, are some complementary approaches being used for this condition. Additional information on these approaches, including precautions, can be found in Appendices A and B. Providers need to assess for the use of complementary approaches as part of the patient's history, as they may impact conventional therapies, and patients may not volunteer this information unless specifically asked. Efficacy of many complementary approaches is not as well documented as that of conventional therapies. Providers need to read the literature before suggesting these complementary approaches.

- Complementary Modalities
  Aromatherapy

References

American College of Obstetrics and Gynecology. (1992). Hormone replacement therapy. *ACOG Technical Bulletin, 166*, 1–7.

Arky, R. (1997). *Physicians' desk reference.* Montvale, NJ: Medical Economics Company.

Belchetz, P.E. (1994). Hormonal treatment of postmenopausal women. *N Engl J Med, 330*(15), 1062–1071.

Bonk, M. (1996). *Controlling hormones naturally.* Minneapolis: MB Publishers.

Butler, R.N., Lewis, M.I., Hoffman, E., & Whitehead, E.D. (1994). Love and sex after 60: How to evaluate and treat the sexually active woman. *Geriatrics, 49*, 33–42.

Carson, D.S. (1994). Postmenopausal hormonal replacement therapy. *Clinical Pharmacy Newswatch, 1*(8), 1–6.

Doughty, S.E.D. (1996). Menopause: A holistic look at an important transition to the last and best third of life. *Topics in Geriatric Rehabilitation, 11*, 7–15.

Eckel, R.H., Krauss, R.M. (1998). American Heart Association call to action: Obesity as a major risk factor for coronary heart disease. *Circulation, 97*(21), 2099–2100.

Felson, D.T., Zhang, Y., Hannan, M.T., et al. (1993). The effect of postmenopausal estrogen therapy on bone density in elderly women. *N Engl J Med, 329*(16), 1141–1146.

Gibaldi, M. (1996). Hormone replacement therapy: Estrogen after menopause. *Pharmacotherapy, 16*(3), 366–375.

Greendale, G.A., & Judd, H.L. (1993). The menopause: Health implications and clinical management. *Journal of the American Geriatric Society, 41*(4), 426–436.

Isaacs, C.J.D., & Swain, S.M. (1994). Hormone replacement therapy in women with a history of breast carcinoma. *Hematology/Oncology Clinics of North America, 8*(1), 179–195.

Lemcke, D.P., Pattison, J., Marshall, L.A., & Cowley, D.S. (1995). *Primary care of women.* Norwalk, CT: Appleton and Lange.

Leppert, P.C., & Howard, F.M. (1997). *Primary care for women.* Philadelphia: Lippincott-Raven.

Lichtman, R. (1996). Perimenopausal and postmenopausal hormone replacement therapy: Part 2. Hormone regimes and complementary and alternative therapies. *Journal of Nurse Midwifery, 41,* 195–210.

Nachtigall, L.E. (1994). A comparative study: Replens versus local estrogen in menopausal women. *Fertility and Sterility, 61,* 178–180.

Northrup, C. (1994). *Women's bodies, women's wisdom.* New York: Bantam Books.

Ojeda, L. (1995). *Menopause without medicine.* Alameda, CA: Hunter House.

Ravnikar, V.A. (1993). Diet, exercise, and lifestyle in preparation for menopause. *Obstetrics and Gynecology Clinics of North America, 20,* 365–378.

Schneider, D.L., Barrett-Connor, E.L., & Morton, D.J. (1997). Timing of postmenopausal estrogen for optimal bone mineral density: The Rancho Bernardo Study. *JAMA, 277*(7), 543–547.

Speroff, L. (1994). The menopause: A signal for the future. In R.A. Lobo (Ed.). *Treatment of the postmenopausal woman: Basic and clinical aspects.* New York: Raven.

Torgerson, D.J., Avenell, A., Russell, I.T., et al. (1987). Factors associated with onset of menopause in women aged 45–49. *Maturitas, 19,* 83–92.

Wilson, J.D., & Foster, D.W. (1992). *Williams' textbook of endocrinology.* Philadelphia: W.B. Saunders.

Wolfson, L., Whipple, R., Derby, C., et al. (1996). Balance and strength training in older adults: Intervention gains and tai chi maintenance. *Journal of the American Geriatrics Society, 44,* 498–506.

Writing Group for the PEPI Trial. (1996). Effects of hormone replacement therapy on endometrial histology in postmenopausal women. *JAMA, 275*(5), 370–375.

Young, L.E., & Koda-Kimble, M.A. (1995). *Applied therapeutics: The clinical use of drugs.* Vancouver, WA: Applied Therapeutics, Inc.

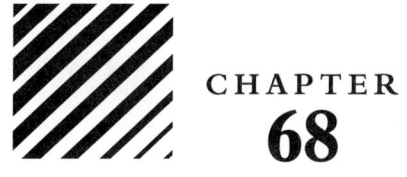

CHAPTER

68

Prostatic Disease

Matthew R. Anderson, MD

Three diagnoses—benign prostatic hyperplasia (BPH), prostate cancer, and prostatitis—represent the core of prostatic disease in primary care. BPH and prostate cancer have assumed increasing importance as the population of North America ages. Prostate cancer is now the most commonly diagnosed noncutaneous tumor and the second leading cause of cancer death in men (American Cancer Society [ACS], 1997).

The field of prostate disease is mired in controversy. It is unclear whether screening for prostate cancer is beneficial; recommendations by professional bodies have been widely divergent. Disagreement exists over which treatment is best for localized prostate cancer. The answers to these questions should become clearer in the next decade. Until then, primary care providers and their patients will have to make difficult decisions based on inadequate data.

Despite these ambiguities, the primary care provider plays a key role in the management of prostatic diseases, even though much of prostate-related care is handled by specialists. Patients come to their primary care provider first with their concerns, symptoms, or anxieties. Despite referral to a specialist, the primary care provider retains an important responsibility to counsel patients and verify that they are receiving accurate advice. In caring for men throughout their life cycle, the primary care provider offers them support in coping with their symptoms, the morbidities of interventions (eg, erectile dysfunction and incontinence), and the realities of a much-feared terminal illness.

ANATOMY, PHYSIOLOGY, AND PATHOPHYSIOLOGY

The base of the prostate lies superiorly against the bladder; the apex lies below, against the urogenital diaphragm. The anterior aspect of the prostate lies against the symphysis pubis, whereas the posterior aspect sits in front of the rectum. Only the posterior aspect of the prostate is palpable.

The prostate contains multiple epithelial glands that produce a thin, milky secretion. This secretion drains via approximately 25 ducts into the back of the urethra. Smooth muscle in both the prostatic capsule and stroma contracts during ejaculation, expelling the secretion into the ejaculate. The prostatic secretion is alkaline, in contrast to the other components of the ejaculate and to the vaginal pH, both of which are acidic. Because sperm are optimally motile at a higher (ie, more alkaline) pH, the prostatic secretion may play a role in maintaining a suitable pH for sperm.

Understanding of the pathophysiology and natural history of prostate conditions is still fragmentary. The relation between the clinical entity of "prostatism" and the prostate gland is obscure. The cause of chronic nonbacterial prostatitis, the most common type of prostatitis, is not clearly known. How to distinguish the prostate cancers that are aggressive from those that are indolent remains a mystery.

DIAGNOSTIC CRITERIA AND HISTORY

Benign Prostatic Hyperplasia

Tradition has divided symptoms of "prostatism" into those of obstruction (hesitancy, poor flow, intermittency, abdominal straining, feeling of not fully emptying bladder, dribbling, and double voiding) and those of irritation (dysuria, nocturia, urgency or urge incontinence, and frequency). A seven-question symptom index was developed by the American Urological Association (AUA) to evaluate the response to therapies for BPH (Table 68-1). The index is used in some settings for making clinical decisions (Barry & O'Leary, 1995).

More recent research has cast doubt on the relation between "prostatism" and the prostate gland. Urodynamic studies and transrectal ultrasound (TRUS) have demonstrated that the AUA symptoms are neither sensitive nor specific for prostatic obstruction. The AUA symptom index is not even statistically related to a number of anatomic and physiologic variables, such as the peak urinary flow rate or the postvoid residual, which are thought to be associated with urinary obstruction. A study of unselected adults age 55 to 79 found no significant differences between AUA symptom scores in men and women (Lepor & Machi, 1993). It would probably be more appropriate to consider these as symptoms of lower urinary tract dysfunction rather than prostate disease. The differential diagnosis for such dysfunction includes cystitis, bladder cancer, ureteral stricture, bladder diverticulae, neurogenic bladder, bladder neck dyssynergia, ureteral stricture, and bladder calculi.

Symptoms of prostatism also need to be evaluated with a sense of how bothersome they are for the patient. Many men find their voiding symptoms tolerable and would prefer not to undergo treatment that has important potential morbidities.

Prostate Cancer

Prostate cancer is often asymptomatic until well advanced. It can cause erectile dysfunction or symptoms of obstruction. More commonly, it presents with metastatic disease. Bony pain is typical in metastatic disease; the pain location depends on the area of tumor spread. Frank spinal cord compression or other neurologic compromise also can occur (Palmer & Chodak, 1996).

Prostatitis

Prostatitis presents with a broad array of symptoms. These may include the classic symptoms of prostatism or symptoms of dyspareunia (painful ejaculation). The patient with bacterial pros-

TABLE 68-1	AUA Symptom Index

Questions To Be Answered	AUA Symptom Score (Circle 1 Number on Each Line)					
	Not At All	Less Than 1 Time in 5	Less Than Half the Time	About Half the Time	More Than Half the Time	Almost Always
1. Over the past month, how often have you had a sensation of not emptying your bladder completely after you finished urinating?	0	1	2	3	4	5
2. Over the past month, how often have you had to urinate again less than 2 hours after you finished urinating?	0	1	2	3	4	5
3. Over the past month, how often have you found you stopped and started again several times when you urinated?	0	1	2	3	4	5
4. Over the past month, how often have you found it difficult to postpone urination?	0	1	2	3	4	5
5. Over the past month, how often have you had a weak urinary stream?	0	1	2	3	4	5
6. Over the past month, how often have you had to push or strain to begin urination?	0	1	2	3	4	5
7. Over the past month, how many times did you most typically get up to urinate from the time you went to bed at night until the time you got up in the morning?	0 (None)	1 (1 time)	2 (2 times)	3 (3 times)	4 (4 times)	5 (5 times or more)

Sum of 7 circled numbers (AUA Symptom Score):
AUA score: Mild (0–7 points); moderate (8–19 points); severe (20–35 points)

Source: Barry, M., & O'Leary, M. (1995). The development and clinical utility of symptom scores. *Urologic Clinics of North America, 22*(2), 299–307.

tatitis may present with fever and septic shock. Prostatodynia refers to a poorly understood symptom complex of pain that can be experienced in the perineal or rectal area or lower back. The prostate gland itself may not be the cause of prostatodynia.

Hematospermia (bloody ejaculate) generally reflects disease of either the prostate or seminal vesicles. Hematuria may suggest prostatic disease but can arise from anywhere in the genitourinary tract. Incontinence is not generally a result of purely prostatic disease.

HISTORY AND PHYSICAL EXAM

The prostate examination (digital rectal examination [DRE]) tends to be uncomfortable for the patient, but it can provide important diagnostic information. Its value as a screening test is controversial.

CLINICAL WARNING:
- Perform DRE very gently in a patient with acute bacterial prostatitis.

As the palpating finger moves superiorly above the anorectal junction, the prostate is felt as a walnut-sized mass.

CLINICAL PEARLS
- Before beginning the exam, inform the patient that it is normal to feel a desire to urinate as the prostate is palpated.
- The median sulcus is easily palpated, as are two lateral lobes. The seminal vesicles lie superior to the prostate and are not normally palpable.

- The examiner can palpate only the posterior surface of the prostate; any anterior lesion will escape detection. This is an important limitation of the DRE.

Several characteristics of the prostate examination have diagnostic importance:

- **Consistency:** The various consistencies of the prostate gland can be illustrated on the hand (Sapira, 1990). The normal consistency of the prostate gland is that of the thenar eminence when contracted—for example, when the thumb is opposed to the little finger. When the muscle is relaxed, it gives the boggy feel of a benign enlarged prostate. Hard nodules are like the bony prominences of the hand; indurated areas are like those of the taut extensor pollices.
- **Symmetry:** Asymmetry of the prostate can indicate carcinoma.
- **Nodularity:** In general, inflammatory nodules are raised; cancerous ones are not. A prostate cancer is often obvious as a hard mass. This mass may extend beyond the capsule of the prostate and fix the organ to the pelvic wall.
- **Size:** The normal size of a prostate is best learned with practice. It is described as being the size of a plum, a golf ball, or a walnut. Urologists often estimate the size in grams. A normal-sized prostate is said to be 20 g, a lemon-sized prostate 35 g, and a baseball-sized prostate 60 g.

CLINICAL PEARL
The size of the prostate on palpation does not correlate with the degree of urethral obstruction. Estimation of prostate size is not particularly useful diagnostically. However, prostate size may influence the choice of therapy for BPH.

Prostatic Massage

Prostatic massage is done to evaluate patients with symptoms of chronic prostatitis. Prostatic massage is not done in acute prostatitis for fear of precipitating bacteremia. Prostatic massage is done either alone or as part of a three-glass test (also known as the four-glass test). This test is described below. Expressed prostatic secretions (EPS) should be cultured for bacteria and mycobacteria. Additional cultures for gonococci and parasites may be appropriate in certain settings.

Prostatic massage is best accomplished by rolling rather than pushing the finger, as this is gentler on the rectum. The basic motion is that of massaging toward the midline of the prostate and down. An occasional patient will have no secretions at the tip of his penis after massage; these patients can be instructed to milk the penis. If no secretions are obtained at this point, the patient should void a few drops of urine, which will contain liquid from the prostate.

Normal prostatic secretions contain lecithin bodies and epithelial cells. The presence of many white cells is diagnostic for prostatitis. Experts disagree on the exact number, but 10 white cells per high-power field is generally accepted as evidence of prostatitis. The presence of fat-laden macrophages is specific for prostatic inflammation (Tanagho & McAninch, 1995).

Estimation of Bladder Size

In patients with prostatic obstruction, it is important to evaluate for possible urinary retention, either acute or chronic. Patients with chronic retention can have massively enlarged bladders and still be relatively or entirely asymptomatic.

Approximately 400 cc of urine must be present in the bladder before it can be palpated suprapubically. A more sensitive method is percussion.

■ ■ ■ ■ CLINICAL PEARLS

- The presence of a dull percussive note one fingerbreadth above the symphysis is a reliable sign that there is at least 100 cc of urine in the bladder (Boyarsky & Goldenberg, 1962).
- An alternate technique uses auscultatory percussion (Guarino, 1985). The diaphragm of the stethoscope is placed just above the symphysis and the finger percusses caudally from the subcostal area. The point at which the auscultatory note changes is a reliable indicator of bladder height. An estimated height 1 cm above the stethoscope's diaphragm corresponds to a bladder volume of approximately 100 cc. Experience and confidence with these techniques can be gained if they are practiced before assessing a postvoid residual.

Postvoid Residual

If there is doubt concerning the size of the bladder, a postvoid residual can be obtained with a Foley catheter or by using ultrasound. Ultrasound is obviously less traumatic for the patient but may not be available in all clinics. In general, postvoid values of more than 50 to 100 cc of urine are considered evidence of retention.

DIAGNOSTIC STUDIES

Evaluation of Urine and Prostatic Secretions

A basic urinalysis and urine culture should be performed in all patients with prostatic symptoms. EPS are generally cultured as part of the three- or four-glass test (Doble, 1994). Patients collect two urine samples before prostatic massage but should not fully empty the bladder at this time. The first two samples are labeled voided bladder 1 (VB1, the first 10 cc of urine voided) and VB2 (a midstream sample). After prostatic massage, an additional two samples are collected: the EPS and VB3 (the first 10 cc of urine voided after the EPS). VB1 is considered a urethral sample, VB2 is a sample of bladder contents, and VB3 is a 1:100 dilution of prostatic secretions. Figure 68-1 describes this test and its significance.

Three general patterns emerge in the three-glass test:

- Bladder infections cause all four samples to show evidence of bacterial infection.
- Urethral infection causes higher colony counts in the VB1 sample than in the EPS or VB3 sample.
- Prostatitis causes the opposite pattern, ie, higher colony counts in EPS and VB3 than VB1 or VB2.

Serum Chemistries

The serum creatinine is used to evaluate kidney function. Acid and alkaline phosphatase played important roles historically in the management of prostate cancer, but these tests have been supplanted by PSA in current practice.

Prostate-Specific Antigen

PSA is a protease that functions to liquefy the ejaculate. It is produced throughout the prostate gland and, for practical purposes, is found nowhere else in the body. As the prostate

	VB1 Voided Bladder 1	VB2 Voided Bladder 2	EPS Expressed Prostatic Secretions	VB3 Voided Bladder 3
How obtained	First 10 mL of voided urine	Midstream sample	Obtained after prostatic massage (see text)	First 10 mL of urine after pro-static massage
Significance	Urethral sample	Bladder sample	Prostatic sample	1:100 dilution of prostatic sample
Urinary tract infection	Abundant leukocytes; positive culture	Abundant leukocytes; positive culture	Abundant leukocytes; positive culture	Abundant leukocytes; positive culture
Urethral infection	Highest colony counts		Lower colony counts	Lower colony counts
Acute bacterial prostatitis	Not generally performed	Abundant leukocytes; positive culture	Not performed because of danger of septicemia	
Chronic bacterial prostatitis	Little or no evidence of infection	Leukocytes may be present; culture may be positive; colony counts at 1/10 level of EPS	Abundant leukocytes and positive culture	Abundant leukocytes and positive culture
Chronic nonbacterial prostatitis	Negative culture	Few to no leukocytes; negative culture	Leukocytes present; culture negative	Leukocytes present; negative culture
Prostatodynia		Negative culture; no leukocytes	Negative culture; no leukocytes	Negative culture; no leukocytes

FIGURE 68-1 The three- (or four-) glass test. (Source: Author)

hypertrophies with age, more PSA is produced. PSA levels tend to increase with age, so the normal range increases as men grow older. Levels also increase in prostatitis and when the prostate is manipulated surgically or by cystoscopy.

Difficulty arises in distinguishing PSA elevations from BPH and those from prostate cancer. This generally occurs with PSA levels in the range of 4 to 10 ng/mL.

CLINICAL WARNING: PSA levels above 10 ng/mL are more specific for cancer.

Four approaches have been proposed for discriminating borderline PSA values (4 to 10 ng/mL) in BPH versus prostate cancer, but none has gained complete acceptance. The approaches are:

- PSA density: determined by dividing the PSA level by the weight of the prostate as determined by TRUS. This theoretically removes the increase in PSA secondary to hypertrophy.
- PSA velocity: the PSA is plotted over time. PSA levels are expected to increase with age, but a change in the velocity of the increase is thought to signal malignant prostatic disease.
- Age-specific PSA values have been published and are used by some laboratories (Oesterling et al, 1993).
- Different molecular forms of PSA may be associated with different types of prostate disease.

CLINICAL PEARL

Finasteride, which is used in the treatment of BPH, decreases PSA values by about half (Gormley et al, 1992).

Urodynamic Studies

Urodynamics includes a variety of techniques, ranging from the simple to the sophisticated. Uroflowmetry is a simple test commonly used for evaluating symptoms of urinary obstruction. It is the urologic equivalent of the pulmonary flow-volume curve. The patient urinates into a special measuring device that produces a curve of flow versus time. The curve permits normal outflow to be distinguished from the decreased pattern characteristic of prostatic obstruction and the plateau characteristic of bladder neck obstruction. Unfortunately, there are limitations to uroflowmetry. Decreased flow can be caused by a lazy detrusor without prostatic obstruction. Normal flow can occur despite obstruction if the detrusor is hypertrophied. Maximum rates of less than 10 mL/second are highly suggestive of obstruction, whereas rates greater than 15 mL/second pretty much rule it out.

Transrectal Ultrasound

TRUS and transrectal biopsy are the current standards for evaluation of a suspicious finding on DRE or PSA. Some experts advocate TRUS as a screening test for prostate cancer. Cancers are usually hypoechoic on TRUS. However, most hypoechoic areas are not cancerous, so all abnormal areas must be biopsied. When no suspicious areas are found, some urologists perform multiple blind biopsies; others prefer to follow serial PSA levels. Bleeding is the main complication of prostatic biopsy.

BENIGN PROSTATIC HYPERPLASIA

The pathogenesis and management of BPH appear straightforward at first glance. As men age, their prostates show areas of hyperplasia or growth of new prostate cells. By the ninth decade, the prevalence of pathologic BPH can reach 90% (Berry et al, 1984). Hyperplasia leads to hypertrophy of the gland, with increases in size and weight. This process results in mechanical obstruction of the urethra as it passes through the prostate. Chronic obstruction leads to dysfunction of the bladder detrusor muscle. The resultant symptoms of "prostatism" can be detected and quantified by symptom scores such as those of the AUA index (Barry & O'Leary, 1995), presented in Table 68-1. These symptom scores can be used to guide management decisions.

Although this sequence of events may occur in some patients, nearly every element in this logical chain is suspect (Abrams, 1995). If hyperplasia is a common finding in elderly men, it might be better thought of as a normal part of aging. Hyperplasia is a microscopic diagnosis and does not necessarily equate with gland hypertrophy, a diagnosis based on TRUS or the physical exam. Hypertrophy of the gland does not necessarily imply obstruction, which is a diagnosis established by urodynamics. To complicate matters further, there appears to be little relation between urodynamically diagnosed obstruction and "obstructive" symptoms (Abrams et al, 1993). Finally, patients who are symptomatic may or may not need or want interventions that carry significant morbidities of their own.

Thus, the provider is left with the difficult task of understanding how a variety of medical diagnoses such as cellular hyperplasia, glandular hypertrophy, and urodynamic obstruction relate to the patient's symptoms. The provider must help the patient decide which, if any, treatments are appropriate for his symptoms (Cassel, 1992).

Epidemiology

Despite the frequency of BPH and the quantity of resources invested in BPH treatment, the epidemiology of the condition remains poorly studied (Guess, 1995). The main risk factors are age and the presence of androgens.

How common BPH is depends on how it is defined: histologically, anatomically, urodynamically, or clinically. Natural history studies have been flawed but have reported that symptoms improve or stabilize in 42% to 86% of untreated patients (Oesterling, 1993). It has been estimated that 31% to 55% of men with BPH will have improvement of symptoms with watchful waiting (Benign Prostatic Hyperplasia Guideline Panel, 1994).

Diagnostic Criteria

Whether volunteered by the patient or elicited by the primary care provider, voiding symptoms usually initiate the workup for BPH. Occasionally, the provider will notice an enlarged bladder that is entirely asymptomatic; this is known as silent prostatism. The AUA symptom index presented in Table 68-1 may be useful at this point to establish a baseline of symptoms against which to judge the effects of therapy.

> **CLINICAL WARNING:** High symptom scores are not diagnostic of prostatic obstruction. However, it may not be strictly necessary to prove that obstruction is the cause of the patient's symptoms before proceeding with therapy.

The size of the prostate on physical exam is of little use diagnostically. Obstruction can occur with small prostates; conversely, large prostates do not necessarily obstruct. Evaluation of bladder size is diagnostically useful. When there is concern about bladder size, postvoid residual should be measured.

The minimum initial evaluation should include a urinalysis and creatinine measurement. These are done primarily to exclude other conditions, including infection or renal damage, rather than to confirm the diagnosis. Whether urodynamics and a PSA are necessary at this stage is controversial. Some providers order these tests routinely, but others do not.

Treatment Options, Expected Outcomes, and Comprehensive Management

Patients who do not meet the criteria for urologic referral can be managed in one of several ways. The choice is largely dictated by patient preference.

WATCHFUL WAITING

Many patients with symptoms of prostatism will improve over a 3- to 6-month waiting period. A frequency–volume chart may teach them to adjust their fluid intake and its timing (Kadow et al, 1988). This is discussed below. Pelvic floor and bladder exercises (Kegel exercises) and control of caffeine and alcohol intake may all be helpful in this setting. Kegel exercises are described in Chapter 34.

> **CLINICAL WARNING:** Watchful waiting is not considered appropriate in men with large postvoid residuals.

MEDICAL THERAPY

There are three approaches to the medical therapy of BPH.

- Alpha-adrenergic blockade relaxes the smooth muscle of the prostate.
- Antiandrogen therapy deprives the prostate of a growth-enhancing factor.
- Combination therapy combines alpha blockade with an antiandrogen.

Selective Alpha$_1$ Blockade

The smooth muscles of the prostate and urinary sphincter respond to alpha-adrenergic stimulation; this is why nasal decongestants have been known to precipitate urinary retention. Selective alpha$_1$-adrenergic blockers cause relaxation of this smooth muscle and can relieve the symptoms of obstruction.

In clinical practice, the four selective alpha-blockers used are prazosin, terazosin, tamsulosin, and doxazosin. The latter

three agents are long-acting and can be given once daily. Prazosin is usually given twice a day. These are all antihypertensive medications and may be the ideal agents in an elderly patient with hypertension. Unfortunately, their hypotensive action is also the source of their side effects, including orthostatic hypotension, headache, and dizziness. Because of these side effects, it is often suggested that these agents be taken at night and titrated up from very low dosages. Overall, about 10% of patients stop taking these medications because of side effects (Elhilai et al, 1996; Lepor et al, 1996) These agents may not help reduce bladder pressure. Tamsulosin is a more selective alpha-blocker that may have less hypotensive effects. Table 68-2 presents one method of initiating terazosin therapy.

Antiandrogen Therapy

Antiandrogens include gonadotropin-releasing hormone analogues, flutamide, and diethylstilbestrol (DES). These agents can reduce the size of the prostate and may affect symptoms. However, antiandrogen therapy has the morbidity associated with castration, including erectile difficulties and decreased libido. These agents are not used in current clinical practice.

Finasteride

Finasteride (Proscar) selectively inhibits 5-alpha-reductase, the enzyme that produces dihydrotestosterone from testosterone. Dihydrotestosterone seems to be the agent responsible for prostatic hyperplasia at the subcellular level. Finasteride, therefore, provides the benefits of antiandrogen therapy without the side effects associated with chemical castration. It is generally tolerated better than the alpha-blockers. Five percent to 10% of patients report a decrease in libido.

Finasteride may take months to achieve a clinical benefit, and less than half the patients experience an improvement in symptoms. However, many patients will improve spontaneously, and slow improvement may be acceptable in a disease with a chronic course.

> **CLINICAL WARNING:** Finasteride is a teratogen. Animal studies have shown that it provokes anomalies of the genital tract in male fetuses. For this reason, pregnant women are advised not to handle broken capsules of finasteride. Men who use finasteride should wear condoms to avoid exposing their sexual partner to finasteride in the ejaculate.

Combination Therapy

The alpha-blockers work rapidly, whereas finasteride generally takes months to achieve its benefits. Some primary care providers combine the two therapies, using alpha-blockers until the

TABLE 68-2	Initiation of Terazosin Therapy
Days 1–3	1 mg at bedtime
Days 4–7	2 mg at bedtime
Days 8–14	5 mg at bedtime
Days 15 forward	10 mg at bedtime

Terazosin is available in tablets or capsules of 1, 2, 5, and 10 mg. Dosages lower than 10 mg may be used in patients experiencing side effects.

finasteride begins to work. However, one large clinical trial found no benefit to adding finasteride to terazosin therapy (Lepor et al, 1996).

PROSTATECTOMY

Prostatectomy can be accomplished transurethrally, suprapubically, or perineally. When surgery is chosen for BPH, transurethral resection of the prostate (TURP) is used in most cases. It produces immediate and dramatic reductions in obstructive symptoms and is considered the gold standard against which other BPH therapies are assessed.

Historically, TURP has been one of the most common operations performed in the United States: in 1987, some 258,000 procedures were performed. Over time, however, it has become clear that TURP is associated with significant morbidities. Newer therapies have been promoted as alternatives, and since the mid-1980s the number of TURPs performed has dropped dramatically, to 168,000 in 1993 (Benign Prostatic Hyperplasia Guideline Panel, 1994; Guess, 1995).

The morbidities of TURP need to be explained carefully to patients (Table 68-3). These morbidities in part reflect the patient population who undergo the procedure—elderly men who often have comorbid conditions.

■ **CLINICAL WARNING:** A significant percentage of men undergoing TURP have prostate cancer diagnosed in the resected tissue.

Transurethral incision of the prostate is an alternative to TURP that is particularly appropriate for men with small prostates. It involves making an incision from the bladder neck to the verumontanum. In properly selected patients, it is as effective as TURP and is associated with fewer side effects, including less retrograde ejaculation.

TABLE 68-3	**Complications of TURP**

Immediate surgical complications (12%)

TURP syndrome
    Dilutional hyponatremia
    Perioperative infection
    Fever
    Urinary retention
    Hemorrhage requiring transfusion
    Myocardial infarction
    Stroke
    Incisional complications
    Mortality at 90 days, 2%

Longer-term complications
    Impotence (13.6%)
    Retrograde ejaculation (73.4%)
    Stress incontinence (2.1%)
    Total incontinence (1.0%)
    Urethral stricture (3.1%)
    Bladder neck contracture (1.7%)

Need for retreatment at 5 years (10%)

Number in parentheses represents an estimation of how many patients are affected.
Source: Benign Prostatic Hyperplasia Guideline Panel, 1994.

NEWER INTERVENTIONAL OPTIONS

Because of the problems associated with medical therapy and with TURP, there has been a search for alternative interventional approaches. A number of modalities are in use, not all of which have been subjected to rigorous and long-term analysis.

The Prostatron, a microwave device placed in the urethra, uses microwave radiation to destroy the periurethral prostatic tissue. The procedure is performed as a single 1-hour outpatient procedure. Sexual dysfunction does not appear to be a problem. Microwave therapy is, however, less effective than TURP. Up to 25% of patients have urinary retention after microwave therapy and require a Foley catheter for an average of 7 days (De la Rosette et al, 1997).

Balloon dilatation of the prostate met with initial enthusiasm as a minimally invasive alternative to TURP. Unfortunately, its efficacy is minimal and it is no longer commonly used.

Several different methodologies involving lasers have been used to resect prostate tissue transurethrally. Lasers can directly burn and coagulate tissue, which then sloughs off in the weeks after the procedure. Lasers can be used to cause tissue evaporation in a procedure called transurethral evaporation of the prostate. These newer interventions also can be incorporated into balloon dilators. All of these techniques are less efficacious than TURP but have fewer side effects.

Additional modalities that are under study include metal stents to open the urethra, high-intensity ultrasound to destroy periurethral tissue, and radiowave ablation of the prostate using transurethral needles. Most of these techniques are still in the experimental stage.

Comprehensive Management

The Agency for Health Care Policy and Research (AHCPR), part of the Department of Health and Human Services, published a set of clinical guidelines for the management of BPH in 1994. A modified version of these guidelines is summarized in Figure 68-2. These guidelines provide a useful framework within which the provider can discuss the management of BPH with patients. The guidelines may be somewhat out-of-date and need to be individualized. Newer interventional options are now available as just discussed, whereas balloon dilatation has fallen out of favor.

A key question for each patient is whether the risks of therapy outweigh the benefit of treating his disease. This is something not easily addressed by the AUA symptom score, whose value lies mainly in terms of monitoring symptoms. Patients need to balance the benefits of improved urination against the real risks associated with surgical and medical therapies.

Teaching and Self-Care

The primary care provider and the patient must work together to ensure that the patient makes a fully informed decision regarding treatment. Patients should understand that the symptoms of prostatism wax and wane with time. There are several simple measures that can be useful to ameliorate them. Patients can keep a log of when and how much they urinate; this is called a frequency–volume log. The data derived from the log can help them to adjust their fluid intake to avoid troublesome nocturia. A bedside urinal can ease the logistical problems associated with nocturia. Kegel exercises and bladder training may also be helpful. If caffeine and alcohol are problems, intake should be minimized or avoided entirely.

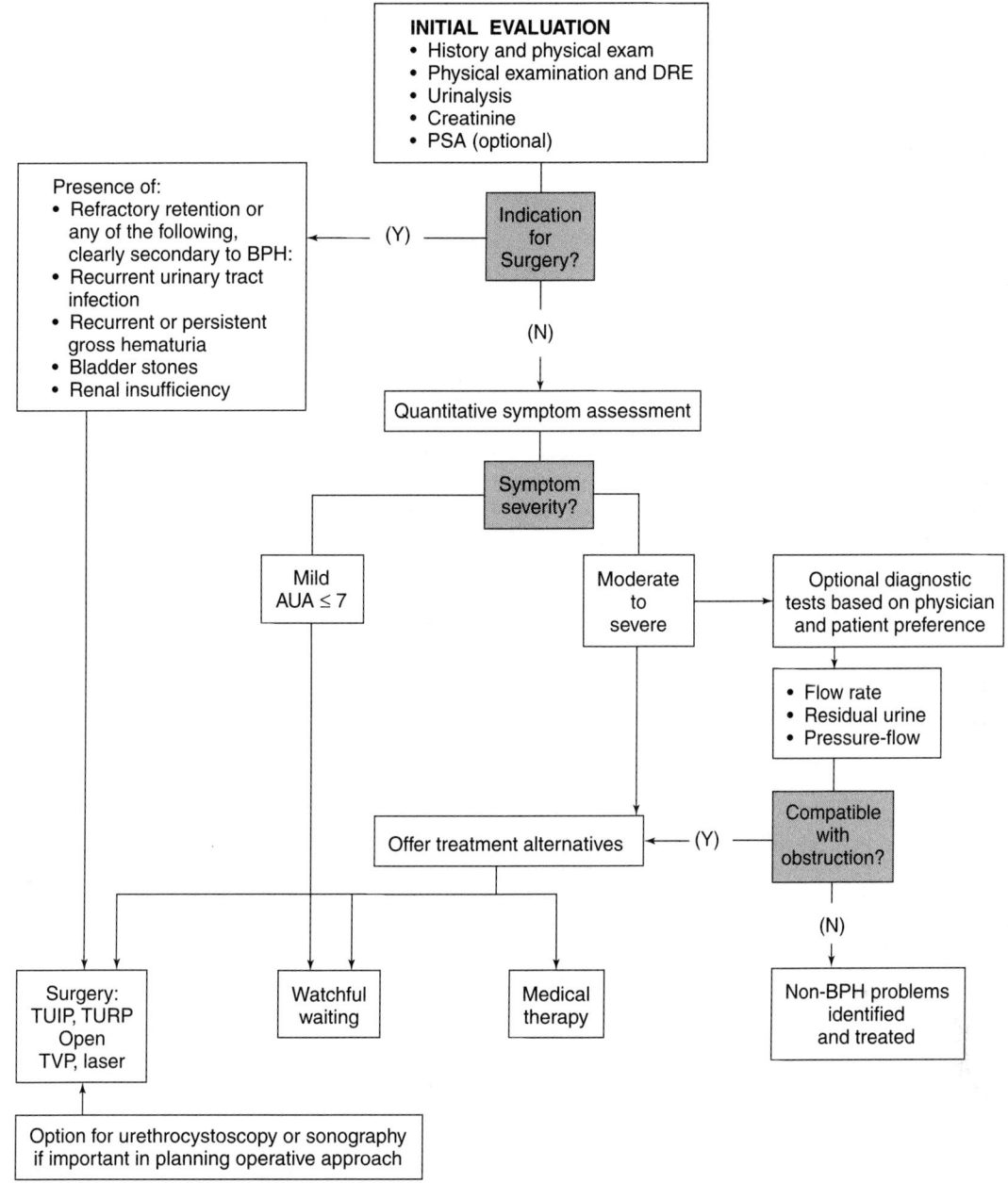

FIGURE 68-2 Treatment algorithm for BPH. (Adapted from McConnell JD, Barry MJ, Bruskewitz RC, et al: Benign prostatic hyperplasia: Diagnosis and treatment. Clinical Practice Guideline, No. 8. ACHCPR Publication No. 94-0582. Rockville, MD. Agency for Health Care Policy and Research, Public Health Service, U.S. Department of Health and Human Services, 1994.)

Referral Points and Clinical Warnings

Referral to a urologist is appropriate in several situations. Acute retention mandates urgent consultation. Stones, recurrent infections, and persistent hematuria should all be given prompt urologic evaluation. Patients with refractory and troublesome symptoms should also be referred to a urologist.

PROSTATE CANCER

Epidemiology

Adenocarcinoma of the prostate is the most common malignancy diagnosed in American men. The ACS estimated that 334,500 men would be diagnosed with prostate cancer in 1997

and that 41,800 would die of this malignancy (ACS, 1997). By way of comparison, the next most common nonskin malignancy in men is lung cancer, of which only 98,000 cases were estimated to occur in 1997, and 94,400 men were anticipated to die of lung cancer. After lung cancer, prostate cancer is the second leading cause of cancer deaths. The diagnosis of prostate cancer has increased dramatically in the past 10 years, reflecting in part the widespread adoption of PSA testing.

As suggested by the comparison with lung cancer, prostate cancer is not one of the more deadly cancers. This is true for several reasons. Prostate cancer tends to be diagnosed in elderly men, many of whom will die of other causes before they become symptomatic from prostate cancer. Most prostate cancers seem to be indolent, growing over years or even decades. It is unclear, therefore, how many newly diagnosed prostate cancers represent clinically important disease destined to affect the health of the men in whom they occur.

Prostate cancer is almost always a disease of men over 50. The prevalence thereafter increases with each decade of life. Prevalence figures for men in this age group based on autopsy studies show prostate cancer in 6% to 30% of cases. There are about 25 million men over 50 years old, so the prevalence of prostate cancer is believed to be 3 million to 7.5 million.

A gene located on the long arm (q) of chromosome 1 has been identified that seems to confer a risk of prostate cancer; it has been named hereditary prostate cancer 1 (Smith et al, 1996).

Diagnostic Criteria

In the era of widespread PSA testing, prostate cancer is now usually asymptomatic at diagnosis. Symptoms generally occur in the context of metastasis. Metastatic prostate cancer presents as bony pain or neurologic compromise. Local extension can cause either urinary obstruction or erectile dysfunction. Prostate cancer can cause local pain and hematuria.

CLINICAL WARNING: Referral to a urologist for a prostate biopsy is necessary to establish the diagnosis.

PROGNOSTIC VARIABLES: STAGING, GRADING, AND SIZE

The urologist can estimate the prognosis for patients with prostate cancer using three variables: staging (where in the body the tumor has spread), grading (how aggressive the tumor appears under the microscope), and size. Different specialists use differing staging protocols. Generally, patients who are diagnosed with prostate cancer will have undergone a TRUS and biopsy. The workup may be stopped at this point in patients with well-differentiated adenocarcinoma, low (<10 ng/mL) PSA levels, and disease that is clinically localized. An intravenous pyelogram and bone scan are additional screening tests obtained routinely by some specialists. Pelvic lymph node dissection is more accurate than computed tomography for detecting metastatic disease to the pelvic nodes.

Two systems are commonly used for the staging of prostate cancer: that of the AUA and that of the American Joint Committee on Cancer. The Gleason system is one of several used to grade the tumor itself. A low Gleason score indicates a well-differentiated tumor, a high Gleason score a poorly differentiated tumor. In general, a low score indicates the patient will do well, and a high score suggests a more aggressive tumor. The predictive value of intermediate scores is less clear.

Diagnostic Studies

Screening for prostate cancer is currently one of the more controversial areas of preventive health care. The ACS and the AUA both recommend annual DREs for men over 40 and DRE combined with PSA in men over 50 (ACS, 1997). The publicity generated by these recommendations and the approval in 1995 by the FDA of PSA as a screening method have generated a demand by male patients for "the prostate test." Nonetheless,

the U.S. Preventive Services Task Force (1995) has recommended against any form of prostate cancer screening. This recommendation has been echoed by the Health Technology Assessment Programme and the Centre for Reviews and Dissemination of the British National Health Service (Woolf, 1997). A third position is that of educating the patient, who is then able to make the decision on screening. This option has been adopted by the American College of Physicians (1997). Arguments for and against screening will be presented.

The criteria for a preventive intervention include addressing an illness with an important burden and whose presymptomatic detection and treatment could reduce morbidity and mortality for patients. Benefits of the intervention must outweigh any harm (Snow, 1996). This is the standard by which to judge screening for prostate cancer.

Undoubtedly, DRE, PSA, and TRUS can all detect asymptomatic prostate cancers, although how well in terms of sensitivity and specificity is not fully known. Asymptomatic cancers are more likely to be localized. Cancers that are confined to the prostate (stages A and B) can be removed by prostatectomy and thus potentially cured. This potential has been the argument for prostate cancer screening.

Nonetheless, there is as yet no evidence that prostate cancer screening results in any improvement in mortality or morbidity. This may be because screening detects primarily the large group of indolent cancers that are not destined to cause problems. Additionally, the process of screening, including the anxiety created by positive results, the process of TRUS with biopsy, and the treatments for cancers that are detected are not without important morbidities. It is hard to justify putting elderly men through these procedures without hard proof that they will benefit from them. This has been the rationale against screening.

A number of clinical trials are underway that address the value of prostate cancer screening. These trials may or may not provide evidence of benefit, but results will not be available for at least another decade. In the interim, the provider must decide if screening is appropriate. Several good references exist for more information (Coley et al, 1997a; Coley et al, 1997b; Oesterling, 1997; Hahn & Roberts, 1993).

Treatment Options, Expected Outcomes, and Comprehensive Management

Several options exist for patients with prostate cancer. The treatment choice will depend on staging and grading of the tumor. As is true for other aspects of prostate disease, the absence of data from well-controlled clinical trials means that management of prostate cancer will continue to be highly controversial.

EXPECTANT MANAGEMENT

Watchful waiting may be an appropriate alternative in patients with localized, well-differentiated disease and a shorter life expectancy. Therapy for localized disease has not been demonstrated to be of benefit. Watchful waiting avoids the problems associated with prostatectomy and radiation therapy (Palmer & Chodak, 1996; Hugosson et al, 1996). The validity of expectant management has been recognized in guidelines published by the AUA in 1995 (Middleton et al, 1995).

SURGERY

Radical prostatectomy is offered to patients with localized disease with the intent of curing their cancer. A number of immediate postoperative complications may occur, including bleeding, rectal damage, deep venous thrombosis or pulmonary embolus, and infection. TURP is occasionally used in patients with advanced disease as symptomatic therapy for urethral obstruction. Incontinence (either total or stress) and erectile dysfunction are the major long-term complications of prostatectomy.

RADIOTHERAPY

Radiotherapy of the prostate is used with curative intent in localized disease. The most commonly used protocol calls for doses of 2 cGy given daily for 7 weeks, for a total dosage of 70 cGy. This treatment is administered by a radiation oncologist. Radiotherapy is used to treat specific symptomatic areas with palliative intent in metastatic disease. Table 68-4 presents selected side effects of total prostatectomy versus those of external-beam radiotherapy in the treatment of prostate cancer.

ENDOCRINE THERAPY

Endocrine therapy is used with palliative intent in symptomatic patients with advanced disease. By depriving the cancer of a necessary growth factor (androgen), hormonal therapies often result in dramatic symptomatic improvement.

■ ■ ■   CLINICAL PEARL

Endocrine therapy does not affect prognosis and is therefore unnecessary in patients without symptoms. Options include DES, orchiectomy, LHRH agonists (leuprolide, goserelin), antiandrogens (flutamide), diethyl-stilbestrol (Stilphostrol), long-acting estrogens (chlorotrianisene [TACE]), megestrol, and drugs that inhibit androgen synthesis (ketoconazole, aminoglutethimide). These treatments may or may not be administered by the primary care provider in conjunction with a specialist.

TABLE 68-4	Selected Side Effects of Therapy for Prostate Cancer
Radical Prostatectomy	**External-Beam Radiation Therapy**
Blood loss of 1–2 L	Acute (30%–50%): proctitis, cystitis, urinary retention, penoscrotal edema.
Impotence (30%–60%)	
Urinary incontinence (5%–15%)	Chronic (4%–7%): proctitis (2%), cystitis (8%), enteritis (3%), impotence (40%–60%), ureteral stricture (4%). Risk of incontinence, <1%.
Vesiculourethral anastomotic stricture (0.6%–25%)	
Rectal injury (0.1%–7%)	
Thromboembolism (1%–12%)	
Wound infection (0.4%–16%)	
Lymphedema (1%–5%)	
Lymphocele (0.4%–2.3%)	

Source: *Catalona.* 1994.

A small improvement in survival has been demonstrated with a strategy of combining LHRH agonists with antiandrogens.

CHEMOTHERAPY

Cytotoxic agents such as cyclophosphamide (Cytoxan), fluorouracil, doxorubicin (Adriamycin), and dacarbazine can provide additional symptomatic relief to patients with advanced symptomatic disease, but they do not affect survival. These treatments are administered by oncologists. Median survival is approximately 36 months in patients with advanced prostate cancer.

Comprehensive Management

It is difficult to provide firm recommendations regarding the therapeutic options for prostate cancer. Recommendations of experts vary greatly (Catalona, 1994).

In December 1995, the AUA published treatment guidelines for clinically localized prostate cancer (Middleton et al, 1995). There are essentially three options for patients with localized disease: waiting, prostatectomy, and radiation. An extensive literature search provided no evidence that any of these three options were superior to the others. Treatment efficacy cannot be used as a criterion for choosing which option is best. The AUA has recommended that treatment decisions be based on the patient's life expectancy and general medical condition and tumor characteristics. Intervention via either prostatectomy or radiation is favored in younger, healthier men with more aggressive tumors.

Whatever the treatment regimen decided on, the primary care provider will need to give comprehensive care to a cancer patient. This will involve more than just careful explanation of different treatment options. Patients who have undergone prostatectomy or radiation therapy will often require care for the sequelae of these procedures, including erectile dysfunction and incontinence. Complications of advanced prostate cancer include anemia, bleeding problems, bony metastatic disease, and neurologic compromise. Patients and their families require compassionate care when faced with terminal illness and the realities of a steadily advancing neoplasm.

Patients with prostate cancer are generally monitored by the urologist with PSA levels. The optimal interval for such monitoring has not been determined. Radical prostatectomy and radiation therapy should cause dramatic drops in PSA levels. Subsequent increases indicate recurrent tumor. In patients receiving antiandrogen therapy, testosterone levels should be at castration levels (generally less than 50 ng/dL).

There are no currently accepted strategies for the prevention of prostate cancer. The National Cancer Institute is currently sponsoring a trial of finasteride as a preventive drug for prostate cancer in healthy men.

Teaching and Self-Care

The patient who presents for a "prostate test" needs to be informed of the risks and benefits of prostate cancer screening. Patients in whom prostate cancer has been diagnosed need to understand their options. Because treatment decisions will generally be made in consultation with a urologist, the primary care provider needs to ensure that the patient is making a fully informed decision. A patient's guide for clinically localized prostate cancer is available from the AUA and is listed in Community-Based Resources below.

Referral Points and Clinical Warnings

Specialist consultation is necessary in the diagnosis and management of prostate cancer. Management of localized disease is typically in the hands of a urologist for prostatectomy or a radiation oncologist for radiotherapy. If no intervention is elected, the primary care provider usually comanages the patient with the specialist. Metastatic disease may be managed by oncologists or urologists, often in conjunction with a radiation oncologist. The need for urologic follow-up for patients in whom no therapy is chosen depends on the provider's experience in managing this disease.

Advanced prostate cancer can present with several oncologic emergencies. Spinal cord compression is typically managed with radiotherapy and steroids. Urinary tract obstruction and uremia may also develop as the cancer grows. These are indications for urgent urologic consultation.

PROSTATITIS

Epidemiology

Prostatitis refers not to a specific entity, but rather to a group of quite distinct clinical syndromes. There are four prostatitis syndromes: acute bacterial prostatitis, chronic bacterial prostatitis, chronic nonbacterial prostatitis, and prostatodynia.

Acute prostatitis is a relatively rare bacterial infection of the prostate. Patients present with acute symptoms that point to a urinary tract problem. Chronic prostatitis is a common urologic complaint with a variety of clinical presentations. Chronic prostatitis is divided into cases in which a bacterial cause is identified (chronic bacterial prostatitis) and those in which cultures are negative (chronic nonbacterial prostatitis, also called abacterial prostatitis or prostatosis). Prostatodynia refers to a poorly understood syndrome of pelvic-centered pain and voiding difficulties for which no cause is found.

There are a number of rare forms of prostatitis, including infections caused by gonorrhea, tuberculosis, parasites, fungi, and granulomatous prostatitis.

Diagnostic Criteria

ACUTE BACTERIAL PROSTATITIS

Patients with acute bacterial prostatitis present with evidence of a systemic illness, including fever and constitutional symptoms. Other symptoms include those that point to a urinary tract location, such as perineal pain and voiding problems. DRE should be performed with care so as not to promote bacteremia. DRE will reveal a swollen, quite tender prostate. The urine will show evidence of infection, typically involving gram-negative gut flora.

 CLINICAL WARNING: EPS is unnecessary because the etiologic agent can be isolated from the urine.

CHRONIC PROSTATITIS

Chronic prostatitis presents a considerable diagnostic challenge. The symptoms are nonspecific and may involve both obstructive and irritative symptoms, including discomfort in the perineal, testicular, or low back regions, and dyspareunia (painful ejaculation). Signs may include hematospermia or hematuria. Chronic prostatitis can also present with persistent or recurrent urinary tract infection despite adequate antibiotic therapy for cystitis. In these cases, the infected prostate serves as a reservoir in which the bacteria persist. The course tends to be indolent, and asymptomatic periods occur.

■ ■ ■ **CLINICAL PEARL**

DRE is not diagnostically useful. The prostate may be either entirely normal or may show asymmetry, enlargement, bogginess, or tenderness.

In patients suspected of having chronic prostatitis, a three-glass test should be done as shown in Figure 68-1. More than 10 to 15 leukocytes per high-power field should be present in the EPS. The presence of fat-laden macrophages is also highly suggestive of chronic prostatitis. Cultures may reveal a bacterial origin (usually gut flora) or may be sterile.

Chronic bacterial prostatitis is occasionally associated with prostatic calculi. Calculi are diagnosed by ultrasound and are common findings in older men. Calculi are usually asymptomatic and can be a nidus of infection in patients with chronic bacterial prostatitis. In these cases, calculi may need to be removed. This can often be accomplished by the urologist with TURP.

PROSTATODYNIA

Patients with prostatodynia have symptoms similar to those of chronic prostatitis, including obstruction, irritation, pain, and dyspareunia. EPS shows no evidence of infection (no leukocytes or fat-laden macrophages), and cultures are negative.

Treatment Options, Expected Outcomes, and Comprehensive Management

ACUTE BACTERIAL PROSTATITIS

Acute bacterial prostatitis is treated with antibiotics that cover intestinal flora (Table 68-5). The antibiotic can be changed when culture results become available. Antibiotics are generally continued for 3 to 4 weeks. Patients who are not candidates for outpatient therapy should be admitted and started on intravenous antibiotics with good gram-negative coverage.

CHRONIC PROSTATITIS

When a bacterial source is identified, chronic prostatitis is treated in much the same way as acute bacterial prostatitis. Antibiotic treatment is generally continued for 12 to 16 weeks. Post-treatment cultures of EPS are necessary to confirm resolution of the infection.

Unfortunately, these regimens are not always successful. For the patient whose disease fails to respond to a prolonged course of antibiotics, two options should be explored. The use of daily suppressive antibiotics (typically sulfamethoxazole–trimethoprim, one single-strength per day) is one option. Surgery is also an option, and various forms of prostatectomy may be offered, depending on the clinical setting.

TABLE 68-5	Prostatitis		
Syndrome	Etiology	Clinical Presentation	Treatment
Acute prostatitis	Bacterial infection of prostate, typically with gram-negative enteric flora	Systemically ill patient with urinary tract symptoms	IV antibiotics may be indicated. Empiric coverage started with sulfamethoxazole–trimethoprim, ciprofloxacin, or doxycycline. Ancillary measures: analgesia, antipyrexia, sitz baths, stool softeners, bed rest.
Chronic bacterial prostatitis	Indolent bacterial infection of prostate. *Escherichia coli* is responsible for approximately 80% of cases.	Nonspecific. Presentation may include irritative or obstructive symptoms, pelvic discomfort, dyspareunia, or recurrent U.T.I.	Antibiotic therapy. Initial agents are those used in acute bacterial prostatitis. Antimicrobial therapy changed when culture results available. Antibiotics continued for 12 to 16 weeks.
Chronic nonbacterial prostatitis	Idiopathic; but link to microbial agents hypothesized but never clearly demonstrated	As for chronic bacterial prostatitis	*Empiric therapy:* 2-week course of doxycycline. Trial of alpha-adrenergic receptor blockers (eg, terazosin). NSAIDs. Sitz baths.
Prostatodynia	Unknown	Similar to chronic prostatitis	Treatment is empiric. Although antibiotics are not used, treatments are similar to those for chronic nonbacterial prostatitis. Diazepam is favored by some authors.

Source: Author

CHRONIC NONBACTERIAL PROSTATITIS (PROSTATOSIS)

The etiology of this disorder is unknown, and treatment is empiric. Some providers give a course of antibiotics (typically doxycycline or erythromycin) on the assumption that *Ureaplasma* or *Chlamydia* is responsible. Antibiotics are not continued beyond 2 weeks unless there is a response. See Chapter 69 for treatment guidelines.

Some authors consider chronic nonbacterial prostatitis to be a consequence of voiding dysfunction, including spasm of the bladder neck and urethra. Treatment recommendations often include alpha-blocking agents (Meares, 1993). Details on the use of these agents can be found in the previous section on BPH.

Other treatments are directed toward the relief of specific symptoms. Pain can be relieved with sitz baths and nonsteroidal anti-inflammatory agents. Some patients find that avoiding alcohol and spicy foods is of benefit. Voiding symptoms may be helped by the use of anticholinergics such as oxybutynin (Ditropan).

■ ■ ■ CLINICAL PEARL

Sexual activity should not be avoided. Some providers advocate frequent ejaculation as a means of turning over prostatic fluids.

PROSTATODYNIA

As with chronic nonbacterial prostatitis, the etiology of prostatodynia is obscure, and treatments are empiric. Antibiotics are not used.

If sphincter dyssynergia is diagnosed, alpha-blocking agents are indicated. Severe problems with the internal sphincter can be dealt with surgically via bladder neck incision. If abnormal tension of the pelvic floor musculature is suspected, benzodiazepines may be prescribed. Other treatments are as for chronic nonbacterial prostatitis.

Comprehensive Management

The care of patients with prostatitis begins with making an accurate diagnosis. For patients with acute bacterial prostatitis, this is usually not a problem. For patients with other forms of prostatitis, however, this requires attention to the subtleties of both symptoms and signs. The provider must be skilled in the methodology of EPS and the three-glass test.

Having established a diagnosis, the primary care provider must then decide if and when further urologic evaluation is necessary. Refractory symptoms, evidence of obstruction, an elevated creatinine level, and recurrent infection are clear indications for referral. Patients with acute bacterial prostatitis need an intravenous pyelogram at some point to evaluate for anatomic abnormalities. Patients with chronic nonbacterial prostatitis and prostatodynia may benefit from video-urodynamic studies to diagnose voiding difficulties.

Teaching and Self-Care

The chronic forms of prostatitis (chronic bacterial prostatitis, chronic nonbacterial prostatitis, and prostatodynia) can be frustrating conditions for both patient and primary care provider.

This is especially so because a clear explanation of the patient's symptoms cannot be given and therapies are empiric.

■ ■ ■ CLINICAL PEARL

Patients need to know that nonbacterial prostatitis and prostatodynia are generally benign conditions that are usually self-limiting.

No specific preventive measures exist for the prostatitis syndromes. A role for sexually transmitted pathogens such as *Chlamydia trachomatis* and *Trichomonas vaginalis* has been postulated for chronic nonbacterial prostatitis, but this has never been clearly demonstrated (Doble, 1994).

■ **CLINICAL WARNING:** Prostatic abscess is a rare complication of bacterial prostatitis. When the prostate exam suggests an abscess (fluctuance or a mass), urologic consultation should be obtained promptly.

COMMUNITY RESOURCES

- AUA publications department, 410-223-4367: The AUA has several publications both for primary care providers and patients. Among them are a guide to the management of localized prostate cancer for practitioners and a patient's guide to prostate cancer.
- AHCPR Publications Clearinghouse, P.O. Box 8547, Silver Spring, MD 20907, 800-358-9295, http://www.ah cpr.gov/.: The AHCPR has published three items of interest for dealing with BPH: clinical practice guidelines (AHCPR Publication No. 94-0582), a quick reference guide for clinicians (Publication No. 94-0583), and a guide for patients (*Treating your enlarged prostate*, Publication No. 94-0584). Individual copies of the latter two documents are available for free. The patient guide provides an excellent basis for patients to make informed decisions. Copies of the patient education material can be downloaded from the Web site.
- ACS, http://www.cancer.org: The ACS's work in the area of reproductive cancers is described in the Community-Based Resources section of Chapters 65, 66, and 70.
- American Foundation for Urologic Disease, Prostate Health Council, 800-242-2383, http://www.auanet. org/pub{ }pat/: Provides educational materials. The foundation has been funded by TAP Pharmaceuticals, the makers of Lupron (injectable leuprolide), to promote prostate cancer screening. Their campaign, "Team Up Against Prostate Cancer," promotes an annual prostate examination in men over 50 years. For providers interested in this type of screening, free educational materials are available by calling 800-319-8633.
- National Kidney and Urologic Diseases Information Clearinghouse, Box NKUDIC, Bethesda, MD 20892, 301-468-4365: Provides information to professionals.
- Urology Department of Princess Margaret Hospital, England, http://ourworld.compuserve.com:80/home pages/SwindonUrol/: Links to many urology-related Web pages, many sponsored by drug companies.

Useful reference sources for the provider include:

- Lepor, H., & Lawson, R. (1993). *Prostate diseases.* Philadelphia: W.B. Saunders. An in-depth discussion of all aspects of prostatic disease.
- Lepor, H. (Ed.). (1995). Advances in benign prostatic hyperplasia. *Urologic Clinics of North America, 22*(2). An entire issue devoted to BPH.
- Tanagho, E., & McAninch, J. (Eds.). (1995) *Smith's general urology*, 14th edition. Norwalk, CT: Appleton & Lange. An outstanding general reference for the primary care provider.

Referral Points and Clinical Warnings

Several situations require urgent evaluation in the patient with bacterial prostatitis. Patients with acute bacterial prostatitis may be septic and need inpatient admission for intravenous antibiotics. Acute bacterial prostatitis can also present with significant bladder obstruction. This must be relieved by a suprapubic tap; the use of a Foley catheter is contraindicated.

EDITOR'S NOTE:
COMPLEMENTARY APPROACHES

A general discussion of complementary approaches can be found in Chapter 3. The following, while not an exhaustive list, are some complementary approaches being used for this condition. Additional information on these approaches, including precautions, can be found in Appendices A and B. Providers need to assess for the use of complementary approaches as part of the patient's history, as they may impact conventional therapies, and patients may not volunteer this information unless specifically asked. Efficacy of many complementary approaches is not as well documented as that of conventional therapies. Providers need to read the literature before suggesting these complementary approaches.

- Vitamins, minerals, herbs, supplements
  Betacarotene
  Saw palmetto

References

Abrams, P. (1995). Managing lower urinary tract symptoms in older men. *British Medical Journal, 310,* 1113–1117.

Abrams, P., Blaivas, J., Griffiths, D., et al. (1993). The objective evaluation of bladder outflow obstruction. In A. Cockett, S. Khury, Y. Aso, et al. (Eds.). *Proceedings of the 2d international consultation on benign prostatic hyperplasia*, pp. 153–209. Jersey: Jersey Scientific Communication.

American Cancer Society. (1997). *Cancer facts & figures, 1997.* Atlanta: Author.

American College of Physicians. (1997). Screening for prostate cancer. *Annals of Internal Medicine, 126,* 465–467.

Barry, M., & O'Leary, M. (1995). The development and clinical utility of symptom scores. *Urologic Clinics of North America, 22*(2), 299–307.

Benign Prostatic Hyperplasia Guideline Panel. (1994). *Benign prostatic hyperplasia: Diagnosis and treatment.* Clinical practice guideline No. 8. AHCPR Publication No. 94-0582. Washington, D.C.: U.S. Department of Health and Human Resources.

Berry, S., Coffey, D., Walsh, P., & Ewing, L. (1984). The development of human benign prostatic hyperplasia with age. *Journal of Urology, 132,* 474–479.

Boyarsky, S., & Goldenberg, J. (1962). Detection of bladder distention by suprapubic percussion. *New York State Journal of Medicine,* 1804–1807.

Cassel, C. (1992). Case commentary: Benign prostatic hypertrophy: Intervene or wait? *Hospital Practice,* 57–73.

Catalona, W. (1994). Management of cancer of the prostate. *N Engl J Med, 331*(15), 996–1004.

Coley, C., Barry, M., Fleming, C., et al. (1997a). Early detection of prostate cancer. I: Prior probability and effectiveness of tests. *Annals of Internal Medicine, 126,* 394–406.

Coley, C., Barry, M., Fleming C., et al. (1997b). Early detection of prostate cancer. II: Estimating the risks, benefits, and costs. *Annals of Internal Medicine, 126,* 468–479.

De la Rosette, J., D'Ancona, F., & Debruyne, F. (1997). Current status of thermotherapy of the prostate. *Journal of Urology, 157,* 430–438.

Doble, A. (1994). Chronic prostatitis. *British Journal of Urology, 74,* 537–541.

Elhilai, E., Ramsey, E., Barkin, J., et al. (1996). A multicenter, randomized, double-blind, placebo-controlled study to evaluate the safety and efficacy of terazosin in the treatment of benign prostatic hyperplasia. *Urology, 47,* 225–342.

Gormley, G., Stoner, E., Bruskewitz, R., et al. (1992). The effect of finasteride in men with benign prostatic hyperplasia. *N Engl J Med, 327,* 1185–1191.

Guarino, J. (1985). Auscultatory percussion of the urinary bladder. *Archives of Internal Medicine, 145,* 1823–1825.

Guess, H. (1995). Epidemiology and natural history of benign prostatic hyperplasia. *Urologic Clinics of North America, 22*(2), 247–261.

Hahn, D., & Roberts, R. (1993). PSA screening for asymptomatic prostate cancer: Truth in advertising. *Journal of Family Practice, 37,* 432–436.

Hugosson, J., Aus, G., & Norlen, L. (1996). Surveillance is not a viable and appropriate treatment option in the management of localized prostate cancer. *Urologic Clinics of North America, 23*(4), 557–573.

Kadow, C., Feneley, R., & Abrams, P. (1988). Prostatectomy or conservative management in the treatment of benign prostatic hypertrophy. *British Journal of Urology, 61,* 432–434.

Lepor, H., & Machi, G. (1993). Comparison of AUA symptom index in unselected males and females between 55 and 79 years of age. *Urology, 42,* 36–40.

Lepor, H., Williford, W., Barry, M., et al. (1996). The efficacy of terazosin, finasteride, or both, in benign prostatic hypertrophy. *N Engl J Med, 335,* 533–539.

Meares, E. (1993). Nonbacterial prostatitis and prostatodynia. In Lepor, H., & Lawson, R. (Eds.). *Prostatic diseases.* Philadelphia: W.B. Saunders.

Middleton, R., Thompson, I., Autenfeld, M., et al. (1995). Prostate cancer clinical guidelines panel summary report on the management of clinically localized prostate cancer. *Journal of Urology, 154,* 2144–2148.

Oesterling, J. (Ed.). (1997). Prostate-specific antigen: The best prostatic tumor marker. *Urologic Clinics of North America, 24.*

Oesterling, J., Jacobsen, S., Chute, C., et al. (1993). Serum prostate-specific antigen in a community-based population of healthy men. *JAMA, 270*(7), 860–864.

Oesterling, J. (1992). Benign prostatic hyperplasia: Its natural history, epidemiologic characteristics, and surgical treatment. *Arch Fam Med 1:* 257–266.

Palmer, S., & Chodak, G. (1996). Defining the role of surveillance in the management of localized prostate cancer. *Urologic Clinics of North America, 23*(4), 551–556.

Sapira, J. (1990). *The art and science of bedside diagnosis.* Baltimore: Williams & Wilkins.

Smith, J., Freije, D., Carpten, J., et al. (1996). Major susceptibility locus for prostate cancer on chromosome 1 suggested by a genome-wide search. *Science, 274,* 1371.

Snow, C. (1996). Guidelines for preventive health care. In D. Dale & D. Federman (Eds.). *Scientific American medicine.* New York: Scientific American, Inc.

Tanagho, E., & McAninch, J. (Eds.). (1995). *Smith's general urology.* Norwalk, CT: Appleton & Lange.

U.S. Preventive Services Task Force. (1995). *Guide to clinical preventive services.* Washington, D.C.: U.S. Government Printing Office.

Woolf, S. (1997). Should we screen for prostate cancer? *British Medical Journal, 314,* 989–990.

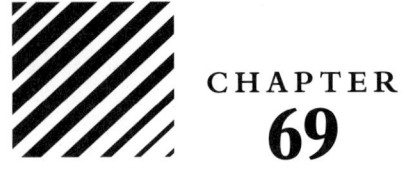
Sexually Transmitted Infections

Carol Buck-Rolland, MS, PNP, OGNP, and Deborah Wachtel, MPH, OGNP

This chapter begins with a discussion of sexually transmitted infections (STIs) in general, followed by sections covering chlamydia, gonorrhea, syphilis, herpes simplex virus, human papillomavirus, bacterial vaginosis, trichomoniasis, and moniliasis. The anatomy and physiology of the male reproductive system are described in Chapters 68 and 70. Female reproductive anatomy is described in Chapter 71. The pathology of each of the STIs is discussed in this chapter. Patient history is not specifically discussed; the provider should ask questions using the standard sexual history and symptom format when screening for STIs. For more specific information on history taking, refer to Chapters 66, 67, and 70. Comprehensive epidemiologic statistics are not provided for trichomoniasis, moniliasis, or bacterial vaginosis because these are not reportable infections; interested readers are referred to current gynecologic texts. Teaching and self-care is covered in the section on STIs in general.

STIs, also known as sexually transmitted diseases (STDs), present a major public health problem in the United States. STIs comprise more than 25 infectious organisms that are transmitted through sexual activity (vaginal, oral, and anal intercourse), along with the dozens of clinical syndromes they cause. Studies show that STIs enhance the risk of sexual transmission of HIV infection (Wasserheit, 1992; Laga et al, 1993, Kreiss, 1994; U.S. Department of Health and Human Services [USDHHS], 1993, 1997). The spectrum of health consequences of STIs ranges from mild acute illness to serious long-term complications (Eng & Butler, 1997).

ANATOMY, PHYSIOLOGY, AND PATHOLOGY

In young female adolescents, the ectocervix has not yet changed from columnar cells to the more protective-type epithelial cells, biologically increasing their vulnerability to the invasion of sexually transmitted infections. Adolescents who initiate intercourse at a young age are more likely to be exposed to multiple partners and risk factors. Any or all of these factors increase the risk of infections over time. Men who are uncircumcised may be at a greater risk (as are their partners) of acquiring certain STIs, such as HIV and chancroid (see Chap. 70). Women who douche are at a higher risk for bacterial vaginosis as well as for later complications of STIs, such as pelvic inflammatory disease (PID). A correlation exists between PID and the frequency of douching (Eng & Butler, 1997) Douching alters the pH of the vaginal mucosa, resulting in an increased susceptibility to transmission of STIs.

STIs are transmitted among all sexually active people, including heterosexuals, bisexuals, and homosexuals. Men who have sex with men are at a greater risk for many life-threatening STIs, including AIDS and hepatitis B and C (American Medical Association, 1995). Women who have sex only with women seem to be at less of a risk for some bacterial STIs. Bacterial vaginosis and genital human papillomavirus infections, however, are not uncommon (Berger et al, 1995).

Certain sexual practices are more likely to facilitate the transmission of STIs. Unprotected receptive rectal intercourse is likely to result in tissue trauma and bleeding, which can facilitate invasion by pathogens. Unprotected vaginal intercourse may also result in tissue trauma, although generally to a lesser degree. Tissue damage facilitates the transmission of both bloodborne pathogens and other viral STIs. Vaginal intercourse during menstruation may facilitate STI transmission. Oral sex is less likely to promote the transmission of STIs.

EPIDEMIOLOGY

Currently, AIDS, syphilis, and gonorrhea are reportable diseases in all 50 states. Primary care providers need to be knowledgeable about the reporting requirements in the areas where they practice. Health departments in many states provide anonymous tracking and notification of partners of patients found to be infected with an STI that falls into the category of a reportable disease. Partner notification can help prevent the spread of reportable infections. According to recent data from the Centers for Disease Control and Prevention (CDC; USDHHS, 1996):

- More than 12 million Americans, including 3 million teenagers, are infected with STIs each year.
- Two thirds of persons who acquire STIs are under age 25.
- 87% of all STI cases reported were among the top 10 most frequently reported diseases in the United States in 1995.
- Since 1980, eight new sexually transmitted pathogens have been recognized in the United States.
- Every year, about $10 billion is spent on major STIs (other than AIDS) and their preventable complications.
- Women and adolescents are disproportionately affected by STIs and their consequences of transmission (Eng & Butler, 1997; USDHHS, 1996).

Risk Factors

Behaviors that place patients at risk for STIs include:

- Initiation of sexual intercourse at an early age
- Greater number of partners
- High-risk partners
- Increased frequency of intercourse

- Certain sexual practices
- Lack of circumcision of male partner
- Vaginal douching
- Lack of barrier contraceptive use (USDHHS, 1996).

TEACHING AND SELF-CARE

Because of the prevalence and consequences of STIs, all primary care providers need to participate actively in prevention efforts. These efforts should focus on preadolescents, before sexual activity begins, and should be driven by current research and surveillance data and re-evaluated frequently. Prevention efforts need to target high-risk populations and provide appropriate messages. These messages must be repeated often and in a variety of ways, altering the strategies depending on the target audience. Clinical services for prevention education as well as for diagnosis and treatment must be available and effective. Local primary care providers can provide such access. STI education should be included in all routine patient encounters. All sexually active patients need to be informed of how sexually transmitted infections are acquired. Primary care providers can work with local health departments and local schools to provide comprehensive STI services. Primary care providers should implement the recommendations of the U.S. Preventive Services Task Force (1996) and the CDC (1993, 1997) for prevention, screening, and management of STIs. The CDC publishes an annual STD surveillance report. Their guidelines for treating STDs are updated every 3 years.

CHLAMYDIA

Infections caused by *Chlamydia trachomatis* are among the most common STIs. Complications in women caused by chlamydia include PID, tubal factor infertility, and ectopic pregnancy. If not adequately treated, 20% to 40% of women infected with chlamydia will develop PID. Pregnant women can transmit the infection to their babies during delivery, potentially causing conjunctivitis or pneumonia. Adolescents and young adults are at a substantial risk of becoming infected with this infection. Unrecognized infection is believed to be highly prevalent in this group (USDHHS, 1993).

Anatomy, Physiology, and Pathology

Infection by chlamydia is insidious. Approximately 70% of chlamydial infections are asymptomatic. The rectum is a common site of initial chlamydial infection for men who engage in receptive anal intercourse. Exposure to chlamydia in females is a result of sexual intercourse. The site of the initial infection is typically the cervix. The urethra and the rectum may also be infected. The infection travels up through the cervix to the vagina, endometrium, and fallopian tubes. This upward migration may induce lower abdominal pain and minor irregular bleeding, such as postcoital bleeding. The proportion of women with chlamydial infection who develop upper reproductive tract infection (endometritis, salpingitis, and pelvic peritonitis) is uncertain. Chlamydia, alone or with other microorganisms, has been isolated from 5% to 50% of women seeking care for symptoms of PID. In 1991, more than 275,000 women were hospitalized and more than 100,000 surgical procedures were performed as a result of PID (USDHHS, 1993). Approxi-

mately 17% of women treated for PID will be infertile; an equal proportion will have chronic pain as a result of infection; and 10% of those who do conceive will have an ectopic pregnancy.

Chlamydial salpingitis may progress to perihepatitis. Chlamydia may be a cause of cystitis in women who have leukouria but negative urine cultures. Pregnant women with chlamydia are at risk for postpartum PID and endometritis (USDHHS, 1993).

Epidemiology

By 1995, 48 states had implemented legislation mandating reporting of chlamydia. The CDC has tracked chlamydial infections since 1984. The sharp increases in the prevalence of infection since 1984 primarily reflect increased screening, recognition of asymptomatic infection (mainly in women), and improved reporting capacity. In 1995, 477,638 chlamydial infections were reported to the CDC. For a second consecutive year, reported cases of chlamydia exceeded the 392,848 reported cases of gonorrhea in 1995. Reported cases of chlamydia for women (290.3 per 100,000 population) exceed those for men (52.1 per 100,000 population) (USDHHS, 1996).

Diagnostic Criteria

Symptoms rarely occur in either gender. When they do occur in females, symptoms include vaginal discharge and dysuria. Most men infected with chlamydia are asymptomatic. Chlamydial infections among heterosexual men may typically induce urethral symptoms of dysuria and discharge. Rectal infections in either gender are generally asymptomatic but may cause symptoms of proctitis (rectal discharge, pain during defecation) or proctocolitis (USDHHS, 1993).

CLINICAL WARNINGS:

- Reiter's syndrome (reactive arthritis, conjunctivitis, and urethritis) is an uncommon complication of untreated chlamydial infection, occurring primarily among men.
- In both genders, chlamydia should be considered in chronic conjunctivitis in adolescents and young adults. Although chlamydia can be detected in the pharynx after inoculation from oral–genital exposure, chlamydia has not been established as a cause of pharyngitis.

History and Physical Exam

Female partners of males with chlamydial infection should be offered a pelvic exam, chlamydia testing, and treatment. The testing and exam of female partners is recommended because:

- A positive test result may mean that additional partners may be infected.
- Asymptomatic women may have signs of PID on examination, requiring more intensive therapy.
- Women may be asymptomatically infected with other STIs.

Male partners of females with chlamydial infection should be evaluated for symptoms of chlamydia and other STIs and for allergy to the treatment medication. A physical exam of male sex partners should be encouraged, but the exam is less important than treatment. The exam is recommended because:

- A positive test may lead to the treatment of additional partners who may be infected.
- Men may be asymptomatically infected with other STIs.
- Male partners may be allergic to the treatment medication.

If it is not possible for a male partner to be examined, the provider must determine that the man does not have symptoms suggestive of another STI and is not allergic to the treatment medication.

Diagnostic Studies

A number of nonculture tests are marketed for the detection of chlamydia. Nonculture tests are easier to perform and are less expensive than cultures. Tests available include:

- Enzyme immunoassays to detect chlamydia antigens
- Fluorescein-conjugated monoclonal antibodies for the direct visualization of chlamydia elementary bodies on smears
- Nucleic acid hybridization tests
- Rapid tests.

CLINICAL WARNING: Nonculture tests have less specificity, leading to false-positive results. All positive nonculture tests should be interpreted as presumptive.

CLINICAL PEARLS

The preferred collection site is the endocervix in women, the urethra in men. Cell culture testing is available and highly specific.

Endocervical specimens should be obtained after obtaining Pap smears or cervical cultures. Urethral specimens should be delayed until 2 hours after the patient has voided. Specific instructions for the various tests must be followed.

The disadvantages of cell cultures include:

- Delayed results (3 to 7 days)
- Only viable organisms are detected, necessitating a special transport medium with control of temperature, and additional cost.

Both enzyme immunoassay and direct fluorescent antibody assay of a first morning urine sample can identify as many infected symptomatic men as does a culture of urethral swabs. Few if any false-positive results are associated with these tests. However, they fail to identify more than 40% of cases in women (Lee et al, 1995).

Urine collection for chlamydia assay uses the nucleic acid amplification method to detect the presence of chlamydia DNA in the specimen. Two methods are the polymerase chain reaction and the ligase chain reaction. Urine collection for detection is less invasive, and early studies have shown a high rate of infection detection, almost 30% greater than that of endocervi-

cal swab culture (Chernesky et al, 1994; Epidemiology Newsletter, 1996; Lee et al, 1995).

The leukocyte estrase test is a dipstick that is applied to urine specimens to screen for urinary tract infection. Data are being collected to determine the role of this tool in the diagnosis of chlamydia.

Culture is the preferred method for detecting chlamydia in rectal specimens. The performance of nonculture tests with conjunctival specimens has been at least as effective as with genital specimens. Chlamydial serology has little value in the routine clinical care of genital tract infections. Chlamydial infections elicit long-lasting antibodies that cannot be easily distinguished from the antibodies produced in a current infection.

CLINICAL PEARL

If a post-treatment test is performed using a nonculture test, the test should be scheduled at least 3 weeks after the completion of antimicrobial therapy.

Everyone with whom the patient has had ongoing sexual exposure within 60 days of the positive test result should be treated. The primary care provider should inform infected patients to have their partners examined and treated. Public health department providers can anonymously contact exposed partners if the patient chooses not to inform them.

Treatment Options, Expected Outcomes, and Comprehensive Management

The recommended antimicrobial agent for uncomplicated urethral, endocervical, or rectal chlamydia in adults is doxycycline or azithromycin. Table 69-1 gives treatment guidelines for both chlamydia and the complication of PID.

TEACHING AND SELF-CARE

Chlamydial infection is especially prevalent among adolescents. Prevention strategies must be targeted toward young people and their sexual partners. Community-based prevention programs should target all sexually active adolescents and young adults. These can include school-based programs, adolescent recreation programs, television programs and ads, and newspaper ads. Posters and patient education materials can be placed in settings where there is a high traffic flow of adolescents and young adults. These measures can help promote increased awareness and vigilant screening and treatment. The principal goal is to prevent both overt and silent chlamydial salpingitis and PID sequelae. Prevention of perinatal and postpartal infection is also critical.

Strategies should target infection prevention. Specific strategies include:

- Recommending behavioral changes that reduce the risk of acquiring or transmitting chlamydia
- Advising teens to delay having intercourse, to decrease the number of sexual partners, and to use barrier contraception
- Identifying and treating patients with genital chlamydial infection before they infect their sexual partners, and infected pregnant women before they infect their infants.

TABLE 69-1	Sexually Transmitted Infections Treatment Guidelines		
Infections	**Symptoms**	**Treatment**	**Partner Treatment**
Chlamydia	Vaginal discharge, postcoital spotting, dyspareunia, dysuria. May be asymptomatic.	Azithromycin 1 g PO, single dose **OR** Doxycycline 100 mg PO BID × 7 days *Alternative:* Erythromycin 500 mg PO QID × 7 days **OR** EES 800 mg PO QID × 7 days **OR** Ofloxacin 300 mg PO BID × 7 days	Male partners should be treated presumptively if exam is not possible. Female partners are encouraged to seek a pelvic exam and treatment.
Pelvic inflammatory disease	Severe cramplike lower abdominal pain, chills and fever, vaginal discharge if chronic. Low-grade fever, dyspareunia, dysmenorrhea, pelvic tenderness, cervical motion tenderness.	Cefotetan 2 g IV BID **OR** Cefoxitin 2 g IV QID **PLUS** Doxycycline 100 mg IV or PO BID (PO × 14 days) *Parenteral therapy may be d/c 24 hrs after clinical improvement.* *Oral regimen:* Ofloxacin 400 mg PO BID × 14 days **PLUS** Metronidazole 500 mg PO BID × 14 days	Treat partner if specific STI diagnosed/suspected as cause of PID.
Gonorrhea	Yellow-green discharge with unpleasant odor, pain, and frequency of urination. Cervix with redness or erosion. Swelling of glands around the vagina. Cervical and pelvic tenderness. Dyspareunia. Rectum may be inflamed and have a discharge. May be febrile.	Cefixime 400 mg PO, single dose **OR** Ceftriaxone 125 mg IM, single dose **OR** Ciprofloxacin 500 mg PO, single dose **OR** Ofloxacin 400 mg PO, single dose **PLUS** Azithromycin 1 g PO, single dose **OR** Doxycycline 100 mg BID × 7 days	Treat current partners and those with known sexual exposure over the previous 60 days.
Syphilis	*Primary stage:* Chancre *Secondary stage:* Generally unwell. Headache and perhaps fever or sore on mouth, nose, throat, genitals, face, palm and soles. *Latent stage:* No symptoms	Benzathine penicillin G 2.4 million units IM **LATENT:** Benzathine penicillin G 7.2 million units, total, given in 3 doses at 1-week intervals *Penicillin allergy:* Doxycycline 100 mg PO BID × 14 days **OR** Tetracycline 500 mg PO QID × 14 days	Sexual contacts should be evaluated and treated presumptively if exposure <90 days ago. If exposure >90 days ago, serologic tests should be done to determine infectivity.
Herpes simplex virus	Painful genital or oral ulcerative lesion(s). Increased vaginal discharge. Enlarged regional lymph nodes.	*Initial occurrence:* Acyclovir 400 mg PO TID × 7–10 days **OR** Acyclovir 200 mg PO 5×/day for 7–10 days **OR** Famciclovir 250 mg PO TID × 7–10 days **OR** Valacyclovir 1.0 g PO BID × 7–10 days *Recurrent episodes:* Acyclovir 400 mg PO TID × 5 days Acyclovir 200 mg PO BID × 5 days Famciclovir 125 mg PO BID × 5 days Valcyclovir 500 mg PO BID × 5 days	
Bacterial vaginosis	Fishy odor, white or yellow-green discharge. Irritation of vagina and vulva.	Metronidazole 500 mg PO BID × 7 days **OR** Clindamycin cream 2%, 5 g intravaginally at bedtime × 7 days **OR** Metronidazole gel 0.75%, 5 g 1 or 2×/day × 5 days	Partners may be treated with metronidazole for recurrent infections.

(continued)

TABLE 69-1	Sexually Transmitted Infections Treatment Guidelines *(Continued)*		
Infections	Symptoms	Treatment	Partner Treatment
Trichomoniasis	Foamy gray or green-yellow discharge. Unpleasant odor. Itching and soreness of vagina and vulva.	Metronidazole 2 g stat **OR** Metronidazole 500 mg BID for 7 days	Treat partner at the same time, same medication and dose.
Moniliasis	Thick, curdlike discharge that smells like yeast. Itching, burning, soreness, and inflammation of vagina or vulva.	Topical butaconazole, clotrimazole, miconazole, nystatin, tioconazole, terconazole as 7-day vaginal cream or 3-day suppository **OR** Fluconazole 150 mg PO, single dose Lotrizome 1% BID, 7–14 days for extreme external symptoms	Treatment not typically recommended. In recurrent infections, treat partner at the same time or if symptoms are present.

Source: U.S. Dept. of Health and Human Services. (1997). Sexually transmitted diseases treatment guidelines. Atlanta: CDC.

■ ■ ■ **CLINICAL PEARL**

Active screening and prompt treatment are necessary because the infections are typically asymptomatic.

Efforts aimed at preventing complications among patients found to be infected with chlamydia include careful screening to identify and treat asymptomatic infection, and treatment of the female partners of men infected with chlamydia.

■ ■ ■ **CLINICAL PEARLS**

■ Early recognition of clinical symptoms suggestive of infection, including mucopurulent cervicitis and urethral symptoms, is important. Treatment is critical for preventing complications.

■ Screening guidelines should reflect prevalence rates within the provider's geographical area.

Because of the high incidence of chlamydial infection among sexually active females, the CDC's screening recommendations include (USDHHS, 1993):

■ Women younger than 20 should be tested when undergoing a pelvic exam, unless sexual activity since the last test for chlamydia has been limited to a single, mutually monogamous partner.

■ All other women who meet the suggested screening criteria:
  Mucopurulent cervical discharge
  Sexually active and younger than 20
  Age 20 to 24 who meet either of the following criteria, or older than 24 who meet both criteria:
    Inconsistent use of barrier contraception
    New or more than one sex partner during the last 3 months.

■ **CLINICAL WARNING:** Young men tend to seek health care less frequently than young women. When men and adolescent males present for health care, screening for chlamydia should be considered.

GONORRHEA

Anatomy, Physiology, and Pathology

Gonorrhea is transmitted almost exclusively sexually, because the gonococcus cannot survive outside the body. Sexual transmission occurs more easily from man to man or man to woman rather than the reverse. Men may have symptoms after a short incubation period of 3 to 7 days. Typically, men note urethritis and a purulent penile discharge. If left untreated, the infection may spread to the urethra, prostate, seminal vesicles, and epididymis. This may result in urethral stricture and obstructive uropathy. Proctitis may result after anal intercourse, although anal transmission is most often asymptomatic. Anoscopy may reveal punctate ulcerations and intraluminal pus. Pharyngitis may occur after oral–genital sex, although these patients are typically asymptomatic.

Conjunctivitis may occur as a result of inoculation into the conjunctiva. Lack of treatment may progress to corneal ulceration. Newborns may acquire gonococcal ophthalmia from contact with infected vaginal discharge during vaginal birth.

In females, the infection ascends to the uterus and fallopian tubes if untreated. This may lead to salpingitis and PID.

Gonococci may disseminate; this occurs more often in women than in men. Gonococcemia manifests as bacteremia, fever, chills, and characteristic hemorrhagic, painful, vesicopustular skin lesions. Frequently seen is tenosynovitis, particularly of the small joints of the hands and feet. Less common manifestations include endocarditis and perihepatic involvement (Fitz-Hugh-Curtis syndrome).

Antimicrobial resistance remains an important consideration in the treatment of gonorrhea. The resistance, caused mainly by the production of a beta-lactamase (penicillinase), affects 5% to 20% of patients in the United States. In 1995, 31.6% of isolates collected by the Gonococcal Isolate Surveillance Project were resistant to penicillin, tetracycline, or both (USDHHS, 1996). Resistance to ciprofloxacin was first identified in 1991 but remains rare (USDHHS, 1996).

Epidemiology

Infections caused by *Neisseria gonorrhoeae* are a major cause of PID, tubal infertility, ectopic pregnancy, and chronic pelvic pain in the United States. Epidemiologic studies provide strong evidence that gonococcal infections facilitate HIV transmission (Eng & Butler, 1997). An estimated 1 million new infections with gonorrhea occur in the United States each year. The rate of gonorrhea has continued to decline since 1975. From 1994 to 1995, the rate decreased from 165.1 per 100,000 population to 149.5. Teens age 15 to 19 had higher rates than the general population; young adults age 20 to 24 from minority populations had the highest rates.

History and Physical Exam

The exam of the external female genitalia may demonstrate swelling and discharge from Bartholin's glands. In men, the exam includes assessing for discharge and regional lymphadenopathy. The prostate should be palpated for signs of acute prostatitis (see Chaps. 68 and 70).

Diagnostic Studies

Cell cultures may be obtained from the sites of exposure (ie, urethra, endocervix, throat, rectum). Microscopic examination of gram-stained specimen discharge may be diagnostic in clinical settings where this is possible, although this method is less sensitive than cell culture. Nonculture tests such as enzyme immunoassays and DNA probes are available and reliable but do not provide information on antibiotic sensitivity (U.S. Preventive Task Force, 1996). Urine tests to detect gonorrhea using the DNA amplification method have a high rate of accurate detection. The directions for specimen collection must be followed carefully.

Treatment Options, Expected Outcomes, and Comprehensive Management

Refer to the general guidelines presented at the beginning of this chapter for the prevention and control of STIs. The CDC recommends screening all pregnant women and all women presenting to STD clinics for gonorrhea (USDHHS, 1993). The U.S. Preventive Task Force (1996) recommends screening all people who are at high risk, including women who have multiple sex partners, a partner with multiple partners, a partner with gonorrhea, or a history of repeated infections. Gonorrhea screening programs have attempted to establish screening criteria that would apply across a variety of provider sites. Frequently used criteria include age (less than 25), marital status, number of recent sexual partners, and repeat clinic visits (Mertz et al, 1997).

When selecting a treatment regimen for gonorrhea infection, the provider must consider the anatomic site of infection, the resistance of gonorrhea strains to the antimicrobials, the possibility of concurrent infection with chlamydia, and side effects and costs. Table 69-1 gives specific treatment guidelines for gonorrhea.

■ **CLINICAL WARNINGS:**

- Because coinfection with chlamydia is common, persons treated for gonorrhea should be treated presumptively with a regimen that is effective against chlamydia (U.S. Preventive Task Force, 1996).
- Any patient treated for gonorrhea should be screened for syphilis.
- Treatment regimens that cover both gonorrhea and chlamydia may treat incubating syphilis, but few data relevant to this topic are available (U.S. Preventive Task Force, 1996).

A test of cure is unnecessary for any of the antimicrobial treatments. Patients with persistent symptoms should be evaluated by culture.

■ **CLINICAL WARNING:** Any gonococci isolated should be tested for antimicrobial resistance.

■ ■ ■ **CLINICAL PEARLS**

- An infection detected after an approved treatment regimen is most likely caused by reinfection. This indicates a need for partner referral for screening and treatment as well as thorough patient education.
- If the patient is symptomatic, all sexual contacts within 30 days of the onset of symptoms should be evaluated and treated for gonorrhea and chlamydia.
- With asymptomatic patients, all sexual contacts within 60 days should be evaluated and treated. If the last sexual contact occurred more than 60 days ago, the most recent sexual contact should be evaluated and treated (U.S. Preventive Task Force, 1996).

SYPHILIS

Anatomy, Physiology and Pathology

Syphilis is a systemic disease caused by *Treponema pallidum*. It progresses through three stages.

Primary syphilis is characterized by a chancre or painless lesion that occurs about 3 weeks after exposure. The chancre is usually a solitary erythematous macule that ulcerates, with a well-defined indurated border. The lesion initially has a clear red base that becomes encrusted. Chancres most frequently occur in the genital area but may occur elsewhere on the body, often near the lips or in the mouth. Systemic symptoms rarely occur during this stage. The chancre often goes unnoticed and resolves without treatment within 3 to 6 weeks.

Secondary syphilis occurs within 6 weeks of the chancre and is characterized by adenopathy and a generalized rash that extends to the palmar and plantar surfaces. The lesions may be macular, maculopapular, or papular and are generally not itchy. The lesions may be accompanied by fever, headache, malaise, fatigue, muscle or joint pain, or lymphadenopathy. The mucous membranes are involved in 20% to 70% of patients with secondary syphilis. Diagnosis at this stage may be difficult because the symptoms frequently mimic those of other conditions, such as psoriasis, tinea corporis, or genital warts. Condylomata lata are secondary syphilis lesions found mainly in the genital and perianal regions; they may be mistaken for genital warts, or condylomata. Pharyngeal erythema without a sore throat occurs in about 25% of patients (Clayton & Krowchuk, 1997).

Tertiary syphilis marks the end of latency and is characterized by neurologic and cardiovascular disease, gumma, auditory or ophthalmic involvement, or cutaneous lesions. Thirty percent to 40% of untreated patients progress to tertiary syphilis in 2 to 30 years after initial infection (Clayton & Krowchuk, 1997).

Epidemiology

The rate of primary and secondary syphilis peaked in 1945, then declined until the 1960s because of penicillin treatment. An increase in incidence occurred in the 1960s because of the "sexual revolution" and dramatic cuts in funding of programs to reduce transmission of STIs. Another upsurge was noted in large cities in 1985 and 1986, among disadvantaged minority populations. Prostitution and drug use appeared to play a role in outbreaks. The most recent increase was in 1990, in women and also in congenital syphilis. Since 1990, a decline in incidence has been observed (Eng & Butler, 1997).

History and Physical Exam

The exam is as described in previous sections. The provider should pay special attention to signs of ulcerative lesions, as well as any generalized rashes that have spread to the palmar and plantar surfaces.

DIAGNOSTIC STUDIES

Dark-field examination and direct fluorescent antibody tests of lesion exudate are the definitive methods for diagnosing early syphilis. Serologic tests provide presumptive diagnosis and should be performed sequentially by the same laboratory. Serologic tests are of two types:

- Nontreponemal (VDRL and RPR): may be negative in 40% of recent infections
- Treponemal (FTA-ABS) antibody tests: positive 5 to 7 days after chancre appears.

CLINICAL WARNINGS:

- False-negative results may occur.
- Abnormal results of serologic testing have been observed among HIV-infected patients. For this reason, additional use of other tests (biopsy or direct microscopy) is recommended.

No single test can be used to diagnosis neurosyphilis. This diagnosis is made using a combination of serologic tests and tests on cerebrospinal fluid.

Treatment Options, Expected Outcomes, and Comprehensive Management

SCREENING

Screening must continue in high-risk populations, including prostitutes and drug users and their partners. Syphilis should be in the differential diagnosis whenever a patient presents with ulcerative lesions or a generalized rash that spreads to the palmar and plantar surfaces. Prevention strategies include discussing with the patient the value of delaying the onset of sexual activity, reducing the number of sexual partners, and using effective barrier methods.

CLINICAL PEARLS

- Patients diagnosed with syphilis need to be considered at high risk for the transmission of HIV.
- Pregnant women should be evaluated for potential infection to prevent the transmission of congenital syphilis.

TREATMENT

Parenteral penicillin G is the preferred pharmacologic treatment for syphilis. The preparation used, the dosage, and the duration of treatment depend on the stage and clinical manifestations. Table 69-1 presents specific treatment guidelines. Parenteral penicillin G is the only therapy with documented efficacy for neurosyphilis and in pregnant women.

CLINICAL WARNINGS:

- Pregnant patients and patients with neurosyphilis who report penicillin allergy should almost always be desensitized to penicillin so that they may be treated with penicillin.
- Nonpregnant patients with penicillin allergy may be treated with doxycycline or tetracycline.

Sexual contacts of patients being treated for syphilis should be evaluated and treated presumptively if their exposure to the patient was less than 90 days ago. If the exposure was more than 90 days ago, serologic tests may be done to determine infection.

COMPREHENSIVE MANAGEMENT AND FOLLOW-UP

No definitive criteria for cure or failure exist. Serologic studies should be done 3 and 6 months after treatment. Patients with persistent symptoms or whose titers sustain a fourfold increase over baseline can be considered to have failed treatment or to have become reinfected. Such patients should be retreated. They should also be evaluated for HIV infection. When patients are retreated, the recommended regimen is benzathine penicillin G 2.4 million units given intramuscularly once a week for 3 weeks, for a total of three doses.

HERPES SIMPLEX VIRUS

Anatomy, Physiology, and Pathology

Genital herpes is acquired through direct contact with virus and can penetrate intact mucous membranes. Viral particles are transported along peripheral sensory nerves to the dorsal root ganglion, where latent infection is established (Clark et al, 1995). The incubation time for herpes simplex virus (HSV) is 3 to 14 days after primary infection. There may be a significant delay in or total absence of symptoms if pre-existing immunity is present. Primary outbreaks are generally more severe than secondary outbreaks and last 2 to 3 weeks.

There are two forms of genital herpes: HSV1 and HSV2. HSV2 causes approximately 80% of infections, manifesting primarily as genital lesions. HSV1 is responsible for the remaining 20%, usually seen as oral lesions. There is significant crossover between the two strains and their locations. Oral herpes is one of the causative organisms in the condition commonly referred to as cold sores; these are intraepidermal vesicles on the lips and buccal mucosa that ulcerate easily and produce tender lesions that crust over before healing without a scar. HSV2 has a much greater propensity toward symptomatic recurrence and asymptomatic shedding then HSV1 (Pereria, 1996). The majority of genital herpes infections are asymptomatic.

Epidemiology

In many countries, successful control of bacterial STIs has coexisted with an increase in the prevalence of viral STIs (Kinghorn, 1996). The continued increase in the incidence of clinical and subclinical genital HSV infections is of particular concern due to the association of increased HIV transmission in the presence of concurrent ulcerative, herpetic lesions. In addition, there is concern that HSV may increase the likelihood of the sexual transmission of hepatitis C (Scott, 1995).

HSV is the most common cause of genital ulcerative disease in industrialized countries (Clayton & Krowchuk, 1997), affecting more than 30 million people in the United States (Eng & Butler, 1997). More than 500,000 new cases of HSV occur in the United States each year (Conant et al, 1996). Genital herpes is generally thought of as an STD, but it should probably be considered an infection transmitted by physical contact (Scott, 1995). Undiagnosed HSV and asymptomatic viral shedding may play a large role in the growing number of new infections. Controlled studies have documented viral shedding between HSV recurrences, asymptomatic shedding in the genitourinary tract, and shedding during the prodromal period that precedes an active outbreak of lesions (Conant et al, 1996). The success of HSV as a pathogen—indeed, its key to survival—is its ability to establish latent infection in the sensory ganglia for the lifetime of the host (Pereria, 1996).

Diagnostic Criteria

Criteria include the presence of fluid-filled lesions on an erythematous base. The selective use of viral culture is an important criterion for diagnosis (Clark et al, 1995).

History and Physical Exam

Clinical diagnosis of genital herpes requires obtaining a standard history for HSV signs and symptoms. Question the patient about past or current presence of the characteristic lesions of HSV. Inquire whether these lesions were accompanied by any of a variety of symptoms, such as superficial to deep pain, burning sensations, and swollen, tender lymph nodes in the area of infection. Note any history of sexual contacts who were possible sources for HSV. Identify whether the patient has a history of HSV1.

Patients with primary infection may experience prodromal flulike symptoms of fever and malaise, headaches, and myalgias and frequently remember pain and pruritus in the area where the lesions emerge. The vesicles rupture within 1 to 2 days of forming, leaving painful superficial ulcers that become crusted until they heal. For men, symptoms tend to be less severe and are often atypical.

The physical exam involves assessing for the presence of fluid-filled vesicles, which appear singly or in groups on an erythematous base. Genital HSV infection can manifest atypically as edema, fissures, erythematous patches, or fleeting irritations. Lesions on the buttocks are frequently misdiagnosed as insect bites or rashes of undetermined significance. Vulvar lesions are often preceded by increased vaginal discharge and irritation, often mistaken for a monilial infection. Other companion symptoms can be lower back pain, pain or aching radiating down one leg, burning with urination, and urinary retention.

Because HSV remains dormant in nerve ganglia, recurrences range from frequent to rare, depending on factors such as endogenous or exogenous stressors and immune system status. Recurrences tend to decrease in frequency over time and may disappear altogether after the primary episode. At the onset of a secondary episode, prodromal symptoms such as aching, burning, and increased vaginal discharge will alert the patient that the eruption of vesicles will follow.

Diagnostic Studies

There are several laboratory methods available to assist with the diagnosis of HSV. Viral culture is the easiest way to separate HSV1 from HSV2. Lesions must be at an early stage; 20% to 30% of culture results are falsely negative (Clark et al, 1995). Results may take 1 to 2 days. If lesions are atypical, equivocal, or old, biopsy or polymerase chain reaction should be considered. Direct immunofluorescence of early vesicular or crusted lesions is as accurate as viral culture and is quicker; results can be available in a few hours (Pereria, 1996)

Treatment Options, Expected Outcomes, and Comprehensive Management

Antiviral medication is started as soon as the diagnosis is established in initial infections, and specific treatment guidelines are given in Table 69-1 during the prodromal period to prevent or shorten recurrent episodes. In recurrent genital herpes, the ulceration is somewhat milder and the associated symptoms are slight or absent, even without pharmacotherapy.

There are three forms of pharmacologic therapies for the treatment of HSV: initial, episodic, and suppressive. Refer to Table 69-1 for specific treatment guidelines.

TEACHING AND SELF-CARE

The treatment of herpes infections includes diet, lifestyle, pharmaceuticals, and attention to psychosocial needs. Genital herpes can have considerable psychological and psychosexual consequences. These may manifest as depression, anger, and lowered self-esteem. The psychological morbidity in patients with a first episode of genital herpes is statistically significantly greater than that occurring in nonherpes patients attending STI clinics (Mindel, 1996). Some patients may express profound regret for poor judgment. They may view this infection as punishment for sexual practices they characterize as promiscuous or unsavory (Conant et al, 1996).

Patients experiencing recurrent episodes have a broad spectrum of concerns. There are questions regarding long-term health issues and future pregnancies. Some patients focus on concerns about disclosure of infection to future partners and family members. People with recurrent genital herpes may experience shame and guilt, withdrawing from intimate relationships for fear of rejection and disapproval. This can lead to self-imposed social isolation (Conant et al, 1996). Treatment must include addressing the issue of self respect. Ideally, this will lead to better management and healing strategies as well as strengthened communication between provider and patient.

HUMAN PAPILLOMAVIRUS

Pathology

Human papillomaviruses (HPVs) are small DNA viruses capable of inducing the proliferation of epithelial cells in the natural hosts (Zheng & Vaheri, 1995). Of the 60 types of HPV that have been identified, 20 are known to cause genital warts. HPV types 6 and 11 are the most prevalent types associated with condylomata acuminata and are not considered to have malignant potential. Types 16, 18, 30, 31, 33, 35, 39, and several more in the 40, 50, and 60 ranges are most frequently associated with genital neoplasia. Genotypes 30 and 40 are associated with laryngeal cancers.

> **CLINICAL WARNING:** Sexual activity is a well-known risk factor for the development of cervical carcinoma. Up to 90% of cervical cancer specimens have been found to harbor DNA of HPV genotypes (Wiener & Walther, 1995).

Epidemiology

As of 1994, the estimated annual incidence of HPV was 500,000 to 1 million (Carson, 1997; Eng & Butler, 1997). It is believed that approximately 40 million Americans are infected with HPV. HPV causes condylomata acuminata (genital warts), considered the leading cause of cervical neoplasia. HPV infection is often subclinical, exhibiting no visible evidence of disease (Eng & Butler, 1997).

Factors that may influence a patient's susceptibility to HPV and the immune system's response to the infection are sexual practices, parity, diet, smoking, other STIs, and immunogenic characteristics. These factors may play a contributory role in the subsequent development of cervical carcinoma (Birley et al, 1995). HPV is transmitted via contact with the virus to sensitive areas of the body. Genital HPV genotypes infect particular membranes such as labial, vaginal, cervical, rectal, oral, and penile tissue. Viral shedding without apparent lesions may occur, but condylomata are highly infectious sources of contact. The role of hand–genital transmission in the etiology of genital warts is unclear. Incubation periods range from 3 to 9 months.

History and Physical Exam

The clinical presentation of genital warts is a diagnostic indicator of HPV. They appear most frequently in the urogenital and rectal areas. Lesions are typically pedunculated or broad-based and mostly papillary, with a lobulated or irregular surface. They may occur as individual lesions, ranging from 0.2 to 1 cm.

When in clusters, they may become confluent and involve large areas of the genitalia. In men who are uncircumcised, lesions are most prevalent on the inner aspect of the prepuce and at the frenulum and coronal sulcus. Conversely, men who have been circumcised often present with involvement of the penile shaft. Lesions may also occur within the urethral meatus (Palefsky & Barrasso, 1996).

During a routine exam in a woman, the provider must perform a careful inspection within the folds of the labia and beneath the clitoral hood; these are classic hiding places for condylomata. Women may be asymptomatic, or they may complain of itching and friability of the lesion. Lesions on the cervix may be flat and endophytic during a routine exam (Palefsky & Barrasso, 1996).

> ■ ■ ■ **CLINICAL PEARL**
>
> Recognition of cervical lesions may require a colposcopic exam. Atypical or subclinical HPV lesions may be identified by draping the genitalia for 3 to 5 minutes with gauze saturated with 5% acetic acid solution (white distilled vinegar) and then examining the area using colposcopy. Abnormal tissue takes on a well-demarcated, whitish hue.

Of all urologic tumors, penile carcinoma is the closest male analogy to cervical cancer. McCance (1994) found HPV in 27 of 53 (51%) penile cancers, and Villa (1997) reported HPV in 8 of 18 cases.

Diagnostic Studies

Laboratory detection of HPV includes cytology, colposcopy, histology, HPV antigen detection, and HPV DNA detection. A Pap smear of the cervix must be performed whenever warts are suspected on the external exam. The Pap smear will detect any evidence of viral damage to the cervical tissue. On microscopic examination, condylomata appear as papillated epidermal hyperplastic lesions showing parakeratosis, koilocytosis, occasional atypia of the nucleus, and hyperemia.

> **CLINICAL WARNING:** A colposcopic exam is considered the standard of care for any lesion appearing on the cervix. Coloposcopy is required for diagnosing cervical changes secondary to HPV.

Treatment Options, Expected Outcomes, and Comprehensive Management

There are a variety of reasons for treating HPV infection, including reduction of viral transmission, prevention of cervical or penile neoplasia, and symptomatic improvement. The management of HPV-induced disease remains rooted to the strategy of repeated local destruction. It is unclear whether treatment affects either the transmission or natural course of the infection. With time, host immunity generally will attain dominance (Reid, 1996). If left untreated, warts resolve spontaneously, proliferate, or remain unchanged.

The usual treatment for warts is cytotoxic or ablative therapy. The CDC's STD treatment guidelines (USDHHS, 1993, 1997) remain current. This document advises cryotherapy with liquid nitrogen or cryoprobe as first-line management for ano-genital warts. This is inexpensive and will not result in scarring if properly applied. The topical chemodestructive agents recommended by the CDC are podophyllin, podofilox, and trichloroacetic acid (TCA). Podophyllin acts by poisoning the mytotic spindle.

■ **CLINICAL WARNING:** Podophyllin must be applied carefully, avoiding healthy surrounding tissue. The patient must be advised to wash off this caustic agent within 3 to 4 hours. Podofilox can be self-administered by women and is not systemically toxic. TCA is a caustic keratolytic agent that acts by precipitation of surface proteins. It produces local burning and a white slough.

Laser therapy has the advantage of precise control and hemostasis and is used primarily for proliferative disease. Electrocautery for small lesions and surgical extirpation for large lesions are also available options. 5-fluorouracil is a pyrimidine antimetabolite that is used as a 5% cream and washed off a few hours after application. A high level of irritation may accompany its use, so this treatment should be used with caution. Interferons may be given intramuscularly, subcutaneously, or intralesionally. Side effects are common but self-limited and for the most part well tolerated.

The only safe recommended treatment during pregnancy includes TCA, cryotherapy, and CO_2 laser.

Teaching and Self-Care

Refer to the section on HSV.

BACTERIAL VAGINOSIS

Anatomy, Physiology, and Pathology

Bacterial vaginosis is thought to occur as a result of an increase in the normal vaginal pH, mediated by the metabolic activity of anaerobic bacteria (Neri et al, 1994). The exact microbes responsible for BV are unknown. The high concentrations of anaerobic gram-negative rods, peptostreptococci, and other opportunistic pathogens in the lower genital tract place women with BV at increased risk for genital infections and adverse pregnancy outcomes (Hill, 1993). Hormonal factors probably play a role, because BV is a condition that typically affects women of reproductive age. BV is a polymicrobial condition distinguished by symptomatic abnormalities of the vaginal secretions. Until recently, BV has not been characterized as an inflammatory process. This has resulted in what may be an underestimation of the long-term consequences to fertility and morbidity. Hillier et al (1996) examined 178 women with PID, looking for the role of BV-associated microorganisms in endometritis; a positive association was found. This suggests an alteration to the historical notion that BV is not an infection but a vaginal inflammation.

Epidemiology

Bacterial vaginosis (BV) is found in up to 25% of women seen in gynecologic and obstetric offices and up to 64% of women seen in STI clinics. Fifty percent of women with BV are asymptomatic (American College of Obstetrics and Gynecology [ACOG], 1996).

Diagnostic Criteria

There are four criteria for the diagnosis of BV:

- pH greater than 4.5
- Clue cells (vaginal epithelial cells studded with a large number of bacteria that obscure the cell border). At least 20% of the epithelial cells must be clue cells for this to be a significant finding.
- Positive whiff test. To perform this test, mix one or two drops of 10% KOH with the vaginal discharge. The test is positive when an amine or fishy odor is produced.
- Homogenous discharge.

The diagnosis of BV is made by finding at least three of these four signs on the vaginal and microscopic exam. Using these criteria will produce a diagnostic accuracy of 90% and will reduce the false-positive rate to less than 10% (ACOG, 1996).

■ **CLINICAL WARNING:** Vaginal cultures are insufficient to diagnose BV without supporting clinical evidence. Gram stain is a useful diagnostic test but is not found in many office practices. As long as BV is confined to the vaginal canal, this is technically not an infection. Thus, there should not be an inflammatory response. The presence of many white blood cells should alert the provider to test for other causative factors, such as chlamydia or gonorrhea.

History and Physical Exam

When confined to the vaginal canal, an overgrowth of normal bacteria typically creates a change in vaginal odor, an increase in discharge, and occasionally labial and urethral irritation. The odor is a result of metabolic byproducts, produced primarily by anaerobic bacteria. It is described as fishy and is exacerbated by contact with semen (ACOG, 1996). The discharge has been described as homogenous, white or gray, soupy, frothy, or milky, adherent to the vaginal walls, and pooling at the introitus.

■ **CLINICAL WARNING:** When the organisms that cause BV ascend into the normally sterile environment of the uterus and tubes, PID may result, causing lower abdominal cramping or pain.

Treatment Options, Expected Outcomes, and Comprehensive Management

All symptomatic infections should be treated. These include grossly apparent cervicitis and PID.

CLINICAL WARNING: Treat all infections before any pelvic instrumentation, such as abortion, endometrial biopsy, IUD insertion, and gynecologic surgery. This is important to prevent ascending infection. Male sex partners should be treated with oral agents if the patient's infection is recurrent. The rationale for male treatment lies in the alkalinity of male spermatic fluid.

Refer to Table 69-1 for specific criteria for managing BV.

Teaching and Self-Care

In general, BV is a result of vaginal imbalance. Women should strive toward healthy lifestyle practices to encourage normal vaginal flora. A diet low in sugar, adequate rest and exercise, and adequate hydration can all help. Other factors may be exposure-based, such as preventing contact with alkaline semen by using condoms. Some women may find that latex or spermicide sensitivity causes BV. They can avoid these substances by using nonlatex condoms without spermicide. Other strategies for self-care in BV are discussed in the subsection on monilial infections.

TRICHOMONIASIS
Anatomy, Physiology, and Pathology

Trichomoniasis is caused by a parasitic protozoan flagellate and is usually sexually transmitted. The infection is typically found in the vagina and urethra in women and the urethra in men.

History and Physical Exam

The physical exam reveals perineal excoriation, erythema, and possible ulcerations. The vaginal exam typically reveals a strawberry-like appearance of the cervix, red papules on the vaginal walls, and a greenish or gray, frothy or bubbly, malodorous discharge. The pH of the discharge is usually more than 5 (5 to 7). Microscopic evaluation reveals motile cells, slightly larger than leukocytes and smaller than epithelial cells. Typically, the white cell count exceeds 10 per high-power field. The whiff test may or may not be fishy.

Treatment and Comprehensive Management

Refer to the treatment guidelines found in Table 69-1.

TEACHING AND SELF-CARE

CLINICAL WARNING: Advise the patient to avoid alcohol for the 24 hours before and after treatment, and sexual intercourse during treatment.

It is important that the provider also treat the patient's sexual partners to prevent reinfection in the patient.

MONILIASIS (CANDIDIASIS, YEAST)
Anatomy, Physiology, and Pathology

Moniliasis is a common STI, usually caused by *Candida albicans*. It may also be caused by *Candida tropicalis*, *Torulopis glabrata*, or other candidal species. These fungi are normal inhabitants of the mouth, gastrointestinal tract, and vagina. Overgrowth occurs as a result of a change in vaginal pH or other changes in the vaginal flora. Systemic antibiotics frequently cause a disruption in the normal balance of the vaginal flora, resulting in a monilial infection. Persistent elevation of the blood glucose level above normal also can cause a monilial infection.

History and Physical Exam

The physical exam in the female typically reveals vulvar and vaginal erythema and irritation. Vaginal discharge is typically thick, odorless, and curdlike, with a pH in the normal range (3.8 to 4.2).

Diagnostic Criteria

Microscopic evaluation reveals hyphae, pseudohyphae, spores, or buds. In male patients, erythema is evident, with satellite lesions.

Treatment Options, Expected Outcomes, and Comprehensive Management

See the treatment guidelines presented in Table 69-1. Many antifungal creams are available over the counter. The patient who self-treats and does not respond to the treatment should be examined to rule out other conditions.

Teaching and Self-Care

Symptom resolution is better ensured if the patient refrains from sexual intercourse during treatment. Women should avoid the use of tampons during this period. Encourage the patient to allow ventilation to the affected area and to avoid tight clothing. Underwear should not be worn when sleeping.

Preventive strategies include wearing cotton rather than nylon underpants. Women should wear cotton underwear underneath their pantyhose. They should reconsider douching and using "feminine hygiene" products; avoiding these products helps maintain healthy vaginal flora.

COMMUNITY RESOURCES

Community-based resources for education and patient support are widely available in all 50 states. Local or regional public health departments offer current information on STI management standards. Public health departments are an excellent resource for patient education posters and brochures as well. They can also provide information about support groups.

- National STD Hotline, 800-227-8922
- American Medical Women's Association, 801 N. Fairfax St., Suite 400, Alexandria, VA 22314, 703-838-0500
- American Social Health Association, P.O. Box 13827, Research Triangle Park, NC 27709
- National Herpes Hotline, 919-361-8488

- The CDC's *Morbidity and Mortality Weekly Report,* mmwr-toc@listserv.cdc.gov
- CDC National Center for HIV, STD, & TB Prevention, Division of STD Prevention, http://www.cdc.gov/nchstp/dstd.html
- Sexually transmitted diseases, http://www.halcyon.com/elf/altsex/stds.html
- Virtual Hospital: What you need to know about sexually transmitted diseases, HIV disease, and AIDS, http://www.vh.org/patients/ihb/intmed/infectious/stds/stdaids.html
- STD Homepage, http://med-www.bu.edu/people/sycamore/std.htm
- *JAMA* Women's Health, Sexually Transmitted Disease Information Center, http://www.amassn.org/special/std/std.htm
- Association of Reproductive Health Professionals, http://www.arhp.org/
- National Women's Health Resource Center, http://www.healthywomen.org/

EDITOR'S NOTE:

COMPLEMENTARY APPROACHES

A general discussion of complementary approaches can be found in Chapter 3. The following, while not an exhaustive list, are some complementary approaches being used for this condition. Additional information on these approaches, including precautions, can be found in Appendices A and B. Providers need to assess for the use of complementary approaches as part of the patient's history, as they may impact conventional therapies, and patients may not volunteer this information unless specifically asked. Efficacy of many complementary approaches is not as well documented as that of conventional therapies. Providers need to read the literature before suggesting these complementary approaches.

- Complementary Modalities
  Aromatherapy

References

American College of Obstetrics and Gynecology. (1996). Vaginitis. *ACOG Technical Bulletin, 226.*

American Medical Association, Council on Scientific Affairs. (1996). Health care needs of gay men and lesbians in the U.S. *JAMA, 275,* 1354–1359.

Berger, B., Kolton, S., Zenilman, J., Cummings, M., Feldman, J., & McCormack, S. (1995). Bacterial vaginosis in lesbians: A sexually transmitted disease. *Clinical Infectious Disease, (21),* 1402–1405.

Birley, H., Hart, C., & Stacey, S. (1995). Human papillomaviruses and the genital tract: Old viruses, new developments [Editorial]. *Journal of Medical Microbiology, 43*(2), 81–84.

Carson, S. (1997). Human papillomatous virus infection update: Impact on women's health. *Nurse Practitioner, 22,* 24–37.

Chernesky, M., Jang, D., Lee, H., et al. (1994). Diagnosis of *Chlamydia trachomatis* infection in men and women by testing first-void urine by ligase chain reaction. *Journal of Clinical Microbiology, 32*(11), 2682–2685.

Clark, J., Tatum, N., & Noble, S. (1995). Management of genital herpes. *American Family Physician, 51*(1), 175–188.

Clayton, B., & Krowchuk (1997). Skin findings and STDs. *Contemporary Pediatrics,* 119–137.

Conant, M., Berger, T., Coates, T., Longo, D., Robinson, J., & Drake, L. (1996). Genital herpes: An integrated approach to management. *Journal of the American Academy of Dermatology, 35*(4), 601–605.

Eng, T., & Butler, W. (Eds.). (1997) *The hidden epidemic: Confronting sexually transmitted diseases.* Washington, D.C.: Institute of Medicine, National Academy Press.

Epidemiology Newsletter. (1996). Chlamydia: New detection methods. Utah Department of Health, Bureau of Epidemiology.

Hill, G. (1993). The microbiology of bacterial vaginosis [Review]. *American Journal of Obstetrics and Gynecology, 169* (2 Pt. 2), 450–454.

Hillier, S., Kiviat, N., Hawes, S., et al. (1996). Role of bacterial vaginosis-associated microorganisms in endometritis. *American Journal of Obstetrics and Gynecology, 175*(2), 435–441.

Kinghorn, G. (1996). Limiting the spread of genital herpes. *Scandinavian Journal of Infectious Diseases, 100,* 20–25.

Laga M, Manoka, A. Kivuvu, M. et al. (1993). Nonulcerative sexually transmitted diseases as risk factors for HIV-1 transmission in women: Results from a cohort study. *AIDS, 7:*95–102.

Lee, H., Chernesky, M., Schachter, J., et al. (1995). Diagnosis of *Chlamydia trachomatis* genitourinary infection in women by ligase chain reaction assay of urine. *Lancet, 345,* 213–216.

McCance, D. (1994). Human papillomaviruses [Review]. *Infectious Disease Clinics of North America, 8*(4), 751–767.

Mertz, K., Levine, W., Mosure, D., Breman, S., Dorian, K., & Hadgu, A. (1997). Screening women for gonorrhea: Demographic screening criteria for general clinical use. *American Journal of Public Health, 87*(9), 1535–1538.

Mindel, A. (1996). Psychological and psychosexual implications of herpes virus infection [Review]. *Scandinavian Journal of Infectious Diseases, 100,* 27–32.

Neri A., Rabinerson, D., & Kaplan, B. (1994). Bacterial vaginosis: Drugs versus alternative treatment [Review]. *Obstetrical & Gynecological Survey, 49*(12), 809–813.

Palefsky, J., & Barrasso, R. (1996). HPV infection and disease in men [Review]. *Obstetrics and Gynecology Clinics of North America, 23*(4), 895–916.

Pereria, F. (1996). Herpes simplex: Evolving concepts. *Journal of the American Academy of Dermatology, 35*(4), 503–516.

Reid, R. (1996). The management of genital condylomas, intraepithelial neoplasia, and vulvodynia [Review]. *Obstetrics & Gynecology Clinics of North America, 23*(4), 917–991.

Scott, L. (1995). Perinatal herpes: Current status and obstetric management strategies. *Pediatric Infectious Disease Journal, 14*(10), 827–830.

U.S. Department of Health and Human Services. (1993). *Recommendations and management of Chlamydia trachomatis infections.* Atlanta, GA: Centers for Disease Control and Prevention.

U.S. Department of Health and Human Services. (1993, 1997). *Sexually transmitted diseases treatment guidelines.* Washington, D.C.: U.S. Government Printing Office.

U.S. Department of Health and Human Services. (1996). *Sexually transmitted disease surveillance 1995.* Atlanta, GA: Centers for Disease Control and Prevention, National Centers for HIV, STD, and TB Prevention.

U.S. Preventive Task Force. (1996). *Guide to clinical preventive services.* Baltimore: Williams & Wilkins.

Villa, L. (1997). Human papillomaviruses and cervical cancer. *Advances in Cancer Research, 71,* 321–341.

Wasserheit, J. (1992). Epidemiologic synergy. Interrelationships between human immunodeficiency virus infection and other sexually transmitted diseases. *Sexually Transmitted Diseases 9,* 61–77.

Wiener, J., & Walther, P. (1995). Human papillomaviruses, biology and role in cervical and penile malignancy. *Infections in Medicine,* 635–641.

Zheng, J., & Vaheri, A. (1995). Human epithelial cells immortalized by human papilloma viruses [Critical Review]. *Oncogenesis, 6*(3–6), 235–250.

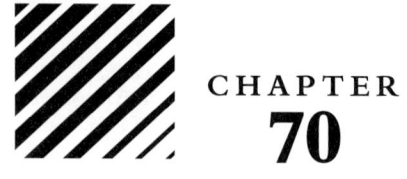

CHAPTER
70

Testicular and Penile Cancer

John Bisson, MD, Carol Green-Hernandez, PhD, RN, CS, ANP/FNP, and
James Tazelaar, MS, FNP, RN, CS

Male genital cancers are not uncommon, and because of their location they may be detected at an early stage. It is important that the primary care provider educate men about the importance of regular self-examination of the testicles and penis. Although cancers of the testes and penis are in close physical proximity, their pathogenesis and management differ so greatly that they will be discussed separately.

TESTICULAR CANCER

Primary cancer of the testis accounts for less than 1% of all malignancies (Gilliland & Key, 1995). With the appropriate use of modern diagnostic and treatment techniques, the long-term disease-free survival rate is 90% or better (van Basten et al, 1997).

Anatomy, Physiology, and Pathology

Germ cells are responsible for sperm production and are the site for 95% of the malignant neoplasms of the testes. Germ cells are arranged in a series of tubules, contained within a dense fascial covering called the tunica albuginea. The testis embryologically originates in the genital ridge and descends from the retroperitoneum during fetal development through the abdomen and inguinal canal into the scrotum (Bosl & Motzer, 1997). Extensions of the peritoneum and abdominal wall cover the testes within the scrotum. These layers include the tunica vaginalis, the internal spermatic fascia, the internal and external cremasteric fascia, and finally the dartos muscle and scrotal wall skin. Testicular neoplasms are contained by the tunica albuginea, resulting in fusiform enlargement of the testis, and metastatic spread via the blood and lymphatic supply is into the retroperitoneal nodes. Tumor spread via the scrotal skin and lymphatics into the groin is not seen unless surgery or other interventions have compromised the tumor itself.

Classification of testicular cancer is based on histologic type; this in turn reflects the major treatment options. Because 95% of testicular neoplasms arise from the germ cells, only their pathology and treatment will be discussed; for others, the provider should consult an oncologist. The two main divisions of germ cell tumors are seminoma and nonseminoma, which are additionally divided into embryonal, teratoma, choriocarcinoma, yolk sac, and mixed-cell tumors.

Right-sided tumors are slightly more common than left-sided ones, corresponding to the increased incidence of right cryptorchidism. The incidence of bilateral primary tumors is 1% to 2%. Asynchronous tumor involvement is more common than synchronous. However, on biopsy, approximately 5% of men with testicular cancer have carcinoma in situ in the contralateral testis. Approximately half of these eventually present

with cancer. This corresponds to the approximately 2% to 5% cumulative risk of developing cancer in the opposite testicle over the initial 25 years after initial diagnosis (Collis et al, 1996).

The most common germ cell tumors are seminomas, which account for about 50%. These malignancies usually present in men between 30 and 40 years of age. There are three types of seminomas: classic, anaplastic, and spermatocytic. Of these, anaplastic is notable for its high mitotic rate. Spermatocytic seminoma presents late in life and has little metastatic potential.

Between 50% and 60% of germ cell tumors are of the nonseminomatous type. This kind of tumor is most common in men up to age 30. Embryonal carcinoma is the most anaplastic of nonseminomatous tumors and may differentiate into any of the other nonseminomatous types. Choriocarcinoma is the rarest type of nonseminomatous tumor and usually shows up in mixed germ cell tumors.

Mixed germ cell tumors can comprise multiple seminomas and nonseminomas. This type of tumor accounts for close to half of tumors identified. In a mixed tumor, it is important to identify the specific type of tumor cell lines and histologic patterns involved, because treatment effectiveness depends on this information. The most difficult cell line identified dictates the treatment to be used.

Epidemiology

Germ cell cancer of the testis is the most common malignancy in males aged 15 to 35 (Devesa et al, 1995; Buetow, 1995). The incidence varies with race and socioeconomic groups. It is highest in northern Europe and New Zealand, intermediate in the United States, and lowest in Africa and Asia (Adami et al, 1994). The worldwide incidence has increased by more than 100% in the past 40 years (Bosl & Motzer, 1997). It is primarily seen in men of European heritage; in developed countries, the incidence in males of European descent is three times that in males of African descent (Feuer, 1995). Testicular cancer is found more often in developed countries than in developing countries, regardless of race. The peak incidence occurs in men age 20 to 40 years, with secondary rate increases in men older than 60 and boys younger than 10. The latter two elevations in occurrence are specific to individual rare histologic types. Primary testis cancer is the most common solid tumor in men aged 20 to 34, and the second most common in men from that point until age 40.

Higher socioeconomic status is connected with an increased frequency of testicular cancer. The relation between prosperity and testicular cancer remains unclear. Henderson et al (1997) postulated that testicular cancer and cryptorchidism are related to in utero estrogen exposure from hyperemesis gravidarum.

The strongest risk factors for hyperemesis gravidarum are early age at pregnancy, nulliparity, and high body weight of the mother.

The primary risk factor for testicular cancer is cryptorchidism. This risk does not appear to be reduced by orchiopexy, although correction of the undescended testicles allows complete palpation. Other factors that appear to increase the risk for testicular cancer are white European heritage, high socioeconomic status, family history, gonadal dysgenesis, fetal exposure to diethylstilbestrol (DES) or oral contraceptives, and a history of orchitis. Lack of descent of the testicles and damage to the testicles appear to be common to all the risk factors listed, but how these link to cancer formation is not clear. Several factors, including orchitis and trauma, may lead to earlier identification of testicular tumors rather than being true risks in and of themselves. No correlations between testicular cancer and nutritional intake or occupational hazards have been established.

Diagnostic Criteria

Testicular cancer is established by pathologic analysis of the testis after inguinal orchiectomy. Diagnosis, staging, and management of malignancies of the testes can be greatly enhanced by the use of tumor markers, discussed below.

DIFFERENTIAL DIAGNOSIS

Torsion, epididymitis, epididymo-orchitis, hydrocele, hernia, hematoma, and spermatocele can in one way or another be confused with testicular cancer. Epididymitis is the most common misdiagnosis. Any solid mass within the testicle should be considered cancer until proven otherwise. If the diagnosis is unclear or examination is hindered by a hydrocele, then ultrasonography should be obtained (Li et al, 1997).

History and Physical Exam

Many, if not most, testicular cancers present with pain or tenderness. The history needs to include assessment of risk factors, including in utero information.

The provider must examine the normal testis first as a baseline. Use the thumb and first two fingers to evaluate the size, consistency, and location of any mass. The scrotal skin should remain normal. In general, any mass within the testis is cancer, and any outside the testis is benign. A hydrocele may be present, making appreciation of a testicular mass more difficult. The abdomen is examined for evidence of retroperitoneal nodal disease; supraclavicular adenopathy suggests advanced disease.

> ■ **CLINICAL WARNING:** Although many, if not most, testicular cancers present with pain, tender gynecomastia may be the only presenting complaint.

Diagnostic Studies

Ultrasound is the single best technique for evaluating testicular pathology and should be performed in all cases of suspected testicular neoplasm. The spread of metastases is predictable, according to the testicle involved. A right testicular tumor tends to metastasize to lymph nodes between the aorta and inferior

vena cava. Metastasis from a left testicular tumor tends to spread to nodes lateral to the aorta (Bosl & Motzer, 1997). Computed tomography (CT) of the pelvis and abdomen will show nodal involvement in these areas much of the time. However, microscopic nodal involvement may still be present with negative CT results. Chest x-ray and CT are used when mediastinal or lung metastasis is suspected. The mediastinum is the source of the primary tumor in rare cases. Brain CT is usually reserved for men who show neurologic impairment.

TUMOR MARKERS

Along with imaging, one of the mainstays of testicular tumor testing is serum tumor markers. Many germ cell cancers of the testis produce useful marker materials in three basic types: oncofetal chemicals (alpha-fetoprotein [AFP]), hormonal substances (the beta subunit of human choriogonadotropin [hCG]), and cellular enzymes (lactase dehydrogenase [LDH]). AFP is produced by the least differentiated nonseminomatous tumors (embryonal carcinoma and yolk sac). The beta-hCG level is elevated in several testicular tumors, including choriocarcinoma, seminoma, and nonseminoma. LDH is not specific to any individual or group of tumor types, but an elevation in the LDH level indicates tissue destruction in advanced disease (Bosl & Motzer, 1997). AFP levels are more often increased in embryonal carcinoma.

> ■ **CLINICAL WARNINGS:**
> ■ Tumor marker elevation is less useful in tumors of mixed germ cell origin, which can include in their mix seminomas, choriocarcinomas, teratomas, embryonal cell carcinomas, and so on.
> ■ Serum marker concentrations should be obtained before initiating therapy, after completion of therapy, and regularly during long-term surveillance. The half-life of AFP and beta-hCG is important in assessing the rate of marker decrease after therapy. Therefore, these markers should begin to fall within a week or two with successful treatment; failure to decline suggests persistent disease or metastases. Tumor marker elevation that persists after radical inguinal orchiectomy is highly correlated with pulmonary metastases or metastatic retroperitoneal involvement.

STAGING

Staging is used to define the extent of testicular cancer before initiating treatment. Staging also helps to guide treatment. Staging of the primary cancer is based on the TMN (tumor, metastasis, node) system, using three stages that correspond to the extent of treatment needed and the prognosis.

Treatment Options, Expected Outcomes, and Comprehensive Management

Testicular self-exam (TSE) is the best known form of early detection. Men at risk need to be educated to do TSE on a regular basis, in addition to having the provider perform the exam.

The following testicular cancer treatment options were taken from the National Cancer Institute's clinician treatment data base (1997). This data base is updated frequently and provides a strong source of current practice standards.

Seminomas are more susceptible to irradiation than non-seminomas. Thus, the treatment of these tumors varies even if they are at the same stage. For this reason, the treatment measures are separated into seminomatous and nonseminomatous sections. In general, mixed tumors are treated as nonseminomatous tumors because these are the more difficult to manage. Patients diagnosed with testicular cancer are referred to a urologist or a uro-oncologist who specializes in the management of this disease. An overview of management is shown in Table 70-1.

Teaching and Self-Care

Rosella (1994) reviewed 11 studies that examined men's knowledge of risk for testicular cancer, knowledge of TSE, and practice of TSE. The results revealed that most men did not know their risk of testicular cancer or how to perform TSE.

Clearly, it is important that the primary care provider teach TSE to all young men at puberty (Table 70-2). Providers should especially target men who are at identified risk for developing testicular cancer.

Monthly TSE has received much attention as a screening method to improve early detection. However, there are no studies showing that TSE leads to earlier identification of testicular carcinomas (Meadus, 1995). Increased surveillance has led to earlier detection of tumors in other at-risk groups (eg, breast cancer, skin cancer). Because most testicular tumors are found by the patient, the more thoroughly prepared a patient is to detect a mass, the more likely he is to succeed. The greatest impediment to tumor identification is the lack of provider teaching of TSE (Rosella, 1994). Because men of this age group often do not seek health care, it is important that the primary care provider take advantage of every opportunity to teach men how to perform TSE.

TABLE 70-1	Testicular Cancer Staging and Management

STAGE 1 SEMINOMA: Cure rate of greater than 95%

1. Standard treatment is removal of the testicle through radical inguinal orchiectomy, followed by medium-dose radiation therapy to retroperitoneal and ipsilateral inguinal lymph nodes.

2. Under clinical evaluation: Radical inguinal orchiectomy followed by a surveillance regimen of frequent serum markers, CT scans, and chest x-rays. It appears that recurrence can be cured with radiation and chemotherapy, yielding an equally high survival rate (NCI, 1997).

STAGE 1 NONSEMINOMA: Cure rate of greater than 95%

1. Standard treatment is removal of the testicle through radical inguinal orchiectomy, followed by retroperitoneal lymphadenectomy (RLA). A nerve-sparing method that in most cases spares antegrade ejaculation has become available and appears to be as effective as non-nerve-sparing RLA.

■ **CLINICAL WARNING:** The presence of lymphatic or vascular invasion appears to increase substantially the likelihood of relapse.

2. An alternative strategy for stage 1 NSGCTT is a surveillance program after radical inguinal orchiectomy with no RLA. The regimen calls for active patient participation because of the need for an intense testing schedule of serum markers, chest x-rays every month, and abdominal CT scans every 2 months for the first 2 years and periodically thereafter.

3. Clinical investigations are ongoing using adjuvant chemotherapy in patients at high risk for relapse based on histologic type and vascular invasion (NCI, 1997).

STAGE 2 SEMINOMA: Divided into bulky and nonbulky disease

1. Bulky stage 2 is defined as tumors greater than 5 cm on CT scan, more than 70% of which are cured with either radiation to the retroperitoneal lymph nodes or chemotherapy (NCI, 1997).

2. For nonbulky stage 2 seminoma, radiation alone has led to a greater than 90% cure rate. Standard treatment is radical inguinal orchiectomy followed by radiation therapy, the extent of which depends on tumor spread (NCI, 1997).

STAGE 2 NONSEMINOMA: Cure rate greater than 95%

1. Radical inguinal orchiectomy followed by RLA with subsequent monthly physical exams, chest x-rays, and serum marker tests. The regimen is most applicable to patients with a low number (<6) and small size (<2 cm) of retroperitoneal lymph nodes at time of dissection. The relapse rate for these patients is moderate (<30%), and most relapses are curable with usual chemotherapy.

2. For patients with more or large lymph nodes: Radical inguinal orchiectomy followed by RLA and chemotherapy and then with subsequent monthly physical exams, chest x-rays, and serum marker tests.

■ **CLINICAL WARNING:** The exact timing of follow-up (eg, every 1 to 2 months) varies from center to center. The provider should be familiar with regional practice.

3. For patients who have lymph node(s) greater than 5 cm that are considered unresectable on lymphangiogram or CT scan, the combination of modalities changes to using chemotherapy first, followed by re-imaging and then consideration of surgical removal of the remnant mass(es) (NCI, 1997).

STAGE 3 SEMINOMA: Usually curable, even with distant metastasis

1. Standard therapy is radical inguinal orchiectomy followed by multidrug cisplatin-based chemotherapy. After chemotherapy, often remnant masses are present. Observation with frequent serum marker and CT scans is used. RLA is often used if individual masses are larger than 3 cm.

STAGE 3 NONSEMINOMA: Cure rate of 70% with standard chemotherapy; cases with a poor prognosis usually have widespread metastasis or mediastinal primary tumors.

1. Standard therapy is radical inguinal orchiectomy followed by multidrug chemotherapy. If the histologic type is aggressive, and CT scan or lymphangiography shows significant residual masses, surgery is done to remove them to avoid regrowth. If viable tumor cells remain, further chemotherapy is indicated. In the case of brain metastasis, along with chemotherapy, whole-brain irradiation and/or surgical excision of solitary lesions may be warranted.

RECURRENT

Treatment and prognosis of patients with refractory or reappearing testicular cancer are governed by the histologic type, the site of recurrence, previous therapies used, as well as many patient-specific variables. In general, the shorter the period of time before recurrence and the more limited the initial disease, the better the prognosis. Chemotherapy as well as surgery may be used (NCI, 1997).

Sources: National Cancer Institute, 1997; Herr et al., 1997.

TABLE 70-2	Testicular Self-Examination

1. TSE must be done in a warm, private place. The shower or bath is ideal. Coldness or privacy concerns can cause the testicles to retract, making a complete exam impossible.

2. The structures of the scrotal sac should be palpated. Each testicle should be palpated between the thumb and fingers of both hands. Testicles should feel smooth and rubbery.

The size and descent of the testicles may vary, with the left often lower than the right. The epididymis is at top rear of the testicle. The epididymis should be soft and slightly tender. Going up from the epididymis in back of the testicle is the spermatic cord. The spermatic cord should be a smooth, firm tube.

3. The exam should be done on the same day every month to make it easy to remember.

4. Any irregularities (eg, a lump in a testicle, heaviness in the scrotum, enlargement of a testicle, a dull ache in the lower abdomen or groin, a sudden collection of fluid in the scrotum) should be brought to the attention of the primary care provider immediately.

Adapted from U.S. Department of Health and Human Services, Public Health Service, National Institutes of Health. Office of Cancer Communications. (1988) *What you need to know about testicular cancer.* NIH Publication No. 88-1565.

■ **CLINICAL WARNING:** TSE is especially important in patients who have undergone an abdominal orchiectomy for testicular cancer. Potential spread to the other testicle needs to be monitored.

For the patient who has been diagnosed with testicular cancer, the education provided depends on the histologic type of tumor, spread of the tumor, and treatment modalities. These patients are typically young men, and treatment options can cause fertility problems. According to cross-cultural studies, the primary care provider should suggest that the patient consider cryobanking his sperm before beginning treatment (Arai et al, 1997; Botchan et al, 1997). The patient should also be evaluated for fertility and emotional concerns. This need may continue even after successful treatment of testicular cancer; psychological referral may be warranted.

Recent studies have demonstrated that many men who undergo treatment for testicular cancer have a decrease in sexual functioning. This decrease is probably the result of retrograde ejaculation difficulties after surgery. Surgery has no anatomic consequences on ejaculation (Jonker-Pool et al, 1997). Neuropathy can result from either retroperitoneal lymph node dissection or chemotherapy. No consistent results as to their effect on sexuality have been found. This may suggest that psychological factors have as much or more to do with sexuality issues after treatment as the therapy itself (Jonker-Pool et al, 1997; Arai et al, 1997).

■ ■ ■ **CLINICAL PEARL**

The provider should discuss with the patient whether referral for infertility or psychological counseling may be warranted. This is especially important if concerns cannot be handled easily or comfortably by the primary provider.

COMMUNITY RESOURCES

- "What You Need to Know About Testicular Cancer," NIH Publication No. 88-1565, June 1988. U.S. Department of Health and Human Services, Public

Health Service, National Institutes of Health, Office of Cancer Communications.

- National Cancer Institute (NCI), Building 31, Room 10A24, Bethesda, MD 20892: "For Men Only: Testicular Cancer and How to Do TSE," (brochure, video), "Cancer Facts for Men" (brochure), other patient information brochures. The NCI's data base (http://wwwicic.nci.nih.gov/clinpdq/) provides information for patients and providers, plus up-to-date abstracts from journal articles for providers.

- American Cancer Society, 1599 Clifton Rd. N.E., Atlanta, GA 30329-4251, 800-ACS-2345, http//www.cancer.org: Contact the local office for patient education brochures, shower cards, and local cancer support groups.

- American Academy of Pediatrics Testicular Tumor Registry, The Cleveland Clinic Foundation, 9500 Euclid Ave., Cleveland, OH 44195: Provides information on specific histologic types and current treatment protocols for providers.

PENILE CANCER

Cancer of the penis occurs in men in their middle to late adult years, typically in the fifth and sixth decades of life. It is usually a squamous cell carcinoma, arising primarily on the foreskin and glans of the penis.

Anatomy, Physiology, and Pathology

Invasive carcinoma of the penis typically presents as an ulcerative or inflammatory lesion that may gradually grow to replace the entire glans, extending into the penile shaft. Dartos fascia and Buck's fascia lie beneath the skin, followed by the tunica albuginea. Penile cancer spreads to the inguinal nodes initially, then to the iliac and femoral nodes.

Penile carcinoma is ordinarily separated into precancerous lesions, carcinoma in situ, and invasive carcinoma.

PRECANCEROUS LESIONS

- Leukoplakia are white, plaquelike lesions on the glans near the meatus.
- Balanitis xerotic obliterans is characterized by atrophic changes in the epidermis.
- Human papillomavirus (HPV) causes penile condylomata, which are wartlike lesions on the surface of the glans and penile shaft. Several specific HPV varieties have been shown to progress into anogenital cancers (Majewski & Jablonska, 1997).
- Penile intraepithelial neoplasia (PIN) consists of flat plaques, found mostly on the inner side of the foreskin, and pigmented papules on the sheath. These are not conspicuous. Only 50% are visible after the application of 3% to 5% acetic acid (Aynaud et al, 1994).

Many authorities consider balanitis xerotic obliterans, HPV, PIN, and Bowen's disease (discussed on the following page) as one entity, because all are caused by HPV (D.B. Rukstalis, personal communication, May 5, 1998).

CLINICAL WARNINGS:

- The importance of PIN as a precursor to penile cancer is significant. As PIN increases in atypia, it correlates increasingly with high-risk HPV infection: 75% of PIN1 samples display potentially oncogenic varieties of HPV, 93% of PIN2, and 100% of PIN3 (Aynaud et al, 1994).

- Multiple studies have shown a high rate of PIN infections in the male partners of women with cervical intraepithelial neoplasia (Monsonego et al, 1993; Hippolainen et al, 1994).

- The detection rate of high-risk HPV infections was similar in circumcised and uncircumcised partners of patients with HPV, but significantly fewer penile lesions were found on the circumcised partners. This suggests that other local factors play a role in the development of PIN lesions from HPV infections (Aynaud et al, 1994).

▪ ▪ ▪ CLINICAL PEARLS

- Men found to have PIN infections should be carefully monitored for progression of the lesions into cancer.

- These patients should be made aware of the cancer risk to their sexual partners.

CARCINOMA IN SITU

Carcinoma in situ of the penis takes the form of bowenoid papulosis and Bowen's disease. Bowenoid papulosis of the penis appears on the glans and usually consists of small, red or brown papules with a smooth surface. They sometimes coalesce and become encrusted. This disease usually occurs in young sexually active adults. It has a normally benign course, with spontaneous regression within several months.

CLINICAL WARNINGS:

- Bowenoid papulosis is highly correlated with high-risk HPVs.

- In older patients, bowenoid papulosis shows no tendency toward spontaneous regression. Because it can develop into cancer, surgical excision is the treatment of choice in older men (Majewski & Jablonska, 1997). Other treatment options include topical chemotherapy and laser ablation (D.B. Rukstalis, personal communication, May 5, 1998).

Bowen's disease differs from bowenoid papulosis by its later age of onset, usually with an enlarging lesion. It has a more chronic course, with no tendency to resolve spontaneously. Bowen's disease typically presents as a single red plaque that is somewhat erythematous and rather flat and noninfiltrative. It is caused by HPV. When localized to the glans, it tends to be ulcerative and takes on a velvety appearance. It is referred to then as erythroplasia of Quyerat.

CLINICAL WARNING: Both Bowen's disease and erythroplasia of Quyerat have been shown to develop into and to coexist

with invasive squamous cell carcinoma of the penis. Topical application of interferon-beta may reduce the relapse rate (Majewski & Jablonska, 1997).

INVASIVE CARCINOMA

Invasive carcinoma of the penis is typically squamous cell carcinoma. It occurs mostly on the glans or the foreskin. Metastatic spread predictably occurs through the inguinal nodes. One specific groin node appears to be the first involved and has been named the sentinel node. Most patients with penile cancer have adenopathy, but in a substantial portion of these patients the adenopathy is a result of inflammation rather than tumor progression (Ayyappan et al, 1994).

Epidemiology

Penile carcinoma represents less than 1% of male cancers seen in the United States and Europe (Wingo et al, 1995; American Cancer Society, 1997). However, in underdeveloped countries, which generally lack indoor plumbing and do not practice neonatal circumcision, the rate can be as high as 20% of adult male cancers (Cold et al, 1997).

CLINICAL WARNING: Neonatal circumcision independent of careful hygiene practices is not a preventive measure. This has been demonstrated by the lower prevalence of penile cancers in Denmark, which has a low circumcision rate, versus the United States, which has a high circumcision rate (Frisch et al, 1995). Poor hygiene appears to be the common factor associated with an increased incidence of cancer in lower socioeconomic groups. The presence of smegma and bacteria and the effects of repeated low-grade infections have been suggested as having a synergistic action with HPV in causing penile cancer (Majewski & Jablonska, 1997). This would help to explain why penile cancer is less common in populations practicing neonatal circumcision, which limits the likelihood of bacterial retention within the foreskin and on the glans.

Table 70-3 lists the risk factors for penile cancer. The greatest risk factor appears to be HPV infection. Penile cancer is

TABLE 70-3	**Risk Factors for Penile Cancer**
History/Activity	Relative Risk vs. No History
Genital warts (HPV)	5.9
Never circumcised	3.2
Circumcised after neonatal period	3.0
History of penile rash (this may be HPV or increase susceptibility to HPV)	9.4
History of penile tear	3.9
Current smoker	2.8
Presence of smegma	2.1
Difficulty retracting foreskin	3.5
History of >30 sexual partners	3.3

Source: Maden et al., 1993.

probably multifactorial, and one causative factor for all cases is unlikely to be found.

Diagnostic Criteria

In addition to the clinical exam, the following determinations should be made:

- Primary tumor (T)
  Incisional/excisional biopsy of lesion and histologic examination for grade and depth of invasion.
  Regional and juxtaregional lymph nodes (N)
  CT scan
  Superficial inguinal node dissection for high-grade or invasive histology
  Lymphangiography and aspiration cytology (optional)
- Distant metastases (M)
  Chest radiograph, CT scan
  MRI, bone scan (optional)
  Biochemical determinations (liver function, calcium).

DIFFERENTIAL DIAGNOSIS

In addition to the precancerous lesions previously described, carcinoma must be differentiated from inflammatory and other benign lesions. Syphilitic chancre is a painless ulcer best diagnosed with dark-field examination. Chancroid is a painful ulcer with *Haemophilus ducreyi* on special culture. Condylomata acuminata are soft, exophytic, wartlike lesions that can occur anywhere on the penis. These are easily distinguished histologically if any doubt exists. Refer to Chapter 69 for more information on their diagnosis and management.

History and Physical Exam

Most patients present with a lesion on the glans, although some may not be aware of a problem because of phimosis. Uncircumcised men are still at risk, so thin white or red plaques should not be discounted without histologic analysis (Cold et al, 1997). The patients should be questioned about a past history of HPV infection of either him or his sexual partners. Past episodes of bowenoid papulosis should be explored. If treatment is not undertaken, many patients return within 1 year with complaints of penile bleeding, discharge, and occasionally pain. Inguinal nodes should be palpated; more than half of patients present with adenopathy.

Diagnostic Studies

Results of the screening laboratory evaluation for men with penile cancer are usually normal. Imaging studies should include chest x-ray, bone scan, and CT scan of the abdomen and pelvis. Anemia and hypercalcemia may be found in extensively metastasized disease. Local secondary infection related to the cancer may cause an elevated white blood cell count. Only a few patients show evidence of distant metastases. Therefore, the provider must determine whether nodal involvement is the result of infection or a neoplasm before referring the patient for nodal biopsy or resection.

■ ■ ▨ **CLINICAL PEARL**

If the patient has received a postsurgical course of antibiotics but the lymph nodes remain palpably enlarged 3 or more weeks after excision of the primary lesion, refer the patient back to the urologic surgeon for consideration of bilateral lymph node excision.

Treatment Options, Expected Outcomes, and Comprehensive Management

The following penile cancer treatment options were taken from the National Cancer Institute's clinician treatment data base (1997). Patients diagnosed with penile cancer should be referred to a urologist or a uro-oncologist who specializes in the management of this disease. An overview of management is presented in Table 70-4.

PROGNOSIS

The National Cancer Institute's Surveillance, Epidemiology, and End Results Program reports that an estimated 1300 new cases of penile cancer and 220 deaths from penile cancer occurred in 1997 (American Cancer Society, 1997). Untreated carcinoma of the penis is characterized by a relentless progressive course, with death from the disease occurring within 2 to 3 years after diagnosis (Ornellas et al, 1994; Lopes et al, 1996). The disease-free and overall 5-year survival rates are most influenced by lymph node metastases, as well as by the degree of tumor differentiation. It has been reported that the survival rate increases when the natural course of the disease is altered with neoplastic lymph node dissection. Stage appears to have no correlation with survival rates except as it relates to metastases. The effect that radiation therapy and chemotherapy may have on these rates is not clear at this time (Ornellas et al, 1994).

Teaching and Self-Care

Because penile cancer tends to occur in the mature population, adult learning principles must be considered in any educational planning. Although neonatal circumcision greatly reduces the risk of penile cancer, there have been cases reported in circumcised men (Cold et al, 1997). Patients who have a history of HPV infection need to be aware of their risk for the development of penile cancer. Because PIN infections tend to develop into cancer, patients with such lesions must be educated about this risk. Because the risk of cervical cancer related to HPV infection is considerably higher than that of penile cancer, female sexual partners of patients need to be made aware of their risk (Monsonego et al, 1993; Hippolainen et al, 1994).

The Danish experience has shown that penile cancer can be reduced in a noncircumcised population through improved hygiene practices such as daily cleaning of the penis after retracting the foreskin (Frisch et al, 1995). Careful teaching of these practices should ideally start with the parents. The provider should reinforce this teaching in uncircumcised boys and men.

TABLE 70-4	**Staging and Treatment of Penile Cancers**

Stage 1: Penile cancer is limited to the glans and the foreskin, not involving the shaft of the penis or substructures. No regional lymph node or distant metastasis. Stage 1 penile cancer is curable.

Treatment options:

Lesions limited to the foreskin can be treated through wide local excision with circumcision.

Carcinoma in situ of the glans (EQ or Bowen's disease) with or without adjacent skin involvement: treat with local applications of fluorouracil cream, or surgery that is microscopically controlled.

For infiltrating tumors of the glans, with or without adjacent skin involvement, the choice of therapy is dictated by tumor size, extent of infiltration, and degree of tumor destruction of normal tissue. Equivalent therapeutic options include penile amputation, external beam radiation, brachytherapy, or microscopically controlled surgery.

Local laser ablation therapy with either YAG or CO_2 lasers is under clinical evaluation, in hopes of preserving cosmetic appearance and sexual function.

Although controversial, elective adjuvant inguinal lymph node dissection for clinically negative lymph nodes is sometimes performed. Its rationale is the high incidence of microscopic nodal metastases.

Stage 2: Penile cancer has invaded the corpora cavernosa but has not spread to lymph nodes on clinical exam. Cure is possible with stage 2 cancers.

Treatment options:

Penile amputation is most often used for local control. Whether the amputation is partial, total, or radical depends on the extent and location of the tumor.

Radiation therapy with surgical salvage is an alternative approach.

In selected cases with small lesions, YAG laser therapy is under clinical trial, with the same advantages as above.

Although controversial, elective adjuvant inguinal lymph node dissection for clinically negative lymph nodes is sometimes performed because there is a high incidence of microscopic nodal metastases.

Stage 3: Penile cancer has spread to the regional lymph nodes in the groin. Cure is related to the number and extent or nodes involved. Inguinal adenopathy in patients with penile cancer is common but may be the result of infection rather than neoplasm. If palpable lymph nodes exist 3 weeks after removal of the infected primary tumor and a course of antibiotic therapy, bilateral inguinal lymph node dissection should be performed.

Treatment options:

Clinically evident regional lymph node metastasis without evidence of distant spread is an indication for bilateral ilioinguinal lymph node dissection after penile amputation.

Radiotherapy may be considered as an alternative for patients who are not surgical candidates.

Postoperative irradiation may decrease the incidence of inguinal recurrences. Several cytotoxic drug combinations are under clinical evaluation for neoadjuvant and adjuvant therapy.

Stage 4: Penile cancer is invasive, causing extensive and inoperable involvement of lymph nodes in the groin and/or distant metastases. There is no standard treatment that is curative. Therapy is directed at palliation.

Treatment options:

Palliative surgery may be considered for control of the penile lesion and for the prevention of the necrosis, infection, and hemorrhage that can result from neglected regional adenopathy.

Radiation therapy may be palliative for primary tumor, regional adenopathy, and bone metastases.

Chemotherapeutic drugs in combination with local controls have shown some efficacy as neoadjuvant and adjuvant therapies in clinical trials.

Recurrent penile cancer: Penile cancer that has recurred in either the primary location or metastases is treated as above, according to location and extent.

Source: National Cancer Institute, 1997.

For patients diagnosed with penile cancer, teaching is needed related to the specific stage and treatments chosen. After treatment, patients should be educated regarding self-surveillance for recurrence. Patients should be taught to inspect the penis and monitor for adenopathy; they should also be taught possible complications of lymphadenectomy. Men who have undergone either radical or total penectomy may benefit from referral for psychological counseling related to their sexual function and identity.

COMMUNITY RESOURCES

There is unlikely to be any form of support group directly related to penile cancer, even in large metropolitan areas, because this form of cancer is so rare.

- American Cancer Society, 1599 Clifton Rd. N.E., Atlanta, GA, 30329-4251, 800-ACS-2345, http://www.cancer.org: The American Cancer Society has a prostate cancer self-help and information group called "Man to Man" that deals with many of the issues pertinent to penile cancer. Contact the local chapter. The ACS also provides information on psychological support, physical rehabilitation, patient education and information, transportation to and from treatment, financial counseling, employment assistance, loaned equipment, and blood programs.

- Internet resource for diagnostic and treatment of testicular cancer can be accessed at http://cancernet.nci.nih.gov/clinpdq/pif/testicular_cancer_patient.html

- Cancer Information Services, 800-4-CANCER: Supplies information about local and regional resources and programs for those interested in psychological, emotional, medical, physical, financial, and employee assistance, support, and education. Publishes educational material.

- Office of Cancer Communications, National Cancer Institute, Bldg. 31, Room 10A24, Bethesda, MD 20829-3100, 800-4-CANCER: Source for current, accurate cancer information on standard and investigational treatment, as well as nutritional and emotional support

- The National Cancer Institute's data base can be accessed at http://www.nci.nih.gov/clinpdq/. NCI has information for both patients and providers, plus a data base of up-to-date abstracts from journal articles for providers. The entire data base is updated frequently and provides a strong source of current practice standards.

- Cancer Care Inc., 1180 Avenue of the Americas, New York, NY 10036, 212-221-3300: Social service agency that provides professional counseling and planning for patients and families. Consultation, education, nursing care, home health care, homemakers, and housekeepers.
- Internet resource for supportive care can be accesssed at http://cancernet.nci.nih.gov/clinpdq/ supportive.html

Referral Points and Clinical Warnings

This information is integrated throughout the chapter.

EDITOR'S NOTE:

COMPLEMENTARY APPROACHES

A general discussion of complementary approaches can be found in Chapter 3. The following, while not an exhaustive list, are some complementary approaches being used for this condition. Additional information on these approaches, including precautions, can be found in Appendices A and B. Providers need to assess for the use of complementary approaches as part of the patient's history, as they may impact conventional therapies, and patients may not volunteer this information unless specifically asked. Efficacy of many complementary approaches is not as well documented as that of conventional therapies. Providers need to read the literature before suggesting these complementary approaches.

- Complementary Modalities
  Aromatherapy

References

Adami, H.O., Bergstrom, R., Mohner, M., et al. (1994). Testicular cancer in nine northern European countries. *International Journal of Cancer, 59*, 33–38.

American Cancer Society Inc. (1997). *Cancer facts and figures, 1997* [Brochure].

Arai, Y., Kawakita, M., Okada, Y., & Yoshida, O. (1997). Sexuality and fertility in long-term survivors of testicular cancer. *Journal of Clinical Oncology, 15*(4), 1444–1448.

Aynaud, O., Ionesco, M., & Barrasso, R. (1994). Penile intraepithelial neoplasia: Specific clinical features correlate with histologic and virologic findings. *Cancer, 74*(6), 1762–1767.

Ayyappan, K., Ananthakrishnan, N., & Sankaran, V. (1994). Can regional lymph node involvement be predicted in patients with carcinoma of the penis? *British Journal of Urology, 73*, 549–553.

Bosl, G.J., & Motzer, R.J. (1997). Testicular germ-cell cancer. *N Engl J Med, 337*(4), 242–253.

Botchan, A., Hauser, R., Yogev, L., et al. (1997). Testicular cancer and spermatogenesis. *Human Reproduction, 12*(4), 755–758.

Buetow, S.A. (1995). Epidemiology of testicular cancer. *Epidemiology Review, 17*, 433–449.

Clore, E.R. (1993). A guide to testicular self-examination. *Journal of Pediatric Health Care, 7*(6), 264–268.

Cold, C.J., Storms, M.R., & Van Howe, R.S. (1997). Carcinoma in situ of the penis in a 76-year-old circumcised man. *Journal of Family Practice, 44*(4), 407–410.

Collis, B.M., Harvey, V.J., Skelton, L., et al. (1996). Bilateral germ-cell testicular tumors in New Zealand: Experience in Auckland and Christchurch, 1978–1994. *Journal of Clinical Oncology, 14*(7), 2061–2065.

Devesa, S.S., Blot, W.J., Stone, B.J., Miller, B.A., Tarone, R.E., & Fraumeni, J.F. Jr. (1995). Recent cancer trends in the United States. *Journal of the National Cancer Institute, 87*, 175–182.

Feuer, E.J. (1995). Incidence of testicular cancer in U.S. men. *Journal of the National Cancer Institute, 86*, 405–406.

Frisch, M., Friis, S., Kjaer, S.K., & Melbye, M. (1995). Falling incidence of penis cancer in an uncircumcised population (Denmark 1943–90). *British Medical Journal, 311*, 1471.

Gilliland, F.D., & Key, C.R. (1995). Male genital cancers. *Cancer, 75*, 295–315.

Henderson, B.E., Ross, R.K., Yu, M.C., & Berstein, L. (1997). An explanation of the increasing incidence of testis cancer: Decreasing age at first full-term pregnancy [letter]. *Journal of the National Cancer Institute, 89*(11), 818–820.

Herr, H.W., Sheinfeld, J., Puc, H.S., et al. (1997). Surgery for a post-chemotherapy residual mass in seminoma. *Journal of Urology, 157*, 860–862.

Hippolainen, M.J., Yliskiski, M., Syrajanen, S., et al. (1994). Low concordance of genital human papillomavirus (HPV) lesions and viral types of HPV-infected women and their male sexual partners. *Sexually Transmitted Diseases, 21*, 76–82.

Jonker-Pool, G., van Basten, J.P., Hoekstra, H.J., et al. (1997). Sexual functioning after treatment for testicular cancer: Comparison of treatment modalities. *Cancer, 80*(3), 454–464.

Li, Y.X., Coucke, P.A., Qian, T.N., et al. (1997). Seminoma arising in corrected and uncorrected inguinal cryptorchism: Treatment and prognosis in 66 patients. *International Journal of Radiation Oncology, Biology, & Physics, 38*(2), 343–350.

Lopes, A., Hidalgo, G.S., Kowalski, L.P., Torloni, H., Rossi, B.M., & Fonseca, F.P. (1996). Prognostic factors in carcinoma of the penis: Multivariate analysis of 145 patients treated with amputation and lymphadenectomy. *Journal of Urology, 156*(5), 1673–1642.

Maden, C., Sherman, K.J., Beckmann, A.M., et al. (1993). History of circumcision, medical conditions, and sexual activity and risk of penile cancer. *Journal of the National Cancer Institute, 85*(1), 19–24.

Majewski, S., & Jablonska, S. (1997). Human papillomavirus-associated tumors of the skin and mucosa. *Journal of the American Academy of Dermatology, 36*(5), 659–685.

Meadus, R.J. (1995). Testicular self-examination (TSE). *Canadian Nurse, 91*(8), 41–44.

Monsonego, J., Zerat, L., Catalan, F., et al. (1993). Genital human papillomavirus infections: Correlation of cytological, colposcopic and histological features with viral types in women and their males partners. *International Journal of Sexually Transmitted Disease and AIDS, 4*, 13–20.

National Cancer Institute. (1997). *Clinician treatment data base*, http://wwwicic.nci.nih.gov/clinpdq/]

Ornellas, A.A., Seixas, A.L.C., Marota, A., Wisnescky, A., Campos, F., & De Moraes, J.R. (1994). Surgical treatment of invasive squamous cell carcinoma of the penis: Retrospective analysis of 350 cases. *Journal of Urology, 151*(5), 1244–1249.

Rosella, J.D. (1994). Testicular cancer health education: An integrative review. *Journal of Advanced Nursing, 20*(4), 666–671.

van Basten, J.P., Koops, H.S., Sleijfer, D.T., Pras, E., van Driel, M.F., & Hoekstra, H.J. (1997). Current concepts about testicular cancer. *European Journal of Surgical Oncology, 23*, 354–366.

Wingo, P.A., Tong, T., & Bolden, S. (1995). Cancer statistics, 1995. *CA, A Cancer Journal for Clinicians, 45*(1), 8–30.

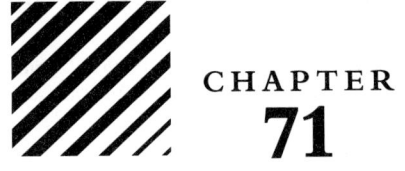

CHAPTER

71

Uterine Bleeding
And Menstruation Disorders

Jane Gannon, MS, CNM

The predictable pattern of the menstrual cycle is easily altered by a breakdown in diverse feedback mechanisms. Activities of daily living such as diet, vigorous exercise, and stress can all have an impact on this cycle. Systemic disorders such as thyroid disease, structural disorders such as fibroids, and pathologic disorders such as endometrial cancer can exert a similar impact.

Dysfunctional uterine bleeding (DUB) describes abnormal uterine bleeding that is not the result of pathology or medical illness. DUB is primarily a diagnosis of exclusion. Between 1984 and 1992, 53 of every 1000 patients aged 18 to 50 reported the presence of a menstrual disorder (Kjerulff et al, 1996). DUB cuts across the reproductive cycle and requires a careful, algorithmic approach to reach an accurate diagnosis.

Medical regimens are gaining favor over long-held surgical approaches such as hysterectomy. When surgery is deemed necessary, less-invasive surgical techniques such as endometrial ablation are replacing hysterectomy. This chapter describes a holistic approach that offers options to patients and involves them in making decisions relevant to their lifestyle.

ANATOMY, PHYSIOLOGY, AND PATHOLOGY

Interaction between the pelvic anatomy and the brain determines the success or failure of the menstrual cycle. Making an accurate diagnosis of DUB requires an understanding of endocrine biochemistry, reproductive neuroendocrinology, the menstrual cycle and its unique phases, and the subsequent impact and response on different organ systems.

The uterus is lined with endometrium, a glandular epithelium. Menstrual flow is the visible result of the fragmentation of the endometrial glands that line the endometrium. The disorganization of cell adhesion molecules within the endometrial lining is associated with this fragmentation and subsequent shedding of the endometrium (Tabibzadeh et al, 1995).

The two ovaries are round glandular tissues covered by a firm fibrous membrane. Each measures about 3.5 by 1.5 by 2 cm. The ovaries are located at the back of the broad ligament on either side of the uterus. On stimulation by luteinizing hormone (LH) and follicle-stimulating hormone (FSH), the ovary produces the sex steroids, estrogen and progesterone.

The functional portions of the pituitary gland, the adenohypophysis and the neurohypophysis, contain cells that secrete a number of peptide hormones, including thyroid-stimulating hormone (TSH), ACTH, FSH, and LH. These specialized cells synthesize and then release hormone through fusion of the secretory granule with the cell surface and exocytosis.

The synthesis and release of the gonadotropic hormones, FSH and LH, are under the control of gonadotropin-releasing hormone (GnRH). GnRH is discharged in a pulsatile pattern from the hypothalamus. The frequency of pulses varies during each menstrual cycle, depending on feedback mechanisms. A disturbance in the pulse pattern of GnRH, merely by stress-induced norepinephrine release, can disrupt ovulation.

Menstruation is controlled by an interacting system of hormones derived mainly from the hypothalamus, the anterior pituitary, and the ovaries. Taken together, these are referred to as the hypothalamus–pituitary–gonad axis. The ovaries and the uterus each have unique cycle phases. The ovaries experience follicular, ovulatory, and luteal phases. The uterus undergoes menstrual, proliferative, and secretory phases (Speroff et al, 1994).

The purpose of the follicular phase is the maturation of one follicle. This phase normally lasts 10 to 14 days. The onset of the follicular phase is stimulated by the falling levels of progesterone and inhibin at the end of the luteal phase of the previous cycle. As a result, GnRH is released from the hypothalamus, resulting in the release of FSH and some LH from the anterior pituitary. The rise in FSH prompts a dramatic response from follicles, and eventually a single, dominant follicle emerges from the maturation process.

By day 5 to 7, the dominant follicle continues the maturation process. By the midfollicular phase, a crucial rise in estrogen determines whether the LH surge will take place. The feedback effect of estrogen on LH production can be either negative or positive, depending on the concentration of estrogen and the duration of that concentration. When a concentration of 200 pg/mL is sustained for 50 hours, positive feedback results and the LH surge is initiated (Speroff et al, 1994). At the same time, a negative feedback on FSH production is occurring.

At this time, the uterine lining has shed as a result of a loss of hormonal support in the previous cycle. By day 7, rising estrogen levels are sufficient to influence secretory changes on the endometrium. By midcycle, the lining is 5 to 10 times its original size.

On initiation of the ovulatory phase, luteinization of the granulosa cells in what is now the preovulatory follicle results in progesterone production. Ovulation occurs approximately 10 to 12 hours after the LH peak and 24 to 36 hours after the estradiol peak (Speroff et al, 1994). The effects on the uterine lining at this stage are notable only for the occasional spotting experienced by some patients as a result of the drop in estrogen that occurs at ovulation.

In the luteal phase, progesterone production peaks by day 22 to 23. The corpus luteum, the remaining structure of the follicle, becomes a significant source of estrogen and progesterone in the postovulatory phase. In the absence of implantation, the corpus luteum develops into the corpus albicans. As it undergoes slow atresia, LH production diminishes, along with estrogen and progesterone production.

The uterus enters the secretory phase during the ovary's luteal phase. Under the influence of progesterone, cell reorganization produces mucus-secreting glands, increased arterial flow into the lining, and numerous thick cell layers. The loss of hormonal support induces both immunoreactive changes and rhythmic vasoconstriction of the spiral arteries within the endometrium. In a normal menstrual cycle, this process results in an orderly separation of the outer layer of the endometrium, and bleeding ensues. The fall in progesterone and inhibin exerts a positive effect on FSH production, and another cycle begins.

The bleeding that occurs in DUB is an extension beyond the processes involved in the normal menstrual cycle. DUB itself is not a pathologic event. DUB is diagnosed when there is no organic cause for the bleeding. The excessive bleeding is thought to be a function of the abnormal hormonal milieu; this affects immunoreactivity and vasoconstriction, both of which play an important role in the normal menstrual cycle. The factors inducing abnormal bleeding may eventually induce pathologic changes.

Approximately 90% of patients with DUB are anovulatory; 10% are ovulatory. Systemic disease, stress, abrupt weight fluctuations, body fat composition, ovarian disease, infection, or medications can induce changes that are crucial in the maturation of an antral follicle. In the case of obesity, that alteration may include extraovarian production of estrogens from androgens in the adipose tissue. The elevated estrogen acts on the feedback mechanisms in the hypothalamus and pituitary, shutting off FSH prematurely and condemning antral follicles to atresia because of the high-androgen environment. Conversely, a direct assault on the pituitary–ovarian axis, as in the case of an ovarian tumor or an endocrine disorder, could disturb steroid hormone production. Anovulation is the result in most cases, setting up the events for abnormal bleeding.

Because a primary follicle fails to emerge despite ongoing recruitment of primordial follicles, the subsequent absence of progesterone production results in absence of ovulation. Anovulation results in chronic stimulation of the endometrium as a result of unopposed estrogen. Endometrial thickening under the influence of estrogen causes its supportive base to become less adhesive. The disorganized estrogen production from failing follicles can lead to intermittent loss of estrogen influence on the endometrium. As a result, the endometrium may begin to slough off. This can happen in an incomplete and irregular fashion or in a prolonged, profuse pattern. This bleeding pattern is referred to as estrogen breakthrough bleeding (Speroff et al, 1994).

The physiology behind these events remains unclear. There is some evidence that elevated levels of prostaglandin E (PGE) may play a role, but the mechanism remains unclear. Early studies on PGE revealed properties that are thought to contribute to menorrhagia, such as its action as an inhibitor of platelet aggregation and adhesiveness, as well as its vasodilatory action.

Recent work suggests that alteration of angiotensin II distribution as well as its receptor levels in the endometrium may play a role in DUB (Li & Ahmed, 1996b). Hyperplastic endometrium, which occurs as a result of unopposed estrogen exposure, has a significantly weaker angiotensin II-like immunoreactivity, in addition to altered angiotensin receptor expression (Li & Ahmed, 1996a).

Early Disease

In the early stages of DUB, the greatest concern is excessive blood loss. Blood loss that requires blood transfusion occurs in some patients.

Late Disease

Chronic proliferation of the endometrial lining as a result of unopposed estrogen exposure leads to simple glandular hyperplasia after many months. The hypertrophied tissue can evolve into a polyp. Hyperplasia may progress from simple changes to adenomatous hyperplasia.

■ **CLINICAL WARNING:** Adenocarcinoma may develop from endrometrial hyperplasia. A study that examined histopathologic endometrial curretages of patients with anovulatory DUB found 446 patients (48%) with endometrial hyperplasia, 412 (42%) with abnormal endometrial proliferation as a result of prolonged persistence of a follicle, and 106 (10%) with deficient endometrial proliferation (Vakiani et al, 1996). Of those with hyperplasia, 72% of the cases of endometrial hyperplasia were (simple) cystic hyperplasias, 26% were (complex) adenomatous hyperplasias, and 2% were atypical hyperplasias (Vakiani et al, 1996).

Alternatively, as in the unique case of the female athlete, ongoing exercise may shift both estrogen and progesterone into low gear; the levels become too low to support the normal menstrual cycle. As a result, rather than progressing toward heavier bleeding, the female athlete is more likely to experience "athletic amenorrhea." Over time, in addition to an absence of menstruation, the female athlete may experience infertility problems (Diaz et al, 1995).

EPIDEMIOLOGY

Reproductive system disorders have a greater incidence in primary care practice than most other medical conditions, including heart disease, hypertension, cancer, allergies, and nonreproductive endocrine problems (Steinberger, 1996). When compared with other gynecologic conditions, menstrual disorders are the most common complaint that brings patients to their primary care provider (Kjerulff et al, 1996; Steinberger, 1996; Wathen et al, 1995). Although adnexal conditions (16.6/1000) and fibroids (9.2/1000) are prominent causes of abnormal bleeding, the most common chronic gynecologic conditions are menstrual disorders (Kjerulff et al, 1996). More than 50% of cases of DUB occur in women older than 45. Steinberger (1996) described common symptoms bringing patients to the provider as an absence of expected menstrual flow or irregular, heavy, or prolonged bleeding. Patients who do no moderate or hard exercise may bleed a quarter of a day longer than patients who engage in moderate exercise.

Women who smoke and use oral contraceptives are 47% more likely to experience abnormal spotting and bleeding than nonsmoking users of oral contraceptives. Smokers also enter menopause earlier because of increased levels of sex hormone-binding globulin and less active estrogen (van der Schouw et al, 1996).

Cultural factors play a greater role in the response of patients to the abnormal bleeding pattern than they do to a cause for DUB. When evaluating the cultural response to abnormal menstruation, a helpful approach is to look at the way communities of people seek health care. In one study, as many as 67% of patients with menstrual disorders had not talked with a health care provider about their experience of DUB (Kjerulff et al, 1996).

Ferguson (1996) provides a model of health care that describes a patient's response to DUB. When a woman experiences an abnormal bleeding pattern, cultural influences are an important consideration in how she responds. Her first response may be to deal with it herself. If she is not a careful historian of her cycles, she may decide she has merely forgotten how recent her last period was. Or she may accept the fact that a cycle or two has been "off," but decides to take a wait-and-see approach. She may also seek information from a bookstore or library.

In some cultures, menstruation imposes restrictions on sexual relations, as well as household and agricultural activities, especially those involving food preparation. Cultural traditions of hot and cold theories dictate how Southeast Asian (Hmong, Cambodian, and Vietnamese) patients cope during menstruation. Warm foods such as rice, chicken, and egg-drop soup with pepper and herbs must be consumed during menstruation (Poirier, 1993). Women must also stay warm, maintain quiet in the house by not allowing visitors, and avoid sexual intercourse. An abnormal bleeding problem thus could lead to social isolation.

If her problem continues, the woman may seek the advice of friends and family. This social support system becomes an important source of help and advice for many patients. Finding that a friend had a similar problem and found relief through a visit to her health care provider may prompt the patient to seek primary professional care. On the other hand, cultural responses to uterine bleeding can be reinforced by family members, further delaying the patient from seeing the primary provider.

The next level of care may find the woman reaching out to self-help networks, such as distant relatives, neighbors, friends of friends, self-help groups, community hotlines, and other self-help resources in the community. With the wide variety of computer resources available, she may also seek help online, perusing news groups, Web pages, list-servers, and forums all devoted to the topic of women's health or abnormal gynecologic conditions.

These informal networks of natural helpers or community medicine can be helpful sources of factual information as well as valuable support systems (Ferguson, 1996). On the other hand, use of lay practitioners may delay the patient's entry into the professional health care system.

When self-care, support systems, and community medicine have not been successful at relieving the woman's symptoms or are not available, she will then usually migrate to a health professional. For some, this may be direct entry into the tertiary level of care—for instance, an emergency room visit with very heavy estrogen breakthrough bleeding.

Consequences of DUB include nonproductivity due to time away from work. Twenty-nine percent of patients report spending 1 or more days in bed as a result of a menstrual irregularity (Kjerulff et al, 1996). Florack et al (1994) found that overall, DUB does not appear to be associated with work-related physical activity or fatigue.

Many concerns are expressed in the lay press about environmental toxins and their effect on health. Many chemicals in use today may mimic the effects of hormones such as estrogen. Much remains unknown, but the theoretical concern postulated by environmental scientists is that exposure to estrogen-mimicking chemicals could add to the estrogenic effects on the endometrium and increase a woman's chance of both breast and endometrial cancer (Renner, 1995). Chemicals known to have an estrogenic effect include phthalates, alkylphenols, and bisphenol A (Warhurst, 1996). Further research is needed in this area to determine the health-related impact of chemicals and preventive measures people need to take to avoid exposure.

DIAGNOSTIC CRITERIA

The postovulatory phase of the menstrual cycle is normally 28 days (range 24 to 35 days), with withdrawal bleeding lasting 4 to 6 days (range 2 to 8 days). Because the preovulatory phase can be unpredictable as a result of individual differences in follicle development, many patients have cycles that are shorter or longer than 28 days. Most blood loss occurs in the first 3 days. Any flow lasting longer than 7 days requires evaluation (Brenner, 1996).

Blood loss can vary. The average amount of blood lost during the menstrual cycle is 30 mL. Blood loss greater than 80 mL per cycle is considered excessive (Gleeson, 1994; Speroff et al, 1994). Some authors believe that quantifying blood loss as accurately as possible is an important part of assessing DUB because of subjectivity (Lee, 1996). Others assert that the woman's perception of blood loss is enough to warrant further investigation (Speroff et al, 1994). Menstrual flow warrants evaluation if it requires two or more sanitary pads per day above the woman's normal pad use, or lasts 3 or more days above normal (Brenner, 1996). A tool such as the pictorial blood loss assessment chart shown in Figure 71-1 has a greater than 80% sensitivity and specificity as a tool for identifying menorrhagia (Higham et al, 1990).

The terms that describe the patterns of abnormal menstrual bleeding are as follows:

- Hypermenorrhea: flow that is excessive in both amount and duration that occurs at regular intervals
- Menorrhagia: prolonged flow
- Metrorrhagia: normal flow occurring at irregular intervals
- Menometrorrhagia: flow that is frequent, excessive, prolonged, and irregular
- Polymenorrhea: bleeding that is frequent and regular but occurs at intervals less than 18 to 21 days
- Intermenstrual bleeding: bleeding that occurs between regular menstrual periods
- Oligomenorrhea: bleeding that occurs at intervals of 35 days to 6 months

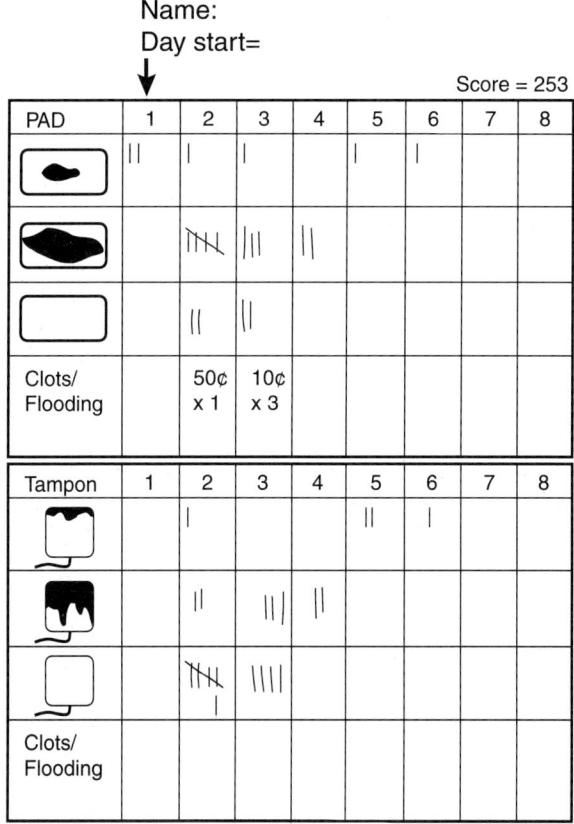

Name:
Day start=

Score = 253

FIGURE 71-1 Tool for identifying menorrhagia (From Higham, JM, O'Brien, PMS, and Shaw, RW. [1990]. Assessment of menstrual loss using a pictorial chart. B J Obstet and Gynaecology, 97. 734–39).

Spotting can be a manifestation of DUB if it occurs at very frequent, prolonged, irregular intervals.

DUB must be differentiated from a pathologic condition or systemic disease of which abnormal bleeding maybe a symptom. Abnormal uterine bleeding can be caused by numerous factors, which can be grouped together into categories (Brenner, 1996):

- Organic gynecologic disease (eg, reproductive tumors, infection, pregnancy complications)
- Systemic disease (eg, hypothyroidism, hepatic disorders, diabetes, adrenal disorders, pituitary tumors)
- Blood dyscrasias (eg, thrombocytopenia, aplastic anemia, Minot–von Willebrand syndrome)
- Iatrogenic causes (eg, contraceptives, androgens, anabolic agents, hypothalamic depressants)
- Trauma (eg, sexual assault, foreign bodies).

HISTORY AND PHYSICAL EXAM

The history should include the woman's age, age at menarche, and a thorough history of menses (flow pattern, frequency, duration). The approximate number of pads or tampons the patient uses should be estimated (see Fig. 71-1). The patient should be questioned about any associated symptoms she experiences with menses or any abnormal bleeding, including molimina (premenstrual syndrome, premenstrual breast tenderness, bloating, cramps).

■ ■ ■ CLINICAL PEARL

The menstrual pattern alone and its related symptoms may help determine quickly if the patient is bleeding in an ovulatory pattern (molimina present) or an anovulatory pattern (molimina absent).

Information about pregnancy and sexual histories and contraceptive use should be obtained. The patient should be asked if she has experienced violence, battering, or sexual assault. Other historical data that should be obtained from the patient and the medical record should include a history of gynecologic problems, including infections and sexually transmitted infections. A surgical history should include an inquiry into whether the patient has experienced excessive bleeding after operative procedures. The family history should be reviewed with a focus on gynecologic conditions, including endometrial cancer. Medication use should be carefully reviewed. The patient's use of contraceptives, hormonal treatments, recreational drugs, prescription drugs, antiretrovirals, nonsteroidal anti-inflammatory drugs (NSAIDs), and vitamins and other over-the-counter drugs or complementary therapies should all be evaluated as possible factors in the abnormal bleeding pattern.

Other lifestyle factors that can help form the differential diagnosis include exercise patterns; alcohol, caffeine, and tobacco use; and stress management and coping mechanisms. Numerous subjective symptoms may help reveal the specific hormonal disorder. Symptoms consistent with hypoestrogenemia include headaches, depression, emotional lability, inability to concentrate, decreased libido, vaginal dryness, breast atrophy, and changes in gastrointestinal or genitourinary symptoms (Steinberger, 1996). Conversely, few of these types of symptoms accompany DUB or other hyperestrogenemia conditions. Subjective symptoms of hypoprogestinemia may include significant molimina, pelvic heaviness (due to cyst formation), and emotional stress.

A thorough physical exam with careful overall visual inspection reveals many clues to the diagnosis. Hyperandrogenic disorders such as polycystic ovary disease are manifested by intensified hair growth on the upper lip, chin, cheeks, and chest and from the pubic crest to the umbilicus. Scalp hair may exhibit asymmetric or patchy balding (alopecia). Acne may be present on the face as well as the back, and skin may be excessively oily. Pale skin may be a clue to the degree of blood loss and subsequent anemia as a result of DUB.

Palpation of the neck may reveal an enlarged thyroid, suggesting a thyroid disorder. Weight should be noted, as well as the patient's overall body type. A patient with a high androgen profile often demonstrates android-type obesity.

A speculum exam should be performed, both to obtain a Pap smear and to view the cervix for evidence of lesions, infection, or polyps. A bimanual exam helps determine uterine size, consistency, contour, and mobility. This assessment will help locate patches of endometriosis, fibroids, pregnancy, and areas of tenderness. The adnexa should be palpated carefully for evidence of masses or pain, which may be an ectopic pregnancy, ovarian cyst, or neoplasm.

DIAGNOSTIC STUDIES

The underlying problem of DUB is one of disruption in the production and metabolism of sex steroids. The diagnostic workup is meant to wade through the different possible causes of DUB. If structural defects, systemic disease, neoplasm, infections, or pregnancy are found during the diagnostic workup, then the abnormal bleeding problem is a symptom of the defect or disease. Presumably, treatment of that disorder will relieve the symptom of abnormal vaginal bleeding. On the other hand, if structural disease and the aforementioned entities are absent, then the diagnosis of DUB is made as a separate entity unto itself. Treatment is aimed at restoring the normal hormonal processes and cyclic uterine bleeding.

The initial laboratory workup should include a pregnancy test. Thyroid function studies (TSH and free To) are ordered if galactorrhea or a palpable thyroid is present on the physical exam. Sexually transmitted infections such as chlamydia can produce bleeding from a friable cervix, so screening should be considered. A more profuse infection such as pelvic inflammatory disease should be evaluated by ordering a complete blood count, erythrocyte sedimentation rate, and C-reactive protein (elevated in infection). If bleeding has been prolonged or heavy, anemia should be ruled out with a complete blood count.

CLINICAL WARNING: If the patient presents with bruising or the sudden onset of a very heavy flow, or reports frequent use of aspirin, NSAIDs, or anticoagulant drugs, investigate whether she has a coagulopathy. Order a prothrombin time, partial thromboplastin time, platelet count, and bleeding time.

Several office procedures can aid in the task of finding a cause for DUB. An endometrial biopsy is used to evaluate the endometrium and is done when the woman has risk factors for endometrial hyperplasia (patients with breakthrough bleeding while receiving hormone replacement therapy, anovulatory bleeding in patients older than 40 or in patients older than 35 with risk factors for endometrial cancer such as obesity, hypertension, and family history). An endometrial biopsy may confirm the suspicion of an anovulatory cycle if simple proliferative hyperplastic endometrium is found. However, if a secretory endometrium is obtained, then uterine disease would be the source of bleeding rather than anovulatory DUB. Endometrial biopsy involves inserting a pipelle into the uterus to the fundus and scraping downward to obtain a sample of the endometrial lining. The sensitivity of pipelle sampling for endometrial carcinoma is excellent, but it is relatively weak for other endometrial diseases because it can fail to detect endometrial polyps and submucosal myomas (Guido et al, 1995). Complications of the procedure include uterine perforation, infection, or damage to other organs.

Both hysteroscopy and transvaginal ultrasonography have been used to rule out pathologic and structural disorders in patients with DUB. Hysteroscopy has been demonstrated to be 79% sensitive and 93% specific in diagnosing intracavitary pathologic disorders; transvaginal ultrasound has 54% sensitivity and 90% specificity (el-Ahmady et al, 1996).

Hysteroscopy allows visual inspection of the endometrial lining. Using a speculum to aid placement, the thin, tubular hysteroscope is inserted directly into the uterus through the cervix. The lighted scope allows the investigator to look for evidence of structural anomalies such as fibroids, adhesions,

polyps, and other neoplastic lesions. Hysteroscopy is both a diagnostic and treatment tool. Fibroids and polyps found during the procedure can be resected at that time. Drawbacks to hysteroscopy include a need for premedication and anesthesia and the risk of postoperative infection and uterine wall perforation. Structural abnormalities on the external surface of the uterus cannot be visualized by hysteroscopy and can be better seen on transvaginal ultrasound.

Transvaginal ultrasonography is used to rule out structural defects of the uterus. Because fibroid tissue displays a greater degree of echogenicity than uterine tissue, the typically thick-walled, fibrous structures can be easily distinguished from normal uterine tissue. Myomas, on the other hand, tend to be less echogenic, and their darker shadows reveal their location. Polycystic ovaries can also be easily seen, with their telltale sign of multiple developing cystic follicles.

Ultrasound can also be used to measure echogenicity and endometrial thickness. The phases of endometrial development can be assessed in this manner using the echo of the endometrial cavity and its surrounding tissue. Because the endometrial thickness varies from the menstrual phase through the secretory phase, abnormal phase changes or an endometrial lining that appears "out of synch" with the hormonal profile might be identified. Excessively thick endometrial measurements or an irregular endometrial cavity echo may indicate endometrial carcinoma or hyperplasia (Sabbagha et al, 1994).

CLINICAL WARNING: An endometrial width of 5 mm or more warrants further investigation to rule out endometrial cancer.

With the diagnostic capabilities of transvaginal sonography, more invasive procedures such as endometrial biopsy may need to be performed only when suspicious endometrial properties are seen on ultrasound. The combination of endometrial biopsy and ultrasound was found to have a sensitivity and specificity of 100% in the diagnosis of endometrial carcinoma (Youssif & McMillan, 1995). Individually, ultrasonography and biopsy have a sensitivity rate around 76% and 60%, respectively (el-Ahmady et al, 1996).

A merger of ultrasound and hysteroscopy has led to a procedure called sonohysterography. Normal saline is infiltrated into the uterine cavity after insertion of the hysteroscope. Transvaginal ultrasound is then directed at the uterus. The acoustic window provided by the normal saline facilitates measurement of the uterine lining.

TREATMENT OPTIONS, EXPECTED OUTCOMES, AND COMPREHENSIVE MANAGEMENT

An orderly, well-planned approach to the management of DUB is likely to bring about a successful resolution of the problem. To a skilled health care provider, the history and physical exam will offer many clues to a working diagnosis. An algorithmic approach such as that in Figure 71-2 helps to clarify the management decisions.

Medical Management

Medical regimens are currently the treatment of choice in the management of DUB. Although some regimens have a risk of side effects, their ability to improve the quality of life for many

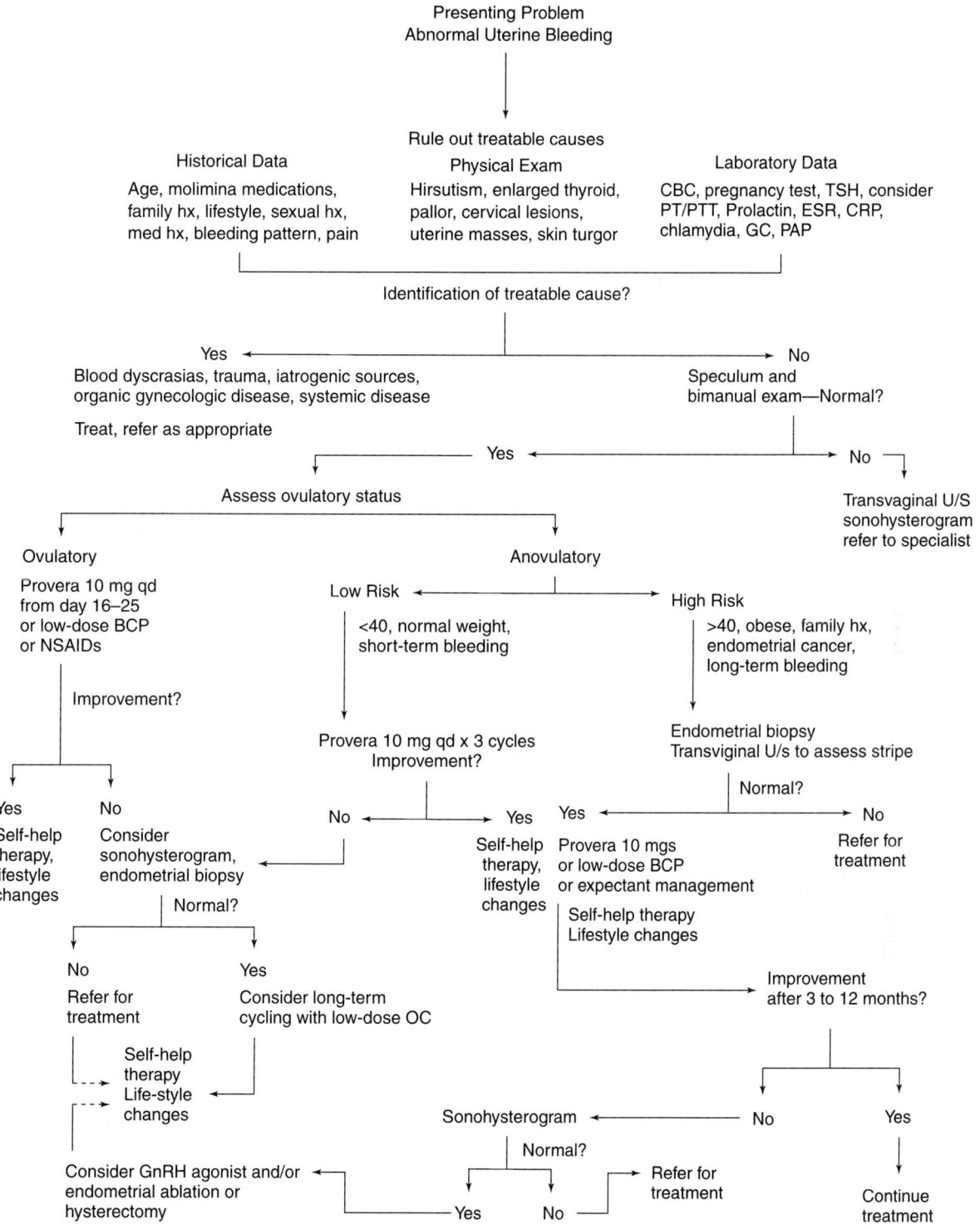

FIGURE 71-2 Uterine bleeding and menstruation disorders. (Source: Author)

patients makes them more desirable than the surgical alternatives. Medical treatment for DUB is geared toward interrupting the proliferation of the endometrium and creating a hormonal environment that is not conducive to endometrial growth. Medical regimens include oral contraceptives, progestins, NSAIDs, antifibrinolytic agents, danazol, and GnRH agonists such as leuprolide acetate and goserelin acetate. The choice of regimen should be based on factors such as desire for fertility,

degree of menorrhagia, accompanying symptoms (eg, dysmenorrhea), accompanying medical conditions, anticipated side effects, cost, patient preference, and provider experience with the regimens (Lee, 1996). Table 71-1 summarizes typical medical regimens used in the treatment of DUB.

For patients not interested in fertility, the first line of treatment usually consists of oral contraceptives, cyclic progesterone, or hormone replacement therapy with estrogen and pro-

TABLE 71-1	Medications in the Treatment of DUB		
Medication	**Dosage**	**Administration**	**Duration**
Cyclic progesterone	10 mg daily for 10 days	Oral: Start on the 16th or 21st day of the menstrual cycle.	3 cycles. May be followed with long-term cycling with oral contraceptives.
Oral contraceptives	1 tablet daily for 28 days	Oral	Long-term if desired
NSAIDs	400 mg Q.I.D. or 600 mg T.I.D.	Oral: Administer during menstrual period only.	
Antifibrinolytic agents (mefenamic acid)	500 mg q8h	Oral: Administer for 5 days from day 1 of menses.	3 consecutive cycles
Danazol	200 mg Q.I.D.	Oral	4–8 weeks
GnRH agonist (goserelin acetate)	3.6 mg	Subcutaneous injection every 28 days	6 months

Source: Claire M. Lintilhac Nurse–Midwifery Center, Fletcher Allen Health Care, Burlington, VT.

gesterone (Wathen et al, 1995). For the 10% of patients who experience ovulatory dysfunctional bleeding (manifested by midcycle spotting or pre- or postmenstrual spotting with regular periods and molimina), treatment is aimed at improving the luteal phase. The drug of choice is medroxyprogesterone (Provera); the typical regimen is 10 mg/day from day 16 through 25 for three cycles. An alternative would be the use of oral contraceptives for 1 or 2 months.

Other medication regimens may be required for the remaining 90% of patients in whom systemic disorders, pregnancy, and endometrial cancer have been ruled out and anovulatory DUB has been diagnosed. Use of medroxyprogesterone can be attempted first. The usual regimen is 5 to 10 mg for 5 to 10 days, ideally administered on the 16th or 21st day of the menstrual cycle. If the anovulatory bleeding returns immediately afterward, then cycling with long-term medroxyprogesterone or oral contraceptives is warranted. This usually decreases menorrhagic bleeding by 50%.

■ ■ ■ CLINICAL PEARL

The use of oral contraceptives is most effective for the typical dysfunctional bleeding seen in teenagers and patients younger than 35 (Gennex Healthcare Technologies, 1996).

■ **CLINICAL WARNING:** Patients receiving oral contraceptives have the added benefit of contraception, but those receiving medroxyprogesterone should use an effective form of birth control.

Antiprostaglandins (NSAIDs) such as naproxen and ibuprofen and antifibrinolytic medications such as mefenamic acid and tranexamic acid have proven effective for some patients, especially for smokers or those who want to attempt pregnancy.

NSAIDs inhibit prostaglandins, including those in the endometrium. They improve platelet aggregation and degranulation. NSAIDs increase uterine vasoconstriction in women with menorrhagia (Rosenfeld, 1996). Many of these medications are well known to patients and well tolerated. Their side effects

are less serious than those of oral contraceptives. Patients with a known sensitivity to aspirin should avoid NSAIDs. NSAIDs should be taken with food or milk to avoid gastrointestinal disturbances. A typical regimen might involve ibuprofen 400 mg four times daily or 600 mg three times daily, taken only during the menstrual period (Rosenfeld, 1996). Antifibrinolytic medications reduce rates of bleeding by 20% for mefenamic acid and 50% for tranexamic acid (Bonner & Sheppard, 1996; Walling, 1996).

NSAIDs and antifibrinolytic medications are less effective at restoring a normal menstrual flow than the GnRH agonists. By constantly stimulating the pituitary, GnRH analogues such as leuprolide acetate and goserelin acetate induce downregulation, and LH and FSH production ceases. The resulting suppression of estrogen and progesterone arrests endometrial growth, and the endometrial mucosa is thinned. Symptom relief usually begins to be noticed 4 weeks after treatment begins. Although the process is reversible, the overall effect is consistent with an induction of menopause and its side effects (eg, hot flashes, vaginal dryness, headaches, emotional lability). More significant side effects can include irreversible osteoporosis, alteration in lipoproteins, and changes in urogenital tissue. Because of the long-term effects of GnRH agonists on bone mass, their use is restricted to short courses (Thomas, 1996). Current strategies to prevent or minimize these side effects include add-back regimens, which add a steroid to the regimen, usually norethindrone, or nonconcurrent estrogen and progestin regimens (Adashi, 1995; Thomas, 1996). Patients who smoke, have excessive alcohol intake or a family history of osteoporosis, or plan concomitant use of medications that have a similar bone-thinning effect need to be informed about the risk of osteoporosis with use of a GnRH analogue.

Despite the alteration in hormone levels and suppression of ovarian function, pregnancy can still occur with GnRH analogues.

■ **CLINICAL WARNING:** The teratogenicity of GnRH medications is unknown, and patients need to be instructed to use a nonhormonal method of birth control. Pregnancy should be delayed for at least 2 months after completing therapy.

Surgical Management

When drug treatments fail to resolve DUB, a surgical approach may be warranted. In the past, hysterectomy for the management of DUB was the most common treatment option offered to patients. Abnormal uterine bleeding is one of the top five reasons for more than 80% of hysterectomies (Hall, 1994).

Surgical loss of the uterus may be a good outcome for patients whose childbearing years are over and those who want a rapid solution to the problem. For those whose bleeding fails to respond to medical regimens, a surgical solution may be the only option. However, for those whose reproductive years are not yet complete and those who want to avoid invasive surgery, new techniques provide a welcome alternative. The provider must be familiar with current surgical techniques and medical regimens to give patients anticipatory guidance before referring them for specialty care.

If a surgical approach is required, endometrial ablation is becoming the treatment of choice in the management of DUB. It can be performed in an outpatient setting, and patients can resume normal activity in 3 to 5 days. Endometrial curettage or ablation strips the endometrium to its bare basal glandular layer. This causes regeneration of a normal endometrial surface and theoretically restores normal menstrual function and flow. In a series of 600 endometrial ablation procedures, immediate resolution of the bleeding problem was obtained in almost all women (Garry et al, 1995). The destruction of the endometrium results in a cessation of menstrual flow. This method is particularly successful for patients with typically heavy estrogen breakthrough bleeding. However, the more time that elapses from the initial surgery, the greater the chance that the patient will require a second procedure.

Endometrial ablation is usually preceded by an endometrial biopsy to rule out a precancerous condition. In addition, danazol, a synthetic form of androgen hormones, or a GnRH analog is often given at least 6 weeks before the operative procedure to thin the endometrium. General or regional anesthesia is required for the procedure. Potential side effects include pulmonary edema, endometriosis, and immediate or delayed hemorrhage. Uterine perforation and the need for further laparoscopy are additional complications, although a series with 600 subjects found no such side effects (Garry et al, 1995).

Patients who undergo this procedure must be warned about the normal postoperative effects of ablation: cramping, vaginal bleeding for up to 14 days, and a profuse watery discharge that can persist for up to 6 weeks. Approximately 50% of patients have no further bleeding; 40% have some bleeding, but the quantity is dramatically reduced from preoperative levels; and 10% require further treatment (Baggish & Sze, 1996; Garry et al, 1995).

A recent study reported that approximately 76% of women who have endometrial ablation can be expected to require a hysterectomy within 10 years (Apgar, 1997).

 CLINICAL WARNING: A reliable form of birth control is necessary after surgery.

Dilatation and curettage (D&C) is indicated for acute heavy bleeding that has not responded to medical management (Lee, 1996). However, its benefit as a treatment for menorrhagia is generally transient. With the recent advances made in endometrial ablation procedures, D&C is falling out of favor as a treatment option for DUB.

 CLINICAL WARNING: Patients need to be counseled regarding the short-term effects of both medication regimens and ablative procedures.

TEACHING AND SELF-CARE

Eliciting the meaning of menstruation for each patient can help determine the impact of the abnormal pattern of menstruation on her overall well-being. A study of American women found that they reported a high level of dissatisfaction with their body image during the perimenstrual phase (Carrnangle et al, 1994). Promoting the patient's involvement in the treatment process can go a long way toward helping her overcome both fear and low self-esteem when dealing with a bleeding problem.

Patients should be encouraged to chart their cycles on a calendar, recording accompanying symptoms and a reliable description of blood loss. Treatment and its impact on the cycle, as well as any untoward effects, should also be monitored by the patient.

Barring any organic disease, some patients may choose to pursue alternative therapies to help them regain hormonal balance and a normally cycling endometrium. However, they may require periodic sampling of the endometrium to rule out pathology if the dysfunctional bleeding pattern does not improve through self-help therapies. Other patients choose complementary health sources as adjunctive therapy to their medical or surgical therapy. Efforts to exercise, eliminate obesity, and manage stress should be strongly encouraged.

For patients whose abnormal bleeding pattern is the result of excessive exercise, a reasonable guideline is to encourage them to limit such activity to the equivalent of running no more than 10 miles a week (American Society for Reproductive Medicine, 1996). This is especially important if they are trying to conceive.

With a long life ahead of them, it is vital that preventive health care options are available to younger patients so that they may reach their maximal level of well-being throughout the life cycle. Unfortunately, many factors may limit a woman's ability to participate in preventive health services. Patients who are living in nontraditional family structures are less likely to seek preventive health services than patients in traditional family structures and patients in double-income families (Harden, 1992). Similarly, patients who are the sole provider for the family are less likely to take preventive measures (Makuc et al, 1989). Low socioeconomic status, for patients of all races and ages, is associated with low use of preventive screening tests (Makuc et al, 1989).

A balance between food intake of the major food groups and energy output through exercise helps to maintain a proper ratio of fat and muscle. Preventing or eliminating obesity is an important part of managing DUB. A diet low in saturated fats, trans-fatty acids, and triglycerides may help maintain hormonal balance. Refer to Chapter 5 for more information on diet and meal planning for good health.

Smoking influences the rate of estrogen metabolism by decreasing midcycle and luteal-phase estradiol levels (Westhoff et al, 1996). The consequences may include an early onset of menopause (Zaldivar et al, 1996). Patients should therefore be strongly cautioned not to smoke.

A moderate amount of exercise should be encouraged. Patients who want to engage in activities such as marathon training should be fully informed about the implications of excess activity on their gynecologic health. Anovulatory cycles and amenorrhea are the most frequently encountered patterns in female athletes who engage in high-impact exercise. This can lead to luteal phase deficiency. The resulting androgen excess has been linked to increases in cardiovascular disease and reproductive site neoplasms (Derman, 1996).

Emotional stress can disrupt the hypothalamic–pituitary axis. The philosophy behind many complementary therapies involves stress reduction, thereby preventing the changes in the hormonal milieu that contribute to disease (Alexander et al, 1996). However, scientific data are lacking about the effectiveness and safety of many alternative therapies. Options that produce no foreseeable harm in patients allow them some control over their health, and this process makes them more responsible users of the health care system.

 CLINICAL WARNING: Health care consumers should be cautioned about the lack of regulation of complementary therapies.

COMMUNITY RESOURCES

Online communication tools such as medical sources, support groups, list-servers, and news groups can be a valuable component in health maintenance by promoting self-care and encouraging personal responsibility for health. Some helpful resources for both consumers and providers include:

- Self-Care Central, www.health.net/selfcare
- Self-help Sourcebook Online, www.cmhc.com/selfhelp/
- HealthWorld Online, www.healthworld.com
- Reuters Health News, www.reutershealth.com
- Melopemene Institute, 2125 E. Hennepin Ave., Minneapolis, MN 55413, 612-378-0545, http://www.bodymatters.com/bodymatters/exchange.html
- Dysmenorrhea Information Page, http://www.uiuc.edu.departments.mckinley/health-info/womenhlt/mencramp.html
- Irregular Menses Information Page, http://www.uiuc.edu.departments.mckinley/health-info/womenhlt/ir-mense.html
- Mayo Health Oasis, http://www.mayohealth.org/mayo/9707/htm/vaginal.htm
- American Medical Women's Association, 801 N. Fairfax St., Suite 400, Alexandria, VA 22314, 703-838-0050

REFERRAL POINTS AND CLINICAL WARNINGS

Three general rules should be considered before making a diagnosis of DUB (Brenner, 1996):

- Abnormal uterine bleeding that occurs in a woman of reproductive age should be considered the result of a complication of pregnancy until proved otherwise.

- Abnormal uterine bleeding occurring in a woman of perimenopausal or postmenopausal age should be considered the result of a malignancy until proved otherwise.
- Menorrhagia occurring in an adolescent should be attributed to a coagulopathy until proved otherwise.

In addition, patients with structural lesions or pelvic masses or those who do not resume normal withdrawal bleeding after treatment with oral contraceptives or other hormone therapy should be referred to a gynecologist for further evaluation and treatment (Lee, 1996; Wathen et al, 1995).

Patients with a bleeding problem brought on by an eating disorder require highly skilled counselors to manage the psychosocial aspects of their illness. This life-threatening illness poses a special challenge to both the young woman and her care providers.

For patients who are highly stressed, both young and old, referral to classes in stress management can be helpful. Some patients may require more intensive counseling and should be referred to appropriate providers in the community.

EDITOR'S NOTE:
COMPLEMENTARY APPROACHES

A general discussion of complementary approaches can be found in Chapter 3. The following while not an exhaustive list, are some complementary approaches being used for this condition. Additional information on these approaches, including precautions, can be found in Appendices A and B. Providers need to assess for the use of complementary approaches as part of the patient's history, as they may impact conventional therapies, and patients may not volunteer this information unless specifically asked. Efficacy of many complementary approaches is not as well documented as that of conventional therapies. Providers need to read the literature before suggesting these complementary approaches.

- Complementary Modalities
  Acupuncture
  Aromatherapy
  Chiropractic

References

Adashi, E.Y. (1995). Long-term gonadotropin-releasing hormone agonist therapy: The evolving issue of steroidal add-back paradigms. *Keio Journal of Medicine, 44*(4), 124–132.

Alexander, D.A., Naji, A.A., Pinion, S.B., et al. (1996). Randomized trial comparing hysterectomy with endometrial ablation for dysfunctional uterine bleeding: Psychiatric and psychosocial aspects. *British Medical Journal, 312*(7026), 280–284.

Apgar, B. (1997). Probability of hysterectomy after endometrial ablation. *American Family Physician, 55*(5), 1891–1893.

Baggish, M.S., & Sze, E.H. (1996). Endometrial ablation: A series of 568 patients treated over an 11-year period. *American Journal of Obstetrics and Gynecology, 174*(3), 908–913.

Bonner, J., & Sheppard, B.L. (1996) Treatment of menorrhagia during menstruation: Randomised controlled trial of ethamsylate, mefenamic acid, and tranexamic acid. *British Medical Journal, 7*(313), 579–582.

Brenner, P. (1996). Differential diagnosis of abnormal uterine bleeding. *American Journal of Obstetrics and Gynecology, 175*(3), 766–769.

Carrnangle, R.E., Johnson, W.G., Bergeron, K.C., & Nangle, D.W. (1994). Body image changes over the menstrual cycle in normal patients. *International Journal of Eating Disorders, 16*(3), 267–273.

Derman, R.J. (1996). Androgen excess in patients. *International Journal of Fertility and Menopausal Studies, 41*(2), 172–176.

Diaz, B., Garcia, R., Colmenero, M.D., Terrados, N., Fernandez, B., & Marin, B. (1995). Melatonin and gonadotropin hormones in pubertal sportsgirls. *Review Espagnol Fisiolgie, 49*(1), 17–22.

el-Ahmady, O., Gad, M., el-Sheimy, R., et al. (1996). Comparative study between sonography, pathology and UGP in patients with perimenopausal bleeding. *Anticancer Research, 16*(4B), 2309–2313.

Ferguson, T. (1996). *Health online: How to find health information, support groups and self-help communities in cyberspace.* New York: Addison-Wesley.

Florack, E.I., Zielhuis, G.A., & Rolland, R. (1994). The influence of occupational physical activity on the menstrual cycle and fecundability. *Epidemiology, 5*(1), 14–18.

Garry, R., Shelley-Jones, D., Mooney, P., & Phillips, G. (1995). Six hundred endometrial laser ablations. *Obstetrics and Gynecology, 85*(1), 24–29.

Gennex Healthcare Technologies. (1996). *Dysfunctional uterine bleeding.* http://www.healthwire.com/patients/dub.htm.

Gleeson, N.C. (1994). Cyclic changes in endometrial tissue plasminogen activator and plasminogen activator inhibitor type 1 in patients with normal menstruation and essential menorrhagia. *American Journal of Obstetrics and Gynecology, 171*(1), 178–183.

Guido, R.S., Kanbour-Shakir, A., Rulin, M.C., & Christopherson, W.A. (1995). Pipette endometrial sampling: Sensitivity in the detection of endometrial cancer. *Journal of Reproductive Medicine. 40*(8), 553–555.

Harden, J. (Ed.). (1992). *The patients's health data book: A profile of patients' health in the United States.* Washington, D.C.: The Jacobs Institute of Patients' Health.

Higham, J.M., O'Brien, P.M.S., & Shaw, R.W. (1990). Assessment of menstrual loss using a pictorial chart. *British Journal of Obstetrics and Gynaecology, 97,* 734–739.

Kjerulff, K.H., Erickson, B.A., & Langenberg, P.W. (1996). Chronic gynecological conditions reported by US patients: Findings from the National Health Interview Survey, 1984 to 1992. *American Journal of Public Health, 86*(2), 195–199.

Lee, J. (1996). *Menorrhagia review questions.* http://www.ices.on.ca/docs/fb1430.htm.

Li, X.F., & Ahmed, A. (1996a). Dual role of angiotensin II in the human endometrium. *Human Reproduction, 11*(2), 95–108.

Li, X.F., & Ahmed, A. (1996b). Expression of angiotensin II and its receptor subtypes in endometrial hyperplasia: A possible role in dysfunctional menstruation. *Laboratory Investigations, 75*(2), 137–145.

Makuc, D.M., Freid, V., & Kleinman, J. (1989) National trends in the use of preventive health care by patients. *American Journal of Public Health, 79,* 21–26.

Poirier, R. (1993). *Cross-cultural midwifery: Working with Southeast Asian patients.* Paper presented at the 38th Annual Meeting of the American College of Nurse-Midwives, Orlando, Florida.

Renner, R. (1995). Endocrine disrupter research strategy completed by EPA. *Environmental Science and Technology, 29,* 494A.

Rosenfeld, J.A. (1996). Treatment of menorrhagia due to dysfunctional uterine bleeding. *American Family Physician, 53*(1), 165–172.

Sabbagha, R., Cohen, L., & Crocker, L. (1994). Sonography of the uterus: Vaginal approach. In R. Sabbagha (Ed.). *Diagnostic ultrasound applied to obstetrics and gynecology,* 3d ed., pp. 627–653. Philadelphia: J.B. Lippincott.

Speroff, L., Glass, R., & Kase, N. (1994). *Clinical gynecologic endocrinology and infertility,* 5th ed. Baltimore: Williams & Wilkins.

Steinberger, E. (1996). *The endocrinologists' approach to ovulatory dysfunction.* In AACE: 1996 Annual Meeting Workshop Abstracts, http://www.aace.com/cmr/workshops/sat7.htm.

Tabibzadeh, S., Babaknia, A., Kong, Q.F., et al. (1995). Menstruation is associated with disordered expression of desmoplakin I/II an d-cadherin/catenins and conversion of F- to G-actin in endometrial epithelium. *Human Reproduction, 10*(4), 776–778.

Thomas, E.J. (1996) Add-back therapy for long-term use in dysfunctional uterine bleeding and uterine fibroids. *British Journal of Obstetrics and Gynaecology, 103*(14), 18–21.

Vakiani, M., Vavilis, D., Agorastos, T., Stamatopoulos, P., Assimaki, A., & Bontis, J. (1996). Histopathological findings of the endometrium in patients with dysfunctional uterine bleeding. *Clinical Experiments in Obstetrics and Gynecology, 23*(4), 236–239.

van der Schouw, Y., van der Graaf, Y., Steyerberg, E., Eijkemans, M., & Dirk, J. (1996). Age at menopause as a risk factor for cardiovascular mortality. *Lancet, 347*(9003), 714–719.

Walling, A. (1996). Effectiveness of medical management of menorrhagia. *American Family Physician, 54*(8), 2533–2535.

Warhurst, M. *Introduction to hormone disrupting chemicals.* (1996). http://easyweb.easynet.co.uk/mwarhurst/oestrogenic.html

Wathen, P.I., Henderson, M.C., & Witz, C.A. (1995). Abnormal uterine bleeding. *Medical Clinics of North America, 79*(2), 329–344.

Westhoff, C., Gentile, G., Lee, J., Zacur, H., & Helbig, D. (1996). Predictors of ovarian steroid secretion in reproductive-age women. *American Journal of Epidemiology, 15*(4), 381–388.

Youssif, S.N., & McMillan, D.L. (1995). Outpatient endometrial biopsy: The pipette. *British Journal of Hospital Medicine, 54*(5), 198–201.

Zaldivar, A., Damm, R., Ruiz, M.R., Lozano, F., Malacara, J.M., & Forsbach, G. (1995). Factors possibly associated with the age at the onset of menopause. Multicenter study. *Gynecologie Obstetric Mexico, 10*(63), 432–438.

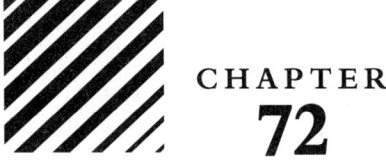

CHAPTER
72

Asthma

Lawrence Glaubiger, MD, and Harry Pomeranz, PA-C

Asthma is a chronic, persistent inflammatory disorder of the airway. It affects people of all ages and is characterized by exacerbations of coughing, wheezing, chest tightness, and difficulty breathing. Asthma is not a specific disease, but rather a syndrome that is triggered by precipitating factors such as allergens and results in reversible airway hyperresponsiveness and narrowing. Complex inflammatory events are responsible for both acute attacks and chronic disease.

New treatment strategies and pharmacologic therapies have developed as a result of an emerging understanding of the pathophysiology of asthma. However, despite an explosion of information concerning the inflammatory cells and mediators involved in asthma, morbidity and mortality rates are on the rise.

ANATOMY, PHYSIOLOGY, AND PATHOLOGY

The human airway consists of a trachea and right and left mainstem bronchi, which divide into ever-narrowing and smaller branches. Nonstriated muscles and fibrous tissue surround the trachea and main bronchi, which are lined with ciliate epithelial cells. These cells remove mucus produced by goblet cells, lymphocytes, and neutrophils. Mast cells are the most important inflammatory cells, followed by helper T cells, eosinophils, and macrophages.

Cholinergic stimulation causes constriction of the bronchi, dilation of the local blood vessels, and increased mucus production. Adrenergic stimulation leads to bronchodilation, mucosal vasoconstriction, and increased ion secretion, resulting in increased ciliary rate and mucus clearance. Bronchodilation results from circulating catecholamines, such as epinephrine and glucocorticoids, which are affected by circadian rhythms, resulting in lower levels at night and early morning (Table 72-1).

The respiratory epithelium has an extensive network of beta-2 receptors that oppose bronchoconstriction. Stimulation of the beta receptors on the mast cells and other inflammatory cells stabilizes them and inhibits the release of inflammatory mediators.

An asthma attack is made up of two phases, an acute phase response and a late phase response. The acute response begins within 5 to 15 minutes of the inciting event and lasts up to an hour. It begins with the interaction of an allergen and a macrophage. The late response occurs within 2 to 6 hours and lasts 12 to 24 hours. It is characterized by the increased infiltration of eosinophils and neutrophils. The sequence of events is summarized in Table 72-2.

Early in an asthma attack, there is increased minute ventilation, which causes hypocarbia. With tiring of the respiratory muscles, there is a reduction in minute ventilation, and hypocarbia is replaced by normocarbia. This should be a signal that the patient is progressing to respiratory failure and might require mechanical ventilation (Fig. 72-1).

Chronic Disease

After repeated attacks and chronic damage to the airways, there are certain classic findings in the biopsy of the bronchial mucosa. There is extensive epithelial cell damage and loss of ciliated mucosa and thickening of the basement membrane. Goblet cell hyperplasia is routinely seen. The bronchial wall is edematous as a result of vascular leakage from swollen and damaged endothelial cells. There is hyperplasia of the bronchial smooth muscle cells rather than hypertropy of the muscle fibers. All these chronic changes thicken the airway walls and narrow the airway diameter. The patient, instead of having only episodic symptoms, could become constantly symptomatic, as in other obstructive lung diseases.

EPIDEMIOLOGY

Asthma is estimated to affect 14 to 15 million persons in the United States, or about 5% of the population. It is the most common chronic disease of childhood, affecting an estimated 4.8 million children. It accounts for 5000 deaths a year. There are 470,000 hospitalizations annually from asthma. The National Health Interviews Survey reported an increase in those affected by asthma from 6.8 million to 10.3 million from 1980 to 1990. The rate for women increased by 50%, with African American women most affected (Asthma, United States, 1992).

In 1990, the cost of care for asthma was estimated at $6.2 billion, nearly 1% of the U.S. health care cost. Nearly half of that, 43%, was spent on emergency department treatment, hospitalization, and fatal asthma.

There are marked geographic differences in mortality rates, with especially high rates in four regions: New York City; Cook County, Illinois; Maricopa County, Arizona; and Fresno County, California. Twenty-one percent of all deaths from asthma occurred in New York City and Cook County, areas that account for only 6.8% of the population at risk. Both New York and Cook County had concentrations of extremely high incidence of asthma in small districts of impoverished inner-city neighborhoods (Weiss et al, 1992).

Race/ethnicity and socioeconomic status affect asthma prevalence but have a greater impact on hospitalization and

TABLE 72-1	Neurogenic Mediators in Asthma
Factors	**Response**
Cholinergic	Stimulation
Bronchoconstriction	Dilatation of blood vessels
Adrenergic	Stimulation
Bronchodilatation	Vasoconstriction

mortality rates. Race-specific hospitalization rates were similar when adjusted for income, suggesting that socioeconomic status is a greater risk for asthma morbidity than race alone.

The physical environment of poor urban centers may also be a contributing factor. Housing in these neighborhoods tends to be deteriorated, with increased exposure to indoor air pollution, including irritant gases, and allergens such as mites, roaches, molds, and animals. Good nutrition is harder to maintain on a limited income, and lower education levels and poor support systems contribute to difficulty in maintaining good health. High-quality, ongoing health care may be difficult to find in underserved areas. Overburdened clinics and emergency departments can delay crucial treatment delivery in acute situations.

DIAGNOSTIC CRITERIA

Diagnosis is usually made clinically with a history of periodic wheezing, breathlessness, and chest tightness. However, asthma can present with just the symptom of cough. Symptoms that increase at night, or especially in the early morning hours, are characteristic of asthma.

Classification of asthma is based on the severity of clinical symptoms and lung function, determined by peak expiratory flow (PEF) measurements. Peak flow meters are inexpensive and easy to use. Improvement or worsening of disease can be documented by having the patient keep a diary of PEF recordings. Nocturnal symptoms and diurnal variability are important in classifying asthma. A drop in PEF to less than 80% of personal best alerts the patient to an impending attack. A PEF of 50% of personal best requires the immediate attention of a health care provider (Table 73-3).

TABLE 72-2	Inflammatory Mediators in Asthma
Phase	**Factors**
Acute phase (15 min. to several hours)	Upregulation of T cells with production of interleukins: IL-3, IL-4, IL-6, IL-13 GM-CSF B-cell stimulation—production of IgE, with mast cell cross-linkage TNF Prostaglandin D$_2$, leukotriene C4
Late response (2–6 hrs.–12–24 hrs.)	Eosinophil infiltration from IL-3, IL-4 production Major basic protein, eosinophilic cationic protein Neutrophil infiltration from GM-CSF Adhesion molecules in response to IL-4, TNF-a, histamine NANC pathways Platelet-activating factor

Lung function tests are a more objective method of diagnosing bronchial hyperactivity. Because of the variable nature of the disease, spirometry cannot be relied on for diagnosing asthma. An increase in the forced expiratory volume in 1 second (FEV$_1$) of 12% or an increase in the forced vital capacity of 300 mL after the use of a beta-2 agonist suggests reversible airflow obstruction, which is seen in asthma.

Airway challenges have been used to make the diagnosis of bronchial hyperactivity. A bronchial provocation test can be done using methacholine or histamine. Doubling concentrations of the drug delivered to the patient from a nebulizer and the concentration which causes a 20% decrease in the initial FEV$_1$ achieved before the challenge is called PC20. Studies using histamine have demonstrated that a PC20 of greater than 8 mg/mL made the diagnosis of bronchial hyperactivity and asthma unlikely. Studies of methacholine also used a similar concept in elucidating bronchial hyperactivity. Starting with 0.1 mg/mL of methacholine, the dose is doubled and the FEV$_1$ is noted with each dose delivered. An FEV$_1$ decrease below 80% of the FEV$_1$ before administration is diagnostic of bronchial hyperactivity and suggestive of asthma if it occurs before or at a concentration of 25 mg/mL of methacholine.

Historically, asthma has been classified by the presence or absence of allergen exposure. Extrinsic asthma refers to symptoms that are triggered by an allergen. A positive skin test to the triggering inhalant and serum studies revealing an elevated IgE would confirm the diagnosis. This type of asthma usually begins in childhood. Intrinsic or nonallergic asthma has no recognizable allergic triggers, nor is there IgE elevation. Acute attacks tend to become more persistent and difficult to control than the extrinsic variety. Intrinsic asthma usually begins in adulthood.

HISTORY AND PHYSICAL EXAM

Factors and conditions known to trigger an asthma attack include:

- Exercise: can trigger an attack within 5 to 20 minutes of onset. Exercise-induced asthma is more common in children and is often precipitated by exposure to cold air.
- Drugs, particularly aspirin and other nonsteroidal anti-inflammatory medications: An association among aspirin-induced asthma, nasal polyps, and perennial rhinitis has been made.
- Irritants such as sulfur dioxide and chemicals such as formaldehyde: Sensitive persons may also be affected by strong odors or perfumes.
- Food additives, particularly metabisulfite, and certain dairy products: Some find this particularly troublesome after eating in restaurants that use monosodium glutamate ("Chinese restaurant syndrome").
- Premenstrual worsening of asthma: common, but usually of little clinical significance
- Pregnancy: The effect on asthma is unpredictable. Some patients improve during pregnancy; others worsen.
- Gastroesophageal reflux: an important trigger of bronchospasm. Acid reflux can cause a reflex vagal stimulation and bronchoconstriction. Concurrent esophageal pH monitoring with peak flow monitoring can determine this cause of asthma.

STEPWISE APPROACH FOR MANAGING ASTHMA IN ADULTS AND CHILDREN OVER 5 YEARS OLD

Goals of Asthma Treatment

- Prevent chronic and troublesome symptoms (eg, coughing or breathlessness in the night, in the early morning, or after exertion)
- Maintain (near) "normal" pulmonary function
- Maintain normal activity levels (including exercise and other physical activity)
- Prevent recurrent exacerbations of asthma and minimize the need for emergency department visits or hospitalizations
- Provide optimal pharmacotherapy with minimal or no adverse effects
- Meet patients' and families' expectation of and satisfaction with asthma care

Classification of Severity: Clinical Features Before Treatment*

	Symptoms**	Nighttime Symptoms	Lung Function
STEP 4 **Severe Persistent**	• Continual symptoms • Limited physical activity • Frequent exacerbations	Frequent	• FEV_1 or PEF ≤60% predicted • PEF variability >30%
STEP 3 **Moderate Persistent**	• Daily symptoms • Daily use of inhaled short-acting beta$_2$-agonist • Exacerbations affect activity • Exacerbations ≥2 times a week; may last days	>1 time a week	• FEV_1 or PEF >60% ≤80% predicted • PEF variability >30%
STEP 2 **Mild Persistent**	• Symptoms >2 times a week but <1 time a day • Exacerbations may affect activity	>2 times a month	• FEV_1 or PEF ≥80% predicted • PEF variability 20%–30%
STEP 1 **Mild Intermittent**	• Symptoms ≤2 times a week • Asymptomatic and normal PEF between exacerbations • Exacerbations brief (from a few hours to a few days); intensity may vary	≤2 times a month	• FEV_1 or PEF ≥80% predicted • PEF variability <20%

* The presence of one of the features of severity is sufficient to place a patient in that category. An individual should be assigned to the most severe grade in which any feature occurs. The characteristics noted in this figure are general and may overlap because asthma is highly variable. Furthermore, an individual's classification may change over time.

** Patients at any level of severity can have mild, moderate, or severe exacerbations. Some patients with intermittent asthma experience severe and life-threatening exacerbations separated by long periods of normal lung function and no symptoms.

FIGURE 72-1 Stepwise approach for managing asthma in adults and children over 5 years old. (From: Highlights of The Expert Panel Report: Guidelines for the Diagnosis and Management of Asthma. NIH Publication N. 97 4051A, May 1997.)

TABLE 72-3	Classification of Asthma		
Classification	Symptoms	PEF Variability	Therapy
Mild intermittent	≤2 times/wk—day ≤2 times/mo—night	<20%/day	Bronchodilators prn
Mild persistent	>2 times/wk but ≤1 time/day—day >2 times/mo—night	20–30% day	Inhaled steroids (low doses) Bronchodilators prn
Moderate persistent	Daily Severe exacerbation >2 times/wk—day >1 time/wk—night	>30%/day Frequent, daily	Bronchodilator Inhaled steroids (high doses) Long-acting bronchodilator (optional) Inhaled chromones (optional)
Severe persistent	Continuous Frequent severe exacerbations—day, several times/wk and every night	>30%/day Frequent, daily	Bronchodilator use Inhaled steroids (high doses) Long-acting bronchodilators Inhaled chromones Antileukotrienes Oral corticosteroids (last resort)

- Cigarette smoking, including passive smoke inhalation
- Household factors (eg, living in a damp house, use of gas for cooking, use of a humidifier)
- Indoor environmental hazards (eg, silica, chemical fragrances [perfume, paint])

Occupational exposures can increase the prevalence of asthma within the general population. If the incidence of asthma within a particular workplace is several times that of the general population, an association can be made between the occupational environment and asthma. Some occupations in which this association has been made are:

- Those who card or spin cotton
- Animal handlers
- Painters using polyurethane, which contains toluene diisocyanate
- Bakers sensitive to cereals, flours, or grain contaminated by insects
- Platinum refiners or those working with the industrial compound trimelitic anhydride
- Pulp and paper workers, who are exposed to chlorine. Chlorine is an irritant gas and vapor that can cause new-onset asthma; this is referred to as reactive airways distress syndrome. Bleach plant workers are also exposed to chlorine.
- Tin and lead solderers. Flux used in tin and lead soldering (colophony) is made of pine resins, a known allergen.
- Printers using acacia and arabic gums, also made of tree resins. Those who work or live near Western red cedar and oak are also at risk.
- Workers processing castor beans in the manufacture of castor bean oil.

Psychosocial factors have also been associated with asthma. Depression can increase the mortality rate from asthma, especially among children. Alcohol abuse, schizophrenia, recent unemployment, and family disruption or loss have also been associated with asthma deaths.

Screening for risk factors should include assessing how asthma is affecting the patient's self-esteem and stress levels. The patient should be encouraged to elicit the reaction of family or friends to the disease and to develop coping mechanisms for physical and emotional stress.

The physical exam of the patient with chronic asthma focuses on the skin, airway, respiratory tract, and chest. Vital signs may show increased respiratory rate, tachycardia, and pulsus paradoxus (a difference of more than 10 mmHg in blood pressure between inspiration and expiration). Eczema on flexor surfaces or other signs of atopy should be noted, as well as the presence of rhinitis, sinusitis, or nasal polyps.

For some, the presence of an upper airway disease can influence the function of the lower airway. Allergic rhinitis or sinusitis may exacerbate asthma, or those with chronic, unremitting asthma may find an association with persistent sinusitis. At times of active allergic rhinitis, the use of topical corticosteroids for allergic rhinitis can decrease the intensity of the asthma symptoms.

Inspection of the chest may reveal signs of hyperinflation of the lungs, such as hunched shoulders or pigeon chest. Intercostal retractions or the use of accessory muscles indicates severe disease. The quality and intensity of breath sounds and the presence of wheezing, rales, or stridor are assessed on auscultation. Mild asthma might reveal wheezing only at end expiration. With increasing severity of disease, wheezing is heard throughout the respiratory cycle. Prolonged expiration or inspiration that equals expiration is also a sign of severe asthma. The absence of wheezing may be a sign of poor air movement and may signal danger and deterioration of the patient's condition. The inability to speak in full sentences or a staccato pattern of speech may also indicate worsening disease.

CLINICAL WARNING: The absence of wheezing may signal a lack of air movement; this may be a danger sign.

DIAGNOSTIC TESTS

Baseline spirometry should be obtained, as well as serial PEF readings. Patients can determine which readings can be expected during symptomatic and asymptomatic periods, given their level of disease. Personal best levels should be known by both the patient and the provider. Complete pulmonary function studies can show other causes of upper airway disorders that simulate asthma.

A chest x-ray can rule out nonasthmatic causes of airway narrowing. A sputum stain may show eosinophilia, which is characteristic of asthma, or neutrophils, which are more common in bronchitis. Stains of nasal secretions can likewise reveal eosinophils, which are more suggestive of asthma, or neutrophils, which are more suggestive of sinusitis.

The presence of an allergic component may be studied by finding eosinophils in a complete blood count or by the presence of specific IgE antibodies. Bronchoprovocation tests with methacholine, histamine, or exercise will elicit a positive reaction. An occupational allergen challenge should be considered in some patients.

Evaluating sinusitis by clinical symptoms alone is often difficult. Patients who regularly use medications and are not improving might benefit from sinus x-rays or a computed tomography scan. An evaluation for gastroesophageal reflux is also important in the diagnostic evaluation.

TREATMENT OPTIONS, EXPECTED OUTCOMES, AND COMPREHENSIVE MANAGEMENT

Prevention

The following precautions should be used to reduce asthmatic flares:

- Exacerbations of rhinitis, sinusitis, and gastroesophageal reflux should be treated quickly.
- Patients should receive an annual influenza vaccine.
- Exercise should be preceded by the use of medication (a short-acting beta-2 agonist, cromolyn, or nedocromil sodium).
- Swimming in an indoor pool with a warm, humidified environment should be encouraged, rather than exercising in cold air.
- Pets (eg, birds, fish, dogs, cats) should be explored as a possible trigger of asthma. Veterinarians have been known to have an increased risk of asthma.
- A supportive partnership between the patient and the primary care provider is important.

The best tool for identifying worsening ventilatory function is twice-daily monitoring of PEF. Morning and evening measurements are recorded each day in a diary, and each reading is compared to the personal best (Table 72-4).

Increased diurnal variability is another indication of an impending attack, so the patient should record daily symptoms as well. Wheezing, cough, nocturnal awakening, chest tightness, increased mucus production, or difficulty walking, talking, or breathing should all be noted. The failure of medications to control symptoms is also important to document.

TABLE 72-4	Evaluation of Peak Expiratory Flow
Level	**Action**
>80% of personal best	Mild exacerbation; inhaled B$_2$ agonist
50%–80% of personal best	Moderate exacerbation; inhaled B$_2$ agonist, oral corticosteroids if not responding
50% of personal best	Severe exacerbation; immediate transportation to the hospital for emergency care

Awareness of weather conditions and air quality may limit acute attacks. Very humid or very cold air affects many patients, as do seasonal changes and climate variations. Autumn is a particular challenge because of the abundance of pollen in the air. It may be prudent to remain inside and use an air conditioner during the summer as well. Preventive measures may include changes in activity in response to weather conditions, adjustments in medications during these periods, and selective immunotherapy where applicable.

The outdoor environment is the major source of pollution. When air pollution is at an unhealthy level, there is often an increase in the irritant sulfur dioxide. Adjusting medications and developing a crisis plan are important factors in limiting the environmental effects on asthma. A permanent change of location may be helpful if it is financially and socially realistic.

Expected Outcomes

Asthma, unlike other airway diseases such as chronic bronchitis, cystic fibrosis, and bronchiectasis, is not necessarily progressive. Even in the absence of treatment, the disease does not necessarily progress from mild to more severe. The clinical course is characterized by exacerbations and remissions. The reasons for this pattern are not clearly defined.

Asthmatics older than 20 years show a lower rate of remissions than children. Atopy has not been useful in predicting relapses or remissions. Allergic rhinitis is not considered a predictor of future asthma. Asthma and allergic rhinitis frequently coexist, but if asthma does not occur within 1 year of the onset of allergic rhinitis, there is only a 5% to 10% chance of developing asthma later in life.

Medical Treatment

Most asthma medications are delivered by a metered-dose inhaler (MDI) mechanism. This is the common form of delivery for bronchodilators and steroid medications. Inhaled therapy for asthma is best because the medication is deposited at the lungs, where its action is most needed. By not taking the medicine orally, the systemic side effects of the medication can be avoided. For adrenergic agonists and anticholinergic medications, cardiac toxicity can be avoided. For corticosteroids, well-known side effects such as hyperglycemia, osteoporosis, immunosuppression, and gastritis can be avoided.

Patients taking inhaled corticosteroids are susceptible to oral candidiasis. This can be avoided by rinsing the mouth after drug administration.

Use of an MDI requires a certain amount of coordination and concentration. Starting at complete exhalation, patients should activate the inhaler with the mouthpiece in the mouth. They should start inspiring and activate the inhaler concurrently. The inhalation must occur slowly; otherwise, the medication will not reach the lungs but will be deposited on the pharyngeal wall. After inhaling slowly and deeply, patients should hold their breath for 5 to 10 seconds before exhaling. These steps are repeated as required.

For patients who have poor coordination or do not breathe slowly enough, a holding chamber may be placed between the mouth and the inhaler. This allows the patient to inhale the medication in the spacer device and allows for greater deposition in the lungs and not on the pharyngeal wall. Large particles of the medication that would have deposited in the oral airways drop out in the spacer device, so that only particles that are small and can reach the small airways are inhaled.

During severe exacerbations, when maximal absorption of medication is needed, the patient might be too anxious and excited to be able to coordinate inhalation efforts appropriately. To prevent a catastrophic event and worsening of the exacerbation, the medication can be given by a hand-held nebulizer. The medication in solution form is placed in a canister. A compressor that can pump air is attached to the canister by a plastic tube. The medication is inhaled through a mouthpiece attached to the canister as a continuous nebulized mist. Thus, the patient can inhale the medicine without much attention to coordinating inhalation, nor is there a need to concentrate on how the inhalation occurs. Elderly or mentally disabled patients might need to take medications only by nebulized form if they lack the coordination and concentration to use an inhaler.

Tables 72-5 and 72-6 summarize oral and MDI asthma medications.

PHARMACOTHERAPY

Beta-Adrenergic Agents

Beta-2 adrenergic agents are the mainstay for relieving acute attacks. They produce bronchodilatation by stimulating sympathetic receptors in the airways. Inhaled beta-2 adrenergic agonists are the first-line agents for an acute asthma exacerbation. Severe attacks might necessitate the use of subcutaneous beta-2 agonists. These medications can precipitate cardiac instability and therefore should be used with caution, especially in older patients.

By attaching to beta-2 receptors, beta-2 agonists act as sympathomimetics and cause smooth muscle relaxation and block mediator release from mast cells. They have little to no effect in preventing the inflammatory reactions of the late airway response. Short-acting beta-2 agonists can be used before exercise or increased activity to prevent exercise-induced asthma. Important side effects include tachycardia, palpitations, tremors, and hypokalemia. The usual duration of a short-acting agent given by MDI is no more than 4 to 6 hours. These may also be an option during an acute attack; nebulization of a short-acting beta-2 agonist might be more appropriate than using

TABLE 72-5	Asthma Medications— Metered-Dose Inhaler
Classification	**Drug**
Corticosteroids	Beclomethasone
	Triamcinolone
	Flunisolide
	Budenoside
	Fluticasone
	Cromones
	Cromolyn sodium*
	Nedocromil sodium
Short-acting B₂ agonists	Albuterol*
	Metaproterenol*
	Pirbuterol
	Bitolterol
	Terbutaline
Long-acting B₂ agonist	Salmeterol
Anticholinergic	Ipratropium bromide*

Also available in nebulized form.

TABLE 72-6	Oral Asthma Medications
Classification	**Drug**
Leukotriene inhibitors	Zafirlukast
	Zileuton
Methylxanthines	Theophylline
Long-acting B₂ agonist	Albuterol (sustained-release)

another drug by MDI because of the coordination challenge for a dyspneic, anxious patient.

New long-acting beta-2 agonists have been used with increasing success. They are especially appropriate for patients with moderate to severe asthma who have nocturnal symptoms or a busy life. However, some studies have found an association between an increased concentration of long-acting beta-2 agonist and an increased mortality rate. This has made the use of long-acting beta-2 agonists controversial. Other studies have suggested that increased beta agonist use causes tachyphylaxis or tolerance, and that the drug loses its bronchoprotective effect. Proponents of long-acting beta-2 agonists claim that most of the patients who use these medications have moderate to severe asthma and, therefore, have a higher degree of morbidity and mortality than the average asthmatic.

Another factor may be that beta-2 agonists give clinical relief that the patient can feel; this may lead to overreliance on them over the use of more important drugs such as steroids and other anti-inflammatory medications. Inflammatory control is more likely to prevent chronic deterioration of the airways. Therefore, beta agonists may not be able to prevent progression of disease in asthmatics.

Subcutaneous epinephrine and terbutaline act within 5 minutes of administration and can usually increase the PEF by 20%. These medications are appropriate only in an emergency setting, where rapid stabilization is needed and adequate monitoring can be achieved.

Anticholinergics

Anticholinergics act as vagolytics and decrease the parasympathetic influence over airway control. Because they do not cause as great a degree of bronchodilatation as sympathomimetics do, they are used only in conjunction with a beta-2 agonist to increase the overall effect. The onset of action begins at 20 minutes, with maximal effect not occurring until 60 to 120 minutes after activation.

Corticosteroids

As the role of inflammation has gained greater recognition in the progression of worsening chronic disease, corticosteroids have become the single most important drug in reducing morbidity and mortality rates. Corticosteroids act by decreasing the production of the most inflammatory mediators of asthma. They inhibit the synthesis of leukotrienes, prostaglandins, arachidonic acid, and platelet activating factor. They directly inhibit the activation of eosinophils, mast cells, and T lymphocytes and decrease their migratory activity. They cause vasoconstriction, decreasing mucosal edema by reducing capillary leakage and mucus production. They also inhibit the production of cytokines.

Corticosteroids interfere mainly with the late phase of asthma; the onset of action is 4 to 8 hours after administration. Because corticosteroids have little effect on bronchoconstriction and dyspnea during the acute phase, many patients do not like them, despite their long-term benefits. Patient education is necessary to stress the importance of steroid use in the prevention of bronchospasm and the maintenance of symptom-free periods.

In an acute setting, parenteral administration of systemic glucocorticoids is used to ensure the rapid absorption of this important medication. Methylprednisolone is usually used (40 to 60 mg intravenously every 6 hours). For asthma exacerbations that are controlled in 48 to 72 hours, the systemic steroid can be abruptly stopped and inhaled corticosteroids substituted. However, if the exacerbation is not controlled after 4 days, and continuous systemic glucocorticoids have been used, then it is wise to taper the steroids slowly (starting with prednisone 40 mg/day orally). This is necessary because suppression of the adrenal–pituitary–hypothalamic axis occurs after this period of use and endogenous steroid production is decreased. Abrupt cessation of exogenous steroids could therefore precipitate shock. Steroids are usually tapered over 2 to 4 weeks.

A daily regimen of inhaled corticosteroids should be considered for all asthmatics who have even mild persistent disease. Although the medication is more expensive than other inhalers, the savings from decreased emergency room visits and hospitalizations more than make up for its cost.

Methylxanthines

Once considered first-line therapy for an acute attack, methylxanthines have been shown to be no more effective than beta agonists for relieving bronchospasm. Indeed, because of their narrow therapeutic window and potential for fatal cardiac arrhythmia and seizures, they are now a second- or third-line medication. However, these medications have been shown to have a weak bronchodilating effect and might inhibit neutrophil chemotactic factor release from mast cells. Therefore, they have some effect in both the early and late phase reactions. Other important benefits include decreased microvascular permeability and enhanced diaphragmatic and respiratory muscle performance, stimulation of mucociliary clearance, and stimulation of the central nervous system respiratory drive. Their action as a phosphodiesterase inhibitor and increaser of cAMP in smooth muscle, and more importantly their ability to sequester and efflux calcium from smooth muscle cells, cause smooth muscle relaxation. Inhibiting adenosine, a potent bronchoconstrictor, and increasing catecholamine release make methylxanthine an important drug.

Because of their potential for fatal side effects, serum levels must be monitored and maintained at 5 to 15 mg/L. Patients with congestive heart failure and cirrhosis should receive a reduced dose. For patients taking medications that affect the cytochrome P-450 system, an alteration in dose should be considered. Inhaled cigarette smoke and charcoal-grilled food can also increase clearance and lower serum levels (Table 72-7).

Although many patients discontinue therapy because of side effects such as nausea, tremors, and anxiety, many improve with methylxanthine administration. As long as toxicity is avoided, it is still a useful drug in some patients with asthma.

Magnesium

Magnesium is thought to inhibit calcium uptake and release from the sarcoplasmic reticulum. This causes smooth muscle relaxation and bronchodilatation. Clinically, its effect is controversial. Studies have shown that magnesium causes either rapid improvement in PEF, especially in status asthmaticus, or no improvement in function. Because of its extremely low side

TABLE 72-7	**Drugs Affecting Theophylline Clearance**
Decreased Clearance	**Increased Clearance**
Cimetidine	Phenytoin
Erythromycin and other macrolides	Phenobarbital
Quinalones	Carbamazepine
Isoniazid	Rifampin
Calcium channel antagonists	Furosemide
Mexiletine	
Allopurinol	
Oral contraceptives	
Caffeine	
Influenza vaccine	

effect profile, it is used for severe asthma attacks in conjunction with other medications.

Cromolyn Sodium

Cromolyn sodium is the foremost noncorticosteroid anti-inflammatory agent used. It blocks mediator release from IgE-stimulated mast cells. It acts by reducing mast cell activity or stabilizing the mast cell membrane. It is especially useful in extrinsic asthma, exercise-induced asthma, or asthma induced by cold dry air. It has wide utility in children with allergic asthma, because inhaled corticosteroids could potentially stunt the growth of a child. It is usually delivered by inhalation as a powder or an aerosol. This medication is not useful for acute exacerbations.

Nedocromil Sodium

Nedocromil sodium is an inhaled anti-inflammatory medication that is 4 to 10 times more potent than cromolyn and has similar indications. Chronic use has shown a decrease in bronchial hyperactivity in nonallergic asthma, with improvement of symptoms, particularly cough. No major side effects have been noted. Like cromolyn, this medication is not useful for acute episodes.

Corticosteroid-Sparing Agents

Many patients with severe asthma taking chronic steroid therapy have suffered considerable side effects, such as glucose intolerance, bone demineralization, immunosuppression, hypertension, and peptic ulcer disease. Among the alternative regimens explored is potent anti-inflammatory therapy used in rheumatologic diseases and in chemotherapy for malignancy.

- Methotrexate, used at a low dose of 15 to 50 mg/wk, reaches maximal effect between 12 and 24 weeks. Although it may reduce or eliminate the need for steroids, it is unclear how potent it is as an antiasthmatic drug. The side effect profile is considerable and includes pulmonary fibrosis, hepatic toxicity, bone marrow suppression, and gastrointestinal disturbance.
- Cyclosporine has been used for its T-lymphocyte inhibitory action. It inhibits the synthesis and release of cytokines, histamines, and leukotrienes and suppresses the function of mast cells, basophils, eosinophils, and neutrophils. Its use has been shown to reduce the dose of corti-

costeroids needed, and improvement in diurnal variability has been documented. This drug also has considerable side effects; the most common are nephrotoxicity, hypertension, paresthesias, and tremor.

- Auranofin or gold has been shown to decrease bronchial hyperactivity and steroid use, although peak activity occurs after 12 weeks. It is postulated to have an effect on the production of leukotrienes and histamine. Side effects chiefly involve mucocutaneous reactions, but diarrhea, bone marrow suppression, nephrotoxicity, and pulmonary fibrosis are also seen.
- Hydroxychloroquine is a known inhibitor of phospholipase A, a decrease in which would correspond to a decrease in the synthesis of leukotrienes, prostaglandins, and platelet activating factor. A dose of 300 to 400 mg/day has been shown to decrease the steroid dosage by 50% to 65%. Gastrointestinal upset, skin rash, and retinal damage have been reported.
- Dapsone can significantly inhibit the action of neutrophils but has toxic side effects, most notably bone marrow suppression. Therapy for 6 to 13 months has been shown to reduce steroid use significantly.

Leukotriene Antagonists

Leukotrienes contribute to smooth muscle contraction, bronchial wall edema and inflammation, and increased mucus secretion. Zafirlukast, which is a direct leukotriene T4 receptor antagonist, and zileuton, which inhibits the conversion of arachidonic acid to leukotrienes, are the primary drugs in this class. These drugs are alternatives to low-dose inhaled corticosteroids and are efficacious for bronchospasm induced by cold air and aspirin-induced attacks. They have been approved for use only in mild to moderate asthma, but the potential benefits of combination therapy of leukotriene antagonists with steroids and other asthma medications are under investigation (McGill & Busse, 1996).

TEACHING AND SELF-CARE

Education and self-management programs begin with a home environment evaluation. Optimally, the primary care provider visits the home and determines the social and financial aspects of the patient's home life, identifies potential allergens or irritants, and meets other family members. Because the cooperation of the entire household is needed to make a change, education and counseling of all family members is needed.

Household modifications include the following:

- Restrict smoking of any household member inside the house, because exposure to second-hand smoke can precipitate bronchospasm. The use of fireplaces, sprays, and aerosols and cooking odors can exacerbate asthma. Exposure to noxious gases, perfumes, detergents, and cleaning solutions can also precipitate an attack.
- Remove plants and rugs from bedrooms; this may relieve nocturnal symptoms.
- Replace feather-filled pillows with synthetic ones.
- Frequent dusting and mopping and conscientious removal of molds may also help control the disease.
- Although the use of chemicals to kill dust mites is no longer routinely recommended, it might be prudent to apply plastic covers over furniture.

- Pets may need to be kept in certain areas of the residence to minimize exposure to allergens in animal fur. An allergist may be needed for skin testing of perennial indoor allergens such as cat dander or dust mites.

Patients with asthma must be wary of all medications that contain beta-blockers, particularly antihypertensives and ophthalmologic preparations. All foods should be checked for metabisulfite, which is often used as a preservative in salads, fruits, potatoes, beer, wine, and shellfish. Aspirin and other nonsteroidal anti-inflammatory medications should be avoided by patients with a known sensitivity to aspirin.

Asthmatics who demonstrate a good understanding of their disease and respect the side effect profile of their medications might be allowed to increase their intake of oral steroids (see treatment section) or increase their use of nebulizer therapy when there is evidence of worsening disease. Providers should weigh the benefits of patient participation in the management of the disease against the possibility that delayed care of an acute episode could lead to death. Guidelines for when the provider should be called must be established and reinforced.

The prevention of chronic long-lasting side effects is mostly related to proper education of the role of inhaled steroids (see treatment). Only inhaled steroids have shown a significant ability to stop the progression of disease. The patient should be counseled that although no immediate symptomatic relief is felt with use of an inhaled steroid, its use is the most important aspect of maintaining ventilatory function and performing normal activities without constraints or disabilities. Preventing severe attacks by treating exacerbations as early as possible will most likely prevent complications as well.

Other lifestyle factors include good nutrition and hydration, weight control, and stabilization of other diseases, especially chronic obstructive pulmonary disease. Physical activity is encouraged and individualized for each patient.

Complementary Treatments

Alternative therapies, including herbal preparations and nonmedication management techniques, appeal to patients who are unsatisfied with orthodox medicine. However, scientific proof of their value is inadequate, and most of the information is anecdotal. Dietary modifications have included reducing intake of dairy products and salt and using magnesium and selenium supplements. Dietary fish oil and polyunsaturated fatty acids may have respiratory benefit. Acupuncture has been used with reports of improvement. Some asthmatics report improvement with goldenseal powder or echinacea.

COMMUNITY RESOURCES

- Atlanta Allergy & Asthma Clinic, http://www.atlallergy.com/rhinitis.html
- Healthline: Allergic Rhinitis, http://www.healthline.com/articles/ap960107.htm and Http://www.health-line.com/articles/ac970102.htm
- American Lung Association, http://www.lungusa.org/noframes/
- Information about Allergies and Asthma, 3554 Chain Bridge Rd., Suite 200, Fairfax, VA 22030, 800-878-4403 or 703-385-4403, fax 703-352-4354
- American College of Allergy, Asthma and Immunology, 85 W. Algonquin Rd., Suite 550, Arlington Heights, IL 60005, 847-427-1294

- National Jewish Medical and Research Center, 1400 Jackson St., Denver, CO 80206, 303-388-4461, 800-222-LUNG

REFERRAL POINTS AND CLINICAL WARNINGS

Certain patients are at greater risk for severe or even fatal asthma as a result of their past history or the findings in a present exacerbation. These warning signs include:

- A history of near-fatal asthma
- A history of prior intubations or intensive care unit admissions
- Trial of steroid therapy with little improvement
- Less than 10% improvement in PEF or FEV_1 in the emergency room
- PEF or FEV_1 less than 25% of predicted
- PCO_2 40 mmHg or more
- A self-report of daily wide fluctuations of PEF
- Recent treatment for acute exacerbation, especially within the past 24 hours
- No audible wheezing on exam
- Obvious fatigue or confusion.

These warning signs should prompt the primary care provider to evaluate the patient for emergency treatment. More aggressive care, even in the primary care setting, may be warranted.

The use of sternocleidomastoid muscles, intercostal muscle retractions, holding on to furniture to maximize the effort of inspiratory muscles, nasal flaring, and cyanosis are all signs of an impending medical catastrophe. The following patients should also be seen immediately by a provider or should go to an emergency department:

Patients with a PEF less than 50% of personal best, with no improvement after short-acting beta-2 agonist therapy delivered via nebulizer or inhaler

Patients unable to say more than a few words at a time.

Patients should also be considered for referral if they have these less-severe warning signs:

- History of an acute, near-fatal attack
- Poor self-management skills
- Difficult family environment
- Atypical signs and symptoms
- Severe episodes with an unclear diagnosis
- Clinical entities such as sinusitis, nasal polyps, severe rhinitis, or aspergillosis that complicate airway disease
- Lack of response to appropriate asthma therapy
- Need for further guidance on environmental control, complications of therapy, or proper medication use.

Patients may also need referral for additional diagnostic testing, such as skin testing, rhinoscopy, bronchoscopy, complete pulmonary function tests, and provocative challenge testing.

After referral, the patient should return to the primary care provider, who will maintain the treatment plan and monitor progress. Some patients may need to be followed by a pulmonologist, although once stabilized they may also return to the primary provider.

EDITOR'S NOTE:

COMPLEMENTARY APPROACHES

A general discussion of complementary approaches can be found in Chapter 3. The following, while not an exhaustive list, are some complementary approaches being used for this condition. Additional information on these approaches, including precautions, can be found in Appendices A and B. Providers need to assess for the use of complementary approaches as part of the patient's history, as they may impact conventional therapies, and patients may not volunteer this information unless specifically asked. Efficacy of many complementary approaches is not as well documented as that of conventional therapies. Providers need to read the literature before suggesting these complementary approaches.

- Complementary Modalities
  Acupuncture
  Aromatherapy
  Biofeedback

References

Asthma, United States, 1980–1990. (1992). *Morbidity and Mortality Weekly Report, 41,* 733.

Weiss, K.B., Gergen, P.J., & Hodgson, T.A. (1992). An economic evaluation of asthma in the United States. *N Engl J Med, 326,* 862.

Bibliography

Barnes, P.J. (1997). Asthma. In R.C. Bone, D.R. Dantzker, R.B. George, R.A. Matthay, & H.Y. Reynolds. (Eds.). *Pulmonary and critical care medicine,* Vol. 1. St. Louis: Mosby.

Buist, A.S., & Vollmer, W.M. (1994). Preventing deaths from asthma. *N Engl J Med, 33,* 1584.

Cockcroft, D.W., & Karla, S. (1996). Outpatient asthma management. *Medical Clinics of North America, 80*(4), 701–718.

George, R.B., Light, W.R., Matthay, M.A., Matthay, M.A., & Matthay, R.A. (Eds.). (1995). *Chest medicine: Essentials of pulmonary and critical care medicine,* 3d ed. Baltimore: Williams & Wilkins.

Geshwin, M.E., & Halpern, M.E. (Eds.). (1993). *Bronchial asthma: Principles of diagnosis and treatment.* Totowa, NJ: Humana Press.

Hunt, L.W., Silverstein, M.D., Reed, C.E., et al. (1993). Accuracy of the death certificate in a population-based study of asthmatic patients. *JAMA, 269,* 1947.

Jagoda, A., Shepherd, S.M., Spevitz, A., & Joseph, M.M. (1997). Refractory asthma, Part 1: Epidemiolgy, pathophysiology, pharmacologic interventions. *Annals of Emergency Medicine, 29*(2), 262–274.

Krishna, M.T., Chauhan, A.J., & Holgate, S.T. (1996). Molecular mediators of asthma: Current insights. *Hospital Practice, 31*(10), 115–130.

Lemiere, C., Malo, J.-L., & Gautrin, D. (1996). Nonsensitizing causes of occupational asthma. *Medical Clinics of North America, 80*(4), 749–774.

McGill, K.A., & Busse, W.W. (1996). Zileuton. *Lancet, 348,* 519–524.

Morris, R.J. (1996). Asthma. *Postgraduate Medicine, 100*(2), 10—5-120.

National Institute of Heart, Lung, and Blood, National Asthma Education and Prevention Program. (1997). *Guidelines for the diagnosis and management of asthma: Second expert panel on the management of asthma.*

Rosenstreich, D.L., and the National Cooperative Inner-City Asthma Study. (1997). The role of cockroach allergy and exposure to cockroach allergen in causing morbidity among inner-city children with asthma. *N Engl J Med, 336*(19), 1356–1363.

Skobeloff, E.M., Spivey, W.H., St. Clair, S.S., et al. (1992). The influence of age and sex on asthma admissions. *JAMA, 268,* 3437.

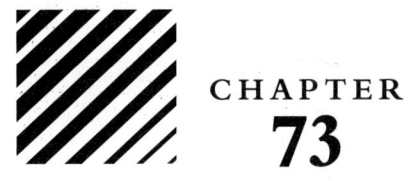

CHAPTER
73

Carcinoma of the Lung

Spiro Demetis, MD, FCCP

Carcinoma arising from cellular elements of the tracheobronchial tree or lung parenchyma accounts for significant morbidity and mortality. The case fatality rate for lung cancer is one of the highest of all malignancies (greater than 90%), and lung cancer accounts for approximately 30% of all cancer deaths in the United States. The most important aspects of epidemiology, diagnosis, treatment, and prevention will be reviewed here.

ANATOMY, PHYSIOLOGY, AND PATHOLOGY

Bronchogenic carcinoma is so named because most lung cancers arise from the tracheobronchial tree. The histologic classification of lung cancer is shown in Table 73-1. The most important task for the pathologist when examining lung specimens is to differentiate between nonsmall cell lung carcinoma (NSCLC) and small cell lung carcinoma (SCLC). This is an important distinction: the staging and the recommended treatment are different for these cancers. NSCLC is more common than SCLC.

Squamous cell (epidermoid) carcinoma is the most common type of NSCLC, closely followed by adenocarcinoma. Squamous cell carcinomas arise from bronchial epithelial cells where squamous metaplasia is present. This cell type is most strongly associated with smoking. The histologic hallmarks of these tumors include keratin "onion pearls" and intercellular bridges. Because 65% of squamous cell cancers arise in the central airways, they present with chronic cough, hemoptysis, or obstructive atelectasis. Squamous cell carcinoma is most often associated with hypercalcemia. After complete resection, local recurrence is most common.

Adenocarcinomas, in contrast, tend to occur most often in the periphery of the lung rather than the central airway. They are more common in women. Tobacco use is a risk factor for this cancer, as is significant exposure to ionizing radiation (eg, mining of uranium). Adenocarcinomas are more likely to metastasize to extrapulmonary sites than are squamous cell cancers. After complete resection of an intrathoracic tumor, distal metastasis to the brain or bone is the most frequent pattern of recurrence. Because of their peripheral location, they are less likely to cause symptoms early in their development. A variable degree of glandular formation and positive staining with mucin carmine are the histologic hallmarks of adenocarcinomas.

Bronchoalveolar carcinoma is a subtype of adenocarcinoma that originates in the terminal bronchioles and extends into the alveolar spaces. The most common radiologic presentation is that of a pneumonic infiltrate. Sputum cytology is usually positive in this type of NSCLC.

SCLC and carcinoid tumors account for about 25% to 30% of all lung carcinomas. Similar to squamous cell cancers, they arise centrally and present clinically with cough, hemoptysis, and obstructive pneumonitis. These tumors have the potential to produce many humoral substances (eg, serotonin, somatostatin, vasoactive intestinal peptide, bombesin) and may produce several neuroendocrine syndromes. Carcinoid syndrome is rarely seen with bronchial carcinoid tumors (2% to 5% incidence).

EPIDEMIOLOGY

The incidence of lung cancer is highest in industrialized nations. The most important risk factor for the development of bronchogenic carcinoma is tobacco smoke. More than 90% of lung cancers in the United States are attributed to smoking; only 2% of lung cancers occur in nonsmokers. The risk for developing lung cancer is directly related to the number of cigarettes smoked daily, years of use, depth of inspiration, cigarette tar content, use of filterless cigarettes, and age of smoking onset. Although the risk for lung cancer is significantly reduced by smoking cessation, it never reaches that of lifelong nonsmokers (Sobue et al, 1991).

Although the data are conflicting, the odds ratio for developing lung cancer with prolonged and significant exposure to environmental tobacco smoke (passive smoking) is 1:34 (National Research Council, 1986). It is believed that 3000 to 5000 lung cancer deaths annually may be caused by exposure to environmental tobacco smoke.

Exposure to potential carcinogens in the workplace increases the risk for the development of lung cancer. Some of these carcinogens are ionizing radiation, asbestos, arsenic, vinyl chloride, nickel, and aromatic hydrocarbons. All of these can act as cocarcinogens with tobacco smoke, and the risk for lung cancer in exposed smokers is multiplicative. Radon produces alpha particles and is directly carcinogenic to the respiratory epithelium. It also acts as a cocarcinogen with tobacco smoke. All homes contain some radon; the concentrations are highest in the basement and lower floors. Lifelong residence in a home with a radon concentration of 8 pCi/L is estimated to result in a lifetime risk for a nonsmoker of about 1 in 100. Although this is controversial, some experts recommend taking remedial measures for homes that consistently test at greater than 4 pCi/L ambient air.

Chronic obstructive pulmonary disease and pulmonary fibrosis are pulmonary diseases that independently increase the risk for the development of bronchogenic carcinoma. Poor clearance of potential carcinogens is the probable mechanism in chronic obstructive lung disease. Persistent chronic inflammation in diseases leading to pulmonary fibrosis is likely to cause the increased incidence of bronchogenic carcinoma.

TABLE 73-1	Histopathology of Lung Cancer
Cell Type	**Frequency (%)**
Nonsmall cell carcinoma	
Squamous cell carcinoma	30–35
Adenocarcinoma (and bronchoalveolar)	25–30
Large cell carcinoma	10–15
Neuroendocrine tumors	
Small cell carcinoma	20–25
Carcinoid (typical or atypical)	2–5
Uncommon primary malignant lung cancers	
Malignant melanoma	
Adenoid cystic carcinoma	
Epithelioid hemangioendothelioma	
Papillomas of the tracheobronchial tree	
Pulmonary blastoma	
Fibrosarcoma and leiomyosarcoma	
Primary pulmonary hemangiopericytoma	

Hurst, J., Willis, ED. (1996). *Medicine for the practicing physician.* Stamford, CT: Appleton and Lange.

The overall incidence of lung cancer in the United States is 80 cases per 100,000 population. There are well-recognized racial, sex, and geographic differences. The incidence is higher in African Americans than in whites. One of the highest rates in the world is seen in African Americans living in the New Orleans area (107 cases per 100,000).

It is likely that the rates of lung cancer in men will plateau by the year 2000. This is mostly attributed to decreasing smoking trends in young white males. On the other hand, the incidence of lung cancer will continue to rise in women because of the considerable increase in tobacco use by females over the last three decades.

DIAGNOSTIC CRITERIA

The definitive diagnosis of lung carcinoma requires the identification of malignant cells in a cytologic specimen (sputum, lung washings, lung brushings, or pleural fluid) or the detection of areas of malignant transformation in a biopsy specimen from the lung parenchyma or bronchi. Lung cancer should be suspected in any patient presenting with a lung nodule or mass on chest x-ray, even in the absence of any symptoms, or when a pneumonia fails to resolve radiologically in 6 to 8 weeks after appropriate antibiotic therapy, especially in a patient with a history of tobacco use. Lung cancer should always be suspected in a smoker who presents with chronic cough, especially when complicated by hemoptysis, even if the chest x-ray is reported as normal.

HISTORY AND PHYSICAL EXAM

The clinical presentation of lung cancer is diverse and depends on the following:

- Location of the primary tumor (central versus peripheral, and its relation to surrounding structures)
- Presence of distant metastases
- Presence of paraneoplastic syndromes or other coexisting diseases.

Although only 15% of lung cancer patients are asymptomatic at the time of diagnosis, the early symptoms are nonspecific and are often ignored for prolonged periods.

The signs and symptoms of lung cancer at the time of diagnosis are summarized in Table 73-2. Cough is by far the most common complaint, followed by dyspnea and hemoptysis. Central (endobronchial) lesions are more likely to be associated with cough early on, and ultimately may lead to hemoptysis. Hemoptysis, when present, is the most alarming symptom to patients, and they usually seek medical attention expeditiously. Critical narrowing of a bronchus by endobronchial tumor or by extrinsic compression may lead to all the symptoms associated with postobstructive pneumonitis (eg, fever, dyspnea, nonproductive cough). Significant weight loss is almost always reported at the time of diagnosis. Localized chest wall pain may be seen secondary to metastases to the thoracic skeletal structures (ribs, sternum, vertebral bodies), muscles, and skin.

The physical exam findings are variable and depend on the extent of intrathoracic spread and the presence and location of distant metastases. The lung exam may be completely normal, even when there is radiologic evidence of tumor. Centrally located (endobronchial) tumors are likely to cause symptoms earlier. The provider may appreciate decreased air entry to a particular lung segment or high-pitched inspiratory sounds over the involved bronchus. Large pleural effusions may also result in compressive atelectasis, along with all the expected physical exam findings (eg, decreased air entry, bronchial breathing, dullness to percussion). The presence of supraclavicular or cervical adenopathy is an important clinical finding and implies advanced inoperable disease.

The presence of significant jugular venous distention suggests involvement of the superior vena cava or pericardial carcinomatosis. All the signs of cardiac tamponade may be seen (eg, enlarged cardiac silhouette, narrow pulse pressure, low cardiac output state, metabolic acidosis), and they should prompt an urgent request for echocardiography, followed by pericardiocentesis or pericardial window. Funduscopic evidence of papilledema, even in the absence of symptoms, should lead to the performance of cranial computed tomography (CT) or magnetic resonance imaging (MRI) to rule out brain metastases. A variety of neurologic findings may be detected on the physical

TABLE 73-2	Symptoms and Signs of Lung Cancer at Initial Presentation
Symptoms/Signs	**Frequency (%) (range)**
No symptoms	15
Cough	75 (30–87)
Dyspnea	46 (8–58)
Hemoptysis	43 (6–57)
Chest pain	35 (30–60)
Weight loss	32 (8–69)
Bone pain	8 (0–25)
Clubbing	7 (0–20)
Hoarseness	7 (1–18)
Superior vena cava syndrome	4 (0–7)

Data from Hyde & Hyde, 1974.

exam, depending on the level of involvement and the presence of paraneoplastic syndromes.

Direct invasion of the brachial plexus, most often associated with apical or superior sulcus tumors, may result in Pancoast's syndrome. This syndrome is characterized by referred pain to the scapula, shoulder, or arm (along with shoulder and upper extremity weakness) and Horner's syndrome (ptosis, myosis, and hemifacial anhidrosis). Hoarseness of voice and dysphagia are ominous signs and indicate direct mediastinal spread by the tumor and advanced nonsurgical disease.

Superior vena cava syndrome may result from mediastinal invasion. Patients with this syndrome report headaches, facial fullness, and edema of the upper extremities. The cause of this syndrome is intraluminal thrombosis of the superior vena cava secondary to extrinsic compression by the tumor. Rarely, lung cancer presents with cardiac tamponade secondary to pericardial infiltration.

Not infrequently, the initial clinical manifestations of lung cancer may be secondary to metastatic disease or paraneoplastic syndromes associated with bronchogenic carcinoma. An exhaustive list of the paraneoplastic syndromes associated with bronchogenic carcinoma is provided in Table 73-3. Headaches, a variety of neurologic deficits, and seizures may be seen with intracranial or spinal cord metastases. Although metastases to

TABLE 73-3	Paraneoplastic Syndromes Associated With Bronchogenic Carcinoma
System	**Syndrome**
Endocrine	Hypercalcemia
	Syndrome of inappropriate ADH secretion
	Cushing's syndrome
	Hypoglycemia
	Galactorrhea
	Gynecomastia
	Carcinoid syndrome
	Hyperthyroidism
Neuromuscular	Eaton-Lambert
	Mononeuritis
	Polymyositis
	Encephalopathy
	Myelopathy
Skeletal	Pulmonary hypertrophic osteoarthropathy
	Digital clubbing
Cutaneous	Acanthosis nigricans
	Erythema multiforme
	Hyperpigmentation
Hematologic	Anemia
	Leukemoid reaction
	Eosinophilia
	Thrombocytopenia
	Dysproteinemia
Other	Nonbacterial endocarditis
	Arterial/venous thrombosis
	Pulmonary embolism
Constitutional symptoms	Fevers
	Anorexia
	Weight loss

Hurst, J., Willis, ED. (1996). *Medicine for the practicing physician.* Stamford, CT: Appleton and Lange.

the adrenals are common, the incidence of adrenal insufficiency is exceedingly rare. Liver metastases are also common and likewise do not frequently result in hepatic failure.

DIAGNOSTIC STUDIES

The chest x-ray is the initial diagnostic tool for lung cancer. Radiologic presentation of lung cancer is diverse and includes:

- Completely normal studies (with small endobronchial lesions)
- An isolated pulmonary nodule (peripheral, <2 cm, and completely surrounded by lung parenchyma)
- Large peripheral masses, either surrounded completely by lung or abutting and invading the chest wall or mediastinum
- Obstructive atelectasis with signs of volume loss (mediastinal or cardiac silhouette shift to the side of atelectasis and ipsilateral elevation of the hemidiaphragm)
- Ill-defined peripheral infiltrates (characteristic of bronchoalveolar cell carcinoma)
- Large pleural effusions
- Evidence of metastasis to the thoracic skeleton, mediastinum, and hilum (White & Templeton, 1993).

Not infrequently, lung tumors present as cavitary lesions on x-ray. Cavitation is secondary to central tumor necrosis (most often associated with squamous cell carcinoma), and secondary colonization with *Aspergillus* species may be seen.

Routine laboratory blood work is rarely of benefit, although hypercalcemia (most often with squamous cell cancer) or hyponatremia (SIADH) may be detected. Some degree of anemia may be seen, especially with small cell carcinomas.

The ultimate diagnosis of bronchogenic carcinoma rests with the presence of malignant cells on cytologic or biopsy specimens. When the disease is limited to the chest, the diagnostic tests available include sputum cytology, fiberoptic bronchoscopy (FOB), and transthoracic needle aspiration (TTNA) (Demetis, 1996). When distal metastases are present, the diagnosis may be made by sampling peripheral sites such as lymph nodes, skin nodules, or bone.

Sputum specimens for cytology should be collected in the morning after brushing the teeth for 5 consecutive days. The yield is highest for squamous cell and bronchoalveolar cell carcinomas, centrally located tumors, and large tumors. Although the test is simple and inexpensive, its sensitivity is low (30% to 40% false-negative rate), and it has a low negative predictive value. Consequently, the diagnosis of lung cancer should never be excluded based on negative sputum cytology results. False-positive results are uncommon (1%).

The decision whether to proceed with FOB or TTNA is based on the size and location of the tumor. FOB, the more commonly performed diagnostic procedure, is used to obtain specimens for diagnosis and to inspect both sides of the tracheobronchial tree. It can also provide information regarding the potential resectability of the lung, as well as the extent of resection required. This test is important because CT has poor sensitivity for the detection or determination of the magnitude of an endobronchial lesion.

The types of specimens that are obtained with this technique include biopsies or brushings (endobronchial or transbronchial), washings, bronchoalveolar lavage, and transbronchial or transtracheal aspiration of lymph nodes. The diagnostic yield of FOB for endobronchial (directly visualized) tumors is extremely high (95% to 100%); for peripheral tumors it is variable (30% to 60%), depending primarily on the size of the tumor and the experience of the bronchoscopist (Arroliga & Matthay, 1993). Although in most cases CT of the chest is not required before FOB is performed, it may be helpful for small peripheral lesions in guiding the bronchoscopist.

Sampling of the hilar, subcarinal, or mediastinal nodes transbronchially with a Wang needle should be attempted in all cases. If the nodes are positive, important staging information is obtained and may spare the patient further invasive procedures such as mediastinoscopy. The yield of this procedure is directly related to the size of the nodes and the expertise of the bronchoscopist.

Potential complications with FOB include bleeding and pneumothorax, as well as worsening of established respiratory failure (in marginal cases), arrhythmias, and rarely myocardial infarction. Some degree of hemorrhage is always expected, especially with biopsies, but it is rarely massive. The incidence of pneumothorax is far less than with TTNA. Pneumothorax is exclusively seen when transbronchial biopsies are performed and is most likely with small peripheral lesions and with the presence of extensive bullous lung disease.

TTNA has the highest yield for small peripheral lesions that are not accessible by transbronchial brushings or biopsies, or when previous FOB failed to provide a diagnosis. Pneumothorax and hemoptysis are the most common complications with TTNA. The likelihood of a pneumothorax is directly related to the distance of the lesion from the lung surface. It may be as high as 30% when a significant amount of lung must be traversed to reach the lesion. Most pneumothoraces are small and clinically insignificant and can be managed conservatively. On occasion, chest tube placement under suction may be required, however.

There is no established role for tumor markers in the diagnosis of bronchogenic carcinoma. Tumor markers may provide some prognostic information in both NSCLC and SCLC. Antibodies to tumor markers may prove valuable in the treatment of bronchogenic carcinoma and other cancers as well.

Rarely, a definitive diagnosis cannot be made, even after using each of these diagnostic tools. Open lung biopsy or thoracoscopy may be considered in these cases. Thoracoscopic biopsy is minimally invasive compared to thoracotomy. Peripheral lesions can be sampled and, if small enough (<3 cm), completely resected with clean margins. The patient can usually be discharged from the hospital the next day. For undiagnosed central lesions, open lung thoracotomy may be required.

Vocal cord paralysis secondary to tumor invasion of the recurrent laryngeal nerve may be detected by indirect laryngoscopy; this finding implies extensive mediastinal spread of tumor. Phrenic nerve paralysis may result in severe dyspnea and can be detected by fluoroscopy.

In evaluating the possible presence of extrathoracic metastases, studies should be ordered based on the patient's symptoms (eg, headache, diplopia, loss of balance, peripheral neurologic deficits, bone pain). "Routine" bone scans and CT scans of the head should not be performed without symptoms to suggest metastases because the yield is very low and does not warrant the overall cost. With large lung tumors, especially adenocarci-

nomas, preoperative CT scans of the head may be done to exclude asymptomatic central nervous system metastases before subjecting the patient to lung resection.

TREATMENT OPTIONS, EXPECTED OUTCOMES, AND COMPREHENSIVE MANAGEMENT

The recommended treatment for established cases of bronchogenic carcinoma depends on the differentiation between NSCLC and SCLC by the pathologist and the stage of the disease. Surgery is the mainstay of therapy for patients with early-stage NSCLC. Other treatment modalities are offered to patients with advanced intrathoracic disease or distant metastases. Surgery is rarely a treatment option for patients with SCLC, and most of these patients are treated with chemotherapy or radiation therapy.

Despite intensive investigation into early detection and aggressive surgical and drug therapies, the case fatality ratio for lung cancer remains greater than 90%, and the 5-year survival rate (13% in 1981 to 1987) has improved only slightly. Survival continues to be low for lung cancer in comparison with other cancers. Prospective studies of the use of regular x-rays and frequent cytologic analyses of sputum in the early diagnosis of lung cancer have not clearly demonstrated a survival benefit.

Prevention

Smoking cessation is by far the most important measure in the prevention of bronchogenic carcinoma. Patient education about methods for smoking cessation is a crucial aspect of the first provider visit. Minimizing potential exposure to carcinogens in the workplace is also important. The potential is immense for improving overall mortality and morbidity rates from lung cancer (as well as other cancers) and from atherosclerotic diseases from smoking. Decreasing the incidence of smoking-related complications would also decrease the overall cost of providing health care nationwide.

Comprehensive Management Recommendations

The most recent staging system for NSCLC, as adopted by the World Health Organization, is shown in Tables 73-4 and 73-5 (Mountain, 1997). The new staging system, compared to

TABLE 73-4	TNM Staging System of Non-Small Cell Lung Cancer		
Occult carcinoma	TX	N0	M0
Stage 0	TIS (carcinoma in situ)		
Stage I	T1	N0	M0
	T2	N0	M0
Stage II	T1	N1	M0
	T2	N1	M0
Stage IIIa	T3	N0, N1	M0
	Any T	N2	M0
Stage IIIb	Any T	N3	M0
	T4	Any N	M0
Stage IV	Any T	Any N	M1 (distant metastases)

Source: Mountain, 1987.

TABLE 73-5	**Definitions of Primary Tumor and Nodal Involvement for NSCLC Primary Tumor (T)**
TX	Positive sputum cytology; tumor cannot be localized by chest x-ray or bronchoscopy
TIS	Carcinoma in situ
T1	Tumor < 3 cm and surrounded by lung or visceral pleura; on FOB, no evidence of invasion proximal to lobar bronchus
T2	Tumor > 3 cm or any size tumor that invades the visceral pleura or has associated atelectasis extending to the hilar region; on FOB, the tumor must be at least 2 cm away from the main carina
T3	Any size tumor with direct extension to the chest wall, diaphragm, mediastinal pleura, pericardium *without invasion* of the heart, great vessels, trachea, esophagus, or vertebral bodies
T4	Any size tumor with invasion of the mediastinum (heart, great vessels, trachea, esophagus, vertebral bodies) or carina, or the presence of a malignant pleural effusion

NODAL INVOLVEMENT

N0	No nodal involvement
N1	Peribronchial and/or ipsilateral hilar nodes
N2	Ipsilateral mediastinal or subcarinal nodes
N3	Contralateral hilar or mediastinal or ipsilateral/contralateral scalene or supraclavicular nodes

Source: Mountain, 1987.

the older system proposed in 1987, accounts for observed differences in survival between T1 and T2 tumors. Patients with T3N0 disease who were classified as stage IIIA under the old classification are now placed into stage IIB. Because these patients have 5-year survival rates similar to those with T2N1 disease, the new staging system is a more practical one.

Staging is done with CT of the chest (extending to the liver and both adrenals). The presence of large (>1 cm) hilar or mediastinal nodes suggests at least stage II disease, although histologic confirmation is necessary. Mediastinoscopy is the diagnostic tool of choice. On occasion, enlarged lymph nodes may be classified as reactive or secondary to a pulmonary inflammatory process such as bacterial pneumonia or other infections. On the other hand, hilar or mediastinal involvement may be documented in the postsurgical staging of the disease, despite a negative CT scan preoperatively. The unequivocal evidence of mediastinal tumor extension on CT indicates that the patient is not a candidate for surgery.

Incidental primary benign adrenal adenomas pose a diagnostic problem. Statistically, adrenal tumors less than 2 cm that are benign by contrast CT criteria are unlikely to represent metastases and should not be addressed further. Contrast MRI studies of the adrenals are rarely of additional benefit and significantly increase health care costs. Larger adrenal tumors with equivocal imaging characteristics should be aspirated by interventional radiology to exclude metastatic involvement.

The best treatment outcomes in NSCLC are seen with surgical resection of early disease limited to the chest. Patients with compromised lung function secondary to chronic obstructive pulmonary disease or pulmonary fibrosis and those expected to undergo complete pneumonectomy should undergo lung perfusion scans preoperatively to predict the postoperative

forced expiratory volume (FEV_1). Usually an estimated postresection FEV_1 of 40% or more of the predicted value should allow the patient to undergo surgery. Preoperative CO_2 retention is a risk factor for perioperative morbidity but is not an absolute contraindication to surgery.

All patients with clinical stages I and II disease should be immediately evaluated for surgical resection. The gold standard is complete lobectomy (regardless of tumor size), along with extensive mediastinal node dissection. Open thoracotomy is the best therapeutic modality for this procedure.

Occasionally the surgeon may realize intraoperatively that larger resection is required (bilobectomy or complete pneumonectomy). This may occur as a result of contiguous tumor spread through a fissure separating two lobes, for example. Therefore, surgeons must understand preoperatively what degree of resection the patient can tolerate. Segmentectomies (simple resection of a tumor with clean margins, without complete lobectomy) may be performed in patients with early-stage disease who have very marginal lung function and cannot undergo more extensive resection. Thoracoscopic resection of small peripheral lesions may also be performed in these patients with marginal lung reserve.

For patients who have limited disease but cannot undergo surgery because of very poor lung reserve or other coexisting diseases, high-dose radiation therapy and chemotherapy are treatment options. SCLCs are more responsive than NSCLCs to these therapies. Platinum-based regimens are the most effective.

Survival may be prolonged with nonsurgical modalities, although the 5-year survival rate is very low (about 6%) when compared to surgical therapy. The 5-year survival rate is 65% for postoperative stage I patients and 50% for postoperative stage II patients. Patients with stage I and II squamous cell carcinoma have a better 5-year survival rate than patients with stage I and II adenocarcinoma. Women have a slightly better outcome.

Because local recurrence can occur postoperatively, especially with squamous cell cancers, mediastinal radiation should follow surgery for most patients with stage II squamous cell carcinoma. Although this practice has been shown to decrease local tumor recurrence, there are no studies that demonstrate an ultimate survival benefit. This is probably because radiation has no effect on distal metastases after surgery and does not prevent deaths from other causes.

Stage IIIa patients should be considered for preoperative chemotherapy or radiation therapy, with follow-up surgery depending on the clinical response (Rusch et al, 1993). The 5-year survival rate is very poor, although a few patients do rather well. There is no established role for surgical therapy in patients with stage IIIB disease, although some survival benefit was seen in a small group of patients inadvertently included in study protocols for stage IIIa treatment modalities.

The treatment of patients with stage IV disease is palliative, and the type of treatment depends on the extent and location of disease and the patient's performance status. Each patient should be well informed about the goals of the proposed therapy and should agree to the risks and benefits inherent in it. A multidisciplinary approach to the care of these patients is pivotal because complications such as bleeding, pneumonia, bone metastases and pathologic fractures, and neurologic and neurosurgical complications are likely.

Bronchoscopic laser therapy or endobronchial stents may be used to relieve obstruction and improve patient comfort. Aggressive surgical therapy may be used for patients who present with a single localized distal recurrence after initial complete resection of intrathoracic tumor. There have been several reports of significant survival with good quality of life after resection of isolated central nervous system metastases.

Most patients with SCLC have extensive disease at presentation. Although the outcome after lung resection in some SCLC patients with limited disease has been good, surgery is rarely an option. The mainstay of therapy is chemotherapy or radiation therapy.

TEACHING AND SELF-CARE

The psychosocial implications that accompany the diagnosis of bronchogenic carcinoma are immense. Most patients realize that there is a substantial risk for death even when diagnosed in the earliest stages of this disease. The behavioral response of patients to these stressful circumstances is variable. Many patients struggle with the notion that their habits, environment, or occupation contributed to the development of lung cancer. This may be true in many cases, but the primary provider should be alert to feelings of despair and low self-worth. Cancer possibly related to spousal second-hand smoke exposure can be a particularly emotional situation. A general discussion regarding the suspected etiology, treatment plan, goals, and prognosis often answers many questions and may correct misconceptions.

Young patients with good lung reserve who have undergone successful lung resection should be encouraged to return to work and resume their usual lifestyle as best they are able. They should be seen several times a year over the next 4 to 5 years to detect possible recurrence early or to detect possible second primary lung tumors. Smoking cessation measures must be addressed and are usually very successful in this motivated group of patients. Pulmonary rehabilitation programs also offer invaluable peer support.

Pulmonary rehabilitation is also important for patients whose surgery results in marginal lung function. Although rehabilitation does not result in objective improvement of pulmonary function, conditioning, stamina, self-image, and overall sense of well-being are often improved with these programs.

Nutritional support is very important for lung cancer patients in all phases of treatment, especially for those with advanced disease who require chronic radiation and chemotherapy. General nutritional counseling should be addressed by the primary care provider or clinical dietitian. Barriers to proper nutrition such as anorexia, oral lesions, fatigue, and perhaps financial concerns need to be addressed and monitored. Oral comfort measures should be managed collaboratively by the oncology specialists involved.

Pain and dyspnea control should also be a top priority. A discussion with the patient regarding the role of pain control and its expected effects, side effects, and complications should occur early in the treatment phase. The patient should be warned about gastrointestinal upset, sedation, breakthrough pain, and constipation. Strategies to minimize side effects should be considered.

Social workers are invaluable members of the team providing care for lung cancer patients. They help educate patients and families about available support services, such as home attendant help and Meals on Wheels, and hospice programs.

Some patients and families may have misconceptions regarding hospice care; for instance, they may not know that hospice care is available in the home. Many terminally ill patients and families agree that hospice care provides the best coordination of medical services and psychosocial support.

The opportunity to meet with a paramedical cancer specialist, such as an oncology clinical nurse specialist, can be quite valuable to patients in providing anticipatory guidance, both at the time of diagnosis and throughout the treatment process.

COMMUNITY RESOURCES

Support groups for lung cancer patients and their families exist in most communities. The American Cancer Society (http://www.cancer.org) and the American Lung Association (800-LUNG-USA) offer literature, support, and transportation to medical appointments.

- Lung Cancer Information Center, http://www.meds.com/lung/lunginfo.html
- Lung Cancer Guide, http://www.meds.com/lung/uindex.html
- Oncolink: Lung Cancer, http://www.oncolink.upenn.edu/disease/lung1/
- National Heart, Lung and Blood Institute, Information Center, P.O. Box 30105, Bethesda, MD 20824-0105, 301-251-1222
- National Cancer Institute, 800-4-CANCER

EDITOR'S NOTE:
COMPLEMENTARY APPROACHES

A general discussion of complementary approaches can be found in Chapter 3. The following, while not an exhaustive list, are some complementary approaches being used for this condition. Additional information on these approaches, including precautions, can be found in Appendices A and B. Providers need to assess for the use of complementary approaches as part of the patient's history, as they may impact conventional therapies, and patients may not volunteer this information unless specifically asked. Efficacy of many complementary approaches is not as well documented as that of conventional therapies. Providers need to read the literature before suggesting these complementary approaches.

- Vitamins, minerals, herbs, supplements
  Betacarotene
  Melatonin
  Vitamin E

References

Arroliga, A.C., & Matthay, R.A. (1993). The role of bronchoscopy in lung cancer. *Clinics in Chest Medicine, 14*(1), 87–98.

Demetis, S. (1996). *Carcinoma of the lung. Medicine for the practicing physician*, pp. 1033–1038. Norwalk, CT: Appleton & Lange.

Hyde, L., & Hyde, C.I. (1974). Clinical manifestations of lung cancer. *Chest, 65*, 299.

Mountain, C.F. (1987). The new international staging system for lung cancer. *Surgical Clinics of North America, 67*(5), 925.

National Research Council Committee on Passive Smoking. (1986). *Measuring and assessing health effects.* Washington, D.C.: National Academy Press.

Sobue, T., Suzuki, T., Fujimoto, I., et al. (1991). Lung cancer rise among ex-smokers. *Japanese Journal of Cancer Research, 82*(3), 273–279.

White, C.S., & Templeton, P.A. (1993). Radiologic manifestations of bronchogenic cancer. *Clinics in Chest Medicine, 14*(1), 55–68.

Bibliography

Mackay, B., Lukeman, J.M., & Ordonez, N.G. (1991). *Tumors of the lung.* In *Major problems in pathology*, Vol. 24. Philadelphia: W.B. Saunders.

Martini, N., & Flehinger, B.J. (1987). The role of surgery in N2 lung cancer. *Surgical Clinics of North America, 67*(5), 1037.

Rusch, V.W., Albain, K.S., et al. (1993). Surgical resection of stage IIIA & stage IIIB NSCLC after concurrent induction chemoradiotherapy. A Southwest Oncology Group Trial. *Journal of Thoracic and Cardiovascular Surgery, 105,* 97.

Samet, J.M., & Hornung, R.W. (1990). Review of radon and lung cancer risk. *Risk Analysis, 10,* 65–75.

Symposium on intrathoracic neoplasms. (1993). *Mayo Clinic Proceedings, 68.*

Chronic Obstructive Pulmonary Disease

Albert Heurich, MD

Chronic obstructive pulmonary disease (COPD) encompasses a number of disorders with the common feature of progressive and irreversible chronic airflow limitation. The two major disease states that make up COPD are chronic bronchitis and emphysema.

Bronchial asthma can be classified as a component of COPD because it often accompanies chronic bronchitis and emphysema. However, the obstructive component in asthma is usually acute and reversible. Asthma is discussed here only in its relation to COPD; further discussion of asthma is found in Chapter 72.

COPD has a long course of slow but progressive disability, with long periods of relatively stable health. The primary care provider can play a key role in maintaining baseline health for as long as possible and in helping the patient cope with the multiple issues this debilitating illness raises.

ANATOMY, PHYSIOLOGY, AND PATHOLOGY

The airway changes in COPD that lead to obstruction include marked enlargement of bronchial mucous glands, gland duct dilation, hypertrophy of airway smooth muscle, and squamous metaplasia of the airway epithelium, causing hypersecretion of mucus and inflammation. The respiratory bronchioles show epithelial hyperplasia, increased numbers of pigmented macrophages, edema, and fibrosis. The membranous bronchioles are obstructed by inflammation, mucus plugs, goblet cell metaplasia, fibrosis, and increased smooth muscle.

The pathology of COPD is evident throughout the lungs, although the disease begins in the small airways. In the large airways there is enlargement of bronchial mucous glands and dilation of gland ducts. The surface lining can show focal squamous metaplasia, and there is an increased frequency of goblet cells. Bronchial smooth muscle shows hypertrophic changes.

Within respiratory bronchioles, inflammation is demonstrated by an increase of mononuclear cells. Additional changes include mucus plugging, increases in smooth muscle, goblet cell metaplasia, and fibrosis. The latter can distort the airway, leading to a further reduction in airflow.

Three forms of emphysema can be found in COPD:

- Centriacinar emphysema initially involves the respiratory bronchioles, with later involvement of the acinus.
- Centrilobular emphysema is associated with cigarette smoking and predominantly involves the upper lobes.
- Panacinar emphysema uniformly affects the acinus and lower lobes.

Paraseptal emphysema occurs in adjacent areas to fibrous septa or pleura. Airflow limitation is mild, but it is implicated as a potential cause of pneumothorax.

Chronic respiratory acidosis, a common sequela to airway obstruction in COPD, is compensated by metabolic alkalosis. Alkalosis reduced respiratory center sensitivity to p_{CO_2}, which normally is the most potent respiratory center stimulus, leaving hypoxemia as the sole chemical stimulus to ventilation in COPD. This creates the conflicting situation of needing to administer oxygen to correct life-threatening hypoxemia and simultaneously removing the remaining stimulus to respiration. However, correction of alveolar hypoxia with oxygen relieves hypoxic pulmonary vasoconstriction in poorly ventilated regions of the lung. This increases pulmonary blood flow to the poorly ventilated areas, causing greater equilibration with the higher alveolar P_{CO_2}. Elimination of the hypoxemic stimulus to ventilation and the worsening of pulmonary ventilation/perfusion ratios from oxygen administration result in further hypercapnia. Minimizing the increase in PA_{CO_2} is accomplished by titration of the oxygen. The use of a device that can deliver high flows of precisely regulated oxygen concentrations usually permits the safe administration of oxygen in this setting.

Respiratory muscles respond to respiratory center drive with a pumping force that produces pulmonary gas exchange. Vagal afferent neural signals transmit information regarding pulmonary mechanics and lung volume, which the respiratory center uses to regulate its output to the muscles of respiration.

Functional residual capacity (FRC) reflects the balance between expiratory lung elastic recoil and inspiratory chest wall elastic recoil. Alveolar pressure is normally zero at FRC. Emphysema reduces lung elastic recoil, causing a new equilibrium of lung and chest wall elastic forces at an increased FRC.

Hyperinflation flattens the contour of the diaphragm and increases its radius of curvature (picture the diaphragm as part of the circumference of a circle that extends over the abdomen). It also shifts the operational lung compliance from the normal region to the low-compliance region, thus increasing pressure requirements for a tidal volume. The increased radius of curvature impairs diaphragmatic contractility and increases respiratory muscle work (Fig. 74-1).

Increased airway resistance prolongs expiration and produces premature airway closure. Premature airway closure results in the trapping of gas volume with positive alveolar pressures at end expiration (PEEP), also called auto-PEEP. This positive pressure must be overcome before inspiration can proceed. This increases the inspiratory work of breathing.

The emphysematous lung is ventilated but not perfused. It forms dead space and areas of low gas diffusion, increasing the work of breathing, although the resting blood gas analysis does not demonstrate this. The patient huffs and puffs to maintain ventilation and has thus been called a "pink puffer."

In chronic obstructive bronchitis, poorly ventilated alveoli remain perfused. This causes hypoxemia with cyanosis and hypercapnia. Chronically elevated pulmonary vascular resistance

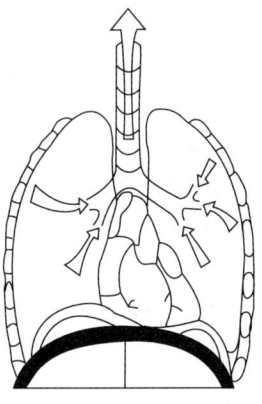

NORMAL
DECREASED RADIUS

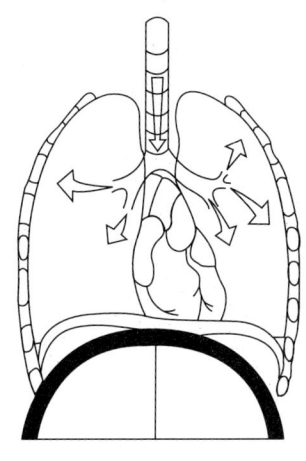

HYPERINFLATION
INCREASED RADIUS

FIGURE 74-1 The normal lung on the left has a small radius of curvature for the diaphragm. The hyperinflated lung of COPD on the right has a large radius of curvature. The pressure generated by the diaphragm is inversely related to the radius of the curvature of the diaphragm.

from hypoxia results in cor pulmonale. This is manifested by tricuspid valve insufficiency, right atrial dilatation, dilated neck veins, hepatic congestion, and pedal edema. The appearance of cyanosis with edema yields the designation "blue bloater" for such patients.

Total ventilation in these patients is high compared to that of normal persons, however. This reflects a high dead space ventilation and an unusually high respiratory drive. Emphysematous patients have a still higher respiratory drive.

The features of asthma, bronchitis, and emphysema are compared in Table 74-1.

EPIDEMIOLOGY

COPD affects 14.6 million Americans. Of these, approximately 12.6 million suffer from chronic bronchitis and 2 million have emphysema. These disorders caused 85,544 deaths in 1991. COPD ranks as the fourth leading cause of death, with a death rate of 18.6 per 100,000 persons. Since 1970, deaths related to COPD have doubled (Celli, 1998).

An increasing number of women are now dying from this disease; the male/female ratio has decreased from 4.3:1 in 1970 to 2.36:1 in 1983. The risk of death from COPD in heavy smokers is 30 times that for nonsmokers.

Alpha-1-antitrypsin (AAT) deficiency plays a relatively small role in the incidence of emphysema in the United States, accounting for less than 1%. The genetic locus responsible for AAT production is termed Pi. The M allele, and phenotype Pi MM, is found in 90% to 95% of the normal white population. Persons homozygous for the phenotype of the Z allele (Pi ZZ) manifest AAT deficiency. Those with disease have AAT levels that average 16% of normal.

DIAGNOSTIC CRITERIA

The diagnosis of COPD is made by clinical symptoms in chronic bronchitis, by anatomic changes in emphysema, and by functional impairment in asthma. The diagnosis of chronic bronchitis is based on the presence of a chronic cough with sputum production for 3 months per year in 2 successive years. The diagnosis

TABLE 74-1	Differential Features in Obstructive Lung Disease		
	Asthma	Bronchitis Type B (Blue Bloater)	Emphysema Type A (Pink Puffer)
FEV₁ Response to Bronchodilator			
Beta-agonist	↑↑↑	↑→	→→
Anticholinergic	↑↑	↑↑↑	→→
Diffusing capacity	N OR ↑	N OR ↓	↓↓ - ↓↓↓
Lung hyperinflation	↑↑↑	↑→	↑↑↑
Lung vascular markings	N	↑↑	↓↓
Heart size	N	↑↑	↓↓
Hematocrit	N	↑↑	N
Lung elastic recoil	N	↓ - N - ↑	↓↓ - ↓↓↓
Static lung compliance	N	↓ - N - ↑	↑↑ - ↑↑↑
Paco₂	N	↑↑ - ↑↑↑	↓ - N
Auscultation	Wheezes	Rhonchi	Reduced or absent breath sounds
Symptom	Cough, dyspnea	Cough, sputum, dyspnea	Dyspnea

N, normal; ↑, increased; ↓, decreased; →, no change.

cannot be made if the patient has another disease explaining these symptoms. Chronic bronchitis accompanied by airway obstruction is called chronic obstructive bronchitis to distinguish it from simple bronchitis, which does not limit airflow.

The diagnosis of emphysema is made by histologic findings of abnormally widened air spaces and destruction of lung tissue distal to the terminal bronchioles. Clinically the diagnosis is made by a combination of history, physical exam, and radiologic and pulmonary function findings. Alveolar destruction transforms the gas-exchanging surface into a nonfunctional air space. This is identified on pulmonary function testing as a decrease in the diffusing capacity of the lung.

The typical patient with COPD presents with overlapping features of more than one of these diseases. Most have a history of cigarette smoking, often exceeding 20 pack-years. However, only 15% of cigarette smokers develop clinically significant COPD. For patients who progress to disease, the long interval between the onset of smoking and the onset of clinical findings reflects the tremendous reserve of lung function that has to be destroyed before a patient becomes symptomatic. This also explains why most patients begin to seek help in their 50s and 60s.

Although most patients with COPD are older, long-time cigarette smokers, an important exception is the young patient with AAT deficiency emphysema. This inherited defect, characterized by a very early onset of emphysema, involves the lower lobes of the lung instead of the upper lobe, found in older patients. Smoking causes an even earlier onset of the disease. This defect can now be corrected with replacement of the deficient AAT, making an accurate diagnosis essential.

HISTORY AND PHYSICAL EXAM

Chronic cough with morning sputum production is the first symptom of chronic bronchitis. Sputum usually has a clear, mucoid appearance but becomes mucopurulent and thick and increases in quantity and frequency during acute exacerbations.

Lung hyperinflation may manifest as an increased anteroposterior diameter of the chest. In the stable patient, auscultation of the lung reveals decreased or absent sounds in emphysema and low-pitched sonorous rhonchi in bronchitis. During exacerbations, higher-pitched wheezes are heard. Dyspnea and tachypnea become more prominent and can progress to both inspiratory and expiratory use of accessory muscles of respiration. Increased intrapleural pressure excursions manifest as inspiratory intercostal muscle retractions, expiratory supraclavicular apical bulging, neck vein distention, and increased tracheal movement.

In severe exacerbations, prominent flaring of the alae nasi occurs. Patients place their elbows on firm surfaces, enabling the shoulder girdles to project away from the chest to enhance the effect of respiratory muscle motion.

During exacerbations of emphysema, patients become tachypneic and may manifest cyanosis if there is significant impairment of alveolar gas exchange. In the chronically hypoxemic patient, signs of cor pulmonale may be present. These include jugular venous distention, hepatomegaly, and pedal edema. Acute and chronic hypercapnia contribute to alveolar hypoxia and produce symptoms of headache and altered mental status.

Hypersomnolence may be an additional complication in the subgroup of COPD patients who have obstructive sleep apnea. This group is also polycythemic and appears plethoric. Patients with AAT deficiency typically present with complaints of cough, sputum production, and shortness of breath.

DIAGNOSTIC STUDIES

Radiologic tests are the chief diagnostic modality used in COPD. Computed tomography (CT) is a very sensitive tool in the detection of COPD and has facilitated early diagnosis, thus enabling intervention early in the disease.

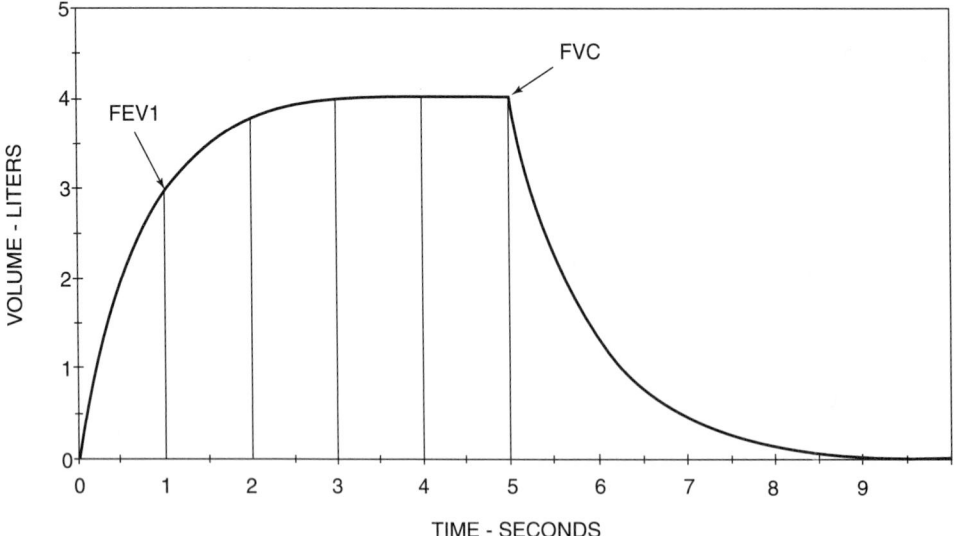

FIGURE 74-2 Normal spiromatic pattern. The expired volume trace rises steeply so that at 1 second, a major part of the volume has already been expired. (FEV_1). The total expired volume is the forced vital capacity (FVC) and is expired in 5 seconds.

OBSTRUCTIVE PATTERN

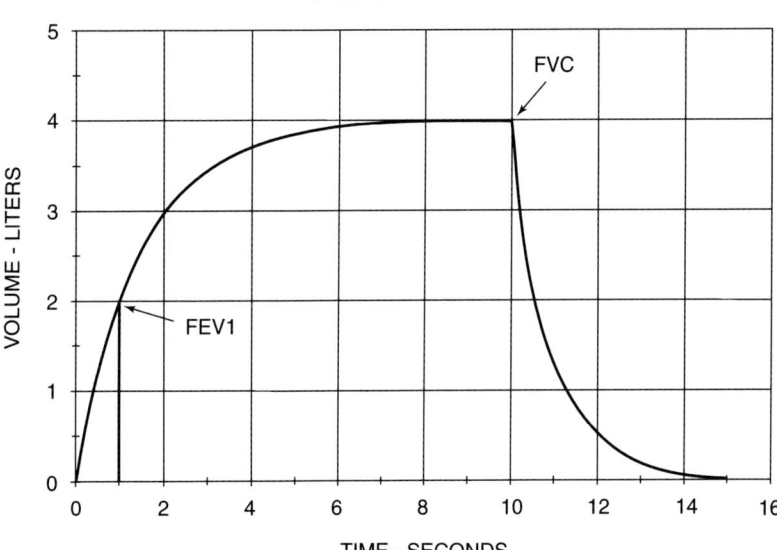

FIGURE 74-3 Obstructive pattern: The expired volume trace rises with a low slope in contrast to the normal spirometric pattern. At 1 second less volume has been expired compared to the normal trace. The total expired volume in this example is comparable to that of the normal but has required 10 seconds to be expired.

Spirometry has also been used to detect COPD in its earliest stages. A commonly used test is the forced expiratory flow, which measures expiratory flow rates between 25% and 75% of the forced vital capacity (FVC), divided by the time between these two points. An isolated decrease in this flow rate may be an early indicator of COPD. At this stage, the abnormality is reversible with bronchodilator therapy.

Spirometric measurement of the ratio of the volume expired in 1 second (FEV_1) divided by the maximal volume that can be exhaled from the lung after a maximal inspiration (FVC) gives a measure of the expiration rate, or the FEV_1/FVC ratio. Airway obstruction is associated with a low FEV_1/FVC ratio (Figs. 74-2, 74-3, and 74-4). This is related to a reduction in the FEV_1. The response of the FEV_1 to the administration of a bronchodilator establishes the degree of reversibility of the obstruction.

The asthmatic airway responds to beta-agonist inhalation, but the airway in COPD does not. The chronic bronchitic airway may respond to inhaled anticholinergic agents such as atropine and ipratropium, whereas the emphysematous airway does not respond at all to inhaled bronchodilators.

The diffusing capacity of the lung for carbon monoxide (DLCO) is useful in differentiating the three main obstructive diseases. It is normal or increased in asthma, normal or slightly decreased in chronic bronchitis, and always significantly decreased in emphysema. A low DLCO is required to establish the diagnosis of emphysema by pulmonary function testing.

SPIROMETRY
NORMAL & OBSTRUCTIVE PATTERNS

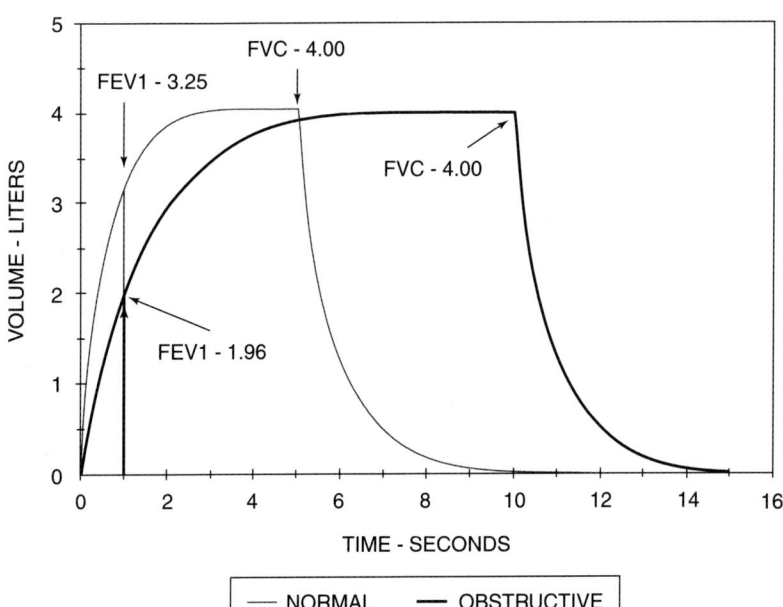

FIGURE 74-4 Comparison of the expiratory volume–time traces for the FVC and FEV_1 in a normal subject and in COPD. Note the difference in volume expired at 1 second and the duration in seconds for full expiration.

Static lung volumes are often increased in COPD. Emphysema shows the largest increases in irreversible lung volume. In asthma, the increased lung volumes are reversible after therapy. Chronic bronchitis may show a slight irreversible increase in lung volume. An increased residual volume/total lung capacity ratio is characteristic of all obstructive diseases.

The shape of the spirometric flow–volume curve in a FVC is useful in assessing airway disease. After peak flow has been attained, normal spirometric flow slopes downward in a linear relation with respect to expired volume. In obstruction, this linearity is transformed into a concave relation of flow to volume. In contrast, in advanced emphysema, the slope is converted into a low peak followed by plateau of flow. The linear and concave slopes reflect a change in diameter of the airway during expiration. The plateau of emphysema reflects a fixed airway diameter due to a result of loss of the tethering effect of elastic fibers in the surrounding lung structures.

TREATMENT OPTIONS, EXPECTED OUTCOMES, AND COMPREHENSIVE MANAGEMENT

The major risk factor for the development of COPD is cigarette smoking, accounting for 80% to 90% of the total risk. The prevalence of COPD increases with age and reflects the cumulative effects of cigarette smoke.

Cigarette smoking has a greater effect on lung function before age 40 than later in life. The number of cigarettes smoked daily is strongly associated with the risk of chronic bronchitis. Among cigarettes, maize leaf cigarettes are associated with the highest risk and filtered cigarettes the lowest.

The FEV_1 in the normal nonsmoking population declines annually by 25 to 30 mL starting at about age 35. The rate of decline is greater in smokers. On cessation of smoking, the rate of FEV_1 decline can revert to that of the nonsmoking population. The slope for rate of decline can thus resume a course parallel to that of nonsmokers, but at a lower level of absolute FEV_1.

Air pollution may be an additional contributor to the development of COPD, but it plays a relatively small role compared to that of cigarette smoking. The combination of tobacco smoke and air pollution appears to increase the risk for development of COPD.

The Dutch hypothesis states that an asthmatic constitution is an underlying factor in patients who develop chronic airflow obstruction. Nonspecific airway hyperreactivity was demonstrated in one study in 85.1% of women and 58.9% of men smokers (Chen et al, 1991). These results support this hypothesis.

FEV_1 and airway hyperreactivity are inversely related, with airway hyperreactivity predictive of an accelerated rate of decline in the lung function of smokers. The diagnosis of COPD must be a consideration in any patient in whom there is a significant history of tobacco use.

Prevention

Prevention of further disease is the first goal of therapy. Smoking cessation is essential as the first step in the management of COPD. After patient education regarding the risks of continued smoking, persons in daily contact with the patient may be enlisted to provide social support to aid the patient in a smoking

cessation program. Group smoking cessation programs and information on smoking cessation are provided by organizations such as the American Lung Association, the American Cancer Society, and the American Heart Association.

The nicotine component in cigarette smoke is addictive and can pose a difficult obstacle in the patient's attempts at smoking cessation. Nicotine is available in the form of chewing gum and transdermal patches; use of these modalities can reduce the symptoms associated with withdrawal. Clonidine and buspirone have been found useful in controlling nicotine withdrawal symptoms.

Preventive therapy includes immunization against pulmonary infection. All COPD patients should receive pneumococcal vaccine and annual influenza vaccines.

Treatment

BRONCHODILATOR THERAPY

Airflow limitation and bronchospasm can be controlled with bronchodilator therapy, customized to the patient's ability to use a particular modality. Inhaled therapy can be delivered via metered-dose inhalers (MDIs), with or without spacer devices, and by nebulization.

The MDI is the preferred method both for immediate relief of bronchospasm in an acute exacerbation and for maintenance therapy. It is portable, and the drug is delivered directly to the airways, where it is needed. Lower drug dosages are needed with this method of delivery, thus avoiding systemic toxicity. The major disadvantage is the need for good patient technique in the use of an MDI. Properly timed activation of the MDI during inspiration, combined with a 10-second breath-hold, can be difficult if not impossible for a dyspneic and tachypneic patient. The addition of a holding chamber device or the use of an MDI activated by patient inhalation can be of help under such circumstances. The patient-activated MDI requires a minimal inspiratory flow of 0.5 L/sec to begin drug delivery, a flow that a patient with severe obstruction may not always be able to generate.

If satisfactory bronchodilator administration cannot be achieved with an MDI, then nebulized drug administration must be considered. The nebulizer delivers the medication over a longer interval (usually 15 minutes) but does not require additional patient effort or expertise. It is, however, more expensive to use. Continuous flow results in the loss of some drug into the environment during patient exhalation, necessitating the use of greater amounts of bronchodilator. This loss can be curtailed with the use of a mouthpiece or face mask.

The power source for nebulization can be electrical or pneumatic. Small, portable electrically powered nebulizers are available that patients can carry with them when traveling. Nebulizers powered by stationary gas sources are used in home, clinic, and hospital settings.

Inhaled bronchodilator agents are either beta agonists or anticholinergic agents. Beta agonists are preferred in an acute exacerbation because of their rapid onset of action, but anticholinergic agents have been found to be more effective in COPD.

Theophylline has been an important oral and parenteral bronchodilating agent but has been partially supplanted by longer-acting inhaled bronchodilators. A major disadvantage of this medication is the narrow range between toxic and therapeutic serum levels, requiring frequent monitoring. However, sustained-release preparations have been useful in the management of nocturnal symptoms, and theophylline remains a helpful agent for patients who cannot effectively use MDIs.

The role of steroids in COPD is less well defined than it is in asthma, where it plays an important role. Airway inflammation is an element in the persistence of airway obstruction in COPD, and short courses of oral or parenteral steroids can be beneficial for patients with an asthmatic component. However, COPD patients have bacterial colonization of airways, recurrent pulmonary infection, and poor airway clearance mechanisms. Using oral steroids to maintain COPD patients provides no added benefit and poses significant risks from side effects and infection. The role of inhaled steroid therapy has not been adequately defined in COPD and is currently under investigation.

Leukotrienes are important agents in the development of pulmonary inflammation, leading to airway obstruction. Drugs that block the production of leukotrienes or antagonize their action are now available for the treatment of asthma. The role of these agents in COPD remains to be determined.

OXYGEN THERAPY

Acute hypoxemia frequently accompanies acute exacerbations of airway obstruction, pneumonia, or congestive heart failure. In the emphysematous patient, exertion commonly produces acute hypoxemia. Chronic hypoxemia develops with chronic CO_2 retention. Supplementary oxygen normalizes arterial P_{O_2} and facilitates tissue oxygenation. Therefore, supplementary oxygen is needed in both acute and chronic conditions that result in hypoxemia.

Supplementary oxygen is most commonly administered at low flow via a nasal cannula. This is generally sufficient to correct hypoxemia. It is well tolerated and has the advantage of allowing the patient to both speak and eat without interrupting oxygen delivery. The disadvantage is that the inspired oxygen concentration (F_{IO_2}) is imprecise and varies inversely with the patient's minute ventilation. If a very precise F_{IO_2} is needed to avoid excess oxygenation, then a venti-mask can be used. A venti-mask has the same disadvantages as any face mask: it limits head mobility and communication, and the patient cannot wear it while eating.

The following are guidelines for the initiation of long-term oxygen therapy:

- Stable patients who on optimized medical therapy and have a Pa_{O_2} of 55 mmHg or less or an oxygen saturation of 88% or less
- Patients with a Pa_{O_2} between 55 and 59 mmHg or an oxygen saturation of 89%
- Patients with evidence of tissue hypoxia such as polycythemia, altered mental status, cor pulmonale, or edema related to right ventricular failure.

The goal of therapy is to maintain a resting oxygen saturation of 90% or greater or a Pa_{O_2} greater than 60 mmHg. The initial prescription for oxygen therapy in the home is determined by a Pa_{O_2} measurement obtained after 30 minutes of breathing at a stable F_{IO_2}. A stable F_{IO_2} is important because the effects of a change are delayed as a result of both the impedance of gas movement into the lung from high airway resistance and the large volume of gas exchange occurring in a hyperinflated lung. Adjustments in the oxygen regimen are made using oximetry as a guide.

CLINICAL WARNING: Excessive F_{IO_2} may be dangerous because it can suppress respiratory drive.

INVASIVE TREATMENT

Thoracoscopy has reintroduced bullectomy as a surgical treatment in the management of severe dyspnea in emphysema. This procedure is indicated when a large bulla occupies at least 30% of a hemithorax, or if there is a history of pneumothorax. It provides relief from dyspnea for several years, but it is likely that symptoms will return. The degree of improvement depends on the condition of the remaining lung.

Reduction pneumoplasty has also been used to reduce hyperinflation in the emphysematous lung. Significant improvement in symptoms and lung function has been demonstrated 2 years after surgery.

Lung transplantation remains an additional surgical option for the patient with advanced disease. However, lung transplantation poses challenges greater than for other organ transplants, because of the limited supply of donor lungs and problems of matching donor and recipient lung size.

Comprehensive Management

The limitations in function of COPD patients can frequently lead to psychological and emotional disorders. Depression occurs in 51% to 74% of COPD patients and may manifest as disturbances in sleep, feelings of hopelessness and despair, poor appetite, lack of energy, a sense of low self-esteem, and thoughts of suicide. Patients tend to withdraw from social contacts. Support groups of COPD patients can be very beneficial in helping a patient adjust to the disease.

Sexual intercourse can present a challenge to the COPD patient but can be overcome with appropriate counseling. It is, in many ways, no more stressful than climbing a flight of stairs. The following may be helpful:

- Identifying intercourse positions that reduce exertion and pressure on the chest
- Planning intercourse for periods when the patient is rested
- Using MDI bronchodilators before intercourse
- Using oxygen, if needed
- Exploring all aspects of intimacy
- Using a waterbed; the fluid movement of the bed can propel the patient without excessive energy expenditure.

Dietary preparations are available that are designed to provide increased calories from a fat source to reduce ventilatory requirements. Such preparations may be particularly useful when attempting to wean a COPD patient from ventilator support. Eating large meals and foods that produce abdominal gaseous distention can increase the work of breathing for the diaphragm. Many COPD patients find that eating six small meals rather than three large meals a day is easier for digestion and reduces diaphragmatic effort.

Expected Outcomes

With the progression of COPD, ventilator support ultimately becomes necessary. Ventilation via a tracheostomy is less desirable than the use of a nasal cannula or face mask. If these options are feasible, the delay of a tracheostomy by using a cannula or mask should be considered.

In the stable patient with hypercapnia, an even more benign and noninvasive treatment, nocturnal positive-pressure ventilation, may allow respiratory muscles to rest and recover from fatigue. The evidence regarding the effectiveness of this modality has been inconclusive, however. Studies have demonstrated the effectiveness of this modality in reversing acute or chronic respiratory failure in acute exacerbations. Positive-pressure ventilation is potentially dangerous, however, and patients receiving such therapy must be closely monitored and managed by specially trained therapists.

Emphysema can be associated with the formation of bullae. A bulla is a distended air space in the lung that is more than 1 cm in diameter. As bullae enlarge, they limit the function of normal adjacent lung areas. They cause hyperinflation, moving the diaphragm downward to a less efficient position for effective contractility. Bullae contribute to increased dyspnea.

Rehabilitation

A program of pulmonary rehabilitation can improve the quality of life for many COPD patients. Although lung function cannot be reclaimed, respiratory muscles and a cardiovascular system that function optimally help the patient tolerate acute exacerbations of COPD. Exercise programs can aid in good muscle tone and promote greater self-sufficiency as well. Selection of patients for participation in a rehabilitation program must be done after a complete evaluation, and the patient should be counseled about the limitations of such a program.

Training in techniques of optimal respiratory muscle use can develop more efficient breathing and lessen dyspnea. In normal persons, approximately 2% to 5% of the total resting body oxygen consumption ($\dot{V}O_2$) is used by the respiratory muscles. With maximal exercise, this percentage increases to 10% to 20%. The ratio of ventilation to $\dot{V}O_2$ is called the ventilatory equivalent ($\dot{V}O_{2eq}$). This is the amount of ventilation required for the consumption of 1 L of oxygen. In healthy persons, this value is 20 to 25 at rest and reaches 30 to 40 at high levels of exercise. In COPD, the resting value can range from 30 to 50. The high $\dot{V}O_{2eq}$ in COPD explains in part the dyspnea experienced by these patients.

Respiratory training programs can help alleviate dyspnea by improving ventilatory muscle function, muscle performance, and muscle coordination, desensitizing the patient to dyspnea, and increasing motivation. Programs are designed to improve both the strength and endurance of the respiratory muscles.

A component of respiratory muscle weakness in COPD relates to the mechanical disadvantage imposed on the diaphragm by a low position and its flattened contour secondary to hyperinflation. Pursed-lip breathing is a technique of exhalation that creates a back-pressure within airways. This prevents or delays airway closure during exhalation, allowing more complete exhalation to a lower FRC.

TEACHING AND SELF-CARE

Patients with COPD should be counseled on smoking cessation, inhaler or nebulizer use, diet, hydration, exercise, and oxygen use. Although only the patient can ultimately stop smoking, the primary care provider should educate, encourage, and support the patient in the effort toward smoking cessation. A variety of behavior modification plans and pharmacologic treatments can be offered, and the patient and provider should together develop a management plan. Frequent follow-up should be scheduled to reassess support and rework the management plan as needed.

Verbal and written inhaler instructions, demonstration of use, and evaluation and feedback on a return demonstration by the patient can be helpful. Use of holding chamber devices can be explained. For patients who use a nebulizer, patients should be instructed to breathe through the mouth if a mouthpiece is used. The treatment should continue until all medication is completed, although this may take as long as 15 minutes.

Nutrition concerns should be addressed in the early stages of the disease to prevent malnutrition later. A well-balanced diet is important to compensate for the extra calories expended on the work of breathing. Overeating should be avoided, and six small meals a day are recommended, with a higher percentage of calories derived from fat than is normally advised.

Patients should maintain adequate hydration to avoid drying and plugging of airway secretions. Large volumes of noncaffeinated fluids will also help prevent constipation, which can cause breathlessness in a patient with COPD.

Pursed-lip breathing should be taught whenever a patient is dyspneic. This technique involves inhaling slowly through the nose to a count of three, then breathing out through pursed lips to a count of six. Patient education that trains patients to cough effectively is useful. During exertion, the patient should first inhale, then exhale while performing the activity.

For patients with copious sputum production or impaired cough mechanisms, postural drainage and chest percussion techniques may be of benefit. Flutter valves and high-frequency oscillation ventilators can also help in the mobilization of secretions.

Exercise regimens should be individualized. This regimen should be reinforced and re-evaluated periodically. Sexual activity should be discussed as above.

For patients using oxygen, instructions on the use of the delivery system should be reinforced. Water-soluble lubricant can be used to prevent dryness and fissuring of the nose and lips. Signs of excessive oxygen intake such as slow or shallow breathing, restlessness, difficulty waking up, headache, and slurred speech should be reported by family members or caregivers. Signs of insufficient oxygen intake should also be monitored, such as irregular breathing, anxiety, drowsiness, confusion, inability to concentrate, and cyanosis.

Environmental humidity should be kept at 40% to 50% with a portable or central humidifier. Extreme cold or heat can precipitate symptoms, and patients should remain indoors during these periods. An air conditioner is advisable during extreme heat.

COMMUNITY RESOURCES

- Cheshire Medical Clinic Programs, http://www.cheshire-med.com
- The National Emphysema Foundation
- National Jewish Center for Immunology and Respiratory Medicine
- The Virtual Hospital
- Lung and Blood Institute
- National Lung Health Education Program (NLHEP)
- COPD: Ask Colorado Health Net

- United Care-Cepts, inc.: COPD, http://www.mediconsult.com/noframes/ucc/pulmonary/40010.html
- American Lung Association, 800-LUNG-USA, http://www.lungusa.org/noframes/
- American Thoracic Society, 1740 Broadway, New York, NY 10019, 212-315-8700

REFERRAL POINTS AND CLINICAL WARNINGS

Consultation with a pulmonologist should be obtained for COPD patients with:

- Signs of worsening respiratory function
- Severe dyspnea
- Bullous disease
- Cardiac, renal, or any other organ impairment
- Pulmonary neoplasia
- Need for ventilatory support
- Perioperative management for surgery
- Sleep apnea.

EDITOR'S NOTE:

COMPLEMENTARY APPROACHES

A general discussion of complementary approaches can be found in Chapter 3. The following, while not an exhaustive list, are some complementary approaches being used for this condition. Additional information on these approaches, including precautions, can be found in Appendices A and B. Providers need to assess for the use of complementary approaches as part of the patient's history, as they may impact conventional therapies, and patients may not volunteer this information unless specifically asked. Efficacy of many complementary approaches is not as well documented as that of conventional therapies. Providers need to read the literature before suggesting these complementary approaches.

- Complementary Modalities
  Aromatherapy

References

Celli, R.C. (1998). Clinical aspects of chronic obstructive pulmonary disease. In G.L. Baum & J.D. Crapo (Eds.). *Textbook of pulmonary diseases*, 6th ed. Philadelphia: Lippincott-Raven.

Chen, Y., Horne, S.L., Dosman, J.A. (1991). Increased susceptibility to lung dysfunction in female smokers. *American Review of Respiratory Disease, 143*, 1224–1230.

Suggested Readings

Belman, M.J. (1993). Ventilatory muscle training and unloading. In R. Casaburi & T.L. Petty (Eds.). *Principles and practice of pulmonary rehabilitation*. Philadelphia: W.B. Saunders.

Benson, M.S., & Pierson, D.J. (1988). Auto-PEEP during mechanical ventilation of adults. *Respiratory Care, 33*, 557–568.

Burrows, B. (1990). Airway obstructive diseases: Pathogenetic mechanisms and natural histories of the disorders. *Medical Clinics of North America, 74*, 547–560.

Emerman, C.L., Connors, A.F., Lukens, T.W., Effron, D., & May, M.E. (1989). Relationship between arterial blood gases and spirometry in acute exacerbations of chronic obstructive pulmonary disease. *Annals of Emergency Medicine, 18*, 523–527.

Higgins, M.W., & Thom, T. (1990). Incidence, prevalence, and mortality: Intra- and inter-county differences. In M.J. Hensley & N.A. Saunders (Eds.). *Clinical epidemiology of chronic obstructive pulmonary disease*, pp. 23–43. New York: Marcel Dekker.

Lodrup Carlsen, K.C., Jaakkola, J.J., Nafstad, P., & Carlsen, K.H. (1997). In utero exposure to cigarette smoking influences lung function at birth. *European Respiratory Journal, 10*(8), 1774–1779.

Lopez-Majano, V., & Dutton, R.E. (1973). Regulation of respiratory drive during oxygen breathing in chronic obstructive lung disease. *American Review of Respiratory Disease, 108*, 232–240.

Postma, D.S., & Sluiter, H.J. (1989). Prognosis of chronic obstructive pulmonary disease: The Dutch experience. *American Review of Respiratory Disease, 140*, S100–S105.

Thurlbeck, W.M. (1990). Pathology of chronic obstructive pulmonary disease. *Clinics in Chest Medicine, 11*, 389–404.

Travis, J. (1989). Alpha-1-proteinase inhibitor deficiency. In M. Massaro (Ed.). *Lung cell biology*, pp. 1227–1246. New York: Marcel Dekker.

CHAPTER
75

Infections

Aymarah M. Robles, MD and Linda S. Efferen, MD, FACP, FCCP

LOWER RESPIRATORY TRACT INFECTIONS

Aymarah M. Robles, MD

Bacterial and viral lower respiratory tract infections are categorized into four groups:

- Acute bronchitis, an acute inflammation of the tracheobronchial tree, is diagnosed by exclusion. Clinically it is characterized by the presence of either a productive or nonproductive cough of 4 to 6 weeks' duration. Chronic bronchitis is part of the spectrum of chronic obstructive pulmonary disease (see Chap. 74).
- Bronchiectasis is the permanent dilatation and subsequent destruction of subsegmental bronchi or bronchioles.
- Lung abscess is the parenchymal destruction caused by an indolent suppurative process.
- Pneumonia is an infection of the distal portion of the lungs, involving the respiratory bronchioles, alveolar ducts, sacs, and alveoli.

Primary care providers frequently evaluate patients with cough, which is the single most common symptom of respiratory illness. All segments of the population will at one time or another be faced with a respiratory infection. Familiarity with the categories of lower respiratory infection and their management is crucial to providing good primary care.

ANATOMY, PHYSIOLOGY, AND PATHOLOGY

The trachea and bronchi are made of a rich epithelial cell surface composed of ciliated cells, secretory goblet cells, subepithelial cells (containing cartilage for structural support of the airways), and inflammatory mediator cells and glands. The amount of cartilage decreases as the respiratory tree branches distally and disappears altogether in the small airways (<2 mm in diameter). Tracheobronchial glands, which secrete mucus, are bigger and more numerous in the proximal airways.

Cells dedicated to airway defense are found scattered within the epithelium and submucosa. Lymphocytes may appear singly or in clusters, especially at branching points or airway bifurcations, and are called bronchus-associated lymphoid tissue. Plasma cells, especially IgA, mast cells, and macrophages, are also found at airway bifurcations. Mast cells increase in the transition zone leading to the distal airway, where gas conduction occurs. Marked branching of the airways continues as surface area is maximized for gas exchange. This architecture helps to keep the area below the main carina sterile.

The lower respiratory tract is uniquely equipped to protect against invading organisms. Aspiration of upper airway flora is the most important risk for infection. Defense mechanisms include a good cough reflex, effective mucociliary clearance (continual upward beating of cilia) to remove bacteria and debris, and angulation of airways, which traps and impinges bacteria at bifurcations. For infection to occur, the following sequential steps are required, especially at oropharyngeal colonization; aspiration of organisms; bacterial attachment to epithelial cell surfaces, preventing normal epithelial cell desquamation; and subsequent removal by expectoration.

The risk of lower airway infection is further increased by both the type of oral microflora present in the airways and host susceptibility. Severely ill patients lose their normal flora and become increasingly susceptible to enteric gram-negative bacilli. Clearance mechanisms progressively malfunction and are associated with abnormalities in mucosal surfaces. A recent viral infection may effectively strip the normal mucosa, causing intense cellular desquamation and loss of mucociliary function and local phagocytic function.

Within the terminal airway, the alveolar macrophage is the primary cellular defense. Alveolar macrophages are capable of overwhelming a challenge of low virulence—for instance, a normal, nocturnal, small-volume aspiration of oropharyngeal secretions. Activated alveolar macrophages also are capable of activating the immune system by recruiting polymorphonuclear leukocytes, found in pulmonary microvasculature reserves.

In addition, alveolar macrophages secrete cytokines, which trigger the intercellular communication systems of the immunologic response. Important lung cytokines include tumor necrosis factor, interleukin 1, and interleukin 8. They are produced in response to alveolar macrophages that activate mononuclear cells to release gamma colony stimulating factor (G-CSF). G-CSF increases myeloid progenitor cells, which trigger polymorphonuclear leukocytes to promote adhesion, chemotaxis, phagocytosis, and phosphorylation at local sites to combat infection.

EPIDEMIOLOGY

Pneumonia ranks as the sixth leading cause of death in the United States and is the leading cause of death attributable to an infectious disease. Current estimates for the United States are 4 million cases annually, with a morbidity rate of 12 per 1000 adults per year. Hospitalizations approach 600,000 per year, at an annual cost of $23 billion (*MMWR*, 1995a,b).

All humans are susceptible to lower respiratory tract infections. Symptoms of acute bronchitis in a previously healthy person implicate common cold viruses: rhinovirus, respiratory syncytial virus, parainfluenza, coronavirus, or adenovirus. Influ-

800

enza A or B may also be a cause. Nonviral agents include *Mycoplasma pneumoniae*, *Chlamydia pneumoniae* (originally described as TWAR), and *Bordetella pertussis*, an increasingly common pathogen in susceptible adults with persistent cough.

Patients with comorbid medical problems, underlying cardiorespiratory illness, immunocompromised status, or impaired cough reflex are at higher risk for infection with the usual respiratory flora and pathogenic bacteria such as *Streptococcus pneumoniae*, *Haemophilus influenzae*, *Staphylococcus aureus*, *Moraxella catarrhalis*, and *Legionella*.

Chronic bronchitis is more common in tobacco users and those exposed to passive smoke. Inhaled irritants in tobacco smoke may decrease ciliary mucosal transport and decrease the phagocytic function of the pulmonary immunologic response. These increase the risk for both colonization and infection, especially by *S. pneumoniae*, *H. influenzae*, and *M. catarrhalis*.

Primary bronchiectasis is associated with multiple insults to the lung and is divided into the following main categories:

- Postinfectious, occurring predominantly in infants and young children or occasionally in adults after upper lobe tuberculous or fungal infection
- Bronchiectasis after aspiration of upper airway flora or gastric contents as a result of impaired consciousness (ie, seizure disorders), neuromuscular disorders, esophageal motility disorders, or general anesthesia or after alcohol or illicit drug use

TABLE 75-1	Epidemiological Clues
Situation	**Organism**
Alcoholism	*S. pneumoniae, Klebsiella pneumoniae, S. aureus*
Bird exposure	*Chlamydia psittaci*
Chronic obstructive lung disease	*S. pneumoniae, Haemophilus influenzae, Moraxella catarrhalis*
Contaminated water source (cooling towers, air conditioners, showers)	*Legionella* species
Diabetes	*S. pneumoniae, S. aureus*, enteric gram negatives
Overcrowding Homeless shelters Incarceration Nursing home	*S. pneumoniae*, influenza A, B, *C. pneumoniae, M. tuberculosis*
Occupational Exposure Construction (excavation) Hunter, Trapper, Veterinarian, Farmer (Parturient cats, cattle, goats, sheep)	*Histoplasma capsulatum* *Blastomycosis* *Coxiella burnetii*
Sickle cell disease	*S. pneumoniae, H. influenzae, Salmonella*
Solid organ transplant recipient	*S. pneumoniae, H. influenzae, Leigionella* species, *Pneumocystis carinii*, cytomegalovirus, *Strongyloides stercoralis*
Travel history (Southeast Asia, Southwestern United States, Mississippi Valley)	*Pseudomonas pseudomallei* (melioidosis) *Coccidiodes immitis* *Histoplasma capsulatum*

TABLE 75-2	Physical Examination Clues

Coexisting illnesses identify patients who may be at higher risk for the development of severe lower respiratory infection requiring hospitalization. These include chronic obstructive pulmonary disease, renal insufficiency, diabetes mellitus, chronic liver disease, congestive heart failure, splenectomy, malnutrition, cancer, abnormal mental status, history of prior hospitalization for pneumonia within the previous year, and age greater than 60 years.

Finding	Organism
Altered mental status, seizure disorder Oral flora anaerobes and aerobic bacteria Bullous myringitis	*Mycoplasma pneumoniae*
Cerebellar ataxia	*M. pneumoniae, L. pneumophila*
Cutaneous nodules (abscesses) and CNS abnormalities	*Nocardia* species *Histoplasma capsulatum*
Ecthyma gangrenosum	*Pseudomonas aeruginosa, Serratia marcescens*
Erythema multiforme	*M. pneumoniae*
Erythema nodosum	*C. pneumoniae, M. tuberculosis*
Encephalitis	*M. pneumoniae, C. burnetii, L. pneumophila*
Periodontal disease with foul-smelling sputum	Anaerobes and aerobes

- Occupational hazards may also predispose to bronchiectasis—for example, inhalation of toxic gases (ammonia, nitrogen or sulfur oxides, and hydrocarbons)
- Foreign body aspiration (eg, nails, tacks, beads, berries, seeds, coins), causing distal obstruction and subsequently leading to bronchiectasis
- Mineral-based oil preparations, such as camphorated oil, are sometimes used inside the nostrils to relieve nasal congestion. The oil may be aspirated, leading to destruction and dilatation of the bronchi.
- Anatomic abnormalities in the airway predispose to bronchiectasis.

Secondary bronchiectasis is associated with inherited or congenital diseases. Cystic fibrosis is the most common; others include immunoglobulin deficiencies and ciliary dyskinetic syndromes.

Predisposing epidemiologic factors leading to lung abscess include events related to impaired consciousness or sensorium, as well as esophageal motility disorders, history of seizures, or the use of alcohol or illicit drugs. These become even more significant in the presence of poor oral hygiene or gingivitis. Anaerobes account for 80% to 90% of all pulmonary suppurative lung abscesses. This is not surprising, given that inflamed gingival surfaces and crevices harbor a large volume of anaerobes (as high as 10^{12} organisms/g).

Evaluation of the epidemiologic setting and the physical exam can yield clues suggesting the most likely pathogen causing pneumonia (Tables 75-1 and 75-2).

DIAGNOSTIC CRITERIA

The diagnosis of both acute and chronic bronchis is based on a constellation of clinical symptoms and findings.

Patients with bronchiectasis present with a prolonged history of recurrent sinopulmonary infections and chronic cough productive of copious amounts of purulent sputum intermittently streaked with blood. The chest radiograph shows hyperlucent cystic areas and peribronchial fibrosis demonstrated by "tram tracks," clearly delineated vertical or parallel lines of a descending bronchus. Thin-section chest computed tomography confirms the diagnosis. When contrast is administered, the so-called "signet ring" sign is seen, showing the diameter of the involved bronchus larger than its accompanying pulmonary artery.

The chest film in lung abscess reveals single or multiple thick-walled cavitary lesions with air-fluid levels. These lesions are generally located at dependent areas of the lungs, especially the superior segments of the lower lobes. Microbiologic diagnosis can be made by Gram stain and culture of sputum specimens.

The clinical spectrum in pneumonia varies, depending on whether the infection is community-acquired. Typical pneumonia presents with fever, productive cough, pleuritic chest pain, and clinical signs of consolidation. In atypical pneumonia, systemic symptoms predominate (eg, fever, headache, myalgias, dry or minimally productive cough, and lack of clinical signs of consolidation).

The chest radiograph demonstrating an infiltrate is the gold standard for the diagnosis of pneumonia. Radiographic abnormalities cannot distinguish bacterial from atypical pneumonia. Chest films can, however, help assess the extent and severity of illness; evaluate complications such as atelectasis, pleural effusion, or multilobar involvement; and assist in planning further diagnostic studies. Difficulties may arise in the interpretation of pneumonia in the presence of coexistent lung diseases or congestive heart failure, as well as in patients who cannot participate in taking standard posteroanterior/lateral films. Suboptimal films must be evaluated within the context of both the clinical presentation and findings. A repeat chest x-ray for diagnostic accuracy may be necessary once the patient can fully participate.

The etiologic diagnosis of pneumonia is based on microbiologic criteria. A definitive diagnosis is made when a pathogenic organism is recovered from a normally sterile site, i.e. blood or pleural fluid, or when an organism that is not a known colonizer is found in respiratory secretions, for example: viral organisms Influenza A or B; respiratory syncytial virus (RSV); herpesvirus (HSV); cytomegalovirus (CMV); *Pneumocystis carinii* Pneumonia (PCP); any fungi; *Legionella; Mycoplasma pneumoniae; Chlamydia pneumoniae* (TWAR); *Bordetella pertussis;* acid fast bacilli: Mycobacterium tuberculosis (MYB) or any atypical pathogenic acid fast bacillus.

Sputum Gram stains are an important diagnostic tool, provided that they are collected appropriately. The specimen must be collected before the initiation of antimicrobial therapy and must contain greater than 25 polymorphonuclear leukocytes and less than 10 epithelial cells per high-power field, demonstrating a true distal airway specimen not contaminated by saliva.

Failure to detect gram-positive clusters or gram-negative bacilli in the initial specimen virtually excludes these organisms from diagnostic consideration. In addition, the Gram stain may allow the detection of penicillin-resistant strains of *S. pneumoniae*. The inability to identify a predominant organism on Gram stain despite the presence of 25 polymorphonuclear leukocytes and less than 10 epithelial cells suggests the possibility of atypical pathogens, such as *Legionella, Mycoplasma, Chlamydia,* or a viral etiology or the use of antimicrobial therapy before obtaining the sputum for diagnostic studies.

HISTORY AND PHYSICAL EXAM

In acute bronchitis, a complete history should be taken, with careful attention to epidemiologic considerations (eg, occupation, recent community outbreak of influenza, overcrowded living conditions, a history of concurrent infections of close contacts). A thorough physical exam focused on the eyes, ears, nose, sinuses, throat, and cardiorespiratory system is crucial. Productive or nonproductive cough, together with retrosternal discomfort with or without wheezing, localizes symptoms to the lower airways. The physical exam is otherwise generally within normal limits. Fever is absent in most viral syndromes responsible for the common cold, most commonly rhinovirus, respiratory syncytial virus, or coronavirus. Fever is a component of influenza A and B, adenovirus, *M. pneumoniae, C. pneumoniae,* and *B. pertussis* infections. Lung auscultation reveals basilar rhonchi or rales that may change or clear with cough. Wheezing is also a nonspecific finding; it may persist long after other symptoms and signs have resolved.

Chronic bronchitis is present in cigarette smokers or persons exposed to chemical or environmental irritants, including passive smoke inhalation. There is a history of progressive exercise intolerance and episodic cough with increased expectoration of mucopurulent sputum. Prolonged recurrences may lead to arterial blood gas derangements, severe hypoxemia, and hypercarbia. In later stages this may lead to pulmonary artery hypertension and right-sided heart failure. The physical exam may reveal coughing and an increased respiratory rate associated with respiratory distress and abnormal breathing patterns. On auscultation, rhonchi and decreased air entry may be heard. Wheezing may be intermittent, especially if associated with acute mucus plugging of a bronchus. In later stages, if pulmonary hypertension ensues, a parasternal right ventricular heave and loud S_2 may be noted. Lower extremity edema may be present if right-sided heart failure occurs.

Bronchiectasis produces copious mucopurulent, often blood-streaked sputum of many years' duration and recurrent sinopulmonary infections. The physical exam reveals a chronically ill-appearing patient and possibly muscle wasting, malnutrition, and failure to thrive. Clubbing of the fingers from chronic hypoxemia may occur. On auscultation, coarse rales with variations in pitch and volume at both inspiration and expiration are often heard, as well as coarse rhonchi representing secretions in large airways.

Patients with lung abscess typically present with an insidious course of a 2- to 4-week duration of fever, purulent fetid blood-streaked sputum, generalized malaise, anorexia, and weight loss. Chest pain is common. On the physical exam, low-grade fever is present. The patient appears chronically ill and pale. The oral exam reveals poor dentition or gingivitis and overall poor dental hygiene. Signs of consolidation may be heard on auscultation, accompanied by amphoric or tubular breath sounds over the site of the lung abscess. When empyema invades the pleural space, pleuritic chest pain may be prominent, and dullness to percussion is encountered.

Symptoms suggestive of pneumonia are nonspecific and include fever, cough, sputum production, shortness of breath, and chest pain. The mean duration of illness before seeking medical attention is usually 5 to 6 days. Fever occurs in approximately 80% of patients. Another 30% have signs of consolidation with egophony. Most patients have at least one of these symptoms.

Those at highest risk for complications of pneumonia are persons with comorbid illness such as chronic obstructive pulmonary disease, congestive heart failure, immunosuppression (including chronic steroid use), diabetes mellitus, renal insufficiency, chronic liver disease, postsplenectomy, or chronic alcohol or illicit drug use and malnutrition, or those older than 60 years.

DIAGNOSTIC STUDIES

The definitive laboratory diagnosis of an upper respiratory viral infection causing acute bronchitis is unnecessary. Chest x-rays should be obtained in all patients who appear ill to exclude a more serious lower respiratory infection.

Chronic bronchitis is also diagnosed primarily on symptoms. Recurrent episodes of clinical deterioration can occur, especially when complicated by upper respiratory infection and fever or increased volume or purulence of sputum. Patients may appear cyanotic and the arterial blood gas analysis may reveal hypoxemia and hypercapnea. Repeated recurrences may lead to permanent blood gas derangements and chronic ventilatory failure characterized by well-compensated respiratory acidosis. This is evidenced by elevated serum bicarbonate levels, confirming renal compensation for the chronic hypercarbia. Erythrocytosis and elevations of hemoglobin and hematocrit are seen on a routine complete blood count as evidence of the compensatory response to chronic hypoxemia. Leukocytosis may be a feature of bacterial infection. An appropriately collected and rapidly processed Gram stain of the sputum with culture will identify the primary bacterial pathogen, or a superinfection after an episode of viral, mycoplasmal, or chlamydial infection. The usual bacterial pathogens include *S. pneumoniae*, *H. influenzae*, and *M. catarrhalis*. Enteric gram-negative organisms, especially *Klebsiella* and *Pseudomonas*, should also be excluded. Electrocardiography may show supraventricular arrhythmias, intraventricular conduction defects, right ventricular strain, right ventricular hypertrophy, right bundle branch block, and morphologic P-wave abnormalities, all related to hypoxemia. Chest radiography is nonspecific and may suggest hyperinflation, bronchial prominence, or other signs of dilatation. If pulmonary hypertension is present, enlarged pulmonary arteries may be seen. In cor pulmonale, an enlarged right ventricle may be seen on chest films. Spirometry indicates signs of airflow obstruction with a decrease in forced expiratory volume in 1 sec (FEV_1) and in the ratio of FEV_1 to forced vital capacity.

In bronchiectasis, hypercarbia with ensuing chronic ventilatory failure is seen in late-stage disease. Additional diagnostic options are tailored to the patient. When an appropriate clinical or family history suggests cystic fibrosis as the etiology for bronchiectasis, a sweat chloride determination with pilocarpine iontophoresis should be performed. Serum protein electrophoresis and IgG subsets may be obtained to evaluate for immunologic abnormalities. If fever and recurrent wheezing are present and central bronchiectasis is found on the chest radiograph, an evaluation for allergic bronchopulmonary aspergillosis should be performed. Sputum Gram stain and culture will identify bacterial pathogens.

Bronchoscopy, percutaneous transthoracic needle aspiration, or diagnostic thoracentesis of pleural fluid have replaced transtracheal aspiration for the diagnosis of a lung abscess. In addition to examining the aspirate, blood cultures are essential. Anemia of chronic disease is usually present. When other conditions coexist, such as alcoholism or malnutrition, an iron or folate deficiency anemia may also be present. A moderate leukocytosis is often found. A computed tomography scan of the chest is often performed to evaluate the parenchyma and distinguish pleural involvement. Additional studies should be tailored to the patient and are used primarily in rapidly worsening disease.

The etiologic diagnosis of pneumonia is based on microbiologic criteria. Accurate identification of a pathogen necessitates that it be present in a normally sterile site, i.e., blood or pleural fluid, and that it not be a known colonizer in respiratory secretions. The most common pathogens for pneumonia include: any fungi, *Histoplasma capsulatum*, *Coccidiodes immitis*, *Blastomyces* dermatitis, *Pneumocystis carinii* pneumonia (PCP); parasites: *Toxoplasma gondii*, strongyloides; viral organisms such as Influenza A or B, respiratory syncytial virus (RSV), Herpesvirus (HSV); *Legionella*, *Mycoplasma pneumoniae*, *Chlamydia pneumoniae* (TWAR), and *Bordetella pertussis*.

In summary, all patients with an increased risk for morbidity or mortality from pneumonia require hospitalization and careful observation. Required studies include chest radiography; arterial blood gas analysis; complete blood count; chemistry profile, including electrolytes and renal and liver function tests; and microbiologic studies (blood cultures, Gram stain and culture of sputum), with additional special studies such as staining and culture for acid-fast bacilli. When *Legionella* is suspected, sputum for both culture and direct fluorescent antibody test (DFA), should be obtained. In addition, a urine sample for *Legionella pneumonia* serogroup 1 radioimmune assay is 80% to 99% sensitive and 99% specific.

Pleural fluid, if present, requires early, aggressive diagnostic thoracentesis and pleural fluid analysis with cell count and differential; pH collected anaerobically and on ice, chemistries, including: glucose, protein, and lactate dehydrogenase; Gram stain and bacterial culture; acid-fast stain; mycobacterial and fungal cultures; and cytology.

TREATMENT OPTIONS, EXPECTED OUTCOMES, AND COMPREHENSIVE MANAGEMENT

Prevention

Annual immunizations with influenza vaccine for susceptible groups, as recommended by the Centers for Disease Control & Prevention, is mandatory to prevent life-threatening illness or death. The influenza vaccine also prevents the secondary development of bacterial pneumonia from *S. pneumoniae*, *H. influenzae*, and *S. aureus* in patients originally infected with influenza. Each year, the influenza vaccine is estimated to be 70% effective in preventing influenza-related pneumonia, hospital admissions, and death. Influenza vaccinations are also recommended for health care workers who care for susceptible patients. Chemoprophylaxis with antiviral agents such as amantadine or rimantadine is also effective against influenza A when used at the initiation of symptoms.

The CDC also recommends vaccination with the polyvalent 23 antigen pneumococcal vaccine. This vaccine is 50% to 70% efficacious, especially against serotypes most likely to cause bacteremic pneumococcal infections. Titers should be checked periodically; if waning, repeat immunization is recommended every 5 to 7 years.

The avoidance of tobacco is crucial for respiratory and cardiac well-being. Good oral hygiene and the avoidance of habits leading to an altered state of consciousness (ie, alcohol and illicit drug use) are important to prevent aspiration syndromes that may lead to severe lower airway respiratory infections.

Age and Economic Considerations

Infection of the lower respiratory tract remains the leading cause of death in persons older than 65 years. As the population ages, the magnitude of this problem will become more acute. Pneumonia in the elderly is a serious clinical dilemma and diagnostic challenge. Atypical presentations with subtle latent symptoms and signs such as confusion, low-grade fever, anorexia, dehydration, mild tachypnea, and worsening of the patient's underlying disease process may confound the clinical presentation and course. Rates of pneumococcal pneumonia in persons older than 65 years are three- to fivefold greater than in young adults and requires hospitalization in approximately 90% of patients.

Morbidity and mortality rates are often higher in persons without adequate medical insurance, who tend to seek assistance late in their course, or those who have no regular access to medical care and who utilize inner-city emergency departments for primary care. Malnourished patients are at increased risk because of the derangements in host defense systems that delay and impair the healing process.

Treatment Options, Expected Outcomes, and Comprehensive Management

Treatment for acute bronchitis is symptomatic: acetaminophen, oral liquids, and bed rest are encouraged when malaise and fever are prominent. Dextromethorphan (15 mg orally every 4 to 6 hours) will suppress a nonproductive cough. Inhaled selective beta-2 agonists (two puffs every 6 hours) may be prescribed when wheezing is present. Antibiotics should be reserved for specific instances where a nonviral etiology is suspected. A trial of oral erythromycin or the newer macrolide antibiotics is useful as first-line therapy for *M. pneumoniae* or *C. pneumoniae.*

Patients with chronic bronchitis should be encouraged to enter a program for smoking cessation. Airflow obstruction is best managed with inhaled ipratropium bromide, with or without inhaled selective beta-2 agonists. Oral theophylline, with careful attention to serum levels, may be considered in selected patients to enhance both diaphragmatic function and mucociliary clearance. The efficacy of inhaled or systemic steroids remains controversial, but they are often used in patients who remain symptomatic despite maximal and appropriate use of inhaled bronchodilator therapy.

Bacterial exacerbations require the use of antibiotic therapy, and a sputum Gram stain should guide the choice of antimicrobial therapy. Common antibiotics used to treat exacerbations include ampicillin, amoxicillin, amoxicillin–clavulanate, trimethoprim–sulfamethoxazole, quinolones, oral second- or third-generation cephalosporins, and erythromycin or other newer macrolides. Home oxygen therapy is required when baseline Pao_2 is less than 55 mmHg. It should be used at least 18 hours per day to ameliorate pulmonary hypertension. Patients with known polycythemia, pulmonary hypertension, or cor pulmonale whose baseline Pao_2 is 56 to 59 mmHg also require supplemental oxygen therapy. Chronic ventilatory failure may be treated by the use of nocturnal noninvasive continuous positive airway pressure.

Antimicrobial therapy of lung abscess is based on the microbiology. Penicillin is acceptable as initial therapy, although high intravenous doses (10 to 20 million U/day) are required. Oral metronidazole added to intravenous penicillin adds efficacy to the regimen (Hammond et al, 1995). In seriously ill patients, intravenous clindamycin is highly efficacious, and a rapid early clinical response is often seen. Once clinically improved, patients require a prolonged course of oral antibiotic therapy until complete resolution of the infiltrate and cavity has occurred. This may necessitate as much as 6 to 12 weeks of therapy.

Chest physiotherapy to promote abscess drainage is an adjunctive therapeutic measure. Bronchoscopic evaluation of the airways may be required to evaluate for foreign body aspiration. Rarely, surgical intervention is required, although it is often related to complications arising from cavity wall vessel erosion that produces massive hemoptysis.

Ideally, therapy for pneumonia should be directed at the causative pathogen. In more than 50% of cases, the etiology is unknown, and empiric, well-informed therapy decisions must be made. The therapy for community-acquired pneumonia is based on the patient's age, the presence or lack of comorbid conditions, and the clinical severity at presentation. Eighty percent of those who develop pneumonia may be treated as outpatients. The most common organisms are *S. pneumoniae, C. pneumoniae, M. pneumoniae,* and respiratory viruses, especially influenza A or B and *H. influenzae.* Initial antimicrobial therapy with a macrolide antibiotic such as erythromycin, clarithromycin, or azithromycin is appropriate. An oral second-generation cephalosporin or trimethoprim–sulfamethoxazole or levofloxacin, the newer extended-spectrum quinolone, may also be used as first-line therapy. Tetracycline may be used if allergy or intolerance to other medications should occur.

Patients older than 60 years or those who have comorbidity are infected with the same organisms as the uncomplicated population. Aerobic gram-negative bacilli, *S. aureus, M. catarrhalis,* and *Legionella* also infect the high-risk group. Initial therapy should reflect the sputum Gram stain results or should empirically cover all the above organisms. Either a second-generation cephalosporin or trimethoprim–sulfamethoxazole or a combination beta-lactamase inhibitor is appropriate for first-line oral therapy. A macrolide antibiotic may be added if infection with *Legionella* is suspected.

Patients who require hospital admission may be infected with any organism, although *S. pneumoniae,* aerobic gram-negative bacilli, and *Legionella* are especially suspect. These pathogens account for a large percentage of severe cases of community-acquired pneumonia. Intravenous second- or third-generation cephalosporins or a β-lactam-inhibitor and the addition of a macrolide is recommended as initial therapy. An alternative regimen combines intravenous therapy with a macrolide antibiotic to cover both *Pneumococcus* and *Legionella* and a third-generation cephalosporin with *Pseudomonas* activity, plus an aminoglycoside or another antipseudomonal antimicrobial, plus an aminoglycoside. All antimicrobial therapy requires re-evaluation and must be individualized once microbiologic confirmation and susceptibilities are available.

In severe pneumonia requiring hospitalization, mortality rates nearing 50% continue to be reported despite effective and appropriate antimicrobial therapy. The high fatality rates may be related to inadequate host defense mechanisms that lead to irreversible physiologic derangements.

TEACHING AND SELF-CARE

All patients with respiratory infections should be encouraged to learn more about their disease process and become active participants in their own care. Teaching is most important in the optimal use of inhaled bronchodilators. Patients with chronic bronchitis or bronchiectasis should carefully monitor the quality, quantity, and characteristics of sputum production. In addition, patients with bronchiectasis may benefit from postural drainage techniques that assist in sputum clearance and improve quality of life.

Nutritional counseling to achieve a balanced diet and an individually tailored exercise program to maintain muscle conditioning and improve overall well-being are highly recommended.

COMMUNITY RESOURCES

An excellent source of information for patients and their families with respiratory disease is the local chapter of the American Lung Association. The American College of Chest Physicians and the CDC can provide additional information about respiratory illness.

- Chronic Lung Disease Information Resource, http://www.cheshire-med.com/programs/pulrehab/rehinfo.html
- American Lung Association, 1-800-LUNG-USA, http://www.lungusa.org/noframes/
- American Thoracic Society, 1740 Broadway, New York, NY 10019, 212-315-8700

REFERRAL POINTS AND CLINICAL WARNINGS

Overall appearance, mental status, and vital signs are the simplest and most important tools for assessing the severity of disease. Detection of the signs in Table 75-3 requires an emergent referral to an acute care setting.

TUBERCULOSIS

Linda S. Efferen, MD, FACP, FCCP

Tuberculosis (TB), a specific disease caused by *Mycobacterium tuberculosis*, can affect almost any tissue or organ of the body, but the most common site of disease is the lung. It is transmit-

TABLE 75-3	Referral Warnings
Abnormal vital signs that help to identify seriously ill patients	■ Respiratory rate greater than 30 breaths per minute ■ Systolic blood pressure less than 90 mmHg ■ Diastolic blood pressure less than 60 mmHg ■ Temperature greater than 101°F (38.3°C) or less than 97°F
Abnormal clinical signs heralding increased severity	■ Impaired level of consciousness ■ Physical findings suggesting extrapulmonary involvement
Laboratory data that predict increased morbidity	■ Leukopenia less than 4,000/cc ■ Leukocytosis greater than 30,000/cc ■ Absolute neutrophil count less than 1,000/cc ■ Severe anemia with a hemoglobin less than 9 g/dL or a hematocrit less than 30% ■ Thrombocytopenia accompanied by increased INR or increased partial thromboplastin time (PTT) ■ Increased fibrin split products greater than 1:40 suggest disseminated intravascular coagulation (DIC) ■ Arterial blood gases obtained on room air demonstrating a Pao$_2$ less than 60 mmHg ■ Paco$_2$ greater than 50 mmHg ■ Abnormal renal function with a serum creatinine greater than 1.2 mg/dL or a blood urea nitrogen greater than 20 mg/dL ■ Anion gap and metabolic acidosis suggesting sepsis and organ dysfunction ■ Serum albumin greater than 30 g/L ■ Bacteriuria
Chest radiograph abnormalities that predict a possibly complicated course	■ Multilobar involvement ■ Cavitary disease ■ Pleural effusion

ted through airborne droplets aerosolized from the lungs of an infectious person. The potential for widespread community contamination is great, and TB epidemics in the past have been a great public health concern. In 1987, it was considered a realistic expectation that TB would be eliminated by the year 2010. Instead, a rising incidence of disease and the emergence of multidrug-resistant disease led to renewed concern on the part of health care providers, consumers, and policy makers. Currently, limited success in re-establishing control of TB has been achieved, but it remains a global health problem. The goal of eradication is no longer considered feasible.

ANATOMY, PHYSIOLOGY, AND PATHOLOGY

Immunopathogenesis

Persons infected with *M. tuberculosis* mount a host defense response that includes both specific and nonspecific mechanisms in an attempt to restrict the growth of the organism and to limit infection. Infected droplet nuclei containing viable mycobacteria, reaching the respiratory bronchioles and alveoli, are generally ingested by alveolar macrophages and removed via the mucociliary system. In addition, macrophages possess some inherent bacteria-killing or growth-inhibiting capabilities. Although generally effective, if these nonspecific defenses are overloaded, the surviving bacilli multiply, causing a localized tuberculous pneumonia. In the presence of a strong specific cell-mediated immune response, this generally heals spontaneously.

During the tissue-invasion phase, transport of the organism through the alveolar wall within macrophages allows access to the bloodstream via the lymphatics, giving rise to a tuberculous bacillemia. Organisms have access to all organs during this phase, which sets the stage for both pulmonary and extrapulmonary disease, which may occur years later.

The principal specific immune response to *M. tuberculosis* is cell-mediated immunity involving T lymphocytes and macrophages. With time, the number of T cells with specificity for antigens and epitopes of *M. tuberculosis* increases, providing a delayed-type hypersensitivity reaction. Persons with strong delayed-type hypersensitivity, whose T cells are sensitized to antigens of the tubercle bacillus, appear to be able to produce more lymphokines capable of activating microbicidal mechanisms in macrophages. They have the ability to organize granulomas, which can then restrict the spread of infection. Activated T cells and macrophages and the production of a variety of lymphokines and cytokines serve a protective function but also result in tissue damage in the form of liquefaction necrosis.

Microbiology

Although there are many mycobacteria, four organisms make up the "tuberculosis complex": *M. tuberculosis, Mycobacterium bovis, Mycobacterium africanum,* and *Mycobacterium microti.* The overwhelming majority of disease is caused by *M. tuberculosis* and *M. bovis. M. africanum* accounts for relatively few cases of TB, and *M. microti* does not cause disease in humans.

Mycobacteria other than tuberculosis, or nontuberculous mycobacteria (NTM), can be broadly categorized as pathogenic or nonpathogenic. These organisms are epidemiologically distinct from tuberculosis. Although they are in many way similar to tuberculosis, the culture of the organism does not necessarily prove disease, treatment regimens differ, and NTM organisms are not considered a public health threat.

The most commonly discussed NTM organism is the *M. avium-intracellulare* complex, which has assumed increasing importance with the HIV epidemic. However, the increasing incidence of NTM infections can be only partly explained by the HIV epidemic.

EPIDEMIOLOGY

In the United States, 22,813 cases of TB were reported in 1995 (8.7 cases/100,000 population), a 6.4% decrease from 1994 and the third consecutive year in which the number of reported cases has decreased. The proportion of cases with resistance to isoniazid decreased from 8.5% to 7.6%, and resistance to isoniazid and rifampin decreased from 1.5% to 1.4% (CDC, 1996a).

Despite some encouraging reports, deaths from TB worldwide rose to 3 million in 1995, which is higher than at any other time in history. The dual epidemic of TB and HIV, which is most serious in Asia, is expected to cause more than 3 million new TB cases in the next 4 years. The percentage of TB cases attributable to HIV disease is expected to rise from 2% in 1990 to 14% by 2000. One third of the world is infected with *M. tuberculosis.* It is estimated that by the year 2005, 12 million new cases of TB will occur annually worldwide (Efferen, 1997).

Screening efforts to reduce the spread of disease within the United States are extremely important. More than 90% of annual foreign arrivals to the United States are nonimmigrant tourists, business visitors, and students who do not receive pretravel TB screening. In addition, each of the five countries from which most documented immigrants come to the United States (Mexico, the Philippines, South Korea, Haiti, and the People's Republic of China) have case rates in excess of 125 per 100,000 (Conference Report, 1996; CDC, 1990). Clearly it will be difficult to eliminate TB within our national borders without efforts to control disease among immigrants and in their countries of origin.

DIAGNOSTIC CRITERIA

Direct microscopy with staining procedures remains the most widely used method to establish the diagnosis of TB once it is clinically suspected. Although direct microscopy is a rapid method of detecting mycobacteria, concern exists regarding its sensitivity and specificity. Culture remains the diagnostic gold standard and is essential for drug sensitivity testing.

Delays in obtaining results from current culturing methods have intensified attempts to create a more sensitive and specific diagnostic test while decreasing the time required to establish a diagnosis. Although numerous diagnostic techniques and strategies continue to be explored, none has yet been identified that can replace direct microscopy and culture techniques (Table 75-4).

Commercially available molecular techniques have been extensively studied. The Mycobacterium Tuberculosis Direct test (Gen-Probe Incorporated, San Diego, CA) is currently approved as an adjunctive test for evaluating acid-fast bacillus smear-positive patients suspected of having TB. This test is performed in conjunction with a mycobacterial culture because *M. tuberculosis* may not be detected in some specimens because of the presence of inhibitors or very low levels of the organism. Also, this test cannot determine drug susceptibility or identify other mycobacterial species that may be clinically significant. The reported sensitivity and specificity of this assay has varied from 78% to 98% and from 96% to 100%, respectively. The Amplicor *M. tuberculosis* test (Roche Diagnostic Systems, Branchburg, NJ) has been similarly evaluated with comparable results.

HISTORY AND PHYSICAL EXAM

Among healthy persons, infection with *M. tuberculosis* is generally clinically silent, detectable only by a positive Mantoux test. The lifetime risk of progression of tuberculous infection to active disease is estimated to be 3% to 10% for healthy persons. In persons coinfected with HIV, this risk may be markedly increased, to 3% to 8% per year (Hopewell & Bloom, 1994).

Symptoms and signs related to TB may be systemic or related to the specific organ system involved. General symptoms of fever, malaise, and weight loss are frequently noted. Hematologic abnormalities, including leukocytosis or leukopenia and anemia, may be present, as well as hyponatremia.

The most common manifestation of pulmonary TB is cough, which characteristically is present for weeks to months

TABLE 75-4	Diagnostic Techniques to Detect Tuberculosis
Technique	**Comments**
Direct microscopy	Sensitivity 25%–70%; specificity may be limited; PPV >90%; inexpensive; rapid; detection limit 5×10^3 bacilli/mL
Culture	
Solid medium	Sensitivity may be as low as 50%; results available in 2–8 weeks; detection limit 10–100 organisms per sample
Liquid (Bactec)	Sensitivity higher, precise estimates unavailable; results available in 1–2 weeks
Gas chromatography, gas chromatography + mass spectrophotometry, high-performance liquid chromatography	Detects specific mycobacterial lipids; equipment expensive; cannot use directly on clinical specimens; not specific
Immunologic assays	Low sensitivity and specificity
Serologic tests (ELISA)	Simple to perform; no test with adequate sensitivity and specificity identified
Nucleic acid probes	High specificity, lack sensitivity; cannot use directly on clinical specimen
Liquid culture + probe	Detection and identification in 4–7 days
Amplification techniques PCR, LCR, TMA, SDA Nested PCR Single-tube nested PCR	See text
Restriction fragment length polymorphism	Ability to fingerprint TB isolates, able to trace spread of specific strain & rapidly recognize MDRTB strains
Pulsed-field gel electrophoresis (PFGE)	Equipment expensive
Luciferase-based reporter mycobacteriophage	Not yet evaluated with clinical specimens

PPV, positive predictive value; ELISA, enzyme-linked immunosorbent assay; PCR, polymerase chain reaction; LCR, ligase chain reaction; TMA, transcription-mediated amplification; SDA, strand displacement amplification; MDRTB, multidrug-resistant tuberculosis.

and may be productive. Hemoptysis, pleuritic chest pain, and shortness of breath may occur. The most commonly involved sites for extrapulmonary TB are the lymphatic system and the pleura, which account for approximately 50% of extrapulmonary sites. In addition to systemic symptoms, site-specific signs may suggest specific organ involvement (Table 75-5).

Before the HIV epidemic, approximately 85% of newly diagnosed cases were limited to the lungs and 15% were extrapulmonary. In HIV-infected populations, the incidence of pulmonary TB is estimated to be approximately 40%, with 30% of patients presenting with extrapulmonary disease and 30% presenting with both pulmonary and extrapulmonary manifestations (Hopewell & Bloom, 1994).

DIAGNOSTIC TESTING

Tuberculin skin testing (5 TU PPD, Mantoux) is a useful means of identifying persons infected with *M. tuberculosis* but does not necessarily indicate active disease. In addition, skin testing can be interpreted as negative in the presence of tuberculous infection, and false-positive reactions may occur as a result of infection with NTM; thus, a positive or negative test cannot be used to establish or rule out tuberculous disease.

Chest radiographs may suggest a diagnosis of TB. In primary TB, or TB occurring after recent infection, a middle- or lower-lobe infiltrate is commonly seen, often in association with ipsilateral adenopathy. Disease that occurs at a time remote from the initial infection, or reactivation TB, characteristically causes cavitary disease in the apical or posterior segments of the upper lobe or superior segment of the lower lobes. In patients with advanced HIV infection, radiographic findings are more atypical; cavitation is uncommon, intrathoracic adenopathy is common, and the radiograph may be more frequently interpreted as normal.

A definitive diagnosis of TB requires the identification of tubercle bacilli in culture. For pulmonary TB, sputum samples are needed. Three separate early-morning sputum specimens are recommended; the diagnostic yield of additional sputum

TABLE 75-5	Extrapulmonary Manifestations of Tuberculosis
Organ System	**Symptoms/Signs**
Pleural	Asymptomatic, pleuritic chest pain, dyspnea
Lymphatic	Painless swelling, sinus tracts
Central nervous system	Headache, decreased sensorium, neck stiffness, cranial nerve abnormalities, focal ischemic syndromes
Pericardial	Pain, cough, dyspnea, orthopnea, ankle swelling
Gastrointestinal	Pain, abdominal swelling, anal fissure, perirectal abscess
Genitourinary	Dysuria, hematuria, frequency, flank pain, prostatitis, orchitis, pelvic pain
Skeletal	Pain, swelling

TABLE 75-6	Diagnosis of Extrapulmonary Tuberculosis		
		Diagnostic Yield (%)	
System	Sample	Smear	Culture
Lymphatic	Lymph node biopsy or aspirate	25–50	70
Pleural	Pleural fluid		20–40
	Pleural biopsy		65–75
Genitourinary	Urine—1st void specimen $\times$ 3*		80–95
Skeletal	Joint fluid	20–25	60–80
	Bone biopsy		>60–80
Central nervous system	Cerebrospinal fluid	10–20	55–80
Abdominal	Ascitic fluid		50
Pericardial	Pericardial fluid		25–30

* May be positive in patients with other form of extrapulmonary TB.

specimens is small. For patients who are not coughing or spontaneously producing sputum, sputum induction can be helpful. Gastric aspirates can also be used but are generally reserved for pediatric patients. If less-invasive tests prove nondiagnostic, fiberoptic bronchoscopy should be considered.

The diagnosis of extrapulmonary TB is difficult to establish, in part because the affected sites are less accessible and the bacillary load is smaller. Specimens from the organ involved are generally indicated and are variably diagnostic (Table 75-6). Blood cultured specifically for *M. tuberculosis* may be positive, especially in disseminated disease or HIV-positive patients.

TREATMENT OPTIONS, EXPECTED OUTCOMES AND COMPREHENSIVE MANAGEMENT

Cultural Factors

As with many other diseases, the diagnosis and effective treatment of TB may be delayed or complicated by the use of "traditional" healers. Unlike other diseases, however, this delay allows for the continued spread of infection to others. Among immigrants, care may be delayed because of fear of deportation, loss of work, and lack of ability to pay for medical services. Language differences between the provider and patient may impede understanding of the need for prompt treatment as well. Concerted efforts must be made to ensure that culturally sensitive education and support are provided throughout the treatment course.

Socioeconomic Factors

More than 90% of the global burden of disease occurs in developing countries. The rise of TB in many industrialized countries, including the United States, has been affected by immigration from high-incidence countries. In 1995, the number of reported cases decreased in U.S.-born persons, whereas the incidence in foreign-born persons increased, accounting for 35.7% of total reported cases. Efforts to develop a global strategy to combat TB are needed.

The traditional association of TB with poverty continues to be a major problem. In the United States, TB is increasingly a focal problem of ethnic minorities in inner-city areas, where the convergence of poverty, homelessness, unemployment, overcrowding, substance abuse, and HIV infection all contribute to TB rates far in excess of the national average. In developing countries with limited resources, population growth, worsening poverty, and the HIV epidemic continue to lead to an increase in the absolute number of cases.

Prevention

Vaccination with bacillus Calmette-Guerin (BCG), first used in 1921, remains the cornerstone of TB control programs throughout most of the world, providing a significant and sustained protective effect with a reasonable safety profile. In the United States, TB control efforts focus on interrupting transmission, performing skin testing on high-risk persons, and administering chemoprophylaxis. Recommendations for BCG are fairly limited; its use is restricted to persons who meet specific criteria when other modalities are not effective (Efferen, 1997a; CDC, 1996b).

Protective immunity against *M. tuberculosis* is presumed to be mediated by T cells that recognize mycobacterial antigens and secrete the T-helper-1 cytokine interferon-gamma. Identification of mycobacterial antigens that stimulate the T-helper-1 response is thought to be critical to the development of effective vaccines. Conversely, antigens that stimulate T-helper-2 cytokines (interleukin 4 and interleukin 10) may suppress cellular immunity and should probably be excluded from a vaccine.

The ideal vaccine should be safe, easily administered, and inexpensive and should provide long-lasting protection. Although BCG fulfills some of these criteria, its protection is not lifelong, its efficacy varies, and methods to allow differentiation between natural versus vaccine-induced immunity are not available. Currently, several different agents are under investigation for possible future use.

CHEMOPROPHYLAXIS

Chemoprophylaxis with isoniazid remains the main intervention in control policies that rely on the identification of active, infectious TB patients or persons at risk for developing disease (Table 75-7). For prophylactic regimens to be effective, appropriate screening and intervention are essential. Screening programs should target persons at high risk for developing disease:

TABLE 75-7	Chemoprophylaxis
Duration	6 months[1]
Agent	Isoniazid[2,3]
Dose	Adult 300 mg QD Pediatric 10–20 mg/kg QD (maximal dose 300 mg)

Indications	PPD >15 mm and age <35 years
	PPD >10 mm, age <35, and:
	    foreign-born from high-prevalence country;
	    medically underserved low-income populations;
	    resident or staff in long-term care facility (nursing
	      home, correctional institution); or
	    staff member in a school, child or health care facility,
	      etc.
	PPD >10 mm, regardless of age, and:
	    recent (within 2 years) converter[4]; or
	    underlying medical condition associated with an
	      increased risk of TB[5]
	PPD >5 mm, regardless of age, and:
	    HIV positive;
	    close contact of recently diagnosed TB case; or
	    fibrotic lesion on chest x-ray

[1] 9–12 months may be more effective and an additional 3–6 months should be considered for compliant patients in the absence of toxicity; 9-month course for pediatric patients generally recommended; 12-month course for HIV-positive individuals or in the presence of a chest x-ray suggestive of previous old healed TB.

[2] With isoniazid-resistant *M. tuberculosis,* consider rifampin with or without ethambutol for 12 months.

[3] Pyridoxine can prevent or reverse peripheral neuropathy, the second most common adverse reaction associated with INH administration. Primarily indicated for patients with other disease that may predispose them to develop neuropathy (ie, diabetes, uremia, alcoholism, malnutrition) or with a pre-existing peripheral neuropathy.

[4] >15 mm increase if age <35 years.

[5] Diabetes mellitus, prolonged therapy with corticosteroids, immunosuppressive therapy, leukemia, Hodgkin's disease, intravenous drug use, end-stage renal disease, chronic malnutrition (including alcoholism)

- Persons with HIV infection
- Close contacts of known infectious TB patients
- Persons with medical risk factors that may increase the risk of TB once infection has occurred
- Foreign-born persons from high-prevalence countries
- Medically underserved, low-income populations
- Alcoholics and intravenous drug users
- Residents and staff of long-term care facilities (eg, correctional institutions and nursing homes)
- Persons in a setting where disease would pose a hazard to a large number of susceptible persons
- Other populations identified locally as having an increased prevalence of TB.

Failure to institute chemoprophylaxis because of a history of BCG vaccination remains a frequent error in treatment. Historically, health care providers' participation in recommended surveillance programs and adherence to isoniazid prophylaxis has been poor. This will ultimately undermine the efficacy of control programs.

Age and Gender Considerations

Case rates for TB in the United States are highest in nonwhite men. In the United States and other developed countries, TB case rates tend to increase with increasing age, reflecting infec-

TABLE 75-8	Regulatory Approach to Occupational TB Control

Engineering Controls
  Ventilation
  HEPA filtration
  Ultraviolet lights
  Negative-pressure respiratory isolation rooms
  Treatment booths/Local exhaust ventilation devices

Administrative and Work Practice Controls
  Early identification and isolation of suspected or confirmed TB patients
  Respiratory isolation policy and procedures
  Education and training of health care workers
  Employee surveillance and treatment policy and procedures

Personal Protective Equipment
  Particulate respirators

tion acquired years before (*MMWR*, 1992, Hopewell & Bloom, 1994).

Nutritional Considerations

Evidence linking malnutrition and immune system deficiency has been demonstrated in other disease states besides TB. Loss of weight in excess of 10% of ideal body weight has traditionally been considered an independent risk factor for developing TB once a person has been exposed. Weight loss secondary to TB is common at the initial presentation. Basic good nutrition, with nutritional supplementation as indicated, should be encouraged.

Occupational Hazards

Health care workers have long been considered to be a high-risk group for occupational exposure to TB and the development of disease. A great deal of attention has been given to the issue of transmission of TB in the workplace, and guidelines for preventing transmission of *M. tuberculosis* in health care facilities were delineated by the CDC in 1994. The regulatory approach to occupational TB control includes engineering controls, administrative and work-practice controls, and personal protective equipment (Table 75-8) (CDC, 1994; McDiarmid et al, 1996). Protective strategies for health care workers include compliance with surveillance programs for occupational exposure and routine PPD testing programs, vaccination, and chemoprophylaxis, in addition to the use of personal protective equipment. Despite published guidelines and algorithms, lack of institutional and employee compliance with recommended standards and policies will undermine the protection afforded by these measures.

TREATMENT OPTIONS, EXPECTED OUTCOMES, AND COMPREHENSIVE MANAGEMENT

The basic tenets of treatment are relatively simple and straightforward, at least in theory (American Thoracic Society, 1994). To avoid the development of resistance, treatment must include more than one drug to which the organism is sensitive, and it must be continued long enough for infection to be eradicated.

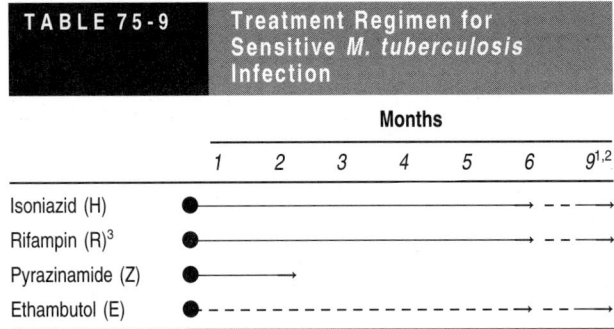

TABLE 75-9 Treatment Regimen for Sensitive *M. tuberculosis* Infection

	Months						
	1	2	3	4	5	6	9[1,2]
Isoniazid (H)	●————————————————→ – – →						
Rifampin (R)[3]	●————————————————→ – – →						
Pyrazinamide (Z)	●————→						
Ethambutol (E)	●– – – – – – – – – – – – –→ – –→						

[1] Intermittent administration of appropriately adjusted doses of drugs after an initial daily phase of treatment equal to daily therapy; intermittent therapy should only be administered via DOT.

[2] Longer course of therapy indicated in HIV-positive patients or treatment regimens not containing Z (ie, pregnancy).

[3] May substitute rifabutin for R in HIV-infected patients to allow concurrent administration of indinavir.

[4] Should add E, or streptomycin, to the initial regimen pending sensitivity testing if rate of H resistance in the community >4%.

Directly observed short-course treatment regimens are outlined in Table 75-9.

The emergence of drug-resistant strains has complicated and prolonged treatment regimens, with an associated increase in morbidity, mortality, and cost (Table 75-10) (Iserman, 1993). Higher rates of treatment failure, relapse, and mortality are known to occur, even in immunocompetent patients. Corticosteroids, surgery, and immunotherapy are important adjuncts in the treatment of select cases of TB.

Comprehensive Management Recommendations

TB is an infectious disease with significant public health implications. Control of TB requires political commitment worldwide and adequate funding to support TB control programs. TB is a preventable and curable disease, but it remains the most lethal infectious disease worldwide, accounting for more than 3 million deaths in 1995, higher than at any other time in history.

Identification, appropriate isolation, and the institution of effective chemotherapy to patients with active disease remains the cornerstone of TB control. Investigation of newly diagnosed cases and secondary prophylaxis for persons infected and at risk for developing TB are integral parts of control programs (Fig. 75-1).

TABLE 75-10 Second-Line Agents for Use in Multidrug-Resistant TB

Streptomycin	Ofloxacin
Kanamycin	Ciprofloxacin
Capreomycin	Amikacin
Para-aminosalicylic acid	Rifabutin
Ethionamide	Clofazimine
Cycloserine	Amoxicillin
Thiacetazone	Rifapentine

Generally none toxic and less efficacious than first-line agents.

TEACHING AND SELF-CARE

Patients should routinely be educated in a culturally sensitive manner regarding their diagnosis, the means by which disease is spread, the need for prolonged therapy, and the consequences of incomplete therapy for themselves and their families and community. Currently, directly observed therapy should be offered to all patients. This does not replace patient education but does provide a means for earlier detection of a nonadherent patient.

The success of TB treatment requires proper medication management and excellent patient participation. Because most treatment regimens last at least 6 months, strategies to encourage full patient commitment for the duration of treatment are crucial. If prophylactic treatment is advised, the risks and benefits should be thoroughly discussed. When a patient has active disease, a discussion regarding contagion, length of treatment, need for following a strict medication regimen, and minimizing side effects should occur at diagnosis.

Adequate rest and fluid intake should be encouraged. Fatigue is common but should improve gradually with treatment. Patients should be discouraged from drinking alcohol because it can increase the risk of hepatotoxicity associated with some anti-TB medications.

Indigent and homeless patients pose specific self-care challenges and require the expertise of the local health department's tuberculosis control programs. Immediate referral at the time of diagnosis is urged. Often such patients require directly observed therapy. They might benefit from incentives such as meal vouchers or bus tokens.

Patients should be warned about harmless but possibly distressing side effects of medications, such as tearing with rifampin or orange-colored urine or stool. Patients should consult their providers before taking other medications.

Rehabilitation

In general, TB is a treatable disease, with full recovery expected. In cases of multidrug-resistant TB, treatment regimens are generally more complex, longer in duration, more toxic, and less efficacious. If pulmonary disease is either extensive or locally destructive, as in the case of spinal TB or central nervous system disease, long-term disability may result. Prevention and early diagnosis and treatment of active disease have the potential to reduce the likelihood of long-term sequelae.

COMMUNITY RESOURCES

Local health departments can provide information regarding local TB clinics or other health care facilities that provide treatment for patients with TB. Many areas have community-based organizations that serve immigrant communities by providing educational materials, support groups, and referrals to health care facilities. Treatment for TB should be provided regardless of the ability to pay, including free medications for the duration of therapy if needed.

REFERRAL POINTS AND CLINICAL WARNINGS

TB is a reportable disease, and all newly diagnosed cases should be reported to the local health department. Treatment should be initiated and supervised by staff with expertise in the treat-

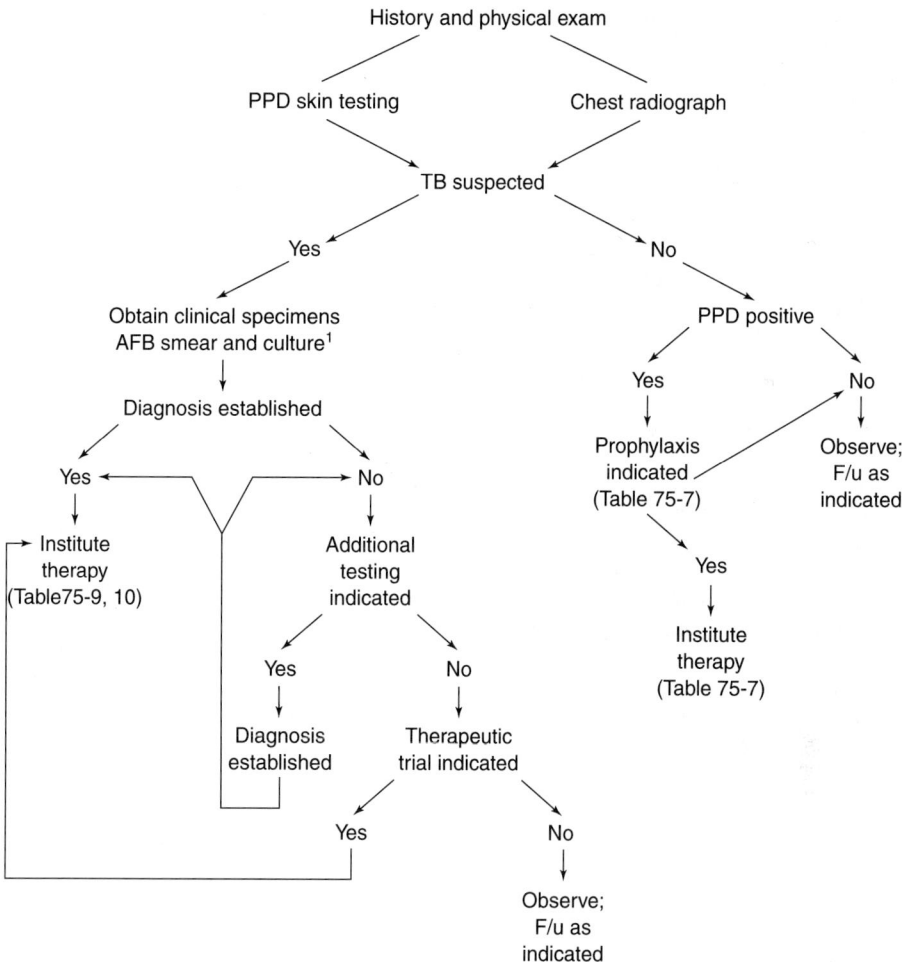

FIGURE 75-1 [1]Sputum × 3, blood, other as indicated; See Table 75-6.

ment of TB. Effective treatment requires the correct and consistent use of medications and a mechanism to ensure that patients follow the prescribed therapeutic regimen. Directly observed therapy should be offered to everyone diagnosed with TB and should be required for patients who do not adhere to therapy. More restrictive measures may need to be considered if a patient does not adhere to the recommended treatment plan. The legitimacy of limiting a person's autonomy to prevent harm to another is well recognized, and although infectious TB patients have been the focus of most control measures, the need to treat patients beyond the period of infectiousness, until cure, has been acknowledged. The nature of the interventions required or desirable to achieve the goal of treatment until cure is not clearly defined. Policies that address the need for local municipalities to provide shelter and psychiatric or drug and alcohol abuse treatment require ongoing evaluation and development, as does the use of inducements, enablers, and ultimately court orders and incarceration (Bayer, 1995; Efferen, 1997b).

Failure of cultures to become negative after 2 months, a high background incidence of multidrug-resistant disease, or a history of previous nonadherence to therapy should alert health care providers to the possibility of multidrug-resistant disease, and treatment regimens should be adjusted accordingly. Failure of the patient to follow recommended therapy or the presence

of adverse drug reactions should initiate a re-evaluation of the treatment regimen.

Significant drug interactions can occur with many of the commonly prescribed anti-TB medications, and a complete medication review should be undertaken when therapy is initiated and periodically thereafter. Rifampin specifically alters the metabolism of numerous drugs, including oral contraceptives, coumadin, digitalis, methadone, and protease inhibitors (antiretroviral agents) among others. Treatment regimens or dosing may need to be adjusted during TB therapy.

FUNGAL INFECTIONS

Linda S. Efferen, MD, FACP, FCCP

Fungal organisms infect the respiratory system through direct inhalation or hematogenous dissemination. The organisms causing histoplasmosis, blastomycosis, and coccidioidomycosis are soil-dwelling and dimorphic (they change form within the mammalian host) and are endemic to North America as well as other areas. Paracoccidioidomycosis, also caused by a soil-dwelling dimorphic organism, is endemic to South America.

Cryptococcosis is caused by a monomorphic organism and has a worldwide distribution. Although inhalation is the route of infection, most clinical cases of cryptococcosis present as chronic meningitis rather than pulmonary infection because of the particular neurotropism of the organism.

Aspergillosis and mucormycosis are caused by soil organisms, occur worldwide, have very low virulence, and usually cause infection only in patients with defective phagocytic function. Likewise, candidiasis, caused by an organism that is part of the normal human flora, is likely to occur only in patients with abnormalities of T-cell function, phagocytosis, or mucosal barriers.

ANATOMY, PHYSIOLOGY, AND PATHOLOGY

The lung is usually the initial and primary site of systemic fungal infection via inhalation of aerosolized environmental fungal forms. Once in the lungs, infection may either be contained by host defense mechanisms or disseminate through the lymphatic system or bloodstream. With *Candida albicans,* an extrapulmonary infection may result in fungemia, and the lungs may be seeded secondarily.

The inhaled infectious organisms elicit an inflammatory reaction, demonstrated by neutrophil and fibrin accumulation within alveolar spaces, resulting in consolidation of lung parenchyma. At this stage, fungal forms can be seen microscopically, highlighted by special stains. Fungal organisms may proliferate and enter the lymphatic system and drain to hilar lymph nodes. Over time, host defenses in immunocompetent persons develop cell-mediated immunity that will contain the infectious process. Necrotizing granulomas result from the accumulation of cells that destroy both fungal organisms and the surrounding tissue. The inflammatory response in candidal infections is predominantly neutrophilic, but granulomatous reactions can occur. In cases of overwhelming infection, diffuse alveolar damage may be seen.

Disseminated fungal infections may cause a miliary pattern, reflecting hematogenous dissemination. Unresolved infections may result in a chronic progressive form of disease with parenchymal destruction characterized by interstitial fibrosis, granulomatous inflammation, cavitation, or bronchiectasis. *Aspergillus* and *Mucor* may cause an invasive form of infection in immunocompromised patients (Davies & Sarosi, 1994; CDC, 1996a; Efferen, 1997a).

EPIDEMIOLOGY

Aspergillus, Mucor, and *Candida* are ubiquitous organisms that rarely cause disease in the absence of impaired host defense mechanisms. *Cryptococcus* is known to occur worldwide. Endemic areas for *Histoplasma, Blastomyces, Coccidioides,* and *Paracoccidioides* are shown in Table 75-11 (Davies, 1994; CDC, 1996a; Efferen, 1997a).

DIAGNOSTIC CRITERIA

The demonstration of fungus in biologic materials, either in culture or on histopathologic exam, in association with an appropriate clinical illness, is the diagnostic gold standard.

HISTORY AND PHYSICAL EXAM

The history and physical exam of patients with endemic fungal infections are generally nonspecific. Symptoms may resemble influenza, with an abrupt onset of fever, chills, and chest discomfort. Some patients demonstrate signs of lung consolidation on auscultation of the chest or present with erythema nodosum if they are infected with histoplasmosis, blastomycosis, or coccidioidomycosis.

Cryptococcal disease may develop in immunocompetent persons but is more common in patients with AIDS, organ transplants, or Hodgkin's disease, or in patients receiving corticosteroid therapy. Symptomatic cryptococcal pulmonary disease is uncommon. Meningitis is the most common clinical manifestation of cryptococcosis. Meningeal involvement may present as a subacute or fulminant illness. Cranial nerve palsies and symptoms of hydrocephalus may be present.

Aspergillosis causes several distinct clinical syndromes, including hypersensitivity pneumonitis, allergic bronchopulmonary aspergillosis, mycetomas, chronic necrotizing pulmonary aspergillosis, and invasive aspergillosis. Allergic bronchopulmonary aspergillosis presents as a characteristic complex of fleeting radiographic infiltrates, wheezing, fever, eosinophilia, and expectoration of brownish plugs. In general, it is characterized by exacerbations and remissions; occasional patients develop chronic respiratory failure. Patients should be closely monitored for evidence of disease exacerbation and treated early.

Aspergillomas are frequently asymptomatic. Patients may present with hemoptysis, which may be life-threatening. Acute

TABLE 75-11	Epidemiology of Fungal Infections	
Infection	**Organism**	**Epidemiology**
Histoplasmosis	*Histoplasma capsulatum*	Endemic midwest and south-central U.S.
Blastomycosis	*Blastomyces dermatitidis*	Endemic central, south-central, and southeast U.S.
Coccidioidomycosis	*Coccidioides immitis*	Endemic southwest U.S.
Paracoccidioidomycosis	*Paracoccidioides braziliensis*	Endemic South America, Central America, and southern Mexico
Cryptococcosis	*Cryptococcus neoformans*	Worldwide
Aspergillosis	*Aspergillus* genus[1]	Ubiquitous saprophytic mold
Mucormycosis	*Mucor, Rhizopus, Absidia* genera	Ubiquitous fungi
Candidiasis	*Candida albicans*	Ubiquitous; normal human flora

[1] Greater than 95% of human illness is caused by *A. fumigatus.*

invasive aspergillosis typically mimics an acute bacterial pneumonia and may be difficult to diagnose.

Both aspergillomas and chronic necrotizing pulmonary aspergillosis occur in patients with underlying lung disease. This may complicate the clinical course or limit the therapeutic options for treatment of the fungal infection. Acute invasive aspergillosis occurs almost exclusively in immunocompromised persons. Early and aggressive treatment may result in cure, but the prognosis is poor.

Mucormycosis and systemic candidiasis similarly occur almost exclusively in immunocompromised persons. Pulmonary mucormycosis usually begins as an acute pneumonia and may progress to hemoptysis and pulmonary infarction and systemic spread to other organs. Candidiasis of the lungs is nonspecific in its clinical presentation, and the diagnosis is often made after death. Positive blood cultures in a patient who is immunocompromised and febrile should be considered presumptive evidence of systemic candidiasis.

DIAGNOSTIC STUDIES

Diagnostic tools that may assist in establishing the diagnosis are listed in Table 75-12. Chest radiographs for the endemic fungal infections are generally nonspecific, and a clinical suspicion for fungal disease is suggested by a history of exposure in an endemic area. Establishing the diagnosis of ubiquitous fungi requires correlation of culture results with the clinical picture. Histopathologic demonstration of tissue invasion is required to prove candidal pneumonia (CDC, 1996a; Efferen, 1997a; Conference Report, 1996).

TREATMENT OPTIONS, EXPECTED OUTCOMES, AND COMPREHENSIVE MANAGEMENT
Health Promotion and Specific Protection

It is often impossible to avoid exposure to fungi, given their ubiquitous nature. In endemic areas where exposure is likely, attempts to avoid or limit inhalation of the mycelia or spores may decrease the likelihood of developing serious disease. Immunocompetent persons may occasionally develop severe, progressive, and potentially life-threatening forms of infection after exposure to endemic fungi. However, immunocompromised persons are at a higher risk for infection from endemic fungi, as well as infection from normally nonpathogenic fungi such as *Mucor* and *Candida*. Efforts to control underlying medical conditions such as diabetes mellitus, iatrogenic immunosup-

TABLE 75-12	Diagnostic Studies			
Infection	Specimens & Technique	Skin Test	Exoantigen Test	Serologic Tests
Histoplasmosis	Sputum, PDH[1] and HIV disease—bone marrow, blood culture; smear, histopathologic examination, culture	y		CF[2], ID[3], RIA[4], antibody or antigen assays
Blastomycosis	10% KOH[5] ingestion of sputum or pus, cytologic or histologic examination, culture	N[a]	y	CF, EIA[6], agar gel double diffusion
Coccidioidomycosis	Direct examination sputum or pus after 10% KOH or staining, histopathologic examination, culture	y	y	TP[7] for IgM antibody, latex particle agglutination test, ID, CF
Paracoccidioidomycosis	Direct exam sputum or tissue after 10% KOH, histopathologic examination, culture[b]	y		CF, agar gel immunodiffusion
Cryptococcosis	Sputum not diagnostic—fungus frequently colonizes airways; CNS culture or latex particle agglutination for antigen, histopathologic examination			Antigen assays
Aspergillosis	APBA[8] clinical criteria: asthma, blood eosinophil count >1000/mm,[3] cutaneous reaction to *Aspergillus* antigen, precipitating antibody to A. antigen, increased total serum IgE and IgG antibody vs A., recurrent pulmonary infiltrates & central bronchiectasis	y		See clinical criteria
	Aspergilloma—radiographic presentation, culture of expectorated sputum	y		Precipitating antibody
	CNPA[9]—culture, histopathologic examination	y		RIA, CIE, EIA[c]
	Invasive—sputum culture may be false +; nasal swab culture; histopathologic examination			
Mucormycosis	Culture, histopathologic examination	N		N
Candidiasis	Histopathologic demonstration of tissue invasion			N

[1] PDH = progressive disseminated histoplasmosis
[2] CF = complement fixation
[3] ID = immunodiffusion
[4] RIA = radioimmunoassay
[5] KOH = potassium hydroxide
[6] EIA = enzyme immunoassay
[7] TP = tube precipitin
[8] ABPA = allergic bronchopulmonary aspergillosis
[9] CNPA = chronic necrotizing pulmonary aspergillosis

[a] Blastomycin skin test limited to investigational purposes
[b] Hazardous to lab personnel
[c] Not established in clinical care

pressive states, or HIV infections may reduce the risk of disseminated or serious disease.

Early Diagnosis, Prompt Treatment, and Disability Limitation

Many patients with acute histoplasmosis, blastomycosis, coccidioidomycosis, and paracoccidioidomycosis are asymptomatic or have self-limiting disease that requires no treatment. For persons presenting with persistent or progressive symptoms or acute overwhelming disease, attempts to establish the diagnosis and institute therapy should be prompt and aggressive to limit morbidity and mortality.

Rehabilitation

Disseminated fungal infections occur more frequently in persons with severe underlying disease, and recovery may require a significant period of convalescence. Both physical and occupational therapy may be employed during the recovery period. Underlying illnesses should be treated aggressively to improve overall function and to limit susceptibility to fungal infection.

Occupational Hazards

Numerous occupations have been identified with an increased risk of exposure to various fungi, especially occupations necessitating close contact with the earth in endemic areas. Agricultural and forestry workers have an increased incidence of paracoccidioidomycosis and blastomycosis, respectively. Construction workers, farm laborers, and workers on archaeologic digs in areas with contaminated soil are at risk for coccidioidomycosis. Similarly, *Histoplasma* contaminates bird and bat droppings, and disturbance of contaminated areas may lead to infection.

 CLINICAL WARNING: Invasive pulmonary aspergillosis, mucormycosis, and systemic candidiasis are potentially life-threatening infections and should be diagnosed and treated emergently.

Treatment Options

Most endemic fungal infections are self-limiting and require no specific therapy. Therapeutic options for persistent, progressive, or severe disease include oral azoles or intravenous ampho-

---

TABLE 75-13	**Clinical Manifestations and Treatment Options**	
Infection	**Clinical Spectrum of Disease**	**Treatment**
Histoplasmosis	Self-limited URI,[1] chronic pulmonary disease, ARDS,[2] PDH[3]	Spontaneous resolution—none; chronic pulmonary disease—oral azoles;[a] ARDS or PDH—AMB[4,b]
Blastomycosis	Influenza-like illness,[c] progressive pulmonary infection,[d] ARDS; extrapulmonary spread	Spontaneous resolution—none; pulmonary or nonmeningeal extrapulmonary—oral anzoles;[a] rapidly progressive or meningeal involvement—AMB[b]
Coccidioidomycosis	Influenza-like illness, occasionally progressive disease, persistent infection	Spontaneous resolution—none; CNS involvement—fluconazole or AMB; ARDS or CD4 count <200—AMB
Paracoccidioidomycosis	Self-limited infection, progressive pneumonia, disseminated disease	Progressive or disseminated disease—oral azoles; critically ill or failed oral therapy—AMB
Cryotococcosis	Self-limited URI, disseminated disease, CNS infection	Isolated pulmonary involvement—oral azoles,[e] meningitis—AMB[b] + 5-flucytosine
Aspergillosis	ABPA,[5] aspergilloma, CNPA,[6] invasive	ABPA—corticosteroids +/− itraconazole; aspergilloma—(BAE[7] or surgery,[f] oral azoles,[g] AMB;[g] CNPA—itraconazole or AMB; invasive—AMB
Mucormycosis	Rhinocerebral or pulmonary mucormycosis	AMB
Candidiasis	Mucocutaneous, candidemia, disseminated candidiasis	Mucocutaneous candidiasis—fluconazole; candidemia—removal of contaminated vascular access lines, fluconazole and/or AMB; disseminated—oral azoles, AMB +/− 5-flucytosine

[1] URI = upper respiratory infection
[2] ARDS = acute respiratory distress syndrome
[3] PDH = progressive disseminated histoplasmosis
[4] AMB = amphotericin B
[5] ABPA = allergic bronchopulmonary aspergillosis
[6] CNPA = chronic necrotizing pulmonary aspergillosis
[7] BAE = bronchial artery embolization

[a] itracomasole preferred
[b] can change to oral azoles once stable
[c] more severe than histoplasmosis
[d] more frequent than histoplasmosis
[e] fluconazole
[f] for life-threatening hemoptysis
[g] case reports, small series

tericin (Table 75-13) (CDC, 1990; Hopewell & Bloom, 1994). Amphotericin B, long considered the standard antifungal therapy, has the potential to cause significant side effects and toxicity, including fever, rigors, hypotension, and nephrotoxicity. Newer formulations of amphotericin B have decreased the risk of nephrotoxicity but still require intravenous administration.

Oral triazole antifungal agents, itraconazole and fluconazole, have a longer half-life, fewer adverse effects, and a broader spectrum of activity than the older imidazole agents, miconazole and ketoconazole. The triazoles have a broad spectrum of activity against endemic mycoses and opportunistic fungal infections, with the exception of mucormycosis and non-albicans *Candida*. However, amphotericin B remains the drug of choice in severe life-threatening infections until the patient is clinically stable.

Itraconazole is especially useful in the treatment of chronic necrotizing pulmonary aspergillosis, progressive disseminated histoplasmosis, pulmonary blastomycosis, and other chronic infections where long-term therapy is required. However, significant drug interactions occur with oral azoles. These include:

- Life-threatening cardiac arrhythmias with the coadministration of terfenadine, astemizole, or cisapride
- Enhanced metabolism of itraconazole, leading to treatment failure with the coadministration of rifampin, phenytoin, phenobarbital, and carbamazepine
- Fluconazole and itraconazole can increase the anticoagulant effect of warfarin and the hypoglycemic effect of oral hypoglycemic agents.

Comprehensive Management Recommendations

The clinical spectrum of disease secondary to endemic fungal infections ranges from asymptomatic infection to severe life-threatening disease. Differentiation of fungal infections from other infectious etiologies such as bacterial or mycobacterial disease or malignancy is important.

The need to institute therapy depends on the patient's symptoms and underlying health status. Management of any condition that predisposes to the development of fungal infections or that limits the ability to eradicate the infection is imperative. The duration of therapy is based at least in part on response to therapy. Treatment of opportunistic fungal infections is usually indicated (see Table 75-13).

TEACHING AND SELF-CARE

Patient education should target management issues of fungal infection. Potential drug toxicities and interactions and the need for relatively long-term therapy are especially important issues.

COMMUNITY RESOURCES

In endemic areas, local health departments can provide the locations of health care facilities or clinics capable of treating suspected endemic mycoses. For patients with diabetes mellitus, HIV infection, or other systemic illnesses that predispose them to severe disease, support groups may exist at the national or local level.

REFERRAL POINTS AND CLINICAL WARNINGS

In general, asymptomatic persons infected with endemic fungal organisms do not require further assessment. The exception is for those who are asymptomatically infected and have an abnormal chest radiograph, where a diagnosis of malignancy is being considered. All patients with cryptococcal disease require lumbar puncture to assess for the presence of meningitis and need for treatment. Anyone with persistent or progressive symptoms should be urgently evaluated and treated if indicated.

EDITOR'S NOTE:
COMPLEMENTARY APPROACHES

A general discussion of complementary approaches can be found in Chapter 3. The following, while not an exhaustive list, are some complementary approaches being used for this condition. Additional information on these approaches, including precautions, can be found in Appendices A and B. Providers need to assess for the use of complementary approaches as part of the patient's history, as they may impact conventional therapies, and patients may not volunteer this information unless specifically asked. Efficacy of many complementary approaches is not as well documented as that of conventional therapies. Providers need to read the literature before suggesting these complementary approaches.

- Vitamins, minerals, herbs, supplements
  Zinc
- Complementary Modalities
  Aromatherapy

References

(1996). Fungus disease of the chest. *Seminars in Roentgenology, 31*(1), 1–83.

(1993). Guidelines for the initial management of adults with community-acquired pneumonia: Diagnosis, assessment of severity, and initial antimicrobial therapy. *American Review of Respiratory Disease, 148,* 1418–1426.

American Thoracic Society & Centers for Disease Control. (1994). Treatment of tuberculosis and tuberculosis infection in adults and children. *American Journal of Respiratory and Critical Care Medicine, 149,* 1359–1374.

Bartlett, J.G., & Mundy, L.M. (1995). Community-acquired pneumonia. *N Engl J Med, 333,* 1618–1624.

Bayer, R., Dupuis, L. (1997). Tuberculosis, public health and civil liberties. *Ann Rev Public Health 16:*307–326.

Centers for Disease Control. (1990). Tuberculosis among foreign-born persons entering the United States. *MMWR 39* (RR18):1–13.

Centers for Disease Control. (1992). Prevention and control of tuberculosis in U.S. communities with at-risk minority populations. *MMWR 41* (RR5):1–11.

Centers for Disease Control. (1994). Guidelines for preventing the transmission of *Mycobacterium tuberculosis* in health care facilities, 1994. *MMWR 43* (RR13):1–132.

Centers for Disease Control. (1996b). The role of BCG vaccine in the prevention and control of tuberculosis in the United States. *MMWR CDC Surveill Summ 45:*1–18.

Centers for Disease Control. (1996a). Tuberculosis morbidity: United States, 1995. *MMWR CDC Surveill Summ 45:*365–370.

Conference Report. 1996. The American Lung Association conference on re-establishing control of tuberculosis in the United States. *Am J Respir Crit Care Med, 154*:251–262.

Davies, S.F. (1994). Fungal pneumonia. *Medical Clinics of North America, 78,* 1049–1065.

Davies, S.F., & Sarosi, G.A. (1994). Fungal infections. In J.F. Murray & J.A. Nadel (Eds.). *Textbook of respiratory medicine.* Philadelphia: W. B. Saunders.

Efferen, L.S. (1997). Tuberculosis update: Will good news become bad news? *Current Opinion in Pulmonary Medicine, 3,* 131–138.

Efferen, L.S. (1997). In pursuit of tuberculosis control: Civil liberty vs public health. *Chest 112*:5–6.

Hammond, J.M., Potgieter, P.D. (1995). The etiology and antimicrobial susceptibility patterns of microorganisms in acute community-acquired lung abscess. *Chest, 108*(4), 937–941.

Hopewell, P.C., & Bloom, B.R. (1994). Tuberculosis and other mycobacterial diseases. In J.F. Murray & J.A. Nadel (Eds.). *Textbook of respiratory medicine.* Philadelphia: W.B. Saunders.

Iseman, M.D. (1993). Treatment of multidrug-resistant tuberculosis. *N Engl J Med, 329,* 784–791.

Kauffman, C.A. (1996). Role of azoles in antifungal therapy. *Clinics in Infectious Disease, 22*(Suppl. 2), S148–153.

Klein, N.C., & Cunha, B.A. (1996). New antifungal drugs for pulmonary mycoses. *Chest, 110,* 525–532.

Marie, T.J. (1994). Community-acquired pneumonia. *Clinics in Infectious Disease, 18,* 501–515.

(1995a). *MMWR*, Oct. 30, *44*(41), 782.

(1995b). *MMWR*, Jul. 21, *44*(28), 535–537.

McDiarmid, M., Gamponia M.J., Ryan, M.A.K., Hirshon, J.M., Gillen N.A., Cox, M. (1996)Tuberculosis in the workplace: OSHA's compliance experience. *Infect Control Hosp Epidemiol 17*:159–169.

New York City Department of Health, Bureau of Tuberculosis Control. (1997). *Protease inhibitors and anti-tuberculosis treatment.* TB Fact Sheet 2i. TB219.

Niederman, M.S., Sarosi, G.A., & Glassroth, J. (1994). *Respiratory infections: A scientific basis for management.* Philadelphia: W.B. Saunders.

Pennington, J.E. (1994). *Respiratory infections: Diagnosis and management.* New York: Raven Press.

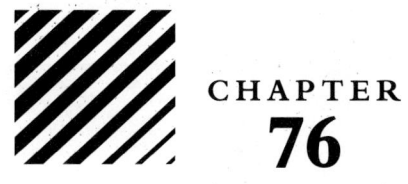

CHAPTER
76

Occupational Lung Disease

Pamela Sass, MD

Primary care providers are in a key position to prevent, identify, and treat occupational illness. First, providers can identify persons at risk of occupational illness because of exposure to a known occupational hazard. Second, primary care providers who care for a multitude of undifferentiated illnesses are also in a position to link an illness and occupational exposure.

The types of occupational pulmonary disorders are listed in Table 76-1. Two of these diseases, occupational asthma and asbestosis, can be adequately diagnosed and treated only if the primary care provider suspects occupational pulmonary disease and elicits a history of a significant workplace exposure.

Occupational asthma is a relatively common medical condition, but the diagnosis could be easily missed without establishing a link between symptoms and the workplace. Asbestosis, an interstitial disease related to asbestos exposure, becomes symptomatic only after a long latency period. An exposure history and knowledge of the early signs and symptoms are essential to diagnose this disease.

The true incidence and prevalence of occupational illness and injury is not known. The annual cost of occupational disease in the United States has been estimated at more than $6 billion (Campos-Outcalt, 1994).

To identify occupationally related disease, primary care providers must maintain a high degree of suspicion and have the following:

- Familiarity with the basic principles of occupational and environmental medicine
- Ability to take an occupational and environmental history
- Understanding of the worker's compensation system
- Awareness of the ethical, legal, and social implications of occupational and environmental-related conditions
- Knowledge of when and how to report hazards to public health and regulatory authorities (Campos-Outcalt, 1994).

Figure 76-1 outlines an initial clinical approach to the recognition of illness caused by occupational exposure. Table 76-2 lists the essential elements of an occupational history.

Workers in small and medium-sized companies may be at higher risk for exposure to occupational hazards because their employers are less likely to know the characteristics of hazardous substances in use (Sattler, 1992). Immigrant workers and others paid lower wages may also be at higher risk for exposure to hazards; there is a relation between low pay and dangerous working conditions (Robinson, 1986).

OCCUPATIONAL ASTHMA

Anatomy, Physiology, and Pathology

Occupational asthma can be defined as a variable airflow limitation caused by a specific agent in the workplace. It can be caused by either allergic or nonallergic injury or inflammation and is manifested by specific or nonspecific airway hyperresponsiveness (Bates et al, 1992). Allergic occupational asthma develops after a period of allergic sensitization to a substance found at work over a period of months to years and is characterized by intermittent airflow limitation. Although the respiratory symptoms are variable, they always occur at work.

Nonallergic occupational asthma is usually the result of high-level exposures to an irritant gas, fume, aerosol, or vapor. It develops without a latency period and is distinguished by persistent nonspecific airway hyperresponsiveness. Although this nonallergic bronchospasm is referred to as reactive airway dysfunction syndrome, it is not true asthma, even though clinically it presents in a similar fashion (Chan-Yeung, 1990).

Epidemiology

Estimates of the prevalence of occupational asthma have ranged between 2% and 15% of all asthmatic adults. The prevalence within industries varies widely and is determined by the agents used in the workplace. The prevalence within a particular industry depends on the type, source, and concentration of the agent, as well as conditions at the workplace (Bates et al, 1992).

Diagnostic Criteria

The task of the primary care provider is twofold. The first is to diagnose asthma, which may present with varied, atypical symptoms such as chest discomfort, cough, or easy fatigability rather than wheezing and breathlessness (Cullen, 1990). The second task is to connect symptomatic episodes to the workplace.

A sound connection to the workplace can be made with serial peak flow measurements at home and work. Another strategy is to perform the "stop–resume" work test, in which the patient measures and records peak flow rates every 2 hours while awake both at home and work. The record should be kept for at least 2 to 3 weeks at work and then for 10 days off work. A graph of the daily maximum, minimum, and mean peak flows is inspected for deterioration at work and improvement away from work (Alberts & Brooks, 1992). If it is not possible to monitor peak flow rates in this detailed way, the patient should be removed from work for 1 to 2 weeks and then carefully monitored for symptoms on return.

Materials in the workplace that are linked to asthma are listed in Table 76-3. There are many agents causing occupational asthma, and new agents are identified every year. If occupational asthma is suspected and a causative agent cannot be identified, an occupational medicine specialist may perform skin

TABLE 76-1	Occupational Pulmonary Disorders

Occupational asthma

Asthma due to allergic sensitization

Other forms of occupational asthma

Pneumoconiosis

Silicosis

Asbestosis

Talcosis

Coal workers' pneumoconiosis

Mixed dust fibrosis

Berylliosis

Hard metal disease

Nonspecific airway disease

Hypersensitivity pneumonitis (extrinsic allergic alveolitis)

Inhaled toxic gases

Respiratory tract cancer

Occupationally linked pulmonary infections

testing, immunologic studies, and bronchial inhalation challenges.

History and Physical Exam

Any adult presenting with new-onset asthma should be evaluated for occupational asthma. The medical history for these patients is detailed in Table 76-4. The primary care provider should look for aggravating agents in the workplace and should attempt to elicit a relation between symptoms and work. Occupational factors that worsen the symptoms of a patient with stable pre-existing asthma should also be sought.

The physical exam should focus on the respiratory tract and skin (see Chap. 72). Rhinitis, nasal polyps, hyperinflation of

TABLE 76-2	Essential Elements of the Occupational History and Questionnaire

Current or Most Recent Work and Exposure History
Job title; type of industry; name of employer
Year work started and year work finished (if not currently employed)
Description of job (what is a typical workday), especially the parts of the job the patient believes may be potentially hazardous
Current work hours and any shift changes
Current exposure to dust, fumes, radiation, chemicals biologic hazards, or physical hazards
Protective equipment used (clothes, safety glasses, hearing protection, respirator, or gloves)
Other employees at the workplace who have similar health problems

Earlier Employment History
Job chronology, working backward from the current or most recent job
The same information as above for each job previously held

Major Types of Exposure Associated With Clinical Illness

Gases	Plastics
Corrosive substances (acids, alkalis)	Solvents
Dyes and stains	Petrochemicals (coal, tar, asphalt,
Dusts and powders	petroleum distillates)
Asbestos, other fibers	Physical factors (noise, lifting,
Infectious agents	thermal stress, vibration, repetitive
Insecticides and pesticides	motion)
Metals and metal fumes	Emotional factors (stress)
Organic dusts (cotton, wood,	Radiation (electromagnetic fields, x-
biologic matter)	ray radiation, ultraviolet radiation)

(Newman, Lee S. (1995). Occupational Illness. New England Journal of Medicine. Volume 333, No. 17:1128–1134.)

the lungs, and a prolonged expiratory phase should be noted. Eczema may suggest the presence of atopy.

Diagnostic Studies

All patients with new onset of asthma-like symptoms should receive a chest radiograph and pulmonary function tests. Other testing was listed in Diagnostic Criteria section.

1. The Quick Survey

Chief Symptom and History of Present Illness
- "What kind of work do you do?"
- "Do you think your health problems are related to your work?"
- "Are your symptoms better or worse when you're at home or at work?"

Review of Systems
- "Are you now or have you previously been exposed to dusts, fumes, chemicals, radiation, or loud noise?"

2. Detailed Questioning Based on Initial Suspicion

Self-Administered Questionnaire for all Patients (Table 76-2)
- Chronology of jobs
- Exposure survey

Review of Exposure. with the Questionnaire as a Guide
- More about the current job: description of a typical day
- Review of job chronology and associated exposures

Examination of the Link between Work and the Chief Symptom
- Clinical clues (Table 76-2)
- Exploration of the temporal link in detail
- "Do others at work have similar problems?"

FIGURE 76-1 The Initial Clinical Approach to the Recognition of Illness Caused by Occupational Exposure. (Newman, Lee S. (1995). Occupational Illness. New England Journal of Medicine. Volume 333, No. 17:1128–1134.)

TABLE 76-3	Materials Causally Linked to Asthma in the Workplace

Vegetable Material	Animal Material
Grain dust	Danders
Flour	Insects
Fig plants	Silkworm larva
Wood dust	Shellfish
Seaweed	Excreta (pigs, chickens)
Green coffee beans	Fish feed
Fungal spores	Animal enzymes
Gum tragacanth	**Metals**
Castor bean	Stainless steel
Tea	Galvanized steel
Tobacco	Aluminum fluoride
Flax	Vanadium
Hemp	Cobalt
Cotton	Tungsten carbide (cobalt)
Hops	Platinum salts
Bacterial enzymes	Nickel
Colophony	Chromium
Plastics/Chemicals	**Pharmaceuticals**
Acid anhydrides	Penicillins
Epoxy resins	Cephalosporins
Diisocyanates (TDI, MDI, HDU)	Piperazine
Persulfate salts	Psyllium
Paraphenylene diamine	Methyldopa
Phthalic anhydride	Spiramycin
Dimethyl ethananolamine	Tetracycline
Azobisformamide	Amprolium
Azodicarbonamide	Cimetidine
Formaldehyde	Isoniazid
Ethylenediamine	Phenylglycine
Acrylates	
Henna	

Cullen, M. Clinical surveillance and management of occupational asthma. Tertiary prevention by the primary practitioner. CHEST, Vol. 98, p. 5.

Treatment Options, Expected Outcomes, and Comprehensive Management

Occupational asthma is treated the same way as is asthma that is not related to the workplace. However, in occupational asthma, an additional goal is to eliminate exposure to the causative agent. If this is not possible, exposure should be minimized.

For patients with occupational asthma secondary to sensitization, removal from the work environment is strongly recommended because even minute exposures to the offending agent may cause fatal bronchospasm (Bates et al, 1992). Worsening asthma is an indication that immediate removal is necessary. Even after removal from the workplace, a patient may continue to be symptomatic from asthma for an indefinite period of time (Chan-Yeung & Malo, 1995).

Recovery from occupational asthma is most likely among patients who initially present with:

- Shorter duration of symptoms before diagnosis
- Relatively normal pulmonary function tests
- A lesser degree of bronchial responsiveness (Alberts & Brooks, 1992).

PREVENTION

In patients who have developed asthma, preventive actions include eliminating exposure to other respiratory irritants such as dusts and cigarette smoke. Medical therapy for asthma should be maximized. Patients with chronic disease should receive annual influenza vaccination and the pneumococcal vaccine.

COMPREHENSIVE RECOMMENDATIONS

Providers who suspect potential exposure to substances linked to asthma can assist the patient by:

- Requesting from the employer Material Data Safety Sheets (MSDS) under the "Right to Know" laws. These sheets are prepared by the manufacturers and include information such as the chemical name, special handling needed, and precautions and hazards.
- Referring the patient to the local department of health, school of public health, or university- or hospital-based occupational medicine referral center.
- Inquiring if the worksite is unionized. The union may be able to offer assistance in minimizing exposure.
- Recommending that the patient consider filing a complaint with the Occupational Safety & Health Administration (OSHA).

The patient may need to find employment in another worksite or in another occupation. The economic and social impacts of this change may result in substantial hardship. Some occupational referral centers have an interdisciplinary team of occupational hygienists, social workers, and occupational physicians to assist the patient in this situation. These specialists can help to facilitate a change in the current workplace, help the patient receive benefits from the worker's compensation system, or help the patient obtain other sources of income. They may also be able to facilitate job training if a change of occupation is recommended.

Many states have laws that mandate provider reporting of various occupational illnesses. The occurrence of occupational asthma (and many other occupational diseases) may be a sentinel event leading to the identification of a hazardous setting, thereby preventing illness in other workers. However, the requirements for reporting are not uniform, and local regulations should be checked with regional health departments (Centers for Disease Control, 1990).

OSHA sets standards for health and safety in the workplace, investigates compliance, and issues citations for violations of safety standards. This agency may be contacted by either the patient or provider for an inspection of the worksite.

Based on OSHA regulations, the patient with occupational disease may be entitled to worker's compensation or legal action. Because some cases are brought to litigation, legal help may be sought, especially if the worker's compensation claim is contested by the employer. Although the worker's compensation system is a no-fault system and workers do not have the right to sue the employer for damages, workers may sue if they can demonstrate willful negligence in exposing workers to a known harmful substance.

Workers can also sue a third party, such as the manufacturer of a harmful substance, if they can establish that the manufacturer knew or should have known that the substance could

TABLE 76-4   Medical History

I. **Symptoms**
   A. Cough, wheezing, shortness of breath, chest tightness, and sputum production (generally of modest degree)
   B. Conditions known to be associated with asthma, such as rhinitis, sinusitis, nasal polyposis, or atopic dermatitis
II. **Pattern of symptoms**
   A. Perennial, seasonal, or perennial with seasonal exacerbations
   B. Continuous, episodic, or continuous with acute exacerbations
   C. Onset, duration, and frequency of symptoms (days per week or month)
   D. Diurnal variation, with special reference to nocturnal symptoms
III. **Precipitating or aggravating factors**
   A. Viral respiratory infections
   B. Exposure to environmental allergens (pollen, mold, house-dust mite, cockroach, animal dander, or secretory product, such as saliva or urine)
   C. Exposure to occupational chemicals or allergens
   D. Environmental change (eg, moving to a new home, going on a vacation, alterations in workplace, work processes, or materials used)
   E. Exposure to irritants, especially tobacco smoke and strong odors, air pollutants, occupational chemicals, vapors, gases, and aerosols
   F. Emotional expressions: fear, anger, frustration, crying, hard laughing
   G. Drugs (aspirin, beta blockers, nonsteroidal anti-inflammatory drugs, others)
   H. Food additives (sulfites) and preservatives
   I. Changes in weather, exposure to cold air
   J. Exercise
   K. Endocrine factors (eg, menses, pregnancy, thyroid diseases)
IV. **Development of disease**
   A. Age of onset, age at diagnosis
   B. Progress of disease (better or worse)
   C. Previous evaluation, treatment, and response
   D. Present management and response, including plans for managing acute episodes
V. **Profile of typical exacerbation**
   A. Prodromal signs and symptoms (eg, itching of skin of the anterior neck, nasal allergy symptoms)
   B. Temporal progression
   C. Usual management
   D. Usual outcome
VI. **Living situation**
   A. Home age, location, cooling and heating (central with oil, electric, gas, or kerosene space heating), wood-burning fireplace
   B. Carpeting over a concrete slab
   C. Humidifier
   D. Description of patient's room, with special attention to pillow, bed, floor covering, and dust collectors
   E. Animals in home
   F. Exposure to cigarette smoke, direct or sidestream, in home
VII. **Impact of disease**
   A. Impact on patient
      1. Number of emergency department or urgent care visits and hospitalization
      2. History of life-threatening acute exacerbation, intubation, or oral steroid therapy
      3. Number of school or work days missed
      4. Limitation of activity, especially sports
      5. History of nocturnal awakening
      6. Effect on growth, development, behavior, school or work achievement, and lifestyle
   B. Impact on family
      1. Disruption of family dynamics, routines, or restriction of activities
      2. Effect on siblings and spouse
      3. Economic impact
VIII. **Assessment of family's and patient's perception of illness**
   A. Patient, parental, and spousal knowledge of asthma and belief in the chronicity of asthma and in the efficacy of treatment
   B. Ability of patient and parents or spouse to cope with disease
   C. Level of family support and patient and parents' or spouse's capacity to recognize severity of an exacerbation
   D. Economic resources
IX. **Family history**
   A. IgE-mediated allergy in close relatives
   B. Asthma in close relatives
X. **Medical history**
   A. General medical history and history of other allergic disorders (eg, chronic rhinitis, atopic dermatitis, sinusitis, nasal polyps, gastrointestinal disturbances, adverse reactions to foods, drugs; in children, history of early life injury to the airways (eg, bronchopulmonary dysplasia, history of pulmonary infiltrates, documented pneumonia, viral bronchiolitis, recurrent croup, symptoms of gastroesophageal reflux, passive exposure to cigarette smoke); in adults, cigarette smoking history
   B. Detailed review of symptoms

National Asthma Education Program; Office of Prevention, Education, and Control; National Heart, Lung and Blood Institute. (1992). *Executive Summary: Guidelines for the diagnosis and management of asthma; National Asthma Education Program, Expert Panel Report.* Bethesda, MD: National Institutes of Health.

cause disease (Bascom, 1992). Compensation and the legal right to sue for damages for occupationally related disease may have a statute of limitations, which begins as soon as any evidence of occupational disease is discovered.

Lastly, the primary care provider should protect the confidentiality of the patient at all times when investigating potential occupational illness. Breaking confidentiality can cause patients to lose their jobs.

Teaching and Self-Care

All patients with asthma should be counseled regarding the signs and symptoms of asthma. The patient and primary care provider should establish a treatment plan that uses peak flow testing and the proper use of bronchodilators and inhaled steroids. Patients should understand when to contact a provider for advice (see Chap. 72).

Patients with asthma should not smoke cigarettes or be exposed to second-hand smoke. The primary care provider should assist the patient in developing a plan to stop smoking.

As with any asthmatic patient, the proper use of metered-dose inhaler medications or other delivery modalities is essential. Peak flow meters are also useful. In occupational asthma, a peak flow meter is used to document airway hyperresponsiveness, aiding in the establishment of the diagnosis.

Patients should be taught how to use protective respiratory equipment. The risks of not using these devices should be stressed.

ASBESTOS-RELATED LUNG DISEASE

Asbestos-related lung disease includes disorders such as benign pleural changes or illnesses such as asbestosis, malignant mesothelioma, and lung cancer. Asbestosis is the pulmonary occupational disease of diffuse interstitial fibrosis caused by asbestos exposure.

Anatomy, Physiology, and Pathology

Asbestos is a group of fibrous minerals that can be woven and that are resistant to heat, acid, and alkali. When crushed, the fibers can be broken into respirable particles that can be deposited in the lung. Fibers that are not cleared tend to accumulate in the lower lobes of the lung and the visceral pleura. If the exposure to asbestos is heavy and prolonged, a diffuse pulmonary fibrosis can develop. Fibrosis begins around the respiratory bronchioles and alveolar ducts in the lower lungs, then progresses in a centrifugal manner upward.

Development of clinical disease usually begins 25 to 40 years after exposure, although radiographic changes may appear before 20 years (Lordi & Reichman, 1993). The probability of developing asbestosis is related to the dose and duration of exposure; however, disease can occur after a brief but massive exposure. The long latency period makes the documentation of the degree of exposure difficult.

Epidemiology

Exposure to large amounts of asbestos occurred in the early part of this century in workers involved in asbestos mining and processing. However, relatively few people were affected until

TABLE 76-5	Some Products That Contain Asbestos	
Cement pipes	Boiler insulation
Roofing shinges	Flowerpots
Textiles	Floor tile
Paper products	Ceiling tiles
Caulk	Brake linings
Wallboard	Clutch plates
Putty	Gaskets
Flooring felt	Pipe coverings
Undercoating	

Orris, P. and Baron, S. A role for the primary care physician. Hospital Practice 1983; 18(3): 195. © 1983 The McGraw Hill Companies, Inc.

the wide-scale use of asbestos during World War II and the 1950s in the ship-building industry. It is estimated that from 1940 to the late 1970s, 27.5 million people were exposed to asbestos in the workplace.

In the late 1970s, federal regulations and industrial hygiene standards led to a major reduction in high exposures to asbestos. However, because asbestos had been used extensively in buildings before the regulations were enacted, exposures still occur in construction workers, electricians, boiler makers, and demolition workers. Although the use of asbestos has decreased dramatically, it still can be found in more than 3000 products (Lordi & Reichman, 1993). Table 76-5 lists some products that may contain asbestos.

Diagnostic Criteria

A diagnosis of asbestosis is made when clinical findings consistent with fibrosis can be linked with an occupational history of significant exposure to asbestos and an appropriate time interval to allow for the development of disease. Table 76-6 highlights the diagnostic criteria.

History and Physical Exam

A thorough medical and occupational history should be taken if a patient is suspected of having asbestosis or past exposure to asbestos. The medical history should focus on a detailed review of respiratory symptoms, as well as other possible causes of pulmonary fibrosis. The occupational history should focus on the duration and intensity of the possible exposure to asbestos.

TABLE 76-6	Clinical Criteria for Diagnosis of Asbestosis

Reliable history of asbestos exposure

Appropriate interval between exposure and disease detection

Abnormal chest radiograph showing fibrosis

Forced vital capacity below normal

Diffusing capacity below normal

Bilateral inspiratory crackles at the posterior lung bases

Lordi, GM, Reichman, LB. Pulmonary complications of asbestos exposure. American Family Physician 1193; 48(8): pp 1474.

Patients with asbestosis first present with fatigue, weight loss, dry cough, and the insidious onset of dyspnea on exertion. As the disease worsens, the dry cough can become productive and the patient may complain of a tight feeling in the chest.

The physical exam should include a thorough auscultatory evaluation of the chest. The first sign of asbestosis my be fine inspiratory rales in the posterior and posterolateral bases of the lung. Late-stage asbestosis is characterized by cyanosis, possible clubbing, and ultimately right-sided heart failure (Westerfield, 1992).

Diagnostic Studies

The chest radiograph initially shows a linear and reticular fibrotic pattern that begins in the lower lobes and spreads upward with more extensive disease. As the fibrosis progresses, cystic changes or honeycombing, as well as various degrees of pleural thickening, plaques, and effusions, may be seen. The presence of pleural thickening and plaques helps distinguish asbestosis from other types of pulmonary fibrosis.

A standardized set of criteria for interpreting radiographs in pneumoconioses has been developed by the International Labor Organization and should be used whenever possible (Harber, 1994; Westerfield, 1992). Radiographs may be helpful in the diagnosis of asbestosis but may not reflect the extent of the fibrosis and pulmonary impairment.

Pulmonary function tests typically demonstrate a restrictive disease pattern with reduced vital capacity and diffusing capacity. The obstructive disease pattern in asbestosis is thought to be the result of other factors, such as cigarette smoking (Lordi & Reichman, 1993).

Treatment Options, Expected Outcomes, and Comprehensive Management

PREVENTION

Asbestosis can be prevented by minimizing the amount of asbestos that becomes airborne. This is especially important when work is done on buildings built before 1979. Most authorities consider that if asbestos within buildings is in good condition and air sampling reveals no release of fibers, it is probably safer to leave the asbestos intact (Mossman et al, 1989). If the asbestos material is in poor condition or must be disturbed for renovation, a certified asbestos abatement company should be used.

Workers in occupations such as the construction trades or automobile repair should be made aware of the potential for exposure to asbestos to minimize workplace exposures (Craighead et al, 1982). Table 76-7 lists occupations that may be associated with asbestos exposure. Because the risk of lung can-

TABLE 76-7	Some Occupations With Current Risk of Asbestos Exposure
Carpenters	Sheet metal workers
Utility workers	Boiler makers
Electricians	Laborers
Pipefitters	Brake mechanics
Steel mill workers	Transmission mechanics

Lordi, GM, Reichman, LB. Pulmonary complications of asbestos exposure. American Family Physician 1193; 48(8): pp 1474.

cer is increased 80- to 90-fold in heavy smokers with significant asbestos exposure (Selikoff et al, 1968; Selikoff et al, 1980), persons with potential exposure to asbestos should receive special attention devoted to smoking cessation.

TREATMENT

Figure 76-2 is a flow chart showing management of asbestos exposure. Patients with asbestosis should stop smoking and receive pneumococcal vaccine and annual influenza vaccinations. Anyone with pulmonary disease should receive prompt and aggressive treatment of pulmonary infections, and patients should be educated to call the provider at the first sign of infection. Late-stage disease with severe fibrosis may require treatment with home oxygen. For patients with advanced asbestosis, pulmonary rehabilitation and stabilization measures should be followed as outlined in Chapter 74.

Teaching and Self-Care

For patients who work in occupations involving asbestos exposure, proper use of protective respiratory equipment should be stressed. Patients should be counseled about the effect of smoking and asbestosis on the risk of pulmonary malignancy.

COMMUNITY RESOURCES

- Agency for Toxic Substances and Disease Registry (ATSDR), 1600 Clifton Rd. N.E., Atlanta, GA 30333, 404-639-6000 (Director of Toxicology), 404-639-6206 (Division of Health Education): To request one or more free self-study cases in environmental medicine, write to the Continuing Education Coordinator at the above address.
- American College of Occupational and Environmental Medicine, 55 W. Seegers Rd., Arlington Heights, IL 60005-3919, 847-228-6850: The college lists physicians who are board-certified in occupational and environmental medicine and are members of the college.
- Association of Occupational and Environmental Clinics, 1010 Vermont Ave., Suite 513, Washington, D.C. 20005, 202-347-4976: This network of academically based occupational and environmental medicine clinics provides exposure and risk assessment, clinical evaluation, and consultation. Clinicians may contact the network to receive a referral assisting in the diagnosis, management, therapy, and prevention of occupational disorders.
- National Institute for Occupational Safety and Health (NIOSH), Robert A. Taft Laboratories, 4676 Columbia Parkway, Cincinnati, OH 45226, 800-356-4674: NIOSH provides information on substance toxicity and workplace hazards. If possible, physicians should have the Material Data Safety Sheet available when calling. The health hazard evaluation program can investigate worksites at which work-related illness and injury are suspected.
- Occupational Safety and Health Administration (OSHA), Department of Labor, 200 Constitution Ave., N.W., Washington, D.C. 20210, 202-219-8148: OSHA determines standards for health and safety in

History of work in high-risk occupation, known history of exposure, or radiographic evidence of asbestos exposure (such as fibrosis and/or pleural plaques)

Detailed occupational history (Table 76-2), Review of the Systems focused on respiratory system (cough, breathlessness, dyspnea on exertion)

Suspect significant asbestos exposure or any respiratory symptoms

History of possible significant asbestos exposure or respiratory symptoms

Do not suspect exposure or no clinical evidence of asbestos exposure

Chest radiograph, pulmonary function tests, diffusing capacity, volumes, and flows

Follow clinically
Educate on development of symptoms
Stop smoking

Consider early referral to occupational medicine specialist for thorough investigation

Normal chest radiograph and pulmonary function

Minimal abnormalities consistent with asbestosis

Moderate to severe abnormalities
Actions listed under minimal abnormalities, plus pulmonary rehabilitation

Stop smoking and further asbestos exposure

Stop smoking, monitor development of dyspnea

Follow respiratory symptoms, serial pulmonary function tests for progression of disease

Refer to occupational medicine specialists for surveillance protocols

Educate about avoiding further exposure to asbestos

Refer for possible legal assistance and workers' compensation

Report to Department of Health and/or Occupational Safety and Health

Consider influenza vaccination

Influenza and pneumococcal vaccines
Treat pulmonary infections aggressively

FIGURE 76-2 Flow diagram for comprehensive management of possible asbestosis.

the workplace, investigates compliance, and issues citations. Call 202-219-4667 for publications about occupational disease. Regional or local offices are listed under local Department of Labor listings.

- Physician Line and LungLine, National Jewish Center for Immunology and Respiratory Medicine, 1400 Jackson St., Denver, CO 80206, 800-652-9555 (Physician Line), 800-222-5864 (LungLine): Telephone consultations for those seeking information on lung and allergic disorders, including those resulting from occupational exposures.
- Patients with asbestosis may want to contact their local White Lung Association, which can provide information and services to persons who have been exposed to asbestos or have asbestos-related disease.

REFERRAL POINTS AND CLINICAL WARNINGS

When the primary care provider suspects a patient's illness is occupationally related, a referral to a specialist is often helpful. Aside from taking a detailed occupational and exposure history, the occupational medicine specialist will investigate the illness of coworkers, help to modify the workplace or change the job description to modify the worker's exposure, and if needed contact specialized social and legal services.

The criteria for referral to an occupational medicine specialist are listed in Table 76-8. The specialist will determine which exams and tests are needed. The specialist may also visit the worksite and confer with industrial hygienists and union leaders to protect all potentially affected workers.

Referral should be made if the diagnosis of asbestosis is considered. The specialist will be able to:

TABLE 76-8	**Criteria for Occupational Medicine Referrals**

1. A patient with a disease that may be related to environmental or occupational factors, for which the primary care physician is unable to make the etiologic diagnosis
2. A group of patients who are all environmentally exposed to a single toxin that is unfamiliar to the primary care physician
3. A patient requiring specialized diagnostic testing
4. A patient requiring expert medical testimony in a compensation case
5. A case involving a request by a lawyer or public health authority for information concerning potential public health effects of environmental pollutants
6. Cases relevant to epidemiologic investigations of potential environmental or industrial hazards

- Make a more accurate estimation of exposure to asbestos in the distant past
- Provide expert radiographic readings
- Order and interpret specialized pulmonary function tests
- Implement or recommend a protocol to monitor for the progression of asbestosis or the development of occupational pulmonary disease.

References

Alberts, W., & Brooks, S. (1992). Advances in occupational asthma. *Clinical Chest Medicine, 13*(2), 281–302.

Bascom, R. (1992). Occupational and environmental respiratory diseases: A medicolegal primer for physicians. *Occupational Medicine: State of the Art Reviews, 7*(2), 331–344.

Bates, D., Gotsch, A., Brooks, S., Hankinson, J., & Merchant, J. (1992). Prevention of occupational lung disease. *Chest, 102*(3, Suppl.), 257S–276S.

Campos-Outcalt, D. (1994). Occupational health epidemiology and objectives for the year 2000. *Primary Care; Clinics in Office Practice, 21*(2), 213–222.

Centers for Disease Control. (1990). Mandatory reporting of infectious disease by clinicians, and mandatory reporting of occupational diseases by clinicians. *MMWR, 39*(No. RR-9), 1–28.

Chan-Yeung, M. (1990). Occupational asthma. *Chest, 98*(5, suppl.), 148S–161S.

Chan-Yeung, M., & Malo, J. (1995). Occupational asthma. *N Engl J Med, 333*(2), 107–112.

Craighead J.E., Mossman B.T. (1982). The pathogenesis of asbestos-associated diseases. *N Engl J Med 306*(24):1446–55.

Cullen, M. (1990). Clinical surveillance and management of occupational asthma, tertiary prevention by the primary practitioner. *Chest, 98*(5, suppl.), 196S–201S.

Harber, P. (1994). Primary care role in preventing occupational and environmental respiratory disease. *Primary Care, 21*(2), 291–310.

Lordi, G., & Reichman, L. (1993). Pulmonary complications of asbestos exposure. *American Family Physician, 48*(8), 1471–1477.

Mossman B., Gee B. (1989) Asbestos-related diseases. *N Engl J Med 320*(26):1721–30.

National Asthma Education Program, Office of Prevention, Education, and Control, National Heart, Lung, and Blood Institute. (1992). *Executive summary: Guidelines for the diagnosis and management of asthma*. National Asthma Educational Program, Expert Panel Report. Bethesda, MD: National Institutes of Health.

Sattler, B. (1992). Rights and realities: A critical review of the accessibility of information on hazardous chemicals. *Occupational Medicine: State of the Art Reviews, 7*(2), 189–196.

Selikoff I.J., Hammond E.C., Churg J. (1968). Asbestos exposure, smoking, and neoplasia. *JAMA 204*:104–10.

Selikoff I.J., Seidman H., Hammond E.C. (1980). Mortality effects of cigarette smoking among amosite asbestos factory workers. *J Natl Cancer Inst 65*:507–13.

Westerfield, B. (1992). Asbestos-related lung disease. *Southern Medical Journal, 85*(6), 616–620.

CHAPTER
77

Pulmonary Thromboembolic Disease

Raffi Calikyan, MD

Venous thromboembolic disease encompasses two closely linked conditions: deep vein thrombosis (DVT) and pulmonary embolism (PE). DVT and PE are significant causes of morbidity and mortality in the United States and in other Western countries. Although the precise incidence in the general population is difficult to determine, it is estimated that venous thromboembolism accounts for approximately 300,000 hospitalizations and as many as 50,000 deaths per year (Anderson & Wheeler, 1991).

Although PE is a frequent, potentially fatal disease, it remains largely underdiagnosed, and the mortality rate has not significantly changed since the 1960s, despite new diagnostic and therapeutic modalities. Efforts to improve this situation should focus on recognizing patients at risk and taking appropriate preventive measures.

ANATOMY, PHYSIOLOGY, AND PATHOLOGY

Anatomy and Physiology

The venous system of the lower extremities can be divided into the superficial and deep vein groups. The superficial venous system includes the greater and lesser saphenous veins and their tributaries. Perforating veins connect the deep and superficial venous systems. The deep veins found in the calf flow into the popliteal vein, which continues into the femoral vein. The femoral vein connects to the iliac venous system and then into the inferior vena cava. The inferior vena cava flows into the right atrium. From the right ventricle the pulmonary artery takes the blood flow into the lungs. Blood supply to the lungs is provided by the pulmonary circulation and by the systemic circulation via the bronchial arteries.

■ ■ ■ **CLINICAL PEARL**

The superficial femoral vein is part of the deep venous system.

The venous flow in the lower extremities is directed from the superficial to the deep veins. Bicuspid valves in the veins of the lower extremity direct the flow centrally. The flow from the periphery into the right side of the heart is aided by the contraction of the skeletal muscles, compressing the veins in the extremities. The greater veins are helped by the negative intrathoracic pressure generated during inspiration.

The normal pulmonary arterial tree consists of large elastic arteries, smaller muscular pulmonary arteries, arterioles, and capillaries. The elastic capacity of the pulmonary circulation allows accommodation of increases in blood flow without increasing pulmonary artery pressures (normal range 25/10

mmHg). However, if a significant obstruction of the pulmonary vascular bed occurs (generally >30%), an abrupt increase in the pulmonary artery pressure results; this may be poorly tolerated by the right ventricle, leading to acute decompensation (Elliott, 1992).

Pathology

DEEP VEIN THROMBOSIS

More than 90% of clinically significant PEs arise from thrombosis of veins in the lower extremities. Thrombi can form in the calf veins, popliteal vein, and more proximal veins of the iliofemoral venous system. In the 19th century Virchow defined the pathophysiologic factors promoting the formation of a thrombus: stasis, abnormalities of the vessel wall, and hypercoagulability. Risk factors for venous thromboembolism are based on these conditions.

DVT usually develops in proximity to the venous valves. Initially a "white thrombus" is formed by platelet aggregation, followed by a "red thrombus" with fibrin deposition. The thrombus propagates by continued fibrin and platelet accretion. Subsequently, it either resolves within hours to days by the fibrinolytic system or undergoes organization with re-endothelization. If there is re-endothelization, the venous lumen narrows and distal venous valves become incompetent because of increased intraluminal pressure. Venous flow is directed into the superficial venous system during leg muscle contraction, leading to edema and impaired viability of subcutaneous tissues, and in the most severe cases to ulceration (post-thrombotic syndrome).

Within 7 to 10 days, the actions of fibrinolysis or organization reach a stable state. Thus, the embolic risk is highest within the first few days of thrombus formation (Hirsh & Hoak, 1996).

PULMONARY EMBOLISM

If the whole thrombus or any portion of it dislodges before it organizes, it may be transported in the venous system to the right side of the heart and into the pulmonary circulation. The acute obstruction of pulmonary vessels by an embolus leads to hemodynamic and respiratory consequences. The most important hemodynamic complication is the acute increase in pulmonary vascular resistance, which in extreme cases can lead to acute right-sided heart failure and death. In addition to mechanical obstruction, vasoconstriction occurs as a result of the release of vasoactive amines (serotonin, thromboxane A_2) and the stimulation of baroreceptors in the pulmonary artery wall.

A major respiratory consequence of PE is increased alveolar dead space, because ventilation continues in lung areas that are not perfused. Both increased dead space and intrapulmonary or intracardiac right-to-left shunting of blood lead to hypoxemia. Tachypnea is caused by the stimulation of juxtacapillary irritant receptors. Release of serotonin may also cause bronchoconstriction, accounting for the wheezing sometimes detected in patients with PE.

Over several hours, atelectasis may develop as a result of loss of surfactant distal to the occlusion. Development of pulmonary infarction is uncommon because of the dual blood supply of the lungs. Infarction occurs in less than 10% of cases, usually only if concomitant heart or lung disease is present (eg, left ventricular failure, mitral stenosis, chronic obstructive lung disease).

After the acute phase, most emboli undergo resolution by fibrinolysis. Some thrombi fail to resolve, presumably as a result of defects in the intrinsic fibrinolytic system or because they were very well organized before embolization (Elliot, 1992).

EPIDEMIOLOGY

Venous thromboembolism is relatively rare in the general population in the absence of predisposing conditions. Numerous factors are associated with an increased risk for venous thromboembolism, including:

- Age older than 40 years
- Prior history of venous thromboembolism
- Major surgery, especially orthopedic surgery of the lower extremities
- Bed rest in excess of 5 days
- Malignancy
- Fracture of the pelvis, hip, or long bones
- Paralytic stroke
- Estrogen treatment, such as high-dose oral contraceptives
- Pregnancy and the puerperium
- Hypercoagulability states (lupus anticoagulant, protein C deficiency, protein S deficiency, antithrombin III deficiency, plasminogen deficiency)
- Obesity
- Congestive heart failure
- Myocardial infarction (Anderson & Wheeler, 1995).

There are some data to suggest that the incidence of venous thromboembolism is higher in African Americans than whites. Asians have the lowest incidence, which may be explained by genetic differences in the control of the coagulation system (Fujimura et al, 1995).

DIAGNOSTIC CRITERIA

Imaging studies establish the diagnosis of DVT or PE. Doppler ultrasound of the legs and nuclear studies of the lungs demonstrate alterations of venous compressibility and lung perfusion, respectively, providing indirect evidence of the presence of a clot. Thrombosis can be demonstrated directly by venography of the lower extremities or by a pulmonary angiogram of the pulmonary arteries.

HISTORY AND PHYSICAL EXAM

In the patient with suspected DVT or PE, the history should focus on risk factors. The most important risk factors are:

- Prior history of thromboembolic disease
- Recent immobilization or long-distance travel
- Estrogen use

- Family history of thromboembolic disease or hypercoagulable states
- Recent trauma.

The most common complaint of the patient with DVT is calf pain. DVT is suggested by unilateral leg swelling, warmth, or erythema. There may be tenderness or increased tissue turgor along the course of the involved vein. Increased resistance or pain during dorsiflexion of the foot (Homan's sign) is an unreliable diagnostic test.

The symptoms of the patient with PE are often nonspecific. Dyspnea and pleuritic chest pain are the most usual symptoms, although apprehension and cough may also be present. Hemoptysis and syncope occur in less than one third of the patients. On the physical exam, the most common presenting signs are tachypnea and tachycardia. The pulmonary component of the second heart sound may be accentuated. In massive PE, signs of acute right ventricular failure, as well as hypotension and cyanosis, are encountered.

DIAGNOSTIC STUDIES

An algorithmic approach to the diagnostic workup for DVT and PE is illustrated in Figures 77-1 and 77-2.

Deep Vein Thrombosis

Routine diagnostic tests available for evaluation of DVT include Doppler ultrasonography, impedance plethysmography (IPG), and contrast venography.

Doppler ultrasonography of the lower extremities is highly sensitive (>90%) for detecting clots in the popliteal and femoral veins but is less sensitive for detecting calf vein thrombosis (about 50%). It is a preferred method because it is noninvasive and can be performed at the bedside.

IPG is a noninvasive test that can detect the changes in blood volume resulting from delayed venous emptying, which occurs if a thrombus is obstructing proximal veins. However, the test is limited in obese or edematous patients, and false-positive results can be seen because of the lack of discrimination between intravascular obstruction and extravascular compression. The sensitivity of IPG is low for nonobstructing or infrapopliteal thrombi. Because of these limitations, ultrasound is a more accurate test for suspected DVT (Burke et al, 1995).

Contrast venography is considered the gold standard for the diagnosis of DVT. However, it is not used as a first-line diagnostic tool because of patient discomfort during venous cannulation and because of the risk of a reaction to the contrast material. Venography is used only if accurate information cannot be obtained with noninvasive tests.

Magnetic resonance imaging can be used to evaluate the pelvic and lower extremity veins. Because of its expense, its use as a first-line test is limited mostly to suspected disease in the upper extremities.

Blood tests for the diagnosis of DVT have not yet been widely adopted. Measurement of plasma levels of D-dimer, a specific product of fibrinolysis, has been used as a complementary test with IPG or ultrasound. If the level of D-dimer is below a certain cutoff point (usually 500 mg/L) and an imaging study is negative, the negative predictive value of the combination is 98.5% (Ginsberg et al, 1997; Bounameux et al, 1994). D-dimer

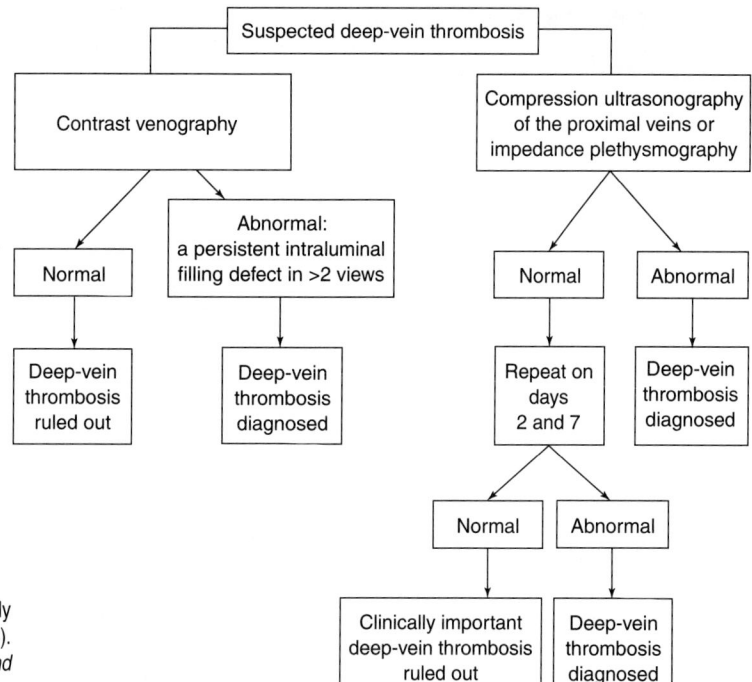

FIGURE 77-1 An approach to patients with clinically suspected deep-vein thrombosis. (J.S. Ginsberg. (1996). Management of venus thromboembolism. *New England Journal of Medicine*, 335(24), 1816–1828.)

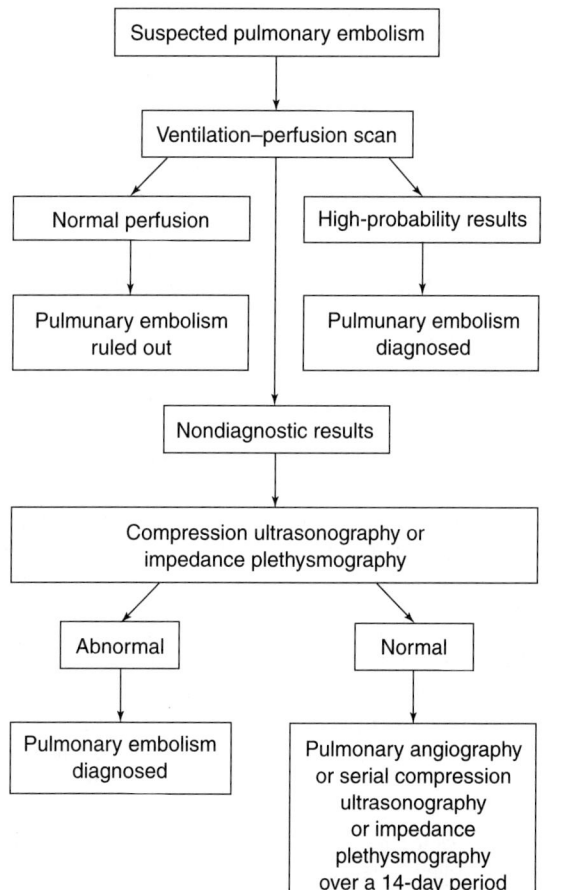

FIGURE 77-2 An approach to patients with clinically suspected pulmonary embolism. Nondiagnostic results are those that indicate an intermediate or low probability of pulmonary embolism, or that do not indicate a high probability. (J.S. Ginsberg. (1996). Management of venus thromboembolism. *New England Journal of Medicine*, 335(24), 1816–1828.)

has also been investigated as a diagnostic tool for PE. Its sensitivity for the diagnosis of PE is 83% to 96.8%, but the specificity is low (45.1% to 68%). This precludes the use of the assay as a screening tool for patients with suspected PE, but it may be useful for patients with inconclusive nuclear scans.

Pulmonary Embolism

Nuclear lung scan is the most widely used imaging technique in the diagnosis of PE. A perfusion scintigraphy is performed with the intravenous administration of labeled microspheres or macroaggregated particles. These particles are trapped in the arteriolar capillary bed during their first passage through the pulmonary circulation. Their nuclear activity is monitored from different views with a camera. Unfortunately, perfusion defects are not specific for embolization. Atelectasis, parenchymal lesions, congenital vascular abnormalities, infectious processes, extravascular compression of pulmonary vessels, reflex vasoconstriction, and increased vascular resistance can all cause a perfusion defect pattern.

The combination of a ventilation scan using radioactive aerosol particles with the perfusion scan is based on the principle that ventilation will be abnormal in areas of consolidation or atelectasis but will not be affected in areas of recent embolization. Simultaneous evaluation of ventilation/perfusion (V/Q) scans can distinguish matched (V/Q defects in the same area) and mismatched defects (a perfusion defect without an associated ventilation defect). Mismatched defects are more suggestive of PE (Weiss, 1996). Abnormal V/Q scans are further classified into high, intermediate, and low probability for PE, according to established criteria. Even with low-probability scans, however, PE may still be likely; including clinical probabilities based on the history and physical exam allows for more individualized decision making (Table 77-1).

Pulmonary angiography is considered the gold standard in the diagnosis of PE. A constant intraluminal filing defect and

TABLE 77-1	Likelihood for PE Based on the Combination of Nuclear Scan and Clinical Exam			
	Clinical Examination Probability			**All Probabilities**
Some Probability	*High*	*Intermediate*	*Low*	
High	96%	88%	56%	87%
Intermediate	66%	28%	16%	30%
Low	40%	16%	4%	14%
Near-normal/Normal	0%	6%	2%	4%

PIOPED Investigators. (1990). Invasive and noninvasive diagnosis of pulmonary embolism. Results of the prospective investigation of pulmonary embolism diagnosis. JAMA, 263, 2753–2759.

vessel cutoffs are considered reliable diagnostic features for PE (Janata-Schwatczek et al, 1996). Pulmonary angiography is an invasive procedure with a 1% risk of major complications (including a 0.5% mortality rate) and a roughly 5% risk of minor complications. Angiography is indicated when noninvasive tests have provided inconclusive data and there is a reasonably high clinical suspicion for PE.

Efforts to increase diagnostic accuracy without the use of invasive imaging studies have resulted in the development of the spiral computed tomography scan. The major drawbacks of this tool for diagnosing PE, as well as for the routine use of magnetic resonance angiography, are lack of availability and high cost.

Respiratory alkalosis and hypoxemia with an increased A-a gradient secondary to shunting and V/Q mismatching are usually found on the arterial blood gas analysis. However, these findings are sufficiently nonspecific that a normal Pao_2 or an A-a gradient cannot rule out PE.

Certain electrocardiographic patterns can suggest the presence of PE. The most frequent abnormality in PE is sinus tachycardia. Other findings, in decreasing order of frequency, are T-wave inversions, nonreciprocal ST depression and elevation in the right precordial leads, and complete or incomplete right bundle branch block. The fourth abnormality, the classically described S1/Q3 pattern, is found in only 12% of the patients.

The chest x-ray is frequently normal. A chest film is useful in patients who have suspected PE and other pathologic conditions, and it can complement the information obtained from a V/Q scan. In the presence of lung infarction, the chest film may reveal a homogenous, wedge-shaped opacity in the periphery of the lung. Other radiographic abnormalities may be related to the distribution of blood vessels. Isolated areas of oligemia, widening of the major pulmonary arteries, and enlargement of the right heart chambers can suggest PE (Stein et al, 1991).

TREATMENT OPTIONS, EXPECTED OUTCOMES, AND COMPREHENSIVE MANAGEMENT

Early Diagnosis, Prompt Treatment, and Disability Limitation

Timely initiation of treatment for PE is crucial: a delay in therapy is associated with a risk of death. The treatment plan must satisfy several goals:

- Improve pulmonary gas exchange
- Maintain adequate cardiac output and systemic circulation

- Prevent extension of the thrombus
- Obtain pulmonary vascular clearance
- Prevent recurrence.

A general approach to the initiation of treatment is shown in Figure 77-3.

Medical Therapy

Anticoagulation is the mainstay of treatment for both DVT and PE unless contraindicated by the presence of active bleeding or a bleeding disorder. Relative contraindications are uncontrolled hypertension, recent surgery or trauma, pericarditis, inadequate facilities to monitor anticoagulation, patients who are prone to falls, and inconsistent patient use (Ewald, 1995). The major risk factors for bleeding are recent surgery or trauma, renal failure, old age, and peptic ulcer disease (Hirsh & Hoak, 1996).

Intravenous heparin is the initial therapy for both DVT and PE. It prevents the extension of an already formed thrombus. Heparin binds with antithrombin III and potentiates the inhibition of thrombin and activated factor X. Its effectiveness is monitored with the activated partial thromboplastin time (aPTT). The target range for aPTT is 1.5 to 2.5 times the upper limit of the control value (Hirsh & Hoak, 1996). Levels that are subtherapeutic are associated with recurrence of PE or extension of DVT. Values in excess of three times the control level increase the risk of bleeding. Other complications of heparin therapy include thrombocytopenia, osteoporosis, hypoaldosteronism, and alopecia (Ginsberg, 1996).

Low-molecular-weight heparin agents offer antithrombotic effects comparable to those of unfractionated heparin, with fewer bleeding-related complications. Compared to unfractionated heparin, they have a lower incidence of thrombocytopenia and osteoporosis. Low-molecular-weight heparin is being used for DVT prophylaxis; however, recent trials have shown promising results for the treatment of DVT with comparable or superior efficacy and safety. Because of the increased bioavailability of low-molecular-weight heparin, treatment regimens with subcutaneous administration once or twice daily are possible, and routine laboratory monitoring is unnecessary. These features facilitate management in the hospital, and certain subsets of patients may be discharged early with continuing outpatient treatment (Tapson & Hull, 1995).

Coumadin derivatives are the oral anticoagulants of choice after initial therapy with heparin. These drugs form inactive coagulation factors by inhibiting the vitamin K-dependent gamma-carboxylation of factors II, VII, IX, and X and proteins C and S. The anticoagulant effect is delayed until normal coagu-

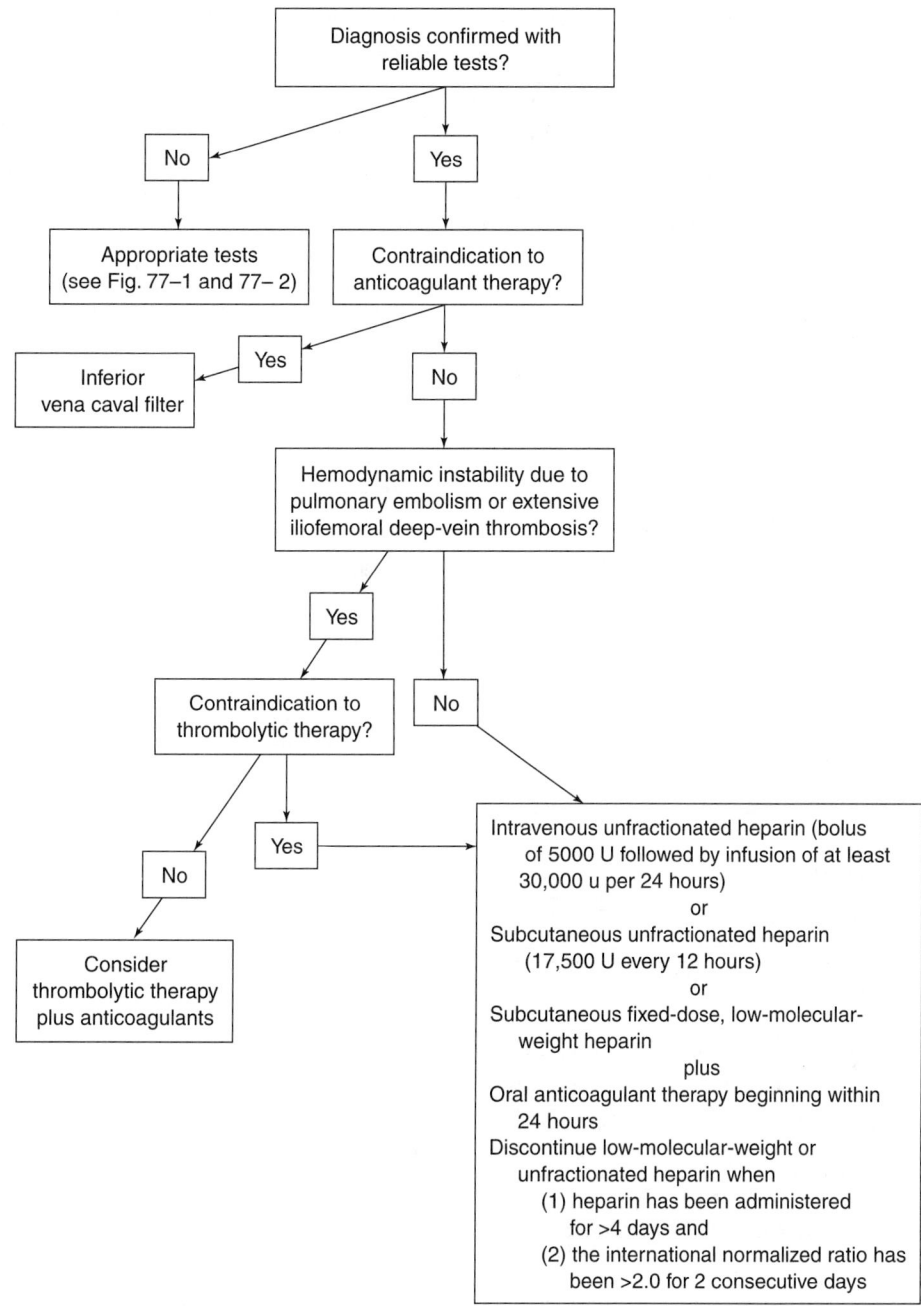

FIGURE 77-3 Initial management of venous thromboembolism. (Ginsberg, J.S. (1996). Management of venous thromboembolism. *New England Journal of Medicine*, 335(24), 1816–1828.)

lation factors are cleared from the plasma. The peak effect does not occur until 36 to 72 hours after the initiation of the treatment. Therapeutic anticoagulation is achieved when an International Normalized Ratio (INR) of 2 to 3 is reached. Oral anticoagulation is usually continued for 3 to 6 months; however, a longer duration of treatment should be considered when underlying risk factors for thromboembolism cannot be eliminated and recurrent thromboembolism occurs.

Complications of oral anticoagulants include bleeding; if underlying protein C or S deficiency is present, coumarin-induced skin necrosis may occur as a result of the occlusion of small skin vessels. This complication can be prevented with overlapping heparin therapy.

Anticoagulation therapy does not resolve the already formed thrombus. Thrombolytic drugs such as streptokinase, urokinase, and recombinant tissue-type plasminogen activator (rt-PA) activate the fibrinolytic system, leading to clot resolution. Bleeding is the major complication of the thrombolytic drugs. Active bleeding, recent cerebrospinal surgery, and an active intracranial process are absolute contraindications to thrombolytic therapy. Diastolic hypertension has been found to be an independent risk factor for intracranial hemorrhage (Kanter et al, 1997).

Selected patients with proximal DVT are candidates for thrombolytic therapy if they have no risk factors for bleeding and the mortality risk of a subsequent PE is very high based on their underlying cardiac and pulmonary reserve (Ginsberg, 1996).

Outcomes associated with anticoagulation treatment are favorable when compared to placebo. Without treatment, DVT is associated with a 40% to 50% risk of clinically detectable PE. The short-term prognosis of proximal DVT after adequate anticoagulation is good. Clinically significant recurrent events occur in 5% to 8% of the cases (Piccioli et al, 1996). Untreated PE carries a mortality rate of 5% to 42%, depending on severity

TABLE 77-2	Three Published Dosing Schemes for Heparin*

WEIGHT-BASED NOMOGRAM

The initial dose is a bolus of 80 U per kilogram of body weight followed by an infusion starting at a rate of 18 U per kilogram per hour. The APTT is measured every 6 hours and the heparin dose adjusted as follows:

Measured Value	Adjustment
PTT <35 sec (<1.2 × control value)	80 U/kg as bolus, then increase infusion rate by 4 U/kg/hr
APTT 35–45 sec (1.2–1.5 × control value)	40 U/kg as bolus, then increase infusion rate by 2 U/kg/hr
APTT 46–70 sec (>1.5–2.3 × control value)	No change
APTT 71–90 sec (>2.3–3 × control value)	Decrease infusion rate by 2 U/kg/hr
APTT >90 sec (>3 × control value)	Stop infusion for 1 hour, then decrease infusion rate by 3 U/kg/hr

5000-U BOLUS DOSE, FOLLOWED BY 1280 U PER HR

APTT (sec)	Bolus (U)	Stop Infusion (min)	Rate of Change (mL/hr)	Repeat APTT
<50§	5000	0	−3	In 6 hr
50–59	0	0	−3	In 6 hr
60–85	0	0	0	Next morning
86–95	0	0	−2	Next morning
96–120	0	30	−2	In 6 hr
>120	0	60	−4	In 6 hr

INTRAVENOUS DOSE-TITRATION NOMOGRAM FOR APTT

The starting dose is a 5000-U bolus, followed by 40,000 U per 24 hours (if the patient has a low risk of bleeding or 30,000 U per 24 hours if there is a high risk of bleeding).

APTT (sec)	Intravenous Infusion		Additional Action
	Rate of Change (mL/hr)	Change in Dose (U/24 hr)	
≤45	+6	+5760	Repeat APTT in 4–6 hr
46–54	+3	+2880	Repeat APTT in 4–6 hr
55–85	0	0	None
86–110	−3	−2880	Stop heparin for 1 hr; repeat APTT 4–6 hr after restarting heparin treatment
>110	−6	−5760	Stop heparin for 1 hr; repeat APTT 4–6 hr after restarting heparin treatment

Ginsberg, S. (1996). Management of venous thromboembolism. New England Journal of Medicine, 335(24)1816–1828.

and underlying cardiopulmonary condition. Anticoagulation reduces the mortality rate from PE to 2.5% to 8% (Stein et al, 1995).

Warfarin is usually initiated at 10 mg daily for 2 days. Subsequent dosage adjustment is made according to INR until stabilization in therapeutic range is achieved. The required maintenance dose varies greatly and may range from 2 to 15 mg daily. Possible regimens for heparin treatment are listed in Table 77-2.

Maintenance of adequate anticoagulation may be deterred by interactions with other drugs, dietary intake and absorption of vitamin K, and alterations of liver function (Hirsh, 1991). Significant drug interactions between warfarin and other drugs are listed in Table 77-3.

Prophylaxis is more cost effective than screening for DVT. Prophylaxis should be aimed at hospitalized patients; recommended regimens are summarized in Table 77-4.

Surgical Intervention

Surgical treatment options include interruption of the vena cava and thrombectomy. Indications for the vena cava interruption are:

- PE with contraindications for anticoagulation or complications from anticoagulants
- Recurrent thromboembolism despite adequate anticoagulation
- Large free-floating vena caval thrombus
- Chronic recurrent embolism with pulmonary hypertension.

Prophylactic use of vena cava interruption with a filter in patients at high risk for PE and bleeding may be warranted. Heparin treatment should be continued after filter placement whenever possible to prevent in situ thrombus formation and embolization from possible collaterals.

Thrombectomy for DVT is rarely used because postoperative recurrence is common. It may be indicated in patients with impending venous gangrene. Indications for pulmonary artery thrombectomy include massive PE in patients with contraindications for thrombolytic therapy and those with chronic thromboembolic pulmonary hypertension. (Simonneau et al, 1995).

Rehabilitation

After DVT, post-thrombotic syndrome with chronic venous insufficiency may develop. In advanced stages, skin ulceration and recurring cellulitis may occur. To minimize these consequences of chronic venous insufficiency, patients should be advised to avoid prolonged standing or sitting. "Stretch breaks" during long trips should be taken. Venous return can be augmented with elastic stockings or sequential compression devices. Foot elevation is helpful, but devices that put pressure on the popliteal area should be avoided, as should crossing the legs. Exercise of the lower extremity muscles may also promote venous return by compression of the veins. These measures should be taken after the stabilization of the thrombus to avoid dislodging emboli.

Most treated PEs resolve over several weeks, and the pulmonary arterial bed is restored to a normal or near-normal status.

TABLE 77-3	Drugs That Alter Prothrombin Time by Interacting With Warfarin, According to Type of Interaction		
Pharmacokinetic (Drugs That Change Warfarin Levels)	**Pharmacodynamic (Drugs That Do Not Change Warfarin Levels)**	**Mechanism Unknown (Drugs Whose Effect on Warfarin Levels Is Unknown)**	
Prolongs prothrombin time	**Prolongs prothrombin time**	**Prolongs prothrombin time**	
Stereoselective inhibition of clearance of *S* isomer	Inhibits cyclic interconversion of vitamin K 2nd- and 3rd-generation cephalosporins	Evidence for interaction convincing	
Phenylbutazone	Other mechanisms	Erythromycin	
Metronidazole	Clofibrate	Anabolic steroids	
Sulfinpyrazone	Inhibits blood coagulation	Evidence for interaction less convincing	
Trimethoprim–sulfamethoxazole	Heparin	Ketoconazole	
Disulfiram	Increases metabolism of coagulation factors	Fluconazole	
Stereoselective inhibition of clearance of *R* isomer	Thyroxine	Isoniazid	
Cimetidine*		Piroxicam	
Omeprazole*		Tamoxifen	
Nonstereoselective inhibitions of clearance of *R* and *S* isomers		Quinidine	
Amiodarone		Vitamin E (megadose)	
		Phenytoin	
Reduces prothrombin time	**Inhibits platelet function**	**Reduces prothrombin time**	
Reduces absorption	Aspirin	Penicillins	
Cholestyramine	Other nonsteroidal anti-inflammatory drugs	Griseofulvin†	
Increases metabolic clearance	Ticlopidine		
Barbiturates	Moxalactam		
Rifampin	Carbenicillin and high doses of other penicillins		
Griseofulvin			
Carbamazepine			

* Causes minimal prolongation of the prothrombin time.

† Has been proposed to cause increased metabolic clearance.

Hirsh, J. (1991). Oral anticoagulant drugs. *NESM 324*(26).

In patients with extensive embolization, residual obstruction may remain and cause persistent pulmonary hypertension. It is essential to prevent recurrent embolization, which could further diminish the effective pulmonary arterial bed.

Both chronic recurrent PE and pulmonary hypertension induce hypoxemia, which can cause further disability. Patients with these disorders benefit from home oxygen therapy to relieve symptoms and to prevent hypoxia-induced increases in pulmonary artery pressures.

Age and Gender Considerations

During pregnancy, the age-adjusted risk for venous thromboembolism is five times higher. Diagnostic modalities should be modified to minimize radiation exposure to the fetus. Heparin is safe during pregnancy, but warfarin should be avoided because of its embryopathic effects and risk of fetal hemorrhage. Treatment can be started with intravenous administration of heparin and continued after 5 to 10 days with weight-adjusted subcutaneous heparin every 12 hours.

◼ ◼ ◼ **CLINICAL PEARL**

Use of low-molecular-weight heparin is safe during pregnancy, and neither heparin nor warfarin is contraindicated during breast-feeding (Toglia & Weg, 1996).

Heparin therapy lasting 1 month or more causes osteoporosis. Although this process is partially reversible after discontinuation of treatment, susceptibility to future fractures might increase by approximately 30%. Low-molecular-weight heparin should be considered for the long-term treatment of patients who are at risk for osteoporosis (Tapson & Hull, 1995).

In elderly patients receiving anticoagulant therapy, fall precautions should be taken and adequate assistance provided. Most elderly patients are anticoagulated for chronic illnesses and tend to be receiving multiple medications. Drug interactions should be considered in the management plan for venous thromboembolism.

Nutritional Considerations

Consumption of a vitamin K-rich diet can impair the efficacy of oral anticoagulants. Foods high in vitamin K include vegetables such as spinach, broccoli, kale, and collards, and soybean and canola oils.

Occupational Hazards

The patient prone to falls or injuries during daily activities or at work should be warned about the risk of excessive bleeding associated with anticoagulation. Patients who must sit for prolonged periods (eg, long-distance drivers, office workers)

TABLE 77-4	Prophylaxis for Deep Venous Thrombosis
Clinical Setting	**Recommended Prophylaxis**
GENERAL SURGERY PATIENTS	
<40 years old, no risk factors	Early ambulation
>40 years old, no additional risk factors	Elastic stockings or low-dose heparin (every 12 h) or intermittent pneumatic compression
>40 years old, with additional risk factors	Low-dose heparin (every 8 h) or low-molecular-weight heparin
>40 years old with additional risk factors and with high potential for wound hematomas or infection	Dextran or intermittent pneumatic compression
>40 years old with multiple risk factors	Intermittent pneumatic compression *plus* low-dose heparin or low-molecular-weight heparin or dextran
ORTHOPEDIC SURGERY	
Hip replacement	Warfarin or low-molecular-weight heparin or low-dose heparin (dose adjusted to aPTT at upper limit of control range)
Hip fracture	Warfarin or low-molecular-weight heparin
Knee surgery	Intermittent pneumatic compression
NEUROSURGERY	Intermittent pneumatic compression
MEDICAL CONDITIONS	
Myocardial infarction	Low-dose heparin if full-dose heparin is not already being administered
Congestive heart failure and/or pulmonary infections	Low-dose heparin
Ischemic stroke with lower extremity paralysis	Low-dose heparin or low-molecular-weight heparin
Nonambulatory patients or patients with venous stasis	Low-dose heparin
Long-term indwelling central venous catheters	Warfarin, 1 mg daily

Ginsberg, S. (1996). Management of venous thromboembolism. New England Journal of Medicine, 335(24)1816–1828.

should be instructed to take breaks every 2 to 3 hours to avoid venous stasis and recurrent thrombosis.

TEACHING AND SELF-CARE

Most patients are discharged on oral anticoagulants (warfarin) after an acute episode of DVT or PE. They should be instructed about the risks and benefits of their medication and the importance of taking them strictly on schedule. The importance of regular monitoring should be emphasized.

The patient may be given a list of common medications that contain aspirin. New drugs and over-the-counter medications should be checked with a pharmacist or other health care provider before the patient takes them.

Medical providers, especially dentists, should be informed that a patient is on oral anticoagulation. A Medic-Alert bracelet or warfarin ID card might be helpful. Patients should be advised to use a soft-bristle toothbrush and to report any blood in the stool or urine, unusual headache, backache, bruising, or bleeding.

Women of childbearing age should be aware of the embryopathic effects of warfarin and should use appropriate contraceptive measures while taking the drug. Foods containing large amounts of vitamin K should be avoided. Limits on athletic activities may need to be discussed with young, active patients. Correct application and care of elastic stockings should be taught.

Any lifestyle changes or new health problems should be discussed during patient visits. New symptoms, especially those related to the lower extremity or respiratory system, should be considered emergency signs.

COMMUNITY RESOURCES

- HealthAnswers: Pulmonary Embolus, http://housecall. orbisnews.com/databases/ami/convert/000132.html
- Multimedia Textbook on the Diagnosis of Pulmonary Embolus, http://www.uni-koeln.de/med-fak/acmcd rom/uiowa/rad/books/ele
- Community Outreach Health System, http://web .bu.edu/COHIS/cardvasc/vessel/vein/pe.htm
- Thrombosis Interest Group of Canada, http:// is.dal.ca/mscully/tig.html
- National Heart, Lung and Blood Institute, Information Center, P.O. Box 30105, Bethesda, MD 20824-0105, 301-251-1222
- American Heart Association, 7272 Greenville Ave., Dallas, TX 75231-4596

REFERRAL POINTS AND CLINICAL WARNINGS

Patients with proven PE should be managed, at least in the initial phase of the illness, by a pulmonologist. The frequency and duration of routine follow-up should be determined by the underlying pathology, as well as the treatment modality used.

Any acute change in symptoms or the development of sudden dyspnea, chest pain, or tachypnea warrants immediate referral. Signs of hemodynamic instability (eg, systolic blood pressure <100 mmHg, heart rate >100/min, signs of hypoxemia) require emergency evaluation in a hospital setting.

Medication side effects such as bleeding or thrombocytopenia should be emergently evaluated by a clinician experienced in the treatment of venous thromboembolism.

EDITOR'S NOTE:
COMPLEMENTARY APPROACHES

A general discussion of complementary approaches can be found in Chapter 3. The following, while not an exhaustive list, are some complementary approaches being used for this condition. Additional information on these approaches, including precautions, can be found in Appendices A and B. Providers need to assess for the use of complementary approaches as part of the patient's history, as they may impact conventional therapies, and patients may not volunteer this information unless specifically asked. Efficacy of many complementary approaches is not as well documented as that of conventional therapies. Providers need to read the literature before suggesting these complementary approaches.

- Vitamins, minerals, herbs, supplements
  Vitamin E

References

Anderson, F.A. Jr., & Wheeler, H.B. (1995). Venous thromboembolism: Risk factors and prophylaxis. *Clinics in Chest Medicine, 16*(2), 235–251.

Anderson, F.A. Jr., Wheeler, H.B., Goldberg, R.J., et al. (1991). A population-based perspective of the hospital incidence and case fatality rates of deep vein thrombosis and pulmonary embolism. The Worcester DVT study. *Archives of Internal Medicine, 151,* 933–938.

Bounameux, H., de Moerloose, P., Perrier, A., et al. (1994). Plasma measurement of D-dimer as diagnostic aid in suspected venous thromboembolism: An overview. *Thrombosis and Haemostasis, 71,* 1–6.

Burke, B., Sostman, D., Caroll, B.A., & Witty, L.A. (1995). The diagnostic approach to deep venous thrombosis: Which technique? *Clinics in Chest Medicine, 16*(2), 253–268.

Elliott, C.G. (1992). Pulmonary physiology during pulmonary embolism. *Chest, 101*(4, Suppl.), 163S–1171S.

Ewald, G.A. (1995) Thromboembolic disorders. *Manual of Medical Therapeutics,* 28th ed., pp. 396–398. Boston: Little, Brown & Co.

Fujimura, H., Kambayashi, J., Monden, M., Kato, H., & Miyata, T. (1995). Coagulation factor V Leiden mutation may have a racial background. *Thrombosis and Haemostasis, 74*(5), 1381–1382.

Ginsberg, J.S. (1996). Management of venous thromboembolism. *N Engl J Med, 335*(24), 1816–1828.

Ginsberg, J.S., Kearon, C., Douketis, J., et al. (1997). The use of D-Dimer testing and impedance plethysmographic examination in patients with clinical indications of deep vein thrombosis. *Archives of Internal Medicine, 157,* 1077–1081.

Hirsh, J. (1991). Oral anticoagulant drugs. *N Engl J Med, 324,* 1867–1875.

Hirsh, J., & Hoak, J. (1996). Management of deep vein thrombosis and pulmonary embolism. A statement for healthcare professionals. *Circulation, 93,* 2212–2245.

Janata-Schwatczek, K., Weiss, K., Riezinger, I., Bankier, A., Domanovits, H., & Seidler, D. (1996). Pulmonary embolism. Diagnosis and treatment. *Seminars in Thrombosis and Hemostasis, 22*(1), 33–52.

Kanter, D.S., Mikkola, K.M., Patel, S.R., Parker, J.A., & Goldhaber, S.Z. (1997). Thrombolytic therapy for pulmonary embolism. Frequency of intracranial hemorrhage and associated risk factors. *Chest, 111*(5), 1241–1245.

Piccioli, A., Prandoni, P., & Goldhaber, S.Z. (1996). Epidemiologic characteristics, management and outcome of deep venous thrombosis in a tertiary care hospital: The Brigham and Women's Hospital DVT registry. *American Heart Journal, 132*(5), 1010–1014.

PIOPED Investigators. (1990). Invasive and noninvasive diagnosis of pulmonary embolism. Results of the Prospective Investigation Of Pulmonary Embolism Diagnosis (PIOPED). *JAMA, 263,* 2753–2759.

Simonneau, G., Azarian, R., Brenot, F., Darteville, P.G., Musset, D., & Duroux, P. (1995). Surgical management of unresolved pulmonary embolism. A personal series of 72 patients. *Chest, 107*(1, Suppl.), 52S–55S.

Stein, P.D., Henry, J.W., & Relyea, B. (1995). Untreated patients with pulmonary embolism. Outcome, clinical and laboratory assessment. *Chest, 107*(4), 931–935.

Stein, P.D., Terrin, M.L., Hales, C.A., Palevsky, H.I., Saltzmann, H.A., Thompson, B.T., & Weg, J.G. (1991). Clinical, laboratory, roentgenographic and electrocardiographic findings in patients with acute pulmonary embolism and no pre-existing cardiac or pulmonary disease. *Chest, 100,* 589–603.

Tapson, V.F., & Hull, R.D. (1995). Management of venous thromboembolic disease. The impact of low-molecular-weight heparin. *Clinics in Chest Medicine, 16*(2), 281–294.

Toglia, M.R., & Weg, J.G. (1996). Venous thromboembolism during pregnancy. *N Engl J Med, 335*(2), 108–114.

Weiss, K. (1996). Pulmonary thromboembolism: Epidemiology and techniques of nuclear medicine. *Seminars in Thrombosis and Hemostasis, 22*(1), 27–32.

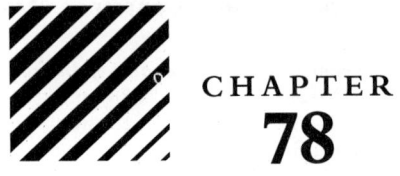

CHAPTER
78

Sarcoidosis

Linda S. Efferen, MD, FACP, FCCP

Sarcoidosis is a multisystem disorder of unknown etiology that is characterized pathologically by the presence of nonnecrotizing granulomatous lesions. It generally affects young, previously healthy adults. Most patients present with typical clinical or radiographic features, but atypical presentations are well known and may mimic other diseases such as tuberculosis or malignancy.

Treatment is nonspecific. Corticosteroids can be used in an attempt to ameliorate significant symptoms and prevent progression of disease in vital organ systems. However, it is unclear if therapy alters the course or eventual outcome of disease (Fanburg & Lazarus, 1994).

ANATOMY, PHYSIOLOGY, AND PATHOLOGY

Pathology

The granulomatous lesion in sarcoidosis is typical but nonspecific and is often found in multiple areas of the body, even in the absence of clinical disease. In the lung, activated T lymphocytes interact with alveolar macrophages infiltrating the air space and interstitium. Interactions among these cells, fibroblasts, and other cells in the lung dictate the course of disease. Alveolar macrophages may amplify inflammation and fibrogenesis by releasing various biochemical markers and cytokines or may suppress or downregulate the inflammatory response.

Resolution of the alveolitis or progression with development of granulomatous lesions may occur. Characteristic microscopic granulomas composed of tightly clustered epithelioid histiocytes may occur, often including multinucleated giant cells. The central core of the granuloma is surrounded by lymphocytes and plasma cells. Central necrosis is rare. The granulomatous lesions may resolve or progress to fibrosis and permanent scarring. These characteristic lesions are not specific for sarcoidosis, however, and can be seen in mycobacterial and fungal infections, berylliosis, extrinsic allergic alveolitis, malignancy, drugs, and foreign body reactions.

EPIDEMIOLOGY

Sarcoidosis has a worldwide distribution, although the reported prevalence of disease varies widely—from 0.04 per 100,000 in Spain to 64 per 100,000 in Sweden. The disease appears to be rare in Africa and Central and South America. The reported rate from North America, Europe, Japan, and the United Kingdom is 10 to 20 per 100,000. In the United States, prevalence ranges from 11 to 71 per 100,000. This large variation may be due in part to variation in medical practice and the frequency with which routine chest radiographs are obtained in a specific region. Based on autopsy, it has been estimated that the true incidence of sarcoidosis may be 10-fold higher than clinical estimates.

Race and gender affect the incidence of disease. African American women experience the highest risk for developing sarcoidosis. In the United States, women are affected more frequently than men, and the prevalence of sarcoidosis among African Americans has been reported to be 8 to 10 times greater than in whites.

DIAGNOSTIC CRITERIA

The diagnosis of sarcoidosis is often suggested by the clinical or radiographic presentation. Sarcoidosis is a disease of young, previously healthy adults; approximately 80% of patients are ages 20 to 40 on initial presentation. Although sarcoidosis can affect any organ system, approximately 90% of patients exhibit signs or symptoms of the disease referable to the chest. When typical clinical and radiographic features are present in a young, previously healthy person, it is highly suggestive of sarcoidosis.

Patients may be asymptomatic on presentation, with characteristic abnormalities found on routine chest radiographs. Symptomatic patients frequently present with an insidious onset of symptoms or findings from pulmonary, ocular, or cutaneous lesions (Table 78-1). Symptoms of fatigue, weakness, malaise, fever, and loss of weight are seen in 40% to 50% of cases. Occasionally patients present with an acute onset of symptoms, including fever, polyarthritis, iritis, and erythema nodosum, suggesting Lofgren's syndrome.

Routine laboratory tests may reveal abnormalities suggestive of sarcoidosis. Hypercalcemia, hypercalciuria, and elevated liver enzymes, especially alkaline phosphatase, may be present. Polyclonal hypergammaglobulinemia is variably reported in 25% to 80% of patients, and leukopenia occurs in 5% to 10%.

The chest radiograph may reveal bilateral hilar or mediastinal adenopathy with or without pulmonary parenchymal involvement. Pulmonary fibrosis and honeycombing may be seen, although a normal chest radiograph is also possible (Table 78-2).

The diagnosis of sarcoidosis requires the exclusion of other diseases that can present with similar clinical, radiographic, and pathologic features. A demonstration of nonnecrotizing granulomatous lesions in pathologic specimens, in an appropriate clinical setting and in the absence of evidence supporting alternative etiologies, would be considered diagnostic. At times, the clinical presentation may be sufficiently typical to preclude the need for tissue confirmation, particularly in an asymptomatic person.

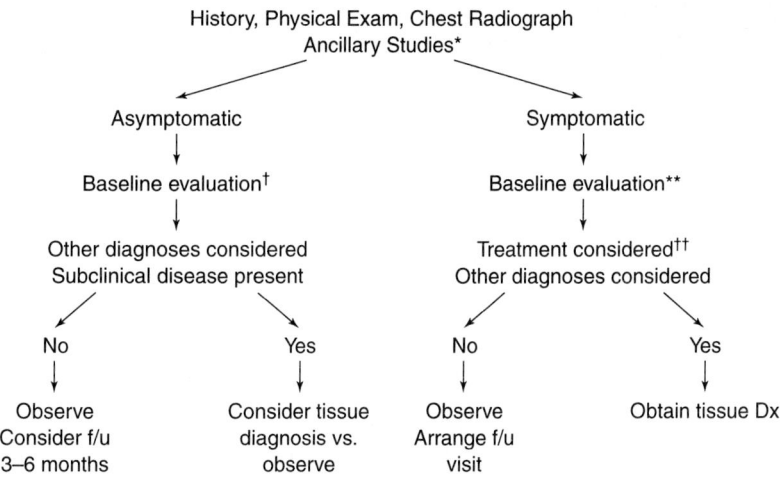

FIGURE 78-1 Initial assessment and diagnosis.

*Anergy panel, serum angiotensin-converting enzyme may be considered
†Pulmonary function testing, ocular screening, liver function tests, serum calcium, urinalysis
**Include other specific organ system evaluation as clinically indicated.
††See Table 78-3.

HISTORY AND PHYSICAL EXAM

Most patients with sarcoidosis are asymptomatic. In symptomatic ones, a subacute or chronic presentation is most often found. The pulmonary system is the most common organ system involved, and symptoms include cough, shortness of breath, dyspnea on exertion, and chest pain. An acute onset of symptoms and physical findings is seen in 10% to 15% of cases.

Findings on the physical exam depend on the organ system involved. The chest exam is usually normal, although end-inspiratory crackles or wheezing may be present. Ocular and cutaneous manifestations of the disease are frequent and fairly characteristic. Unusual signs or symptoms from commonly affected organ systems or from less frequently involved systems may lead to an initial delay in considering the diagnosis.

DIAGNOSTIC STUDIES

An initial evaluation including pulmonary function tests, ocular screening, liver function tests, and serum calcium levels should be performed to evaluate the presence of occult, multiorgan system disease and to serve as a baseline for subsequent evaluation and testing (Fig. 78-1). In symptomatic patients, evaluation specific to the organ system involved should also be included. Tuberculin skin testing is usually performed and often demonstrates cutaneous anergy.

The most frequent abnormality detected on pulmonary function testing is a restrictive lung pattern characterized by decreased lung volumes and diffusing capacity. Reduced expiratory air flow rates, indicative of airflow obstruction, occur in approximately 20% of cases. Airway hyperreactivity to metha-

TABLE 78-1	Clinical Manifestations of Sarcoidosis
Organ System	**Symptoms/Signs**
Intrathoracic—lungs and/or lymph nodes (90%)*	Asymptomatic, shortness of breath, nonproductive cough, chest pain, wheezing, radiographic abnormalities
Ocular (20%–30%)	Iridocyclitis, chorioretinitis, keratoconjunctivitis, glaucoma, cataract, blindness, Heerfordt's syndrome†
Cutaneous (20%–30%)	Erythema nodosum, lupus pernio, nodular or flat plaques, subcutaneous nodules
Reticuloendothelial system	Peripheral lymphadenopathy (40%), hepatosplenomegaly (20%)
Musculoskeletal (10%–15%)	Polyarthritis, bone cysts, myositis
Myocardial (5%)	Palpitations, syncope, dizziness, chest pain, arrhythmia, sudden death
Nervous system (5%)	Seizures, basal granulomatoid meningitis, hypothalamic hypopituitarism or hypothyroidism, cranial nerve palsies, hydrocephalus
Exocrine glands (4%)	Painless swelling of the parotid glands, keratoconjunctiva sicca**
Renal	Hypercalcemia (10%–20%), hypercalciuria (20%–25%), nephrocalcinosis

* Percent of patients with involvement

† Anterior uveitis, parotid gland enlargement, facial palsy, fever

** Lacrimal gland enlargement, xerostomia, xerophthalmia

TABLE 78-2	Chest Radiographic Stages in Sarcoidosis	
Description		**Frequency at Presentation**
0.	Normal film	10%
I.	Bilateral hilar adenopathy; paratracheal adenopathy possible	50%
II.	Adenopathy with pulmonary parenchymal involvement	30%
III.	Pulmonary parenchymal involvement without adenopathy	10%
IV.*	Pulmonary fibrosis with honeycombing	

* Variably delineated separately from stage III.

choline challenge is demonstrable in a smaller percentage of patients. In general, pulmonary function testing is not a reliable means for detecting disease or estimating the extent of disease and does not correlate with clinical or radiographic findings. However, sequential measurements may allow assessment of change in individual patients.

The need for tissue diagnosis should be determined clinically. In an asymptomatic patient with characteristic radiographic findings in whom treatment is not being considered, tissue diagnosis may be unnecessary unless an alternative diagnosis such as tuberculosis or lymphoma is clinically suspected. When tissue diagnosis is required, fiberoptic bronchoscopy with transbronchial biopsies is the method most frequently used. It is diagnostic in 75% to 90% of patients with abnormal chest radiographs (stage I to III) and in up to 50% of patients with a normal radiograph (stage 0).

Alternatively, if other organ involvement is present, such as the skin or conjunctiva, tissue biopsy from other organs can be considered. Mediastinal lymph node biopsies are reported to be diagnostic in up to 95% of patients with intrathoracic lymphadenopathy, and liver biopsy may be positive in 75% to 90% of patients. However, these procedures are not generally required or routinely used. Similarly, open lung biopsy to establish a diagnosis of sarcoidosis is rarely necessary.

Numerous ancillary tests have been used in an attempt to establish a diagnosis of sarcoidosis. The Kveim test has limited utility because it produces variable results based on the source of antigen, and there is a long delay (4 to 6 weeks) in obtaining the results.

Serum angiotensin-converting enzyme measurement and gallium-67 scanning have been used extensively but have not proved to be as reliable as noninvasive diagnostic tests. Serum angiotensin-converting enzyme determinations are neither sensitive or specific. In clinically active untreated cases, levels are reported to be elevated in 33% to 88% of patients. Elevated levels are nonspecific and have been associated with a variety of other diseases, including infections (tuberculosis, fungal, HIV), intravenous drug use, Gaucher's disease, and liver cirrhosis. They can be found in normal persons as well. Gallium scans are positive in 60% to 80% of patients but are also nonspecific. A pattern of bilateral hilar uptake is suggestive and most commonly seen in sarcoidosis, whereas extrathoracic lymph node uptake is more common in lymphoma. However, overlap exists, limiting the overall diagnostic utility of this test.

Bronchoalveolar lavage (BAL) in sarcoidosis characteristically demonstrates a lymphocytic alveolitis. In BAL from normal subjects, there is a preponderance of macrophages, with lymphocytes making up less than 10% of the cell population, 90% of which are T cells. In sarcoidosis there is a marked increase in the percentage of lymphocytes, due almost exclusively to an increase in helper T cells. Although a great deal of information has been obtained from BAL studies in sarcoid patients, its precise role in diagnosis and treatment remains to be determined. Persistence of alveolitis appears to be a poor prognostic indicator but is neither diagnostic nor an established indication for treatment independent of clinical and physiologic correlation.

High-resolution computed tomography provides a more definitive description of alveolar architecture and adenopathy than conventional radiography. It may play a role in predicting the patient's response to therapy by demonstrating evidence of active alveolitis as opposed to end-stage fibrosis. However, it is not a diagnostic tool, and its role in the clinical management of sarcoidosis requires further study.

TREATMENT OPTIONS, EXPECTED OUTCOMES, AND COMPREHENSIVE MANAGEMENT

In the absence of a known cause for sarcoidosis, primary prevention is impossible. Therapy to ameliorate symptoms and to limit the progression of disease may not be successful in altering the clinical outcome. Attempts to minimize morbidity related to treatment should be stressed, and exposure to prolonged or unnecessary therapy should be avoided.

Cultural Considerations

The diagnosis and treatment of sarcoidosis in heterogenous patient groups can be a challenge. Among immigrants, diagnosis and treatment may be delayed or complicated by the use of nontraditional health providers or reliance on home remedies. Other patient populations may prefer nontraditional medical models as well, resulting in similar delays. The bureaucratic nature of the current health care system, as well as sociocultural and language differences, may further impede access to and use of health care resources.

Nutritional Considerations

Glucocorticoid-induced osteoporosis is a significant potential complication in patients requiring prolonged corticosteroid therapy for sarcoidosis. With the advent of dual-energy x-ray absorptiometry, bone density can be readily assessed and therapeutic strategies developed to minimize or reverse ongoing bone resorption. Adherence to general nutritional guidelines for calcium intake should be encouraged.

Treatment Options

No definitive therapy for sarcoidosis exists, and one is unlikely to be developed in the absence of an identifiable cause for the disease. Corticosteroids have been used in an attempt to ameliorate symptoms and prevent progression of disease and are considered the mainstay of therapy. They are effective in suppressing the clinical and physiologic manifestations of disease in 70% to 90% of patients. Relapse is common when treatment is stopped, however, and the long-term benefit is unclear. The potential side effects and complications of systemic corticosteroids are well known.

Estimation of treatment efficacy has been favorably biased by the overall benign clinical course of the disease and the high rate of remission even in the absence of therapy. More recently, investigators have begun to question whether the use of corticosteroids in sarcoidosis may actually prolong the clinical course of disease. In the absence of any clear long-term benefit, treatment should be reserved for patients with significant symptoms not controlled with other therapy or with evidence of vital organ involvement (eg, cardiac, central nervous system, ocular). Asymptomatic patients with progressive deterioration of lung function may be considered for therapy as well (Table 78-3).

An initial observation period before the initiation of therapy, or after a relapse, is reasonable in anticipation of possible spontaneous resolution. The duration of observation is not well defined. Lack of improvement over 6 months may be considered an indication for treatment. Alternatively, continued observation of a stable patient may be reasonable (Gottlieb et al, 1997; Gibson et al, 1996; Hunninghake et al, 1994).

The optimal dose and duration of corticosteroids are not well defined. A maximum dose of 1 mg/kg is generally recommended for potentially life-threatening organ system involvement. Lower doses of 30 to 40 mg/day for non–life-threatening disease can be used. Therapy for 1 year or longer has been recommended but may unnecessarily prolong the exposure to corticosteroids.

A more rational approach may be to follow the patient's response to therapy, with gradual withdrawal and discontinuation of corticosteroids when the patient is clinically and physiologically stable (Fig. 78-2). Should relapse occur, reinstitution of therapy can be considered. If prolonged corticosteroid therapy is required, conversion to alternate-day dosing should be considered.

Systemic corticosteroids are not always required. Inhaled corticosteroids have relatively low toxicity and when used in relatively high doses (budesonide 1600 μg/day or equivalent) may suppress markers of alveolitis. This form of therapy may be useful in patients with mild pulmonary disease, especially if cough, wheezing, or bronchial hyperreactivity is present. Ocular involvement manifested by anterior uveitis may be managed with topical corticosteroids. Cutaneous involvement may be managed with hydroxychloroquine or topical therapy. Hypercalcemia may also be controlled with hydroxychloroquine in some cases.

TABLE 78-3	Indications for Systemic Corticosteroid Therapy*

Vital organ involvement
    Ocular—not amenable to topical therapy
    Cardiac
    Central nervous system
    Upper airway (laryngeal)

Symptomatic pulmonary involvement with moderate to severe physiologic abnormalities**

Asymptomatic pulmonary involvement with progressive deterioration in physiologic function**

Hypercalcemia or hypercalciuria not responsive to other treatment modalities

Relapse of disease after withdrawal of corticosteroids**

Dermatologic involvement unresponsive to other therapies

Hyperplenism producing thrombocytopenia

* Tissue diagnosis generally recommended.

** Observation period before initiation of therapy in anticipation of spontaneous resolution may be considered.

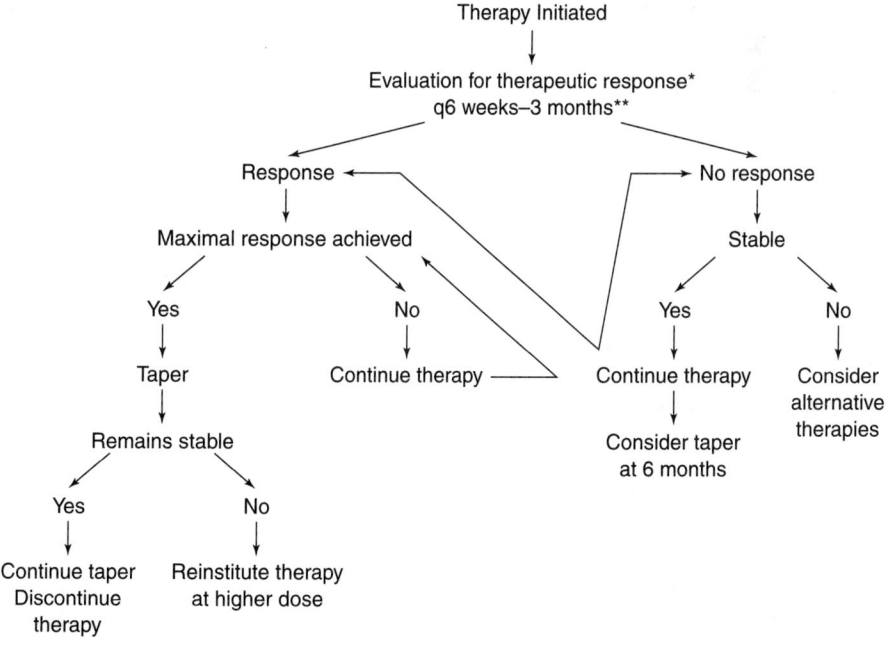

FIGURE 78-2 Evaluation of response to therapy.

*Response should be determined based on predetermined objective markers.
**Frequency of follow-up should be determined clinically.

TABLE 78-4	Therapeutic Alternatives in Refractory Disease	
Agent	Dose	Major Toxicity
Methotrexate	10 mg/wk–20 mg twice weekly	Liver
Azathioprine	200 mg/d	Bone marrow
Cyclophosphamide	1–2.5 mg/kg/d	Bone marrow, bladder, malignant neoplasms**
Chlorambucil	4–12 mg/d	Bone marrow, hematologic malignancies**
Cyclosporin A	5–7 mg/kg/d	Renal, hypertension
Chloroquine	250–500 mg OD*	Ocular
Hydroxychloroquine	200 mg BID	Ocular

* May be administered BID.

** Dose-dependent increased risk.

CLINICAL WARNING: Any sign or symptom consistent with adrenal insufficiency should be emergently evaluated.

Other agents have been used for patients with refractory disease or intolerance to corticosteroids (Table 78-4). These agents have been used in anecdotal cases or small clinical trials or based on presumed benefit due to the drug's mechanism of action. No strong recommendation for any particular agent can be made, although methotrexate and azathioprine appear to have gained more support based on their risk/benefit ratios and clinical experience. These drugs may be considered for use in select cases as an adjunct or alternative to corticosteroid therapy (Lynch & McCune, 1997; Muthiah & Macfarlane, 1990).

Transplantation may be considered in appropriate candidates with progressive deterioration in organ function of the heart, liver, or lung. Recurrence of disease in transplanted organs occurs, despite treatment with corticosteroids and immunosuppressive agents, but is not currently considered a contraindication to transplantation.

Expected Outcomes

In most instances, sarcoidosis follows a benign clinical course. Although estimates vary, up to 80% of patients have a mild to moderate course with resolution of disease even in the absence of therapy. Severe, unremitting disease with progressive organ dysfunction occurs in approximately 20% of patients. Treatment may ameliorate symptoms and laboratory evidence of disease, but alteration in the eventual outcome may not be possible.

Predicting the course an individual patient will experience is difficult. Older age at onset, multisystem involvement, and radiographic stage III have been associated with a worse prognosis, however (Takada et al, 1993).

TEACHING AND SELF-CARE

A well-informed patient is an invaluable component in the therapeutic strategy. Patients should be apprised of their diagnosis, possible course and response to therapy, and potential complications. Knowledge regarding the rationale for the use of medications and the limitations of therapy will allow patients to participate in and follow their plan of care. Patients should notify the health care provider of disease exacerbations or side effects from medications in a timely fashion. Patients should be advised of potential effects of corticosteroid use, such as impaired glucose tolerance, osteoporosis, decreased ability to fight infection, peptic ulcer formation, psychological changes, and suppression of the hypothalamic–pituitary–adrenal axis. Bone density scanning and additional measures to combat osteoporosis (adequate calcium and vitamin D intake, estrogen replacement therapy, weight-bearing activity) may be necessary.

Patients should be taught that sarcoidosis is a restrictive lung disease that may require changes in activity based on progression of symptoms. Fatigue and dyspnea may preclude extensive physical activities, but patients should be encouraged to maintain their daily activity at the highest level of function possible.

Patients should remain alert to extrapulmonary involvement. They should report any new visual symptoms, such as red or painful eyes or blurred vision, which may indicate iritis. Signs of additional organ system involvement may include facial nerve weakness or paresthesias, peripheral neuropathies, cutaneous lesions, abdominal pain, jaundice, palpitations, and arthritis. Patients should be counseled regarding their medication regimens, including dosages and proper application of topical cutaneous and ophthalmic corticosteroids. The patient should be cautioned not to stop taking corticosteroids abruptly and to return for follow-up and re-evaluation of therapy.

Patients should be encouraged to ask questions regarding any aspect of their care. Referral to support groups and services should be made as needed.

COMMUNITY RESOURCES

Sarcoidosis is often referred to as a hidden disease or a medical mystery, but it should be neither. It is not a rare disease, and in most patients it is not a difficult diagnosis to establish. However, it has not garnered much public attention, so it is unfamiliar to most patients, and patients are not usually aware of others with the disease. Recently, concerted efforts have been made to increase the public's and the medical community's awareness of sarcoidosis. Local support groups may exist within the community.

- The National Sarcoidosis Resource Center (NSRC), P.O. Box 1593, Piscataway, NJ 08855-1593, 908-699-0733, fax 908-699-0882: A resource guide and directory, written by Sandra Conroy, president of the

NSRC, provides a directory of physicians, support groups, government resources, and other information.

- The Sarcoidosis HelpNet, 191 Melvin Ave., Staten Island, NY 10314, 718-982-7118
- Sarcoidosis National Network, The American Lung Association, 1726 M Street, N.W., Suite 902, Washington, D.C. 20036, 202-785-3355
- Sarcoid Research Institute, 3475 Central Ave., Memphis, TN 38111, 901-766-6951
- The National Sarcoidosis Foundation at St. Michael's Medical Center, 268 Martin Luther King Blvd., Newark, NJ 07102, 800-223-6429, fax 201-877-2850
- The American Lung Association, 1740 Broadway, New York, NY 10019-4374, 800-LUNG-USA or 212-315-8700, http://ovchin.uc.edu/htdocs/ala/sarcoidosis.html
- Sarcoidosis Research Institute, http://www.netten.net/soskelnt/
- National Jewish Medical and Research Center, http://njc.org/MSUhtml/MSU   Sarcoidosis.html
- Sarcoidosis Worldwide Support Group, http://members.aol.com/swsg2/index.htm

REFERRAL POINTS AND CLINICAL WARNINGS

A patient with active sarcoidosis should be managed jointly with a specialist of the organ systems involved, unless the primary care provider has developed significant expertise in the disease. The frequency of routine follow-up should be determined by the degree of clinical acuity.

Progressive deterioration in functional status or any acute change in symptoms should be evaluated. Treatment with corticosteroids may unmask previously occult diabetes or hypertension or exacerbate pre-existing clinical diseases. Corticosteroids may impair immunity, and patients should be monitored for signs and symptoms of infection. Patients should be advised never to discontinue taking corticosteroids abruptly due to suppression of endogenous cortisol production from chronic exogenous corticosteroid use.

References

Fanburg, B.L., & Lazarus, D.S. (1994). Sarcoidosis. In J.F. Murray & J.A. Nadel (Eds.). *Textbook of respiratory medicine.* Philadelphia: W.B. Saunders.

Gibson, G.J., Prescott, R.J., Muers, M.F., et al. (1996). British Thoracic Society Sarcoidosis study: Effects of long-term corticosteroid treatment. *Thorax, 51,* 238–247.

Gottlieb, J.E., Israel, H.L., Steiner, R.M., et al. (1997). Outcome in sarcoidosis; The relationship of relapse to corticosteroid therapy. *Chest, 111,* 623–631.

Hunninghake, G.W., Gilbert, S., Pueringer, R., et al. (1994). Outcome of the treatment for sarcoidosis. *American Journal of Respiratory and Critical Care Medicine, 149,* 893–898.

Lynch, J.P., & McCune, W.J. (1997). Immunosuppressive and cytotoxic pharmacotherapy for pulmonary disorders. *American Journal of Respiratory and Critical Care Medicine, 155,* 395–420.

Muthiah, M.M., & Macfarlane, J.T. (1990). Current concepts in the management of sarcoidosis. *Drugs, 40*(2), 231–237.

Takada, K., Ina, Y., Noda, M., et al. (1993). The clinical course and prognosis of patients with severe, moderate or mild sarcoidosis. *Journal of Clinical Epidemiology, 46,* 359–366.

Vitamins, Minerals, Herbs, and Supplements

Steven J. Lowy, MD

This appendix is intended to aid the provider whose patients are using supplements; it includes only the most basic information for each supplement. It is not meant to be a definitive reference. *The provider is urged to do further research before recommending any of the substances discussed.*

There are hundreds of supplements sold in health food stores. Space does not allow discussion of all these compounds; only the most commonly used are included. Supplements without published documentation for their use were excluded from this list, except as noted. However, exclusion from this chapter does not mean a supplement is ineffective, but that it either is not among the most commonly used or lacks appropriate experimental proof of its usefulness.

- **Note 1**: Use of most supplements by children or pregnant women is not well researched. Use in pediatrics and pregnancy thus cannot be recommended
- **Note 2**: Particular care should be taken with herbal products because many of them are tinctures and should therefore be avoided in patients who should not be ingesting alcohol.
- **Note 3**: There is little or no governmental regulation of the manufacture of most supplements. As with any products, some brands are more reputable and reliable than others. Choosing a good brand takes research and sometimes experimentation.
- **Note 4**: In general, natural supplements are slower-acting than artificially engineered drugs. For most of the supplements, it is prudent to observe their use for up to 2 months before making decisions on their efficacy.

Beta-Carotene

There has been much recent controversy about beta-carotene's value and possible adverse affects. It has been included here because it is still one of the most commonly used supplements, and the provider should be aware of its potentials for harm and good.

Beta-carotene is one of a large group of compounds called carotenoids, found mostly in fruits and vegetables. Although often considered interchangeable with vitamin A (particularly in product labeling), it is merely a precursor and is metabolized to vitamin A by the body in a rate-limited fashion.

Effects

Most of its actions are considered to be due to its antioxidant capacity.

Uses

Dermatologic

Patients with skin cancer have lower-than-normal levels of beta-carotene. It is possible, but unproven, that supplementation would help prevent or treat these cancers (Engle et al, 1991).

Oncologic

Some research shows a protective effect against cancer in general (Pool-Zobel et al, 1997) and cancer of the lung, prostate, bladder, esophagus (Harris et al, 1991), and cervix in particular (Engle et al, 1991). However, evidence is conflicting and inconclusive at this time.

Precautions

Some studies using beta-carotene alone have shown increased incidences of lung cancer and stroke, particularly in smokers. Other studies using beta-carotene in combination with other antioxidants (eg, vitamin A, vitamin C, and selenium) have shown only beneficial effects (Blot, 1997). Pending definitive studies, it may be prudent for smokers to avoid large doses of beta-carotene, especially if not taken in combination with other antioxidant supplements.

All carotenoids are not the same. Care should be taken not to lump them all together; rather, they should be considered individually and researched individually with regard to supplementation. Whole foods often contain several or many individual carotenoids, so results from dietary carotenoids cannot be extrapolated easily to the use of individual carotenoids such as beta-carotene. There is conflicting evidence as to whether supplementation with beta-carotene alone results in a depletion of other carotenoids and loss of their beneficial effect (Albanes et al, 1997; Nierenberg et al, 1997; Knekt et al, 1997).

Toxicity of beta-carotene, except as mentioned above, is very low. Consumption of high doses can cause a temporary and completely reversible elevation of beta-carotene in the blood and skin (carotenemia), causing the skin to take on an orange hue.

See also Notes 1, 2, 3, and 4 at the beginning of the appendix.

References

Albanes, D., Virtamo, J., Taylor, P.R., Rautalahti, M., Pietinen, P., & Heinonen, O.P. (1997). Effects of supplemental beta-carotene, cigarette smoking, and alcohol consumption on serum carotenoids in the Alpha-Tocopherol, Beta-Carotene Cancer Prevention Study. *American Journal of Clinical Nutrition, 66*(2), 366–372.

Blot, W.J. (1997). Vitamin/mineral supplementation and cancer risk: International chemoprevention trials. *Proceedings of the Society for Experimental Biology in Medicine, 216*(2), 291–296.

Engle, A., Muscat, J.E., & Harris, R.E. (1991). Nutritional risk factors and ovarian cancer. *Nutrition & Cancer, 15*(3-4), 239–247.

Harris, R.W., Key, T.J., Silcocks, P.B., Bull, D., & Wald, N.J. (1991). A case-control study of dietary carotene in men with lung cancer and in men with other epithelial cancers. *Nutrition & Cancer, 15*(1), 63–68.

Hsueh, Y.M., Chiou, H.Y., Huang, Y.L., et al. (1997). Serum beta-carotene level, arsenic methylation capability, and incidence of skin cancer. *Cancer Epidemiology Biomarkers & Prevention, 6*(8), 589–596.

Knekt, P., Jarvinen, R., Seppanen, R., et al. (1997). Dietary flavonoids and the risk of lung cancer and other malignant neoplasms. *American Journal of Epidemiology, 146*(3), 223–230.

Nierenberg, D.W., Dain, B.J., Mott, L.A., Baron, J.A., & Greenberg, E.R. (1997). Effects of 4 g of oral supplementation with beta-carotene on serum concentrations of retinol, tocopherol, and five carotenoids. *American Journal of Clinical Nutrition, 66*(2), 315–319.

Pool-Zobel, B.L., Bub, A., Muller, H., Wollowski, I., & Rechkemmer, G. (1997). Consumption of vegetables reduces genetic damage in humans: First results of a human intervention trial with carotenoid-rich foods. *Carcinogenesis, 18*(9), 1847–1850.

Cabbage Juice (Glutamine)

A remedy with little documentation since 1950. Still, it is described in most texts on alternative therapies and has no side effects.

Effects

Mode of action unknown; perhaps due to its large content of the amino acid glutamine, which has been shown to reduce ulcer formation in humans and laboratory animals.

Uses

Gastrointestinal

Treatment and prevention of peptic ulcers

Precautions

Glutamine contains more nitrogen than most amino acids and may form more ammonia on metabolism. Therefore, its use is not recommended in the presence of hepatic or renal dysfunction, or any other disease where excess ammonia buildup is possible.

See also Notes 1, 2, 3, and 4 at the beginning of this appendix.

References

Cheney, G. (1949). Rapid healing of peptic ulcers in patients receiving fresh cabbage juice. *California Medicine, 70,* 10–14.

Hung, C.R., & Neu, S.L. (1997). Acid-induced gastric damage in rats is aggravated by starvation and prevented by several nutrients. *Journal of Nutrition, 127,* 630–666.

Shive, W., (1957). Glutamine in treatment of peptic ulcer. *Texas State Journal of Medicine, 53,* 840–843.

Carnitine (L-Carnitine)

Carnitine is structurally similar to amino acids but is not a building block for proteins. It is a transporter of fatty acids and is essential for the metabolism of fats for energy.

Effects

Most of carnitine's usefulness comes from its enhancement of fat metabolism in muscle and, in particular, myocardium (Gaby, 1995).

Uses

Cardiovascular

- When used after myocardial infarction (MI), it has been shown to reduce mortality, the size of the infarct, and the incidence of post-MI angina.

- Lowers serum lipids; improves cardiac function and general well-being in patients taking standard antihypertensive drugs (Digiesi et al, 1994)
- Shown to improve survival dramatically after cardiogenic shock (Corbucci & Loche, 1993)
- In patients with severe lower limb arterial insufficiency, carnitine reduces claudication and increases walking distance (Brevetti et al, 1995).

Precautions

Very low toxicity. Can cause mild gastrointestinal upset.

See also Notes 1, 2, 3, and 4 at the beginning of this appendix.

References

Brevetti, G., Perna, S., Sabbá, C., Martone, V.D., Condorelli, M. (1995). Propionyl-L-carnitine in intermittent claudication: Double-blind, placebo-controlled, dose titration, multicenter study. *Journal of the American College of Cardiology, 26*(6), 1411–1416.

Corbucci, G.G., & Loche, F. (1993). L-carnitine in cardiogenic shock therapy: Pharmacodynamic aspects and clinical data. *International Journal of Clinical Pharmacologic Research, 13*(2), 87–91.

Digiesi, V., Cantini, F., Bisi, G., Guarino, G., & Brodbeck, B. (1994). L-carnitine adjuvant therapy in essential hypertension. *Clinical Therapy, 144*(5), 391–395.

Gaby, A.R. (1995). *Nutrition and Healing,* April, 3.

Singh, R.B., Niaz, M.A., Agarwal, P., Beegum, R., Rastogi, S.S., & Sachan, D.S. (1996). A randomised, double-blind, placebo-controlled trial of L-carnitine in suspected acute myocardial infarction. *Postgraduate Medicine, 72*(843), 45–50.

Coenzyme Q10

Also known as ubiquinone and CoQ10, this naturally occurring compound is essential for energy production in the mitochondria. Serum levels of CoQ10 have been found to be significantly lowered in several forms of cancer (including breast cancer and melanoma); similar lowered levels have been found in cardiac failure and ischemia. This deficiency has sparked interest in the use of CoQ10 in the treatment of cancer and heart disease.

Effects

Improves energy production in the mitochondria and improves the function of cardiac and skeletal muscle

Uses

Cardiovascular

- Strengthens the failing heart
- Lowers blood pressure (Langsjoen et al, 1994; Digiesi et al, 1994)
- Improves cardiac function and survival of patients with dilated cardiomyopathy
- Reduces the frequency of anginal attacks.

Oncologic

- May protect myocardium against chemotherapy-induced damage
- Has caused regression and "disappearance" of metastatic breast cancer.

Precautions

No known toxicities. Important to obtain from a reputable source; essentially all quality CoQ10 is imported from Japan. May be better absorbed in oil-based form.

See also Notes 1, 2, 3, and 4 at the beginning of this appendix.

References

Cortes, E.P., Gupta, M., Chou, C., Amin, V.C., & Folkers, K. (1978). Adriamycin cardiotoxicity: Early detection by systolic time interval and possible prevention by coenzyme Q10. *Cancer Treatment Reports, 62*(6), 887–891.

Digiesi, V., Cantini, F., Oradei, A., et al. (1994). Coenzyme Q10 in essential hypertension. *Molecular Aspects of Medicine, 15* Suppl, S257–263.

Domae, N., Sawada, H., Matsuyama, E., Konishi, T., & Uchino, H. (1981). Cardiomyopathy and other chronic toxic effects induced in rabbits by doxorubicin and possible prevention by coenzyme Q10. *Cancer Treatment Reports, 65*(1-2), 79–91.

Gaby, A.R. (1994). *Nutrition and Healing,* August, 3.

Ishiyama, T., Morita, Y., Toyama, S., Yamagami, T., & Tsukamoto, N. (1976). A clinical study of the effect of coenzyme Q on congestive heart failure. *Japan Heart Journal, 17*(1), 32–42.

Kamikawa, T., Kobayashi, A., Yamashita, T., Hayashi, H., & Yamazaki, N. (1985). Effects of coenzyme Q10 on exercise tolerance in chronic stable angina pectoris. *American Journal of Cardiology, 56*(4), 247–251.

Langsjoen, P.H., Folkers, K., Lyson, K., Muratsu, K., Lyson, T., & Langsjoen, P. (1988). Effective and safe therapy with coenzyme Q10 for cardiomyopathy. *Klin Wochenschr, 66*(13), 583–590.

Langsjoen, P.H., Langsjoen, P.H., & Folkers, K. (1990). A six-year clinical study of therapy of cardiomyopathy with coenzyme Q10. *International Journal of Tissue Reactions, 12*(3), 169–171.

Langsjoen, P., Langsjoen, P., Willis, R., & Folkers, K. (1994). Treatment of essential hypertension with coenzyme Q10. *Molecular Aspects of Medicine, 15* Suppl, S265–272.

Lockwood, K., Moesgaard, S., Hanioka, T., & Folkers, K. (1994). Apparent partial remission of breast cancer in "high risk" patients supplemented with nutritional antioxidants, essential fatty acids and coenzyme Q10. *Molecular Aspects of Medicine, 15* Suppl, S231–240.

Lockwood, K., Moesgaard, S., Yamamoto, T., & Folkers, K. (1995). Progress on therapy of breast cancer with vitamin Q10 and the regression of metastases. *Biochemical & Biophysical Research Communications, 212*(1), 172–177.

Morisco, C., Trimarco, B., & Condorelli, M. (1993). Effect of coenzyme Q10 therapy in patients with congestive heart failure: A long-term multicenter randomized study. *Clinical Investigations, 71*(8, Suppl), S134–136.

Echinacea

Echinacea is a common purple flower used medicinally by the American Indians.

Effects

Enhances natural killer cell activity in mononuclear cells (See et al, 1997) and stimulates phagocytosis by granulocytes (Bauer et al, 1988)

Uses

Immunologic

Although human and animal experiments have demonstrated its stimulatory actions on the cellular immune system (See et al, 1997; Bauer et al, 1988; Roesler et al, 1991), there is no definitive documentation of echinacea's efficacy in preventing viral or bacterial disease. Nonetheless, this botanical is used extensively by the general population, and the provider should be aware of it. In theory, its stimulation of immune cells could be of help in the treatment of AIDS, but no studies are available to prove or disprove this possibility.

Precautions

No known toxicities. Theoretically, because it stimulates the immune system, it may aggravate conditions associated with autoimmunity.

See also Notes 1, 2, 3, and 4 at the beginning of this appendix.

References

Bauer, V.R., Jurcic, K., Puhlmann, J., & Wagner, H. (1988). Immunologic in vivo and in vitro studies on Echinacea extracts. *Arzneimittelforschung, 38,* 276–281.

Roesler, J., Emmendörffer, A., Steinmüller, C., Luettig, B., Wagner, H., & Lohmann-Matthes, M.L. (1991). Application of purified polysaccharides from cell cultures of the plant *Echinacea purpurea* to test subjects mediates activation of the phagocyte system. *International Journal of Immunopharmacology, 13,* 931–941.

See, D.M., Broumand, N., Sahl, L., & Tilles, J.G. (1997). In vitro effects of echinacea and ginseng on natural killer and antibody-dependent cell cytotoxicity in healthy subjects and chronic fatigue syndrome or acquired immunodeficiency syndrome patients. *Immunopharmacology, 35,* 229–235.

Fish Oils (Omega-3 Unsaturated Fatty Acids)

The best dietary sources are fatty fish such as salmon, mackerel, and sardines, as well as certain vegetable oils. Commercial supplements are a mixture of two of the omega-3 fatty acids, EPA and DHA.

Effects

- Decreases platelet aggregation
- Decreases blood lipids
- Reduces arterial spasm, particularly that induced by high-fat meals.

Uses

Cardiovascular

- Decreases the incidence of anginal pain and the need for nitroglycerin
- Hypertension
- Reduced afterload may help in congestive heart failure.
- Reduces serum lipids.

Dermatologic

Treatment of chronic inflammatory diseases of the skin such as atopic dermatitis, acanthosis nigricans, and psoriasis

Gastrointestinal

Reduces symptoms and clinical findings of ulcerative colitis

Musculoskeletal

Reduces symptoms of rheumatoid arthritis; may even allow discontinuation of nonsteroidal anti-inflammatories (Kremer et al, 1995; van der Tempel et al, 1990)

Precautions

Oils must be kept cool to prevent oxidation and rancidity. Unsaturated fats can increase vitamin E requirements. Because they can increase bleeding times, they should be used with care in conjunction with anticoagulants.

See also Notes 1, 2, 3, and 4 at the beginning of this appendix.

References

Adler, A.J., & Holub, B.J. (1997). Effect of garlic and fish-oil supplementation on serum lipid and lipoprotein concentrations in hypercholesterolemic men. *American Journal of Clinical Nutrition, 65*(2), 445–450.

Escobar, S.O., Achenbach, R., Iannantuono, R., & Torem, V. (1992). Topical fish oil in psoriasis—a controlled and blind study. *Clinical Experiments in Dermatology, 17,* 159–162.

Isseroff, R.R. (1988). Fish again for dinner! The role of fish and other dietary oils in the therapy of skin disease. *Journal of the American Academy of Dermatology, 19,* 1073–1080.

Kremer, J.M., Lawrence, D.A., Petrillo, G.F., et al. (1995). Effects of high-dose fish oil on rheumatoid arthritis after stopping nonsteroidal antiinflammatory drugs. Clinical and immune correlates. *Arthritis & Rheumatism, 38,* 1107–1114.

McCarty, M.F. (1996). *Medical Hypotheses, 46*(4), 400–406.

Salachas, A., Papadopoulus, C., Sakadamis, G. (1994). Effects of a low-dose fish oil concentrate on angina, exercise tolerance time, serum triglycerides, and platelet function. *Angiology, 45,* 1023–1031.

Salomon, P., Kornbluth, A.A., & Janowitz, H.D. (1990). Treatment of ulcerative colitis with fish oil n-3-omega-fatty acid: An open trial. *Journal of Clinical Gastroenterology, 12*(2), 157–161.

Sherertz, E.F. (1988). Improved acanthosis nigricans with lipodystrophic diabetes during dietary fish oil supplementation. *Archives of Dermatology, 124,* 1094–1096.

Siyland, E., Funk, J., Rajka, G., et al. (1994). Dietary supplementation with very long-chain n-3 fatty acids in patients with atopic dermatitis. A double-blind, multicentre study. *British Journal of Dermatology, 130,* 757–764.

van der Tempel, H., Tulleken, J.E., Limburg, P.C., Muskiet, F.A., & van Rijswijk, M.H. (1990). Effects of fish oil supplementation in rheumatoid arthritis. *Annals of Rheumatic Disease, 49,* 76–80.

Folic Acid

There has been increased interest in this B vitamin due to its ability to lower elevated homocysteine levels and prevent certain birth defects.

Uses

Cardiovascular

There is increasing evidence that elevated homocysteine levels are at least a risk factor for, and possibly a cause of, arteriosclerotic cardiovascular disease. Folate has been shown to lower serum homocysteine levels (Franken et al, 1994). Homocysteine levels will probably become a routine screening test; folic acid may become an important weapon against arteriosclerotic cardiovascular disease.

Obstetric

Studies have shown the importance of folic acid supplementation (in doses still higher than the newly revised RDA) in the prevention of congenital neural tube birth defects (Mills & Conley, 1996).

Precautions

There is no known toxicity; however, large doses may mask symptoms of vitamin B_{12} deficiency.

See also Notes 1, 2, 3, and 4 at the beginning of this appendix.

References

Franken, D.G., Boers, G.H., Blom, H.J., Trijbels, F.J., & Kloppenborg, P.W. (1994). Treatment of mild hyperhomocysteinemia in vascular disease patients. *Arteriosclerosis & Thrombosis, 14*(3), 465–470.

Mills, J.L., & Conley, M.R. (1996). Folic acid to prevent neural tube defects: Scientific advances and public health issues. *Current Opinion in Obstetrics & Gynecology, 8,* 394–397.

Garlic

One of the most useful and beneficial of all supplements. It has a wide variety of therapeutic effects.

Effects

- Antithrombotic
- Inhibits platelet aggregation
- Lowers elevated cholesterol and serum lipid levels
- Protects against atherosclerosis
- Antihypertensive
- Protects against cancer and may have cancer-treating effects
- Antibacterial and antifungal. Its mode of action, the inhibition of certain enzymes present in a wide variety of bacteria, fungi, and viruses, has been recently identified.

Uses

Cardiovascular

- Treatment of hyperlipidemia
- Prevention and possible treatment of arteriosclerotic cardiovascular disease
- Antihypertensive.

Gastroenterologic

Peptic ulcer treatment and prevention and gastric cancer prevention through inhibitory action on *Helicobacter pylori.*

Dermatologic

Antidermatophytic

Oncologic

Cancer prophylaxis

Urologic

Possible bladder cancer treatment

Precautions

Antithrombotic, so care must be taken when garlic is used with other anticoagulants and perioperatively. Anticlotting actions are decreased with cooking. Making "odorless" preparations removes some of the effective ingredients in garlic, reducing its antibacterial activity.

See also Notes 1, 2, 3, and 4 at the beginning of this appendix.

References

Adler, A.J., & Holub, B.J. (1997). Effect of garlic and fish-oil supplementation on serum lipid and lipoprotein concentrations in hypercholesterolemic men. *American Journal of Clinical Nutrition, 65,* 445–450.

Agarwal, K.C. (1996). Therapeutic actions of garlic constituents. *Medical Research Review, 16*(1), 111–124.

Ankri, S. (1997). *Antimicrobial Agents and Chemotherapy, 41*(10), 2286–2288.

Bordia, T., Mohammed, N., Thomson, M., & Ali, M. (1996). An evaluation of garlic and onion as antithrombotic agents. *Prostaglandins, Leukotrienes & Essential Fatty Acids, 54,* 183–186.

Bordia, A., Verma, S.K., & Srivastava, K.C. (1996). Effect of garlic on platelet aggregation in humans: A study in healthy subjects and patients with coronary artery disease. *Prostaglandins, Leukotrienes & Essential Fatty Acids, 55*(3), 201–205.

Naganawa, R., Iwata, N., Ishikawa, K., Fukuda, H., Fujino, T., & Suzuki, A. (1996). Inhibition of microbial growth by ajoene, a sulfur-containing compound derived from garlic. *Applied Environmental Microbiology, 62*(11), 4238–4242.

Orekhov, A.N., Tertov, V.V., Sobenin, I.A., & Pivovarova, E.M. (1995). Direct anti-atherosclerosis-related effects of garlic. *Annals of Medicine, 27*(1), 63–65.

Riggs, D.R., DeHaven, J.I., & Lamm, D.L. (1997). *Allium sativum* (garlic) treatment for murine transitional cell carcinoma. *Cancer, 79*(10), 1987–1994.

Silagy, C.A., & Neil, H.A. (1994). A meta-analysis of the effect of garlic on blood pressure. *Journal of Hypertension, 12*(4), 463–468.

Sivam, G.P., Lampe, J.W., Ulness, B., Swanzy, S.R., & Potter, J.D. (1997). *Helicobacter pylori*—in vitro susceptibility to garlic (*Allium sativum*) extract. *Nutrition & Cancer, 27*(2), 118–121.

Steiner, M., Khan, A.H., Holbert, D., & Lin, R.I. (1996). A double-blind crossover study in moderately hypercholesterolemic men that compared the effect of aged garlic extract and placebo administration on blood lipids. *American Journal of Clinical Nutrition, 64*(6), 866–870.

Ti-Pai, S.T., & Platt, M.W. (1995). Antifungal effects of *Allium sativum* (garlic) extract against the *Aspergillus* species involved in otomycosis. *Letters in Applied Microbiology, 20*, 14–18.

Venugopal, P.V., & Venugopal, T.V. (1995). Antidermatophytic activity of garlic (*Allium sativum*) in vitro. *International Journal of Dermatology, 34*, 278–279.

Ginger

The active ingredients in ginger are found in its root. The root can be taken as a powder, an extract, or a tea.

Effects

The following are proven effects of ginger; the mechanisms of action are unclear but probably partially involve an antiprostaglandin effect:

- Antiemetic
- Anti-inflammatory
- Reduction of platelet aggregation.

Uses

Gastrointestinal

- Prevention of anesthesia-related nausea and vomiting
- Prevention of motion sickness.

Musculoskeletal

Treatment of rheumatoid arthritis, osteoarthritis, and myositis

Precautions

Although there is evidence for the efficacy and safety of ginger in the treatment of the nausea during pregnancy, there is some evidence of mutagenicity for the fetus. Until this question is definitively answered, the use of ginger in pregnancy cannot be recommended. Other than this potential but unproven risk, ginger has no known side effects.

See also Notes 1, 2, 3, and 4 at the beginning of this appendix.

References

Bone, M.E., Wilkinson, D.J., Young, J.R., McNeil, J., & Charlton, S. (1990). Ginger root—a new antiemetic. The effect of ginger root on postoperative nausea and vomiting after major gynaecological surgery. *Anaesthesia, 45*(8), 669–671.

Grontved, A., Brask, T., Kambskard, J., & Hentzer, E. (1988). Ginger root against seasickness. A controlled trial on the open sea. *Acta Otolaryngology (Stockholm), 105*(1-2), 45–49.

Phillips, S., Ruggier, R., & Hutchinson, S.E. (1993). *Zingiber officinale* (ginger)—an antiemetic for day case surgery. *Anaesthesia, 48*(8), 715–717.

Srivastava, K.C., & Mustafa, T. (1992). Ginger (*Zingiber officinale*) in rheumatism and musculoskeletal disorders. *Medical Hypotheses, 39*(4), 342–348.

Ginkgo

Preparations are made from the leaf of the ginkgo tree, an Asian tree now found extensively in American cities.

Effects

- Vasodilator
- Inhibitor of platelet-activating factor
- Free radical scavenger.

Uses

Neurologic

Treatment of tinnitus and Alzheimer's disease

Precautions

Because of its antiplatelet function, ginkgo should be used with caution in patients receiving anticoagulant therapy. Side effects can include restlessness, irritability, and headache.

See also Notes 1, 2, 3, and 4 at the beginning of this appendix.

References

Hoffmann, F., Beck, C., Schutz, A., & Offermann, P. (1994). Ginkgo extract EGb 761 (tenobin)/HAES versus naftidrofuryl (Dusodril)/HAES. A randomized study of therapy of sudden deafness. *Laryngorhinootologie 3*(3), 149–152.

Kanowski, S., Herrmann, W.M., Stephan, K., Wierich, W., & Horr, R. (1996). Proof of efficacy of the *Ginkgo biloba* special extract EGb 761 in outpatients suffering from mild to moderate primary degenerative dementia of the Alzheimer type or multi-infarct dementia. *Pharmacopsychiatry, 29*(2), 47–56.

Meyer, B. (1986). Multicenter randomized double-blind drug vs. placebo study of the treatment of tinnitus with *Ginkgo biloba* extract. *Presse Medicale, 15*(31), 1562–1564.

Ginseng

Ginseng is an herb with enormous, almost cult, popularity, especially among Asians. There are several different varieties (American, Asian, Siberian) varying mostly in potency. It is widely used as a general tonic and performance enhancer. The literature on ginseng's efficacy is widely split, with European studies showing effectiveness and American studies disputing that. Ginseng is one of the supplements with potentially serious side effects. This potential for harm, coupled with its wide use, requires its mention here.

Precautions

Ginseng has been reported to cause hypertension. Experimental evidence shows that it has both vasodilatory and vasoconstrictive effects, depending on the dosage. It can cause restlessness and irritability. Rare cases of the induction of occupational asthma and postmenopausal bleeding have also been reported.

References

Chen, X., Gillis, C.N., & Moalli, R. (1984). Vascular effects of ginsenosides in vitro. *British Journal of Pharmacology, 82*(2), 485–491.

Hopkins, M.P., Androff, L., & Benninghoff, A.S. (1988). Ginseng face cream and unexplained vaginal bleeding. *American Journal of Obstetrics & Gynecology, 159*(5), 1121–1122.

Subiza, J., Subiza, J.L., Escribano, P.M., et al. (1991). Occupational asthma caused by Brazil ginseng dust. *Journal of Allergy & Clinical Immunology, 88*(5), 731–736.

Glucosamine Sulfate

Glucosamine is a compound found naturally in the body, mostly in connective tissues and bone.

Effects

It has chondrometabolic, antireactive, and antiarthritic properties, without effects on prostaglandin synthesis. It is not a strong anti-inflammatory agent but its toxicity is so low that its therapeutic index as an anti-inflammatory is quite high.

Uses
Musculoskeletal

Treatment of osteoarthritis and gonococcal arthritis

Precautions

No significant toxicity; occasional gastrointestinal upset

References

Giordano, N., Nardi, P., Senesi, M., et al. (1996). The efficacy and safety of glucosamine sulfate in the treatment of gonarthritis. *Clinical Therapy, 147*(3), 99–105.

Reichelt, A., Forster, K.K., Fischer, M., Rovati, L.C., & Setnikar, I. (1994). Efficacy and safety of intramuscular glucosamine sulfate in osteoarthritis of the knee. A randomised, placebo-controlled, double-blind study. *Arzneimittelforschung, 44*(1), 75–80.

Setnikar, I. (1992). Antireactive properties of "chondroprotective" drugs. *International Journal of Tissue Reactivity, 14*(5), 253–261.

Setnikar, I., Cereda, R., Pacini, M.A., & Revel, L. (1991). Antireactive properties of glucosamine sulfate. *Arzneimittelforschung, 41*(2), 157–161.

Setnikar, I., Pacini, M.A., & Revel, L. (1991). Antiarthritic effects of glucosamine sulfate studied in animal models. *Arzneimittelforschung, 41*(5), 542–545.

Glutamine (See Cabbage Juice)
Hawthorn (*Crataegus*)

Berries, flowers, and leaves of the plant have been used extensively in Europe as a cardiac tonic. It is considered one of the most effective supplements for use in heart disease.

Effects

In animal models, hawthorn dilates coronary vessels, improves myocardial contractility and metabolic efficiency, and is an antiarrhythmic and an angiotensin-converting enzyme inhibitor.

Uses
Cardiovascular

Treatment of congestive heart failure

Precautions

Very low toxicity. Large doses may cause hypotension.

See also Notes 1, 2, 3, and 4 at the beginning of this appendix.

References

Pöpping, S., Rose, H., Ionescu, I., Fischer, Y., & Kammermeier, H. (1995). Effect of a hawthorn extract on contraction and energy turnover of isolated rat cardiomyocytes. *Arzneimittelforschung, 45*(11), 1157–1161.

Schüssler, M., Hölzl, J., & Fricke, U. (1995). Myocardial effects of flavonoids from *Crataegus* species. *Arzneimittelforschung, 45*, 842–845.

Uchida, S., Ikari, N., Ohta, H., et al. (1987). Inhibitory effects of condensed tannins on angiotensin-converting enzyme. *Japanese Journal of Pharmacology, 43*, 242–245.

Weikl, A., Assmus, K.D., Neukum-Schmidt, A., et al. (1996). *Crataegus* Special Extract WS 1442: Assessment of objective effectiveness in patients with heart failure. *Fortschr Med, 114*(24), 291–296.

Kava-Kava

Used for thousands of years as a recreational drink by South Pacific islanders. Now available in extract and capsule form.

Effects

Changes GABA receptor binding in the brain

Uses
Neurologic

Anticonvulsive

Psychological

Effective anxiolytic; treatment alternative to tricyclic antidepressants and benzodiazepines in anxiety disorders. No loss of concentration or cognition, as opposed to oxazepam.

Precautions

- Potentiating effects of ethanol shown in rats but not in humans
- Hematogenous contact eczema. Heavy kava drinkers may acquire kava dermopathy (reversible ichthyosiform eruption).

References

Gleitz, J., Friese, J., Beile, A., Ameri, A., & Peters, T. (1996). Anticonvulsive action of (+ / -)-kavain estimated from its properties on stimulated synaptosomes and Na + channel receptor sites. *European Journal of Pharmacology, 315*(1), 89–97.

Herberg, K.W. (1993). Effect of Kava-Special Extract WS 1490 combined with ethyl alcohol on safety-relevant performance parameters. *Blutalkohol, 30*(2), 96–105.

Jamieson, D.D., & Duffield, P.H. (1990). Positive interaction of ethanol and kava resin in mice. *Clinical & Experimental Pharmacology & Physiology, 17*(7), 509–514.

Jussofie, A., Schmiz, A., & Hiemke, C. (1994). Kavapyrone-enriched extract from *Piper methysticum* as modulator of the GABA binding site in different regions of rat brain. *Psychopharmacology (Berlin), 116*(4), 469–474.

Kinzler, E., Kromer, J., & Lehmann, E. (1991). Effect of a special kava extract in patients with anxiety, tension, and excitation states of non-psychotic genesis. Double-blind study with placebos over 4 weeks. *Arzneimittelforschung, 41*(6), 584–588.

Munte, T.F., Heinze, H.J., Matzke, M., & Steitz, J. (1993). Effects of oxazepam and an extract of kava roots (*Piper methysticum*) on event-related potentials in a word recognition task. *Neuropsychobiology, 27*(1), 46–53.

Norton, S.A., & Ruze, P. (1994). Kava dermopathy. *Journal of the American Academy of Dermatology, 31*(1), 89–97.

Suss, R., & Lehmann, P. (1996). Hematogenous contact eczema caused by phytogenic drugs exemplified by kava root extract. *Hautarzt, 47*(6), 459–461.

Volz, H.P., & Kieser, M. (1997). Kava-kava extract WS 1490 versus placebo in anxiety disorders—a randomized placebo-controlled 25-week outpatient trial. *Pharmacopsychiatry, 30*(1), 1–5.

Licorice (Deglycyrrhizinated Licorice, DGL)

The root of the plant contains the active chemicals. Most licorice candies in the United States contain little or no actual licorice. Imported licorice, especially from England, contain much more of the active ingredients in licorice root.

Effects

Licorice exerts a significant antiulcer effect through stimulation of mucus secretion by goblet cells without change in acid production. Thus, it does not cause nutritional malabsorption problems related to low acid and may also be used in conjunction with acid-lowering drugs, if needed.

Uses

Gastrointestinal

- Treatment and prevention of peptic ulcer disease
- Prevention of gastric and duodenal erosions from aspirin use.

Precautions

One of the components of licorice root, glycyrrhizin, can cause symptoms and signs of pseudohyperaldosteronism: hypokalemia, edema, and hypertension. Reports of rhabdomyolysis and paralysis from sustained high licorice intake are in the literature. Deglycyrrhizinated licorice (DGL) is free of these dangerous metabolic side effects but has unaltered antiulcer properties. Preparations of DGL are readily available in health food stores.

References

Berlango Jimenez, A., Jimenez Murillo, L., Montero Perez, F.J., Munoz Avila, J.A., Torres Murillo, J., & Calderon de la Barca Gazquez, J.M. (1995). Acute rhabdomyolysis and tetraparesis secondary to hypokalemia due to ingested licorice. *Annals Medica Interna, 12*(1), 33–35.

Brailski, K.H., Kadiian, K.H., & Bozhiianov, V. (1975). Clinical trial of the preparation Caved S in treating peptic ulcer. *Vutr Boles, 14*(4), 101–106.

Dehpour, A.R., Zolfaghari, M.E., Samadian, T., & Vahedi, Y. (1994). The protective effect of liquorice components and their derivatives against gastric ulcer induced by aspirin in rats. *Journal of Pharmacy & Pharmacology, 46*(2), 148–149.

Larkworthy, W., & Holgate, P.F. (1975). Deglycyrrhizinized liquorice in the treatment of chronic duodenal ulcer. A retrospective endoscopic survey of 32 patients. *Practitioner, 215*(1290), 787–792.

Rees, W.D., Rhodes, J., Wright, J.E., Stamford, L.F., & Bennett, A. (1979). Effect of deglycyrrhizinated liquorice on gastric mucosal damage by aspirin. *Scandinavian Journal of Gastroenterology, 14*(5), 605–607.

Schambelan, M. (1994). Licorice ingestion and blood pressure-regulating hormones. *Steroids, 59*(2), 127–130.

Magnesium

Magnesium is a safe and inexpensive supplement with many uses. Stress, diuretic use, alcoholism, and the typical Western diet of highly refined foods can deplete magnesium. Magnesium depletion has been correlated with a number of entities, including latent tetany, migraine headaches, allergies, and mitral valve prolapse.

Effects

- Lowers blood pressure by relaxing arterial smooth muscle, especially in magnesium-depleted persons
- Inhibits platelet function and arterial thrombus formation

- Is a general antiarrhythmic; specifically reduces arrhythmias from digitalis toxicity.

Uses

Cardiovascular

- Reduces mortality from myocardial infarction (MI) if given early in the event; deaths from acute MI have been shown to be inversely proportional to the levels of magnesium in drinking water, and oral supplementation of magnesium may reduce MI risk.
- Antiarrhythmic actions, particularly for digitalis toxicity
- Antihypertensive
- Can reduce symptoms secondary to mitral valve prolapse without affecting the prolapse itself.

Neurologic

Effective in prophylaxis and treatment of migraine headaches

Precautions

Serum magnesium levels may not accurately reflect total body magnesium; intracellular (erythrocyte) magnesium levels should also be tested. Oral magnesium in large quantities can cause diarrhea. Oral calcium and magnesium may inhibit the absorption of each other; therefore, magnesium supplementation should be considered for the many people taking calcium supplements. Magnesium may be better absorbed as an amino acid chelate such as aspartate than the less-expensive salt forms. Toxicity, although rare, may occur with laxative abuse and, especially, impaired renal function.

See also Notes 1, 2, 3, and 4 at the beginning of this appendix.

References

Heesch, C.M., & Eichhorn, E.J. (1994). Magnesium in acute myocardial infarction. *Annals of Emergency Medicine, 24*(6), 1154–1160.

Lfuderitz, B., & Manz, M. (1994). The value of magnesium in intensive care medicine. *Z Kardiol, 83*(Suppl 6), 121–126.

Lichodziejewska, B., Klos, J., Rezler, J., et al. (1997). Clinical symptoms of mitral valve prolapse are related to hypomagnesemia and attenuated by magnesium supplementation. *American Journal of Cardiology, 79*(6), 768–772.

Mauskop, A., Altura, B.T., Cracco, R.Q., & Altura, B.M. (1995). Intravenous magnesium sulfate relieves cluster headaches in patients with low serum ionized magnesium levels. *Headache, 35*, 597–600.

Ravn, H.B., Kristensen, S.D., Vissinger, H., & Husted, S.E. (1996). Magnesium inhibits human platelets. *Blood Coagulation & Fibrinolysis, 7*(2), 241–244.

Rubenowitz, E., Axelsson, G., & Rylander, R. (1996). Magnesium in drinking water and death from acute myocardial infarction. *American Journal of Epidemiology, 143*(5), 456–462.

Sanjuliani, A.F., de Abreu Fagundes, V.G., & Francischetti, E.A. (1996). Effects of magnesium on blood pressure and intracellular ion levels of Brazilian hypertensive patients. *International Journal of Cardiology, 56*, 177–183.

Taubert, K. (1994). Magnesium in migraine. Results of a multicenter pilot study. *Fortschr Med, 112*, 328–330.

Thomas, J., Thomas, E., & Tomb, E. (1992). Serum and erythrocyte magnesium concentrations and migraine. *Magnesium Research, 5*(2), 127–130.

Zehender, M., Meinertz, T., Faber, T., et al. (1997). Antiarrhythmic effects of increasing the daily intake of magnesium and potassium in patients with frequent ventricular arrhythmias. *Journal of the American College of Cardiology, 29*(5), 1028–1034.

Melatonin

Melatonin is a hormone secreted by the pineal gland and a regulator of diurnal rhythms. Melatonin release seems to be adversely affected by electromagnetic fields, leading to hypotheses that decreased melatonin may be an important link in the causative relation between electromagnetic fields and cancer, particularly breast cancer.

Effects

- Is an immune system regulator and stimulator
- Is present in larger-than-normal quantities in the sera and tumors of cancer patients, particularly those with breast cancer. Works synergistically with other antineoplastic drugs as well as possessing oncostatic properties of its own. Effects may be due to reversal of the immunosuppressive effects of the neoplasms.
- Modulates circadian rhythms and especially sleep patterns.

Uses

Neurologic

Treatment of jet lag and other sleep disorders

Oncologic

Effective in treatment of a wide variety of tumors, including breast cancer, lung cancer, melanoma, and glioblastoma. Not only assists in regression of tumor, but also reduces side effects of other therapeutic agents.

Precautions

Very low toxicity. Optimal dosage not fully researched. Improperly timed use can cause sleep pattern disturbances. One report of reversible disorientation and lethargy after overdose (10 to 20 times normal dose).

See also Notes 1, 2, 3, and 4 at the beginning of this appendix.

References

Arendt, J., & Deacon, S. (1997). Treatment of circadian rhythm disorders: Melatonin. *Chronobiology International, 14*(2), 185–204.

Chase, J.E., & Gidal, B.E. (1997). Melatonin: Therapeutic use in sleep disorders. *Annals of Pharmacotherapy, 31*(10), 1218–1226.

Conti, A., & Maestroni, G.J. (1995). The clinical neuroimmunotherapeutic role of melatonin in oncology. *Journal of Pineal Research, 19*(3), 103–110.

Holliman, B.J., & Chyka, P.A. (1997). Problems in assessment of acute melatonin overdose. *Southern Medical Journal, 90*(4), 451–453.

Maestroni, G.J., & Conti, A. (1996). Melatonin in human breast cancer tissue: Association with nuclear grade and estrogen receptor status. *Laboratory Investigations, 75*(4), 557–561.

Panzer, A., & Viljoen, M. (1997). The validity of melatonin as an oncostatic agent. *Journal of Pineal Research, 22*(4), 184–202.

Stevens, R.G., & Davis, S. (1996). The melatonin hypothesis: Electric power and breast cancer. *Environmental Health Perspectives, 104*(Suppl 1), 135–140.

Wichmann, M.W., Zellweger, R., DeMaso, A.A., & Chaudry, I.H. (1996). Melatonin administration attenuates depressed immune functions in trauma-hemorrhage. *Journal of Surgical Research, 63*(1), 256–262.

Milk Thistle

The active agent is silymarin, a compound found mostly in the seeds.

Effects

- Selective inhibition of leukotriene formation by Kupffer cells
- Increases levels of glutathione (a potent protective antioxidant) in liver cells
- Inhibits the endogenous tumor promoter tumor necrosis factor-alpha.

Uses

Gastrointestinal

Improves liver function in a wide range of disease states, including cirrhosis and chronic hepatitis

Precautions

No known significant side effects. Because it is a choleretic, it may cause loose stools.

See also Notes 1, 2, 3, and 4 at the beginning of this appendix.

References

Dehmlow, C., Erhard, J., & de Groot, H. (1996). Inhibition of Kupffer cell functions as an explanation for the hepatoprotective properties of silibinin. *Hepatology, 23*(4), 749–754.

De Martiis, M., Fontana, M., Assogna, G., D'Ottavi, R., & D'Ottavi, O. (1980). Milk thistle (*Silybum marianum*) derivatives in the therapy of chronic hepatopathies. *Clinical Therapy, 94*(3), 283–315.

Ferenci, P., Dragosics, B., Dittrich, H., et al. (1989). Randomized controlled trial of silymarin treatment in patients with cirrhosis of the liver. *Journal of Hepatology, 9*(1), 105–113.

Lirussi, F., & Okolicsanyi, L. (1992). Cytoprotection in the nineties: Experience with ursodeoxycholic acid and silymarin in chronic liver disease. *Acta Physiology Hungary, 80*(1-4), 363–367.

Murray, M.T. (1992). *The healing power of herbs*, p. 71. Rocklin, CA: Prima Publishers.

Valenzuela, A., Aspillaga, M., Vial, S., & Guerra, R. (1989). Selectivity of silymarin on the increase of the glutathione content in different tissues of the rat. *Planta Med, 55*(5), 420–422.

Zi, X., Mukhtar, H., & Agarwal, R. (1997). Novel cancer chemopreventive effects of a flavonoid antioxidant silymarin: Inhibition of mRNA expression of an endogenous tumor promoter TNF alpha. *Biochemical & Biophysical Research Communications, 239*(1), 334–339.

Niacin (See Vitamin B₃)

Omega-3 Unsaturated Fatty Acids (See Fish Oils)

Peppermint

Used as a digestive aid for thousands of years. One of its main active ingredients is menthol. Usually taken as a tea or an enteric-coated capsule.

Effects

Antispasmodic actions on intestinal smooth muscle

Uses

Gastrointestinal

- Symptomatic relief of irritable bowel syndrome and other spasmodic intestinal illnesses
- Relief of dyspepsia, nausea
- Reduces spasm during and after barium enema.

Neurologic

Relief of tension headache

Precautions

Because peppermint relaxes smooth muscle, it relaxes the gastroesophageal sphincter; therefore, it can exacerbate symptoms of hiatal hernia with reflux.

Many of the active ingredients are absorbed high in the gastrointestinal tract. To obtain relief from colonic spasm, peppermint must be taken as an enteric-coated preparation. For high gastrointestinal tract relief, teas are adequate.

References

Dew, M.J., Evans, B.K., & Rhodes, J. (1984). Peppermint oil for the irritable bowel syndrome: A multicentre trial. *British Journal of Clinical Practice, 38*(11-12), 394–398.

Friedman, G. (1991). Diet and the irritable bowel syndrome. *Gastroenterologic Clinics of North America, 20,* 313–324.

Gobel, H., Fresenius, J., Heinze, A., Dworschak, M., & Soyka, D. (1996). Effectiveness of *Oleum menthae piperitae* and paracetamol in therapy of headache of the tension type. *Nervenarzt, 67*(8), 672–681.

Gobel, H., Schmidt, G., & Soyka, D. (1994). Effect of peppermint and eucalyptus oil preparations on neurophysiological and experimental algesimetric headache parameters. *Cephalalgia, 14*(3), 228–234.

Hills, J.M., & Aaronson, P.I. (1991). The mechanism of action of peppermint oil on gastrointestinal smooth muscle. An analysis using patch clamp electrophysiology and isolated tissue pharmacology in rabbit and guinea pig. *Gastroenterology, 101*(1), 55–65.

May, B., Kuntz, H.D., Kieser, M., & Köhler, S. (1996). Efficacy of a fixed peppermint oil/caraway oil combination in non-ulcer dyspepsia. *Arzneimittelforschung, 46*(12), 1149–1153.

Rees, W.D., Evans, B.K., & Rhodes, J. (1979). Treating irritable bowel syndrome with peppermint oil. *British Medical Journal, 2*(6194), 835–836.

Sparks, M.J., O'Sullivan, P., Herrington, A.A., & Morcos, S.K. (1995). Does peppermint oil relieve spasm during barium enema? *British Journal of Radiology, 68*(812), 841–843.

Pyridoxine (See Vitamin B₆)

Saw Palmetto (*Serenoa*)

Active ingredients found in the berry of a shrub native to coastal areas of the southeast United States. Often combined with another herb, *Pygeum*, in products designed to treat prostatism.

Effects

Exerts an antiandrogenic effect by blocking receptors in prostatic cells and other tissues as well. Interferes with conversion of testosterone to dihydrotestosterone.

Uses

Gynecologic

Potential treatment for hirsutism and virilism in women

Urologic

Prevention and treatment of benign prostatic hypertrophy

Precautions

Mild side effects of nausea and abdominal discomfort have been reported. Patients taking this botanical for symptoms of prostatism should be reminded that they need to be followed by a physician even if their symptoms subside.

See also Notes 1, 2, 3, and 4 at the beginning of this appendix.

References

Carilla, E., Briley, M., Fauran, F., Sultan, C., & Duvilliers, C. (1984). Binding of Permixon, a new treatment for prostatic benign hyperplasia, to the cytosolic androgen receptor in the rat prostate. *Journal of Steroid Biochemistry, 20*(1), 521–523.

el-Sheikh, M.M., Dakkak, M.R., & Saddique, A. (1988). The effect of Permixon on androgen receptors. *Acta Obstetrics & Gynecology Scandinavica, 67*(5), 397–399.

Plosker, G.L., & Brogden, R.N. (1996). *Serenoa repens* (Permixon). A review of its pharmacology and therapeutic efficacy in benign prostatic hyperplasia. *Drugs & Aging, 9*(5), 379–395.

Sultan, C., Terraza, A., Devillier, C., et al. (1984). Inhibition of androgen metabolism and binding by a liposterolic extract of *Serenoa repens B* in human foreskin fibroblasts. *Journal of Steroid Biochemistry, 20*(1), 515–519.

St. John's Wart (*Hypericum*)

Recently repopularized botanical; used for centuries as a folk remedy for insomnia and anxiety. Taken as tea, tincture, powder, or extract.

Effects

Multiple modes of action, including upregulation of serotonin receptors in the brain and inhibition of serotonin uptake by postsynaptic receptors.

Uses

Psychological

- Treatment of seasonal affective disorder
- Treatment of depression—perhaps as effective and safer than prescription antidepressants.

Precautions

Very low toxicity. Photosensitivity has been reported, although at least one study shows no such problem (Brockmoller et al, 1997; Golsch et al, 1997). A study involving 3250 patients reported an incidence of less than 0.6% for each of the following side effects: gastrointestinal irritation, allergic reactions, tiredness, and restlessness (Woelk et al, 1994).

See also Notes 1, 2, 3, and 4 at the beginning of this appendix.

References

Brockmoller, J., Reum, T., Bauer, S., Kerb, R., Hubner, W.D., & Roots, I. (1997). Hypericin and pseudohypericin: Pharmacokinetics and effects on photosensitivity in humans. *Pharmacopsychiatry, 30*(Suppl 2), 94–101.

Czekalla, J., Gastpar, M., Hubner, W.D., & Jager, D. (1997). The effect of hypericum extract on cardiac conduction as seen in the electrocardiogram compared to that of imipramine. *Pharmacopsychiatry, 30*(Suppl 2), 86–88.

Golsch, S., Vocks, E., Rakoski, J., Brockow, K., & Ring, J. (1997). Reversible increase in photosensitivity to UV-B caused by St. John's wort extract. *Hautarzt, 48*(4), 249–252.

Kasper, S. (1997). Treatment of seasonal affective disorder (SAD) with hypericum extract. *Pharmacopsychiatry, 30*(Suppl 2), 89–93.

Linde, K., Ramirez, G., Mulrow, C.D., Pauls, A., Weidenhammer, W., & Melchart, D.. (1996). St. John's wort for depression—an overview and meta-analysis of randomised clinical trials. *British Medical Journal, 313*(7052), 253–258.

Perovic, S., & Muller, W.E. (1995). Pharmacological profile of hypericum extract. Effect on serotonin uptake by postsynaptic receptors. *Arzneimittelforschung, 45*(11), 1145–1148.

Teufel-Mayer, R., & Gleitz, J. (1997). Effects of long-term administration of hypericum extracts on the affinity and density of the central serotonergic 5-HT1 A and 5-HT2 A receptors. *Pharmacopsychiatry, 30*(Suppl 2), 113–116.

Volz, H.P. (1997). Controlled clinical trials of hypericum extracts in depressed patients—an overview. *Pharmacopsychiatry, 30*(Suppl 2), 72–76.

Woelk, H., Burkard, G., & Grunwald, J. (1994). Benefits and risks of the hypericum extract LI 160: Drug monitoring study with 3250 patients. *Journal of Geriatric Psychiatry & Neurology, 7*(Suppl 1), S34–S38.

Taurine

An amino acid that can be synthesized by the liver; highly concentrated in specific organs such as skeletal muscle, myocardium, and the central nervous system, especially the brain. It is also highly concentrated in the bile.

Effects

Exact nature of action is unknown, but it probably acts to stabilize membranes, especially the sarcolemma, by regulating ionic balance and transfer, especially calcium.

Uses
Cardiovascular

Shown to improve heart function significantly in congestive heart failure.

Precautions

No known toxicities.

See also Notes 1, 2, 3, and 4 at the beginning of this appendix.

References

Azuma, J., Hasegawa, H., Sawamura, A., et al. (1983). Therapy of congestive heart failure with orally administered taurine. *Clinical Therapy, 5*(4), 39800-408.

Gaby, A.R. (1997). *Nutrition and Healing*, p. 3.

Vitamin B₃ (Niacin)

This water-soluble vitamin is most commonly used for lowering serum cholesterol levels.

Effects
Uses
Cardiovascular

Lowers serum cholesterol and raises serum high-density lipoprotein levels

Precautions

Causes flushing and skin reactions, which can be minimized with "nonflush" preparations. More serious side effects (elevation of blood glucose, hepatic dysfunction) seem to be dose-related. Sustained-release preparations of niacin, although more effective in lipid lowering and better tolerated by patients, may be severely hepatotoxic and should be avoided.

See also Notes 1, 2, 3, and 4 at the beginning of this appendix.

References

Luria, M.H. (1988). Effect of low-dose niacin on high-density lipoprotein cholesterol and total cholesterol/high-density lipoprotein cholesterol ratio. *Archives of Internal Medicine, 148*, 2493–2495.

McKenney, J.M., Proctor, J.D., Harris, S., & Chinchili, V.M.A. (1994). Comparison of the efficacy and toxic effects of sustained- vs. immediate-release niacin in hypercholesterolemic patients. *JAMA, 271*, 672–677.

Vitamin B₆ (Pyridoxine)

There is increasing interest in this water-soluble vitamin due to its ability to lower elevated homocysteine levels.

Effects
Uses
Cardiovascular

There is increasing evidence that elevated homocysteine levels are at least a risk factor for and possibly a cause of arteriosclerotic cardiovascular disease. Vitamin B₆ has been shown to lower serum homocysteine levels. Homocysteine levels should soon become a routine screening test, and B₆ may become an important weapon against arteriosclerotic cardiovascular disease.

Precautions

Large doses have been reported to cause nerve damage.

See also Notes 1, 2, 3, and 4 at the beginning of this appendix.

References

Franken, D.G., Boers, G.H., Blom, H.J., Trijbels, F.J., & Kloppenborg, P.W. (1994). Treatment of mild hyperhomocysteinemia in vascular disease patients. *Arteriosclerosis & Thrombosis, 14*(3), 465–470.

Schaumber, H. (1983). Sensory neuropathy from pyridoxine abuse; a new megavitamin syndrome. *N Engl J Med, 309*, 445–448.

Vitamin B₁₂ (Cyanocobalamin)

Perhaps more controversy surrounds this vitamin than any other supplement. For many years, providers have given intramuscular doses of vitamin B₁₂ to patients with no documentable B₁₂ deficiency. Usually the supplementation is given for vague symptoms of fatigue and "feeling run down." There is little in the recent literature to defend this practice other than anecdotal experience.

Effects

- Essential for proper metabolism of fats and carbohydrates
- Essential for normal erythrocyte development
- Involved in the production of myelin. Helps maintain the health of nervous tissue, including the brain. Low or borderline-low serum B₁₂ levels have been found in several types of dementia, especially in the elderly.

Uses
Musculoskeletal

Controversial use as a general tonic for fatigue, listlessness, and other nonspecific symptoms

Psychiatric

Possible use in several forms of dementia, including Alzheimer's, as well as mood disorders and psychoses

Precautions

No known toxicity. Probably needs to be given parenterally for best effect. This may account for the variability of effectiveness in clinical studies.

References

Dommisse, J. (1991). Subtle vitamin B₁₂ deficiency and psychiatry: A largely unnoticed but devastating relationship? *Medical Hypotheses, 34*(2), 131–140.

Fine, E.J., & Soria, E.D. (1991). Myths about vitamin B$_{12}$ deficiency. *Southern Medical Journal, 84*(12), 1475–1481.

Gaby, A.R. (1995). The story of vitamin B$_{12}$. *Nutrition and Healing,* p. 3.

Gottfries, C.G. (1988). Dementia: Classification and aspects of treatment. *Psychopharmacol Ser, 5,* 187–195.

Thompson, W.G., & Freedman, M.L. (1989). Vitamin B$_{12}$ and geriatrics: Unanswered questions. *Acta Haematology, 82*(4), 169–174.

Vitamin C

A water-soluble vitamin found in many fruits and vegetables; citrus fruits are the best source. May work synergistically with vitamin E. Since Dr. Linus Pauling championed vitamin C as the cure for the common cold, among other things, debate has raged about the value of large doses—in part because a large percentage of each dose is quickly excreted in the urine.

Effects

- A very potent antioxidant
- Maintains the integrity of collagen
- Bacteriostatic agent, notably to *Helicobacter pylori*
- Immune system booster
- Inverse relation between vitamin C intake and risk of some cancers
- Reduction in low-density lipoprotein oxidation
- Uricosuric
- Facilitates iron absorption
- Retards progression of clinical osteoarthritis
- Eradicates rheumatoid arthritis cells in vitro.

Uses

Cardiovascular

May have protective effect for coronary artery disease. Data indicate that vitamin C deficiency is a risk factor for coronary artery disease, but there are no solid data to date showing a preventive effect of vitamin C supplementation.

Gastroenterologic

Prevention and healing of peptic ulceration due to *H. pylori*; protection against gastric cancer

Musculoskeletal

Treatment of osteoarthritis and, perhaps, rheumatoid arthritis

Oncologic

Although it shows promise, data are inconclusive on the efficacy of intravenous vitamin C in the treatment of advanced cancer.

Ophthalmologic

Prevention of cataracts

Urologic

Already in the traditional medical armamentarium for urinary antisepsis and acidification of urine for treatment of some renal calculi

Precautions

Few serious side effects, except it can precipitate renal stone formation in patients with abnormal oxalate metabolism or elevated uric acid levels. Best taken as a chelated salt or esterized form to avoid dyspepsia. Most common side effects are temporary flatulence, bloating, and diarrhea with high doses; symptoms respond quickly to reduction in dosage. Increased iron absorption may be an unwanted side effect because iron is a powerful oxidizing agent. Can cause false-negative results in slide tests for fecal occult blood.

See also Notes 1, 2, 3, and 4 at the beginning of this appendix.

References

Cameron, E., & Pauling, L. (1976). Supplemental ascorbate in the supportive treatment of cancer: Prolongation of survival times in terminal human cancer. *Proceedings of the National Academy of Science USA, 73*(10), 3685–3689.

Comstock, G.W., Alberg, A.J., Huang, H.Y., et al. (1997). The risk of developing lung cancer associated with antioxidants in the blood: Ascorbic acid, carotenoids, alpha-tocopherol, selenium, and total peroxyl radical absorbing capacity. *Cancer Epidemiology Biomarkers & Prevention, 6*(11), 907–916.

Jacques, P.F., Taylor, A., Hankinson, S.E., et al. (1997). Long-term vitamin C supplement use and prevalence of early age-related lens opacities. *American Journal of Clinical Nutrition, 66*(4), 911–916.

La Vecchia, C., Braga, C., Negri, E., et al. (1997). Intake of selected micronutrients and risk of colorectal cancer. *International Journal of Cancer, 73*(4), 525–530.

McAlindon, T.E., Jacques, P., Zhang, Y., et al. (1996). Do antioxidant micronutrients protect against the development and progression of knee osteoarthritis? *Arthritis & Rheumatism, 39,* 648–656.

Mosca, L., Rubenfire, M., Mandel, C., et al. (1997). Antioxidant nutrient supplementation reduces the susceptibility of low-density lipoprotein to oxidation in patients with coronary artery disease. *Journal of the American College of Cardiology, 30*(2), 392–399.

Nyyssonen, K., Parviainen, M.T., Salonen, R., Tuomilehto, J., & Salonen, J.T. (1997). Vitamin C deficiency and risk of myocardial infarction: Prospective population study of men from eastern Finland. *British Medical Journal, 314*(7081), 634–638.

Wilkins, E.S., & Wilkins, M.G. (1979). Effect of aspirin and vitamins C and E on synovial rheumatoid arthritic and other cells. *Experientia, 35,* 244–246.

Zhang, H.M., Wakisaka, N., Maeda, O., & Yamamoto, T. (1997). Vitamin C inhibits the growth of a bacterial risk factor for gastric carcinoma: *Helicobacter pylori. Cancer, 80*(10), 1897–1903.

Vitamin E

One of the fat-soluble vitamins. Long thought of as significant only when deficient. Now receiving much attention and research, especially in regard to prevention of coronary artery disease. May work synergistically with vitamin C.

Effects

- Vitamin E's beneficial effects are mostly due to its activity as an antioxidant.
- One of the most powerful natural antioxidants. Prevents oxidation of low-density lipoprotein cholesterol: this is probably the mechanism of vitamin E's protective effect against coronary artery disease and perhaps cancer.
- Lowers platelet adhesiveness without effect on platelet aggregation.

Uses

Cardiovascular

- In pharmacologic doses, it lowers the incidence of myocardial infarction. Protection against other forms of atherosclerotic disease is likely but unproven to date.
- Potential for prevention of thromboembolic events
- Has been used perioperatively to lessen the incidence of pulmonary embolism.

Oncologic

Low serum vitamin E levels have been shown to be an indicator for development of cancer, particularly lung, colon, and breast cancer, and higher rates for colon cancer have been correlated with lower dietary vitamin E intake. Definitive studies proving the cancer-protective effect of vitamin E supplementation are lacking. Still, the available evidence, coupled with the low toxicity of vitamin E, makes a good case for its use.

Ophthalmologic

May protect against cataract formation

Precautions

Pharmacologic (10 to 20 times RDA) doses are required for antiarteriosclerotic effects; lower doses are probably ineffective. Little toxicity. Poorly documented side effects are idiosyncratic hypertension and vitamin K antagonism; extra vigilance is prudent with patients taking both vitamin E and coumarin.

See also Notes 1, 2, 3, and 4 at the beginning of this appendix.

References

Bostick, R.M., Potter, J.D., McKenzie, D.R., et al. (1993). Reduced risk of colon cancer with high intake of vitamin E: The Iowa Women's Health Study. *Cancer Research, 53,* 4230–4237.

Kanofsky, J.D., & Kanofsky, P.B. (1981). Prevention of thromboembolic disease by vitamin E. *N Engl J Med, 305*(3), 173–174.

Knekt, P. (1993). Vitamin E and smoking and the risk of lung cancer. *Annals of the New York Academy of Science, 686,* 280–288.

Knekt, P. Aromaa, A., Maatela, J., et al. (1991). Vitamin E and cancer prevention. *American Journal of Clinical Nutrition, 53,* 283S–286S.

Rimm, E.B., & Stampfer, M.J. (1997). The role of antioxidants in preventive cardiology. *Current Opinion in Cardiology, 12*(2), 188–194.

Robertson, J.M., Donner, A.P., & Trevithick, J.R. (1989). Vitamin E intake and risk of cataracts in humans. *Annals of the New York Academy of Science, 570,* 372–382.

Steiner, M. (1991). Influence of vitamin E on platelet function in humans. *Journal of the American College of Nutrition, 10*(5), 466–473.

Stephens, N.G., Parsons, A., Schofield, P.M., Kelly, F., Cheeseman, K., & Mitchinson, M.J. (1996). Randomised controlled trial of vitamin E in patients with coronary disease. *Lancet, 347*(9004), 781–786.

Zinc

A trace mineral, zinc is involved in a broad range of enzymatic and other chemical processes in the body. Mild dietary deficiency is common.

Effects

Essential for healing and for maintaining a healthy immune system

Uses

Dermatologic

Treatment of acne, especially when used in conjunction with erythromycin

Otorhinolaryngologic

Treatment of tinnitus

Respiratory

Treatment of the common cold

Precautions

Zinc overload can suppress the immune system, just as zinc deficiency can. Zinc supplementation may cause a copper deficiency, so copper should be added to the regimen if zinc is to be used on a long-term basis. Best absorbed as an amino acid chelate such as zinc picolinate.

See also Notes 1, 2, 3, and 4 at the beginning of this appendix.

References

Eby, G.A., Davis, D.R., & Halcomb, W.W. (1984). Reduction in duration of common colds by zinc gluconate lozenges in a double-blind study. *Antimicrobial Agents & Chemotherapy, 25*(1), 20–24.

Favier, A. (1993). Current aspects about the role of zinc in nutrition. *Rev Prat, 43*(2), 146–151.

Ochi, K., Ohashi, T., Kinoshita, H., et al. (1997). The serum zinc level in patients with tinnitus and the effect of zinc treatment. *Nippon Jibiinkoka Gakkai Kaiho, 100*(9), 915–919.

Okada, A., Takagi, Y., Nezu, R., & Lee, S. (1990). Zinc in clinical surgery—a research review. *Japanese Journal of Surgery, 20*(6), 635–644.

Paaske, P.B., Pedersen, C.B., Kjems, G., & Sam, I.L. (1991). Zinc in the management of tinnitus. Placebo-controlled trial. *Annals of Otology, Rhinology, & Laryngology, 100*(8), 647–649.

Schachner, L., Eaglstein, W., Kittles, C., & Mertz, P. (1990). Topical erythromycin and zinc therapy for acne. *Journal of the American Academy of Dermatology, 22*(2 Pt 1), 253–260.

Complementary Modalities

Philip Grover, DC, Holly Nadal, LMT, Yoshiaki Omura, MD, ScD, FACA, FICAE, Ellen Rich, PhD, RN, CS, FNP, Certified Biofeedback Therapist, Margaret Rowlett, ARNP, BS, Certified Clinical Aromatherapist, and Tad Wanveer, LMT, Craniosacral Therapist

Acupuncture
Suggested Reading
Omura, Y. (1975). Pathophysiology of acupuncture treatments: Effects of acupuncture on cardiovascular and nervous systems. *Acupuncture & Electrotherapeutic Research, 1,* 51–141.

Omura, Y. (1996). *Acupunture medicine: Its historical and clinical background.* Elmsford, NY: Cognizant Communication Corp.

Aromatherapy
Cardiovascular

- Coronary artery disease: Rosemary (*Rosmarinus officinalis*)
- Hyperlipidemia: Immortelle (*Helichrysum italicum*), lemongrass (*Cymbopogon citratus*), rosemary
- Heart failure: Eucalyptus (*Eucalyptus globulus*), geranium (*Pelargonium graveolens*), mandarin (*Citrus reticulata*)
- Arrhythmia: Rosemary, ylang ylang (*Cananga odorata* var. *genuina*), eucalyptus
- Hypertension: Clary sage (*Salvia sclarea*), juniper (*Juniperus communis*), lavender (*Lavandula angustifolia*), lemon (*Citrus limon*), mandarin, lemon balm (*Melissa officinalis*), sweet marjoram (*Origanum marjorana*)

Dermatology

- Eczema: German chamomile (*Matricaria recutitia*), Roman chamomile (*Chamaemelum nobile*), bergamot (*Citrus bergamia*), juniper, geranium, lavender
- Psoriasis: Palma rosa (*Cymbopogon martinii* var. *motia*), bergamot
- Papilloma: Tea tree (*Melaleuca alternifolia),* lemon
- Acne: Geranium, mandarin, lemon, petigrain (*Citrus aurantium ssp. amara fol*), juniper
- Vitiligo: Angelica (*Angelica archangelica*)
- Impetigo: Tea tree, palma rosa
- Tinea corporis: Geranium, tea tree
- Skin cancer: Frankincense (*Boswellia carteri*)

Respiratory

- Emphysema: Eucalyptus
- Asthma: Frankincense, lavender, lavendin (*Lavandula intermedia*), rosemary, angelica, sweet marjoram, basil (*Ocimum basilicum*), Pine (*Pinus sylvestris*)
- Infections: Bergamot, eucalyptus, juniper, ravansara (*Ravansara aromatica*)
- Tuberculosis: Eucalyptus, basil, sweet marjoram, tea tree

Musculoskeletal

Temporomandibular joint disease (TMJ), chondromyalgia, fibromyalgia, low back pain, osteoarthritis: Eucalyptus, black pepper (*Piper nigrum*), German chamomile, Roman chamomile, clary sage, ginger (*Zingiber officinalis*), lavender, lemongrass, peppermint (*Mentha piperita*), ylang ylang, sweet marjoram

Gastroenterology

- Gallbladder: Rosemary
- Hepatitis: Rosemary, myrrh (*Commiphora molmol*)
- Cirrhosis: Rosemary
- Obstructive bowel disease: Sweet marjoram
- Peptic ulcer disease: Roman chamomile, geranium
- Inflammatory bowel disease: Palma rosa
- Hemorrhoids: Cypress (*Cupressus sempervirens*), juniper

Cancer Treatment

- Nausea: Ginger, peppermint
- Diarrhea: Sandalwood (*Santalum album*)
- Depression: Bergamot, angelica
- Pain: Peppermint, German chamomile, lemongrass, cypress

Genitourinary

Urinary tract infection: Juniper, pine, sandalwood, lemongrass

Neurologic

- Headaches: Lavender, lemongrass, rosemary, Roman chamomile, eucalyptus, sweet marjoram, lemon balm, peppermint
- Multiple sclerosis: Rosemary
- Dementia: Basil, rosemary
- Dizziness: Basil, black pepper, peppermint
- Cardiovascular accident: Basil, lavender, peppermint, rosemary

Endocrine

- Hypothyroidism: Myrrh
- Diabetes mellitus: eucalyptus, geranium, juniper, clary sage, frankincense

Psychiatric

- Eating disorders: Roman chamomile, cardamom (*Elettaria cardamomum*), fennel (*Feoniculum vulgaris*)
- Sleep disorders: Lavender, mandarin, petigrain, clary sage, ravansara, sandalwood, sweet marjoram

- Depression: Bergamot, angelica, basil, Roman chamomile, patchouli (*Pogostemon cablin*)
- Drug addiction: Angelica, ylang ylang
- Anxiety/panic: Bergamot, ylang ylang

Reproductive

- Dysmenorrhea: German chamomile, clary sage, lemon balm, juniper
- Amenorrhea: Clary sage, fennel, juniper, myrrh
- Menorrhagia: Cypress, damask rose (*Rosa x damascena*)
- Premenstrual syndrome: Lavender, geranium, clary sage
- Menopause: Clary sage, geranium, Roman chamomile, cypress

Sexually Transmitted Diseases

- Herpes simplex virus: Tea Tree, bergamot, eucalyptus
- HIV/AIDS: Rosemary, angelica, ravansara, tea tree, bergamot, palma rosa
- Candida: Tea tree, angelica, bergamot, eucalyptus, geranium, peppermint, lemongrass

Contraindications and Possible Adverse Reactions

- Angelica: Possible phototoxicity
- Basil: Avoid use of basil with high estrogen content.
- Bergamot: Possible phototoxicity
- Black pepper: Avoid use on face; may be irritant.
- Chamomile, German: Avoid if allergic to ragweed.
- Chamomile, Roman: Avoid if allergic to ragweed.
- Clary sage: Avoid in oncology.
- Frankincense: The absolute may cause skin irritation.
- Geranium: Avoid in oncology.
- Lavender: Can act as powerful stimulant if used in large doses; less equals more
- Lemongrass: Can cause skin irritation
- Mandarin: Possible phototoxicity
- Melissa: Possible skin sensitization
- Peppermint: Can cause skin irritation; can act as powerful stimulant. Do not use with cardiac patients. Do not use with G6PD deficiency.
- Pine: Avoid in allergic skin conditions.
- Rosemary: Avoid in hypertension and epilepsy.
- Tea tree: Avoid in hot baths. May cause severe itching.
- Ylang ylang: Avoid in oncology. Avoid with use of 5-fluorouracil.

Suggested Reading

Buckle, J. (1997). *Clinical aromatherapy in nursing*. San Diego: Singular Publishing.

Davis, P. (1988). *Aromatherapy: An A–Z*. Essex, England: C.W. Daniel Company Limited.

Price, S. (1994). *Practical aromatherapy*. London: Harper-Collins.

Tisserand, R., & Balacs, T. (1995). *Essential oil safety*. New York: Churchill Livingstone.

Tisserand, R. (1997). *The art of aromatherapy*. Rochester, VT: Healing Arts Press.

Ulla-Maija, G. (1996). *Aromatherapy for practitioners*. Essex, England: C.W. Daniel Company Limited.

Valnet, J. (1980). *The practice of aromatherapy*. Rochester, VT: Healing Arts Press.

Williams, D. (1997). *The chemistry of essential oils*. Port Washington, NY: Micelle Press, Scholium International.

Worwood, V. (1991). *The complete book of essential oils and aromatherapy*. San Raphael, CA: New World Library.

Biofeedback
Suggested Reading

Runck, B. (1983). *Biofeedback*. U.S. Department of Health and Human Services (ADM) 82-1273.

Chiropractic
Suggested Reading

Bigos, S., Bowyer, O. (1994). *Acute low back pain in adults*. Clinical Practice Guideline Number 14. Rockville, MD: U.S. Department of Health and Human Services, Public Health Sevice, Agency for Health Care Policy and Research, AHCPR Pub. No. 95-0642.

Blunt, D.C. (1997). Chiropractic management of fibromyalgia. *Journal of Manipulative and Physiological Therapeutics, 20*(6), 389–399.

Boline, P.D., & Kassak, K. (1995). Spinal manipulation vs. amitriptyline for the treatment of chronic tension-type headaches: A randomized clinical trial. *Journal of Manipulative and Physiological Therapeutics, 18*(3), 148–154.

Koes, B.W., Bouter, L.M. (1992). Randomized clinical trial of manipulative therapy and physiotherapy for persistent back and neck complaints: Results of one-year follow-up. *British Medical Journal, 304*(6827), 601–605.

Kokjohn, D., Schmid, D.M., et al. (1992). The effect of spinal manipulation on pain and prostaglandin levels in women with primary dysmenorrhea. *Journal of Manipulative and Physiological Therapeutics, 15*(5), 279–285.

Meade, T.W., Dyer, S., et al. (1995). Randomized comparison of chiropractic and hospital outpatient management for low-back pain: Results from extended follow-up. *British Medical Journal, 311*(7001), 349–351.

Yates, R.G., & Lamping, D.L. (1988). Effects of chiropractic treatment on blood pressure and anxiety: A randomized, controlled trial. *Journal of Manipulative and Physiological Therapeutics, 11*(6), 484–488.

Craniosacral Therapy
Suggested Reading

Magoun, H.I. (1966, 1976). *Osteopathy in the cranial field*, 3d ed. Kirksville, MO: Journal Publishing

Upledger, J.E. (1987). *CranioSacral Therapy II: Beyond the dura*. Vista, CA: Eastland Press.

Upledger, J.E. (1990). *SomatoEmotional Release and beyond*. Palm Beach Gardens, FL: UI Enterprises.

Upledger, J.E. (1991). *CranioSacral Therapy, SomatoEmotional Release: Your inner physician and you*. Palm Beach Gardens, FL: UI Enterprises.

Upledger, J.E. (1996). *A brain is born*. Berkeley, CA: North Atlantic Books and UI Enterprises.

Upledger, J.E., & Vredevoogd, M.F.A. (1983). *Craniosacral Therapy*. Vista, CA: Eastland Press.

Massage Therapy

Massage can be performed on persons with the following conditions, but the massage therapist must be advised of this. Sometimes a primary care provider's supervision must be sought; in other cases, the massage therapist's technique should be adapted with the condition in mind.

- Hypertension
- Infections

- Osteoporosis
- Cancer
- Renal failure
- Coagulopathies
- HIV/AIDS

Suggested Reading

Bei, Y. (1993). Clinical observation on the treatment of 98 cases of peptic ulcer by massage. *Journal of Traditional Chinese Medicine, 13*(1), 50–51.

Beck, M. (1994). *Milady's theory and practice of therapeutic massage,* 2d ed. Albany, NY: Delmar.

Ferrell-Torry, A., & Glick, O. (1993). The use of therapeutic massage as a nursing intervention to modify anxiety and the perception of cancer pain. *Cancer Nursing, 16*(2), 93–101.

Field, T., Ironson, G., Scafidi, F., et al. (1996). Massage therapy reduces anxiety and enhances EEG pattern of alertness and math computations. *International Journal of Neuroscience, 86*(3-4), 197–205.

Field, T., Quintino, O. Henteleff, T., Wells-Keife, L., & Delvecchio-Feinberg, G. (1997). Job stress reduction therapies. *Alternative Therapies in Health & Medicine, 3*(4), 5.

Fryback, P., & Reinert, B. (1997). Alternative therapies and control for health in cancer and AIDS. *Clinical Nurse Specialist, 11*(2), 64–69.

Ironson, G., Field, A., Scafidi, F., et al. (1996). Massage therapy is associated with enhancement of the immune system's cytotoxic capacity. *International Journal of Neuroscience, 84*(1-4), 205–217.

Labyak, S., & Metzger, B. (1997). The effects of effleurage massage on the physiological components of relaxation: A meta-analysis. *Nursing Research, 46*(1), 59–62.

Shulman, K., & Jones, G. (1996). The effectiveness of massage therapy intervention on reducing anxiety in the workplace. *Journal of Applied Behavioral Science, 32*(2), 160.

Preoperative Evaluation

Dennis E. Frierman, MD, PhD, Maria Procopio-Dugan, DO, Samuel A. Sandowski, MD

Surgery involves a continuum of medical care to which the primary care provider, anesthetist, and surgeon contribute. It is difficult, if not impossible, for any single specialty to be knowledgeable of all medical issues applicable to the perioperative management of a patient. Therefore, they must work together to obtain the ultimate goal: reduction in surgical morbidity and mortality.

The primary care provider must "optimize" any pre-existing medical conditions to ensure the best possible outcome. Many procedures that previously required overnight hospitalization are now done on an outpatient basis. Most patients are admitted to the hospital on the day of surgery. This, in many ways, hampers the provider's ability to address complicated medical problems in the preoperative period. The primary care provider, therefore, must do preoperative optimization on an outpatient basis.

This appendix is not intended to be comprehensive; rather, it is intended to stress the importance of communication among the primary care provider, surgeon, and anesthetist. Several common coexisting diseases are briefly addressed because the primary care provider will often need to educate the patient as to how to be optimized for surgery. The patient must realize that being optimized does not guarantee risk-free surgery, but it reduces the risk. Benefits and risks of both the surgery and the anesthesia must always be discussed.

Risk Assessment

The term "clearance for surgery" is a misnomer. Patients who are "cleared" are those who have had their medical conditions evaluated and treated as best as possible. They are optimized. Even the healthiest patient has some surgical risk; no one should be considered risk-free. The word "cleared" implies that surgical risks have been assessed, medical issues have been addressed, appropriate intervention has been completed, and the patient has been informed of the risks and benefits of surgery.

The American Society of Anesthesiologists (ASA) classification is commonly used to assess the patient's physical status (Table C-1). Several large studies have found a direct correlation between physical status and morbidity and mortality (Vacanti et al, 1970; Prause et al, 1997). This classification scheme, however, is not an absolute predictor of anesthesia risk. For example, deaths due to airway mishaps are not necessarily related to the patient's underlying medical conditions. Further, the classification system lacks precision; the same patient could conceivably be classified in different ASA classes by different anesthesiologists (Owens et al, 1978).

Disease-Specific Considerations

Cardiac

Probably the most significant information in the preoperative evaluation is the history of a recent myocardial infarction (MI). MI in the perioperative period is associated with a highly signifi-

cant mortality rate (>20%) (Mangano, 1993). A recent (<6 months) history of MI increases the risk of another MI in the perioperative period by 6% to 37% (Tarhan et al, 1972; Rao et al, 1983). However, if the cardiac event is greater than 6 months old and the patient is medically optimized without recurrent symptoms, there is no need to delay the surgery.

The Goldman multifactorial index (Table C-2) is used to evaluate the risk of a perioperative cardiovascular complication in patients undergoing noncardiac surgery (Goldman et al, 1977). The history, physical findings, or laboratory data are used to classify the patient's risk. The greatest risk occurs in the patient with decompensated congestive heart failure, recent MI, or arrhythmias. Table C-3 shows the risk stratification based on the Goldman criteria. Patients with a class II or greater may benefit from a consultation with a specialist such as a cardiologist.

Pulmonary

Pre-existing pulmonary disease may increase the patient's risk for perioperative complications, postoperative pneumonia, and prolonged intubation. Patients with chronic obstructive pulmonary disease (COPD) may be dependent on either hypoxic or hypercarbic drive, both of which may be blunted by general anesthesia. This places the patient at risk in the postoperative period for respiratory failure. Regional anesthesia, however, may not necessarily diminish this postoperative risk: many patients with obstructive pulmonary disease are dependent on accessory muscles of respiration, and regional anesthesia may impede the patient's ability to use these muscles. Additionally, when the regional anesthesia wears off, the patient will need appropriate pain control; this will probably include narcotics, which can diminish both hypoxic and hypercarbic drive.

Patients with COPD and asthma may benefit from spirometry (FEV_1/FVC) to help assess their disease state. Complete pulmonary function tests are not usually warranted unless the patient is undergoing a lung resection. An arterial blood gas determination is useful to assist in risk stratification (Goldman criteria) and to assist in ventilation management. A referral to a pulmonologist should be sought in patients with moderate to severe pulmonary disease.

Hepatic

General anesthesia and regional anesthesia both diminish liver blood flow. This is further exacerbated when the operative site is near the liver (Gelman, 1976). Pre-existing hepatic dysfunction may be exacerbated by anesthesia. Further, blood product transfusions are associated with the risk of hepatitis.

Renal

Renal insufficiency can be associated with several other abnormalities that, if not properly investigated, may put a patient at additional risk. For example, low hematocrit levels, reduced

TABLE C-1	American Society of Anesthesiologist (ASA) Classification of Physical Status
ASA Classification	**Physical Status**
I	Healthy, no systemic disorder
II	Mild systemic disease
III	Severe systemic disease but not incapacitating
IV	Life-threatening systemic disease
V	Morbid patient unlikely to survive 24 hours with or without surgery

Adapted from Owens et al, 1978.

TABLE C-3	Risk Stratification for the Goldman Criteria		
Class	**Points**	**Risk of Major Complication**	**Risk of Cardiac Death**
I	0–5	0.7%	0.2%
II	6–12	5%	2%
III	13–25	11%	2%
IV	>25	22%	56%

Adapted from Goldman et al., 1977.

intravascular volume, and electrolyte abnormalities are frequently associated with chronic renal insufficiency. Reduced hematocrit values place the patient at risk for myocardial ischemia secondary to decreased oxygen delivery. Decreased blood volume places the patient at risk for hypotension with induction of general or regional anesthesia (secondary to decreased vascular or sympathetic tone/stimulation). Electrolyte abnormalities are associated with arrhythmias.

Preoperative Evaluation Note

The preoperative evaluation should include a complete history and physical exam to estimate the risk of surgery, identify specific medical issues that may affect risk, and serve to establish a baseline to help in postoperative assessment. It may include medical management recommendations to minimize risk; it also serves as an opportunity to update routine health care maintenance.

Before surgery, a clearance note should reach the anesthetist (Table C-4). The physical exam should include evaluation of the following systems: cardiovascular, pulmonary, liver, kidney, central nervous system, endocrine, and gastrointestinal, in addition to disease- and operation-specific organs. Laboratory studies should be specific to the disease and are described below.

What useful information should be addressed in the preoperative evaluation note? Moreover, what information is not

useful? The latter question is probably easier to answer. Not infrequently, the preoperative evaluation contains recommendations such as, "Avoid hypoxia and hypotension." This states the obvious and does not add to the care of the patient. Statements such as "Patient is cleared for surgery under spinal anesthesia" or "Patient is cleared for surgery under local anesthesia" are also of little value. Not uncommonly, procedures that are to be performed under local or regional anesthesia are converted to general anesthesia, and preoperatively all patients are informed of this. The anesthetist, surgeon, and patient should determine the choice of anesthetic technique; however, the choices are heavily influenced by the information provided by the patient's primary care provider.

Abnormal Laboratory Results and Physical Findings

Laboratory tests should be ordered only when indicated. In fact, the ASA's position on preoperative blood tests is that "no routine laboratory or diagnostic screening test is necessary for the pre-anesthetic evaluation of patients" (ASA, 1994). However, many hospitals still have protocols requiring routine preoperative testing. Table C-5 lists several common preoperative screening laboratory tests. Specific tests should be ordered for patients with certain medical conditions and those in specific age groups.

Some guidelines may cause providers to cancel elective cases. Most of these guidelines are not based on experimental or prospective studies but rather on what is believed to be good medical practice. A recent history of cardiac chest pain, a common cold, wheezing, or rales may lead to the cancellation of surgery.

TABLE C-2	Goldman Criteria for Cardiac Risk in Noncardiac Surgery	
Criteria		**Points**
Congestive Heart Failure, JVD, gallop (S_3)		11
Myocardial infarction within past 6 months		10
Rhythm other than sinus or PAC on ECG		7
PVC 5/minute		7
Age >70		5
Emergency operation		4
Aortic stenosis		3
Thoracic, abdominal, or aortic surgery		3
Poor general health*		3

* Po_2 60 mmHg, Pco_2>50, K^+ <3.0 mEq/L, HCO_3<20 mEq/L, BUN > 50 mg/dL, creatinine > 3 mg/dL, abnormal SGOT, signs of chronic liver disease, bedridden from noncardiac cause.
Adapted from Goldman et al, 1977.

TABLE C-4	The Preoperative Clearance Note

- Surgical procedure
- History of the present illness
- Present medical problems
- Past surgical history, including complications related to anesthesia
- Review of specific systems
- List of all medications prescribed and used
- Allergies to medicines
- Social history (smoking, ethanol use, recreational and illicit drug use)
- Physical exam
- Pertinent laboratory results
- Mention of appropriate consultations obtained before surgery
- Perioperative and postoperative recommendations

TABLE C-5	Laboratory Testing and Suggested Applications	
Test	Specific Requirements	Common Practices
Complete blood count (CBC)	Hematocrit/hemoglobin in menstruating women; operations with potentially large blood loss, most pre-existing medical conditions	All patients over age 18
Electrolytes	Genitourinary surgery, renal dysfunction, any medical condition requiring the use of diuretics or digoxin, diabetes, cardiac dysfunction or surgery	All patients over age 18
Liver function test	Liver disease, any surgery involving the liver	All patients over age 18
Prothrombin time/ partial thromboplastin time (PT/PTT)	Liver disease, surgery, or medical conditions requiring anticoagulation disease	All patients over age 18
Pregnancy test	All women menstruating or of childbearing age	
Urinalysis (UA)	Rule out infection or surgery for implantation of a prosthesis, genitourinary surgery	All patients over age 18
Electrocardiogram (ECG)	Age greater than 35, HTN, diabetes, coronary artery disease	All patients over age 35–40
Chest x-ray	Pulmonary disease or over age 65	
Cervical spine x-ray	Diseases affecting the cervical-spine, paresthesia with neck movement	Specific indications
Pulmonary function tests (PFTs)	Thoracic surgery (lung resection)	Specific indications

A diastolic blood pressure of more than 110 mmHg also may lead to the cancellation of surgery (Goldman & Caldera, 1979). Laboratory abnormalities such as a glucose level of more than 300 mg/dL, a sodium level of less than 130 or more than 150 mEq/L, a potassium level of less than 3 or more than 5.5 mEq/l (Cheung & Chernow, 1992; Stoelting & Dierdorf, 1993), or liver transaminase values more than two to three times the upper limit of normal would probably be a reason to cancel surgery. It is controversial whether elective surgery should proceed in the presence of potassium concentrations of less than 3.5 mEq (Harrington et al, 1982). Some studies have shown no increase in the incidence of arrhythmias in patients with a potassium level of 2.6 to 3.5 mEq (Hirsch et al, 1988); however, a potassium level of less than 3 mEq needs to be investigated and corrected. Abnormal electrocardiograms or chest x-rays should be addressed preoperatively. Elective surgery should be postponed until the above abnormalities have been addressed and corrected. If correction is not possible due to the underlying medical problem or necessary medications, then the risks and benefits of the surgery must be addressed.

Preparation of the Patient and Recommendations

After the patient has been evaluated preoperatively by the primary care provider and the patient is optimized, what additional preparations are necessary? Questions that need to be addressed are:

■ When does the patient need to stop eating or drinking? The NPO status of a patient before surgery has undergone changes in the past several years. The general rule is that all solids and nonclear liquids are stopped at least 8 hours before surgery. Most patients are allowed to drink clear liquids up to 3 hours before surgery (Goresky & Maltby, 1990). There are exceptions to this; also, regulations at some hospitals may call for the patient to be NPO for 8 hours. Obese patients

or patients with diabetes or any medical disorder that might interfere with gastric emptying should be NPO for 8 or more hours. Patients receiving drugs that delay gastric emptying (eg, narcotics) should be NPO for 8 or more hours.

■ Should patients continue to take their usual medications before and on the day of surgery? Should diabetics take all their insulin or oral hypoglycemic agents before surgery? Most medications should be continued up to and including the morning of surgery (Green & Pandit, 1995; Roizen, 1994). Oral medications may be taken with a small sip of water the morning of surgery. Diabetics are at risk for poor wound healing and hyperglycemia or hypoglycemia. It is generally recommended that oral hypoglycemics be stopped 24 hours before surgery. Metformin should be held on the morning of surgery and should not be restarted until 48 hours after surgery. Half of the usual morning dose of long-acting insulin is given on the morning of surgery, and the blood sugar level is monitored during the procedure. Insulin-dependent diabetics should not receive any regular insulin on the morning of surgery.

Almost all antihypertensive and cardiac medications should be continued. The two most common exceptions are coumadin and diuretics. Patients receiving coumadin are usually admitted to the hospital 2 to 3 days before surgery and switched to heparin, which is discontinued on the morning of surgery. Some providers prefer to withhold diuretics on the morning of surgery because of the risk of volume depletion or electrolyte abnormalities. Aspirin should be stopped 5 to 7 days before surgery because it irreversibly inhibits platelet function. Most other nonsteroidal anti-inflammatories are reversible inhibitors of cyclo-oxygenase and need to be stopped only 1 or 2 days before surgery.

■ Which patients need prophylaxis against endocarditis? Prophylaxis is recommended for patients who are at higher risk for endocarditis than the general population and for certain high-risk procedures. Patients with prosthetic heart valves, previous bacterial endocarditis, and complex congenital heart disease (eg, tetralogy of Fallot) are considered to be in the high-risk category. Those with acquired valvular disease (eg, rheumatic fever, aortic stenosis and regurgitation), mitral valve prolapse with mitral regurgitation or thickened leaflets, ventricular septal defect, coarctation of the aorta, and bicuspid aortic valve are in the moderate-risk category. Prophylaxis is not indicated in patients with prior coronary artery bypass graft, mitral valve prolapse without regurgitation, isolated atrial septal defect, functional or innocent murmurs, or cardiac pacemakers.

The American Heart Association recommends prophylaxis against endocarditis in at-risk patients undergoing dental extractions, periodontal procedures, or any dental procedure where significant bleeding is expected. Also included are surgical procedures involving the respiratory or intestinal mucosa, tonsillectomy, rigid bronchoscopy, esophageal or urethral dilation, surgery of the biliary tract or the prostate, endoscopic retrograde cholangiography with biliary obstruction, and cystoscopy. Common procedures in which prophylaxis is not recommended are restorative dentistry, endotracheal intubation, flexible bronchoscopy, cardiac catheterization, angioplasty, and incision or biopsy of surgically scrubbed skin. Endocarditis prophylaxis during transesophageal echocardiography, endoscopy with and without biopsy, and vaginal hysterectomy is optional for patients with the highest risk (Dajani et al, 1997).

The recommendations for endocarditis prophylaxis were revised in 1997 (Tables C-6 and C-7) (Dajani et al, 1997). In most cases, antibiotics are now given only preoperatively. The newly recommended oral dose in adult patients not allergic to penicillin is 2 g amoxicillin administered 1 hour before the procedure. In penicillin-allergic patients, clindamycin or vancomycin can be given, depending on the procedure.

- How can postoperative thrombosis be prevented? Prophylactic anticoagulation with 5000 heparin U subcutaneously every 12 hours reduces the incidence of thrombosis, embolism, and thromboembolic death by 40% to 70% without increasing the risk of fatal bleeding (Kelley, 1997). Low-molecular-weight heparin may be used, though this may increase the risk of epidural hematones with regional anesthesia (Porterfield, 1997). Elastic stockings placed perioperatively are also effective in preventing thromboembolic complications. In high-risk procedures such as hip and knee replacements, low-dose coumadin is started perioperatively.

- How can the risk of postoperative pneumonia be minimized? In patients with pulmonary disease, the use of beta agonists and anti-inflammatory agents should be optimized preoperatively. Patients receiving bronchodilators should use their medications the morning of surgery. In a patient with intermittent bronchospasm or asthma, beta agonists should be started 1 or 2 days before surgery and continued for several days afterward. Deep-breathing and coughing exercises should be initiated several days before surgery in patients with COPD, and patients with chronic purulent sputum production should receive broad-spectrum antibiotics for 5 to 7 days preoperatively to decrease the quantity and purulence of secretions (Barker et al, 1991). All patients who smoke should be encouraged to stop 5 to 7 days before surgery. Incentive spirometry should be used in all patients who have had abdominal surgery or pelvic surgery or will be on prolonged bed rest.

- When should stress doses of corticosteroids be given? Patients who are currently taking a pharmacologic dose of corticosteroids (the equivalent of more than 20 to 30 mg/day hydrocortisone), who have been taking a pharmacologic dose of corticosteroids for 2 or more weeks in the past year, or who take replacement doses for adrenal insufficiency are at risk for developing adrenal insufficiency or crisis from the stress of surgery. These patients should receive additional

TABLE C-6	Prophylactic Regimens for Dental, Oral, Respiratory Tract, or Esophageal Procedures	
Situation	**Agent**	**Regimen***
Standard general prophylaxis	Amoxicillin	Adults: 2.0 g; children: 50 mg/kg orally 1 h before procedure
Unable to take oral medications	Ampicillin	Adults: 2.0 g IM or IV; children: 50 mg/kg IM or IV within 30 min before procedure
Allergic to penicillin	Clindamycin or	Adults: 600 mg; children: 20 mg/kg orally 1 h before procedure
	Cephalexin† or cefadroxil† or	Adults: 2.0 g; children; 50 mg/kg orally 1 h before procedure
	Azithromycin or clarithromycin	Adults: 500 mg; children: 15 mg/kg orally 1 h before procedure
Allergic to penicillin and unable to take oral medications	Clindamycin or	Adults: 600 mg; children: 20 mg/kg IV within 30 min before procedure
	Cefazolin†	Adults: 1.0 g; children: 25 mg/kg IM or IV within 30 min before procedure

* Total children's dose should not exceed adult dose.

† Cephalosporins should not be used in individuals with immediate-type hypersensitivity reaction (urticaria, angioedema, or anaphylaxis) to penicillins.

Source: Dajan, A.S. et al. (1997). *JAMA 277*(22):1794.

TABLE C-7	Prophylactic Regimens for Genitourinary Gastrointestinal (Excluding Esophageal) Procedures	
Situation	**Agents***	**Regiment**
High-risk patients	Ampicillin plus Gentamicin	Adults: ampicillin 2.0 g IM or IV plus gentamicin 1.5 mg/kg (not to exceed 120 mg) within 30 min of starting the procedure; 6 h later, ampicillin 1 g IM/IV or amoxicillin 1 g orally Children: ampicillin 50 mg/kg IM or IV (not to exceed 2.0 g) plus gentamicin 1.5 mg/kg within 30 min of starting the procedure; 6 h later, ampicillin 25 mg/kg IM/IV or amoxicillin 25 mg/kg orally
High-risk patients allergic to ampicillin/amoxicillin	Vancomycin plus Gentamicin	Adults: vancomycin 1.0 g IV over 1–2 h plus gentamicin 1.5 mg/kg IV/IM (not to exceed 120 mg); complete injection/infusion within 30 min of starting the procedure Children: vancomycin 20 mg/kg IV over 1–2 h plus gentamicin 1.5 mg/kg IV/IM; complete injection/infusion within 30 min of starting the procedure
Moderate-risk patients	Amoxicillin or Ampicillin	Adults: amoxicillin 2.0 g orally 1 h before procedure, or ampicillin 2.0 g IM/IV within 30 min of starting the procedure Children: amoxicillin 50 mg/kg orally 1 h before procedure, or ampicillin 50 mg/kg IM/IV within 30 min of starting the procedure
Moderate-risk patients allergic to ampicillin/amoxicillin	Vancomycin	Adults: vancomycin 1.0 g IV over 1–2 h; complete infusion within 30 min of starting the procedure Children: vancomycin 20 mg/kg IV over 1–2 h; complete infusion within 30 min of starting the procedure

* Total children's dose should not exceed adult dose.

† No second dose of vancomycin or gentamicin is recommended.

Source: Dajan, A.S. et al. (1997). *JAMA 277*(22):1794.

corticosteroids in the perioperative period. Patients should take their usual dose the day before surgery. On the day of surgery, the patient should receive hydrocortisone 100 mg intravenously in the early morning, and then a 100-mg dose intravenously every 6 hours for the first 24 hours after surgery. The dose is decreased to 50 mg every 6 hours and then 25 mg every 6 hours in the second and third postoperative day, respectively. At this point, the preoperative dosage may be resumed. This regimen assumes that there is no prolonged stress after surgery that may necessitate continued high doses of steroid. For minor procedures, the patient may return to the usual dose in 24 to 48 hours.

- When should the patient on hemodialysis be dialyzed? Patients with end-stage renal disease should undergo hemodialysis before elective surgery. Patients with severe anemia and end-stage renal disease can be transfused with their hemodialysis without the risk of fluid overload (Prough & Foreman, 1992).

- Is there anything additional I can do for the very anxious patient? Patients who are extremely anxious can be given medications to relieve their anxiety. Some common anxiolytics used preoperatively are diazepam (Valium) and lorazepam (Ativan), given orally on the morning of surgery. Caution should be used if the patient is elderly or taking multiple medications; in this case, the response to these medications may be exaggerated or unpredictable. Geriatric patients are at higher risk for postoperative delirium. Consent for the planned procedure must be received before the administration of any anxiolytic that may alter thinking or consciousness in any way.

- What about patients of childbearing age? Women of childbearing age should have a pregnancy test. The pregnant patient should have an obstetric consultation and should be told of the risks and benefits of the procedure.

Types of Anesthesia

General Anesthesia

The components of general anesthesia are usually described to include amnesia, analgesia, muscle relaxation, and modulation of the autonomic nervous system. There are three phases to general anesthesia: induction, maintenance, and emergence.

Numerous medications are at the anesthetist's disposal to induce and maintain these components. Some are complete anesthetics that induce and maintain all the components of anesthesia—for example, the potent inhaled anesthetics (isoflurane). Others are used for a specific objective or to augment or maintain individual components of anesthesia. For example, thiopental is used for induction of general anesthesia, fentanyl is used for analgesia, and curare is used for muscle relaxation. Many anesthetists use a combination of these. This would include a short-acting induction agent, an opioid combined with a low dose of a potent inhaled agent, and a neuromuscular blocking agent for muscle relaxation.

Regional Techniques

Regional, or conduction block, anesthesia usually refers to a spinal (direct injection of local anesthetic into the spinal fluid), epidural (injection of local anesthetic around the dural sac), or caudal block (epidural performed in the sacral area). These techniques are usually reserved for perineal, lower abdominal, or lower extremity surgery and are contraindicated in patients with bleeding disorders. Peripheral nerve blocks can be used for surgery of the neck, shoulder, and upper or lower extremity. Field blocks ("local") are usually used for relatively superficial surgery confined to a small area. All of the above techniques are often supplemented with various sedating medications.

In a significant percentage of patients, a procedure begun with nongeneral anesthesia will be converted to one using general anesthesia. This may be due to failure of the technique, patient anxiety, or an unexpected complication. Epidural anesthesia fails in 2% to 5% of cases (Asato, 1990). Regional anesthesia is not applicable to all types of surgical procedures. Other limitations of regional anesthesia include the following:

- It requires different skills than general anesthesia.
- It is often associated with a slower onset.
- It may be associated with a prolonged recovery, especially in ambulatory settings.

However, several studies suggest that regional anesthesia may reduce the incidence of some perioperative complications, such as thromboembolic events and cardiovascular or pulmonary complications (Modig, 1985; Prins & Hirsh, 1991). Because the numbers of patients in these studies are small, additional studies will be required to substantiate these benefits of regional anesthesia.

Combined Techniques

Occasionally patients undergo combined techniques. One of the most common combined techniques is the epi-general. This technique makes use of the advantages of both of these techniques. For example, the use of the epidural lowers the anesthetic requirement to maintain general anesthesia. Also, the patient is not awake for the procedure. At the end of a long surgical procedure, the patient is less sedated and is in the less pain. Further, the epidural can be used for postoperative pain control.

References

American Society of Anesthesiologists. (1994). *Statement on routine preoperative laboratory and diagnostic screening*, p. 775.

Asato, F., Kirakawa, N., Oda, M. et al. (1990). A midline epidural septum is not a common cause of unilateral epidural blockade. *Anesthesia & Analgesia, 71*, 427–429.

Barker, L.R., Burton J.R., & Zieve, P.D. (1991). *Principles of ambulatory medicine*, 3d ed., pp. 1191–1207. Baltimore: Williams & Wilkins.

Cheung, A.T., & Chernow, B. (1992). Perioperative electrolyte disorders. In J.L. Benumof & L.J. Saidman (Eds.). *Anesthesia: Perioperative complications*. St. Louis: Mosby

Dajani, A.S., Taubert, K.A., Wilson, W., et al. (1997). Prevention of bacterial endocarditis recommendations by the American Heart Association. *JAMA, 277*(22), 1794–1801.

Gelman, S.I. (1976). Disturbances in hepatic blood flow during anesthesia and surgery. *Archives of Surgery, 111*, 881.

Goldman, L., & Caldera, D.L. (1979). Risks of general anesthesia in elective operation in the hypertensive patient. *Anesthesiology, 50*, 285, 1979.

Goldman, L., Caldera, D.L., Nussbaum, S.R., et al. (1977). Multifactorial index on cardiac risk in noncardiac surgical procedures. *N Engl J Med, 297*, 845.

Goresky, G.V., & Maltby, J.R. (1990). Fasting guidelines for elective surgical patients. *Canadian Journal of Anaesthesia, 37*, 493.

Green, C.R., & Pandit, S.K. (1995). Preoperative preparation. In R. Twersky (Ed.). *The ambulatory anesthesia handbook*. St. Louis: Mosby.

Harrington, J.T., Isner, J.M., & Kassirer, J.P. (1982). Our national obsession with potassium. *American Journal of Medicine, 73*, 159.

Hirsch, I.A., Tomlinson, D.L., Slogoff, S. et al. (1988). The overstated risk of preoperative hypokalemia. *Anesthesia & Analgesia, 67*, 131.

Kelley, W.M. (1997). *Textbook of internal medicine*, 3d ed., pp. 241–243. Philadelphia: Lippincott-Raven.

Mangano, D.T. (1993). Preoperative assessment of cardiac risk. In J.A. Kaplan (Ed.). *Cardiac anesthesia*, 3d ed. Philadelphia: W.B. Saunders.

Modig, J. (1985). The role of lumbar epidural anesthesia as antithrombic prophylaxis in total hip replacement. *Acta Chirurgica Scandinavica, 151*, 589.

Owens, W.D., Felts, J.A., & Spitznagel, E.L. (1978). ASA physical status classifications: A study of consistency of ratings. *Anesthesiology, 49*, 239.

Porterfield, W.R., Wu, C.L. (1997). Epidural hematoma in an ambulatory surgical patient. *Journal of Clinical Anesthesia 9*; 74–77.

Prause, G., Ratzenhofer-Comenda, B., Pierrer, G., Smolle-Juttner, F., Glanzer, H., & Smolle, J. (1997). Can ASA grade or Goldman's cardiac risk index predict perioperative mortality? A study of 16,227 patients. *Anaesthesia, 52*(3), 203–206.

Prins, M.H., & Hirsh, J. (1991). A critical review of the evidence supporting a relationship between impaired fibrinolytic activity and venous thromboembolism. *Archives of Internal Medicine, 151*, 1721.

Prough, D.S., & Foreman, A.S. (1992). Anesthesia and the renal system. In P.G. Barash, B.F. Cullen, & R.K. Stoelting (Eds.). *Clinical anesthesia*, 2d ed. Philadelphia: J.B. Lippincott.

Rao, T.K., Jacobs, K.H., & El-Etr, A.A. (1983). Reinfarction following anesthesia in a patient with myocardial infarction. *Anesthesiology, 59*, 499.

Roizen, M.F. (1994). Anesthetic implications of current diseases. In R.D. Miller (Ed.). *Anesthesia*, 4th ed. New York: Churchill Livingstone.

Stoelting, R.K., & Dierdorf, S.F. (1993). Renal disease. In *Anesthesia and co-existing disease*, 3d ed. New York: Churchill Livingstone.

Tarhan, S., Moffitt, E., Taylor, W.F., et al. (1972). Myocardial infarction after general anesthesia. *JAMA, 220*, 1451.

Vacanti, C.J., VanHouten, R.J., & Hill, R.C. (1970). A statistical analysis of the relationship of physical status to postoperative mortality in 68,388 cases. *Anesthesia & Analgesia, 49*, 564.

Index

Note: Page numbers followed by *f* indicate figures; numbers followed by *t* indicate tables.